PRACTICAL

ORTHOPAEDIC

SPORTS

MEDICINE

AND

ARTHROSCOPY

PRACTICAL ORTHOPAEDIC SPORTS MEDICINE AND ARTHROSCOPY

■ **DONALD H. JOHNSON, MD, FRCS**

Associate Professor
University of Ottawa
Ottawa, Ontario, Canada

■ **ROBERT A. PEDOWITZ, MD, PHD**

Professor and Chairman
Department of Orthopaedic Surgery
University of South Florida College of Medicine
Tampa, Florida

Wolters Kluwer | Lippincott Williams & Wilkins
Health

Philadelphia · Baltimore · New York · London
Buenos Aires · Hong Kong · Sydney · Tokyo

Acquisitions Editor: Robert A. Hurley
Developmental Editor: Eileen Wolfberg
Project Manager: Jennifer Harper
Manufacturing Coordinator: Kathleen Brown
Marketing Director: Sharon Zinner
Art Director: Risa Clow
Production Services: GGS Book Services
Printer: R.R. Donnelley, Willard

Library of Congress Cataloging-in-Publication Data

Johnson, Donald (Donald Hugh)
    Practical orthopaedic sports medicine & arthroscopy / Donald H. Johnson, Robert A Pedowitz.
      p. ; cm.
    ISBN-13: 978-0-7817-5812-3
    ISBN-10: 0-7817-5812-2
1. Sports injuries—Surgery.   2. Arthroscopy.   3. Sports medicine. I. Pedowitz, Robert A. II. Title.
III. Title: Practical orthopaedic sports medicine and arthroscopy.
    [DNLM: 1. Athletic Injuries—surgery. 2. Arthroscopy—methods. 3. Orthopedic Procedures—methods. 4. Sports Medicine—methods. QT 261 J66p 2007]
    RD97.P7344 2007
    617.1'027—dc22

                                                                            2006034170

DEDICATIONS

I would like to dedicate this book to my family: my wife Carole, who put up with me spending long hours working on the computer; my three sons Mike, Chris, and Paul, who were all active in sports and fortunately did not require the expertise of some of these sports medicine experts; and my grandchildren, Sarah, Julia, and Ryely, who will probably benefit from the advances in sports medicine. Finally, I also dedicate this book to my mentor Bob Jackson, who taught me arthroscopy and stimulated my longstanding interest in teaching and education.
DHJ

I present this book as a toast to the influential forces of my life. To my dedicated parents, who taught me that everything is possible. To my loving wife, Loraine, and our wonderful children, Rachel and Jason, who manage when things are impossible. To my friends, who remind me of what is really worthwhile. And to Wayne Akeson, MD, a mentor, a gentleman, and a friend, who amazes with the brilliance and foresight to ask the really important questions.
RAP

Wayne H. Akeson, MD
Emeritus Professor
Department of Orthopaedics
University of California, San Diego
San Diego, California

Chief
Department of Orthopaedics and Surgery
VA San Diego Health Care System
San Diego, California

Amro Al-Hibshi, MBChB, FRCSC
Fellow, Department of Orthopaedics
Dalhousie University
Halifax, Nova Scotia, Canada

Ali Alsuwaidi, MD, FRCSI, FRCSC
Head, Section Shoulder and Sports Medicine
Department of Surgery
Sheikh Khalifa Medical City
Abu Dhabi, United Arab Emirates

Annunziato Amendola, MD
Department of Orthopaedics and Rehabilitation
University of Iowa Hospitals and Clinics
Iowa City, Iowa

David Amiel, PhD
Professor
Department of Orthopaedic Surgery
University of California, San Diego
La Jolla, California

John G. Anderson, MD
Orthopaedic Associates of Grand Rapids
Grand Rapids, Michigan

Steven P. Arnoczky, DVM, Dipl ACVS
Director
Laboratory for Comparative Orthopaedic
  Research
Michigan State University
East Lansing, Michigan

Michael S. Aronow, MD
Associate Professor
Department of Orthopaedic Surgery
University of Connecticut Health Center
Farmington, Connecticut

George K. Bal, MD, FACS
Assistant Professor
Department of Orthopaedics
West Virginia University
Morgantown, West Virginia

Assistant Professor
Department of Orthopaedics
West Virginia University Hospital
Morgantown, West Virginia

Rahul Banerjee, MD
Clinical Instructor
Department of Orthopaedic Surgery
Texas Tech University Health Sciences
  Center
El Paso, Texas

Interim Chief of Orthopaedic Trauma
Department of Orthopaedic Surgery
William Beaumont Army Medical Center
El Paso, Texas

F. Alan Barber, MD, FACS
Fellowship Co-Director
Plano Orthopaedic and Sports Medicine
  Center
Plano, Texas

Aaron A. Bare, MD
Department of Orthpaedics
Central DuPage Hospital
Winfield, Illinois

Ronnie Barnes, ATC
Vice President and Head Trainer
New York Football Giants
New York, New York

Wael K. Barsoum, MD
Assistant Professor of Surgery
Cleveland Clinic Lerner College of Medicine
Cleveland, Ohio

Vice Chairman
Department of Orthopaedic Surgery
The Cleveland Clinic Foundation
Cleveland, Ohio

Carl J. Basamania, MD
Department of Orthopaedic Surgery
Duke University Medical Center 3531
Durham, North Carolina

Jack M. Bert, MD
Adjunct Clinical Professor
University of Minnesota, School of Medicine
Minneapolis, Minnesota

Medical Director
Summit Orthopedics, Ltd.
St. Paul, Minnesota

Thomas M. Best, MD, PhD, FACSM
Professor, Chief
Division of Sports Medicine
Department of Family Medicine
The Ohio State University
Columbus, Ohio

Donald R. Bohay, MD, FACS
Associate Clinical Professor
Department of Orthopaedic Surgery
Michigan State University
Orthopaedic Associates of Grand Rapids
Grand Rapids, Michigan

Lori A. Bolgla, PT, PhD, ATC
Department of Physical Therapy
Medical College of Georgia
Augusta, Georgia

Mark D. Bracker, MD
Clinical Professor
Department of Family and Preventive Medicine
University of California, San Diego
La Jolla, California

Michael P. Bradley, MD
Teaching Fellow
Department of Orthopaedics
Brown University School of Medicine
Rhode Island Hospital
Providence, Rhode Island

Paul C. Brady, MD
Arthroscopic Shoulder Specialist
Tennessee Orthopaedic Clinics
Knoxville, Tennessee

Patrick S. Brannan, MD
Department of Orthopaedic Surgery
Wilford Hall Med Center/MCSO
Lackland Air Force Base, Texas

John A. Brown, MD
Director
Division of Sports Medicine

The C.O.R.E. Institute
Sun City West, Arizona

William Bugbee, MD
Associate Adjunct Professor
Department of Orthopaedics
University of California, San Diego
San Diego, California

Orthopaedic Surgeon
Division of Orthopaedics
Scripps Clinic
La Jolla, California

Steven S. Burkhart, MD
Director of Orthopaedic Education
The San Antonio Orthopaedic Group
San Antonio, Texas

Clinical Associate Professor
Department of Orthopaedic Surgery
The University of Texas
    Health Sciences Center at San Antonio
San Antonio, Texas

J.W. Thomas Byrd, MD
Orthopaedic Surgeon
Nashville Sports Medicine and Orthopaedic
    Center
Nashville, Tennessee

Aaron Campbell, MD
Assistant Professor
Department of Orthopaedic Surgery
Queen's University
Kingston, Ontario, Canada

Henry G. Chambers, MD
Clinical Assistant Professor
Department of Orthopaedic Surgery
University of California, San Diego
San Diego, California

Director of Sports Medicine
Department of Pediatric Orthopaedic Surgery
Rudy Children's Hospital
San Diego, California

Donald Chow, MD, FRCSC, Dipl Sports Med
Assistant Professor
Department of Surgery
Division of Orthopaedics
University of Ottawa
Ottawa, Ontario, Canada

Orthopaedic Spine Surgeon
Spine Surgery Unit
Department of Orthopaedics
Ottawa Hospital, Civic Campus
Ottawa, Ontario, Canada

Steven B. Cohen, MD
Rothman Institute Orthopaedics
Director of Sports Medicine Research
Assistant Professor
Thomas Jefferson University
Philadelphia, Pennsylvania

Jonathan P. Cornelius, MD
Clinical Instructor
Grand Rapids Orthopaedic Surgery
  Residency Program
Michigan State University
Grand Rapids, Michigan

John G. Costouros, MD
Clinical Instructor
Harvard Shoulder Service
Department of Orthopaedic Surgery
Harvard Medical School
Massachusetts General Hospital
Boston, Massachusetts

Chief
Center for Shoulder Disorders
Department of Orthopaedic Surgery
Kaiser-Permanente Medical Group,
  Santa Teresa
San Jose, California

Jeffrey R. Counts, DO
Kentucky Sports Medicine Clinic
Lexington, Kentucky

Marjorie Delo, MD

Michael H. Dienst, MD
Department of Orthopaedic Surgery
University Hospital
Homburg/Saar, Germany

Douglas P. Dietzel, DO
Department of Orthopaedic Surgery
MSU Health Team
Mid-Michigan Orthopaedic Institute
East Lansing, Michigan

Julie A. Dodds, MD
Clinical Associate Professor
Section of Sports Medicine
Michigan State University
East Lansing, Michigan

Active Staff
E.W. Sparrow Hospital
Lansing, Michigan

Craig J. Edson, MHS, PT, ATC
Geisinger Medical Center
Danville, Pennsylvania

Wylie S. Elson, MD
Senior Researcher
Taos Orthopaedic Institute
Taos, New Mexico

Director
Medical Education and Communications, Inc.
Taos, New Mexico

James C. Esch, MD
Assistant Clinical Professor
Department of Orthopaedics
University of California, San Diego School of
  Medicine
San Diego, California

Tri-City Orthopaedics
Oceanside, California

Paul D. Fadale, MD
Associate Professor
Department of Orthopaedic Surgery
Brown Medical School
Providence, Rhode Island

Chief, Division of Sports Medicine
Department of Orthopaedic Surgery
Rhode Island Hospital
Providence, Rhode Island

Gregory C. Fanelli, MD
Sports Injury Clinic
Danville, Pennsylvania

Scott P. Fischer, MD
Orthopaedic Specialty Institute of Orange County
Orange, California

Ramces A. Francisco, MD
Associate Orthopaedic Surgeon
Orthopaedic Arthroscopic Surgery International
Milan, Italy

Jan Fronek, MD
Clinical Instructor
Department of Orthopaedic Surgery
University of California, San Diego
San Diego, California

Sport Medicine Section, Chief
Department of Orthopaedic Surgery
Scripps Clinic Medical Group
La Jolla, California

Freddie H. Fu, MD
David Silver Professor of Orthopaedic Surgery
Chairman, Department of Orthopaedic Surgery
University of Pittsburgh Medical Center
Chairman, Department of Orthopaedic Surgery
University of Pittsburgh School of Medicine
Pittsburgh, Pennsylvania

Price A.M. Gallie, MB, BS, FRACS
Staff Surgeon
Department of Orthopaedics
Gold Coast Hospital
Southport, Australia

Michael S. George, MD
KSF Orthopaedic Center
Houston, Texas

Michael B. Gerhardt, MD
Director
Center for Hip and Groin Disorders
Division of Sports Medicine
Santa Monica Orthopaedic and Sports Medicine Group
Santa Monica, California

Eric Giza, MD
Director
Foot and Ankle Center
Santa Monica Orthopaedic and Sports Medicine Group
Santa Monica, California

Mark A. Glazebrook, MD, MSc, PhD, Dip Sports Med, FRCS(C)
Assistant Professor
Department of Surgery
Dalhousie University
Halifax, Nova Scotia, Canada

Staff
Department of Surgery
Queen Elizabeth II Health Science Centre
Halifax, Nova Scotia, Canada

Alberto Gobbi, MD
Director
Department of Sports Medicine
Orthopaedic Arthroscopic Surgery International
Milan, Italy

Elise T. Gordon, DO, CDR, MC, USN

Carlos A. Guanche, MD
Southern California Orthopedic Institute
Van Nuys, California

Dan Guttmann, MD
Taos Orthopaedic Institute
Taos, New Mexico

Jeffrey Halbrecht, MD
Institute for Arthroscopy and Sports Medicine
San Francisco, California

Private Practice
San Francisco, California

Justin D. Harris, MD
Geisinger Medical Center
Danville, Pennsylvania

George F. (Rick) Hatch, III, MD
Assistant Professor
Department of Orthopaedic Surgery
USC/Keck School of Medicine

Assistant Professor
Department of Orthopaedic Surgery
USC University Hospital
Los Angeles, California

Richard Hawkins, MD
Principal
Steadman Hawkins Clinic of the Carolinas
Spartanburg, South Carolina

Clinical Professor
Department of Orthopaedics
University of Colorado
Denver, Colorado

Team Physician
Colorado Rockies Baseball Organization
Denver, Colorado

Team Physician
Denver Broncos Baseball Organization
Denver, Colorado

Lorraine Hendry, BSc(PT), MCPA, FCAMT
Joint Appointee/Physiotherapist
School of Rehabilitation Sciences
    Physiotherapy Program
University of Ottawa
Ottawa, Ontario, Canada

Carlos A.M. Higuera, MD
Resident
Department of Orthopaedic Surgery
The Cleveland Clinic Foundation
Cleveland, Ohio

Heinz R. Hoenecke, MD
Scripps Clinical Medical Group
La Jolla, California

John Hung, MD
Center of Athletic Medicine
Chicago, Illinois

University of Illinois, Chicago
Chicago, Illinois

Graham R. Hurvitz, MD
Medical Director
Summit and Premier Surgery Centers
Santa Barbara, California

Private Practice
Santa Barbara, California

Mark R. Hutchinson, MD
Professor of Orthopaedics
Department of Orthopaedics
University of Illinois, Chicago
Chicago, Illinois

Helen D. Iams, MD, MS
Clinical Assistant Professor of Medicine
Family Practice Residency at Cheyenne
University of Wyoming
Cheyenne, Wyoming

Active Medical Staff
Family Medicine
Cheyenne Regional Medical Center
Cheyenne, Wyoming

Mary Lloyd Ireland, MD
President/Director and Orthopaedic Surgeon
Kentucky Sports Medicine Clinic
Lexington, Kentucky

Donald H. Johnson, MD, FRCS
Associate Professor
University of Ottawa
Ottawa, Ontario, Canada

Director
Sports Medicine Clinic Carleton University
Ottawa, Ontario, Canada

Attending Staff
The Ottawa Hospital
Ottawa, Ontario, Canada

Paul Johnson, MD
Physician
Sports Medicine Clinic Carleton University
Ottawa, Ontario, Canada

Christopher C. Kaeding, MD
Orthopedic Surgery and Sports Medicine
University Hospital
Ohio State Medical Center
Columbus, Ohio

Serge Kaska, MD
Department of Orthopaedic Surgery
Orange, California

Viktor E. Krebs, MD
Head
Section of Adult Reconstruction
Department of Orthopaedic Surgery
The Cleveland Clinic Foundation
Cleveland, Ohio

Bernie Lalonde, MD
Carleton Sports Medicine Clinic
Carleton University
Ottawa, Ontario, Canada

Scott E. Lawrance, MS, PT, ATC, CSCS
Physical Therapist
The Shelbourne Clinic at Methodist Hospital
Indianapolis, Indiana

John K. Locke, MD
Assistant Clinical Professor
Department of Surgery
Uniformed Services University of the Health
    Sciences
Bethesda, Maryland

Orthopaedic Surgeon
Bone and Joint Sports Medicine Institute
Naval Medical Center, Portsmouth
Portsmouth, Virginia

James H. Lubowitz, MD
Clinical Assistant Professor
Department of Orthopaedic Surgery
University of New Mexico School of
    Medicine
Albuquerque, New Mexico

Director
Research Foundation and Sports Medicine Fellowship
    Training Program
Taos Orthopaedic Institute
Taos, New Mexico

Anthony C. Luke, MD, MPH
Assistant Professor
Director Primary Cares Sports Medicine
Department of Orthopaedics, Department of Family and
    Community Medicine
University of California, San Francisco
San Francisco, California

Andrew T. Mahar, MS
Director
Department of Orthopedics
Orthopedic Biomechanics Research Center
Rady Children's Hospital, San Diego
San Diego, California

Research Scientist
Department of Orthopaedic Surgery
University of California, San Diego
San Diego, California

Eric C. McCarty, MD
Associate Professor
Department of Orthopaedics
University of Colorado School of Medicine
Denver, Colorado

Chief of Sports Medicine and Shoulder Surgery
Department of Orthopaedics
University of Colorado Health Sciences Center
Denver, Colorado

Peter J. Millett, MD, MSc
Assistant Professor
Harvard Medical School
Boston, Massachusetts

Director of Shoulder Surgery
Steadman Hawkins Clinic
Vail, Colorado

Keith D. Nord, MD, MS
Fellowship Director
Shoulder Arthroscopy and Sports Medicine
Sports, Orthopedics & Spine
Jackson, Tennessee

Stephen J. O'Brien, MD, PLLC
Hospital for Special Surgery
New York, New York

Daniel R. Orcutt, MD
Geisinger Medical Center
Danville, Pennsylvania

Mark A. Palumbo, MD
Orthopedic Surgeon
University Orthopedics
Providence, Rhode Island

Anastasios Papadonikolakis, MD
Resident in Orthopaedic Surgery
Department of Orthopaedic Surgery
Wake Forest University
Winston-Salem, North Carolina

Resident in Orthopaedic Surgery
Department of Orthopaedic Surgery
North Carolina Baptist Medical Center
Winston-Salem, North Carolina

Andrew D. Pearle, MD
Instructor
Department of Orthopaedic Surgery
New York Presbyterian Hospital
New York, New York

Assistant Attending Orthopaedic Surgeron
Department of Shoulder and Sports Medicine Service
Hospital for Special Surgery
New York, New York

David I. Pedowitz, MD, MS
Chief Resident
Department of Orthopaedic Surgery
University of Pennsylvania School of Medicine
Philadelphia, Pennsylvania

Robert A. Pedowitz, MD, PhD
Professor and Chairman
Department of Orthopaedic Surgery
University of South Florida College of Medicine
Tampa, Florida

Walter J. Pedowitz, MD
Clinical Professor
Department of Orthopaedic Surgery
Columbia University
New York Presbyterian Hospital
New York, New York

Murray J. Penner, MD, FRCSC
Clinical Assistant Professor
Department of Orthopaedics
University of British Columbia
Vancouver, British Columbia, Canada

Orthopaedic Foot and Ankle Surgeon
Vancouver Bone and Joint Clinic
Vancouver, British Columbia, Canada

Camiron Pfennig, MD
Resident
Department of Orthopaedic Surgery
Indiana University School of Medicine
Indianapolis, Indiana

Andrew Pickle, MD, FRCS(C)
Private Practice
Orthopedic Surgery and Sports
    Medicine
Belleville, Ontario, Canada

Joshua M. Polster, MD
Staff Radiologist
Department of Radiology
The Cleveland Clinic Foundation
Cleveland, Ohio

Chadwick Prodromos, MD
Assistant Professor
Department of Orthopaedic Surgery
Rush University Medical Center
Chicago, Illinois

President
Illinois Sports Medicine and Orthopaedic
    Centers
Glenview, Illinois

Benjamin D. Rubin, MD, MS
Orthopaedic Specialty Institute
Orange, California

Richard K.N. Ryu, MD
Private Practice
Santa Barbara, California

Marc R. Safran, MD
Associate Professor
Department of Orthopaedic Surgery
University of California, San Francisco
San Francisco, California

Chief
Division of Sports Medicine
Department of Orthopaedic Surgery
University of California, San Francisco
San Francisco, California

Sakae Sano, MD, PhD
Orthopaedic Surgeon
Department of Orthopaedic Surgery
Graduate School of Medicine,
    Chiba University
Chiba, Japan

Judy R. Schauer, DO, CDR, MC, USN

Ronald M. Selby, MD
Clinical Assistant Professor
Department of Orthopaedic Surgery
New York Medical College
Valhalla, New York

Attending
Department of Orthopaedic Surgery
Saint Vincent's Catholic Medical Center
Saint Vincent's Hospital Manhattan
New York, New York

K. Donald Shelbourne, MD
Associate Clinical Professor
Department of Orthopaedic Surgery
Indiana University School of Medicine
Indianapolis, Indiana

Orthopaedic Surgeon
The Shelbourne Clinic at Methodist Hospital
Indianapolis, Indiana

Walter R. Shelton, MD
Fellowship Co-Director
Mississippi Sports Medicine and Orthopaedic
    Center
Jackson, Mississippi

Mississippi Baptist Hospital
Jackson, Mississippi

Jian Shen, MD
Resident
Department of Orthopaedics
Wake Forest University Medical Center
Winston-Salem North Carolina

Joel J. Smith, MD
Department of Orthopaedic Surgery
University of California, San Diego
San Diego, California

R. Lance Snyder, MD
Dickson/Diveley Orthopaedic Clinic
Kansas City, Missouri

Tim Spalding, MB, BS, FRCS Orth
Specialist Knee Surgeon
Department of Trauma and Orthopaedic Surgery
University Hospital Coventry and Warwickshire
    NHS Trust
Coventry, West Midlands, England

Kurt P. Spindler, MD
Professor, The Kenneth D. Schermerhorn
Vice Chairman, Orthopaedics & Rehabilitation
Vanderbilt Medical School
Nashville, Tennessee

Director, Vanderbilt Sports
    Medicine Orthopaedic Patient Care Center
Orthopaedics & Rehabilitation
Vanderbilt Medical Center
Nashville, Tennessee

William D. Stanish, MD, FRCSC, FACS
Professor
Department of Surgery
Dalhousie University
Halifax, Nova Scotia, Canada

Director
Orthopaedic & Sports Medicine Clinic
    of Nova Scotia
Halifax, Nova Scotia, Canada

James Starman, MD
Department of Orthopaedic Surgery
University of Pittsburgh School of Medicine
Pittsburgh, Pennsylvania

James W. Stone, MD
Medical College of Wisconsin
Milwaukee, Wisconsin

Dawn L. Swarm, MD
Orthopaedic Surgeon
Department of Orthopaedic Surgery
Kaiser Medical Center
Woodland Hills, California

Michael P. Swords, DO
Assistant Clinical Professor
Department of Surgical Specialties
Michigan State University College of Orthopaedic
    Medicine
East Lansing, Michigan

Department of Surgery, Orthopaedic Section
Sparrow Health System
Lansing, Michigan

Robert Talac, MD, PhD
Orthopedic Surgery Resident
Department of Orthopaedic Surgery
University of California, San Diego
San Diego, California

Orthopedic Surgery Resident
Department of Orthopaedic Surgery
UCSD Medical Center
San Diego, California

Jeffrey W. Tamborlane, MD
Staff Physician
Orthopedics
Kaiser-Permanente Moanalua Medical Center
Honolulu, Hawaii

James Patrick Tasto, MD
Clinical Professor
Department of Orthopaedics
University of California, San Diego
San Diego, California

Orthopedic Surgeon
Department of Orthopedic Surgery
San Diego Sports Medicine & Orthopaedic
    Center
San Diego, California

Walter A. Thomas, MD
Department of Orthopaedics
Scripps Hospital
Chula Vista, California

Monika Volesky, MD
Assistant Professor
McGill University
Division of Orthopaedic Surgery
Jewish General Hospital
Montreal, Quebec, Canada

Jon J.P. Warner, MD
Professor
Department of Orthopaedic Surgery
Massachusetts General Hospital
Boston, Massachusetts

Chief, The Harvard Shoulder Service
Department of Orthopaedics
Massachusetts General Hospital

Russell F. Warren, MD
Professor of Orthopaedic Surgery
Weill Medical College of Cornell University
New York, New York

Attending Orthopaedic Surgeon
Hospital for Special Surgery
New York, New York

Surgeon-in-Chief Emeritus
Department of Orthopaedics
Hospital for Special Surgery
New York, New York

Derek W. Weichel, BS
Medical Student
University of Virginia School of Medicine
Charlottesville, Virginia

Ethan R. Wiesler, MD
Assistant Professor
Department of Orthopaedic Surgery
Wake Forest University School of Medicine
Winston-Salem, North Carolina

Faculty
Department of Orthopaedic Surgery
North Carolina Baptist Hospital
Winston-Salem, North Carolina

James Williams, MD
Department of Orthopaedic Surgery
Cleveland Clinic Foundation
Cleveland, Ohio

John J. Wilson, MD
Sports Medicine Fellow, Research Fellow
Department of Family Medicine
University of Wisconsin School of Medicine and
    Public Health
Madison, Wisconsin

Clinical Instructor
Department of Family Medicine
University of Wisconsin Hospitals and Clinics
Madison, Wisconsin

Kevin J. Wing, MD, FRCSC
Clinical Assistant Professor
Department of Orthopaedic Surgery
University of British Columbia
Vancouver, British Columbia, Canada

Consultant
Department of Orthopaedic Surgery
St. Paul's Hospital
Vancouver, British Columbia, Canada

Alastair Younger, MSc, MBChB, FRCSC
Clinic Director
Orthopaedic Surgeon
Burrard Medical Centre
Vancouver, British Columbia, Canada

Horacio Yepes, MD
Lecturer, Department of Orthopaedics
Dalhousie University
Halifax, Nova Scotia, Canada

David Zijerdi, MD
Geisinger Medical Center
Danville, Pennsylvania

The aim of our text is to present the practical aspects of orthopaedic sports medicine in a format that enables the ever-busy orthopaedic residents and surgeons to absorb the most information in the least amount of time. The text covers all career phases: certification, review for recertification, and daily clinical practice. To provide a global perspective, we have tapped the knowledge of the top innovators in orthopaedic sports medicine from around the world.

HIGHLIGHTS:

- Key points in each chapter outline the concepts to be covered and serve as a review to prepare for Boards.
- Opening section presents basic science in detail.

- Chapters are organized by anatomy, that is, treatment of the athlete from head to toe.
- A section is dedicated to special needs of the athlete, such as stress fractures, special needs of the female athlete, pediatric challenges, and team physician issues.
- Copious original illustrations enhance the understanding of anatomy and operative techniques.
- Rehabilitation is emphasized.

The goal of our approach is to get the injured player back in the game as quickly as possible and in top physical condition. The techniques we present will help our fellow surgeons achieve the best results for all athletes, from young players with dreams of going professional to the professionals themselves.

ACKNOWLEDGMENTS

This book was made possible by the energy and commitment of many individuals. We would like to thank our Executive Editor, Bob Hurley, for establishing the concept and for his steady support of the work. Jennifer Harper was the Project Manager, coordinating all phases of production, and was essentially the unsung hero of this enterprise. We especially thank our fearless and tireless Developmental Editor, Eileen Wolfberg, who nurtured the book like it was her baby. Last, and certainly not least, we would like to sincerely thank all of the authors and coauthors for giving their time, effort, and expertise to the project. This textbook would be nothing without their selfless contributions.

CONTENTS

■ SECTION 11
APPENDICES

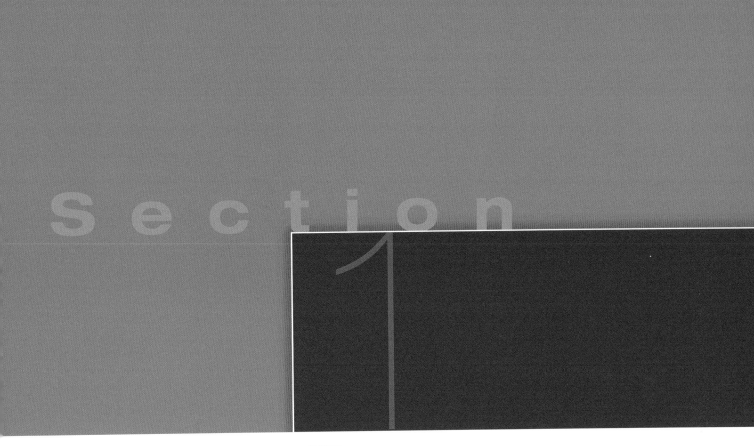

BASIC SCIENCE

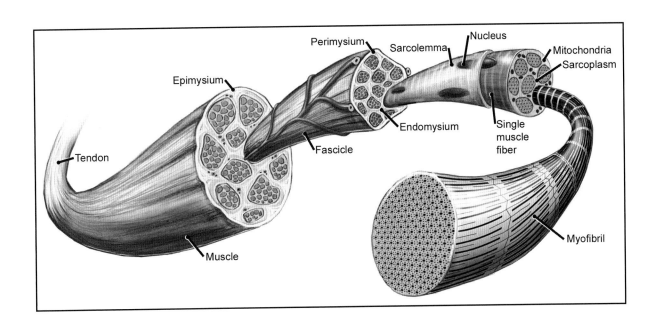

PERIARTICULAR LIGAMENTOUS TISSUE: A BIOCHEMICAL AND PHYSIOLOGIC ASSESSMENT

DAVID AMIEL, PhD, SAKAE SANO, MD, PhD

■ KEY POINTS

- Although tendons and ligaments are composed primarily of fibrillar collagens, they have entirely different functions. Tendons are a conduit, connecting muscle to bone. Ligaments are short bands of fibrous tissue that bind bone to bone.
- Collagen is the single most abundant animal protein in mammals. Collagen molecules assemble into characteristic fibers responsible for the functional integrity of tissues such as bone, cartilage, skin, ligament, and tendon.
- The medial collateral ligament (MCL) of the knee is notable for rod-shaped and spindle-shaped cells that are intermediate in length compared with patellar tendon and anterior cruciate ligament (ACL) cells. The cellular morphological characteristics of the MCL are those of all fibroblasts, whereas the ACL cellular characteristics are similar to fibrocartilage cells.
- A distinct form of collagen in cartilage, now known as Type II collage, was discovered about 30 years ago. Since then, many other unique molecular species have been observed. Types I, II, III, V, and XI collagen are categorized as fiber-forming collagens. They all exhibit lengthy, uninterrupted collagenous domains and are first synthesized as biosynthetic precursors (procollagens).
- Proteoglycans consist of small amounts of protein bound to negatively charged polysaccharide chains referred to as glycosaminoglycans (GAGs). In articular cartilage, proteoglycans form a large portion of the macromolecular framework, but in ligaments they form only a small portion of this framework.

The ligaments of the knee are well-designed for their role in the maintenance of normal joint kinematics, with each ligament oriented in the direction needed to provide joint stability. Ligaments are well-designed connective tissues. Their densely packed collagen fiber bundles are arrayed in parallel along the length of the tissue substance to allow for the most efficient resistance of tensile loads.

Ligament insertions to bone are also well-adapted to their intended function. Force dissipation is achieved through a gradual transition from ligament to fibrocartilage to bone. Disruption is less likely to occur in this transition region than in the bone or peri-insertional tissue substance (1–3). For many years, tendons and ligaments have been classified together as dense, regularly arranged connective tissue (4–6). Although tendons and ligaments are composed primarily of fibrillar collagens, they have entirely different functions. Tendons are a conduit, connecting muscle to bone, thereby allowing movement of a joint complex through muscle contraction or relaxation. Ligaments are short bands of fibrous tissue that bind bone to bone and provide support for internal organs. In concert with the bony geometry and the dynamic effects of muscle and tendon (7,8) ligaments limit and guide joint motion.

Collagen is the single most abundant animal protein in mammals, accounting for up to 30% of all proteins (9). Collagen molecules assemble into characteristic fibers responsible for the functional integrity of tissues such as bone, cartilage, skin, ligament, and tendon (10). They contribute a structural framework for most organs. Crosslinks between adjacent molecules are a prerequisite for the collagen fibers to withstand the physical stresses to which they are exposed. A variety of human conditions, normal and pathologic, involve the ability of tissues to repair and regenerate their collagenous framework. Many disabling conditions result from changes in the nature and organization of collagen (9).

■ STRUCTURE

The histology of periarticular tendons and ligaments is a much-neglected area of investigation. Although many histology texts combine these two tissues as "dense, regular connective tissue" (11–14), certain ligaments and tendons are sufficiently characteristic to be distinguishable from each other based upon their histological appearance (15).

The variables considered are collagen bundle width, cell morphology and size, as well as "crimp." Crimp is a feature of tendons and ligaments; it represents a regular sinusoidal pattern in the matrix. The periodicity and amplitude of crimp appear to be structure-specific features, and they are best evaluated under polarized light. A simple functional explanation for this accordionlike pattern in the matrix is that it provides a "buffer" in which slight longitudinal elongation may occur without fibrous damage. It also provides a mechanism for control of tension and acts as a "shock absorber" along the length of the tissue. When physiologic mechanical limits of this crimp are exceeded, however, irreversible damage occurs and the physical properties of the tissue are changed (16).

Although tendons and ligaments have crimping within their fascicles, there appear to be differences in the crimp pattern between these two structures (17). In the canine anterior cruciate ligament (ACL) and patellar tendon, two patterns of crimping are noted. The centrally located fascicles in the ACL are either straight or undulated in a planar wave pattern, whereas those located at the periphery are arranged in a helical wave pattern. In the patellar tendon, all the fascicles are found to undulate in the helical wave pattern.

The following histological description refers to rabbit tendons and ligaments unless otherwise specified. Microscopic examination of patellar tendon sections that have been stained with hematoxylin and eosin or evaluated directly under polarized light reveals the presence of longitudinally oriented bundles of collagenous tissue. These bundles are approximately 20 micrometers (μm) in width and have the characteristic crimp pattern of regular connective tissue. In patellar tendon, the crimp period is approximately 120 μm in length, with a corresponding amplitude of about 15 μm. On either side of the bundles or fascicles are spindle-shaped fibroblasts that are approximately 25 μm long. They are aligned longitudinally. Cytoplasm is indistinct, and only nuclei can be seen. More cellular areas within areolar connective tissue are observed. These sites, which are actually investing layers of tissue, are called "peritendineum" **(Fig 1-1)** and have been previously described as a site of reserve cells (18). They also mark the site of nerve and blood supply to the tendon.

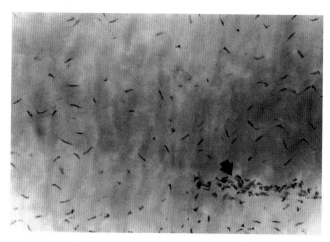

Fig 1-1. Histology of normal patellar tendon [H&E stain, original magnification 50×]. Note spindle-shaped fibroblasts, coarse fibrillar crimp, and peritendineum (*arrow*).

Rabbit Achilles tendon demonstrates cell morphology, cell size, bundle width, and crimp period that are similar to those of patellar tendon. The crimp amplitudes of these tissues are different, with the Achilles tendon having almost three times (40 μm) the wave height relative to the patellar tendon. This difference may be related to an increased margin of shock absorbance for the Achilles tendon.

Histological assessment of the ACL demonstrates longitudinally oriented bundles of collagen with a width of about 20 μm as seen in the patellar tendon. The crimp period in the ACL, however, is considerably shorter (45 to 60 μm), and the amplitude is less than 5 μm. Fibroblasts are located on either side of the collagenous bundles, but the ligament is considerably more cellular than the tendon **(Fig 1-2)**. ACL fibroblasts are round to ovoid and are substantially different in appearance from the fibroblasts in the patellar tendon. They measure about 5 to 8 μm in diameter and 12 to 15 μm in length. Cells are arranged longitudinally along the borders of the fascicles.

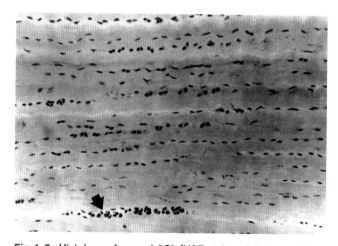

Fig 1-2. Histology of normal ACL [H&E stain, original magnification 50×]. Note rounded fibroblasts, fine fibrillar crimp, and cluster of potential reserve cells (*arrow*).

TABLE 1-1	Summary of Histologic Observations of Rabbit Periarticular Connective Tissue				
Tissue width	Collagen bundle (μm)	Crimp period (μm)	Crimp amplitude (μm)	Cell shape	Cell size (μm $\times$ μm)
Patellar tendon	20	120	15	Spindle	3–5 $\times$ 15
Achilles tendon	20	120	40	Spindle	3–5 $\times$ 15
Anterior cruciate ligament (ACL)	20	45–60	<5	Round to ovoid	5–8 $\times$ 12–15
Medial collateral ligament (MCL)	20	45	10	Rod to spindle	3–5 $\times$ 15

Like the patellar tendon, groups of cells, which concentrate in areolar connective tissue, are observed (Fig 1-2). These may be the ligamentous correlates to the peritendineum areas.

The medial collateral ligament (MCL) of the knee is notable for rod-shaped and spindle-shaped cells that are intermediate in length compared with patellar tendon and ACL cells. The MCL has cells that are 15 μm long and 25 μm wide. The crimp period measures approximately 45 μm, with a 10 μm amplitude, and the collagen bundle width is approximately 20 μm, as seen in the other structures discussed. Measurements of cell size, shape, crimp specifics, and bundle width of the tendons and ligaments are provided in **Table 1-1**.

These substantial differences in morphology and ultrastructure may reflect the functional and environmental differences between these two periarticular ligaments, the ACL and MCL. The cellular morphological characteristics of the MCL are those of all fibroblasts, whereas the ACL cellular characteristics are similar to fibrocartilage cells. These observations lead to a series of profound and important questions concerning the differences in function, homeostasis, and repair between the ACL and MCL.

The biochemical parameters used to assess the constitutional properties of collagenous tissue include collagen structure and type, collagen reducible and nonreducible crosslink analysis, proteoglycan content, and glycoprotein. The value of each of these variables is related to its importance in the study of both (a) soft tissue injury and healing and (b) the response to exercise and the deleterious effects of immobilization. A more complete understanding of these problems could improve various treatment modalities and place them on firm scientific ground. This is particularly the case because most investigations of tissue injury and healing involve skin, not tendons or ligaments (19–21).

■ COLLAGEN IN TENDONS AND LIGAMENTS

Collagen is the major protein in ligaments and tendons, and it is not a single entity. It is the single most abundant animal protein in mammals, accounting for up to 30% of all proteins. The collagen molecules, after being secreted by the cells, assemble into characteristic fibers responsible for the functional integrity of tissues such as bone, cartilage, skin, ligaments, and tendon (22). They contribute a structural framework to other tissues such as blood vessels and most organs. Crosslinks between adjacent molecules are a prerequisite for the collagen fibers to withstand the physical stresses to which they are exposed. Significant progress has been made toward understanding the functional groups on the molecules that are involved in the formation of such crosslinks, their nature, and location. A variety of human conditions, normal and pathologic, involve the ability of tissues to repair and regenerate their collagenous framework. Some of these conditions are characterized by excessive deposition of collagen (e.g., cirrhosis, scleroderma, keloid, pulmonary fibrosis, diabetes, etc.). After trauma or surgery, abnormal deposition of collagen may impair function (adhesions following repair of long tendons, scar formation during healing, etc.). In addition, many disabling conditions result from changes in the nature and organization of collagen (heart-valve lesions, osteoarthritis, rheumatoid arthritis, and congenital collagen diseases such as Marfan's and Ehlers-Danlos syndromes, osteogenesis imperfecta, etc.).

The Collagen Molecule

The arrangement of amino acids in the collagen molecule is shown schematically in **Figure 1-3**. Every third amino acid is glycine. Proline and hydroxyproline follow each other relatively frequently, and the (gly, pro, hyp) sequence makes up about 10% of the molecule. This triple helical structure generates a symmetrical pattern of three left-handed helical chains that are, in turn, slightly displaced to the right, superimposing an additional "supercoil" with a pitch of approximately 8.6 nanometers (nm). These chains, known as α-chains, have a molecular weight of around 100 k Daltons and contain approximately 1,000 amino acids for the interstitial collagen Types I, II, and III **(Fig 1-4)**. The amino acids within each chain are displaced by a distance h = 0.201 nm with a relative twist of 100 degrees, making the number of

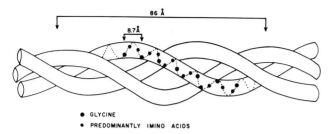

Fig 1-3. The collagen triple helix. The individual α chains are left-handed helices with approximately three residues per turn. The chains are in turn coiled around each other following a right-handed twist. The hydrogen bonds which stabilize the triple helix (not shown) form between opposing residues in different chains (interpeptide hydrogen bonding) and are therefore quite different from α helices which occur between amino acids located within the same polypeptide.

TYPE I

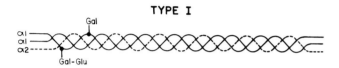

TYPE II

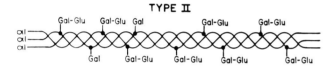

TYPE III

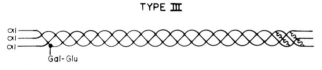

Fig 1-4. Diagram of the three interstitial types of collagen. Type I is present in skin, bone, ligaments, tendons, etc.; Type II is present in cartilage; and Type III is present in blood vessels and developing tissues and as a minor component in skin and other tissues. There are differences in the chain composition and degrees of glycosylation. Disulfide crosslinks are only seen in Type III collagen.

residues per turn 3.27, and the distance between each third glycine 0.87 nm. The individual residues are nearly fully extended in the collagen structure, since the maximum displacement within a fully stretched chain would be approximately 0.36 nm. This separation is such that it will not allow *intrachain* bonds to form (as does occur in the alpha helix), and only interchain hydrogen bonds are possible. The exact number of hydrogen bonds that stabilize the triple helical structure has not been determined. One model describes two hydrogen bonds for every three amino acids, whereas another assumes one.

In addition to these intramolecular conformational patterns, there seems to exist a supermolecular coiling. Microfibrils, possibly representing intermediate stages of packing, have been described.

A process of *self assembly* causes the collagen molecules to organize into fibers. The thermodynamics of such a system involve changes in the state of the water molecules, many of which are associated with nonpolar regions of the collagen molecule (23).

Biosynthesis: Procollagen

In order for the organism to develop an extracellular network of collagen fibers, the cells involved in the biosynthetic process must first synthesize a precursor known as procollagen. This molecule is later enzymatically trimmed of its nonhelical ends, giving rise to a collagen molecule that spontaneously assembles into fibers in the extracellular space. Procollagen molecules have been identified as precursors of the three interstitial collagens (Types I, II, and III). Several of the N- and C-terminal peptides (propeptides) have been characterized and the primary sequences determined.

The carboxyterminal propeptides of both pro α1 and pro α2 chains have molecular weights of 30,000 to 35,000 Daltons and globular conformations without any collagenlike domain. These peptides contain asparagines-linked oligosaccharide units composed of N-acetylglucosamine and mannose. Once the molecule is completed and translocated to the cell surface, the extensions are enzymatically removed from those collagens, which then form fibrils. Enzymes that selectively remove these extensions can be found in a variety of connective tissues, and in the culture media derived from collagen-secreting cells.

Gene Expression

Since the discovery about 30 years ago of a distinct form of collagen in cartilage, now known as Type II collagen, many other unique molecular species have been observed. Types I, II, III, V, and XI collagen are categorized as *fiber-forming collagens*. They all exhibit lengthy, uninterrupted collagenous domains and are first synthesized as biosynthetic precursors (procollagens). Gene cloning experiments have demonstrated that the Group I collagen genes are evolutionarily related, for they share a common ancestral gene structure. Human chromosome number 17 contains the coding information for the α1 chain of Type I collagen, while chromosome 7 codes for its complementary α2 chain. A comparison of the five fibrillar collagens described shows that, with one exception [Types III and α2 (V) are located on chromosome 2], all other genes are located on different chromosomes.

The genes coding for fiber-forming collagens are large, about 10 times the size of the functional mRNA. Many of the exons (coding sequences) are 54 base pairs (bp) in length and are separated from each other by large intervening sequences (introns) that range in size from about 80 to 2,000 bp. The gene itself contains 38,000 bp and is very complex. The finding that most exons of these genes have identical lengths suggests that the ancestral gene for collagen was assembled by multiple duplications of single genetic units containing an exon of 54 bp **(Fig 1-5)**. It is likely that a primordial exon this

ASSEMBLY OF THE ANCESTRAL COLLAGEN GENE

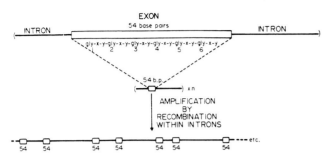

Fig 1-5. The collagen gene is made up of multiple units containing 54 base pairs, each of which corresponds to sequences of 18 amino acids. The conservation of this minimum sequence and the fact that it is repeated in such an exacting fashion provide valuable information to investigators interested in the process of evolution of proteins.

size could have encoded for a gly-pro-pro tripeptide repeated six times ($3 \times 3 \times 6$). Such a polypeptide of 18 amino acids probably had the minimum length needed to form a stable triple helical structure.

Translational, Cotranslational, and Early Post-translational Events

After the gene is transcribed, it is spliced to remove introns and to yield a functional mRNA that contains about 3,000 bases. Specific mRNAs for each chain and collagen type are translocated to the cytoplasm and translated into proteins in the rough endoplasmic reticulum (RER) on membrane-bound polysomes. As the collagen polypeptide is synthesized in the RER, it is modified in important ways. Two major constituents of collagen are the modified amino acids hydroxyproline and hydroxylysine, but neither of these can be directly incorporated into proteins. Instead, proline and lysine are incorporated and then modified by two hydroxylating enzymes, prolyl and lysyl hydroxylases. These enzymes require ferrous iron, ascorbate, and α-ketoglutarate for their activity. The degree of hydroxylation differs from tissue to tissue and depends on availability of substrate, rate of synthesis, turnover, and the time during which the molecule remains in the presence of the hydroxylating enzymes. The time required for the synthesis of a complete pro α chain is about 6.7 min.

As lysyl residues in the newly synthesized pro α chains are hydroxylated, sugar residues are added to the resulting hydroxylysyl groups. Glycosylation is catalyzed by two specific enzymes, a galactosyltransferase and glucosyltransferase. Once the translation, modifications, and additions are completed, the individual pro α chains become properly aligned for the triple helix to form.

Intracellular Translocation of Procollagen and Extrusion into the Extracellular Space

The procollagen molecules, now detached from the ribosome, emerge from the endoplasmic reticulum (ER) and move toward the Golgi apparatus (G) through the microsomal

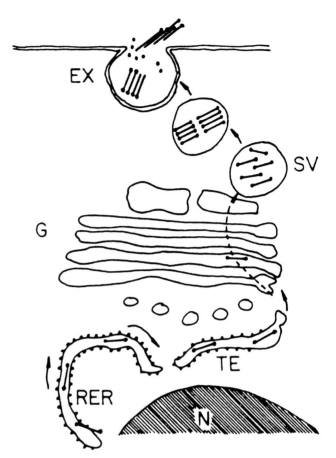

Fig 1-6. Movement of procollagen through the cisternae of the rough endoplasmic reticulum (*RER*) and through a transitional endoplasm *(TE)* to the Golgi apparatus (*G*), where it is packaged into secretory vesicle (*SV*) prior to extrusion (*EX*) by exocytosis. N, Nucleus.

lumen. In the Golgi, the C-terminal mannose-rich carbohydrate extensions are remodeled, the molecules are packaged in vesicles, and subsequently carried towards the cellular membrane **(Fig 1-6)**.

The small aggregates of oriented procollagen molecules are probably trimmed of their nonhelical amino and carboxyl extensions by specific peptidases when they reach the extracellular space. In the case of Type I collagen, the first peptidase to act seems to be the amino protease; this is followed by a carboxyprotease. In Type III collagen the sequence of removal may be reversed.

Lysyl Oxidase

Recently formed microfibrils seem to be recognized by the enzyme lysyl oxidase, which converts certain peptide-bound lysines and hydroxylysines to aldehydes. The enzyme is an extracellular amine oxidase, which has been purified from a variety of connective tissues. It requires Cu^{2+} and probably pyridaxal as cofactors; molecular oxygen seems to be the cosubstrate, and hydrogen acceptor. It is irreversibly inhibited by the lathyrogen BAPN (β-amino pro-pronitrile, a substance found in the flowering sweet-pea, lathyrus

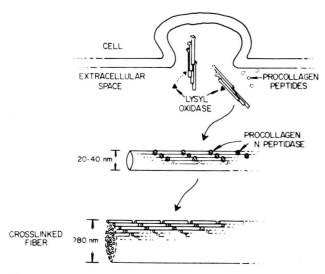

Fig 1-7. Fibrillogenesis: Microfibrils in a quarter-staggered configuration have lost their carboxy-terminal nonhelical extensions, part of their amino (N)-terminal nonhelical extensions, and part of their amino (N)-terminal extensions. In this form, they seem to organize readily into small-diameter fibrils which retain part of the amino-terminal nonhelical extensions. After being relieved of these peptides by a procollagen peptidase, fibrils are able to grow in diameter by apposition of microfibrils or by merger with other small-diameter fibrils.

odoratus). This enzyme exhibits maximal activity when acting on collagen fibrils rather than upon monomeric collagen.

Fibrillogenesis

The tendency of collagen molecules to form macromolecular aggregates is well-known. This tendency is common with most fibrous proteins that form filaments with helical symmetry and which occupy equivalent or quasiequivalent positions.

The exact mode in which the collagen molecules pack into microfibrils (precursors of the larger fibrils) still remains a subject for speculation. A five-stranded microfibril was first suggested to account for such a substructure, one that would satisfy the condition that adjacent molecules were quivalently related by a quarterstagger **(Fig 1-7)**.

When monomeric collagen is heated to 37°C it progressively polymerizes, generating a turbidity curve that reflects the presence of intermediate aggregates. The lag phase (persistence of monomers), the nucleation and appearance of turbidity (microfibrils), and the rapid increase in turbidity (fiber formation) have been equated to how the cell may handle this process.

Different Types of Collagen

Almost 3 decades have passed since we first realized that all collagen fibers within a particular organism are not made up of identical molecules. The different collagen types are usually identified using Roman numerals, assigned as they are purified and characterized.

Since this paper focuses on ligaments, we shall only describe the major characteristics of the two collagen types present in the ACL, namely Types I and III. Type V collagen seems to be present at less than one percent.

Type I Collagen

Before 1969, Type I collagen was the only mammalian collagen known. It is composed of three chains: two identical, termed α1 chains, and one different from the other two, called α2. Type I collagen is most abundant in skin, tendon, ligament, bone, cornea, etc.; it comprises between 80% to 99% of the body's total collagen. Bone matrix is essentially all Type I collagen.

Type III Collagen

When human dermis is digested with pepsin under conditions in which the collagen molecules retain their helical conformation, Type I molecules can be separated from Type III by differential salt precipitation at pH 7.5. The Type III molecules are composed of three identical chains. Characteristic of this collagen is the presence of intramolecular disulfide bonds involving two cysteine residues close to the C-terminal region of the triple helix. Because the ratio of Type I and Type III collagen changes with age, Type III being predominant in fetal skin, this type of collagen is many times referred to as *fetal* or *embryonic collagen*.

Formation of intermolecular disulfide bridges by Type III collagen could be of great advantage during early development and wound healing, where collagen is deposited at a rapid rate in order to fill a gap.

Normal bone matrix may be the only tissue containing Type I collagen that lacks Type III collagen. Blood vessels are particularly rich in Type III collagen.

Collagen Metabolism

Collagen is the most abundant of all body proteins. Tissues such as bone, which are involved in active remodeling, are responsible for the major turnover. Other less dynamic tissues in the full-grown individual, such as skin and tendons, may exhibit slow and almost negligible turnover. The collagen synthesizing activity of cells is usually assessed by their ability to synthesize hydroxyproline or by the activities of specific enzymes such as the proline and lysyl hydroxylases.

Degradation: Collagenases, Bacterial, and Mammalian

Because of its triple helical structure stabilized by hydrogen bonds, the collagen molecules are quite resistant to enzymatic degradation in their native configuration. They can be degraded by collagenases. The first of these to be isolated were of bacterial origin, specifically, Clostridium Histolyticum. These enzymes are quite specific for collagen but will also degrade gelatin, which is denatured collagen. They are inhibited by cysteine and other SH-compounds and by EDTA, a chelator for divalent cations. These enzymes are specific for peptide bonds involving glycine in a collagen helix conformation. Because of the abundance of this amino acid in collagen (every third residue) this enzyme generates a large number of small peptides.

The first enzyme derived from animal tissue capable of degrading collagen at neutral pH was isolated from the

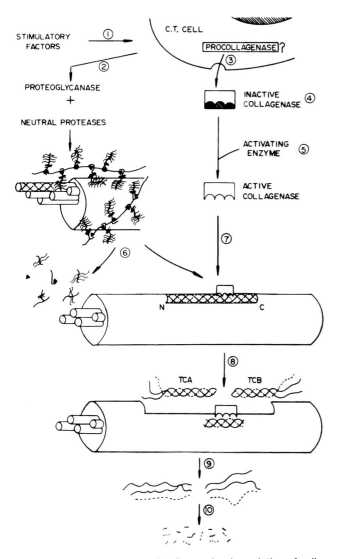

Fig 1-8. Sequence of events leading to the degradation of collagen fibers by the enzyme collagenase. (1) A variety of factors stimulate connective tissue (CT) cells to synthesize collagenase, glycosidases, and neutral proteases. (2) The proteoglycan-degrading enzymes remove the mucopolysaccharides which surround collagen fibers and expose them to collagenase. (3) Inactive collagenase is secreted. (4) The enzyme is usually found in the extracellular space bound to an inhibitor. (5) An activating enzyme removes the inhibitor. (6) Glycosidases complete the degradation of the proteoglycans. (7) The active collagenase binds to fibrillar collagen. (8) Collagenase splits the first collagen molecule into two fragments (TCA and TCB), which denature and begin to unfold at body temperature. The enzyme now moves on to an adjacent molecule. (9) The denatured collagen fragments are now susceptible to other proteases. (10) Nonspecific neutral proteases degrade the collagen polypeptides.

culture fluid of tadpole tissue. It cleaves the native molecule into two fragments in a highly specific fashion at a temperature below that of substrate denaturation. Since then, collagenolytic enzymes have been obtained from a wide range of animal tissues. In general, these enzymes have fundamental properties in common; they all have a neutral pH optima and are not stored within the cell, but rather are secreted either in an inactive form or bound to inhibitors. **Figure 1-8** summarizes schematically the fundamental aspects of these enzymes and their mode of action. They appear to be zinc metalloenzymes requiring calcium, and are not inhibited by agents that block serine or sulphydryl-type proteinases. Nearly all the collagenases studied so far have a molecular mass that ranges from 25,000 to 60,000 Daltons. Mammalian collagenases display a great deal of specificity, cleaving bands between Gly-Leu or Gly-Ile. There are slight differences in the amino acid sequences surrounding the scission site; these may account for the differences in the rates at which various collagens are degraded.

The enzymes interact tightly with the collagen fibers and appear to remain bound to the macromolecular aggregate during the degradation process. Approximately 10% of the collagen molecules in reconstituted collagen fibrils appear accessible for binding, in close agreement with the theoretical number of molecules estimated to be present near the surface of the fiber. The *in vitro* data obtained seem to indicate that digestion proceeds to completion by hopping from one molecule to another without returning to the solution. Collagen from older individuals is more resistant to enzymatic digestion.

Crosslinking

Intramolecular and Intermolecular Crosslinks
Crosslinking renders the collagen fibers stable and provides them with a degree of tensile strength and visco-elasticity adequate to perform their structural role. The degree of crosslinking, the number and density of the fibers in a particular tissue, and the orientation and diameter combine to provide this function. Crosslinking begins with the oxidative deamination of the ϵ-carbon of lysine or hydroxylysine to yield the corresponding semialdehydes, and is mediated by the enzyme lysyl oxidase **(Fig 1-9)**. Enzymatic activity is inhibited by β-aminoproprionitrile, chelating agents, isonicotinic acid hydrazide, and other carbonyl reagents. Lysyl oxidase exhibits particular affinity for the lysines and hydroxylysines present in the nonhelical extensions of collagen, but can, at a slower pace, also alter residues located in the helical region of the molecule.

In general, lysine-derived crosslinks seem to predominate in soft connective tissues such as skin and tendon, whereas hydroxylysine-derived crosslinks are prevalent in the harder connective tissues such as bone, cartilage, and dentine, which are less prone to yield soluble collagens.

Several other crosslinks have been identified and their location established. These more complex polyfunctional

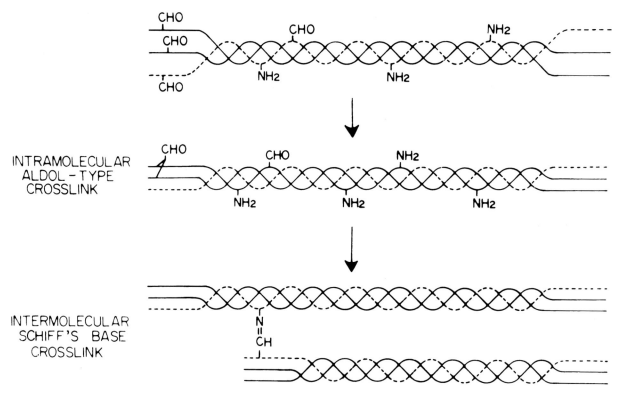

Fig 1-9. Formation of intramolecular and intermolecular crosslinks in Type I collagen. Intramolecular crosslinks occur in the nonhelical regions and involve a condensation reaction between lysine- or hydroxylysine-derived aldehydes within a single molecule. Intermolecular crosslinks, on the other hand, involve aldehydes and ε-amino groups of lysine present in different molecules.

crosslinks can contain histidine or can result in the formation of naturally fluorescent pyridinium ring structures.

Inhibition of Collagen Crosslinking: Amino Nitriles and D-Penicillamine

Lathyrism is a connective tissue disorder associated with the ingestion or injection of BAPN (β-amino propionitrile and its chemical analogues), extracts of the sweet pea, or other members of the lathyrus family usually consumed during periods of great famine. The skeletal changes observed differ among species and vary with age, being much more pronounced in younger animals. The epiphyseal plate is a prime target.

The connective tissue abnormalities are associated with crosslinking defects in collagen and elastin. They are revealed by an increased solubility in hypertonic neutral salt solutions, due to an inhibition of lysyl oxidase activity. Since Cu^{2+} deficiency also inhibits the enzymatic activity, the similarities of the defects induced by these two mechanisms are readily explainable.

Administration of penicillamine to animals and humans also causes an accumulation of neutral salt soluble collagen in skin and various soft tissues. Two of the more characteristic properties of penicillamine, namely the ability to trap carbonyl compounds and to chelate heavy metals, are of primary significance in impairing collagen crosslinking.

The former property manifests itself in all effective dose ranges, whereas the latter occurs only at dosages far higher than those administered to humans.

The collagen extracted from tissues of animals treated with D-penicillamine is able to form stable fibers *in vitro* and is not deficient in aldehydes, as is that from BAP-treated animals. In fact, its aldehyde content is even higher than normal, suggesting that the mechanisms of action of BAPN and penicillamine are different.

■ THE PROTEOGLYCANS

Proteoglycans consist of small amounts of protein bound to negatively charged polysaccharide chains referred to as GAGs. In articular cartilage, proteoglycans form a large portion of the macromolecular framework (commonly about 30% to 35% of the tissue dry weight), but in ligaments they form only a small portion of this framework, usually less than 1% of the dry weight (15,24,25). Nonetheless, proteoglycans may have an important role in organizing the extracellular matrix and in interacting with the tissue fluid (26–33).

Like tendon, meniscus, and articular cartilage, ligaments contain two known classes of proteoglycans: large articular cartilage type proteoglycans containing long, negatively charged chains of chondroitin and keratin sulfate (syndecan) and smaller proteoglycans that contain dermatan sulfate (28–30). Because of their long chains of negative charges, the articular cartilage type proteoglycans tend to expand to their maximum domain until restrained by the collagen fibril network. As a result, they maintain water within the tissue, alter fluid flow within the tissue during loading, and exert a swelling pressure, thereby contributing to the mechanical properties of the tissue and filling the regions between collagen fibrils.

Small dermatan sulfate proteoglycans (decorin and biglycan) usually lie on the surface of collagen fibrils and seem to affect the formation, organization, and stability of the extracellular matrix, including collagen fibril formation and diameter (34,35). These molecules may also affect the ability of mesenchymal cells to repair ligament injuries. They can inhibit fibroblast adhesion to other matrix macromolecules (especially the noncollagenous protein fibronectin) and thereby may limit the ability of the cells to bind to the matrix and form new tissue (36).

The concentration of GAGs present in rabbit knee ligaments differs significantly from that present in tendinous tissue (15,24). The ACL has the highest proportion of GAGs, two to four times the amount observed in tendons (15,24). Although the functional importance of these differences is unknown, it is clear that the higher the GAG content, the more water that is associated with the complex. This naturally alters the viscoelastic properties of these tissues and may represent an additional "shock-absorbing" feature in ligaments (optimized in the cruciate ligaments) that is less important in tendon.

■ THE NONCOLLAGENOUS PROTEINS (GLYCOPROTEINS)

These molecules consist primarily of protein, but many of them also contain a few monosaccharides and oligosaccharides (25,28,30). Although noncollagenous proteins such as fibronectin contribute only a few percentage points to the dry weight of ligaments, they have an important role in the complex interaction of ligament cells and their environment during growth, healing, and remodeling. However, this role is poorly understood.

Fibronectins are important in an array of cellular functions, particularly those involving a cell's interaction with its surrounding extracellular matrix. They are high-molecular-weight extracellular glycoproteins whose functions include (modulating?) intra- and extracellular matrix morphology, cellular adhesion (both cell-to-cell and cell-to-substratum), and cell migration. Examined by electron microscopy, fibronectins appear as fine filaments or granules coating the surface of fibrillar collagens or associated with cell membranes. Fibronectins have an adhesive domain specific to fibrin, actin, hyaluronic acid, cell surface factors, and collagen. They function to attract and couple key elements in normal healing and in growing tissue.

Quantitative studies of fibronectin concentrations in rabbit ligaments demonstrate significantly (two to three times) higher amounts of fibronectin in the cruciate ligaments as compared to the collateral ligaments (15). This difference may reflect the fact that the cruciate ligaments are surrounded by a synovial sheath, and therefore have a higher degree of cellularity as compared to the extraarticular ligaments.

The maintenance of ligament tissue and its ability to respond to changes in loading depend on interactions between the cells and matrix. Normally the matrix macromolecules are slowly but continually degraded and replaced. The cells must synthesize new macromolecules to balance the losses due to normal degradation or microtrauma. The matrix provides to the cells protection from mechanical injury during normal loading and transmits signals generated by loading to the cells.

Cells bind to the matrix primarily through a family of cell surface proteins called integrins. These molecules mechanically link the matrix macromolecules, including fibronectin, to the internal cell cytoskeleton. They participate in cell adhesion, migration, and proliferation and in regulation of cell synthesis of new matrix macromolecules.

■ GROWTH FACTORS

A vast and rapidly growing literature abounds on a class of peptides commonly called growth factors. Accelerated healing of skin wounds has been reported after local application of several growth factors (37–39).

After injury, the platelets travel to the wound site, form a clot, and hemostasis is obtained. Platelets secrete peptides such as platelet-derived growth factor (PDGF) and transforming growth factor-beta (TGF-β). Both PDGF and TGF-β play an important role in the initiation of repair processes after injury. These factors are chemotoxic for inflammatory cells and appear to regulate proliferation and differentiation of fibroblasts (40–44). Inflammatory cells at the wound site then release other peptides such as basic fibroblast growth factor (bFGF) and epidermal growth factor (EGF). bFGF is multifunctional, since it can either stimulate proliferation and induce or delay differentiation (45). Most importantly, bFGF has demonstrated stimulatory effects on angiogenesis, urokinase-type plasminogen activator (implicated in the neovascular response), and wound healing (46).

Because the synovial fluid washes clots away from the ligament injury site, it is hypothesized that a deficiency of growth factor exists at the wound site. Without the necessary stimulus from growth factors and other clot-derived substances, the response to injury is poor.

■ ACKNOWLEDGMENTS

The authors would like to acknowledge the support of National Institutes of Health grants AR33097 and AG07996.

■ REFERENCES

1. Noyes FR, DeLucas JL, Torvik PJ. Biomechanics of anterior cruciate ligament failure: an analysis of strain rate sensitivity and mechanisms of failure in primates. *J Bone Joint Surg.* 1974;56A: 236–253.

2. Noyes FR, Grood ES. The strength of the anterior cruciate ligament in humans and rhesus monkeys: age-related and species-related changes. *J Bone Joint Surg.* 1976;58A:1074–1082.

3. Noyes FR, Grood ES, Butler DL, et al. Clinical biomechanics of the knee-ligament restraints and functional stability. In: Funk FJ Jr, ed. *Surgical repair and reconstruction.* Am Acad Orthop Surg Symp on the Athlete's Knee. St Louis: Mosby; 1980:1–55.

4. Bloom W, Fawcett DW, eds. *A Textbook of Histology.* 8th ed. Philadelphia: WB Saunders; 1962.

5. Copenhaver WM, Bunge RP, Bune MP, eds. *Bailey's Textbook of Histology.* 16th ed. Baltimore: Williams & Wilkins; 1971.

6. Ham AW, ed. *Histology.* 6th ed. Philadelphia: JB Lippincott Co; 1974.

7. Grood ES, Stowers SF, Noyes FR. Limits of motion in the human knee. Effect of sectioning the posterior cruciate ligament and posterolateral structures. *J Bone Joint Surg.* 1988;70A: 88–97.

8. Palmer I. On injuries to the ligaments of the knee joint. *Acta Chir Scand.* 1938;53(suppl):1.

9. Amiel D, Nimni ME. The collagen in normal ligaments. *Iowa Orthop J.* 1993;13:49–55.

10. Nimni ME, Harkness RD. Molecular structures and functions of collagen. In: Nimni ME, ed. *Collagen: biochemistry.* Boca Raton, FL: CRC Press; 1988.

11. Amenta P, ed. *Histology.* 3rd ed. New Hyde Park, NY: New York Medical Examination Publishing Company; 1983.

12. Bailey FR. In: Kely DE, Wook RL, Enders AC, eds. *Bailey's textbook of microscopic anatomy.* 18th ed. Baltimore: Williams & Wilkins; 1984.

13. Leeson CR, Leeson TS, eds. *Textbook of Histology.* 5th ed. Philadelphia: WB Saunders; 1985.

14. Snell RS, ed. *Clinical and Functional Histology for Medical Students.* 1st ed. Boston: Little, Brown and Company; 1984.

15. Amiel D, Frank CB, Harwood FL, et al. Tendons and ligaments: a morphological and biochemical comparison. *J Orthop Res.* 1984;1(3):257–265.

16. Viidik A. Simultaneous mechanical and light microscopic studies of collagen fibers. *Z Anat Entwicklungsgesh.* 1972;136:204.

17. Yahia LH, Drouin G. Microscopical investigation of canine anterior cruciate ligament and patellar tendon: collagen fascicle morphology and architecture. *J Orthop Res.* 1989;7:243–251.

18. Leeson TS, Leeson CR, eds. *A Brief Atlas of Histology.* Philadelphia: WB Saunders; 1979.

19. Clore JN, Cohen K, Diegelmann RF. Quantitation of collagen types I and III during wound healing in rat skin. *Proc Soc Exp Biol Med.* 1979;161:337.

20. Dunphy JE. *Wound Healing.* New York: Medcom Press; 1974.

21. Gay S, Viljanto J, Rackallio J, et al. Collagen types in early phases of wound healing in children. *Acta Chir Scand.* 1978;144:205.

22. Nimni ME, Harkness RD. Molecular structures and functions of collagen. In: Nimni ME, ed. *Collagen: biochemistry.* Boca Raton: CRC Press; 1988:1–77.

23. Nimni ME. Collagen: structure, function, and metabolism in normal and fibrotic tissues. *Semin Arthritis Rheum.* 1983;13:1–86.

24. Amiel D, Billings E, Akeson WH. Ligament structure, chemistry, and physiology. In: Daniel D, Akeson W, O'Connor J, eds. *Knee ligaments: structure, function, injury, and repair.* New York: Raven Press; 1990:77–91.

25. Frank CB, Woo SL-Y, Andriacchi T, et al. Normal ligament: structure, function and composition. In: Woo SL-Y, Buckwalter JA, eds. *Injury and repair of the musculoskeletal soft tissues.* Park Ridge, IL: American Academy of Orthopaedic Surgeons; 1988.

26. Bray DF, Frank CB, Bray RD. Cytochemical evidence for a proteoglycan-associated filamentous network in ligament extracellular matrix. *J Orthop Res.* 1990;8:1–12.

27. Buckwalter JA. Cartilage. In: Dulbecco R, ed. *Encyclopedia of human biology.* 2nd ed. San Diego: Academic Press; 1991:201–215.

28. Buckwalter JA, Cooper RR. The cells and matrices of skeletal connective tissues. In: Albright JA, Brand RA, eds. *The scientific basis of Orthopaedics.* Norwalk, CT: Appleton & Lange; 1987:1–29.

29. Buckwalter JA, Cruess R. Healing of musculoskeletal tissues. In: Rockwood CA, Green DP, eds. *Fractures in adults.* Philadelphia: Lippincott; 1991:181–222.

30. Buckwalter JA, Maynard JA, Vailas AC. Skeletal fibrous tissues: tendon, joint capsule, and ligament. In: Albright JA, Brand RA, eds. *The scientific basis of orthopaedics.* Norwalk, CT: Appleton & Lange; 1987.

31. Hardingham TE. Proteoglycans: their structure, interactions, and molecular organization in cartilage. *Biochem Soc Trans.* 1981; 9:489–497.

32. Hascall VC. Interactions of cartilage proteoglycans with hyaluronic acid. *J Supremol Structure.* 1977;7:101–120.

33. Muir H. Proteoglycans as organizers of the extracellular matrix. *Biochem Soc Trans.* 1983;11:613–622.

34. Poole AR, Webbed C, Pidoux I, et al. Localization of a dermatan sulfate proteoglycan (DSPGII) in cartilage and the presence of an immunologically related species in other tissues. *J Histochem Cytochem.* 1986;34:619–625.

35. Rosenberg LH, Choi HU, Neame PJ, et al. Proteoglycans of soft connective tissues. In: Leadbetter WB, Buckwalter JA, Gordon SL, eds. *Sports induced inflammation - basic science and clinical concepts.* Park Ridge, IL: American Academy of Orthopaedic Surgeons; 1990.

36. Rosenberg LC, Choi HU, Poole AR, et al. Biological roles of dermatan sulfate proteoglycans. *Ciba Found Symp.* 1986;124: 47–61.

37. Kowalewski K, Yong S. Effect of growth hormone and an anabolic steroid on hydroxyproline in healing dermal wounds in rats. *Acta Endocrinol.* 1968;59:53.

38. Laato M, Niinikoski J, Lebel L, et al. Stimulation of wound healing by epidermal growth factor. *Ann Surg.* 1986;203:379–381.

39. Prudden JF, Nishihara G, O'Campo L. Studies on growth hormone. III. The effect on wound tensile strength of marked postoperative anabolism induced with growth hormone. *Surg Gynecol Obstet.* 1958;107:481.

40. Deuel TF, Senior M, Huang JS, et al. Chemotaxis of monocytes and neutrophils to platelet-derived growth factor. *J Clin Invest.* 1982;69:1046–1049.

41. Roberts AB, Anzano MA, Lamb LC, et al. New class of transforming growth factors potentiated by epidermal growth factor: isolation from non-neoplastic tissues. *Natl Acad Sci.* 1981;78: 5339–5343.

42. Roberts AB, Sporn MB, Assoian RK, et al. Transforming growth factor type β. Rapid induction of fibrosis and angiogenesis *in vivo* and stimulation of collagen formation *in vitro. Proc Natl Acad Sci.* 1986;83:4167–4171.

43. Seppa H, Grotendorst G, Seppa S, et al. Platelet-derived growth factor is chemotactic for fibroblasts. *J Cell Biol.* 1982;92:584.

44. Sporn MB, Roberts AB, Wakefield LM, et al. Transforming growth factor β: biological function and chemical structure. *Science.* 1986;233:532–534.

45. Hemler ME, Huang C, Schwartz L. The VLA protein family. *J Biol Chem.* 1987;262:3300–3309.

46. Montesano R, Vassalli JD, Baird A, et al. Basic fibroblast growth factor induces angiogenesis *in vitro. Proc Natl Acad Sci.* 1986; 83:7297.

MENISCUS

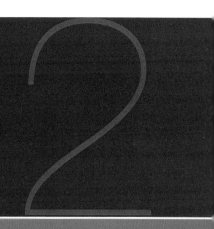

JULIE A. DODDS, MD, STEVEN P. ARNOCZKY, DVM, Dipl ACUS

■ KEY POINTS

■ Once described as functionless remains of leg muscle, the menisci are now realized to be integral components in the complex biomechanics of the knee joint.

■ The menisci are extensions of the tibia, serving to deepen the articular surfaces of the tibial plateau to better accommodate the condyles of the femur.

■ The functions of the menisci include load bearing, shock absorption, joint stability, lubrication, and proprioception. Loss of the meniscus significantly alters these functions and predisposes the joint to degenerative changes.

■ The vascular supply of the meniscus is the essential element in determining its potential for repair. This blood supply must have the ability to support the inflammatory response characteristics of wound repair. The peripheral meniscal blood supply is capable of producing a reparative response similar to that in other connective tissue.

■ When examining injured menisci for potential repair, lesions are often classified by the location of the tear relative to the blood supply of the meniscus and the "vascular appearance" of the peripheral and central surfaces of the tear.

■ Because no perfect substitute has been created to eliminate the problems seen after meniscal removal, the goal remains meniscal preservation through repair.

The menisci of the knee are C-shaped wedges of fibrocartilage interposed between the condyles of the femur and tibia. Once described as functionless remains of leg muscle (1), the menisci are now realized to be integral components in the complex biomechanics of the knee joint (2–10). Knowledge of the form, function, and biology of these unique structures

is an important prerequisite to applying the various clinical procedures available to treat, preserve, and replace the menisci of the knee joint. It is the purpose of this chapter to review the basic science aspects of the menisci in order to provide a sound, fundamental basis for the care and treatment of meniscal injuries.

■ ANATOMY

The menisci of the knee joint are actually extensions of the tibia, which serve to deepen the articular surfaces of the tibial plateau to better accommodate the condyles of the femur. The peripheral border of each meniscus is thick and convex and attached to the joint capsule, while the inner border tapers to a thin, free edge (11). The proximal surfaces of the menisci are concave and in contact with the condyles of the femur; their distal surfaces are flat and rest on the tibial plateau (Fig 2-1).

The medial meniscus is somewhat semicircular in form. It is approximately 3.5 cm in length and considerably wider posteriorly than it is anteriorly. The anterior horn of the medial meniscus is attached to the tibial plateau in the area of the anterior intercondylar fossa, anterior to the anterior cruciate ligament (ACL) (Fig 2-2). The posterior fibers of the anterior horn merge with the transverse ligament, which connects the anterior horns of the medial and lateral menisci (11). The posterior horn of the medial meniscus is firmly attached to the posterior intercondylar fossa of the tibia between the attachment of the lateral meniscus and the posterior cruciate ligament (PCL). The periphery of the medial meniscus is attached to the joint capsule throughout its length. The tibial portion of the capsular attachment is referred to as the

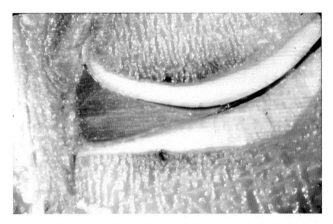

Fig 2-1. Frontal section of the medial compartment of a human knee, illustrating the articulation of the menisci with the condyles of the femur and tibia. (From Warren R, Arnoczky SP, Wickiewicz TL. Anatomy of the knee. In: Nicholas JA, Hershman EB, eds. *The lower extremity and spine in sports medicine.* St. Louis: Mosby; 1995:591; with permission.)

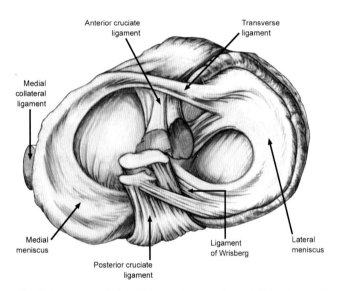

Fig 2-2. Human tibial plateau showing the relative size and attachments of the medial and lateral menisci.

coronary ligament. At its midpoint, the medial meniscus is more firmly attached to the femur and tibia through a condensation in the joint capsule known as the deep medial collateral ligament (MCL) (11).

The lateral meniscus is more circular in shape and covers a larger percentage of the articular surface of the tibial plateau than the medial meniscus. The anterior and posterior horns are approximately the same width (Fig 2-2). The anterior horn of the lateral meniscus is attached to the tibia anterior to the intercondylar eminence and posterior to the attachment of the ACL, with which it partially blends (11). The posterior horn of the lateral meniscus is attached posterior to the intercondylar eminence of the tibia, anterior to the posterior horn of the medial meniscus. In addition to this posterior attachment to the tibia, two ligaments may run from the posterior

horn of the lateral meniscus to the medial femoral condyle, passing either in front of or behind the origin of the PCL (11). These attachments are known as the anterior meniscofemoral ligament (ligament of Humphrey) and the posterior meniscofemoral ligament (ligament of Wrisberg). Although there is no attachment of the lateral meniscus to the lateral collateral ligament, there is a loose peripheral attachment to the joint capsule (11). Posteriorly, the meniscocapsular continuity is interrupted by the popliteal hiatus, a 1.3 (+/− 0.1) cm opening, which allows passage of the popliteus tendon through the knee joint (12). Occasionally, fascicles attach the popliteus tendon to the meniscus (13).

■ ULTRASTRUCTURE

Histologically, the meniscus is a fibrocartilaginous tissue composed primarily of an interlacing network of collagen fibers interposed with cells (3). The cells of the meniscus are responsible for synthesizing and maintaining the extracellular matrix. There is still some debate as to whether the cells of the meniscus are fibroblasts, chondrocytes, or a mixture of both and whether the tissue should be classified as fibrous tissue or fibrocartilage (14). The cells have been termed fibrochondrocytes because of their chondrocytelike appearance and their ability to synthesize a fibrocartilage matrix **(Fig 2-3)**. Two basic types of fibrochondrocytes have been described within the meniscus: a fusiform cell found in the superficial zone of the meniscus and an ovoid or polygonal cell found throughout the remainder of the tissue (14). Although the fusiform cells resemble fibroblasts, they are situated in well-formed lacunae and resemble the chondrocytes found in the superficial (tangential) zone of articular cartilage (14). Both cell types contain abundant endoplasmic reticulum (ER) and Golgi

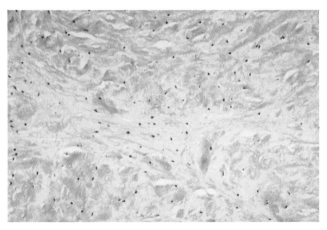

Fig 2-3. Photomicrograph of a longitudinal section of human meniscus showing the histologic appearance of meniscal fibrocartilage (hematoxylin and eosin ×100). (From Crawford MF, Dodds JA, Arnoczky SP. Healing of knee menisci. In: Scott WN, ed. *Surgery of the knee.* Philadelphia: Elsevier Science; 2007:482; with permission.)

complexes. Mitochondria are only occasionally visualized, suggesting that, as in articular chondrocytes, the major pathway for energy production for the fibrochondrocytes in their avascular surroundings is probably anaerobic glycolysis (15,16).

The extracellular matrix of the meniscus is composed primarily of collagen (60% to 70% of the dry weight) (14–18). It is mainly Type I collagen (90%), although Types II, III, V, and VI have been identified within the meniscus (15–18). The circumferential orientation of these collagen fibers appears to be most directly related to the function of the meniscus. In a classic study describing the orientation of the collagen fibers within the menisci, it was noted that although the principal orientation of the collagen fibers is circumferential, a few small, radially disposed fibers appear on both the femoral and tibial surfaces of the menisci as well as within the substance of the tissue **(Figs 2-4, 2-5)** (19). It is theorized

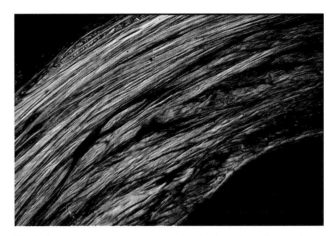

Fig 2-6 Photomicrograph of a longitudinal section of a meniscus under polarized light, demonstrating the orientation of the coarse, deep, circumferentially oriented collagen fibers.

that these radial fibers act as "ties" to provide structural rigidity and help resist longitudinal splitting of the menisci resulting from undue compression. Subsequent light and electron microscopic examinations of the menisci have revealed three different collagen framework layers: a superficial layer composed of a network of fine fibrils woven into a mesh-like matrix, a surface layer just beneath the superficial layer composed in part of irregularly aligned collagen bundles, and a middle layer in which the collagen fibers are larger and courser and are oriented in a parallel, circumferential direction (20,21) **(Fig 2-6)**. It is this middle layer that allows the meniscus to resist tensile forces and function as a transmitter of load across the knee joint.

In addition to collagen, the extracellular matrix of the meniscus also consists of proteoglycans, matrix glycoproteins, and elastin (3,14–17). The proteoglycan content of the adult meniscus is approximately 10% of the amount found in hyaline cartilage, although this has been shown to vary with age and location within the tissue. A study in the porcine meniscus has shown a higher (two to four times) content of hexosamine and uronic acid in the inner third of the meniscus as compared to the outer two thirds (1,14). These substances have also been known to be more prevalent in the anterior horn as compared to the posterior horn in both the medial and lateral meniscus (1,8). The glycosaminoglycan (GAG) profile of the adult human meniscus has been reported to consist of chondroitin 6-sulfate (40%), chondroitin 4-sulfate (10% to 20%), dermatan sulfate (20% to 30%), and keratan sulfate (15%) (3,14–16).

Matrix glycoproteins, such as the link proteins that stabilize the proteoglycan-hyaluronic acid aggregates, and a 116-k Dalton protein of unknown consequence, have also been identified within the extracellular matrix (3,14–16). In addition, adhesive glycoproteins, such as Type VI collagen, fibronectin, and thrombospondin, have been isolated from the meniscus (15,16). These macromolecules have the property to bind to other matrix macromolecules and/or cell surfaces and may play a role in the supramolecular organization of the extracellular molecules of the meniscus (15,16).

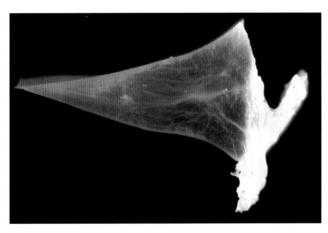

Fig 2-4. Cross-section of a lateral meniscus showing the radial orientation of fibrous ties within the substance of the meniscus. (From Arnoczky SP, Torzilli PA. The biology of cartilage. In: Hunter LY, Funk FJ Jr, eds. *Rehabilitation of the Injured Knee*. St. Louis: Mosby; 1984:148; with permission.)

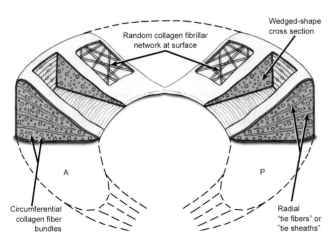

Fig 2-5. Collagen fiber ultrastructure of the meniscus. Note the predominant circumferential orientation of the large collagen fiber bundles on the interior of the tissue. The fibers of the surface layer have no preferred orientation. Also within the interior of the meniscus are radially oriented collagen "tie" fibers.

■ MENISCAL FUNCTION

While the term "shock absorber" has often been used to describe the meniscus, the menisci actually serve many functions in the human knee. Additional functions are theorized to be load bearing, lubrication, and proprioception. The meniscal function of load bearing may be clinically inferred by the degenerative changes that accompany meniscectomy. Fairbank (22) described radiographic changes following meniscectomy, which included narrowing of the joint space, flattening of the femoral condyle, and the formation of osteophytes. These changes were attributed to the loss of the weight bearing function of the meniscus. Biomechanical studies have demonstrated that at least 50% of the compressive load of the knee joint is transmitted through the meniscus in extension, and approximately 85% of the load is transmitted in 90 degrees of flexion (23). In the totally meniscectomized knee, the contact area is reduced approximately 50% (23,24). This significantly increases the load per unit area and results in articular damage and degeneration. Partial meniscectomy has also been shown to significantly increase contact pressures (25). In an experimental study, resection of as little as 15% to 34% of the meniscus increased tibiofemoral contact pressures by more than 350% (26). Thus, even partial meniscectomy can affect the ability of the meniscus to function in load transmission across the knee (5,6,25,27–32).

Another proposed function of the meniscus is that of shock absorption. By examining the compressive load-deformation response of the normal and meniscectomized knee, it has been suggested that the viscoelastic menisci may function to attenuate the intermittent shock waves generated by impulse loading of the knee during gait (26,33). Studies have shown that the normal knee has a shock-absorbing capacity about 20% higher than knees that have undergone meniscectomy (33). As the inability of a joint system to absorb shock has been implicated in the development of osteoarthritis (34), the shock absorption mechanism would appear to play a role in maintaining the health of the knee joint.

In addition to the role of the meniscus in load transmission and shock absorption, the menisci are thought to contribute to knee joint stability (9,35–37). Although medial meniscectomy alone does not significantly increase anterior-posterior joint stability, several studies have shown that medial meniscectomy in association with ACL insufficiency significantly increases the anterior laxity of the knee (9,35–37). However, lateral meniscectomy, alone or in association with ACL insufficiency, has not been shown to increase knee joint laxity (9).

Because the menisci serve to increase the congruity between the condyles of the femur and tibia, they contribute significantly to overall joint conformity. It has been suggested that this function assists in the overall lubrication of the articular surfaces of the knee joint. Posterior translation of the menisci (lateral greater than medial) during knee flexion has been demonstrated in magnetic resonance imaging (MRI) studies **(Fig 2-7)** (38,39). Additionally, the anterior

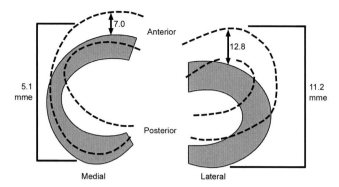

Fig 2-7. Diagram of mean meniscal excursion (mme) along the tibial plateau. The ratio of posterior to anterior translation (P/A) was significant (*p <0.05). (From Thompson WO, Thaete FL, Fu FH, et al. Tibial meniscal dynamics using three-dimensional reconstruction of magnetic resonance images. *Am J Sports Med.* 1991;19:210–216; with permission.)

and posterior translation of the menisci during flexion and extension is hypothesized to protect the articular surfaces from injury (40).

Finally, the menisci have been suggested as proprioceptive structures providing a feedback mechanism for joint position sense. Neural elements have been identified within the meniscal tissue (41–47). While the anterior and posterior horns of the menisci appear to be the most richly innervated, myelinated and unmyelinated nerve fibers have been identified within the peripheral body of the meniscus (44–46). These nerve fibers originate in the highly innervated perimeniscal tissue and radiate into the peripheral third of the meniscus. Many of these fibers accompany the vascular network of the meniscus; however, some neural elements are not exclusively paravascular in position, suggesting a function other than vasomotor or vasosensory.

Studies of human specimens have identified three morphologically distinct mechanoreceptors within the medial meniscus: Ruffini endings, Golgi tendon organs, and Pacinian corpuscles (44,45). These neural elements were found in greatest concentration in the horns of the meniscus, particularly the posterior horn (44,45). The presence of these neuroreceptors in the meniscus has led to the hypothesis that the menisci may serve an important afferent role in the sensory feedback mechanism of the knee (3,42,44,45,47). During extremes of knee flexion and extension, the horns of the menisci become more taut. This increase in tension would activate the mechanoreceptors located in the meniscal horns and provide the central nervous system with information regarding joint position. This may, in turn, contribute to a reflex arc that stimulates protective or postural muscular reflexes. It is theorized that the greatest concentration of neural elements found in the anterior and posterior horns of the meniscus reflects the need for afferent feedback at the extremes of flexion and extension (44).

In summary, the proposed functions of the menisci include load bearing, shock absorption, joint stability, lubrication, and proprioception. Loss of the meniscus, partially or totally, significantly alters these functions and predisposes the joint to degenerative changes.

■ MENISCAL MOTION

As the knee passes through a range of motion, the menisci move with respect to the tibial articular surface. A classic study demonstrated that from 0 degrees to 120 degrees of knee flexion the mean meniscal excursion (defined as the average anteroposterior displacement of the anterior and posterior meniscal horns along the tibial plateau in the midcondylar, parasagittal plane) of the medial meniscus was 5.1 (±0.96) mm while that of the lateral meniscus was 11.2 (±3.27) mm (39) (Fig 2-7). The lack of bony opposition (i.e., convex femoral condyle and tibial plateau), an unconstrained peripheral margin, and the close approximation of its central tibial attachment appear to allow the lateral meniscus a greater degree of movement.

Rotation of the knee joint also has an effect on meniscal motion with a greater effect being observed in the lateral meniscus. The posterior oblique fibers of the MCL appear to limit the movement of the medial meniscus in rotation, which may place it at increased risk of tear during tibiofemoral rotation (48).

In addition to their anterior-posterior translation, the menisci deform to remain in constant congruity with the tibial and femoral articular surfaces throughout the full range of joint motion. This allows the meniscus to provide additional joint stability (48). The anterior horn segments of the medial and lateral menisci demonstrate differing mobility compared with posterior horn segments. This differential allows the menisci to assume a decreasing radius with flexion that correlates with a decreasing radius of curvature of the posterior femoral condyle. The change in radius enables the menisci to maintain congruity with the articulating surfaces throughout flexion. The greatest deformation appears to occur at the anterior horn of the medial meniscus as it moves onto the tibial plateau with flexion and is manifested as an increase in the concavity of the superior articulating meniscal surface. This is probably due to the increasing load resulting from femoral flexion (48).

■ BASIC SCIENCE OF MENISCAL REPAIR

Thomas Annandale was credited with the first surgical repair of a torn meniscus in 1883 (49). It was not until 1936, when King published his classic experiment on meniscus healing in dogs, that the actual biological limitations of meniscus healing were set forth. King demonstrated that for meniscal lesions to heal, they must communicate with the peripheral blood supply (50). Enhancing vascularity at or near the site of meniscal injury has remained a major focus in the techniques of

surgical repair. In addition, advances in cellular and molecular biology now allow researchers to investigate the role of specific growth factors and cytokines in the cellular response to injury. Further application of these findings will continue to provide for means of enhancing meniscal repairs.

Vascular Anatomy of the Meniscus

The vascular supply to the medial and lateral menisci originates predominantly from the medial and lateral genicular arteries (inferior and superior branches) (51). Branches from these vessels give rise to a perimeniscal capillary plexus within the synovial and capsular tissues of the knee joint. The plexus is an arborizing network of vessels that supplies the peripheral border of the meniscus about its attachment to the joint capsule **(Figs 2-8, 2-9)** (51). These perimeniscal vessels are oriented in a predominantly circumferential pattern, with radial branches being directed toward the center of the joint **(Fig 2-10)**. Anatomic studies have shown that the degrees of peripheral vascular penetration are 10% to 30% of the width of the medial meniscus and 10% to 25% of the width of the lateral meniscus (51). The middle genicular artery, along with a few terminal branches of the medial and lateral genicular vessels, also supplies vessels to the menisci through the vascular synovial covering of the anterior and posterior horn attachments (51). These synovial vessels penetrate the horn attachments and give rise to smaller vessels that enter the meniscal horns for a short distance and end in terminal capillary loops.

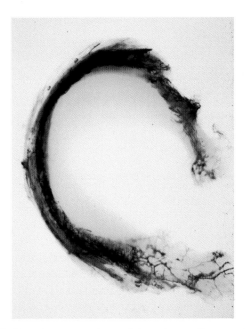

Fig 2-8. Superior aspect of a medial meniscus after vascular perfusion with India ink and tissue-clearing with a modified Spalteholz technique. Note the vascularity at the periphery of the meniscus as well as at the anterior and posterior horn attachments. (From Arnoczky SP, Warren RF. Microvasculature of the human meniscus. *Am J Sports Med.* 1982;10:90; with permission.)

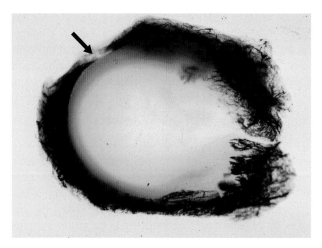

Fig 2-9. Superior aspect of a lateral meniscus after vascular perfusion with India ink and tissue-clearing with a modified Spalteholz technique. Note the absence of vascularity at the posterior lateral aspect of the meniscus *(arrow)*. This is adjacent to the popliteal hiatus. (From Arnoczky SP, Warren RF. Microvasculature of the human meniscus. *Am J Sports Med.* 1982;10:90; with permission.)

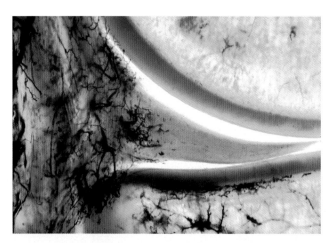

Fig 2-10. A 5-mm-thick frontal section of the medial compartment of a human knee (Spalteholz' preparation). Branching radial vessels from the perimeniscal capillary plexus (PCP) penetrate the peripheral border of the medial meniscus. RR, red-red zone; RW, red-white zone; WW, white-white zone. (From Arnoczky SP, Warren RF. Microvasculature of the human meniscus. *Am J Sports Med.* 1982;10:90; with permission.)

A small reflection of the vascular synovial tissue is also present throughout the peripheral attachment of the medial and lateral menisci on the femoral and tibial articular surfaces (51). This "synovial fringe" extends for a short distance over the peripheral surfaces of the meniscus and contains small, terminally looped vessels. Although the synovial fringe is adherent to the articular surfaces of the menisci, it does not contribute vessels to the meniscus per se (50). The clinical significance of these fringe vessels lies in their potential

contribution to the reparative response of the meniscus, as seen in "synovial abrasion" techniques (52–75).

Vascular Response to Injury

The vascular supply of the meniscus is the essential element in determining its potential for repair. This blood supply must have the ability to support the inflammatory response characteristic of wound repair. Clinical and experimental observations have demonstrated that the peripheral meniscal blood supply is capable of producing a reparative response similar to that in other connective tissue (65,76–91).

Following injury within the peripheral vascular zone, a fibrin clot forms that is rich in inflammatory cells. Vessels from the perimeniscal capillary plexus proliferate through this fibrin "scaffold," accompanied by the proliferation of undifferentiated mesenchymal cells (76). Eventually, the lesion is filled with a cellular, fibrovascular granulation tissue that "glues" the wound edges together and appears to be continuous with the adjacent normal meniscal fibrocartilage (75,78). The initial strength of this repair tissue, as compared with the normal meniscus, is minimal. Increased collagen synthesis within the granulation tissue slowly results in a fibrous scar **(Fig 2-11)**.

Experimental studies have shown that radial lesions of the meniscus, extending to the synovium, are completely healed with fibrovascular scar tissue by 10 weeks **(Fig 2-12)** (74,76). Modulation of this scar into normal-appearing fibrocartilage, however, requires several months (78). The initial strength of this repair tissue, as compared to the normal meniscus, has been found to be significantly decreased during this time (33% at 8 weeks, 52% at 4 months, and 62% at 6 months) (79). Further study is required to

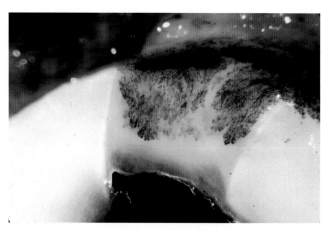

Fig 2-11. A meniscus 6 weeks following the creation of a radial lesion. The fibrovascular scar tissue has filled the defect, and vascular proliferation from the synovial fringe can be seen. (From Arnoczky SP, Warren RF. Microvasculature of the meniscus and its response to injury: an experimental study in the dog. *Am J Sports Med.* 1983;11:131; with permission.)

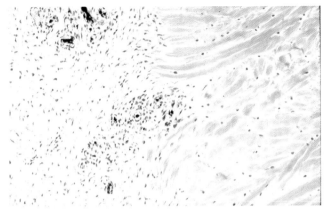

Fig 2-12. Photomicrograph of the junction of the meniscus and the fibrovascular repair tissue at 10 weeks (hematoxylin and eosin ×100). (From Arnoczky SP, Warren RF. Microvasculature of the meniscus and its response to injury: an experimental study in the dog. *Am J Sports Med.* 1983;11:131; with permission.)

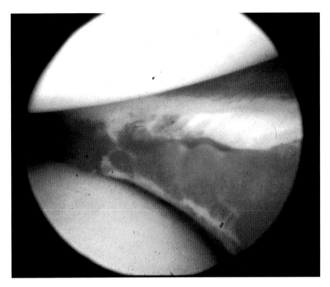

Fig 2-13. Arthroscopic view of a peripheral tear of a human meniscus. Note the vascular granulation tissue present at the margin of the lesion. This is classified as a red-white tear. Also note the proliferation of the synovial fringe over the femoral surface of the meniscus. (From Arnoczky SP, Torzilli PA. The biology of cartilage. In: Hunter LY, Funk FJ Jr, eds. *Rehabilitation of the injured knee.* St. Louis: Mosby; 1984:148; with permission.)

delineate the biomechanical properties at each stage of the repair process.

The ability of meniscal lesions to heal has provided the rationale for the repair of peripheral meniscal injuries, and many reports have demonstrated excellent results following primary repair of peripheral meniscal injuries (69,80,83,84,88–93). Follow-up examinations of these peripheral repairs have revealed a process of repair similar to that noted in the experimental models.

When examining injured menisci for potential repair, lesions are often classified by the location of the tear relative to the blood supply of the meniscus and the "vascular appearance" of the peripheral and central surfaces of the tear (Fig 2-10) (77). The so-called *red-red* tear (peripheral capsular detachment) has a functional blood supply of the capsular and meniscal side of the lesion and obviously has the best prognosis for healing. The *red-white* tears (meniscus tears through the peripheral vascular zone) have an active peripheral blood supply; however, the central (inner) surface of the lesion is devoid of functioning vessels **(Fig 2-13)**. These lesions have sufficient vascularity to heal by the aforementioned fibrovascular proliferation. The *white-white* tears (meniscus lesions completely in the avascular zone) are without blood supply and theoretically cannot heal (77). In an effort to "extend" the level of repair into these avascular areas, techniques such as synovial abrasion, fibrin clot placement, and vascular access channels have been developed to attempt to provide vascularity to these *white-white* tears.

Cellular Response to Injury

The ability of fibrochondrocytes within a meniscus to mount a reparative response is dependent in part upon cellular activity. Cytokines and growth factors present during the inflammatory response to injury may promote meniscal healing through enhancement of cell migration, cell division, and the production of extracellular matrix. While no specific growth factor has been shown to enhance meniscus healing, researchers are beginning to identify how the meniscal fibrochondrocyte responds to various growth factors (94–100). Meniscal repair augmentation methods such as fibrin clot and platelet rich plasma (PRP) are based upon the concept that growth factors positively impact meniscal healing. Understanding which growth factors positively impact the healing potential of the meniscal fibrochondrocyte matrix will undoubtedly provide future strategies for treating meniscal injuries.

■ SUMMARY

Understanding the structure of the meniscus and its process of repair has been critical in advancing surgical techniques and increasing healing rates following meniscal repair. Knowledge of the circumferential orientation of the collagen fibers has lead to the preferred position of sutures—vertical mattress. Increasing knowledge of normal meniscal healing and meniscal vascularity has lead to the application of vascular enhancement techniques, and the ability to extend meniscal repair into the *white-white* zone.

Further understanding of basic science and the understanding of meniscal healing have allowed us to expand the potential for meniscal repair. In the treatment of difficult fractures and non-unions, growth factors, such as the bone morphogenic proteins, have had a dramatic impact in increasing healing rates. Similarly, the future of meniscal repair will likely utilize growth factors as well as innovative vascular enhancement techniques to improve healing. Considering that no perfect substitute has been created to eliminate the problems seen after meniscal removal, we must continue to strive for meniscal preservation through meniscal repair.

■ REFERENCES

1. Sutton JB. *Ligaments: Their Nature and Morphology.* London: MK Lewis & Co.; 1897.
2. Arnoczky SP, Warren RF, Spivak JM. Meniscal repair using an exogenous fibrin clot. An experimental study in dogs. *J Bone Joint Surg Am.* 1988;70A:1209–1217.
3. Arnoczky SP, Adams ME, DeHaven K, et al. Meniscus. In: Woo SL-Y, Buckwalter JA, eds. *NIAMS/AAOS Workshop on the Injury and Repair of the Musculoskeletal Soft Tissues.* Park Ridge: American Academy of Orthopaedic Surgeons; 1988:487–537.
4. Burr DB, Radin EL. Meniscal function and the importance of meniscal regeneration in preventing late medial compartment osteoarthrosis. *Clin Orthop Relat Res.* 1982;171:121–126.
5. Cox JS, Nye CE, Schaeffer WW, et al. The degenerative effects of partial and total resection of the medial meniscus in dogs. *Clin Orthop Relat Res.* 1975;109:178–183.
6. Cox JS, Cordell LD. The degenerative effects of medial meniscal tears in dog's knees. *Clin Orthop Relat Res.* 1977;125:236–242.
7. Fairbank TJ. Knee joint changes after meniscectomy. *J Bone Joint Surg.* 1948;30B:664–670.
8. Krause WR, Pope MH, Johnson RJ, et al. Mechanical changes in the knee after meniscectomy. *J Bone Joint Surg.* 1976;58A:599–604.
9. Levy IM, Torzilli PA, Warren RF. The effect of medial meniscectomy on anterior-posterior motion of the knee. *J Bone Joint Surg.* 1982;64A:883–888.
10. Mow VC, Fithian DC, Kelly MA. Fundamentals of articular cartilage and meniscus biomechanics. In: Ewing JW, ed. *Articular cartilage and knee joint function.* New York: Raven Press; 1989:1–18.
11. Warren R, Arnoczky SP, Wickiewicz TL. Anatomy of the knee. In: Nicholas JA, Hershman EB, eds. *The lower extremity and spine in sports medicine.* St. Louis: Mosby; 1986:657.
12. Cohn AK, Mains DB. Popliteal hiatus of the lateral meniscus. Anatomy and measurement at dissection of 10 specimens. *Am J Sports Med.* 1986;7:221–226.
13. Last R. The popliteus muscle and the lateral meniscus. *J Bone Joint Surg.* 1950;32B:93.
14. Ghadially FN. *Fine Structure of Synovial Joints: A Text and Atlas of the Ultrastructure of Normal and Pathological Articular Tissues.* London: Butterworths; 1983:103–144.
15. McDevitt CA, Miller RR, Spindler P. The cells and cell matrix interactions of the meniscus. In: Mow VC, Arnoczky SP, Jackson DW, eds. *Knee meniscus: basic and clinical foundations.* New York: Raven Press; 1992:29–36.
16. McDevitt CA, Webber RJ. The ultrastructure and biochemistry of meniscal cartilage. *Clin Orthop.* 1990;252:8–18.
17. Adams ME, Hukins DWL. The extracellular matrix of the meniscus. In: Mow VC, Arnoczky SP, Jackson DW, eds. *Knee meniscus: basic and clinical foundations.* New York: Raven Press; 1992:15–28.
18. Eyre DR, Koob TJ, Chun LE. Biochemistry of the meniscus: unique profile of collagen types and site dependent variations in composition. *Trans Orthop Res.* 1983;8:56.
19. Bullough PG, Munuera L, Murphy J, et al. The strength of the menisci of the knee as it relates to their fine structure. *J Bone Joint Surg Br.* 1970;52:564–567.
20. Aspden RM, Hulkins DWL. Structure, function, and mechanical failure of the meniscus. In: Yettram AL, ed. *Material properties and stress analysis in biomechanics.* Manchester: Manchester University Press; 1989:109–122.
21. Aspden RM, Yarker YE, Hukins DW. Collagen orientations in the meniscus of the knee joint. *J Anat.* 1985;140(Pt 3): 371–380.
22. Fairbank TJ. Knee joint changes after meniscectomy. *J Bone Joint Surg Br.* 1948;30:644.
23. Ahmed AM, Burke DL. In-vitro measurement of static pressure distribution in synovial joints—part I: tibial surface of the knee. *J Biomech Eng.* 1983;105:216–225.
24. Fukubayashi T, Kurosawa H. The contact area and pressure distribution pattern of the knee. A study of normal and osteoarthritic knee joints. *Acta Orthop Scand.* 1980;51:871–879.
25. Baratz ME, Fu FH, Mengato R. Meniscal tears: the effect of meniscectomy and of repair on intraarticular contact areas and stress in the human knee. A preliminary report. *Am J Sports Med.* 1986;14:270–275.
26. Seedhom BB, Hargreaves DJ. Transmission of the load in the knee joint with special reference to the role of the menisci. *Eng Med.* 1979;8:220.
27. Andersson-Molina H, Karlsson H, Rockborn P. Arthroscopic partial and total meniscectomy: a long-term follow-up study with matched controls. *Arthroscopy.* 2002;18:183–189.
28. Chatain F, Adeleine P, Chambat P, et al. A comparative study of medial versus lateral arthroscopic partial meniscectomy on stable knees: 10-year minimum follow-up. *Arthroscopy.* 2003;19:842–849.
29. Scheller G, Sobau C, Bulow JU. Arthroscopic partial lateral meniscectomy in an otherwise normal knee: clinical, functional, and radiographic results of a long-term follow-up study. *Arthroscopy.* 2001;17:946–952.
30. Jorgensen U, Sonne-Holm S, Lauridsen F, et al. Long-term follow-up of meniscectomy in athletes. A prospective longitudinal study. *J Bone Joint Surg Br.* 1987;69:80–83.
31. Fauno P, Nielsen AB. Arthroscopic partial meniscectomy: a long-term follow-up. *Arthroscopy.* 1992;8:345–349.
32. Kruger-Franke M, Siebert CH, Kugler A, et al. Late results after arthroscopic partial medial meniscectomy. *Knee Surg Sports Traumatol Arthrosc.* 1999;7:81–84.
33. Voloshin AS, Wosk J. Shock absorption of meniscectomized and painful knees: a comparative in vivo study. *J Biomed Eng.* 1983;5:157–161.
34. Radin EL, Rose RM. Role of subchondral bone in the initiation and progression of cartilage damage. *Clin Orthop Relat Res.* 1986;213:34–40.
35. Markolf KL, Kochan A, Amstutz HC. Measurement of knee stiffness and laxity in patients with documented absence of the anterio cruciate ligament. *J Bone Joint Surg.* 1984;66A:242–252.
36. Allen CR, Wong EK, Livesay GA, et al. Importance of the medial meniscus in the anterior cruciate ligament-deficient knee. *J Orthop Res.* 2000;18:109–115.
37. Papageorgiou CD, Gil JE, Kanamori A, et al. The biomechanical interdependence between the anterior cruciate ligament replacement graft and the medial meniscus. *Am J Sports Med.* 2001; 29:226–231.
38. Kawahara Y, Uetani M, Fuchi K, et al. MR assessment of movement and morphologic change in the menisci during knee flexion. *Acta Radiol.* 1999;40:610–614.
39. Thompson WO, Thaete FL, Fu FH, et al. Tibial meniscal dynamics using three-dimensional reconstruction of magnetic resonance images. *Am J Sports Med.* 1991;19:210–215.
40. Kawahara Y, Uetani M, Fuchi K, et al. MR assessment of meniscal movement during knee flexion: correlation with the severity

of cartilage abnormality in the femorotibial joint. *J Comput Assist Tomogr.* 2001;25:683–690.

41. Wilson AS, Legg PG, McNeur JC. Studies of the innervation of the medial meniscus in the human knee joint. *Anat Rec.* 1969; 165:485–492.

42. Kennedy JC, Alexander IJ, Hayes KC. Nerve supply of the human knee and its functional importance. *Am J Sports Med.* 1982;10:329–335.

43. Gardner E. The innervation of the knee joint. *Anat Rec.* 1948;101:109–130.

44. Zimny ML, Albright DJ, Dabezies E. Mechanoreceptors in the human medial meniscus. *Acta Anat (Basel).* 1988;133:35–40.

45. Day B, Mackenzie WG, Shim SS, et al. The vascular and nerve supply of the human meniscus. *Arthroscopy.* 1985;1:58–62.

46. Wilson AS, Legg PG, McNeur JC. Studies on the innervation of the medial meniscus in the human knee joint. *Anat Rec.* 1969; 165:485–492.

47. O'Connor BL. The structure and innervation of cat knee menisci, and their relation to a "sensory hypothesis" of meniscal function. *Am J Anat.* 1987;153:431–442.

48. Mow VC, Ratcliffe A, Chern KY, et al. Structure and function relationships of the menisci of the knee. In: Mow VC, Arnoczky SP, Jackson DW, eds. *Knee meniscus: basic and clinical foundations.* New York: Raven Press; 1992:37–57.

49. Annandale T. An operation for displaced semilunar cartilage. *Br J Med.* 1885;1:1885.

50. King D. Regeneration of the semilunar cartilage. *Surg Gynecol Obstet.* 1936;62:167.

51. Arnoczky SP, Warren RF. Microvasculature of the human meniscus. *Am J Sports Med.* 1982;10:90–95.

52. Cannon WD Jr, Vittori JM. The incidence of healing in arthroscopic meniscal repairs in anterior cruciate ligament-reconstructed knees versus stable knees. *Am J Sports Med.* 1992;20:176–181.

53. Hashimoto J, Kurosaka M, Yoshiya S, et al. Meniscal repair using fibrin sealant and endothelial cell growth factor. An experimental study in dogs. *Am J Sports Med.* 1992;20:537–541.

54. Henning CE, Lynch MA, Yearout KM, et al. Arthroscopic meniscal repair using an exogenous fibrin clot. *Clin Orthop.* 1990;64–72.

55. Henning CE. Arthroscopic repairs of meniscus tears. *Orthopedics.* 1983;6:1130–1132.

56. Henning CE. Current status of meniscus salvage. *Clin Sports Med.* 1990;9:567–576.

57. Henning CE, Lynch MA. Current concepts of meniscal function and pathology. *Clin Sports Med.* 1984;4:259–265.

58. Klompmaker J, Jansen HW, Veth RP, et al. Porous polymer implant for repair of meniscal lesions: a preliminary study in dogs. *Biomaterials.* 1991;12:810–816.

59. Lipscomb AB, Anderson AF. Tears of the anterior cruciate ligament in adolescents. *J Bone Joint Surg Am.* 1986;68:19–28.

60. Miller DB Jr. Arthroscopic meniscus repair. *Am J Sports Med.* 1988;16:315–320.

61. Mooney MF, Rosenberg TD. Arthroscopic reattachment of the meniscus. *Orthopade.* 1994;23:143–152.

62. Okuda K, Ochi M, Shu N, et al. Meniscal rasping for repair of meniscal tear in the avascular zone. *Arthroscopy.* 1999;15: 281–286.

63. Ritchie JR, Miller MD, Bents RT, et al. Meniscal repair in the goat model. The use of healing adjuncts on central tears and the role of magnetic resonance arthrography in repair evaluation. *Am J Sports Med.* 1998;26:278–284.

64. Barrett GR, Treacy SH, Ruff CG. Preliminary results of the T-fix endoscopic meniscus repair technique in an anterior cruciate ligament reconstruction population. *Arthroscopy.* 1997;13: 218–223.

65. Shelbourne KD, Rask BP. The sequelae of salvaged nondegenerative peripheral vertical medial meniscus tears with anterior cruciate ligament reconstruction. *Arthroscopy.* 2001;17:270–274.

66. Shelbourne KD, Heinrich J. The long-term evaluation of lateral meniscus tears left in situ at the time of anterior cruciate ligament reconstruction. *Arthroscopy.* 2004;20:346–351.

67. Tetik O, Kocabey Y, Johnson DL. Synovial abrasion for isolated, partial thickness, undersurface, medial meniscus tears. *Orthopedics.* 2002;25:675–678.

68. Talley MC, Grana WA. Treatment of partial meniscal tears identified during anterior cruciate ligament reconstruction with limited synovial abrasion. *Arthroscopy.* 2000;16:6–10.

69. Henning CE, Lynch MA, Clark JR. Vascularity for healing of meniscus repairs. *Arthroscopy.* 1987;3:13–18.

70. Henning CE, Clark JR, Lynch MA, et al. Arthroscopic meniscus repair with a posterior incision. *Instr Course Lect.* 1988; 37:209–221.

71. Uchio Y, Ochi M, Adachi N, et al. Results of rasping of meniscal tears with and without anterior cruciate ligament injury as evaluated by second-look arthroscopy. *Arthroscopy.* 2003;19: 463–469.

72. DeHaven KE, Arnoczky SP. Meniscus repair: basic science, indications for repair, and open repair. *Instr Course Lect.* 1994;43: 65–76.

73. O'Meara PM. Surgical techniques for arthroscopic meniscal repair. *Orthop Rev.* 1993;22:781–790.

74. Schmitz MA, Rouse LM Jr, DeHaven KE. The management of meniscal tears in the ACL-deficient knee. *Clin Sports Med.* 1996; 15:573–593.

75. Henning CE, Yearout KM, Vequist SW, et al. Use of the fascia sheath coverage and exogenous fibrin clot in the treatment of complex meniscal tears. *Am J Sports Med.* 1991;19:626–631.

76. Arnoczky SP, Warren RF. The microvasculature of the meniscus and its response to injury. An experimental study in the dog. *Am J Sports Med.* 1983;11:131–141.

77. Arnoczky SP. Meniscus healing. *Contemp Orthop.* 1985;10:31.

78. Cabaud HE, Rodkey WG, Fitzwater JE. Medical meniscus repairs. An experimental and morphologic study. *Am J Sports Med.* 1981;9:129–134.

79. Cassidy RE, Shaffer AJ. Repair of peripheral meniscus tears. A preliminary report. *Am J Sports Med.* 1981;9:209–214.

80. Curtis RJ, Delee JC, Drez DJ Jr. Reconstruction of the anterior cruciate ligament with freeze dried fascia lata allografts in dogs. A preliminary report. *Am J Sports Med.* 1985;13:408–414.

81. Danylchuk KD, Finlay JB, Krcek JP. Microstructural organization of human and bovine cruciate ligaments. *Clin Orthop Relat Res.* 1978;131:294–298.

82. Roeddecker K, Muennich U, Nagelschmidt N. Meniscal healing: a biomechanical study. *J Surg Res.* 1994;56:20–27.

83. DeHaven KE. Peripheral meniscus repair: an alternative to meniscectomy. *J Bone Joint Surg Br.* 1981;63:463.

84. Hamberg P, Gillquist J, Lysholm J. Suture of new and old peripheral meniscus tears. *J Bone Joint Surg Am.* 1983;65: 193–197.

85. Heatley FW. The meniscus—can it be repaired? An experimental investigation in rabbits. *J Bone Joint Surg Br.* 1980;62:397–402.

86. Jakob RP, Staubli HU, Zuber K, et al. The arthroscopic meniscal repair. Techniques and clinical experience. *Am J Sports Med.* 1988;16:137–142.

87. King D. The healing of the semilunar cartilage. *J Bone Joint Surg.* 1936;64:883.

88. Lynch MA, Henning CE, Glick KR Jr. Knee joint surface changes. Long-term follow-up meniscus tear treatment in stable anterior cruciate ligament reconstructions. *Clin Orthop Relat Res.* 1983; 172:148–153.

89. Rosenberg TD, Scott SM, Coward DB, et al. Arthroscopic meniscal repair evaluated with repeat arthroscopy. *Arthroscopy.* 1986;2:14–20.

90. Scott GA, Jolly BL, Henning CE. Combined posterior incision and arthroscopic intra-articular repair of the meniscus. An

examination of factors affecting healing. *J Bone Joint Surg Am.* 1986;68:847–861.

91. Stone RG, VanWinkle GN. Arthroscopic review of meniscal repair: assessment of healing parameters. *Arthroscopy.* 1986;2: 77–81.

92. DeHaven KE. Meniscus repair in the athlete. *Clin Orthop.* 1985;198:31–35.

93. DeHaven KE. Meniscus repair—open vs. arthroscopic. *Arthroscopy.* 1985;1:173–174.

94. Spindler KP, Mayes CE, Miller RR, et al. Regional mitogenic response of the meniscus to platelet-derived growth factor (PDGF-AB). *J Orthop Res.* 1995;13:201–207.

95. Lietman SA, Yanagishita M, Sampath TK, et al. Stimulation of proteoglycan synthesis in explants of porcine articular cartilage by recombinant osteogenic protein-1 (bone morphogenetic protein-7). *J Bone Joint Surg Am.* 1997;79:1132–1137.

96. Lietman SA, Hobbs W, Inoue N, et al. Effects of selected growth factors on porcine meniscus in chemically defined medium. *Orthopedics.* 2003;26:799–803.

97. Bhargava MM, Attia ET, Murrell GA, et al. The effect of cytokines on the proliferation and migration of bovine meniscal cells. *Am J Sports Med.* 1999;27:636–643.

98. Collier S, Ghosh P. Effects of transforming growth factor beta on proteoglycan synthesis by cell and explant cultures derived from the knee joint meniscus. *Osteoarthritis Cartilage.* 1995;3:127–138.

99. Kumagae Y. Proteoglycan and collagen synthesis of cultured fibrochondrocytes from the human knee joint meniscus. *Nippon Seikeigeka Gakkai Zasshi.* 1994;68:885–894.

100. Webber RJ, Harris MG, Hough AJ Jr. Cell culture of rabbit meniscal fibrochondrocytes: proliferative and synthetic response to growth factors and ascorbate. *J Orthop Res.* 1985;3:36–42.

ARTICULAR CARTILAGE: A BRIEF REVIEW OF ITS STRUCTURE, FUNCTION, AND REPAIR

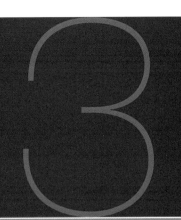

■ WAYNE H. AKESON, MD, WILLIAM BUGBEE, MD

■ KEY POINTS

- Few mechanical devices even remotely approach the durability and efficiency of cartilage.
- The typical response to cartilage injury in which the subchondral plate is fractured is the formation of fibrocartilage, a scarlike tissue unsuited to the support of compressive loads and shear forces.
- The pattern of collagen fibrils within articular cartilage is well suited to the functional requirements of the tissue.
- Loss of the densely packed collagen mat at the surface of cartilage in weight-bearing regions is the prelude to fibrillation, accelerated wear, and ensuing degenerative arthritis.
- Collagen is the key protein in musculoskeletal stability. It provides the mechanical properties to connective tissue, and it constitutes 65% to 80% of the mass by dry weight of such connective tissues as tendons, ligaments, skin, joint capsules, and cartilage.
- Attempts to achieve cartilage repair, as in surgical arthroplasty, do not successfully regenerate cartilage and seldom produce completely satisfactory clinical results. The collagen fiber architecture of the arthroplasty repair tissue is disordered throughout the deep layers and lacks the membranelike characteristics so important to the surface layer of articular cartilage. These are major factors contributing to failure of cartilage regeneration.

Cartilage is a unique tissue that unless injured, provides virtually frictionless mechanical motion throughout the latter decades of life. Few mechanical devices even remotely approach the durability and efficiency of cartilage. The purpose of this chapter is to provide a brief account of the structure, composition, and mechanical properties of articular cartilage. Such an account is basic to understanding both the function of cartilage and the therapeutic goals of cartilage restoration by any of the present (and future) attempts at surgically induced regeneration.

The typical response to cartilage injury in which the subchondral plate is fractured is the formation of fibrocartilage, a scarlike tissue unsuited to the support of compressive loads and shear forces (1,2). If the subchondral plate is not fractured, attempts at healing rely on articular cartilage cells, the response of which to injury is consistently and completely ineffectual (3).

Given the elegant precision of the morphological and compositional interdependence of articular cartilage, it is not surprising that attempts at effective regeneration of articular cartilage have frustrated clinicians and basic scientists alike. Mature mammalian cartilage cells, which constitute only 2% of the total volume of the tissue, have lost the ability to dedifferentiate. This property of cartilage cells is shared with the universe of other mammalian cells resulting from evolutionary progress. This circumstance likely is a controlling factor in the limitation of the biological response of articular cartilage to injury.

As mentioned, articular cartilage is a unique tissue in many respects, but especially with regard to its structural, metabolic, and functional interactions. Articular cartilage possesses unparalleled biomechanical functional efficiency, and this efficiency is derived from design features that are marveled at by physicians and engineers attempting to design artificial substitutes for diseased joints. For example, the articular cartilage lubrication efficiency is an order of magnitude superior to the best bearing surfaces known to modern engineering. Such efficiencies are achieved in spite of stringent limitations imposed on the tissue, such as the lack of blood supply and a tissue thickness that measures a few millimeters at most. Couple these points with a limited repair capability and the consequent requirement that the tissue survive a lifetime of use and then the question becomes, "How can synovial joints survive as long as they do?" The thrust of this chapter will be to describe the morphological, biochemical, and physiological interactions of the cartilage matrix to provide insight regarding the basis for successful long-term survival of cartilage and the requirements for its successful repair or regeneration.

A useful phenomenological concept that is helpful in understanding the function is air tent, which is a structure used as a cover for recreational areas, such as swimming pools and tennis courts, or as a temporary cover for exhibitions (4) **(Fig 3-1)**. The functional requirements for the air tent are (a) an inflation pump or fan, (b) an intake tube for the inflation medium, (c) the inflation medium (air), and (d) the fabric required to contain the pressurization and to provide the cover. The pump must be working constantly to maintain expansion of the system because of inevitable leaks through the fabric. In the case of cartilage, the surface membrane (i.e., the fabric) consists of the fine collagen fibril network concentrated at the articular surface. The inflation pump of cartilage is the proteoglycan molecular structure, and the inflation medium is an ultrafiltrate of synovial fluid. Cartilage, of course, has no single intake vent for the inflation medium to enter. Rather, fluid inflating the tissue enters through a myriad of microscopic pores at the surface; these are the same pores from which the fluid exits when compressed. These elements are interrelated, and a deficiency in any of them will result in failure of the system. In the case of the air tent, a tear in the fabric for which the pump is not able to compensate will result in collapse of the tent. Or, if the pump fails, the tent will gradually collapse as pressurized air leaks through the pores of the fabric.

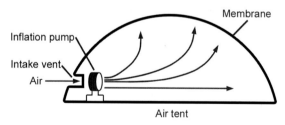

Fig 3-1. Air-tent analogy with articular cartilage. Articular cartilage is a pressurized structure that is similar conceptually to an air tent. The air-tent system requires a pump that must be constantly operating to maintain inflation of the tent because of leaks in the fabric. In the case of cartilage, the surface "membrane" is the lamina splendens, consisting of a fine fibrillar network concentrated at the articular surface. The inflation pump mechanism of articular cartilage is served by the proteoglycan molecules, and the inflation medium is an ultrafiltrate of the synovial fluid. Articular cartilage has no single intake vent for the inflation medium; rather, the fluid that inflates the structure enters through the same myriad of fine surface pores from which it exits when compressed (see text).

More specifically, the fabriclike structure at the cartilage surface, consisting of fine collagen fibrils packed tightly in a matted pattern parallel to the surface, is much different from that seen in the deeper layers, where fibers become thicker, their orientation becomes more vertical, and the spaces between the fibers increase. The surface "fabric" of cartilage has tiny pores that permit fluid and small molecules access to and egress from the tissue but that block the movement of large molecules. The inflation medium in articular cartilage is, of course, fluid rather than air. The cartilage fluid is in equilibrium with the synovial fluid, which is essentially an ultrafiltrate of plasma. The fluid in articular cartilage is significantly pressurized. Calculations by Ogston (5) led him to conclude that articular cartilage is inflated to the equivalent of "motor tire pressure." The pump for this pressurized system is not intuitively obvious, but its presence has been established without doubt by modem techniques of rheology and biophysics. The pump for the articular cartilage system is chiefly aggrecan, a proteoglycan molecule that becomes linked to hyaluronan to form a huge molecule designated as a proteoglycan aggregate. This huge macromolecule is locked within the articular cartilage fibrillar matrix by its large size and volume.

In its state of equilibrium, the expansion pressure in the articular cartilage system is in balance with the resisting tension of the collagen fibers; however, the balance can be upset by an externally applied load. If the external pressure exceeds the internal pressure, fluid will flow outward until a new equilibrium is reached. As the proteoglycan molecules become compressed, their charges become more concentrated, and this causes the fluid pressure within the cartilage to be increased until a new equilibrium is reached. The theoretical analysis of the fluid flow patterns and viscoelastic properties under various loading conditions has been studied extensively. This fluid movement is of great interest, because it explains the mechanism of several fundamental properties of the articular cartilage system, including lubrication, load bearing, and nutrition.

As indicated above, the proper evaluation of attempts at repair requires fundamental knowledge of articular cartilage form, composition, and biomechanical characteristics. The collagen matrix of normal articular cartilage, its proteoglycan and proteoglycan aggregate, and the movement of fluid within cartilage are described in greater detail in the following sections with respect to its morphologic, biochemical, and functional features.

■ COLLAGEN

Morphology of the Collagen Framework

The pattern of collagen fibrils within articular cartilage is well suited to the functional requirements of the tissue. The air-tent analogy described earlier requires that a pressurized internal medium be constrained from expansion by a membrane. A matted surface layer of collagen fibrils provides this membranelike function.

The collagen pattern in the deeper layers of the cartilage surface is morphologically quite different from the surface pattern. In 1925, Benninghoff (6) described an arcade pattern of organization for articular cartilage collagen **(Fig 3-2)**. This pattern has subsequently been challenged with respect to the precise accuracy of the proposed scheme (7–9). The concept is at least partially correct, however, and it is useful in understanding the function of cartilage. The surface fibrillar pattern clearly differs from that of fibers in deeper layers (10). The surface collagen fibrils are smaller (diameter, 30–32 nm) and more closely packed than in the middle and deeper layers. The surface pattern of the collagen framework as described has been recognized implicitly for decades by the term "armor plate" layer, referring to the tough, resilient, skinlike cartilage surface. The collagen concentration is greatest at the surface, where the small fibrils are compacted tangentially. This arrangement creates a small pore size, which has been calculated by McCutchen (11) to be approximately 6 nm. The largest molecule that can traverse a pore of this dimension is hemoglobin. Small ions and glucose, for example, easily traverse these pores, but larger molecules, such as most proteins and hyaluronan (hyaluronic acid), do not enter cartilage in significant amounts under normal conditions.

Collagen fibers in the intermediate layers are no longer oriented tangentially to the surface but, rather, are directed obliquely or randomly. They are larger than the surface fibrils, with most ranging between 40 and 100 nm. The deepest fibrils are the largest in cartilage. They are disposed perpendicularly relative to the joint surface, and they perforate the calcified basal layers of cartilage through the tidemark regions and, eventually, enter the subchondral bone layer,

where they are firmly attached, much as in the attachment of the Sharpey fibers of ligament to cortical bone. This feature is crucial for cartilage to be able to resist shearing forces, which otherwise would tend to peel the cartilage away from the subchondral surface.

It has been well demonstrated clinically that loss of the densely packed collagen mat at the surface of cartilage in weight-bearing regions is the prelude to fibrillation, accelerated wear, and degenerative arthritis. This seems completely logical, because the coarse, widely spaced fibrils in deeper layers that are principally oriented vertically are poorly suited for constraining the swelling forces that are generated by the matrix proteoglycans. The term fibrillation describes the tendency of these fibrils to be split vertically all the way to their subchondral attachment, much as wood splits along the grain of its fibers. The villuslike strands so exposed collectively resemble a shag rug, and the individual strands are prone to tear off at the base when mechanically loaded and exposed to shear stresses. Clearly, the description of an "armor plate" applies well to the normal surface mat of collagen fibrils, and loss of this layer no longer permits the cartilage to function as a pressurized unit suited to weight-bearing.

Evidence supporting the fibril pattern of collagen orientation derives from several types of observation, including routine histology, transmission-electron microscopy, scanning-electron microscopy, and the demonstration of Hultkrantz lines (12). Hultkrantz lines typically are observed on the surface of cartilage and are analogous to the Langer lines of skin (13). These lines become visible when the surface of cartilage is pricked with a pin. Coating the cartilage surface with India ink and then wiping it dry best demonstrates the puncture defects. Hultkrantz noted many years ago that the puncture holes appeared as slits rather than round holes. Furthermore,

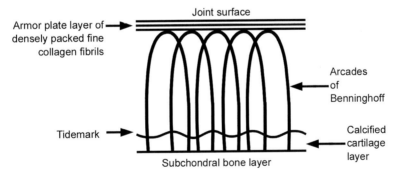

Fig 3-2. Benninghoff arcades. This schematic diagram shows the collagen fibril orientation within articular cartilage. The fibrils are tightly packed near the articular surface in a tangential layer that has been termed the lamina splendens, or the "armor plate" layer. Fibrils in the deeper layers become progressively larger as they progress toward the subchondral bone layer. The fibrils also are more widely spaced in the deeper layers of cartilage. The diagram shown is an idealized conception, and the fibrils of cartilage are not all ordered so precisely. However, the concept is useful in visualizing the fundamental interaction of the fibrils with other constituents of cartilage. The collagen fibrils anchor into the subchondral bone layer after traversing the calcified cartilage, which is demarcated by a change in staining properties termed the tidemark line. The anchoring of these fibrils into bone is analogous to the continuation of ligamentous attachments into bone termed the Sharpey fibers.

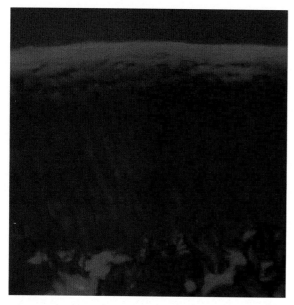

Fig 3-3. Polarized light microscopy of articular cartilage. This micrograph of an articular cartilage surface observed under polarized light shows the differences in refractility of the surface layer compared with the deeper layers. The preferred tangential orientation of the collagen fibrils at the surface creates refractile differences from the deeper layers and is seen here as a bright line. Original magnification, 45×.

these slits have axes that generally are perpendicular to the principal axis of movement of the joint. Hultkrantz lines therefore are different for each joint of the body. Mechanical tensile tests have confirmed that the Hultkrantz lines indicate the preferred orientation of the collagen fibrils at the surface of the joint resists tensile forces. Bullough and Goodfellow (14) have shown this characteristic of joint surfaces in polarized-light experiments illustrated in **Figure 3-3.** For interested readers, the pattern of matrix and cellular organization of articular cartilage has been described in greater detail by Wong and Hunziker (10).

Collagen Chemistry

The molecular structure of collagen has been of considerable interest for more than a century, because it is the principal structural protein (by mass) for all mammals. It constitutes 65% to 80% of the mass by dry weight of such specialized connective tissues as tendons, ligaments, skin, joint capsules, and cartilage. It is the only protein with significant tensile force–resisting properties with the exception of elastin, the functional role of which is quite different. Therefore, collagen is the key protein in musculoskeletal stability, providing the mechanical properties that impart the "connect" to connective tissue.

The tensile force–resisting properties of cartilage derive from the precise molecular configuration of the collagen macromolecule. This molecule is one of the largest in the body, forming a rodlike structure 300 nm in length and

1.5 nm in diameter. These rods are termed tropocollagen (15). They are assembled in a three-dimensional array in the extracellular environment, being influenced, somehow, by environmental stresses and additional biological factors of which the full details regarding their nature are still unclear. The sum of the extracellular influences somehow affects the orientation and size of fibrils that are assembled from the tropocollagen units (15–19). The tropocollagen assembly typically is patterned in a quarter stagger.

The α chains are not identical among species or within a single species. Early data regarding mammalian skin collagen demonstrated two types of α chains, α_1 and α_2, which were present in a ratio of 2:1 (15). Miller and Matukas (20) were the first to show that cartilage possesses a collagen that is different in composition from that in most fibrous connective tissues. This collagen contains a different type of α_1 chain, which they termed α_1, type II. The collagen in most cartilages consists of three such identical chains, and the abbreviated nomenclature is now $\alpha 1 [II]_3$, or type II collagen (21).

At least 27 different types of collagen products of 40 genes have been described in vertebrates (21). These collagens can be divided into two major classes on the basis of their primary structure and supramolecular assembly: the fibril-forming collagens, and the non–fibril-forming collagens. The fibril-forming collagens include types I, II, III, V, and XI (22). Each of these types has a long, central, triple-helix domain without any interruptions in the glycine-x-y sequence, where x and y are amino acids. The rest of the collagens belong to the non–fibril-forming class. Although they vary in size, they share the feature of having imperfections in the glycine-x-y sequence. Within this class, type IX, XII, and XIV collagens form a subgroup called the fibril-associated collagens with interrupted triple helices (FACIT). They are associated with type I or II collagen fibrils, and they play a role in the interaction of these fibrils with other matrix components. Although their sizes and primary structures vary, they share several common structural features. Type XVI collagen appears to be a member of this group (23). Summaries of the makeup and distribution of the collagen types accepted at present have been provided in several recent review articles (22–25).

The significance of the type II collagen to cartilage is not yet known. It is a heteropolymer with type IX collagen molecules covalently linked at the surface and type XI collagen molecules forming a filamentous template at the core. The principal differences between this collagen and the more common type I collagen that is found in fibrous connective tissue involve the number of hydroxylysine molecules and the presence of a small number of residues of cysteine. The type II collagen fibrils are thinner near the articular surface and the tangential zone than that are in the deeper zones, and the collagen concentration is greater at the surface. Evidence is accumulating that type IX and XI collagens make critical contributions to the organization and mechanical stability of the type II collagen fibrillar network **(Fig 3-4)**.

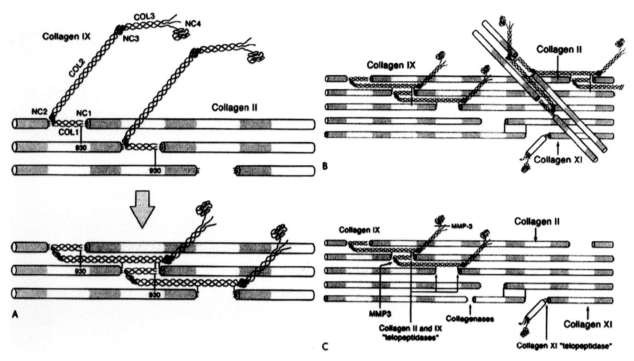

Fig 3-4. The collagens of articular cartilage. The assembly of tropocollagen II units into fibers and fibrils in cartilage is controlled, in part, by the minor collagens. Type IX collagen is a surface molecule that binds to type II collagen and to itself. Its side arms interfere with further growth of the fiber by steric interference with the addition of more type II molecules. Type XI collagen is located in the core of the fiber and is thought to be important in the determination of ultimate fiber size. Type XI collagen is present in the largest quantities in small fibers. Type X collagen is found in growth plate cartilage, not in articular cartilage. **A:** How the type IX collagen molecule is predicted to fold and to interact with molecules on the surface of type II collagen fibrils to accommodate all known cross-linking reactions. **B:** The potential for the fibril-to-fibril cross-links in a network. **C:** The known site of cleavage in the type II collagen triple helix by collagenases implicated in pathologic degradation in osteoarthritis (OA) and inflammatory arthritis. (Adapted from Eyre DR. Collagens and cartilage matrix homeostasis. *Clin Orthop Relat Res.* 2004;vol: S118–S122; with permission.)

Type IX collagen makes up approximately 10% of the collagen protein in fetal mammalian articular cartilage, but the amount decreases to approximately 1% in adult tissue. The molecule also is categorized as a proteoglycan, because it was originally demonstrated in chicks that single site for attachment of chondroitin sulfate exists on the type IX collagen molecule. Type IX collagen also is characterized by the presence of four globular domains in the triple-helix structure (26). In bovine articular cartilage, type IX collagen is found on the surface of type II collagen and appears to be linked covalently to at least one molecule of the type II collagen triple helix (26). From this evidence, type IX collagen is believed to provide a covalent interface between the surface of the type II collagen fibril and the interfibrillar proteoglycan domain. Another theory is that type IX collagen provides interfibrillar linkages between type II collagen fibrils and, therefore, may enhance the mechanical stability of the fibrillar network.

Type XI collagen makes up approximately 3% of mature articular cartilage collagen. It has a single globular domain on one end of the triple helix, and it is located within the type II collagen fibrils (21). Diagrams illustrating the Type II/IX/XI

collagen heteromer is shown in Figure 3-4. Other fibrous collagens found in articular cartilage are type VI and X collagens. Both have a short helix. Type X collagen is found only in hypertrophic zones of growth plates. Type VI collagen has a globular domain on each end (21). Type VI collagen is unique in that it has no aldehyde cross-link and has arginine–glycine–aspartic acid (RGD) sequences in each α chain; these sequences are important in cell attachment (27). It binds to hyaluronan (28) and to fibronectin (29), and it has been identified in the perilacunar matrix surrounding chondrocytes.

The fundamental process of collagen formation the chondroblasts and chondrocytes is nearly identical to its synthesis by the fibroblast and fibrocyte. The collagen turnover in cartilage proceeds at a rate not unlike that seen in connective tissue of the fibrous type. Because significant collagen synthesis occurs in adult cartilage, the control processes for spatial orientation of the product, although poorly understood, clearly are of crucial importance.

It is a source of frustration to surgeons and their patients that attempts to achieve cartilage repair, as in surgical arthroplasty, do not successfully regenerate cartilage and seldom produce completely satisfactory clinical results. The collagen fiber architecture of the arthroplasty repair tissue is disordered throughout the deep layers and lacks the membranelike characteristics that are so important to the surface layer of articular cartilage. These are major factors contributing to the failure of cartilage regeneration. Details regarding the biology of the cartilage repair process are described later in this chapter.

Collagen Cross-Links

Stabilization of collagen occurs extracellularly, after its assembly into the quarter-stagger arrays that make up filaments, fibrils, and fibers. The stabilization and ultimate tensile strength of the fiber structure are thought to result mainly from the development of intramolecular and intermolecular cross-links. The former occur between α chains of the individual tropocollagen molecule and the latter between adjacent tropocollagen molecules. The cross-links result from enzyme-mediated reactions involving mainly lysine and hydroxylysine. The details of the bifunctional, trifunctional, or quadrifunctional cross-links so created are beyond the scope of this discussion but are available in several relevant reviews (30–39).

■ PROTEOGLYCANS OF ARTICULAR CARTILAGE

Sulfated proteoglycan macromolecules constitute 12% of articular cartilage dry weight. The proteoglycans of articular cartilage serve as the "pump" of the highly pressurized cartilage system. As mentioned earlier, the characteristics of the proteoglycan molecules that permit this crucial function include their very large size and resulting immobility within the collagen fibril meshwork; their densely concentrated, fixed, negative sulfate and carboxyl charges; and the large number of hydroxyl groups contained. These characteristics collectively serve to attract water and small positively charged ions into the cartilage. Donnan osmotic pressure results from this process. The negative charges on the proteoglycan molecules naturally create repulsive forces between each other, which are termed chemical expansive stresses. The sum of the Donnan osmotic pressure and the chemical expansive stress constitutes the cartilage swelling pressure (17). Ogston (5) noted the rough equivalence of the pressure within articular cartilage with "motor tire pressure"!

The extraordinary size of the proteoglycan aggregate molecules of articular cartilage is achieved by supra-assembly of three different types of linear-chain molecular species: sulfated glycosaminoglycans, a core protein, and hyaluronan (a nonsulfated glycosaminoglycan). The purpose of this section is to describe briefly the chemical structure of the functionally vital proteoglycan and its proteoglycan aggregate and to illustrate the manner in which the functional role derives from the chemical structure.

Glycosaminoglycans

Figure 3-5 shows the repeating disaccharide unit for the glycosaminoglycans of articular cartilage: chondroitin-4-sulfate, chondroitin-6-sulfate, hyaluronan, and keratan sulfate. In most of the glycosaminoglycan molecules, hexosamine alternates with another sugar polymerized in a repeating disaccharide pattern. The predominance of the amine group

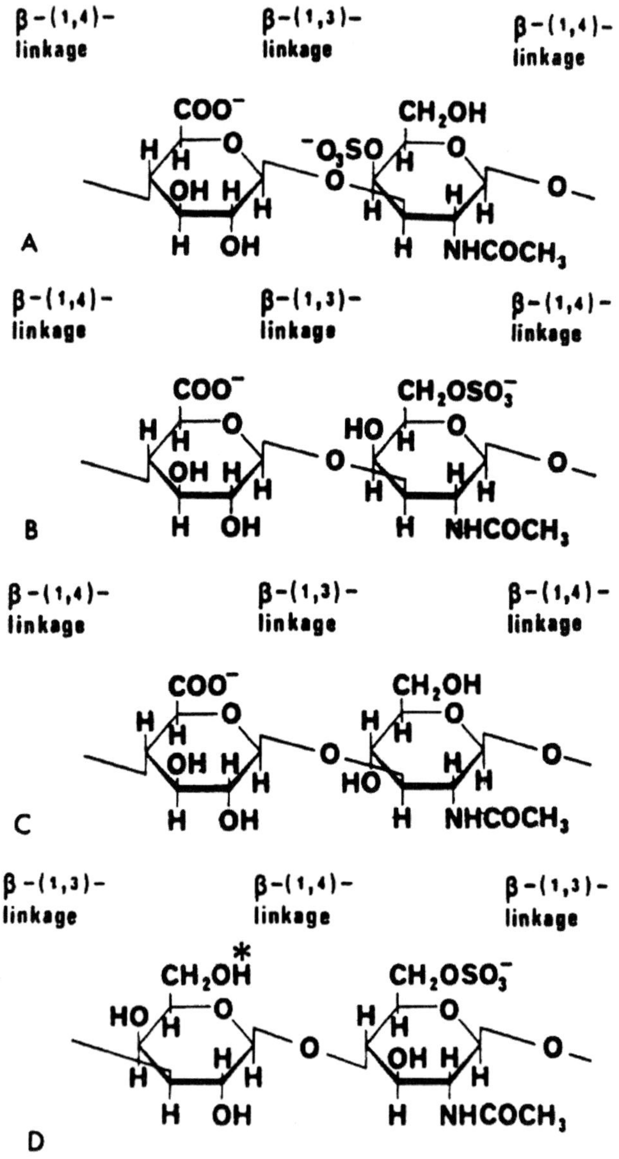

Fig 3-5. The disaccharide configuration of the principal glycosaminoglycans of the proteoglycan constituents of articular cartilage. A: The molecular configuration of chondroitin-4-sulfate. This configuration differs from that of chondroitin-6-sulfate only in the location of the sulfate group on the hexosamine molecule. Both contain alternating glucuronic acid and galactosamine sugars. B: Chondroitin-6-sulfate. C: Hyaluronan. This disaccharide contains alternating molecules of glucosamine and glucuronic acid, but it lacks a sulfate group. D: Keratan sulfate. This disaccharide contains galactose rather than a uronic acid moiety. The hexosamine is glucosamine, which is sulfated in the C6 position.

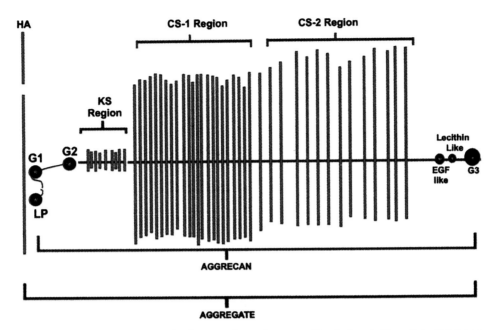

Fig 3-6. Aggrecan molecule. This diagram shows the assembly of chondroitin sulfate (CS-1 and CS-2) and keratan sulfate molecules onto a protein core linear structure, which in turn becomes fixed to hyaluronan via specialized G-1 and LP regions. The various specialized linkage regions are composed of highly specific molecular configurations (see text). The attachment of the core protein and its polysaccharide side chains (aggrecan) to hyaluronan to create the aggregate structure is shown. Typically, a high concentration of keratan sulfate, with its smaller number of disaccharide units near the attachment site of the core protein to hyaluronan, is present. (The CS-1 and CS-2 regions are not drawn to scale; usually, they are twice as long as shown.)

in this configuration is the reason for the use of "amino-" in the term glycosaminoglycan. The common features of the group are obvious at first glance. In particular, the location of the *N*-acetylamine group at the C2 of the hexosamine is common to all the disaccharides shown. The hexosamine is galactosamine in three of the four cases; keratan sulfate possesses glucosamine as the alternating hexosamine. All except hyaluronan are sulfated at the C4 or C6 position of the hexosamine. Each disaccharide contains at least three hydroxyl groups. All except keratan sulfate contain uronic acid as the second element of the disaccharide, with a carboxyl terminal at C6. Keratan sulfate possesses galactose rather than uronic acid as the second half of the disaccharide (17).

Aggrecan

The glycosaminoglycans are covalently bound to core protein to form aggrecan in a structure that locates keratan sulfate side arms preferentially close to the linkage region to hyaluronan. The keratan sulfate–rich region of the aggrecan protein polysaccharide is illustrated in **Figure 3-6**. The keratan sulfate molecules characteristically are of lower molecular weight than the chondroitin sulfate chains (Fig 3-6). The core protein molecule has three globular domains, called G1, G2, and G3. The G1 region is the point of attachment of proteoglycan to hyaluronan to create aggregate, G2 is located near the keratan sulfate rich region, and G3 is located at the opposite terminal end of

the core protein (40). Phosphorylation of serine residues occurs adjacent to the chondroitin sulfate–containing peptides of the core protein (41).

Aggregate

The ability of proteoglycan to contribute to an even larger molecular structure by combining with hyaluronan originally was described by Hardingham and Muir (42). Those authors elaborated on the dissociation and association experiments of Sajdera and Hascall (43) to establish the mechanism of formation of the larger molecule, termed proteoglycan aggregate **(Fig 3-7)**. Much attention has been given to the degree of aggregate formation in various tissues and in various pathologic conditions (44–48). Clearly, the ability of the proteoglycan molecule to form aggregates of great molecular size amplifies its physiological functional properties as the "pump" of the articular cartilage system.

Lohmander (49) has noted that the molecular weight of aggregate is 100,000,000 to 200,000,000 Da, whereas for a common protein, such as insulin, the molecular weight is only 6,000 Da. Because of its much greater size, the aggregate formed will impose even greater fixation of the proteoglycan molecules, locking them more securely within the interstices of the collagen framework of the tissue and ensuring fixation of the negative charges needed to maintain swelling pressure for expansion of the articular cartilage matrix.

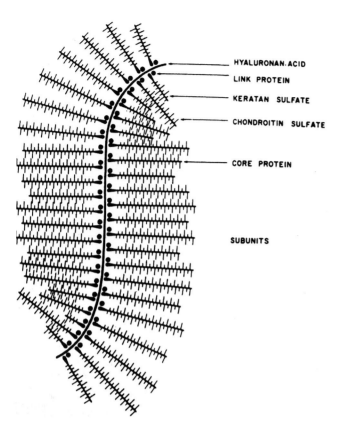

HYALURONAN. ACID
LINK PROTEIN
KERATAN SULFATE
CHONDROITIN SULFATE

CORE PROTEIN

SUBUNITS

Fig 3-7. Aggregate molecule. Here, the aggrecan is expanded from the single unit shown in Figure 3-6 to its more fully expanded state, in which dozens of aggrecan molecules are linked to the hyaluronan linear chain. The spectacular augmentation in molecular weight from the original glycosminoglycan weight of approximately 50,000 Da to that of aggrecan with a molecular weight in the millions to that of aggregate with a molecular weight of many millions is well seen.

Nature of the Aggregate Linkage

The linkage of proteoglycan subunit, aggrecan, to hyaluronan is noncovalent, which contrasts with the covalent linkage of glycosaminoglycans to core protein in aggrecan. The aggregate linkage is facilitated and strengthened by low-molecular-weight proteins termed link proteins (50–54). The linkage can occur without the presence of a link protein, but such proteins have been found in all cartilages so far examined. The noncovalent linkage of aggrecan and hyaluronan can be dissociated by concentrated solutions of guanidinium hydrochloride, calcium chloride, or magnesium chloride (42,43,55–60). The dissociated components can be reassociated by a reduction in the concentration of the dissociative solvents. Under conditions of approximately 0.5 M guanidinium hydrochloride, the three elements hyaluronan, link protein, and aggrecan reassociate to form the aggregate once again. This process has been the key technique in unraveling the chemical structure of aggrecan and aggregate, in understanding the nature of their association, and in deciphering the role of link proteins. Cartilages from different sources possess different percentages of aggregation of proteoglycan, but the factors controlling this process are not yet fully understood.

Small Proteoglycans of Articular Cartilage

Small proteoglycan molecules consisting of biglycan, decorin, and fibromodulin represent approximately 5% of the proteoglycan of articular cartilage. Dermatan sulfate proteoglycans were first observed in articular cartilage by Rosenberg (61) in 1985. The small proteoglycans each consist of a protein core and glycosaminoglycan chain branches. The core protein of the small proteoglycans is only one fourth the length of the core protein of aggrecan and is very similar in the three molecules. The horseshoe-shaped protein is linked near the open end by a disulfide bond. The glycosaminoglycan side chains are limited in number, consisting of a single chondroitin sulfate/dermatan sulfate side chain in decorin, two such chains in biglycan, and as many as four keratan sulfate side chains in the case of fibromodulin (61–63). Decorin (64) and fibromodulin (65) are located in the superficial zones of articular cartilage in association with collagen fibers. Smaller amounts of decorin are found in deeper cartilage layers (65). Biglycan (65) and decorin (66) are both found in the pericellular lacunar regions of chondrocytes.

The small proteoglycans have critical functional roles. Decorin and fibromodulin are associated with collagen fibers. Decorin inhibits type I and II collagen formation (67–69), however, and fibromodulin inhibits collagen enesis (70). Both biglycan and decorin possess properties of competitive binding with transforming growth factor (TGF)-β, thereby inhibiting the role of this growth factor in repair processes in cartilage (71,72). Because TGF-β is considered to be the "conductor of the symphony" in connective tissue repair (27), the modulation of its role by biglycan and decorin has great significance in the control of repair processes in connective tissue. Both decorin and biglycan also bind with other adhesion proteins, including fibronectin (73,74), thrombospondin (75), and type VI collagen (76). Each of these so-called adhesion proteins have the RGD amino acid sequences originally described by Ruoslahti and Pierschbacher (27) as playing key roles in cell adhesion. Decorin or biglycan binding to the adhesion proteins inhibits the cellular attachment of fibroblasts, another key step in the control of connective tissue healing (74). These small proteoglycan roles most certainly are relevant to the questions of limitations of repair potential of articular cartilage. Fibronectin, type VI collagen, thrombospondin, and the adhesion proteins have complex roles, binding to collagen (27,77), serving as bridges between cells and matrix (27,78) and between themselves (79), and binding to hyaluronan (28). These molecules undoubtedly possess functional roles far greater than the quantitative measures of their content in connective tissue matrix suggest, and their functional roles must be understood more completely to provide a comprehensive understanding of normal articular cartilage as well as its repair processes. Facilitation of the biological repair of articular cartilage by surgical procedures may not be made more feasible by this understanding, however, given the complexity of the processes involved, but at the same time, this facilitation is unlikely to be achieved without such an understanding.

■ FLUID OF ARTICULAR CARTILAGE

As noted earlier in the air-tent analogy, the inflation medium of articular cartilage is synovial fluid, which essentially is an ultrafiltrate of plasma plus hyaluronan. The hyaluronan molecules are too large to enter cartilage through its surface pores (diameter, 6 nm), but most of the remaining ions and molecules of normal synovial fluid, such as water, sodium, potassium, and glucose, are sufficiently small to pass easily through these pores (11,80). Movement of fluid into and out of cartilage occurs, to some extent, by diffusion, but diffusion does not seem adequate in and of itself to provide for cartilage health. The percentage of water in cartilage ranges from more than 60% to nearly 80% (81–83). The water is bound by a variety of weak forces, such as hydrogen bonding to proteoglycan and collagen or simple hydration shell formation, but is relatively mobile.

Net flow into and out of cartilage is induced by the normal weight-bearing function of synovial joints. Maroudas et al. (84,85) has calculated that for normal articular cartilage, the sum of swelling pressures is greatly exceeded (10-fold) by loading conditions, such as walking. The implications would seem to be that under loading conditions, cartilage would be compressed rapidly and completely, much as a wet sponge is compressed by weight. The rate of fluid movement permitted by the small pore size and the cartilage microarchitecture is sufficiently slow, however, that cartilage is only partially compressed even after loading for hours.

Other experiments have illustrated this point well (86–88). Those investigators used an apparatus designed to fit into a centrifuge capable of forcing fluid out of cartilage and into a receptacle. The cartilage fits into a porous, basketlike container into which a plunger rests. The unit is placed into a centrifuge, and the faster the centrifuge revolves, the greater the pressure on the cartilage in the basket. In this way, the effect of varying loads over varying periods of time on the rate of fluid expression from cartilage can be evaluated. These experiments showed that the amount of fluid that can be expressed (~30%) is extremely small in relation to the total water content **(Fig 3-8)**.

Subsequent experiments using an animal joint demonstrated the processes of fluid movement in cartilage more directly; the device constructed for that experiment was termed an arthrotripsometer **(Fig 3-9)**. By developing the necessary design criteria, it was possible to vary loading conditions with respect to amplitude of load and to stationary versus cyclic conditions. The joint was immersed in synovial fluid during testing, and deformation versus time was seen to be greater for stationary than for cyclic loads. The explanation

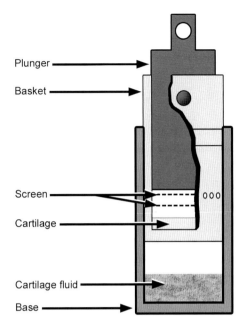

Fig 3-8. This device, used by Linn and Sokoloff to express fluid from articular cartilage, consists of a perforated basket within a centrifuge collection system. A plunger within the basket effectively compresses cartilage at the bottom of the basket when the system is spun in the centrifuge. Time and pressures can be controlled by the duration and speed of the operation. This technique permits the amount and composition of the expressed cartilage fluid to be analyzed. (From Linn FC, Sokoloff LH. Movement and composition of interstitial fluid of cartilage. *Arthritis Rheum.* 1965;8:481; with permission.)

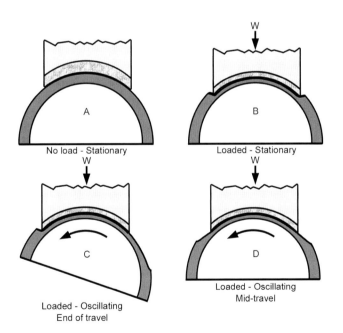

Fig 3-9. Effect of loading on articular cartilage. A stationary load **(B)** produces significant compression after some time. When oscillation occurs using the same loading condition, however, the compressive effect for a given time is considerably less, because the cartilage is unloaded for a portion of the time and resorbs some of the fluid that had been expressed. (Adapted from Linn FC. Lubrication of animal joints. *J Bone Joint Surg Am.* 1967;49:1079; with permission.)

for this observation is that in the cyclic condition, partial recovery occurs because of the effect of swelling pressure in pulling fluid back into cartilage during the phase of the cycle when the cartilage is unloaded. The effectiveness of this unparalleled system of load bearing by articular cartilage depends on functional integrity and detailed interaction of each architectural, biomechanical, and biochemical element within the system. Details of viscoelastic properties of articular cartilage, including the Poisson ratio and compressive modulus, have been concisely summarized in recent reviews (85,89–92).

The fluid movement that occurs during the loading process as described appears to be important for lubrication of the joint surfaces as well as for load carriage. On the basis of calculations obtained from complex mathematical models, Mow et al. (89,93) have proposed that fluid is expressed out of cartilage in front of the advancing contact surfaces of cartilage. This process provides a fluid film that minimizes cartilage–cartilage contact, thus also minimizing wear. Indeed, if this analysis is correct, then in a sense, we walk on water.

Issues of cartilage nutrition and metabolism are beyond the scope of this chapter. However, it its notable that the cellular population of articular cartilage is sparse and that the metabolic domain of a single chondrocyte is huge. Wong and Hunziker (10) and Hunziker et al. (94,95) have calculated the volume of matrix that must be maintained by a single chondrocyte to be 180,000 μm. Given the turnover of matrix components at a level not dissimilar to that of other connective tissues, the miracle of articular cartilage continues to amaze all students of the subject.

Cartilage Healing

It generally is agreed that intrinsic healing of cartilage lesions does not occur (1,96–98). There may be a response of the chondrocyte to injury, but this response does not result in cartilage repair. The obvious example is seen in degenerative arthritis [degenerative joint disease (DJD) osteoarthrosis, and osteoarthritis (OA)], in which chondrocytes often form clones of cells that demonstrate an increased rate of synthesis of matrix components in an attempt to repair damaged surfaces (99–104). The synthesized components are not retained within the matrix, however, and newly synthesized molecules, such as proteoglycans, are reduced in concentration despite the increased rate of synthesis. In reported experimental studies of mammalian joints, linear incisions created on articular cartilage surfaces remained indefinitely. Efforts at surgical reconstruction of articular defects therefore have shifted focus to allografts or cartilage autografts developed from cultured cells. These techniques will be addressed in subsequent chapters.

Historically, most surgical attempts at cartilage healing involved exposure of marrow cells to mount a repair response. This was achieved by subchondral bone resection (e.g., cup arthroplasty) or by drilling, abrasion, or microfracture of the

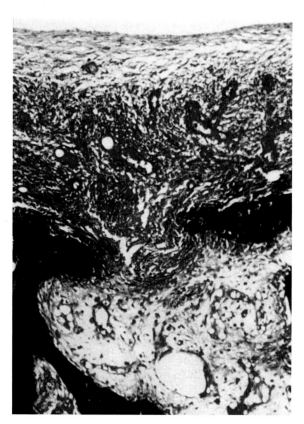

Fig 3-10. Photograph of a section of the femoral head 10 days after a cup arthroplasty procedure. The hip was denuded of cartilage and subchondral bone, and a vitalium cup was placed between the head of the femur and the acetabulum. Grossly and histologically, the tissue at this stave was very soft and highly vascular. The repair tissue has all the characteristics of the granulation tissue typical of soft tissue repair at other sites. The proliferative response is derived from primitive cellular elements in the subchondral bone marrow.

subchondral plate (1,102,105–112). When examined histologically a few days after surgery, the response to injury mounted by primitive marrow cells produces an outgrowth of a granulation-type tissue (1) **(Fig 3-10)**. This cellular response consists for the most part of immature vascular cells, fibroblasts, and macrophages. With the passage of time, maturation of the surface into fibrocartilage occurs, provided that the surface is protected from compressive and shear forces during the early stages of repair **(Fig 3-11)**.

The fibrocartilage so formed is remarkably different from hyaline articular cartilage. The fibrocartilage surface is deficient in both the precise morphology and the composition of normal articular cartilage, as documented earlier in this chapter. The fibrocartilage cells vary in shape from place to place in the matrix. Occasionally, they are seen as round cells in a lacunalike structure, but they tend more commonly to be spindle shaped (1) (Fig 3-11). The fibrous matrix lacks both the precise morphology of arcades in the deeper layers and the packing of thin, parallel fiber organization at the surface, and it is not anchored securely into the subchondral plate.

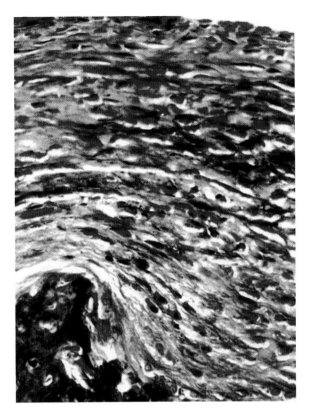

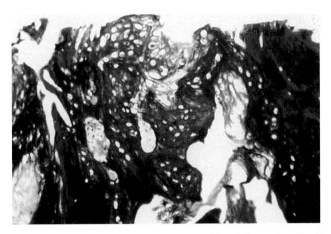

Fig 3-12. Micrograph of a canine femoral head 4 months after a cup arthroplasty procedure performed as described in Figure 3-10. This section is from the superior weight-bearing surface. The repair elements that had grown out from the underlying marrow have been worn away by contact with the opposing surface. Below the surface is residual repair tissue between trabecular bone struts. The remaining fibrocartilage cells are surrounded by matrix that stains metachromatically. The fiber pattern of the matrix appears to be random rather than highly ordered. The failure of the repair surface is related to its poor load-bearing characteristics and is predicted by its low proteoglycan content and disordered fiber pattern.

Fig 3-11. Micrograph of the canine femoral head 1 month after a cup arthroplasty procedure was performed as described in Figure 3-10. Cellular elements in the non–load-bearing area shown have survived and undergone metaplasia into fibrocartilage. Note the coarse nature of the collagen architecture, which has little resemblance to the fibrous architecture of normal articular cartilage. Nothing resembling the architecture of normal hyaline cartilage was seen. Notably, only sparse metachromasia is observed. Metachromatic staining indicates glycosaminoglycan molecules in the tissue. This type of repair response is typical of that seen after abrasion arthroplasty or its variants; such tissue has poor loading characteristics. Original magnification, 120×.

Strikingly, the proteoglycan content is only a fraction of that in normal articular cartilage (1,113,114). Not surprisingly, this reconstituted surface is not an efficient load-bearing organ. Mechanical tests done on experimental arthroplasty surfaces show a resistance to compression of only one third that of normal articular cartilage (2,115–117). As a result, the durability of regenerated arthroplasty surfaces of this type is limited, and the fibrocartilage surface is gradually worn away (1,113,118–120) **(Fig 3-12)**.

The consequence of the unsatisfactory outcome of the biological healing response was the relatively rapid abandonment of procedures such as cup arthroplasty of the hip in the late 1960s and early 1970s in favor of total hip replacement constructs using artificial components. Similarly, arthroscopic debridement of degenerative knee joints using abrasion techniques on exposed bone to stimulate fibrocartilage formation is presently being applied principally as a temporizing procedure to defer total knee replacement.

A related problem encountered surgically is the localized osteochondral defect exemplified by osteochondritis dissecans

of the knee or ankle. Frequently, the necrotic fragment with its overlying cartilage is damaged and/or displaced and is not suitable for replacement and fixation in the cavity from which it originated. In such cases, the surgeon is confronted with a defect of sufficient size to jeopardize long-term survival of the joint because of incongruity of the opposing surfaces. In the past, this defect was "repaired" by curettage of the cavity and drilling the base of the exposed bone. The expectation was that the cavity would be filled with repair tissue and that a new surface would be regenerated.

The rationale for this approach was partially derived from experimental studies with small animals that indicated drill holes in articular cartilage could heal. The model commonly used in such experiments was the rabbit knee joint in which a 1- to 2-mm drill hole was created that penetrated the subchondral plate. However, the absolute geometry of the larger defects in the human knee—often 2 cm in diameter—respond quite differently from the response seen in size of defects studied in the small animal models. Experiments performed in large animals, however, represent a more realistic model. The experiments of Convery et al. (120) on the horse's knee, in which defects of 1.5 to 2.5 cm diameter were created, demonstrated grossly imperfect healing in all cases (120) **(Fig 3-13)**. Other studies have confirmed the limitation of healing large osteochondral defects (117,121). Such results motivated the search for more realistic solutions, such as allografting, to the Osteochondritis Dessicans (OCD) lesion in humans. Some of the newer surgical approaches to this question are reviewed in a later chapter.

The implication of the evolving knowledge of normal articular cartilage is the recognition of its phenomenal

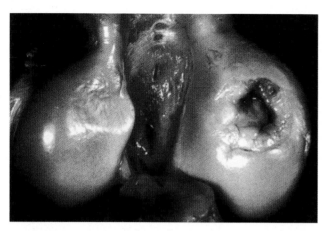

Fig 3-13. Photograph of the knee of a horse 4 months after drilling a 4-mm and a 2-cm, full-thickness defect in the medial femoral condyle. This experiment illustrates the futility of drilling the base of an osteochondritis defect with the expectation of complete repair. Although the 4-mm defect is difficult to see 4 months later (superior and medial to the larger defect), the 2-cm defect has achieved only partial filling. The repair tissue that survives is present only at the margin, is fibrocartilaginous, and could not be expected to perform effectively as a functional weight-bearing surface. Therefore, allografting or mosaicplasty techniques are preferred over simple drilling procedures of such lesions when primary healing has failed and the original bone-cartilage fragment has been damaged too severely to be replaced.

genius as a biologically engineered construct. It follows that all the evolving surgical attempts at reconstruction are faced with the daunting challenge of the precise requirements for replicating articular cartilage. Normal articular cartilage remains the exacting benchmark against which all new therapeutic concepts must be measured. Current efforts seeking a biological solution to repair are exciting. Clearly, however, the hurdles that remain are large, and the race to the ultimate biological solution has just begun.

■ REFERENCES

1. Akeson WH, Miyashita C, Taylor TK, et al. Experimental arthroplasty of the canine hip. Extracellular matrix composition in cup arthroplasty. *J Bone Joint Surg Am.* 1969;51:149–164.
2. Coletti JM Jr, Akeson WH, Woo SL. A comparison of the physical behavior of normal articular cartilage and the arthroplasty surface. *J Bone Joint Surg Am.* 1972;54:147–160.
3. Mankin H. Current concepts review. The response of articular cartilage to mechanical injury. *J Bone Joint Surg Am.* 1982;64:460–466.
4. Akeson W, Amiel D, Gershuni D. Articular cartilage physiology and metabolism. In: Resnick D, ed. *Diagnosis of bone and joint disorders.* Philadelphia: WB Saunders; 1994:23-1–23-31.
5. Ogston A. The biological functions of the glycosaminoglycans. In: Balazs E, ed. *Chemistry and molecular biology of the intercellular matrix,* Vol 3. London: Academic Press; 1970:1231.
6. Benninghoff A. Form und bau der gelenkknorpel in ihren beziehungen zur funktion. *Z Anat Entwicklungsgesch.* 1925;76:43.
7. Weiss C, Rosenberg L, Helfet AJ. An ultrastructural study of normal young adult human articular cartilage. *J Bone Joint Surg Am.* 1968;50:663–674.
8. Clark JM. The organization of collagen in cryofractured rabbit articular cartilage: a scanning electron microscopic study. *J Orthop Res.* 1985;3:17–29.
9. Little K, Pimm L, Trueta J. Osteoarthritis of the hip: an electron microscope study. *J Bone Joint Surg Br.* 1958;40:123.
10. Wong M, Hunziker E. Articular cartilage biology and mechanics. *Sports Med Arthros Rev.* 1998;6:4–12.
11. McCutchen C. The frictional properties of animal joints. *Wear.* 1962;5:1.
12. Hultkrantz W. Uber die spaltrichtungen der gelenkknorpel. *Verhandlungen der Anatomischen Gesellschaft.* 1898;12:248.
13. Langer C. Zur anatomie und physiologie der haut. *Sitzungsb d k acad wissensch.* 1861;45:223.
14. Bullough P, Goodfellow J. The significance of the fine structure of articular cartilage. *J Bone Joint Surg Br.* 1968;50:852–857.
15. Piez KA. Characterization of a collagen from codfish skin containing three chromatographically different α chains. *Biochemistry.* 1965;4:2590–2596.
16. Mayne R. Preparation and applications of monoclonal antibodies to different collagen types. *Clin Biochem.* 1988;21:111–115.
17. Mathews MB. Connective tissue. Macromolecular structure and evolution. *Mol Biol Biochem Biophys.* 1975;19:1–318.
18. Eyre DR. The specificity of collagen cross-links as markers of bone and connective tissue degradation. *Acta Orthop Scand Suppl.* 1995;266:166–170.
19. Amiel D, Billings EJ, Akeson W. Ligament structure, chemistry, and physiology. In: Daniel D, Akeson W, O'Connor J, eds. *Knee ligaments: structure, function, injury, and repair.* New York: Raven Press; 1990:77.
20. Miller EJ, Matukas VJ. Chick cartilage collagen: a new type of α_1 chain not present in bone or skin of the species. *Proc Natl Acad Sci U S A.* 1969;64:1264–1268.
21. Eyre DR. Collagens and cartilage matrix homeostasis. *Clin Orthop Relat Res.* 2004;S118–S122.
22. Van der Rest M, Garrone R. Collagen family of proteins. *FASEB J.* 1991;5:2814–2823.
23. Pan TC, Zhang RZ, Mattei MG, et al. Cloning and chromosomal location of human α_1(XVI) collagen. *Proc Natl Acad Sci U S A.* 1992;89:6565–6569.
24. Cremer MA, Rosloniec EF, Kang AH. The cartilage collagens: a review of their structure, organization, and role in the pathogenesis of experimental arthritis in animals and in human rheumatic disease. *J Mol Med.* 1998;76:275–288.
25. Prockop DJ. What holds us together? Why do some of us fall apart? What can we do about it? *Matrix Biol.* 1998;16:519–528.
26. Van der Rest M, Mayne R. Type IX collagen proteoglycan from cartilage is covalently cross-linked to type II collagen. *J Biol Chem.* 1988;263:1615–1618.
27. Ruoslahti E, Pierschbacher MD. New perspectives in cell adhesion: RGD and integrins. *Science.* 1987;238:491–497.
28. McDevitt CA, Marcelino J, Tucker L. Interaction of intact type VI collagen with hyaluronan. *FEBS Lett.* 1991;294:167–170.
29. McDevitt D, Francois P, Vaudaux P, et al. Identification of the ligand-binding domain of the surface-located fibrinogen receptor (clumping factor) of *Staphylococcus aureus. Mol Microbiol.* 1995;16:895–907.
30. Piez KA. Cross-linking of collagen and elastin. *Annu Rev Biochem.* 1968;37:547–570.
31. Kang AH, Gross J. Relationship between the intra- and intermolecular cross-links of collagen. *Proc Natl Acad Sci U S A.* 1970;67:1307–1314.
32. Gallop PM, Blumenfeld OO, Seifter S. Structure and metabolism of connective tissue proteins. *Annu Rev Biochem.* 1972;41:617–672.

33. Tanzer ML, Fairweather R, Gallop PM. Isolation of the cross-link, hydroxymerodesmosine, from borohydride-reduced collagen. *Biochim Biophys Acta.* 1973;310:130–136.

34. Tanzer ML, Housley T, Berube L, et al. Structure of two histidine-containing cross-links from collagen. *J Biol Chem.* 1973;248:393–402.

35. Vuorio E, de Crombrugghe B. The family of collagen genes. *Annu Rev Biochem.* 1990;59:837–872.

36. Wu JJ, Eyre DR. Cartilage type IX collagen is cross-linked by hydroxypyridinium residues. *Biochem Biophys Res Commun.* 1984;123:1033–1039.

37. Wu JJ, Eyre DR. Identification of hydroxypyridinium cross-linking sites in type II collagen of bovine articular cartilage. *Biochemistry.* 1984;23:1850–1857.

38. Wu JJ, Lark MW, Chun LE, et al. Sites of stromelysin cleavage in collagen types II, IX, X, and XI of cartilage. *J Biol Chem.* 1991;266:5625–5628.

39. Wu JJ, Eyre DR. Structural analysis of cross-linking domains in cartilage type XI collagen. Insights on polymeric assembly. *J Biol Chem.* 1995;270:18865–18870.

40. Yanagishita M. Function of proteoglycans in the extracellular matrix. *Acta Pathol Jpn.* 1993;43:283–293.

41. Anderson RS, Schwartz ER. Phosphorylation of proteoglycans. Identification of phosphorylation sites in chondroitin sulfate-rich region of core protein. *Arthritis Rheum.* 1985;28:804–812.

42. Hardingham TE, Muir H. The specific interaction of hyaluronic acid with cartilage proteoglycans. *Biochim Biophys Acta.* 1972;279:401–405.

43. Sajdera SW, Hascall VC. n-Polysaccharide complex from bovine nasal cartilage. A comparison of low and high shear extraction procedures. *J Biol Chem.* 1969;244:77–87.

44. Gregory JD. Multiple aggregation factors in cartilage proteoglycan. *Biochem J.* 1973;133:383–386.

45. Hascall VC, Sajdera SW. Protein-polysaccharide complex from bovine nasal cartilage. The function of glycoprotein in the formation of aggregates. *J Biol Chem.* 1969;244:2384–2396.

46. Hascall VC, Heinegard D. Aggregation of cartilage proteoglycans. II. Oligosaccharide competitors of the proteoglycan-hyaluronic acid interaction. *J Biol Chem.* 1974;249:4242–4249.

47. Hascall VC, Heinegard D. Aggregation of cartilage proteoglycans. I. The role of hyaluronic acid. *J Biol Chem.* 1974;249:4232–4241.

48. Heinegard D, Hascall VC. Aggregation of cartilage proteoglycans. 3. Characteristics of the proteins isolated from trypsin digests of aggregates. *J Biol Chem.* 1974;249:4250–4256.

49. Lohmander S. Proteoglycans of joint cartilage. Structure, function, turnover, and role as markers of joint disease. *Baillieres Clin Rheumatol.* 1988;2:37–62.

50. Buckwalter JA, Rosenberg LC. The effect of link protein on proteoglycan aggregate structure. An electron microscopic study of the molecular architecture and dimensions of proteoglycan aggregates reassembled from the proteoglycan monomers and link proteins of bovine fetal epiphyseal cartilage. *J Biol Chem.* 1984;259:5361–5363.

51. Fife RS, Myers SL. Evidence for an interaction between canine synovial cell proteoglycans and link proteins. *Biochim Biophys Acta.* 1985;843:238–244.

52. Fife RS. Identification of link proteins and a 116,000-dalton matrix protein in canine meniscus. *Arch Biochem Biophys.* 1985;240:682–688.

53. Choi HU, Tang LH, Johnson TL, et al. Proteoglycans from bovine nasal and articular cartilages. Fractionation of the link proteins by wheat germ agglutinin affinity chromatography. *J Biol Chem.* 1985;260:13370–13376.

54. Fife RS, Caterson B, Myers SL. Identification of link proteins in canine synovial cell cultures and canine articular cartilage. *J Cell Biol.* 1985;100:1050–1055.

55. Rosenberg LC, Pal S, Buckwalter JA. Structural changes related to malignancy in proteoglycans from cartilage neoplasms. *Ala J Med Sci.* 1980;17:283–292.

56. Campo RD, Tourtellotte CD. The composition of bovine cartilage and bone. *Biochim Biophys Acta.* 1967;141:614–624.

57. Buckwalter JA, Pita JC, Muller FJ, et al. Structural differences between two populations of articular cartilage proteoglycan aggregates. *J Orthop Res.* 1994;12:144–148.

58. Hedlund H, Hedbom E, Heinegard D, et al. Association of the aggrecan keratan sulfate-rich region with collagen in bovine articular cartilage. *J Biol Chem.* 1999;274:5777–5781.

59. Roughley PJ, Lee ER. Cartilage proteoglycans: structure and potential functions. *Microsc Res Tech.* 1994;28:385–397.

60. Poole AR, Rizkalla G, Ionescu M, et al. Osteoarthritis in the human knee: a dynamic process of cartilage matrix degradation, synthesis, and reorganization. *Agents Actions Suppl.* 1993;39:3–13.

61. Rosenberg LC, Choi HU, Tang LH, et al. Isolation of dermatan sulfate proteoglycans from mature bovine articular cartilages. *J Biol Chem.* 1985;260:6304–6313.

62. Roughley PJ, White RJ. Dermatan sulfate proteoglycans of human articular cartilage. The properties of dermatan sulfate proteoglycans I and II. *Biochem J.* 1989;262:823–827.

63. Fisher LW, Termine JD, Young MF. Deduced protein sequence of bone small proteoglycan I (biglycan) shows homology with proteoglycan II (decorin) and several nonconnective tissue proteins in a variety of species. *J Biol Chem.* 1989;264:4571–4576.

64. Poole AR, Webber C, Pidoux I, et al. Localization of a dermatan sulfate proteoglycan (DS-PGII) in cartilage and the presence of an immunologically related species in other tissues. *J Histochem Cytochem.* 1986;34:619–625.

65. Poole AR, Rosenberg LC, Reiner A, et al. Contents and distributions of the proteoglycans decorin and biglycan in normal and osteoarthritic human articular cartilage. *J Orthop Res.* 1996;14:681–689.

66. Roughley PJ, White RJ, Cs-Szabo G, et al. Changes with age in the structure of fibromodulin in human articular cartilage. *Osteoarthritis Cartilage.* 1996;4:153–161.

67. Vogel KG, Fisher LW. Comparisons of antibody reactivity and enzyme sensitivity between small proteoglycans from bovine tendon, bone, and cartilage. *J Biol Chem.* 1986;261:11334–11340.

68. Vogel KG, Meyers AB. Proteins in the tensile region of adult bovine deep flexor tendon. *Clin Orthop.* 1999;S344–S355.

69. Vogel K, Paulson M, Heinegaard R. Specific inhibition of type I and type II collagen fibrillogenesis by the small proteoglycan of tendon. *Biochem J.* 1984;223:587–597.

70. Scott J. Proteoglycan-fibrillar collagen interactions. *Biochem J.* 1988;252:313–323.

71. Yamaguchi Y, Mann D, Ruoslahti E. Negative regulation of transforming growth factors by the proteoglycan decorin. *Nature.* 1990;346:381–384.

72. Ruoslahti E. Proteoglycans in cell regulation. *J Biol Chem.* 1989;264:13369–13372.

73. Winnemoller M, Schmidt G, Kresse H. Influence of decorin on fibroblast adhesion to fibronectin. *Eur J Cell Biol.* 1991;54:10–17.

74. Lewandowska K, Choi HC, Rosenberg LC, et al. Fibronectin-mediated adhesion of fibroblasts: inhibition by dermatan sulfate proteoglycan and evidence for a cryptic glycosaminoglycan-binding domain. *J Cell Biol.* 1987;105:1443–1454.

75. Winnemoller M, Schon P, Vischer P, et al. Interactions between thrombospondin and the small proteoglycan decorin: interference with cell attachment. *Eur J Cell Biol.* 1992;59:47–55.

76. Bidanset DJ, Guidry C, Rosenberg LC, et al. Binding of the proteoglycan decorin to collagen type VI. *J Biol Chem.* 1992;267:5250–5256.

77. Watkins SC, Lynch GW, Kane LP, et al. Thrombospondin expression in traumatized skeletal muscle. Correlation of appearance with posttrauma regeneration. *Cell Tissue Res.* 1990;261:73–84.

78. Marcelino J, McDevitt CA. 1995. Attachment of articular cartilage chondrocytes to the tissue form of type VI collagen. *Biochim Biophys Acta.* 1995;1249:180–188.

79. Bornstein P. Diversity of function is inherent in matricellular proteins: an appraisal of thrombospondin 1. *J Cell Biol.* 1995; 130:503–506.

80. Maroudas A. Transport of solutes through cartilage: permeability to large molecules. *J Anat.* 1976;122:335–347.

81. Eichelberger L, Akeson W, Roma M. Biochemical studies of articular cartilage. 1. Normal values. *J Bone Joint Surg.* 1958;40:142.

82. Mankin HJ, Thrasher AZ. Water content and binding in normal and osteoarthritic human cartilage. *J Bone Joint Surg Am.* 1975; 57:76–80.

83. Jaffe FF, Mankin HJ, Weiss C, et al. Water binding in the articular cartilage of rabbits. *J Bone Joint Surg Am.* 1974;56:1031–1039.

84. Maroudas A, Bullough P, Swanson SA, et al. The permeability of articular cartilage. *J Bone Joint Surg Br.* 1968;50:166–177.

85. Maroudas A. Biophysical chemistry of cartilaginous tissues with special reference to solute and fluid transport. *Biorheology.* 1975;12:233–248.

86. Linn F, Sokoloff L. Movement and composition of interstitial fluid of cartilage. *Arthritis Rheum.* 1965;8:481.

87. Linn FC. Lubrication of animal joints. I. The arthrotripsometer. *J Bone Joint Surg Am.* 1967;49:1079–1098.

88. Linn FC, Radin EL. Lubrication of animal joints. 3. The effect of certain chemical alterations of the cartilage and lubricant. *Arthritis Rheum.* 1968;11:674–682.

89. Mow VC, Wang CC, Hung CT. The extracellular matrix, interstitial fluid, and ions as a mechanical signal transducer in articular cartilage. *Osteoarthritis Cartilage.* 1999;7:41–58.

90. Mow VC, Ateshian GA, Spilker RL. Biomechanics of diarthrodial joints: a review of twenty years of progress. *J Biomech Eng.* 1993;115:460–467.

91. Mow VC, Ratcliffe A, Poole AR. Cartilage and diarthrodial joints as paradigms for hierarchical materials and structures. *Biomaterials.* 1992;13:67–97.

92. Nordin M, Frankel V. *Basic Biomechanics of the Musculoskeletal System.* Philadelphia: Lea & Febiger; 1989.

93. Mow VC, Holmes MH, Lai WM. Fluid transport and mechanical properties of articular cartilage: a review. *J Biomech.* 1984;17: 377–394.

94. Hunziker EB, Herrmann W. In situ localization of cartilage extracellular matrix components by immunoelectron microscopy after cryotechnical tissue processing. *J Histochem Cytochem.* 1987;35:647–655.

95. Hunziker EB, Wagner J, Studer D. Vitrified articular cartilage reveals novel ultra-structural features respecting extracellular matrix architecture. *Histochem Cell Biol.* 1996;106:375–382.

96. Mankin HJ. The response of articular cartilage to mechanical injury. *J Bone Joint Surg Am.* 1982;64:460–466.

97. Hunziker EB. Articular cartilage repair: are the intrinsic biological constraints undermining this process insuperable? *Osteoarthritis Cartilage.* 1999;7:15–28.

98. DePalma AF, McKeever CD, Subin DK. Process of repair of articular cartilage demonstrated by histology and autoradiography with tritiated thymidine. *Clin Orthop.* 1966;48:229–242.

99. Mankin HJ, Laing PG. Protein and ribonucleic acid synthesis in articular cartilage of osteoarthritic dogs. *Arthritis Rheum.* 1967; 10:444–450.

100. Mankin HJ, Lippiello L. Biochemical and metabolic abnormalities in articular cartilage from osteoarthritic human hips. *J Bone Joint Surg Am.* 1970;52:424–434.

101. Mankin HJ. The reaction of articular cartilage to injury and osteoarthritis (second of two parts). *N Engl J Med.* 1974;291: 1335–1340.

102. Mankin HJ. The reaction of articular cartilage to injury and osteoarthritis (first of two parts). *N Engl J Med.* 1974;291: 1285–1292.

103. Mankin HJ. Biochemical changes in articular cartilage in osteoarthritis. In: *Symposium on osteoarthritis.* St. Louis: Mosby; 1976:1–22

104. Mankin HJ. Alterations in the structure, chemistry, and metabolism of the articular cartilage in osteoarthritis of the human hip. *Hip.* 1982;126–145.

105. Buckwalter J, Mankin H. Articular cartilage. Part II: degeneration and osteoarthrosis, repair, regeneration, and transplantation. *J Bone Joint Surg.* 1997;79:612.

106. Cheung HS, Lynch KL, Johnson RP, et al. In vitro synthesis of tissue-specific type II collagen by healing cartilage. I. Short-term repair of cartilage by mature rabbits. *Arthritis Rheum.* 1980; 23:211–219.

107. Insall JN. Intra-articular surgery for degenerative arthritis of the knee. A report of the work of the late K. H. Pridie. *J Bone Joint Surg Br.* 1967;49:211–228.

108. Insall J. The Pridie debridement operation for osteoarthritis of the knee. *Clin Orthop.* 1974;101:61–67.

109. Magnuson P. Technique for debridement of the knee joint for arthritis. *Surg Clin North Am.* 1946;24:249.

110. Gomar-Sancho F, Gastaldi-Orquin E. Repair of osteochondral defects in articular weight-bearing areas in the rabbit's knee. The use of autologous osteochondral and meniscal grafts. *Int Orthop.* 1987;11:65–69.

111. Shapiro F, Koide S, Glimcher MJ. Cell origin and differentiation in the repair of full-thickness defects of articular cartilage. *J Bone Joint Surg Am.* 1993;75:532–553.

112. Sprague NF. Arthroscopic debridement for degenerative knee joint disease. *Clin Orthop.* 1981;118–123.

113. Wei X, Gao J, Messner K. Maturation-dependent repair of untreated osteochondral defects in the rabbit knee joint. *J Biomed Mater Res.* 1997;34:63–72.

114. Wei X, Messner K. Maturation-dependent durability of spontaneous cartilage repair in rabbit knee joint. *J Biomed Mater Res.* 1999;46:539–548.

115. Nelson BH, Anderson DD, Brand RA, et al. Effect of osteochondral defects on articular cartilage. Contact pressures studied in dog knees. *Acta Orthop Scand.* 1988;59:574–579.

116. Wayne JS, Woo SL, Kwan MK. Finite element analyses of repaired articular surfaces. *Proc Inst Mech Eng [H].* 1991;205: 155–162.

117. Landells J. The reaction of injured human articular cartilage. *J Bone Joint Surg Br.* 1957;39B:548.

118. Ghadially FN, Ghadially JA, Oryschak AF, et al. Experimental production of ridges on rabbit articular cartilage: a scanning electron microscope study. *J Anat.* 1976;121:119–132.

119. Mitchell N, Shepard N. The resurfacing of adult rabbit articular cartilage by multiple perforations through the subchondral bone. *J Bone Joint Surg Am.* 1976;58:230–233.

120. Convery FR, Akeson WH, Keown GH. The repair of large osteochondral defects. An experimental study in horses. *Clin Orthop.* 1972;82:253–262.

121. Ghadially JA, Ghadially R, Ghadially FN. Long-term results of deep defects in articular cartilage. A scanning electron microscope study. *Virchows Arch B Cell Pathol.* 1977;25: 125–136.

SKELETAL MUSCLE AND TENDON

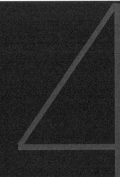

■ THOMAS M. BEST, MD, PhD, FACSM, JOHN J. WILSON, MD

■ KEY POINTS

■ Skeletal muscle has a complex organization of nerves, blood vessels, and connective tissue matrix that protects against injury and organizes individual cellular elements into functional contractile units of muscle.

■ Muscle fibers range a few millimeters to several centimeters in length. Fibers are arranged into larger units known as fascicles. Perimysium, a connective tissue sheath, surrounds fascicles. Whole muscles, made of numerous fasciculi, are surrounded by epimysium.

■ Tendon is juxtaposed between muscle and bone and is responsible for transmitting muscular forces to the skeletal system during limb locomotion.

■ The majority of skeletal muscle injuries that occur in sports are the result of indirect strain or direct blunt force trauma. Lacerations, ischemia, and infections are less common in athletics.

■ Indirect muscle strain injuries usually occur at the myotendinous junction during a stereotypical eccentric contraction. Certain muscles are more likely to sustain this type of injury (e.g., hamstrings during the rapid acceleration found in football, sprinting, and soccer).

■ Delayed muscle soreness (DMS) usually occurs at least 24 hours after exercise. Eccentric exercises, especially unfamiliar and repetitive ones, are more likely to predispose patients to DMS. Patients with DMS complain of pain, stiffness, and swelling in the muscles.

■ Direct trauma can occur at any point in the muscle. The quadriceps is the most common site of athletic muscle contusion, especially in football players. Under sufficient force, disruption of the muscle tissue and architecture can occur, often resulting in a hematoma.

Skeletal muscle accounts for nearly 45% of an average person's body weight, making it the largest organ in the human body. Although it can be thought of as a single organ, skeletal muscle is highly compartmentalized into separate entities, each with its own unique role within a functional muscle. Muscle has a complex organization of nerves, blood vessels, and connective tissue matrix that protects against injury and organizes individual cellular elements into functional contractile units of muscle. Skeletal muscle generates forces that result in bodily movement, steady posture, joint stabilization, and heat production through normal contractile functioning. This chapter begins with a discussion of the cellular structure and architecture of muscle, including myofibrillar contractile proteins, and then proceeds to the larger subunits and, ultimately, to skeletal gross anatomy. A detailed knowledge of the muscle structure will aid in understanding the biomechanics and physiology of normal skeletal muscle described here as well.

Because muscles must exert their force on the human skeleton, the tendons that accomplish this task are discussed as well. Tendons are positioned between muscles and bones, so the tension generated by muscle contraction can be conveyed to the bone trigger locomotion. The myotendinous junction is the transition point between muscle and tendon, and the osteotendinous junction (OTJ) is the point of tendon insertion into bone. Like the muscles they serve, tendons have an intricate cellular structure of collagen fibrils, elastin proteins, extracellular ground substance, and fibroblast cells. Tendons also have a rich vascular supply and innervation, which are important for normal functioning. The biomechanical properties of tendons make them suitable for transmitting muscular forces to bone with minimal loss of energy or stretch.

■ STRUCTURE AND ARCHITECTURE OF SKELETAL MUSCLE

Histology

Understanding the structure and architecture of skeletal muscle begins at the level of the muscle cell, or fiber, itself. Muscle fibers are multinucleated cells with a cylindrical shape, and they have diameters ranging between 10 to 100 μm. Fibers range a few millimeters to several centimeters in length. This wide variation in muscle fiber structure has important implications for their contractile mechanics. A covering of endomysium surrounds individual muscle fibers, and fibers are arranged into larger units, visible to the naked eye, known as fascicles. A connective tissue sheath known as the perimysium surrounds fascicles. Finally, whole muscles made of numerous fasciculi are surrounded by the epimysium (1) **(Fig 4-1)**. The connective tissue surrounding muscle carries the vast array of blood vessels supplying the tissue with a rich vascular network. The membranes are intimately, but loosely, associated with muscle to allow the changes in length and diameter that occur with muscle contraction. The epimysium, perimysium, and endomysium also provide a broad attachment surface for muscles to join with tendons. The perimysium becomes continuous with the endotenon sheath of tendon at the myotendinous junction (2), and it allows the tendon to transmit the force that is generated by muscle contraction to result in limb locomotion. Tendons are considered more fully later in the chapter.

The arrangement of muscle fibers and fascicles in muscles varies, and this is apparent on gross inspection of muscle anatomy. Fibers can be arranged either parallel or at an angle to the longitudinal axis of muscle; the latter predominates and includes the unipennate, bipennate, fusiform, and multipennate types **(Fig 4-2)**. The specific orientation of muscle fibers within a muscle affects a muscle's physiological cross-sectional area (i.e., the estimated sum of the cross sectional areas of all the fibers).

Orientation of muscle fibers plays an important role in determining the contractile properties of a given muscle. Force production is proportional to the physiological cross sectional areas of muscles and fiber orientation, but the speed and absolute amount of shortening are proportional to the muscle fiber length. Shorter fibers have a lower velocity of shortening and a greater force production compared to longer fibers. Although a pennate arrangement of fibers results in a small reduction of the contractile force conducted to the tendon, pennate muscles have a greater number of fibers acting in parallel. Therefore, a pennate muscle will be more powerful (i.e., have a greater force of contraction) than a muscle of equal mass with a parallel arrangement. Contraction of the pennate muscle–tendon unit causes the tendon to move along the axis of force, increasing pennation of the muscle fibers.

Skeletal Muscle Cytology

Each muscle fiber is surrounded by its plasma membrane, or sarcolemma. Within this sarcolemma lie quiescent satellite cells that are essential for the repair of muscle after injury. Following muscle injury, inflammatory substances are thought to stimulate these satellite cells to undergo proliferation and differentiation into new muscle fibers (3,4). Fibers are further divided into smaller units called myofibers or myofibrils, which are made of sarcomeres arranged in series alignment. Sarcomeres are the basic unit of muscle contraction; they are made of myosin, actin, tropomyosin, and troponin proteins. Muscle fibers contain

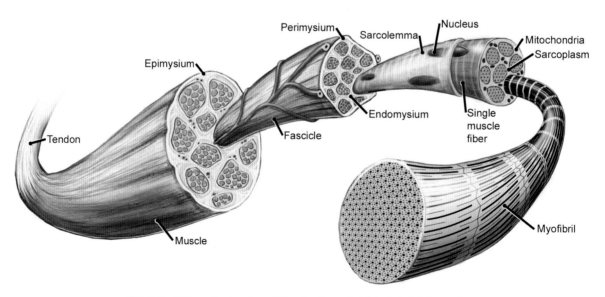

Fig 4-1. Schematic drawing of the structure of striated skeletal muscle.

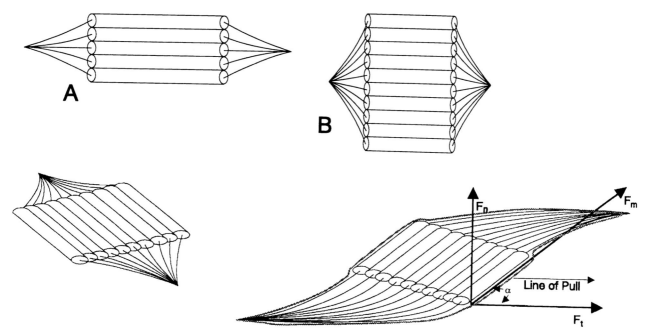

Fig 4-2. The role of muscle architecture in force production. (From Garrett WE, Best TM. Anatomy, physiology, and mechanics of skeletal muscle. In: Simon SR, Einhorn TA, Buckwalter JA, eds. *Orthopaedic basic science.* Rosemont, IL: American Academy of Orthopaedic Surgeons; 1994: 89–126; with permission.)

a number of other intracellular organelles that are important for normal function as well. Each fiber has hundreds to thousands of nuclei that are found peripherally. Nuclei are the regulatory control centers of the cell, determining cellular material and distribution (e.g., synthesis). The amount and type of proteins to be synthesized is determined by the nuclear DNA, and it is carried out by ribosomes in response to mRNA encoding. Because of their ability to quickly up- and down-regulate protein synthesis, muscles are fairly adaptable. Depending on the type of muscle fiber, cellular mitochondria may account for nearly 20% of total cell volume (5), being most abundant in highly oxidative, slow-twitch fibers. Mitochondria are responsible for production of adenosine triphosphate (ATP) through oxidative metabolism. This ATP is the crucial energy source for skeletal muscle force production as well as most other cellular tasks. Muscle fibers also contain various amounts of enzymes, lipids, and glycogen.

Motor Unit

Muscle fibers are arranged into discrete entities known as motor units. The muscle fiber motor unit is the most basic neuromuscular contractile unit, and it is composed of a single α-motor neuron and all the muscle fibers that it innervates (6,7). A single motor neuron can innervate as few as 10, or as many as several thousand, muscle fibers (8). As a motor neuron enters its muscle at the motor point, the nerve

axons branch many times, and each muscle fiber in the motor unit is contacted by a single nerve ending at the motor end plate (typically at the fiber midsection) **(Fig 4-3)**. Adjacent muscle fibers do not typically belong to the same motor unit, because fibers from a single unit usually are distributed throughout the muscle (9). Also, fibers belonging to the same motor unit share similar fiber type and contractile characteristics (10,11). As few as 10 fibers may be seen per motor unit in areas such as ocular muscles, where fine motor control is necessary. In large, force-generating muscles such as the quadriceps, however, there may be thousands of fibers per motor unit (12).

Contraction of a motor unit is initiated by an action potential arising from the nerve cell body that lies in the anterior horn of the spinal cord. The action potential reaches the muscle at a synapse known as the motor end plate or neuromuscular junction. Nerve action potentials pass efficiently and rapidly from the spinal cord to peripheral muscle because of a myelin sheath surrounding the axon that serves as an electrical insulator. The myelin sheath surrounds peripheral nerves until they reach their destination with the motor end plate. At the motor end plate, the axon loses its myelin sheath and expands into a Schwann cell–enveloped synaptic terminal. The nerve terminal of the presynaptic axon forms many terminal folds that include thousands of synaptic vesicles containing the neurotransmitter acetylcholine (ACh). The ACh-containing vesicles congregate in specialized release sites called active zones, which are

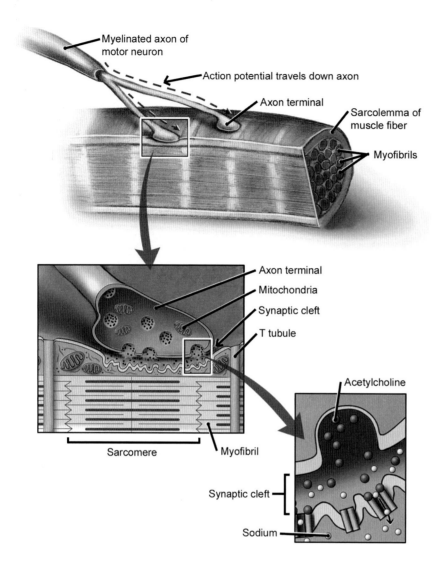

Fig 4-3. Schematic drawing of the motor end plate.

adjacent to the postsynaptic folds of the muscle membrane known as the sole plate. The sole plate is a specialized region of the muscle sarcolemma that is characterized by numerous junctional folds containing ACh receptors and chemically gated ion channels. An action potential reaching the terminal axon will stimulate an influx of calcium ions through voltage-gated calcium channels into the presynaptic cell. The increased intracellular calcium concentration mediates the fusion of synaptic vesicles with the axon membrane and the release of ACh into the neuromuscular cleft. ACh diffuses across the cleft, then binds to the ACh receptors of the postsynaptic muscle membrane that mediate depolarization of the muscle sarcolemma, thereby initiating an action potential in the muscle. This action potential rapidly spreads along the muscle fiber to trigger calcium release and subsequent excitation–contraction coupling and, thereby, muscle contraction. ACh released by the axon terminal and bound to the muscular ACh receptors is rapidly deactivated by acetylcholinesterase enzymes in the synaptic cleft bound to the postsynaptic membrane. One byproduct of this enzymatic inactivation, choline, is then reabsorbed by the

terminal axon and resynthesized to ACh for future transmitter release.

Sarcoplasmic Reticulum

Activation of skeletal muscle contraction is triggered through the release of calcium ions from a system of membranous sacs within the cell known as the sarcoplasmic reticulum (SR). Release of calcium from the SR is accomplished through rapid propagation of the muscle action potential throughout the muscle fiber via a complex system of membranes. The muscle membrane system ensures that the muscle action potential initiated at the superficially located muscle end plate rapidly reaches the depths of the fiber and is then transmitted from one cell to the next with great velocity. The SR is made up of the longitudinal tubules and the transverse tubules (T tubules). The action potential is carried the length of the fiber's surface by the longitudinal tubule and lateral sac system and to the inner fiber by T tubules. The T tubules penetrate the muscle fibers near the Z line perpendicular to the depths of the muscle fiber. Each T tubule is closely associated with two lateral sacs, which in turn are connected with the longitudinal tubules. The two lateral sacs and their related T tubule are collectively known as a triad.

The SR has a highly specialized membrane system for actively sequestering calcium and maintaining a low resting calcium concentration in the myoplasm. The maintenance of low myoplasmic calcium concentrations is accomplished by calcium adenosine triphosphatase (ATPase) pumps that transport calcium ions against a concentration gradient via cleavage of one ATP molecule. When a muscle action potential is transmitted along the surface of the sarcolemma and into the T tubule and longitudinal tubule system, the SR becomes more permeable to Ca^{2+}, and Ca^{2+} is released from the SR into the myoplasm. Most of the free calcium binds to troponin to initiate contraction. Relaxation of the muscle occurs when the low myoplasmic Ca^{2+} concentration is restored via the Ca^{2+} ATPase pumps. This process is commonly referred to as excitation–contraction coupling.

Structural Proteins of Muscle

Myosin, actin, tropomyosin, and troponin are the four major structural proteins that make up muscle **(Table 4-1)**. These proteins form the foundation of the basic contractile unit known as the sarcomere. The banding pattern seen in striated skeletal muscle comes from the repeating arrangement of two myofibrillar filaments, thick filaments and thin filaments.

Thick filaments are composed primarily of a large protein, myosin [~470,000 Daltons (Da)]. Myosin accounts for approximately 55% of the total percentage of structural protein in muscle. The myosin molecule is hexameric, being composed of two heavy chains and four light chains. Trypsin can cleave the heavy chains to yield fragments of heavy meromysin (HMM), and light meromysin, (LMM) which

account for the head and tail, respectively, of the myosin molecule **(Fig 4-4)**. The HMM can be further divided into smaller fragments by papain cleavage to yield subfragments 1 and 2 (S1 and S2, respectively). The S1 fragment of HMM is responsible for the ATPase activity of myosin, allowing actin–myosin cross-bridging during muscle contraction. The thick filament also contains C protein, M protein, and titin. The C protein is involved in cross-bridge regions of the thick filament, and the M protein contains the creatine phosphokinase enzyme. Titin is an elastic protein that is thought to provide resistance to elongation of the sarcomere and to protect against overstretch (13).

Thin filaments contain primarily actin, along with lesser amounts of tropomyosin and troponin proteins, which form an α-helical cylinder. The actin of thin filaments is anchored at the end of the sarcomere to the Z line. Thin filaments measure approximately 1.0 μm in length and are arranged in a hexagonal pattern around each thick filament **(Fig 4-5)**. Actin thin filaments also are associated with troponin and tropomyosin proteins, which serve a regulatory function during contraction and are discussed later in this section. Nebulin is a cytoskeletal protein that has been proposed to regulate the length of the thin filament during contraction and stretch.

Myofibrils demonstrate a regular, repeating arrangement of dark and light bands every 2 to 3 μm when viewed with an electron microscope. The regular arrangement of striations in skeletal muscle results from the organization of thick and thin filament proteins within the sarcomere **(Fig 4-6)**. The sarcomere extends from one Z band to another, with I bands and A bands in between. The Z band, or Z disk (from *Zwishen-Schieben*, which is German for "interim disk"), anchors thin filaments at either end of the sarcomere. The I (isotropic) band, which is made of actin, troponin, and tropomyosin, is less densely packed with proteins and, therefore, appears lighter under a polarizing microscope. The A (anisotropic) band is composed of myosin and the actin–tropomyosin complex and corresponds with the thick filaments. It is more densely packed with proteins, giving it a darker appearance when viewed with a polarizing microscope. In the center of the A band is a protein-dense band known as the H (Heller) zone that contains the center of the sarcomere, the M (Middle) line.

TABLE 4-1	Relative Proportions of Myofibrillar Proteins in Rabbit Skeletal Muscle

Protein	% of total structural protein
Myosin	55
Actin	20
Tropomyosin	7
Troponin	2
C-protein	2
M-protein	<2
α-Actinin	10
β-Actinin	2

From Carlson FD, Wilkie DR. *Muscle Physiology*. Englewood Cliffs, NJ: Prentice-Hall; 1974; with permission.

Sliding Filament Model of Contraction

The length of the thick and thin filaments remains constant during contraction, but the overall sarcomere length becomes shorter. The I band becomes shorter with contraction as the thick filaments slide past the thin filaments in a process known, appropriately, as the sliding filament model of muscle contraction. The sliding filament model was proposed by both Huxley and Simmons (14) and by Huxley (15) in 1971 and is still the guiding hypothesis for the molecular basis of muscle contraction.

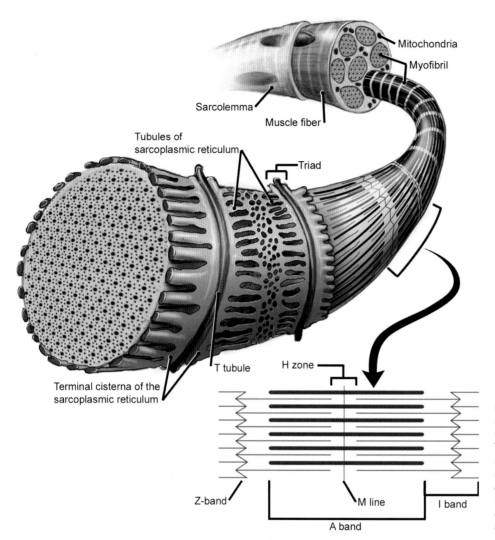

Fig 4-4. Schematic drawing of myosin molecule showing subunit structure. (From Garrett WE, Best TM. Anatomy, physiology, and mechanics of skeletal muscle. In: Simon SR, Einhorn TA, Buckwalter JA, eds. *Orthopaedic basic science.* Rosemont, IL: American Academy of Orthopaedic Surgeons; 1994: 89–126; with permission.)

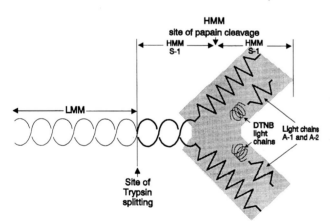

Fig 4-5. Schematic drawing of the sarcoplasmic reticulum (SR). An action potential spreads throughout the membranous SR, down the transverse tubules (T tubules), and causes calcium release from the SR.

Our current understanding of molecular contraction begins with the hydrolysis of ATP by myosin on the thick filament. This hydrolysis of ATP results in a conformational change of myosin, flexing it approximately 45°. The myosin binds to the active site on the actin thin filament, forming a cross-bridge. Once cross-bridge formation has occurred, ADP and phosphate are released from the myosin head, facilitating cross-bridge flexion during the myosin molecule conformation, pulling the thin filaments a short distance past the thick filaments. To continue the contraction, myosin must release its bond with the actin molecule. This occurs when another molecule of ATP is bound by the myosin ATPase-binding site. The ATP molecule is then cleaved, repeating the process numerous times in rapid succession to cause a single contraction. This process produces a ratcheting phenomenon that causes sarcomere shortening.

Sarcomere contraction is regulated by troponin and tropomyosin. Troponin is intimately associated with tropomyosin along the actin thin filament, and it serves as a regulatory protein for contraction **(Fig 4-7)**. Troponin has three subunits: I, T, and C. Troponin I is inhibitory and is able to block actin–myosin interaction. Troponin T enables binding of troponin and tropomyosin. Troponin C binds calcium. When myoplasmic calcium concentrations are low, the troponin–tropomyosin complex is situated on the actin

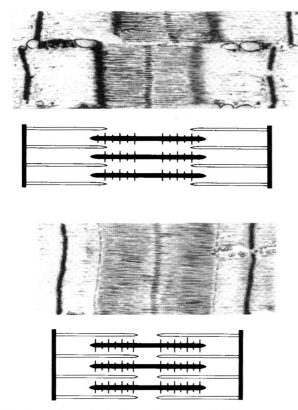

Fig 4-6. Schematic drawing of sarcomere lattice arrangement. (From Carlson FS, Wilkie DR. *Muscle Physiology.* New Jersey: Prentice Hall; 1974; with permission.)

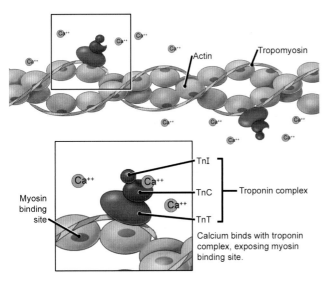

Fig 4-7. Thin filament with associated troponin–tropomyosin complex.

filament in a way that prevents actin–myosin cross-bridge formation. A rise in myoplasmic calcium concentration allows Ca^{2+} to bind with troponin C. The binding of Ca^{2+} to troponin causes a conformational change in the troponin I molecule complex that removes the troponin–

tropomyosin complex from the actin-binding sites. This change permits myosin–actin cross-bridge cycling. Even a small increase in the cellular Ca^{2+} concentration results in a troponin–tropomyosin conformational change. This ensures that many cross-bridges are formed with only small changes in intracellular Ca^{2+} concentrations. When Ca^{2+} concentrations are returned to normal resting levels, troponin I reverts to its inhibitory conformation, and the actin-binding sites are again blocked from forming cross-bridges.

Muscle Twitch and Tetanus

The molecular events during the process of muscle contraction just described can now be considered in more detail (i.e., at the level of the entire muscle). In response to a single stimulus of adequate strength, a momentary rise in tension known as a twitch is produced. A muscle twitch has three phases. The latent period is defined as the brief delay, lasting approximately 15 milliseconds, during which the muscle maintains a constant length without force production. This is the period of muscle depolarization, Ca^{2+} release from the SR, and cross-bridge formation before sarcomere shortening occurs. The contraction period is that period during which sarcomere shortening occurs because of rapid succession of myosin–actin cross-bridge cycling. The relaxation phase is defined by restoration of resting myoplasmic Ca^{2+} concentrations, release of cross-bridges, and relaxation of muscle to its original length.

If a second stimulus reaches the muscle fiber after the relaxation phase of a twitch, no increase in muscle tension occurs, and another twitch of identical tension takes place **(Fig 4-8)**. If, however, a second stimulus of adequate intensity

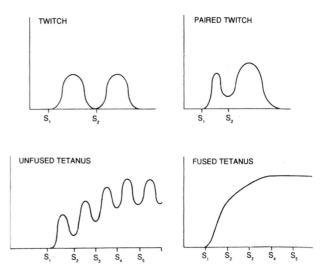

Fig 4-8. Twitch, paired twitch, unfused tetanus, and fused tetanus. As the frequency of stimulation increases, the generation of muscle force rises until the point of fused tetanus. (From DeLee JC, Drez DM, Miller MD. *DeLee & Drez's Orthopaedic Sports Medicine. Principles and Practice.* 2nd ed. Philadelphia: Elsevier Science; 2003; with permission.)

reaches the fiber before completion of the relaxation phase, an increase in tension above that of the first twitch is possible. This summation is known as an unfused tetanus. The temporal summation of twitch tension increases proportionately with the stimulation frequency. As the stimulation frequency increases, the amount of tension produced is increased proportionally until reaching a maximum level known as a fused tetanus.

The rate of muscle shortening depends on both the muscle fiber type and the weight of the load being lifted. Fibers can be Type I (red, or slow twitch) or Type II (white, or fast twitch). Type I fibers have a relatively long time period before they reach peak tension, whereas Type II fibers have a short time to peak tension. If the force that is generated by the contraction is greater than the resisting load, the muscle shortens. Another term for a shortening contraction is a concentric contraction. If the resisting load is greater than the amount of tension being produced, there will be a lengthening contraction, which is commonly referred to as eccentric contraction. The force of the muscle contraction depends not only on the frequency of motor unit stimulation but also on the absolute number of motor units that are stimulated for contraction. The quantity of motor units being stimulated with each contraction is adjustable through a method known as recruitment. The two entities, stimulation frequency and recruitment, are believed to act in concert with each other to effect an optimal combination for force production and limb movement.

■ BIOMECHANICS OF SKELETAL MUSCLE

Fiber Types and Muscle Adaptability

As mentioned, muscle fibers vary in type and can be differentiated by their histological, biochemical, and physiologic properties. Muscle fiber types can be divided into at least three separate entities based on these criteria. Each motor unit possesses fibers that are all of a similar fiber type, but some overlap of muscle fiber types is found within whole muscles. Determination of fiber type is dependent on the type of myosin ATPase activity and, therefore, contraction velocity. This protein occurs in several varieties, each with different abilities to generate tension at different velocities. Large fibers tend to produce tension at a faster rate, because they tend to express rapid myosin ATPase. Smaller fibers are inclined to produce tension more slowly, because they usually express a slower form of myosin ATPase. The rates of ATPase activity help to classify muscle fiber types into three different profiles: Type I, Type IIA, and Type IIB **(Table 4-2)**. Some overlap certainly occurs, which allows other types to be considered.

Type I fibers are slow oxidative fibers that have slower contraction and relaxation times compared to those of Type II fibers. They are very fatigue resistant because of the high concentration of mitochondria and myoglobin they contain. Type IIA fibers, or fast oxidative glycolytic fibers, are an intermediate fiber type, because they contain forms of myosin ATPase that are present in both Type I and Type IIB fibers. Therefore, their contraction velocity is faster than that of Type I fibers but slower than that of Type IIB fibers. Similarly, Type IIA fibers are more fatigue resistant than Type IIB fibers, but less so than Type I fibers. The Type IIB fibers are fast glycolytic fibers that are the least resistant to fatigue, but they have the fastest contraction velocity.

Human skeletal muscle is composed of a combination of the fiber types discussed above, with most muscles having 50% of slow-twitch fibers and 50% fast-twitch fibers. The relative percentage of Type I or Type II fibers generally is accepted to be determined genetically and, therefore, are not subject to change through training. A study by Gollnick et al. (16) in 1972 demonstrated a preponderance of one fiber type or another in trained athletes that would be

TABLE 4-2	Characteristics of Human Skeletal Muscle Fiber Types		
	Type I	**Type IIA**	**Type IIB**
Other Names	Red, slow twitch (ST) Slow oxidative (SO)	White, fast twitch (FT) Fast oxidative glycolytic (FOG)	Fast glycolytic (FG)
Speed of contraction	Slow	Fast	Fast
Strength of contraction	Low	High	High
Fatigability	Fatigue-resistant	Fatigable	Most fatigable
Aerobic capacity	High	Medium	Low
Anaerobic capacity	Low	Medium	High
Motor unit size	Small	Larger	Largest
Capillary density	High	High	Low

From Garrett WE, Best TM. Anatomy, physiology, and mechanics of skeletal muscle. In: Simon SR, Einhorn TA, Buckwalter JA, eds. *Orthopaedic basic science.* Rosemont, IL: American Academy of Orthopaedic Surgeons; 1994:89–126; with permission.

advantageous for their event. The endurance athletes who were studied had higher percentages of fatigue-resistant, Type I fibers, whereas nonendurance athletes had higher percentages of Type II fibers. Despite this knowledge, athletic ability is certainly dependent on more than just fiber type predominance, so muscle biopsy for selecting sport-specific athletes generally is not accepted.

Although muscle fiber type usually is fixed under normal physiologic conditions, various forms of overload stimulation can cause adaptation of muscle fibers, especially within the Type II fibers (17). For example, prolonged endurance training seems to increase the percentage of Type IIA fibers at the expense of Type IIB fibers, making the muscle more fatigue resistant. Conversely, strength training may increase the percentage of Type IIB fibers.

Length–Tension Relationship

Experiments studying the relationship between muscle length and the tension produced at a fixed length during passive stretch and active isometric contraction have demonstrated that force generation depends on the length of the muscle **(Fig 4-9)**. The passive curve was determined by measuring the tension in muscle at a series of different lengths. The increasing tension with greater passive stretch is a result of the connective tissue and fascial components surrounding muscle fibers and, possibly, to some extent, even the myofibrillar proteins. In fact, passive stretch tensions can exceed

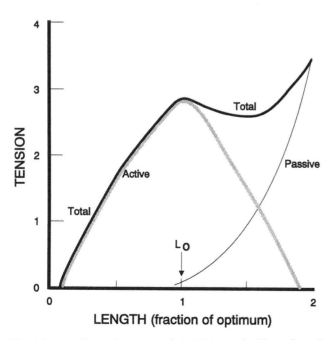

Fig 4-9. Length–tension curve of skeletal muscle. (From Garrett WE, Best TM. Anatomy, physiology, and mechanics of skeletal muscle. In: Simon SR, Einhorn TA, Buckwalter JA, eds. *Orthopaedic basic science.* Rosemont, IL: American Academy of Orthopaedic Surgeons; 1994:89–126; with permission.)

maximal isometric contraction tensions at the limits of mechanical failure of muscle. The active tension curve was determined by measuring the tension of isometric tetanic contractions at various fixed lengths. This curve demonstrates that an isometric contraction generates maximal force at a certain length (L_o) at which the maximal number of mechanical couplings of thick and thin filaments occurs. The linear decrease in force production at greater lengths is proportional to the lesser number of actin–myosin cross-bridges that can be formed as the overlap of thick and thin filaments decreases with the increased sarcomere length. At muscle lengths shorter than L_o, tension development is not maximal because of excessive overlap of thick and thin filaments, resulting in disordered cytoskeletal geometry.

Force–Velocity Relationship

Shortening velocities are dependent on several independent factors. As discussed earlier, shortening velocity is proportional to fiber length. Shortening velocity also is dependent on the load being placed on the muscle. Classic studies of muscle physiology have shown that the velocity of muscle shortening is related to the load being moved by the muscle. The rate of myosin ATPase induced cross-bridge flexion between thick and thin filaments is reduced as the stress placed on the cross-bridges increases. Heavier loads increase the amount of time that is required for cross-bridge cycling, thereby reducing the shortening velocity of the muscle. As the load increases, the velocity of shortening approaches zero, and the isometric force being generated approaches a maximum. Conversely, an unloaded muscle can generate maximum shortening velocity. Again, the maximum shortening velocity of any given muscle is dependent on the fiber type and myosin ATPase that are unique to that muscle.

■ TENDON

Tendon Structure and Architecture

Tendon is juxtaposed between muscle and bone and is responsible for transmitting muscular forces to the skeletal system during limb locomotion. It is a dense, regularly arranged connective tissue that is well suited for resisting tensile loads with minimal elongation during muscle contraction. Approximately 85% of a tendon's dry weight is composed of Type I collagen, which serves to provide the tendon with most of its tensile strength. Tendon gets most of its elasticity from the protein elastin, which accounts for less than 5% of a tendon's total mass. Surrounding the collagen fibers and elastin proteins is an extracellular matrix, or ground substance, that is rich in proteoglycans, glycosaminoglycans (GAGs), and a variety of other lipids and proteins. The extracellular matrix is important, both because it provides a structural support for the collagen framework and

Tendon Hierarchy

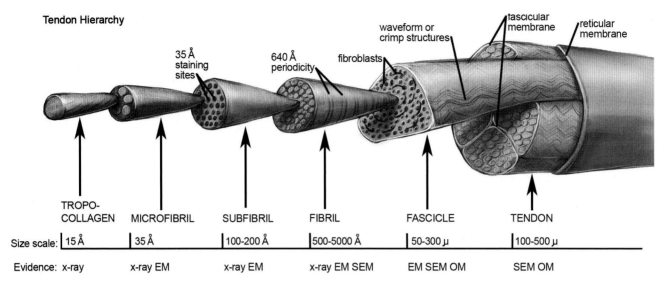

Fig 4-10. Schematic drawing of tendon organization.

because its viscoelastic properties help to reduce the frictional and shear stresses that are placed on the tendon. Fibroblasts can be found within the tendon ground substance and also are important, because they are capable of producing new collagen and ground substance materials, which are essential for maintenance and repair of the tendon.

The hierarchical arrangement of collagen fibers is similar to that of muscles described earlier in this chapter. Tendons are composed of densely organized collagen at various levels of complexity **(Fig 4-10)**. Tropocollagen is the basic building block of the Type I collagen found in tendon. The triple-helix polypeptide chain of tropocollagen is further organized into microfibrils, fibrils, fascicles, tertiary bundles, and

finally, tendon itself. The entire tendon is sheathed in its epitenon that carries the nerve's rich neurovascular supply. A mesh of loose areolar connective tissue known as the paratenon often surrounds the epitenon, and together, they are known as the peritendon **(Fig 4-11)**. Occasionally, tendons that traverse areas of increased frictional stress will possess a double-layer covering that is lined by synovial cells instead of the paratenon. This synovial-lined covering is known as a tenosynovium. The flexor tendons in the forearm are examples of tendons possessing a tenosynovium. The endotenon lining of the tendon bundles is continuous with the perimysium of muscle at the myotendinous junction, and it adjoins the periosteum at the OTJ. Four zones in the

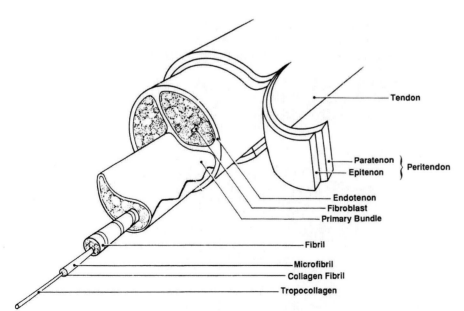

Fig 4-11. Schematic drawing of tendon structure. (From DeLee JC, Drez DM, Miller MD. *DeLee & Drez's Orthopaedic Sports Medicine. Principles and Practice.* 2nd ed. Philadelphia: Elsevier Science; 2003; with permission.)

direct insertion of tendon at the OTJ are recognizable microscopically (2):

1 Tendon (fibers of Sharpey)
2 Fibrocartilage
3 Mineralized fibrocartilage
4 Bone

These four distinct zones are thought to reduce tendon loads by distributing the forces over a greater surface area of bone.

Collagen

The fibroblast cells in the tendon ground substance produce collagen, but first, they produce a large intracellular collagen precursor, procollagen. Once the procollagen has been secreted into the extracellular matrix, it can be cleaved by procollagen peptidases to form the triple-helix molecule known as tropocollagen. The tropocollagen molecules are then aligned in an orderly fashion in the extracellular environment and undergo polymerization with each other to form collagen fibrils.

The architecture of collagen has been studied extensively (18–22) and is responsible for the physical properties and tensile strength of tendon. When viewed with electron microscopy, collagen fibrils exhibit a regularly repeating, band-like pattern every 64 to 68 nm. This banding pattern is a result of an organized, repetitive packing of individual triple-helix collagen molecules into an overlapping arrangement that results in a rigid, rodlike fibril. Type I collagen accounts for the vast majority of human tendon mass. The collagen molecule spans approximately 280 nm and is 1.5 nm in thickness (20). Individual collagen molecules are composed of three primary amino acids: glycine, which accounts for every third amino acid in the chain (~33%); proline (15%); and hydroxyproline (15%) (19). Three α-peptide chains make up the triple-helix structure of the Type I collagen molecule: two α_1 chains, and a single α_2 chain. The polymerization of these three chains into a triple-helix arrangement gives the molecule greater rigidity than either of the two types of collagen α-chains alone. The collagen fibrils are arranged into fibers that run parallel to the long axis of the tendon, imparting excellent tensile strength to the tissue.

Elastin

As its name implies, elastin provides tendons with elasticity, stretch, and recoil. When viewed with light microscopy, tendon has a crimped appearance **(Fig 4-12)** because of the presence of elastin. The small amount of elastin in tendons allows them to undergo a small, protective amount of deformation and stretch in response to increasing loads while minimizing the amount of contractile energy loss (23).

Ground Substance

Tendon acquires much of its viscoelastic properties from the extracellular matrix, or ground substance, surrounding the

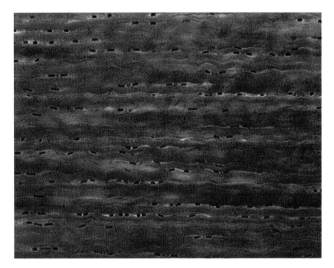

Fig 4-12. Light micrograph of tendon. Note the crimped appearance.

collagen fibers. Human tendons contain limited amounts of ground substance by total dry weight (~1%). The ground substance is rich with (GAGs) linked to proteoglycans at the molecular level. These GAGs are long, unbranched, polysaccharide chains of repeating disaccharide units that are covalently linked to the proteoglycan core as side chains. Currently, researchers hypothesize that these molecules are critical for stabilizing the collagen fiber arrangement in tendons—in effect, acting as an extracellular cytoskeleton. The proteoglycans have a high affinity for water, imparting a gellike consistency to the extracellular matrix. The high viscosity that this provides is important for reducing shear and compressive forces in areas of mechanical stress.

■ BIOMECHANICS OF TENDON

Tendon possesses unique linear and viscoelastic properties, allowing it to transmit high muscular forces to the skeleton with minimal elongation during muscle contraction. Subjecting tendons to various tensile loads and examining tendon response can help to define tendon biomechanical properties.

A classic load–elongation curve **(Fig 4-13)** results from lengthening a tendon at a constant rate under tensile stress (22). Initially, little force is required to elongate the tendon as the wavy collagen pattern becomes straight because of fiber reorientation in the direction of stress. The first concave portion of the curve, which is known as the "toe" region, represents this phenomenon. The second portion of the curve is linear as the tendon becomes stiffer and elongates at the molecular and fibrillar levels. Progressive failure of collagen begins in the third region, until complete failure and tendon rupture occur in an unpredictable, sudden episode. The vast majority of physiologic tensile loads are well below the maximal force that is required to rupture

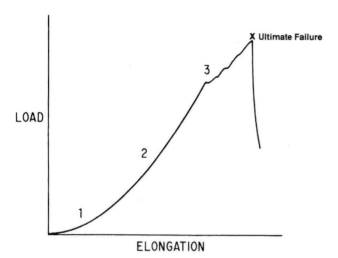

Fig 4-13. Load–elongation curve of tendon. (From DeLee JC, Drez DM, Miller MD. *DeLee & Drez's Orthopaedic Sports Medicine. Principles and Practice.* 2nd ed. Philadelphia: Elsevier Science; 2003; with permission.)

tendon, but athletes occasionally sustain higher loads and may experience tendon rupture.

Tendon also is viscoelastic, and it exhibits different behaviors at different rates of tensile loading (22). Tendons exhibit properties known as load relaxation and creep **(Fig 4-14)**. Load relaxation occurs when a submaximal load is held at a fixed length in the "toe" region of the load–elongation curve. Tensile stress will diminish rapidly at first, then stabilizes with time. Tendon creep occurs when load is held constant and tendon length is variable. Tendon elongation will

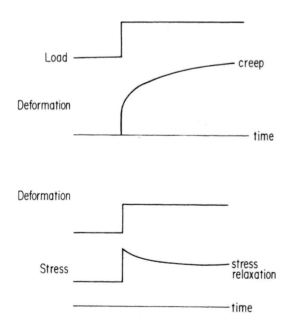

Fig 4-14. Biomechanical properties of tendon. (From DeLee JC, Drez DM, Miller MD. *DeLee & Drez's Orthopaedic Sports Medicine. Principles and Practice.* 2nd ed. Philadelphia: Elsevier Science; 2003; with permission.)

increase rapidly before eventually stabilizing over time. These concepts also are important clinically. For example, a patient with Achilles tendinitis will develop a plantar flexion contracture requiring casting in a neutral position to regain range of motion through the creep model.

■ MYOTENDINOUS JUNCTION

The myotendinous junction is the interface between muscle and tendon, and it allows the force generated by muscle contraction to be exerted on the skeleton to enact limb locomotion. To maximize the junctional surface area, a region of highly folded membranes in a fingerlike arrangement exists **(Fig 4-15)**. This increases the surface area between the muscle and tendon by 10- to 20-fold, which considerably reduces the applied force per surface unit area during contraction. The increased surface area displaces stress, but in addition, the longitudinal arrangement of the membrane invaginations reorients stresses in a parallel orientation to the longitudinal axis of the muscle. This orientation creates a shearing stress alignment rather than a tensile load alignment. Despite the well-developed molecular structure, the myotendinous junction remains the weak link in the muscle–tendon unit, making it more susceptible to injury and rupture compared to the muscle belly, tendon, or OTJ.

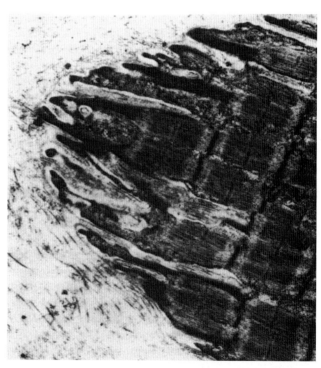

Fig 4-15. Electron micrograph of a myotendinous junction sectioned longitudinally. Myofilaments distal to the terminal Z disk end in a series of filaments that are bounded by a folded plasmalemma. (From Tidball JG. Myotendinous junction: morphological changes and mechanical failure associated with muscle cell atrophy. *Exp Mol Pathol.* 1984;40:1–12.)

■ MYOTENDINOUS INJURY AND REPAIR

The majority of skeletal muscle injuries that occur in sports are the result of indirect strain or direct blunt force trauma. Other forms of muscular injury, such as lacerations, ischemia, and infections, are not commonly seen in athletics. The amount of research in the area of muscle injury and repair is growing, but we do not yet fully understand the precise mechanisms behind the molecular changes that occur during muscle injury or the exact biochemical regulation of the healing response. It appears that the postinjury release of soluble proinflammatory cytokines, growth factors, and certain free radicals from injured muscle is a central component to muscle tissue damage and repair.

Indirect muscle strain injuries usually occur at the myotendinous junction during a stereotypical eccentric contraction. Such injuries are common in athletics during the active contraction with muscle lengthening that occurs during impact absorption (24). Certain muscles that perform primarily eccentric contractions during sports are more likely to sustain this type of injury. The hamstrings are particularly vulnerable during bursts of rapid acceleration, as are found in football, sprinting, and soccer. The hamstrings function to decelerate the leg extension phase during running, combining an activated lengthening muscle contraction that predisposes these athletes to muscle strain injury. Despite the frequency of this problem in athletics, research in this area has been limited until lately. Most research models of muscle injury are patterned after this muscle activation and stretch mechanism.

Delayed muscle soreness (DMS) is a common but separate entity from pain resulting from indirect muscle strain. Onset of DMS usually occurs at least 24 hours after exercise, reaching a maximum at 48 to 72 hours. In contrast, acute muscle strain causes pain immediately. Eccentric exercises, especially unfamiliar repetitive ones, are more likely to predispose patients to DMS. Patients often will complain of painful, stiff, and swollen muscles. A significant loss of maximal force generation often persists for up to 1 week after the original injury and for several days after the muscles are no longer painful. Histological evidence of muscle disruption may help to explain the source of pain and the reversible loss of force generation. The exact cause of DMS pain is not known, but it appears to be related to mechanical tissue damage, not lactic acid buildup (25).

Direct trauma to muscles can occur at any point in the muscle. The quadriceps is the most common site of athletic muscle contusion, especially in tackle football. With sufficient force, disruption of the muscle tissue and architecture can occur, often resulting in a hematoma. Quadriceps contusions can result in significant morbidity to athletes because of swelling and pain (26,27). Not uncommonly, calcification or ossification can occur at the site of previously contused muscle. Myositis ossificans, as it is known, is heterotopic bone formation in previously damaged muscle. One prospective study found that approximately 20% of patients with quadriceps hematoma develop myositis ossificans (28). The bone formations of myositis ossificans often will regress or even disappear over time, but sometimes, it will enlarge before eventually stabilizing.

Shortly after a muscle injury, a series of events occur that produce chemoattractant signals to invading neutrophils and macrophages. In muscle strain injuries, a disruption occurs in normal fiber architecture and calcium homeostasis, leading to functional deficits as well as chemotactic substances being released from the tissue. As quickly as 1 hour after an inciting injury, neutrophils begin migrating to the tissue, and their presence at elevated levels can last for as long as 5 days (29). Neutrophil presence following injury is important for removal of necrotic tissue and debris through phagocytosis (30); however, the neutrophils also release enzymes, such as myeloperoxidase, that promote free radical formation in the tissues during times of neutrophil invasion. Highly reactive free radicals, such as superoxide, may directly cause damage to the surrounding tissues and cell membranes, actually promoting further damage and not repair. In fact, recent research has demonstrated that superoxide produced by activated neutrophils is capable of sarcolemma lysis in vitro, and the addition of superoxide dismutase (SOD) inhibits this muscle cell membrane lysis (31). Inflammatory cytokines and trophic substances also may be produced by local endothelial tissue, macrophages, myoblasts, damaged myofibrils, and activated fibroblasts. The expression and importance of these cytokines and substances in vivo, as well as the role they play in skeletal muscle after muscle injury, remain unknown. Ongoing research will play a key role in developing new and improved strategies for the prevention and treatment of these common problems.

■ REFERENCES

1. Ishikawa H. Fine structure of skeletal muscle. *Cell Muscle Motil.* 1983;4:1–84.
2. Cooper RR, Misol S. Tendon and ligament insertion. *J Bone Joint Surg Am.* 1970;52:1–19.
3. Bischoff R. The satellite cell and muscle regeneration. In: Engel AE, Franzini-Armstrong C, eds. *Myology: basic and clinical.* 2nd ed. New York: McGraw-Hill; 1994:97–118.
4. Schultz E. Satellite cell behavior during skeletal muscle growth and regeneration. *Med Sci Sports Exer.* 1989;21:S181–S186.
5. Eisenberg BR. Quantitative ultrastructure of mammalian skeletal muscle. In: Peachey LD, Adrian RH, eds. *Handbook of physiology: Section 10, Skeletal muscle.* Baltimore, MD: Williams & Wilkins; 1983:73–112.
6. Buchtal F, Schmalbruch H. Motor unit of mammalian muscle. *Physiol Rev.* 1980;60:90–142.
7. Burke RE, Edgerton VE. Motor unit properties and selective involvement in movement. *Exerc Sport Sci Rev.* 1975;3:31–81.
8. Feinstein B, Lindegard B, Nyman E, et al. Morphologic studies of motor units in normal human muscles. *Acta Anat.* 1955;23:127–142.
9. Eisen A, Karpati G, Carpenter S, et al. The motor unit profile of the rat soleus in experimental myopathy and reinnervation. *Neurology.* 1974;24:878–884.

10. Garnett RA, O'Donovan MJ, Stephens JA, et al. Motor unit organization of human medial gastrocnemius. *J Physiol (Lond).* 1978;287:33–43.
11. Kugelberg E. Histochemical composition, contraction speed and fatigability of rat soleus motor units. *J Neurol Sci.* 1973;20: 177–198.
12. Buchtal F, Schmalbruch H. Motor unit of mammalian muscle. *Physiol Rev.* 1980;60:90–142.
13. Wang K. Titin/connectin and nebulin: giant protein rulers of muscle structure and function. *Adv Biophys.* 1996;33:123–134.
14. Huxley AF, Simmons RM. Proposed mechanism of force generation in striated muscle. *Nature.* 1971;233:533–538.
15. Huxley HE. The structural basis of muscular contraction. *Proc R Soc Biol (Lond).* 1971;178:131–149.
16. Gollnick PD, Armstrong RB, Saubert CW IV, et al. Enzyme activity and fiber composition in skeletal muscle of untrained and trained men. *J Appl Physiol.* 1972;33:312–319.
17. Burke RE, Edgerton VE. Motor unit properties and selective involvement in movement. *Exerc Sports Sci Rev.* 1975;3:31–81.
18. Ramachandran GN. Molecular structure of collagen. *Int Rev Connect Tissue Res.* 1963;1:127–182.
19. Ramachandran GN, Kartha G. Structure of collagen. *Nature (Lond).* 1954;174:269–270.
20. Rich A, Crick FHC. The structure of collagen. *Nature.* 1955; 176:915–916.
21. Rich A, Crick FHC. The molecular structure of collagen. *J Mol Biol.* 1961;3:483–506.
22. Abrahams M. Mechanical behavior of tendon in vitro: a preliminary report. *Med Biol Eng.* 1967;5:433–443.
23. Kannus P. Structure of the tendon connective tissue. *Scand J Med Sci Sports.* 2000;10:312–320.
24. Zarins B, Ciullo JV. Acute muscle and tendon injuries in athletes. *Clin Sports Med.* 1983;2:167–182.
25. Schwane JA, Watrous BG, Johnson SR, et al. Is lactic acid related to delayed-onset muscle soreness? *Physician Sport Med.* 1983; 11:124–131.
26. Jackson DW, Feagin JA. Quadriceps contusions in young athletes. *J Bone Joint Surg Am.* 1973;55:95–101.
27. Ryan JB, Wheeler JH, Hopkinson WJ, et al. Quadriceps contusions: West Point update. *Am J Sports Med.* 1991;19: 299–304.
28. Rothwell AG. Quadriceps hematoma: a prospective clinical study. *Clin Orthop.* 1982;171:97–103.
29. Fielding RA, Manfredi TJ, Ding W, et al. Acute phase response in exercise. III. Neutrophil and IL-1β accumulation in skeletal muscle. *Am J Physiol Regul Integr Comp Physiol.* 1993;265: R166–R172.
30. Lowe DA, Warren GL, Ingalls CP, et al. Muscle function and protein metabolism after initiation of eccentric contraction-induced injury. *J Appl Physiol.* 1995;79:1260–1270.
31. Nguyen HX, Tidball JG. Interactions between neutrophils and macrophages promote macrophage killing of muscle cells in vitro. *J Physiol.* 2003;547:125–132.

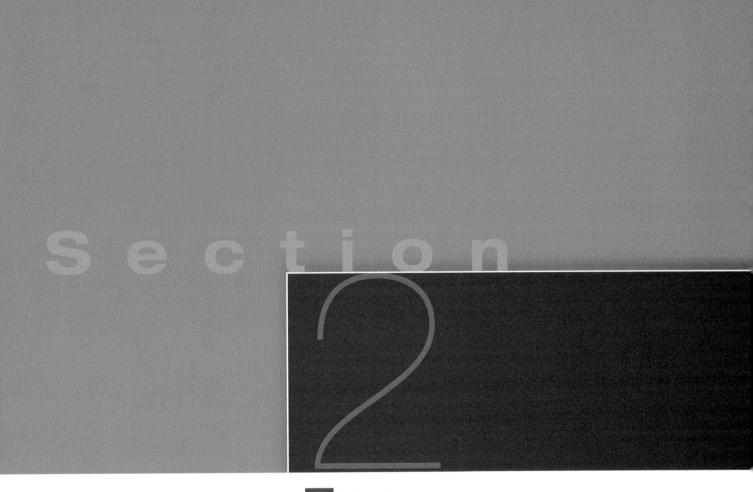

Section

2

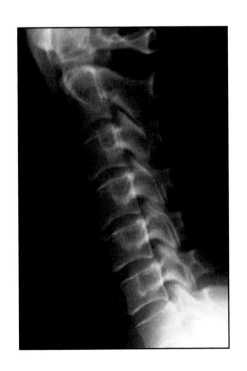

5

CERVICAL SPINE INJURIES IN THE ATHLETE

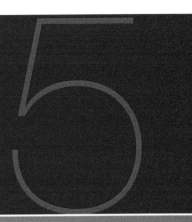

RAHUL BANERJEE, MD, MICHAEL P. BRADLEY, MD, MARK A. PALUMBO, MD, PAUL D. FADALE, MD

KEY POINTS

- Football, ice hockey, rugby, skiing, snowboarding, and equestrian athletes have been identified as being at an increased risk of spinal cord injury. Athletic injuries are the fourth most common cause of spinal cord injury. The risk is small, but such an injury can be devastating to a young player's career and life.
- Equipment and rule changes, as well as education of coaches, have helped to reduce the risk of injury.
- If the space available for the spinal cord is reduced because of a narrow canal, an athlete is at greater risk. Cord compression can be anticipated when the diameter of the midsagittal cervical spinal canal is 10 mm or less.
- Cervical spine injuries can be classified as either catastrophic or noncatastrophic.
- Catastrophic injuries can be defined as a structural distortion of the cervical spinal column associated with actual or potential damage to the spinal cord. Such injuries include unstable fractures and dislocations, transient quadriplegia, and acute central disc herniation.
- The vast majority of injuries are noncatastrophic. These injuries include neuropraxia of the cervical root or brachial plexus (known as a "stinger" or "burner"), paracentral intervertebral disc herniation, stable fractures, spinal ligament injury, and intervertebral disc injury.
- In football and hockey, the injury vector most frequently associated with cervical spinal cord injury is compression (axial loading).
- During competition, sports medicine staff should make efforts to monitor play. A visual image of the traumatic event can be useful in attempting to determine both the type and the severity of injury.
- The initial evaluation follows the ABCDE sequence of trauma care: A, airway maintenance with cervical spine protection; B, breathing and ventilation; C, circulation; D, disability (i.e., neurological status); and E, exposure of the athlete.
- Regardless of the etiology, the primary objective when respiratory compromise exists is to rapidly identify hypoxia and then intervene by providing proper ventilation for the injured player. This must be accomplished without causing any further injury to the spinal and neurological structures.
- Protective equipment should be removed before transport only in select cases.
- Unless an emergency exists that requires removal of the helmet and/or shoulder pads, initial screening radiographs can be obtained with the protective equipment in place. Lateral computed tomography (CT) scout films have been used effectively in this case.

Cervical spine injuries in the athlete continue to present a small but inherent risk and may devastate a young player's career and life. The injured athlete must be handled cautiously until the extent of skeletal and neurological injury can be defined. Athletic injuries are the fourth most common cause of spinal cord injury (behind motor vehicle accidents, violence, and falls) and account for approximately 7.5% of the total injuries since 1990 (1). Sports-related spinal cord injuries occur at a much younger age (mean age, 24 years) compared with other causes of this injury (2). Furthermore, sports injuries are the second most common cause of spinal cord injury under the age of 30 years (3). Several sports, including football, ice hockey, rugby (4,5), skiing (6,7), snowboarding (6,7), and equestrian (8), have been identified as carrying an increased risk for athletes to sustain spinal cord injury. American football and ice hockey, which are the most popular collision sports around the country, account for most these cervical spine injuries. In addition, these sports have been, perhaps, most influenced by changes in injury and prevention secondary to their popularity and high visibility worldwide.

Defining the spectrum of cervical spine injuries can range from temporary, fully recoverable injuries to permanent, catastrophic injuries. **A catastrophic cervical spine injury can be defined as a structural distortion of the cervical spinal column associated with actual or potential damage to the spinal cord**. As mentioned, these catastrophic injuries not only can instantly change an athlete's life but also leave them with irreversible and devastating neurological consequences. Many advances in protective equipment, including helmet design and modifications in rules of play, have helped to decrease the rate of these injuries in collision sports. Recognizing and quantifying injury data on a national level have helped to drive several changes in these collision sports; however, this clinical problem challenges the sports medicine physician during early, on-field decision making. Furthermore, because of the overall low incidence of catastrophic cervical spine injuries, few physicians develop the extensive experience and essential skills that are necessary for the emergency care of cervical spine injuries. Perhaps the single most important primary decision deals with handling of the cervical spinal column on the field and during transport. Many authors now agree that improper handling of the spine during the early stabilization period can worsen spinal cord dysfunction. An athlete's cardiac and respiratory status can be significantly compromised with improper management of the cervical spine. Furthermore, the initial management of a collision sport athlete versus that of a typical trauma victim with an injured cervical spine is very different. Specifically, the protective helmet and shoulder pads worn by the player complicate the medical evaluation and immobilization process during initial management; however, the consensus currently is to leave helmets and shoulder pads in place unless specific circumstances exist. Many clinical scenarios will be reviewed at the end of this chapter.

In this chapter, we will review the epidemiology, functional anatomy, and diagnostic considerations that are relevant to cervical spine trauma in the athlete. We will consider specific injury patterns and clinical syndromes. Although a number of different sports have been associated with spine injuries, we will focus primarily on the collision sports of American football and ice hockey. The unique aspects of the protective gear (i.e., helmet and shoulder pads) in these sports will be described. We also will provide the reader with a concise protocol for on-field diagnosis and management of the athlete with an injured spine. Finally, we will review initial management of the spine-injured athlete on transfer to the emergency room.

■ EPIDEMIOLOGY

Equipment modifications, rule changes, and educational efforts directed at athletes, coaches, and parents have helped to decrease the incidence of cervical spine injuries. The potential for catastrophic injuries in collision sport athletes, however, continues to exist.

American Football

Roughly 1.8 million athletes per year participate at various levels in the collision sport of football. Approximately 1.5 million participate at the junior/senior high school level. Additionally, approximately 75,000 play in college, and approximately 2,000 are in professional football (9). Although spinal cord injury is uncommon in this sport, a significant burden of cervical trauma exists. Despite the fact that football has a lower rate of catastrophic cervical spine injuries (per 100,000 players) compared with ice hockey or gymnastics, the large number of participants has resulted in football being associated with the largest overall number of catastrophic cervical spine injuries in the United States (9,10).

In football, specific patterns of injury to the cervical spine have evolved over time. From 1959 to 1963, Schneider (11) documented 56 cases (1.36 per 100,000 participants) of cervical fracture/dislocation, of which 30 cases (0.73 per 100,000) were associated with permanent quadriplegia. From 1971 to 1975, the National Football Head and Neck Injury Registry compiled 259 cases (4.14 per 100,000) cervical fracture/dislocations and 99 cases (1.58 per 100,000) of quadriplegia (12). This disturbingly high rate of cervical spine injury was thought to be influenced by the introduction of modern football helmets. Techniques that incorporated the helmet top as the initial point of contact during tackling had been implemented, and it became apparent that using this initial point of contact for blocking or tackling placed the cervical spine at increased risk of injury.

This important realization helped to shape major rule modifications in American football. Head-first contact was banned by the National Collegiate Athletic Association (NCAA) Football Rules Committee and high school football governing bodies early in 1976. Penalties for "spearing" behavior were adapted by the National Federation of High Schools (9,13,14). These important rule changes forced players and coaches to adhere to techniques in tackling that helped to decrease the incidence of spinal cord injury in football for close to a decade. From 1976 to 1987, the rate of cervical injuries decreased by 70%, from 7.72 per 100,000 to 2.31 per 100,000, at the high school level (13). Additionally, traumatic quadriplegia decreased by approximately 82% over the same time period, from an annual rate of 2.24 per 100,000 to 0.38 per 100,000 in high school football and from 10.66 per 100,000 to 0 per 100,000 in college football (9). The yearly incidence of permanent cervical quadriplegia from 1975 to 1995 is shown in **Figure 5-1**.

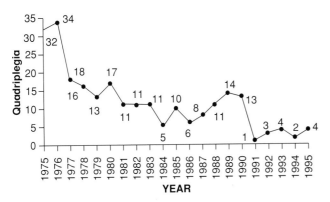

Fig 5-1. Annual incidence of permanent quadriplegia for all levels of participation in American football, 1975–1995. (From Torg JS, Vegso JJ, O'Neill MJ, et al. The epidemiologic, pathologic, biomechanical, and cinematographic analysis of football-induced cervical spine trauma. *Am J Sports Med.* 1990;18:50–57; with permission.)

Most recent data indicate a continued plateau in the incidence of traumatic quadriplegia from approximately 1991 to present. In 2002, the incidence of this injury was 0.33 per 100,000 in high school football and 1.33 per 100,000 in college football (9).

The incidence of catastrophic spine injuries in American football from 1977 to 2001 was reviewed by Cantu and Mueller (10). In their review of this 25-year period, the authors reported 223 football players sustained a catastrophic cervical spine injury with either no or incomplete recovery. In summary, 183 injuries occurred in high school athletes, 29 in college athletes, 7 in professional athletes, and 4 injuries in recreational players. The incidence rates, therefore, over the past 25 years are 0.52 in high school, 1.55 in college, and 14 in professional football. Interestingly, more defensive players were affected (71% versus 29%), and most of these injuries resulted from tackling (69%). Fracture/dislocations accounted for almost 80% of these catastrophic injuries.

Ice Hockey

Ice hockey continues to be increasingly popular throughout the United States and Canada. In contrast to American football, hockey experienced a marked increase in the occurrence of cervical spine injuries since 1980. The Canadian surveys performed by Tator et al. (15) from 1966 to 1993 reported a total of 241 spinal fracture and dislocations related to hockey. Almost 90% of these injuries were neck related and occurred between C1 and the cervicothoracic junction. An alarmingly increased rate had been documented from 1982 to 1993, with an average of 16.8 fractures/dislocations per year. Of the 207 athletes in the Canadian registry with adequate documentation of neurological status, 108 (52.2%) sustained a permanent spinal cord injury, and in 52 (25.1%), the cord lesion was complete. Eight players died as a result of complications of their spinal cord injury.

The annual incidence of spinal cord damage with paralysis is *at least* threefold greater in Canadian hockey than in American football (9,15). We have noted before that overall total catastrophic neck injuries are reportedly higher in football, but this is attributed to increased participation. Hockey seems to pose a much higher rate and total number of permanent paralysis and death because of spinal injury.

Checking an opponent from behind ("boarding") has been identified as an important causative factor of cervical spine trauma in hockey. This playing tactic typically produces a head-first collision of the checked player with the boards (15,16). In an effort to prevent these injuries, rule changes have been adopted that prohibit both checking from behind and checking of an opponent no longer controlling the puck. Data from the Canadian registry suggest that fewer cases of major spinal column trauma and complete quadriplegia have been caused by illegal playing techniques since the institution of these rule changes (15). Furthermore, educational programs, such as the Safety Toward Other Players (STOP) program, have helped to decrease injury by providing a visual reminder (in the shape of a Stop sign) on the back of players' jerseys to prevent checking from behind (17) **(Fig 5-2)**.

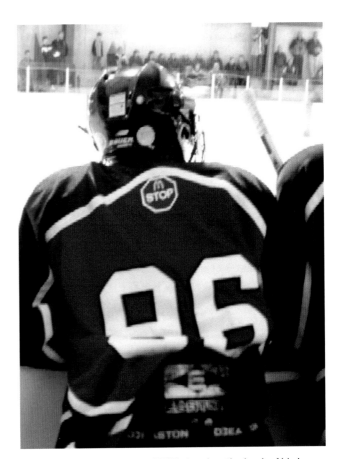

Fig 5-2. Player wearing the STOP signal on the back of his jersey.

■ CLINICAL ANATOMY

Understanding the structure of the cervical spine and the pathoanatomy of characteristic patterns of injury is essential for initial, effective management. Simply stated, the cervical spine supports the head and protects the neural elements; but motion about the cervical spine can be quite complex. Many agree that distinct regional differences exist between the upper cervical spine and the lower cervical spine. In this section, we will briefly explore some of these important characteristics.

The occiput and the first two vertebrae make up the **upper cervical spine (Fig 5-3)**. The atlas (C1) is a bony ring that articulates with the occipital condyles. The major function of the atlanto-occipital joint is motion in the sagittal plane. In fact, 40% of all cervical flexion and extension occurs above the axis (C2). In contrast, only 5° to 10° of lateral bending occurs at the atlanto-occipital joint. The axis (C2) has a true vertebral body, from which the odontoid process, or dens, projects. The major stabilizing force at this joint is the transverse atlantal ligament (TAL). The ligament crosses posterior to the dens and attaches to C1 on both sides; this prevents anterior translation of the atlas on the axis. This specialized osseoligamentous anatomy allows C1 to rotate on C2 in a highly unconstrained manner, providing 60% of all cervical rotation (18).

The **lower cervical spine** consists of the C3 through C7 vertebrae. These joints account for the remaining arc of neck motion, including flexion, extension, lateral bending, and rotation. Two contiguous vertebrae and supporting soft tissues make up a motion segment, and these motion segments can be separated into an anterior and a posterior column **(Fig 5-4)**. Stability of a cervical motion segment is derived

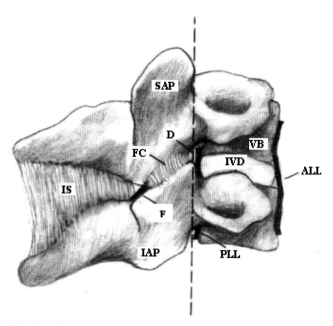

Fig 5-4. Anatomy of the lower cervical spine. The elements of the anterior column include the posterior longitudinal ligament and all structures ventral to it. The posterior column consists of those structures dorsal to the posterior longitudinal ligament. ALL, anterior longitudinal ligament; D, division between anterior and posterior column; F, facet articulation; FC, facet joint capsule; IAP, inferior articular process; IS, interspinous ligament; IVD, intervertebral disc; PLL, posterior longitudinal ligament; SAP, superior articular process; VB, vertebral body.

mainly from the anterior column elements. The vertebral bodies and intervertebral discs provide the majority of resistance to compression. In contrast, it is the surrounding paraspinal musculature and ligaments that resist shear forces.

Of course, the coronal orientation of the articular processes of the facet joints in the cervical spine provides additional resistance to anterior translation. Distraction and tensile forces are resisted by the annulus fibrosus and longitudinal ligaments. Secondary support structures include the supraspinous and interspinous ligaments, the ligamentum flavum, and the facet capsules (18).

The **spinal cord** lies within, and is protected by, the upper and lower spinal columns. From the foramen magnum to the cervicothoracic junction, the osseoligamentous structures of the cervical spine provide a protective space described as the **cervical spinal canal**. This spinal canal occupies a funnel shape from cephalad to caudal (19) **(Fig 5-5)**. In fact, the cord occupies less than half the canal's cross-sectional area at the level of the atlas, but this space reduces significantly in the lower cervical spine. Almost 75% of the cross-sectional area of the canal is occupied by the larger spinal cord between C4 and C7 (19).

The dimensions of the lower cervical spine remain relatively consistent among most patients (20), but some important, distinct differences exist. For instance, the diameter of the midsagittal cord averages between 8 and 9 mm; however, a range of 14 to 23 mm exists for the vertebral canal at the

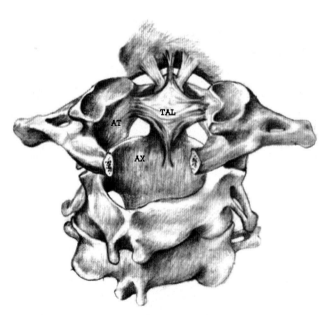

Fig 5-3. Anatomy of the atlantoaxial complex. The transverse atlantal ligament (*TAL*) stabilizes the median atlantodens articulation. The dens acts as a pivot about which the atlas rotates. AT, atlas; AX, axis.

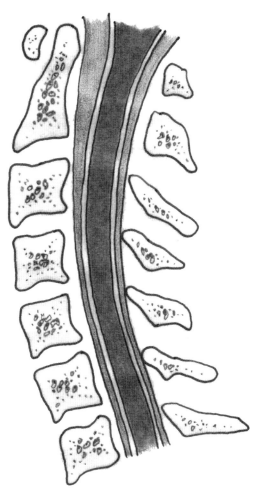

Fig 5-5. The diameter of the spinal canal progressively narrows in a cranial-to-caudal direction, with the space available for the spinal cord being at a minimum between C4 and C7.

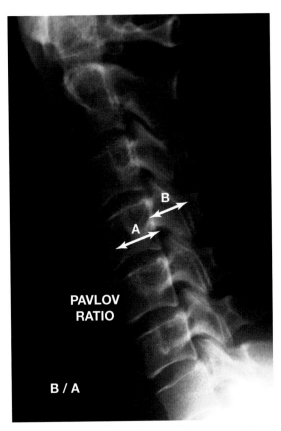

Fig 5-6. At each cervical level, the sagittal diameter of the spinal canal is measured from the middle of the posterior vertebral body cortex to the nearest point on the spinolaminar line. The Pavlov ratio is calculated by dividing the anteroposterior width of the vertebral body into the diameter of the spinal canal. Cervical stenosis is indicated when the canal diameter measures less than 13 mm or the Pavlov ratio is less than 0.8.

corresponding level. Criteria for radiographic stenosis are anteroposterior dimensions measuring less than 13 mm on a lateral radiograph (21). Additionally, a Pavlov ratio of less than 0.8 has been used to describe stenosis **(Fig 5-6)**. Even without radiographic criteria for a stenotic canal, the potential for increased risk at the time of injury exists secondary to anatomical variation.

In summary, if the space available for the spinal cord is reduced because of a narrow canal, an important risk factor and predictor of acute neurological dysfunction is present (22). When the diameter of the midsagittal cervical spinal canal is 10 mm or less, cord compression can be anticipated (21). Cervical canal stenosis has been implicated as a risk factor for the burner phenomenon (see Fig 5-13) in college football players (23).

■ CLASSIFICATION OF INJURY

Cervical spine injuries can be classified, as described previously, as either catastrophic or noncatastrophic. The vast majority of injuries are noncatastrophic. Catastrophic cervical spine injuries include unstable fractures and dislocations, transient quadriplegia, and acute central disc herniation. Additionally, some congenital spinal anomalies can place an athlete at increased risk for injury. All these conditions typically produce neurological symptoms and signs that involve the extremities in a **bilateral** distribution.

As mentioned, only a very small percentage of football and hockey players sustain a catastrophic cervical spine injury. Most cervical spine injuries and injury patterns associated with collision sports do not involve spinal cord injury. In contrast to catastrophic injuries, these common syndromes usually do not affect the extremities in a bilateral fashion. Most neck-injured athletes display clinical findings in (a) a single upper extremity, (b) the neck and arm, or (c) the neck only. These syndromes include neuropraxia of the cervical root or brachial plexus (the "stinger" or "burner"), paracentral intervertebral disc herniation, stable fractures, spinal ligament injury, or intervertebral disc injury.

The sports medicine physician's initial evaluation of an injured athlete's signs and symptoms may help to distinguish between catastrophic and noncatastrophic injuries on the basis of the structural patterns of injury.

■ CATASTROPHIC CERVICAL SPINE INJURIES

In this section, we will review the four most common catastrophic cervical spine injuries (unstable fractures and dislocations, transient quadriplegia, acute central disc herniation, and congenital spinal anomalies) experienced by the sports medicine physician and specific concerns in each scenario.

Unstable Fractures and Dislocations

As expected, unstable fractures and/or dislocations make up the majority of catastrophic spinal injuries in athletes. An osseous or ligament injury is considered to be unstable when it results in loss of the ability of the spine, under physiological loads, to maintain its premorbid patterns of motion, so there

is no initial or additional damage to the spinal cord or nerve roots, no major deformity, and no incapacitating pain (24).

Spinal column damage occurs when the force and resistance balance of the normal motion of the spine is exceeded. Injury patterns often can help to illustrate the mechanism of cervical motion and damage. In football and hockey, the injury vector most frequently associated with cervical spinal cord injury is compression (axial loading) (13,15,25). A smaller percentage of injuries result from excessive flexion. Finally, extension, lateral stretch, and congenital instability also have been reported in cervical spine injury (26).

Initial loading most often occurs at the vertex of the collision athlete's helmet. The cervical spine is then left to compress between the mass of the oncoming body, which represents the instantly decelerated head, and the mass of the remaining body. Perhaps most influential in determining specific injury patterns is the neck position at the time of impact. Neutral alignment leaves the cervical spinal column slightly extended because of the normal lordotic posture. Compressive forces in this position are dissipated by the

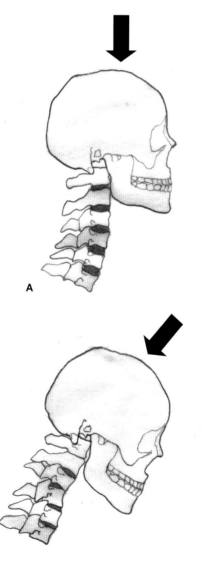
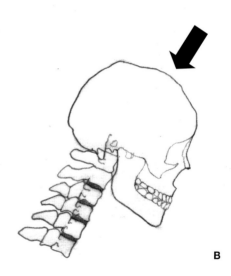

Fig 5-7. A: With the neck in neutral alignment, the vertebral column is extended. The compressive force can be dissipated by the spinal musculature and ligaments. **B:** With the neck in a flexed posture, the spine straightens out and becomes colinear with the axial force. **C:** At the time of impact, the straightened cervical spine undergoes a rapid deformation and buckles under the compressive load.

anterior paravertebral musculature and vertebral ligaments (anterior longitudinal ligament) **(Fig 5-7A)**. Slight flexion will eliminate cervical lordosis and direct force along the spine's longitudinal axis. This will result in large forces being transferred directly to the vertebrae as opposed to the surrounding soft tissues (13) **(Fig 5-7B)**. Cadaveric studies have shown that the cervical spine, when straight and colinear with the applied load, responds to compression by buckling (27) **(Fig 5-7C)**.

Most fractures and dislocations in injured athletes occur in the lower cervical spine. Two major patterns of compressive spinal column damage exist. Most often, evidence of a compressive–flexion injury is present as a result of a combination of axial force and a bending moment. The anterior column shortens under loading. We then see compressive failure of the vertebral body and tensile failure of the posterior spinal ligaments **(Fig 5-8A)**. This pattern can be highly unstable both anteriorly and posteriorly, with displacement of the anterior fracture and widening of the posterior elements, and it often may be associated with spinal cord injury (28).

Pure vertical compression (the cervical spine is slightly flexed, eliminating the normal lordosis) results in equal force on the anterior and posterior columns, which may result in an axial loading fracture ("burst") (29) **(Fig 5-8B)**. Intradiscal pressure rises such that the adjacent end plate fractures and fails. Bone fragments often can displace in all directions secondary to forced, extruded disc material within the vertebral body. In fact, these burst fractures are notable for retropulsion of osseous material into the spinal canal.

During most normal neck motion, the cervical spine remains in slight extension (or lordosis). Flexion vectors, however, can be created either by a direct blow to the occipital region or by a rapid deceleration of the torso. In this situation, spine flexion subjects the posterior ligamentous structures of the involved motion segment to tensile forces. These are characterized as flexion–distraction injuries, and the most common specific injury pattern to result in spinal cord dysfunction is a bilateral facet dislocation (30–32) **(Fig 5-9A)**. An axial rotation force in conjunction with the flexion–distraction injury may produce a unilateral facet dislocation (spinal cord injury in up to 25% of cases) (30) **(Fig 5-9B)**.

The spectrum of neurological dysfunction with cervical fractures or dislocations often can be highly variable. Syndromes include complete quadriplegia, with total loss of sensory or motor function below the level of the cord lesion, versus partial spinal cord injury, with incomplete loss of sensory or motor function in the extremities and torso. The most common clinical entity of partial spinal cord injury is central cord syndrome, followed by anterior cord syndrome. Maroon et al. (33) and Wilberger et al. (34) reported a variant of the central cord lesion that was characterized by dysesthesias in both hands without loss of strength or sensation. Although the etiology is not entirely clear, this "burning hands" syndrome is thought to result from a vascular insufficiency. This may affect the medial portion of the somatotopically arranged spinothalamic tracts.

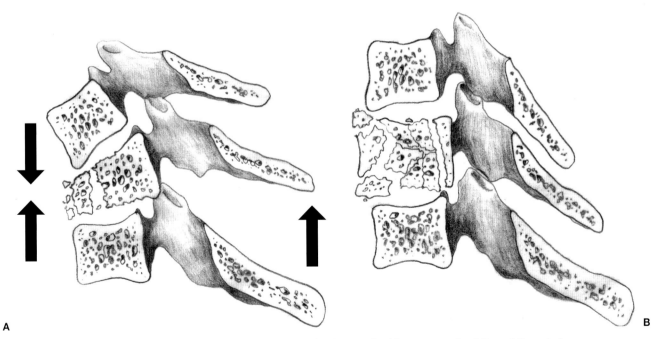

A   B

Fig 5-8. A: The "teardrop" fracture variant is characterized by compressive failure of the anterior column with a coronal plane fracture extending through the vertebral body. Tensile forces cause disruption of the posterior spinal ligaments. **B:** In the "burst" fracture variant, comminution of the vertebral body can be associated with retropulsion of osseous fragments into the spinal canal.

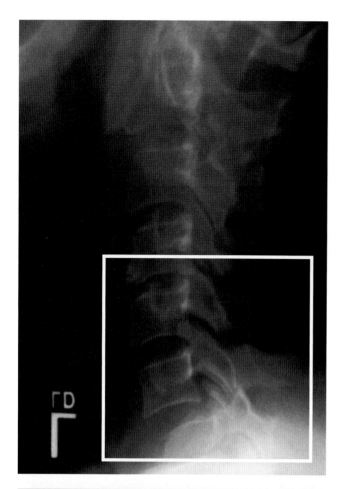

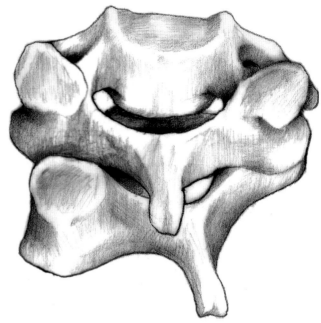

B

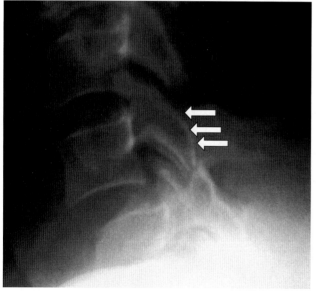

A

Fig 5-9. A: Lateral cervical spine radiographs showing bilateral facet dislocation of C6 on C7. This pattern of injury results from disruption of the supraspinous and interspinous ligament, facet capsules, ligamentum flavum, posterior longitudinal ligament, and the dorsal portions of the annulus fibrosus. The soft tissue damage can be associated with fractures of the superior articular processes. **B:** Unilateral facet dislocation usually is caused by the combination of flexion and rotational forces. The addition of shear or compressive forces can cause fracture of the articular process.

Upper cervical spinal fractures and dislocations, although significant injuries, rarely cause spinal cord damage. The spinal canal in the upper cervical region has a much greater proportion of space to spinal cord. Therefore, even with displacement, cord compression is unlikely in relation to upper cervical spinal injury. In fact, a burst fracture of the atlas (Jefferson fracture) and traumatic spondylolisthesis of the axis (Hangman fracture) expand the dimensions of the spinal canal, making cord compression and neurological injury improbable. Some scenarios may place the upper cervical cord at increased risk for injury. Odontoid fractures or ruptures of the transverse ligament will destabilize the atlantoaxial joint. Typically, high cervical cord injuries can cause respiratory compromise secondary to high-cord/low-brainstem injury as well as diaphragmatic paralysis from trauma to the anterior horn cells of the phrenic nerve.

Thus far, we have discussed primarily upper motor neuron damage from cervical injury. Occasionally, a lower motor neuron finding will be the only sign. For instance, a unilateral facet dislocation may compress the dislocated side at the foraminal opening. This phenomenon certainly can cause isolated nerve root symptoms (monoradiculopathy).

Transient Quadriplegia

The clinical syndrome of neuropraxia often can help to explain more complex clinical syndromes of the cervical spinal cord. Transient quadriplegia has been estimated to occur in 7 per 10,000 football players (35). As mentioned previously, congenital cervical stenosis may predispose athletes to cord compression (36). In one study, a Pavlov ratio of less than 0.8 was documented in 93% of football players with cervical cord neuropraxia (37). The phrase "pincer mechanism" has been used by Penning (38) to describe a momentary cord compression at the extremes of neck extension or flexion.

As illustrated in **Figure 5-10**, this forced hyperextension of a lower cervical motion segment causes an impingement on the posterior margin of the end plate of the more cranial vertebral body. Therefore, the spinolaminar line of the subjacent vertebra is disturbed. The soft-tissue structures that lie along this radiographic spinolaminar line (posterior longitudinal ligament and the ligamentum flavum) will then displace and

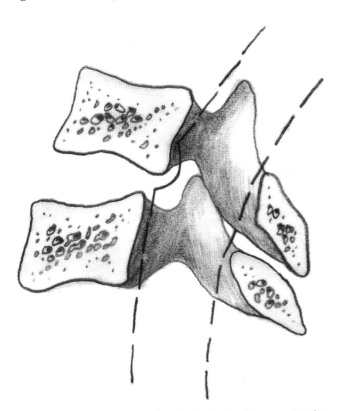

Fig 5-10. The "pincer mechanism" effect of hyperextension causes dynamic compression of the spinal cord between the end plate of the cranial vertebral body and the spinolaminar line of the subjacent vertebra.

make the spinal canal narrower. Most experts now agree that the pathophysiology associated with this phenomenon is less an anatomical disruption and more a physiological conduction block. The conduction block, or neuropraxia, in this case relates to possible segmental demyelination and increasing refractory period of the long tract axons (39). Describing this postconcussive state, Torg et al. (40) theorized that local anoxia and increased intracellular calcium concentration are responsible for the temporary disturbance of spinal cord function.

Signs and symptoms of transient quadriplegia include pain, tingling, or loss of sensation bilaterally in the upper and/or lower extremities. A mild quadriparesis usually exists, but motor weakness does not need to be present. Of course, complete quadriplegia also is possible. Limited range of motion and neck pain/tenderness usually are absent. Although transient in nature, this syndrome may last from 15 minutes to 48 hours, but full recovery often is expected. Certain players have risk factors (spinal canal stenosis) for developing transient quadriplegia, and recurrence rates as high as 56% have been reported (41).

Intervertebral Disc Herniation

Although rare, acute cervical disc herniation can occur in collision sport athletes. Extrusion of the nucleus pulposus posteriorly can cause acute cord compression. Unlike the more common lower lumbar disc herniations, cervical disc herniations can produce permanent cord injury. Posterior neck pain, paraspinal muscle spasm, and either transient or permanent acute paralysis are the most common symptoms. Radiating (radicular) pain or referred pain unilaterally down the shoulder and arm also may be present.

Congenital Spinal Anomalies

Anatomical variants and congenital anomalies predispose athletes to certain forms of spinal cord injury. For example, Klippel-Feil syndrome, which reduces the number of motion segments in the spine, may lead to progressive instability or degenerative stenosis. Multiple fusions in the cervical spine in this condition make it difficult to dissipate loads that are applied to the cervical spine **(Fig 5-11)**.

Hypoplasia of the dens (i.e., a failure of formation involving the second vertebra) and developmental os odontoideum can both result in atlantoaxial instability **(Fig 5-12)**. Many of these conditions are completely asymptomatic, and too often, the realization of their existence is appreciated only at the time of injury.

■ NONCATASTROPHIC CERVICAL SPINE INJURIES

Noncatastrophic injuries include neuropraxia of the cervical root or brachial plexus (the "stinger" or "burner"), paracentral intervertebral disc herniation, stable fractures, spinal

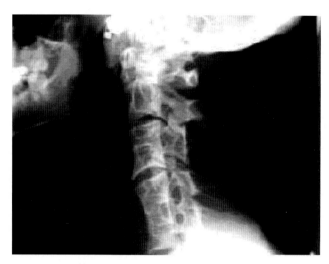

Fig 5-11. Lateral radiograph showing multiple levels of cervical fusion.

ligament injury, and intervertebral disc injury. These more common syndromes make up the majority of injuries encountered by sports medicine physicians.

Unilateral upper extremity involvement usually represents **neuropraxia of a cervical nerve root or the brachial plexus**. Many descriptions and explanations for this well-known "stinger" or "burner" phenomenon exist. Foraminal compression of a nerve root from forceful neck extension and rotation toward the affected side are thought to be involved. Alternatively, traction (tensile forces) may injure the brachial plexus, resulting in a neuropraxia **(Fig 5-13)**.

Direct compression of the upper trunk between the shoulder pad and the ipsilateral scapula has been reported (42). Again, the signs and symptoms include burning pain, weakness, or paresthesias in the shoulder girdle and arm.

Neck tenderness usually is absent, and range of motion often is full (43). Transient motor, sensory, and/or reflex deficit can occur, but these symptoms resolve within several minutes. Some athletes, however, may not gain full strength until 24 to 48 hours later. Although muscle weakness is variable, it is unlikely to represent permanent motor loss. The lifetime incidence of a "burner" in college football players has been reported to be 65% (44).

Paracentral disc herniation also can cause unilateral upper limb and neck symptoms associated with nerve root compression. Causes range from high-energy impact loading to a minor twisting injury to the neck. Typically, a tear in the posterolateral aspect of the annulus fibrosus allows the nucleus pulposus to protrude posteriorly. Monoradiculopathy, paresthesias, and/or weakness in the upper extremity often are present. Careful, initial evaluation of the nerve symptoms and deficits should allow a presumptive determination of the affected disc level (45). Spasm and neck pain almost always are present.

Localized neck symptoms usually signify more minor injuries: stable fractures, spinal ligament injuries (cervical sprains), or intervertebral disc injury. **Stable fractures** of the anterior column generally are secondary to compressive forces. In contrast, fractures of the posterior elements typically result from a hyperextension injury vector. During minor **spinal ligament injuries** or **intervertebral disc injuries**, the stability of the spinal column is not compromised; therefore, the integrity of the neural elements is maintained. Typically, however, these injuries present with tenderness to palpation over the affected area and limited range of motion.

Figure 5-14 summarizes the diagnostic algorithm for initial evaluation of an athlete with a suspected injury to the cervical spine (46).

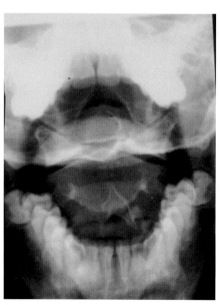

A

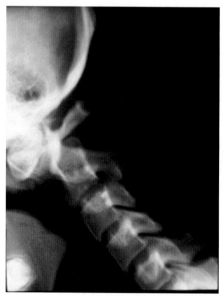

B

Fig 5-12. Anteroposterior and dynamic lateral radiograph of the cervical spine (*flexion view*) demonstrating atlantoaxial instability because of os odontoideum.

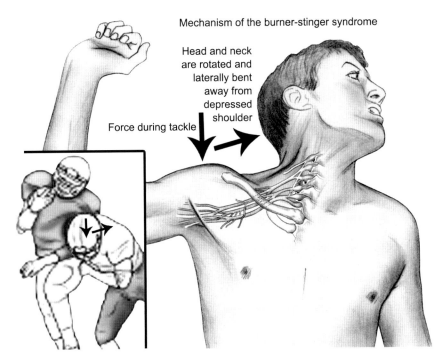

Mechanism of the burner-stinger syndrome

Head and neck are rotated and laterally bent away from depressed shoulder

Force during tackle

Fig 5-13. The mechanism of the burner-stinger syndrome. The shoulder is depressed while the head and neck are rotated and laterally bent away from the affected shoulder, as may occur during a football tackle. This same mechanism, combined with extension of the neck, may result in compression of the nerves on the contralateral shoulder, also resulting in a burner and stinger. (From Safran MR. Nerve injury about the shoulder in athletes. Part 2: Long thoracic nerve, spinal accessory nerve, burners/stingers, thoracic outlet syndrome. *Am J Sports Med.* 2004; 32:1063–1076; with permission.)

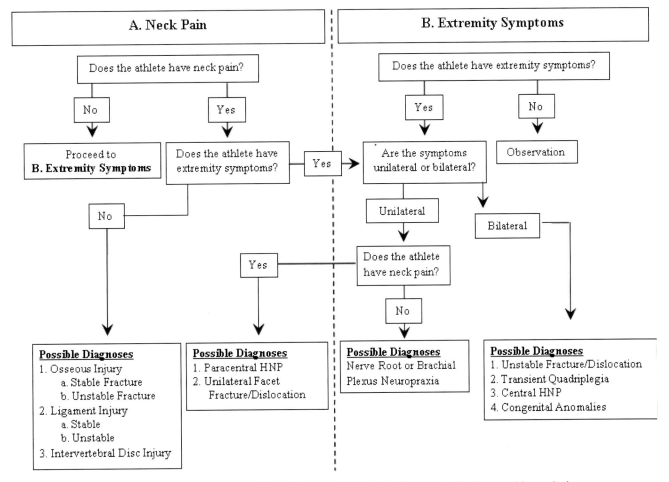

Fig 5-14. Diagnostic algorithm. (From Banerjee R, Palumbo MA, Fadale PD. Catastrophic cervical spine injuries in the collision sport athlete. Part II. Principles of emergency care. *Am J Sports Med.* 2004;32:1760–1764; with permission.)

■ PREGAME PLANNING

Personnel and staff who are responsible for the care of athletes need to ensure that necessary pre-event planning and preparations are accomplished. These tasks may be summarized as follows: (a) establish a protocol for prehospital care of the injured athlete, (b) organize all necessary equipment for on-field management, and (c) select a hospital system for the transfer of care.

A well-devised diagnostic and therapeutic protocol allows all staff to be effective team members in the execution of an emergency plan. A standard chain of command exists, with the sports medicine physician or head athletic trainer responsible for on-field direction. The protocol should be easily understood by each member.

Necessary emergency equipment includes items for airway management and cardiopulmonary resuscitation. A backboard and means for rapid immobilization of the cervical spine must be available. Additionally, face mask shears and other tools for the removal of protective athletic gear should be available as well.

Emergency medical technicians are essential team members when transport of the athlete is necessary. Working relationships and clear communication are essential between these health care providers and the on-field medical team. A standard protocol for ambulance transport, including which personnel should accompany the athlete, should be decided as well. Optimally, the medical facility chosen for transfer will have expertise in definitive treatment of cervical spinal cord injuries.

All hospital systems will have the services necessary for initial resuscitation of a critically injured athlete. Early consultation with a spine surgeon, however, will be essential, because early definitive care of cervical spine injuries has been demonstrated to improve patient outcomes.

■ INJURY PREVENTION AND EDUCATION

Instruction and education of athletes, although often overlooked, remain the most crucial elements in preventing cervical spine injuries. The majority of cervical spine injuries occurring in football, as demonstrated by Torg et al. (13), happen when the athlete uses an improper tackling technique with the neck in flexion during axial loading. As mentioned previously, rule modifications have banned techniques such as "spearing"; however, a recent survey showed that football players had poor knowledge regarding the dangers of "spearing" (47). A less dangerous technique encourages the player to assume a natural lordotic cervical posture such that their face mask is placed directly into the number on the opponent's jersey (48). These techniques, although simple in concept, are increasingly important for preventing injuries caused by improper tackling and blocking.

Data from the ice hockey injuries have indicated checking from behind as a potential cause of cervical spine injury (49). Again, instruction and education in proper techniques could aid in decreasing potential scenarios that may lead to cervical spine injuries. The STOP program, as cited previously, is one example of a visual aid accompanied by an educational program to help reduce spine injuries.

■ MANAGEMENT OF CERVICAL SPINE INJURIES

During competition, the sports medicine staff should be knowledgeable about available medical equipment, and they should make every effort to monitor play. A visual image of the traumatic event can be useful in attempting to determine both the type and the severity of injury. Any player suspected of having sustained a serious spinal injury should receive immediate attention by the athletic trainer and/or team physician.

Primary Survey

On reaching the injured player, the primary objectives are to assess for immediately life-threatening conditions and to prevent further injury. The initial evaluation follows the ABCDE sequence of trauma care: A, airway maintenance with cervical spine protection; B, breathing and ventilation; C, circulation; D, disability (i.e., neurological status); and E, exposure of the athlete. During this primary survey, appropriate resuscitation procedures are instituted for any identified alteration of vital functions. The emergency medical system should be activated immediately after recognizing a life-threatening problem or serious spinal injury.

The findings of the primary survey will determine how the player is subsequently treated. In this regard, one of three clinical scenarios will become apparent (50) **(Table 5-1)**. The first—and least likely—scenario involves the life-threatening problem of actual or impending cardiorespiratory collapse. The second scenario involves the athlete with an altered mental status but no compromise of the cardiovascular or respiratory system. In the third—and most common—scenario involves a neck-injured player with a normal level of consciousness and normal cardiopulmonary function. When selecting the appropriate management procedure for a specific scenario, the athlete's body position on the playing surface must be taken into account as well.

Scenario 1: Cardiorespiratory Compromise

Life-threatening alteration of cardiopulmonary function is a rare event in the collision sport athlete. Respiratory distress from obstruction of the airway can result by a foreign body, facial fractures, or direct injury to the trachea or larynx. The ability to maintain airway patency also can be lost secondary to a depressed level of consciousness. In the absence of upper

TABLE 5-1	Cervical Spine Trauma: Potential Clinical Scenarios	
Scenario	**Consciousness**	**Cardiorespiratory status**
1	Abnormal	Compromised
2	Abnormal	Normal
3	Normal	Normal

airway compromise, problems with respiration may develop in association with an upper cervical spinal cord injury as a result of paralysis of the diaphragm and accessory breathing muscles. Other possible causes of altered pulmonary function include pneumothorax, asthma, and anaphylaxis. If not rapidly recognized and treated, any of these conditions may progress to frank respiratory failure with the potential to degenerate into cardiac arrest. Circulatory collapse from a primary cardiac event is distinctly uncommon in this setting.

Regardless of the etiology of respiratory compromise, the primary objective is to rapidly identify hypoxia and then intervene by providing proper ventilation of the injured player. This must be accomplished without causing any further injury to the spinal or neurological structures. In this regard, any athlete with a life-threatening condition is assumed to have a catastrophic cervical spine injury until proven otherwise. Protection of the cervical spine is an important underlying principle.

When airway obstruction is identified during the primary survey, immediate steps to reestablish patency of the upper respiratory tract are taken. While maintaining manual stabilization of the neck in a neutral position, the mouthpiece is extracted. The athlete who is lying prone on the playing surface must be carefully log-rolled into a supine position (see *Protocol for Positioning and Helmet Removal*). Once supine, the face mask is rapidly removed. A chin-lift, jaw-thrust maneuver is performed to move the tongue away from the back of the throat, thereby opening the airway; the head-tilt technique should be avoided because of potential alteration of cervical spine alignment. In the player who is unresponsive or has altered mental status, an oral airway may need to be inserted to prevent occlusion of the oropharynx. Removal of the helmet is *not* routinely indicated unless it interferes with resuscitation of the patient.

Once the airway has been opened and protected, the next priority is to maintain adequate ventilation and perfusion. Patency of the airway does not assure adequate alveolar gas exchange, however, and ventilation also is dependent on appropriate function of the diaphragm, chest wall musculature, and lungs. The initial assessment of respiratory function involves observation of chest excursions along with feeling and listening for air movement at the mouth or nares. Auscultation of breath sounds with a stethoscope should be performed early during the evaluation process. Assisted ventilation is required if breathing is of insufficient depth or rate. In general, on-field ventilatory support involves use of a bag-valve device and a face mask. Indications for definitive airway control by endotracheal intubation include apnea, inability to maintain oxygenation with face mask supplementation, protection from aspiration, and severe closed head injury.

Circulation is the third issue to consider during the primary survey. The peripheral and central pulses should be evaluated in terms of quality, rate, and rhythm. Diminished amplitude of the peripheral pulses in combination with bradycardia often signifies neurogenic shock as a result of cervical spinal cord injury. A rapid, thready pulse of normal rhythm is consistent with hypovolemic shock; this unusual finding in the collision sport athlete can be related to rapid internal blood loss, such as with a splenic injury. An irregular pulse rhythm should raise suspicion of potential cardiac dysfunction. Inability to palpate the femoral or carotid pulses indicates the need to initiate cardiopulmonary resuscitation. In most cases, the front of the shoulder pads can be opened to allow chest compressions and, when necessary, defibrillation. If the helmet has been removed, however, the shoulder pads also should be removed to maintain the neutral alignment of the cervical spine.

Scenario 2: Altered Mental Status without Cardiorespiratory Compromise

Care of the cervical spine in the collision athlete with altered mental status presents a challenging problem for the sports medicine physician. After a rapid primary survey, a brief neurological assessment is performed to determine the athlete's level of consciousness. Important aspects of the on-field neurological examination include assessment of mental status (i.e., Glasgow Coma Scale), pupillary response, assessment of eye movements and visual fields, and gross motor and sensory examination of the extremities. The prone athlete should be carefully log-rolled into a supine position (see *Protocol for Positioning and Helmet Removal*). Altered mental status is an indication for early and rapid removal of the face mask.

Complete loss of consciousness in this scenario usually is related to a closed head injury. Other causes include, but are not limited to, hypoglycemia, hyperthermia, and drug overdose. Closed head injury also may alter the athlete's state of awareness and his or her ability to respond to questioning and/or a neurological examination. Therefore, any athlete with altered mental status is considered to have a cervical spine injury until proven otherwise. The unconscious athlete is always assumed to have a cervical spine injury.

Scenario 3: Normal Mental Status without Cardiorespiratory Compromise

The most common clinical scenario encountered by the sports medicine physician is the athlete with normal mental status and without cardiorespiratory compromise. Catastrophic cervical spine injury, however, can still occur in this scenario often insidiously.

After the primary survey, a neurologic assessment should be performed. Catastrophic cervical trauma should be assumed in the player with symptoms or signs referable to cord damage. In the absence of neurological abnormalities, an unstable spinal column injury with potential cord compromise is suggested by significant cervicothoracic pain, focal spinal tenderness, or restricted neck motion.

Any athlete with a suspected cervical spine injury should be carefully immobilized and prepared for transport. Once the decision to transport has been made, the face mask should be carefully removed.

In preparation for transport, the athlete should be immobilized on a backboard. Emergency medical personnel should be briefed regarding the injury and the patient's current status and examination findings. During transport, ongoing assessment of the patient's vitals, mental status, and neurological status is important.

■ MANAGEMENT OF PROTECTIVE EQUIPMENT

Collision sports, such as football and ice hockey, further complicate the risk of cervical spine injury because of the protective equipment associated with each athlete. Helmets and shoulder pads aim to protect athletes from contact, but they often provide little additional support for motion of the spine and, quite frankly, make it difficult to assess the patient completely.

In 1998, the National Athletic Trainers' Association (NATA) formed the Inter-Association Task Force for Appropriate Care of the Spine-Injured Athlete to develop guidelines for the proper management of the athlete with a catastrophic spine injury (51). Unlike motorcycle helmets, which limit force distribution for impact, most recent designs for football and ice hockey helmets work with the shoulder pads to prevent excessive motion of the spine. Although this topic has been the subject of much debate historically, these recent advances in design recognize the importance of keeping protective equipment on during the initial evaluation. This increased, if limited, stability of the cervical spine in neutral position is more important than full exposure, because even small amounts of abnormal motion during a suspected cervical spine injury may cause damage (52).

Numerous cadaveric and human studies were used to formulate a consensus, and formal regulations are now in place (49,53–59). Basic science studies support the idea that helmets and pads give support and alignment to the injured cervical spine. In the study by Palumbo et al. (54), the removal of the helmet or the shoulder pads from a cadaveric model significantly changed the cervical lordosis in a spine with C5-C6 instability. Clinically, LaPrade et al. (49) again demonstrated by computed tomography (CT) that removal of the helmet or the shoulder pads in ice hockey players resulted in a significant increase in cervical spine extension (lordosis). Furthermore, Waninger et al. (55) demonstrated that during transport and backboard-immobilization, an athlete's helmet effectively limits cervical motion.

Understandably, leaving protective equipment in place is not possible in all scenarios. The safety of the athlete may, in fact, rely on removal of the helmet or shoulder pads. Specific protocols have been developed by the

TABLE 5-2	Equipment Removal Guidelines

The following situations warrant helmet removal in the injured athlete:

1 If after a reasonable period of time, the face mask cannot be removed to gain airway access.
2 If the design of the helmet and chin strap is such that even after removal of the face mask, the airway cannot be controlled or ventilation provided.
3 If the helmet and chin straps do not hold the head securely such that immobilization of the helmet does not also immobilize the head.
4 If the helmet prevents immobilization for transport in an appropriate position.
5 If the shoulder pads are removed.

The following situations warrant shoulder pad removal in the injured athlete:

1 Multiple injuries requiring full access to the shoulder area
2 Ill-fitting shoulder pads causing inability to maintain spinal immobilization.
3 Cardiopulmonary resuscitation requiring access that is inhibited by shoulder pads.
4 If the helmet is removed.

From Kleiner DM, Almquist JL, Bailes J, et al. *Prehospital care of the spine-injured athlete: a document from the Inter-Association Task Force for Appropriate Care of the Spine-Injured Athlete.* Dallas: National Athletic Trainers' Association; 2001; with permission.

Inter-Association Task Force for Appropriate Care of the Spine-Injured Athlete to emphasize the importance of using multiple care providers for equipment removal. Donaldson et al. (53) used cadaver models to measure motion and technique during helmet removal of specimens with C1-C2 instability. Their study, along with the advent of digital fluoroscopy, helped to establish a more accepted protocol of using four providers, as recommended by NATA, that limits cervical motion (60). Guidelines for equipment removal before transport are outlined in **Table 5-2**. Our preferred technique for cervical spine stabilization and equipment removal are detailed below.

■ PROTOCOL FOR POSITIONING AND HELMET REMOVAL

The Prone Athlete

1 If an athlete is found in the prone position after an injury, cervical spine injury should be assumed. The team physician and the training staff should complete their initial evaluation (i.e., primary survey) without moving the athlete.

2 The team physician and athletic trainer position themselves by the patient. The trainer stabilizes the cervical spine while the physician completes the primary survey.

3 The athlete's cervical spine is stabilized by placing one hand on each side of the player's helmet. The trainer's hands are crossed, which will facilitate turning the athlete.

4 Once the primary survey is completed, turn the patient to a supine position to complete the evaluation and prepare the patient for transport. This step requires a minimum of four members of the athletic training team. One member is positioned above the athlete and is solely responsible for control of the head and neck. The other three members position themselves as shown above, kneeling next to the patient. The athlete's body is held at the torso, hip, and legs to facilitate turning.

5 The patient is turned slowly on the command of the person who is stabilizing the cervical spine. Take care to maintain a neutral position of the body relative to the cervical spine.

6 The patient may be rolled directly onto a spine board to prepare for transport. Alternatively, the patient may be rolled first to a supine position to allow completion of the medical evaluation; once the decision to transport the athlete has been made, the patient is then rolled onto the spine board.

7 Once the patient is positioned supine on the spine board, the cervical spine is immobilized with foam blocks, and straps are placed across the helmet and the body. The cervical spine should be manually stabilized until it is securely immobilized.

Removal of Helmet and Shoulder Pads

1 Manual stabilization of the cervical spine is maintained by placing one hand on each side of the athlete's helmet.

2 The chin strap is cut, and all accessible internal padding is removed.

3 The second care provider (team physician) then slides his or her hands along each side of the mandible and stabilizes the cervical spine.

4 The team physician now assumes responsibility for manual stabilization of the cervical spine. The athletic trainer gently removes the helmet by first spreading the area over the cheeks. Next, the helmet is gently removed. The helmet may be rolled forward slightly to allow easy removal. Once the helmet is removed, the first care provider reassumes manual stabilization.

5 Removal of the shoulder pads begins with cutting the jersey and all other shirts from the neck to the waist and from the midline to the end of each arm sleeve. All straps holding the shoulder pads in place should be cut, as opposed to unbuckled, to avoid unnecessary movement. Most shoulder pad systems use lacing or strapping over the sternum to connect the two halves of the shoulder pad unit. This lacing should be cut, after which the anterior half of the shoulder pads can be opened.

6 Manual stabilization of the cervical spine is then shifted such that the team physician maintains stabilization by placing his or her forearms on the athlete's chest. One hand is placed on each side of the patient's mandible, with the fingers directed posteriorly around the base of the occiput.

7 With several assistants, the injured athlete is then carefully lifted while manual stabilization is maintained. The athletic trainer gently removes the shoulder pads by pulling the unit superiorly, and the athlete is gently lowered onto the spine board.

8 The athlete is secured to the spine board. Manual stabilization of the cervical spine is maintained until the athlete's head is stabilized with foam blocks.

Management in the Emergency Room

After safe transport, the care of the athlete is transferred to the hospital emergency room personnel. If possible, a member of the on-field medical team should accompany the athlete during transport. This provides an accurate, knowledgeable briefing to the emergency room physicians, which may be essential during the early management of the case. Furthermore, the on-field medical team member may be the only one who is familiar with proper techniques of helmet removal in this setting.

At this point, initial primary and secondary surveys are completed by the emergency room physician. The emergency room physician specifically documents a full neurological examination and any changes from previous examinations.

Radiographic examination should then be performed. Initially, these include an anteroposterior, lateral, and odontoid view of the cervical spine. Removal of protective equipment for these initial films is controversial (see below).

In any case of suspected catastrophic cervical spine injury, appropriate consultation with the hospital's spine surgeon should be rapidly obtained.

■ CURRENT CONTROVERSIES

Removal of Protective Equipment

Although most prehospital personnel now accept the recommendations of the Inter-Association Task Force for Appropriate Care of the Spine-Injured Athlete (51), some concern exists on the part of prehospital care providers regarding the inability to fully evaluate the helmeted head and neck before transport to the hospital.

Historically, cervical spine protocols were designed for motorcycle helmets; thus, they reflected the nature and energy of these injuries (61–63). Prehospital care protocols may still reflect these injuries. Given the higher energy and severity of motorcycle injuries to the head and neck, it may be reasonable to remove helmets in these cases for better evaluation of the patient.

Unlike motorcycle helmets, however, the combination of football helmets and shoulder pads helps to maintain a neutral alignment of the cervical spine. Furthermore, athletic injuries from collision sports are of much lower energy and have a lower incidence of severe head or neck injury.

In light of this, there is a consensus regarding the removal of protective gear during the initial on-field assessment of the spine-injured athlete. The current NCAA guidelines for football helmet management state that unless special circumstances exist (Table 5-2), protective equipment (helmet and shoulder pads) should not be removed on the field (64).

This consensus may not be reflected at the level of local and community emergency medical services, however, which may lead to compromise of cervical spine care. Proper communication and cooperative education with local emergency medical services, hospitals, and on-field care providers should be undertaken to improve prehospital care.

Initial Radiographic Imaging

On transport to the emergency room, the initial imaging modality to evaluate the cervical spine is plain-film radiography.

Both the NCAA (64) and the Inter-Association Task Force for Appropriate Care of the Spine-Injured Athlete (51) have recommended that initial radiographs be obtained with the helmet and shoulder pads in place (but with the face mask removed). After the initial radiographic screening has been performed, the helmet and shoulder pads can be removed as described above. Standard anteroposterior, lateral, and odontoid views of the cervical spine are effective screening radiographs for patients with suspected cervical spine injury (65).

Helmets and shoulder pads, however, have been shown to interfere with adequate imaging of the cervical spine, particularly at the cervicothoracic junction (66,67,68). In a small study using volunteers, Davidson et al. (66) demonstrated that the upper cervical spine and the cervicothoracic junction were poorly depicted when radiographs were obtained with protective gear in place. The designs of hockey and football helmets differ, however, such that the initial lateral cervical spine scout film may be adequate with the equipment in place for ice hockey players (69).

Given the problems with plain-film radiographs, several authors have suggested use of CT as the initial screening modality (70–73). Lateral CT scans have been used to effectively depict the entire cervical spine with protective equipment in place (49). As CT technology improves, this modality may become the primary choice for initial radiographic screening of athletes with a cervical spine injury.

We recommend that initial screening radiographs be obtained with the protective equipment in place. If these films are inadequate, perform additional imaging. In the athlete with a high suspicion of a cervical spine injury (e.g., severe neck pain or a neurological deficit), we recommend proceeding directly to CT with the protective equipment in place. If urgent CT is unavailable, remove the protective gear to obtain adequate films. In lower-risk cases, the helmet and shoulder pads can be carefully removed using the protocol described above; plain-film radiographs can then be obtained with the neck immobilized.

■ CONCLUSION

Cervical spine injury is a challenging problem, and it can be an overwhelming event in an athlete's life. Effective management of these injuries requires a concerted effort by the sports medicine physician, athletic trainers, emergency medical services, and the hospital emergency room.

In this chapter, we have reviewed the multiple aspects of the care of cervical spine injuries in the athlete. The following list is provided for the reader's review:

■ The rate of catastrophic cervical spine injuries decreased after the institution of rules and educational programs to minimize these injuries in both American football and ice hockey.
■ The diameter of the spinal canal progressively narrows in a cranial to caudal direction, with the space available for the spinal cord being at a minimum between C4 and C7. Injuries to the lower cervical spine therefore may have a greater potential of spinal cord injury.
■ A catastrophic cervical spine injury can be defined as a structural distortion of the cervical spinal column associated with actual or potential damage to the spinal

cord. Catastrophic injuries include unstable fractures and dislocations, transient quadriplegia, acute central disc herniation, and congenital spinal anomalies. These are distinguished by their presentation with **bilateral** signs and symptoms.

■ Pre-event training and athlete education are important adjuncts in the care of athletes with a cervical spine injury.

■ Protective gear (helmets and shoulder pads) should not be removed before transport except in select cases (Table 5-2).

■ When protective gear is interfering with the urgent care of the athlete, the helmet and shoulder pads must be removed according to a careful, coordinated protocol to minimize secondary injury.

■ Initial radiographic evaluation with plain films should be performed with protective gear in place. If these films are inadequate, CT may be an option; otherwise, protective equipment must be carefully removed to ensure that adequate radiographs are obtained.

■ REFERENCES

1. National Spinal Cord Injury Statistical Center (NSCISC). *Spinal Cord Information Network—facts and figures at a glance.* Birmingham, AL: University of Alabama at Birmingham; 2003. (Available online at www.ncddr.org/rpp/hf/hfdw/mscis/nscisc.html.)

2. DeVivo MJ. Causes and costs of spinal cord injury in the United States. *Spinal Cord.* 1997;35:809–813.

3. Nobunga AI, Go BK, Karunas RB. Recent demographic and injury trends in people served by the model spinal cord injury care systems. *Arch Phys Med Rehabil.* 1999;80:1372–1382.

4. Quarrie KL, Cantu RC, Chalmers DJ. Rugby union injuries to the cervical spine and spinal cord. *Sports Med.* 2002;32:633–653.

5. Wetzler MJ, Akpata T, Laughlin W, et al. Occurrence of cervical spine injuries during the rugby scrum. *Am J Sports Med.* 1998;26:177–180.

6. Levy AS, Smith RH. Neurologic injuries in skiers and snowboarders. *Semin Neurol.* 2000;20:233–245.

7. Tarazi F, Dvorak MFS, Wing PC. Spinal injuries in skiers and snowboarders. *Am J Sports Med.* 1999;27:177–180.

8. Schmitt H, Gerner HJ. Paralysis from sport and diving accidents. *Clin J Sport Med.* 2001;11:17–22.

9. National Center for Catastrophic Sport Injury Research (NCCSIR). *Twentieth Annual Report: Fall 1982–Spring 2002.* Chapel Hill, NC: University of North Carolina; 2003. (Available online at www.unc.edu/depts/nccsi/.)

10. Cantu RC, Mueller FO. Catastrophic spine injuries in American football, 1977–2001. *Neurosurg.* 2003;53:358–363.

11. Schneider RC. Serious and fatal neurosurgical football injuries. *Clin Neurosurg.* 1964;12:226–236.

12. Torg JS, Quedenfeld TC, Burstein A, et al. National football head and neck injury registry: report on cervical quadriplegia, 1971 to 1975. *Am J Sports Med.* 1979;7:127–132.

13. Torg JS, Vegso JJ, O'Neill MJ, et al. The epidemiologic, pathologic, biomechanical, and cinematographic analysis of football-induced cervical spine trauma. *Am J Sports Med.* 1990;18:50–57.

14. Martin V. Football rules seek to curb head blocking. *Phys Sportsmed.* 1980;8:119.

15. Tator CH, Carson JD, Edmonds VE. Spinal injuries in ice hockey. *Clin Sports Med.* 1998;17:183–194.

16. Molsa JJ, Tegner Y, Alaranta H, et al. Spinal cord injuries in ice hockey in Finland and Sweden from 1980 to 1996. *Int J Sports Med.* 1999;20:64–67.

17. Waninger KN. Management of the helmeted athlete with suspected cervical spine injury. *Am J Sports Med.* 2004;32: 1331–1350.

18. Ghanayem AJ, Zdeblich TA, Dvorak J. Functional anatomy of joints, ligaments, and discs. In: The Cervical Spine Research Society, eds. *The cervical spine,* 3rd ed. Philadelphia: Lippincott–Raven Publishers; 1998:45–52.

19. Parke WW. Correlative anatomy of cervical spondylotic myelopathy. *Spine.* 1988;13:831–837.

20. Okada Y, Ikata T, Katoh S, et al. Morphologic analysis of the cervical spinal cord, dural tube, and spinal canal by magnetic resonance imaging in normal adults and patients with cervical spondylotic myelopathy. *Spine.* 1994;19:2331–2335.

21. Eismont FJ, Clifford S, Goldberg M, et al. Cervical sagittal spinal canal size in spine injury. *Spine.* 1984;9:663–666.

22. Kang JD, Figgie MP, Bohlman HH. Sagittal measurements of the cervical spine in subaxial fractures and dislocations. An analysis of two hundred and eighty-eight patients with and without neurological deficits. *J Bone Joint Surg Am.* 1994;76:1617–1628.

23. Kelly JD, Aliquo D, Sitler MR, et al. Association of burners with cervical canal and foraminal stenosis. *Am J Sports Med.* 2000; 28:214–217.

24. White AA, Panjabi MM. *Clinical biomechanics of the spine.* 2nd ed. Philadelphia: JB Lippincott Co; 1990.

25. Torg JS: *Athletic Injuries to the Head, Neck, and Face.* Philadelphia: Lea & Febiger; 1982.

26. Funk FJ, Wells RE. Injuries of the cervical spine in football. *Clin Orthop.* 1975;109:50–58.

27. Wong WB, Panjabi MM, White AA. Mechanisms of injury in the cervical spine. In: The Cervical Spine Research Society, eds. *The cervical spine.* 3rd ed. Philadelphia: Lippincott–Raven Publishers; 1998:45–52.

28. Torg JS, Pavlov H, O'Neill MJ, et al. The axial load teardrop fracture. A biomechanical, clinical and roentgenographic analysis. *Am J Sports Med.* 1991;19:355–364.

29. Allen BL Jr, Ferguson RL, Lehmann TR, et al. A mechanistic classification of closed, indirect fractures and dislocations of the lower cervical spine. *Spine.* 1982;7:1–27.

30. Coelho DG, Brasil AV, Ferreira NP. Risk factors of neurological lesions in low cervical spine fractures and dislocations. *Arq Neuropsiquiatr.* 2000;58:1030–1034.

31. Razack N, Green BA, Levi AD. The management of traumatic cervical bilateral facet fracture-dislocations with unicortical anterior plates. *J Spinal Disord.* 2000;13:374–3781.

32. Wolf A, Levi L, Mirvis S, et al. Operative management of bilateral facet dislocation. *J Neurosurg.* 1991;75:883–890.

33. Maroon JC, Abla AA, Wilberger JI, et al. Central cord syndrome. *Clin Neurosurg.* 1991;37:612–621.

34. Wilberger JE, Abla A, Maroon JC. Burning hands syndrome revisited. *Neurosurgery.* 1986;19:1038–1040.

35. Torg JS, Guille JT, Jaffe S. Injuries to the cervical spine in American football players. *J Bone Joint Surg Am.* 2002;84:112–122.

36. Thomas BE, McCullen GM, Yuan HA. Cervical spine injuries in football players. *J Am Acad Orthop Surg.* 1999;7:338–347.

37. Torg JS, Naranja RJ Jr, Palov H, et al. The relationship of developmental narrowing of the cervical spinal canal to reversible and irreversible injury of the cervical spinal cord in football players. *J Bone Joint Surg Am.* 1996;78A:1308–1314.

38. Penning L. Some aspects of plain radiography of the cervical spine in chronic myelopathy: *Neurology.* 1962;12:513–519.

39. Zwimpfer TJ, Bernstein M. Spinal cord concussion. *J Neurosurg.* 1990;72:894–900.

40. Torg JS, Thibault L, Sennett B, et al. The pathomechanics and pathophysiology of cervical spinal cord injury. *Clin Orthop.* 1995;321:259–269.

41. Torg JS, Corcora TA, Thibault LE, et al. Cervical cord neuro-praxia: classification, pathomechanics, morbidity, and management guidelines. *J Neurosurg.* 1997;87:843–850.

42. Robertson WC Jr, Eichman PL, Clancy WG. Upper trunk brachial plexopathy in football players. *JAMA.* 1979;241:1480–1482.

43. Vegso JJ, Lehman RC. Field evaluation and management of head and neck injuries. *Clin Sports Med.* 1987;6:1–15.

44. Sallis RE, Jones K, Knopp W. Burners: offensive strategy for an underreported injury. *Physician Sportsmed.* 1992;20:47–55.

45. Scherping SC Jr. Cervical disc disease in the athlete. *Clin Sports Med.* 2002;21:37–47.

46. Banerjee R, Palumbo MA, Fadale PD. Catastrophic cervical spine injuries in the collision sport athlete. Part II. Principles of emergency care. *Am J Sports Med.* 2004;32:1760–1764.

47. Lawrence DW, Stewart GW, Christy DM, et al. High school football-related cervical spine injuries in Louisiana: the athlete's perspective. *J La State Med Soc.* 1997;149:27–31.

48. Cross KM, Serenelli C. Training and equipment to prevent athletic head and neck injuries. *Clin Sports Med.* 2003;22:639–667.

49. LaPrade RF, Schnetzler KA, Broxterman RJ, et al. Cervical spine alignment in the immobilized ice hockey player: a computed tomographic analysis of the effects of helmet removal. *Am J Sports Med.* 2000;28:800–803.

50. Banerjee R, Palumbo MA, Fadale PD. Catastrophic cervical spine injuries in the collision sport athlete. Part I. Epidemiology, functional anatomy, and diagnosis. *Am J Sports Med.* 2004;32:1077–1087.

51. Kleiner DM, Almquist JL, Bailes J, et al. *Prehospital Care of the Spine-injured Athlete: A Document from the Inter-Association Task Force for Appropriate Care of the Spine-Injured Athlete.* Dallas: National Athletic Trainers' Association; 2001.

52. DeLorenzo RA, Olson JE, Boska M, et al. Optimal positioning for cervical immobilization. *Ann Emerg Med.* 1996;28:301–308.

53. Donaldson WF, Lauerman WC, Heil B, et al. Helmet and shoulder pad removal from a player with suspected cervical spine injury. *Spine.* 1998;23:1729–1732.

54. Palumbo MA, Hulstyn MJ, Fadale PD, et al. The effect of protective football equipment on alignment of the injured cervical spine. *Am J Sports Med.* 1996;24:446–453.

55. Waninger KN, Richard JG, Pan WT, et al. An evaluation of head movement in backboard-immobilized helmeted football, lacrosse, and ice hockey players. *Clin J Sports Med.* 2001;11:82–86.

56. Aprahamian C, Thompson BM, Darin JC. Recommended helmet removal techniques in a cervical spine injured patient. *J Trauma.* 1984;24:841–842.

57. Gastel JA, Palumbo MA, Hulstyn MJ, et al. Emergency removal of football equipment: a cadaveric cervical spine injury model. *Ann Emerg Med.* 1998;32:411–417.

58. Metz CM, Kuhn JE, Greenfield ML. Cervical spine alignment in immobilized hockey players: radiographic analysis with and without helmets and shoulder pads. *Clin J Sports Med.* 1998;8:92–95.

59. Prinsen RKE, Syrotuik DG, Reid DC. Position of the cervical vertebrae during helmet removal and cervical collar application in football and hockey. *Clin J Sports Med.* 1995;5:155–161.

60. Peris MD, Donaldson WF III, Towers J, et al. Helmet and shoulder pad removal in suspected cervical spine injury: human control model. *Spine.* 2002;27:995–999.

61. Branfoot T. Motorcyclists, full-face helmets, and neck injuries: can you take the helmet off safely, and if so, how? *J Accid Emerg Med.* 1994;11:117–120.

62. Gallup DA, Boker JR, Hartz L. Helmet types and removal. *Emerg Med Serv.* 1981;10:91–92.

63. Hafen BQ, Karren KJ. Helmet removal. In: *Prehospital Emergency Care and Crises Intervention.* Englewood Cliffs, NJ: Prentice Hall; 1992:285–288.

64. National Collegiate Athletic Association. Guideline 4-F: guidelines for helmet fitting and removal in athletes. In: Schluep C, ed. *2003–2004 NCAA sports medicine handbook.* 16th ed. Indianapolis: National Collegiate Athletic Association; 2003:79–81.

65. Mower WR, Hoffman JR, Pollack CV, et al. Use of plain radiography to screen for cervical spine injuries. *Ann Emerg Med.* 2001;38:1–7.

66. Davidson RM, Burton JH, Snowise M, et al. Football protective gear and cervical spine imaging. *Ann Emerg Med.* 2001;38:26–30.

67. Hollenberg GM, Beitia AO, Tan RK, et al. Imaging of the spine in sports medicine. *Curr Sports Med Rep.* 2003;2:33–40.

68. Waeckerle JF, Kleiner DM. Protective athletic equipment and cervical spine imaging. *Ann Emerg Med.* 2001;38:26–30.

69. Veenema K, Greenwald R, Kamali M, et al. The initial lateral cervical spine film for the athlete with a suspected neck injury: helmet and shoulder pads on or off? *Clin J Sports Med.* 2002;12:123–126.

70. Hanson JA, Blackmore CC, Mann FA, et al. Cervical spine injury: a clinical decision rule to identify high-risk patients for helical CT screening. *AJR Am J Roentgenol.* 2000;174:713–717.

71. Li AE, Fisherman EK. Cervical spine trauma: evaluation by multidetector CT and three-dimensional volume rendering. *Emerg Radiol.* 2003;10:34–39.

72. Quencer RM, Nunez D, Green BA. Controversies in imaging acute cervical spine trauma. *AJNR Am J Neuroradiol.* 1997;18:1866–1868.

73. Schleehauf K, Ross SE, Civil ID, et al. Computed tomography in the initial evaluation of the cervical spine. *Ann Emerg Med.* 1989;18:815–817.

THE THORACOLUMBAR SPINE

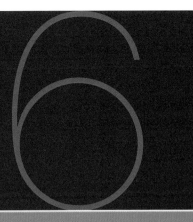

■ DONALD CHOW, MD, FRCSC, Dipl Sports Med

■ KEY POINTS

- The majority of thoracolumbar spine injuries arising from low-velocity sports usually are less catastrophic than some of the athletic injuries involving the more vulnerable cervical spine. The thoracic spinal cord is protected by the relatively larger and less mobile thoracic vertebra and rib cage.
- The sports physician may be required to assess for a spinal problem in situations varying from an unconscious athlete on a steep ski slope to a preparticipation examination in a sports medicine clinic.
- If the patient has any disorientation or depressed level of consciousness, the spine should be protected with a cervical collar and with log-roll precautions for the lumbar spine.
- The primary concern of a sports physician for a severely traumatized athlete should be to assess the airway once the cervical spine has been immobilized, followed by a rapid survey of respiratory and circulatory function.
- The initial investigation for the majority of athletes with thoracolumbar pain includes plain-film anteroposterior (AP) and lateral radiographs. The AP view will depict the sagittal alignment as well as congenital anomalies at the thoracolumbar and lumbosacral junction.
- The use of computed tomography (CT) enhances the evaluation of osseous structures. This modality better depicts the contents of the spinal canal and any small, lytic lesions in the bone.
- Magnetic resonance imaging (MRI) is now the modality of choice to evaluate soft tissues of the thoracolumbar spine. An MRI can depict nerve root compression with various degrees of disc degeneration, ligamentous injury, hematoma formation, and soft-tissue tumors.
- The use of blood work, such as a complete blood count (CBC), erythrocyte sedimentation rate (ESR), C-reactive protein, and blood cultures, may be useful to confirm and follow spinal infections.

Management of the athletic spine by the sports physician may vary from the preparticipation examination of an asymptomatic athlete to on-field stabilization of an acute injury in an athlete with neurological deficits. The majority of thoracolumbar spinal injuries may be relatively minor and self-limiting. The incidence of these injuries may vary greatly, ranging from 7% to 27% (1). Serious thoracolumbar injuries may be relatively rare; however, the fear of major neurological loss or mechanical instability may make return to play a difficult task for the athlete. Several comprehensive reference texts are available to the spinal specialist (2,3), so the goal of this chapter is to provide the sports physician with the basic tools for assessing and managing the athlete's spine.

■ ANATOMY AND BIOMECHANICS

A good background in the anatomy and clinical biomechanics of the thoracolumbar spine will provide the basis for understanding the mechanisms of injury and the principles of management (4). The majority of thoracolumbar spine injuries arising from low-velocity sports usually are less catastrophic than some of the athletic injuries involving the more vulnerable cervical spine. The thoracic spinal cord is protected by the relatively larger and less mobile thoracic vertebra and rib cage. The spinal cord has outer white matter, which contains the myelinated nerve fibers that form the ascending sensory and descending motor tracts. The gray matter within the spinal cord contains the cell bodies of the nerve roots and is vulnerable to irreversible damage if compressed. The cord ends with the conus medullaris at the level of the L1 vertebra. The spinal nerves, which arise from the cord, usually can re-innervate after a compression injury similar to a peripheral nerve after a compression injury. The cauda equina is a collection of spinal nerves below the level of the conus. The cord and spinal nerve roots are suspended in cerebrospinal fluid contained within the dura mater (5) **(Fig 6-1)**.

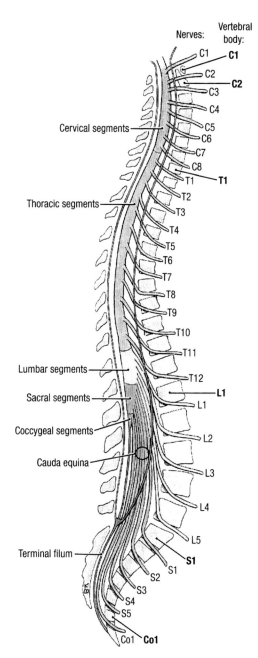

Fig 6-1. This sagittal section of the adult spine shows the conus of the spinal cord containing the sacral segments at the level of the L1 vertebra. The cauda equina is formed below this level by the remaining spinal nerves. (Adapted from Agur AMR, Dalley AF, eds. *Grants Atlas of Anatomy.* 11th ed. Baltimore: Lippincott Williams & Wilkins; 2005; with permission.)

The human body has 12 thoracic and 5 lumbar vertebrae, which consist of the vertebral bodies that support the trunk and the neural arch that protects the neural elements. Transverse and spinous processes act as lever arms to attach the stabilizing muscles and ligaments. The thoracic vertebrae provide attachment of the supporting rib cage at the costovertebral and costotransverse junctions. This buttressing by the "nonfloating" ribs on the neural arch may protect the posterior half of the thoracic vertebral body from axial loading, thus explaining the relatively small incidence of burst fractures in the T1 to T10 levels (6).

The vertebrae articulate with each other by means of a fibrocartilagenous intervertebral disc, two facets joints, and numerous intervertebral ligaments. The avascular disc has an outer, fibrous annulus and an inner, gelatinous nucleus pulposus. The end plates are hyaline cartilage that distributes the pressure of axial loading and allows the diffusion of nutrients into the discs from the adjacent subchondral bone. The disc annulus has innervation only to the outermost layer. This explains the asymptomatic, degenerative tears of the inner annulus layers and the severe pain and reflex spasms that occur with outer annular tears and disc herniations, even when the nerve roots are not being compressed.

The facets are synovial joints on the posterior neural arch that are oriented along the coronal plain in the thoracic spine and the more sagittal orientation in the lumbar spine. This orientation of the thoracic spine facets is more suitable for flexion and rotation, whereas the lumbar facets may allow relatively more flexion and extension as well as lateral bending (4).

The area of bone that connects the lamina to the pedicles and is between the superior and inferior facets is called, appropriately, the pars interarticularis. This portion of the bony neural arch forms the roof of the neural foramina for the exiting nerve roots. A defect in the pars is known as a spondylolysis. This pseudoarthrosis may become painful when compressed between the inferior facet of the cephalad vertebra and the superior facet of the vertebra caudal to the pars involved. The soft tissue of the defect may be a fibrous or a pseudosynovial junction, which may enlarge and compress the exiting nerve root beneath it.

Spondylolisthesis is the forward translation of one vertebral body over another. In athletes, it usually is related to a spondylolysis, because the supporting posterior facets have lost the osseous continuity with the vertebral body. In the older population, degeneration of the facets may lead to an unstable forward translation despite having an intact pars interarticularis. This condition is known as a degenerative spondylolisthesis.

The intervertebral ligaments and thoracolumbar musculature receive the least clinical attention but are the most responsible for providing dynamic stability (7). These well-innervated soft tissues also are the structures involved in the majority of symptomatic spinal injuries, which can be classified as minor strains or sprains. The anterior longitudinal ligament resists hyperextension, whereas the intraspinous,

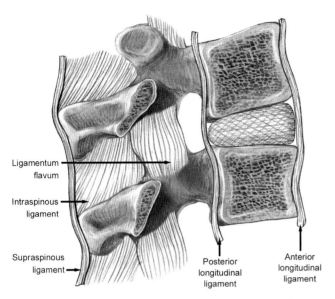

Ligamentum flavum

Intraspinous ligament

Supraspinous ligament

Posterior longitudinal ligament

Anterior longitudinal ligament

Fig 6-2. This sagittal section of the lumbar spine shows the two longitudinal ligaments against the body and the various ligaments between the neural arches. (Adapted from An HS, ed. *Principles and Techniques of Spinal Surgery.* Baltimore: Williams & Wilkins; 1998; with permission.)

TABLE 6-1	Checklist for the Diagnosis of Clinical Instability of the Thoracic and Lumbar Spine

Element involved	Points[a]
■ Anterior elements destroyed or unable to function	2
■ Posterior elements destroyed or unable to function	2
1. Disruption of the costovertebral articulations	1
■ Radiographic criteria	2
2. Sagittal plane displacement of >2.5 mm	
■ Relative sagittal plane angulation of >5°	2
■ Spinal cord or cauda equina damage	2
■ Dangerous loading anticipated	1

[a]A total of five or more points indicates instability.
Adapted from White AA, Panjabi MM. *Clinical Biomechanics of the Spine.* 2nd ed. Philadelphia:JB Lippincott Co; 1990; with permission.

supraspinous, and facet capsular ligaments resist hyperflexion forces. The ligamentum flavum, which connects the adjacent lamina, is unique in that it contains elastin fibers that allow a tension spring action instead of the fixed-length rope restraints of other ligaments containing predominately collagen fibers **(Fig 6-2)**.

The musculature of the thoracolumbar spine can be divided into three groups: superficial, intermediate, and deep. The superficial group consists of the trapezius, latissimus dorsi, the levator scapulae, and the rhomboids, and it helps to stabilize the shoulder girdles. The intermediate muscles of the back consist of the serratus posterior, both superior and inferior, that assist in respiration. The deep muscles of the spine are known as the intrinsic muscle; these include the erector spinae and transversospinalis group of muscles. The intrinsic muscles stabilize the local vertebrae for movements such as extension, rotation, and lateral bending of the spine.

The abdominal muscles of the thoracolumbar spine can be divided into the anterior and posterior groups. The abdominal muscles along with the diaphragm help to stabilize the mobile lumbar vertebra. The rectus abdominis, external oblique, internal oblique, and transversus abdominis muscles form the anterior lateral group. The posterior group includes the psoas, iliacus, and quadratus lumborum muscles (4).

White and Panjabi (7) have defined clinical instability as "the loss of ability of the spine under physiological loads to maintain relationships between vertebra in such a way that there is either damage or subsequent irritation to the spinal cord or nerve roots. In addition there is development of incapacitating deformity or pain due to structural changes." Clinical instability may result from trauma, degeneration, surgery, or pathologic disease, such as neoplastic or infectious conditions. White and Panjabi (7) also have developed a checklist for thoracic and thoracolumbar instability **(Table 6-1)**.

■ CLINICAL EVALUATION

History

The sports physician may be required to assess for a spinal problem in situations varying from an unconscious athlete in a difficult environmental presentation, such as on a steep ski slope or in a crumpled racecar, to a preparticipation examination in a sports medicine clinic. The history may be the most important aspect of a clinical evaluation; however, the details of the incident may have to come from on-field officials or other participants if the athlete has a diminished level of consciousness. Occasionally, the true story is not known until videotapes of the incident reveal the directions and magnitude of the force vectors to which the athlete's spinal column was exposed. Finding or excluding the presence of a spinal injury is much simpler in an alert, awake patient with no other distracting injuries. If the patient has any disorientation or a depressed level of consciousness, the spine should remain protected with a cervical collar and with log-roll precautions for the lumbar spine. Even when the athlete regains consciousness, he or she may have retrograde amnesia of the accident. The firm spine board used for immobilization during patient transport should be removed as soon as possible to prevent serious decubitus ulcers (8).

The most common symptom following injuries to the thoracolumbar spine is pain, and the details regarding the time of onset, quality, location, alleviating and aggravating factors must be obtained. Associated symptoms, such as weakness and numbness, are important in localizing the area of injury. Constitutional symptoms, such as fever, fatigue, unexplained weight loss, or night pain, may raise flags to investigate for other diseases, such as infections or neoplasms, that may lead to a pathologic fracture of the spine during a session of athletic activity. The location of the predominant pain will be important in determining the neurological status of the condition. The sharp, electrical pain shooting down a single dermatome to the toes is a classical sign of nerve root irritation and is known as radicular pain. When this occurs with nerve roots that form the sciatic nerve (L4, L5, and S1), the term **sciatica** is used. The term **femoratica** describes the radicular pain in the dermal distribution of the nerve roots forming the femoral nerve (L2, L3, and L4). If low back pain is predominant with a diffuse, dull aching in the buttocks or upper thighs, this is likely to be referred mechanical back pain. This type of referred pain is best explained to the patient using the classical left arm pain of coronary angina as an example. The converse also is possible, in that conditions in the hips, pelvis, and abdomen may refer pain to the thoracolumbar spine area. Renal calculi, which may be more common in athletes who experience frequent dehydration, may first present with episodes of severe lumbar pain.

The classical neurogenic claudication symptoms of leg pain and weakness brought on by activities with the spine extended and relieved with flexion of the lumbar spine are suggestive of spinal stenosis. Although this usually is seen in elderly patients, the problem also can occur in younger adults who have the underlying condition of shorter pedicles (commonly reported by radiologists as having congenital spinal stenosis). Typically, these athletes may have difficulty walking more than 100 meters yet will be able to bike more than 10 kilometers. The diagnosis can be confirmed with further spinal imaging.

The patient's past medical, surgical, family, and social history may be very helpful. This can be especially true in cases of nontypical mechanical or radicular back pain.

Myelopathy resulting from spinal cord compression or vascular insufficiency may involve little or no back pain. Neurological deficits, such as loss of balance, weakness, and numbness, may be the first symptoms. Painless myelopathy needs further investigation to check for neuropathies, such as multiple sclerosis, amyotrophic lateral sclerosis (Lou Gerhig's disease), or transverse myelitis.

Physical Examination

The examination of the injured athlete's spine initially may be limited to a cursory four-limb sensory and voluntary motor assessment along with palpation of the entire spine for point tenderness during the log-roll onto a spine board for transport off the playing field. The primary concern of the sports physician with a severely traumatized athlete should be to assess the airway with cervical spine immobilization, followed by a rapid survey of the respiratory and circulatory function. If immediately life-threatening injuries are identified, these are attended to as part of the primary survey (8). The initial palpation of the spine may reveal the location of point tenderness or a deformity, such as a step or gap between spinous processes. A definite motor or sensory level on the trunk indicates a significant spinal injury, and urgent transfer to a medical center capable of investigating and comprehensively treating spinal injuries is required. Gentle testing for hip flexion power with resistance to contraction of the iliopsoas muscle may lead to inhibition of pain if a thoracolumbar fracture is present.

Once a patient is off the field and stabilized hemodynamically, a detailed examination documenting the neurological status is required. The *Standard Neurological Classification of Spinal Cord Injury* form, which is available from the American Spinal Injury Association, provides easy charting of the patient's neurological status **(Fig 6-3)**.

The ambulatory athlete with a thoracolumbar spinal injury will include tests to determine neurological deficit, signs of nerve root irritation, any loss of spinal range of motion, and the exact location of tenderness, pain radiation, or paresthesias. Special maneuvers to reproduce the pain also should be carried out (2).

Inspection of the spine for deformity and loss of sagittal trunk balance can be carried out with the standing patient. Also, bruising, café-au-lait spots, or abnormal hair tufts may indicate other underlying pathology. Paraspinal spasm may cause a postural scoliosis and limitation of forward flexion because of pain. Structural scoliosis involves a rotation of the vertebrae and can be detected on the forward-bending test **(Fig 6-4)**. Range-of-motion testing may indicate the location of the source of pain. Pain with trunk extension may be an indication that pain is coming from the posterior elements of the neural arch, such as degenerative facets or a pars defect of spondylolysis. Severe reproduction of shooting pain with forward bending may indicate disc herniation. Reproduction of the shooting pain with straight-leg raise test (the Leseque test) along with the Cram test (positive bowstring sign) indicates irritation of the nerve roots that form the sciatic nerve. Similarly, the femoral nerve stretch test, which flexes the knee while the hip is extended, will detect irritation of the upper lumbar roots that form the femoral nerve **(Fig 6-5)**. The neurological examination will match the clinical relationships with deficits of sensory, reflexes, and motor testing to determine the neurological level. For example, the S1 level deficits will have numbness to the lateral aspect of the foot with weakness of the gastrocnemius muscle and either a diminished or absent Achilles tendon reflex. The patellar tendon reflex may be affected by L3 or L4 nerve root compression. It should be noted that the L5 nerve root does not have a reliable reflex test, but the tibialis posterior tendon may show a slight response (9). The Babinski test is useful in detecting myelopathy. However, it may be positive in patients with brain injury. The rectal examination may be used to check for sacral nerve root or sacral cord segment involvement. In a paraplegic patient

STANDARD NEUROLOGICAL CLASSIFICATION OF SPINAL CORD INJURY

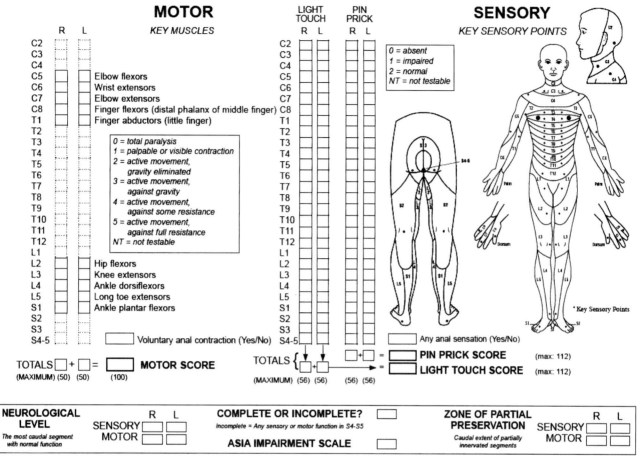

This form may be copied freely but should not be altered without permission from the American Spinal Injury Association.

2000 Rev.

A

B

ASIA IMPAIRMENT SCALE

☐ **A** = **Complete:** No motor or sensory function is preserved in the sacral segments S4-S5.

☐ **B** = **Incomplete:** Sensory but not motor function is preserved below the neurological level and includes the sacral segments S4-S5.

☐ **C** = **Incomplete:** Motor function is preserved below the neurological level, and more than half of key muscles below the neurological level have a muscle grade less than 3.

☐ **D** = **Incomplete:** Motor function is preserved below the neurological level, and at least half of key muscles below the neurological level have a muscle grade of 3 or more.

☐ **E** = **Normal:** motor and sensory function are normal.

CLINICAL SYNDROMES

☐ Central Cord
☐ Brown-Sequard
☐ Anterior Cord
☐ Conus Medullaris
☐ Cauda Equins

Fig 6-3. Standard Neurological Classification of Spinal Cord Injury form for documenting neurologic status. (From International Standards for Neurologic Classification of Spinal Cord Injury. Atlanta, GA: American Spinal Injury Association; 2002.

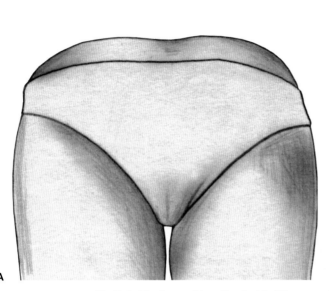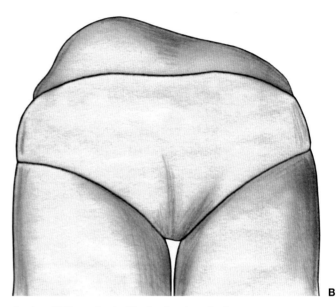

Fig 6-4. The forward-bending test in **(A)** a normal patient and **(B)** a patient with structural scoliosis, showing the rotational deformity in the rib prominence. (From An HS, ed. *Principles and Techniques of Spinal Surgery.* Baltimore: Williams & Wilkins; 1998; with permission.)

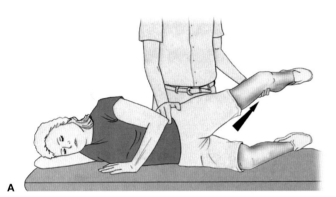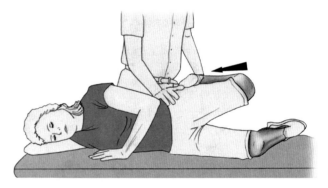

Fig 6-5. Femoral nerve stretch test. The patient is either on the side or is prone with the hip extended **(A)**, then flexion of the knee reproduces the femoral neuritis **(B)**. (From Watkins RG, ed. *The Spine in sports.* St. Louis: Mosby–Year Book; 1996; with permission.)

lacking both power and sensation in the lower extremities, the presence of perianal sensation and voluntary contraction of the anal sphincter is an indication of a partial cord injury known as sacral sparing.

Cauda equina syndrome occurs with the acute severe compression of the spinal nerves in the lumbar spinal canal and is characterized by bowel and bladder dysfunction. The loss of anal sphincter tone leads to fecal incontinence, and the loss of the bladder tone leads to urinary retention. Severe nerve root irritation signs are found on physical examination.

Examination of the pelvis, with particular attention to the sacroiliac and hip joints, should be performed. The range of motion of the sacroiliac joints is minimal because of the extensive fibrous anterior and posterior ligaments as well as the irregular articular surfaces. In relatively high-velocity impact trauma, the athlete may sustain unstable pelvic injuries that result in open-book or closed-book movement

of the iliac wings relative to each other. If vertical shifting of a hemipelvis is present, this indicates a major disruption of the posterior hemipelvis, which would be very unstable for any weight bearing on the ipsilateral limb. These severe pelvic injuries may be associated with spinal fractures as well as hemodynamic instability resulting from massive bleeding into the retroperitoneum.

Most injuries of the lumbar spine may involve tenderness over one or both sacroiliac joints, because the majority of the intrinsic muscles of the lumbar spinal area have their origin on the posterior capsule and/or the bones adjacent to the sacroiliac joints. Stressing of the sacroiliac joints to reproduce pain originating from within the joint can be done with the Patrick test, which involves flexion, abduction, and external rotation of the hip while counterpressure is applied on the contralateral iliac wing. When the sacroiliac joint is inflamed or unstable after trauma, reproduction of the severe

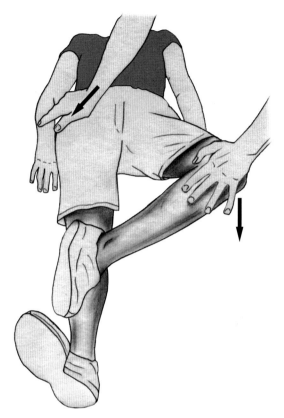

Fig 6-6. The Patrick test uses flexion, abduction, and external rotation of the hip, with the ankle on the opposite knee, while counter pressure is applied on the opposite iliac wing. (From Hoppenfeld S. *Physical Examination of the Spine and Extremities.* London: Appleton-Centurey-Crofts; 1976; with permission.)

low back pain can occur with this maneuver. In patients with inflammation of the hip joint itself, the pain that is produced by the Patrick test may be referred to the anterior hip and groin region **(Fig 6-6)**.

■ DIAGNOSTIC IMAGING

For the majority of athletes presenting with thoracolumbar pain, the initial investigation is still the plain-film anteroposterior (AP) and lateral radiographs. The AP view will depict the sagittal alignment as well as congenital anomalies at the thoracolumbar and lumbosacral junctions. The architecture of the bodies, spinous processes, transverse processes, lamina, and pedicles also are depicted on the AP radiograph. The absence of pedicles in the painful spine is highly suggestive of neoplasia. Sclerotic bone in the area of the pars interarticularis indicates a healing attempt of a pars defect of a spondylolysis. Sclerotic lesions with a painful scoliosis in an adolescent or young adult is suggestive of an osteoid osteoma, a type of benign bone tumor. Abnormal alignment of the spinous processes will indicate a rotatory or lateral translation of the vertebral bodies. If this occurs after a high-energy trauma, one may suspect a significant degree of instability of the

spine. Direct blows to the lumbar spine may result in fracturing of the transverse processes. The AP radiographs will depict a loss of vertebral height in both anterior compression fractures and burst fractures. The burst fractures may show a splaying of the pedicles. The interpedicular distance gradually increases with each caudal vertebra. A sudden widening followed by a narrower normal vertebra is a classical sign of a burst fracture, which involves both the anterior and posterior halves of the vertebral body.

If an athlete sustains a sudden deceleration with his or her abdomen against a narrow restraint, such as a lap seatbelt or a guardrail, the resulting flexion–distraction forces to the spinal column may lead to a vertical separation of the spinal processes seen on the AP radiograph. If the distraction force passes through the pedicles and the transverse processes, the fragments appear as double pedicles and double transverse processes. Any abrupt, lateral translation of the vertebral column at a fracture site on the AP radiograph would indicate a fracture dislocation injury pattern. These relatively unstable fracture dislocations have a high incidence of neurological deficits because of shearing force across the spinal canal. Additional imaging, such as magnetic resonance imaging (MRI), usually is indicated to further delineate the status of the neural elements.

The lateral radiograph will depict the thoracic kyphosis and the lumbar lordosis as well as the contour of the vertebral bodies and the intervertebral disc spaces. The lateral view also helps to differentiate the fracture types. Compression of the anterior half of the vertebral body with axial load but without collapse of the posterior vertebral body results in fractures known as anterior compression fractures. Loss of both anterior and posterior vertebral body height (relative to the vertebral bodies adjacent to the fracture) is indicative of a burst fracture pattern. The acute angular deformity can be measured on the lateral radiographs focused at the level of the injuries. Any translation forward or backward in the sagittal plane of an acutely fractured vertebrae is considered to be a fracture dislocation (6).

The standing lateral view is helpful in following the degree of spondylolisthesis to determine if the deformity has progressed. The disc space may show progressive narrowing in the formation of significant disc degeneration. These signs include sclerotic end plates with osteophytes and the vacuum sign within the disc. With multiple levels of disc degeneration and narrowing, the posterior elements will assume an extended position to maintain the trunk in an erect position. The subsequent abutting of the spinous processes have been labeled "kissing spines" (10). If a single level of severe disc degeneration is seen in an otherwise healthy-looking spine on the lateral radiograph, the possibility of an infective discitis should lead to further investigations, such as a labeled white-cell bone scan and further blood work for infection.

The oblique plain-film radiographs of the lumbar spine demonstrate the facets and pars interarticularis area. The posterior elements form a "Scottie dog" image. The presence of a radiolucent collar indicates a defect in the pars interarticularis known as a spondylolysis. If the collar is sclerotic, a healed pars defect or an undisplaced hypertrophic defect may be present. Further computed tomography (CT) scanning will confirm the presence of a defect. A bone scan may indicate if the defect is new or recently irritated.

The use of CT has greatly enhanced the evaluation of osseous structures. In fact, the development of the current classifications of thoracolumbar fracture was a direct result of this technology (6). The degree of canal compromise by bony fragments as well as determination of the angular deformities now can be done using the various reconstruction views of the spinal column from the CT data. Plain-film radiographs do not visualize the spinal canal contents or small lytic lesions in the bone as well as CT scans do (11).

In trauma cases, CT scans of the thoracolumbar spine may be derived from the trauma CT series of the thorax, abdomen, and pelvis; however, CT scans should not be used as a screening tool for the entire spine. The spinal CT study should focus on the area of clinical pathology as determined by the history, physical examination, plain-film radiographs, or bone scan (12). The use of CT is especially helpful in examining spondylolytic lesions in athletic patients (13), and use of sagittal and coronal CT reconstructions has made planar tomography obsolete in many centers.

Although CT initially was very useful in finding disc bulges and herniations, the use of MRI is now the investigation of choice to evaluate the soft tissues of the thoracolumbar spine. The MRI uses varying amounts of water content in various tissues to generate the different shades of gray that are seen in the image. This is in contrast to CT, which relies on the radiodensity of tissue to create the scans. Adjacent soft tissues, such as the disc annulus and the nucleus pulposis, may have similar radiodensities on a CT scan; however, the nucleus may contain much more water than the annulus, allowing definition of the nucleus material to be more precise. The presence of a new, extruded disc nucleus may have different prognostic and management factors compared with those of an old, bulging annulus or postoperative epidural scar tissue. The MRI can depict very well nerve root compression with various degrees of disc degeneration, ligamentous injury, hematoma formation, and soft-tissue tumors (14). The new, high-resolution MRI can depict extremely well details such as conjoint nerve roots and small syringomyelia. Intravenous gadolinium acts as an MRI contrast agent to delineate vascular scar tissue from avascular disc material in the canal.

The use of myelography followed by CT has decreased with the advent of the noninvasive MRI. In patients with contraindications to MRI, myelography followed by CT may be the best alternative for imaging of the neural canal. Contraindications to MRI may include having a cardiac pacemaker, an implanted neurostimulator, nonsurgical metal foreign bodies, older lens implants containing metal, as well as extreme claustrophobia.

Discography is used as a technique for pain reproduction to confirm the source of pain. The volume of dye, the pressure to dye insertion, and the containment or leakage of the dye from the nucleus will illustrate the competency of the annulus. Follow-up CT can demonstrate the location of annular tears and disc herniations.

Nuclear imaging, such as the use of bone scans and white cell–labeled scans, are very useful when fresh stress fractures, infections, or tumors are suspected in the athlete presenting with thoracolumbar spine pain. A focused radiographic correlation, usually with CT of any areas presenting with increased uptake, generally will confirm the diagnosis. The use of a more sophisticated imaging technique known as single-photon emission CT (SPECT) allows the data to be reformatted in axial images similar to CT scans. The SPECT image localizes well the presence of recently developed spondylolytic defects.

■ OTHER DIAGNOSTIC TOOLS

Blood work, such as a complete blood count (CBC), erythrocyte sedimentation rate (ESR), C-reactive protein, and blood cultures, may be useful to confirm and to follow spinal infections. A rheumatological workup may be ordered if seronegative spondyloarthropathy, such as ankylosing spondylitis, is suspected.

The use of electrophysiological testing can confirm a clinical diagnosis, such as multiple sclerosis or amyotrophic lateral sclerosis (Lou Gehrig's disease). These tests include nerve conduction studies and electromyelography, which may help to localize nerve injury lesions, to determine the extent of injury, and to assist in prognosis (15).

■ DECISION MAKING AND CLASSIFICATION

The primary decision that a sports physician must make when confronted with a thoracolumbar condition is whether the athlete has a significant mechanical and/or neurological instability requiring urgent or emergent stabilization. The spinal problem can be categorized initially as a high-energy injury, a low-energy injury, or even a no-injury situation. In turn, high-energy injuries to the spine may be classified as spinal traumatic conditions, whereas low-energy injuries and no-injury situations may be classified as nontraumatic back pain. The athlete presenting with major neurological deficits but with no history, or a very minor history, of trauma must raise a red flag the sports physician's mind. The suspicion of an underlying pathology, such as neoplasia, demyelinating disease, infection, or a peripheral neuropathy, must be investigated promptly.

High-energy injuries are more prevalent in sporting activities such as horseback riding, parachuting, motor sports, downhill skiing, and the recent popular extreme sports, such as skateboarding, snowboarding, freestyle skiing, and BMX cycling. Spinal fractures must be suspected when a first responder attends these fallen athletes, especially if the athlete has a depressed level of consciousness or other major distracting injury (16). Life-threatening injuries are dealt with first, and precautions to minimize movement of the spinal column are taken. Plain-film radiographs are obtained, and focused CT is performed on areas of clinical suspicion. Fractures are classified to assist with the treatment and prognostication and to help standardize research into therapeutic options. Ideally, the classification system should be simple yet precise as well as logical yet comprehensive (17).

The Denis classification system (18) was based on the analysis of plain-film radiographs and CT scans of spinal fractures. This system uses the concept of dividing the spine into three columns. The anterior column includes the anterior longitudinal ligament and the anterior half of both the vertebral body and the intervertebral disc. The middle column includes the posterior longitudinal ligament and the posterior half of both the vertebral body and the intervertebral disc. The posterior column comprises the elements of the posterior bony arch and the attached ligamentous structures. Denis classifies the types of injuries as compression fractures, burst fractures, seatbelt-type injuries, and fracture dislocations. The subgroups are based on the mechanism of injuries (Tables 6-2 and 6-3).

Another recent classification is the modified AO/ASIF classification of thoracolumbar injuries (17). This system describes three main types of fractures: compression, distractions, and multidirectional with translation. Each type is then subdivided into three groups as outlined in Table 6-4.

Follow up examinations for comparison with the baseline neurological assessment are done to ensure detection of any neurological deterioration. Consultation and transfer to a spinal surgery center for definitive care is carried out properly if the clinical examination and investigations reveal any significant fractures or neurological deficits (8). The differentiation by a sports physician between a burst fracture and a fracture dislocation is not as crucial to the patient as ensuring that the spinal fracture is promptly recognized and appropriately referred for definitive management.

If the injury has a relatively low-energy etiology or is recurrent in nature, the detailed history and physical examination will determine if any significant neurological instability exists. If a cauda equina syndrome or myelopathy is found, prompt referral for decompression management is required after appropriate emergent imaging. The majority of low-energy injuries are classified as soft-tissue injuries requiring no further investigation but, rather, prompt rehabilitation after a short period of rest to minimize the deconditioning and stiffening that occurs with inactivity. The soft tissues involved are the musculotendinous strains or ligamentous sprains with associated contusions, spasms, and inflammation. The pain usually is nonradiating, and the

TABLE 6-2	Denis Three-Column Classification: Basic Types of Spine Fractures and Their Mechanisms
Type of fracture	**Mechanism**
Compression	Flexion
A. Anterior	**A.** Anterior flexion
B. Lateral	**B.** Lateral flexion
Burst	
A. Both end plates	Axial load
B. Superior end plates	Axial load plus flexion
C. Inferior end plate	Axial load plus flexion
D. Rotation	Axial load plus rotation
E. Lateral Wedging	Axial load plus lateral flexion
Seatbelt	Flexion–distraction
Flexion–rotation	Flexion–rotation
Flexion–distraction	Flexion–distraction

From Denis F. The three-column spine and its significance in the classification of acute thoracic and lumbar spinal injuries. *Spine.* 1983;8:817–831; with permission.

TABLE 6-3	Denis Three-Column Classification: Basic Types of Spinal Fractures and the Columns Involved in Each

Type of fracture	Anterior column	Middle column	Posterior column
Compression	Compression	None	None or distraction in severe fractures
Burst	Compression	Compression	None or distraction
Seatbelt	None or compression	Distraction	Distraction
Fracture–dislocation	Compression and/or rotation/shear	Distraction and/or rotation shear	Distraction and/or rotation shear

From Denis F. The three-column spine and its significance in the classification of acute thoracic and lumbar spinal injuries. *Spine.* 1983;8:817–831; with permission.

TABLE 6-4	Modified AO/ASIF. Classification of Thoracolumbar Injuries		
Type	**Group**		
A. Compression	**1.** Impaction (wedge) **2.** Split (coronal) **3.** Burst (posterior ligaments intact)		
B. Distraction	**1.** Through the posterior soft tissue **2.** Through the posterior bony arch **3.** Through the anterior disc (extension spondylolysis)		
C. Multidirection with translation	**1.** Anteroposterior (dislocation) **2.** Lateral (lateral shear) **3.** Rotational (rotational burst)		

From Gertzbein SD. Spine update. Classification of thoracic and lumbar fractures. *Spine.* 1994;19:626–628; with permission.

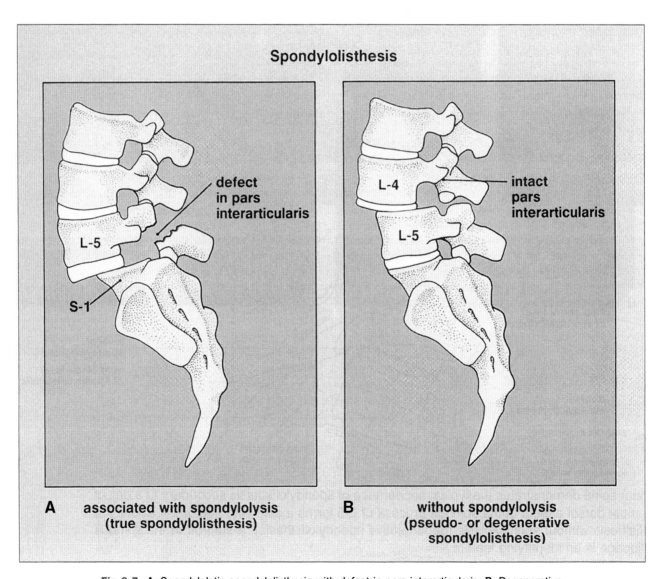

Fig 6-7. A: Spondylolytic spondylolisthesis with defect in pars interarticularis. **B:** Degenerative spondylolisthesis with intact pars interarticularis. (Adapted from Greenspan A. *Orthopedic Radiology: A Practical Approach.* Philadelphia: JB Lippincott Co; 1988; with permission.)

exact etiology generally is not identified. Predisposing factors include inadequate conditioning, poor posture, overuse activity, and improper mechanics for lifting or performing the sport.

The classification of these acute nontraumatic back pains developed by Dr. Hamilton Hall is based on the clinical presentation of the pain and has been very useful in planning initial treatment (19). The classification does not focus on the exact pathology of the pain generator but, rather, on the history and concordant physical examination. Hall's classification system involves four different patterns, and the nomenclature specifically does not assign blame to any one anatomical structure as the pain generator.

Pattern 1 pain is a back-dominant pain, usually in the low back or buttock, which is aggravated by activities that flex the thoracolumbar spine, such as bending forward or prolonged sitting. The physical examination reproduces the pain with forward flexion, and two pattern 1 subsets exist based on the physical examination. Pattern 1 fast responders have alleviation of the pain with spinal extension, whereas pattern 1 slow responders either have no change in the pain or have equal or more pain with spinal extension. The neurological exam is normal for pattern 1. This pain likely originates from the outer aspect of the annulus fibrosis or the adjacent ligaments or end plates, but the exact pathology is not required to start treatment.

Pattern 2 pain also is a back-dominant pain that is worsened with extension but not with flexion activities. On physical examination, the pain is reproduced with extension but is either improved or not affected by flexion. The neurological examination of pattern 2 pain also is normal. The pain generators likely are in the ligaments and joints of the posterior neural arch complex.

Pattern 3 pain is a leg-dominant pain that is aggravated by spinal movement. Patients also may report pain in the back. As with pattern 1 pain, pattern 3 patients fall into two subsets, as determined by the physical examination. Pattern 3 fast responders will have some reduction of their leg symptoms by specific postures. Pattern 3 slow responders will have no change in pain with some postures and will have aggravation of pain with other postures; no pain-alleviating postures found. The neurological examination will be positive for signs of nerve root irritation, such as straight-leg raising or the femoral nerve stretch test. Reproduction of the patient's pain will occur with testing for signs of nerve root irritation. The most common pain generator for pattern 3 patients is an acute herniated disc.

Pattern 4 pain is a leg-dominant pain that is intermittent and brought on by activities or postures that maintain spinal extension. Relief occurs soon after the patient changes his or her posture to a flexed position. The physical examination usually is negative for neurological deficits or signs of nerve root irritation. Classically, pattern 4 pain is a neurogenic claudication type of pain. The cause of this neurogenic claudication usually is spinal stenosis, but not all patients with spinal stenosis depicted on their radiographs will have

neurogenic claudication (19). In athletes with pattern 4 pain, the neurological claudication may have been associated with developmentally short pedicles, leading to a smaller, trefoil-shaped spinal canal.

Recurrent or persistent mechanical back pain in an athlete without signs of nerve root irritation should signal the possibility of a spondylolysis, which is considered to be a type of stress fracture of the pars interarticularis (20). Forward subluxation of the vertebral body over another vertebrae is termed a spondylolisthesis. A spondylolisthesis can occur without a pars defect in which the facets are severely degenerated, fractured, or surgically removed, resulting in segmental instability (Fig 6-7). The pars defect is the radiolucent "collar" on the "Scottie dog" that is seen on plain oblique radiographs of the lumbar spine (Figs 6-8 and 6-9). The incidence of spondylolytic spondylolisthesis varies in different sporting activities (Table 6-5).

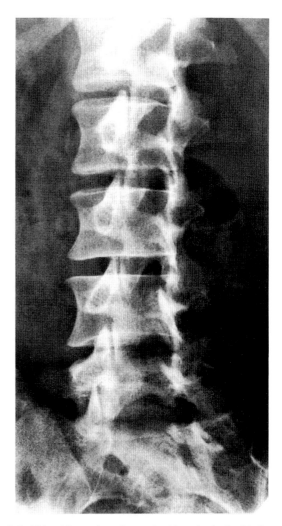

Fig 6-8. This oblique view shows the "Scottie dog" with the pars interarticularis defect of L5 compared to the intact L4 pars interarticularis. (From Greenspan A. *Orthopedic Radiology: A Practical Approach.* Philadelphia: JB Lippincott Co; 1988; with permission.)

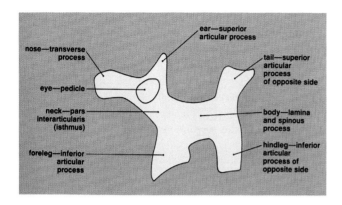

Fig 6-9. The anatomical elements of the "Scottie dog" as seen on oblique radiographs of the lumbar spine. (From Greenspan A. *Orthopedic Radiology: A Practical Approach.* Philadelphia: JB Lippincott Co; with permission.)

TABLE 6-5	Incidence of Spondylolisthesis in Sports
Type	**Incidence (%)**
Judo	12
Gymnastics	11–32.8
Wrestling	12–33
Weight lifting	15–36.2
Football	15.2–21
Diving	63.3

From Hambly MF, Wilstse LL, Peek RD. Spondylolisthesis. In: Watkins RG, ed. *The spine in sports.* St. Louis: Mosby–Year Book; 1996:157–163.

The grading of the degree of spondylolisthesis is based on the percentage of the AP diameter of the vertebral body that has slipped forward. Grade 1 slips are up to 25%, grade 2 spondylolisthesis are between 26% and 50%, and so on **(Fig 6-10)**. The clinical presentation usually is a pattern 2 type of pain; however, a pattern 3 nerve root irritation may develop because of compression of the nerve root exiting beneath the pseudoarthrosis of the pars defect. Imaging with CT delineates the defect well. If the injury was a high-energy hyperextension force, an acute fracture of the pars interarticularis may occur. The CT scan will show an acute fracture without sclerosis at the fracture site, and a bone scan will show increased uptake 2 to 3 days after the injury and lasting for 6 to 9 months. The defect may be unilateral on both the CT and the bone scan. A consultation with a sports medicine physician may take place several weeks to months after the initial onset, and by this time, the CT and bone scans may show sclerotic healing or pseudoarthrosis and the bone scan still shows some increased activity at the defect site.

If the bone scan is normal, then the defect or sclerotic area is an old lesion. Patient compliance with the rehabilitation scheme is the key to conservative treatment, and reassurance that the painful back can be controlled is paramount in obtaining compliance. The knowledge that these athletes cannot only perform with these defects but also excel usually provides a vote of confidence in the rehabilitation program. Surgery may be required if neurological signs develop or the pain becomes unremitting.

Nonpainful back conditions, such as scoliosis or kyphosis, can be followed by three foot-standing AP and lateral

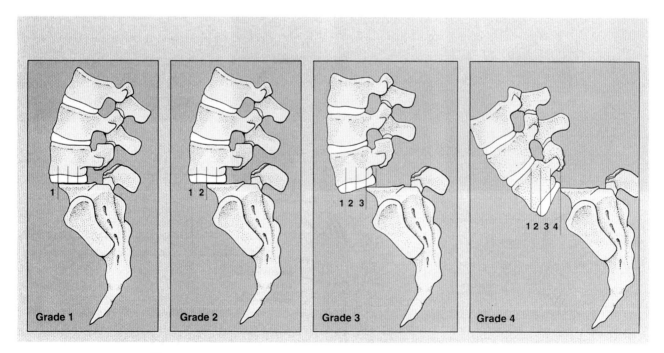

Fig 6-10. The grading of spondylolisthesis. (Adapted from Greenspan A. *Orthopedic Radiology: A Practical approach.* Philadelphia: JB Lippincott Co; 1988; with permission.)

radiographs using the Cobb technique of measuring the deformity. Most scoliotic deformities will not require surgical correction. Standard back-conditioning exercises specific to the sport in which athlete is participating will help to minimize the usual incidence of back pain that similar athletes with normal-contoured spines will experience. In adolescents, the deformity should be followed every 6 to 12 months clinically, with radiographs being obtained if the structural curve is increasing on the physical examination. Bracing may be recommended for moderate-sized curves if the adolescent athlete is still in the growth spurt. For curves that are rapidly progressing past 45° of scoliosis in a skeletally immature adolescent, surgical treatment to stabilize the curve may be warranted.

■ TREATMENT

Nonoperative

The goal of treatment is return to play by the athlete. Athletes can perform a certain level of activity if they have conditioned themselves both physically and mentally. Patient education is the key to obtaining compliance in the rehabilitation of the athlete. Although the pathology of a spinal problem appears to be complex, the athlete may better understand the rehabilitation of an injury if described using a simple analogy of a fractured long bone in the leg. The bone will heal with either nonoperative (casting) or operative (plate and screw fixation) treatment. Once the bone heals solid after a predetermined length of time, the athlete likely will have subpar performance on the first game day, with a much greater chance of injury to another part of the body, if he or she returns to a competitive sport without general fitness conditioning of the body as well as specific range-of-motion, strengthening, and proprioceptive training of the healed "lower limb." The bottom line is that the athlete will need intensive rehabilitation regardless of whether surgery is performed for the injury. The specifics for rehabilitation of the spine will be dealt with elsewhere in this book; however, the basic goals of regaining range of motion with stretching exercises, trunk strengthening of the paraspinal and abdominal muscle groups, as well as cardiovascular training for general fitness should be achieved before an athlete's return to sport-specific practice.

The use of narcotic analgesics should be limited to a few weeks after the traumatic injuries or surgery. Non-narcotic analgesia, either acetaminophen or nonsteroidal anti-inflammatory agents, should be the analgesia of choice during the rehabilitation period.

The use of physical modalities can help with pain relief during physical rehabilitation. The choice of one modality over another, however, is based solely on the athlete's response or lack thereof to the treatment modality. Remember that many nontraumatic pains are self-limiting and will heal despite the treatment modality. A back support can be used after an acute traumatic injury. A thoracolumbosacral orthosis

(TLSO) is basically a removable body cast, and it can be used for stable fractures of the thoracolumbar spine. For acute spondylolytic defects, a lumbosacral orthosis can be used until symptoms subside. Lumbosacral supports also have been used in nontraumatic conditions, and if it reduces the pain, such a support may be temporarily helpful. It does not act as body protection from recurrent injury, however, nor does it immobilize the spine during athletic activities. If the lumbar support gives an athlete the confidence to perform his rehabilitation exercises better, he should begin to wean himself out of the brace as soon as appropriate trunk reconditioning has been started.

Operative Treatment

Spinal surgery can be directed toward three main goals:

1 Decompression of compressed neural elements.
2 Realignment of a spinal deformity.
3 Stabilization of an unstable mobile segment.

Patient selection for surgery is extremely important to achieving favorable outcomes. The patient's expectations must be realistic and consider what type of rehabilitation he or she must endure postoperatively. Return to play in many cases is a bonus, and the successful outcome of the decompression of the spinal cord or spinal nerves may simply be the alleviation of pain with partial return of neural function. The athlete may wish for completely normal neurological function, but that surgical outcome may be unrealistic.

Indications and Timing

A positive correlation between the history, physical examination, and diagnostic imaging is needed to confirm the presence of a surgically amenable lesion. The patient must have failed conservative therapy or have a lesion that would have a poor outcome if left to nonoperative care, such as a cauda equina syndrome in a weight-lifting bodybuilder (21). Neurological deficits, especially those with progression of neurological sign, usually are an indication for urgent decompression; generally, these are associated with high-velocity spinal injuries. Emergent imaging, ideally with MRI, will delineate the location of the lesion. Decompression of the lesion should be done as soon as the patient is stable enough for an anaesthetic and surgery. Resuscitation of any life-threatening respiratory or cardiac injuries must be done first, because a decompressed spinal cord with inadequate perfusion will still do poorly.

Decompression of individual nerve roots without cord or cauda equina compression can be done on an elective basis if nonoperative treatment has failed. Despite the minimally invasive incisions being used to protect the soft-tissue structures or the dramatic pain relief postoperatively, the athlete must comply with the rehabilitation program to be fit enough for return-to-play consideration.

Indications for spinal realignment procedures of the unstable spine include burst fractures and fracture dislocations. In some cases, realignment of the spine will decompress the spinal canal without need for the surgical removal of bone from the canal. The need to reduce a spondylolisthesis is not as important as stabilization of the spinal segment to prevent the defect from progressing. The same is said for scoliosis surgery in adults, in whom the goal is to prevent further deformity. Partial correction of the scoliotic deformity with instrumentation is an added benefit. Except in the cases of severe neurological deficits, the need for realignment alone usually is an elective consideration.

Stabilization with bony fusion of a spinal mobile segment is unphysiological, in that the end result is, hopefully, a complete loss of motion. If the unstable motion is causing intermittent nerve compression and unremitting mechanical back pain refractory to nonoperative treatment, the stiff, painfree segment would be ideal. The athlete must realize that all spinal surgery will have some pain from the soft-tissue dissection, and as minimally invasive as the newer surgical techniques are, muscle stripping and dissection are still incurred in every fusion. The patient may want a "quick fix," but the natural history of a slow responder with patterns of mechanical or nerve irritation pain may still resolve nonsurgically if given adequate time. The length of rehabilitation can be estimated from the prognostic factors that are found during the early assessments.

■ TECHNIQUES

The details of spinal surgery can fill entire textbooks (3–24), and the details of these surgical techniques are beyond the scope of this chapter. Major changes in techniques are constantly and rapidly evolving, and dissection has become extremely "respectful" of the soft tissues that are encountered. The small-incision trend of arthroscopy is now entering the spinal surgery environment. Adequate decompression, prevention of further malalignment, and obtaining a solid fusion are still the basic goals of spinal surgery intervention. The number of mobile segments needing to be immobilized has decreased, however, as the use of the Harrington rods and hooks has given way to the stronger pedicle screws and rod systems. Now, most fracture surgeries will fuse only the mobile segments that are immediately involved with the unstable fractured vertebrae, compared with the historical rod and hook placements of three levels above and three levels below. The use of bone graft substitutes, such as coraline hydroxyapatite, in fusions has reduced the incidence of chronic pain at the posterior iliac crest graft site from approximately 20% to 0%. The dissection involving the bone graft donor site would increase intraoperative blood loss and injury to local sensory nerves. As well, stripping of a portion of the gluteus maximus, which later would have to reattach to the raw cancellous iliac crest, will leave some painful dysfunction,

at least temporarily in the hip extensors. The use of electrocautery, autologous blood banking preoperatively, and the Cell-Saver has decreased the need for transfusions during spinal surgeries.

■ COMPLICATIONS

When obtaining consent for spinal surgery, the possibilities of complications must be discussed with the athlete. Again, the details of the complications of spinal surgery could fill a book (25), and they are beyond the scope of this chapter. In general, however, the possible complications include wound infections, postoperative bleeding that requires transfusion, nonunion of the fusion site, loosening or breaking of the spinal instrumentation (if used), chronic pain despite adequate decompression or solid fusion, nerve root or spinal cord injury intraoperatively, excessive epidural scar tissue formation, arachnoiditis, and perianesthetic risks. If a discotomy is carried out, the patient has a risk of disc reherniation (because not all of the disc nucleus is removed), recurrent spinal stenosis above or below the level of decompression, or accelerated mobile segment degeneration above and below a fusion segment, leading to recurrent mechanical pain or other recurrent leg-dominant pain.

■ CONCLUSIONS AND FUTURE DIRECTIONS

Every sport has its own kinetics applied to the spine, ranging from the twisting of golfing to the possible sudden deceleration of motor sports. In his book on the spine in sports, Watkins (2) provides individual chapters for 29 different sports. Special considerations, especially regarding the rehabilitation for the athlete's individual sport, must be made to ensure that the treating physician and the athlete have a realistic set of outcome goals. The sports physician must understand the basic principles of resuscitation of spinal injuries and the need for prompt initial referral to a spinal surgical center for treatment if significant neurological deficits and/or major mechanical instability are found. Prompt rehabilitation and reassurance is required for nontraumatic back pain. Elective referral of the patient with spinal deformities and minor instabilities to a spine specialist may assist in patient education and planning of elective surgery for conditions not responding to adequate physical rehabilitation.

In the future, spinal surgery may be performed with biological materials only and using minimally invasive techniques. Will areas of instability be stabilized with an injection of a biological "bone glue"? Studies concerning replacement discs are underway, with an emphasis on repairing mobility rather than on fusion for significant instability. As sports become more extreme, the care of the spine in the athlete also becomes more complex. The sports physician must watch for differing injury patterns and, hopefully, help to develop preparticipation conditioning programs as well as safety standards to prevent major injuries of the spine in addition to treating the injured spine appropriately.

■ REFERENCES

1. Watkins RG. Lumbar spine injuries. In: Watkins RG, ed. *The spine in sports.* St. Louis: Mosby–Year Book; 1996:137–145.
2. Watkins RG, ed. *The Spine in Sports.* St. Louis: Mosby–Year Book; 1996.
3. An HS, ed. *Principles and Techniques of Spinal Surgery.* Baltimore: Williams & Wilkins; 1998.
4. An HS. Anatomy of the spine. In: An HS, ed. *Principles and techniques of spinal surgery.* Baltimore: Williams & Wilkins; 1998:1–30.
5. Agur AMR, Dalley AF, eds. *Grants Atlas of Anatomy.* 11th ed. Baltimore: Lippincott Williams & Wilkins; 2005.
6. Denis F. The three-column spine and its significance in the classification of acute thoracic and lumbar spinal injuries. *Spine.* 1983;8:817–831.
7. White AA, Panjabi MM. *Clinical Biomechanics of the Spine.* 2nd ed. Philadelphia: JB Lippincott Co; 1990.
8. American College of Surgeons Committee on Trauma. *Advanced Trauma Life Support for Doctors. Student Course Manual.* 7th ed. Chicago: American College of Surgeons; 2004.
9. Hoppenfeld S. *Physical Examination of the Spine and Extremities.* London: Appleton-Centurey-Crofts; 1976.
10. Hazlett J. Kissing spine. *J Bone Joint Surg Am.* 1964;46: 1368–1369.
11. Hellstrom M, Jacobsson B, et al. Radiographic abnormalities of the thoracolumbar spine in athletes. *Acta Radiol.* 1990;31:127–132.
12. Rosenthal DF, Manken HJ, Bauman RA. Musculoskeletal application for computed tomography. *Bull Rheum Dis.* 1983;33:1.
13. Rothman SL, Glenn WJ Jr. CT multiplanar reconstruction: 253 cases of lumbar spondylolysis. *AJNR Am J Neuroradiol.* 1984;5:81.
14. Haughton VM. MR imaging of the spine. *Radiology.* 1988; 166:297.
15. Press JM, Young JL, Herring SA. Electrodiagnostic evaluation of spinal problems. In: Watkins RG, ed. *The spine in sports.* St. Louis: Mosby–Year Book; 1996:61–70.
16. Stanislas MJ, Latham JM, Porter KM, et al. A high-risk group for thoracolumbar fractures. *Injury.* 1998;29:15–18.
17. Gertzbein SD. Spine update. Classification of thoracic and lumbar fractures. *Spine.* 1994;19:626–628.
18. Denis F. Spinal instability so defined by the three-column spine concept in acute spinal trauma. *Clin Orthop.* 1984;189:65.
19. Wilson L, Hall H, McIntosh G, et al. Intertester reliability of a low back pain classification system. *Spine.* 1999;24:248–254.
20. Hambly MF, Wilstse LL, Peek RD. Spondylolisthesis. In: Watkins RG, ed. *The spine in sports.* St. Louis: Mosby–Year Book; 1996:157-163.
21. Fortin JD. Weightlifting. In: Watkins RG, ed. *The spine in sports.* St. Louis: Mosby–Year Book; 1996:484–498.
22. Hitchon PW, Traynelis VC, Rengachary S, eds. *Techniques in Spinal Fusion and Stabilization.* New York: Thieme Medical Publishers; 1995.
23. Marguilies JY, Aebi M Farcy JP, eds. *Revision Spine Surgery.* St. Louis: Mosby; 1999.
24. Torrens MJ, Dickson RA. *Operative Spinal Surgery.* London: Churchill Livingstone; 1991.
25. Garfin S, ed. *Complications of Spine Surgery.* Philadelphia: Williams & Wilkins; 1988.

FUNCTIONAL SPINAL REHABILITATION

LORRAINE HENDRY, BSc(PT), MCPA, FCAMT

■ KEY POINTS

- Low back pain affects up to 80% of the population at least once in their lifetime.
- The term core stabilization is used to describe the management of low back pain through training of the deep stabilizing muscles of the trunk to protect the spine and to allow improved motor control of the spine.
- The spinal stability system features passive, active, and control subsystems, each of which is interdependent but capable of compensating for a deficit in another (1).
- The multifidus is the most medial and largest of the paraspinal muscles. It has an origin and insertion from one vertebra to another within the lumbar spine and between the lumbar and sacral vertebrae.
- The anterior, middle, and posterior layers of the thoracolumbar fascia create an envelope for the muscles of the lumbar spine.
- The transversus abdominis is the deepest muscle of the abdominal muscle complex. It originates from the lateral one-third of the inguinal ligament, the anterior two-thirds of the inner lip of the iliac crest, the lateral raphe of the thoracodorsal fascia, and the internal aspect of the lower six costal cartilages interdigitating with the costal fibers of the diaphragm.
- Pain can be significantly decreased and functional ability increased with lumbar stabilization exercises.
- Proprioception may be assisted by postural retraining and stabilization exercises in neutral postures progressing to unstable surfaces in functional movements.
- The supine active straight-leg raise test (ASLR) is a valid tool for assessing the load transfer between the trunk and lower extremities. When functioning normally and with adequate stability, the patient should be able to raise his or her straight leg from the table without a great deal of effort and without movement of the pelvis in relation to the thorax and lower extremity. This test combines observations by the patient and the doctor.
- Functional exercise programs should be directed towards retraining the motor control in as many potential lumbar spine stabilizers, while in erect weight-bearing postures to stimulate day-to-day activities.

Low back pain is a common complaint and reportedly affects up to 80% of the population at least once in their lifetime (2). A recurrence of low back pain or chronic low back pain is seen in 10% to 40% of this population (2,3). "Eighty-five percent of low back pain patients are classified as 'non-specific' because a definitive diagnosis cannot be achieved by current radiological methods" (2).

The terms core stabilization and motor control have been used to describe the management of low back pain through training of the deep stabilizing muscles of the trunk to protect the spine and to allow improved movement of the spine in functional tasks (4,5).

Impairment to the lumbopelvic and hip regions requires integration and coordination of treatment approaches to allow effective load transfer between the lower extremity, the trunk, and the upper extremity. There must be a clear understanding of the causes of dysfunction when evaluating the lower quadrant, including the lumbar spine, pelvis, and lower extremity, to determine the causes of dysfunction. Optimal function requires both mobility and stability (6) in the joints and muscles of the lumbar spine and pelvis. A lack of identification of the areas of dysfunction, and lack of follow-up with appropriate treatment, may lead to recurrence of low back pain in both daily and sporting activities. Athletes require coordination, strength, endurance, and flexibility between the trunk and extremities to be effective in achieving rapid and precise movements. Research has focused on the factors contributing to low back pain and on the treatment used to improve stability through improved motor control of the lumbar spine. This chapter reviews the literature concerning stabilization of the lumbar spine and current exercise programs.

■ DEFINITIONS

Panjabi (5) introduced a spinal stability system that includes passive, active, and control subsystems. The passive subsystems involve the osteoarticular and ligamentous components, which provide restraint primarily in the end range of motion. The active subsystems are of great interest in the research and clinical fields for looking at the role of muscle and fascia and their ability to control the mechanical components of the spine segments. The control subsystems introduce neurological function as well as its effect and timing on motor control. The role of the neural subsystem is to coordinate feedback from the active and passive subsystems, with appropriate levels of muscular contraction to balance against destabilizing forces between the subsystems (7). The emotional or psychological subsystem (8) has been added to account for psychological and social factors influencing the patients' pain and "their capacity to increase the central nervous system mediated drive of pain via the forebrain" (9–11).

The passive, active, and control subsystems are interdependent, with each one being capable of compensating for a deficit in another (1,5,12). Back pain may be related to a deficit in control of one subsystem and to an inability of the remaining subsystems to compensate for this deficit (4). A deficit in one subsystem may produce back pain as a result of decreased control of a spinal segment, with compression of neural and articular structures (1) **(Fig 7-1)**.

Panjabi (1) described articular motion in the lumbar spine with the terms neutral and elastic zones: "The neutral zone is a region of intervertebral motion around the neutral posture where little resistance is offered by the passive spinal column" (1). The elastic zone is the part of the motion "from the end of the neutral zone up to the joint's physiological limit" (1). He used the concept of a ball in a bowl to describe the neutral and elastic zones. The ball resting in the center of the bowl represents the neutral zone within a joint that has a higher degree of laxity **(Fig 7-2)**. As the ball rolls toward the ends of the bowl, increasing resistance from the soft tissue is seen, as at the end of physiological range of motion in a joint with a stiffening effect. "The neutral zone of the spinal segment is dependent on the muscles for control and proprioceptive feedback" (13). Research indicates that the "lumbar spine's vulnerability to instability is greatest

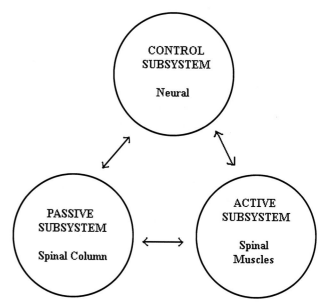

Fig 7-1. Spinal stability systems. (Adapted from Panjabi MM. The stabilizing system of the spine. Part II. Neutral zone and instability hypothesis. *J Spinal Disord.* 1992;5:390–396.)

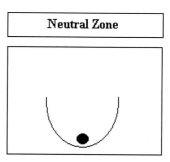

Fig 7-2. Neutral zone. (Adapted from Hodges PW. Science of stability: clinical application to assessment and treatment of segmental spinal stabilization for low back pain. Course Notes; 2000.)

in the neutral zone of motion, under low load conditions and where motor control of the spine is compromised" (14). The risk of injury in the elastic zone increases as the motor system relaxes to allow passive systems to provide restraint in the spinal segment (13).

Hypomobility is described as restricted movement within the articular surfaces of a joint. Hypermobility is described as excessive movement within a joint that is beyond a normal degree of movement before the stabilizing structures provide restraint.

According to Panjabi (1), "Clinical instability is a significant decrease in the capacity of the stabilizing system to maintain the intervertebral neutral zone within physiological limits so that there is no neurological dysfunction, no major deformity and no incapacitating pain." He describes clinical instability as a lack of motor control within the neutral zone (1). Motor control also has been described as "the way in which a task is performed. Altered motor control describes the manner by which the movement or posture has changed" (13). Clinical instability at a segmental level is seen with increased movement in the neutral zone and excessive motion at the end of range (15). "Instability of the lumbar motion segments is closely related to deep muscles which support and control intersegmental movement during functional tasks" (15). The size of the neutral zone may increase with disc degeneration, spinal injury, or poor muscle control, which will all affect stability (1).

Bergmark (16) introduced the concept of two muscle classifications. These are the local and global stabilizing systems.

The local muscle groups provide specific segmental spinal stability through their attachment directly to the lumbar vertebrae. These muscles provide control of intersegmental motion and position of the lumbar spine (16). This group would include the transversus abdominis (TrA) (6,17,18), multifidus (19,20), and internal oblique (fiber insertion into thoracolumbar fascia) (16,21). Additional studies have found that the pelvic floor muscles (6,18,22–24), the diaphragm (18,25,26), and the intertransversarii, interspinales, longissimus thoracis pars lumborum, iliocostalis lumborum pars lumborum, and medial fibers of the quadratus lumborum (16) also are included as local stabilizing muscles. The TrA and internal oblique muscles provide stability for the lumbar spine through the thoracolumbar fascia along with the control of the intra-abdominal pressure. (27–31) **(Fig 7-3)**.

The global muscle groups provide large trunk movements and general trunk stability through their attachments between the thorax and pelvis and/or pelvis and legs, with no specific attachment to the lumbar spine (27). This group would include the rectus abdominis, external oblique, and thoracic erector spinae muscles, longissimus thoracis pars thoracis, iliocostalis lumborum pars thoracis, quadratus lumborum lateral fibers, and internal oblique (16). The global muscle group also has been described as being divided into four slings between the thorax, pelvis, and lower extremity (6,32–34). The posterior oblique sling would include the latissimus dorsi and the gluteus maximus via the thoracolumbar fascia. The anterior oblique sling would include the external oblique, the anterior abdominal fascia, the contralateral internal oblique abdominal muscle, and adductors of the lower extremity. The longitudinal sling involves connections between the peroneii, the biceps femoris, the sacrotuberous ligament, the deep lamina of the thoracodorsal fascia, and the erector spinae. The lateral sling includes the gluteus medius and minimus, the tensor fascia latae, and the lateral stabilizers of the thoracopelvic region (6,32–34). The integration between and within these slings provides stability and effective transfer of loads between the spine and the extremities. The local stabilizing muscle system sometimes is referred to in the literature as the inner unit, with the global stabilizing system being referred to as the outer unit **(Fig 7-4)**.

A significant neurophysiological difference exists in the timing of the contraction of these two local and global muscular systems. Motor control refers to the "timing of specific muscle action and inaction" (6). When loads are predictable, the local system contracts in anticipation before the movement, regardless of the direction of movement (17–20, 35,36). The global system contracts later and is direction dependent (6,18,37,38). Local muscles are controlled independently of the global system (4,12).

With low-load situations, the local muscle system is associated with low levels of intra-abdominal pressure and relaxed respiration. Activity is seen in the muscles of the pelvic floor, the transverse abdominal wall, the psoas, and the multifidus. The psoas acts synergistically with the lumbar multifidus to control the position of the pelvis on the hips and lordosis (13). The global muscle system is involved in posture and initiation of movement and is associated with low levels of intra-abdominal pressure and relaxed respiration (13). With high-load situations, the local and global systems co-contract, in association with higher levels of intra-abdominal pressure, to act as a splint and to restrict the movement of the pelvis and thorax (13).

Lee (6) has focused on the local system of the lumbopelvic region, including the pelvic floor, diaphragm, multifidus, and TrA, in looking closely at the evaluation and treatment of pelvic girdle dysfunction. Sapsford et al. (39) reported that "in healthy subjects, voluntary activity in the

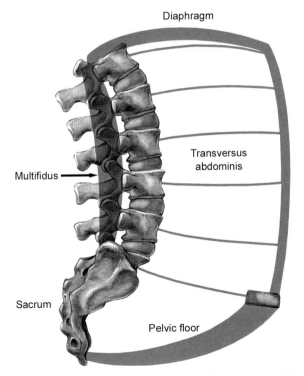

Diaphragm

Transversus abdominis

Multifidus

Sacrum

Pelvic floor

Fig 7-3. The local system of the lumbopelvic region consists of the muscles of the pelvic floor, the transversus abdominus, and the diaphragm as well as the deep fibers of the multifidus. (From Lee D. *The Pelvic Girdle: An Approach to the Examination and Treatment of the Lumbopelvic-hip Region.* 3rd ed. New York: Churchill Livingstone; 2004; with permission.)

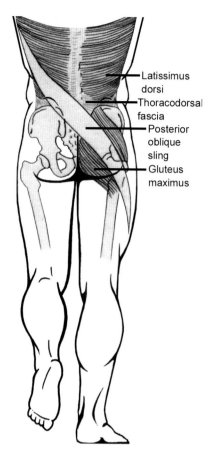

Fig 7-4. The posterior oblique sling of the global system includes the latissimus dorsi, the gluteus maximus, and the intervening thoracodorsal fascia. (From Lee D. *The Pelvic Girdle: An Approach to the Examination and Treatment of the Lumbopelvic-hip Region.* 3rd ed. New York: Churchill Livingstone; 2004; with permission.)

abdominal muscles results in increased pelvic floor muscle activity." Difficulties in establishing a stable base within the pelvic girdle will affect stabilization strategies of the lumbar spine and, therefore, need to be addressed concurrently.

◼ ANATOMY OF THE LUMBAR BACK MUSCLES

Multifidus

The multifidus is the most medial and largest of the paraspinal muscles. It has an origin and insertion of vertebra to vertebra attachments within the lumbar spine and between the lumbar and sacral vertebrae (12,40).

The multifidus is composed of repeating fascicles, which originate from the laminae and spinous processes of the lumbar vertebrae and insert in a caudal direction. The shortest (deepest) fascicles (laminar fibers) of the multifidus arise from the vertebral laminae and insert on the mamillary process of the vertebrae two levels caudal. The L5 fibers insert on an area of the sacrum just above the first dorsal

sacral foramen (12). "The other fascicles arise from the spinous process and are longer than the laminar fibers. Each lumbar vertebra gives rise to one group of fascicles which overlap those of the other levels. The fascicles from a given spinous process insert onto mamillary processes of the lumbar and sacral vertebrae three, four, or five levels inferiorly. The longest fascicles, from L1, L2, and L3, have some attachment to the posterior superior iliac spine" (12). The fascicles in each group diverge caudally to assume separate attachments to mamillary processes, the iliac crest, and the sacrum. Some of the deeper fibers of these fascicles attach to the capsules of the zygapophyseal joints next to the mamillary process. "The attachment of the muscles of the thoracolumbar fascia represents a raphe separating the multifidus from the gluteus maximus muscle" (41) **(Fig 7-5)**.

Moseley et al. (19) reported that the deep and superficial fibers of multifidus are "differentially active from single and repetitive movements of the arm." They concluded that the "superficial multifidus contributes to the control of spine orientation, and that the deep multifidus has a role in controlling intersegmental motion" (19). Biomechanical research by Wilke et al. (42) found that multifidus acts to increase lumbar segmental stability by increasing the stiffness in the motion segment. Multifidus works in co-contraction with the transversus abdominus to control the neutral zone (13).

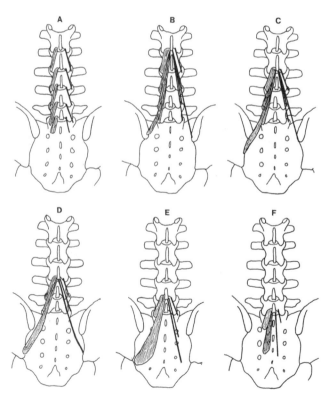

Fig 7-5. The component fascicles of multifidus. **A:** The laminar fibers of the multifidus. **B–F:** The fascicles from the L1 **(B)**, L2 **(C)**, L3 **(D)**, L4 **(E)**, and L5 **(F)** spinous processes. (From Bogduk N. *Clinical Anatomy of the Lumbar Spine and Sacrum.* 3rd ed. New York: Churchill Livingstone; 1997; with permission.)

Thoracolumbar Fascia

The thoracolumbar fascia has three layers—anterior, middle, and posterior—creating an envelope for the muscles of the lumbar spine. The anterior layer originates from the anterior surfaces of the transverse processes of the lumbar spine and intertransverse ligaments, and it covers the anterior surface of the quadratus lumborum. The middle layer is attached to the tips of the lumbar transverse processes and intertransverse ligaments before it passes behind the quadratus lumborum. The posterior layer "arises from the lumbar spinous processes in the middle posteriorly and wraps around the back muscles to blend with the outer layers of the thoracolumbar fascia" (43). The posterior layer consists of two laminae: superficial which are oriented in a caudomedial direction and deep layer which are oriented in a caudolateral direction (43). The three layers, particularly the middle and posterior layers, blend laterally to the quadratus lumborum to form the lateral raphe (43). The posterior layer provides indirect attachment for the TrA to the lumbar spine through the lateral raphe (43). The thoracolumbar fascia gives attachment to the middle fibers of the TrA, the posterior fibers of the internal oblique, the latissimus dorsi, the gluteus maximus, the lower trapezius, and the hamstrings (13) **(Figs 7-6 and 7-7)**.

When the TrA contracts, tension of the thoracolumbar fascia increases via the lateral raphe (30,43). Pressure in the abdominal cavity also increases (28).

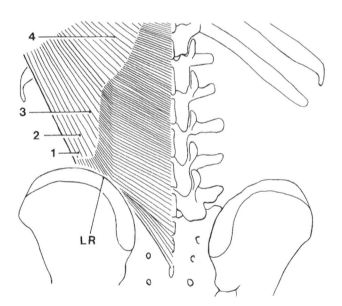

Fig 7-6. The superficial lamina of the posterior layer of thoracolumbar fascia. **1:** Aponeurotic fibers of the most lateral fascicles of latissimus dorsi insert directly into the iliac crest. **2:** Aponeurotic fibers of the next most lateral part of latissimus dorsi glance past the iliac crest and reach the midline at the sacral levels. **3:** Aponeurotic fibers from this portion of the muscle attach to the underlying lateral raphe (*LR*), then deflect medially to reach the midline at the L3 to L5 levels. **4:** Aponeurotic fibers from the upper portions of latissimus dorsi pass directly to the midline at thoracolumbar levels. (From Bogduk N. *Clinical Anatomy of the Lumbar Spine and Sacrum.* 3rd ed. New York: Churchill Livingstone; 1997; with permission.)

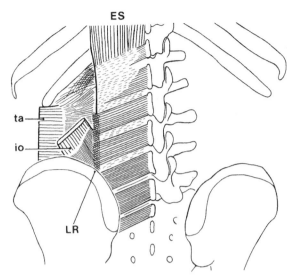

Fig 7-7. The deep lamina of the posterior layer of thoracolumbar fascia. Bands of collagen fibers pass from the midline to the posterior superior iliac spine to the lateral raphe (*LR*). Those bands from the L4 and L5 spinous processes form alarlike ligaments that anchor these processes to the ilium. Attaching laterally to the lateral raphe are the aponeurosis of transversus abdominis (ta) and a variable number of the most posterior fibers of the internal oblique (io). ES, erector spinae. (From Bogduk N. *Clinical Anatomy of the Lumbar Spine and Sacrum.* 3rd ed. New York: Churchill Livingstone; 1997; with permission.)

Richardson et al. (12) have suggested that the TrA contributes to support the abdominal contents. They also have suggested that it provides contributions to respiration and to movements in the lumbar spine of extension and rotation.

Transversus Abdominis

The TrA is the deepest muscle of the abdominal muscle complex, with the internal and external oblique being more ventral and the rectus abdominis in the center with a fascial envelope encased with a bilaminar aponeurosis **(Fig 7-8)**. The TrA is the deepest muscle of the abdominal muscle complex, with the internal and external oblique being more

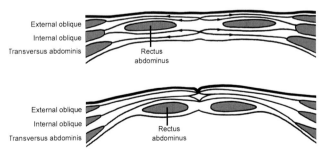

Fig 7-8. The pattern of decussation of the anterior fascia of the external oblique, internal oblique, and transversus abdominis above **(top)** and below **(bottom)** the umbilicus. (From Lee D. *The Pelvic Girdle: An Approach to the Examination and Treatment of the Lumbopelvic-hip Region.* 3rd ed. New York: Churchill Livingstone; 2004; with permission.)

ventral and the rectus abdominis in the centre within a fascial envelope encased with a bilaminar aponeurosis (6).

The TrA originates from the "lateral one-third of the inguinal ligament, the anterior two-thirds of the inner lip of the iliac crest, the lateral raphe of the thoracodorsal fascia, and the internal aspect of the lower six costal cartilages interdigitating with the costal fibers of the diaphragm. The muscle runs transversely around the trunk where its upper and middle fibers bend with the fascial envelope of the rectus abdominis. Superior to the umbilicus, the aponeurotic fibers of the transversus abdominis pass posterior to the rectus abdominis in either [a] superior or an inferior direction to blend with aponeurotic fibers of contralateral transversus abdominis and internal oblique. Below the umbilicus, all of the aponeurotic fibers run inferiorly with the anterior laminae passing anterior to the rectus abdominis and the posterior laminae passing posterior to the rectus abdominis. Caudally, the posterior laminar fibers gradually pass anterior to the rectus abdominis along with the anterior laminar fibers" (6). The TrA has stabilizing and respiratory functions (13). With contraction of the TrA, a drawing in or hollowing of the abdominal wall occurs, which produces tension of the thoracolumbar fascia through the lateral raphe and increased abdominal pressure (12) **(Fig 7-9)**.

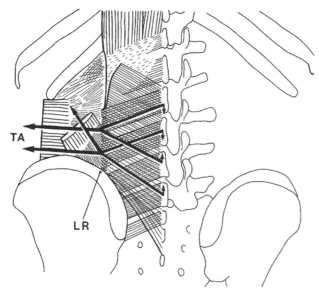

Fig 7-9. The mechanics of the thoracolumbar fascia. From any point in the lateral raphe (*LR*), lateral tension in the posterior layer of thoracolumbar fascia is transmitted upward, through the deep lamina of the posterior layer, and downward, through the superficial layer. Because of the obliquity of these lines of tension, a small downward vector is generated at the midline attachment of the deep lamina, and a small upward vector is generated at the midline attachment of the superficial lamina. These mutually opposite vectors tend to approximate or oppose the separation of the L2 and L4 and the L3 and L5 spinous processes. Lateral tension on the fascia can be exerted by the transversus abdominis (*TA*) and, to a lesser extent, by the few fibers of the internal oblique when they attach to the lateral raphe. (From Bogduk N. *Clinical Anatomy of the Lumbar Spine and Sacrum.* 3rd ed. New York: Churchill Livingstone; 1997; with permission.)

External Oblique

The external oblique originates from the inferior border and outer surfaces of the lower eight ribs. It interdigitates with the serratus anterior and latissimus dorsi, with upper, middle, and lower attachments (6). The upper and middle fibers attach into the abdominal aponeurosis (6). The posterior attachments descend to insert on the anterior half of the iliac crest. Rizk (44) and Lee (6) have described the external oblique as being bilaminar, with the two layers blending with the fascia of the opposite side and the contralateral internal oblique. The external oblique muscle has been identified as part of the global stabilizing system (16).

Internal Oblique

The internal oblique is the largest muscle of the abdominal wall (13) **(Fig 7-10)**. The internal oblique forms the middle layer of the abdominal wall between the TrA and the external oblique. It originates from the "lateral two-thirds of the inguinal ligament, anterior two-thirds of the iliac crest, and the lateral raphe of the thoracolumbar fascia in a band 2–3 cm wide, attaching to fibers of the deep lamina arising from the L3 spinous process" (12). The posterior layer of the fascia passes posterior to the rectus abdominis and is continuous with the TrA, whereas the anterior fibers are anterior to the rectus abdominus and continuous with the contralateral external oblique (12). The internal oblique has been recognized as a global muscle, although some portions appear to function in the local support system, according to Bergmark (16), because of the posterior fibers attaching to the lateral raphe. The lower anterior fibers compress and work with the TrA to support the lower abdominal viscera. The upper anterior and lateral fibers, when acting bilaterally, flex the vertebral column and assist in respiration. When acting unilaterally, along with the external oblique on the opposite side, rotate the vertebral column and bring the thorax backward or pelvis forward (45).

Quadratus Lumborum

The quadratus lumborum consists of medial and lateral fibers that are enclosed by the anterior and middle layers of the thoracolumbar fascia (43,46). The medial fibers attach "from the ilium to the anterior surface of the transverse processes of the lumbar vertebrae and other fibers travel from the transverse processes to anchor onto the twelfth rib. The lateral portion of the muscle, which belongs to the global system, spans the lumbar area, attaching on the lateral ilium to insert into the twelfth rib without attachment to any vertebrae" (12). Because of the attachments of the medial portion of the muscle to the vertebrae, it may be capable of providing some segmental stability (47). McGill et al. (47) provided evidence of increased muscle activity with increasing spinal compression during a symmetrical bucket-holding task. Andersson et al. (48) found increased

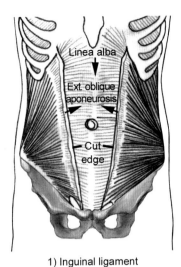

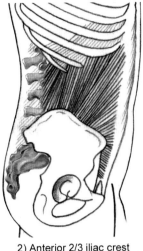

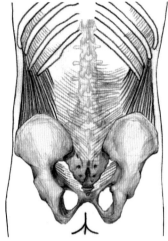

1) Inguinal ligament

2) Anterior 2/3 iliac crest
Origins of the Internal oblique

3) Lateral raphe of thoracolumbar fascia

Fig 7-10. Internal oblique. Ext., external. (Redrawn from Kendall FP, McCreary EK, Provorce PA. *Muscle Testing and Function.* Baltimore: Williams & Wilkins; 1993; with permission.)

activity of the muscle during full forward flexion. The medial fibers of the quadratus lumborum are considered to be part of the local stabilizing system (16) because of its segmental attachments and, therefore, are able to provide segmental stability (12). The lateral fibers of the quadratus lumborum are considered to be part of the global stabilizing system (16), because there is no attachment to any vertebrae (12). McGill et al. (47) provided evidence of the quadratus lumborum being "more active than other muscles during isometric side support postures." He has suggested the use of "horizontal side support" or side bridging as an exercise to incorporate for training. The quadratus lumborum provides lateral stabilization of the lumbopelvic region (13).

■ LITERATURE REVIEW

Patients with chronic low back pain have been found to have specific motor dysfunctions (40,49–52). Hodges and Richardson (52,53) found that those with a history of low back pain and dysfunction had poor motor control. The local system dysfunction developed after the onset of pain and pathology (12).

With the occurrence of pain and dysfunction, it is believed that the pain may resolve but that the dysfunction may persist (12,49,55). Research has concentrated on the decrease in function of muscles found in patients with low back pain and on exercise programs that have been found to be effective and to provide improved stability. They reported "early activation of the transversus abdominis (TrA) and obliquus internus abdominis (OI) with upper limb movement at both fast and intermediate speeds for the control group" (53). Those with low back pain "failed to recruit transversus abdominis or obliquus internus abdominis in

advance of fast movement, and no activity of the abdominal muscle was recorded in the majority of intermediate speed trials" (53). It was found that "muscle recruitment associated with limb movement is altered in people with low back pain with movement at a variety of speeds" (53), and it is believed that exercise should focus on changes in motor control rather than on strength training (53). Hodges and Richardson (55) also found that the TrA "does not produce trunk movement but contributes to the control of spinal stiffness in a non-direction specific manner."

O'Sullivan et al. (56) looked at those patients with clinical instability resulting in chronic low back pain and diagnosed radiologically with spondylolysis and spondylolisthesis. Those authors were able to significantly decrease the pain and increase the functional ability through a specific exercise program aimed at lumbar stabilization. No change was found in the pain level or in the function of the control group, who were treated conservatively by their treating practitioner. They had continued with their regular weekly exercises such as swimming, walking, and gym work.

O'Sullivan et al. (14) directed some of their research toward patients with a clinical diagnosis of lumbar spine instability in the flexion pattern, and those authors found that they demonstrated an inability to find and to maintain a neutral posture of their lumbar spine when sitting. This loss of position sense or proprioceptive awareness may lead to abnormal loading of the joint surfaces, followed by injuries and degenerative changes over time (14,57–59). It is hypothesized that a deficit or delay in the timing and ability of the muscle contractions to protect joints from excessive movement in clinical instabilities leads to recurrent injury (14). Development of proprioception may be assisted by postural retraining (27) and stabilization exercises in neutral postures progressing to unstable surfaces in functional movements and sports. It is beneficial to incorporate proprioception in the treatment of patients with back pain related to lumbar segmental instabilities.

O'Sullivan et al. (27) further researched the activity of lumbar spine musculature with common postures seen in a painfree population. The passive postures of slumped sitting or sway standing showed a decrease in activity of the lumbopelvic stabilizing muscles. Conversely, there was an increase in activity of lumbopelvic stabilizing muscles of thoracic erector spinae and internal oblique found in erect sitting and standing postures in the same population. Postural retraining in conjunction with specific exercise stabilization programs of the lumbar spine is supported by research concerning the treatment of low back pain (21,60,61).

O'Sullivan et al. (27) also found that erect posture in weight-bearing positions would increase the strength of the muscles that provides stability of the lumbopelvic region. "In contrast, facilitation of muscle activity in non-weightbearing or poorly aligned positions may hinder the transfer of improved lumbo-pelvic muscle function into everyday activities" (27). Strengthening of the lumbopelvic muscle groups would be better achieved in weight-bearing and erect postures to simulate everyday and sporting activities (27).

Research indicates that deep trunk muscles, including the TrA, the multifidus, the internal oblique, and the diaphragm, will be activated in advance of limb and trunk movement to reduce intervertebral motion in the spine and, therefore, increase spinal stability (17,19,35,62,63). A delay in onset of activation of the TrA with rapid limb movement also was found in those with recurrent low back pain (49,52,53,64). Researchers have indicated that contraction of the abdominal muscles before movement of the limbs or the trunk may contribute to stabilization of the lumbar spine against forces associated with the limb movement (55). The transversus abdominis is activated independent of the direction of trunk movement and activation is continuous (28). Exercise for the abdominal muscles may facilitate the maintenance of coordination, strength, support, and endurance for the muscles of the pelvic floor (39). Exercise progressions for the TrA will improve lumbar stabilization.

Lumbar multifidus provides stabilization and control in the lumbar spine (19). During voluntary arm movements, it was found that the "superficial fibers of multifidus were responsible for the control of spine orientation and the deep fibers of multifidus contributed in the control of intervertebral motion" (19). The multifidus, lumbar longissimus, and iliocostalis "contribute to the support and control of the orientation of the lumbar spine and the support or stabilization of the lumbar segments" (12).

Those patients with a first-time episode of lumbar back pain having no radiological pathology were found to have a reduced cross-sectional area of the multifidus at the level of pain as well as dysfunction in the lumbar spine as demonstrated by ultrasound. A specific exercise program with cocontraction of the TrA and the multifidus produced an increased cross-sectional area of the multifidus and reduced recurrence rate of low back pain as followed over the course of a year. The control group had no improvement in the cross-sectional area of the multifidus with the continuation of normal activities (54,61,65).

Kavcic et al. (64) found that "as loads are applied to the spine there is an integration of the many different muscles in order to balance the stability and moment demands, and these patterns change as the spine loading patterns change." They concluded that the focus should not be directed toward one or two single muscle groups to provide the stability of the lumbar spine. Instead, the exercise programs should be directed toward training many of the potential lumbar spine stabilizers for improved motor patterns, which will change with the functional task. "The role of each individual lumbar muscle changes as the loads placed on the spine changes" (64). They also concluded that "the smaller muscles have a stabilizing role and that as loads increase, the need for the stronger global muscles is required" (64).

The supine active straight-leg raise test (ASLR) has been introduced as a valid tool for assessing the load transfer between the trunk and lower extremities (66–69). When the lumbopelvic-hip region is functioning optimally, the leg should rise effortlessly from the table. There should be no movement of the pelvis in relation to the thorax and lower extremity (5), but there should be adequate contraction of the muscles in the local and global systems to stabilize the thorax, lumbar spine, and pelvis while moving the lower extremity (5). Mens et al. (67) have researched the specific relationship between impairment of the ASLR and the increase in pelvic mobility as depicted radiographically and the resulting pelvic pain disorders.

With the ASLR, the patient is in the supine position and is asked to actively raise one straight leg 5 cm above the table without bending the knees. The patient reports the subjective findings, and the examiner observes the movement between the pelvis and lower extremity. A four-point scale is used to rank the weakness observed:

0 = the patient feels no weakness, and the examiner sees no abnormal pattern
1 = the patient feels weakness, but the examiner sees no abnormal moving pattern
2 = the patient feels weakness, and the examiner assesses that raising the leg causes difficulties
3 = the patient is unable to raise the leg

A patient with a difference of one or more points between the left leg and right leg is classified as having an asymmetrical weakness (64).

This test demonstrates the importance of core stabilization in providing a stable base within the trunk, from which the lower extremities can move with the speed, coordination, and strength required in sports.

■ CONCLUSION

The term core stabilization is used to describe the management of low back pain through training of the deep stabilizing muscles of the trunk to protect the spine and to allow improved motor control of the spine (4). "Strength, coordination and timing of motor control in the lumbar spine are required to improve stability" (70). The role of the physiotherapist is to assess the patient for dysfunction in any of the active, passive, and control subsystems and to determine the appropriate exercise programs to be used in treatment. Progressions on stable and unstable surfaces incorporating functional tasks and sporting activities are used when the patient is ready.

The multifidus (along with the TrA in the local muscle system) has been identified as playing a key role in providing spinal stability. The internal oblique also may function along with the TrA to provide further support. Specific exercise programs done in weight-bearing positions along with postural retraining can be used in the treatment of low back pain, both to reduce pain and to improve the stability of the lumbar segments over the long term. Proprioceptive training can be incorporated with the use of unstable surfaces in the specific exercise programs.

The local and global systems need to be progressed to account for individual differences in motor control dysfunction and to address the changing muscle requirements that are needed to adapt to the changing loads on the spine. These exercise programs need to be incorporated into functional tasks and sporting activities as the patient progresses to maintain stability and motor control of the lumbar spine. Core stabilization exercises (Appendix 7-1) may assist in the prevention of lower extremity injuries by providing a stable base from which to function. Lumbar stabilization exercise programs become essential in preventing low back pain, averting the progression from acute to chronic injury, and ensuring the rehabilitation process for both situations.

■ ACKNOWLEDGEMENTS

The author would like to thank Karen LeValliant and Adam Eikenberry for their assistance in the preparation and research for this chapter. The author also would like to acknowledge the invaluable instruction and support of Dr. Don Johnson, Erl Pettman, and Diane Lee.

■ REFERENCES

1. Panjabi MM. The stabilizing system of the spine. Part II. Neutral zone and instability hypothesis. *J Spinal Disord.* 1992;5:390–396.
2. Dillingham T. Evaluation and management of low back pain: an overview. *State of the Art Reviews.* 1995;9:559–574.
3. Croft P, Macfarlane G, Papageorgiou A, et al. Outcome of low back pain in general practice: a prospective study. *BMJ.* 1998; 2:1356–1359.
4. Hodges PW. Science of stability: clinical application to assessment and treatment of segmental spinal stabilization for low back pain. Course Notes; 2000.
5. Panjabi MM. The stabilizing system of the spine. Part I: function, dysfunction, adaptation, and enhancement. *J Spinal Disord.* 1992; 5:383–389.
6. Lee D. *The Pelvic Girdle: An Approach to the Examination and Treatment of the Lumbopelvic-hip Region.* 3rd ed. New York: Churchill Livingstone; 2004.
7. Kavcic N, Grenier S, McGill SM. Quantifying tissue loads and spine stability while performing commonly prescribed low back stabilization exercises. *Spine.* 2004;29:2319–2329.
8. Lee D. Treatment of pelvic instability. In: Vleeming A, Mooney V, Dorman T, et al., eds. *Movement, stability, and low back pain.* Edinburgh: Churchill Livingstone; 1997.
9. Linton S. A review of psychological risk factors in back and neck pain. *Spine.* 2000;25:1148–1156.
10. Zusman M. Forebrain-mediated sensitization of central pain pathways: 'non-specific' pain and a new image for MT. *Man Ther.* 2002;7:80–88.
11. Waddell G. *The Back Pain Revolution.* Edinburgh: Churchill Livingstone; 2004.
12. Richardson CA, Jull GA, Hodges PW, et al. *Therapeutic Exercise for Spinal Segmental Stabilization in Low Back Pain—Scientific Basis and Clinical Approach.* Edinburgh: Churchill Livingstone; 1999.
13. O'Sullivan P. The changing face of physiotherapy: diagnosis and management of chronic low back pain disorders from a bio-psycho-social perspective (level 1). Course Notes; 2005.
14. O'Sullivan PB, Burnett A, Floyd AN, et al. Lumbar repositioning deficit in a specific low back pain population. *Spine.* 2003;28: 1074–1079.
15. Hodges P, Moseley L. Motor control and the neurophysiology of pain in lumbopelvic stability training: integration of motor control training and the bio-psycho-social model in clinical assessment and training techniques for lumbopelvic pain. Course Notes; 2001.
16. Bergmark A. Stability of the lumbar spine. A study in mechanical engineering. *Acta Ortho Scand.* 1989;230:1–54.
17. Hodges PW, Richardson CA. Contraction of the abdominal muscles associated with movement of the lower limb. *Phys Ther.* 1997;77:132–144.
18. Hodges PW. Neuromechanical Control of the Spine. PhD thesis. Stockholm, Sweden; Karolinska Institute; 2003.
19. Moseley GL, Hodges PW, Gandevia SC. Deep and superficial fibers of the lumbar multifidus muscle are differentially active during voluntary arm movements. *Spine.* 2002;27:E29–E36.
20. Moseley GL, Hodges PW, Gandevia SC. External perturbation of the trunk in standing humans differentially activates components of the medial back muscles. *J Physiol.* 2003;547:581–587.
21. O'Sullivan PB. Lumbar segmental 'instability': clinical presentation and specific stabilizing exercise management. *Man Ther.* 2000;5:2–12.
22. Constantinou CE, Govan DE. Spatial distribution and timing of transmitted and reflexly generated urethral pressures in healthy women. *J Urol.* 1982;127:964–969.
23. Bo K, Stein R. Needle EMG registration of striated urethral wall and pelvic floor muscle activity patterns during cough, Valsalva, abdominal, hip adductor, and gluteal muscles contractions in nulliparous healthy females. *Neurourol Urodyn.* 1994;13:35–41.
24. Sapsford RR, Hodges PW, Richardson CA, et al. Coactivation of the abdominal and pelvic floor muscles during voluntary exercises. *Neurourol Urodyn.* 2001;20:31–42.
25. Hodges PW, Gandevia SC. Changes in intra-abdominal pressure during postural and respiratory activation of the human diaphragm. *J Appl Physiol.* 2000;89:967–976.
26. Hodges PW, Gandevia SC. Activation of the human diaphragm during a repetitive postural task. *J Physiol.* 2000;522:165–175.

27. O'Sullivan PB, Grahamslaw KM, Kendell M, et al. The effect of different standing and sitting postures on trunk muscle activity in a pain-free population. *Spine*. 2002;27:1238–1244.

28. Cresswell A, Grundstrom H, Thorstensson A. Observations on intra-abdominal pressure and patterns of abdominal intramuscular activity in man. *Acta Physiol Scand*. 1992;144:409–418.

29. Hodges PW. Is there a role for transversus abdominis in lumbopelvic stability? *Arch Phys Med Rehabil*. 1999;80:1005–1012.

30. Tesh K, Dunn J, Evans J. The abdominal muscles and vertebral stability. *Spine*. 1987;12:501–508.

31. Comerford MJ, Mottram SL. Functional stability retraining: principles and strategies for managing mechanical dysfunction. *Man Ther*. 2001;6:3–14.

32. Vleeming A, Pool-Goudzwaard AL, Stoeckart R, et al. The posterior layer of the thoracolumbar fascia: its function in load transfer from spine to legs. *Spine*. 1995;20:753.

33. Vleeming A, Snijders CJ, Stoeckart R, et al. A new light on low back pain. In: *Proceedings from the second interdisciplinary world congress on low back pain*. San Diego: 1995:149–168.

34. Snijders, CJ, Vleeming A, Stoeckart R. Transfer of lumbosacral load to iliac bones and legs. 1: biomechanics of self-bracing of the sacroiliac joints and its significance for treatment and exercise. *Clin Biomech*. 1993;8:285–294.

35. Hodges PW, Richardson C. Feedforward contraction of transversus abdominis is not influenced by the direction of arm movement. *Exp Brain Res*. 1997;114:362–370.

36. Hodges PW, Cresswell AG, Thorstensson A. Preparatory trunk motion accompanies rapid upper limb movement. *Exp Brain Res*. 1999;124:69–79.

37. Radebold A, Cholewicki J, Panjabi MM, et al. Muscle response pattern to sudden trunk loading in healthy individuals and in patients with chronic low back pain. *Spine*. 2000;25:947–954.

38. Radebold A, Cholewicki J, Polzhofer GK, et al. Impaired postural control of the lumbar spine is associated with delayed muscle response times in patients with chronic idiopathic low back pain. *Spine*. 2001;26:724–730.

39. Sapsford RR, Hodges PW. Contraction of the pelvic floor muscles during abdominal maneuvers. *Arch Phys Med Rehabil*. 2001;82:1081–1088.

40. MacIntosh JE, Valencia F, Bogduk N, et al. The morphology of the human lumbar multifidus. *Clin Biomech*. 1986;1:196–204.

41. Willard FH. The muscular, ligamentous, and neural structure of the low back and its relation to back pain. In: Vleeming A, Mooney V, Dorman T, et al., eds. *Movement, stability, and low back pain*. Edinburgh: Churchill Livingstone; 1997:3–35.

42. Wilke HJ, Wolf S, Claes LE, et al. Stability increase of the lumbar spine with different muscle groups. A biomechanical in vitro study. *Spine*. 1995;20:192–198.

43. Bogduk N. *Clinical Anatomy of the Lumbar Spine and Sacrum*. 3rd ed. New York: Churchill Livingstone; 1997.

44. Rizk NN. A new description of the anterior abdominal wall in man and mammals. *J Anat*. 1980;131:373–385.

45. Kendall FP, McCreary EK, Provorce PA. *Muscle testing and function*. Baltimore: Williams & Wilkins; 1993.

46. Williams PL, Warwick R, Dyson M, et al., eds. *Gray's Anatomy*. 37th ed. Edinburgh: Churchill Livingstone; 1989.

47. McGill SM, Juker D, Kropf P. Quantitative intramuscular myoelectric activity of quadratus lumborum during a wide variety of tasks. *Clin Biomech*. 1996;11:170–172.

48. Andersson EA, Oddsson LIE, Grundstrom OM, et al. EMG activities of the quadratus lumborum and erector spinae muscle during flexion-relaxation and other motor tasks. *Clin Biomech*. 1996;11:392–400.

49. Hodges PW, Richardson CA. Inefficient muscular stabilization of the lumbar spine associated with low back pain. A motor control evaluation of transversus abdominis. *Spine*. 1996;21:2640–2650.

50. O'Sullivan PB, Twomey L, Allison GT. Altered abdominal muscle recruitment in patients with chronic back pain following a specific exercise intervention. *J Orthop Sports Phys Ther*. 1998;27:114–124.

51. Richardson CA, Jull GA. Muscle control–pain control. What exercises would you prescribe? *Man Ther*. 1995;1:2–10.

52. Hodges PW, Richardson CA. Delayed postural contraction of transversus abdominis associated with movement of the lower limb in people with low back pain. *J Spinal Disord*. 1998;11:46–56.

53. Hodges PW, Richardson CA. Altered trunk muscle recruitment in people with low back pain with upper limb movement at different speeds. *Arch Phys Med Rehabil*. 1999;80:1005–1012.

54. Hides JA. Multifidus muscle recovery in acute low back patients. PhD thesis. Brisbane, Australia; Department of Physiotherapy, University of Queensland; 1996.

55. Hodges PW, Richardson CA. Transversus abdominis and the superficial abdominal muscles are controlled independently in a postural task. *Neurosci Lett*. 1999;265:91–94.

56. O'Sullivan PB, Phyty GD, Twomey LT, et al. Evaluation of specific stabilizing exercise in the treatment of chronic low back pain with radiologic diagnosis of spondylolysis or spondylolisthesis. *Spine*. 1997;22:2959–2967.

57. Gross MT. Effects of recurrent lateral ankle sprains on active and passive judgments on joint position. *Phys Ther*. 1987;67:1505–1509.

58. Forwell LA, Carnahan H. Proprioception during manual aiming in individuals with shoulder instability and controls. *J Orthop Sports Phys Ther*. 1996;23:111–119.

59. Cholewicki J, McGill S. Lumbar posterior ligament involvement during extremely heavy lifts estimated from fluoroscopic measurements. *J Biomech*. 1992;25:17–28.

60. O'Sullivan P, Twomey L, Allison G. Dynamic stabilization of the lumbar spine. *Crit Rev Phys Rehabil Med*. 1997;9:315–330.

61. Hides JA, Richardson CA, Jull GA. Multifidus muscle recovery is not automatic following resolution of acute first episode low back pain. *Spine*. 1996;21:2763–2769.

62. Hungerford B, Gilleard W, Hodges P. Evidence of altered lumbopelvic muscle recruitment in the presence of sacroiliac joint pain. *Spine*. 2003;28:1593–1600.

63. Cholewicki J, Panjabi M, Khachatryan A. Stabilizing function of trunk flexor-extensor muscles around neutral spine posture. *Spine*. 1997;22:2207–2212.

64. Kavcic N, Grenier S, McGill SM. Determining the stabilizing role of individual torso muscles during rehabilitation exercises. *Spine*. 2004;29:1254–1265.

65. Hides J, Stokes M, Saide M, et al. Evidence of lumbar multifidus muscle wasting ipsilateral to symptoms in patients with acute/subacute low back pain. *Spine*. 1994;19:165–172.

66. Mens JMA, Vleeming A, Snijders CJ, et al. Active straight leg raising test: a clinical approach to the load transfer function of the pelvic girdle. In: Vleeming A, Mooney V, Dorman T, et al., eds. *Movement, stability, and low back pain*. Edinburgh: Churchill Livingstone; 1997:425–431.

67. Mens JMA, Vleeming A, Snijders CJ, et al. The active straight-leg raising test and mobility of the pelvic joints. *Eur Spine J*. 1999;8:468–473.

68. Mens JMA, Vleeming A, Snijders CJ, et al. Reliability and validity of the active straight-leg raise test in posterior pelvic pain since pregnancy. *Spine*. 2001;26:1167.

69. Mens JMA, Vleeming A, Snijders CJ, et al. Validity of the active straight-leg raise test for measuring disease severity in patients with posterior pelvic pain after pregnancy. *Spine*. 2002;27:196.

70. Lee D, Lee L-J. *An integrated approach to the assessment and treatment of the lumbopelvic-hip region* [DVD]. Vancover, BC: DV Media, Inc.; 2004.

■ BASIC EXERCISES

Neutral Spine: Anterior or Posterior Pelvic Tilt

Position: The patient is supine (lying on back), with a towel underneath the back. The physiotherapist assists the patient with moving into anterior pelvic tilt. Palpate the lumbar multifidus contraction with anterior tilt of the pelvis. Remove the towel, and assist the patient into a posterior pelvic tilt. The patient needs to find neutral lordosis or position.

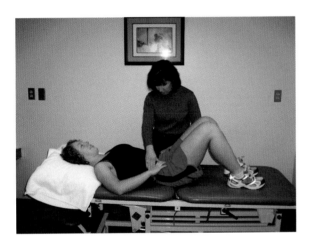

Position: Repeat with prone-lying (lying on front).

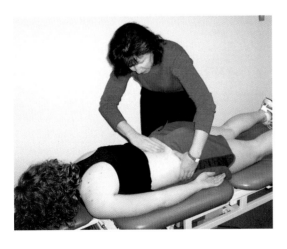

Transverse Abdominal Wall with Co-contraction of Lumbar Multifidus and Pelvic Floor

Position: Supine. Palpate medial to ASIS and lower abdomen:

■ Maintain the spine in neutral position with co-contraction of lumbar multifidus.
■ Draw the pelvic floor up and in.

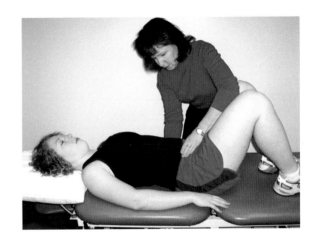

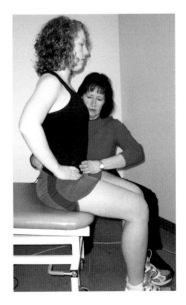

- Slowly draw in the lower abdomen away from the physiotherapist's fingers (a light tensioning can be felt when contracted).
- Isometric hold, and breath normally with controlled lateral costal diaphragmatic breathing.
- Maintain independence of the lower abdominal wall from upper abdominal wall; no joint movement and no pain.

Avoid breath-holding, thoracic flexion, and upper abdominal bracing that restricts breathing.

Progression:

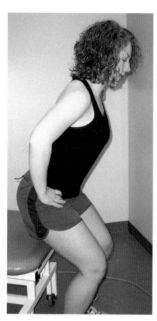

Sit to stand

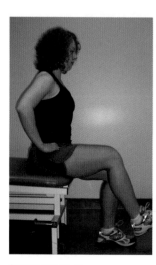

Sitting hip flexion

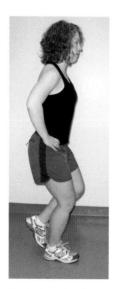

Single-leg standing

Bent-knee fall out:

- Allow one bent leg to fall to the side while maintaining muscle contraction. Return to upright bent-knee position. Repeat for opposite leg. Relax, and repeat.

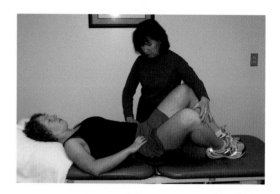

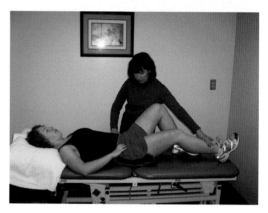

Single-Leg heel slide:

- Slowly straighten one leg, sliding the heel forward on the floor, while maintaining muscle contraction. Return to the bent-knee position. Repeat for opposite leg. Relax, and repeat.

Position: Four-point kneeling with feet over the edge of the bed:

- Shoulders over hands, and hips over knees.
- Maintain spine in neutral position.

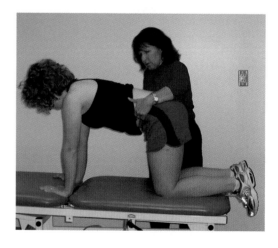

- Tension transverse abdominal wall and lumbar multifidus as above.
- Hold, and breath normally.

Progressions:

- Slowly raise one arm up, keeping it in line with the trunk. Relax slowly to lower the arm down, and repeat with other arm.
- Slowly raise one leg up, keeping it in line with the trunk. Relax slowly to lower the leg down, and repeat with other leg.

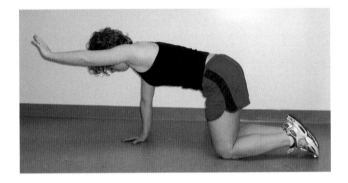

■ ADVANCED EXERCISES

Transverse Abdominal Wall

Progression: Sitting to standing (single leg).

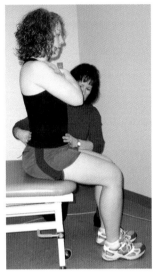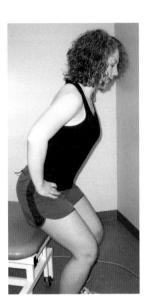

Bridging in Supine (Back Bridge)

Position: Supine with knees bent:

- Contract transversus abdominal wall and multifidus as described above while breathing gently.
- Lift hips and back off the floor to straight-line position of knees, hips, and shoulders. Hold.
- Relax slowly to lower the hips down onto the bed. Repeat.

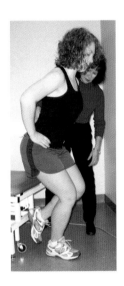

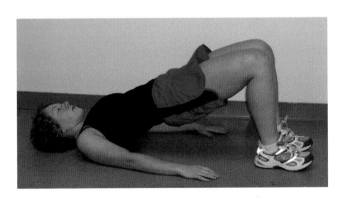

Multifidus (with co-contraction of gluteal muscles)

Progression:

- Simultaneously raise one leg and the opposite arm up and in line with the trunk. Hold.
- Relax, and repeat for opposite side.

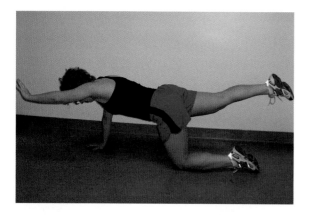

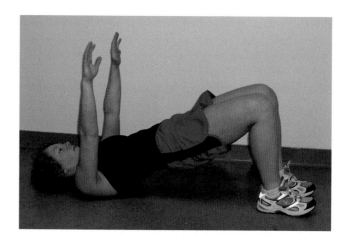

Progressions using ball:

- Position: Lying on stomach on the ball, with equal weight between arms and legs.
- Arm raises: Slowly raise one arm up, keeping it in line with the trunk. Relax slowly to lower the arm down, and repeat with other arm.
- Leg raises: Slowly raise one leg up, keeping it in line with the trunk. Relax slowly to lower the leg down, and repeat with other leg.
- Simultaneously raise one leg and the opposite arm up and in line with the trunk. Hold, and repeat for opposite side.

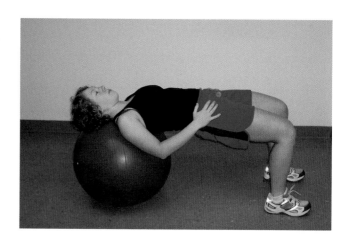

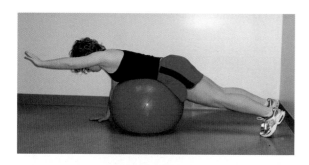

- One-leg bridging: Lift hips off floor first, then release a leg and keep it in line with body.
- Sitting on ball, walk out slowly until the shoulders and head rest comfortably on the ball. Ensure the knees are above the feet for support. Raise hips up to maintain a straight-line position through knees, hips, and shoulders. Hold. Relax slowly, and repeat.
- Progress slowly to narrowing base of support, bringing feet and knees closer together.

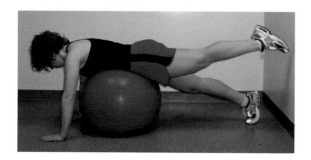

Front Bridge (from knees)

Position: Lying on stomach, flat on the floor:

- Bring elbows under shoulders and bend knees.
- Raise hips off the floor to a straight-line position of knees, hips, shoulders, and neck while contracting the transverse abdominal wall and breathing gently. Hold.
- Relax slowly to lower body back to floor. Repeat.

Progressions:

- Position as above: Support from feet (wide) and elbows.
- Position as above: Support from feet (narrow) and elbows.

Back Bridge

Progressions:

- Narrow the base of support, bringing the knees and feet together.
- Arm raises: To vertical positions to remove support.

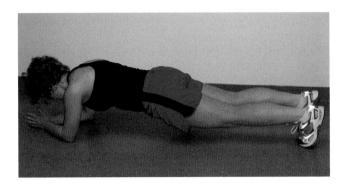

- Lying on stomach on the ball, slowly walkout onto the hands, releasing support of the feet, until the ball rests under the thighs (above the knees). Hold, maintaining a straight-line position through the hips, trunk, and shoulders. Relax slowly, and repeat.
- Progress slowly to ball resting on shins (lower leg).

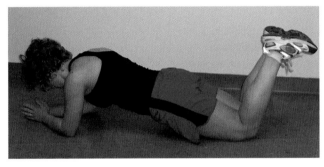

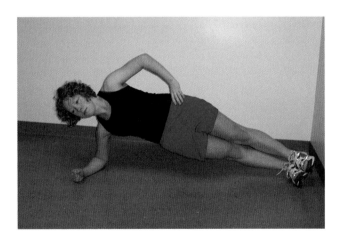

Side Bridge (from knees)

Position: Lying on side, resting on one elbow, with knees bent.

- Position elbow under the shoulder. Keep the knees together. The hips can be flexed (bent) slightly for the starting position on the floor.
- Rest the top arm on the hip.
- Raise the hips off floor to a straight-line position through the knees, hips, shoulders, and neck while contracting the transversus abdominis and breathing gently. Hold.
- Relax slowly to lower the entire body down flat on the floor. Repeat.
- Repeat sequence on opposite side.

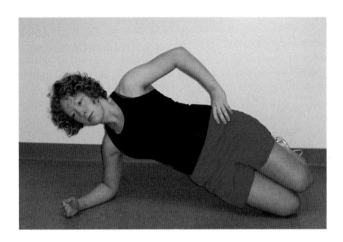

Progressions:

- Position as above: Support from feet and elbow.

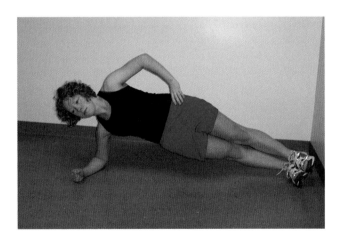

THORACIC AREA

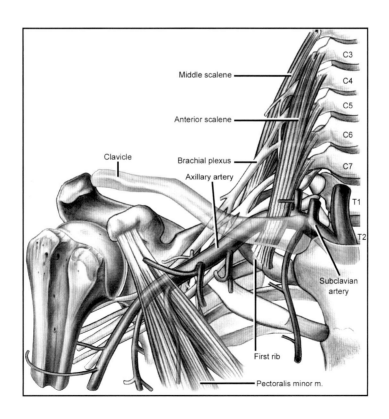

C3

C4

C5

C6

C7

T1

T2

Middle scalene

Anterior scalene

Clavicle

Brachial plexus

Axillary artery

Subclavian artery

First rib

Pectoralis minor m.

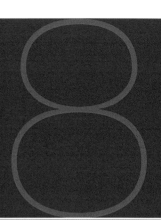

SCAPULOTHORACIC DYSFUNCTION, BURNERS, STINGERS, THORACIC OUTLET SYNDROME, AND MISCELLANEOUS NERVE INJURIES

■ MARC R. SAFRAN, MD, ANTHONY C. LUKE, MD, MPH

■ KEY POINTS

■ The scapula is a triangular, flat bone that lies along the posterior thoracic wall. The stability of the scapula depends mainly on the 17 muscles that are attached to it.

■ The scapula is an essential structure for proper biomechanics for the shoulder, because it offers a stable foundation for movement. Disorders of the scapula and the nerves surrounding the glenohumeral joint can result in significant dysfunction and pain involving the shoulder.

■ Scapular "dyskinesis" describes loss of the normal motion and positioning of the scapula.

■ The patient with a scapular problem often presents with a history of shoulder impingement or pain. Common complaints among throwing athletes are difficulties generating force and pain over the posterior aspect of the shoulder.

■ Blunt trauma or repetitive microtrauma from nerve traction or compression are the common causes of neurogenic winging encountered in athletes. The long thoracic nerve is vulnerable to direct injury because of its subcutaneous location as it exits the pectoralis muscle at the fourth and fifth ribs and travels along the rib cage.

■ Brachial plexus neuropathy presents with temporary burning, stinging, or tingling that occurs when the head is forcefully bent sideways. These injuries are commonly referred to as stingers or burners. Symptoms typically last for seconds to minutes, but in 5% to 10% of cases, a neurological deficit can last for hours, days, or even weeks. When treating the symptoms, it is important to rule out underlying factors that may predispose the athlete to more serious injury.

■ Nerve compression, nerve traction, or a direct blow to the brachial plexus are the three main mechanisms for a stinger or burner.

■ Thoracic outlet syndrome (TOS) refers to a symptom complex of upper extremity pain and paresthesias involving compressions of neurovascular structures.

■ A subtle cause of shoulder pain and weakness involves compression or traction of the suprascapular nerve. Overhead and throwing athletes often are affected because of repetitive trauma. A diagnosis of suprascapular nerve entrapment often is made clinically, based on a thorough history and physical examination.

Apart from the pathology of the glenohumeral joint, disorders of the surrounding nerves and scapula can result in significant dysfunction and pain involving the shoulder. The scapula is an essential structure for proper biomechanics of the shoulder, because it offers a stable foundation for movement. Proper coordination and positioning of the scapula and glenohumeral joint is necessary for efficient and effective shoulder motion. Nerve injuries around the shoulder can cause weakness of the scapular stabilizers and the rotator cuff muscles, which can result in improper and symptomatic mechanics of the shoulder. This chapter reviews problems involving the scapula and the nerves around the shoulder that often are overlooked and, possibly, underdiagnosed. The concept of scapulothoracic dysfunction or dyskinesis is introduced, and specific nerve injuries around the neck and shoulder are discussed.

■ SCAPULOTHORACIC PROBLEMS

Scapular "dyskinesis" describes loss of the normal motion and positioning of the scapula (1). Several specific pathologies are associated with abnormal function of the scapula.

Scapular dyskinesis, scapular crepitus or "snapping scapula," and scapular bursitis are discussed in this section, and scapular winging caused by nerve injuries are discussed in the following section.

Basic Science

Anatomy

The scapula is a triangular, flat bone that lies along the posterior thoracic wall. The "plane of the scapula" at rest is approximately 30 to 40 degrees in the frontal plane and is tipped anteriorly by approximately 10 to 20 degrees (2). Its attachment to the axial skeleton involves the acromioclavicular and sternoclavicular joints and the clavicle, which acts as a strut (3). The stability of the scapula depends mainly on the muscle attachments and their dynamic stabilizing functions. Seventeen muscles have their origin or insertion on the scapula (4). The subscapularis and the serratus anterior muscles lie between the scapula and the thoracic wall. Several bursae also exist around the scapula, between it and the chest wall. Anatomical bursae include the infraserratus and supraserratus bursa, and adventitial bursae can develop, particularly around the superomedial angle and the inferior angle (5) (Fig 8-1). Some experts believe that these occur as an adaptation to repetitive movements or abnormal mechanics around the scapula. Cadaveric studies have demonstrated anatomical variants involving the superomedial border and the inferior pole of the scapula, which may or may not contribute to clinical symptoms (6).

Biomechanics

The scapula is a functional link that stabilizes the shoulder and allows a longer lever arm for force generation (7).

Scapular movement allows the articular surface of the head of the humerus to remain relatively centered with respect to the glenoid. During abduction of the upper extremity, the scapula moves laterally for the first 30 to 50 degrees of glenohumeral joint abduction, followed by rotation about a fixed axis in abduction, resulting in approximately 65 degrees of rotation through full abduction of the shoulder (3,8).

Abnormal scapular motion can result in subacromial impingement in patients with an inability to position the acromial arch away from the humeral head. Several muscles attaching to the scapula work as force couples to stabilize the scapula during movements of the upper extremity. For proper acromial elevation, the appropriate force couples are the lower trapezius and the serratus muscles, working together, paired with the upper trapezius and rhomboid muscles (3). Nerve injuries, such as those to the spinal accessory nerve innervating the upper trapezius or long thoracic nerve supplying the serratus anterior, have been estimated to cause abnormal scapular function in less than 5% of cases (3). Consequently, the more common cause of scapular dysfunction is felt to be from muscle inhibition or weakness caused by painful conditions of the shoulder (1).

"Snapping scapula" is an unusual condition described as a "tactile-acoustic phenomenon occurring as a consequence of some anomalous condition existing between the thoracic wall and the undersurface of the scapula" (9). Friction between the scapula and the chest wall is a normal, physiological phenomenon that results from muscle action and typically is asymptomatic. The snapping scapula is associated, however, with a louder, grating or snapping sound, which can be pathologic. The underlying causes can be divided into bony and soft-tissue problems (Table 8-1). Although rare, osteochondroma is the most common scapular tumor and may

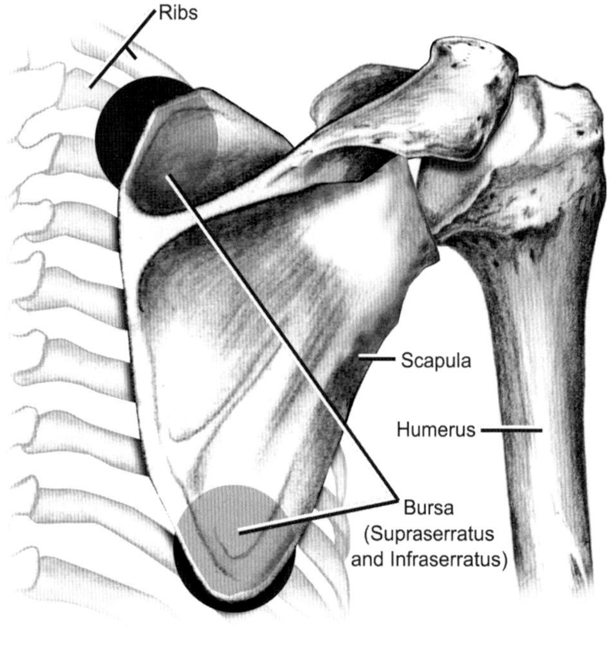

Fig 8-1. Scapulothoracic bursae (supraserratus and infraserratus bursas).

TABLE 8-1	Reported Causes of Snapping Scapula Syndrome

Bony alterations
  Abnormal curvature of the superior angle of the scapula
  Tubercle of Luschka
  Prominence or Hook from the lateral inferior pole
    of the scapula
  Omovertebral bone
  Curling of the vertebral border
  Irregularities of the subscapular ribs
  Exostosis of the subscapular ribs
  Osteogenic sarcoma
  Osteochondroma

Soft tissue
  Bursae
  Exostosis bursata
  Interstitial myofibrosis of surrounding muscles
  Atrophy of surrounding muscles (or imbalance)
  Chondrosarcoma

Elastofibroma
No obvious cause

present as a mass on the deep surface that projects into the scapulothoracic space. A Sprengel deformity, which is a congenital abnormality causing a dysplastic scapula; a Lushka tubercle, which is an exostosis over the superomedial border of the scapula; and scapular or rib fracture malunion are other bony causes of a snapping scapula (9,10).

Evaluation

History

The patient with a scapular problem often presents with a history of shoulder impingement or pain around the scapula. Difficulties in generating force and pain over the posterior aspect of the shoulder are common complaints among throwing athletes. Previous history of shoulder or neck problems should be clarified to identify potential underlying structural or nerve pathologies. Some individuals may report crepitus around the back of the shoulder. Scapular sounds occur in from 8% to 70% of the normal population (10) and do not always represent symptomatic pathology. The intensity of the sound does not parallel the severity of symptoms, nor does it suggest a specific underlying cause (11).

Physical Examination

A postural evaluation should examine for cervical hyperlordosis, thoracic kyphosis, or scoliosis. Signs of atrophy should be noted in the trapezius, supraspinatus, infraspinatus, and inferior trapezius areas, suggesting either a peripheral nerve injury or disuse—in turn suggesting a chronic problem. Scapular motion can be observed for asymmetry by having the patient perform repeated flexion of the shoulder (e.g., 10 times), because abnormalities may not appear until the patient's muscles fatigue. Tightness of the posterior capsule may be suggested by decreased internal rotation of the affected arm with the shoulder at 90 degrees of flexion and the elbow flexed to 90 degrees, similar to the Hawkin test but in abduction **(Fig 8-2)**. Wall push-ups can be used to assess for weakness of the serratus anterior, which is demonstrated by elevation of the inferior and/or medial border of the scapula. Kibler (3) has suggested three scapular tests. The scapular assistance test involves manually stabilizing the inferior scapula and elevating it as the arm is flexed. The scapular retraction test involves manual stabilization of the medial border of the scapula with flexion of the arm. A decrease in impingement symptoms is considered to be a positive in both tests. The lateral scapular slide test assesses any asymmetrical differences in distances from the spine to the medial border of the scapula in three positions: the hands at the side, the hands on the hips, and the arms abducted at or below 90 degrees with glenohumeral internal rotation. A difference of 1.5 cm between measurements suggests weakness with scapular retraction and most commonly is seen during testing with the patient's arms abducted (3). Pseudo-winging represents a scapular prominence that is forced out by a deep surface lesion characterized by a palpable mass, scapular grating, prominence at rest, and presence of normal scapulohumeral rhythm (12).

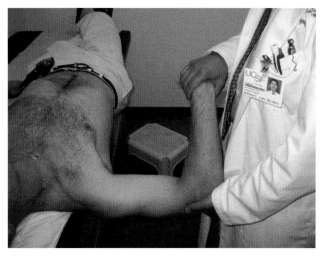

Fig 8-2. Assessment of posterior capsule tightness. The shoulder is abducted to 90 degrees, and the arm is internally rotated. Compare the abducted and internally rotated arm with the other arm to identify any asymmetry or internal rotation deficit. (From Levine MJ, Albert TJ, Smith MD. Cervical radiculopathy: diagnosis and nonoperative management. *J Am Acad Orthop Surg.* 1996;4:305–316; with permission.)

Imaging

Radiographs of the scapula and chest wall may demonstrate bony abnormalities of the scapula, such as osteochondroma growth from the scapula or the ribs or previous scapular fracture malunion (13). Osteochondromata can be difficult to see on anteroposterior (AP) radiographs. A tangential scapulolateral view or computed tomographic (CT) scan often is needed to demonstrate the bony lesion. Magnetic resonance imaging (MRI) is the preferred test to evaluate for a soft-tissue mass, such as an elastofibroma, or to identify scapular bursitis, although it may not necessarily demonstrate pathology in all cases.

Additional Studies

Electromyography (EMG) can be considered 3 months after the injury to rule out injuries, particularly to the spinal accessory nerve and the long thoracic nerve. Follow-up EMGs should be performed at 6- to 12-week intervals to assess for improvements if changes in denervation are observed (13).

Management

Nonoperative Management

Management of scapulothoracic dysfunction involves addressing, if possible, the underlying problem, whether that problem is an internal derangement of the shoulder, glenohumeral joint instability, rotator cuff tendinopathy, or scapular lesion. Restoration of muscle activation patterns is the next step to recover normal, asymptomatic movement. Postural exercises are important to re-establish proper, stable positioning of the scapula for better glenohumeral joint movement. Rehabilitation exercises often focus on improving shoulder range of motion and muscular flexibility and on strengthening the scapular stabilizers, especially the serratus anterior, rhomboids, levator scapulae, and all three portions of the trapezius muscles (2,14).

Adjuncts for treatment include nonsteroidal anti-inflammatory medications and injection therapy, mainly when symptoms of pain are affecting rehabilitation. A local injection of a long-acting anesthetic and a corticosteroid into the area of maximal tenderness (i.e., the bursa) can be helpful, but care must be taken to stay in the proper plane to avoid the risk of pneumothorax. Extension, internal rotation, and adduction of the shoulder, similar to the lift-off test position (15), can elevate the scapula to facilitate injection at the superomedial angle of the scapula. Placing the arm into abduction to 60 degrees and forward flexion to 30 degrees may assist with injection of the inferomedial scapular bursa. A figure-eight bandage may help to remind patients to maintain proper posture. Taping the scapula from the proximal aspect of the clavicle over the upper trapezius toward the thoracic spine in the orientation of the lower trapezius muscle is a common adjunct in rehabilitation. In normal patients, no changes in EMG activity have occurred with taping (16); however, taping may provide benefits for patients with abnormal shoulder function. A new tool in the armamentarium of proprioceptive rehabilitation of scapulothoracic function is the "Alignmed S3" brace, and although scientific studies are lacking, early clinical experience with this brace by the senior author and other clinicians is promising for relieving symptoms and improving scapulothoracic function.

Operative Management

Snapping scapula and painful scapulothoracic problems can be managed surgically by decompressing this articulation through removal of the documented bony prominences into the scapulothoracic space from the scapula or ribs and excision of thickened bursa. Bony resection of the medial scapular border, particularly the superomedial scapular border, even without definitively identified bony deformity, has been recommended (6,13). Although these procedures have been commonly performed as open procedures with good success (17), anatomical feasibility studies and subsequent clinical success has been reported with endoscopic surgical decompression of bony prominences in patients with snapping scapula syndrome (18,19). Galinat (18) reported 66% good to excellent results in six patients with 2-year follow-up who were treated with excision of a 3-cm triangle of bone from the superomedial angle of the scapula after failing nonoperative treatment. Recently, Ciullo (20) used isolated endoscopic resection of bursal adhesions, a more conservative approach, in those with subscapular snapping scapula syndrome with good success.

Return to Play

The literature is lacking when it comes to scientific evidence for return-to-play criteria for athletes with scapular problems who have been treated conservatively or operatively. Thus, athletes may return to play on an individual basis. Most clinicians suggest that if symptoms are mild enough, athletes can continue participation in their sport and be released to play. If the pain is persistent, clinical signs of soft-tissue injury are observed, and/or the athlete is ineffective in performing his or her activity, then consider withdrawal from play—or at least modification of his or her training until adequate treatment can be done and symptoms improve.

■ SCAPULAR WINGING

Scapular winging, like "scapular dyskinesis," describes dysfunction of the scapula, usually as a consequence of nerve injury causing weakness or paralysis to one of the scapular muscles. The most common cause of neurogenic winging is injury to the long thoracic nerve, resulting in paralysis of the serratus anterior muscle. Other causes of winging are injury to the spinal accessory nerve, causing trapezius nerve palsy, and damage to the dorsal scapular nerve, causing rhomboideus palsy.

Basic Science

Anatomy

The long thoracic nerve is formed by the C5, C6, and C7 nerves distal to the scalene muscles (Fig 8-2). The long thoracic nerve is approximately 22 to 24 cm in length (21,22). The nerve passes under the brachial plexus, below the clavicle, and under the first or second rib. The nerve runs along the chest wall in the midaxillary line to the outer border of the serratus anterior, where it sends branches to each of serratus anterior muscular digitations.

The serratus anterior is the primary upward rotator of the scapular during abduction of the arm, and it stabilizes the shoulder during scapular protraction. The muscle arises from the first through ninth ribs, and it inserts onto the costomedial border of the scapula. The upper fibers of the serratus anterior insert onto the superior angle of the scapula and stabilize the scapula during the initial stages of abduction, whereas the middle fibers insert onto the vertebral border of the scapula. The lower fibers of the serratus anterior insert onto the inferior angle of the scapula.

The spinal accessory nerve is the 11th cranial nerve and provides the motor innervation to the trapezius muscle (23). The nerve passes from the base of the skull via the jugular foramen into the upper third of the sternocleidomastoid muscle. The nerve then travels subcutaneously, along the floor of the posterior cervical triangle, to innervate the trapezius muscle, which is a large, flat muscle that is divided into the upper, middle, and lower groups of muscle fibers. The upper fibers work to elevate and rotate the scapula, the middle fibers function in retracting and stabilizing the shoulder blade, and the lower fibers depress and rotate the scapula downward (24). Therefore, the trapezius muscle has important roles in the proper function of the shoulder, including abducting the shoulder, stabilizing and rotating the scapula during overhead activities, and preventing drooping of the shoulder (25).

The dorsal scapular nerve originates from the C5 nerve root. This nerve travels deep into or, in some cases, through the levator scapulae to supply the rhomboid muscles (13).

Biomechanics

Blunt trauma and repetitive microtrauma from nerve traction or compression are the common mechanisms causing neurogenic winging encountered in athletes. The long thoracic nerve is vulnerable to direct injury because of its subcutaneous location, because it exits the pectoralis muscle at the fourth or fifth ribs and travels along the rib cage (26). Also, repeated tilting and lateral rotation of the head away from the affected extremity with the arm raised overhead, such as during the serving motion in tennis, may cause stretching of the long thoracic nerve (27). This nerve has several points of fixation, including the scalene medius muscle and the superior aspect of the serratus anterior, which can result in traction to the nerve with certain repetitive movements and possible vascular intimal injury (22). Areas of potential compression include the scalene muscles (medius and posterior), the first rib, between the clavicle and the second rib, between the second rib and the coracoid, the inferior angle of scapula, or inflamed bursae along the course of the long thoracic nerve (13,21,22,28). Traction over a fascial band from the inferior aspect of the brachial plexus extending to the proximal aspect of the serratus anterior has been postulated as another potential cause, because in cadavers, the nerve has been shown to bowstring over this band with the arm in abduction and external rotation, accentuated by proximal and medial migration of the scapula (29). Poor epineural blood supply may make the nerve susceptible to damage from repeated traction and compression (22).

Open injury to the long thoracic nerve is unusual without penetrating trauma or a complication of surgical procedures in the axillary region (e.g., surgery for breast cancer or to relieve thoracic outlet compression) (30–32).

Other reported causes of nerve injury include viral illnesses and immunizations, but the pathology is not clearly understood (21). Horwitz (28) suggested that a viral etiology might affect the multiple bursae noted along the course of the nerve, resulting in transient nerve injury that usually disappears spontaneously. Brachial neuritis or neuralgic myotrophy, also known as Parsonage–Turner syndrome, is a condition affecting the brachial plexus. The exact etiology is still unknown, but an autoimmune cause is suspected. Tsairis et al. (33) found that 25 of 99 patients affected with brachial neuritis reported a history of antecedent or concurrent upper respiratory tract infection or flulike symptoms.

Because of its subcutaneous location in the neck, the spinal accessory nerve is mainly damaged. In sports, this can occur with blunt trauma (e.g., contact with a hockey or lacrosse stick) (34). Otherwise, penetrating trauma, such as a stab wound or ballistic injury, is needed to injure the nerve. Injury to this nerve has been a reported complication following surgical procedures including radical neck dissection for tumor, carotid endarterectomy, excision of subcutaneous mass or cyst, or cervical lymph node biopsy.

Seddon (35) introduced a classification for peripheral nerve injury that has been applied to injuries to the brachial plexus by Clancy et al. (36). Neurapraxia involves a reversible axonal dysfunction with focal demyelinization following minor injury. The axon continuity is preserved, and the nerve does not undergo distal degeneration (37). Typically, this is seen in compression nerve injuries, and it most likely represents the majority of burners and stingers. Axonotmesis has more variable recovery, because there loss of continuity of axons and damage to the tissue elements of the nerve occur (37). Finally, neurotmesis involves "physiologic disruption of the entire nerve" (37). Wallerian degeneration results from deterioration of myelin, and axons become disorganized distal to the point of injury. With denervation, the associated muscle atrophy reaches a relatively stable state at 60% to 80% weight loss by approximately 4 months (37). Ideally, function can improve if reinnervation of the motor end plates can be achieved within approximately 12 months of denervation; earlier reinnervation has better outcomes (37).

Evaluation

History

Athletes with a long thoracic nerve injury often complain of pain or discomfort about the shoulder, neck, and/or scapular area. Most often, athletes will complain of an insidious onset of weakness. They may present with shoulder impingement symptoms or pain around the scapula. Overhead activity usually is difficult, and they may demonstrate weakness with forward elevation and overhead motions. Especially early in the process, the pain may not be severe enough to stop sports. Athletes may note a loss of serving speed or power. Affected athletes may be involved in a sport requiring repetitive use of the upper extremity, or they may describe blunt trauma and traction on the neck or shoulder or landing on their side with the arm outstretched. Isolated serratus anterior paralysis may result from direct injury or after carrying objects on the shoulder without any significant injury. Traction injury to the long thoracic nerve has been identified in tennis as well as other sports, including volleyball, archery, golf, gymnastics, bowling, weight lifting, soccer, hockey, and riflery.

Athletes with injury to the spinal accessory nerve similarly complain of disabling pain, weakness, and deformity. These athletes also cite the inability to fully elevate or abduct their upper extremity overhead. Weakness is noted with forward elevation, particularly above the shoulder level. Drooping of the shoulder and loss of normal shoulder function also can result in painful symptoms of shoulder impingement.

Physical Examination

On physical examination, decreased active forward elevation and loss of power/strength often are noted (56). On examination from behind, the subject will have winging, especially

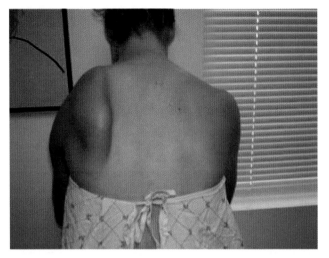

Fig 8-3. Long thoracic nerve palsy. Winging of an 18-year-old female with a 3-year history of left shoulder pain caused by a long thoracic nerve palsy sustained during a water-skiing accident. (From Thomas BE, McCullen GM, Yuan HA, et al. Cervical spine injuries in football players. *J Am Acad Orthop Surg.* 1999;7: 338–347; with permission.)

of the inferior border and particularly with forward elevation and/or wall push-ups **(Fig 8-3)**. The subject also may have uncoordinated scapulohumeral rhythm. A thin or muscular subject may have wasting or atrophy of the serratus anterior.

Injury to the spinal accessory nerve [cranial nerve (CN) XI] should be ruled out, because it also can produce scapular

winging clinically, asymmetry of the neckline, winging of the scapula, and weakness in abduction as a result of the resultant paralysis of the trapezius. The trapezius will have weakness and atrophy, and the sternocleidomastoid also can be involved. Typically, the patient has difficulty abducting the extremity above the horizontal plane and often is unable to shrug the affected shoulder, although rested levator scapulae can produce a normal shrug test (38). Winging will involve the superomedial aspect of the scapula as it is displaced laterally, rotating both downward and outward **(Fig 8-4)**, and will occur with the arms in abduction but not with the arms in forward elevation.

Imaging

Plain radiographs often are nondiagnostic but still should be obtained in cases of trauma and to assess for a cervical rib injury, which can be a cause of long thoracic nerve injury. Radiographs demonstrate marked inferior subluxation of the humeral head 2.5 weeks after the onset of symptoms in a patient with paralytic brachial neuritis affecting the deltoid and rotator cuff. Other imaging studies, such as CT and MRI, are not particularly helpful unless other cervical pathology is present, although the latter may demonstrate atrophy and denervation of the muscle on T_2-weighted films (39).

Additional Studies

Both EMG and NCV studies are helpful to confirm the etiology of neurogenic scapular winging and to document the

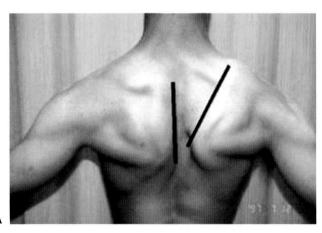

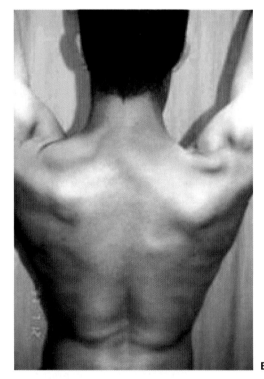

Fig 8-4. Spinal accessory nerve palsy in a 17-year-old male with a 1-year history of shoulder pain. **A:** Winging of the superior medial angle of the scapula with abduction. A line drawn along the medial border of the normal (left) shoulder is to be compared with the symptomatic (right) shoulder. **B:** Forward elevation does not result in winging in this patient, differentiating winging caused by spinal accessory nerve palsy from that caused by long thoracic nerve palsy.

severity of nerve injury. These studies can be performed as early as 3 weeks and can be repeated every 3 to 6 months to follow recovery. For spinal nerve pathology, conditions of the trapezius, sternocleidomastoid, and potentially transferable muscles (e.g., levator scapulae, rhomboideus major, and rhomboideus minor) usually are assessed.

Management

Nonoperative Management

Nonoperative treatment for scapular winging includes activity modification, symptomatic management, physical therapy (including maintaining shoulder range of motion and strength of compensatory muscles), and possibly, bracing. Athletes should be reassured and informed that most cases of atraumatic long thoracic nerve injury subside within 6 to 9 months (21) and that almost all cases resolve satisfactorily within 12 months (27,33,40,41). The athlete should avoid lifting heavy objects or participating in activities that exacerbate symptoms and place the nerve at risk. Nonsteroidal anti-inflammatory or other medications for neurogenic pain can be useful for control of symptoms. It should be stressed to the patient that he or she could maintain full glenohumeral range of motion. Furthermore, strengthening exercises should focus on the scapular stabilizers, particularly the trapezius, rhomboids, and levator scapulae, which will be stressed more to compensate for the dysfunctional serratus anterior. Taping commonly is used to support the scapula. Use of an orthosis has been recommended to help hold or support the scapula to the chest wall (42), but success is inconsistent. This has been reported to relieve pain, to control the stability of the scapula, and to prevent overstretching of the serratus anterior (32).

Because of the relatively good prognosis for spontaneous recovery, the mainstay of initial management is a nonoperative program. The natural history of atraumatic long thoracic nerve palsy is resolution within 1 year (43); however, cases resulting from Parsonage–Turner syndrome (brachial plexitis) may take as long as 2 to 3 years to resolve (21). Even so, it has been reported that conservative treatment will not be successful in approximately one-quarter of patients with a long thoracic nerve injury (40).

Return to Play

Return-to-play recommendations should be made on an individual basis (44). Hershman et al. (45) recommended that an athlete who has recovered a plateau in of adequate strength may be allowed to return to sports; however, if full strength has not been recovered, the athlete may need to limit his or her activities, particularly in contact sports.

Operative Management

The indications for surgery in patients with scapular winging caused by long thoracic nerve injury include penetrating trauma or persistent pain and symptoms that persist beyond 1 to 2 years despite adequate conservative treatment and failure of documented EMG improvement in nerve function. Because they are amenable to primary repair and have

improved function if the repair is successful, penetrating injuries resulting in long thoracic nerve laceration should be treated with nerve exploration and, possibly, nerve repair. Options for delayed surgical repair of nerve laceration or direct injury include neurolysis and/or nerve grafting when patients show evidence of loss of nerve function (13).

Serratus anterior palsy resulting from chronic long thoracic nerve palsy traditionally has been treated surgically with muscle transfers, scapulopexy, and/or scapulothoracic fusion (46–48). Unfortunately, these surgical options for chronic injury to the long thoracic nerve rarely allow an athlete to return to most competitive sports that require arm strength and motion. A variety of muscles have been used as a musculotendinous transfer to control scapular winging, including the pectoralis major (49–54), pectoralis minor (55–57), rhomboids and teres minor (58–60). The senior author's preference to use the pectoralis major as the muscle transfer for scapular winging caused by long thoracic nerve injury (61).

Recently, reports have appeared of small series or patients treated for long thoracic nerve dysfunction without using a muscle transfer or scapulothoracic fusion. Disa et al. (62) reported excellent results with supraclavicular neurolysis of the long thoracic nerve that was dysfunctional because of nerve compression within the scalene muscles. These same authors also reported excellent results in all four patients who underwent neurolysis 10 to 35 months after the onset of symptoms. Transfer of the thoracodorsal nerve or medial pectoral nerve to the long thoracic nerve has been reported to have good functional results in patients with symptomatic long thoracic nerve injury (63,64).

■ STINGERS AND BURNERS

Brachial plexus neuropathy presents with temporary stinging, burning, or tingling that occurs when the head is forcefully bent sideways. These injuries commonly are referred to as stingers or as burners. The incidence of these injuries is uncertain, because they occur so commonly and are so familiar to athletes and coaches that most do not present for medical care. Symptoms from this syndrome typically last for seconds to minutes; however, in 5% to 10% of cases, the neurological deficit can last for hours, days, or even weeks (65,66). Controversy remains whether damage occurs at the nerve root or at the brachial plexus itself. Management typically involves symptomatic treatment, because the condition usually is self-limited. The important consideration, however, is to rule out underlying factors that may predispose the athlete to more serious, persistent injury.

Basic Science

Anatomy

At each segmental level, the dorsal and ventral roots exit the spinal cord and join to form the cervical (or spinal) nerve root. The ventral (or anterior) roots are formed by the motor

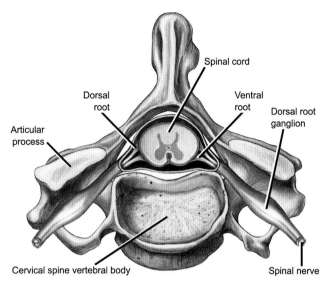

Fig 8-5. Neural structures of the cervical spine. (From Levine MJ, Albert TJ, Smith MD. Cervical radiculopathy: diagnosis and non-operative management. *J Am Acad Orthop Surg.* 1996;4:305–316; with permission.)

nerve fibers leaving the anterior horns cells of the anterior gray area of the spinal cord, whereas the dorsal roots consist of the cell bodies of the sensory fibers. The cervical nerve root enters the neuroforamen, where it forms the dorsal root ganglion (67) **(Fig 8-5)**. Distal to the foramen, the cervical root then divides into a posterior primary ramus, which innervates the paraspinal muscles, posterior elements of the spine and overlying skin, and anterior primary ramus. Several nerves come off the spinal nerves as small branches, such as the dorsal scapular nerve (from the C5 spinal nerve), the long thoracic nerve (C5–C7), and the phrenic nerve (C3–C5). The cervical roots then form the brachial plexus, which supplies motor function and sensation to the upper extremities.

The cervical nerve roots are more susceptible to injury as a result of traction injury compared with the brachial plexus. The cervical roots do not have the protective epineurium, perineurium, fascicular structure, and fascicular plexiform arrangement that protects the brachial plexus from stretch and compression (68). The plexiform structure of the brachial plexus, with its compliant, surrounding soft-tissue structures, can tolerate a greater amount of tension compared with the cervical nerve roots (69), which pass through bony, rigid canals that can be narrowed by anatomical factors.

Biomechanics

Three main mechanisms have been described that may result in a burner or stinger: (a) nerve compression, (b) nerve traction, or (c) a direct blow to the brachial plexus, resulting in upper trunk or cervical root symptoms, particularly involving C5 and C6. Lower cervical roots are less susceptible to damage, but injury can occur with the shoulder either

abducted or fully extended. Controversy remains regarding whether a burner is primarily a brachial plexus or a cervical root injury, a situation that is compounded by the lack of clear demarcation about where the cervical nerve root ends and the brachial plexus begins. Permanent nerve damage can result from recurrent brachial plexus injuries.

Narrowing of the intervertebral foramen occurs with neck extension and with lateral bending, especially when the two motions are combined (70). The narrowing is most pronounced at the C4–C5 and C5–C6 levels. Published series suggest that the extension–lateral compression mechanism is predominately the cause of burners (83% to 85% of cases) (71–73). It appears that compression injuries occur in adult populations, whereas traction injuries are more common in children. Burners associated with these mechanisms are seen in athletes with pre-existing (though may be asymptomatic) cervical spine pathology, such as cervical disc disease or degenerative change.

A second mechanism of a burner is nerve traction as the shoulder is depressed and the nerves are fixed proximally. The traction forces are transmitted to the upper trunk of the brachial plexus, especially the upper cervical nerve roots (C5–C6), stretching and injuring these structures (74–76). The shoulder can be driven downward, and the head and neck in the opposite direction, while blocking or tackling in football or while landing on the shoulder in wrestling, the second most common sport in which this injury occurs (77). This is suggested to be the most frequent mechanism in younger athletes without cervical stenosis or arthritic change (36,76,77).

Finally, the third mechanism is a direct blow to the Erb point, which lies superior and deep to the medial clavicle, just lateral to the sternocleidomastoid muscle (25). In football, the upper trunk of the brachial plexus can be compressed between the shoulder pad and the superior medial scapula following direct trauma (78,79).

Athletes with recurrent cervical nerve root neurapraxia were found to have disc disease and narrowing of the intervertebral foramen in 93% of cases (71). Several papers have identified an association between the incidence of burners and developmentally narrowed spinal canals. In two series, 47% (72) and 53% (71) of athletes had a Pavlov ratio of less than 0.8, and a significant difference was found between measurements among individuals with a previous history of a burner and controls (80) **(Fig 8-6)**.

Evaluation

History

The athlete with a burner usually complains of a traumatic episode with transient numbness, weakness, and/or electrical pain that shoots down the arm to the hand and that lasts for seconds to minutes. Complaints are almost always unilateral, and the athlete rarely complains of neck pain. It most commonly occurs following blocking or tackling; thus, it more commonly affects those athletes participating in

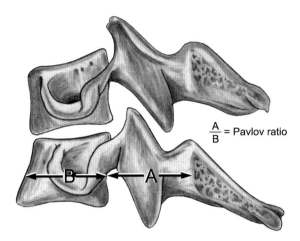

Fig 8-6. Pavlov ratio. (From Thomas BE, McCullen GM, Yuan HA, et al. Cervical spine injuries in football players. *J Am Acad Orthop Surg.* 1999;7:338–347; with permission.)

American football who play as a defensive back, linebacker, and/or lineman (81). Up to 65% of collegiate football players are noted as having had a burner or stinger during their 4-year college career (36,77,79).

Physical Examination

The athlete with a burner may come off the field shaking his or her arm and hand. If significant neck pain exists, or when neurological symptoms involve two or more extremities, cervical spine precautions should be taken with the athlete until the player is cleared from having a cervical spine injury. A typical examination of a burner includes observation and palpation of the neck region for tenderness, swelling, or deformity. The athlete may hold the neck flexed to alleviate pressure on the cervical root. Palpation around the affected nerve root may cause local pain and aggravate symptoms. The shoulder, clavicle, sternoclavicular, and acromioclavicular joints also should be evaluated for deformity and swelling to rule out any other injury. The range of motion in the neck should be assessed by observing active movement through full motion, including flexion, extension, lateral bending, and rotation. If the range of motion is not significantly restricted and little apprehension is noted with movement of the neck, a Spurling maneuver may be performed by gently, laterally bending and extending the head with mild downward pressure (82). A positive sign is reproduction of symptoms down the arm. In cases of traction injury, lateral bending of the neck away from the symptomatic side may cause stretching of the brachial plexus, reproducing symptoms. A careful examination of sensation and motor strength should be performed on the upper extremities. The most common pattern of symptoms is over the lateral aspect of the arm, along the radial nerve distribution (C5–C6). Special attention should be taken to assess upper trunk function (deltoid, rotator cuff, and biceps) to evaluate the burner and recovery from the injury and to assess the lower

trunk (ulnar nerve) to rule out other significant injuries that may be masquerading as a burner. A Tinel sign may be elicited by tapping in the region of the Erb point (superior and deep to the medial clavicle, just lateral to the sternocleidomastoid muscle). With a mild injury, symptoms often resolve quickly (within minutes).

Imaging

For any significant neck injury, radiography of the cervical spine should be performed, including AP, lateral, bilateral oblique, lateral flexion, and extension views. Imaging may be deferred in cases of recurrent burners in which symptoms resolve, but radiography should be considered for any athlete with first-time symptoms. Radiographs should be evaluated for loss of cervical lordosis, spinal stenosis, foraminal stenosis, and instability. Meyer et al. (72) and Kelly et al. (80) have reported that players with a Pavlov ratio of less than 0.8 have an increased risk of experiencing a burner. It should be noted that although athletes with a Pavlov ratio of less than 0.80 demonstrate a higher risk of recurrent stingers, but not of first-time stingers, the level of stenosis did not correlate with the level of stinger symptoms (83).

Magnetic resonance imaging can be helpful in identifying nerve root injuries. In one series, 11 patients with MRIs demonstrating root avulsion had the diagnosis confirmed during surgery, with no false positives (84). Edema in the spinal cord was suggestive of root avulsion. The sensitivity of MRI to detect nerve root avulsions has been reported to be from 81% to 92.9% (84,85). Also, MRI can rule out structural pathologies (86), such as herniated discs, ligamentous injuries, facet injuries, and nondisplaced fractures. Magnetic resonance neurography remains investigational, however, and its role in brachial plexus problems is still being evaluated (87).

Additional Studies

Electrodiagnostic studies can be useful in localizing the site of nerve injury and in quantifying the degree of neurological damage (88). However, EMG and nerve conduction studies are considered only with prolonged neurological symptoms. Continued muscular weakness at 72 hours has been shown to correlate with positive electrodiagnostic testing at 4 weeks (66). EMG may not demonstrate accurate changes until at least 14 days (86). Thus, electrodiagnostic studies have not been helpful in making return-to-play decisions; cases have been reported in which the EMG remained abnormal for more than 4 years after the injury even after full clinical recovery (66,89).

Management

Nonoperative Management

The athlete with no sign of cervical spine injury should be removed from play and observed on the sidelines. Symptoms usually are self-limited and mild. Athletes with prolonged burner symptoms are treated with removal from play, modification of activities, ice, and nonsteroidal anti-inflammatory medications. A soft neck collar can be used for severe symptoms. Physical therapy includes neck range of motion; strengthening of the neck stabilizers, shoulder, and periscapular muscles; stretching; gentle traction; and soft-tissue myofascial techniques.

The common practice is that an athlete can return to full contact activities dependent on painfree, full passive and active range of motion of the neck and shoulders and a normal neurological examination, including full and symmetrical strength of the shoulders and neck. If underlying neck pathology must be ruled out, the athlete should be investigated first before being cleared to play. Because most athletes have resolution of symptoms and a normal examination within minutes, most can return to play during the same game in which they were injured. The natural history of athletes who have sustained burners has not been studied.

The key to management of a burner is the prevention of recurrence. Prevention is initiated by practicing proper tackling technique from a more vertical, upright position rather than by dropping the shoulder and rotating the head, which can result in lateral bending and extension of the neck. Tackling with the crown of the helmet or "spearing" must be avoided, because axial load to the neck is particularly dangerous. The shoulder pads should be checked for appropriate fit (73). A protective neck-roll or collar that limits neck extension is anecdotally useful in preventing recurrence of burners.

Operative Management
Recurrent burners rarely require surgical intervention. Nerve root avulsions are serious injuries, and treatment is controversial. Surgical options for nerve root avulsions include nerve repair or grafts.

■ THORACIC OUTLET SYNDROME

Thoracic outlet syndrome (TOS) refers to a symptom complex of upper extremity pain and paresthesias involving compression neurovascular structures (90,91). It has been subdivided into: (a) vascular (arterial and venous), (b) true neurological, and (c) nonspecific or "disputed" neurological categories. The exact incidences of these categories are unclear. The true neurological TOS is rare and involves compression of the brachial plexus, typically involving the lower trunk and/or C8 to T1 anterior primary rami, by a cervical rib or a fibrous band from the tip of the transverse process (92). Neurogenic TOS may present with atrophy in the abductor pollicis brevis, whereas the vascular TOS is the result of compression of the subclavian blood vessels as they emerge from the thorax and enter the upper limb (93). The disputed, nonspecific entity is the most common presentation. The physician must have a suspicion for this diagnosis clinically, because investigations often are nondiagnostic and the diagnosis is made by exclusion.

Basic Science

Anatomy
The thoracic outlet may be considered as a space between the relatively fixed, immobile thorax, particularly the first rib and clavicle, extending to the anterior and middle scalene muscles and under the pectoral tendon and coracoid process laterally.

The brachial plexus forms from the fifth cervical to the first thoracic nerves after they exit from their respective intervertebral foramen. The anterior and middle scalene muscles take their origin from the transverse processes of the upper cervical spine and insert on the first rib. The brachial plexus and the subclavian artery, which leaves the chest off the aortic arch, travel between these two muscles, over the first rib, and beneath the clavicle **(Fig 8-7)**. The subclavian vein travels over the first rib anterior to the anterior scalene before joining the subclavian artery and brachial plexus.

Biomechanics
Compression of the neurovascular structures can occur with any factor that increases angulation of the nerves or vessels around features in the thoracic outlet or that causes narrowing of the outlet. Possible causes of compression of the brachial plexus and/or the subclavian vasculature can be related to the scalene muscles (94), a cervical rib, a clavicle fracture (nonunion, malunion, or abundant callus formation) (95,96), and accessory neck muscles and fibrous bands at the interscalene region. Hyperabduction syndrome has been described as compression or traction of the neurovascular structures under the pectoral tendon and coracoid when the arm is abducted.

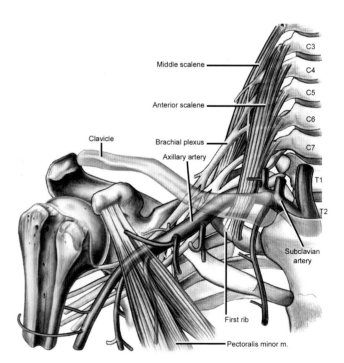

Fig 8-7. Anatomy of the thoracic outlet syndrome. The pertinent anatomy of the brachial plexus and subclavian vessels, which may get compressed, resulting in thoracic outlet compression syndrome, is shown.

Abduction of the arm to an overhead position, excessive shoulder girdle depression (90), and overly developed trapezius and neck musculature have been associated with TOS. Affected athletes often perform repetitive motions involving abduction of the arm to 180 degrees or pulling the shoulders down and back, such as with the cocking phase of serving in tennis. Muscle swelling from trauma, exercise, or hypertrophy is thought to initiate TOS, as seen in some tennis players and baseball pitchers, especially those with greater muscle development of the dominant arm, increased scapular depression, and failure to maintain adequate scapular stabilization (97). Muscle weakness, trauma, arteriosclerosis, abnormal anatomy, and poor posture may play a role as well.

Evaluation

The treatment algorithm for TOS is shown in **Figure 8-8**.

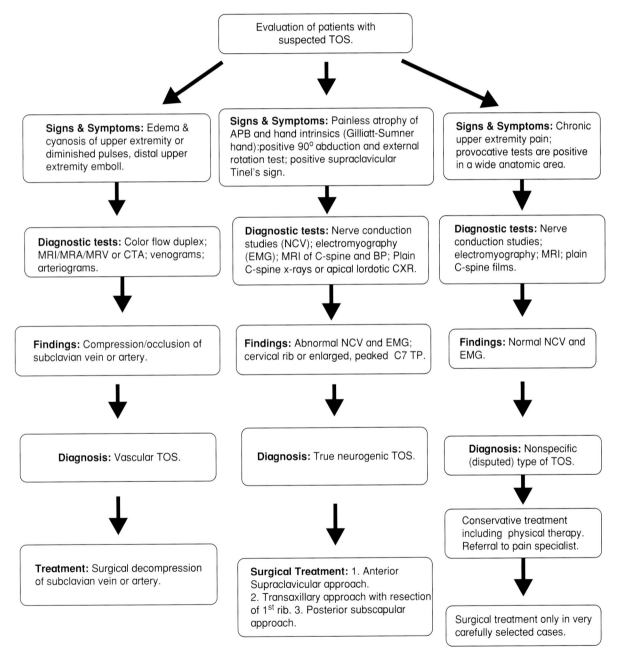

Fig 8-8. Treatment algorithm for thoracic outlet syndrome. APB, abductor pollicis brevis; MRI, magnetic resonance imaging; MRA, magnetic resonance angiography; MRV, magnetic resonance venography; CTA, computed tomographic angiography; BP, brachial plexus; C-spine, cervical spine; CXR, chest x-ray; TP, transverse process. (From Huang JH, Zager EL. Thoracic outlet syndrome. *Neurosurgery.* 2004;55:897–903; with permission.)

History

The subjective complaints and objective findings depend on which structures are being compressed (arterial, venous, or neurological). Symptoms are exacerbated by repetitive overhead movements and are present during or after activities. The syndrome is more prevalent in women (98). Most patients (95% to 97%) complain of neurological symptoms (99–102). Paresthesias with overhead activities are noted, sometimes involving the entire upper extremity but more often in the lower trunk or ulnar nerve distribution (C8–T1). As many as 50% of patients will complain of weakness (103), especially involving the intrinsic muscles, as well as pain and paresthesia. Athletes with arterial compromise may present with complaints of ischemia, such as numbness, tingling, aching, pain, pallor, and coolness of the involved extremities. Symptoms of venous involvement produce complaints of swelling, heaviness, mottled or blotchy or purple discoloration, engorgement of the superficial veins, as well as numbness and/or tingling. Most patients note some history of trauma temporally associated with the onset of symptoms (94,102).

Physical Examination

Inspect the arm for symmetry with regard to size, color, and skin temperature. Palpation of the cervical spine, the scalenes, and the clavicle can be used to look for structural causes of TOS. A Tinel sign may be elicited over the supraclavicular fossa. A careful neurovascular examination should include strength testing of the muscles and checking sensation, especially in areas supplied by the lower brachial plexus.

A few provocative maneuvers have been described to test for TOS, but their use and specificity for establishing the diagnosis of TOS are unclear (104,105). For each of the following maneuvers, a positive test involves the decrease or elimination of a palpable pulse or reproduction of symptoms, such as paresthesias, sensation of heaviness, and/or

fatigue, which are consistent with the diagnosis of TOS and that may not occur on the asymptomatic, contralateral side. During the Adson maneuver, the examiner palpates the ipsilateral radial pulse, while the patient rotates the head toward the side being tested and extends the neck **(Fig 8-9)**. The subject inhales to further compress the structures of the thoracic outlet. The Wright test (106) is performed with the subject's arm being progressively hyperabducted and externally rotated while assessing for ipsilateral radial pulse diminution and reproduction of paresthesias **(Fig 8-10)**. With the Roos stress test or the elevated arm stress test, the patient is asked to repeatedly open and close the hands for several minutes, holding the shoulders in abduction and external rotation of 90 degrees while the elbows are flexed at 90 degrees **(Fig 8-11)**.

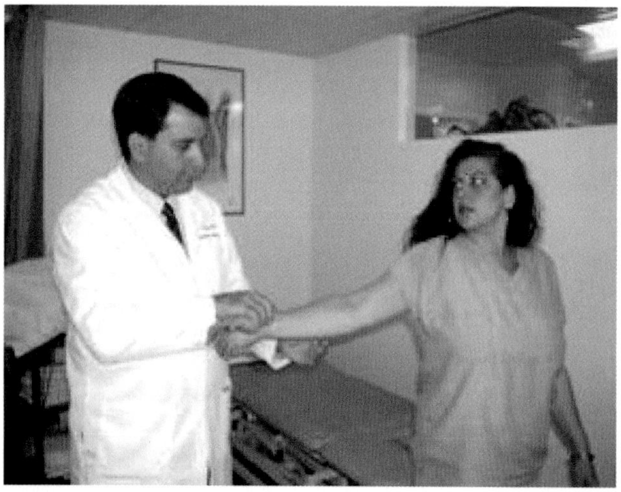

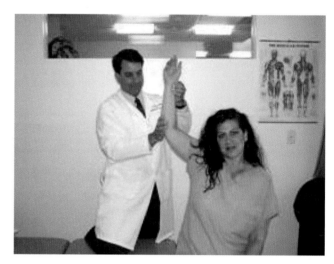

Fig 8-10. The Wright test. The examiner palpates the radial pulse and hyperabducts the patient's arm.

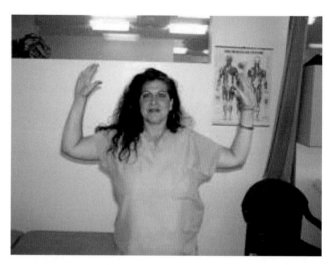

Fig 8-11. The Roos test. The Patient is asked to abduct and externally rotate both shoulders. The patient repetitively opens and closes the hands for 1 minute to exacerbate the symptoms of thoracic outlet syndrome.

Fig 8-9. The Adson test. The examiner palpates the radial pulse and extends the patient's arm. The patient turns the head toward examiner and takes a full breath.

Imaging

Cervical spine and chest radiographs are useful to rule out the uncommon cervical rib (107), long transverse process of C7, abnormal clavicle fracture healing, cervical spondylolysis, narrowed intervertebral space, and osteophytes impinging on the neural foramina. Accessory ribs are found in approximately 0.27% of the general population and are more common in women (77%) (108,109). Color-flow duplex may demonstrate abnormalities in venous or arterial flow, and MRI can be useful to rule out nerve or cord compression from degenerative changes in the cervical spine or herniated discs. Magnetic resonance angiography is useful in establishing the diagnosis of the rare vascular compromise subset of TOS (97).

Additional Studies

Electrodiagnostic studies may only be abnormal in some cases (91,110), because the compression of the brachial plexus often is quite proximal and difficult to test for accurately. Therefore, electrodiagnostic testing, such as EMG and NCV, is useful when the test is positive, but a negative electrodiagnostic test result does not rule out TOS (110). Somatosensory-evoked potentials (SSEP) show less sensitivity for TOS (111).

Management

Nonoperative Management

Conservative treatment is almost always the initial management, provided that no severe vascular compromise is present. Success rates for nonoperative treatment have been reported to range from 67% to 90% (103,104). Nonoperative management includes relative rest and nonsteroidal anti-inflammatory medications to reduce repetitive irritation and swelling around the nerve that may be causing the symptoms. Postural exercise is necessary, because slouching may decrease the space that is available for the neurovascular structures. Physical therapy should focus on improving posture using postural feedback, strengthening the scapular stabilizers and depressors of the shoulder girdle and modalities. Several modalities, including ultrasound and transcutaneous nerve stimulation and biofeedback, have been recommended (90,104,112).

Operative Management

If patients fail conservative management of TOS and have severe and persistent symptoms or progressive neurological dysfunction, surgery often is recommended (108). Surgical intervention bypassing conservative treatment usually is indicated for patients with acute vascular insufficiency. A variety of surgeries have been recommended for the treatment of TOS; however, because TOS may result from a variety of causes, the specific recommended surgery is based on the underlying pathology. Thus, surgery often involves the release or removal of the structures that appear to be causing the compression, and it may involve releasing the scalene

muscles, resection of the first rib or cervical rib, claviculectomy and/or resection of anomalous fibromuscular bands, or some combination of these procedures. The surgical approach can be transaxillary, anterior supraclavicular, posterior subclavicular, or some combination of these (113). Series of surgical decompression of TOS have reported success rates ranging from 70% to 90%, with poorer results in patients having work-related TOS (100,107,114,115).

■ SUPRASCAPULAR NERVE INJURY

A subtle cause of shoulder pain and weakness involves compression or traction of the suprascapular nerve. Overhead and throwing athletes often are affected because of repetitive trauma (e.g., tennis players, baseball players, and weight lifters) (98,116–120). Volleyball players are particularly affected, with one series reporting up to 45% of athletes having clinical and neurophysiological evidence of infraspinatus muscle impairment (121–124). The diagnosis of suprascapular nerve entrapment often is made clinically, based on a careful and thorough history and physical examination.

Basic Science

Anatomy

The suprascapular nerve originates from the fifth and sixth anterior cervical roots, which are part of the upper trunk of the brachial plexus. The suprascapular nerve typically is a motor nerve with no cutaneous sensory capabilities. It travels laterally, across the posterior cervical triangle, deep to the posterior belly of the omohyoid muscle and the anterior border of the trapezius muscle, along the posterior border of the clavicle. The nerve then reaches the upper border of the scapula, where it passes through the suprascapular notch, which can have various shapes (e.g., "U" or "V") and can be either deep and narrow or shallow and wide. While the nerve travels under the transverse scapular ligament as it passes through the notch, the suprascapular artery and vein travel over the ligament (Fig 8-12). Beyond the transverse scapular ligament, the suprascapular nerve sends off one or two motor branches to the supraspinatus muscle, and it receives several sensory fibers from the glenohumeral joint, the acromioclavicular (AC) joint, the coracohumeral ligament (125) and in 15% of patients, cutaneous sensory fibers from the upper lateral arm (deltoid patch) (126). The nerve continues obliquely under the supraspinatus muscle along the floor of supraspinous fossa toward the rim of the glenoid. The nerve then enters the infraspinatus fossa via the spinoglenoid notch, which lies at the lateral margin of the base of the scapular spine. The spinoglenoid notch may be covered by the spinoglenoid ligament, also known as the inferior transverse scapular ligament (127–129). After the nerve passes around the spinoglenoid notch, the nerve divides into two or more branches to supply the infraspinatus muscle.

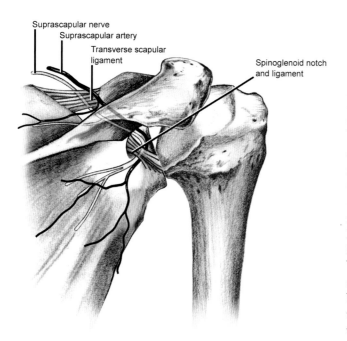

Fig 8-12. Anatomy of the suprascapular nerve.

Biomechanics

During sports, repetitive microtrauma can damage the nerve in several ways, including entrapment and compression, traction and friction, direct trauma, as well as conditions affecting the brachial plexus in general. Besides direct effects on the nerve, intimal damage to the axillary or suprascapular artery has been proposed to result from direct trauma or friction that, in turn, can result in ischemic injury to the nerve (119), particularly at the suprascapular notch.

Because the suprascapular nerve is relatively fixed regarding its position under the rotator cuff and ligaments, it is susceptible to compression by ganglion cysts, lipomas, the transverse scapular ligament (129–131), enlarged spinoglenoid notch veins, or the spinoglenoid ligament (119,124, 132–134). The more frequent sites of compression are the suprascapular notch and the spinoglenoid notch. Between these two, the more common area of entrapment is at the spinoglenoid notch, especially in elite athletes who are involved in overhead sports. The spinoglenoid ligament inserts into the posterior glenohumeral capsule. The ligament has been demonstrated to tighten with cross-body adduction and internal rotation, which can compress the nerve (e.g., during the follow-through phase of throwing a ball or serving in tennis) (128). Also, with extreme abduction and full external rotation, the medial tendinous margin of the infraspinatus and supraspinatus muscles has been shown to be able to impinge strongly against the lateral edge of the scapular spine, compressing the infraspinatus branch of the suprascapular nerve (124). Because the injury to the nerve at the spinoglenoid notch occurs more distally, the supraspinatus muscle and approximately 30% to 40% of the infraspinatus function are left intact (117,118,122). Only the innervation to the infraspinatus is affected, so asymptomatic sports activity may still be possible, because partial function of the muscle may remain and the teres minor can help to compensate for the infraspinatus dysfunction.

A second mechanism of injury to the suprascapular nerve involves traction or mechanical stretching of the nerve, with or without friction, because it travels sharply around critical points (135,136). The nerve can be fixed in several areas: (a) the origin from the upper trunk at the Erb point, (b) the suprascapular notch (under the transverse scapular ligament), (c) the insertion into the infraspinatus muscle, and (d) the spinoglenoid notch or lateral spine of the scapula. Studies have shown that altered conduction can be identified within a nerve when it is stretched 6% beyond its resting length. Stretching the nerve more than 15% beyond its resting length leads to irreversible nerve damage (137,138). With overhead activities in sports, such as the cocking, acceleration, and follow-through phases of serving in volleyball and tennis, the extreme torques and angular velocity that are placed on the shoulder can result in repetitive, undue tensile stresses to the nerve.

The suprascapular nerve also is susceptible to direct injury (120,135,13). Cases with direct nerve injury have been described following dislocation of the glenohumeral joint, fracture of the proximal humerus or scapula, and penetrating injury (98,120,140–142). Injury to the suprascapular nerve also has been a reported complication following surgical procedures, such as distal clavicle resection, shoulder stabilization, or open rotator cuff repair (125,143–145).

Evaluation

History

The presentation of an athlete with a suprascapular nerve palsy can be quite variable. The athlete usually is involved in overhead, repetitive-use sports or heavy labor. Symptoms can be similar to those of atraumatic glenohumeral instability. The history of symptoms tends to be vague, with an insidious onset, but infrequently, there may be an incident of direct impact on the shoulder or of indirect trauma, such as a fall on an outstretched arm (98). The patient may describe poorly localized pain over the lateral and posterior shoulder that usually is exacerbated by activity, which feels like a "dull ache" or a "burning" sensation. Over time, the pain may become constant and can even awaken the patient at night. The athlete may complain about weakness of external rotation and abduction with overhead activity. This is not always the case, however, because injuries involving the distal nerve branches to the infraspinatus often can be incomplete, leaving the supraspinatus unaffected and sparing 30% to 40% of the infraspinatus (122). Certain scapular movements may be painful, which may lead to restriction of shoulder motion, simulating a stiff shoulder.

Physical Examination

The physical examination findings of the athlete depend on the degree of nerve dysfunction and the chronicity of the injury. Athletes presenting early in the process often have an examination that is nonfocal and nonspecific. Patients with chronic problems will demonstrate wasting or atrophy of the involved muscles. If the nerve is injured or entrapped at the suprascapular notch, atrophy of the supraspinatus and infraspinatus muscles occurs, while if the pathology occurs at the spinoglenoid notch, atrophy of the only infraspinatus muscle occurs. The atrophy of the infraspinatus is more obvious than wasting of the supraspinatus muscle, because the supraspinatus atrophy may be partly hidden by the overlying trapezius muscle. With underlying pathology or if the injury to the nerve is localized, tenderness at the affected area often is noted on deep palpation, such as at the suprascapular notch or the spinoglenoid notch. The rotator cuff should be tested carefully for weakness of involved muscles, which can suggest the level of nerve injury. If the nerve is injured at the suprascapular notch, weakness of external rotation typically is noted, especially in adduction but also in abduction, as is weakness of abduction in the scapular plane (particularly the empty can test) because of the involvement of innervation to the infraspinatus and the supraspinatus muscles (146). If the nerve is injured at the spinoglenoid notch, these athletes are more likely to have painless wasting (122,147) and weakness only with external rotation (especially in adduction). Cross-body adduction with the arm extended or internally rotated may exacerbate the posterior shoulder pain.

Imaging

Imaging techniques to help in the evaluation of suprascapular nerve injury include the standard radiographic shoulder series, including an AP radiograph in which the beam is directed caudally by 15 to 30 degrees (131,136). The suprascapular notch also may be seen on the Stryker notch view. Although plain radiographs usually are nondiagnositic, they can be useful both in assessing the morphology of the notch and in assessing for a calcified transverse scapular ligament or in revealing a callus after scapular or clavicle fracture that may irritate, tether, or compress the nerve. CT scans also may reveal osseous abnormalities affecting the nerve, including shape assessment of the notch, calcified ligament, or fracture callus (148). MRI is best to define the anatomy of the soft tissues, to identify the course of the suprascapular nerve, and to determine the presence of any cysts or lesions compressing the nerve (133,149–152). The MRI is also useful to demonstrate rotator cuff atrophy and to rule out other internal derangement of the shoulder or causes of shoulder pain (e.g., rotator cuff tears). Ganglion cysts around the shoulder causing suprascapular nerve compression are estimated to be associated with labral tears, seen either arthroscopically or by MRI, in nearly 90% of cases (153–155).

Additional Studies

EMG and NCV may be helpful in confirming the diagnosis, but limitations remain regarding their applications in suprascapular nerve injury (98,142,156,157). A positive EMG for suprascapular nerve dysfunction demonstrates motor loss in the affected muscles, depending on the location of the lesion, with signs of denervation potentials, fibrillations, spontaneous activity, and prolonged motor latencies. Often, delayed conduction velocity from the Erb point to the supraspinatus or infraspinatus muscle is noted. Normal mean latencies of 3.3 m per second have been recorded from the Erb point to the infraspinatus muscle (158,159). Scapular nerve dysfunction, however, may still exist even with normal nerve studies. Also, nerve studies do not always define the exact nature of the pathologic changes, nor can they routinely localize the exact site of compression. The delay in nerve conduction does not always correlate to clinical or symptomatic dysfunction. An increasing delay in suprascapular nerve conduction was shown in baseball players as the season progressed (119); however, the increasing delay in conduction did not correlate to performance on the field. Chronic neuropathy also can result in false-positive results in some patients (160).

Another test is a diagnostic injection or nerve block. A positive result that is consistent with suprascapular nerve injury at the suprascapular notch is relief of shoulder pain, which is dramatic but of brief duration, following an injection of 1% local anesthetic without epinephrine (131,161, 162). To inject the suprascapular notch, a posterosuperior approach is taken using a 25-gauge needle. A negative test, however, does not rule out suprascapular nerve entrapment, because one cannot be certain that the injection was in the exact location of the nerve.

Management

Nonoperative Management

The initial management of suprascapular nerve injuries usually is nonoperative (117,120,132,163,164). Most authors have found that resolution of symptoms occurs within 6 to 12 months after diagnosis. This is particularly true if the patient has no evidence of a space-occupying lesion (cyst) (117). Because most of these injuries in athletes are thought to be related to traction or repetitive microtrauma, activity modification often is necessary. Specific activities, such as overhead motions and weight lifting, should be avoided if they cause symptoms. Nonsteroidal anti-inflammatory medications may help to relieve nerve inflammation associated with irritation as well as pain. An appropriate therapy program consists of maintaining full shoulder motion and strengthening of the shoulder using proper posture and proprioceptive exercises. Particular attention should be directed toward stretching the posterior capsule of the shoulder and adequate strength of the serratus anterior, trapezius, and rhomboids. Theoretically, stretching the posterior capsule, especially in abduction, because this is the insertion of the spinoglenoid ligament, will reduce tension on the ligament during overhead sports activities. The goal of a strengthening program is to enhance the compensatory muscles and to regain muscular balance about the shoulder. Several authors recommend at least 4 to 6 months of nonoperative management, with follow-up electrodiagnostic testing to determine whether recovery is progressing if deficits or symptoms continue (132).

Operative Management

Surgical decision making is first dependent on whether a cyst is causing suprascapular nerve compression. If a ganglion cyst is present, then the cyst is a result of intra-articular pathology; in athletes, this frequently is because of a labral tear. The natural history of ganglion cysts about the shoulder is not known; however, it commonly is thought that these cysts persist and may enlarge over time (153). Even so, reports of spontaneous cyst resolution have appeared (149). Approximately 90% of ganglion cysts about the shoulder that cause suprascapular nerve compression are associated with labral tears (153–155). In these cases, the current recommendation is arthroscopic debridement or repair of the labrum (153,154,165–167). Some surgeons recommend direct decompression of the cyst while also addressing the labral pathology (154). Multiple approaches to cyst decompression have been reported to have good success; these approaches include arthroscopy (153,167), open cyst excision (122,131,168), and percutaneous aspiration under CT or ultrasound guidance (93,153,169). Ganglion cyst decompression about the shoulder without also addressing the intra-articular pathology has been associated with a failure rate of up to 50%, whereas the inability to aspirate the cyst has been reported to occur in 18% of cases (93,153). It is worth noting, however, that excellent results have been reported with open decompression/excision of the cyst without exploration of the glenohumeral joint (53,56,170).

Controversy exists with regard to the timing of surgery if suprascapular nerve dysfunction is present but no periarticular cyst is identified. Some authors (including the senior author) use the criteria of no improvement in comfort and strength despite 6 months of nonoperative management and/or no improvement of EMG findings as an indication for surgical decompression of the suprascapular nerve. Other authors advocate immediate surgical intervention once the diagnosis has been made to prevent progressive and, potentially, irreversible muscle atrophy and, because it is felt that the pathology, if not the symptoms, likely have been present for at least 6 months by the time the diagnosis has been established (102,170). Still other clinicians and surgeons recommend surgical decompression of the nerve at the first evidence of any muscle wasting to enhance the possibility of maximal muscle recovery (171). On the other hand, some surgeons recommend surgery only after one full year of nonoperative management (provided no cyst present) (172).

Techniques

The technique and approach of surgical decompression of the suprascapular nerve is dependent on the location of the presumed etiology of the nerve dysfunction. If the pathology is at the suprascapular notch, then the transverse scapular ligament and suprascapular notch may be approached anteriorly, superiorly, or posteriorly (171). The anterior approach uses a saber-type incision, just medial to the coracoid (173, 174). Generally, however, the anterior approach is recommended because of the complexity and risk of this dissection as well as poor visualization (56,171). The superior approach is a relatively quick procedure, with minimal morbidity (171). The transverse scapular ligament is easily identified using the superior approach and splitting the trapezius in line with its fibers; this approach is more difficult in muscular patients and in those without atrophy of the supraspinatus (171). Anatomical studies have identified the topographical landmarks for the superior approach (175). The transverse scapular ligament is situated 1.3 cm posterior to the posterior clavicular edge, 2.9 cm medial to the acromioclavicular joint, and 4 cm below the skin (175). The trapezius is elevated from the spine of the scapula and separated from the supraspinatus with the posterior approach (56). Alternatively, the trapezius may be split in line, with its fibers superior to the scapular spine, to avoid trapezial detachment (176,177). Splitting the trapezius muscle posteriorly risks injury to the spinal accessory nerve. The senior author prefers trapezius muscle elevation from the scapular spine when a posterior approach is indicated; using the posterior approach, the transverse scapular ligament and ganglion are easily identified (Fig 8-7).

Regardless of the approach that is used, the principles of suprascapular nerve decompression with or without cyst excision are the same. Initially, the transverse scapular ligament is cut, taking care to protect vascular structures that rest on the ligament. Sectioning of the transverse scapular ligament should occur at its medial insertion to minimize the risk of injury to the suprascapular nerve and vessels that are positioned more laterally on the ligament and taking care to protect the superficial artery. The suprascapular notch can be narrow or sharp ("V"-shaped) because of development or trauma. When the notch is narrow, a notchplasty can be performed by resecting the medial notch wall using Kerrison rongeurs, a burr, and/or curette (24,66,171,176,178). If a notchplasty is required, the surgeon should smooth the cut bony edges of the notch with bone wax. Recently, endoscopic division of the transverse scapular ligament, decompressing the suprascapular nerve, has been suggested and discussed.

If the nerve is compressed at the spinoglenoid notch, then the posterior surgical approach is used. Frequently, the spinoglenoid ligament can be exposed just by retracting the deltoid and elevating the infraspinatus. Some surgeons recommend partial deltoid detachment from the scapular spine to enhance visualization. Once the infraspinatus is elevated, the spinoglenoid ligament is identified and sectioned. Frequently, a notchplasty is performed with a burr when the etiology is felt to be traction of the nerve or tethering at the base of the spine of the scapula, but this is somewhat controversial (102,179). Occasionally, a Kerrison rongeur or curette may be useful to assist in performing the notchplasty. Following the notchplasty, the surgeon needs to be sure the raw edge of bone is smoothed, using bone wax to reduce friction to and scarring of the nerve.

It is the philosophy of some surgeons to release the transverse scapular ligament in conjunction with posterior release, even if the physical examination and EMG findings suggest that the offending area of compression is at the spinoglenoid notch (102). The logic behind this approach is to address potential double-crush situations. Both ligaments can be cut through the same posterior approach, but the trapezius must be detached from the spine of the scapula to reach the transverse scapular ligament. To detach and reattach the trapezius to get to the transverse scapular ligament requires an increased length of postoperative immobilization and carries the potential for increased morbidity. Endoscopic visualization and sectioning of the spinoglenoid ligament have been discussed recently, but to our knowledge, no studies have been published.

Assessment of the results of surgery is difficult, because most published series are small and retrospective, with only short-term follow up and no control group. Assessment is further complicated by the lack of natural history studies for comparison. One complicating factor is the difficulty of knowing how long after the onset of suprascapular nerve injury the patient presents; another is difficulty quantifying the degree of atrophy at presentation, producing difficulty in measuring postoperative change. Anecdotally, following surgery, most patients note immediate relief of the pain that they felt preoperatively. In most cases, surgical decompression of the nerve generally does not help with regeneration of the nerve or with resolution of the atrophy.

Following surgery, muscular strengthening exercises should be performed to restore balance to the rotator cuff musculature. With appropriate rehabilitation, muscle function can be maximized to provide the balance needed for overhead sports.

Return to Play
Fortunately, despite persistent atrophy, most athletes are able to return to full athletic function (169,180).

■ AXILLARY NERVE INJURY

Axillary nerve injuries generally are uncommon in sports and have been estimated to represent less than 1% of all nerve injuries (181). Most of the problems are associated with a trauma, such as an anterior shoulder dislocation or a combined brachial plexus injury. Postoperative complications also have been reported. Another uncommon syndrome involves compression of the axillary nerve within the quadrilateral space. This clinical entity initially was identified in overhead athletes, particularly baseball players, but has since been identified following trauma to the upper extremity or fall on an outstretched hand (182–184).

Basic Science

Anatomy
The main function of the axillary nerve is to provide the motor supply to the deltoid. The axillary nerve originates from the spinal cord at the C5 and C6 levels, with occasional contribution from the C4 level. The nerve travels below the coracoid process, then obliquely along the anterior surface of the subscapularis. Approximately 3 to 5 mm medial to the musculotendinous junction of the subscapularis, the axillary nerve receives a sensory branch from the anterior articular capsule of the shoulder and dives to the inferolateral border of subscapularis (185) **(Fig 8-13)**. The nerve then takes a posterior course, adjacent to inferomedial capsule, and passes through the quadrilateral space (148).

The borders of the quadrilateral space include the long head of the triceps medially, the humeral shaft laterally, the teres minor muscle superiorly, the teres major and latissimus dorsi muscles inferiorly, and the subscapularis muscle anteriorly **(Fig 8-14)**. The axillary nerve enters the quadrilateral space with the posterior circumflex humeral artery, then courses around the posterolateral humeral neck (surgical neck). Finally, the nerve branches into anterior and posterior branches supplying the deltoid muscle. Forty-five percent of the strength of external rotation is from the teres minor, whereas the deltoid generally is identified as the prime mover of the shoulder (186).

Biomechanics
The most common mechanism of injury to the axillary nerve is closed trauma involving a traction injury to the shoulder,

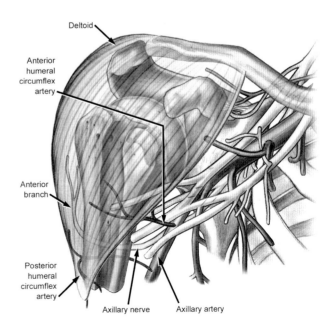

Fig 8-13. Anatomy of the axillary nerve. The axillary nerve comes from the posterior cord of the brachial plexus and travels on the subscapularis tendon before going under the joint and posteriorly with the posterior circumflex humeral artery.

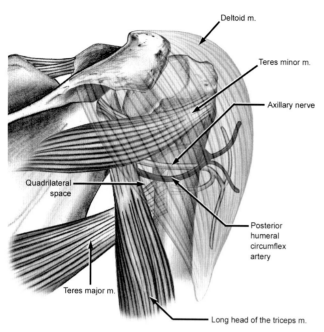

Fig 8-14. The quadrilateral space (posterior view of shoulder). With the arm in adduction, there is no compression of the axillary nerve and posterior circumflex humeral artery. m, muscle.

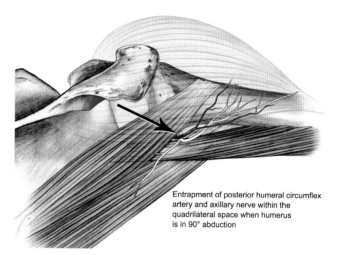

Entrapment of posterior humeral circumflex artery and axillary nerve within the quadrilateral space when humerus is in 90° abduction

Fig 8-15. Proposed mechanism of quadrilateral space syndrome. With abduction of the arm, intermittent compression of the nerve and artery results from shearing and closing down of the space by the teres major and teres minor.

such as stretching of the nerve over the humeral head during an anterior shoulder dislocation. The incidence of axillary nerve injury has been reported to be between 19% and 55% following an anterior shoulder dislocation (187–189) and up to 58% following proximal humeral fractures (190). Several of these injuries may go unnoticed, because the pain of a shoulder fracture or dislocation may mask symptoms (187). Risk factors associated with axillary nerve injury after shoulder dislocation include advancing patient age at the time of dislocation (especially >40 years of age), length of time the shoulder is left unreduced (>12 hours), and amount of trauma required to cause the dislocation (188,191,192).

Otherwise, blunt trauma to the anterolateral aspect of the shoulder has been reported to be a possible cause of isolated axillary nerve injury (192). Traumatic causes that affect the nerve at the quadrilateral space include direct trauma to the posterior shoulder, traction injury to the upper extremity, and a deep posterior shoulder intramuscular injection.

In quadrilateral space syndrome, compression of posterior circumflex humeral artery and axillary nerve results from nontraumatic causes within confines of the quadrilateral space. Fibrous bands frequently have been seen during surgery within the quadrilateral space of patients with this problem (193). Unfortunately, the origin of these bands is unknown. Other suggested causes for compression of these structures have been shearing forces between the teres major and teres minor **(Fig 8-15)**, friction or irritation of the nerve as it passes around posterior glenoid, compression by a hypertrophied portion of subscapularis muscle that inserts onto the humerus just inferior to lesser tuberosity, dilated veins within the quadrilateral space, or a paralabral cyst (148,194). Overuse

conditions of the shoulder causing repetitive microtrauma or abnormal biomechanics may lead to this pathologic syndrome.

Evaluation

History
Surprisingly, many athletes with axillary nerve injury may be asymptomatic with complete or incomplete lesions (195). Often, however, affected athletes may fatigue quickly when they exercise, especially with overhead activity and heavy lifting. If pain is present, the athlete usually complains of a poorly localized, dull aching or burning pain over the lateral and posterior aspects of the shoulder. The pain is exacerbated by overhead activities, particularly with the arm in abduction, external rotation, and extension. Athletes involved in repetitive-use overhead sports, such as baseball, tennis, and volleyball, and some football players appear to get this condition. They may note numbness of the lateral arm; however, complete deltoid muscle deficit may occur with normal sensation of the upper lateral arm and shoulder (187). Affected individuals also may notice reduced abduction strength or inability to raise their arm. A history of trauma, dislocation, or fracture should be documented. Quadrilateral space syndrome tends to affect young, active adults between the ages of 20 and 40 years. Because the presentation of axillary nerve conditions is nonspecific, patients with this syndrome may have had previous operations, with persistent pain even after the other surgical procedures.

Physical Examination
The physical examination of athletes with axillary nerve injury should include evaluation for range of motion (passive and active) as well as strength (abduction, forward elevation, external rotation, and internal rotation). Patients with a chronic history of the problem may demonstrate atrophy or

asymmetry of the deltoid muscle mass. A neurovascular examination should be performed to assess sensation over the upper lateral arm and to rule out other lesions, such as TOS, and brachial plexus and cervical spine lesions. It is important to note that complete deltoid muscle deficit may occur with normal sensation of the upper lateral arm and shoulder.

Identification of the quadrilateral space syndrome is difficult, because many signs are nonspecific. Some patients may have tenderness of the posterior shoulder in the area of the quadrilateral space. Symptoms are most likely to be reproduced with the FABER (forward elevation, abduction, and external rotation) test of the shoulder, which is held for more than 1 minute. Wasting or atrophy of the deltoid and/or teres minor muscles may be noted when evaluating the patient with the shirt off. Resisted muscle strength testing of the shoulder should be performed with the shoulder in abduction, forward flexion, and extension to assess deltoid muscle strength. External rotation strength also should be tested to assess the teres minor, although the patient may not appear to have weakness because of the function of the infraspinatus muscle. Pulses in the upper extremities should be normal.

Imaging

Several tests may be necessary to rule out other causes of shoulder pain, because isolated axillary nerve injury and quadrilateral space syndrome are rare. Plain radiographs typically are ordered, but these are useful in these cases only with a history of trauma that is consistent with a possible proximal humerus fracture, scapular neck fracture, or anterior shoulder dislocations.

Cervical spine radiography may be considered to rule out neck pathology, such as cervical spondylosis or osteoarthritis, which may be causing radiculopathy and subsequent deltoid weakness and/or atrophy. CT may reveal osseous abnormalities affecting the nerve, such as excessive callus formation following a scapular neck or proximal humeral fracture. MRI can help to identify the course of the axillary nerve and any associated soft-tissue lesions. A paralabral cyst or venous dilation compressing the nerve has been reported (148,194). In advanced cases, atrophy of the deltoid and/or teres minor can be seen with MRI (196), whereas while fatty replacement of the muscle suggests a poor prognosis for recovery of function (134). Finally, MRI is helpful to rule out other pathologies, such as rotator cuff tears. The role of magnetic resonance neurography is still being determined.

To diagnose quadrilateral space syndrome, the classic test is arteriography. During arteriography, the vessel of interest is the posterior circumflex humeral artery, which travels through the quadrilateral space with the axillary nerve. With the arm in adduction, normal flow typically will be seen in the posterior circumflex humeral artery and should be seen passing around the posterolateral humeral neck. When the arm is held in abduction and external rotation, however, contrast flow is lost within the posterior circumflex humeral

artery distal to the quadrilateral space (Fig 8-15). Angiography can be performed as an angio-MRI; however, this test can demonstrate occlusion of the posterior circumflex humeral artery with the shoulder in abduction in up to 80% of asymptomatic patients (197).

Additional Studies

Nerve studies, such as EMG and NCV, are helpful to confirm the diagnosis, to determine the severity of the nerve injury to guide prognosis and expected timeline for recovery, and to establish a baseline from which to follow recovery of the nerve. These studies also may rule out other causes of axillary nerve injury. EMG should be obtained 3 weeks after injury to document the injury (because earlier 3 weeks, it may still be normal), to confirm the diagnosis, and to serve as a baseline value with which to follow recovery. Nerve studies are less useful for the diagnosis of quadrilateral space syndrome because of the intermittent nature of the nerve compression, especially early in the process. With prolonged compression of the axillary nerve at the quadrilateral space and development of muscular atrophy in long-standing situations, however, EMG may reveal chronic atrophic changes (194).

Another test that may help to confirm quadrilateral space syndrome is a diagnostic nerve block. The diagnostic injection of 1% local anesthetic (without epinephrine) in the area of the quadrilateral space syndrome is useful if it positively produces relief of the shoulder pain. A negative test or no relief of pain symptoms, however, cannot absolutely rule out the condition, because it is difficult to confirm the proper positioning of the needle into the quadrilateral space.

Management

Nonoperative Management

Nonoperative management of an axillary nerve injury includes reassurance, activity modification, symptomatic management, and physical therapy. As the nerve recovers, active, passive-, and active-assisted range of shoulder motion should be performed to maintain motion, and electrical stimulation and strengthening exercises may help to reduce atrophy of the deltoid. The athlete should be reassured of nerve recovery, because the prognosis after shoulder fracture, dislocation, or direct trauma generally is good. Full recovery of axillary nerve injury caused by dislocation or fracture is expected in 85% to 100% of cases managed conservatively within 6 to 12 months from the time of injury (187,188, 191). Even if the deltoid paralysis persists, return to sports like football and rugby is possible—and quite likely. Specifically, nonoperative treatment of quadrilateral space syndrome, which should be tried initially, should include aggressive stretching of the posterior shoulder, especially the teres minor, as well as assessment of biomechanics during sports, such as a patient's throwing, serving, or hitting, which should be corrected if possible. Most cases of quadrilateral space syndrome are thought to be self-limiting, and symptoms resolve with nonoperative treatment. Athletes should avoid lifting heavy objects or participating in activities that exacerbate symptoms (usually overhead movements) until symptoms improve.

Return to Play

Axillary nerve injury caused by a direct blow to the anterolateral shoulder has a less optimistic prognosis for recovery. Surprisingly, athletic function often remains good except in sports such as tennis and baseball.

Operative Management

For axillary nerve injury resulting from penetrating trauma or iatrogenic causes, management is immediate repair. When axillary nerve injury results from causes other than penetrating trauma or surgery (i.e., those with closed trauma), surgery is indicated for symptomatic patients with no clinical or EMG/NCV evidence of recovery 3 to 6 months following injury (126,198). The best functional results occur when surgery is performed within 6 months of injury; patients can expect excellent return of strength and function. Surgery after 6 months results in more modest gains. Functional improvement can be expected with surgery up to 1 year after injury (59,126,199). Surgery performed more than 1 year after the injury in symptomatic patients has an even poorer prognosis for functional recovery (59,126,198,199). Surgical approaches include neurolysis, neurorrhaphy, nerve grafting, nerve transfer, and neurotization (68,181,200–202). After 1 year, tendon transfers may be undertaken, but these are salvage procedures and are not designed for return to sports.

Reviewing the literature does not help in determining the outcome for athletes. Most series do not report their results of athletes independently from the general population. Furthermore, most series combine the results of surgery in patients with axillary nerve injury from many different etiologies.

The symptoms of quadrilateral space syndrome are thought to result from intermittent compression of the axillary nerve at the quadrilateral space, but EMG/NCV studies are almost uniformly negative. No studies have determined the natural history, but many suggest that this syndrome may resolve with nonoperative management provided the patient has no space-occupying lesion, such as a cyst, or bony abnormality causing this syndrome. One investigator has suggested that only 30% of patients experience symptoms warranting surgical intervention (71).

The indication for decompression of the quadrilateral space for quadrilateral space syndrome is persistent symptoms beyond 6 months despite nonoperative management. Cahill and Palmer (193) recommend surgery only if the diagnosis is confirmed by angiography, the patient is point tender at the quadrilateral space of the posterior shoulder, and the patient has failed 6 months of conservative management. The surgical approach requires splitting the deltoid in line with its fibers posteriorly (95), but some advocate detaching part of the origin of the deltoid (144,193). The axillary nerve and posterior circumflex artery are readily

identified and isolated. Often, fibrous bands are identified, and if so, they are sectioned or excised. Some surgeons also recommend releasing part of the teres major to further relieve pressure on the nerve (71); however, the senior author has not found this to be necessary. Once the nerve and artery have been released, digital palpation of the arterial pulse with the arm in abduction and external rotation will confirm adequate decompression.

Looking to the literature, no large series of quadrilateral space syndrome have appeared since the initial report of 18 patients by Cahill and Palmer (193). Of these 18 patients, eight had dramatic relief of symptoms, eight were improved (with some persistence of night pain), and two were no better following surgery. In the experience of the senior author as well as that of others, however, patients with arteriogram-proven quadrilateral space syndrome usually have immediate relief of symptoms after release of fibrous bands (55,71, 144,149,193).

■ REFERENCES

1. Warner JJ, Micheli LJ, Arslanian LE, et al. Scapulothoracic motion in normal shoulders and shoulders with glenohumeral instability and impingement syndrome: a study using Moire topographic analysis. *Clin Orthop.* 1992;285:191–199.
2. Manske RC, Reiman MP, Stovak ML. Nonoperative and operative management of snapping scapula. *Am J Sports Med.* 2004;32: 1554–1565.
3. Kibler WB. The role of the scapula in athletic shoulder function. *Am J Sports Med.* 1998;26:325–337.
4. Kuhn JE. Scapulothoracic crepitus and bursitis in athletes. In: DeLee JC, Drez D Jr, Miller MD, eds. *DeLee & Drez's orthopaedic sports medicine.* 2nd ed. Philadelphia: WB Saunders; 2003: 1006–1014.
5. Kuhn JE, Plancher KD, Hawkins RJ. Symptomatic scapulothoracic crepitus and bursitis. *J Am Acad Orthop Surg.* 1998;6: 267–273.
6. Edelson JG. Variations in the anatomy of the scapula with reference to the snapping scapula. *Clin Orthop.* 1996;322:111–115.
7. Kibler WB, McMullen J. Scapular dyskinesis and its relation to shoulder pain. *J Am Acad Orthop Surg.* 1995;3:319–325.
8. Poppen NK, Walker PS. Normal and abnormal motion of the shoulder. *J Bone Joint Surg Am.* 1976;58:195–201.
9. Milch H. Partial scapulectomy for snapping in the scapula. *J Bone Joint Surg Am.* 1950;32:561–566.
10. Milch H. Snapping scapula. *Clin Orthop.* 1961;20:139–150.
11. Percy EC, Birbraeger D, Pitt MJ. Snapping scapula: a review of the literature and presentation of 14 cases. *Can J Surg.* 1988;31: 248–250.
12. Cooley LH, Torg JS. "Pseudowinging" of the scapula secondary to subscapular osteochondroma. *Clin Orthop.* 1982;162:119–124.
13. Kuhn JE, Plancher KD, Hawkins RJ. Scapular winging. *J Am Acad Orthop Surg.* 1995;3:319–325.
14. Safran MR. Management of scapulothoracic problems. *Curr Opin Orthop.* 1997;8:67–74.
15. Greis PE, Kuhn JE, Schultheis J, et al. Validation of the lift-off test and analysis of subscapularis activity during maximal internal rotation. *Am J Sports Med.* 1996;24:589–593.
16. Cools AM, Witvrouw EE, Danneels LA, et al. Does taping influence electromyographic muscle activity in the scapular rotators in healthy shoulders? *Man Ther.* 2002;7:154–162.

17. Sisto DJ, Jobe FW. The operative treatment of scapulothoracic bursitis in professional pitchers. *Am J Sports Med.* 1986;14:192–194.
18. Galinat BJ. Endoscopic scapuloplasty: a minimum 2-year follow-up. In: *Transactions of the 64th Annual Meeting of the American Academy of Orthopaedic Surgeons.* Rosemont, IL: AAOS;1997:204.
19. Ruland LJ, Ruland CM, Matthews LS. Scapulothoracic anatomy for the arthroscopist. *Arthroscopy.* 1995;11:52–56.
20. Ciullo JV. Subscapular bursitis: treatment of "snapping scapula syndrome" or "washboard syndrome." *Arthroscopy.* 1992;8:412–413.
21. Foo CL, Swann M. Isolated paralysis of the serratus anterior: a report of 20 cases. *J Bone Joint Surg Br.* 1983;65:552–556.
22. Kauppila LI. The long thoracic nerve: possible mechanisms of injury based on autopsy study. *J Shoulder Elbow Surg.* 1993;2:244–248.
23. Footnote A 7, 81, 105.
24. Basmajian JV. *Primary Anatomy.* 8th ed. Baltimore: Williams & Wilkins; 1982.
25. Safran MR. Nerve injury about the shoulder in athletes. Part 2. Long thoracic nerve, spinal accessory nerve, burners/stingers, thoracic outlet syndrome. *Am J Sports Med.* 2004;32:1063–1076.
26. Overbeck D, Grormley R. Paralysis of the serratus magnus muscle. *JAMA.* 1940;114:1904–1906.
27. Gregg JR, Labosky D, Harty M, et al. Serratus anterior paralysis in the young athlete. *J Bone Joint Surg Am.* 1979;61:825–832.
28. Horwitz MT, Tocantins LM. An anatomic study of the role of the long thoracic nerve and the related scapular bursae in the pathogenesis of local paralysis of the serratus anterior. *Anat Rec.* 1938;71:375–385.
29. Hester P, Caborn DNM, Nyland J. Cause of long thoracic nerve palsy: a possible dynamic fascial sling cause. *J Shoulder Elbow Surg.* 2000;9:31–35.
30. Wood VE, Frykman GK. Winging of the scapula as a complication of first rib resection. *Clin Orthop.* 1980;149:160–163.
31. Wood VE, Verska JM. The snapping scapula in association with the thoracic outlet syndrome. *Arch Surg.* 1989;124:1335–1337.
32. Vastimaki M. Pectoralis minor transfer in serratus anterior paralysis. *Acta Orthop Scand.* 1984;55:293–295.
33. Tsairis P, Dyck PJ, Mulder DW. Natural history of brachial plexus neuropathy. Report on 99 patients. *Arch Neurol.* 1972;27:109–117.
34. Vastamaki M, Solonen KA. Accessory nerve injury. *Acta Orthop Scand.* 1984;55:296–299.
35. Seddon HJ. *Surgical disorders of the peripheral nerves.* Baltimore: Williams & Wilkins; 1972:68–88.
36. Clancy WG, Brand RL, Bergeld JA. Upper trunk brachial plexus injuries in contact sports. *Am J Sports Med.* 1977;5:209–214.
37. Lee SK, Wolfe SW. Peripheral nerve injury and repair. *J Am Acad Orthop Surg.* 2000;8:243–252.
38. Barron OA, Levine WN, Bigliani LU. Surgical management of chronic trapezius dysfunction. In: Warner JJP, Iannotti JP, Gerber C, eds. *Complex and revision problems in shoulder surgery.* Philadelphia: Lippincott–Raven Publishers; 1997:377–384.
39. Helms CA, Martinez S, Speer KP. Acute brachial neuritis (Parsonage–Turner syndrome): MR imaging appearance—report of three cases. *Radiology.* 1998;207:255–259.
40. Fery A. Results of treatment of anterior serratus paralysis. In: Post M, Morrey BF, Hawkins RJ, eds. *Surgery of the shoulder.* St. Louis: Mosby–Year Book; 1990:325–329.
41. Parsonage MJ, Turner JWA. Neuralgic amyelotrophy: the shoulder girdle syndrome. *Lancet.* 1948:973–978.
42. Marin R. Scapula winger's brace: a case series on the management of long thoracic nerve palsy. *Arch Phys Med Rehab.* 1998;79:1226–1230.
43. Leffert RD. Neurological problems. In: Rockwood CA Jr, Matsen FA III, eds. *The shoulder.* Vol 2. Philadelphia: WB Saunders; 1990:750–790.
44. McCarty EC, Tsairis P, Warren RF. Brachial neuritis. *Clin Orthop.* 1999;368:37–43.
45. Hershman EB, Wilbourn AJ, Bergfeld JA. Acute brachial neuropathy in athletes. *Am J Sports Med.* 1989;17:655–659.
46. Atasoy E, Majd M. Scapulothoracic stabilization for winging of the scapula using strips of autogenous fascia lata. *J Bone Joint Surg Br.* 2000;82:813–817.
47. Copeland SA, Howard RC. Thoracoscapular fusion for fascioscapulohumeral dystrophy. *J Bone Joint Surg Br.* 1978;60:547–551.
48. Whitman A. Congenital elevation of scapula and paralysis of the serratus magnus muscle. *JAMA.* 1932;99:1332–1334.
49. Dickson FD. Fascial transplants in paralytic and other conditions. *J Bone Joint Surg.* 1937;19:405–412.
50. Gozna ER, Harris WR. Traumatic winging of the scapula. *J Bone Joint Surg Am.* 1979;61:1230–1233.
51. Iceton J, Harris WR. Treatment of winged scapula by pectoralis major transfer. *J Bone Joint Surg Br.* 1987;69:108–110.
52. Marmor L, Bechtal CO. Paralysis of the serratus anterior due to electric shock relieved by transplantation of the pectoralis major muscle. A case report. *J Bone Joint Surg Am.* 1963;45:156–160.
53. Noerdlinger MA, Cole BJ, Stewart M, et al. Results of pectoralis major transfer with fascia lata autograft augmentation for scapula winging. *J Shoulder Elbow Surg.* 2002;11:345–350.
54. Post M. Pectoralis major transfer for winging of the scapula. *J Shoulder Elbow Surg.* 1995;4:1–9.
55. Chaves JP. Pectoralis minor transplant for paralysis of the serratus anterior. *J Bone Joint Surg Br.* 1951;33:228–230.
56. Rapp IH. Serratus anterior paralysis treated by transplantation of the pectoralis minor. *J Bone Joint Surg Am.* 1954;36:852–854.
57. Vastamaki M. Pectoralis minor transposition in serratus anterior paralysis. In: Vastimaki M, ed. *Surgery of the shoulder.* Burlington, VT: BC Decker; 1984:252–254.
58. Herzmark MH. Traumatic paralysis of the serratus anterior relieved by transplantation of the rhomboidei. *J Bone Joint Surg Am.* 1951;33:235–238.
59. Lindstrom N, Danielsson L. Muscle transposition in serratus anterior paralysis. *Acta Orthop Scand.* 1962;32:369–373.
60. Zeier FG. The treatment of winged scapula. *Clin Orthop.* 1973;91:128–133.
61. Safran MR, Warner JJP. Paralysis. Functional restoration. In: Herndon JH, ed. *Reconstruction of the upper extremity.* Stamford, CT: Appleton & Lange; 1998:141–174.
62. Disa JJ, Wang B, Dellon AL. Correction of scapular winging by supraclavicular neurolysis of the long thoracic nerve. *J Reconstr Microsurg.* 2001;17:79–84.
63. Novak CB, Mackinnon SE. Surgical treatment of a long thoracic nerve palsy. *Ann Thorac Surg.* 2002;73:1643–1645.
64. Tomaino MM. Neurophysiologic and clinical outcome following medial pectoral to long thoracic nerve transfer for scapular winging: a case report. *Microsurgery.* 2002;22:254–257.
65. Archambault JL. Brachial plexus stretch injury. *J Am Coll Health.* 1983;31:256–260.
66. Speer KP, Bassett FH. The prolonged burner syndrome. *Am J Sports Med.* 1990;18:591–594.
67. Levine MJ, Albert TJ, Smith MD. Cervical radiculopathy: diagnosis and nonoperative management. *J Am Acad Orthop Surg.* 1996;4:305–316.
68. Rockett FX. Observations on the burner: traumatic cervical radiculopathy. *Clin Orthop Rel Res.* 1982;164:18–19.
69. Wall EJ, Massie JB, Kwan MK, et al. Experimental stretch neuropathy. Changes in nerve conduction under tension. *J Bone Joint Surg Br.* 1992;74:126–129.
70. Yoo JU, Zou D, Edwards WT, et al. Effect of cervical spine motion on the neuroforaminal dimensions of the human cervical spine. *Spine.* 1992;17:1131–1136.
71. Levitz CI, Reilly PJ, Torg JS. The pathomechanics of chronic, recurrent cervical nerve root neurapraxia. The chronic burner syndrome. *Am J Sports Med.* 1997;25:73–76.

72. Meyer SA, Schulte KR, Callaghan JJ, et al. Cervical spinal stenosis and stingers in collegiate football players. *Am J Sports Med.* 1994;22:158–166.

73. Watkins RG. Neck injuries in football players. *Clin Sports Med.* 1986;5:215–246.

74. Bateman JE. Nerve injuries about the shoulder in sports. *J Bone Joint Surg Am.* 1967;49:785–792.

75. Hoyt W. Etiology of shoulder injuries in athletes. *J Bone Joint Surg Am.* 1967;49:755–766.

76. Robertson WC Jr, Eichman PL, Clancy WG. Upper trunk plexopathy in football players. *JAMA.* 1979;241:1480–1482.

77. Sallis RE, Jones K, Knopp W. Burners: offensive strategy for an under-reported injury. *The Phys Sportsmed.* 1997; 20:47–55.

78. DiBenedetto M, Markey K. Electrodiagnostic localization of traumatic upper trunk brachial plexopathy. *Arch Phys Med Rehab.* 1984;65:15–17

79. Markey KL, DiBennedetto M, Curl WW. Upper trunk brachial plexopathy: the stinger syndrome. *Am J Sports Med.* 1993;21:650–655.

80. Kelly JD IV, Aliquo D, Sitler MR, et al. Association of burners with cervical canal and foraminal stenosis. *Am J Sports Med.* 2000;28:214–217.

81. Hershman EB. Brachial plexus injuries. *Clin Sports Med.* 1990;9:311–329.

82. Vikari-Juntura E, Porras M, Laasonen EM. Validity of clinical tests in the diagnosis of root compression in cervical disc disease. *Spine.* 1989;14:253–257.

83. Castro FP Jr, Ricciardi J, Brunet ME, et al. Stingers, the Torg ratio, and the cervical spine. *Am J Sports Med.* 1997;25:603–608.

84. Hems TEJ, Birch R, Carlstedt T. The role of magnetic resonance imaging in the management of traction injuries to the adult brachial plexus. *J Hand Surg Br.* 1999;24:550–555.

85. Doi K, Otsuka K, Okamoto Y, et al. Cervical nerve root avulsion in brachial plexus injuries: magnetic resonance imaging classification and comparison with myelography and computerized tomography myelography. *J Neurosurg Spine.* 2002;96:277–284.

86. Cantu RC. Stingers, transient quadriplegia, and cervical spinal stenosis: return to play criteria. *Med Sci Sports Exerc.* 1997; 29[Suppl]:233–235.

87. Zhou L, Yousem DM, Chaudhry V. Role of magnetic resonance neurography in brachial plexus lesions. *Muscle Nerve.* 2004;30:305–309.

88. Wilbourn AJ, Hershman EB, Bergfeld JA. Brachial plexopathies in athletes: The EMG findings. *Muscle Nerve.* 1986;9:254.

89. Bergfeld JA, Hershman EB, Wilbourn A. Brachial plexus injury in sports: a five-year follow-up. *Orthop Trans.* 1988;12:743–744.

90. Karas SE. Thoracic outlet syndrome. *Clin Sports Med.* 1990;9:297–310.

91. Wilbourn A. Thoracic outlet syndromes. *Neurol Clin.* 1999;17:477–497.

92. Le Forestier N, Moulonguet A, Masionobe T, et al. True neurogenic thoracic outlet syndrome: electrophysiological diagnosis in six cases. *Muscle Nerve.* 1998;21:1129–1134.

93. Toby ED, Koman LA. Thoracic outlet compression syndrome. In: Szabo RM, ed. *Nerve compression syndromes: diagnosis and treatment.* Winsdale, ON, Canada: Slack Publishers; 1989:209–226.

94. Sanders RJ, Pearce WH. The treatment of thoracic outlet syndrome: a comparison of different operations. *J Vasc Surg.* 1989;10:626–634.

95. Fujita K, Matsuda K, Sakai Y, et al. Late thoracic outlet syndrome secondary to malunion of the fractured clavicle: case report and review of the literature. *J Trauma.* 2001;50:332–335.

96. Kay SP, Eckardt JJ. Brachial plexus palsy secondary to clavicular nonunion. Case report and literature survey. *Clin Orthop Rel Res.* 1986;206:219–222.

97. Esposito MD, Arrington JA, Blackshear MN, et al. Thoracic outlet syndrome in a throwing athlete diagnosed with MRI and MRA. *J Magn Reson Imaging.* 1997;7:598–599.

98. Yoon TN, Grabois M, Guillen M. Suprascapular nerve injury following trauma to the shoulder. *Trauma.* 1981;21:652–655.

99. Hempel GK, Rusher AH Jr, Wheeler CG, et al. Supraclavicular resection of the first rib for thoracic outlet syndrome. *Am J Surg.* 1981;141:213–215.

100. Hempel GK, Shutze WP, Anderson JF, et al. 770 Consecutive supraclavicular first rib resections for thoracic outlet syndrome. *Ann Vasc Surg.* 1996;10:456–463.

101. Sanders RJ, Monsour JW, Gerber WF, et al. Scalenectomy versus first rib resection for treatment of the thoracic outlet syndrome. *Surgery.* 1979;85:109–121.

102. Sellke FW, Kelly TR. Thoracic outlet syndrome. *Am J Surg.* 1988;156:54–57.

103. McGough EC, Pearce MB, Byrne JP. Management of thoracic outlet syndrome. *J Thorac Cardiovasc Surg.* 1979;77:169–174.

104. Roos DB. Congenital anomalies associated with thoracic outlet syndrome: anatomy, symptoms, diagnosis, and treatment. *Am J Surg.* 1976;132:771–778.

105. Adams JT, DeWeese JA. "Effort" thrombosis of the axillary and subclavian veins. *J Trauma.* 1971;11:923–930.

106. Wright IS. The neurovascular syndrome produced by hyperabduction of the arms. *Am Heart J.* 1945;29:1–19.

107. Sanders RJ, Hammond SL. Management of cervical ribs and anomalous first ribs causing neurogenic thoracic outlet syndrome. *J Vasc Surg.* 2002;36:51–56.

108. Roos DB. Thoracic outlet syndrome is underdiagnosed. *Muscle Nerve.* 1999;22:130–136.

109. Firsov GI. Cervical ribs and their distinction from underdeveloped first ribs. *Arkh Anat Gistol Embriol.* 1974;67:101–103.

110. Leiberman JL, Taylor RG. Electrodiagnosis in upper extremity nerve compression. In: Szabo RM, ed. *Nerve compression syndromes: diagnosis and treatment.* Winsdale, ON, Canada: Slack Publishers; 1989:67–88.

111. Veilleux M, Stevens JC, Campbell JK. Somatosensory evoked potentials: lack of value for diagnosis of thoracic outlet syndrome. *Muscle Nerve.* 1988;11:571–575.

112. Leffert RD. Thoracic outlet syndrome. In: Gelberman RH, ed. *Operative nerve repair and reconstruction.* Philadelphia: JB Lippincott Co; 1991:1177–1195.

113. Huang J, Zager EL. Thoracic outlet syndrome. *Neurosurgery.* 2004;55:897–903.

114. Sharp WJ, Nowak LR, Zamani T, et al. Long-term follow-up and patient satisfaction after surgery for thoracic outlet syndrome. *Ann Vasc Surg.* 2201;15:32–36.

115. Urschel HC Jr, Razzuk MA. Neurovascular compression in the thoracic outlet: changing management over 50 years. *Ann Surg.* 1998;228:609–617.

116. Agre JC, Ash N, Cameron MC, et al. Suprascapular neuropathy after intensive resistive exercise: case report. *Arch Phys Medial Rehabil.* 1987;68:236–238.

117. Black KP, Lombardo JA. Suprascapular nerve injuries with isolated paralysis of the infraspinatus. *Am J Sports Med.* 1990;18:225–288.

118. Bryan WJ, Wild JJ. Isolated infraspinatus atrophy: a common cause of posterior shoulder pain and weakness in throwing athletes. *Am J Sports Med.* 1986;17:130–131.

119. Ringel SP, Treihaft M, Carry M, et al. Suprascapular neuropathy in pitchers. *Am J Sports Med.* 1990;18:80–86.

120. Weaver HL. Isolated suprascapular nerve lesions. *Injury.* 1983;15:117–126.

121. Eggert von S, Holzgraefe M. Compression neuropathy of the suprascapular nerve in high performance volleyball players. *Sportverl Sportschad.* 1993;7:136–142.

122. Ferretti A, Cerullo G, Russo G. Suprascapular neuropathy in volleyball players. *J Bone Joint Surg Am.* 1987;69:260–263.

123. Holzgraefe M, Kukowski B, Eggert S. Prevalence of latent and manifest suprascapular neuropathy in athletes. *Br J Sports Med.* 1994;28:177–179.

124. Sandow MJ, Ilic J. Suprascapular nerve rotator cuff compression syndrome in volleyball players. *J Shoulder Elbow Surg.* 1998;7:516–521.

125. Warner JJP, Krushell RJ, Masquelet A, et al. Anatomy and relationships of the suprascapular nerve: anatomical constraints to mobilization of the supraspinatus and infraspinatus muscles in the management of massive rotator cuff tears. *J Bone Joint Surg Am.* 1992;74:36–45.

126. Ajmani ML. The cutaneous branch of the human suprascapular nerve. *J Anat.* 1994;185:439–442.

127. Demaio M, Drez DJ, Mullins RC. The inferior transverse scapular ligament as a possible cause of entrapment of neuropathy of the nerve to the infraspinatus. *J Bone Joint Surg Am.* 1991;73:1061–1063.

128. Demirhan M, Imhoff AB, Debski RE, et al. The spinoglenoid ligament and its relationship to the suprascapular nerve. *J Shoulder Elbow Surg.* 1998;7:238–243.

129. Ticker JB, Djurasovic M, Strauch RJ, et al. The incidence of ganglion cysts and other variations in anatomy along the course of the suprascapular nerve. *J Shoulder Elbow Surg.* 1998;7:472–478.

130. Alon M, Weiss S, Fishel B, et al. Bilateral suprascapular nerve entrapment syndrome due to an anomalous transverse scapular ligament. *Clin Orthop Rel Res.* 1988;234:31–33.

131. Garcia G, McQueen D. Bilateral suprascapular nerve entrapment syndrome: case report and review of the literature. *J Bone Joint Surg Am.* 1981;63:491–492.

132. Drez D Jr. Suprascapular neuropathy in the differential diagnosis of rotator cuff injuries. *Am J Sports Med.* 1976;4:43–45.

133. Inokuchi W, Ogawa K, Horiuchi Y. Magnetic resonance imaging of suprascapular nerve palsy. *J Shoulder Elbow Surg.* 1998;7:223–227.

134. Ogino T, Minami A, Kato H, et al. Entrapment neuropathy of the suprascapular nerve by a ganglion: a report of three cases. *J Bone Joint Surg Am.* 1991;73:141–147.

135. Hadley MN, Sonntag VKH, Pittman HW. Suprascapular nerve entrapment. a summary of seven cases. *J Neurosurg.* 1986;64:843–848.

136. Rengachary SS, Burr D, Lucas S, et al. Suprascapular entrapment neuropathy: a clinical, anatomical, and comparative study. Part 2. Anatomical study. *J Neurosurg.* 1979;5:447–451.

137. Bora FW, Pleasure DE, Didizian NA. A study of nerve regeneration and neuroma formation after nerve suture by various techniques. *J Hand Surg.* 1976;1:138–143.

138. Sunderland S. The anatomy and physiology of nerve injury. *Muscle Nerve.* 1990;13:771–784.

139. Rengachary SS, Neff JP, Singer PA, et al. Suprascapular entrapment neuropathy: a clinical, anatomical, and comparative study. Part 1. Clinical study. *J Neurosurg.* 1979;5:441–445.

140. Boerger TO, Limb D. Suprascapular nerve injury at the spinoglenoid notch after glenoid neck fracture. *J Shoulder Elbow Surg.* 2000;9:236–237.

141. Edland H, Zachrisson B. Fracture of the scapular notch associated with lesion of the suprascapular nerve. *Acta Orthop Scand.* 1975;46:758–763.

142. Zoltan JD. Injury to the suprascapular nerve associated with anterior dislocation of the shoulder: case report and review of the literature. *J Trauma.* 1979;19:203–206.

143. Bigliani LU, Dalsey RM, McCann PD, et al. An anatomical study of the suprascapular nerve. *Arthroscopy.* 1990;6:301–305.

144. Mallon WJ, Bronec PR, Spinner RJ, et al. Suprascapular neuropathy after distal clavicle excision. *Clin Orthop Rel Res.* 1996;329:207–211.

145. Shaffer BS, Conway J, Jobe FW, et al. Infraspinatus muscle splitting incision in posterior shoulder surgery: an anatomic and electromyographic study. *Am J Sports Med.* 1994;22:113–120.

146. Kelly BT, Kadrmas WR, Speer KP. The manual muscle examination for rotator cuff strength. An electromyographic investigation. *Am J Sports Med.* 1996;24:581–588.

147. Montagna P, Colonna S. Suprascapular neuropathy restricted to the infraspinatus muscle in volleyball players. *Acta Neurol Scand.* 1993;87:248–250.

148. Safran MR. Nerve injury about the shoulder in athletes. Part 1. Suprascapular nerve and axillary nerve. *Am J Sports Med.* 2004;32:803–819.

149. Fritz RC, Helms CA, Steinbach LS, et al. Suprascapular nerve entrapment: evaluation with MR imaging. *Radiology.* 1992;182:437–444.

150. Gersovich EO, Greenspan A. Magnetic resonance imaging in the diagnosis of suprascapular nerve syndrome. *Can Assoc Radiol J.* 1993;44:307–309.

151. Goss TP, Aronow MS, Coumas JM. The use of MRI to diagnose suprascapular nerve entrapment caused by a ganglion. *Orthopedics.* 1994;4:359–362.

152. Ludig T, Walter F, Chapuis D, et al. MR imaging evaluation of suprascapular nerve entrapment. *Eur Radiol.* 2001;11:2161–2169.

153. Hawkins RJ, Piatt BE, Fritz RC, et al. Clinical evaluation and treatment of spinoglenoid notch ganglion cysts [abstract]. *J Shoulder Elbow Surg.* 1999;8:551.

154. Moore TP, Fritts HM, Quick DC, et al. Suprascapular nerve entrapment caused by supraglenoid cyst compression. *J Shoulder Elbow Surg.* 1997;6:455–462.

155. Tirman PFJ, Feller JF, Janzen DL, et al. Association of glenoid labral cysts with labral tears and glenohumeral instability: radiographic findings and clinical significance. *Radiology.* 1994;190:653–658.

156. Clein LJ. Suprascapular entrapment neuropathy. *J Neurosurg.* 1975;43:337–342.

157. Vastamaki M, Goransson H. Suprascapular nerve entrapment. *Clin Orthop Rel Res.* 1993;297:135–144.

158. Khalili AA. Neuromuscular electrodiagnostic studies in entrapment neuropathy of the suprascapular nerve. *Orthop Rev.* 1974;3:27–28.

159. Kraft GH. Axillary, musculocutaneous, and suprascapular nerve latency studies. *Arch Phys Medial Rehab.* 1972;53:383–387.

160. Post M, Grinblat E. Suprascapular nerve entrapment. diagnosis and results of treatment. *J Shoulder Elbow Surg.* 1993;2:190–197.

161. Rask MR. Suprascapular nerve entrapment: a report of two cases treated with suprascapular notch resection. *Clin Orthop Rel Res.* 1977;123:73–75.

162. Solheim L, Roaas A. Compression of the suprascapular nerve after fracture of the suprascapular notch. *Acta Orthop Scand.* 1978;49:338–340.

163. Jackson DL, Farrage J, Hynninen BC, et al. Suprascapular neuropathy in athletes: case reports. *Clin J Sports Med.* 1995;5:134–136.

164. Zuckerman JD, Polonsky L, Edelson G. Suprascapular nerve palsy in a young athlete. *Bull Hosp Joint Dis.* 1993;53:11–12.

165. Chochole MH, Senker W, Meznik C, et al. Glenoid-labral cyst entrapping the suprascapular nerve: dissolution after arthroscopic debridement of an extended SLAP lesion. *Arthroscopy.* 1997;13:753–755.

166. Fehrman DA, Orwin JF, Jennings RM. Suprascapular nerve entrapment by ganglion cysts: a report of six cases with arthroscopic findings and review of the literature. *Arthroscopy.* 1995;11:727–734.

167. Iannotti JP, Ramsey ML. Arthroscopic decompression of a ganglion cyst causing suprascapular nerve compression. *Arthroscopy.* 1996;12:739–745.

168. Callahan JD, Scully TB, Shapiro SA, et al. Suprascapular nerve entrapment. *J Neurosurg.* 1991;74:893–896.

169. Biedert RM. Atrophy of the infraspinatus muscle caused by a suprascapular ganglion. *Clin J Sports Med.* 1996;6:262–264.

170. Post M, Mayer J. Suprascapular nerve entrapment. diagnosis and treatment. *Clin Orthop Rel Res.* 1987;223:126–136.
171. Vastamaki M, Kauppila LI. Etiologic factors in isolated paralysis of the serratus anterior muscle. A report of 197 cases. *J Shoulder Elbow Surg.* 1993;2:240–243.
172. Merrell GA, Barrie KA, Katz DL, et al. Results of nerve transfer techniques for restoration of shoulder and elbow function in the context of a meta-analysis of the English literature. *J Hand Surg [Am].* 2001;26:303–314.
173. Neviaser TJ, Ain BR, Neviaser RJ. Suprascapular nerve degeneration secondary to attenuation by a ganglionic cyst. *J Bone Joint Surg Am.* 1986;68:627–628.
174. Simeone FA. Neurologic complications of closed shoulder injuries. *Orthop Clin North Am.* 1975;6:499–506.
175. White AM, Witten CM. Long thoracic nerve palsy in a professional ballet dancer. *Am J Sports Med.* 1993;21:626–628.
176. Carroll KW, Helms CA, Otte MT, et al. Enlarged spinoglenoid notch veins causing suprascapular nerve compression. *Skel Radiol.* 2003;32:72–77.
177. Narakas AO. Operative management of lesions of the axillary nerve, isolated or combined with other nerve lesions. *Clin Neurol Neurosurg.* 1992;94[suppl]:S64–S66.
178. Rayan GM. Lower trunk brachial plexus compression neuropathy due to cervical rib in young athletes. *Am J Sports Med.* 1988;16:77–79.
179. Hama H, Ueba Y, Morinaga T, et al. A new strategy for treatment of suprascapular entrapment neuropathy in athletes: shaving of the base of the scapular spine. *J Shoulder Elbow Surg.* 1992;1:253–260.
180. Leung YF, Chung OM, Ip PS, et al. An unusual case of thoracic outlet syndrome associated with long distance running. *Br J Sports Med.* 1999;33:279–281.
181. Pollack LJ, Davis L. Peripheral nerve injuries. *Am J Surg.* 1932;17:462–471.
182. Cormier PJ, Matalon MAS, Wolin PM. Quadrilateral space syndrome: a rare cause of shoulder pain. *Radiology.* 1988;167:797–798.
183. Nuber GW, McCarthy WJ, Yao JST, et al. Arterial abnormalities of the shoulder in athletes. *Am J Sports Med.* 1990;18:514–519.
184. Redler MR, Ruland LJ, McCue FC. Quadrilateral space syndrome in a throwing athlete. *Am J Sports Med.* 1986;14:511–513.
185. Levy HJ, Uribe JW, Delaney LG. Arthroscopic assisted rotator cuff repair: preliminary results. *Arthroscopy.* 1990;6:55–60.
186. Saha AK. Surgery of the paralyzed and flail shoulder. *Acta Orthop Scand Suppl.* 1967;97:5–90.
187. Blom S, Dahlback LO. Nerve injuries in dislocations of the shoulder joint and fractures of the neck of the humerus. *Acta Chir Scand.* 1970;136:461–466.
188. Toolanen G, Hildingsson T, Hedlund T, et al. Early complications after anterior dislocation of the shoulder in patients over 40 years. An ultrasonographic and electromyographic study. *Acta Orthop Scand.* 1993;64:549–552.
189. Visser CPJ, Brand R, et al. The incidence of nerve injury in anterior dislocation of the shoulder and its influence on functional recovery. A prospective clinical and EMG study. *J Bone Joint Surg Br.* 1999;81:679–685.
190. Visser CPJ, Napoleon L, et al. Nerve lesions in proximal humeral fractures. *J Shoulder Elbow Surg.* 2001;10:421–427.
191. Gumina S, Postacchini F. Anterior dislocation of the shoulder in elderly patients. *J Bone Joint Surg Br.* 1997;79:540–543.
192. Perlmutter GS, Apruzzese W. Axillary nerve injury in contact sports: recommendations for treatment and rehabilitation. *Sports Med.* 1998;26:351–361.
193. Cahill BR, Palmer RE. Quadrilateral space syndrome. *J Hand Surg.* 1983;8:65–69.
194. Sanders TG, Tirman PFJ. Paralabral cyst: an unusual cause of quadrilateral space syndrome. *Arthroscopy.* 1999;15:632–637.
195. Palmer SH, Ross AC. Recovery of shoulder movement in patients with complete axillary nerve palsy. *Ann R Coll Surg Engl.* 1998;80:413–415.
196. Linker CS, Helms CA, Fritz RC. Quadrilateral space syndrome: findings at MR imaging. *Radiology.* 1993;188:675–676.
197. Mochizuki T, Isoda H, Masui T, et al. Occlusion of the posterior circumflex humeral artery: detection with MR angiography in healthy volunteers and in a patient with quadrilateral space syndrome. *AJR Am J Roentgenol.* 1994;163:625–627.
198. Burkhead WZ Jr, Scheinberg RR, Box G. Surgical anatomy of the axillary nerve. *J Shoulder Elbow Surg.* 1992;1:31–36.
199. Kopell HP, Thompson WAL. Pain and the frozen shoulder. *Surg Gynecol Obstet.* 1959;109:92–96.
200. Alnot JY, Valenti PH. Surgical reconstruction of the axillary nerve. In: Post M, Morrey BF, Hawkins RJ, eds. *Surgery of the shoulder.* St. Louis: Mosby–Year Book; 1990:330–333.
201. Colachis SC, Strom BR. Effect of suprascapular and axillary nerve blocks on muscle forces in the upper extremity. *Arch Phys Med Rehabil.* 1971;52:22–29.
202. Mestdagh H, Drizenko A, Ghestem P. Anatomical bases of suprascapular nerve syndrome. *Anat Clin.* 1981;3:67–71.

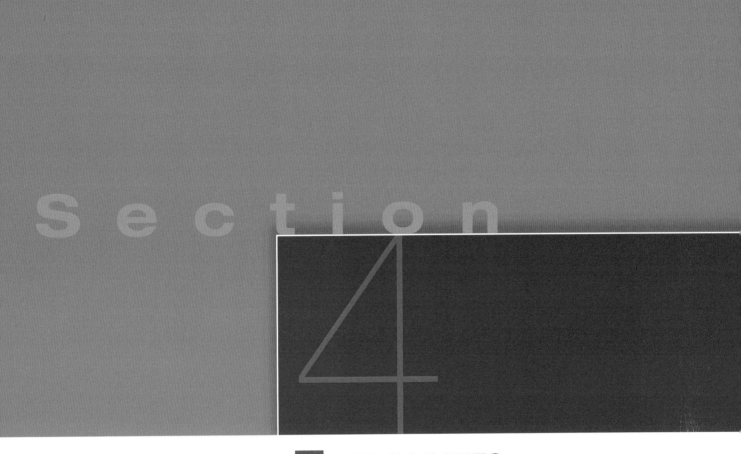

H EAD INJURIES

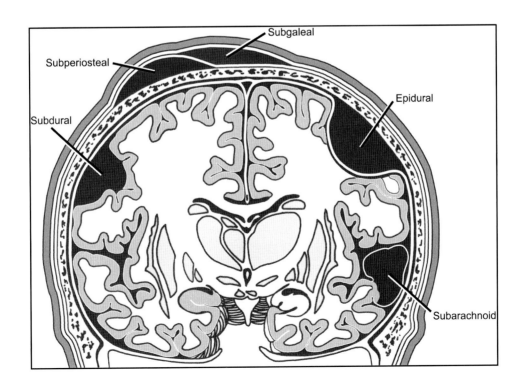

HEAD INJURIES AND CONCUSSION

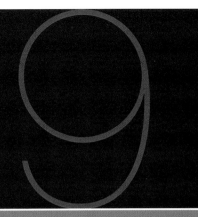

ANDREW D. PEARLE, MD, RONNIE BARNES, ATC, RUSSELL F. WARREN, MD

■ KEY POINTS

■ Traumatic events can lead to both primary injuries [e.g., scalp lacerations, intracranial bleeds, skull fractures, concussion, and diffuse axonal injury, (DAI)] and later, secondary injuries (e.g., herniation syndromes, diffuse edema, and hypoxic/ischemic injuries).

■ Initial evaluation and treatment should progress through the ABCs (airway, breathing, and circulation) of trauma resuscitation. Glasgow Coma Scale is a standard measure of level of consciousness.

■ Orientation (time, place, and person), retrograde amnesia, dizziness, visual changes, nausea, tinnitus, pupils, and head/neck pain should also be assessed.

■ Physical examination should include detailed head and neck assessment for crepitus/deformity, bruising (e.g., the Battle sign), blood or fluid leakage [e.g., cerebrospinal fluid (CSF) leak], and tenderness. A careful neurologic examination, including cranial nerve assessment, is important; mini-mental status examinations can be helpful in the evaluation of neurocognitive function.

■ Intracranial hemorrhage can be divided into epidural, subdural, and subarachnoid.

■ The most common definition of concussion is a "clinical syndrome characterized by immediate and transient posttraumatic impairment of neural functions, such as alteration of consciousness, disturbance of vision, equilibrium, etc. due to brain stem involvement." A concussion is sometimes called mild traumatic brain injury (MTBI).

■ Any head trauma associated with a loss of consciousness is a concussion. Headache (46%), dizziness (42%), and blurred vision (16%) are the most common symptoms.

■ It is estimated that 20% of patients with head trauma will suffer postconcussive symptoms (impaired memory and concentration, persistent headache, fatigue, mood and sleep disturbances, and dizziness).

■ Second-impact syndrome is a rare, potentially life-threatening event that results when a second impact occurs before complete recovery from the initial concussion. It can occur with a relatively minor impact. Clinically, the athlete appears to be stunned, then collapses within minutes. Pupils become dilated, and patient is semicomatose and develops respiratory distress.

■ Dementia puglistica (ataxia, pyramidal tract dysfunction, tremor, impaired memory, dysarthria, and behavioral changes) is a chronic brain injury that results from multiple concussions. Chronic traumatic brain injury (CTBI) is the term that has been used more recently. It includes decreased processing speed, short-term memory impairment, concentration deficit, irritability or depression, fatigue and sleep disturbance, a general feeling of fogginess, and academic difficulties.

■ The management of concussions has three crucial components: identifying neurologic emergencies, preventing second-impact syndrome, and avoiding the effects of repetitive concussions.

■ Once an athlete is asymptomatic, progression of activity is instituted over several days and is followed with continued monitoring. Each step takes a minimum of 1 day. The recommended steps from the 2001 Vienna Conference on Concussions in Sport are (a) no activity, rest until asymptomatic; (b) light aerobic activity; (c) sport-specific training; (d) noncontact training drills; (e) full-contact training; and (f) game play.

131

Head injuries are a major concern to the team physicians, and these injuries represent a wide spectrum of trauma. Concussion remains the most common type of sports-related head injury and is the focus of this chapter. However, more severe intracranial lesions, such as intracranial hemorrhage, cerebral contusion, and related complications, must be considered with any head injury.

Primary injuries arise from an initial traumatic event and include scalp and skull injuries, extraparenchymal hemorrhage, cortical contusion, concussion, and diffuse axonal injury. As with any trauma, patients are at risk of subsequent secondary injury, which in the setting of head injury can be particularly devastating because of the limited and fixed cranial space and the inability of cerebral tissue to repair or to regenerate. Secondary injury includes herniation syndromes, secondary infarcts and bleeds, diffuse cerebral edema, hypoxic and ischemic injuries, and hydrocephalus. The fundamental goals in treating head injury are to recognize primary injuries and to prevent secondary lesions.

PATHOPHYSIOLOGY OF HEAD INJURIES

Athletic head injuries usually result from direct impact and/or deceleration-rotational events. Classic principles of brain contusions include the concept of coup injury, in which a forceful blow to a stationary head imparts maximal brain injury directly beneath the point of impact. On the other hand, contrecoup injuries occur when the energy of impact is transferred to the mobile brain, such that it glides against the fixed, sharp surfaces of the dural reflection or skull base ridges, thus resulting in a contusion at a site opposite that of the initial external trauma. The effect of forces on the brain parenchyma normally are buffered by the cerebrospinal fluid (CSF), which serves as a shock absorber, protecting the brain by converting focal stresses to more uniformly distributed compressive stress. The contrecoup injury pattern occurs because, in the moving head, the floating brain lags behind the leading skull edge, diminishing the protective CSF in the trailing surface and creating a thickened layer of CSF at the leading cranial surface. In the setting of skull fractures, the depressed fragment may directly injure the adjacent parenchyma.

Three types of stresses commonly are imparted to brain tissue—compression, tensile, and shear—and these types may occur in combination. Compressive forces result in direct impact to the brain parenchyma, as in the case of depressed skull fractures. Tensile and compressive forces may occur with linear acceleration injuries, such as in the coup/contrecoup injury patterns. Shearing injuries are often caused by rotational forces and are poorly tolerated by brain parenchyma. These injuries are thought to be related to differences in the physical properties of gray matter and axonal fibers (density differences), such that they decelerate at different velocities; thus, shearing injuries typically occur at gray matter–white matter junctions (1).

CLINICAL EVALUATION OF HEAD INJURIES

On-the-Field Evaluation

The initial on-the-field evaluation is directed toward assessing the levels of consciousness and of associated injuries, particularly cervical spine trauma. The medical personnel must first assess the patient's airway, breathing, and circulation (i.e., ABCs). If the patient is unconscious, the initial respondent must assume that an associated cervical spine injury has occurred, and the neck should be stabilized immediately. A rapid assessment must be made concerning the need for possible emergent transport to a hospital setting.

The standard method for assessing the level of consciousness is the Glasgow Coma Scale (Table 9-1). In addition to observing the patient's motor, eye opening, and verbal responses, medical personnel should assess for orientation to person, place, and time and for the presence of retrograde amnesia.

Symptoms such as dizziness, visual changes, and head or neck pain must be ascertained before removing the athlete

TABLE 9-1	Glasgow Coma Scale
Eye opening	
Spontaneous	4
To voice	3
To pain	2
None	1
Verbal response	
Oriented	5
Confused	4
Inappropriate words	3
Incomprehensible sounds	2
None	1
Motor response	
Obeys commands	6
Purposeful movement	5
Withdraw to pain	4
Flexion to pain	3
Extension to pain	2
None	1

Eye opening + verbal response + motor response = 3−15

- GCS ≥13 = *possible* mild brain injury
- GCS 9–12 = moderate injury
- GCS 8 = severe brain injury
- GCS ≤7 = Coma
- 90% of those ≤8 are in coma
- **GCS ≥11 = usually excellent prognosis**

from the field. If the athlete is able to understand and follow commands, he or she may be assisted to a seated position. If the initial respondent is confident that the athlete has sufficient strength and coordination, the patient can be helped to his or her feet and assisted off the field. Medical personnel should consider the use of a motorized cart or stretcher if the athlete cannot maintain balance in the seated or standing position.

On-the-Bench Evaluation

Athletes should be questioned for specific symptoms when they are taken off the field. In particular, athletes should be questioned about dizziness, visual changes (e.g., photophobia, double vision, or blurriness), headache, nausea, vertigo, and tinnitus. Many of these symptoms may not be present immediately but may occur in a delayed fashion. Vomiting may be indicative of a significant head injury with elevated intracranial pressure.

Physical examination should be directed at careful inspection and palpation of the head and neck. Facial bones should be evaluated carefully for crepitus and fracture. Mandibular fractures can be detected based on pain or malorientation with teeth clenching and grinding. Nasal fractures can be determined by palpation or visualization of deformity.

Certain findings are indicative of specific fracture patterns. Leakage of cerebral spinal fluid from the nose is suggestive of a cribiform plate fracture of the skull. Spinal fluid adjacent to the tympanic membrane is suggestive of a fracture in the temporal bone. The Battle sign (i.e., ecchymosis posterior to the ear in the mastoid region) is indicative of a posterior skull fracture.

A careful cranial nerve examination should be performed. Salient features of this examination include changes in pupil size, which can suggest increased intracranial pressures or a unilateral sympathetic nerve response; deficient oculomotor function caused by injury to the third cranial nerve from a skull fracture or subdural hematoma; asymmetric upward case because of infraorbital blow-out fractures resulting in entrapment of the inferior rectus muscle; and cranial nerve VII palsy from basilar skull fractures. In addition, transient nystagmus often is seen after shearing or rotatory injury to the brainstem. A complete neurologic examination, including assessment for strength, sensation, and coordination, should be performed.

A neurocognitive assessment should include the athlete's orientation to person, place, and time; recent memory, new learning, and delayed recall can be tested using short word recalls. Concentration can be evaluated by having the patient say the months of the year in reverse or by subtracting with serial sevens. The Mini-Mental Status Exam is a formalized, brief screening tool that discriminates patients with moderate or severe deficits (2). Other structured sideline assessments of neurocognitive dysfunction may be employed to standardize evaluation after head trauma (Appendix 1) (3–5).

■ SPECTRUM OF HEAD INJURIES

Intracranial hemorrhage can be divided into three types: epidural, subdural, and subarachnoid **(Fig 9-1)**. Each type of intracranial hemorrhage is potentially devastating, so prompt, accurate assessment and appropriate treatment must be instituted. The initial presentation ranges from headache to neurologic deficits to loss of consciousness. Blood is an irritant to brain tissue and may precipitate a seizure.

Arterial epidural hematomas often are associated with temporal bone fractures and may rapidly enlarge. The bleeds frequently are the result of middle meningeal arterial injuries. Blood rapidly accumulates between the skull and dura, and the amount of blood may reach a fatal accumulation in 30 to 60 minutes. Classically, patients are described as having a lucid interval after an initial loss of consciousness, but this only occurs in approximately one third of patients (6). Early diagnosis and rapid evacuation of large or expanding hematomas are essential in many cases. A good outcome can occur with appropriate craniotomy and evacuation, whereas an unrecognized bleed may be fatal.

Subdural hematomas occur between the dura and arachnoid and often are the result of torn bridging veins. Subdural hematomas are a leading cause of death in athletes, and they are approximately threefold more common than epidural hematomas (7). Unlike epidural hematomas, subdural hematomas commonly are associated with insult to brain tissue that can make recovery guarded. Acute subdural hematomas can lead to herniation-induced brainstem dysfunction with a high mortality rate, even with neurosurgical intervention (8). Subdural hematomas can present with rapid-onset, focal neurologic signs, including hemiparesis, aphasia, and a "blown pupil." Chronic subdural hematomas, on the other hand, may present in a delayed

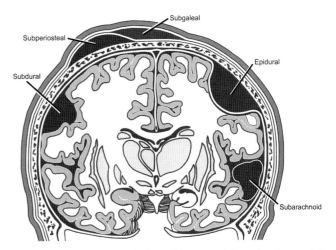

Fig 9-1. Anatomic depiction of intracranial and extracranial hemorrhages.

fashion, with persistent symptoms of headache and subtle changes in mental, motor, or sensory function.

Finally, subarachnoid hematomas are hemorrhages confined to the CSF space along the surface of the brain, usually as a result of rupture of the small, surface brain vessels. Nuchal rigidity may be present because of the meningeal irritation. Subarachnoid hemorrhage, even if posttraumatic, can irritate the meninges and cause vascular spasm, leading to infarcts.

Cerebral contusion is a "bruise" of the brain parenchyma. These lesions may occur in the setting of a depressed skull fracture or when acceleration–deceleration forces cause the brain to impact with the inner table of the skull. Cerebral contusions most commonly are supratentorial and are associated with concussion. They may progress to focal neurologic deficits over the first 24 to 48 hours; close monitoring with serial computed tomographic (CT) evaluation is essential.

Diffuse axonal injuries occur with high-velocity rotational forces. In this injury, multifocal microhemorrhages and edema may occur that can be detected with CT scanning, although magnetic resonance imaging (MRI) is more sensitive. Common locations for the hemorrhages include the gray matter–white matter junctions, deep gray matter, upper brainstem, corpus callosum, and internal capsule.

■ CONCUSSION

Overview

Now commonly referred to as mild traumatic brain injury (MTBI), concussion is clearly the most common athletic head injury, but agreement on its definition remains elusive. The most commonly cited definition, proposed by the Committee on Head Injury Nomenclature of the Congress of Neurologic Surgeons, is a "clinical syndrome characterized by immediate and transient posttraumatic impairment of neural functions, such as alteration of consciousness, disturbance of vision, equilibrium, etc. due to brain stem involvement" (9). The cardinal features of concussion are an alteration of mental status after head injury, a Glasgow Coma Scale ranging from 13 to 15, and negative findings on neuroimaging; these features may or may not be accompanied by a loss of consciousness (10).

Although most athletes fully recover from a concussion, an unknown percentage of patients will have persistent sequelae that can be disabling and, in some cases, permanent. Most physicians are aware of the dangers of second-impact syndrome, which is the catastrophic scenario of a second head trauma in a patient who remains symptomatic from a previous concussion (11); however, more subtle chronic sequelae of repetitive concussive episodes, such as impairment of cognitive processes, mood, and behavior as well as increased risk of subsequent MTBIs, are less understood (12–15). At present, we have no treatment for acute

concussions or the chronic sequelae, no established means to predict chronicity, and no definitive guidelines for return to play. However, early diagnosis of concussion and postconcussive symptoms and utilization of preventative strategies are likely to result in better treatment of athletes with head injuries.

Cerebral Pathophysiology of Concussion

Concussion injuries are thought to result from diffuse axonal injuries caused by rapid acceleration/deceleration of the head, which results in stretching of nerve fibers (16). During the past decade, significant insight has been gained regarding the pathophysiology of concussion. The postconcussive defects clearly do not occur with significant anatomic perturbation and do appear to resolve over time. This has led to the concept that MTBI results in temporary neuronal dysfunction rather than cell death. However, whereas brain cells are not irreversibly destroyed by MTBI, neural cells remain in a vulnerable state before recovery. The neurometabolic events after experimental concussive brain injury have been elucidated, yielding insight concerning the etiology of postconcussive symptomatology and vulnerability (17).

Experimental animal models have demonstrated metabolic dysfunction to be the key physiological event after a concussive event. Disorganized release of neurotransmitters results in poorly regulated neuronal depolarizations and abnormal ionic shifts. The altered cellular physiology causes a hypermetabolism of glucose and a "cellular energy crisis" that is exacerbated by a decrease in cerebral blow flow (18). This cellular energy crisis is thought to cause the increased vulnerability to a second concussive event (19). After the initial period of hypermetabolic glucose consumption, the concussed brain is thought to enter a period of depressed metabolism that may impair posttraumatic neural connectivity, leading to lasting changes in cognitive potential (17). Cerebral metabolic function can be adversely affected for days in animals, but the time course appears to be significantly longer in humans (17). As the clinical significance and duration of the neurometabolic events after MTBI are defined further, more appropriate guidelines for return to play will be established.

Epidemiology

Overall, it is estimated that approximately 300,000 sports-related concussive events occur in the United States annually (20). It has been estimated that 3.9% to 7.7% of high school and college athletes sustain a concussion each year (21). Contact sports in particular place athletes at risk for head trauma. Football is recognized as having the highest risk; however, basketball, softball, soccer, baseball, rugby, and ice hockey also have a moderate to high risk of concussion [9].

The incidence of concussion among high school and collegiate football players is approximately 3% to 20%. In a recent study using comprehensive concussion assessment to investigate the incidence of concussion among 17,500 football players, Guskiewicz et al. (9) found that 5.1% of athletes sustained a concussion in a single season; the greatest incidence of concussion was found at the high school level, followed by the division III college level. Recent data from the National Football League collected between 1996 and 2001 demonstrated a concussion rate of 0.41 concussions per NFL game (22).

Recent studies have highlighted an increased predisposition to future concussive events after an initial MTBI. Guskiewicz et al. (23) found a threefold increase in concussive risk if a player had suffered three or more MTBIs during a period of 7 years. In a separate study, the incidence of a recurrent concussion within a single football season was 14.7% (9). Recurrent concussive events also may be associated with slower recovery severe and more severe symptoms. Players with two or more previous concussions require a longer time for symptom resolution (23), and athletes with three or more previous concussions have an eightfold increased risk of experiencing loss of consciousness after MTBI (14). The increased risk of repeat MTBI is thought to result from postconcussive neurometabolic changes that produced increased cerebral vulnerability to recurrent injury.

Mechanism of Injury

A committee of representatives from the NFL Team Physicians Society and the NFL Athletic Trainers Society, NFL equipment managers, and scientific experts in the area of traumatic brain injury recently investigated the location and direction of helmet impacts in the NFL using sophisticated acquisition of high-speed video impact data and biomechanical reconstruction to determine impact velocity, change in head velocity, and acceleration forces (22,24,25). Data from this study group have demonstrated the striking observation that concussed players in the NFL experienced average head impacts of approximately 21 mph. The change in head velocity of injured players averaged 16 mph, which was significantly higher than the change in head velocity for the uninjured players involved in the collision (average, 9 mph) (25). The majority of concussions occurred by impact with another player's helmet (24). Interestingly, concussion occurred with the lowest head acceleration if a player was struck on the side of the face mask as compared with impacts to other areas of the helmet. Those authors suggest that impacts to the face mask twist the head in addition to accelerating it, and this combination of rotation coupled with translation may influence concussion tolerance (25). These data provide initial information regarding the biomechanics of athletic concussion in football and begin to provide insight regarding the forces that are required to cause MTBI.

Diagnosis of Concussion

The signs and symptoms of concussion vary, but any change in an athlete's behavior should be recognized as an indication

TABLE 9-2	Signs and Symptoms of Concussion

Concussion signs observed by medical staff

Appears dazed
Confused about play
Moves clumsily
Answers question slowly
Personality/behavior change
Forgets plays prior to hit
Retrograde amnesia (forgets plays after hit)
Anterograde amnesia (loses consciousness)

Concussion symptoms reported by athlete

Headache
Nausea
Balance problems
Double vision
Photosensitivity
Feeling sluggish
Feeling foggy
Change in sleep pattern
Cognitive changes

From Collins MW, Lovell MR, McKeag DB. Current issues in managing sports-related concussion. *JAMA.* 1999;282:2283–2285; with permission.

of altered neurologic functioning. Common signs and symptoms of concussion are shown in **Table 9-2**. Typical features of concussion are headache, disorientation, blank stare, slurred speech, delayed verbal responses to questions, slow and uncoordinated motor function, dizziness, emotional lability, and short-term memory deficits; any head trauma associated with a loss of consciousness is a concussion (26).

Recent studies have documented the prevalence of various signs and symptoms of concussion. The most common symptoms of concussion in NFL players were headaches (55%), dizziness (42%), and blurred vision (16%). The most common signs of concussion found on physical examination in these players were problems with immediate recall, retrograde amnesia, and information-processing problems. Loss of consciousness occurred in 9% of players, and hospitalization was required in 2.4% of cases (22).

Postconcussion Syndrome

It has been estimated that 20% of patients will suffer postconcussive symptoms after concussion (27). Characteristics of postconcussion syndrome include impaired memory and concentration, persistent headache, fatigue, mood and sleep disturbances, and dizziness. Many of these symptoms are short-lived, and they usually resolve spontaneously. Treatment includes nonnarcotic analgesics and rest. Recent neurocognitive testing protocols have begun to objectify the evaluation of postconcussion syndrome and likely will refine return-to-play guidelines (12,28–33). Postconcussive symptoms are thought to represent the clinical manifestation of the neurometabolic derangements that are seen in experimental models of concussion.

■ SECOND-IMPACT SYNDROME

An extremely rare but life-threatening consequence of premature return-to-play is the second-impact syndrome. This occurs when an athlete who has not completely recovered from an initial concussive event sustains a second head trauma. The second event may be relatively minor, but a catastrophic increase in intracranial pressure can occur because of dysregulation of cerebral blood flow, which can result in vascular engorgement, cerebellar herniation, and death.

The clinical scenario of this syndrome is unique: The athlete may appear to be stunned and often does not lose consciousness. Within seconds to minutes, the patient collapses, becomes semicomatose, and develops dilated pupils as well as evidence of respiratory failure. Demise occurs much more quickly than in patients with intracranial hemorrhage syndromes. The mortality rate for this condition is approximately 50%, and the morbidity rate is nearly 100% (1).

At present, at least 17 deaths have been reported as a result of second-impact syndrome (1). In each case, athletes returned to sports before full resolution of their symptoms (34). Second-impact syndrome has been shown to occur up to 2 weeks postinjury and is thought to occur most often in athletes younger than 21 years of age.

Chronic Traumatic Brain Injury

The long-term sequelae of multiple concussive events remain unclear. In boxers, dementia puglistica or punch drunk syndrome, which includes a pattern of ataxia, pyramidal tract dysfunction, tremor, impaired memory, dysarthria, and behavioral changes, has long been recognized as a result of the cumulative effects of concussions (35). More recently, the term chronic traumatic brain injury (CTBI) has been applied to the long-term neurologic consequences of repetitive concussive and subconcussive blows to the brain (36). The proposed symptoms of CTBI include decreased processing speed, short-term memory impairment, concentration deficit, irritability or depression, fatigue and sleep disturbance, a general feeling of fogginess, and academic difficulties. Although CTBI has been described primarily in boxers, with up to 17% of retired fighters exhibiting symptoms (36), more subtle forms of CTBI may be seen after repetitive MTBI from other sports. Recent studies have implicated repeated concussions in cognitive impairments among college football players (29). In addition, diminished neuropsychological functioning has been seen in amateur soccer players suffering from multiple concussions (37). Two studies

have demonstrated a cumulative effect of concussion on neuropsychological performance (14,15).

Management of Concussion

The management of concussion has three crucial considerations. First, immediate neurologic emergencies must be identified. Second, the devastating scenario of second-impact syndrome must be prevented, and the risk of recurrent concussive episodes should be minimized. Finally, the cumulative effects of repeated concussion, which may lead to CTBI, must be avoided (38). The identification of neurologic emergencies may be possible with a careful patient history and physical examination, but algorithms to prevent second-impact syndrome, recurrent MTBI, and CTBI remain ill-defined.

Current guidelines for concussion management are based on parameters that lack a rigorous, evidence-based foundation. This results, in large part, from a traditional lack of markers to diagnose the severity of brain injury or to prognosticate recovery. At this time, which of the signs and symptoms of concussion predict the most ominous outcome is unclear. Recent research, for example, has disputed the commonly held assumption that loss of consciousness is the most severe symptom of concussion (39). As such, much research has been directed toward identifying empirical markers of recovery from concussion (28–30,40,41). A goal of this research is to determine the acute recovery curves for specific signs and symptoms that occur with concussion.

The movement toward evidence based concussion management with a foundation of more empirical markers includes the use of standardized assessment of concussion scoring forms, neuropsychological testing, and functional MRI. The correlation between symptoms and markers such as neuropsychological function as well as the relationship between neurocognitive function, postconcussive symptoms, and chronic sequelae remain unknown. For example, recent work has demonstrated the persistence of neurocognitive derangement in the setting of postconcussive patients who are free of symptoms. However, it is difficult to generalize the results of these studies, because there may be different recovery patterns and risks in different age groups and patient populations. Thus, the clinical application of this emerging data remains unclear.

Current Grading Systems

More than 15 grading systems and return-to-play parameters have been published to guide the team physician, trainer, and coach in the evaluation and management of concussion. However, because of a lack of scientific foundation, these recommendations and grading systems are relatively arbitrary guides. For example, most concussion grading systems determine return-to-play decisions based on the

TABLE 9-3	Concussion Grading Scales		
	Grade 1 (mild)	**Grade 2 (moderate)**	**Grade 3 (severe)**
Cantu	No LOC or posttraumatic amnesia <1 hr	LOC <5 min or posttraumatic amnesia 1–24 hours	LOC >5 min or posttraumatic amnesia >24 hr
Colorado Medical Society	No LOC, confusion without amnesia	No LOC, confusion with amnesia	LOC
American Academy of Neurology	No LOC, symptoms <15 min	No LOC, symptoms >15 min	LOC

LOC, loss of consciousness.

presence and duration of loss of consciousness or amnesia, but neither symptom is necessary for an injury to be classified as a concussion (30).

Table 9-3 lists the most common grading systems. The Cantu guidelines (42) are based on the experience of a clinical neurosurgeon as well as a review of the literature. The Colorado guidelines (43) were generated by members of the Colorado Medical Society after the death of an athlete from an on-field head injury. These criteria mandate that any loss of consciousness is considered to be a grade 3 concussion and should be treated as a severe injury. The Colorado guidelines were amended by the American Academy of Neurology (AAN) in 1997 (38); these criteria permit return-to-play following a grade 1 concussion if the athlete is asymptomatic 15 minutes after the episode.

These grading systems have promoted consistent terminology and a framework to assess severity of concussion, but concern remains that little data support the criteria established by the grading systems (31). Because the concussion guidelines are not evidence based, concussion is difficult to categorize, and reliable return-to-play decisions are challenging.

Standardized Assessment of Concussion

Standardized concussion assessment forms have been developed for initial evaluation of the concussed athlete (3–5, 18,44) (Appendix 9-1). While standardized assessment is not a substitute for a physician evaluation or a formal neurologic or neuropsychological examination, it does help to detect and quantify initial cognitive deficits, and it provides an objective and standardized mental status examination directed toward the concussed athlete (4,5,18,44). The utility of a standardized concussive assessment is maximized when individual baseline test data are available. These types of forms have allowed longitudinal and multicenter studies to better define the significance of postconcussion symptomatology. Using these types of standardized assessment instruments, it was shown that amnesia is up to 10-fold more predictive of

outcome following sports concussion relative to brief loss of consciousness in high school and college athletes (30).

Neuropsychological Testing

Neuropsychological tests are functional cognitive instruments that are used to assess changes in attention, concentration, memory, information-processing speed, and motor speed or coordination (12). These tests provide a validated means to quantify cognitive weakness (45,46), and it is increasingly clear that neuropsychological assessment is a useful tool for measuring both the initial and recovery stages of athletes after concussive events (47). Traditionally, these tests have been administered to a patient by a neuropsychologist or technician. More recently, computerized neurocognitive assessment tools have been developed that facilitate large-scale testing and tracking of athletes. Neuropsychological data should be interpreted by a board-certified neuropsychologist.

Neuropsychological tests are most useful when baseline data on the athlete exist and can be longitudinally compared to serial tests after concussive episodes. For example, Kutner et al. (47) have used a computerized neurocognitive assessment to track concussive injuries for the New York Giants football team since 1995 and have compared postinjury test results with baseline data to help with return-to-play decision making **(Fig 9-2)**.

Large-scale studies using standardized baseline and postconcussive neuropsychological tests have begun to elucidate the neurocognitive manifestations of postconcussive symptoms as well as the time course of neurocognitive dysfunction after MTBI. It was demonstrated that high school athletes with the postconcussive symptom of headache had significantly worse performance on reaction time and memory neurocognitive scores compared to athletes without headache after concussion (28). Lovell et al. (33) found that high school athletes with an AAN grade 1 concussion demonstrated a decline in memory and a dramatic increase in self-reported symptoms at 36 hours after injury compared to a preinjury evaluation. Neuropsychological testing completely

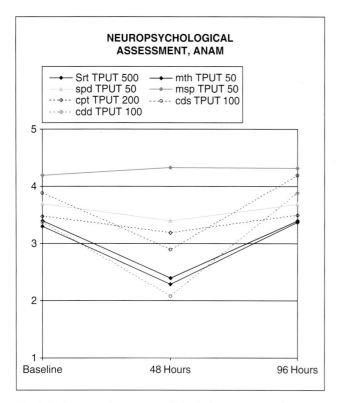

NEUROPSYCHOLOGICAL ASSESSMENT, ANAM

Legend:
- Srt TPUT 500
- mth TPUT 50
- spd TPUT 50
- msp TPUT 50
- cpt TPUT 200
- cds TPUT 100
- cdd TPUT 100

(x-axis: Baseline, 48 Hours, 96 Hours; y-axis: 1 to 5)

Fig 9-2. An example neuropsychological assessment of a player who sustained a concussion. The graph shows the player's baseline cognitive status on the neuropsychological test ANAM. His 48-hour baseline revealed impaired cognitive functioning in comparison to his baseline. The player's test results revealed that he returned to baseline by 96 hours. srt, simple reaction time accuracy; spd, simple reaction time speed; mth, mathematic reasoning accuracy; msp, matching to sample; cpt, continuous performance accuracy; cds, continuous performance speed; cdd, continuous performance total.

normalized by 6 days after the concussion. These data suggest that some current return-to-play recommendations, which allow athletes with grade 1 concussions to return to the game after the symptoms resolve, may be too liberal and permit athletes to return to competition before complete recovery from injury.

Functional MRI

Because concussion is believed to represent a functional neural perturbance rather than a structural one, use of structural neuroimaging modalities, such as MRI and CT, is normal in cases of concussion. Functional MRI examines the metabolic/physiological state of the brain and, thus, has been proposed as an empirical means to assess and monitor concussion (48). Functional MRI provides task-specific information about neural function, and it detects defects in neural function during cognitive load. Using this technique, specific neural signatures of concussion have been demonstrated in selected individuals by comparing postconcussion results with the preconcussion baseline (49). In the future, this tool may allow mapping of neural injury patterns to

quantify injury load and more accurately direct return-to-play guidelines.

Return to Play

At present, two basic approaches are used to manage concussion and to make return-to-play decisions. One approach is to grade the concussion using, for example, the Cantu or AAN Concussion Grading Scale (Table 9-3) at the time of the event and within 15 minutes of the concussion. This gives an immediate estimation of the injury severity; however, many MTBIs behave differently than expected based on the initial evaluation. Guidelines established by this type of approach were published in 1999 by the AOSSM Concussion Workshop Group (4,5,18,44):

Return to Play (Same Day)

1 Signs and symptoms cleared within 15 minutes or less both at rest and with exertion
2 Normal neurologic evaluation
3 No documented loss of consciousness

Delayed Return to Play (Not the Same Day)

1 Signs and symptoms did not clear within 15 minutes at rest or with exertion
2 Documented loss of consciousness

These guidelines stipulate that new symptoms arising after an asymptomatic period should preclude play. In addition, symptoms that last for 20 to 30 minutes should be considered as prolonged symptoms and disqualify the athlete from returning to competition on the same day. The guidelines recommend that asymptomatic athletes be subject to a provocative test before a return to play. The objective of the provocative test is to raise the intracranial pressure with physical stress and determine if symptoms occur. Common provocative tests include a 40-yard dash, five sit-ups, five push-ups, five deep knee bends, or reclining in a supine position with the legs elevated for several seconds (18). Return to play must always be accompanied by serial examination to assess for recurrence of symptoms.

A second approach is to forgo the use of a grading system and, instead, monitor the athlete's recovery based on symptoms, serial neurocognitive testing, and postural-stability testing (50). With this approach, no attempt is made at grading the concussion to prognosticate the athlete's return to play. Instead, the athlete's symptoms are closely monitored; once the athlete is asymptomatic, a progression of activities is instituted that increases demands over several days in a stepwise fashion (50). This type of approach was endorsed in a recent consensus statement from the 2001 Vienna Conference on Concussion in Sport (51), which recommended an incremental increase in exercise duration and intensity when the athlete is completely asymptomatic and has normal neurologic and cognitive evaluations. Each step in this approach takes a minimum of 1 day, and a recurrence of symptomatology mandates that the athlete drop back to the previous asymptomatic level and then try to progress again after 24 hours. The return-to-play protocol endorsed by the Vienna Conference (51) is as follows:

1 No activity, complete rest; once asymptomatic, proceed to level 2
2 Light aerobic exercise, such as walking or stationary cycling
3 Sport-specific training, such as staking in hockey or running in soccer
4 Noncontact training drills
5 Full-contact training after medical clearance
6 Game play

Although multiple return-to-play guidelines have been written, none has been systematically researched. Whatever guidelines are utilized, the physician must integrate the athlete's self-report of symptoms, the trainer's assessment, the athlete's neurocognitive functioning, and the results of physical and neurologic examinations in return-to-play decisions.

■ CONCLUSIONS

Head injuries are a major concern to team physicians, and concussions remain the most common type of sports-related head injury. Initial evaluation should be directed toward identifying the extent of primary injury. Management is then focused on preventing secondary injury, with immediate neurosurgical consultation in cases of intracranial hemorrhage or appropriate return-to-play precautions in cases of concussion.

Recovery after concussion is an emerging area of intense research. Neuropsychological testing and functional MRI are beginning to add objectivity to the treatment of concussions. In addition to more empirical grading and return-to-play criteria, future research may help to better predict the long-term effects of concussion.

■ ACKNOWLEDGMENTS

Special thanks to Kenneth C. Kutner, PhD, and Sherri Birchansky, MD, for providing assistance with manuscript and figures.

■ REFERENCES

1. Cantu RC. Head injuries in adults. In: DeLee JC, Drez D Jr, eds. *Orthopaedic sports medicine: principles and practice*, Vol 1. 2nd ed. Philadelphia: WB Saunders; 2003.
2. Folstein MF, Folstein SE, McHugh PR. "Mini-mental state." A practical method for grading the cognitive state of patients for the clinician. *J Psychiatr Res.* 1975;12:189–198.
3. Kutner KC, et al. Sports-related head injury—sideline concussion checklist-B. *The National Academy of Neuropsychology Bulletin.* 1998;14:19–23.
4. McCrea M, et al. Standardized assessment of concussion in football players. *Neurology.* 1997;48:586–588.
5. McCrea M, et al. Standardized assessment of concussion (SAC): on-site mental status evaluation of the athlete. *J Head Trauma Rehabil.* 1998;13:27–35.
6. Bruno LA, Gennarelli TA, Torg JS. Management guidelines for head injuries in athletics. *Clin Sports Med.* 1987;6:17–29.
7. Warren WL Jr, Bailes JE. On the field evaluation of athletic head injuries. *Clin Sports Med.* 1998;17:13–26.
8. Cantu RC. Return to play guidelines after a head injury. *Clin Sports Med.* 1998;17:45–60.
9. Guskiewicz KM, et al. Epidemiology of concussion in collegiate and high school football players. *Am J Sports Med.* 2000;28:643–650.
10. Rimel RH, Eisenberg, Boll T. Disability caused by minor head injury. *Neurosurgery.* 1981;9:221–228.
11. Kelly J. Concussion. In: Torg JS, Shephard RJ, eds. *Current therapy in sports medicine.* 3rd ed. St. Louis: Mosby; 1995.
12. Lovell MR, Collins MW. Neuropsychological assessment of the college football player. *J Head Trauma Rehabil.* 1998;13:9–26.
13. DeRoss AL, et al. Multiple head injuries in rats: effects on behavior. *J Trauma.* 2002;52:708–714.
14. Collins MW, et al. Cumulative effects of concussion in high school athletes. *Neurosurgery.* 2002;51:1175–1181.
15. Iverson GL, et al. Cumulative effects of concussion in amateur athletes. *Brain Inj.* 2004;18:433–443.
16. Povlishock JT, Coburn TH. Morphological change associated with mild head injury. In: Levin HS, Eisenberg HM, Benton AL. *Mild head injury.* New York: Oxford University Press; 1989.
17. Giza CC, Hovda DA. The neurometabolic cascade of concussion. *J Athl Train.* 2001;36:228–235.
18. Wojtys EM, et al. Concussion in sports. *Am J Sports Med.* 1999;27:676–687.
19. Bergsneider M, et al. Cerebral hyperglycolysis following severe traumatic brain injury in humans: a positron-emission tomography study. *J Neurosurg.* 1997;86:241–251.
20. Centers for Disease Control and Prevention. Sports-related recurrent brain injuries. *MMWR Morb Mortal Wkly Rep.* 1997;46:224–227.
21. Powell JW, Barber-Foss JD. Traumatic brain injury in high school athletes. *JAMA.* 1999;282:958–963.
22. Pellman EJ, et al. Concussion in professional football: epidemiological features of game injuries and review of the literature—part 3. *Neurosurgery.* 2004;54:81–96.
23. Guskiewicz KM, et al. Cumulative effects associated with recurrent concussion in collegiate football players: the NCAA Concussion Study. *JAMA.* 2003;290:2549–2555.
24. Pellman EJ, et al. Concussion in professional football: location and direction of helmet impacts—part 2. *Neurosurgery.* 2003;53:1328–1341.
25. Pellman EJ, et al. Concussion in professional football: reconstruction of game impacts and injuries. *Neurosurgery.* 2003;53:799–814.
26. Stevenson KL, Adelson PD. Pediatric sports-related head injuries. In: DeLee JC, Drez D Jr, eds. *Orthopaedic sports medicine: principles and practice*, Vol. 1. 2nd ed. Philadelphia: WB Saunders; 2003.
27. Wrightson P, Gronwall D. Time off work and symptoms after minor head injury. *Injury.* 1981;12:445–454.
28. Collins MW, et al. Relationship between postconcussion headache and neuropsychological test performance in high school athletes. *Am J Sports Med.* 2003;31:168–173.
29. Collins MW, et al. Relationship between concussion and neuropsychological performance in college football players. *JAMA.* 1999;282:964–970.

30. Collins MW, et al. On-field predictors of neuropsychological and symptom deficit following sports-related concussion. *Clin J Sport Med.* 2003;13:222–229.
31. Collins MW, Lovell MR, McKeag DB. Current issues in managing sports-related concussion. *JAMA.* 1999;282:2283–2285.
32. Lovell MR, et al. Recovery from mild concussion in high school athletes. *J Neurosurg.* 2003;98:296–301.
33. Lovell MR, et al. Grade 1 or "ding" concussions in high school athletes. *Am J Sports Med.* 2004;32:47–54.
34. Cantu RC. Second-impact syndrome. *Clin Sports Med.* 1998;17:37–44.
35. Marland HS. Punch-drunk. *JAMA.* 1928;19:1103–1107.
36. Rabadi MH, Jordan BD. The cumulative effect of repetitive concussion in sports. *Clin J Sport Med.* 2001;11:194–198.
37. Matser EJ, et al. Neuropsychological impairment in amateur soccer players. *JAMA.* 1999;282:971–973.
38. Practice parameter: the management of concussion in sports (summary statement). Report of the Quality Standards Subcommittee. *Neurology.* 1997;48:581–585.
39. Lovell MR, et al. Does loss of consciousness predict neuropsychological decrements after concussion? *Clin J Sport Med.* 1999;9:193–198.
40. Guskiewicz KM, et al. No evidence of impaired neurocognitive performance in collegiate soccer players. *Am J Sports Med.* 2002;30:157–162.
41. Johnston KM, et al. New frontiers in diagnostic imaging in concussive head injury. *Clin J Sport Med.* 2001;11:166–175.
42. Cantu RC. *The Exercising Adult.* New York: MacMillan; 1987.
43. *Report of the Sports Medicine Committee: guidelines for the management of concussion in sports.* Denver: Colorado Medical Society; 1991.
44. McCrea M, et al. Immediate neurocognitive effects of concussion. *Neurosurgery.* 2002;50:1032–1042.
45. Boll T. Developing issues in neuropsychology. *J Clin Exp Neuropsychol.* 1985;5:473–485.
46. Barth JT, et al. Neuropsychological sequelae of minor head injury. *Neurosurgery.* 1983;13:529–533.
47. Kutner KC, Warren RF, Barnes R. Computerized neuropsychological assessment in the NRF. In: *NFL physician society sports symposium.* Indianapolis; 1997.
48. Chen JK, et al. Functional abnormalities in symptomatic concussed athletes: an fMRI study. *Neuroimage.* 2004;22:68–82.
49. Jantzen KJ, et al. A prospective functional MR imaging study of mild traumatic brain injury in college football players. *AJNR Am J Neuroradiol.* 2004;25:738–745.
50. Guskiewicz KM, et al. National Athletic Trainers' Association Position Statement: Management of sport-related concussion. *J Athl Train.* 2004;39:280–297.
51. Aubry M, et al. Summary and agreement statement of the First International Conference on Concussion in Sport, Vienna 2001. Recommendations for the improvement of safety and health of athletes who may suffer concussive injuries. *Br J Sports Med.* 2002;36:6–10.

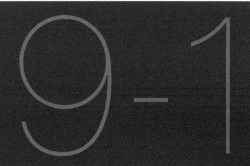

Player_____   Date ___/___/___

    LOC No___   **Yes ___ Length ____**   **Time of Injury _____**
    Respiration: **Normal _____ Apnea _____ Irregular _____**

Trial	#1	#2	#3	#4
Time	__:__	__:__	__:__	__:__

1. Unequal Pupils ≥2mm

	y __ n __	y __ n__	y __ n__	y __n__

2. Orientation: *If on sidelines turn player away from field.*

	#1	#2	#3	#4
Opponent	y __ n __	y __ n __	y __ n __	y __n__
Current Date	y __ n __	y __ n __	y __ n __	y __n__
Current Quart	y __ n __	y __ n __	y __ n __	y __n__
Current Score	y __ n __	y __ n __	y __ n __	y __n__
Play Injured	y __ n __	y __ n __	y __ n __	y __n__

3. Fine Motor: thumb to fingertip sequencing

	#1	#2	#3	#4
Right	intact__	intact__	intact__	intact__
	impair__	impair__	impair__	impair__
Left	intact__	intact__	intact__	intact__
	impair__	impair__	impair__	impair__

4. Vomiting:

	y __ n__	y __ n __	y __ n__	y __n__

5.

	0 = None	1 = Mild	2 = Moderate	3 = Severe
Headache:	_____	_____	_____	_____
Dizziness:	_____	_____	_____	_____
Nausea:	_____	_____	_____	_____

6. Dysmetria: Have player touch examiner's finger then his nose at right, left and midline.

	#1	#2	#3	#4
Right	intact__	intact__	intact__	intact__
	impair__	impair__	impair__	impair__
Left	intact__	intact__	intact__	intact__
	impair__	impair__	impair__	impair__

7. Diplopia: Examine with eyes open with central fixation. Have player count lines or fingers.

	y __ n __	y __ n __	y __ n __	y __n__

Trial	#1	#2	#3	#4

8. Tandem: Heel-toe for 10 steps

   Gait:

	intact__	intact__	intact__	intact__
	impair__	impair__	impair__	impair__

   Right

	intact__	intact__	intact__	intact__
	impair__	impair__	impair__	impair__

   Left

	intact__	intact__	intact__	intact__
	impair__	impair__	impair__	impair__

9. Cognition:

   ST Memory—shirt, car, apple

	y __ n __	y __ n __	y __ n__	y __n__

Digit Span:

Forward

	63716	63716	63716	63716
	y __ n __	y __ n __	y __ n__	y __n__

Backward

	8517	8517	8517	8517
	y __ n __	y __ n __	y __ n__	y __n__

Oral Trail B: Alternate numbers and letters
1 – A –2 – B – 3 – C – 4 – D – 5 – E – 6 – F- 7 –G-8 –H- 9- I- 10- J

	y __ n __	y __ n __	y __ n__	y __n__

Remote Memory: *Player explains coach-provided play*

	y __ n __	y __ n __	y __ n__	y __n__

LT Memory—shirt, car, apple

	y __ n __	y __ n __	y __ n__	y __n__

10. Exertion Stress Test

   Asymptomatic_____   Symptomatic_____

   Other:

	y __ n __	y __ n __	y __ n__	y __n__

   i.e. Lethargy
      Agitation

Examiner:_____

Kutner, K., Relkin, N., Barth, J., Barnes, R., Warren, R., & O'Brien, S. 8/1/97

Section

5

SHOULDER

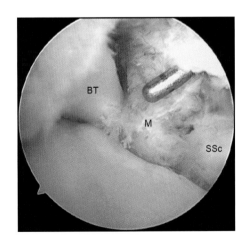

SHOULDER ANATOMY AND BIOMECHANICS

■ DAWN L. SWARM, MD, ANDREW T. MAHAR, MS, DEREK W. WEICHEL, BS, ROBERT A. PEDOWITZ, MD, PhD

■ KEY POINTS

- The shoulder complex is composed of three bones—the clavicle, the scapula, and the humerus—as well as four articulations—the acromioclavicular (AC), the sternoclavicular (SC), the scapulothoracic, and the glenohumeral (GH) joints.
- The clavicle serves a variety of functions. It acts as a rigid base for muscular attachments of the shoulder, neck, and chest. It also provides protection for the major vessels at the base of the neck and for the nerves and vessels supplying the upper limb. In addition, it forms a strut that holds the GH joint in the parasagittal plane.
- The scapula is a flat, triangular-shaped bone that serves as the articulating surface for the head of the humerus as well as provides areas for 17 muscle attachments.
- The proximal humerus is composed of the humeral head, the lesser and greater tuberosities, the bicipital groove, and the proximal humeral shaft.
- The AC joint is a diarthrodial joint and the only articulation between the clavicle and the scapula. The motion of the AC joint is minimal, involving small translations and, mainly, rotation between the clavicle and the acromion with arm movement.
- The SC joint is the only true joint that connects the upper extremity to the axial skeleton. It is a gliding joint with little inherent bony stability.
- The scapulothoracic articulation is not a true joint, but it represents the space between the concave surface of the anterior scapula and the convex surface of the posterior chest wall. The muscular and ligamentous attachments provide the stability of this articulation as the scapula retracts, protracts, and rotates along the posterior chest wall.

- The GH joint is a diarthrodial joint with minimal bony constraint, allowing it the largest range of motion of any major diarthrodial joint in the body.
- The glenoid labrum provides another static restraint to GH motion. The labrum is a fibrous ring that is attached to the glenoid articular surface through a fibrocartilagenous transition zone.
- The GH ligaments function as static restraints to shoulder motion.
- The rotator cuff (RTC) muscles, as well as the scapular rotators, contribute to GH stability by enhancing the concavity–compression mechanism. Contraction of the long head of the biceps tendon, coordinated scapulothoracic rhythm, and proprioceptive mechanoreceptors in the joint capsule also contribute to the stability.
- The RTC is composed of the supraspinatus, the infraspinatus, the subscapularis, and the teres minor muscles. The RTC often serves more than one function simultaneously. The muscles act as prime movers if the line of action is within the intended direction of motion.
- Nerve injuries can occur with both arthroscopic and open shoulder procedures.
- RTC repair using an open technique has been clinically successful in terms of repair, although arthroscopic techniques are now more common.

The shoulder is a complex joint that has the greatest degree of mobility of all major joints in the human body. The osseous and ligamentous structures that comprise the joint, as well as the surrounding musculature, interact to provide a wide range of motion as well as stability. Under normal conditions, four articulations move in synchrony, allowing smooth, unhindered motion of the arm. The control of glenohumeral (GH) stability is achieved by the complex interaction between the static restraints (i.e., the ligament and tendons) and the dynamic restraints (i.e., muscular contraction acting across the joint).

■ OSSEOUS STRUCTURES AND STATIC RESTRAINTS

The shoulder complex is composed of three bones—the clavicle, the scapula, and the humerus—as well as four articulations—the acromioclavicular (AC), the sternoclavicular (SC), the scapulothoracic, and the GH joints **(Fig 10-1)**.

Clavicle

The clavicle, an "S"-shaped bone, is the only long bone that ossifies by an intramembranous process. It is the first bone in the body to ossify (fifth week of fetal gestation) and is the last bone to fuse (medial epiphysis at 25 years of age). The clavicle consists of cancellous bone surrounded by an outer layer of compact bone, and it is unique in that it does not have a medullary cavity (1,2).

The clavicle serves a variety of functions. First, it acts as a rigid base for muscular attachments of the shoulder, neck, and chest. It also provides protection for the major vessels at the base of the neck and for the nerves and vessels supplying the upper limb. In addition, it forms a strut that holds the

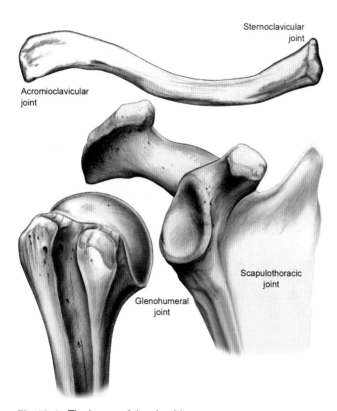

Fig 10-1. The bones of the shoulder.

GH joint in the parasagittal plane, increasing the range of motion of the shoulder as well as the power of the arm in motions above the horizontal (1).

The clavicle articulates with the manubrium of the sternum through the SC joint and with the acromion at the AC joint. It is attached to the coracoid by the coracoclavicular ligaments, the conoid medially and the trapezoid laterally.

Scapula

The scapula is a flat, triangular-shaped bone that serves as the articulating surface for the head of the humerus as well as provides areas for 17 muscle attachments. With the arm at the side, the scapula overlaps the dorsal surfaces of the second to seventh ribs. It has three prominent projections: the spine, the coracoid process, and the acromion. The scapular spine divides the posterior aspect of the scapula into two depressions, the supraspinatus fossa and the infraspinatus fossa. In addition, the spine serves as a site for insertion of the trapezius muscle and as the origin for the posterior third of the deltoid muscle (2,3).

The coracoid process is a hooklike projection that curves anteriorly, upward, and outward in front of the glenoid cavity. The base of the coracoid is the attachment site of the coracoclavicular ligaments. The tip serves as the origin of the short head of the biceps and the coracobrachialis muscles and as the insertion site of the pectoralis minor muscle. The coracoid also serves as the anterior limit of the coracoacromial arch and is a palpable landmark during rotator cuff (RTC) surgery (2,3).

The acromion serves as an attachment site for the trapezius muscle above and the deltoid muscle below, and it articulates with the distal clavicle. The acromion usually forms from two or three ossification centers that appear during puberty and that fuse between 18 and 25 years of age. These three ossification centers are described as the preacromion, the mesoacromion, and the meta-acromion. The os acromiale, an unfused secondary ossification, occurs with an incidence of 1% to 15%, and 60% of cases involve bilaterality (4–7). The most common location is at the junction of the meso- and meta-acromion (4,7). An os acromiale can be identified on an axillary radiograph or magnetic resonance image (MRI) and should not be mistaken for a fracture.

In addition, the acromion has been classified into three morphologic patterns as viewed on a scapular outlet radiograph: flat (Type I), curved (Type II), and hooked (Type III) (8). A Type III morphology has been implicated in impingement and RTC pathology (9,10). Investigators have further classified the acromion based on thickness: Type A, <8 mm; Type B, 8–12 mm; and Type C, >12 mm (11).

Differences in the size of the acromion have been observed between men and women. Nicholson et al. (7) observed in men that the average length was 48.5 mm, the average anterior width was 19.5 mm, and the average anterior thickness was 7.7 mm. In women, the acromial length averaged 40.6 mm, the anterior width averaged 18.4 mm, and the anterior thickness averaged 6.7 mm (7). That study also determined that basic acromial morphology is a primary anatomical characteristic independent of age and, in contrast, that anterior acromial spurs were dependent on age, because they were present in only 7% of patients <50 years and in 30% of patients >50 years.

The acromion contributes to the coracoacromial arch, or supraspinatus outlet, which consists of the coracoid process, the acromion, and the coracoacromial ligament. This arch marks the superior boundary of the subacromial space. Interest has been focused on the structure and function of the coracoclavicular ligament and the importance of the coracoacromial arch (12–15). Although commonly described as having a "Y"-shaped configuration, other morphological types of the coracoclavicular ligament have been described (13–16). Soslowsky et al. (15) identified four types: quadrangular (48%); "Y"-shaped, with a broader lateral band and thinner medial band (42%); broad banded (8%); and with multiple bands (2%). The length of the coracoid attachment averaged 32 mm and the length of the acromial attachment averaged 19 mm. The average midpoint thickness was 1.3 mm. The length of the lateral band was significantly shorter, and the cross-sectional area was significantly larger, in specimens with a tear in the RTC (15).

The role of the coracoacromial arch as a secondary restraint to anterosuperior migration of the humeral head also has become of interest (17–19). The coracoacromial ligament has been shown to provide a static restraint to the GH joint as well as significantly contributing to anterior GH stability at 30 degrees of abduction (20,21). Release of the coracoacromial ligament has been suggested to increase both anterior and superior translation of the humeral head. It is important to maintain the integrity of the coracoacromial arch in the cuff-deficient shoulder, because the arch is the last restraint to anterosuperior migration (12,20,22).

The scapula also gives rise to the glenoid cavity, which is situated laterally, below the acromion. This lateral thickening of the scapula provides the bony articulation with the humeral head. The articular surface of the glenoid is concave and covered with hyaline cartilage, which is thinner in the center and thicker toward the periphery. A bare spot exists in the center of the inferior glenoid, which is equidistant to the anterior, posterior, and inferior glenoid rim when viewed with an arthroscope (23,24).

Glenoid version has been examined in several studies (25–28). In most, the glenoid displayed from 2 to 10 degrees of retroversion in relation to the long axis of the scapula, with an average of superior tilt of 5 degrees (26–31). In a study measuring the glenoid version in relation to the supraspinatus fossa, 40% were retroverted, 38% neutral, and 22% anteverted (32).

In addition, the shape of glenoid also changes from superior to inferior (28,33–36). Inui et al. (34,37) have shown that the superior part of glenoid surface is retroverted and that the inferior portion may be anteverted. In an MRI study of 40 subjects, Inui et al. (34) showed the upper aspect has a large radius of curvature, is convex, and subsequently, becomes flat and then concave in the lower portion with a small radius of curvature.

The shape of the glenoid resembles a pear, being 20% narrower superiorly than inferiorly (23,26,38). The reported average vertical diameter ranges from 33 to 39 mm (24,26, 30,35) and the average transverse diameter from 23 to 29 mm (24,26,30,35,39). The distance from the anteroinferior margin of the glenoid to the bare area averages 12.8 mm (23,24).

The articular surface of the glenoid is one-third to one-fourth the area of the articular surface of the humeral head, whereas the radius of curvature of the glenoid is 2.3 mm greater than the radius of curvature of the humeral head (26,27,35,39).

Humerus

The proximal humerus is composed of the humeral head, the lesser and greater tuberosities, the bicipital groove, and the proximal humeral shaft, and it is highly variable. The anatomical neck lies at the junction of the articular surface of the head and the greater tuberosity and humeral shaft. The surgical neck lies below the greater and lesser tuberosities. The major blood supply to the humeral head is through the ascending branch of the anterior humeral circumflex artery, which penetrates the head at the bicipital groove and becomes the arcuate artery. This artery crosses under the tendon of the long head of the biceps, runs proximally just adjacent to the lateral aspect of the bicipital groove, and enters the humeral head at the proximal end of transition from the greater tuberosity to the bicipital groove. The posterior circumflex artery supplies the posterior portion of the greater tuberosity and a small posteroinferior part of the humeral head (2,3).

The bicipital groove lies on the anterior proximal humerus, just below the articular surface, and it is defined by the greater and lesser tuberosities. The long head of the biceps tendon lies in this groove and is covered by the transverse humeral ligament.

Both the greater and lesser tuberosities provide attachment for the RTC tendons. The supraspinatus, infraspinatus, and teres minor insert on the greater tuberosity from superior to posterior.

The subscapularis tendon attaches to the lesser tuberosity, also overlying the bicipital groove, and provides additional support to the long head of the biceps tendon (2,3).

Multiple studies have been performed to determine the head–neck ratio, the central axis of the humerus, and the anatomical relationships of the greater tuberosity and the bicipital groove assist in prosthetic replacement and design (22,26,40,41). The articular surface of the humeral head has an average radius of from 42 to 46 mm, whereas the average thickness of the humeral head is 19 mm. The thickness of the humeral head is proportional to both the length of the humerus and the head radius (41,42). The humeral head is retroverted from −6.5 to 35 degrees relative to the transepicondylar axis of the distal humerus (31,40,41). The angle formed by the neck and shaft axes varies from 114 to 147 degrees (28, 42,43). No significant differences between genders have been reported; however, a difference in the retroversion angle has been found between dominant and nondominant sides, with a measure of 33 degrees on the dominant side and 29 degrees on the nondominant side (22).

The humeral head center is offset from the humeral axis by 7 mm medial and 2 mm posterior. A predictable relationship has been found between the central axis of the humeral head and the bicipital groove. In an evaluation of 18 cadavers, the average distance between the central axis of the humeral head and biceps tendon was 9 mm posterior to the posterior margin of the bicipital groove (44). The superior aspect of the humeral head is 6 mm higher than the superior aspect of the greater tuberosity (40). Iannotti et al. (26) reported that the mean distance between the greater tuberosity and the humeral head was 10 mm or less and that this distance was not correlated with other parameters. Takase et al. (45), however, found a significant correlation between the size of the humeral head and the neck shaft angle regardless of gender or age.

The bicipital groove rotates internally along its course between the upper and lower aspects of the proximal humerus. The mean change in rotation of the lateral lip from the proximal to distal groove was 15.9 degrees (40,46). Rotation of the bicipital groove in the proximal-to-distal direction is relevant to shoulder fracture work, particularly fracture arthroplasty, because the groove can assist with proper orientation of humeral head version.

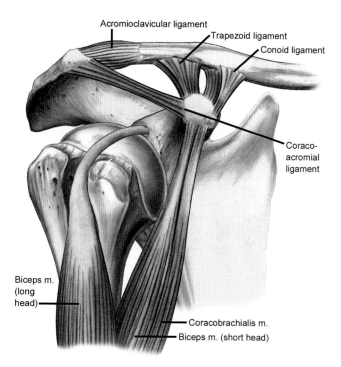

Fig 10-2. Orientation of the acromioclavicular joint, the coracoclavicular and acromioclavicular ligaments, and the biceps tendon. m., muscle.

Acromioclavicular Joint

The AC joint is a diarthrodial joint and the only articulation between the clavicle and scapula. Variable inclinations exist, with being nearly vertical to angled downward and medially accounting for up to 50 degrees (2,3). The AC joint has an incomplete fibrocartilagenous intra-articular disc, potentially predisposing it to degenerative changes.

Degenerative changes have been shown to occur as early as the second decade of life, with loss of articular cartilage, eburnation of subchondral bone, and formation of marginal osteophytes; however, these changes do not necessarily produce symptoms (47).

The motion of a normal AC joint is minimal, involving small translations and, mainly, rotation between the clavicle and the acromion with arm movement. The AC ligaments prevent anteroposterior instability **(Fig 10-2)**. Biomechanical studies have shown that the inferior AC capsular ligaments represent the major restraint against anterior joint translations, whereas the superior and posterior ligaments provide the most stability against posterior translations (56% and 25%, respectively) (48,49). Therefore, the posterior and superior capsular ligaments should be spared during distal clavicle excision to prevent excessive posterior clavicle translations after resection (49,50). The coracoclavicular ligaments

(the trapezoid and the conoid) together resist superior displacement of the joint, but with larger amounts of displacement and induced loads, the conoid ligament contributes the major share (48,49).

Sternoclavicular Joint

The SC joint is the only true joint that connects the upper extremity to the axial skeleton. It is a gliding joint with little inherent bony stability. Substantial incongruity exists between the two articular surfaces, but the interposition of an intra-articular disc compensates for this (2,3). This disc has not shown severe degenerative alterations until the seventh decade of life, but even then, the joint seems to be well preserved (47).

The SC joint is enveloped in a loose, fibrous capsule that blends with the margin of the disc (47). The stability of the joint, which is provided mainly by the surrounding ligaments, protects the important underlying vasculature, pleural domes, trachea, and esophagus. The SC ligaments consist of the anterior and posterior SC and capsular ligaments, the interclavicular ligaments, and the anterior and posterior costoclavicular ligaments (47,51). These allow motion in all planes, including rotation. The SC ligaments prevent upward displacement of the medial clavicle caused by downward forces on the lateral end of the clavicle. The posterior capsular ligament is the most important stabilizer (51). These ligaments allow the clavicle to move 30 degrees upward, 30 degrees in an anteroposterior direction, and rotate 45 degrees about its long axis (47,51).

Scapulothoracic Articulation

The scapulothoracic articulation is not a true joint; rather, it represents the space between the concave surface of the anterior scapula and the convex surface of the posterior chest wall. The muscular and ligamentous attachments provide the stability of this articulation as the scapula retracts, protracts, and rotates along the posterior chest wall (2,3).

Williams et al. (52) divided the anatomical structures of this articulation into three layers: superficial, intermediate, and deep. The trapezius and latissimus dorsi muscles and an inconsistent bursa between the latissimus and inferior angle of the scapula comprise the superficial layer. The intermediate layer is composed of the rhomboid major and the rhomboid minor, the levator scapulae muscles, and the spinal accessory nerve and bursa between the superomedial scapula and trapezius muscle. The spinal accessory nerve travels closely along this bursa at an average of 2.7 cm lateral to the superomedial scapular angle. Finally, the deep layer consists of the serratus anterior and subscapularis muscles and the corresponding scapulothoracic and subscapularis bursa (52,53).

Glenohumeral Joint

The GH joint is a diarthrodial joint with minimal bony constraint, allowing it the largest range of motion of any major diarthrodial joint in the body (2,3,31,54). The GH joint has been described as being similar to a golf ball on a tee, with a large humeral head balanced on a smaller glenoid. The GH joint approximates ball-and-socket kinematics, with only one-third of the humeral head being covered by the glenoid in any position of rotation, and the articular surface of the humeral head is threefold that of the glenoid (2,43,55).

In most shoulders, the glenoid and humerus have similar radii of curvature, providing a basically congruent articulation with less than 2 mm of mismatch between the glenoid and the humeral head. This matched concavity–convexity of the articulation provides stability when muscle forces act across the joint. This provides the foundation for the RTC musculature to establish a concavity–compression effect (33,54–57).

The combined version of the glenoid and humeral head results in a retroversion of approximately 30 to 40 degrees (2,28,31,57). In normal shoulders, the center of the humeral head is usually within 1 mm of the plane of the scapular spine (58). The spherical humeral articular surface articulates with the spherical concavity of the glenoid, whereas the proximal humeral convexity articulates with the spherical concavity of the coracoacromial arch (55).

A negative intra-articular pressure exists within the GH joint, creating a vacuumlike effect. The joint acts as a closed compartment with a flexible diaphragm. The weight of the arm tends to pull the joint surfaces away from each other, creating negative pressure (59,60). In addition, an adhesion–cohesion effect exists secondary to the viscous and intermolecular properties of the synovial fluid, similar to water keeping two glass surfaces together (55).

Glenoid Labrum

The glenoid labrum provides another static restraint to GH motion. The labrum is a fibrous ring attached to the glenoid articular surface through a fibrocartilagenous transition zone. The labrum functions as an anchor point for the GH ligaments and the biceps tendon; it also deepens the glenoid socket and enhances stability (2,3,39).

This wedge-shaped, fibrous structure consists of densely packed collagen bundles in a woven pattern within the hyaline cartilage (61). It is firmly attached to the glenoid rim below the equator, where it appears as a rounded, fibrous elevation. Above the glenoid equator, the glenoid is more mobile and meniscal-like, with a triangular shape (62). The superior labrum inserts directly into the biceps tendon distal to the insertion of the tendon at the supraglenoid tubercle. The biceps tendon anchor and the superior glenoid cover approximately 1.5 cm of the superior rim of the glenoid (35).

In addition to greatly increasing the depth of the glenoid socket, the labrum enhances the concavity–compression mechanism that is created as the humeral head is compressed in the glenoid during RTC contraction (56). Excision of the glenoid labrum decreases the depth of the socket by 50% and reduces the resistance to instability by 20% (33,39,63).

Branches of the suprascapular artery, the circumflex scapular branch of the subscapular artery, and the posterior circumflex artery supply the glenoid labrum as it is vascularized throughout its peripheral attachment to the joint capsule. The superior and anterosuperior portions of the labrum, however, are less vascular than the posterior and inferior parts (62). This decreased vascularity of the superior labrum may explain the vulnerability of this area to disruption.

Glenohumeral Ligaments and Joint Capsule

The GH joint capsule consists mainly of Type I collagen, with smaller amounts of Types II and III. Localized thickenings of the capsule make up the GH ligaments, which are named according to their attachments on the glenoid rim. **(Fig 10-3)**. The GH ligaments function as static restraints to shoulder motion. These discrete, capsular thickenings function as checkreins at the limits of rotation, preventing excess GH translation and becoming taut at varying positions of abduction and humeral rotation. Because of the orientation of these ligaments, portions of the capsule reciprocally tighten and loosen as the GH joint rotates, thus limiting translation and rotation by load sharing. Their function is dependent on the arm position and on the direction of the applied force on the joint.

Variation exists in the presence and size of these ligaments. The anatomical configuration of the inferior glenohumeral ligament (IGHL) is fairly consistent, but the configuration of the superior glenohumeral ligament (SGHL) and the middle glenohumeral ligament (MGHL) is variable. In a study of 84 cadaveric shoulders, the MGHL was separate from the origin of the SGHL in 56%, and the remaining

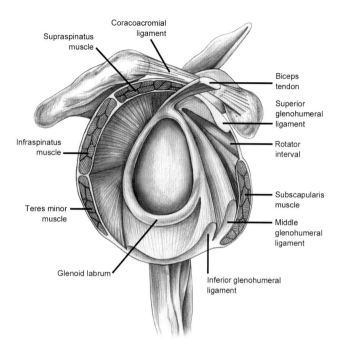

Fig 10-3. Ligaments of the shoulder, demonstrating the superior, middle, inferior, and posterior glenohumeral (GH) ligaments and the rotator interval (RTI).

34%, the MGHL originated at the same location as the SGHL (64). Overall 94% of the specimens had a SGHL. Only 63% had a discrete MGHL, however, and of these, 17.9% had cordlike MGHL.

Normal variants, such as a sublabral foramen, a cordlike MGHL, and a Buford complex, have been reported. A sublabral foramen or sulcus in which the labrum is not attached to the anterosuperior glenoid can be confused with a labral detachment (62,64,65). The prevalence of a sublabral foramen has been reported to be between 12% and 19% (66,67). In addition, the medial and lateral edges of the MGHL can appear to be rolled in a cordlike fashion. The Buford complex is a cordlike MGHL originating directly from the superior labrum and crossing the subscapularis tendon to insert on the humerus. With a Buford complex, no anterosuperior labrum is present, and this can be confused with a Bankart lesion. The reported prevalence of a Buford complex has ranged from 1.5% to 6% (66,67). It is important to recognize these anatomical variants and not to confuse them with a pathologic lesion.

Superior Glenohumeral Ligament
The SGHL originates on the supraglenoid tubercle, just anterior to the origin of the long head of the biceps, and it inserts on the proximal tip of the lesser tuberosity, on the medial ridge of the intertubercular groove. The SGHL is present in more than 90% of individuals. In an anatomical study, Steinbeck et al. (68) found the SGHL to be missing in 6% of the specimens, and in 17% of the specimens, the SGHL had a common origin with the MGHL, at the one-o'clock position on the glenoid labrum.

The SGHL runs parallel to the coracohumeral ligament (CHL), and it reflects around the biceps tendon, serving as an internal pulley at the floor of the rotator interval (RTI) (69,70). During a selective sectioning study, the SGHL was found to be an important inferior stabilizer of the adducted shoulder (70). In addition, it limits posterior translation with the arm in forward flexion, adduction, and internal rotation, and it prevents anterosuperior migration of the humeral head.

Coracohumeral Ligament
The CHL originates on the dorsolateral base of the coracoid process and blends with the capsule to the greater and lesser tuberosities (69). The CHL is present in more than 90% of individuals, and it runs parallel to the SGHL, blending with the superior border of the SGHL inferiorly. Portions of the CHL form the tunnel for the biceps tendon on the anterior side of the joint, and reinforces the RTI. In addition, the CHL reinforces the supraspinatus and infraspinatus tendon insertions as the RTC cable (71).

The CHL has been reported to have multiple functions, limiting external rotation in the adducted arm as well as inferior translation and preventing anterosuperior migration of the humeral head (29,59,69,70). In a study of 11 cadaveric specimens that tested the static restraints of the GH joint, however, found that the CHL does not play a suspensory role (69,70).

Middle Glenohumeral Ligament
The MGHL originates on the supraglenoid tubercle or anterosuperior labrum, and it inserts on the lesser tuberosity running obliquely to the SGHL and the CHL. It is present between 60% and 80% of individuals as a discrete band or thickening of the anterior capsule confluent with the IGHL.

The MGHL becomes taut at 45 degrees of abduction and 10 degrees of extension and external rotation (69,72). Selective sectioning of the MGHL resulted in increased translation at the joint, and abducting the arm to 45 degrees increased the strain in the MGHL (73,74). Therefore, the overall function of the MGHL is to support the arm, to limit both anterior and posterior translation of the arm at 45 degrees of abduction and 45 degrees of external rotation, and to provide anterosuperior stability (69,70).

Inferior Glenohumeral Ligament
The IGHL originates on the inferior half of the glenoid neck or anterior inferior labrum, and it inserts inferior to the MGHL on the lesser tuberosity (64). Various descriptions have been used to define this large, ligamentous structure that undergoes reciprocal tightening and loosening, depending on the position of the arm. Some have used the terms superior band, anterior axillary pouch, and posterior axillary pouch to describe the three regions of this ligament; others have described its anatomy as resembling a hammock, with a thick anterior band and a thin posterior band, surrounding the axillary pouch. The axillary pouch runs from the inferior

one-third of the humeral head to the inferior two-third of the anterior glenoid. In external rotation, the IGHL complex moves in the anterior direction, whereas with internal rotation, the complex moves in the posterior direction (69,70).

In a cadaveric study by Steinbeck et al. (68), the IGHL was a clearly defined structure in 72% of the specimens and only a thickening of the inferior joint capsule in 21%. The superior band was the thickest, with an average size of 2.8 mm, whereas the posterior portion was thinner (mean thickness, 1.7 mm). In addition, that study revealed that the IGHL is thicker at the glenoid origin (mean thickness, 2.3 mm) than at the humeral insertion (mean thickness, 1.6 mm). The length and width of the anterior band have been reported to average of 37 and 13 mm, respectively (75,76). Histologically, the collagen fibers are predominantly radial fibers that are linked to each other by circular elements (68,75–77).

The IGHL complex functions as the primary restraint to anterior, posterior, and inferior GH translation with the arm at 45 to 90 degrees of abduction and external rotation (69,70). The anterior band and axillary pouch are anterior stabilizers, resisting anterior and inferior translation at 45 to 90 degrees degrees of abduction and external rotation, whereas the posterior band resists posterior translation of the humeral head in shoulder flexion and internal rotation (69,72,78,79).

At the neutral position (0 degrees of abduction, 30 degrees of horizontal extension), the anterior band of the IGHL becomes the primary stabilizer. Sectioning of the anterior band of the IGHL and the anterior half of the axillary pouch resulted in significant increases in anterior, posterior, and total translation at −30 and 0 degrees of flexion and extension, respectively (80).

The posterior capsule of the GH joint lies proximal to the superior portion of the posterior band of the IGHL. It is the thinnest part of the capsule, being approximately 1 mm in width. It often is blamed for poor results after surgery for posterior instability, and it functions to limit posterior translation of the humeral head with the arm in forward flexion, adduction, and internal rotation (58,81).

Rotator Interval

The RTI is an area of shoulder capsule that is bounded by the supraspinatus superiorly, the subscapularis inferiorly, the coracoid process medially, and the long head of the biceps tendon laterally. The floor of the RTI is variably bridged by the GH capsule, the SGHL, the CHL, and occasionally, the MGHL (82,83). This area serves as safe portal for arthroscopic entry into the GH joint, because it does not violate the muscles of the RTC.

In a cadaveric study comparing the RTI of fetuses with those of adults, the RTI capsule was found, histologically, to be made of a disorganized system of collagen fibers, and it often contained a congenital hole or defect between the supraspinatus and subscapularis muscles (82). This evidence suggests that an RTI capsular defect is a normal anatomical variant and not an acquired lesion (82–84).

The RTI can thus contribute to inferior instability of the adducted arm. A persistent sulcus sign that does not lessen or disappear with external rotation of the arm suggests a loose or deficient RTI capsule. In patients with multidirectional instability, the RTI is characteristically thinned or absent, and a defect in this area can disrupt the negative intra-articular pressure system that normally exists in the shoulder and contribute further to instability. In contrast, a tight RTI is associated with adhesive capsulitis or postoperative stiffness and may need to be released in order to regain adequate range of motion (82–84).

In a biomechanical study using cadaveric specimens, a transverse incision in the RTI allowed for statistically significant increases in humeral head translation in all planes tested. Subsequent imbrication of the RTI decreased inferior translation in adduction and posterior translation in flexion (85).

■ DYNAMIC RESTRAINTS

Many dynamic factors contribute to GH stability. The RTC muscles as well as the scapular rotators contribute to stabilization by enhancing the concavity–compression mechanism. In addition, contraction of the long head of the biceps tendon, coordinated scapulothoracic rhythm, and proprioceptive mechanoreceptors in the joint capsule contribute to the dynamic stabilization of the GH joint.

Long Head of the Biceps

The long head of the biceps tendon has a variable origin, with 30% to 40% originating at the supraglenoid tubercle, 45% to 60% directly from the labrum, and 25% to 30% from both (62,86,87). It travels obliquely within the shoulder joint, then turns sharply to exit inferiorly beneath the transverse humeral ligament along the bicipital groove. It decreases in size and shape along its course. The tendon becomes more flat as it progresses over the humeral head and more triangular in the bicipital groove (88,89). In abduction, the tendon deforms to follow the shape of the bicipital groove; in adduction, the proximal portion regains its original shape as it exits the groove (60,88,90). The long head of the biceps tendon is covered by a reflection of the synovial sheath, which ends as a blind pouch at the distal part of the bicipital groove, thus making the tendon an intra-articular, but extrasynovial, structure. The tendon has an average length of 102 mm (86).

The role of the biceps in shoulder function continues to be a topic of debate. Neer (91) and others have suggested that it functions as a humeral head depressor and, thus, that tenodesis should be avoided, especially in patients with an RTC tear (92). Electromyographical (EMG) studies have shown that the biceps is extremely active in throwing athletes when the shoulder is placed in the vulnerable position of abduction and external rotation, as during the late cocking phase of pitching (93,94). These studies also have shown an even higher rate of activity of the biceps during this phase in pitchers with anterior instability (90,95–97). In addition, biomechanical studies have shown that the long head of the biceps increased the torsional rigidity of the GH joint by 32%, thus providing greater anterior stability and also serving a protective role by decreasing the load required by the IGHL (90,95–97).

More recent EMG studies, however, have suggested that the biceps shows little action during shoulder motion, acts mainly to control the elbow, and is not active during simple shoulder abduction (98,99). This is an important concept, because it has been suggested that the biceps may prevent superior displacement of the humeral head in the case of a massive RTC tear. In contrast, Walch et al. (100) have had success with tenodesis of the biceps tendon even in patients with RTC tears, and those authors have not observed instability in these patients. It also is possible that the long head of the biceps serves a proprioceptive function and that it may play a role in neuromuscular control and coordination of shoulder motion in relation to the elbow, because the muscle–tendon unit crosses both joints. This theoretical role is supported by the interesting analogy to all the major proximal long bones, because two articulation muscles are a consistent finding in the human body (i.e., triceps in the upper arm and rectus femoris/hamstrings in the thigh). Research concerning—and the debate regarding—the function of the long head biceps tendon will surely continue.

Rotator Cuff Muscles

The RTC is composed of the supraspinatus, the infraspinatus, the subscapularis, and the teres minor muscles **(Table 10-1)**. The tendinous portion of the supraspinatus interdigitates with the subscapularis and the infraspinatus to form a common, continuous insertion on the humeral head, enveloping approximately 75% of the GH articulation and with a mean area of insertion on the greater tuberosity of approximately 6 cm². The mean distance across the insertion is 14.7 mm, and the thickness of the terminal 2 cm of the

RTC ranges from 9 to 12 mm (101,102). The size and area of supraspinatus insertion (1.55 cm²) is less than that of the infraspinatus insertion (1.76 cm²) (101,103,104).

The RTC often serves more than one function simultaneously. The muscles act as prime movers if their line of action is within the intended direction of motion. In addition, they act as joint stabilizers by opposing the action of the deltoid, thereby centering the humeral head against the glenoid during shoulder motion. Loss of RTC function, either from fatigue or from frank tears, can lead to superior translation of the humeral head during arm elevation, because the deltoid is left unopposed (105).

The thin, crescent-shaped sheet of RTC comprising the distal portions of the supraspinatus and infraspinatus insertions is termed the rotator crescent, and it is bounded on its proximal margin by a thick bundle of fibers called the rotator cable (2,71). The rotator cable averages 2.6-fold the thickness of the rotator crescent that it surrounds, and it shields the RTC tendons from excessive stress and is readily seen arthroscopically from within the GH joint.

The supraspinatus muscle is active with any motion involving elevation, and it is the most commonly torn tendon of the cuff (102,106,107). Investigators have described distinct anterior and posterior portions of the supraspinatus tendon. The anterior portion has a larger physiological cross-sectional area, making it better suited to withstand greater mechanical loads (102,108). The supraspinatus tendon inserts as a footprint, thickening at its insertion, with an average of 1.55 mm of bone between the cartilage edge and the tendon insertion approximately 2 mm medial to the greater tuberosity. This is important in determining the size of partial-thickness RTC tears (101,109).

The posterior portion of the RTC is made up of the infraspinatus and teres minor muscles. The infraspinatus has a pennate architecture with a central raphe that should not be confused with the intermuscular interval between it and the teres minor (110).

The subscapularis internally rotates the humerus and acts as a passive stabilizer to anterior subluxation and external

TABLE 10-1	Muscles of the Rotator Cuff				
Muscle	**Origin**	**Insertion**	**Nerve**	**Arterial supply**	**Action**
Supraspinatus	Supraspinous fossa of scapula	Superior facet of greater tuberosity	Suprascapular	Suprascapular artery	Abduction of arm
Infraspinatus	Infraspinous fossa	Middle facet of greater tuberosity	Suprascapular	Suprascapular and/or circumflex scapular artery	External rotation of arm
Subscapularis	Subscapular fossa	Lesser tuberosity	Upper and lower subscapular	Subscapular artery	Internal rotation and adduction of arm
Teres minor	Upper portion of lateral border of scapula	Lower facet of greater tuberosity	Axillary	Circumflex and scapular artery	Rotation of arm laterally

TABLE 10-2	Scapulothoracic and Additional Shoulder Muscles				
Muscle	Origin	Insertion	Nerve	Arterial supply	Action
Deltoid	Lateral third of clavicle/acromion/ scapular spine	Deltoid tuberosity	Axillary	Posterior, humeral, circumflex	Arm abduction, flexion, extension
Teres major	Dorsal surface of inferior angle of scapula	Medial lip of bicepetal groove	Lower subscapular	Subscapular	Arm adduction, internal rotation
Latissimus dorsi	Spines of T7–L5 iliac crest	Floor of bicipital groove	Thoracodorsal	Thoracodorsal	Arm adduction, internal rotation
Serratus anterior	Ribs 1–9	Inferior angle of scapula	Long thoracic	Supreme thoracic/ thoracodorsal	Protraction, upward rotation
Pectoralis major	Sternum, ribs, clavicle	Lateral lip of bicipital groove	Medial and lateral pectoral	Pectoral	Flexion, adduction, internal rotation
Pectoralis minor	Ribs 3–5	Coracoid process	Medial pectoral	Pectoral	Protraction
Levator scapulae	Transverse process of C1–C4	Superior angle of scapula	Dorsal scapular	Dorsal scapular	Elevation, rotation of scapula
Rhomboid major	Spines of T2–T5	Medial border of scapula	Dorsal scapular	Dorsal scapular	Retraction
Rhomboid minor	Spines of C7–T1	Base of scapular spine	Dorsal scapular	Dorsal scapular	Retraction

rotation (3,111–113). The lower fibers of the subscapularis also contribute to GH stability, resisting the shear forces and superior pull of the deltoid (114). Tears in the upper portion of the subscapularis can result in dislocation of the long head of the biceps tendon because other structures composing the sling are torn as well.

Multiple vessels contribute to the vascularity of the RTC (115–118) (Table 10-1). In addition, the deltoid muscle and scapular rotators play a role in shoulder motion and stability (Table 10-2).

Several bursae lie within the soft tissues surrounding the shoulder joint. The subacromial and subdeltoid bursae are found superficial to the tendons and separate it from deltoid. The bursae vary in size and extend laterally from the subacromial space to the proximal humeral metaphysis. The subacromial bursa becomes thickened in disease states, and it has numerous free nerve endings, indicating that it may be involved with pain perception in pathologic conditions. The subscapularis bursa lies between the tendon and neck of the scapula, just inferior to coracoid process, and protects the tendon as it courses along the scapular neck and coracoid. This bursa communicates with the GH joint capsule and can harbor intra-articular loose bodies (2,119,120).

Proprioception

The perception of joint motion and position, or proprioception, is mediated by mechanoreceptors that transduce mechanical deformation into electric neural signals. Highly specialized nerve endings have been found in the joint capsule,

GH lie, and tendon surrounding the shoulder joint. Capsular stretch produces an afferent signal that produces an efferent signal, causing a protective muscular contraction that enhances the stability of the joint when the shoulder joint suddenly rotates to extreme position or translation (121,122). In patients with shoulder instability, this mechanism is disrupted but is restored after capsulolabral repair (121).

■ NERVE INJURIES/ENTRAPMENT

Nerve injuries can occur with both arthroscopic and open shoulder procedures. The axillary nerve courses from anterior to posterior from the posterior cord of the brachial plexus, 3 to 5 mm medial to musculotendinous junction of the inferior lateral border of the subscapularis muscle. It lies in contact with the GH joint capsule until it exits the quadrangular space and then reflects anteriorly, running deep to the surface of the deltoid from posterior to anterior (123). Adduction and internal rotation of the arm during an open anterior approach will help to displace the axillary nerve away from the surgical field. In addition, the nerve can be injured during suture placement through the inferior capsule, capsular release for adhesive capsulitis, and retraction of the subscapularis medially and the deltoid laterally (124,125). To avoid injury to the posterior branch of the nerve, incisions on the lateral aspect of the shoulder should not extend more than 5 cm below the acromion.

The posterior branch of the anterior circumflex branch of the axillary nerve courses medially along the posterior aspect of the inferior glenoid rim for an average distance of 18 mm before entering the muscle at its inferior border. The motor branch to the teres minor arises from the posterior branch of the axillary nerve, just adjacent to the inferior aspect of the capsule at the level of the glenoid rim (126). The superolateral brachial cutaneous branches of the axillary nerve also arise from the posterior branch. Therefore, sensory loss over the deltoid may be associated with dysfunction of the teres minor (126).

The musculocutaneous nerve enters the coracobrachialis muscle 3.1 to 8.2 cm from the coracoid; therefore, excessive traction of the conjoined tendon should be avoided. The long thoracic nerve is at risk where it is draped over the second rib and can be injured indirectly by positioning the patient improperly (2,3).

The suprascapular nerve is a mixed peripheral nerve that supplies motor innervation to the supraspinatus and infraspinatus and sensation to the AC and GH joints (127–129). The suprascapular nerve lies within 2 cm of the superior glenoid rim and as close as 1 cm to the posterior middle glenoid (124,125,130). This nerve can be entrapped or injured at the suprascapular notch and the spinoglenoid notch by tumors, cysts, excessive traction in overhead athletes, and direct trauma. The suprascapular nerve first passes through the suprascapular notch, which is bordered by the transverse scapular ligament; the suprascapular artery passes over this ligament (129,131,132). In addition to entrapment in the notch, hypertrophy of the subscapularis muscle can cover the entire anterior surface of the suprascapular notch and lead to nerve compression (128). After innervating the supraspinatus, the nerve passes around the base of the glenoid and scapular spine through the spinoglenoid notch, another site of entrapment (128,131,133). The projected distance from the most medial edge of the acromion to the spinoglenoid notch averages 14.5 mm (27).

■ BIOMECHANICAL FACTORS SPECIFIC TO ROTATOR CUFF REPAIR

RTC repair using an open technique has been clinically successful in terms of repair, although arthroscopic techniques are now more common. Arthroscopy for RTC repair is popular for several reasons: (a) exploration of the joint space for degenerative disease and loose bodies; (b) lower patient morbidity, with earlier relief of pain and return to activity; and (c) ability to be performed on an outpatient basis. Despite these advantages and good to excellent outcomes (134–138), postoperative imaging studies indicate that improvements can still be made to this technique (139). Whether open or arthroscopic, the quality of the cuff repair depends on the blood supply and the quality of the tendon–bone interface (140), and it also is affected by the type of suture material used, the type of anchor, and the placement of the anchor (141). These latter factors have come under

close scrutiny to determine differences that may affect the repair.

It is intuitive that a more stable knot construct should provide improved biomechanics compared to a knot that may be subjected to slippage, and recently, a variety of knots have been devised to maximize such security (141–147). Surgeons should choose the knot that they feel is most stable, but also they should choose the knot with which they are most facile. It is apparent from the literature that mechanical differences exist between knots (148). Examination of knot security typically is conducted by using cyclic biomechanical tests followed by a failure test **(Fig 10-4)**. These data provide information regarding knot slippage during physiological loading and maximal knot security during high loads while also elucidating construct behavior in terms of failure mechanisms (136). Knot security should not be confused with loop security, however, which can be defined as the ability to maintain a secure loop while the knot is being tied and the ability to resist high deformation (loop elongation) during the cyclic physiological loads that occur during the rehabilitation period. Improving loop security recently was addressed by the use of new suture materials, such as Fiberwire (Arthrex, Naples, FL) or ForceFiber (Teleflex Medical, Mansfield, MA). Historically, Ethibond (Ethicon, Inc., Somerville, NJ) has been the suture of choice, but it is more flexible than the more recent materials (149). The Fiberwire and ForceFiber materials have been shown to better resist cyclic deformation and to have nearly 200% greater failure strength. The design of such materials does not come without a cost, of course, and this cost has been discovered to be early knot loosening and construct slippage during cyclic submaximal loading, potentially caused by a sliding core within an outerwoven sheath (Fiberwire) or, perhaps, by the "slippery" polymer coating of the suture (ForceFiber) **(Fig 10-5)**. Surgeons should not ignore

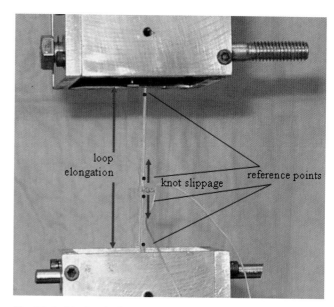

Fig 10-4. Mechanical test setup for analysis of suture material and arthroscopic knots.

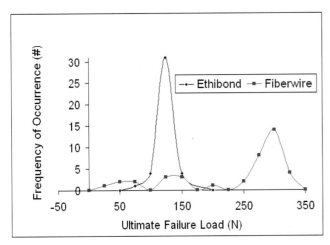

Fig 10-5. Results of mechanical analysis of two material types, demonstrating submaximal failure (slippage) of the stiffer but more "slippery" Fiberwire material.

the potential effects not only of knot selection but also of material selection on the potential for healing.

Benchtop studies can evaluate different material–knot constructs, but another chronic failure of the repair occurs in the tendon–suture interface (150–154). Soft-tissue structures of poor quality (because of degenerative or atrophic reasons) are susceptible to the sutures cutting through the tissue. It would seem that a more forgiving material would lessen the chances of cutting through the tendon. As discussed above, however, a more flexible material may come at the cost of limiting tendon–bone apposition. Whereas the suture may cut through the tendon on one side of the repair, the suture also may be susceptible to failure at the suture–anchor interface. Previous investigations have shown that the ultimate weak link of the repair lies, in fact, with the suture–anchor interface (155,156). In these instances, and despite a strong knot/loop security, the suture bears significant load as it exits the anchor eyelet **(Fig 10-6)**. The suture may fray because of abrasive wear at the eyelet, which is

yet another reason to develop a stronger suture material. Because of this weak link, the anchor eyelet also has come under scrutiny to improve stabilization, and surgeons have attempted new surgical techniques designed, in part, to protect the suture–eyelet interface.

The operating surgeon has the opportunity to deliver a suture anchor in a deeper-than-recommended position. This may be because of error, poor bone quality, or intentionally (either to maximize anchor purchase or to protect the suture–eyelet interface). This may seem to be an attractive option, but an anchor delivered to twice the recommended depth (6 mm) below the cortical surface was found to experience early construct elongation (157). On closer examination, it was noted that the suture material had cut a path through the cortical bone in the direction of physiological loading **(Fig 10-7)**. This phenomenon was further supported by another study that found the same result with deeper anchors (158). Thus, current clinical opinion is to avoid deliberately delivering the anchors into a deep position.

Osteoporotic bone may entice the surgeon to place a deep anchor out of concern for anchor migration into a proud position that could cause subsequent damage to opposing structures. Questions remain, however, regarding how an osteoporotic humeral head may affect anchor stability. It has been noted during in vitro investigations that the anchor can translate within the humeral head (159), but the amount of translation was not described. Quantifying the amount of translation and rotation of the anchor recently

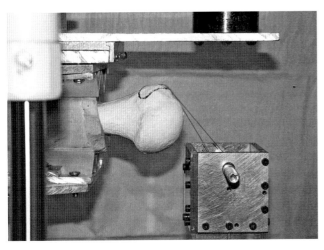

Fig 10-6. Mechanical test setup for in vitro investigation of different types of suture anchors and surgical techniques.

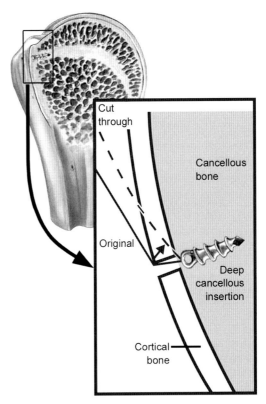

Fig 10-7. Representation of potential "cut-through" of suture material through the cortical margin at the insertion point.

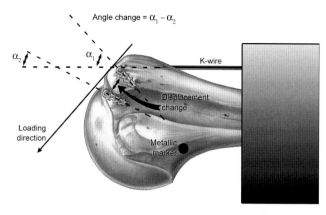

Fig 10-8. Method of fluoroscopic analysis to quantify the magnitudes of suture anchor translation/rotation during physiological cyclic loading.

was attempted using fluoroscopy during biomechanical testing (160) **(Fig 10-8)**. Surprisingly, fluoroscopic measurements after 500 cycles of physiological loading reported translations of between 1 and 2 mm and rotations of between 12 and 21 degrees for a variety of anchors. Considering that 3 mm of construct displacement has been used previously to describe failure of RTC repair (136), anchor movement may contribute significantly to these reported losses. Clearly, anchor position and design significantly influence the potential repair. In an attempt to alleviate these concerns with bone quality, some anchor designs have focused on an intracortical placement to maximize stability; with these designs, the anchor eyelet is flush with the cortical surface. These anchors appear to have some biomechanical advantages (160), but they too suffer from anchor movement. Thus, translation of an already-flush anchor means that the device would then be within the joint space, potentially causing degenerative changes to the articular surfaces.

Overall, surgeons should concern themselves with each component to the RTC repair. Each suture material, knot type, and anchor design have "pearls and pitfalls" associated with them. No combination will necessarily be ideal, but a surgeon's awareness of all biomechanical factors may assist with an optimal selection to maximize the quality of the arthroscopic RTC repair.

■ REFERENCES

1. Moseley HF. The clavicle: its anatomy and function. *Clin Orthop.* 1968;58:17–27.
2. O'Brien S, Arnoczsky S, Warren R, et al. Developmental anatomy of the shoulder and anatomy of the glenohumeral joint. In: Rockwood C, Matsen F, eds. *The shoulder.* Philadelphia: WB Saunders; 1990:1–33.
3. Jobe CM. Anatomy and surgical approaches. In: Jobe F, ed. *Operative techniques in upper extremity sports medicine.* St. Louis: Mosby; 1996:124–160.
4. Edelson JG, Zuckerman J, Hershkovitz I. Os acromiale: anatomy and surgical implications. *J Bone Joint Surg Br.* 1993;75:551–555.

5. Mudge MK, Bernardino S, Wood VE, et al. Rotator cuff tears associated with os acromiale. *J Bone Joint Surg Am.* 1984;66:427–429.
6. Neer CS. Rotator cuff tears associated with os acromiale. *J Bone Joint Surg Am.* 1984;66:1320–1321.
7. Nicholson GP, Goodman DA, Flatow EL, et al. The acromion: morphologic condition and age-related changes: a study of 420 scapulas. *J Shoulder Elbow Surg.* 1996;5:1–11.
8. Bigliani LU, Morrison DS, April EW. The morphology of the acromion and its relationship to rotator cuff tears. *Orthop Trans.* 1986;10:216.
9. Gill TJ, McIrvin E, Kocher MS, et al. The relative importance of acromial morphology and age with respect to rotator cuff pathology. *J Shoulder Elbow Surg.* 2002;11:327–330.
10. Toivonen DA, Tuite MJ, Orwin JF. Acromial structure and tears of the rotator cuff. *J Shoulder Elbow Surg.* 2001;10:434–437.
11. Snyder SJ, Wuh HCK. Arthroscopic evaluation and treatment of the rotator cuff superior labrum anterior posterior lesion. *Op Tech Orthop.* 1991;1:212–213.
12. Edelson JG, Luchs J. Aspects of coracoacromial ligament anatomy of interest to the arthroscopic surgeon. *Arthroscopy.* 1995;11:715–719.
13. Holt EM, Allibone RO. Anatomic variants of the coracoacromial ligament. *J Shoulder Elbow Surg.* 1995;4(5):370–375.
14. Salter EG, Nasca RJ, Shelley BS. Anatomical observations on the acromioclavicular joint and supporting ligaments. *Am J Sports Med.* 1987;15:199–206.
15. Soslowsky LJ, An CH, Johnston SP, et al. Geometric and mechanical properties of the coracoacromial ligament and their relationship to rotator cuff disease. *Clin Orthop.* 1994;304:10–17.
16. Soslowsky LJ, An CH, DeBano CM, et al. Coracoacromial ligament: in situ load and viscoelastic properties in rotator cuff disease. *Clin Orthop.* 1996;330:40–44.
17. Gohlke F, Barthel T, Gandorfer A. The influence of variations of the coracoacromial arch on the development of rotator cuff tears. *Arch Orthop Trauma Surg.* 1993;113:28–32.
18. Matsen FI, Thomas S, Rockwood CJ. Anterior glenoid instability. In Rockwood C, Matsen F, eds. *The shoulder.* Philadelphia: WB Saunders; 1990:526–622.
19. Wiley AM. Superior humeral dislocation. A complication following decompression and debridement for rotator cuff tears. *Clin Orthop.* 1991;263:136–141.
20. Lee SB, Itoi E, O'Driscoll SW, et al. Contact geometry at the undersurface of the acromion with and without a rotator cuff tear. *Arthroscopy.* 2001;7:365–372.
21. Lee TQ, Black AD, Tibone JE, et al. Release of the coracoacromial ligament can lead to glenohumeral laxity: a biomechanical study. *J Shoulder Elbow Surg.* 2001;10:68–72.
22. Kronberg M, Bromstrom LA, Soderlund V. Retroversion of the humeral head in the normal shoulder and its relationship to the normal range of motion. *Clin Orthop.* 1990;253:113–117.
23. Burkhart SS, DeBeer JF, Tehrany AM, et al. Quantifying glenoid bone loss arthroscopically in shoulder instability. *Arthroscopy.* 2002;18:488–491.
24. DeWilde LF, Berghs BM, Audenaert E, et al. About the variability of the shape of the glenoid cavity. *Surg Radiol Anat.* 2004;26:54–59.
25. Friedman RJ, Hawthorne KB, Genez BM. The use of computerized tomography in the measurement of glenoid version. *J Bone Joint Surg Am.* 1992;74:1032–1037.
26. Iannotti JP, Gabriel JP, Schneck SL, et al. The normal glenohumeral relationships. *J Bone Joint Surg Am.* 1992;74:491–500.
27. Mallon WJ, Brown HR, Vogler JB, et al. Radiographic and geometric anatomy of the scapula. *Clin Orthop.* 1992;277:142–154.
28. Saha AK. Dynamic stability of the glenohumeral joint. *Acta Orthop Scand.* 1971;42:491–505.

29. Basmajian JV, Bazant FJ. Factors preventing downward dislocation of the adducted shoulder joint in an electromyographic and morphological study. *J Bone Joint Surg Am.* 1986;41:1182–1186.

30. Churchill RS, Brems JJ, Kotschi H. Glenoid size, inclination, and version: an anatomic study. *J Shoulder Elbow Surg.* 2001;10:327–332.

31. DeWilde LF, Berghs BM, Van de Vyver F, et al. Glenohumeral relationship in the transverse plane of the body. *J Shoulder Elbow Surg.* 2003;12:260–267.

32. Tetreault P, Krueger A, Zurakowski D, et al. Glenoid version and rotator cuff tears. *J Orthop Res.* 2004;22:202–207.

33. Halder AM, Kuhl SG, Zobitz ME, et al. Effects of the glenoid labrum and glenohumeral abduction on stability of the shoulder joint through concavity-compression. *J Bone Joint Surg Am.* 2001; 83:1062–1069.

34. Inui H, Sugamoto D, Miyamoto T, et al. Evaluation of three-dimensional glenoid structure using MRI. *J Anat.* 2001;199: 323–328.

35. Lehtinien JT, Tingart MJ, Apreleva M, et al. Anatomy of the superior glenoid rim: repair of superior labral anterior to posterior tears. *Am J Sports Med.* 2003;31:257–260.

36. Wong AS, Gallo L, Kuhn JE, et al. The effect of glenoid inclination on superior humeral head migration. *J Shoulder Elbow Surg.* 2003;12:360–364.

37. Inui H, Sugamoto K, Miyamoto T, et al. Glenoid shape in atraumatic posterior instability of the shoulder. *Clin Orthop.* 2002;403: 87–92.

38. Lo IKY, Parten PM, Burkhart SS. The inverted pear glenoid: an indicator of significant glenoid bone loss. *Arthroscopy.* 2004;20: 169–174.

39. Frich LH, Odgaard A, Dalstra M. Glenoid bone architecture. *J Shoulder Elbow Surg.* 1998;7:356–361.

40. Boileau P, Walch G. The three dimensional geometry of the proximal humerus: implications for surgical technique and prosthetic design. *J Bone Joint Surg Br.* 1997;79:857–865.

41. Robertson DD, Yuan J, Bigliani LU, et al. Three-dimensional analysis of the proximal part of the humerus: Relevance to arthroplasty. *J Bone Joint Surg Am.* 2000;82:1594–1602.

42. Hertel R, Knothe U, Ballmer FT. Geometry of the proximal humerus and implications for prosthetic design. *J Shoulder Elbow Surg.* 2002;11:331–338.

43. Walch G, Boileau P, Levigne C, et al. Arthroscopic stabilization for recurrent anterior shoulder dislocation: result of 59 cases. *Arthroscopy.* 1995;11:173–179.

44. Tillett E, Smith M, Fulcher M, et al. Anatomic determination of humeral head retroversion: the relationship of the central axis of the humeral head to the bicipital groove. *J Shoulder Elbow Surg.* 1993;2:255–256.

45. Takase K, Imakiire A, Burkhead WZ. Radiographic study of the anatomic relationship of the greater tuberosity. *J Shoulder Elbow Surg.* 2002;11:557–561.

46. Itamura J, Dietrick T, Roidis N, et al. Analysis of the bicipital groove as a landmark for humeral head replacement. *J Shoulder Elbow Surg.* 2002;11:322–326.

47. DePalma AF. Surgical anatomy of the acromioclavicular and sternoclavicular joints. *Surg Clin North Am.* 1963;43:1541–1550.

48. Fukuda K, Craig EV, An KN, et al. Biomechanical study of the ligamentous system of the acromioclavicular joint. *J Bone Joint Surg Am.* 1986;68:434–440.

49. Lee K-W, Debski RE, Chen C-H, et al. Functional evaluation of the ligaments at the acromioclavicular joint during anteroposterior and superoinferior translation. *Am J Sports Med.* 1997;25:858–862.

50. Klimkiewicz JJ, Williams GR, Sher JS, et al. The acromioclavicular capsule as a restraint to posterior translation of the clavicle: a biomechanical analysis. *J Shoulder Elbow Surg.* 1999;8:119–124.

51. Bearn JG. Direct observations on the function of the capsule of the sternoclavicular joint in clavicular support. *J Anat.* 1967; 101:159–170.

52. Williams GR, Shakil M, Klimkiewicz J, et al. Anatomy of the scapulothoracic articulation. *Clin Orthop.* 1999;359:237–246.

53. Ruland RJ III, Ruland CM, Matthews LS. Scapulothoracic anatomy for the arthroscopist. *Arthroscopy.* 1995;11:52–56.

54. Kelkar R, Wang VM, Flatow EL, et al. Glenohumeral mechanics: a study of articular geometry, contact, and kinematics. *J Shoulder Elbow Surg.* 2001;10:73–84.

55. Matsen FA III, Lippitt SB. Principles of glenohumeral stability. In: Matsen FA III, Lippitt SB, eds. *Shoulder surgery: principles and procedures.* Philadelphia: WB Saunders; 2004:80–117.

56. Lippitt SB, Vanderhooft JE, Harris SL, et al. Glenohumeral stability from concavity–compression: a quantitative analysis. *J Shoulder Elbow Surg.* 1993;2:27–35.

57. McMahon PJ, Debski RE, Thompson WO, et al. Shoulder muscle forces and tendon excursions during glenohumeral abduction in the scapular plane. *J Shoulder Elbow Surg.* 1995;4:199–208.

58. Tung GA, Hou DD. MR arthrography of the posterior labrocapsular complex: relationship with glenohumeral joint alignment and clinical posterior instability. *AJR Am J Roentgenol.* 2003; 180:369–375.

59. Harryman DT II, Sidles JA, Clark JM, et al. Translation of the humeral head on the glenoid with passive glenohumeral motion. *J Bone Joint Surg Am.* 1990;72:1334–1343.

60. Itoi E, Motzkin NE, Browne AO, et al. Intra-articular pressure of the shoulder. *Arthroscopy.* 1993;9:406–413.

61. Debski RE, Moore SM, Mercer JL, et al. The collagen fibers of the anteroinferior capsulolabrum have multiaxial orientation to resist shoulder dislocation. *J Shoulder Elbow Surg.* 2003;12:247–252.

62. Cooper DE, Arnoczky SP, O'Brien SJ, et al. Anatomy, histology, and vascularity of the glenoid labrum. *J Bone Joint Surg Am.* 1992;74:46–52.

63. Pagnani MJ, Deng XH, Warren RF, et al. Effect of lesions of the superior portion of the glenoid labrum on glenohumeral translation. *J Bone Joint Surg Am.* 1995;77:1003–1010.

64. Ide J, Maeda S, Takagi K. Normal variations of the glenohumeral ligament complex: an anatomic study for arthroscopic Bankart repair. *Arthroscopy.* 2004;20:164–168.

65. Rao AG, Kim TK, Chronopoulos E, et al. Anatomical variants in the anterosuperior aspect of the glenoid labrum. *J Bone Joint Surg Am.* 2003;85:653–659.

66. Ilahi OA, Labbe MR, Cosculluela P. Variants of the anterosuperior glenoid labrum and associated pathology. *Arthroscopy.* 2002;18:882–886.

67. Williams MM, Synder SJ, Buford D Jr. The Buford complex: "cord-like" middle glenohumeral ligament and absent anterosuperior labrum complex: a normal anatomic capsulolabral variant. *Arthroscopy.* 1994;10:241–247.

68. Steinbeck J, Liljenqvist U, Jerosch J: The anatomy of the glenohumeral ligamentous complex and its contribution to anterior shoulder stability. *J Shoulder Elbow Surg.* 1998;7:122–126.

69. Burkart AC, Debski RE. Anatomy and function of the glenohumeral ligaments in anterior shoulder instability. *Clin Orthop.* 2002;400:32–39.

70. Warner JJP, Deng X, Warren RF, et al. Static capsuloligamentous restraints to superior-inferior translation of the glenohumeral joint. *Am J Sports Med.* 1992;20:675–685.

71. Burkhart SS, Esch JC, Jolson RS. The rotator crescent and rotator cable: an anatomic description of the shoulder's "suspension bridge." *Arthroscopy.* 1993;9(6):611–616.

72. Turkel SJ, Panio MW, Marshall JL, et al. Stabilizing mechanisms preventing anterior dislocation of the GH joint. *J Bone Joint Surg Am.* 1981;63:1208–1217.

73. O'Connell PW, Nuber GW, Mileski RA, et al. The contribution of the glenohumeral ligaments to anterior stability of the shoulder. *Am J Sports Med.* 1990;18:579–584.

74. Schwartz E, Warren RF, O'Brien SF, et al. Posterior shoulder instability. *Orthop Clin North Am.* 1987;18:409–419.

75. McMahon PJ, Dettling J, Sandusky MD, et al. The anterior band of the inferior glenohumeral ligament: assessment of its permanent deformation and the anatomy of its glenoid attachment. *J Bone Joint Surg Br.* 1999;81:406–413.

76. McMahon PJ, Tibone JE, Cawley PW, et al. The anterior band of the inferior glenohumeral ligament: biomechanical properties from tensile testing in the position of apprehension. *J Shoulder Elbow Surg.* 1998;7:467–471.

77. Eberly VC, McMahon PJ, Lee TQ. Variation in the glenoid origin of the anteroinferior glenohumeral capsulolabrum. *Clin Orthop.* 2002;400:26–31.

78. Soslowsky LJ, Flatow EL, Bigliani LU, et al. Quantitation of in situ contact areas at the glenohumeral joint: a biomechanical study. *J Orthop Res.* 1992;10:524–534.

79. Urayama M. Hatakeyama Y, Pradhan RL, et al. Function of the three portions of the inferior glenohumeral ligament: a cadaveric study. *J Shoulder Elbow Surg.* 2001;10:589–594.

80. O'Brien SJ, Schwartz RS, Warren RF, et al. Capsular restraints to anterior-posterior motion of the abducted shoulder: a biomechanical study. *J Shoulder Elbow Surg.* 1995;4:298–308.

81. Burkhart SS, Morgan CD, Kibler WB. The disabled throwing shoulder: spectrum of pathology. Part I: pathoanatomy and biomechanics. *Arthroscopy.* 2003;19:404–420.

82. Cole BJ, Rodeo SA, O'Brien SJ, et al. The anatomy and histology of the rotator interval capsule of the shoulder. *Clin Orthop.* 2001; 390:129–137.

83. Fitzpatrick MJ, Powell SE, Tibone JE, et al. The anatomy, pathology, and definitive treatment of rotator interval lesions: current concepts. *Arthroscopy.* 2003;19:70–79.

84. Kolts I, Busch LC, Tomusk H, et al. Macroscopical anatomy of the so called "rotator interval": a cadaver study on 19 shoulder joints. *Ann Anat.* 2002;184:9–14.

85. Harryman DT, Sidles JA, Harris SL, et al. The role of the rotator interval capsule in passive motion and stability of the shoulder. *J Bone Joint Surg Am.* 1992;74:53–66.

86. Werner A, Mueller T, Boehm D, et al. The stabilizing sling for the long head of the biceps tendon in the rotator cuff interval: a histoanatomic study. *Am J Sports Med.* 2000;28:28–31.

87. Vangsness CT Jr, Jorgenson SS, Watson T, et al. The origin of the long head of the biceps from the scapula and glenoid labrum. An anatomical study of 100 shoulders. *J Bone Joint Surg Br.* 1994; 76:951–954.

88. Heers G, O'Driscoll SW, Halder AM, et al. Gliding properties of the long head of the biceps brachii. *J Orthop Res.* 2003;21: 162–166.

89. McGough RL, Debiski RE, Taskiran E, et al. Mechanical properties of the long head of the biceps tendon. *Knee Surg Sports Traumatol Arthrosc.* 1996;3:226–229.

90. Healey JH, Barton S, Noble P, et al. Biomechanical evaluation of the origin of the long head of the biceps tendon. *Arthroscopy.* 2001;17:378–382.

91. Neer CS. Anterior acromioplasty for the chronic impingement syndrome in the shoulder: a preliminary report. *J Bone Joint Surg Am.* 1972;54:41–50.

92. Kumar VP, Satku K, Balasubramaniam P. The role of the biceps brachii in the stabilization of the head of the humerus. *Clin Orthop.* 1989;244:172–5.

93. Glousman R, Jobe F, Tibone J, et al. Dynamic electromyographic analysis of the throwing shoulder with glenohumeral instability. *J Bone Joint Surg Am.* 1988;70:220–226.

94. Gowan ID, Jobe FW, Tibone JE, et al. A comparative electromyographic analysis of the shoulder during pitching: professional versus amateur pitchers. *Am J Sports Med.* 1987;15: 586–90.

95. Itoi I, Kuechle DK, Newman SR, et al. Stabilizing function of the biceps in stable and unstable shoulders. *J Bone Joint Surg Br.* 1993;75:546–550.

96. Itoi E, Newman SR, Kuechle DK, et al. Dynamic anterior stabilizers of the shoulder with the arm in abduction. *J Bone Joint Surg Br.* 1994;76:834–836.

97. Rodosky MW, Harner CD, Fu FH. The role of the long head of the biceps muscle and superior glenoid labrum in anterior stability of the shoulder. *Am J Sports Med.* 1994;22:121–131.

98. Levy AS, Kelly BT, Lintner SA, et al. Function of the long head of the biceps at the shoulder: electromyographic analysis. *J Shoulder Elbow Surg.* 2001;10:250–255.

99. Yamaguchi K, Riew DK, Galatz IM, et al. Biceps activity during shoulder motion: an electromyographic analysis. *Clin Orthop.* 1997;336:122–129.

100. Walch G, Edwards B, Boulahia A, et al. Arthroscopic tenotomy of the long head of the biceps in the treatment of rotator cuff tears: clinical and radiographic results of 307 cases. *J Shoulder Elbow Surg.* 2005;14:238–245.

101. Fallon J, Blevins FT, Vogel K, et al. Functional morphology of the supraspinatus tendon. *J Orthop Res.* 2002;20:920–926.

102. Ruotolo C, Fow JE, Nottage WM. The supraspinatus footprint: an anatomic study of the supraspinatus insertion. *Arthroscopy.* 2004;20:246–249.

103. Dugas JR, Campbell DA, Warren RF, et al. Anatomy and dimensions of rotator cuff insertions. *J Shoulder Elbow Surg.* 2002;11: 498–503.

104. Poppen NK, Walker PS. Forces at the glenohumeral joint in abduction. *Clin Orthop.* 1978;135:165–170.

105. Sharkey NA, Marder RA. The rotator cuff opposes superior translation of the humeral head. *Am J Sports Med.* 1995;23: 270–275.

106. Howell SM, Imobersteg AM, Seger DH, et al. Clarification of the role of the supraspinatus muscle in shoulder function. *J Bone Joint Surg Am.* 1986;68:398–404.

107. Yamaguchi K, Tetro AM, Blam O, et al. Natural history of asymptomatic rotator cuff tears: a longitudinal analysis of asymptomatic tears detected sonographically. *J Shoulder Elbow Surg.* 2001;10:199–203.

108. Volk AG, Vangsness CT. An anatomic study of the supraspinatus muscle and tendon. *Clin Orthop.* 2001;384:280–285.

109. Poppen NK, Walker PS. Normal and abnormal motion of the shoulder. *J Bone Joint Surg Am.* 1976;58:195–201.

110. Mura N, O'Driscoll SW, Zobitz ME, et al. The effect of infraspinatus disruption on glenohumeral torque and superior migration of the humeral head: a biomechanical study. *J Shoulder Elbow Surg.* 2003;12:179–184.

111. Gamulin A, Pizzolato G, Stern R, et al. Anterior shoulder instability: histomorphometric study of the subscapularis and deltoid muscles. *Clin Orthop.* 2002;398:121–126.

112. Halder AM, Halder CG, Zhao KD, et al. Dynamic inferior stabilizers of the shoulder joint. *Clin Biomech.* 2001;16:138–143.

113. Halder AM, Zhae KD, O'Driscoll SW, et al. Dynamic contributions to superior shoulder stability. *J Orthop Res.* 2001;19:206–212.

114. Boon JM, de Beer MA, Botha D, et al. The anatomy of the subscapularis tendon insertion as applied to rotator cuff repair. *J Shoulder Elbow Surg.* 2004;13:165–169.

115. Brooks Ch, Revell WJ, Heatley FW. A quantitative histological study of the vascularity of the rotator cuff tendon. *J Bone Joint Surg Br.* 1992;74:151–153.

116. Gerber C, Schneeberger AG, Vinh TS. The arterial vascularization of the humeral head: an anatomic study. *J Bone Joint Surg Am.* 1990;72:1486–1494.

117. Moseley HF, Goldie IG. The arterial pattern of the rotator cuff of the shoulder. *J Bone Joint Surg Br.* 1963;45:780–789.

118. Rothman RH, Parke WW. The vascular anatomy of the rotator cuff. *Clin Orthop.* 1965;41:176–186.

119. Colas F, Nevoux J, Gagey O. The subscapular and subcoracoid bursae: descriptive and functional anatomy. *J Shoulder Elbow Surg.* 2004;13:454–458.

120. Duranthon LD, Gagey OJ. Anatomy and function of the subdeltoid bursa. *Surg Radiol Anat.* 2001;23:23–25.

121. Lephart SM, Warner JJP, Borsa PA, et al. Proprioception of the shoulder joint in healthy, unstable, and surgically repaired shoulders. *J Shoulder Elbow Surg.* 1994;3:371–380.

122. Warner JJ, Lephart S, Fu FH. The role of proprioception in pathoetiology of shoulder instability. *Clin Orthop.* 1996;330: 35–39.

123. Lo IKY, Lind CC, Burkhart SS. Glenohumeral arthroscopy portals established using an outside-in technique: neurovascular anatomy at risk. *Arthroscopy.* 2004;20:596–602.

124. Boardman ND, Cofield RH. Neurologic complications of shoulder surgery. *Clin Orthop.* 1999;368:44–53.

125. Ho E, Cofield RH, Balm MR, et al. Neurologic complications of surgery for anterior shoulder instability. *J Shoulder Elbow Surg.* 1999;8:266–270.

126. Ball CM, Steger T, Galatz LM, et al. The posterior branch of the axillary nerve: an anatomic study. *J Bone Joint Surg Am.* 2003;85: 1497–1501.

127. Andary JL, Petersen SA. The vascular anatomy of the glenohumeral capsule and ligaments: an anatomic study. *J Bone Joint Surg Am.* 2002;84:2258–2265.

128. Bayramoglu A, Demiryurek D, Tuccar E, et al. Variations in anatomy at the suprascapular notch possibly causing suprascapular nerve entrapment: an anatomical study. *Knee Surg Sports Traumatol Arthrosc.* 2003;11:393–398.

129. Weinfeld AB, Cheng J, Nath RK, et al. Topographic mapping of the superior transverse scapular ligament: a cadaver study to facilitate suprascapular nerve decompression. *Plast Reconstr Surg.* 2002;110:774–779.

130. Mair SD, Hawkins RJ. Open shoulder instability surgery: complications. *Clin Sports Med.* 1999;18:719–736.

131. Ide J, Maeda S, Takagi K. Does the inferior transverse scapular ligament cause distal suprascapular nerve entrapment? An anatomic and morphologic study. *J Shoulder Elbow Surg.* 2003;12: 253–255.

132. Shishido H, Kikuchi S. Injury of the suprascapular nerve in shoulder surgery: an anatomic study. *J Shoulder Elbow Surg.* 2001;10:372–376.

133. Demirkan AF, Sargon MF, Erkula G, et al. The spinoglenoid ligament: an anatomic study. *Clin Anat.* 2003;16:511–513.

134. Burkhart SS, Danaceau SM, Pearce CE Jr. Arthroscopic rotator cuff repair: analysis of results by tear size and by repair technique—margin convergence versus direct tendon-to-bone repair. *Arthroscopy.* 2001;17:905–912.

135. Kim SH, Ha KI, Park JH, et al. Arthroscopic versus mini-open salvage repair of the rotator cuff tear: outcome analysis at 2 to 6 years' follow-up. *Arthroscopy.* 2003;19:746–754.

136. Lo IKY, Burkhart SS, Chan KC, et al. Arthroscopic knots: determining the optimal balance of loop security and knot security. *Arthroscopy.* 2004;20:489–502.

137. Park JY, Chung KT, Yoo MJ. A serial comparison of arthroscopic repairs for partial- and full-thickness rotator cuff tears. *Arthroscopy.* 2004;20:705–711.

138. Wolf EM, Pennington WT, Agrawal V. Arthroscopic rotator cuff repair: 4- to 10-year results. *Arthroscopy.* 2004;20:5–12.

139. Galatz LM, Ball CM, Teefey SA, et al. The outcome and repair integrity of completely arthroscopically repaired large and massive rotator cuff tears. *J Bone Joint Surg Am.* 2004;86: 219–224.

140. Reilly P, Amis AA, Wallace AL, et al. Supraspinatus tears: propagation and strain alteration. *J Should Elbow Surg.* 2004;12: 134–138.

141. Kim SH, Ha KI, Kim SH, et al. Significance of the internal locking mechanism for loop security enhancement in the arthroscopic knot. *Arthroscopy.* 2001;17:850–855.

142. DeBeer JF, van Rooyen K, Boezaart AP. Nicky's knot—a new slip knot for arthroscopic surgery. *Arthroscopy.* 1998;14:109–110.

143. Field MH, Edwards TB, Savoie FH. Technical note: a "new" arthroscopic sliding knot. *Orthop Clin North Am.* 2001;32: 525–526.

144. Fleega BA, Sokkar SH. The giant knot: a new one-way self-locking secured arthroscopic slip knot. *Arthroscopy.* 1999;15: 451–452.

145. Kim SH, Ha KI. The SMC knot—a new slip knot with locking mechanism for loop security enhancement in the arthroscopic knot. *Arthroscopy.* 2000;16:563–565.

146. Pallia CS. The PC knot: a secure and satisfying arthroscopic slip knot. *Arthroscopy.* 2003;19:558–560.

147. Rolla PR, Surace MF. The double-twist knot: a new arthroscopic sliding knot. *Arthroscopy.* 2002;18:815–820.

148. Abbi G, Espinosa L, Odell T, et al. Evaluation of 5 knots and 2 suture materials for arthroscopic rotator cuff repair: very strong sutures can still slip. *Arthroscopy.* 2006;22:38–43.

149. Mahar AR, Moezzi DM, Serra-Hsu F, et al. Comparison and performance characteristics of 3 different knots when tied with 2 suture materials used for shoulder arthroscopy. *Arthroscopy.* 2006;22(6):610–614.

150. Barber FA, Cawley P, Prudich JF. Suture anchor failure strength—an in vivo study. *Arthroscopy.* 1993;9:647–652.

151. Meyer DC, Nyffeler RW, Fucentese SF, et al. Failure of suture material at suture anchor eyelets. *Arthroscopy.* 2002;18:1013–1019.

152. Meyer DC, Gerber C. Failure of anterior shoulder instability repair caused by eyelet cutout of absorbable suture anchors. *Arthroscopy.* 2004;20:521–523.

153. Rupp S, George T, Gauss C, et al. Fatigue testing of suture anchors. *Am J Sports Med.* 2002;30:239–247.

154. Schneeberger AG, von Roll A, Kalberer F, et al. Mechanical strength of arthroscopic rotator cuff repair techniques: an in vitro study. *J Bone Joint Surg Am.* 2002;84:2152–2160.

155. Burkhart SS, Diaz Pagan JL, Wirth MA, et al. Cyclic loading of anchor-based rotator cuff repairs: tension overload as a possible cause of failure. *Arthroscopy.* 1997;13:172–176.

156. Burkhart SS, Johnson TC, Wirth MA, et al. Cyclic loading of transosseous rotator cuff repairs: confirmation of the tension overload phenomenon and comparison of suture anchor fixation with transosseous fixation. *Arthroscopy.* 1997;13:720–724.

157. Bynum KC, Lee S, Mahar A, et al. Failure mode of suture anchors as a function of insertion depth. *Am J Sports Med.* 2005; 33:1030–1034.

158. Mahar A, Tucker B, Upasani V, et al. Increasing the insertion depth of suture anchors for rotator cuff repair does not improve biomechanical stability. *J Shoulder Elbow Surg.* 2005;14(6):626–630.

159. Roth CA, Bartolozzi AR, Ciccotti MG, et al. Failure properties of suture anchors in the glenoid and the effects of cortical thickness. *Arthroscopy.* 1998;14:186–191.

160. Mahar A, Allred DW, Wedemeyer M, et al. A biomechanical and radiographic analysis of standard and intracortical suture anchors for arthroscopic rotator cuff repair. *Arthroscopy.* 2006; 22(2):130–135.

11

SHOULDER IMPINGEMENT

JAMES PATRICK TASTO, MD, JOHN K. LOCKE, MD

■ KEY POINTS

- In clinical frequency, shoulder pain is exceeded only by low back pain and neck pain. The most common source of shoulder pain originates in the subacromial space, with the most prevalent diagnosis being impingement syndrome.
- Without treatment, symptoms will persist and usually progress.
- Shoulder impingement has been described as "symptomatic mechanical irritation of the rotator cuff tendons from direct contact at the anterior edge of the coracoacromial arch."
- In the normal shoulder, the coordinated muscle tension within the rotator cuff compresses the humeral head, keeping it centered within the glenoid fossa. By coupling with the force of the deltoid, a fulcrum is created, generating strength through a wide arc of motion.
- Any process that interferes with the rotator cuff's capability to keep the humeral head centered or that compromises the normal coracoacromial arch, including calcium deposits, thickened bursae, and an unfused os acromiale, can lead to impingement of the rotator cuff.
- Functional overload, intrinsic tendonopathy, and internal anatomic impingement have also led to shoulder impingement.
- It is important to rule out other potential sources of shoulder pain, including: acromioclavicular arthrosis, rotator cuff tear, instability, adhesive capsulitis, biceps tendonitis, labral pathology, and cervical radiculopathy.
- The x-ray views that are most helpful are anterior-posterior view, supraspinatous outlet view, and axillary lateral. A 15-degree cephalic view of the Acromioclavicular (AC)

joint and an anterior posterior (AP) view with humeral internal rotation can also be helpful.

- Nonoperative care is tried before surgical intervention is considered. The majority of patients can be treated conservatively. Treatment consists of physical therapy, activity modification, anti-inflammatory medications, and steroid injections into the subacromial space.
- When nonoperative treatment fails, the procedure of choice is arthroscopic subacromial decompressions (ASAD). The advantages of arthroscopy include minimally invasive surgery without detachment of the deltoid.
- Conventional postoperative pain control can generally be obtained with oral medications. Stiffness can be avoided when early motion is emphasized.
- Through progressive steps in exercises, full active range of motion can usually be achieved within three to four weeks. Athletes using overhead motions should avoid sports for at least 3 months, and complete recovery can take 6 months.

The concept of mechanical impingement on the rotator cuff was popularized by Neer (1). He noted that with forward elevation of the arm, the rotator cuff tendons were subject to repeated mechanical insult by the overlying coracoacromial arch. He observed that impingement was a result of bony spurs at the anterior third of the acromion and the coracoacromial ligament. This concept of anterior impingement as opposed to lateral acromial impingement has been generally accepted.

Neer (2) reported the cause of most impingement to be due to an inadequate "outlet" and described this phenomenon as outlet impingement. The outlet is the space beneath

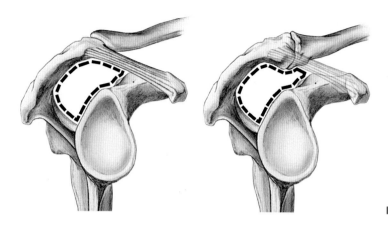

Fig 11-1. The supraspinatus outlet.

the anterior acromion, coracoacromial ligament, and acromioclavicular (AC) joint. Within this space, the rotator cuff tendons pass to their insertions on the tuberosities of the humerus. The superior border of the outlet forms an arch known as the coracoacromial arch. Any prominence that affects this arch may encroach on the outlet causing outlet impingement (3). In addition to outlet impingement, the terms subacromial, primary or external impingement are also used. The definition has more recently been described as "symptomatic mechanical irritation of the rotator cuff tendons from direct contact at the anterior edge of the coracoacromial arch" (4) **(Fig 11-1)**.

■ ANATOMY AND PATHOPHYSIOLOGY

In the normal shoulder, the coordinated muscle tension within the rotator cuff compresses the humeral head, keeping it centered within the glenoid fossa (3). By coupling with the force of the deltoid, a fulcrum is created that allows strength through a wide arc of motion (5). The overlying subacromial bursae reduces friction between the tendonous cuff and the coracoacromial arch. With normal overhead movement, the bursae facilitates smooth gliding of the tendons within this limited space.

In most individuals, the space between the greater tuberosity and the undersurface of the acromion is approximately 7 to 14 mm while standing with the arm at the side (6). There is little room for clearance, and during normal overhead shoulder function light contact between the rotator cuff and coracoacromial arch may occur. Any process that interferes with the rotator cuff's capability to keep the humeral head centered or compromises the normal coracoacromial arch can lead to impingement of the rotator cuff. This can include calcium deposits, thickened bursae, and an unfused os acromiale (7).

Specific acromial morphologies affect the size of the outlet. Bigliani (8) described three types of acromia. Type I is flat, Type II is curved, and Type III is hooked. A curved or

hooked acromion decreases the space available for tendons to glide and they have been associated with impingements symptoms and rotator cuff tears. Outlet impingement may also occur from hypertrophy or calcification of the coracoacromial ligament. Osteophytes at the acromioclavicular joint or at the lateral acromion may cause impingement in these areas **(Fig 11-2)**.

Other Causes of Impingement

In addition to outlet impingement, recent clinical and lab investigations have led to other mechanisms of impingement. These include functional overload, intrinsic tendonopathy, and internal anatomic impingement (9). Functional overload results from excessive strain within the tendon from repetitive overuse or a one-time overload. The subsequent inflammation and tendonitis can lead to a continuous cycle, which leads to further impingement symptoms. Eventually, partial thickness cuff tears may result. These tears can occur within the tendon, or at the tendon-bone interface. The worst case of functional overload is a traumatic complete rotator cuff tear.

Intrinsic tendonopathy or tendonosis is a degenerative process that occurs over time. As such, it is seen more commonly in the elderly (10). Histological studies have shown that with aging, tendon collagen fibers increase in diameter and become less organized (11). Biochemical changes include an increase in collagen, a decrease in mucopolysaccharides and a decrease in water content (12). A lower level

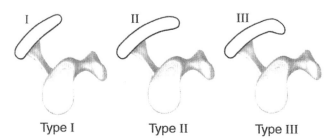

Fig 11-2. Acromial morphology.

of vascularity is also observed in the aged tendon (13). This combination of loss of cellular integrity and decreased vascularity predisposes the older tendon to an increased incidence of injury.

It should be noted that the term internal or secondary impingement refers to a different condition. Due to arthroscopy, it has only recently been described as a source of pain and dysfunction (14). Internal impingement occurs in the overhead position with abduction and maximal external rotation (throwing position). In this position the supraspinatus and infraspinatous tendons impinge on the posterior superior aspect of the glenoid labrum (15). In overhead athletes, repetitive internal impingement can lead to labral injury and rotator cuff tears. The cuff tears created by this mechanism are typically partial thickness articular sided tears (16).

At arthroscopy, kissing lesions can often be identified between the superior labrum and undersurface cuff when the arm is placed in abduction and external rotation. Anterior capsular laxity as well as posterior capsular contracture often coexist and can exacerbate the symptoms. When conservative measures fail to improve symptoms, surgical intervention should be considered. Arthroscopic debridement alone has had a success rate of approximately 70 to 80% (17–19). Capsular imbrication, either open or arthroscopic, has also been recommended as a treatment to address the anterior capsular laxity. Success for this operation has ranged from 68% (20) to 97% (21). In addition, a tight posterior band of the inferior glenohumeral ligament complex (PIGHL) has recently been identified as contributing to the pathology. Arthroscopic release of this thickened structure has been shown to be effective in the 10% of patients who do not respond to posterior capsular stretching (22).

■ INCIDENCE AND NATURAL HISTORY

Shoulder pain is a common presenting complaint for patients of all ages and activity levels. In clinical frequency it is exceeded only by low back pain and neck pain (23). About 50% of the adult population will have at least one episode of shoulder pain each year (24). The most common source of shoulder pain originates in the subacromial space, with the most prevalent diagnosis being impingement syndrome (25). The spectrum of pathologies includes rotator cuff tendonosis, calcific tendonitis, and subacromial bursitis.

The natural course of subacromial impingement varies somewhat. Long term outcome suggests that it is not self limiting and without treatment, symptoms will persist and usually progress (26). The impingement process has been described as having three chronologic stages (27). Stage 1 is characterized by acute bursitis with subacromial edema and hemorrhage. As the irritation continues, the bursae loses its capability to lubricate and protect the underlying cuff and tendonitis of the rotator cuff develops. This leads to stage II,

which is characterized by inflammation and possible partial thickness tears of the rotator cuff. As the process continues the wear on the tendon results in a full thickness tear (stage III). Several authors have shown that this progressive process can be interrupted with surgical acromioplasty (28–30).

Patient Presentation

Although impingement symptoms may arise following trauma, the pain more typically develops insidiously over a period of weeks to months (31). The patient's history will usually consist of pain with overhead activity, reaching, lifting, and throwing. They may have a job or recreational activity that involves repetitive overhead movement (painting, assembly work, tennis). A long day of overhead activity may increase symptoms to the point where the patient seeks medical attention.

The pain usually occurs over the anterolateral aspect of the shoulder, and the patient may point to this specific area. It may radiate down to the deltoid insertion. Very often the patient may report pain at night, exacerbated by lying on the involved shoulder or sleeping with the arm overhead. A complete history and physical is essential to making a diagnosis of subacromial impingement.

Physical Exam

A thorough physical examination should include careful evaluation of the cervical spine to rule out a neurologic problem such as a herniated cervical disc that can mimic shoulder pathology. This is especially true if a patient presents with bilateral symptoms.

If subacromial impingement is suspected, specific tests should be used and documented. The Neer and Hawkins signs for impingement are used commonly and have been found to be reproducible and helpful. In attempting to elicit a positive Neer sign the examiner stabilizes the patient's scapula while raising the arm passively in forward flexion (27). This decreases room available in the subacromial space, thus causing the rotator cuff and overlying bursae to be compressed under the coracoacromial arch. In attempting to elicit a positive Hawkins sign the patient's arm is passively flexed to 90 degrees. The elbow is also bent to 90 degrees and the arm is forcibly internally rotated (32). This brings the greater tuberosity under the acromion, compressing the cuff and bursae. Individually, both exams have been shown to be sensitive but not very specific for diagnosing subacromial impingement. When combined, however, these two tests have a negative predictive value greater than 90% (33) **(Figs 11-3 and 11-4)**.

Differential Diagnosis

It is important to carefully evaluate for other sources of shoulder pain. These may include acromioclavicular arthrosis,

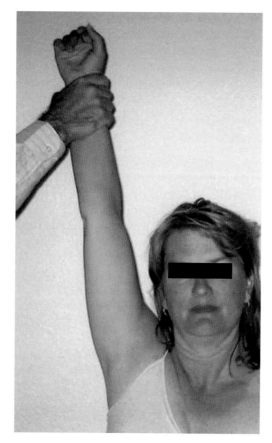

Fig 11-3. Neer sign for impingement.

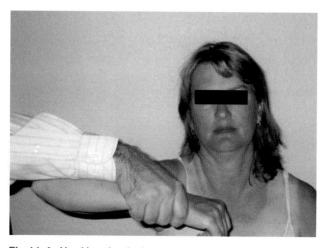

Fig 11-4. Hawkins sign for impingement.

rotator cuff tear (partial or complete), instability, adhesive capsulitis, glenohumeral arthritis, biceps tendonosis, labral pathology (34), and cervical radiculopathy. It is also important to remember that there can be more than one source of pain. The two most common coexisting conditions are AC arthrosis and rotator cuff tears.

Patients with AC arthrosis often point directly at the AC joint as the source of pain. They are point tender over this area and have pain with cross arm adduction. An injection into this joint may result in a decrease in symptoms and x-rays will often show joint degeneration.

Full thickness tears of the rotator cuff result in weakness of the particular muscle group involved. Isolated muscle strength testing with comparison to the asymptomatic extremity can pick up even subtle differences. Active range of motion in forward flexion and abduction may be less than passive range of motion. In chronic conditions, muscle atrophy is often present.

Differential injections can be helpful in making the diagnosis of impingement syndrome. Injections may be given in the subacromial space, AC joint, or glenohumeral joint. The original impingement injection test was described as a valuable method for separating impingement lesions from other causes of shoulder pain. This test involves injection of 10 ml of 1% lidocaine into the subacromial bursae. If after injection, "the painful arc is considerably reduced or abolished, it establishes the anatomic site of the lesion but does not give an indication of the precise pathology or extent of the lesion" (35).

The most common indication for selective injection involves differentiating subacromial and AC joint pain. These injections may also be used in the biceps tendon sheath. They typically contain a local anesthetic and often a corticosteroid. The effect of the local anesthetic should begin almost immediately. It is important to have the patient move their arm and document what percentage of pain relief was obtained. The effect of the steroid can be determined at a follow up visit quantifying amount and duration of pain relief.

Imaging Evaluation

X-ray films are an integral part of the work up and necessary to gain additional information. The views that are the most valuable are anterior-posterior (AP) view, supraspinatous outlet view, and axillary lateral. A 15-degree cephalic view of the AC joint, and an AP view with humeral internal rotation can also be helpful.

It is essential to evaluate acromial morphology and thickness on the outlet film. The AC joint is closely evaluated for bony pathology (best seen on the AP or 15 degree cephalic). Arthritis of the glenohumeral joint and the presence of an os acromiale are best seen on the axillary lateral.

Magnetic resonance imaging (MRI) examination can be helpful to rule out associated pathology. It can give an excellent picture of the rotator cuff tendons and presence of tendonosis, partial, or complete tear. It is also useful for looking at the rotator cuff muscles and the presence or absence of fatty infiltration. Within the shoulder joint, the biceps tendon, labrum, and chondral surfaces can be assessed. The osseous anatomy can be further evaluated for edema secondary to contusions and for the presence of avascular necrosis **(Fig 11-5)**.

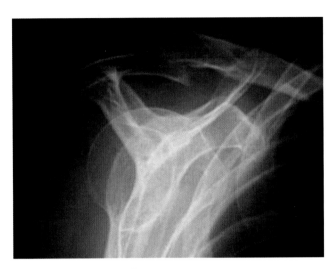

Fig 11-5. Type III Acromion.

Nonoperative Treatment

A trial of nonoperative care is implemented before surgical intervention is considered. The majority of patients with impingement syndrome can be managed conservatively. The treatment program consists of formal physical therapy, activity modification, anti-inflammatory, and the judicious use of steroid injections into the subacromial space. By emphasizing the importance of following the rehabilitation protocol and working closely with a skilled therapist, the majority of patients should have a satisfactory result and not require surgery.

The physical therapy program includes soft tissue stretching and strengthening of the humeral head depressors. These are the internal and external rotators. Strengthening these muscles helps to depress the humeral head and decrease impingement. Passive capsular stretching is used to return the normal rolling-gliding of the glenohumeral joint. As range of motion increases, pain levels should decrease.

The scapular stabilizers should also be strengthened. These include the upper and lower trapezius, seratus anterior, and rhomboids. These muscles contribute to optimal positioning of the scapula during overhead activities. If these muscles fatigue, the scapula is no longer able to keep up with the humerus (36). The humeral head continues to translate anteriorly and superiorly worsening impingement symptoms. Strengthening of the deltoid muscle is counterproductive as its action promotes elevation of the humeral head. In a recent large study based on the above therapy program, an overall 70% success rate was obtained in treating patients with chronic subacromial impingement (37). In this study the acromial morphology was shown to affect the outcome of conservative treatment. Patients with a Type I acromion had a 91% successful result. Patients with Types II and III had less success with 68% and 64%, respectively.

The majority of orthopedic surgeons find the occasional use of corticosteroid injections helpful in the treatment of impingement syndrome; however, several studies have shown no significant improvement when compared with placebo in terms of pain or range of motion (38,39). A recent randomized and blinded study found patients to have decreased pain at 1 month post-injection, but no difference 3 months after injection (40). If used, injections should be individualized and done in conjunction with an exercise program.

Operative Treatment

For patients who fail nonoperative treatment, the procedure of choice is arthroscopic subacromial decompression (ASAD). The advantages of the arthroscopic approach include minimally invasive surgery without detachment of the deltoid. This leads to a more comfortable postoperative recovery and the capability to accelerate rehabilitation. Arthroscopy also allows complete evaluation of the glenohumeral joint and the ability to address other pathology as identified.

As with the open procedure, general anesthesia is usually used. To decrease bleeding, the systolic blood pressure is kept below 100 mmHg unless there is a medical contraindication. Prior to final positioning, an examination under anesthesia is performed of both shoulders. This is done to detect any signs of occult instability as well as any palpable or audible signs of labral tears.

The ASAD procedure can be performed in the lateral decubitus or beach chair position. If conversion to an open procedure is necessary, this can be done easily from either position. With either position, care is taken to protect the patient's head and neck during positioning. It is then firmly secured in a neutral position avoiding hyperflexion or extension **(Fig 11-6)**.

We have generally used the lateral position and will describe our preferred technique. It is important to roll the patient back approximately 30 degrees from the perpendicular. If one starts with the patient too vertical, the shoulder tends to fall anterior and away from the surgeon. The patient is stabilized with a beanbag and an axillary roll is appropriately positioned. The arm is placed in 30 degrees of

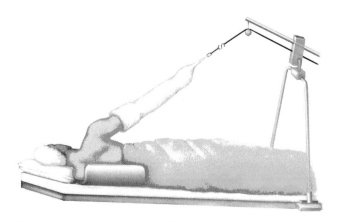

Fig 11-6. Lateral decubitus position.

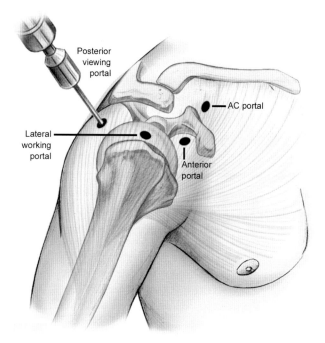

Fig 11-7. Arthroscopy portals.

abduction and 20 degrees of forward flexion. After prepping and draping, approximately 10 lbs of weight is applied to suspend the arm.

The osseous landmarks are clearly identified with a marking pen. The anterior, posterior, and lateral edges of the acromion, the clavicle, AC joint, and coracoid are clearly marked. This helps in establishing portals initially and more importantly later when shoulder swelling can make landmarks more difficult to identify. The posterior portal is placed first. It is located at the soft spot 2 cm inferior and 2 cm medial to the posterolateral corner of the acromion. A pop will be felt as the cannula enters the capsule **(Fig 11-7)**.

After in the glenohumeral joint complete diagnostic arthroscopy is carried out, a 14-gauge spinal needle can be placed anteriorly to allow for outflow. If no glenohumeral pathology is encountered, it may not be necessary to place an anterior cannula. If an anterior portal is necessary, it can be established in the rotator interval with either an outside in technique following the path of the spinal needle or inside out using the cannula and blunt obturator to drive through the interval. Any glenohumeral surgery is carried out at this time with additional portals as needed.

Following this, one withdraws the arthroscope completely and, with the blunt obturator, redirects the cannula into the subacromial space. It may be helpful to drive the metal cannula through to the anterior portal and bring another cannula over the top. This clearly identifies your location and a shaver can be brought from the front. Under direct visualization, bursal tissue is removed and a space is created. It is important to maintain correct orientation to avoid inadvertent injury to the rotator cuff. The scope is

positioned such that the acromion is superior and the cuff inferior throughout.

The lateral portal is placed next. It is positioned 1.5 to 2 cm inferior to the lateral border of the acromion. A spinal needle can be used to verify position prior to portal placement. The needle should be seen coming in parallel to the undersurface of the acromion and in line with the anterior portion of the acromion to be removed. Correct position of this portal is necessary for correct bone resection. If the portal is misplaced in any direction, an angled cut of the undersurface of the acromion will result. If the portal is placed in such a way that a precise cut can not be done easily, it is better to make another portal than try to complete the resection from one that is poorly placed.

The shaver is used from the lateral portal to perform a partial bursectomy. A bipolar radiofrequency device is helpful to ablate the periosteum and fascia. The coracoacromial ligament is subperiosteally dissected off the acromion but is not resected. Adequate flow and pressure are maintained throughout the procedure. Good visualization is essential. If any bleeding is encountered, it is addressed immediately with the radiofrequency device for coagulation. After the periosteum has been removed, the bony anatomy is clearly identified. A thorough examination of the rotator cuff's bursal surface is critical to determine the presence of cuff pathology **(Fig 11-8)**.

Bone resection is begun only after all soft tissue preventing visualization is removed. It is critical to expose the anterolateral corner to prevent inadequate resections. This is the site at which most contact pressure is applied to the rotator cuff during elevation and abduction. An arthroscopic burr is brought in from the lateral portal and a step cut at the anterolateral corner is performed. The preoperative x-rays should be used to gauge how much resection is to be performed. The diameter of the burr is known and can be used to evaluate the depth of this initial resection. Generally we take 6 to 12 mm from the undersurface of the anterior acromion.

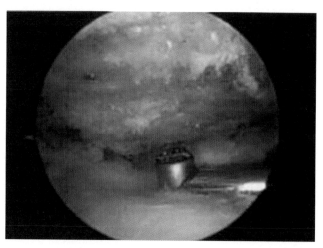

Fig 11-8. Debridement of soft tissue with radiofrequency device.

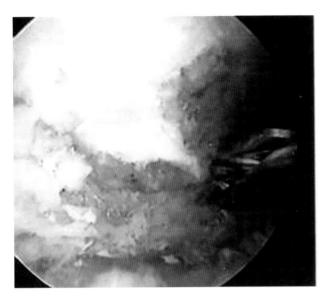

Fig 11-9. "Step-Cut" technique.

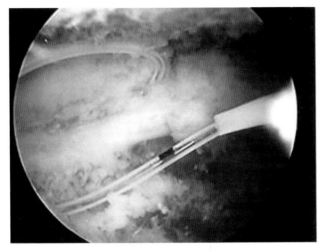

Fig 11-11. Insertion of pain pump catheter.

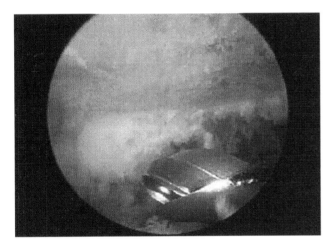

Fig 11-10. Verify adequate decompression.

After the step cut is created and the appropriate amount of anterior resection is confirmed, we proceed to the rest of the acromion from lateral to medial. The anterior acromial resection is usually performed to keep the newly resected surface in line with the anterior surface of the AC joint. The initial step cut can always be used as a reference to ensure a flat line of resection. Care is taken to smooth the anterior surface and prevent detachment of the deltoid **(Fig 11-9)**.

The entire procedure can be done working through the lateral portal, viewing from the posterior portal, and using the anterior portal for outflow. We do not employ a posterior cutting block technique. This technique is dependent on the morphology of the posterior acromion and has the potential for inadequate or excessive bone removal. Following completion of decompression, the surgeon may want to place the

arthroscope in the lateral portal to get an "outlet" perspective of what was done. Thorough irrigation should follow resection to remove all bony debris.

If distal clavicle resection is going to be performed, a bipolar radiofrequency device is again used to remove soft tissue and delineate the anatomic landmarks underneath the distal clavicle and AC joint. The arthroscopic Mumford procedure can then be performed with the burr brought in from the anterior portal. A step cut is again helpful followed by completion of resection. If no AC surgery is to be performed we prefer not to violate or destabilize this area and do not perform a coplaning **(Fig 11-10)**.

A pain pump can be placed into the subacromial space, particularly if concominant AC resection or rotator cuff repair is performed. The portals are closed and a sterile bulky dressing is applied. The patient is placed into a sling and usually discharged home within 2 hours. Neurovascular status is assessed and documented prior to discharge from the recovery room **(Fig 11-11)**.

■ RESULTS

The results of arthroscopic subacromial decompression have been well documented. Ellman (41) was one of the first to publish results comparable with the previous good results seen with an open technique. His subsequent 2 to 5 year results yielded on overall 89% satisfaction (42). These excellent results have been reproduced and expanded upon in terms of patient numbers and length of follow-up by numerous authors validating arthroscopic decompression as an effective treatment for subacromial impingement (43–45). Successful outcomes can be expected in approximately 90% of cases.

ASAD for impingement symptoms in the face of mild to moderate glenohumeral degenerative joint disease has been shown to be effective in improving shoulder function (46);

therefore, these changes should not be considered a contraindication for decompression. Radiographically severe degenerative joint disease has, however, had less predictable results (47). A limited subacromial decompression has also been recommended by several authors in patients with a massive irreparable rotator cuff tear (48,49). A reverse decompression or tuberoplasty has also yielded good results in patients with massive rotator cuff tears (50).

■ POSTOPERATIVE MANAGEMENT

Generally, patients tolerate ASAD well and do not report significant postoperative pain. Conventional pain control can be obtained with oral medications. The patient may have the dressing removed in approximately 48 hours. A formal therapy program is then employed. Stiffness can be avoided when early motion is emphasized and any problems are recognized early.

Pendulum exercises are started within 2 days after surgery. This is followed by passive range of motion and active-assisted motion. Full active range of motion can usually be achieved by 3 to 4 weeks. Light weights and strengthening can begin at 6 weeks. The overhead athlete should avoid these sports until at least 3 months. It is not unusual to take 6 months for complete recovery.

Complications

Surgical complications related to ASAD are similar to those of other shoulder procedures. They can be separated into complications related to inaccurate or incomplete diagnosis and those related to incorrect technique. An incomplete diagnosis can occur from failure to recognize and address coexisting pathology such as a labral tear or partial rotator cuff tear. These can be minimized with a thorough preoperative work-up and after in the operating room, a meticulous and complete diagnostic arthroscopy.

The most common technical errors are usually related to excessive or inadequate bone resection. Iatrogenic fractures of the acromion have been reported after aggressive acromioplasty and surgical disorientation. Some series have reported postoperative AC joint symptoms after excessive coplaning during surgery. Inadequate bone resection is most common anteriorly or laterally.

Infections are uncommon and have an incidence of less than 1%. Reflex sympathetic dystrophy is rare but may occur in patients who have reported prodromal radicular symptoms. Postoperative stiffness is a relatively common problem after all shoulder surgery. Early range of motion and a supervised therapy program are beneficial in order to minimize the risk of permanent stiffness. Operating on a shoulder that is stiff preoperatively may lead to a very stiff shoulder post-op. Performing an ASAD on a patient that has early adhesive capsulitis is a potential complication that can be avoided.

■ REFERENCES

1. Neer CS II. Anterior acromioplasty for the chronic impingement syndrome in the shoulder. *J Bone Joint Surg Am.* 1972;54A:41–50.
2. Neer CS II, Poppen NK. Supraspinatus outlet. *Orthop Trans.* 1987;11:234.
3. Neer CS II. Shoulder Reconstruction. Philadelphia: WB Saunders; 1990:43–48.
4. Nordt WE, Garretson RB, Plotkin E. The measurement of subacromial contact pressure in patients with impingement syndrome. *Arthroscopy.* 1999;15:121–125.
5. Saha AK. Dynamic stability of the glenohumeral joint. *Acta Orthop Scand.* 1971;42:491–505.
6. Weiner DS, Macnab I. Superior migration of the humeral head. A radiological aid in the diagnosis of tears of the rotator cuff. *J Bone Joint Surg Br.* 1970;52:524–527.
7. Mudge MK, Wood, VE, Frykman GK. Rotator cuff tears associated with os acromiale. *J Bone Joint Surg Am.* 1984;66A:427–429.
8. Bigliani LU, Morrison, DS, April EW. The morphology of the acromion and its relationship to rotator cuff tears. *Orthop Trans.* 1986;10:216.
9. Morrison DS, Greenbaum BS, Einhorn A. Shoulder impingement. *Orthop Clinic North Am.* 2000;31:285–293.
10. Ingelmark BE. The Structure of tendons at various ages and under different functional conditions. *Acta Anatomy.* 1948;6:193–225.
11. Ippolito E, Pier Giorgio N, Postacchini F, et al. Morphological, immunochemical and biochemical study of rabbit achilles tendon at various ages. *J Bone Joint Surg.* 1980;62A:4.
12. Uhthoff, HK, Sarkar, K. Classification and definition of tendinopathies, basic science and clinical application in the athlete's shoulder. *Clin Sports Med.* 1991;10(4):707–720.
13. Ahmed IM, Lagopoulos M, Soames RW, et al. Blood supply of the achilles tendon. *J Orthop Res.* 1998;16:591–596.
14. Walch G, Boileau P, Noel E. Impingement of the deep surface of the supraspinatus tendon on the posterosuperior glenoid rim: an arthroscopic study. *J Shoulder Elbow Surg.* 1992;1:238–245.
15. Perry J. Anatomy and biomechanics of the shoulder in throwing, swimming, gymnastics and tennis. *Clin Sports Med.* 1983;2:247–270.
16. Krishnan SG., Hawkins RJ., Warren RF. The Shoulder and the Overhead Athlete. Philadelphia: Lipincott; 2004:125–134.
17. Andrews, JR, Broussard TS, Carson WG. Arthroscopy of the shoulder in the management of partial tears of the rotator cuff: a preliminary report. *Arthroscopy.* 1985;1(2):117–122.
18. Altcheck DW, Warren RF, Wickiewicz TL. Arthroscopic labral debridement. *Am J Sports Med.* 1992;20(6):702–706.
19. Sonny-Cottet B, Edwards TB, Noel E. Results of arthroscopic treatment of posterosuperior glenoid impingement in tennis players. *Am J Sports Med.* 2002;30(2):227–232.
20. Jobe FW, Ciangarra CE, Kvitne RS. Anterior capsulolabral reconstruction of the shoulder in athletes in overhead sports. *Am J Sports Med.* 1991;19(5):428–434.
21. Montgomery WH, Jobe FW. Functional outcomes in athletes after modified anterior capsulolabral reconstruction. *Am J Sports Med.* 1994;22(3):352–358.
22. Morgan CD. Operative Arthroscopy. Philadelphia: Lippincott; 2003:570–584
23. Calliet R. Shoulder Pain. Philadelphia: FA Davis Co; 1991:1–50.
24. Brox JI. Regional musculoskeletal conditions: shoulder pain. *Best Pract Clin Rheumatol.* 2003;17:33–56.
25. Morison DS, Greenbaum BS, Einhorn A. Shoulder impingement. *Orthop Clin North Am.* 2000;31:285–293.
26. Chard MD, Satelle LM, Hazelman BL. The long term outcome of rotator cuff tendonitis: a review study. *Br J Rheumatology.* 1988; 27:385–389.
27. Neer CS II. Impingement lesions. *Clin Orthop.* 1983;173:70–77.

28. Altcheck DW, Warren RF, Wickiewicz T L, et al. Arthroscopic acromioplasty. Technique and results. *J Bone Joint Surg*. 1990; 72A:1198–1207.

29. Matsen FA, Arntz CT. The Shoulder Vol 2, Philadelphia: WB Saunders; 1990:662–646.

30. Tibone JE, Jobe FW, Kerlan RK, et al. Shoulder impingement syndrome in young athletes treated by an anterior acromioplasty. *Clin Orthop*. 1985;198:134–140.

31. Koester MC, George MS, Kuhn JE. Shoulder Impingement Syndrome. *Am J of Med*. 2005;118:452–455.

32. Hawkins RJ, Brock RM, Abrams JS, et al. Acromioplasty for impingement with an intact rotator cuff. *J Bone Joint Surg Br*. 1988;70:795–797.

33. MacDonald PB, Clark P, Sutherland K. An analysis of the diagnostic accuracy of the Hawkins and Neer subacromial impingement signs. *J Shoulder Elbow Surg*. 2000;9:299–301.

34. Andrews JR, Carson WG, Mcleod WD. Glenoid labral tears related to the long head of the biceps. *Am J Sports Med*. 1985; 13(5):337–341.

35. Kessel I. Clinical disorders of the shoulder. Edinburgh: Churchill Livingstone, 1982.

36. Scovazzo ML. The painful shoulder during freestyle swimming: An electromyographic analysis of twelve muscles. *Am J Sports Med*. 1991;19:577–587.

37. Morrison DS, Fragmeni AD, Woodworth P. Conservative management of subacromial impingement syndrome. *J Bone Joint Surg Am*. 1997;79:732–737.

38. Vecchio PC, Hazleman BL, King RH. A double-blind trial comparing subacromial methylprednisone and lidocaine in acute rotator cuff tendonitis. *Br J Rheumatology*. 1993;Aug 32(8):743–745.

39. Berry H, Fernandes L, Bloom B, et al. Clinical study comparing acupuncture, physiotherapy, injection and oral anti-inflammatory therapy in shoulder-cuff lesions. *Curr Med Res Opin*. 1980;7: 121–126.

40. Akgun K, Birtane M, Akarirmak U. Is local subacromial injection beneficial in subacromial impingement syndrome? *Clin Rheumatology*. 2004;23(6):496–500.

41. Ellman H. Arthroscopic subacromial decompression: analysis of one to three year results. *Arthroscopy*. 1987;3:173–181.

42. Ellman H, Kay SP. Arthroscopic subacromial decompression for chronic impingement. Two to five year results. *J Bone Joint Surg Br*. 1991;73:8:482–487.

43. Esch JC. Arthroscopic subacromial decompression and postoperative management. *Orthop Clin North Am*. 1993;24:161–171.

44. Roye RP, Grana WA, Yates CK. Arthroscopic subacromial decompression: two to seven year follow-up. *Arthroscopy*. 1995;11: 301–306.

45. Speer KP, Lohnes J, Garrett WE. Arthroscopic subacromial decompression: results in advanced impingement syndrome. *Arthroscopy*. 1991;7:291–296.

46. Stephens SR, Warren RF, Payne LZ et al. Arthroscopic acromioplasty: a six to ten year follow-up. *Arthroscopy*. 1998;14:382–388.

47. Guyette TM, Bae H, Warren RF, et al. Results of arthroscopic subacromial decompression in patients with subacromial impingement and glenohumeral degenerative joint disease. *J Shoulder Elbow Surg*. 2002;4:299–304.

48. Burkart S. Arthroscopic treatment of massive rotator cuff tears. *Clin Orthop*. 1991;267:45–56.

49. Gartsman GM. Massive irreparable tears of the rotator cuff: results of operative debridement and subacromial decompression. *J Bone Joint Surg Am*. 1997;79:715–721.

50. Scheibel M, Lichtenberg S, Habermeyer P. Reversed arthroscopic subacromial decompression for massive rotator cuff tears. *J Shoulder Elbow Surg*. 2004;13,3:272–278.

SHOULDER LABRAL TEARS AND INSTABILITY

12

GEORGE F. (RICK) HATCH, III, MD, JOHN G. COSTOUROS, MD, PETER J. MILLETT, MD, MSc, JON J.P. WARNER, MD

■ KEY POINTS

- The goal of therapeutic approaches to glenohumeral joint instability is the restoration of anatomy.
- The glenohumeral joint is inherently unstable, with the large humeral head articulating with the small and shallow glenoid.
- The labrum acts as the anchor point for the capsuloligamentous structures, increases the depth of the glenoid socket, and facilitates the concavity-compression mechanism as the humeral head is compressed in the glenoid during rotator cuff contraction.
- Bankart lesions have been considered the primary pathology leading to recurrent anterior dislocation. These lesions were originally described as injuries to the labrum corresponding to the detachment of the anchoring point of the inferior glenohumeral (IGHL) and middle glenohumeral (MGHL) ligaments from the glenoid rim.
- Traumatic intra-substance injury of the joint capsule is commonly associated with anterior dislocation. Depending on the magnitude of the anterior shear force, either plastic deformation or a complete tear of the joint capsule can occur.
- The most common bony lesion associated with traumatic glenohumeral instability is a compression fracture at the posterolateral margin of the humeral head. Commonly known as a Hill-Sachs lesion, this fracture occurs as the humeral head impacts the glenoid edge during dislocation.
- Shoulder instability is categorized on the basis of four criteria: frequency, etiology, degree, and direction.
- The degree of instability–dislocation, subluxation, or microinstability–is also important in determining appropriate treatment options.
- Many athletes with ligamentous laxity have instability that is primarily posterior in nature. These patients suffer recurrent posterior subluxation and have a history of posterior shoulder pain rather than complaints of rank instability.
- A true anteroposterior (AP) view with an axillary lateral view is the minimum radiographic workup necessary for evaluation of an acute dislocation or suspected subluxation.
- The goal of treatment in both open and arthroscopic surgery is to restore the labrum to its anatomic attachment site and to establish the appropriate tension to the inferior capsuloligamentous complex of the joint.
- Interscalene regional blockade has been effective in providing early postoperative pain relief and in decreasing overall narcotic requirements following surgery.
- Strong indications for open stabilization procedures include significant degrees of glenoid or humeral bone loss, capsular deficiencies, or irreparable rotator cuff tears, particularly those of the subscapularis. In individuals with significant anterior glenoid erosion, an osseous reconstruction should be performed.
- Revision instability surgery is the most technically challenging of all open shoulder surgery. When attempting to salvage failed anterior instability cases, surgeons should be prepared to face challenging scenarios such as distorted anatomic tissue planes, severe scarring, capsular deficiencies from multiple prior surgeries or thermal capsulorrhaphy, bony deficiencies due to erosion or fracture, and subscapularis deficiencies.

The treatment of shoulder instability has evolved rapidly in recent years due to a better understanding of shoulder biomechanics and pathoanatomy, advancements in imaging technology, and improvements in surgical implants and techniques. The goal of contemporary therapeutic approaches to glenohumeral joint instability is the restoration of anatomy. This requires a thorough and clear understanding of the anatomy and biomechanics of the glenohumeral articulation.

This chapter will summarize the relevant basic science, evaluation, and treatment of patients with labral pathology with an emphasis on shoulder instability, including discussion of those rare patients with instability secondary to bony abnormalities or posterior labral pathology. This chapter will also include a section on special considerations in revision surgery for failed stabilization procedures, complications, and future directions.

■ BASIC SCIENCE

Anatomy

The glenohumeral joint is formed by a unique articulation between a larger and nearly spherical humeral head with a shallow and much smaller glenoid. Minimal bony constraints combined with a unique anatomical architecture and functional arrangements allow the shoulder joint to have the largest range of motion in the body. Despite its minimally constrained nature, the glenohumeral joint can carry both small and large loads at various speeds of arm motion while maintaining stability due the joint's tremendous reliance on soft tissue support. Instability is defined as abnormal or painful excessive movement of the humeral head out of the glenoid during active shoulder motion and must be distinguished from laxity, which is asymptomatic instability in both normal and unstable shoulders.

Glenohumeral stability is achieved by the complex interactions between static and dynamic constraints. Static constraints include the capsule, ligaments, and tendons; dynamic constraints are obtained by active muscle contraction. In the middle range of rotation, joint stability is provided by the dynamic action of the rotator cuff and the biceps muscles through compression of the humeral head in the glenoid socket (1) **(Fig 12-1)**. The ligamentous structures provide passive restraints at the extremes of rotation, preventing excessive translation of the humeral head on the glenoid **(Fig 12-2)**. Contraction of the muscles around the shoulder may also have the secondary effect of protecting the smaller ligamentous structures from injury at the end-range positions (2,3). Authors have demonstrated differences in rotator cuff and scapular muscle firing patterns between patients with stable and unstable shoulders (4).

The osseous anatomy, capsuloligamentous structures, negative intra-articular pressure, synovial fluid adhesion-cohesion, the rotator cuff, scapular stabilizers, and biceps tendon all play roles in providing stability (1,5,6). Additional

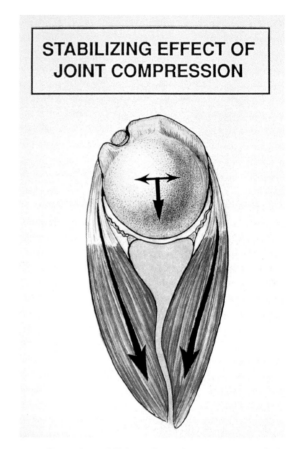

Fig 12-1. Dynamic stabilizing effect of the rotator cuff. (Adapted with permission from Matsen FA III, Lipitt SB. *Principles of stability*. In: *Shoulder surgery: principles and procedures*. Philadelphia: Saunders; 2004, Fig 8-7.)

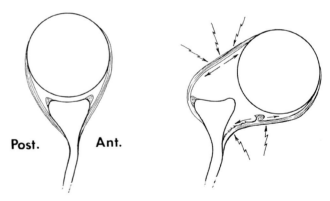

Fig 12-2. Illustration of the ligamentous structures preventing excessive translation of the humeral head on the glenoid. (Adapted from Matsen FA III, Lipitt SB. *principles of glenoid concavity*. In: *Shoulder surgery: principles and procedures*. Philadelphia: Saunders; 2004, Fig 9-24.)

factors that contribute to stability are patient age and gender, capsular integrity, and strength and conditioning of the rotator cuff, and scapular stabilizing muscles of the shoulder complex.

■ BIOMECHANICS OF SHOULDER STABILITY

Static Stability Factor

The glenohumeral joint is inherently unstable, with the large humeral head articulating with the small and shallow glenoid. Static stability is provided by the orientation of the articular surfaces, the articular conformity of humerus and the glenoid, the glenoid labrum, the negative intra-articular pressure, the adhesion-cohesion of synovial joint fluid, and the glenohumeral joint capsule and its ligaments (1,7–9).

The glenoid labrum is a wedge-shaped fibrous ring attaching to the glenoid articular surface through a fibrocartilaginous transition zone. Below the glenoid equator, the inferior labrum is firmly continuous with the articular cartilage; above the equator it is more mobile and meniscal in nature.

The contribution of the labrum to glenohumeral stability has been clearly established: It acts as the anchor point for the capsuloligamentous structures, increases the depth of the glenoid socket, facilitates the concavity-compression mechanism as the humeral head is compressed in the glenoid during rotator cuff contraction (10) **(Fig 12-3)**. Loss of the labrum (Bankart lesion) has been reported to result in a 50% decrease in the glenoid depth. Lippit et al. (9) demonstrated that the translational force required to dislocate the humeral head was 20% smaller after removal of the glenoid labrum. Although the functional anatomy of the glenoid labrum is becoming better understood, its role in the glenohumeral restraining mechanism, particularly at the extremes of motion, remains unclear.

Discrete thickenings of the joint capsule have traditionally been described as the glenohumeral ligaments **(Fig 12-4)**. The nomenclature is based on their attachment from superior to inferior and anterior to posterior. Improved understanding of the anatomy and biomechanics of the glenohumeral ligaments has resulted from numerous cadaveric studies and intraoperative observations. Because of the orientation of these ligaments, portions of the capsule reciprocally tighten

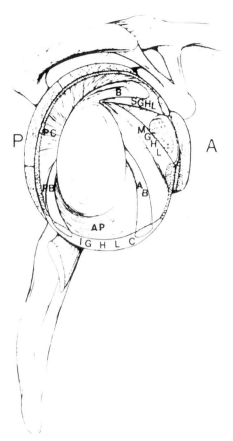

Fig 12-4. The discrete thickenings of the joint capsule described as the glenohumeral ligaments. SGHL, superior glenohumeral ligament; MGHL, middle glenohumeral ligament; IGHLC, inferior glenohumeral ligament complex; AB, Anterior band of the inferior glenohumeral ligament; PB, posterior band of the inferior glenohumeral ligament. (Adapted from O'Brien SJ, Neves MC, Arnoczky SP, et al. The anatomy of and histology of the inferior glenohumeral complex of the shoulder. *Am J Sports Med.* 1990; 18:449.)

and loosen as the glenohumeral joint rotates, thus limiting translation and rotation by load sharing (11–13) **(Table 12-1)**. In the middle range of motion, these structures are relatively lax with a surface area two times that of the humeral head (14,15); therefore, stability in the midrange rotation is maintained primarily by the action of the rotator cuff muscles compressing the humeral head into the conforming glenoid socket (16).

Superior Glenohumeral Ligament

The superior glenohumeral ligament (SGHL) and coracohumeral ligament (CHL) originate on the supraglenoid tubercle and coracoid process, respectively, and both insert on the lesser tuberosity. Both make up the reinforcing structures of the rotator interval and are present in over 90% of individuals (17). These structures both provide resistance to inferior translation and external rotation when the arm is adducted (18). Additionally, both structures limit posterior translation when the arm is forward flexed, adducted,

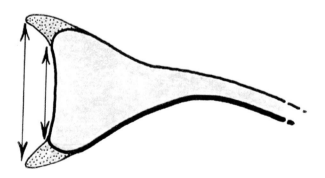

Fig 12-3. The labrum's contribution to increasing the depth of the glenoid socket. (Adapted from Warner JJP, Carbon DM. Overview of shoulder instability. *Crit Rev Phys Rehabil Med.* 1992;4:145–198.)

TABLE 12-1	Anatomy and Function of the Glenohumeral Ligaments and Capsule				
	Structure	**Origin**	**Insertion**	**Anatomic Relationships**	**Function**
Coracohumeral ligament (CHL)	Dense, fibrous, 1- to 2-cm wide; thin structure	Lateral surface of the coracoid process	Greater and lesser tuberosities adjacent to the bicipital groove	Extra-articular intermingled with the edges of the supraspinatus and subscapulans tendons; reinforcement of the rotator interval	Limits interior translation and external rotation when the arm is adducted and posterior translation when the shoulder is in a position at forward flexion, adduction, and internal rotation
Superior glenohumeral ligament (SGHL)	Variable in size; present in 90% of individuals	Superior glenoid tubercle just inferior to the biceps tendon	Superior aspect of the lesser tuberosity just medial to the bicipital groove	Intra-articular, ties deep to the CHL: reinforcement of the rotator interval	Same as the CHL
Middle glenohumeral ligament (MGHL)	Great variation in size and presence; absent or poorly defined in 40% of individuals	Superior glenoid tubercute and anterosuperior labrum, often along with the SGHL	Anterior to the lesser tuberosity	Intra-articular, blending with the posterior aspect of the subscapularis tendon	Passive restraint to both anterior and posterior translation when the arm is adducted in the range of 60° to 90° in external rotation and limits inferior translation when the arm is adducted at the side
Inferior glenohumeral complex (IGHLC)	Consists of three components: anterior band, posterior band, axillary pouch: decreases in thickness from anterior to posterior	Anteroinferior labrum neck of the glenoid adjacent to the labrum	Inferior to the MGHL at the humeral neck	Can be sheetlike and confluent with the SGHL or cordlike with a luraminal separation between it and the anterior band of the IGHL complex	Functions as a hammock of the humeral head: in adduction, it acts as a secondary restraint, limiting large inferior translations; in abduction, it becomes taut under the humeral head, limiting inferior translation; in internal rotation, it moves posteriorly, and in external rotation, it moves interiorly, forming a barrier to posterior and anterior dislocation, respectively
Posterior capsule	Thinnest region of the joint capsule without discrete ligamentous reinforcements	Posterior band of the IGHLC posterosuperior labrum to the insertion of the biceps	Posterior humeral neck	Blends with the posterior aspect of the infraspinatus and teres minor	Limits posterior translation when the arm is forward flexed, adducted, and internally rotated

Reproduced with permission from Norris TR. OKU: Shoulder and Elbow Update 2. Rosemont, IL: American Academy of Orthopaedic Surgeons; 2002.

and internally rotated. Lastly, the SGHL and the CHL are believed to prevent anterior-superior migration of the humeral head.

Middle Glenohumeral Ligament

The middle glenohumeral ligament (MGHL) is a highly variable structure between individuals. It presents as either a discrete band or a thickening of the anterior capsule confluent with the inferior glenohumeral ligament (IGHL) complex in 60% to 80% of the population (17,19). The MGHL originates from the glenoid tubercle or the anterior labrum and inserts on the lesser tuberosity, coursing oblique to the SGHL and CHL. The MGHL statically limits rotation of the adducted humerus, inferior translation of the adducted humerus and externally rotated humerus. In addition, the MGHL also limits anterior and posterior translation of the partly abducted (45 degree) and externally rotated arm.

Inferior Glenohumeral Ligament

The IGHL functions as the primary restraint to anterior, posterior, and inferior glenohumeral translation between 45 degree and 90 degree elevation of the arm (20). The IGHL originates from the inferior half of the glenoid neck or the anterior-inferior labrum, to insert inferior to the MGHL on the lesser tuberosity. The IGHL forms a hammocklike structure with discrete anterior and posterior bands with an interposed pouch. This formation allows for reciprocal tightening and loosening, depending on arm position **(Fig 12-5)**. In external rotation, the complex moves anteriorly; in internal rotation, the complex moves posteriorly (18).

Posterior Capsule

The posterior capsule starts just proximal to the posterior band of the IGHL. The posterior capsule is the thinnest portion of the shoulder capsule, measuring less than 1 mm in thickness (average thickness 1.5 mm), and as a result is believed to be the cause of poor results following posterior instability surgery (21). The posterior capsule limits posterior translation when the arm is in the forward flexed, adducted, and internally rotated position.

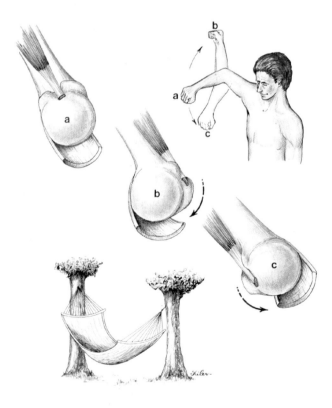

Fig 12-5. The inferior glenohumeral ligament complex functions like a hammock that supports the humeral head. With the arm in neutral, the ligament complex is relatively static (*a*). In external rotation (*b*) and internal rotation (*c*), the IGHLC rotates to the front and back of the shoulder acting like a checkrein against dislocation. (Adapted from Warner JJP, Carbon DM. Overview of shoulder instability. *Crit Rev Phys Rehabil Med.* 1992;4:145–198.)

Rotator Interval

The rotator interval is the region of the shoulder defined by the borders of the supraspinatus superiorly, the subscapularis inferiorly, the corcoid process medially, and biceps laterally. The SGHL, CHL, and MGHL reinforce the rotator interval region. As a result, this region is highly variable among individuals (22). The rotator interval may be completely devoid of tissue or composed solely of loosely arranged collagen tissue; in a stable shoulder, this likely represents a normal variant. The rotator interval functions to limit inferior translation in the adducted arm, and tightens when the adducted arm is externally rotated (1). Laxity in the rotator interval may contribute to inferior and posterior glenohumeral instability. At the other end of the spectrum, an excessively tight rotator interval is associated with both adhesive capsulitis and post-operative stiffness (23).

Dynamic Stability Factors

Glenohumeral stability is mainly achieved through dynamic factors. Active contraction of the rotator cuff contributes to joint stabilization by coordinated muscular activity and by secondary tightening of the ligamentous constraints. This effect works in combination with the concavity-compression mechanism, in which muscle contraction causes compression of nearly congruent articular surfaces into one another.

The rotator cuff consists of the subscapularis, supraspinatus, infraspinatus, and teres minor muscles. The tendons of the rotator cuff muscles almost completely surround the humeral head as they blend together at their insertions on the greater and lesser tuberosities of the humerus. Because the rotator cuff muscles insert very close to the center of rotation of the axis of rotation of the humerus, the rotator cuff provides a joint compression force at the glenohumeral articulation. This coordinated compressive function of the rotator cuff muscles is required to counteract the upward shearing force of the strong deltoid muscle during abduction and/or flexion. The rotator cuff, therefore, maintains stability and allows for a spinning motion of the humerus on the glenoid by counteracting the shearing motion of the deltoid. Ligament and capsulolabral sectioning studies have demonstrated that muscle action of the rotator cuff and deltoid provided joint stability even after a large Bankart lesion was created or the entire capsule and glenohumeral ligaments were sectioned (21,24,25). Dynamic stability of the glenohumeral joint is also provided for by the contraction of the long head of the biceps, coordinated scapulothoracic rhythm, and the proprioceptive modulation of all dynamic factors (26).

The scapular rotators include the trapezius, rhomboids, the serratus anterior, and the levator scapulae. Of these, scapulothoracic rotation is primarily achieved by the serratus anterior and trapezius muscles, which provide the overall rhythm of the shoulder motion. The ratio of normal glenohumeral to scapulothoracic motion is 2:1 (glenohumeral

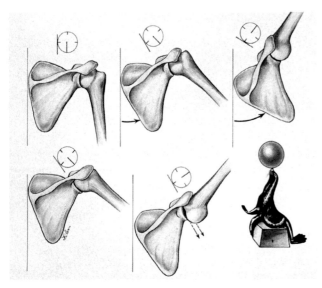

Fig 12-6. The effect of scapulothoracic motion on stability of the shoulder. Analogous to a ball balancing on the nose of a seal in the circus. (Adapted from Warner JJP, Carbon DM. Overview of shoulder instability. *Crit Rev Phys Rehabil Med.* 1992;4:145–198.)

rotation to scapulothoracic rotation) **(Fig 12-6)**. This normal relationship is important because it maintains the glenoid as a stable platform underneath the humeral head as the shoulder rotates into positions required for overhead motions such as throwing. Because the axioscapular muscles (scapular rotators) tend to fatigue first during repetitive overhead motions such as throwing and swimming, a lag in normal scapulothoracic rotation has been implicated as a contributing factor for instability and pain during shoulder motion in these sports activities (27).

The serratus anterior acts as a scapular rotator and protractor, therefore normal positioning of the scapula and glenoid is dependent on proper serratus anterior function (28). Several authors have noted an association between altered serratus anterior function and anterior instability (2,29,30). Decreased serratus anterior function in unstable shoulders may cause decreased upward scapular rotation with shoulder abduction, scaption, or flexion which would alter the position of the humerus relative to the glenoid. This could be important in unstable shoulders where this altered scapulothoracic rhythm may act to increase shear forces across the glenohumeral joint via inefficient glenoid positioning.

The possible association between glenohumeral and scapulothoracic problems has been investigated by several authors, who have demonstrated scapular malpositiong or abnormal scapular function in patients with instability (2,4,30). However, although scapular malpositioning, or muscle dysfunction, is associated with shoulder instability (4,30–32), whether this represents a primary phenomenon or if painful conditions such as instability inhibit the scapulothoracic muscles secondarily is still unknown. The association between the scapular dyskinesias and instability form the rationale for supplementing rotator cuff strengthening

with an axioscapular strengthening program when treating shoulder instability.

■ LESIONS AND THE BIOMECHANICS OF INSTABILITY

Bankart Lesions

For the humeral head to escape the glenoid fossa, the soft-tissue restraint must be disrupted. The location of the disruption depends on several factors such as the direction of the force applied to the shoulder; the position of the arm at the time of injury; and most importantly, the age of the patient. In older patients the more common lesion is a tear of the rotator cuff, the "posterior mechanism" of dislocation, with or without labral pathology; however, in patients younger than age 40 years, the predominant finding is a tear of the anteroinferior labrum, a Bankart lesion.

Bankart lesions have been considered the primary and most common pathology leading to recurrent anterior dislocation (33,34) **(Fig 12-7)**. These lesions were originally described as injuries to the labrum corresponding to the detachment of the anchoring point of the IGHL and MGHLs from the glenoid rim. Taylor and Arciero (35) reported the arthroscopic findings in 63 patients who sustained an initial anterior dislocation. All patients in the study were younger than 24 years of age. Sixty-one of the 63 patients (93%) had an avulsion of the anteroinferior glenoid labrum (Bankart lesion) with no evidence of intracapsular injury. Fourteen of the 63 (22%) had an associated osseous lesion of the glenoid

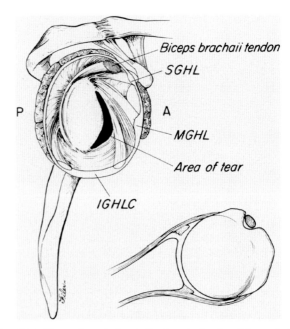

Fig 12-7. Illustration of classic Bankart lesion involving anterior-inferior glenolabrum. (Adapted from Matsen FA III, Lipitt SB. *Principles of Glenohumeral Ligaments and Capsule.* Philadelphia: Saunders; 2004; Fig 10-7.)

rim. In addition, there were six superior labral tears, two included the biceps origin. There were no full-thickness rotator cuff tears.

Skeletal Lesions

The limited constraint provided by the glenoid is further decreased by bony lesions of the anterior or posterior glenoid rim. These lesions may result from an osseous (anterior or posterior) Bankart lesion, a displaced glenoid fracture, or wear and erosion of the glenoid rim as a result of multiple recurrent dislocations **(Fig 12-8)**. Burkhart and De Beer (36) reported on 194 consecutive arthroscopic Bankart repairs using a suture anchor technique with an average of 27 months follow-up. The 173 patients without significant bone defects sustained 4% recurrence rate, whereas 21 patients with significant bone defects (either glenoid rim fractures resulting in inverted-pear shaped glenoids or humeral engaging Hill-Sachs lesions) sustained a 67% recurrence rate. The authors concluded that restoring bony anatomy is imperative for preventing recurrence and that arthroscopic Bankart repairs should not be performed in patients with the aforementioned significant bone defects.

Gerber et al. (37) have reported their clinical experience, which suggests that if a defect involves more than 25% of the glenoid surface, it should be repaired with intra-articular bone grafting. Gerber and Nyffeler (38) demonstrated a method for quantifying the degree of glenoid bone loss with computed tomography (CT) scan by measuring the glenoid surface on either an oblique sagittal image or a three-dimensional reconstruction. Through biomechanical testing, they determined that the force required for anterior dislocation is reduced by 70%, compared with that required when the glenoid is intact, if the length of the glenoid defect exceeds the radius **(Fig 12-9)**. The goal of surgery is to increase the glenoid constraint and provide support for the joint capsule; however, in cases of excessive glenoid bone loss, standard Bankart repairs (arthroscopic or open) are likely to fail, and osseous augmentation is recommended (39).

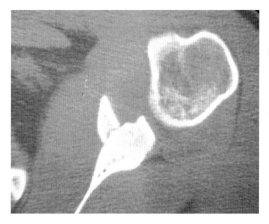
Fig 12-8. CT scan of large fracture involving anterior glenoid.

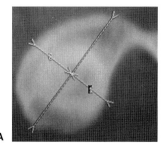 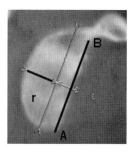
Fig 12-9. Equation for calculating stability: If A − B > r, then the force for dislocation is reduced 70%. Sagittal CT of normal Glenoid **(A)**, and osseous lesion anterior glenoid **(B)**.

Capsular Lesions

Traumatic intra-substance injury of the joint capsule is commonly associated with anterior dislocation. Depending on the magnitude of the anterior shear force, either plastic deformation or a complete tear of the joint capsule can occur. The recognition of a concomitant posttraumatic capsular laxity or rupture and a Bankart lesion is essential in order to select the correct surgical procedure. A traumatic capsular rupture or open rotator interval leads to venting of the joint, which increases glenohumeral translation. A positive sulcus sign in external rotation is the clinical sign for an open rotator interval.

Wolf et al. (40) described an intra-articular lesion associated with anterior instability where the glenohumeral ligaments are disruptive from the humerus and not the glenoid as in the case of a classic Bankart lesion. The authors coined the term a humeral avulsion of the glenohumeral ligaments, or HAGL lesion (40). Although the entity appears to be rare, the authors concluded that the diagnosis must be kept in mind particularly in cases of traumatic anterior dislocations in the absence of Bankart lesions. Boker et al. (41) reported on the largest series (41 cases) so far in the literature of HAGL lesions in contact athletes. The authors demonstrated that the surgeon must keep a high suspicion for a HAGL lesion in patients who have sustained a traumatic anterior dislocation and fail to have evidence of a Bankart lesion at arthroscopic examination. Although there is debate as to the best way to address the HAGL lesion, either open or arthroscopically, the current consensus appears to be that the lesion must be addressed in some way if surgical intervention is chosen (42).

Rarely, HAGL lesions may occur in conjunction with a Bankart lesion. Thus, appreciation of the humeral capsular insertion is important at the time of surgery. Tensioning of the capsule in the midrange can potentially overtighten and constrain the joint limiting rotation. In extreme cases, this can lead to posterior subluxation of the humeral head and arthritis (43,44).

Superior Labral Lesions

Lesions of the superior labrum have been associated with glenohumeral instability. Hinterman and Gachter (45) noted

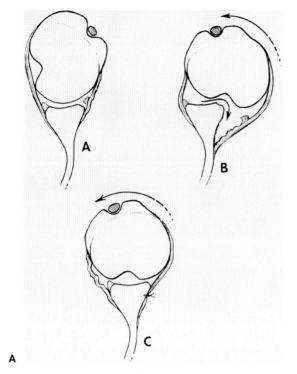

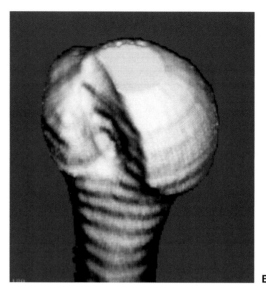

Fig 12-10. Hill Sachs lesion **(A)**, three-dimensional CT reconstruction of large Hill Sachs lesion **(B)**.

that 7% of their patients (14 of 212) with traumatic anterior instability requiring surgery had lesions of the superior labrum. Taylor and Arciero (35) reported 10% (6 of 63) of their patients had superior labral lesions associated with an initial anterior dislocation. Pagnani et al. (46) showed in a cadaver study that superior labral lesions contributed to instability of the glenohumeral joint if the biceps attachment was destabilized.

Hill-Sachs Lesions

The most common bony lesion associated with traumatic glenohumeral instability is a compression fracture at the posterolateral margin of the humeral head **(Fig 12-10)**. Commonly known as a Hill-Sachs lesion, this fracture occurs as the humeral head impacts the glenoid edge during dislocation. The lesion is present in 80% of anterior dislocations, 25% of anterior subluxations, and almost 100% of cases of recurrent anterior instability (19). With posterior instability, a *reverse* Hill-Sachs lesion results from impaction of the articular surface when the humeral head dislocates over the posterior glenoid rim. These articular humeral lesions rarely contribute to instability, as they are usually small; however, when the lesion includes more than 30% of the articular surface and associated with instability, it may be an important indication for surgery (17). Such large lesions occur only after recurrent dislocations. Gerber and Lambert (47) have demonstrated that one option of treating these kinds of injuries is restoration of normal articular cartilage conformity by allograft reconstruction.

■ CLINICAL EVALUATION

Instability

We use a classification system originally proposed by the Hospital of Special Surgery **(Table 12-2)**. This system categorizes shoulder instability on the basis of four criteria: frequency, etiology, degree, and direction.

Frequency

The *instability* itself may be acute or chronic, the differentiating feature being whether the event occurred within the

TABLE 12-2	Classification of Shoulder Instability
Frequency	Degree
Acute (primary)	Dislocation
Chronic	Subluxation
Recurrent	Microinstability
Fixed	
	Direction
Etiology	Unidirectional
Traumatic	Anterior
(macrotrauma)	Posterior
Atraumatic	Inferior
Voluntary (muscular)	Bidirectional
Involuntary	Anterior-inferior
Acquired (microtrauma)	Posterior-inferior
	Multidirectional

previous 24 hours. The number of recurrences (frequency of instability) is also critical in the classification scheme because it contributes to the level of damage to anatomic structures. This characteristic is extremely important when considering the degree and cause of instability. This component of the history is critical in determining the appropriate treatment.

Etiology

Etiology can be subdivided into traumatic, microtraumatic, or atraumatic groups also includes congenital and neuromuscular causes. The atraumatic group includes patients who exhibit a voluntary component of their instability. In this classification, these patients can be further subdivided into *group I*: voluntary instability, which is arm-position dependent and usually posterior; and *group II*: voluntary instability exhibited by the ability to selectively contract muscles, causing dislocation. Although patients in group I can voluntarily demonstrate instability, they chose to avoid dangerous arm positions. This condition subsequently affects activities of daily living (48). Conversely, patients in group II tend to have an underlying psychiatric problem, using their instability as a means to control their environment (49).

Degree of Instability

The *degree of instability* (dislocation, subluxation, and micro-instability) is also important in determining appropriate treatment options. Dislocation refers to complete dissociation of the articular surfaces of the humeral head and the glenoid cavity. Subluxation describes increased humeral head translation within the glenoid cavity, where the humeral head translates to the edge of the glenoid without true dislocation. Microinstability in the shoulder joint is a more subtle instability pattern.

Recurrent subluxation may manifest as pain rather than instability. Repetitive, high-energy, overhead activities can cause progressive attenuation of the capsular, ligamentous, and labral structures (50–52). As these static stabilizers fail and the dynamic stabilizers weaken, anterior subluxation occurs leading to impingement symptoms. This results from recurrent microtrauma which can ultimately lead to rotator cuff tearing and destabilization of bicep-labral complex.

Direction of Instability

The *direction of instability* has been a critical component of most classification systems. Traditionally, there was an assumption that 95% of shoulder instability was anterior (53). It has become increasingly apparent, however, that many athletes with ligamentous laxity have instability that is primarily posterior in nature (54–57). These patients suffer recurrent posterior subluxation and have a history of posterior shoulder pain rather than complaints of frank instability. This category of patients is more prevalent than previously recognized but should be distinguished from the rare true posterior dislocation that results from an acute traumatic event (58,59).

Traumatic posterior shoulder dislocation is notoriously overlooked on initial patients presentation. Hawkins et al. (60) reported on a series of 40 patients with 41 locked posterior shoulder dislocations. The initial physician missed the diagnosis in the majority of the cases reviewed. In this often quoted series, the causes of posterior dislocation were motor-vehicle accidents, seizures, alcohol-related injuries, or electroshock therapy.

History

The history can raise suspicion of shoulder instability. A patient's age, occupation, employment status, activity level, hand dominance, and other medical problems ate helpful in classifying the nature of the instability. Certain circumstances, such as work-related injuries or those with associated litigation, might affect patients' perception of their disabilities as well as their expectations for recovery and compliance (61).

The clinician should seek out specific complaints. For example, a patient who is a contact athlete may indicate that the arm "went dead" during a football tackle or ice-hockey check (62). This symptom is likely associated with a traumatic subluxation of the joint and the presence of a Bankart lesion. Another example is the patient who gives a history of having a seizure and then awaking with the sensation of the joint "out of place." This situation suggests posterior dislocation or subluxation as the result of unchecked internal rotation forces overcoming the weak external rotators of the shoulder.

A careful history and physical exam will provide information about the onset, direction, degree, duration, frequency of symptoms, and previous surgical treatments. Determining the presence of a traumatic cause will provide clues about the pathoanatomy that can be expected. Arm position, at the time of initial injury and during symptoms, can help differentiated the direction of the instability.

If pain is a major component of the patient's complaint, which activities cause the pain? When examining athletes, the clinician should always question as to the type of sports, the position played, and the duration, frequency and level of involvement. For example, throwers, swimmers, and tennis players may develop excessive capsular laxity as a result of subjecting their shoulders to repetitive microtrauma (63,64). The result is recurrent shoulder subluxation, which can create a sense of "looseness" or "slipping" with activity. In addition, secondary "non-outlet" impingement can occur as anterior instability decreases the subacromial space, causing pain with over-head activities. Furthermore, these same subluxations can create damage to the superior labral area, creating a SLAP lesion, especially in the setting of a contracted posterior capsule (65).

In recent years the existence of posterior instability has become better recognized. Posterior subluxation has been well documented in athletes who require repetitive arm motion in front of the body, such as offensive-line football players, volleyball, softball, and baseball players (54,56,57). Throwing sports in particular lead to posterior shoulder pain during late-cocking and follow-through phases, which has been associated with posterior subluxation and resultant microtrauma to the posterior capsulolabral complex (65,66).

Physical Findings

A systematic evaluation includes observation for abnormal motion patterns and atrophy, palpation to localize painful areas, assessment of both active and passive range of motion, measurement of strength of the rotator cuff, deltoid and scapular stabilizer muscles, neurovascular examination, and finally provocative testing maneuvers for instability. It is important to examine the opposite shoulder for comparison.

In evaluating shoulder motion, the examiner must carefully document any scapulothoracic substitution for glenohumeral motion, scapular winging, and other abnormal muscle patterns. Atrophy of the spinatus muscles may indicate longstanding associated rotator cuff tear or injury to the suprascapular nerve. Similarly, atrophy of the deltoid may indicate axillary nerve injury.

In addition, patients should always be assessed for findings of generalized ligamentous laxity, including the ability to hyperextend their elbows more than 10 degrees, apply the thumb to the forearm, hyperextend the metacarpalphalangeal joints more than 90 degree, or touch the palm of each hand to the floor while keeping the knees extended (Fig 12-11). While there is no direct relationship between generalized laxity and shoulder instability, there is some association between hyperlaxity and glenocapsular development (61).

The patient with an acute, unreduced anterior shoulder dislocation typically holds the arm in slight abduction and internal rotation (20,50). Before attempting any reduction maneuvers, carefully perform a neurovascular examination

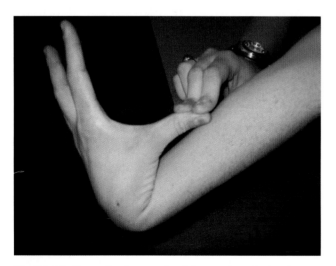

Fig 12-11. Example of generalized ligamentous laxity, demonstrating the ability to apply the thumb to the forearm.

to rule out brachial plexus injury, and specifically an axillary nerve injury (67,68). The latter condition may sometimes escape detection, as decreased sensation over the lateral deltoid is not always present with an injury to this nerve. In patients older than 60 years of age or younger patients involved in severe trauma, be aware of the possibility of an associated fracture of the humerus (69). Therefore, proper radiographic imaging is particularly important before attempting closed reduction in such cases.

Regardless of the particular closed reduction maneuver employed, perform all maneuvers as a gradual and gentle technique with appropriate analgesia (either intravenous or intra-articular) to ensure muscle relaxation. A method of gentle traction in line with the arm using counter-traction is usually successful.

Always be alert to the possibility of an unrecognized chronic (fixed) dislocation. The direction is typically posterior, however a chronic anterior dislocation is also possible. Many of these patients are poor historians secondary to dementia or chronic alcohol abuse (60). On exam, a patient with a fixed posterior dislocation will have severe limitation of external rotation compared to their opposite shoulder. Upon inspection, there is typically a flattening of the anterior aspect of the shoulder with an associated prominence of the coracoid process and possibly some prominence and rounding of the posterior aspect of the shoulder. The application of excessive force in attempting to close reduce such an injury risks neurovascular injury and/or fracture.

Athletes with instability are typically first seen by an orthopedic surgeon in the office, or in the training room, not in the emergency department. They may have had a documented episode of instability, or an injury with pain, but no true sense of shoulder instability. After a careful neurovascular examination, it is important to assess both active and passive range-of-motion. A discrepancy between active and passive motion may indicate either an associated rotator cuff tear or a nerve injury.

It is particularly important to identify a subscapularis tear in the setting of shoulder instability, a condition that is frequently missed (70,71). Patients with such tears can passively increase externally rotation with the arm adducted at the side, as well as associated apprehension in this position. Strength assessment is also important. Significant external rotation weakness may indicate a rotator cuff tear.

A subscapularis tear also typically demonstrates internal rotation weakness. In this situation, the patient has an associated *lift-off sign* and *belly-press test*. The belly-press test maneuver is very useful in situations when the patient lacks adequate internal rotation to perform a lift-off test. To perform the belly-press test, the patient places their hand on their abdomen, with their elbow flexed at 90 degree, and attempts to bring their elbow anterior to the coronal plane of their body, while keeping the hand on their abdomen at all times. If the elbow remains posterior to the anterior aspect of the mid-abdomen (i.e., the coronal plane of their body), there is likely a subscapularis tendon tear.

Specific tests for shoulder instability allow the clinician to classify the instability pattern. The apprehension test was originally described by Neer and Foster (72). With the patient seated or standing, place the symptomatic shoulder into a position of 90 degree of abduction and maximum external rotation. The patient's withdrawing from the examiner or complaining about a sense of shoulder instability demonstrates apprehension.

Pain as a chief complaint is not specific for shoulder instability. Other shoulder conditions such as arthritis and rotator cuff disease commonly present with shoulder pain. Kvitne and Jobe (73) proposed a modification of the apprehension maneuver to increase specificity for subtle anterior instability. Place the patient in a supine position, and perform the apprehension test as described above. Ask whether the patient has a sense of instability or simply pain. Place posterior pressure on the humerus, and ask whether this pressure relieves the sense of apprehension or pain. This "relocation maneuver" increases specificity of the diagnosis of instability if the patient reports decreased apprehension. If this maneuver simply reduces pain, it is not diagnostic of instability and may be associated with a variety of other diagnoses, including a SLAP lesion or impingement syndrome (74).

Inconsistencies in the apprehension test led Gerber and Ganz (75) to develop the anterior and posterior drawer test to assess the shoulder for excessive translation compared with the contralateral side. Others have found merit in this method of examination and have developed grading scales for the degree of shoulder laxity (76–78). These tests may offer some insight into the degree and direction of the instability. If one assesses laxity of the shoulder in the office setting, it is important to determine whether translation of the humeral head is greater on the painful side and whether this translation causes symptoms (55). Laxity testing assessment in the office setting can be of limited value if pain is causing the patient to guard the affected shoulder. Instead, this method is best used during examination under anesthesia to confirm the suspected degree and direction of shoulder instability.

Altchek et al. (76) and Hawkins et al. (78) proposed a grading scale for translation of the humeral head on the glenoid. Instability is graded on a scale of 0 − 3+ for all three directions (anterior, posterior, and inferior). For anterior and posterior drawer testing, a grade of 0 represents no humeral head translation, while movement of the humeral head up to but not over the glenoid rim represents 1+ instability. Translation of the humeral head over the glenoid rim with an associated spontaneous reduction with relief of pressure represents 2+ instability. Frank dislocation and locking of the humeral head over the glenoid rim is graded as 3+ instability. Whether in the office or under anesthesia, when performing drawer tests, it is important to bear in mind that the position of the arm determines the degree of tension in the glenohumeral ligaments. With the arm at the side in adduction, the IGHL is relatively lax, and anterior and posterior drawer testing may be of limited value. In abduction, the IGHL comes underneath the humeral head and forms a hammock that passively limits anterior, posterior, and inferior translation (79,80). Perform anterior drawer testing with the shoulder positioned in abduction in the plane of the scapula. Maintain the arm in neutral rotation while using one hand to place an axial load along the humerus and the other hand to apply an anterior or posterior force to the humerus. Often the examiner can feel the humeral head move back into the glenoid rather than out of the glenoid during the maneuver. The patient may note a painful click with such a maneuver. This can be particularly helpful in identifying posterior instability.

Posterior apprehension can be elicited by a modification of the posterior drawer test. To perform this modification, place the patient's arm in 90 degree of forward flexion and adduction while applying an axial load down the shaft of the humerus. Pain and a palpable shift and click suggests posterior labral injury and instability (61).

A modification of this test, termed the *jerk test*, has been described for posterior instability (81,82). With the patient seated, load the adducted shoulder axially into the glenoid with one hand, and with the other hand, palpate the posterior aspect of the shoulder. Then bring the arm into horizontal abduction anterior to the plane of the scapula; the humeral head may sublux posteriorly. Then bring the humerus posterior to the plane of the scapula; the humeral head may suddenly reduce into the glenoid. A palpable shift and pain accompany a positive test.

The *sulcus sign* is basically an inferior drawer test **(Fig 12-12)**. Originally described by Neer and Foster (72), it was initially believed to be pathognomonic for inferior and multidirectional instability. Unfortunately, a common misconception has been that a large sulcus sign that is asymptomatic, thus indicates inherent joint laxity, is a positive finding. The key point is that this maneuver should be associated with pain and should reproduce the patient's symptoms to be clinically relevant as a finding of inferior instability. A positive

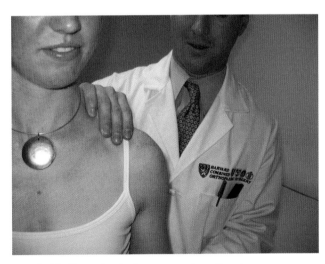

Fig 12-12. Example of a large asymptomatic sulcus.

sulcus sign in the absence of clinical symptoms is diagnostic only for inferior laxity, not inferior instability.

To perform the *sulcus test*, have the patient seated and the arm adducted at the side. Rotation of the shoulder is very important in assessing the degree of inferior instability. First, with the arm in neutral rotation, pull the humerus inferiorly, and estimate the amount of separation between the acromion and the humeral head. Grade is based on a scale of 0 − 3+ (76): A separation of 1 cm is a 1+ sulcus sign, 2 cm is a 2+ sulcus sign, and 3 cm is a 3+ sulcus sign. Anatomically, a sulcus sign greater than 2+ indicates a capacious capsule and specific laxity of the anterosuperior capsular region (rotator interval).

The *sulcus* sign should always be repeated with the arm placed in external rotation. If the sulcus sign remains greater than 2+ with the arm in external rotation, there is a marked deficiency of the superior capsule, and a large rotator interval defect in the capsule is likely (61). This is the result of damage to the superior and MGHLs, as well as the CHL. With this information before surgical repair, the surgeon then knows that surgical reconstruction of this region (rotator interval closure) with a capsular shift must be a component of the operation (83,84).

The *Gagey test* or *Hyperabduction test* measures the range of passive abduction (RPA) of the shoulder joint with the scapula stabilized **(Fig 12-13)**. Anatomical and clinical findings have demonstrated that when passive abduction occurs in the glenohumeral joint only, the abduction is controlled by the IGHL. An RPA of more than 105 degree is associated with lengthening and laxity of the IGHL. Gagey and Gagey (85) demonstrated a high association of an RPA of over 105 degree and instability.

Since the description of superior labral pathology by Andrews et al. (86) in 1985 and of the SLAP lesion by Snyder et al. (87) in 1990, several examination techniques

have evolved to diagnose this pathology. Andrews reported increased pain in patients during full shoulder flexion and abduction, with noticeable catching and popping. Snyder reported pain in patients with resisted shoulder flexion with elbow extension and forearm supination (biceps tension test).

Another useful diagnostic test is the *compression-rotation test*. With the patient supine, abduct the shoulder 90 degree, with the elbow flexed 90 degree. Apply compression force to the humerus to trap the torn labrum (in the same manner as McMurray's test for the knee is performed). O'Brien et al. (80) also described a maneuver testing for the presence of superior labral injuries. Commonly known as the *O'Brien's Test*, it is performed by placing the patient's shoulder in 90 degree of forward flexion and then adducting it across the body. Ask the patient to flex the arm further against resistance when the shoulder is first internally rotated and then externally rotated. If pain occurs when the shoulder is rotated internally but not when it is rotated externally, the test is positive. With the *O'Brien Test*, pain arising from acromioclavicular joint (AC) disease versus pain from a superior labral tear can be differentiated by where the patient localizes the pain with a positive test during internal rotation. If the pain localizes to the acromialclavicular joint or "on top" of the shoulder the test is diagnostic for AC joint disease; whereas pain or painful clicking described by the patient as "inside" the shoulder is indicative of labral pathology (88).

Unfortunately, independent examination of several of the popular existing physical exam tests for SLAP lesions have failed to demonstrate high accuracy, sensitivity, or specificity. Therefore, the results of such tests should be interpreted with caution when considering surgery, and therefore used as one of several pieces of information (along with appropriate history and radiological studies) which may point to a suspected superior labral anterior-posterior lesion (89,90).

Imaging

The minimum radiographic workup necessary for evaluation of an acute dislocation or suspected subluxation is a true anteroposterior (AP) view and an axillary lateral view. These images will allow accurate determination of the position of the humeral head relative to the glenoid. A true AP radiograph is obtained by angling the x-ray beam 45 degree relative to the sagittal plane of the body. A scapular Y or transcapular view can also give information about the position of the humeral head, but it is not as accurate as an axillary view. If a standard axillary view cannot be obtained, a Velpeau axillary view without removing the patient's arm from the sling will suffice.

In the office setting, a true AP view of the shoulder with the arm in internal rotation may demonstrate a Hill-Sachs lesion. A Stryker notch view is a special view that will also demonstrate a Hill-Sachs lesion (91,92).

West Point axillary view may prove helpful in a patient suspected of having had an episode of instability. Take the

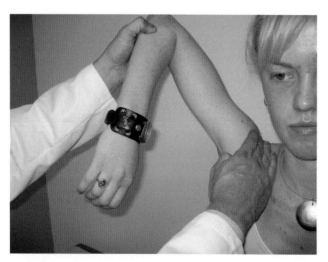

Fig 12-13. Example of the Gagey test or Hyperabduction test that measures the range of passive abduction (RPA) of the shoulder joint with the scapula stabilized.

image with the patient prone so the anterior glenoid is shown in profile without an overlying acromial shadow. This view demonstrates the glenoid rim better.

Adjuvant imaging techniques add vital information about the three-dimensional relationship and architecture of the joint or confirmation of the presence of a Bankart lesion, either bony or soft-tissue. Computed tomography (CT) demonstrates bony injuries or abnormalities including glenoid dysplasia, congenital version anomalies, acquired version abnormalities from erosion, and glenoid rim fractures (Fig 12-8). In addition, it allows measurement of the size of a humeral head defect (Hill-Sachs lesion) in cases of chronic instability (93). When combined with intra-articular dye, CT arthrography also demonstrates Bankart lesions and articular erosions.

Magnetic resonance imaging (MRI) with or without gadolinium has enormous popularity, although unfortunately it is often used as a screening tool in the evaluation of patients. Its role should instead be to confirm the presence of lesions that may need surgical treatment. MRI or CT with contrast are valuable for identifying labral tears, capsular injuries, or bony deficiencies.

Although the arthroscope can be used for diagnostic purposes, we prefer to identify coexisting pathology (rotator cuff tears), the degree of capsular laxity, and the extent of labral pathology with the appropriate imaging studies preoperatively, so that the appropriate surgical procedure can be selected and planned. In some cases, however, where the quality of capsular tissue is questionable by imaging studies or concomitant pathology is highly suspected but not found preoperatively, a diagnostic arthroscopy performed at the start of a planned open procedure can help add additional information, and possible arthroscopic treatment) regarding intra-articular pathology. A prolonged arthroscopic evaluation and/or treatment done immediately prior to performing an open procedure can distort tissue planes, and in some cases add no new information but only create technical problems for the planned open procedure.

Recent studies show MRI arthrography to be highly sensitive and specific for detecting capsulolabral lesions (94,95). CT is preferred if osseous pathology is suspected. CT is particularly helpful in the evaluation of glenoid retroversion in patients with posterior instability. CT arthrography can also be used to show chondral erosion, labral detachment, or excessive capsular redundancy (96,97).

Treatment Options

Successful treatment requires a correct diagnosis and performance of the appropriate procedure with excellent technique followed by a closely monitored and sound postoperative rehabilitation protocol. An error at any step will result in a poor clinical outcome. A successful outcome begins with an accurate diagnosis followed by the specific treatment required for the particular patient.

Nonoperative Care

Studies on the natural history of traumatic shoulder instability demonstrate a high rate of recurrence with nonoperative treatment (98–100). Rowe and Sakellarides (101) reported a recurrence rate of 58% in 398 patients with 53% follow-up. A strong correlation was noted between patient age and recurrence, with an incidence of recurrence of 94% in patients younger than 20 years, 79% in patients between 20 and 40 years, and 14% in patients older than 40 years. Subsequent studies verified this finding (69,102,103). A large Scandinavian study also confirmed the findings that recurrence rate appears to be inversely proportional to age of initial dislocation. Hovelius et al. (99) reported on a 10-year follow-up of 247 primary dislocations in patients younger than 40 years. Although the group was somewhat mixed in terms of diagnosis, including "spontaneous" dislocations and dislocations with associated greater tuberosity fracture, the study is important purely on the basis of the duration and percentage of follow-up. Of the 247 shoulders, 52% sustained further dislocations, while 23% required later surgical stabilization. For patients younger than 25 years of age, the risk of recurrence was greater than 60%, with the recurrence rate rapidly decreasing with the initial dislocation after 25 years of age. Important conclusions from this landmark study: (a) recurrence rate is inversely correlated with the age of initial dislocation; (b) the rate of dislocation arthropathy is 20% and is unrelated to surgical treatment or number of recurrences; (c) recurrence rate is not affected by initial treatment. Recurrence rates appear to be even higher in the pediatric age groups. Marans et al. (104) reported one or more recurrent episodes in all of the children in their study.

Thus, it is clear that the most important factors in determining recurrence of instability after a traumatic injury are age and activity level. Surgical intervention for a patient with an initial dislocation has become more accepted in recent years. In theory, these patients have better-defined pathology and healthier tissue, making them prime candidates for surgical repair, particularly with arthroscopic techniques. Arciero et al. (105), in a prospective study among students at the U.S. Military Academy at West Point, comparing the results of nonsurgical management and arthroscopic repair in patients with initial dislocations, the recurrence rate in this high-demand patient population was 80% in the non-surgical group and 14% in the surgical group. Kirkley et al. (100) in 1999, randomized patients younger than 30 years with initial dislocations into two groups: those treated with immobilization and rehabilitation and those treated with arthroscopic Bankart repair. At follow-up of 33 months, those who had arthroscopic stabilization had a recurrence rate 15.9%, compared with 47% in the nonsurgical. Based on the available data for young patients and particularly, young contact athletes (i.e., contact athletes and military recruits) younger than 25 years of age should be strongly considered for an arthroscopic Bankart repair in the off-season. For any patient younger than 25 years of age who sustains a first-time dislocation, the advantages and disadvantages of immediate arthroscopic Bankart repair should be discussed, and this treatment should be offered as a viable option. Open Bankart repair also may be an option, but because no significant difference in surgical ease or outcome between early and late open Bankart repair has been demonstrated, arthroscopic repair is probably indicated for first-time dislocations. The authors, preference is for arthroscopic repair in all young, active, high-demand patients including contact athletes.

Nonoperative SLAP treatment

Treatment of SLAP lesions is typically conservative at first, as many patients respond to rest and rehabilitation in the acute period. However, after the inflammation has subsided, and if patient has completed course of rehabilitation and is still unable to resume athletic activities, serious consideration must be made for surgical intervention.

■ TECHNIQUE

SLAP Surgical Techniques

Surgical treatment of symptomatic SLAP lesions consists of shoulder arthroscopy, which frequently demonstrates a positive "drive-through" sign, a displaceable biceps vertex and, in up to 60% of cases, associated rotator cuff pathology, mostly partial-thickness undersurface tears (106). If the biceps-labral anchor is avulsed, it is partially debrided and secured back to the glenoid with suture anchors or tacks, followed by a post-operative rehabilitation program for posterior capsular stretching. If small tearing and fraying is present, but no true avulsion of the anchor, a simple labral debridement is performed.

Principles of Instability Surgery

The goal of treatment in both open and arthroscopic instability surgery is twofold: to restore the labrum to its anatomic attachment site and to re-establish the appropriate tension to the inferior capsuloligamentous complex of the joint. Cadaveric studies have shown that both the labrum and the capsule must be injured for a dislocation to occur (107). If the labrum is torn (Bankart or posterior/reverse Bankart lesion), it should be repaired anatomically to the rim of the glenoid. Capsular laxity can be addressed by the superior and medial shift of the capsule. Plication can be used to increase the tension in the capsule and decrease laxity. In situations in which labral tears are not present and the principal pathology is redundant capsule, a plication should be performed on the appropriate side of the joint to decrease capsular volume and prevent translation. In patients with MDI, the plication is performed inferiorly, posteriorly, and anteriorly. The rotator interval should always be closed in patients with MDI or posterior instability.

Associated injuries to the rotator cuff or superior labrum should be repaired surgically. In rare instances, midcapsular ruptures of the glenohumeral capsule or humeral avulsions of the glenohumeral ligaments (HAGL lesions) are discovered. If these lesions cannot be effectively treated arthroscopically, the surgeon should convert to an open procedure.

Anesthesia and Positioning for Arthroscopy

Interscalene regional blockade has been effective in providing early postoperative pain relief and in decreasing overall narcotic requirements following surgery (108). Following adequate preoperative anesthesia, the choice of patient position (either beach-chair or lateral decubitus) must be tailored to the surgeon such that comprehensive visualization and repair of the pathologic structures are not compromised.

Lateral decubitus is preferred for patients with MDI or posterior instability because this position eases access to the axillary pouch and posteroinferior capsule because of the lateral traction that is applied. The patient is positioned on a long beanbag, and the arm held in a longitudinal arm-traction device with 20 degrees of abduction and 20 degrees of flexion. A second, laterally directed force is also applied to the proximal humerus using 2 to 5 kg of traction. If the beach-chair position is chosen for a posteroinferior labral repair, an accessory trans-rotator cuff portal may be used to enable direct visualization of the postero-inferior glenohumeral joint (108a).

Examination under Anesthesia

Examination of the glenohumeral joint with the arm in various degrees of abduction and external rotation allows the surgeon to assess the degree and direction of glenohumeral laxity. Side-to-side comparisons can be particularly helpful in patients with subtle instability patterns or for those with global laxity. As described earlier in the chapter, laxity is graded from 0 to 3+, and the sulcus is measured and quantified by the distance between the lateral border of the humeral head and the acromion. The examination under anesthesia should confirm the preoperative diagnosis that was established through a careful history, physical, and imaging studies.

■ PORTALS

Anterior Instability

Two anterior portals (superior and inferior) are established using an "outside-in" technique with a spinal needle. These portals function as utility portals for instrument passage, glenoid preparation, suture management, and knot tying. It is important to separate these anterior cannulas widely so cannula crowding in the joint is not a problem **(Fig 12-14)**. The second cannula is placed as low as possible in the rotator interval typically entering just superior to the subscapularis

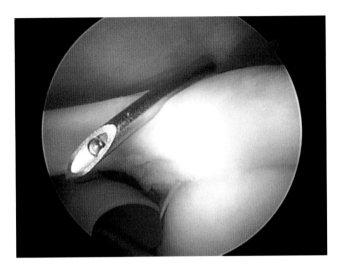

Fig 12-14. Intra-operative photograph of proper portal placement for instability repair. Spinal needle is used to localize anterior superior portal behind bicep tendon. Portals must be spaced widely apart to prevent crowding.

tendon and usually placed a centimeter inferior and lateral to the palpable coracoid process so that it enters the joint aiming slightly lateral to medial. The first anchor is placed at the five o'clock position with the proper medial orientation. The anchor must be placed at the corner of the anterior glenoid rim or even a couple of millimeters onto the articular face of the glenoid to incorporate the labrocapsuloligametous sleeve as a prolongation of the glenoid cavity. It is imperative to ensure the avoidance of medial placement of the anchors on the scapular neck. Alternately, a transsubscapularis approach can be used to improve inferior access if needed.

Posterior Instability and MDI

One to two posterior arthroscopic portals are used for the suture anchor placement/capsular advancement and suture shuttling. The arthroscope remains in the anterior superior portal for the majority of the case. The posterior portal needs to be more lateral than usual to allow better access to the posterior glenoid rim and posterior inferior capsule. A high anterior portal is placed lateral and superior to the coracoid process and is used for the arthroscopic viewing and inflow. The shift begins in the six o'clock position.

Capsulolabral Repair with Suture Anchors

For capsulolabral repair with suture anchors, the 30 degree arthroscope should be placed in the posterior viewing portal. It also can be placed in the anterosuperior portal ("bird's eye" portal) to view the anterior labrum. Working instruments can be then placed in the anteroinferior portal. In some instances, it is helpful to use a 70 degree arthroscope to visualize the glenoid rim while mobilizing the capsulolabral sleeve. The IGHL complex is mobilized from the glenoid

neck as far inferiorly as the six o'clock position using electrocautery or a small elevator. The capsulolabral sleeve must be mobilized until it can be shifted superiorly and laterally onto the glenoid rim. The release should proceed until the muscle fibers of the underlying subscapularis are seen. Next, the glenoid neck is decorticated with a motorized shaver to facilitate healing of the repaired labrum and capsule.

Anchors are placed on the articular rim, or a few millimeters on the articular surface, through the anterior-inferior cannula at an angle that avoids skiving across the articular cartilage. They should not be placed inadvertently along the medial scapular neck. The anchor should be assessed for security and the suture for slideability.

The labrum is repaired and the capsule is shifted superiorly. The authors prefer using a shuttling device [arthrex suture lasso (Arthrex, Naples, FL) or linvatec spectrum (Linvatec, Largo, FL)], and a shuttle relay [linvatec (Linvatec, Largo, FL)] or monofilament suture is placed through the device and retrieved out the superior cannula (while viewing from posterior portal), or the posterior cannula (while viewing from anterosuperior portal). The suture limb that exits the anterosuperior cannula (while viewing from the posterior portal) is the suture that will ultimately pass through the soft tissue and becomes the "post" suture down which the sliding arthroscopic knot will move. It is advisable to have the knot on the soft tissue capsulolabral side of the repair. Standard arthroscopic sliding knots are then tied. The knot is cut leaving a 3- to 4-mm tail. These steps are repeated for each subsequent anchor.

Capsular Plication

Capsular plication is used to tension abnormally lax or redundant tissue that is often found in patients with MDI or atraumatic anterior or posterior instability. For posterior instability and MDI, the joint is visualized through the anterior cannula while the posterior cannula is used for instrumentation. Using the motorized shaver on reverse without suction, the posterior capsule is abraded to promote healing. The shift begins at the six o'clock position. Using an angled shuttling instrument, the capsule is grasped and the sharp tip of the instrument is passed through it and through the labrum. The shift begins about 1.5 cm lateral to the glenoid rim. When working on the posterior capsule, the angled shuttling instrument usually has a curve in the opposite direction of the side of shoulder being worked on (i.e., in a right shoulder posterior capsule, use a left-curved shuttling instrument). This is the opposite scenario than what is encountered when working on the anterior capsule, where the instrument curve is the same as the side of the shoulder being worked on (i.e.,. right shoulder anterior capsule, right curved shuttling instrument). A monofilament suture or shuttle relay (Linvatec, Largo, FL) is then passed through the capsule and labrum. A sliding, locking knot is used to fold the capsule over itself and create a "bumper" of capsulolabral tissue. The same steps are repeated at the seven, eight, and nine o'clock positions to complete the inferior and posterior capsular shifts. After the posterior capsular

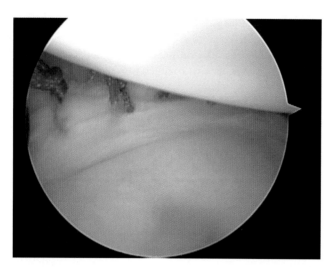

Fig 12-15. Intra-operative photograph (right shoulder) looking from posterior portal at anterior capsular suture anchor placement.

capsulorraphy, the capsular shift is repeated at the five and four o'clock positions to tighten the anteroinferior capsule **(Fig 12-15)**. In MDI cases with global placement of anchors and plication, sometimes it can be helpful to place and tie the anterior five o'clock anchor first before moving to complete the posterior capsule plications. In this situation the rest of the anterior anchors are then placed after completion of the posterior capsule. Placing the anterior five o'clock anchor prior to the posterior capsular plication can sometimes be helpful because this anterior-inferior position can be very hard to reach after a complete posterior capsule plication has been performed.

In the case of a posterior Bankart lesion, the lesion is released and mobilized as described for anterior instability. With the use of the motorized shaver, electrocautery, and small elevator, the capsulolabral tissue is released mobilized and the glenoid rim abraded. Here again, drill holes are made on the edge of the glenoid rim, or a few millimeters on the glenoid face. The anchors are inserted through a posterior portal. In some cases it may be helpful to place an accessory posteroinferior portal (and slightly more lateral than a standard posterior portal) that provides a better angle and approach to the inferior capsule and glenoid rim. While viewing from the anterosuperior portal or from the standard anterior portal. The same steps as described previously are repeated to tension the posterior capsule superiorly to nine o'clock position. Complete repair is assessed from both the anterior and the posterior portals.

Rotator Interval Closure

If after repair of the labrum and IGHL and MGHLs, the shoulder shows persistent inferior or inferoposterior translation, rotator interval closure is performed. The authors close the rotator interval in all patients with MDI and posterior instability.

The arthroscope is inserted posteriorly to visualize the rotator interval. The arm should be placed in external rotation

and a curved shuttling device (example, spectrum, Linvatec, Largo, FL), suture hook, spinal needle, or penetrating instrument (penetrator, Arthrex, Naples, FL) is placed directly through the anterosuperior cannula or percutaneously through the portal without the cannula. The instrument is then advanced through the robust capsular tissue immediately superior to the subscapularis tendon. The suture or shuttle is then advanced into the joint. The cannula is backed out of the joint, the penetrating instrument is then passed through the strong tissue just anterior to the supraspinatus tendon. The suture or shuttle is then grasped. Both sutures limbs are then retrieved out of the anterosuperior cannula. A crochet hook can help can help in this retrieval. The sutures are then tied blindly and extra-articularly. Additional sutures may be added as needed.

Open Surgery

Open surgery for instability remains an acceptable method of treatment when the surgeon lacks the equipment, experience, or technical expertise to perform an arthroscopic repair. Furthermore, open surgery is indicated in situations where current arthroscopic methods are likely to fail—namely, in the setting of large bone or soft tissue deficiencies or in the context of revision surgery.

The degree of bony deficiency or capsular laxity that obviates an open procedure continues to be debated in the literature. Rowe's (109) suggestion that glenoid loss of up to 30% was amenable to a soft-tissue procedure was largely based on qualitative visual inspection and anecdotal experience. Burkhart and DeBeer (36,110) have reported that significant bony loss of the anterior glenoid at the time of arthroscopy, termed an "inverted pear glenoid," was associated with a high failure rate after arthroscopic stabilization.

A growing body of evidence is bringing attention to the significance of alterations in biomechanical stability brought about by glenoid and or/humeral bone loss or dysplasia (111–116). For instance, Gerber (117) has provided a method to quantify the risk of dislocation based on the degree of glenoid bone loss using three-dimensional CT scan to assist in operative planning. Specifically, if the length of the glenoid defect exceeds the maximum radius of the glenoid, the force required for anterior dislocation is reduced by 70%. Based on this criteria, Gill and Warner (39) has reported favorable results (ASES 2004, Neer award paper), on surgical reconstruction of patients with recurrent instability using intra-articular tricortical iliac crest bone graft contoured to restore the bony architecture of the deficient glenoid.

Most open procedures employ a combination of "anatomic" and "non-anatomic" repair based largely on Speer's work that indicated in a cadaveric model that injury to both the labrum and capsule was a necessary prerequisite for complete dislocation (107). For this reason, most open procedures involve, for example, a classic Bankart repair (anatomic) in conjunction with a capsular shift (non-anatomic).

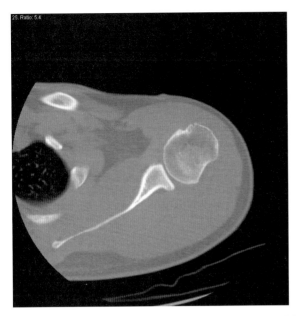

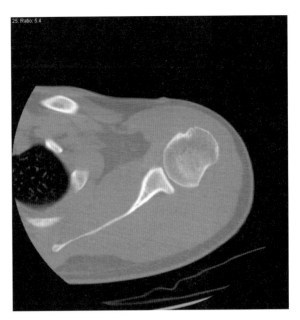

Fig 12-16. MRI T2-weighted image of a humeral avulsion of the glenohumeral ligament. Because the capsule and ligaments insert beneath the humeral head, arthroscopic repair often is not possible.

Fig 12-17. Axial CT scan demonstrating marked anterior bone loss.

Nonanatomic surgical procedures utilize a bony or soft-tissue checkrein to block excessive translation and substitute for capsulolabral or bony injury. The Bristow and Latarjet, for instance, transfer either the tip or entire coracoid process to the anterior glenoid to buttress the humerus from subluxating anteriorly (118,119). The Magnuson-Stack procedure (120) is an advancement of the subscapularis that was popularized by DePalma. Finally, the Putti-Platt procedure, which was reported by Osmond-Clarke in 1948 (121), is an imbrication and shortening of the subscapularis. Many series (122–126) have reported excellent outcomes with non-anatomic type stabilizations, but the reported complications such as loss of motion, recurrent instability, and premature arthritis (120,127–131) have led many North American surgeons to avoid them as an initial form of treatment (127,132–134).

Relative Indications for Open Surgery

Despite advancements in surgical technique and implants, certain clinical scenarios are prone to failure by arthroscopic methods. These include HAGL lesions and capsular ruptures **(Fig 12-16)**. Other relative indications for open surgery include failed prior arthroscopic or open repairs. In the setting of failed thermal capsulorrhaphy, the surgeon is often faced with residual casulolabral tissue that is of poor quality or completely necrotic and absent that can only be addressed by open methods.

The treatment of the contact or high-demand athlete with anterior instability remains controversial. For some surgeons, shoulder instability in a contact athlete is a clear indication for open surgery, and excellent results have certainly been

reported (135). Other skilled arthroscopists believe that with careful patient selection, arthroscopic approaches can yield similar results. Burkhart and DeBeer (36) reported on a group of 194 patients who had undergone arthroscopic Bankart repair of the shoulder. One hundred and one of these patients were contact athletes. Although the recurrence rate was 87% in those contact athletes who had significant bone defects, in those who did not have bone defects the recurrence rate was only 6.5%.

Absolute Indications for Open Surgery

Absolute indications for open stabilization procedures include significant degrees of glenoid or humeral bone loss, capsular deficiencies, or irreparable rotator cuff tears, particularly those of the subscapularis. In individuals with significant anterior glenoid erosion, an osseous reconstruction should be performed **(Fig 12-17)**. In the rare case where a large humeral head defect (Hill-Sachs lesion) plays a role in the recurrence of instability, open surgery is performed. More commonly, however, when there is a large Hill Sachs defect, anterior glenoid bone loss plays the critical role in instability. When there is a chronic disruption of the subscapularis, usually in the setting of prior surgery, an open repair is performed.

Contraindications for Open Instability Surgery

In cases of concomitant severe arthritis, open instability repair may not be effective. Depending on the status of the osseous glenoid and surrounding rotator cuff, arthroplasty or arthrodesis may be better options. Paralysis may also be associated with chronic instability and in such cases arthrodesis may be more successful in eliminating pain (136–139). Relative contraindications for open repair of anterior instability include voluntary or psychogenic instability (49,140,141) and the presence of active infection.

■ TECHNIQUES

Open Anatomic Repair

The classic open Bankart repair, Neer capsular shift, and multiple subsequent modifications have been reported for many years (109,132,142,143). In the appropriate patient population and while adhering to meticulous surgical technique, the results are consistently very good. With Rowe et al. (109) and Gill et al. (132) reporting 97% and 95% success rates respectively with open anterior stabilization, it is not surprising that open techniques such as the Bankart are heralded as the "gold standard." The Bankart procedure restores normal anatomy by reattaching the labrum to its anatomic position at the anterior articular margin of the joint (33,144). The concept of a "selective capsular shift" was introduced as a refinement to this technique **(Fig 12-18)**. The selective shift is based on the observation that the capsuloligamentous static stabilizers function at predictable positions of rotation and act as checkreins to excessive rotation

and translation (142,145) and that the pathoanatomy involves injury to both the labrum and the capsule (107). The Bankart lesion is anatomically repaired and then the capsule is shifted to tighten the joint while avoiding over-constraint.

Glenoid Bone Deficiency

Although osteoarticular pathology rarely is a cause of anterior instability, it is essential that it be ruled out prior to proceeding with any soft-tissue stabilization procedure or in the revision setting. A small subset of patients may be predisposed to instability due to developmental glenoid dysplasia, or pathologic flattening or hypoconcavity of the glenoid as well as abnormal glenoid version. More commonly, significant loss of normal glenohumeral bony anatomy is the result of traumatic dislocation or recurrent episodes of instability. The anterior glenoid rim can actually become rounded and flattened from recurrent dislocations (146). Experience has shown that when such defects are present there is an increased risk of failure when only soft-tissue repairs are performed (9,10,38,114). Burkhart and DeBeer (110), for example, noted that in patients with recurrent anterior instability treated arthroscopically, there was a recurrence rate of 4% in subjects with normal bony

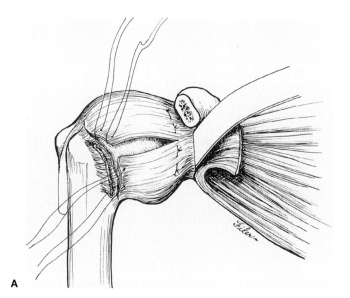

A

C

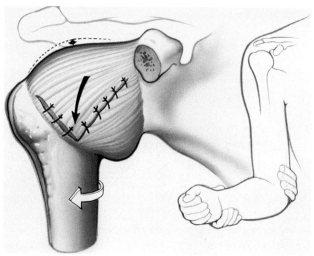

B

Fig 12-18. Demonstration of the concept of the selective capsular shift. The Bankart lesion is repaired anatomically **(A)**, the arm is then placed in the desired position (approximately 30 degrees of glenohumeral abduction and 30 degrees external rotation) **(B)**, and the capsule is then shifted laterally to the humerus to the remove the capsular redundancy **(C)**. (Adapted from Clavert PH, Millett PJ, Warner JJP. Traumatic anterior instability: open solutions. In: Warner JJP, Iannotti JP, Flatow EL, eds. *Complex and revision problems in shoulder surgery*. Philadelphia: Lippincott Williams & Wilkins; 2005; Figs 2.22–23.)

anatomy compared to 67% in those with significant bony defects.

Fortunately, many surgeons now recognize the need to reconstruct or compensate for anterior or posterior glenoid bone loss by open methods (38,110,114,147). The surgical options include either an anatomic reconstruction of the glenoid with bone graft or a coracoid process transfer, such as the Bristow or Latarjet procedures. The authors use the patient's symptoms and Gerber's biomechanical work to form a framework under which glenoid bone grafting is considered (38). If (a) the patient has recurrent instability, particularly with mid-range symptoms; (b) if the patient has symptoms of instability during sleep, or with decreasing degrees of trauma; (c) if a bone defect is seen on x-ray; (d) or if the patient has failed a prior arthroscopic procedure; a CT scan is obtained. If the CT scan demonstrates an osseous defect that is longer in the sagittal plane than the maximum radius of the glenoid, then an anatomic glenoid reconstruction is performed (39) (Fig 12-9).

Glenoid Reconstruction with Iliac Crest Bone Graft

Glenoid reconstruction with iliac crest bone graft restores bone to recreate the arc of the glenoid **(Fig 12-19)**. Bodey et al. (148) were the first to report on this technique in 1983 in 16 shoulders for recurrent anterior dislocation with all patients able to return to their prior level of work and sporting activities. Others have reported good to excellent results with a low rate of recurrence and a high level of patient satisfaction (149,150).

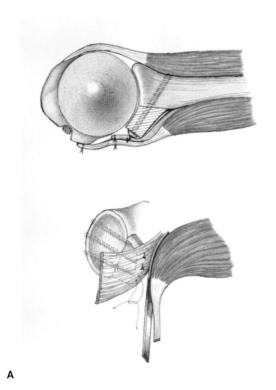

A

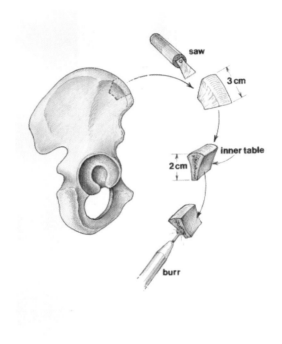

B

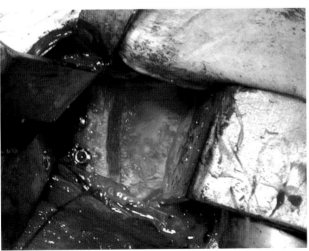

C

Fig 12-19. **A:** Illustrations demonstrating an anatomic glenoid reconstruction with autogeneous iliac bone graft. The graft restores the articular arc and glenohumeral stability. (Adapted from Clavert PH, Millett, PJ, Warner JJP. Traumatic anterior instability: open solutions. In: Warner JJP, Iannotti JP, Flatow EL, eds. *Complex and revision problems in shoulder surgery.* Philadelphia: Lippincott Williams & Wilkins; 2005: 35–36.) **B:** Illustration demonstrating harvest and preparation of tricortical autogeneous iliac crest bone graft. **C:** Intra-operative photograph demonstrating the graft in position. (Drawing from Clavert PH, Millett, PJ, Warner JJP. Traumatic anterior instability: open solutions. In: Warner JJP, Iannotti JP, Flatow EL, eds. *Complex and revision problems in shoulder surgery.* Philadelphia: Lippincott Williams & Wilkins; 2005: 42.)

Open Nonanatomic Repairs

Latarjet was the first to describe the technique of using a portion of the coracoid transferred to the anterior glenoid as a buttress to anterior humeral translation in 1958 (119). In this procedure, the transfer includes a portion of the coracoacromial ligament that is sutured to the capsular tissue through a short horizontal incision made in the subscapularis. The Latarjet procedure reconstructs the glenoid depth and width with the bone block and creates a dynamic reinforcement of the inferior capsule through the coracobrachialis muscle, particularly while the arm is abducted and externally rotated. In the Bristow procedure, popularized by Helfet, only the tip of the coracoid process and attached coracobrachialis is transferred to the anterior glenoid (118). Even though these nonanatomic techniques fail to address the essential lesion, they do provide reliable and durable anterior stabilization (122–126). Recurrence rates vary from

0% [0 out of 58 procedures for Allain et al. (123)] to 6% [7 recurrences out 111 patients for Hovelius et al. (151); 3 cases out 52 patients for Levigne et al. (152)].

Humeral Bone Deficiency

Humeral head defects are commonly present in patients with shoulder instability. The defects are usually small and carry the eponym Hill-Sachs lesion when secondary to anterior instability and reverse Hill-Sachs lesions when secondary to posterior instability. Although quite ubiquitous in recurrent anterior shoulder instability, the management of large Hill-Sachs defects remains controversial especially in the absence of an associated glenoid defect.

When the glenohumeral joint dislocates, the Hill-Sachs defect can occur at any of a variety of angles as determined by the position of the humerus at the time of dislocation.

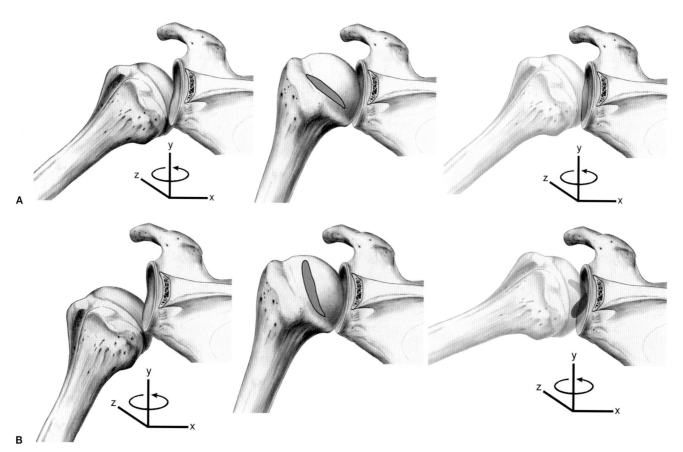

Fig 12-20. A: The engaging Hill-Sachs lesion. In a functional position of abduction and external rotation, the long axis of this lesion is parallel to the anterior glenoid and engages its anterior corner. Creation of lesion with the arm in abduction and external rotation (*left*); orientation of Hill-Sachs lesion (*middle*); and engagement of Hill-Sachs lesion in functional position of abduction and external rotation (*right*). The orthogonal three-dimensional Cartesian system is represented by xyz. **B:** The nonengaging Hill-Sachs lesion. This lesion was created with the arm at the side and in some extension, and will engage only with the arm at the side with external rotation and extension, which is not a functional position (*left*). Orientation of the Hill-Sachs lesion (*middle*). In a functional position of abduction and external rotation, the Hill-Sachs lesion is diagonal to the anterior margin of the glenoid and does not engage (*right*). The orthogonal three-dimensional Cartesian coordination system is represented by xyz.

Some Hill-Sachs lesions will engage the anterior glenoid rim when the glenohumeral joint is in a position of abduction and external rotation. Burkhart has described these as "engaging" Hill-Sachs lesions (36). They can be defined as defects in which the long axis of the humeral head defect aligns parallel to the anterior glenoid rim, when the shoulder is in a position of abduction and external rotation **(Fig 12-20)**. Such configurations have been found to be particularly prone to recurrent dislocation and subluxation after arthroscopic repair. Furthermore, if a large Hill-Sachs lesion is combined with a glenoid defect, they can be particularly problematic **(Fig 12-21)**. Hovelius et al. (99) found significant Hill-Sachs defects in 54% of his study population of 247 individuals with primary anterior instability, and he also found a significantly higher risk of recurrence when a Hill-Sachs defect was present. Rowe et al. (127) also suggested that a Hill-Sachs lesion could be a reason for failure after open surgical repair. Other authors however have found that the presence and magnitude of a Hill-Sachs lesion did not influence the outcome after open Bankart repair (153).

With the "nonengaging" Hill-Sachs lesion, the long axis of the Hill-Sach's defect crosses diagonally across the glenoid rim with the arm in abduction and external rotation so that it never "engages" the glenoid rim. In these types of defects, there is a continuous smooth articular contact throughout the range of motion. According to Burkhart, such shoulders with nonengaging Hill-Sachs lesions are not at significant risk for recurrence when repaired arthroscopically, and therefore

patients with these types of humeral lesions are good candidates for arthroscopic repair (36).

Clinically significant, large humeral head defects are fortunately quite rare. They are usually diagnosed by recurrent symptoms of instability, by locking, or by three-dimensional imaging studies. The morphology of the Hill-Sachs defect has been suggested by some as a prognostic factor for the degree of instability (154). Burkhart and Danaceau (155) have suggested that the mismatch in the articular arc that occurs with a Hill-Sachs lesion is the important pathoanatomic feature. Most Hill-Sachs lesions are simply ignored at the time of surgery and the anterior capsule and labrum are addressed with an anatomic repair, as discussed previously. When the bone defect is large, however, the bone defect may need to be addressed. There are unfortunately no guidelines from the literature about what size defect needs surgical treatment. The authors do become concerned when the defect exceeds 20 to 30% of the humeral head as measured on CT scan or when a Hill-Sachs lesion is combined with a glenoid defect.

Surgical options for management of humeral head defects (Hill-Sachs lesions) include reconstructing the humerus with an allograft to restore the humeral articular arc, reconstructing the glenoid with an anterior bone graft to lengthen the glenoid articular arc and prevent the humeral defect from engaging the glenoid rim, or rotating the humeral head with an osteotomy to move the defect so that it does not come in contact with the anterior glenoid. If there is an associated glenoid defect, the authors recommend

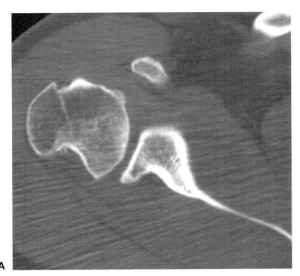

A

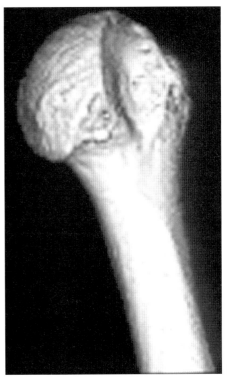

B

Fig 12-21. **A:** Axial CT scan demonstrating massive Hill-Sachs lesion, notice concomitant anterior glenoid erosion. **B:** Three-dimensional CT reconstruction of Hill-Sachs lesion.

that the glenoid be reconstructed first; if the humeral defect is still significant, it can be reconstructed with an allograft. Unfortunately, the evidence for each of these approaches is largely anecdotal and based on small series or case reports (155–157).

Salvage Procedures

In rare cases, individuals will continue to complain of instability despite attempted surgical reconstructions. In certain settings, glenohumeral arthrodesis may be the only option available (138,158,159). A sobering observation was presented by Richards (159), who found that many subjects had subjective sensations of instability despite radiographic evidence of solid arthrodeses. Moreover, some of these patients developed problems with their scapulothoracic joint due to severe posturing, secondary scapular winging, pseudowinging, and snapping scapula. These symptoms may occur as a result of the arthrodesis or may be aggravated by the fusion (159). Despite the concerns about arthrodeses, there may be no other reasonable option in this difficult subcategory of patients.

Revision and Complex Problems

Revision instability surgery is the most technically challenging of all open shoulder surgery. Nevertheless, it can also be the most satisfying, if basic principles are observed. When nonanatomic repairs need to be revised, the normal tissue planes are often distorted. This adds significant technical complexity to the procedure and increases the potential risk for complications. When attempting to salvage failed anterior instability cases, surgeons should be prepared to face challenging scenarios such as distorted anatomic tissue planes, severe scarring, capsular deficiencies from multiple prior surgeries or thermal capsulorrhaphy (160,161), bony deficiencies due to erosion or fracture, and subscapularis deficiencies.

Capsular Deficiency

Fortunately, capsular deficiency is a rare condition. There is a paucity of literature that deals with soft tissues deficiency in relation to instability (162–165). It is more common in revision settings and after thermal capsulorraphy. The soft-tissue deficiency may also include the subscapularis. There are several reasonable surgical options and choices for soft tissue augmentation for the unstable shoulder with a deficient capsule.

Lazarus et al. (166) presented a method of using hamstrings for repair of such deficiencies. Good outcomes, using a modification of this technique, have been reported by Warner et al. (165) **(Fig 12-22)**. Gallie et al. (167) described the use of the iliotibial band for capsular reconstruction to treat glenohumeral instability associated with an irreparable capsule. More recently Iannotti et al. (162) have reported their experience in seven cases using this technique. Results were generally good with no recurrences or problems with persistent apprehension. Moekel et al. (163) have described the use of Achilles allograft in the setting of anterior instability after shoulder arthroplasty. The researchers reported on 10 patients with persistent anterior shoulder instability from a series of 236 total shoulder arthroplasties. The results were generally fair to good with some loss of motion but restoration of stability.

Subscapularis Tears

Rupture of the subscapularis in association with primary anterior shoulder instability is more common after a prior open instability repair and should be suspected in those who have had prior anterior stabilization procedures in which the subscapularis was released for exposure (43). Failure to recognize and treat a subscapularis tear in a proper and timely fashion can result in a poor outcome. A careful physical examination to assess the subscapularis is necessary. Individuals with subscapularis deficiency will have increased passive external rotation and positive belly press and lift off

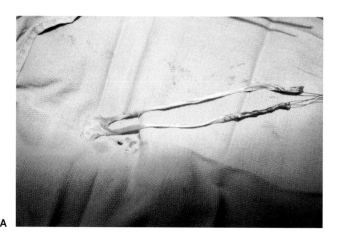
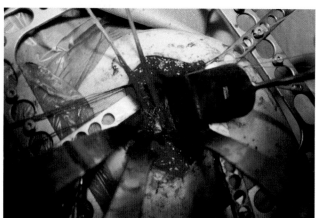

A   B

Fig 12-22. Intra-operative photographs demonstrating anterior capsular reconstruction with hamstring autograft for repair of capsular deficiency.

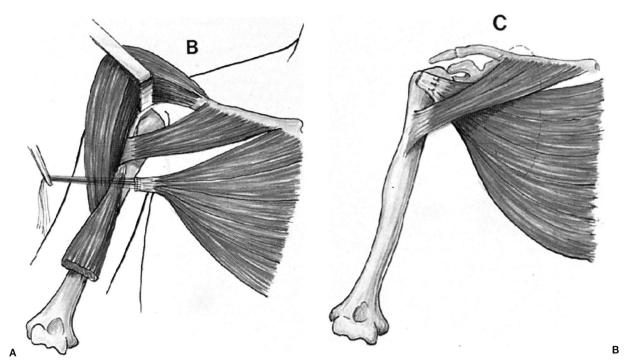

Fig 12-23. Illustration of split pectoralis major transfer. **A:** Harvest of sternal head. **B:** Transfer of sternal head to greater tuberosity. (Adapted from Warner JJP. Management of massive irreparable rotator cuff tears: the role of tendon transfer. *Instr Course Lect.* 2001;50:63.)

signs (70,168). A CT-arthrogram or MRI-arthrogram can also be helpful when evaluating the structural integrity of the subscapularis tendon. Three-dimensional imaging allows for the quantification of muscle atrophy, best observed on the axial and sagittal oblique views (169). On rare occasions, individuals who have had prior surgery may have subscapularis dysfunction due to denervation of the muscle, and in such settings an EMG may be helpful.

There are several published studies on rupture of the subscapularis tendon in association with instability (71,164, 170–175). Hauser (171) was the first to describe an isolated tear of the subscapularis tendon in association with anterior instability. Neviaser et al. (176) have emphasized that a rupture of the subscapularis tendon should be suspected in all cases of recurrent instability and in older patients after an initial anterior dislocation of their shoulder. Results of surgical treatment for subscapularis tendon tears are less successful than those reported for supraspinatus tears. Gerber and Krushell (70) have emphasized the importance of timely diagnosis and early surgical management. Results are significantly better if the duration between the traumatic event and the repair is short. Delay in diagnosis leads to retraction of the tendon and atrophy of the muscle such that tendon mobilization becomes difficult. Results of surgical repair are usually good for pain and instability, but many patients continue to have mild to moderate internal rotation weakness (70,71).

When the subscapularis tendon is deficient or irreparable, a pectoralis major muscle transfer may be used to augment or substitute for the subscapularis. Gerber et al. (70) originally described the surgical technique for the mobilization and repair of the subscapularis tendon and recommended that the inferior portion of the subscapularis tendon be repaired so that the pectoralis major transfer can be used simply to augment the function of the deficient upper part of the tendon **(Fig 12-23)**. There are several reports of transfer of the pectoralis major tendon for anterior shoulder instability in the literature (70,145,164,177–179). Decreased pain and restored stability are the main benefits of this surgery. Usually functional gains in term of mobility are variable and unfortunately more limited. Even when motion is improved in flexion and abduction, many individuals remain limited in overhead activities. In the majority of instances, the lift off test and the belly-press test remain positive post-operatively.

■ COMPLICATIONS AND PITFALLS

Recurrence

Recurrence is the most frequently reported complication after open and arthroscopic surgery for anterior instability (127–129,166,180–184). Recurrence may be secondary to new trauma or to atraumatic events (44,180,185). Patients with traumatic recurrence of their instability usually have better post-operative results after revision surgery than patients with atraumatic recurrence (140). The recurrence rate is related to the number of prior surgeries. For example,

Levine et al. (140) have shown that the recurrence rate in subjects who had one prior surgery was 17%, while in individuals with multiple failed prior surgeries it was 44%. The repetitive damage to the subscapularis and the capsule undoubtedly compromises further surgery and ultimate outcome.

A variety of factors can contribute to failure after open anterior instability surgery. The most common are incorrect diagnosis, incorrect or technically inaccurate surgical procedure, bone defect with loss of glenoid concavity, and anterior capsular deficiency. Examples of misdiagnosis are failure to recognize posterior or multidirectional instability patterns (38,129,180,184,186), failure to diagnose a significant voluntary component to the instability (49,187) or failure to recognize and treat associated injuries. Inaccurate or technically imprecise surgical procedures can also lead to recurrence. Subscapularis rupture is one such complication that can be devastating. Numerous studies have shown that residual Bankart lesions (188), under-corrected anterior capsular redundancy, and unrecognized laxity of the rotator interval (127–129,133,140,181,188) will result in recurrent instability. As discussed previously, defects in the glenoid concavity due to a bony Bankart lesion or an anterior glenoid rim erosion lead to an increased risk of recurrence (9,10,38,114).

Stiffness

Stiffness after surgery for open anterior instability is infrequently noted in literature and the incidence of this complication is probably under-reported (10,44,189). Certain repairs were designed to limit external rotation and hence the risk of recurrence, so loss of motion was not considered a complication. In some settings (e.g., capsular reconstruction or revision surgery), limited external rotation may be an expected outcome, and this should be conveyed to patients preoperatively. While loss of 10 degrees of external rotation may have little functional consequence for most individuals, it may be devastating for an overhead athlete. This is an important point that should be considered when selecting the procedure and when selectively shifting the capsule. Over-tightening should be avoided, as the over-constrained joint develops abnormal kinematics with shear across the articular cartilage, altered joint reactive forces, and premature degenerative arthrosis (190). Harryman et al. (191) have shown that passive motion of the glenohumeral joint is coupled reproducibly to translation of the humeral head on the glenoid. When the anterior capsule is overly tight, the humeral head has excessive posterior translation with external rotation. This posterior translation creates shearing forces on the posterior glenoid rim that may result in cartilage erosion and early osteoarthrosis (44,186,192). This phenomenon has been called "capsulorrhaphy arthropathy" or "arthritis of dislocation" and results from loss of motion with subsequent cartilage deterioration and joint arthrosis.

Unfortunately, there is no clear threshold beyond which these biomechanical consequences become realized. A loss of external rotation of greater than 30%, as compared with the controlateral shoulder, increases the risk of capsulorrhaphy arthropathy (44,186,192) and is a reasonable indication for a capsular release with or without a subscapularis lengthening.

Motion loss is best prevented at the time of surgical repair by physiologically tensioning the capsule while the arm is in abduction and external rotation. A rule of thumb is 30 degrees of external rotation and 30 degrees of abduction. This avoids over-constraint. Furthermore, proper rehabilitation postoperatively can prevent the development of excessive stiffness. When refractory motion loss persists, formal capsular release may be considered (190).

Subscapularis Deficiency

Rupture of the subscapularis after an anterior open instability repair causes significant functional disability, which may or may not be associated with recurrence of instability. Often such tears go unrecognized when patients present postoperatively with weakness and pain but no clear evidence of recurrent instability. A high index of suspicion and a careful physical examination is necessary in order to detect this problem.

When a subscapularis rupture occurs, repair poses a significant surgical challenge and risk for the surrounding neurovascular structures (193–195). Unless it is detected and addressed quickly, the subscapularis muscle and tendon are often retracted and adherent to the surroundings structures. The axillary nerve, musculocutaneous nerve, and brachial plexus are at risk. This problem is best avoided by meticulous repair of the tendon. If subscapularis rupture occurs, successful revision repair is often possible with direct repair of the tendon. In chronic cases, tendon transfer of the pectoralis is necessary as previously described (145).

Arthrosis

Glenohumeral arthrosis has been a well-described complication of various surgical procedures to correct shoulder instability (122,123,196–201). Over-tightening of the anterior structures, can result in stiffness, and drive the humeral head posteriorly, creating shear on the cartilage and early arthrosis. Some patients paradoxically may have instability and stiffness. They feel unstable because of excessive laxity in the axillary pouch and an untreated IGHL detachment, yet they are stiff because the MGHL, the rotator interval, and sometimes subscapularis are excessively tight. Complex releases with revision capsular shift may be required. An example might be Z-plasty subscapularis lengthening combined with an anterior-inferior selective capsular shift. Fortunately, such scenarios are rare.

Other causes of premature osteoarthrosis are iatrogenic, such as anterior impingement from a coracoid bone block that is placed too far laterally along the glenoid rim (122, 123,151,202), impingement on local hardware such as a screw, or incorrect intra-articular placement of metal anchors (200).

Hardware Problems

Any surgical implant has the potential to break, loosen, and migrate. Zuckerman et al. (200) have emphasized that loose hardware in the shoulder can migrate and may threaten the vital structures of the thorax. They also reported that most patients with hardware problems required additional surgery and had significant iatrogenic chondral defects. Moreover, when hardware needs to be removed, the potential always exists for significant bone defects that require grafting.

Neurovascular Injuries

The axillary nerve, musculocutaneous nerve, and brachial plexus are at risk during open surgery for anterior instability. Injuries may occur by excessive tissue retraction, especially retraction of the coracobrachialis, by direct laceration, or by suture entrapment. Fortunately, most are transient neurapraxias. Shoulder surgeons should be comfortable locating and isolating the axillary nerve, the musculocutaneous nerve, and the Brachial plexus, especially in revision settings. Of all the procedures described, the Bristow and Latarjet procedures have the highest reported risk of injury to the axillary and musculocutaneous nerves (152,193,195,203). Revision surgery after a failed Bristow or Latarjet can be quite challenging and exposing the axillary nerve in such instances can be quite difficult in open posterior instability surgery.

■ CONCLUSIONS

Although arthroscopic capsulolabral repair is becoming the standard of care for the treatment of traumatic recurrent shoulder instability, open approaches are still reliable, time tested options that in many instances remain the "gold standard." Despite tremendous advances in arthroscopic technique, significant bone loss, soft tissue deficiencies, and revision situations often require open approaches. As arthroscopic techniques continue to evolve, surgeons should carefully and continuously define their indications based on their surgical skill and on the spectrum of relevant pathology that may be faced. As detailed in this chapter, there are many instances in both primary and revision anterior instability shoulder surgery where open surgery remains the preferred method of treatment. A surgical approach that combines careful preoperative and intra-operative evaluation with a thoughtful and skillful technique will ensure the highest possibility of good and excellent surgical outcomes.

■ REFERENCES

1. Harryman DT II, Sidles JA, Harris SL, et al. The role of the rotator interval capsule in passive motion and stability of the shoulder. *J Bone Joint Surg Am.* 1992;74:53–66.
2. Glousman RE, Jobe F, Tibone J. et al. Dynamic electomyographic analysis of the throwing shoulder with glenohumeral jont instability. *J Bone Joint Surg Am.* 1988;70:220–226.
3. Joseph TA, Brems JJ. Multidirectional and posterior shoulder instability. In: Norris TR, ed. *Orthopaedic knowledge update: shoulder and elbow 2.* Rosemont, IL: American Academy of Orthopaedic Surgeons; 2002:91–102.
4. McMahon PJ, Jobe FW, Pink MM, et al. Comparative electromyographic analysis of shoulder muscles during planar motions: anterior glenohumeral instability versus normal. *J Shoulder Elbow Surg.* 1996;5(2 Pt 1):118–123.
5. Debski, RE, Wong EK, Woo SL-Y, et al. Contributions of the passive properties of the rotator cuff to glenohumeral stability during anterior-posterior loading. *J Shoulder Elbow Surg.* 1999; 8:324–329.
6. Warner JJ, McMahon PJ. The role of the long head of the biceps brachii in superior stability of the glenohumeral joint. *J Bone Joint Surg Am.* 1995;77:366–372.
7. Turkel SJ, Panio MW, Marshall JL, et al. Stabilization mechanisms preventing anterior dislocation of the glenohumeral joint. *J Bone Joint Surg Am.* 1981;62:1208–1217.
8. Kumar VP, Balasubramaniam P. The role of atmospheric pressure in stabilizing the shoulder: An experimental study. *J Bone Joint Surg Br.* 1985;67:719–721.
9. Lippit SB, Vanderhooft JE, Harris SL. Glenohumeral stability from concavity-compromise: a qualitative analysis. *J Shoulder Elbow Surg.* 1993;2:27–35.
10. Lazarus MD, Sidles JA, Harryman DT, et al. Effect of a chondral-labral defect on glenoid cavity and glenohumeral stability: a cadaveric model. *J Bone Joint Surg Am.* 1996;78:94–102.
11. Brenneke SL, et al. Glenohumeral kinematics and capsulo-ligamentous strain resulting from laxity exams. *Clin Biomech* (Bristol, Avon), 2000;15:735–742.
12. Bigliani LU, et al. Glenohumeral stability. Biomechanical properties of passive and active stabilizers. *Clin Orthop.* 1996;330:13–30.
13. McMahon PJ, et al. Shoulder muscle forces and tendon excursions during glenohumeral abduction in the scapular plane. *J Shoulder Elbow Surg.* 1995;4:199–208.
14. Debski RE, et al. In situ force distribution in the glenohumeral joint capsule during anterior-posterior loading. *J Orthop Res.* 1999;17:769–776.
15. Wulker N, et al. [Measurement of glenohumeral joint translation with a dynamic shoulder model]. *Z Orthop Ihre Grenzgeb.* 1996;134:67–72.
16. Karduna AR, et al. Kinematics of the glenohumeral joint: influences of muscle forces, ligamentous constraints, and articular geometry. *J Orthop Res.* 1996;14:986–993.
17. Cole BJ, Katolik LI. The shoulder. In: Miller MD, Cooper DE, Warner JJ, eds. *Review of sports medicine and arthroscopy.* Philadelphia: WB Saunders; 2002:142–218.
18. Warner JJ, et al. Static capsuloligamentous restraints to superior-inferior translation of the glenohumeral joint. *Am J Sports Med.* 1992;20:625–685.
19. Cole BJ, Warner JJ. Anatomy, biomechanics, and pathophysiology of glenohumeral instability. In: Iannotti JP, Williams GR, eds. *Disorders of the shoulder: diagnosis and management.* Philadelphia: Lippincott Williams & Wilkins; 1999:207–231.
20. Warner JJ, Caborn DN. Overview of shoulder instability. *Crit Rev Phys Rehabil Med.* 1992;4:145–198.
21. Blasier RB, et al. Posterior glenohumeral subluxation: Active and passive stabilization in a biomechanical model. *J Bone Joint Surg Am.* 1997;79:433–440.

22. Cole BJ, et al. The anatomy and histology of the rotator interval capsule in the shoulder. *Clin Orthop.* 2001;390:129–137.

23. Fitzpatrick MJ, et al. Instructional course lecture 106: the anatomy, pathology, and definitive treatment of rotator interval lesions: current concepts. *Arthroscopy.* 2003;19:70–79.

24. Apreleva M, et al. A dynamic analysis of the glenohumeral motion after simulated capsulolabral injury: a cadaver model. *J Bone Joint Surg Am.* 1998;80:474–480.

25. Soslowsky LJ, Malicky DM, Blasier RB. Active and passive factors in inferior glenohumeral stabilization: a biomechanical model. *J Shoulder Elbow Surg.* 1997;6:371–379.

26. Warner JJ, et al. Effect of joint compression on inferior stability of the glenohumeral joint. *J Shoulder Elbow Surg.* 1999;8:31–36.

27. Glousman R. Electromyographic analysis and its role in the athletic shoulder. *Clin Orthop.* 1993;288:27–34.

28. Basmajian JV. The upper limb. In: Muscles Alive. 4th ed. Baltimore: Williams & Wilkins; 1974;189–212.

29. Cools AM, et al. Scapular muscle recruitment patterns: trapezius muscle latency with and without impingement symptoms. *Am J Sports Med.* 2003;31:542–549.

30. Warner JJ, Micheli LJ, Arslanian LE, et al. Scapulothoracic motion in normal shoulders and shoulders with glenohumeral instability and impingement syndrome. *Clin Orthop.* 1992;285:191–199.

31. Warner JJ, Micheli LJ, Arslanian LE, et al. Patterns of flexibility, laxity, and strength in normal shoulders and shoulders with instability and impingement. *Am J Sports Med.* 1990;18:366–75.

32. Kibler WB. The role of the scapula in athletic shoulder function. *Am J Sports Med.* 1998;26:325–337.

33. Bankart ASB. The pathology and treatment of recurrent dislocations of the shoulder joint. *Br J Surg.* 1939;26:23–29.

34. Bankart ASB. Recurrent or habitual dislocation of the shoulder joint. *BMJ.* 1923;2:1132–1133.

35. Taylor DC, Arciero RA. Arthroscopic and physical examination findings in first-time, traumatic anterior dislocations. *Am J Sports Med.* 1997;25:306–311.

36. Burkhart SS, De Beer JF. Traumatic glenohumeral bone defects and their relationship to failure of arthroscopic Bankart repairs: Significance of the inverted-pear glenoid and the humeral engaging Hill-Sachs lesion. *Arthroscopy.* 2000;16:677–694.

37. Gerber C, Nyffeler RW. Abstract: Pathology of dislocated Bankart facture: Experimental and clinical assessment. *J Bone Joint Surg Br.* 1999;81:133–134.

38. Gerber C, Nyffeler RW. Classification of glenohumeral joint instability. *Clin Orthop.* 2002;400:65–76.

39. Gill TJ, et al. Glenoid reconstruction for recurrent anterior shoulder instability. In: *Read at Annual Meeting of the Academy of Orthopaedic Surgeons.* San Francisco; CA: Mar 10–14, 2004.

40. Wolf EM, Cheng JC, Dickson K. Humeral avulsion of the glenohumeral ligaments as a cause of anterior shoulder instability. *Arthroscopy.* 1995;11:600–607.

41. Boker DJ, Conboy VB, Olson C. Anterior instability of the glenohumeral joint with humeral avulsion of the glenohumeral ligaments: a review of 41 cases. *J Bone Joint Surg Br.* 1999; 81:93–96.

42. Millett PJ, Clavert P, Warner JJ. Arthroscopic management of anterior, posterior, and multidirectional shoulder instability: pearls and pitfalls. *Arthroscopy.* 2003;19:86–93.

43. Lazarus MD, Harryman DT II. Complications of open anterior stabilization of the shoulder. *J Am Acad Orthop Surg.* 2000;8:122–132.

44. Hawkins RJ, Angelo RL. Glenohumeral osteoarthrosis: A late complication of the Putti-Platt repair. *J Bone Joint Surg Am.* 1990;72:1193–1197.

45. Hintermann B, Gachter A. Arthroscopic findings after shoulder dislocation. *Am J Sports Med.* 1995;23:545–551.

46. Pagnani MJ, et al. Role of the long head of the biceps brachii in glenohumeral stability: a biomechanical study in cadavera. *J Shoulder Elbow Surg.* 1996;5:255–262.

47. Gerber C, Lambert SM. Allograft reconstruction of segmental defects in the humeral head for the treatment of chronic locked posterior dislocation of the shoulder. *J Bone Joint Surg Am.* 1996;78:376–382.

48. Silliman JF, Hawkins RJ. Classification and physical diagnosis of instability of the shoulder. *Clin Orthop.* 1993;291:7–10.

49. Rowe CR, Pierce DS, Clark JG. Voluntary dislocation of the shoulder: A preliminary report on a clinical, electromyographic, and psychiatric study of twenty-six patients. *J Bone Joint Surg Am.* 1973;55:445.

50. Allen AA, Warner JJ. Shoulder instability in the athlete. *Orthop Clin North Am.* 1995;26:487–490.

51. Jobe FW, et al. Anterior capsulolabral reconstruction of the shoulder in athletes in overhand sports. *Am J Sports Med.* 1991; 19:428–434.

52. Treacy SH, Field LD, Savoie FH. Rotator interval capsular closure: an arthroscopic technique. *Arthroscopy.* 1997;13:103–105.

53. Cave RB, Rowe CR. Capsular repair for recurrent dislocation of the shoulder: pathologic findings and operative technique. *Surg Clin North Am.* 1947;27:1289–1292.

54. Fronek J, Warren RF, Bowen MK. Posterior subluxation of the glenohumeral joint. *J Bone Joint Surg Am.* 1989;71:205–208.

55. Gerber C. Observations on the classification of instability. In: Warner JJ, Iannotti JP, Gerber C, eds. *Complex and revision problems in shoulder surgery.* Philadelphia: Lippincott-Raven Publishers; 1997:9–12.

56. Tibone JE, Bradley JP. The treatment of posterior subluxation in athletes. *Clin Orthop.* 1993;291:124–126.

57. Warren RF. Subluxation of the shoulder in athletes. *Clin Sports Med.* 1983;2:339–342.

58. Boyd HB, Sisk TD. Recurrent posterior dislocation of the shoulder. *J Bone Joint Surg Am.* 1972;54:779–780.

59. Noble W. Posterior traumatic dislocation of the shoulder. *J Bone Joint Surg Am.* 1962;44:523–524.

60. Hawkins RJ, et al. Locked posterior dislocation of the shoulder. *J Bone Joint Surg Am.* 1987;69:9–11.

61. Jones D, Warner JJ. Shoulder instability. In: Chapman MW, ed. *Chapman's orthopaedic sugery.* Philadelphia: Lippincott Williams & Wilkins; 2001.

62. Townley CO. The capsular mechanism in recurrent dislocation of the shoulder. *J Bone Joint Surg Am.* 1950;32:370–373.

63. Jobe CM, et al. Anterior instability, impingement, and rotator cuff tear. In: Jobe FW, et al., eds. *Operative techniques in upper extremity sports injuries.* St. Louis, MO: Mosby-Year Book; 1996: 164–177.

64. Jobe FW, Jobe CM. Painful athletic injuries of the shoulder. *Clin Orthop.* 1983;173:117–124.

65. Grossman MG, et al. A cadaveric model of the throwing shoulder. Possible etiology of SLAP lesions. In: *Orthopaedic research society.* New Orleans, LA: 2003.

66. Kuhn JE, et al. Failure of the biceps superior labral complex: A cadaveric biomechanical investigation comparing late cocking and early deceleration positions of throwing. *Arthroscopy.* 2003;19:373–379.

67. De Laat EA, et al. Nerve lesions in primary shoulder dislocations and humeral neck fractures: a prospective clinical and EMG study. *J Bone Joint Surg Br.* 1994;76:381–384.

68. Groh GI, Rockwood CA. The terrible triad: Anterior dislocation of the shoulder with rupture of the rotator cuff and injury to the brachial plexus. *J Shoulder Elbow Surg.* 1995;4:51–54.

69. Hawkins RJ, et al. Anterior dislocation of the shoulder in the older patient. *Clin Orthop.* 1986;206:192–196.

70. Gerber C, Kuechle DK. Isolated rupture of the tendon of the subscapularis muscle: clinical features of six cases. *J Bone Joint Surg Br.* 1991;73:389–391.

71. Warner JJ, Allen AA, Gerber C. Diagnosis and management of subscapularis tendon tears. *Oper Tech Orthop.* 1994;9:116–119.

72. Neer CS, Foster CR. Inferior capsular shift for involuntary instability and multidirectional instability of the shoulder: a preliminary report. *J Bone Joint Surg Am*. 1980;62:897–899.

73. Kvitne RS, Jobe FW. The diagnosis and treatment of anterior instability in the throwing. *Clin Orthop*. 1993;291:107–110.

74. Speer KP, et al. An evaluation of the shoulder relocation test. *Am J Sports Med*. 1994;22:177–180.

75. Gerber C, Ganz R. Clinical assessment of instability of the shoulder: with special reference to anterior and posterior drawer tests. *J Bone Joint Surg Br*. 1984;66:551–553.

76. Altchek DW, et al. T-plasty modification of the Bankart procedure for multidirectional instability of the anterior and inferior types. *J Bone Joint Surg Am*. 1991;73:105–109.

77. Cofield RH, Nessler JP, Weinstabl R. Diagnosis of shoulder instability by examination under anesthesia. *Clin Orthop*. 1993;291:45–47.

78. Hawkins RH, et al. Translation of the glenohumeral joint with the patient under anesthesia. *J Shoulder Elbow Surg*. 1996;5:286–289.

79. O'Brien SJ, et al. The anatomy and histology of the inferior glenohumeral ligament complex of the shoulder. *Am J Sports Med*. 1990;18:449–453.

80. O'Brien SJ, et al. Capsular restraints to anterior-posterior motion of the abducted shoulder: a biomechanical study. *J Shoulder Elbow Surg*. 1995;4:298–301.

81. Lerat JL, et al. Dynamic anterior jerk of the shoulder: a new clinical test for shoulder instability: a preliminary study. *Rev Chir Orthop Reparatrice Appar Mot*. 1994;80:461–462.

82. Blasier RB, et al. Posterior glenohumeral subluxation: Active and passive stabilization in a biomechanical model. *J Bone Joint Surg Am*. 1997;79:433–435.

83. Romeo AA. *Rotator Interval: Anatomy, pathology, and treatment options*. In: *AANA Fall Course*. Palm Springs, CA; 2002.

84. Hawkins RH. Arthroscopic staple repair for shoulder instability: a retrospective study of fifty patients. *Arthroscopy*. 1989;5:122–124.

85. Gagey OJ, Gagey N. The hyperabduction test. *J Bone Joint Surg Br*. 2001;83:69–74.

86. Andrews JR, Carson WGJ, McLeod WD. Glenoid labrum tears related to the long head of the biceps. *Am J Sports Med*. 1985;19:428–434.

87. Snyder SJ, et al. SLAP lesions of the shoulder. *Arthroscopy*. 1990;6:274–276.

88. O'Brien SJ, et al. The active compression test: a new and effective test for diagnosing labral tears and acromioclavicular joint abnormality. *Am J Sports Med*. 1998;26:610–613.

89. Stetson WB, Templin K. The crank test, the O'Brien test, and routine magnetic resonance imaging scans in the diagnosis of labral tears. *Am J Sports Med*. 2002;30:806–809.

90. McFarland EG, Kim TK, Savino RM. Clinical assessment of three common tests for superior labral anterior-posterior lesions. *Am J Sports Med*. 2002;30:810–815.

91. Pavlov H, et al. Roentgenographic evaluation of anterior shoulder instability. *Clin Orthop*. 1985;194:153–154.

92. Engebretsen L, Craig EV. Radiographic features of shoulder instability. *Clin Orthop*. 1993;291:29–31.

93. Goss TP. Fractures of the glenoid cavity. *J Bone Joint Surg Am*. 1992;74:299–302.

94. Green M, Christensen K. Magnetic resonance imaging of the shoulder. Sensitivity, specificity, and predictive value. *J Bone Joint Surg Am*. 1994;22:493–498.

95. Iannotti JP, Zlatkin M, Esterhai J. Magnetic resonance imaging of the shoulder. *J Bone Joint Surg Am*. 1991;73:17–29.

96. Kinnard P, Tricoire J, Levesque J. Assessment of the unstable shoulder by computed tomography: a preliminary report. *Am J Sports Med*. 1983;11:157–159.

97. Singson R, Feldman F, Bigliani LU. CT arthrographic patterns in recurrent glenohumeral instability. *Am J Roentgenol*. 1987;149:749–753.

98. Burkhead WZ, Rockwood CA, Treatment of instability of the shoulder with an exercise program. *J Bone Joint Surg Am*. 1992;74:890–894.

99. Holevius L, et al. Primary anterior dislocation of the shoulder in young patients: A ten-year prospective study. *J Bone Joint Surg Am*. 1996;78:1677–1684.

100. Kirkley A, et al. Prospective randomized clinical trial comparing the effectiveness of immediate arthroscopic stabilization versus immobilization and rehabilitation in first time traumatic anterior dislocations of the shoulder. *Arthroscopy*. 1999;15:507–514.

101. Rowe CR, Sakellarides H. Factors related to recurrence of anterior dislocations of the shoulder. *Clin Orthop*. 1961;20:40–48.

102. Holevius L. Anterior dislocation of the shoulder in teen-agers and young adults: five-year prognosis. *J Bone Joint Surg Am*. 1987;69:393–396.

103. Micheli LJ. Sports injuries in children and adolescents: questions and controversies. *Clin Sports Med*. 1995;14:727–730.

104. Marans HJ, et al. The fate of the traumatic anterior dislocation of the shoulder in children. *J Bone Joint Surg Am*. 1992;74:1242–1246.

105. Arciero RA, et al. Arthroscopic Bankart repair versus nonoperative treatment for acute, initial anterior shoulder dislocation. *Am J Sports Med*. 1994;22:589–594.

106. Burkhart SS, Morgan CD, Kibler WB. Current concepts: the disabled shoulder: spectrum of pathology Part I. Pathoanatomy and biomechanics. *Arthroscopy*. 2003;19:404–420.

107. Speer KP, Deng X, Borrero S. A biomechanical evaluation of the Bankart lesion. *J Bone Joint Surg Am*. 1994;76:1819–1826.

108. D'Alession JG, Rosenblum M, Shea KP. A retrospective comparison of interscalene block and general anesthesia for ambulatory shoulder surgery. *Reg Anesth*. 1995;20:62–68.

108a. Costouros JG, Clavert P, Warner JJ. Trans-cuff portal for arthroscopic posterior capsulorrhaphy. *Arthroscopy*. 2006;22(10):1138.

109. Rowe CR, Patel D, Southmayd WW. The Bankart procedure: a long-term end-result study. *J Bone Joint Surg Am*. 1978;60:1–16.

110. Burkhart SS, et al. Quantifying glenoid bone loss arthroscopically in shoulder instability. *Arthroscopy*. 2002;18:488–491.

111. Edelson JG. Bony changes of the glenoid as a consequence of shoulder instability. *J Shoulder Elbow Surg*. 1996;5:293–298.

112. Greis PE, et al. Glenohumeral articular contact areas and pressures following labral and osseous injury to the anteroinferior quadrant of the glenoid. *J Shoulder Elbow Surg*. 2002;11:442–451.

113. Habermeyer P, Gleyze P, Rickert M. Evolution of lesions of the labrum-ligament complex in posttraumatic anterior shoulder instability: a prospective study. *J Shoulder Elbow Surg*. 1999;8:66–74.

114. Itoi E, et al. The effect of a glenoid defect on anteroinferior stability of the shoulder after Bankart repair: a cadaveric study. *J Bone Joint Surg Am*. 2000;82:35–46.

115. Itoi E, et al. A new method of immobilization after traumatic anterior dislocation of the shoulder: a preliminary study. *J Shoulder Elbow Surg*. 2003;12:413–415.

116. Lazarus MD, et al. Effect of a chondral-labral defect on glenoid concavity and glenohumeral stability. A cadaveric model. *J Bone Joint Surg Am*. 1996;78:94–102.

117. Gerber A, Apreleva M, Warner JJ. The basic science of glenohumeral instability. In: Norlin R, ed. *Orthopaedic knowledge update: shoulder and elbow 2*. Rosemont, IL: American Academy of Orthopaedic Surgeons; 2002:13–22.

118. Helfet AJ. Coracoid transplantation for recurring dislocation of the shoulder. *J Bone Joint Surg Br*. 1958;40B:198–192.

119. Latarjet M. Technic of coracoid preglenoid arthroereisis in the treatment of recurrent dislocation of the shoulder. *Lyon Chir*. 1958;54:604–607.

120. Magnuson PB, Stack JK. Recurrent dislocation of the shoulder. *JAMA*. 1943;123:889–892.

121. Osmond-Clarke H. Habitual dislocation of the shoulder. *J Bone Joint Surg Br*. 1948;30:19–25.

122. Walch G, et al. L'opération de Trillat pour luxation définitive antérieure de l'épaule. Résultats à long terme de 250 cas avec un recul moyen de 11,3 ans. *Lyon Chir.* 1989;85:25–31.

123. Allain J, Goutallier D, Glorion C. Long-term results of the Latarjet procedure for the treatment of anterior instability of the shoulder. *J Bone Joint Surg Am.* 1998;80:841–852.

124. Barry TP, et al. The coracoid transfer for recurrent anterior instability of the shoulder in adolescents. *J Bone Joint Surg Am.* 1985;67:383–387.

125. Lombardo SJ, et al. The modified Bristow procedure for recurrent dislocation of the shoulder. *J Bone Joint Surg Am.* 1976;58:256–261.

126. Dewaal Malefijt J, Ooms AJ, Vanrens TJ. A comparison of the results of the Bristow-Latarjet procedure and the Bankart/Putti-Platt operation for recurrent anterior dislocation of the shoulder. *Acta Orthop Belgica.* 1985;51:831–842.

127. Rowe CR, Zarins B, Ciullo JV. Recurrent anterior dislocation of the shoulder after surgical repair. Apparent causes of failure and treatment. *J Bone Joint Surg Am.* 1984;66:159–168.

128. Hovelius L, Thorling J, Fredin H. Recurrent anterior dislocation of the shoulder. Results after the Bankart and Putti-Platt operations. *J Bone Joint Surg Am.* 1979;61:566–569.

129. McAuliffe TB, Pangayatselvan T, Bayley I. Failed surgery for recurrent anterior dislocation of the shoulder. Causes and management. *J Bone Joint Surg Br.* 1988;70:798–801.

130. Cadenat FM. The treatment of dislocations and fractures of the outer end of the clavicle. *Int Clinics.* 1917;1:145–169.

131. Karadimas J, Rentis G, Varouchas G. Repair of recurrent anterior dislocation of the shoulder using transfer of the subscapularis tendon. *J Bone Joint Surg Am.* 1980;62:1147–1149.

132. Gill TJ, et al. Bankart repair for anterior instability of the shoulder. Long-term outcome. *J Bone Joint Surg Am.* 1997;79(6):850–857.

133. Zabinski SJ, et al. Revision shoulder stabilization: 2- to 10-year results. *J Shoulder Elbow Surg.* 1999;8:58–65.

134. Young DC, Rockwood CA Jr. Complications of a failed Bristow procedure and their management. *J Bone Joint Surg Am.* 1991;73:969–981.

135. Hubbell JB, et al. Comparison of shoulder stabilization using arthroscopic transglenoid sutures versus open capsulolabral repairs: a 5-year minimum follow-up. *Am J Sports Med.* 2004;32:650–654.

136. Clare DJ, et al. Shoulder arthrodesis. *J Bone Joint Surg Am.* 2001;83A:593–600.

137. Gonzalez-Diaz R, Rodriguez-Merchan EC, Gilbert MS. The role of shoulder fusion in the era of arthroplasty. *Int Orthop.* 1997;21:204–209.

138. Diaz JA, et al. Arthrodesis as a salvage procedure for recurrent instability of the shoulder. *J Shoulder Elbow Surg.* 2003;12:237–241.

139. Rouholamin E, Wootton JR, Jamieson AM, Arthrodesis of the shoulder following brachial plexus injury. *Injury.* 1991;22:271–274.

140. Levine WN, et al. Open revision stabilization surgery for recurrent anterior glenohumeral instability. *Am J Sports Med.* 2000;28:156–160.

141. Hattrup SJ, Cofield RH, Weaver AL. Anterior shoulder reconstruction: prognostic variables. *J Shoulder Elbow Surg.* 2001;10:508–513.

142. Warner JJ, et al. Technique for selecting capsular tightness in repair of anterior-inferior shoulder instability. *J Shoulder Elbow Surg.* 1995;4:352–364.

143. Cole BJ, et al. Comparison of arthroscopic and open anterior shoulder stabilization. A two to six-year follow-up study. *J Bone Joint Surg Am.* 2000;82A:1108–1114.

144. Rowe CR. Dislocation of the shoulder. In: Rowe CR, ed. *The shoulder.* New York: Churchill Livingstone; 1988:165–291.

145. Gerber C, et al. Effect of selective capsulorrhaphy on the passive range of motion of the glenohumeral joint. *J Bone Joint Surg Am.* 2003;85A:48–55.

146. Sugaya H, et al. Glenoid rim morphology in recurrent anterior glenohumeral instability. *J Bone Joint Surg Am.* 2003;85A:878–884.

147. O'Brien SJ, Warren RF, Schwartz E. Anterior shoulder instability. *Orthop Clin North Am.* 1987;18:395–408.

148. Bodey WN, Denham RA. A free bone block operation for recurrent anterior dislocation of the shoulder joint. *Injury.* 1983;15:184–188.

149. Haaker RG, Eickhoff U, Klammer HL. Intraarticular autogenous bone grafting in recurrent shoulder dislocations. *Mil Med.* 1993;158:164–169.

150. Hutchinson JW, Neumann L, Wallace WA. Bone buttress operation for recurrent anterior shoulder dislocation in epilepsy. *J Bone Joint Surg Br.* 1995;77:928–932.

151. Hovelius L, et al. The coracoid transfer for recurrent dislocation of the shoulder. Technical aspects of the Bristow-Latarjet procedure. *J Bone Joint Surg Am.* 1983;65:926–934.

152. Levigne C. Long-term results of anterior coracoid abutments: apropos of 52 cases with homogenous 12-year follow-up. *Rev Chir Orthop Reparatrice Appar Mot.* 2000;86(suppl 1):114–121.

153. Ungersbock A, Michel M, Hertel R. Factors influencing the results of a modified Bankart procedure. *J Shoulder Elbow Surg.* 1995;4:365–369.

154. Ito H, Takayama A, Shirai Y. Radiographic evaluation of the Hill-Sachs lesion in patients with recurrent anterior shoulder instability. *J Shoulder Elbow Surg.* 2000;9:495–497.

155. Burkhart SS, Danaceau SM. Articular arc length mismatch as a cause of failed Bankart repair. *Arthroscopy.* 2000;16:740–744.

156. Yagishita K, Thomas BJ. Use of allograft for large Hill-Sachs lesion associated with anterior glenohumeral dislocation. a case report. *Injury.* 2002;33:791–794.

157. Weber BG, Simpson LA, Hardegger F. Rotational humeral osteotomy for recurrent anterior dislocation of the shoulder associated with a large Hill-Sachs lesion. *J Bone Joint Surg Am.* 1984;66:1443–1450.

158. Richards RR, et al. Shoulder arthrodesis using a pelvic-reconstruction plate. A report of eleven cases. *J Bone Joint Surg Am.* 1988;70:416–421.

159. Richards RR, Beaton D, Hudson AR. Shoulder arthrodesis with plate fixation: functional outcome analysis. *J Shoulder Elbow Surg.* 1993;2:225–239.

160. McFarland EG, et al. Histologic evaluation of the shoulder capsule in normal shoulders, unstable shoulders, and after failed thermal capsulorrhaphy. *Am J Sports Med.* 2002;30:636–642.

161. Wong KL, Williams GR. Complications of thermal capsulorrhaphy of the shoulder. *J Bone Joint Surg Am.* 2001;83(suppl 2): 151–155.

162. Ianotti JP, et al. Iliotibial band reconstruction for treatment of glenohumeral instability associated with irreparable capsular deficiency. *J Shoulder Elbow Surg.* 2002;11:618–623.

163. Moeckel BH, et al. Instability of the shoulder after arthroplasty. *J Bone Joint Surg Am.* 1993;75:492–497.

164. Resch H, et al. Transfer of the pectoralis major muscle for the treatment of irreparable rupture of the subscapularis tendon. *J Bone Joint Surg Am.* 2000;82:372–382.

165. Warner JJ, et al. Management of anterior capsular deficiency of the shoulder. Report of one case following manipulation for adhesive capsulitis. *Clin J Sports Med.* 1992;2:71–72.

166. Lazarus MD, Harryman DT. Open repair for anterior instability. In: Warner JJ, Ianotti JP, Gerber C, eds. *Complex and revision problems in shoulder surgery.* Philadelphia: Lippincott Raven Publishers; 1997:47–63.

167. Gallie WE, Le Menuisier AB. Recurring dislocation of the shoulder. *J Bone Joint Surg Br.* 1948;30B:9–18.

168. Gerber C, Hersche O, Farron A. Isolated rupture of the sub-scapularis tendon. *J Bone Joint Surg Am.* 1996;78:1015–1023.
169. Goutallier D, et al. Fatty muscle degeneration in cuff ruptures. Pre- and postoperative evaluation by CT scan. *Clin Orthop Relat Res.* 1994;304:78–83.
170. Wirth MA, Blatter G, Rockwood CA Jr. The capsular imbrication procedure for recurrent anterior instability of the shoulder. *J Bone Joint Surg Am.* 1996;78:246–259.
171. Hauser ED. Avulsion of the tendon of the subscapularis muscle. *J Bone Joint Surg Am.* 1954;36A:139–41.
172. Ticker JB, Warner JJ. Single-tendon tears of the rotator cuff. Evaluation and treatment of subscapularis tears and principles of treatment for supraspinatus tears. *Orthop Clin North Am.* 1997;28:99–116.
173. Deutsch A, et al. Traumatic tears of the subscapularis tendon. Clinical diagnosis, magnetic resonance imaging findings, and operative treatment. *Am J Sports Med.* 1997;25:13–22.
174. Gerber C, Fuchs B, Hodler J. The results of repair of massive tears of the rotator cuff. *J Bone Joint Surg Am.* 2000;82:505–515.
175. Nove-Josserand L, et al. Isolated lesions of the subscapularis muscle. Apropos of 21 cases. *Rev Chir Orthop Reparatrice Appar Mot.* 1994;80:595–601.
176. Neviaser RJ, Neviaser TJ, Neviaser JS. Concurrent rupture of the rotator cuff and anterior dislocation of the shoulder in the older patient. *J Bone Joint Surg Am.* 1988;70:1308–1311.
177. Wirth MA, Rockwood CA Jr. Operative treatment of irreparable rupture of the subscapularis. *J Bone Joint Surg Am.* 1997;79:722–731.
178. Warner JJ. Management of massive irreparable rotator cuff tears: the role of tendon transfer. *Instr Course Lect.* 2001;50:63–71.
179. Galatz LM, et al. Pectoralis major transfer for anterior-superior subluxation in massive rotator cuff insufficiency. *J Shoulder Elbow Surg.* 2003;12:1–5.
180. Burkhead WZ, Richie MF. Revision of failed shoulder reconstruction. *Contemps Orthop.* 1992;24:126–133.
181. Norris TR. Complications following anterior instability repairs. In: Bigliani LU, ed. *Complications of shoulder surgery.* Baltimore: Williams & Wilkins; 1993:98–116.
182. Norris TR, Thomas SC, Rockwood CA Jr. Anterior glenohumeral stability. In: Rockwood CA Jr, Matsen FA III, eds. *The shoulder.* Philadelphia: WB Saunders; 1990:547–551.
183. Norris TR, Bigliani LU. Analysis of failed repair for shoulder instability: a preliminary report. In: Bateman JE, Welch RP, eds. *Surgery of the shoulder.* Philadelphia: BC Decker; 1984:111–116.
184. Hawkins RH, Hawkins RJ. Failed anterior reconstruction for shoulder instability. *J Bone Joint Surg Br.* 1985;67:709–714.
185. Youssef JA, et al. Arthroscopic Bankart suture repair for recurrent traumatic unidirectional anterior shoulder dislocations. *Arthroscopy.* 1995;11:561–563.
186. Matsen FA, et al. Practical evaluation and management of the shoulder. Philadelphia: WB Saunders; 1994.
187. Fuchs B, Jost B, Gerber C. Posterior-inferior capsular shift for the treatment of recurrent, voluntary posterior subluxation of the shoulder. *J Bone Joint Surg Am.* 2000;82:16–25.
188. Rowe CR, Zarins B. Recurrent transient subluxation of the shoulder. *J Bone Joint Surg Am.* 1981;63:863–872.
189. Lusardi DA, et al. Loss of external rotation following anterior capsulorrhaphy of the shoulder. *J Bone Joint Surg Am.* 1993;75:1185–1192.
190. Werner CM, et al. The effect of capsular tightening on humeral head translations. *J Orthop Res.* 2004;22:194–201.
191. Harryman DT II, et al. Translation of the humeral head on the glenoid with passive glenohumeral motion. *J Bone Joint Surg Am.* 1990;72:1334–1343.
192. Walch G, et al. Static posterior subluxation of the humeral head: an unrecognized entity responsible for glenohumeral osteoarthritis in the young adult. *J Shoulder Elbow Surg.* 2002;11:309–314.
193. Flatow EL, Bigliani LU, April EW. An anatomic study of the musculocutaneous nerve and its relationship to the coracoid process. *Clin Orthop Relat Res.* 1989;244:166–171.
194. McFarland EG, et al. Prevention of axillary nerve injury in anterior shoulder reconstructions: use of a subscapularis muscle-splitting technique and a review of the literature. *Am J Sports Med.* 2002;30:601–606.
195. Bryan WJ, Schauder K, Tullos HS. The axillary nerve and its relationship to common sports medicine shoulder procedures. *Am J Sports Med.* 1986;14:113–116.
196. Morrey BF, Janes JM. Recurrent anterior dislocation of the shoulder. Long-term follow-up of the Putti-Platt and Bankart procedures. *J Bone Joint Surg Am.* 1976;58:252–256.
197. O'Driscoll SW, Evans DC. Long-term results of staple capsulorrhaphy for anterior instability of the shoulder. *J Bone Joint Surg Am.* 1993;75:249–258.
198. Rosenberg BN, Richmond JC, Levine WN. Long-term followup of Bankart reconstruction. Incidence of late degenerative glenohumeral arthrosis. *Am J Sports Med.* 1995;23:538–544.
199. Cameron ML, et al. The prevalence of glenohumeral osteoarthrosis in unstable shoulders. *Am J Sports Med.* 2003;31:53–55.
200. Zuckerman JD, Matsen FA III. Complications about the glenohumeral joint related to the use of screws and staples. *J Bone Joint Surg Am.* 1984;66:175–180.
201. Trevlyn DW, Richardson MW, Ranelli GC. Degenerative joint disease following extraarticular anterior shoulder reconstruction. *Contemp Orthop.* 1992;25:151–156.
202. Torg JS, et al. A modified Bristow-Helfet-May procedure for recurrent dislocation and subluxation of the shoulder. Report of two hundred and twelve cases. *J Bone Joint Surg Am.* 1987;69:904–913.
203. Burkhead WZ, Scheinberg RR, Box G. Surgical anatomy of the axillary nerve. *J Shoulder Elbow Surg.* 1992;1:31–36.

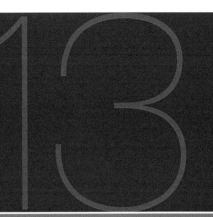

THE ROTATOR CUFF

RICHARD K.N. RYU, MD, GRAHAM R. HURVITZ, MD

■ KEY POINTS

- The majority of symptomatic rotator cuff disease patients respond to a nonoperative program emphasizing the restoration of normal biomechanics, unrestricted motion, and functional force couples.
- Early surgical management should be considered for acute rotator cuff tears in physiologically young and very active individuals.
- The ability to recognize the complex layered anatomy in addition to the tear configuration is critical if an anatomic repair is to be achieved.
- The rotator cuff muscles centralize the humeral head and permit a single center of rotation while providing stability and strength. During active shoulder elevation, the rotator cuff muscles depress the humeral head, allowing efficient elevation of the extremity.
- When surgery is necessary, the goal should be to properly and anatomically restore the balanced forces of the supraspinatus and deltoid muscles so that their counteraction is maintained.
- Tearing of the rotator cuff as a function of age is a common occurrence. Many of these tears may be clinically silent.
- Mechanical impingement is the most common recognizable source of recurring rotator cuff pain and disability in the active population. When impingement-type symptoms present in a younger patient, great care must be taken to avoid overtreating because the impingement may be internal or may be secondary to instability which effectively moves the cuff closer to the arch.
- The unaffected shoulder can serve as a "normal" template for comparison during physical examination. One

should survey for atrophy or asymmetry, especially in the supra- and infraspinatus fossae. Long-standing rotator cuff tears are often accompanied by significant, visible atrophy.
- The initial evaluation of the painful shoulder should include quality plain radiographs. The standard radiographs should include a true anterior-posterior view with the shoulder in the internal and neutral position, an axillary view and the outlet (supraspinatus) view described by Neer and Poppen which is used to evaluate and classify acromial morphology and arch anatomy.
- Magnetic resonance imaging (MRI) is the test of choice when evaluating the soft tissues of the shoulder. T1 weighted images revealing increased signal in the rotator cuff, combined with a focal defect or loss of continuity of the cuff on the T2 weighted image, is a common finding when a full or partial-thickness tear is encountered.
- MRI scans for those anticipating shoulder surgery can be helpful in evaluating tears, assessing possible atrophy, and establishing the presence of co-morbidities.

Injuries to the rotator cuff occur commonly. Treatment for these common disorders is most effective when a management algorithm can be developed based on a keen understanding of pertinent anatomy, pathology, and outcomes studies supporting specific treatment. Suffice to say that the majority of patients with symptomatic rotator cuff disease respond to a well-planned, nonoperative program emphasizing the restoration of normal biomechanics, unrestricted motion, and functional force couples. Clearly there will be

201

those patients in whom the pathology has progressed to a point where surgical intervention may be appropriate.

This chapter is organized into three sections: The first details the anatomy, biology, function, and pathoanatomy; the second section focuses on the physical exam and diagnostic testing; the final section considers treatment alternatives and selected techniques.

■ BASIC SCIENCE

Anatomy and Biology

The rotator cuff consists of the supraspinatus, infraspinatus, teres minor, and subscapularis muscles, all of which arise from the scapula and insert into the proximal humerus. The subscapularis muscle is innervated by the upper and lower scapular nerves, and arises from the anterior surface of the scapula, inserting into the lesser tuberosity. The nerve supply to the supraspinatus is provided by the suprascapular nerve, and the muscle originates from the supraspinatus fossa, inserting into the greater tuberosity. The infraspinatus muscle is also innervated by the suprascapular nerve after it passes around the spinoglenoid notch. The muscle arises from the infraspinatus fossa and inserts into the posterolateral aspect of the greater tuberosity. The axillary nerve innervates the teres minor, which originates from the inferior and lateral aspect of the scapula, inserting into the inferior portion of the greater tuberosity.

Another important and under appreciated feature of the rotator cuff is its distinct layered makeup (1–3). The first layer is a superficial one extending from the coracoid process to the greater tuberosity following the course of the coracohumeral ligament. The second layer consists of the supraspinatus and infraspinatus tendinous fibers. Layer three is composed of the same muscle groups, but the fibers are oriented obliquely and interconnect with the adjacent rotator cuff fibers including the subscapularis. The deep fibers of the coracohumeral ligament make up the fourth layer extending into the supraspinatus and infraspinatus junction laterally. Layer five represents the actual capsular layer of the joint. The ability to recognize the complex layered anatomy in addition to the tear configuration is critical if an anatomic repair is to be achieved. Furthermore, collagen organization is more robust on the bursal aspect of the rotator cuff as compared to articular-sided fibers (4,5), a pertinent fact when evaluating partial thickness tears. It is also worth noting that a significant contribution to the vascular environment of the rotator cuff, when considering healing potential, may arise from adjacent subacromial structures including the bursa (6,7).

Investigators have further refined the insertional anatomy of the rotator cuff components (8,9). Each segment of the rotator cuff has a specific "footprint" that can be quantified. This is particularly important when assessing partial thickness cuff tears (Fig 13-1). The depth of the tear, as judged by the amount of exposed "footprint," allows the clinician to not only estimate the severity of the tear, but to also choose the most effective treatment (10–12).

The vascular anatomy of the rotator cuff has been well described. The anterior humeral circumflex, the subscapular, and the suprascapular arteries provide the primary blood

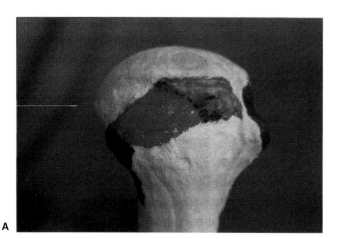

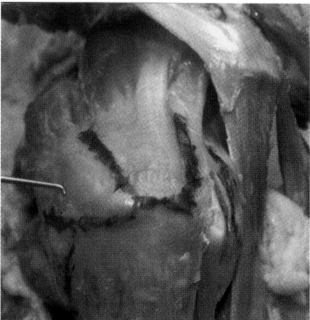

A   **B**

Fig 13-1. A: The insertional anatomy of the rotator cuff depicted on model. Green represents supraspinatus footprint; infraspinatus footprint shown in red. **B:** Cadaveric representation of distinct insertional anatomy for the rotator cuff.

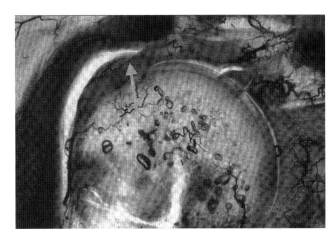

Fig 13-2. Arrow points to zone of diminished vascularity on coronal photomicrograph.

supply to the rotator cuff (13–15). Lindblom has described an area of avascularity in the supraspinatus tendon proximal to its insertion into the greater tuberosity (16,17) **(Fig 13-2)**. Other authors have reported a dynamic reason for the decreased vascularity within the supraspinatus tendon, citing a "wringing out" effect with supraspinatus tension (18). Benjamin (19) described the histological transition that takes place from tendon to calcified fibrocartilage to bone, accounting for the vascular differences at the insertion site. The zone of uncalcified fibrocartilage is more avascular with respect to the other zones and may be vulnerable to delayed or incomplete healing when traumatized.

The subacromial arch is defined as the space between the distal clavicle and acromion superiorly and the humeral head inferiorly. This space between the acromion and humeral head averages 8 to 12 millimeters on plain x-ray, and can be further divided into the coracoacromial arch which is formed by the acromion, coracoacromial ligament and the coracoid process. As the rotator cuff passes beneath this arch, contact between the tendons and the arch can occur, leading to tendon pathology as well as secondary changes to the arch in the form of traction-based ossification within the coracoacromial ligament at the acromial attachment site (20–26) **(Fig 13-3)**.

Function

The rotator cuff muscles centralize the humeral head and permit a single center of rotation while providing stability and strength. During active shoulder elevation, the rotator cuff muscles depress the humeral head, allowing efficient elevation of the extremity while the head remains reduced in the glenoid (27–30). Studies have been performed evaluating the individual rotator cuff muscles and their respective contribution to shoulder strength. The supraspinatus and infraspinatus provide approximately 45% of abduction strength and the infraspinatus contributes nearly 90% of external rotation power (31,32). The supraspinatus and deltoid muscles

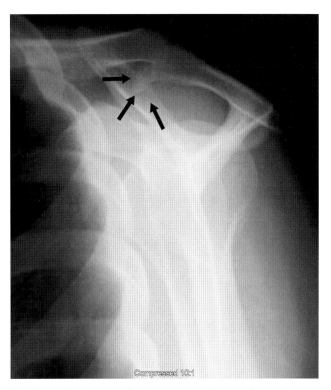

Fig 13-3. Radiograph of subacromial outlet reveals sharp, bony excresence *(arrows)* originating from coracoacromial ligament attachment site.

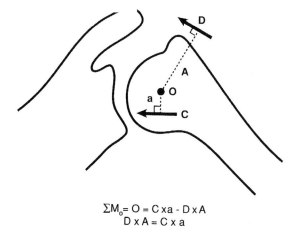

$$\Sigma M_o = O = C \times a - D \times A$$
$$D \times A = C \times a$$

Fig 13-4. Coronal plane force couple. The inferior portion of the rotator cuff (below the center of rotation) creates a moment that must balance the deltoid moment. *(C)*, resultant rotator cuff forces; *(D)*, deltoid muscle force; *(O)*, center of rotation; *(a)*, moment arm of the inferior portion of the rotator cuff; *(A)*, moment arm of the deltoid. (From Lo IK, Burkhart SS. Current concept in arthroscopic rotator cuff repair. *Am J Sports Med.* 2003;31:308-324; reprinted with permission.)

provide balancing forces in the coronal plane of motion (33) **(Fig 13-4)**.

The importance of balanced force couples cannot be overemphasized, and the goal of surgery, when necessary, should be to properly and anatomically restore these forces such that their counteraction is maintained. Furthermore, the importance of the transverse force couple and the need for balanced function in this plane was further emphasized by Burkhart (34–38) **(Fig 13-5)**. Loss of greater than half of the infraspinatus or loss of subscapularis function leads to superior humeral head migration, a phenomenon often detected on plain films as the acromial-humeral head distance diminishes to less than 7 millimeters **(Fig 13-6)**.

If the coronal and transverse force couples remain functional and balanced, the end result is a properly centered humeral head and surprisingly good function even if a significant, possibly irreparable tear is present. Burkhart remains a

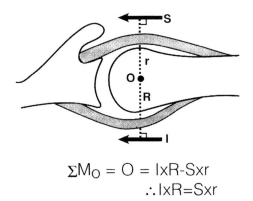

$$\Sigma M_O = O = IxR - Sxr$$
$$\therefore IxR = Sxr$$

Fig 13-5. Transverse plane force couple *(axillary view)*. The subscapularis tendon anteriorly is balanced against the infraspinatus and teres minor tendons posteriorly. *(I)*, infraspinatus; *(S)*, subscapularis; *(o)*, center of rotation; *(r)*, moment arm of the subscapularis tendon; *(R)*, moment arm of the infraspinatus and teres minor tendons. (From Lo IK, Burkhart SS. Current concept in arthroscopic rotator cuff repair. *Am J Sports Med.* 2003;31;308-324; reprinted with permission.)

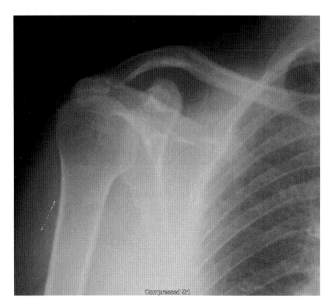

Fig 13-6. Loss of interval between humeral head and acromion indicates massive rotator cuff tear and compromised humeral head containment.

pioneer in helping us recognize that torn rotator cuffs can be very functional and that attempting to "cover the humeral head" utilizing nonanatomic tissue re-approximation is an approach that must be avoided (35). Burkhart's concept of partial repairs in an effort to restore force couples has been successfully applied in lieu of tendon transfers that may serve only to weaken the balanced force couple (36–40).

Although there has been speculation that the biceps serves as a humeral head depressor and maintains an active role in shoulder function, comparative anatomic studies (41) as well as electromyographic data indicate that the biceps probably does not function as a humeral head depressor (42), and that the hypertrophy often encountered in the massive rotator cuff tear may be inflammatory in origin (43) as opposed to a reflection of intrinsic strengthening (44). There is some evidence from EMG studies that the biceps may serve as an additional shoulder stabilizer in those with anterior shoulder instability (45,46).

Pathoanatomy

Before describing the mechanics of rotator cuff pathology, post-mortem studies provide an interesting backdrop to the issue of etiology. There is little doubt that rotator cuff tearing is a function of age among other factors. Post-mortem studies have indicated an incidence of full or partial thickness tears ranging from 5% to nearly 40% (47–51). Fukuda et al. (52) reported a 13% incidence of partial rotator cuff tears in a cadaveric study of 249 anatomic specimens. The prevalence of these partial thickness tears appears to increase with age. DePalma (53) studied 96 shoulders of patients aged 18 to 74 years without a history of shoulder dysfunction and found an incidence of partial ruptures of the supraspinatus tendon in 37%. Petersson (54) reported on 27 asymptomatic patients ranging from 55 to 85 years of age with a nearly 50% incidence of full or partial thickness tears based on arthrographic studies. Suffice to say that tearing of the rotator cuff as a function of age is clearly a common occurrence. Furthermore, many of these tears, both full thickness and partial, may be clinically silent (10,49,55). As clinicians, we must be cautious in attributing causation to findings detected during diagnostic testing as these results may simply reflect the senescence process without significant clinical sequelae.

After a tear is noted, its natural history deserves attention. Several authors have reported on the progression of partial to full thickness tears (49,56,57). There is also evidence that full thickness tears are unable to heal spontaneously although an ineffective healing response may occur (58,59). Codman (60) believed that spontaneous healing of partial tears might occur, yet histological studies of partial thickness rotator cuff tears has yielded no evidence of active repair (61). Yamanaka (56) studied 40 patients with symptomatic articular-sided partial rotator cuff tears treated nonoperatively with serial arthrography. Repeat arthrography revealed that 10% of the tears had presumably healed, 10% had decreased in size while enlargement of tear size occurred in 51%, and 28% progressed to a full thickness tear. A study comparing operative and nonoperative treatment for full-thickness rotator cuff tears concluded that larger rotator cuff tears in older individuals most likely progress in size although they can remain clinically quiescent (48). The study also concluded that the results of rotator cuff repair are clearly superior to that achieved with nonoperative measures only.

In a compelling longitudinal study of the natural course of rotator cuff tears, Yamaguchi et al. (49) reported on the risk of progression of asymptomatic rotator cuff tears detected by ultrasound in 58 patients with unilateral symptoms and bilateral rotator cuff tears. Fifty-one percent of asymptomatic tears became symptomatic over a three-year follow-up period. Nine of 23 patients restudied with ultrasound clearly demonstrated an increase in tear size, and no patient showed evidence of healing.

Etiology

When considering the possible causes of rotator cuff disease, mechanical impingement of the rotator cuff is considered the most common recognizable source of recurring pain and disability in the active population. Neer's classic work (20,62) served to organize the clinician's approach to rotator cuff disease and, most importantly, to define rotator cuff pathology as a spectrum of disease ranging from reversible edema to cuff fiber failure.

Primary impingement occurs at the anterior one third of the acromion and coracoacromial arch (24,63–68). The mechanical stresses endured by the rotator cuff, as well as its poor vascular design, both dynamic and static, have been well documented (13–17). Additional factors influencing rotator cuff pathology include acromial shape (20,22,24, 69–71), slope (21,72–75), coracoacromial ligament size (76,77), postfracture deformity, os acromiale (78–82) and acromioclavicular joint spurring (24,83). Snyder (72) has recently reported on the "keeled" acromion, a particularly pernicious acromial variant associated with rotator cuff injury.

Functional abnormalities, such as asynchronous shoulder motion, posterior capsular contractures, scapular dyskinesia, glenohumeral instability, and distant neurological injury leading to weakness can also adversely affect the rotator cuff on a secondary basis with increased impingement forces concentrated in the subacromial space (84,85,86,87).

Impingement may occur from a direct mechanical insult, usually the result of an acromial excrescence excoriating the bursal aspect of the rotator cuff **(Fig 13-7)**. However, another plausible injury cascade begins with intrinsic cuff failure, leading to insufficient humeral head depression and subsequent superior migration with creation of a traction spur within the coracoacromial ligament as a secondary phenomenon (24,26,68,71). The cause for intrinsic cuff failure can range from fatigue on an overuse basis to underlying shoulder instability or superior labral pathology, injuries that have

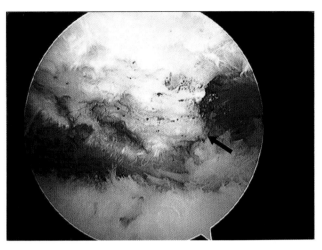

Fig 13-7. Arthroscopic view of a symptomatic acromial spur (*arrows*) after coracoacromial ligament release in subacromial space of a left shoulder.

been associated with internal impingement and articular sided cuff failure (88–93). Regardless of etiology, a narrowed or stenotic supraspinatus outlet poses continued risk to the rotator cuff.

■ CLINICAL EVALUATION

History

Rotator cuff disease, especially that related to the impingement phenomenon, is usually evident from the history alone. A painful range of motion beginning at 70 degrees of forward flexion through 120 degrees is commonplace with pain localizing to the anterior-superior shoulder, often radiating down the lateral upper arm into the deltoid insertion. Overhead activities are the most provocative, and in instances where the rotator cuff has actually torn, night pain and difficulty sleeping are common complaints. Motion is usually not restricted, other than that due to pain; however, for longer standing injuries, a secondary adhesive capsulitis pattern can be encountered, especially in the older population. Most often the onset of pain is insidious and takes place over a longer period of time, but for those with an acute injury, a tearing sensation associated with profound early weakness may be the presenting history.

Because rotator cuff disease reflects a spectrum of pathology, the history and physical findings may overlap. There may be little difference in the presentation and findings of patients with isolated impingement, partial and even small full thickness rotator cuff tears.

Physical Examination

After completing a detailed history, a focused examination can be undertaken. It is critical to compare extremities as the unaffected shoulder can serve as a "normal" template to

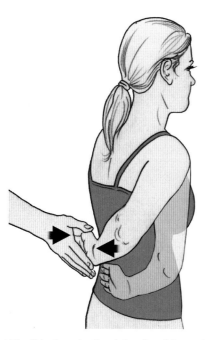

Fig 13-8. Lift-off test evaluating integrity of the subscapularis. May be difficult position to achieve in patients limited by pain and motion restrictions.

which one can compare. One should survey for atrophy or asymmetry, especially in the supra and infraspinatus fossae. Long-standing rotator cuff tears are often accompanied by significant, visible atrophy. Examination should include assessment of range of motion, both active and passive, observing forward flexion, abduction in the scapular plane, internal rotation, and external rotation both in abduction and with the elbow at the side. Careful evaluation of scapular tracking should be included as poor scapulo-thoracic mechanics can lead to secondary subacromial pathology. In some instances of suspected impingement, simply treating scapular dyskinesia can alleviate secondary subacromial space symptoms (84,86,87). Strength testing should be performed in an attempt to isolate the different components of the rotator cuff to assess weakness. The "lift-off" test can help to assess subscapularis integrity (94) **(Fig 13-8)**.

Although clinically useful, placing the arm in the testing position can be provocative and difficult to achieve, especially in the older population. The "belly-press" test (or Napolean sign) can also help determine integrity of the subscapularis, is less provocative than the "lift-off" test and can actually be quantified to assess partial tears as well (95,96) **(Fig 13-9)**.

Resisted external rotation with the elbow by the side is useful in detecting tears extending into the infraspinatus

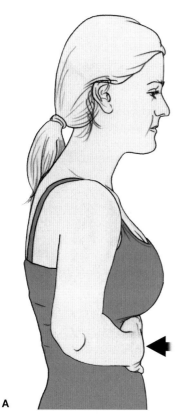
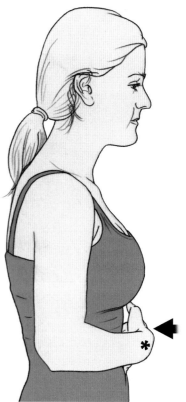

A   **B**

Fig 13-9. A: Alternative belly-press test for subscapularis integrity. Subscapularis considered intact if wrist and elbow remain in straight line (no wrist flexion) while pressing into abdomen. **B:** Positive belly-press test for injured subscapularis as wrist flexion substitutes for subscapularis while pressing against abdomen.

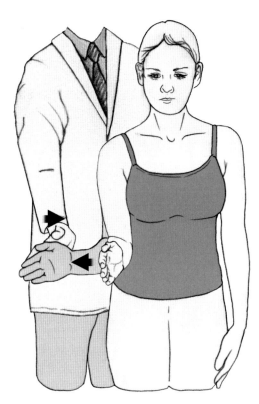

Fig 13-10. External rotation testing evaluates infraspinatus and teres minor integrity. Weakness indicates loss of posterior transverse force couple.

(Fig 13-10). This manual test is critical for assessing the posterior transverse force couple while the "belly-press" test determines subscapularis function. If significant weakness is noted in either or both muscle groups, loss of humeral head containment is imminent if not already present. Loss of the normal distance between the humeral head and acromion

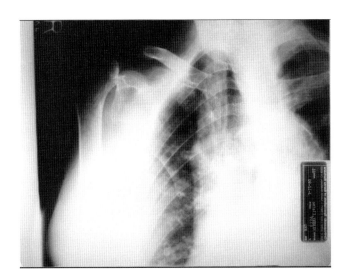

Fig 13-11. Loss of humeral head containment and anterior-superior subluxation can result from acromioplasty if transverse force couples are compromised. Humeral head can erode through the thinned acromion.

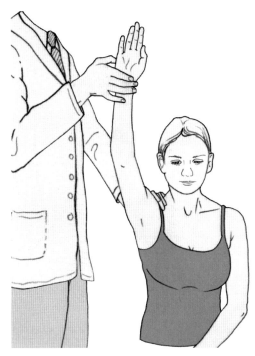

Fig 13-12. Neer sign for impingement. Neer test utilizes the same maneuver following a subacromial injection of anesthetic. Amelioration of pain confirms diagnosis of impingement.

should be evident, and one must proceed with great caution if a decompression is undertaken. Violation of the arch in conjunction with inadequate transverse force couples may ultimately lead to erosion of the acromion by the humeral head and subsequent anterior-superior humeral head migration (97–99) **(Fig 13-11)**.

The impingement sign **(Fig 13-12)** as originally described by Neer involves stabilizing the scapula while elevating the shoulder in the scapular plane. Pain elicited in the arc from 70 to 120 degrees is indicative of the impingement phenomenon. Confirmation of this finding in the form of the impingement test consists of complete resolution of pain during the painful arc of motion after an anesthetic has been injected into the subacromial space.

A variation of the impingement sign is the Hawkin's test **(Fig 13-13)** in which the shoulder is placed in 90 degrees of forward flexion, the elbow is flexed 90 degrees and the shoulder is then internally rotated. Rotation of the greater tuberosity under the arch in this position decreases space for the rotator cuff leading to impingement pain.

Diagnostic Imaging

It is essential that the initial evaluation of the painful shoulder include quality plain radiographs. The standard radiographs should include a true anterior-posterior view with the shoulder in the internal and neutral position, an axillary view, and the outlet (supraspinatus) view described by Neer and Poppen (100), which is used to evaluate and classify acromial morphology and arch anatomy. Bigliani et al. (69)

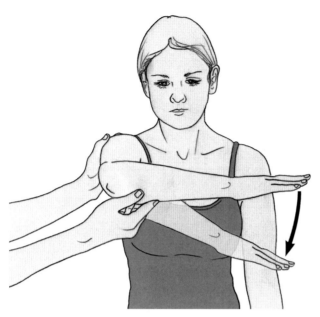

Fig 13-13. Positive Hawkins sign, indicative of subacomial impingement, is elicited when pain occurs as the shoulder is internally rotated with the shoulder forward flexed 90 degrees.

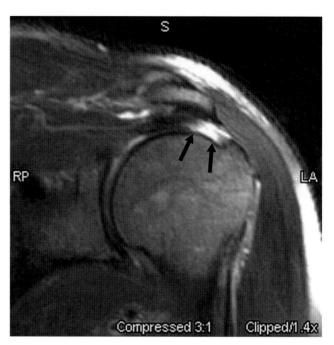

Fig 13-15. Coronal MR T-2 weighted image depicting full-thickness rotator cuff tear (*arrows*); fluid filling the gap is enhanced on T-2 imaging.

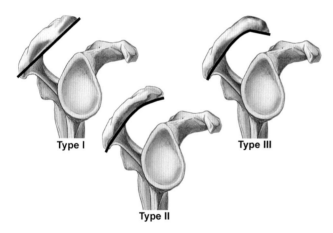

Fig 13-14. Acromial shape can be categorized into Type I: flat, Type II: curved, and Type III: hooked. Type III associated with impingement anatomy.

have classified the types into I flat, II curved, and III hooked (**Fig 13-14**). In addition to establishing morphology, the thickness of the acromion should also be assessed and if surgery is recommended, a pre-operative decision can be made regarding the amount of bone to be resected so as to prevent excessive thinning or inadequate bone resection.

The standard anterior-posterior views may show superior migration of the humeral head consistent with a cuff tear and potential subscapularis involvement. Cystic and/or sclerotic change in the greater tuberosity may also signal tendon pathology. The axillary view is most helpful in assessing concomitant glenohumeral degenerative changes, but is

most helpful in establishing the presence of an os acromiale (78,79).

Magnetic resonance imaging is the current test of choice when evaluating the soft tissues of the shoulder (101,102). T1 weighted images revealing increased signal in the rotator cuff combined with a focal defect or loss of continuity of the cuff on the T2 weighted image is a common finding when a full or partial- thickness tear is encountered (**Fig 13-15**). The addition of a contrast agent such as gadolinium significantly enhances the positive predictive value for diagnosing a full thickness tear, and can also aid in detecting and quantifying partial tears of the cuff as well (103,104). Several studies have demonstrated a poor correlation between arthroscopic findings and MRI abnormalities (105,106). The combination of fat suppressed images combined with contrast has been reported to significantly improve the sensitivity and specificity for detecting full and partial thickness cuff tears (107).

One must exercise caution when interpreting MR findings because asymptomatic individuals may have significant rotator cuff findings on MRI, but may remain completely asymptomatic (55). Magnetic resonance imaging continues to demonstrate its greatest utility and potential when combined with a thorough and reliable history and physical examination.

Although an MRI scan is not essential for every patient with shoulder pain, for those anticipating a surgical procedure, a pre-operative MRI scan can be helpful for the following reasons: evaluating whether a cuff tear accompanies a suspected impingement syndrome, the presence of which would alter the post-operative regimen, allowing the patient to properly plan for post-operative care; determining the size and potential tear configuration, including retraction, delamination, and thinning, factors that need to be considered in the surgical planning; assessing the presence or absence of atrophy **(Fig 13-16)** or fatty infiltration **(Fig 13-17)**, both

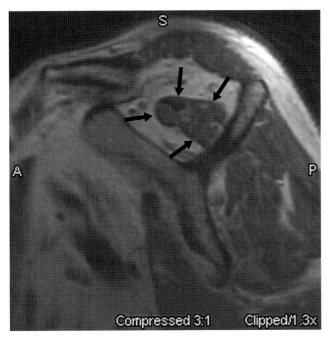

Fig 13-16. Oblique sagittal view through supraspinatus fossa demonstrates atrophic changes (*arrows*) within the supraspinatus muscle belly which should completely fill the fossa.

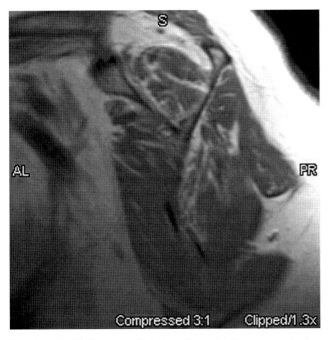

Fig 13-17. Oblique sagittal view through the supraspinatus fossa demonstrating fatty infiltration within the substance of the muscle belly. Fatty streaks within the subscapularis and infraspinatus are also visible.

important prognostic factors (108–110); and establishing the presence of co-morbidities such as partial biceps or labral tears.

■ DECISION-MAKING AND TREATMENT

Because rotator cuff pathology can represent as a wide spectrum of disease, there is some utility to compartmentalizing the most common entities in an effort to develop algorithms which guide treatment. The management of impingement with or without associated cuff tearing, partial thickness-tears and full-thickness rotator cuff injuries will be the primary topics of this section.

Impingement: Primary

Impingement of the tendinous portion of the rotator cuff as it passes under the coracoacromial arch is a classic cause of rotator cuff injury. The impingement syndrome, as originally described by Neer (20), encompasses a spectrum of pathologic changes involving the rotator cuff and associated bony changes within the coracoacromial arch, affecting primarily those 40 years of age and older. When impingement-type symptoms present in a younger population, great care must be taken to avoid over-diagnosing and over-treating as the impingement may be internal or secondary to instability, which effectively moves the cuff closer to the arch (87,90,93). Middle-aged to older patients presenting with impingement symptoms are generally recreational overhand athletes or individuals whose occupation requires repetitive, forceful overhead work. These patients present with chronic, low-level shoulder pain that is exacerbated with overhead activity or motions that necessitate internal rotation of the humerus in the abducted position, such as reaching behind a car seat. The pain usually localizes to the anterosuperior shoulder with radiation into the deltoid insertion region, following the course of the underlying bursa and capsule. Frequently, the primary reason for presenting to the orthopaedic surgeon is sleep disturbance.

Treatment of impingement syndrome is patient specific. After the diagnosis has been made, the varying degrees of pathology and patient expectations must be considered. To assist in developing a treatment plan, Neer (20) described the three stages of rotator cuff involvement: Stage 1: reversible edema and inflammation; Stage 2: tendon fibrosis and chronic inflammation, a stage that has been further subcategorized (74) into Type 1 without a cuff tear and Type 2 associated with a partial thickness tear; and Stage 3 complete fiber failure with a full thickness tear. Knowing the status of the rotator cuff is critical in making therapeutic decisions.

If impingement is diagnosed, the initial treatment should be conservative. Great care should be taken to evaluate the scapula and to diagnose any associated dyskinesia. In addition

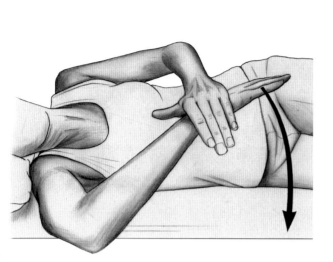

A

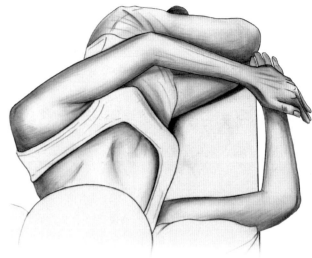

B

Fig 13-18. A: "Sleeper" stretch to combat glenohumeral internal rotation deficit. Shoulder abducted 90 degrees with patient in 60 to 70 degrees of lateral decubitus (this helps maintain scapular stability to prevent substitution). Elbow maintained in 90 degrees of flexion while internal rotation generated with opposite extremity. **B:** "Sleeper" stretch from superior view.

to proper activity modification, physical therapy exercises can be of great benefit, focusing not only on rehabilitating the rotator cuff musculature, but also on re-establishing a full, pain-free range of motion and normal scapulo-thoracic rhythm and strength. The net effect of a proper rehabilitation program should result in decreased inflammation and thickening in the subacromial space as well as an increase in the interval between the humeral head and acromion.

The younger overhand athlete with impingement-type pain should be carefully examined for a functional loss of internal rotation. A tight posterior capsule tends to shift the humeral head in a posterior-superior direction leading to rotator cuff symptoms. By simply stretching the posterior capsule using the "sleeper" stretch **(Fig 13-18)**, resolution of symptoms can often be achieved in this population of patients. Nonsteroidal anti-inflammatory medication is appropriate to assist in decreasing associated soft tissue swelling while, on occasion, the judicious use of a steroid can be very helpful when introduced into the subacromial space (110).

For those who fail conservative care, surgery may be appropriate. Most patients who respond to a nonoperative program will do so within a six-month period (10,48). If surgery is indicated, an MRI may prove useful to determine whether or not there is concomitant significant cuff pathology. If the cuff is intact, a simple subacromial decompression should be performed **(Fig 13-19)**. If the impingement has resulted in associated cuff tearing, the tear may need to be repaired in addition to the decompression.

In the properly selected patient, the results of subacromial decompression have been reliable and durable (66,67, 111–114). Although there are several described surgical techniques for subacromial decompression (115), the "cutting block" approach may be the most reliable with regard to

referencing the final result against known anatomic guidelines (116) **(Fig 13-20)**. Furthermore, pre-operative planning should include the shape and width of the acromion such that over or under-resection is avoided (117).

Subacromial decompression has become one of the most common procedures performed by the orthopaedist, and although a success rate of nearly 90% has been reported for isolated decompressions, a word of caution is warranted. Failures can and do occur. Authors have reported failure rates ranging from 5% to 40% (118–120). Despite appropriate treatment, complications and unsatisfactory results can occur (118,121–123). When a failed acromioplasty is encountered, it is incumbent upon the treating surgeon to invoke a systematic, thorough analysis of the failed acromioplasty. The work-up should attempt to answer the follow questions: Was the initial diagnosis correct? Was the appropriate operation chosen? Was the procedure performed technically correctly? Was associated pathology recognized? Was the postoperative rehabilitation timely and appropriate?

As these questions are answered during the re-evaluation, the cause for failure can be established and categorized as initial diagnostic error, treatment failure, or a complication of treatment, and then appropriately treated.

Impingement: Secondary

Individuals with shoulder instability or other underlying pathology can develop significant abnormal mechanics that can lead to rotator cuff functional disability, eventual fatigue and loss of humeral head containment. When this occurs, rather than the coracoacromial arch moving toward the cuff, the cuff migrates cephalad as containment is compromised. In addition to articular-sided internal impingement-type

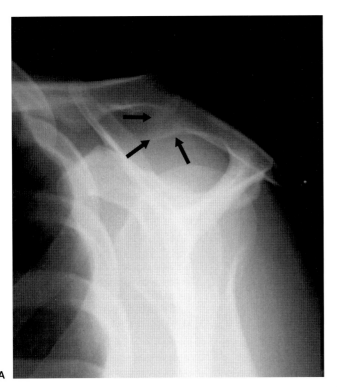
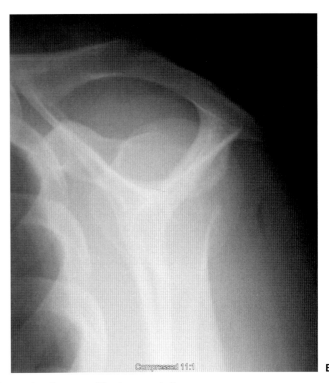

Fig 13-19. **A:** Type III acromion (*arrows*) contributing to classic external impingement phenomenon. **B:** Appearance of acromial outlet after acromioplasty.

rotator cuff tearing, secondary changes, including traction spurring of the CA ligament and abrasive changes of the bursal aspect of the cuff can be encountered.

Several investigators have described partial articular-sided rotator cuff tears resulting from internal impingement (68,88,90–93). This entity represents contact between the undersurface of the cuff and the posterior-superior glenoid and labrum. There exist a plethora of potential causes for

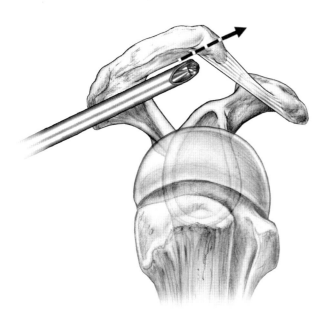

Fig 13-20. Cutting-block technique for precision acromioplasty.

internal impingement including physiologic to pathologic change from repetitive intra-articular contact, torsional forces created by loss of humeral head retroversion, ligamentous insufficiency and abnormal mechanics, especially with regard to scapular dyskinesia. These patients are younger, and often complain of pain localizing to the posterior shoulder. They also complain of early fatigue and loss of control in the throwing motion. Fatigue of the dynamic stabilizers and excessive external rotation secondary to overstretching of the anterior capsule may predispose individuals to development of internal impingement. A subset of patients, usually baseball pitchers, develop a glenohumeral internal rotation deficit (GIRD syndrome) with a significant loss of internal rotation on the affected side (93) **(Fig 13-21)**. This contracture initiates a cascade of kinematic abnormalities that can result in increased torsional strain within the cuff, labral abnormalities and tertiary capsular insufficiency, all implicated in the secondary articular-sided partial cuff tears. In later stages, the ability to discriminate between primary and secondary impingement may be challenging. Even if a primary instability is present and treatment is directed toward correcting the primary pathology, consideration of subacromial debridement up to and including bony resection must be considered as part of the overall treatment regimen if changes such as bursal-sided cuff tearing and fraying of the coaracoacromial ligament are witnessed. The real challenge for the clinician is to carefully evaluate these patients to assign the correct diagnosis before proceeding with surgical treatment. Performing a subacromial decompression without treating

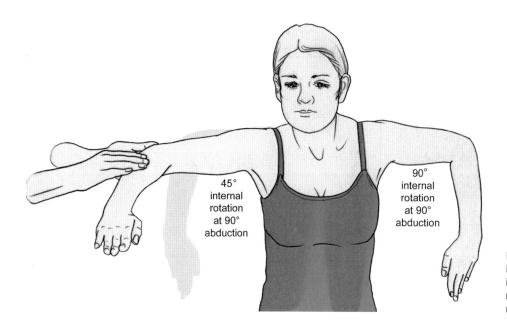

45°
internal
rotation
at 90°
abduction

90°
internal
rotation
at 90°
abduction

Fig 13-21. Typical physical findings in patient with glenohumeral internal rotation deficit. Scapula must be stabilized while testing range of motion.

instability in those with underlying symptomatic shoulder laxity can serve to worsen the degree of instability (124).

Partial Thickness Rotator Cuff Tears: Treatment

Partial thickness rotator cuff tears can result from intrinsic cuff degeneration and tendinopathy absent an injury or impingement. The lack of uniformity of collagen bundles and the paucity of vascular supply contributes to weakness, especially along the articular aspect of the rotator cuff (4,5, 9–13,125). These degenerative tears often exit the articular surface and can be well visualized at surgery, but sometimes can be entirely contained within the cuff (intrasubstance), and therefore easily missed.

As noted earlier, extrinsic impingement due to narrowing of the supraspinatus outlet can result in chronic cuff abrasion leading to a partial cuff tear. Histological changes consistent with trauma have been found on the undersurface of cadaveric acromion specimens with bursal surface tears but not in those with articular surface tears (126). This suggests that bursal-surface tears may be more likely to be related to abrasion of the cuff by the acromion. Furthermore, extrinsic impingement due to coracoacromial arch narrowing has been postulated to cause partial tears on the articular side as well as the bursal surface of the cuff based on transmural shear stress (127) leading to fiber failure of the laminated cuff.

Trauma, absent impingement, can cause a partial thickness tear, usually leading to a partial avulsion of the articular surface of the cuff. This can be the result of repetitive microtrauma or simply a single high-energy episode. This type of avulsion injury has been named the "PASTA" lesion (partial articular sided tendon avulsion) (128).

The symptoms of partial thickness rotator cuff tears are nonspecific and may overlap with impingement, rotator cuff tendonitis, and small, full thickness rotator cuff tears. Similar to the impingement population, most patients have a painful arc of motion between 60 and 120 degrees of elevation. They may also have loss of motion with posterior capsular tightness and resultant restriction of internal rotation.

The impingement signs described by Neer (pain with forced passive forward elevation) and Hawkins (pain with passive internal rotation of the arm placed in 90 degrees of forward flexion) are positive in nearly all patients with symptomatic partial thickness rotator cuff tears. Strength is usually preserved on clinical examination; however, pain inhibition may result in an apparent loss of strength and in a decrease in active range of motion in these patients with a partially torn rotator cuff.

The clinical course of patients with partial thickness rotator cuff tears is often indistinguishable from that of patients with impingement syndrome, tendonitis, or small, full thickness rotator cuff tears. Symptoms may also be difficult to differentiate from bicipital tendonitis, labral or SLAP lesions, and mild cases of adhesive capsulitis.

There is currently no universally accepted classification system for partial thickness rotator cuff tears. Evaluating the results of treatment has been challenging due to this lack of conformity. Although the classification of partial tears continues to be refined, the system most commonly used is that proposed by Ellman (129) in which the depth of the tear is estimated: Grade I: 1-3 mm, Grade II: 3-6mm, and Grade III: 6mm or greater **(Table 13-1)**.

Anatomic knowledge of the "footprint" makes this assessment more uniform and reproducible. If the average supraspinatus "footprint" is approximately 12 mm in size, it is possible to grade the percentage of tearing. Using the "footprint" as a guide, if more than 6 mm of the footprint is exposed, a greater than 50% tear of the supraspinatus insertion has

Table 13-1	Ellman Classification for Partial-thickness Rotator Cuff Tears

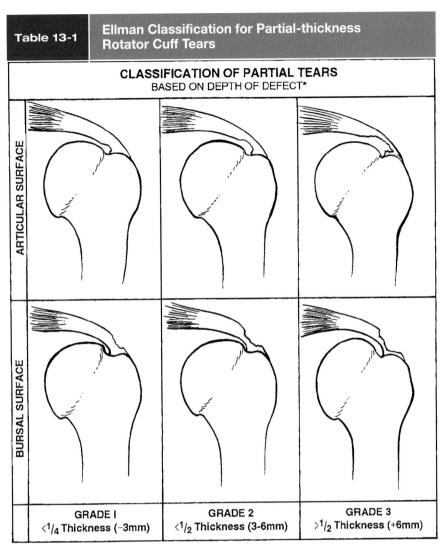

CLASSIFICATION OF PARTIAL TEARS
BASED ON DEPTH OF DEFECT*

ARTICULAR SURFACE

BURSAL SURFACE

GRADE I	GRADE 2	GRADE 3
$<1/4$ Thickness (−3mm)	$<1/2$ Thickness (3–6mm)	$>1/2$ Thickness (+6mm)

*Indicate <u>AREA OF DEFECT</u>: Base of tear × maximum retraction = mm^2

occurred (8). Snyder (10) has proposed a grading system in which the articular and bursal sides of the cuff are evaluated separately in an effort to be more precise in judging severity **(Table 13-2)**.

Individuals with a suspected partial tear due to extrinsic impingement or intrinsic tendinopathy are treated in a similar fashion as those with impingement syndrome. Subacromial bursal inflammation is controlled with activity modification, nonsteroidal anti-inflammatory medication, and the judicious use of injectable corticosteroids. The role of rehabilitation to restore normal joint mechanics and strengthen the rotator cuff and parascapular musculature has been proposed to reduce the progression of rotator cuff disease in those with both external and internal impingement. The role of the external rotators which act as humeral head depressors may play a role in reducing external impingement thus reducing further mechanical impingement of the cuff from the cora-coacromial arch.

Partial thickness tears that fail to respond to conservative measures usually require surgical intervention, including debridement alone, debridement in conjunction with a subacromial decompression, and decompression combined with a rotator cuff repair, either mini-open or arthroscopic.

Arthroscopic debridement alone of partial tears has led to mixed results (113,130,131). One study evaluating the results for decompression alone recorded failure rates exceeding 50% (132). Furthermore treating a partial tear without addressing potential underlying causes such as instability has also been associated with a high failure rate (88).

Arthroscopic subacromial decompression combined with arthroscopic debridement of partial tears has also led to mixed results. Several investigators have described failure rates ranging from 20 to 30% in this treatment group (133–135). Ryu (66) reported on 35 patients treated with an arthroscopic subacromial decompression and debridement with a follow-up of 23 months and had 86% good results with

Table 13-2	Snyder Classification System for Grading Partial-thickness Rotator Cuff Tears
Location of Tears	
A	Articular surface
B	Bursal surface
Severity of Tear	
0	Normal cuff, with smooth coverings of synovium and bursa
I	Minimal, superficial bursal or synovial irritation or slight capsular fraying in a small, localized area; usually <1 cm
II	Actually fraying and failure of some rotator cuff fibers in addition to synovial, bursal, or capsular injury; usually <2 cm
III	More severe rotator cuff injury, including fraying and fragmentation of tendon fibers, often involving the whole surface of a cuff tendon (most often the supraspinatus); usually <3 cm
IV	Very severe partial rotator tear that usually contains, in addition to fraying and fragmentation of tendon tissue, a sizable flap tear and often encompasses more than a single tendon

bursal sided tears exhibiting a more favorable result as compared to articular-sided lesions.

Because of concerns about cuff integrity and tear progression, repair of extensive partial rotator cuff tears has been recommended (52,57,134,135). Ellman (134) was one of the first to recommend arthroscopic subacromial decompression along with open repair of significant, partial tears of the rotator cuff. Fukuda (61), reporting on 66 patients with partial tears treated with an open acromioplasty and repair, achieved satisfactory results in 94% of his patients.

Weber (136) has documented the clear advantage of repairing separate partial thickness tears in conjunction with subacromial decompression. His re-operation rate was significantly lower for those treated with a concomitant repair versus those who simply underwent a debridement. In another study, Weber (137) determined that by completing the articular-sided tear, excising unhealthy tissue and advancing healthy tendon back to its attachment site, an all-arthroscopic approach led to results equal to those reported with the mini-open technique.

Bursal-sided partial tears of the rotator cuff are usually a direct result of mechanical impingement occurring at the arch. These injuries are readily visualized at surgery and the depth of the tear can be accurately estimated in most cases. For those with a Grade I or II partial tear in conjunction with impingement, a simple debridement in association with a subacromial decompression may be the most appropriate treatment. For those individuals who have a significant

partial tear, Grade III, and higher post-operative expectations of their shoulder, a more aggressive approach including repair of the partial tear in addition to the decompression may be more suitable.

The articular-sided tears occur two to three times more commonly than bursal-sided tears, and may not necessarily be associated with the impingement phenomenon. Repetitive traction forces or underlying primary pathology such as a superior labral injury or symptomatic capsular redundancy can result in articular-sided cuff tears. Additionally in some instances, internal impingement may be the source of the tearing. The GIRD syndrome (glenohumeral internal rotation deficit) has been established as a common pathway for articular-sided partial rotator cuff injuries. Loss of internal rotation leads to abnormal joint mechanics with subsequent loss of the normal cam effect on the glenohumeral joint. This permits pathologic hyper-external rotation, superior labral pathology and cuff tearing on a tensile failure basis (93). Others have postulated a direct contact lesion occurring between the articular surface of the cuff and the posterior-superior glenoid and labrum (88,90).

Grade I and II articular-sided partial thickness tears should be debrided. Careful consideration to an underlying primary pathology, especially instability, must be given, and if discovered, treated concomitantly. A Grade III articular-sided partial tear deserves a repair, either trans-tendon or by completing the tear and converting to a full thickness lesion. Whether a decompression is warranted or not should be determined by the presence or absence of subacromial changes. Those lacking pathologic changes in the subacromial space such as coacoacromial ligament fraying should not be treated with a decompression as further instability is potentially incurred.

If a repair of a partial tear is performed, the arthroscopic trans-tendon technique for treating significant partial articular sided rotator cuff tears ('PASTA' lesion: partial articular-sided tendon avulsion) has been described (138) **(Fig 13-22)**.

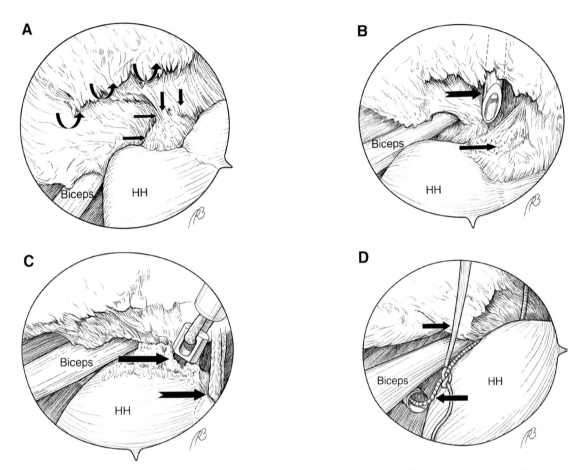

Fig 13-22. A: Identify and quantitate the tear (*curved arrows*) using the anatomic "footprint" (*straight arrows*) as the reference point. Prepare the exposed footprint with a motorized shaver using a standard anterior portal. Debride the partial articular-sided tear. **B:** Pass a percutaneous spinal needle lateral to the edge of the acromion (*large arrow*). This needle will traverse through the substance of the remaining attached rotator cuff into the exposed footprint (*small arrow*). This will serve as a guide for anchor insertion. Rotation of the shoulder may facilitate accurate needle placement. **C:** A narrow diameter sleeve or instrument specific cannula is passed percutaneously through the rotator cuff (transtendon) and the appropriate instrumentation is used to place 1 or 2 anchors (*arrows*), each double-loaded, depending on the size of the tear. **D:** For each anchor in sequence, a suture limb of the anchor is grasped through the anterior portal. A loaded spinal needle (No.1 absorbable suture) is then passed through the bursal side of the cuff, aiming for the edge of the partial tear. The suture is introduced into the joint and grasped through the anterior portal and will serve as a suture shuttle. A simple loop is tied in the absorbable suture and one of the limbs from the anchor, which has been brought through the anterior portal, is loaded on the shuttle outside the joint by tightening the loop. The shuttle (*arrow pointing right*) and accompanying anchor suture (*arrow pointing left*) are then pulled retrograde, in order, through the cannula, the tear edge, and into the subacromial space. **E:** After the shuttle is brought through the cuff (*left arrow*), the remaining sutures are passed in a similar fashion and eventually tied in the subacromial space to reproduce the anatomic footprint (*double arrow*) to the humeral head *(HH)*. **F:** The arthroscope is introduced into the subacromial space. Color-coded sutures facilitate identification of matched sutures. The appropriate suture pairs (*curved arrows*) are separated and then tied through the lateral or anterior cannula. **G:** The arthroscope is reintroduced into the glenohumeral joint and the edge of the partial tear should be contiguous with the articular margin, completely effacing the previously exposed footprint (*arrows*). (From Stetson WB, Ryu RKN, Bittar ES. Arthroscopic treatment of partial rotator cuff tears. *Oper Tech Sports Med.* 2004; 12:135-148; reprinted with permission.)

Fig 13-22. *(continued)*

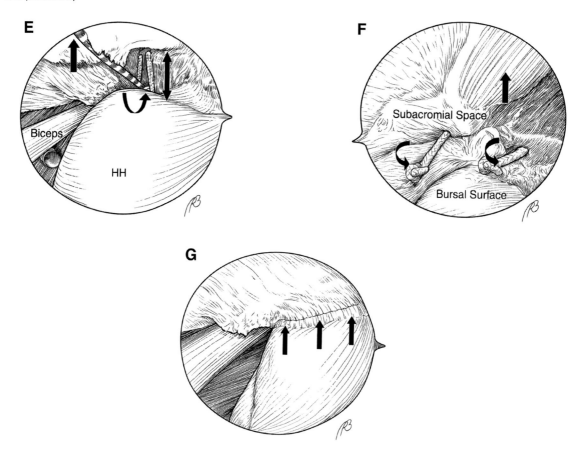

This method seeks to replace the partially torn tendon to its native "footprint" on the tuberosity, preserving the remaining fiber attachment. It is an alternative technique to the arthroscopic approach championed by Weber (137) in which the tear is first converted to a full-thickness injury and then repaired arthroscopically.

Full-thickness Rotator Cuff Tears: Treatment

It is important to understand that not all full thickness rotator cuff tears are alike, and that some complete tears are compatible with excellent function and minimal discomfort. Armed with biomechanical models, basic engineering principles, and kinematic studies of patients with known rotator cuff tears, Burkhart (35,40) defined the "functional rotator cuff tear." His reasoning was based on intact force couples in the transverse and coronal planes despite tearing. With the humeral head well-centered, the anatomically deficient rotator cuff tear can still provide functional integrity. A biomechanically functioning torn rotator cuff must spare a portion of the infraspinatus as well as the subscapularis. Alterations in this relationship can cause the centroid to move superiorly, thereby allowing the humeral head to translate superiorly and limiting shoulder elevation and normal kinematics.

Because not all tears are symptomatic, are there indications for the nonsurgical management of full-thickness tears? Yamaguchi has proposed three categories of risk: Group 1: those not at risk for irreversible changes to the rotator cuff in the near future; Group II: those at risk for irreversible changes with prolonged nonsurgical management; and Group III: those already with irreversible changes (139).

Irreversible changes include fatty infiltration, muscle atrophy, degenerative joint disease, and morphologic changes to the cuff including retraction and thinning. These irreversible changes in turn reflect the pre-operative risk factors portending a poorer outcome including larger tears, delay in treatment, and advanced age (141-143).

The size of the tear, degree of retraction, the presence or absence of fatty infiltration or atrophy, patient age, and activity level help the clinician determine the appropriate category, and then decisions can be made regarding the duration of nonsurgical management versus early surgical intervention. If a small tear can progress during the course of nonsurgical management but the results of treatment are not jeopardized, a prolonged conservative course may be worthwhile without posing a significant risk to the final outcome.

As noted earlier, the clinical presentation of a full-thickness rotator cuff tear can mimic findings consistent with simple impingement or with a partial thickness tear. The most common physical finding that distinguishes those with full thickness tears from impingement is weakness upon stress testing. Although weakness may be an indication of inhibitory pain, the Neer test can help document actual tendon weakness. After pain is relieved with the subacromial injection, significant weakness on stress testing is indicative of a full thickness injury. Often in those with large, chronic tears, visible atrophy within the supraspinatus and infraspinatus fossa may be present.

Small Tears Less Than 1 Centimeter

Smaller tears are easily missed as patients present with findings and symptoms consistent with impingement. Occasionally weakness is present, but even following the Neer test, significant weakness may not be detected. These tears usually involve the supraspinatus tendon insertion, and pain is the primary presenting complaint. Examination usually reveals normal motion and strength.

After the diagnosis has been confirmed, usually by MR testing, definitive treatment can be individualized. Several authors have shown that small tears treated with decompression alone can achieve significant pain relief while maintaining good function (66,113,135,143,144). In an older patient unable or unwilling to undergo the more arduous rehabilitation associated with a full thickness repair, the simple decompression alternative is a realistic one. In the younger, more active population, obvious concern regarding propagation of the tear is a legitimate one. The study by Yamaguchi et al. (49), revealing a 51% incidence of asymptomatic to symptomatic tearing over a five-year period raises doubts about a simple decompression resulting in a lasting and durable outcome for those who lead a vigorous lifestyle. For those individuals, a decompression in conjunction with a repair is the treatment of choice.

Although the open acromioplasty and rotator cuff repair technique has been associated with a high success rate, the technique has been supplanted by the arthroscopically assisted mini-open and the all-arthroscopic techniques (145–157). Several studies have validated these two newer approaches with success rates equal to those achieved through an incision alone (146,152). Furthermore, the mini-open and all-arthroscopic techniques have demonstrated little or no difference when compared in clinical studies (152).

The all-arthroscopic approach relies on meticulous technique and a well-patterned step-wise approach to a successful outcome. Arthroscopy is particularly helpful in allowing a panoramic view of the torn rotator cuff. After the tear pattern is recognized, an anatomic repair can be achieved. The goal of rotator cuff surgery is to achieve an anatomic repair in which the tendon is stressed appropriately and can function as originally intended.

Using standard anterior, posterior, and lateral portals, the tear is identified and the tear pattern recognized **(Fig 13-23)**. Small tears are generally crescentic in nature with minimal retraction due to their small size. Associated pathology is identified such as biceps fraying or tearing, and treated. A subacromial decompression is accomplished if there are

findings of impingement such as coracoacromial ligament fraying.

The actual rotator cuff repair begins with mobilization of the cuff, if necessary, and using a grasper to reapproximate the torn edge of the cuff back to the greater tuberosity. Simply mobilizing the cuff tendon in larger, retracted tears from a medial to lateral position and re-attaching to bone is usually an oversimplified approach and one that usually leads to structural failure. Chronic tears often have a specific pattern of retraction, and diagonal reduction maneuvers recreate the original anatomic attachment. The bony bed of the greater tuberosity can be prepared with the shaver blade or a curette in an attempt to minimize bone loss and to maximize the pullout strength of the implants. The suture anchors are placed 5 to 7 mm from the articular margin and are separated by at least 1 cm **(Fig 13-24)**. The insertion angle

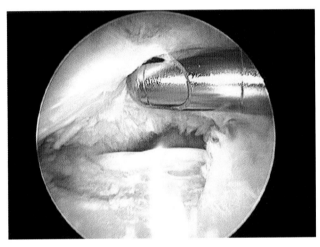

Fig 13-23. Small full-thickness rotator cuff tear with crescent pattern and minimal retraction visualized from the lateral portal of a right shoulder.

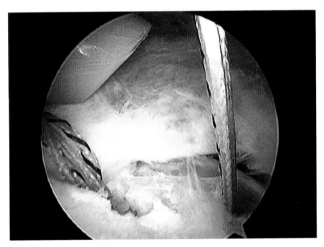

Fig 13-24. Double-loaded anchors inserted into the greater tuberosity approximately one centimeter apart and 1 to 2 cm from the articular margin. An insertion angle of 45 degrees or less improves pull-out characteristics of the implants.

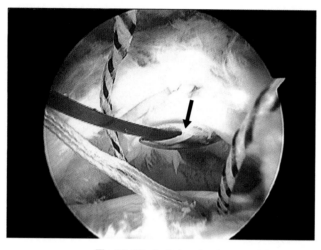

A

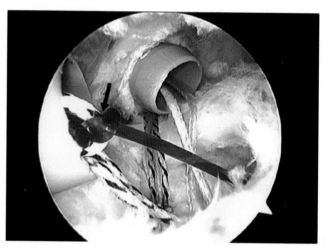

B

Fig 13-25. A: Suture hook passed through the free edge of the rotator cuff tear (*arrow*). The No.1 absorbable suture functions as a suture shuttle. **B:** No. 1 absorbable suture is retrograded through the free edge of the rotator cuff tear after loading with a suture limb (*arrow*) from one of the anchors.

approximates 45 degrees from the long axis of the humerus to maximize pull-out characteristics (54).

There exists a multitude of implant devices intended for rotator cuff repair, and for all, satisfactory bone purchase is essential. After the anchors are inserted, the sutures must be either ante- or retrograded through the free edge of the torn tendon **(Fig 13-25)**. Numerous ingenious instruments and devices are available to assist the surgeon in accomplishing this portion of the procedure. Several accessory portals are also available which can facilitate retrograde suturing of the rotator cuff.

After the sutures have been passed, careful, meticulous knot-tying is required during which both knot and loop security must be maintained, loop security referring to the tension with the suture itself as it passes through tissue. The final result should consist of an anatomic repair with excellent coaptation of tissue to the bony bed **(Fig 13-26)**. As the shoulder is ranged, no undue tension on the repair site should be present. Satisfactory clearance in the subacromial space should be verified as well.

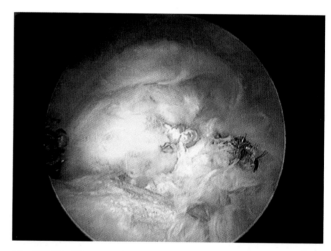

Fig 13-26. After completion of arthroscopic repair, knot and loop security must be maintained. Shoulder is ranged to assess undue tension, as anatomic repair should obviate premature fixation failure.

Medium to Large Size Tears 1 to 4 Centimeters

When larger tears are encountered, the option of a simple decompression becomes less compelling. Some authors have described satisfactory early results with this approach only to discover progressive deterioration, especially in the larger tears (113,135,143). Although the possibility of an isolated decompression in a low demand individual with limited goals remains an option, patients with sizeable tears are more likely to benefit from a formal repair of the torn tendon.

The goals and steps outlined for smaller tears is applicable for tears of all sizes. There are, however, several technical "pearls" that can improve the ease of the procedure as well the final result in the larger and more challenging tears. Again,

initial accurate identification of the tear configuration is the key step in achieving an anatomic repair. In those with a chronic, retracted U-shaped tear, the principle of margin convergence can be used with great effect on the final construct. Converging the free margin of the retracted tear to the greater tuberosity by placing side to side sutures not only facilitates the tendon to bone repair, but also relieves the forces at the repair site as well (98,158) **(Fig 13-27)**.

For those chronically retracted L-shaped tears with an anterior extension, an interval release (147,159) that divides the coracohumeral ligament can be very effective in gaining length and satisfactory mobilization such that an anatomic repair can be performed consisting of a side to side repair followed by tendon to bone **(Fig 13-28)**. This same approach

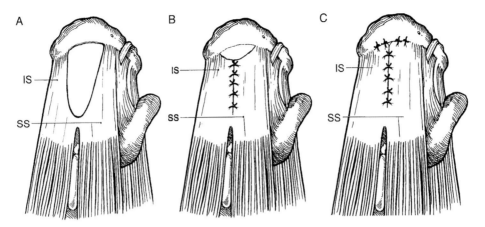

Fig 13-27. U-shaped cuff tear. **A:** Superior view of a U-shaped rotator cuff tear involving the supraspinatus *(SS)* and infraspinatus *(IS)* tendons; **(B)**, U-shaped tears demonstrate excellent mobility from an anterior-to-posterior direction and are initially repaired with side-to-side sutures using the principle of margin convergence; **(C)**, the repaired margin is then repaired to bone in a tension-free manner. (From Lo IK, Burkhart SS. Current concept in arthroscopic rotator cuff repair. *Am J Sports Med.* 2003;31:308-324; reprinted with permission.)

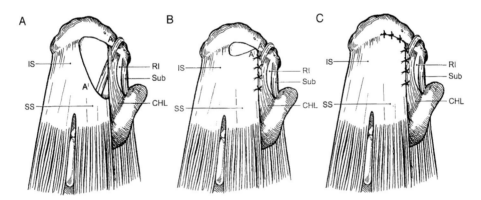

Fig 13-28. Chronic L-shaped tear. **A:** superior view of a chronic L-shaped tear, which has assumed a U-shaped configuration. **B:** L-shaped tears demonstrate excellent mobility from an anterior-to-posterior direction; however, one of the tear margins (usually the posterior leaf) is more mobile. These tears should be initially repaired using side-to-side sutures A' → A) by using the principle of margin convergence. **C:** The converged margin is then repaired to bone in a tension-free manner. *IS,* infraspinatus tendon; *SS,* supraspinatus tendon; *RI,* rotator interval; *Sub,* subscapularis tendon; *CHL,* coracohumeral ligament. (From Lo IK, Burkhart SS. Current concept in arthroscopic rotator cuff repair. *Am J Sports Med.* 2003;31:308-324; reprinted with permission.)

can be utilized for those L-shaped tears that exhibit a posterior extension with a diagonal retraction pattern.

Massive Rotator Cuff Tears

These tears usually exceed 4 to 5 cm in dimension, but can be deceiving. Clearly a tear retracted in a lateral to medial direction of 5 cm presents as a very challenging repair whereas a tear extending 5 cm in an anterior to posterior direction without significant retraction is a much easier surgical problem to solve. In general, massive tears refer to those chronic, retracted tears that are usually accompanied by fatty infiltration, muscle belly atrophy as well as thinning and scarring of

the torn end of the rotator cuff. The approach to these massive, retracted tears can be difficult, and requires that the clinician gather as much information as possible before embarking on a therapeutic course.

These patients often present with pain as their overwhelming symptom, and on examination can exhibit significant motion restriction. Not uncommonly, if motion is restored with a well-supervised physical therapy program, the pain can be significantly reduced. If functioning force couples are in effect, restoration of motion may be all that is required to attain a satisfactory result without surgery.

For those with significant strength deficits, the prospect of a repair has to be considered. Certainly concomitant fatty infiltration and muscle atrophy are poor prognostic factors, and patients must be counseled accordingly. Achieving re-attachment of the rotator cuff may not result in significant functional improvement if the rotator cuff is significantly diseased in advance of surgery.

Simple debridement and acromial "contouring" have been described as salvage-type procedures that may palliate some of the pain (66,144); however, the risk of violating the coracoacromial arch and of losing anterior-superior head containment must be carefully considered before embarking on a debridement-only approach. Clearly, if such an approach is selected, minimizing bone resection is of utmost importance. If the rotator cuff cannot keep the humeral head centered, the coracoacromial arch becomes a fulcrum for shoulder elevation. If the arch is violated and an aggressive bone resection is performed, the humeral head can erode through what remains of the acromion (Fig 13-11).

The technical principles guiding the repair of massive rotator cuff tears remain consistent with the techniques previously described. As the tear patterns become more complex, additional surgical maneuvers become applicable such as the double-interval slide described by Burkhart and Lo (159). When a complete repair of a massive tear is not technically feasible, consideration of a partial repair must be entertained. Restoring balanced force couples in a massive tear may provide enough stability for a functional outcome.

A discussion of post-operative rotator cuff integrity and its effect on the final outcome is relevant (160). Utilizing ultrasound, Harryman et al. (161) reported on a 65% incidence of intact rotator cuffs post-operatively. In his study, the results were directly correlated with the integrity of the final repair, namely pain relief and strength were better in those with an intact cuff. Galatz et al. (162) reported on the outcome of large and massive rotator cuffs repaired arthroscopically. Seventeen of 18 tears recurred as documented by post-operative ultrasound. Although at 12 months following surgery, the results were impressive from a pain relief and functional perspective, at 2 years and greater follow-up, two-thirds of the patients exhibited deterioration in both categories. Klepps et al. (163) described an experience with post-operative MR evaluation of open cuff repairs and noted that 74% had an intact cuff post-operatively if the initial tear was smaller while those with larger tears had an intact cuff in 62% of the cases. In this study, the end result was not affected by the integrity of the repair, and furthermore, improved strength, as well as pain relief, was noted in those who exhibited a recurrent tear based on post-operative imaging. Jost (164) reported similar findings with their patient population in which an intact cuff did not correlate with better results.

Perhaps the partial repair concept may be the best explanation. Burkhart et al. (89,90) has proposed a unified rationale for the treatment of rotator cuff tears, including partial repairs based on maintaining functional force couples. An arthroscopic approach to partial repairs in large and massive tears has also been reported as an alternative to tissue transfer (91,92). A proponent of partial repair of otherwise massive, irreparable tears of the rotator cuff, Burkhart has argued that maintaining force couples is of greater concern than closing the defect. Although the repair is not water tight, and although a defect may be present post-operatively as judged by MR or ultrasound, the restoration of balanced force couples keeps the humeral head well-centered thereby allowing the extrinsic musculature to function efficiently.

■ CONCLUSIONS

Understanding the anatomy, biology, and pathoanatomy of the rotator cuff is of utmost importance if skilled treatment of rotator cuff injuries is the objective. Recognizing the spectrum of disease and the various etiologies takes effort and experience. After the injury is understood, the pathoanatomy well-visualized, and the patient's specific needs acknowledged, treatment of the rotator cuff injury can be well-formulated with every expectation of a satisfactory outcome for both patient and surgeon.

■ REFERENCES

1. Clark JM, Harryman DT. Tendons, ligaments, and capsules of the rotator cuff. *J Bone Joint Surg Am.* 1992;74:713–725.
2. Harryman DT, Clark JM Jr. Anatomy of the rotator cuff. In: Burkhead WZ, ed. *Rotator cuff disorders.* Philadelphia: Williams & Wilkins; 1996:23–25.
3. Sonnabend DH, Yu Y, Howlett R, et al. Laminated tears of the human rotator cuff: a histologic and immunochemical study. *J Shoulder Elbow Surg.* 2001;10:109–115.
4. Williams GR, et al. Anatomic, histologic, and magnetic resonance imaging abnormalities of the shoulder. *Clin Orthop.* 1996; 330:66–74.
5. Lee SB, Nakajima T, Luo ZP, et al. The bursal and articular sides of the supraspinatus tendon have a different compressive stiffness. *Clin Biomech.* 2000;15:241–247.
6. Montenegro S. Arthroscopic cuff repair with and without bursal incorporation-second look. Presented at the 21st Annual San Diego Shoulder Meeting, San Diego, CA: July 2004.
7. Ishii H, Brunet JA, Welsh RP, et al. "Bursal reactions" in rotator cuff tearing, the impingement syndrome, and calcifying tendinitis. *J Shoulder Elbow Surg.* 1997;6:131–136.
8. Ruotolo C, Fow JE, Nottage WM. The supraspinatus footprint: An anatomic study of the supraspinatus insertion. *Arthroscopy.* 2004;20:246–249.
9. Dugas JR, Campbell DA, Warren RF, et al. Anatomy and dimensions of rotator cuff insertions. *J Shoulder Elbow Surg.* 2002;11: 498–503.
10. Stetson WB, Ryu RKN. Evaluation and arthroscopic treatment of partial rotator cuff tears. *Sports Med Arthrosc Rev.* 2004;12: 114–123.
11. Gartsman GM, et al. Articular surface partial-thickness rotator cuff tears. *J Shoulder Elbow Surg.* 1995;4:409–415.
12. Curtis A. Arthroscopic repair of partial rotator cuff tears, indications, and technique. Presented at the Arthroscopy Association of North America Fall Course, Palm Desert; 2002.
13. Moseley HF, Goldie I. The arterial pattern of the rotator cuff of the shoulder. *J Bone Joint Surg Br.* 1963;45:780–789.

14. Rathbun JB, Macnab I. The microvascular pattern of the rotator cuff. *J Bone Joint Surg Br.* 1970;52:540–553.

15. Rothman RH, Parke WW. The vascular anatomy of the rotator cuff. *Clin Orthop Relat Res.* 1965;173:78–91.

16. Lindblom K. Arthrography and roentgenography in rupture of the tendon of the shoulder joint. *Acta Radiol.* 1939;54:548–554.

17. Lindblom K. On pathogenesis of rupture of the tendon aponeurosis of the shoulder joint. *Acta Radiol.* 1939;54:563–577.

18. Nixon JE. Ruptures of the rotator cuff. *Orthop Clin North Am.* 1976;6:423–447.

19. Benjamin M. The histology of tendon attachments to bone in man. *J Anat.* 1986;149:89–100.

20. Neer CS II. Anterior acromioplasty for the chronic impingement syndrome in the shoulder: a preliminary report. *J Bone Joint Surg Am.* 1972;54:41–50.

21. Tuite MJ, Toivonen DA, Orwin JF, et al. Acromial angle on radiographs of the shoulder: correlation with the impingement syndrome and rotator cuff tears. *AJR Am J Roentgenol.* 1995;165:609–613.

22. Bigliani LU, Ticker JB, Flatow EL, et al. The relationship of acromial architecture to rotator cuff disease. *Clin Sports Med.* 1991;10:823–838.

23. Ozaki J, Fujimoto S, Nakagawa Y, et al. Tears of the rotator cuff of the shoulder associated with pathological changes in the acromion. *J Bone Joint Surg Am.* 1988;70:1224–1230.

24. Gohlke F, Barthel T, Gandorfer A. The influence of variations of the coracoacromial arch on the development of rotator cuff tears. *Acta Orthop Trauma Surg.* 1993;113:28–32.

25. Ogata S, Uhthoff HK. Acromial enthesopathy and rotator cuff tear: a radiologic and histologic postmortem investigation of the coracoacromial arch. *Clin Orthop.* 1990;254:39–48.

26. Ozaki J, Fujimoto S, Nakagawa Y, et al. Tears of the rotator cuff of the shoulder associated with pathological changes in the acromion: a study in cadavera. *J Bone Joint Surg Am.* 1988;70: 1224–1230.

27. Basmajian JV. Factors preventing downward dislocation of the adducted shoulder joint: an EMG; morphologic study. *J Bone Joint Surg Am.* 1959;41:1182–1186.

28. DePalma AF, Cooke AJ, Prabhaker M. The role of the subscapularis in recurrent anterior dislocations of the shoulder. *Clin Orthop.* 1967;54:35–49.

29. Saha AK. Dynamic stability of the glenohumeral joint. *Acta Orthop Scand.* 1972;42:476–483.

30. Symeonides PP. The significance of the subscapularis muscle in the pathogenesis of recurrent anterior dislocation of the shoulder. *J Bone Joint Surg Br.* 1972;54:476–483.

31. Colachis SC, Strohom BR. Effects of axillary nerve blocks and muscle force in the upper extremity. *Arch Physiol Med Rehab.* 1969;50:647–654.

32. Colachis SC. The effect of suprascapular and axillary nerve blocks and muscle force in the upper extremity. *Arch Physiol Med Rehab.* 1971;53:22–29.

33. Inman VT, Saunders JB, Abbott LC. Observations on the function of the shoulder joint. *J Bone Joint Surg.* 1944;26:1–30.

34. Burkhart SS. Current concepts: A stepwise approach to arthroscopic rotator cuff repair based on biomechanical principles. *Arthroscopy.* 2000;16:82–90.

35. Burkhart SS. Reconciling the paradox of rotator cuff repair versus debridement. A unified biomechanical rationale for the treatment of rotator cuff tears. *Arthroscopy.* 1994;10:4–19.

36. Burkhart SS. Arthroscopic debridement and decompression for selected rotator cuff tears: clinical results, pathomechanics, and patient selection based on biomechanical parameters. *Orthop Clin North Am.* 1993;24:111–123.

37. Burkhart SS. Partial repair of massive rotator cuff tears: the evolution of a concept. *Orthop Clin North Am.* 1997;28:125–132.

38. Burkhart SS. Shoulder arthroscopy. New concepts. *Clin Sports Med.* 1996;15:635–653.

39. Burkhart SS, Nottage WM, Ogilvie-Harris DJ, et al. Partial repair of irreparable rotator cuff tears. *Arthroscopy.* 1994;10:363–370.

40. Burkhart SS. Fluoroscopic comparison of kinematic patterns in massive rotator cuff tears: a suspension bridge model. *Clin Orthop.* 1992;284:144–152.

41. Hitchcock HH, Bechtol CH. Painful shoulder: observations on the role of the tendon of the long head of the biceps brachii in its causations. *J Bone Joint Surg Am.* 1948;30:263–273.

42. Yamaguchi K, Riew KD, Galatz, LM, et al. Biceps activity during shoulder motion: an electromyographic analysis. *Clin Orthop.* 1997;336:122–129.

43. Goldfarb C, Yamaguchi K. The biceps tendon: dogma and Controversies. *Sports Med and Arthro Rev.* 1999;7:93–103.

44. Leffert RD, Rowe CR. Tendon rupture. In: Rowe CR, ed. *The shoulder.* New York: Churchill-Livingstone; 1988:131–163.

45. Jobe FW, Moynes DR, Tibone JE, et al. An EMG analysis of the shoulder in pitching. A second report. *Am J Sports Med.* 1984;12:218–220.

46. Glousman R, Jobe F, Tibone J, et al. Dynamic electromyographic analysis of the throwing shoulder with glenohumeral instability. *J Bone Joint Surg Am.* 1988;70(2):220–226.

47. Tempelhof S, Rupp S, Seil R. Age-related prevalence of rotator cuff tears in asymptomatic shoulders. *J Shoulder Elbow Surg.* 1999; 8:296–299.

48. Ruotolo C, Nottage WM. Surgical and non-surgical management of rotator cuff tears. *Arthroscopy.* 2002;18:527–531.

49. Yamaguchi K, Tetro AM, Blam O, et al. Natural history of asymptomatic rotator cuff tears: a longitudinal analysis of asymptomatic tears detected sonographically. *J Shoulder Elbow Surg.* 2001;10:199–203.

50. Cotton RE, Rideout DF. Tears of the humeral rotator cuff. A radiological and pathological necropsy survey. *J Bone Joint Surg Br.* 1964;46B:314–328.

51. Lehman C, Cuomo F, Kurnmer CJ, et al. The incidence of full thickness rotator cuff tears in a large cadaveric population. *Bull Hosp Jt Dis.* 1995;54:30–31.

52. Fukuda H, et al. Partial thickness of the rotator cuff: a clinico-pathological review based on 66 surgically verified cases. *Clin Orthop.* 1996;20:257–265.

53. DePalma AF. *Surgery of the shoulder.* Philadelphia: JB Lippincott Co;950:108.

54. Pettersson G. Rupture of the tendon aponeurosis of the shoulder joint in anterior inferior dislocation. *Acta Chir Scand.* 1942; 77(suppl):1–184.

55. Sher JS, et al. Abnormal findings on magnetic resonance images of asymptomatic shoulders. *J Bone Joint Surg Am.* 1995;77:10–15.

56. Yamanaka, K. The joint side of the rotator cuff: a follow-up study by arthroscopy. *Clin Orthop.* 1994;304:68–73.

57. Fukuda M, Mikasa M, Yamanaka K. Incomplete thickness rotator cuff tears diagnosed by subacromial bursography. *Clin Orthop.* 1987;223:51–55.

58. Gartsman GM. Arthroscopic treatment of rotator cuff disease. *J Shoulder Elbow Surg.* 1995;4:228–241.

59. Carpenter JE, Thomopoulos J, Flanagan CL, et al. Rotator cuff defect healing: a biomechanical and histologic analysis in animal models. *J Shoulder Elbow Surg.* 1998;7:599–605.

60. Codman EA. *The Shoulder.* Boston: Thomas Todd; 1934.

61. Fukuda H, Hamada K, Nakajima T, et al. Pathology and pathogenesis of the intratendinous tearing of the rotator cuff viewed from en bloc histologic sections. *Clin Orthop.* 1994;304:60–67.

62. Neer CS II. Impingement lesions. *Clin Orthop.* 1983;173:70–77.

63. Burns WC, Whipple TL. Anatomic relationships in the shoulder impingement syndrome. *Clin Orthop.* 1993;294:96–102.

64. Rockwood CA, Lyons FR. Shoulder impimgement syndrome: diagnosis, radiographic evaluation, and treatment with a modified Neer acromioplasty. *J Bone Joint Surg Am.* 1993;74:409–424.

65. Zuckerman JD, Klummer FJ, Cuomo F, et al. The influence of the coracoacromial arch anatomy on rotator cuff tears. *J Shoulder Elbow Surg.* 1992;1:4–14.

66. Ryu RKN. Arthroscopic subacromial decompression: a clinical review. *Arthroscopy.* 1992;8:141–147.

67. Altchek DW, Warren RF, Wickiewicz TL, et al. Arthroscopic acromioplasty: technique and results. *J Bone Joint Surg Am.* 1990; 72:1198–1207.

68. Payne LZ, Deng XH, Craig EV, et al. The combined dynamic and static contributions to subacromial impingement: a biomechanical analysis. *Am J Sports Med.* 1997;25:801–808.

69. Bigliani LU, Morrison DS, April EW. The morphology of the acromion and its relationship to rotator cuff tears. *Orthop Trans.* 1986;10:228(abst).

70. Morrison DS, Bigliani LU. The clinical significance of variations in acromial morphology. *Orthop Trans.* 1987;11:234(abst).

71. Tucker T, Snyder SJ. The keeled acromion: an aggressive acromial variant-A series of 20 patients with associated rotator cuff tears. *Arthroscopy.* 2004;20:744–753.

72. Banas MP, Miller RJ, Totterman S. Relationship between the lateral acromion angle and rotator cuff disease. *J Shoulder Elbow Surg.* 1995;6:454–461.

73. Jobe FW. Impingement problems in the athlete. *AAOS Instruct Course Lect.* 1989;38:205–209.

74. Hawkins RJ, Kennedy JC. Impingement syndrome in athlete. *Am J Sports Med.* 1980;8:151–158.

75. Aoki M, Ishii S, Usui M. Clinical application for measuring the slope of the acromion. In: Post M, Morrey B, Hawkins R, eds. *Surgery of the shoulder.* St. Louis: Mosby-Year Book; 1990:200–203.

76. Soslowsky LJ, An CH, DeBano CM, et al. Coracoacromial ligament: in situ load and viscoelastic properties in rotator cuff disease. *Clin Orthop.* 1996;330:40–44.

77. Harris JE, Blackney MC. The anatomy and function of the coracoacromial ligament. *J Shoulder Elbow Surg.* 1993;2:56–60.

78. Ryu RKN, Fan R, Dunbar WH. The treatment of symptomatic os acromiale. *Orthopedics.* 1999;22:325–328.

79. Warner JJP, Beim GM, Higgins L. The treatment of symptomatic os acromiale. *J Bone Joint Surg Am.* 1998;80:1320–1326.

80. Bigliani LU, Norris TR, Fischer J. The relationship between the unfused acromial epiphysis and subacromial impingement lesions. *Orthop Trans.* 1981;7:138(abst).

81. Mudge MK, Wood VE, Frykman GK. Rotator cuff tears associated with os acromiale. *J Bone Joint Surg Am.* 1984;66:427–429.

82. Hutchinson MR, Veenstra MA. Arthroscopic decompression of shoulder impingement secondary to os acromiale. *Arthroscopy.* 1993;9:28–32.

83. Peterson CJ, Gentz CF. Ruptures of the suprespinatus tendon: the significance of distally pointing acromioclavicular osteophytes. *Clin Orthop.* 1983;174:143–147.

84. Kibler WB, Livingston BP. Closed chain rehabilitation for the upper and lower extremity. *J Am Acad Orthop Surg.* 2001;9: 412–421.

85. Warner JP, Micheli LJ, Arslanian LE, et al. Scapulothoracic motion in normal shoulders and shoulders with glenohumeral instability and impingement syndrome: a study using Moire topographic analysis. *Clin Orthop.* 1992;285:191–199.

86. Kibler WB. The role of the scapula in athletic shoulder function. *Am J Sports Med.* 1998;26:325–337.

87. Burkhart SS, Morgan CD, Kibler WB. The disabled throwing shoulder: spectrum of pathology part III: the sick scapula, scapular dyskinesis, the kinetic chain and rehabilitation. *Arthroscopy.* 2003;19:641–661.

88. Walch G, Boileau P, Noel E, et al. Impingement of the deep surface of the supraspinatus tendon on the posterosuperior glenoid rim: an arthroscopic study. *J Shoulder Elbow Surg.* 1992;1: 238–245.

89. Davidson PA, Elattrache NS, Jobe CM, et al. Rotator cuff and posterior-superior glenoid labrum injury associated with increased glenohumeral motion: a new site of impingement. *J Shoulder Elbow Surg.* 1995;4:384–390.

90. Jobe CM. Posterior superior glenoid impingement: expanded spectrum. *Arthroscopy.* 1995;11:530–536.

91. Paley KJ, Jobe FW, Pink MM, et al. Arthroscopic findings in the overhand throwing athlete: Evidence for posterior internal impingement of the rotator cuff. *Arthroscopy.* 2000;16:35–40.

92. Morgan CD, Burkhart SS, Palmeri M, et al. Type II SLAP lesions: three subtypes and their relationship to superior instability and rotator cuff tears. *Arthroscopy.* 1998;14:553–565.

93. Burkhart SS, Morgan CD, Kibler WB. The disabled throwing shoulder: Spectrum of pathology. Part I: pathoanatomy and Biomechanics. *Arthroscopy.* 2003;19:404–420.

94. Tokish JK, Decker MS, Ellis HB, et al. The belly-press test for the physical examination of the subscapularis muscle: electromyographic validation and comparison to the lift-off test. *J Shoulder Elbow Surg.* 2003;12:427–430.

95. Burkhart SS, Tehrany AM. Arthroscopic subscapularis tendon repair: technique and preliminary results. *Arthroscopy.* 2002;18: 454–463.

96. Warner JJ, Higgins L, Parsons IM IV, et al. Diagnosis and treatment of anterosuperior rotator cuff tears. *J Shoulder Elbow Surg.* 2001;10:37–46.

97. Burkhart SS. Fluoroscopic comparison of kinematic patterns in massive rotator cuff tears. A suspension bridge model. *Clin Orthop.* 1992;284:144–152.

98. Burkhart SS, Athanasiou KA, Wirth MA. Margin convergence: A method of reducing strain in massive rotator cuff tears. *Arthroscopy.* 1996;12:335–338.

99. Burkhart SS, Danaceau SM, Pearce CE Jr. Arthroscopic rotator cuff repair: analysis of results by tear size and by repair technique-margin convergence versus direct tendon-to-bone repair. *Arthroscopy.* 2001;17:905–912.

100. Neer CS, Poppen NK. Supraspinatus outlet. *Orthop Trans.* 1987; 11:234.

101. Stoller DW, Wolf EM. The Shoulder. In: Stoller DW, ed. *Magnetic resonance imaging in orthopaedics and sports medicine.* 2nd ed. Philadelphia: Lippincott-Raven Publishers; 1997:597–742.

102. Crues JV, Ryu RKN. Magnetic resonance imaging of the shoulder. In: Stark D, Bradley W, eds. *Magnetic resonance imaging.* Baltimore: Williams & Wilkins; 1991:2424–2458.

103. Hodler J, et al. Rotator cuff disease: assessment with MR arthrography versus standard MR imaging in 36 patients with arthroscopic confirmation. *Radiology.* 1992;182:431–436.

104. Lee R, et al. Horizontal component of partial-thickness tears of rotator cuff: imaging characteristics and comparison of ABER view with oblique coronal view at MR arthrography-intial results. *Radiology.* 224:470–476.

105. Reinus WR, et al. MR diagnosis of rotator cuff tears of the shoulder. Value of using T2-weighted fat-saturated images. *AJR American J Roentgenol.* 1995;164:1451–1455.

106. Traughber PD, et al. Shoulder MRI: arthroscopic correlation with emphasis on partial tears. *J Comput Assist Tomogr.* 1992;16: 129–133.

107. Quinn SF, et al. Rotator cuff tendon tears: Evaluation with fat-suppressed MR imaging with arthroscopic correlation in 100 patients. *Radiology.* 1995;195:497–500.

108. Goutallier D, Postel J, Gleyze P, et al. Influence of cuff muscle fatty degeneration on anatomic functional outcome after simple suture of full-thickness tears. *J Shoulder Elbow Surg.* 2003;12: 550–554.

109. Thomazeau H, Boukobza E, Morcet N, et al. Prediction of rotator cuff repair results by magnetic resonance imaging. *Clin Orthop.* 1997;344:275–283.

110. Blair B, Rokito AS, Cuomo F, et al. Efficacy of injections of corticosteroids for subacromial impingement syndrome. *J Bone Joint Surg Am.* 1996;78:1685–1689.

111. Neer CS. Anterior acromioplasty for the chronic impingement syndrome in the shoulder: a preliminary report. *J Bone Joint Surg Am.* 1972;54:41–50.

112. Roye RP, Grana WA, Yates CK. Arthroscopic subacromial decompression: two-to seven-year follow up. *Arthroscopy.* 1995;11:301–306.

113. Esch JC, Ozerkis LR, Helgager JA, et al. Arthroscopic subacromial decompression: results according to the degree of rotator cuff tear. *Arthroscopy.* 1988;4:241–249.

114. Olsewski JM, Depew AD. Arthroscopic subacromial decompression and rotator cuff debridement of Stage II and Stage III impingement. *Arthroscopy.* 1994;1:61–68.

115. Ellman H. Arthroscopic subacromial decompression: analysis of one- to three-year results. *Arthroscopy.* 1987;3:173–181.

116. Sampson TD, Nisbet JK, Click JM. Precision acromioplasty in arthroscopic subacromial decompression of the shoulder. *Arthroscopy.* 1991;7:301–307.

117. Snyder SJ, Wuh HCK. A modified classification of the supraspinatus outlet view based on the configuration and the anatomic thickness of the acromion. *Orthop Trans.* 1992;16:767.

118. Seltzer DG, Wirth MA, Rockwood CA. Complications and failures of open and arthroscopic acromioplasties. *Oper Tech Sports Med.* 1994;l2:136–150.

119. Hawkins RJ, Chris T, Bokor D. Failed anterior acromioplasty: a review of 51 cases. *Clin Orthop.* 1989;243:106–111.

120. Hawkins RJ, Saddemi SR, Mor JT. Analysis of failed arthroscopic subacromial decompression. *Arthroscopy.* 1991;7:315–316(abst).

121. Matthews LS, Burkhead WZ, Gordon S, et al. Acromial fracture: a complication of arthroscopic subacromial decompression. *J Shoulder Elbow Surg.* 1994;3:256–261.

122. Dennis DH, Ferlic DC, Clayton ML. Acromial stress fractures associated with cuff tear arthropathy: a report of three cases. *J Bone Joint Surg Am.* 1986;68:937–940.

123. Flugstad D, Masten FA, Larry I, et al. Failed acromioplasty etiology and prevention. *Orthop Trans.* 1986;10:229(abst).

124. Lee TQ, Black AD, Tibone JE, et al. Release of the coracoacromial ligament can lead to glenohumeral laxity: a biomechanical study. *J Shoulder Elbow Surg.* 2001;10:68–72.

125. Sano H, Ishii H, Trudeo G, et al. Histologic evidence of degeneration at the insertion of three rotator cuff tendons: a comparative study with cadaveric shoulders. *J Shoulder Elbow Surg.* 1999;8:574–579.

126. Fukuda H, Hamada K, Yamanaka K. Pathology and pathogenesis of bursal-sided rotator cuff tears viewed from en bloc histologic section. *Clin Orthop.* 1990;254:75–80.

127. Luo ZP, Hsu HC, Grabowski JJ, et al. Mechanical environment associated with rotator cuff tears. *J Shoulder Elbow Surg.* 1998;7:616–620.

128. PASTA.

129. Ellman H, Gartsman GM. *Arthroscopic Shoulder Surgery and Related Procedures.* Philadelphia: Lea & Febiger; 1993.

130. Snyder SJ, Pachelli AF, Pizzo WD, et al. Partial thickness rotator cuff tears: results of arthroscopic treatment. *Arthroscopy.* 1991;1:1–7.

131. Andrews JR, Broussard TS, Carson WG. Arthroscopy of the shoulder in the management of partial tears of the rotator cuff: a preliminary report. *Arthroscopy.* 1985;1:117–122.

132. Ogilvie-Harris DJ, Wiley AM, Sattarian J. Failed acromioplasty for impingement syndrome I. *Bone Joint Surg Br.* 1990;72:1070–1072.

133. Cordasco FA. The partial thickness rotator cuff tear: Is acromioplasty without repair sufficient? *Am J Sports Med.* 2002;30:257–260.

134. Ellman H. Diagnosis and treatment of incomplete rotator cuff tears. *Clin Orthop.* 1990;254:64–74.

135. Levy HJ, Gardner RD, Lemak LJ. Arthroscopic subacromial decompression in the treatment of full-thickness rotator cuff tears. *Arthroscopy.* 1991;7:8–13.

136. Weber SC. Arthroscopic debridement and acromioplasty versus mini-open repair in the management of significant partial thickness tears of the rotator cuff. *Ortho Clin North Am.* 1997;28:79–82.

137. Weber SC. Arthroscopic repair of partial thickness rotator cuff tears: The safety of completing the repair. Presented at the 22nd Annual Meeting of the Arthroscopy Association of North America, Phoenix, AZ; 2003.

138. Stetson WB, Ryu RKN, Bittar ES. Arthroscopic treatment of partial rotator cuff tears. *Oper Tech Sports Med.* 2004;12:135–148.

139. Lashgari CJ, Yamaguchi K. Natural history and non-surgical treatment of rotator cuff disorders. In: Norris T. ed. *Orthopedic knowledge update: shoulder and elbow.* Chicago: American Academy of Orthopedic Surgeons; 2002:155–161.

140. Kronberg M, Wahlstrom P, Brostrom LA. Shoulder function after surgical repair of rotator cuff tears. *J Shoulder Elbow Surg.* 1997;6:125–130.

141. Iannotti JP, Bernot MP, Kuhlmann JR, et al. Postoperative assessment of shoulder function: a prospective study of full-thickness rotator cuff tears. *J Shoulder Elbow Surg.* 1996;5:449–457.

142. Mansat P, Cofield RH, Kersten TE, et al. Complications of rotator cuff repair. *Orthop Clin North Am.* 1997;28:205–213.

143. Ellman H, Say SP, Wirth M. Arthroscopic treatment of full-thickness rotator cuff tears: 2 to 7 year follow-up study. *Arthroscopy.* 1993;9:195–200.

144. Rockwood CA Jr, Williams GR, Burkhead WZ. Debridement of degenerative, irreparable lesions of the rotator cuff. *J Bone Joint Surg Am.* 1995;77:857–866.

145. Paulos LE, Kody MH. Arthroscopically enhanced "mini-approach" to rotator cuff repair. *Am J Sports Med.* 1994;22:19–25.

146. Liu SH, Baker CL. Arthroscopically-assisted rotator cuff repair: correlation of functional results with integrity of the cuff. *Arthroscopy.* 1994;10:54–60.

147. Tauro J. Arthroscopic "Interval Slide" in the repair of large rotator cuff tears. *Arthroscopy.* 1999;15:527–530.

148. Snyder SJ, Heat DP. Arthroscopic repair of rotator cuff tears with miniature suture screw anchors and permanent mattress sutures. *Arthroscopy.* 1994;10:345(abst).

149. Jones C, Savoie F. Arthroscopic repair of large and massive rotator cuff tears. *Arthroscopy.* 2003;19:564–571.

150. Lo IK, Burkhart SS. Arthroscopic repair of massive, contracted, immobile rotator cuff tears using single and double interval slides: technique and preliminary results. *Arthroscopy.* 2004;20:22–33.

151. Bennett W. Arthroscopic repair of full-thickness supraspinatus tears (small to medium): a prospective study with two- to four-year follow up. *Arthroscopy.* 2003;19:249–256.

152. Severud E, Ruotolo C, Abbott D, et al. All-arthroscopic versus mini-open rotator cuff repair: a long-term retrospective outcome comparison. *Arthroscopy.* 2003;19:234–238.

153. Wilson F, Hinov V, Adams G. Arthroscopic repair of full-thickness tears of the rotator cuff: two- to four-year follow-up. *Arthroscopy.* 2002;18:136–144.

154. Bennett W. Arthroscopic repair of massive rotator cuff tears: a prospective cohort with two- to four-year follow-up. *Arthroscopy.* 2003;19:380-390.

155. Gartsman GM, Khan M, Hammerman SM. Arthroscopic repair of full thickness tears of the rotator cuff. *J Bone Joint Surg.* 1998;80:832–840.

156. Tauro JC. Arthroscopic rotator cuff repair; analysis of technique and results at two- and three-year follow-up. *Arthroscopy.* 1998;14:45–51.

157. Murray TF, Lajtai G, Mileski RM, et al. Arthroscopic repair of medium to large full-thickness rotator cuff tears: outcome at two- to- six-year follow-up. *J Shoulder Elbow Surg.* 2002;11:19–24.

158. Burkhart SS. Arthroscopic treatment of massive rotator cuff tears: clinic results and biomechanical rationale. *Clin Orthop.* 1991;267:45–56.

159. Lo IK, Burkhart SS. Current concept in arthroscopic rotator cuff repair. *Am J Sports Med.* 2003;31:308–324.

160. Rokito AS, Cuomo F, Gallagher MA, et al. Long-term functional outcome of repair of large and massive chronic tears of the rotator cuff. *J Bone Joint Surg.* 1999;81:991–997.

161. Harryman DT, Mack LA, Wang KY, et al. Repairs of the rotator cuff: correlation of functional results with integrity of the cuff. *J Bone Joint Surg.* 1991;73:982-989.

162. Galatz LM, Ball CM, Teefy SA, et al. The outcome and repair integrity of completely arthroscopically repaired large and massive rotator cuff tears. *J Bone Joint Surg.* 2004;86:219–224.

163. Klepps S, Bishop J, Lin J, et al. Prospective evaluation of the effect of rotator cuff integrity on the outcome of open rotator cuff repairs. *Am J Sports Med.* 2004;32:1716–1722.

164. Jost B, Pfirrmann CW, Gerber C. Clinical outcome after structural failure of rotator cuff repairs. *J Bone Joint Surg.* 2000;82: 304–314.

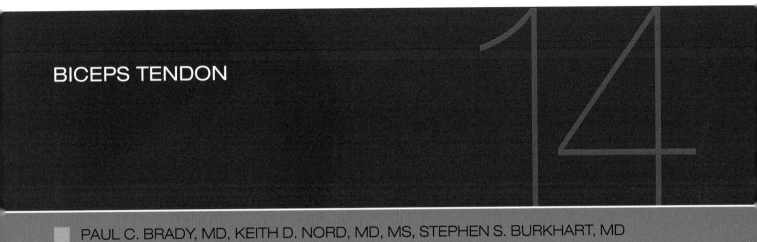

BICEPS TENDON

14

■ PAUL C. BRADY, MD, KEITH D. NORD, MD, MS, STEPHEN S. BURKHART, MD

■ KEY POINTS

■ The long head of the biceps (LHB) originates at and around the supraglenoid tubercle. Although it is intra-articular, it is extrasynovial.

■ Although acute ruptures of the LHB do occur, LHB ruptures are more commonly the result of chronic biceps tendonitis.

■ There is such a close association between subacromial impingement and biceps tendonitis that the two conditions have closely overlapping symptoms. They can be difficult to distinguish and more often than not occur in tandem.

■ The hallmark of biceps tendon related pathology is point tenderness in the bicipital groove.

■ Given the close relationship between biceps tendon pathology and concomitant subacromial impingement and/or rotator cuff tear, it is important to examine the remainder of the shoulder. Specific tests for range of motion, impingement, rotator cuff integrity, and instability should be performed.

■ Ultrasound and arthrography are equally effective for the diagnosis of biceps tendon and rotator cuff problems, but ultrasound is superior when evaluating the biceps tendon.

■ Complications of the biceps tenotomy primarily involve the anticipated 21% risk of a "Popeye" deformity of the biceps muscle as it retracts distally. Arthroscopic biceps tenotomy is otherwise a relatively safe procedure with very minor risks of infection, blood clots, or neurovascular injury. Biceps tenodesis may be appropriate for younger, more active patients to maximize shoulder and elbow function.

The long head of the biceps (LHB) tendon . . . what does it do? What symptoms does it cause? What is the etiology of its pathology? What is the best treatment of biceps associated disorders? These are just a few of the questions concerning the biceps tendon for which opinions are abundant but firm conclusions are elusive. In our understanding of the shoulder, the LHB is still somewhat of an enigma. There are many beliefs and a plethora of data which provide much information but little clarity on the biceps tendon.

This chapter will attempt to provide a comprehensive overview regarding the biceps tendon. It will discuss both the undisputed aspects such as its anatomy as well as more controversial topics such as its function, pathophysiology, and treatment. The goal is to present a balanced and succinct overview of the biceps tendon and its pathology and treatment.

■ BASIC SCIENCE

Anatomy

The anatomy of the LHB has been thoroughly examined and little controversy exists in this realm. The LHB originates at and around the supraglenoid tubercle. Although it is intra-articular, it is extrasynovial. Its blood supply is dependant on the portion of tendon in question. The proximal and middle portions receive blood supply from branches of the anterior humeral circumflex artery and the distal third of the tendon receives nourishment from branches of the deep brachial artery. The blood supply is markedly reduced in the portion of the tendon which slides in the bicipital groove.

Habermayer et al. (1) demonstrated LHB origin from the supraglenoid tubercle in 20% of specimens, origin from the posterosuperior labrum in 48%, and origin from both the labrum and tubercle in 28%. Pal et al. (2) demonstrated the major origin from the supraglenoid tubercle in 25% and from the posterosuperior labrum in 70%. The association between the biceps tendon and the superior labrum was further examined by Vangsness et al. (3) who classified the origin into four types. Type I (22% of specimens) demonstrated origin entirely from the posterior labrum; Type II (33%) demonstrated primarily posterior attachment with small anterior labral component; Type III (37%) demonstrated equal anterior and posterior labral components; and Type IV (8%) demonstrated only anterior labral contribution. The close relationship between the biceps and the labrum was further supported by Cooper et al. (4) who demonstrated an intimate relationship between the collagen fibrils of the two structures.

The length of the tendinous portion of the LHB measures approximately 9 cm and the musculotendinous junction is at the level of the deltoid and pectoralis major insertions. Its shape is relatively flat at its origin, becoming more tubular as it proceeds distally and into the intertubercular groove (5). McGough et al. (5) examined the tensile properties of the LHB and demonstrated that it is weakest at the midpoint—where all his experimental specimens ruptured.

The course of the LHB is from the posterosuperior aspect of the glenoid obliquely over the top of the humeral head. It then enters the bicipital (intertubercular) groove. This groove is formed by the confluence of the lesser tuberosity (anteriorly) and the greater tuberosity (superiorly). Anatomic studies have demonstrated varying depths of the groove (average = 4.3 mm) and varying inclination of the walls of the groove (6). Ueberham et al. (7) described a ridge on the upper portion of the lesser tuberosity (termed a supratubercular ridge) in 45% of anatomic specimens, which was postulated to "push" the biceps anteriorly. Although some authors have suggested that a shallow inclination of the groove predisposes to dislocation (1,8), others have found no such association (6).

The most critical anatomical consideration to understand regarding the LHB is that of its stabilizing structures. Specifically, a thorough understanding of the rotator interval is essential. The rotator interval is the triangular interval bordered superiorly by the anterior margin of the supraspinatus, inferiorly by the superior margin of the subscapularis, and medially by the anterior aspect of the glenoid. Within this triangular space exists anterior glenohumeral capsule as well as the coracohumeral ligament (CHL) and the superior glenohumeral ligament (SGHL). The SGHL and the medial head of the CHL join to form a medial sling for the LHB and this is the major restraint to medial subluxation/dislocation of the LHB (10,11) **(Fig 14-1)**.

The CHL originates from the base of the coracoid process and divides into two bands—a superior band, which inserts into the anterior supraspinatus, and an inferior band whose medial head inserts into the superior subscapularis

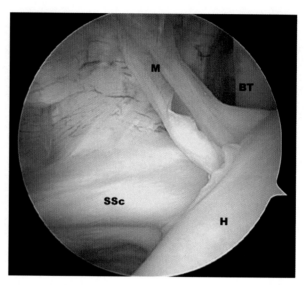

Fig 14-1. Posterior view of the right shoulder demonstrating the medial sling *(M)* of the biceps tendon *(BT)* and its confluence with the superolateral border of the subscapularis *(SSc)*.

and then onto the superior aspect of the lesser tuberosity. The SGHL also contributes to this medial sling as it courses from the anterior labrum (just anterior to the biceps origin) and inserts onto the superior aspect of the lesser tuberosity. The fibers of the medial head of the CHL are much more robust and structurally important to the medial sling than the fibers of the SGHL. This sling is critical in preventing the LHB from displacing medially onto the lesser tuberosity. In this way, the sling protects the proximal insertion of the subscapularis from the stresses that would result from a medially displaced LHB.

The medial sling and its relationship to the biceps tendon has been described as "the comma sign" (9). This comma sign is an arthroscopic description of the aforementioned anatomy of the medial sling and was so named because of its arthroscopic appearance. The comma sign consists of the medial head of the CHL and SGHL (medial sling of the biceps) intersecting with the superior border of the subscapularis. Although the comma sign is visible in the absence of pathology, it is much more prominent, recognizable, and useful in the presence of a torn and retracted subscapularis tendon. When the subscapularis is torn from its insertion on the lesser tuberosity, the medial sling of the biceps is also pulled off and its association maintained with the subscapularis. Identification of this comma structure is critical when searching for the subscapularis tendon because it is always located at the superolateral border of the subscapularis tendon **(Fig 14-2)**.

Historically, it was felt that the transverse humeral ligament was the vital structure in regards to retaining the biceps within the bicipital groove (12); however, this view has been challenged (13–15). Paavolainen et al. (15) cut the transverse humeral ligament in cadaver specimens but were still unable to dislocate the biceps tendon. Also, Gross

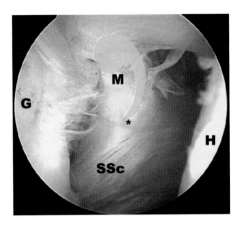

Fig 14-2. Posterior view of a right shoulder with a torn subscapularis (SSc) tendon. The comma sign is created by the intersection of the medial sling *(M)* and the subscapularis. The asterisk (*) represents the superolateral corner of the subscapularis.

[Ruotolo et al. (16)] reported on a technique of arthroscopic release of the sheath of the biceps tendon. In this technique the transverse humeral ligament was divided yet postoperative dislocation or subluxation of the biceps tendon did not occur. Gross emphasized that the CHL be preserved with this technique to prevent biceps instability.

Biomechanics

Few would dispute the critical role of the biceps brachii at the elbow joint and its function has been well documented at this position (17). It is with the LHB's role at the shoulder where the arguments intensify. Many authors have suggested that the LHB has a role in humeral head depression—particularly with shoulder external rotation (18). Andrews et al. (19) observed the biceps arthroscopically while electrically stimulating the biceps muscle and saw lifting of the labrum superiorly and compression of the glenohumeral joint. Likewise Kumar et al. (20) reported significant upward and anterior migration of the humeral head when the LHB was sectioned and then the biceps muscle was electrically stimulated. In another study, however, Lippmann (21) saw no humeral head motion with active biceps contraction.

Electromyography (EMG) studies have also demonstrated varying findings. Basmajian (22) demonstrated that the LHB did have EMG activity during active shoulder flexion. The LHB was estimated to contribute 7% of the power of shoulder flexion (23,24). Jobe et al. (25,26) showed peak biceps activity during follow-through and deceleration in the throwing motion. In separate studies, however, Yamaguchi et al. (27,28) and Levy et al. (29) modified the EMG experiment to control (limit) elbow flexion and both studies showed minimal to no EMG activity during isolated shoulder flexion. Another intriguing EMG finding has been an increase in EMG activity of the LHB in patients with rotator cuff deficiency (30). This increased activity may

result in the increased tendon diameter, which was observed by Rowe (31). Overall, although still somewhat controversial, there is some current literature supporting that the LHB has a depressing function in the shoulder and helps stabilize the humeral head in the glenoid. Even so, these effects are not dramatic.

Pathophysiology

Multiple classification schemes have been developed to describe disorders of the LHB tendon. These divisions have been only marginally useful in regards to diagnosis and treatment decisions. More important is to understand the various pathological processes involving the biceps tendon and how to treat each process accordingly. The three biceps tendon pathologies that we will discuss are biceps tendinitis, rupture, and instability. Lesions involving the biceps origin (SLAP lesions) will be discussed in greater detail elsewhere.

■ BICEPS TENDINITIS

Biceps tendinitis has been partitioned into primary tendinitis versus secondary tendinitis. Primary tendinitis involves inflammation of the tendon within the bicipital groove. To be considered primary, no other pathological findings (such as impingement, bony abnormalities within the groove, or biceps subluxation) should be present. It is considered an uncommon condition (32) and should be thought of as a diagnosis of exclusion (33). Habermayer and Walch (34) noted that this diagnosis can only be made during arthroscopy.

Much more common is the condition of secondary biceps tendinitis. As the LHB has an intimate relationship with its adjacent rotator cuff structures—most notably the anterior supraspinatus and superior subscapularis—it is affected by the same forces that produce pathology in these areas. Although subacromial impingement produces undue forces on the anterior rotator cuff, it also compresses the underlying LHB and produces concomitant pathology (and thereby symptoms) in this structure (33–39). In fact, the impingement upon the LHB worsens as a rotator cuff tear progresses and increased contact between the LHB and the coracoacromial arch occurs.

Another potential cause of secondary biceps tendinitis is the presence of bony anomalies of the proximal humerus. Most commonly these bony anomalies are secondary to malunion or nonunion of a proximal humerus fracture. If a fracture extends into the bicipital groove, significant irritation of the LHB can occur. DePalma and Callery (40) suggested that younger patients with biceps tendinitis are more likely to have groove anomalies such as narrowing or osteophytes, but it is difficult to determine the sequence of events in such conditions. Do the groove anomalies cause the tendinitis or the tendinitis cause resultant groove anomalies?

Biceps Tendon Rupture

Although acute ruptures of the LHB do occur, they are more commonly the end result of chronic biceps tendinitis. Acute ruptures can occur with a violent force placed on the LHB such as with a fall on an outstretched hand. Another traumatic event, which can cause significant damage to the LHB, is rapid deceleration of the arm during throwing activities (41). In this case the deceleratory force can result in trauma to the origin of the LHB resulting in a SLAP lesion. If the force is great enough in a single traumatic event or on a repetitive basis, it can result in LHB rupture with an associated SLAP tear (42).

Chronic biceps tendinitis is a more common etiology resulting in eventual LHB rupture. The LHB becomes attenuated and weakened by the continued impingement between the humeral head and the coracoacromial arch. In these cases of impingement causing rupture, the rupture typically occurs around the area of the rotator cuff interval (a weak point for the LHB) rather than at its origin (33).

Biceps Instability

Biceps instability takes the form of either frank dislocation or more subtle subluxation. As noted previously, the primary restraining structures holding the LHB in the bicipital groove are the medial sling and subscapularis tendon. Habermayer and Walch (34) divided LHB dislocations into extra-articular or intra-articular. The much less common extra-articular dislocations dislodge from the bicipital groove and travel over (anterior to) an intact subscapularis tendon. According to Habermayer and Walch (34), as well as in our experience, these dislocations are extremely uncommon. More commonly a LHB dislocation from within the bicipital groove is associated with a partial or complete tear of the subscapularis tendon, allowing the LHB to dislocate posterior to the subscapularis. The medial sling remains attached to the superolateral border of the subscapularis tendon—even when that tendon retracts medially. This arthroscopic anatomic landmark has been termed the "comma sign" (9). It is a critical arthroscopic finding because the comma easily guides the surgeon to the superolateral border of the subscapularis tendon thereby assisting in anatomic arthroscopic repair of the tendon back to the lesser tuberosity bone bed (9).

Biceps tendon subluxation can be a much more subtle diagnosis and we believe it is frequently missed even during arthroscopy. Again the critical anatomic components to prevent biceps subluxation are the medial sling and subscapularis tendon. In the early phases of biceps subluxation, the medial sling structures may remain largely intact while creating mechanical wear to the anteromedial portion of the LHB, which resides in the bicipital groove. It is therefore quite important to thoroughly examine the anteromedial portion of the LHB by pulling the structure intra-articularly with a probe while visualizing "over the top." This maneuver

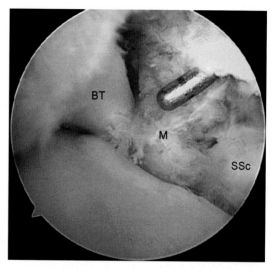

Fig 14-3. Posterior view of the left shoulder demonstrating fraying of the medial sling *(M)* of the biceps tendon *(BT)*. This we define as a "pre-comma" sign. Note that the biceps appears to be cutting posterior to the anterior plane of the subscapularis tendon *(SSc)*.

often requires a 70-degree arthroscope to adequately visualize these structures. As the pathology progresses, the medial sling becomes detached from its insertion on the superior aspect of the lesser tuberosity and the LHB begins to act as a knife cutting its way through the subscapularis tendon insertion, causing it to become detached from the lesser tuberosity. Early findings of this phenomenon can only be seen with the 70 degree scope visualizing "over the top" to look down at the bone bed of the lesser tuberosity. The senior author has described this view with the 70-degree scope as the "aerial view" (9). Fraying may also be appreciated on the medial sling. This finding is termed a "pre-comma sign" **(Fig 14-3)**.

As the humerus is internally and externally rotated the biceps tendon can be seen "breaking" posterior to the plane of the anterior border of the subscapularis (Fig 14-3). As a normal biceps tendon should remain anterior to the plane of the subscapularis, this "broken plane" phenomenon is a sure sign of early biceps instability. If not recognized, this will likely progress to LHB dislocation and complete tearing of the upper subscapularis insertion.

■ CLINICAL EVALUATION

History

Anterior shoulder pain (particularly in the region of the bicipital groove) is the hallmark of biceps tendon associated problems. With biceps tendinitis the pain is usually described as a chronic aching pain, which is worsened by lifting and overhead activities. The pain frequently radiates distally to approximately the mid arm level but seldom radiates proximally. Inciting events include repetitive activities involving

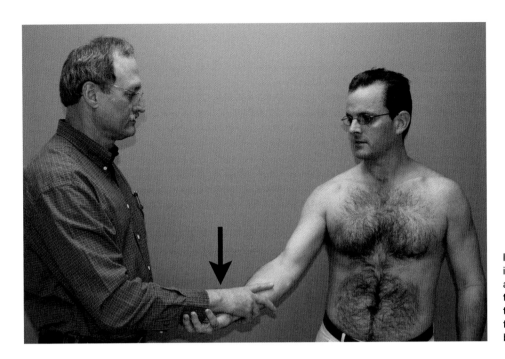

Fig 14-4. Photograph demonstrating the Speed's test. The examiner applies a downward force (*arrow*) to the patient's extended arm while the patient resists the downward force. Pain in the region of the biceps tendon is positive.

lifting and overhead activities. There is such a close association between subacromial impingement and biceps tendonitis that the two conditions have closely overlapping symptoms. They can be very difficult to distinguish and more often than not occur in tandem.

Patients who present with rupture of the LHB are usually much easier to diagnose. These patients complain of a history of chronic anterior shoulder pain consistent with biceps tendinitis and/or impingement. They then usually report an episode of a painful "pop" in the shoulder, followed by partial or complete relief of their impingement symptoms. Subsequently they may develop ecchymosis in the arm and an associated muscular deformity in the arm, frequently termed the Popeye muscle. Sometimes the Popeye deformity does not develop secondary to the LHB becoming incarcerated in a stenotic bicipital groove.

Physical Findings

Distinguishing anterior shoulder pain caused by biceps tendon disorders as opposed to subacromial impingement can be difficult, as these two entities usually co-exist. Although there are some exam maneuvers, which attempt to isolate the biceps tendon, there is still a fair amount of overlap and the definitive diagnosis of isolated biceps tendon pathology is extremely difficult based on history and physical exam alone. Often selective injections are helpful in differentiating the etiology of the pain.

The hallmark of biceps tendon related pathology is point tenderness in the bicipital groove. Without this finding it is extremely unlikely the LHB is involved in the patient's symptoms. The bicipital groove is best palpated approximately three inches below the acromion with the arm in 10 degrees of internal rotation (43). As the arm is internally and externally rotated, the pain should move with the arm. This is distinct from subacromial bursitis where the pain location remains relatively constant despite the position of the arm. Burkhead et al. (33) reports this "tenderness in motion" sign was quite specific for biceps tendon disorders. In the situation in which it is unclear whether the pain is secondary to the LHB or to possible impingement/bursitis, selective injections of these areas can help make the diagnosis.

There are several provocative tests that can be helpful in the diagnosis of LHB pathology; however, the sensitivity/specificity of these tests are questionable. These tests are intended for the diagnosis of LHB pathology. Tests for the diagnosis of SLAP lesions are covered elsewhere in this textbook.

- Speed's test (44) **(Fig 14-4)**—With the elbow in extension, the patient flexes the shoulder against resistance from the examiner. Pain in the bicipital groove is considered positive.
- Yergason test (45)—The patient attempts to supinate the wrist against resistance (with the elbow flexed at the side). Pain in the bicipital groove is considered positive.
- Bear Hug test (46) **(Fig 14-5)**—This test was developed by Barth et al. (46) to better isolate upper subscapularis lesions. Because these lesions are almost always associated with LHB instability, it is a good test for LHB pathology. The patient places the open palm of the affected extremity on the contralateral shoulder. In so doing, the ipsilateral elbow is held well anterior to the plane of the patient's body. As the examiner tries to lift the hand off the shoulder (resisted internal rotation), the patient tries to keep the palm on the shoulder. Weakness (in comparison to the

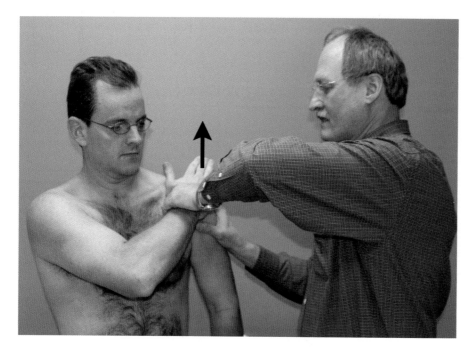

Fig 14-5. Photograph demonstrating the Bear Hug test. The patient places the palm of the affected extremity on the contralateral shoulder with the fingers held straight and the elbow kept in front of the patient. The examiner applies an upward force (*arrow*) to the extremity while the patient resists this force and tries to keep the palm on the shoulder. If the examiner is able to lift the palm off the shoulder this is a positive test.

- Napoleon test (47,48) **(Fig 14-6)**—This test also attempts to assess the integrity of the subscapularis for the reasons noted in the previous bullet point. The patient pushes on the abdomen with the palm of the affected extremity and tries to keep the wrist completely straight. If the patient is unable to keep the wrist straight but rather flexes the wrist to perform the test, this is considered a positive or intermediate test and suggestive of a subscapularis tear.
- Belly-Press test (48,49)—This test is similar to the Napoleon test in that the patient places the palm on the abdomen with the wrist held straight. The physician then tries to pull the hand off of the abdomen. If the physician is able to pull the hand off easily, this is considered a positive test and suggestive of a subscapularis tear.
- Lift-off test (50) **(Fig 14-7)**—This is the fourth test to assess subscapularis integrity. The patient places the back of the hand of the affected extremity on the ipsilateral buttock. The examiner then lifts the hand posteriorly and asks the patient to hold it in that position. Weakness or inability to lift the hand off the lower back is considered positive and suggestive of a subscapularis tear.

Other tests have been described, such as the Ludington test (51), biceps instability test (52), and the deAnguin's test (53); however, we do not utilize these tests and have therefore not described them. The described tests can be useful in assisting the clinician with the diagnosis of biceps tendon disorders. As noted previously, however, the sensitivity/specificity of most of these tests has not been examined. The exceptions include the Speed test, which Bennett (54) determined to be 90% sensitive for shoulder pain, but only 13% specific for bicipital pathology. Its positive predictive value was 23% while its negative predictive value was 83%. The Bear Hug test was determined to have a sensitivity of 60% and specificity of 92% for tears of the upper subscapularis (46).

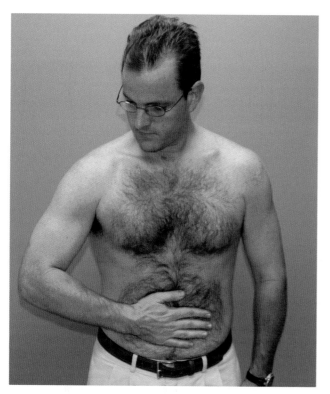

Fig 14-6. Photograph demonstrating the Napoleon test. The patient places the hand of the affected extremity on the abdomen and tries to keep the wrist straight. Inability to keep the wrist straight while performing this test is a positive finding

contralateral side) is a positive test and indicative of a tear of the upper subscapularis (and thereby likely LHB instability). In general, the examiner should not be able to lift the hand off the contralateral shoulder unless there is tearing of the upper subscapularis, in which case there is usually concomitant subluxation of the biceps tendon.

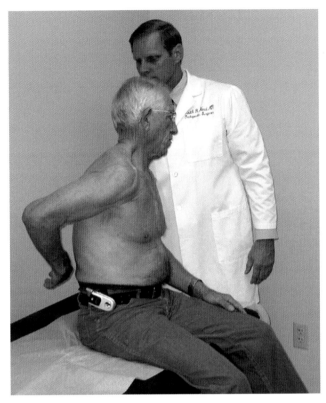

Fig 14-7. Photograph demonstrating the Lift-off test. The patient is asked to place the hand behind the back and then lift the dorsum of the hand off the back. Inability to do so is considered a positive test.

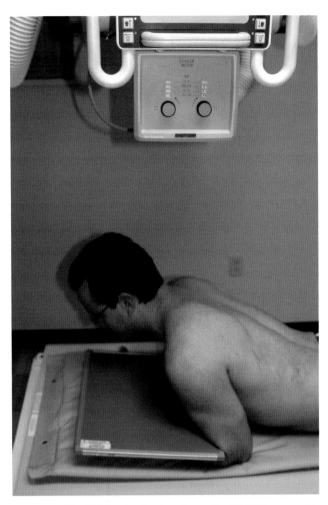

Fig 14-8. The Fisk projection has the patient hold the cassette while leaning forward on their elbows. The beam is projected perpendicular to the x-ray cassette.

Findings associated with complete rupture of the LHB are usually much more obvious. Examination reveals an alteration of the contour of the biceps such that a portion of the biceps feels (and appears) "balled up" at the mid arm level. This is termed the "Popeye" muscle. Rupture of the LHB is also often accompanied by ecchymosis, which migrates down the anterior surface of the arm.

Given the intimate relationship between biceps tendon pathology and concomitant subacromial impingement and/or rotator cuff tear it is important to examine the remainder of the shoulder in this patient population. Specific tests for range of motion, impingement, rotator cuff integrity, and instability should be performed.

■ IMAGING

As with almost every other orthopaedic condition, the clinician should begin by obtaining a complete series of plain film radiographs. For the shoulder, these should include an anteroposterior (AP) view, axillary view, and outlet view (or scapular-Y view). We also include a 30-degree caudal tilt view to better assess the acromioclavicular (AC) joint. Others have described radiographic projections, which are more specific for the bicipital groove region of the proximal humerus. These include the Fisk projection (55) and the bicipital

groove view (56). The Fisk method has the patient hold the cassette while leaning forward on their elbows and the beam projected perpendicular to the floor (and cassette) **(Fig 14-8)**. This view looks down the bicipital tunnel.

The bicipital groove method has the patient lie prone with the shoulder slightly abducted and the arm in external rotation. The cassette is placed on the top of the shoulder and the beam is directed up the patient's axilla (parallel to the long axis of the humerus) and perpendicular to the plate **(Fig 14-9)**. This view can elucidate the depth of the bicipital groove, the inclination of the walls of the groove, as well as any associated spurs within the groove.

Prior to the advent of magnetic resonance imaging (MRI), arthrography was a commonly utilized method of evaluation of the rotator cuff. It was also useful in the evaluation of the biceps tendon. The loss of a sharp delineation of the tendon can indicate biceps tendon pathology (57). Arthrography remains an invasive technique with possible contrast complications and this constitutes its main disadvantage.

Ultrasound has emerged as a potentially effective and noninvasive technique in the evaluation of biceps tendon

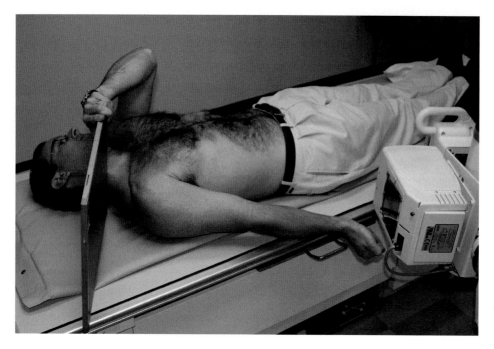

Fig 14-9. The bicipital groove view is obtained by having the patient lie supine with the arm in slight external rotation. The x-ray cassette is held on top of the patient's shoulder and the x-ray beam is aimed perpendicular to the cassette along the axis of the patient's humerus.

pathology. Middleton et al. (58,59) compared ultrasound to arthrography for the diagnosis of biceps tendon and rotator cuff pathology. They found the two modalities equally effective in the diagnosis of rotator cuff problems, but ultrasound was superior in the evaluation of the biceps tendon. Another study performed a biceps subluxation test and demonstrated 86% sensitivity in the diagnosis of LHB subluxation (as confirmed surgically) with ultrasound (60). Ultrasound has the added benefit of being a dynamic study. This allows easy evaluation with shoulder motion. In comparison to other imaging modalities, ultrasound is more operator dependent and therefore a well-trained technician is essential to obtain meaningful and helpful studies.

As with the evaluation of most other shoulder disorders, MRI has become increasingly popular. The anatomy (or patho-anatomy) of the biceps tendon and the bicipital groove is well delineated with MRI and associated findings such as rotator cuff pathology are also easily identified. Making the diagnosis of biceps tendon rupture or dislocation is relatively simple with MRI; however, biceps tendinitis and degenerative changes within the tendon are difficult to determine via MRI. Although some authors have suggested that increased fluid around the biceps is suggestive of biceps tendinitis (12), others report low sensitivity and specificity using this criterion (61).

■ TREATMENT

Nonoperative

The initial treatment of bicipital tendinitis is conservative using the traditional methods of rest, ice, and nonsteroidal anti-inflammatory medications. As symptoms improve, range

of motion exercises and strengthening can be added. The actual treatment is frequently directed more toward the treatment of underlying rotator cuff pathology. Subacromial injections or bicipital sheath injections may also be utilized. Caution should be exercised in injecting the bicipital sheath. Intratendinous injection should be avoided due to the risk of tendon rupture or atrophic changes. Although DePalma (62) reported on injection of the tendon directly, other authors (63) recommend sheath injections with 74% good to excellent results. It can be difficult to inject directly into the bicipital sheath, and therefore intra-articular injections have been advocated by some (64) because the proximal portion of the tendon is directly accessible and some of the fluid can track down the bicipital groove.

We prefer an intra-articular injection using a standard posterior portal approach. The joint line is palpated and entered approximately 4 cm inferior and 4 cm medial to the postero-lateral corner of the acromion. A 22-gauge 1.5-inch needle is aimed toward the coracoid and a pop is felt as the needle perforates the posterior capsule. This is the same direction as inserting a posterior cannula for glenohumeral arthroscopy. Four ml of Betamethasone (6 mg per ml) and six ml of 0.5% lidocaine HCL are instilled into the glenohumeral joint. In addition to the rapid therapeutic effects of bupivicaine on the intra-articular portion of the biceps, its added volume aids in travel of the mix down the bicipital groove.

Injections of a corticosteroid should be limited to two or three injections due the risk of tendon rupture, fluid retention, and weight gain. The patient is seen back at monthly intervals for re-evaluation and possible repeat injection. If symptoms progress or the condition worsens, further work-up with MRI, ultrasound, or CT arthrogram may be indicated. If symptoms improve with initial conservative therapy, gradual increase in activities is allowed, still limiting any inciting activity until the patient is relatively symptom free. If no other pathology is present, greater than 80% of patients can be expected to achieve good results with nonoperative treatment (65). If patients continue to have significant pain and further work-up including MRI is negative, other sources of pain must be considered such as cervical radiculopathy, instability, glenohumeral or acromioclavicular arthritis, coracoid impingement, adhesive capsulitis, lung conditions with referred pain such as Pancoast tumor (malignancy in the upper lobe of the lung), or medical conditions including cardiac or gallbladder referred pain.

Associated SLAP tears may be present, but little information regarding success rates with nonoperative treatment of SLAP lesions is available. The same conservative treatments may be employed, but many SLAP tears may ultimately require surgical intervention or may not be definitively diagnosed until arthroscopy is performed. The important subject of SLAP tears will be addressed elsewhere in this text.

Instability lesions of the biceps including subluxations or dislocations are frequently associated with rotator cuff tears. Treatment should be directed toward treatment of the rotator cuff tear and such treatment is frequently operative. Conservative treatment strategies should initially be employed but surgical intervention is often necessary. Ruptures of the LHB tendon typically do not require surgical intervention. Patients with proximal biceps ruptures regain function and have substantial pain relief. Many patients with pain before a biceps rupture will report pain relief once the rupture occurs. An associated cosmetic defect may be present in approximately 21% of proximal biceps ruptures (66), and patients should be provided information regarding the minimal strength loss if surgical intervention is avoided. Mariani et al. (67) reported on 26 patients (27 shoulders) undergoing biceps tenodesis vs. 30 patients undergoing nonsurgical treatment. Residual arm pain was minimal in both groups. Biomechanical analysis showed a 21% loss of forearm supination strength and 8% loss of elbow flexion strength in the nonsurgical group. The nonsurgical group had no weakness in pronation, elbow extension, or grip. The surgically treated patients had no loss of strength in elbow flexion, extension pronation, supination, or grip. Additionally, surgically treated patients returned to work later than nonsurgical patients, but 11 in the nonsurgical group were not able to return to full work capacity with weakness as their primary complaint. Only two patients in the surgically treated group could not return to full work capacity. Warren (68) tested 10 patients with chronic biceps ruptures and reported no loss of flexion strength and 10% loss of supination strength. Phillips et al. (69) used Cybex testing to compare nonoperative vs. operative intervention in 19 patients and found no significant difference in elbow flexion or supination strength.

■ OPERATIVE

Indications

After conservative treatment measures have failed, if the patient continues to have biceps associated symptoms, surgical management should be considered. The imaging studies previously discussed should be utilized prior to considering surgical treatment because of the significant overlap of biceps disorders and other shoulder conditions.

Biceps tendinitis is commonly associated with impingement syndrome and rotator cuff tendinitis or tears (70–74). Ruptures of the biceps tendon can result from trauma often with associated rotator cuff tears or SLAP lesions (75–77). Overload flexion force or flexion with forced extension may cause rupture of the biceps tendon (78). Other maladies associated with the biceps tendon involve medial dislocation (78–80), spontaneous dislocation (81,82), and pathologic lesions (83).

Basically there are only three treatments for biceps tendon disorders. They are debridement of the LHB, biceps tenotomy, or biceps tenodesis. The decision regarding tenotomy vs. tenodesis is a controversial subject. A tenotomy of the proximal biceps has been reported to carry a 21% incidence of a Popeye deformity with distal retraction of the biceps resulting in a larger muscle mass contracted distally and loss of the proximal muscle bulk (66).

Simple debridement of the biceps tendon is of questionable value. If fraying or partial tearing of the biceps tendon is encountered during arthroscopy its cause should be thoroughly explored. Even a small amount of fraying is suggestive of a mechanical abnormality within the shoulder joint and likely needs further arthroscopic evaluation and treatment. Although some have advocated biceps tendon debridement for tears of less than 50% (84), we feel tendon debridement is in essence treating the end result of the mechanical problem and not addressing the source of the problem.

The debate over biceps tenotomy vs. tenodesis will not be fully explored in this chapter, as the subject is quite controversial. We weigh many factors when making the decision to perform tenotomy or tenodesis. These factors include the patient's age, body habitus, activity level, and extent of biceps tendon degeneration. Typically tenotomy is reserved for elderly patients, sedentary patients with a larger body habitus, or patients with significant tendon degeneration which extends into the bicipital groove. Tenodesis in the latter situation may result in persistent pain due to pathology extending distal to the tenodesis site.

In general the authors opt for arthroscopic biceps tenodesis in almost every situation other than those mentioned earlier in this chapter. Many open techniques have been implemented in the tenodesis of the LHB. One commonly used open procedure is the keyhole technique (85). Alternative methods of open tenodesis involve soft tissue/periosteal tenodesis within the bicipital groove (86). For chronic retracted

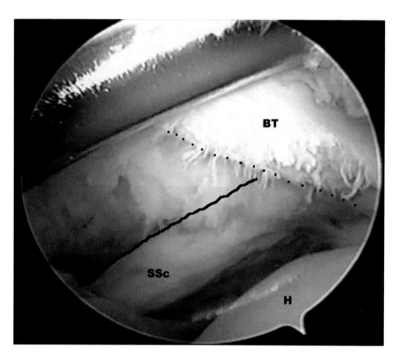

Fig 14-10. Aerial view of the right shoulder demonstrating an abnormal relationship between the biceps tendon *(BT)* and the subscapularis *(SSc)*. The biceps tendon *(outlined by the dotted line)* is seen cutting posterior to the plane of the anterior subscapularis *(outlined by the solid line)*.

ruptures of the LHB, open techniques are usually required although Richards and Burkhart (87) reported an arthroscopic assisted tenodesis technique (the Cobra procedure) for dealing with selected retracted tears of the biceps tendon. The remainder of this article will describe several arthroscopic biceps tenodesis techniques.

Technique

Operative intervention for biceps pathology begins with arthroscopic inspection and debridement. The proximal biceps tendon is easily visualized during standard glenohumeral arthroscopy. The tendon is first visualized thoroughly from the posterior portal. The tendon should be inspected from its origin on the superior glenoid tubercle and/or superior labrum all the way into the bicipital sheath. It is examined for fraying, degenerative changes, thickening or synovitis. The tendon from inside the bicipital sheath should be pulled into the joint with a probe to assess the integrity of the tendon. This can be facilitated by flexing the elbow, supinating the forearm, externally rotating and abducting the arm (70). This decreases the tension on the biceps and lengthens the amount of tendon that can be brought into the joint. This can expose lesions of the biceps that might otherwise be missed. This step is important to assess the integrity of the tendon. If the surgeon notices any fraying of the biceps tendon adjacent to the medial sling, this can be an important clue to early tendon subluxation. Arthroscopic biceps tenodesis can obviate the need for a repeat surgery to deal with a much more difficult problem such as tendon dislocation with associated subscapularis tears.

The next important portion of the diagnostic arthroscopy is the assessment of the medial sling. This is best done using a 70 degree arthroscope. The scope is directed to obtain an "aerial" view of the confluence of the subscapularis, the biceps tendon, and the medial sling of the biceps (composed of the medial head of the CHL and the SGHL). This view is maintained while an assistant internally and externally rotates the humerus. Special attention is paid to the relationship of the biceps to the anterior border of the subscapularis. In a normal shoulder, the biceps tendon should never cut posterior to the plane of the anterior subscapularis tendon during arm rotation. If the biceps does slip posterior to this plane it is a sure sign of early biceps instability **(Fig 14-10)**. If the biceps is not addressed by tenotomy or tenodesis, the patient may eventually develop frank biceps instability and an associated subscapularis tear.

At the completion of the diagnostic arthroscopy, if biceps pathology exists the surgeon must make the decision between biceps tenotomy vs. tenodesis as outlined previously. Tenotomy can easily be performed using arthroscopic scissors or electrocautery. The tendon should be cut at its base being sure not to damage the superior glenoid labrum during this procedure. The tendon will usually retract into the bicipital sheath; however, if it does not, the shaver should be used to excise the intra-articular portion of the biceps tendon so it does not impinge during shoulder motion.

The Bio-Tenodesis Screw System

We perform all arthroscopic shoulder procedures in the lateral decubitis position under general anesthesia. Five to 10 pounds of balanced suspension are used with the arm in 20 degrees to 30 degrees of abduction and 20 degrees of forward flexion (Star Sleeve Traction System, Arthrex, Inc., Naples, FL). Diagnostic glenohumeral arthroscopy is performed through

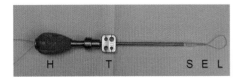

Fig 14-11. Bio-Tenodesis cannulated driver (Arthrex, Inc., Naples, FL) with driver handle *(H),* reverse threaded sleeve and thumbpiece *(T),* bioabsorbable Bio-Tenodesis screw *(S),* and a loop of suture *(L)* loaded through the cannulated tip. Turning the handle (H) and holding the thumbpiece *(T)* advances the screw *(S)* by means of the reverse-threaded sleeve that advances on the driver shaft while the driver end *(E)* remains stationary at the base of the bone socket. The measuring guides on the thumbpiece *(T)* are used to size the biceps tendon.

a standard posterior portal with an arthroscopic pump maintaining pressure at 60 mmHg. An anterosuperolateral portal is created using a spinal needle to localize the portal site. A cannula is inserted above the biceps at the superior edge of the safe zone bordered by the biceps superiorly, subscapularis tendon inferiorly and the glenoid medially. The biceps/labrum complex and the LHB are assessed. A complete assessment of the biceps tendon is performed by pulling the intertubecular

portion of the biceps tendon intra-articularly and assessing the amount of degeneration, partial tearing, and instability.

The technique described by Lo and Burkhart (88) utilizes a Bio-Tenodesis Screw system (Arthrex, Inc., Naples, FL), which uses a uniquely designed driver for inserting an interference screw. The cannulated driver **(Fig 14-11)** is specially designed with a reverse threaded sleeve and thumb piece on the driver shaft. The pitch of the threads on the sleeve are equal and opposite in direction to the pitch of the threads on the Bio-Tenodesis screw. This design allows the biceps tendon to be maintained at the bottom of the bone socket under tension as the Bio-Tenodesis screw is advanced in the bone socket by the hex-driver and by the reverse threaded pitch of the thumb sleeve. Fixation is achieved using a bioabsorbable PLLA (poly-L-lactic acid) cannulated screw. These BioTenodesis interference screws are available in three diameters (7 to 9 mm) and are 23 mm in length.

After completion of diagnostic arthroscopy, any tendon degeneration is debrided. If a concomitant rotator cuff tear is present, a lateral portal is established directly through the defect created by the torn rotator cuff. Two racking stitches are placed into the biceps tendon **(Fig 14-12)**. Sutures are placed approximately 1 to 1.5 cm distal to the biceps origin from

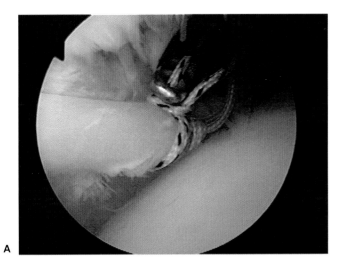

A

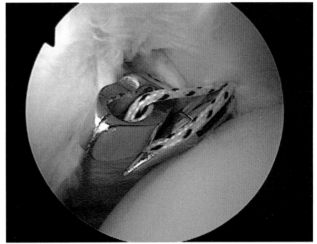

B

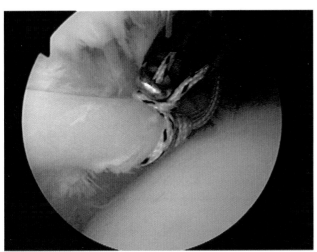

C

Fig 14-12. Arthroscopic view of the right shoulder biceps tendon demonstrating two racking sutures being placed. **A:** A Penetrator (Arthrex, Inc., Naples, FL) is used to penetrate the biceps tendon. Another suture retriever is used to hold the suture while the Penetrator is retracted. **B:** The Penetrator then grabs the suture and the loop is pulled out of the canula. **C:** The free ends of the suture are brought through the looped end and the free ends are pulled which creates a tight racking suture around the biceps tendon. The knot pusher allows the racking suture to be tightened.

the superior labrum and are then retrieved through the lateral or anterosuperolateral portal. The racking sutures tightly grip the degenerative biceps tendon. The biceps tendon is then severed from the superior labrum using electrocautery or arthroscopic scissors **(Fig 14-13)**.

The tendon is then exteriorized extra-corporeally through the anterosuperolateral portal. Flexion of the elbow allows a greater length of tendon to be pulled through the skin. The

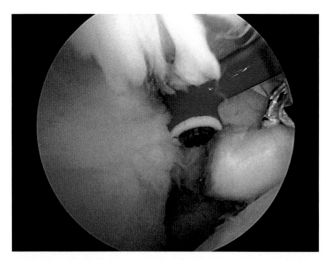

Fig 14-13. The biceps tendon is cut from its origin on the superior labrum/glenoid with the cautery device. If increased length is needed, the pencil tip cautery allows maximal retention of biceps tendon length.

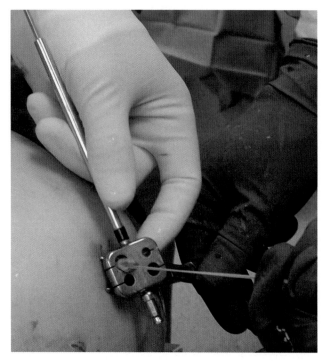

Fig 14-14. The tendon is exteriorized and measured. The thumb piece from the BioTenodesis driver (Arthrex, Inc. Naples, FL) will be used to size the tendon.

diameter of the tendon is then measured using the slotted measuring plate on the BioTenodesis driver **(Fig 14-14)**. Typically the tendon measures approximately 8 mm in men and 7 mm in women. If the tendon will not fit easily through the 8 mm hole, the end of the tendon is tapered such that it will fit through the 8 mm slotted measuring plate **(Fig 14–15)**. It is important that the tendon fit rather easily through the plate, as this will make insertion into the bone socket much easier later in the case. A Krakow whip stitch is placed in the tendon such that the suture ends exit the superior surface of the tendon 5 mm from its free end and then the racking sutures are removed **(Fig 14-16)**.

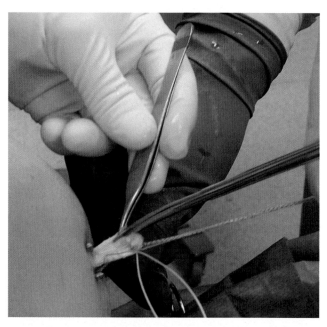

Fig 14-15. If the tendon does not fit easily through an 8 mm slot on the measuring device, the end of the tendon is tapered with scissors.

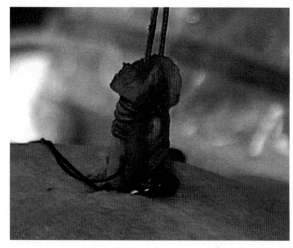

Fig 14-16. The biceps stump is seen here exteriorized. A Krakow whip stitch is placed in the tendon and the racking sutures will be removed.

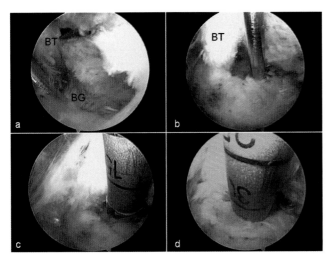

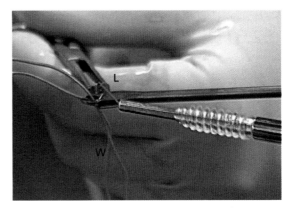

Fig 14-18. The whip stitch *(W)* from the biceps tendon is then passed through the loop of suture *(L)* passing through the BioTenodesis driver (Arthrex, Inc. Naples, FL).

Fig 14-17. A: The biceps tendon *(BT)* is seen within the bicipital groove *(BG)*. **B:** The guide wire is placed at the top of the bicipital groove in this case (without an associated rotator cuff tear). **C:** The cannulated reamer is then advanced over the guidewire. **D:** The reamer is advanced to a depth of 25 mm.

Next, a bone socket is created in the greater tuberosity, approximately 5 mm posterolateral to the top of the bicipital groove. A 2.4 mm guide wire is initially placed and is then over-reamed with a cannulated headed reamer (Arthrex Inc; Naples, FL). The bone socket is reamed to the size of biceps tendon previously measured (usually 7 or 8 mm in diameter) and to a depth of 25 mm to accommodate a screw length of 23 mm **(Fig 14-17)**. If there is not an associated rotator cuff tear involving the supraspinatus tendon, the bone socket should be drilled at the top of the bicipital groove. After the biceps tenodesis portion of the procedure, two or four suture

tails (depending on the technique) will be exiting the Bio-Tenodesis screw construct.

The whip-stitch sutures are then passed through a loop of suture at the end of the cannulated driver **(Fig 14-18)**.

The driver tip is advanced to the end of the tendon (on its superior surface). In this position, the biceps tendon can be manipulated and controlled by the cannulated driver tip. Alternatively, the whip-stitch sutures can be threaded through the cannulated driver. This has the advantage of making manipulation of the biceps tendon easier and has become our preferred method. The disadvantage is that only two suture strands (rather than four) will protrude from the BioTenodesis screw.

The driver tip is used to push the biceps tendon down to the base of the previously drilled bone socket **(Fig 14-19)**. A BioTenodesis screw (the same size as the drilled socket) is

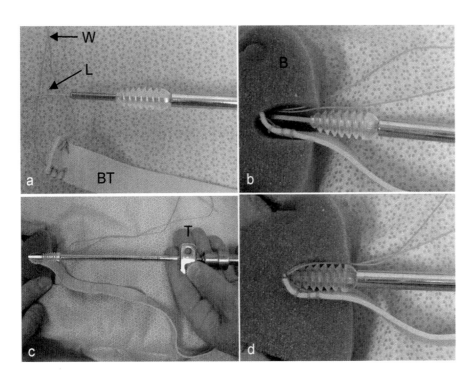

Fig 14-19. This is a dry lab demonstration of the BioTenodesis system. **A:** The whip-stitch *(W)* from the biceps tendon is then passed through the loop of suture *(L)* passing through the BioTenodesis driver (Arthrex, Inc. Naples, FL). **B:** The biceps tendon is pushed to the base of the prepared bone socket with the tip of the BioTenodesis driver. **C:** The screw is advanced by holding onto the thumbpiece while turning the driver clockwise. **D:** The screw is advanced until it is flush with the bone surface.

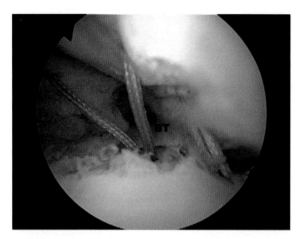

Fig 14-20. The BioTenodesis screw is advanced to the point it is flush with the bone surface. The biceps tendon *(BT)* is now secure in the bone socket.

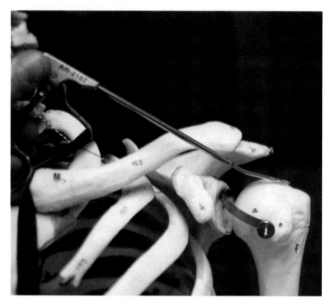

Fig 14-21. Skeleton demonstrating the proper orientation for the subclavian portal passing anterior and inferior the acromioclavicular (AC) joint and into the subacromial bursa. The penetrator (Arthrex, Inc., Naples, FL) is utilized in this fashion to retrieve sutures through the supraspinatous tendon. For insertion of an anchor during biceps tenodesis, the anchor is aimed slight caudal. The exact location is identified with a spinal needle prior to insertion of the anchor.

then advanced by turning the driver handle while holding the thumb plate that is attached to the reverse threaded sleeve. This allows the screw to be advanced while the tendon is maintained in a stationary position at the base of the bone socket.

This assures an adequate bone-tendon-screw interface within the bone socket **(Fig 14-20)** and eliminates the need for transosseous drilling. We prefer to avoid transosseous drilling (89,90) to eliminate any potential risk to the axillary nerve. The two or four sutures exiting the BioTenodesis screw should be used in place of a suture anchor to augment the rotator cuff repair or can simply be cut if no cuff tear is present.

Suture Anchor Technique

Tenodesis with suture anchors was first described by Gartsman and Hammerman (91) and subsequently by Nord et al. (92). Each used suture anchors inserted in different locations to obtain fixation to the proximal humerus or the greater tuberosity. Two suture anchors are inserted through the subclavian portal (Nord) or from the anterior portal (Gartsman). The method described by Gartsman requires debridement of the CHL and requires more extensive anterior debridement to allow insertion of the anchors into the intertubercular groove.

The Nord Technique

Glenohumeral arthroscopy is performed in the lateral decubitus position under 10 lbs. of traction as described in the preceding paragraphs. The arm is suspended at approximately a 45-degree angle of abduction and 10 degree forward flexion and distraction of the shoulder joint is accomplished with 10 lbs. of traction. This allows for external and internal rotation of the shoulder while distracted. This technique can be performed in the beach chair position if the surgeon

desires. Four to six portals are utilized during the procedure. The anterosuperior, posterior, and lateral portals are made to obtain visualization of anatomical structures and defects. These portals are also used as working portals and cannulas are utilized. When a rotator cuff repair is necessary, the subclavian, anterolateral and modified Neviaser portals are utilized as necessary for passing suture through the tendon. Anchors for rotator cuff repair are typically inserted through an anterolateral portal without a cannula. To facilitate biceps tenodesis, the subclavian portal is used for anchor insertion. The subclavian portal is located 1 to 2 cm medial to the AC joint, above and slightly medial to the coracoid, and directly inferior to the clavicle **(Fig 14-21)**. A cannula is not needed or recommended for this portal. Instruments or anchors are passed inferior and anterior to the AC joint before entering the subacromial bursa. Subacromial decompression optimizes the use of the subclavian portal.

The scope is introduced into the glenohumeral joint through a standard posterior portal. An anterosuperolateral portal is made following the path of a spinal needle. The anatomical structures are visualized and any abnormalities are assessed. Treatment of other pathology is performed as indicated. The shoulder is evaluated for rotator cuff tears. If present, the rotator cuff defect facilitates access to the biceps tendon. A lateral portal is created and subacromial decompression is performed, which relieves shoulder impingement and facilitates the use of the subclavian portal. The scope is utilized through the posterior portal below the rotator cuff to gain visualization of the biceps tendon. Using a burr

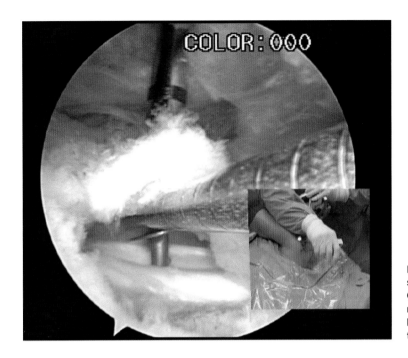

Fig 14-22. Arthroscopic view looking from posterior showing anchor passing through the rotator interval/CHL and directly through the biceps tendon just proximal to the bicipital groove. The area under the biceps has been abraded with a shaver to improve healing of the tendon to bone.

through the lateral portal, a small area of the articular and bony surface is abraded under the biceps tendon, just proximal to the bicipital groove. A spinal needle is inserted through the subclavian portal in order to identify the tract through the CHL to the biceps tendon. A 3 mm incision is made for the subclavian portal and no cannula is used. A suture anchor, 5 mm (preferred) or 3.5 mm, is passed through the subclavian portal entering the joint through the rotator interval. The suture anchor is then placed through the biceps tendon slightly proximal to the bicipital groove. Lifting the biceps tendon with a probe will help facilitate visualization of the anchor through the biceps tendon and embedding into bone **(Fig 14-22)**.

The subclavian approach allows fixation of the tendon "in-situ" just proximal to the point at which the tendon enters the bicipital groove. The anchor can be placed directly through the biceps or adjacent to it. Sutures are passed with a penetrating suture grasper such as the Penetrator or Bird Beak (Arthrex, Inc. Naples, FL) or with suture passers such as the Viper or Scorpion (Arthrex, Inc. Naples, FL). The sutures can be passed via the subclavian or anterosuperolateral portal—whichever provides a better angle. The biceps is left attached while the suture anchor is inserted through the tendon. If a rotator cuff tear is present, the sutures through the biceps may be tied through the lateral portal; however, if a rotator cuff tear is not present, sutures are tied through the anterior portal. One limb of the suture is pulled underneath and over the biceps tendon, and then out the appropriate portal with a crochet hook. The sutures are each tied. Knot security and loop security are assessed. A second suture anchor is introduced into the subclavian portal, passed through the biceps tendon slightly proximal to the other suture anchor, and sutures retrieved. The biceps tendon is

found to be firmly attached by testing the tenodesis with a hook probe. The residual intra-articular biceps tendon is released from a site just proximal to the sutures using a basket cutter and the remaining stump is excised at the point of attachment at the superior glenoid labrum utilizing a basket cutter and shaver. Arthroscopic rotator cuff repair is performed as necessary after the completion of the biceps tenodesis. The tenodesis will not add any significant bulk beneath the rotator cuff repair and allows for normal shoulder motion. During range of motion testing of the shoulder and elbow, stability of the biceps tenodesis is arthroscopically assessed.

Soft Tissue Tenodesis Technique

Suture tenodesis to soft tissue has been advocated due to its simplicity. Two methods have been described. One involves open treatment of suturing the biceps tendon to the transverse humeral ligament and the arthroscopic technique involves suturing the tendon to the CHL or the anterior supraspinatus tendon.

The arthroscopic suture tenodesis technique begins with standard glenohumeral arthroscopy. Any associated pathology is treated appropriately. An anterosuperior portal is made for introduction of a suture passing device or alternatively a spinal needle can be used to pass PDS suture through the biceps after passing the needle through the rotator cuff through an anterolateral portal. If the tendon is of poor quality, racking sutures provide better purchase on the tendon. A second suture can then be placed in a similar manner. The biceps is then released from its attachment to the labrum and supraglenoid tubercle. This is accomplished with a radiofrequency device or arthroscopic scissors. The edge of the superior labrum is smoothed. After the tendon is released from the labrum, it retracts slightly and the sutures are passed through the CHL or anterior supraspinatus with a penetrating suture device such as the Penetrator or Bird Beak (Arthrex, Inc. Naples, FL). If a spinal needle was used with #1 PDS, the sutures are already passed through the supraspinatus. The camera is then directed into the subacromial space, the sutures retrieved through the lateral cannula and are then securely tied. This anchors the biceps to the supraspinatus or the CHL. The authors seldom perform this soft tissue tenodesis technique, but rather prefer to securely anchor the biceps to bone. The senior author (SSB) uses this technique only in the case of extremely degenerative tendon. In such cases, BioTenodesis interference fixation is sometimes not secure, and two racking sutures in the degenerative biceps provide relatively secure purchase on the tendon.

■ COMPLICATIONS AND SPECIAL CONSIDERATIONS

Complications of the biceps tenotomy primarily involve the anticipated 21% risk of a Popeye deformity of the biceps muscle as it retracts distally. Most men may not be concerned about this deformity, but it may not be cosmetically acceptable to women or bodybuilders. Patients should be counseled on these risks if this treatment modality is elected. If this is unacceptable to the patient, a tenodesis should be performed.

Arthroscopic biceps tenotomy is otherwise a relatively safe procedure with very minor risks of infection, blood clots or neurovascular injury. The portals used for a tenotomy are the standard arthroscopy portals and the risks are comparable to diagnostic shoulder arthroscopy risks. Pain relief is generally very good although occasionally a patient may have some residual pain or cramping with activities involving forceful elbow flexion. Risks of shoulder arthroscopy include infection, blood vessel or nerve injury, upper extremity deep venous thrombosis, neuropraxia of ulnar nerve secondary to compression of the nerve at the cubital tunnel, and brachial plexus traction injuries which are usually a result of head and neck position.

Complications associated with the BioTenodesis screw technique as described by Lo and Burkhart (88) include the same associated risks as tenotomy except a Popeye deformity would not be expected unless failure of fixation occurred. Prominence of the BioTenodesis screw could potentially cause impingement upon the acromion if it were not adequately seated in the bone bed. Therefore the surgeon must advance the screwhead until it is flush with the bone surface. The tendon may not pull down into the drill hole resulting in a lax tendon or fixation of the tendon down with sutures alone. Close attention to technique will prevent this problem. Fractures could potentially occur depending on the location of screw insertion but we have not seen this complication. Osteoporotic bone may not allow rigid fixation but

the BioTenodesis screw would be expected to have better fixation than suture anchors in osteoporotic bone. If the BioTenodesis screw appears somewhat loose after insertion into osteoporotic bone, its stability may be improved by inserting a 5 mm BioCorkscrew suture anchor directly adjacent to it, thereby achieving an interference fit of the anchor against the BioTenodesis screw.

Complications associated with suture anchors carry all the standard arthroscopy risks. Additionally, failure of fixation can occur in the form of anchor pullout or suture breakage. When postoperative anchor pullout occurs an additional procedure is required to retrieve the anchor if a metallic anchor is used. Failure of fixation of the biceps tendon results in a biceps tenotomy with the potential Popeye deformity, so the surgeon should discuss this possibility with the patient.

■ CONCLUSIONS AND FUTURE DIRECTIONS

The LHB tendon is a fascinating structure that, in many respects, remains somewhat perplexing. A plethora of literature regarding the function, pathology, and treatment of the biceps tendon exists. As the science of our specialty progresses we will continue to discover the truths behind the LHB. Long-term patient outcome studies comparing alternative treatment modalities will also be crucial. As is the trend with most orthopedic shoulder cases, arthroscopic treatment strategies will continue to advance and will likely become the standard of care for the treatment of disorders of the biceps tendon.

■ REFERENCES

1. Habermayer P, Kaiser E, Knappe M, et al. Functional anatomy and biomechanics of the long biceps tendon. *Unfallchirurg.* 1987;90:319–329.
2. Pal GP, Bhatt RH, Patel VS. Relationship between the tendon of the long head of biceps brachii and the glenoid labrum in humans. *Anat Rec.* 1991;229:278–280.
3. Vangsness CT Jr, Jorgenson SS, Watson T, et al. The origin of the long head of the biceps from the scapula and glenoid labrum. *J Bone Joint Surg Br.* 1994;76:951–954.
4. Cooper DE, Arnoczky SP, O'Brien SJ, et al. Anatomy, histology and vascularity of the glenoid labrum. An anatomical study. *J Bone Joint Surg Am.* 1992;74:46–52.
5. McGough R, Debski RE, Taskiran E, et al. Tensile properties of the long head of the biceps tendon. *Knee Surg Sports Traumatol Arthrosc.* 1996;3:226–229.
6. Cone RO, Danzig L, Resnick D, et al. The bicipital groove: Radiographic, anatomic, and pathologic study. *AJR Am J Roentgenol.* 1983;41:781–788.
7. Ueberham K, Le Floch-Prigent P. Intertubercular sulcus of the humerus: biometry and morphology of 100 dry bones. *Surg Radiol Anat.* 1998;20:351–354.
8. Hitchcock HH, Bechtol CO. Painful shoulder. Observations on the role of the tendon of the long head of the biceps brachii in its causation. *J Bone Joint Surg Am.* 1948;30:263–273.

9. Lo IK, Burkhart SS. The Comma Sign: An arthroscopic guide to the torn subscapularis tendon. *Arthroscopy*. 2003;19(3):334–337.

10. Bennett WF. Visualization of the anatomy of the rotator interval and bicipital sheath. *Arthroscopy*. 2001;17:107–111.

11. Bennett WF. Subscapularis, medial and lateral head coracohumeral ligament insertion anatomy: arthroscopic appearance and incidence of "hidden" rotator interval lesions. *Arthroscopy*. 2001;17:173–180.

12. Patton WC, McCluskey GM. Biceps tendonitis and subluxation. *Clin Sports Med*. 2001;20(3):505–529.

13. Paynter KS. Disorders of the long head of the biceps tendon. *Phys Med Rehabil Clin N Am*. 2004;15:511–528.

14. Meyer AW. Spontaneous dislocation and destruction of the tendon of the long head of the biceps brachii. *Arch Surg*. 1928;17:493–506.

15. Paavolainen P, Bjorkenheim JM, Slatis P, et al. Operative treatment of severe proximal humeral fractures. *Acta Orthop Scand*. 1983;54:374–379.

16. Ruotolo C, Nottage WM, Flatow EL, et al. Controversial topics in shoulder arthroscopy. *Arthroscopy*. 2002;18(2):65–75.

17. Basmajian JV, Latif MA. Integrated actions and function of the chief flexors of the elbow. *J Bone Joint Surg Am*. 1957;39:1106–1118.

18. Lucas DB. Biomechanics of the shoulder joint. *Arch Surg*. 1973;107:425–432.

19. Andrews J, Carson W, McLeod W. Glenoid labrum tears related to the long head of the biceps. *Am J Sports Med*. 1985;13:337–341.

20. Kumar VP, Satku K, Balasubramaniam P. The role of the long head of biceps brachii in the stabilization of the head of the humerus. *Clin Orthop*. 1989;244:172–175.

21. Lippmann RK. Frozen shoulder, periarthritis, bicipital tenosynovitis. *Arch Surg*. 1943;47:283–296.

22. Basmajian JV. *Muscles Alive*, 5th ed. Baltimore: Williams & Wilkins; 1985.

23. Laumann U. Decompression of the subacromial space: an anatomical study. In: Bayley I, Kellel L, eds. *Shoulder surgery*. Berlin: Springer–Verlag; 1982:12–21.

24. Laumann U. Kinesiology of the shoulder joint. In: Kolbel R, Bado H, Blauth W, eds. *Shoulder replacement*. New York: Springer-Verlag; 1987.

25. Jobe FW, Tibone JE, Perry J, et al. An EMG analysis of the shoulder in throwing and pitching a preliminary report. *Am J Sports Med*. 1983;11:3–5.

26. Jobe FW, Tibone JE, Tibone JE, et al. An EMG analysis of the shoulder in pitching. A second report. *Am J Sports Med*. 1984;12:218–220.

27. Yamaguchi K, Riew KD, Galatz LM, et al. Biceps function in normal and rotator cuff deficient shoulders: an electromyographic analysis. *Orthop Trans*. 1994;18:191.

28. Yamaguchi K, Riew KD, Galatz LM, et al. Biceps during shoulder motion. *Clin Orthop*. 1997;336:122–129.

29. Levy AS, Kelley BT, Lintner SA, et al. Function of the long head of the biceps at the shoulder: electromyographic analysis. *J Shoulder Elbow Surg*. 2001;10:250–255.

30. Ting A, Jobe FW, Barto P, et al. An EMG analysis of the lateral biceps in shoulders with rotator cuff tears. Paper presented at the Third Open Meeting of the Society of American Shoulder and Elbow Surgeons, California 1987.

31. Rowe CR, ed. *The Shoulder*. New York: Churchill Livingstone; 1988:145.

32. Walch G. La pathologie de la longue portion du biceps. Conference d'enseignement de la SOFCOT, Paris 1993.

33. Burkhead WZ, Arcand MA, Zeman C, et al. The biceps tendon. In: Rockwood CA Jr, Matsen FA, eds. *The shoulder*, 3rd ed, Philadelphia: WB Saunders; 2004:1059–1119.

34. Habermayer P, Walch G. The biceps tendon and rotator cuff disease. In: Burkhead WZ Jr, ed. *Rotator cuff disorders*. Media, PA: Williams & Wilkins; 1996:142.

35. Yamaguchi K, Bendra R. Disorders of the biceps tendon. In: Iannotti JP, Williams GR Jr, eds. *Disorders of the shoulder: diagnosis and management*. Philadelphia: Lippincott Williams & Wilkins; 1999:159–190.

36. Post D, Benca P. Primary tendonitis of the long head of the biceps. *Clin Orthop*. 1989;246:117–125.

37. Neviaser RJ. Lesions of the biceps and tendonitis of the shoulder. *Orthop Clin North Am*. 1980;11:343–348.

38. Dines D, Warren RF, Inglis AE. Surgical treatment of lesions of the long head of the biceps. *Clin Orthop*. 1982;164:165–72.

39. Sethi J, Wright R, Yamaguchi K. Disorders of the long head of the biceps tendon. *J Shoulder Elbow Surg*. 1999;8:644–654.

40. DePalma AF, Callery GE. Bicipital tenosynovitis. *Clin Orthop*. 1954;3:69–85.

41. Andrews JR, Carson WG Jr, McLeod WD. Glenoid labrum tears related to the long head of the biceps. *Am J Sports Med*. 1985;13:337–342.

42. Burkhart SS, Fox DL. SLAP lesions in association with complete tears of the long head of the biceps tendon: a report of two cases. *Arthroscopy*. 1992;8:31–35.

43. Neer CS II. Impingement lesions. *Clin Orthop*. 1983;173:70–77.

44. Gilcreest EL, Albi P. Unusual lesions of muscles and tendons of the shoulder girdle and upper arm. *Surg Gynecol Obstet*. 1939;68:903–917.

45. Yergason RM. Rupture of biceps. *J Bone Joint Surg*. 1931;13:160.

46. Barth JR, Burkhart SS, deBeer JF. The bear hug test: the most sensitive test for diagnosing a subscapularis tear. *Arthroscopy*. In Press.

47. Schwamborn T, Imhoff AB. Diagnostik und klassifikation der rotatorenmanchettenlasionen. In: Imhoff AB, Konig U, eds. *Schulterinstabilitat-Rotatorenmanschette*. Darmstadt: Steinkopff Verlag; 1999:193–195.

48. Burkhart SS, Tehrany AM. Arthroscopic subscapularis tendon repair: technique and preliminary results. *Arthroscopy*. 2002;18(5):454–463.

49. Gerber C, Hersche O, Farron A. Isolated rupture of the subscapularis tendon. *J Bone Joint Surg Am*. 1996;78(7):1015–23.

50. Gerber C, Krushell RJ. Isolated rupture of the tendon of the subscapularis muscle: clinical features in 16 cases. *J Bone Joint Surg Br*. 1991;73:389–394.

51. Ludington NA. Ludington test. *Am J Surg*. 1923;77:358.

52. Abbott LC, Saunders LB de CM. Acute traumatic dislocation of the tendon of the long head of biceps brachii: report of 6 cases with operative findings. *Surgery*. 1939;6:817–840.

53. Walch G, Nove-Josserand L, Boileau P, et al. Subluxations and dislocations of the tendon of the long head of the biceps. *J Shoulder Elbow Surg*. 1998;7:100–108.

54. Bennett WF. Specificity of the Speed's test: arthroscopic technique. *Arthroscopy*. 1998;14:789–796.

55. Fisk C. Adaptation of the technique for radiography of the bicipital groove. *Radiol Technol*. 1965;37:47–50.

56. Cone RO, Danzig L, Resnick D, et al. The bicipital groove: Radiographic, anatomic, and pathologic study. *AJR Am J Roentgenol*. 1983;41:781–788.

57. Neviaser TJ. Arthrography of the shoulder. *Orthop Clin North Am*. 1980;11:205–217.

58. Middleton WD, Reinus WR, Trotty WG, et al. Ultrasonographic evaluation of the rotator cuff and biceps tendon. *J Bone Joint Surg Am*. 1986;68:440–450.

59. Middleton WD, Reinus WR, Trotty WG, et al. US of the biceps tendon apparatus. *Radiology*. 1985;157:211–215.

60. Farin PU, Jaroma H, Harju A, et al. Medial displacement of the biceps brachii tendon: evaluation with dynamic sonography during maximal external shoulder rotation. *Radiology*. 1995;195:845–848.

61. Spritzer CE, Collins AJ, Cooperman A, et al. Assessment of instability of the long head of the biceps tendon by MRI. *Skeletal Radiol*. 2001;30:199–207.

62. DePalma AF. *Surgery of the Shoulder*. Philadelphia: JB Lippincott Co; 1950.
63. Kennedy JC, Willis RB. The effects of local steoid injection on tendons: a biomechanical and microscopic correlative study. *Am J Sports Med.* 1976;4:11–21.
64. Rockwood CA, Matsen FA. *The Shoulder*. 2nd Ed. Philadelphia: WB Saunders; 1998.
65. Yamaguchi K, Bindra R. Disorders of the biceps tendon. In: Ianotti JP, Williams GR, eds. *Disorders of the shoulder: diagnosis and management*, Philadelphia: Lippincott Williams & Wilkins; 1999.
66. Cameron ML. The Incidence of "Popeye" Deformity and Muscle Weakness following Biceps Tenotomy for Recalcitrant Biceps Tendonitis. Poster presentation (P240) at 70th AAOS meeting in New Orleans, LA; Feb 2003; (http://www.aaos.org/wordhtml/anmt2003/poster/p240.htm).
67. Mariani EM, Cofied RH, Askew LJ, et al. Rupture of the tendon of the long head of the biceps brachii. Surgical versus nonsurgical treatment. *Clin Orthop.* 1988;228:233–239.
68. Warren RF. Lesions of the long head of the biceps tendon. *AAOS Instr Course Lect.* 1985;34:204–209.
69. Phillips BB, Canale ST, Sisk TD, et al. Ruptures of the proximal biceps tendon in middle-aged patients. *Orthop Rev.* 1993;22:349–353.
70. Bennett GE. Shoulder and elbow lesions of professional baseball pitcher. *JAMA.* 1941;117:510–514.
71. Neviaser TJ. The role of the biceps tendon in the impingement syndrome. *Orthop Clin of North Am.* 1987;18:383–386.
72. Neviaser TJ. Lesions of the biceps and tendonitis of the shoulder. *Orthop Clin of North Am.* 1980;11:343–348.
73. Becker DA, Cofield RH. Tenodesis of the long head of the biceps brachii for chronic bicipital tendonitis. *J Bone Joint Surg.* 1989;376–380.
74. Murthi AM, Vosburgh CL, Neviaser TJ. The incidence of pathological changes of the long head of the biceps tendon. *J Shoulder Elbow Surg.* 2000;382–384.
75. Gilcreest EL. The common syndrome of rupture, dislocation and elongation of the long head of the biceps brachii. *Surg Gynecol Obstet.* 1948;30:263–273.
76. Burkhart SS, Fox DL. SLAP lesions in association with complete tears of the long head of the biceps tendon: a report of two cases. *Arthroscopy.* 1992;8:31–35.
77. Grauer JD, Paulos LE, Smutz WP. Biceps tendon and superior labral injuries. *Arthroscopy.* 1992;8:488–497.
78. Slatis P, Aalto K. Medial dislocation of the tendon of the long head of the biceps brachii. *Acta Orthop Scand.* 1979;50:73–77.
79. Hitchcock HH, Becthol CO. Painful shoulder: observations on the role of the tendon of the long head of the biceps brachii in its causation. *J Bone Joint Surg.* 1948;30:263–273.
80. O'Donoghue DH. Subluxing biceps tendon in the athlete. *Clin Orthop.* 1982;164:26–29.
81. Meyer AW. Spontaneous dislocation and destruction of tendon of long head of biceps brachii. *Arch Surg.* 1928;17:493–506.
82. Petersson CJ. Spontaneous medial dislocation of the tendon of the long biceps brachii: an anatomic study of prevalence and pathomechanics. *Clin Orthop.* 1986;211:224–227.
83. Refior HJ, Sowa D. Long tendon of the biceps brachii: sites of predilection for degenerative lesions. *J Shoulder Elbow Surg.* 1995;4:436–440.
84. Barber FA, Byrd JT, Wolf M, et al. How would you treat the partially torn biceps tendon? *Arthroscopy.* 2001;17(6):636–639.
85. Froimson AI, Oh I. Keyhole tenodesis of biceps origin at the shoulder. *Clin Orthop.* 1975;112:245–249.
86. Hitchcock HH, Bechtol CO. Painful shoulder. Observations on the role of the tendon of the long head of the biceps brachii in its causation. *J Bone Joint Surg Am.* 1948;30:263–273.
87. Richards DP, Burkhart SS. Arthroscopic-assisted biceps tenodesis for ruptures of the long head of the biceps brachii: the Cobra procedure. *Arthroscopy.* 2004;20(6):201–207.
88. Lo IK, Burkhart SS. Arthroscopic biceps tenodesis using bioabsorbable interference screw. *Arthroscopy.* 2004;20:85–95.
89. Boileau P, Krishnan SG, Coste JB, et al. Arthroscopic biceps tenodesis: a new technique using bioabsorbable interference screw fixation. *Techniques Shoulder Elbow Surg.* 2001;2:153–165.
90. Boileau P, Walch G. A new technique for tenodesis of the long head of the biceps using bioabsorbable screw fixation. *J Shoulder Elbow Surg.* 1999;8:557.
91. Gartsman GM, Hammerman, SM. Arthroscopic biceps tenodesis: operative technique. *Arthroscopy.* 2000;16(5):650–652.
92. Nord KD, Smith GB, Mauck BM. Arthroscopic biceps tenodesis: using suture anchors through the subclavian portal. *Arthroscopy.* 2003;19:24.

15

CARTILAGE

CARLOS A. GUANCHE, MD

■ KEY POINTS

- Full-thickness articular cartilage defects have a limited capacity to heal. Thus, articular cartilage lesions and osteochondral defects in any joint present a challenging problem.
- Cartilage lesions are less likely to be seen in the glenohumeral joint than in the knee, therefore there has not been extensive research on shoulder cartilage repair.
- Making the diagnosis without the benefit of an arthroscopic visualization of the joint can be problematic.
- Mechanical injuries include direct trauma to the cells and matrix, causing an acute disruption of the surface, or more subtle changes attributable to damage of the matrix macromolecules.
- Biologic injuries include metabolic abnormalities, most commonly osteoarthritis, but also avascular necrosis and a variety of osteochondral injuries.
- Although the use of gadolinium-enhanced arthrograms has improved diagnosis, a significant portion of lesions are not identified prospectively.
- The goal of treatment is often to restore durable hyaline cartilage through a practical and minimally invasive approach (preferably arthroscopic), which is associated with minimal morbidity postoperatively and in the long term.
- The end-stage management of many cartilage lesions is a replacement procedure. A titanium coated shaft portion with an articular bearing surface of cobalt-chrome alloy is implanted in the central articular defect and recreates the circumference of the humerus.
- The goals of arthroscopic debridement are primarily to relieve pain and secondarily to improve function. The removal of loose tissues that cause pain and impingement helps to achieve these goals.

- The decision making process for arthroscopic debridement is radiographic analysis. The proper views are critical to allow an appropriate diagnosis. These include an anteroposterior (AP) view in internal rotation, an AP view in the scapular plane with the arm in external rotation and slight abduction and an axillary view.

Articular cartilage lesions and osteochondral defects in any joint present a challenging problem to both patient and physician. The critical issue is that full-thickness articular cartilage defects have a limited capacity to heal at any age. Many procedures have been described to improve the joint alignment, induce reparative tissue proliferation or provide cartilage tissue that is more nearly normal. The bulk of this work has occurred in lesions about the knee, with very little research in any other joints. The use of autogenous and allograft reconstruction of focal defects has been extensively studied in the knee (1–3). Other techniques including abrasion arthroplasty, drilling, and microfracture have been described for smaller lesions (4–6). There is a paucity of research that discusses the problem of cartilage lesions about the glenohumeral joint and provides treatment recommendations, with the exception of a few case reports and small series of patients.

Certainly, the problem is less likely to be seen about the glenohumeral joint and therefore impacts the lack of need for extensive research. Complicating the problem is that unlike the knee, there is significant difficulty with access to the joint when a lesion is identified. Furthermore, the management options are not as obvious as a result of the lack of large-scale research.

There is a spectrum of pathology encountered with the lesions ranging from simple chondral delamination injuries to more extensive osteochondral injuries and culminating in arthritic degeneration of the glenohumeral joint. All of these lesions can be encountered in the typical active population commonly seen in the average sports medicine practice.

Making the diagnosis can also be problematic without the benefit of arthroscopic visualization of the joint. Several series point to the need for improved imaging techniques that allow better determination of the articular surfaces in a prospective fashion and this area also requires further study (7,8). In addition, the concurrent association of cartilage defects with the status of other areas of the joint, specifically, the rotator cuff and impingement is poorly understood both with respect to etiology and treatment (9,10).

After the diagnosis has been made, there are many options available for treatment if the management algorithms follow those historically applied to knee pathology. There are a variety of autogenous techniques including osteoarticular harvest with subsequent transplantation as well as the more complex technique of biologic regeneration of cartilage (2). Allograft applications are also available and those include fresh and preserved specimens. In addition to the biologic resurfacing techniques, there are also devices that allow for resurfacing using metallic and other materials. Finally, in cases of limited damage or sometimes in the face of extensive degeneration of the cartilage surfaces, arthroscopic techniques can be employed primarily for symptom amelioration (9,11–13).

■ IMPACT OF CARTILAGE LESIONS

The spectrum of pathology includes a gradation in the severity of cartilage damage beginning with simple delamination of a small area and ending with complete degeneration of the articular surfaces, i.e., osteoarthritis.

Although the glenohumeral joint surface geometry historically has been considered less of a stabilizing factor as a result of the smaller surface area of the glenoid in comparison with the humeral head and the apparent shallowness of the glenoid, technology has now given us a new perspective. Classically, most studies of the joint have analyzed congruency with radiographs, thus underestimating the degree of congruity afforded by the articular cartilage because only the bony surfaces were visualized and assessed (14). If only the subchondral bone is analyzed, there appears to be less conformity within the joint. With the addition of the articular cartilage, the effective congruence of the joint is much greater.

As an example, Kelkar et al. (14) analyzed a group of glenohumeral cadaveric joints. In their analysis, the average radii of the humeral head and glenoid articular surfaces were 25.5 and 27.2 mm, respectively. The average difference between the two radii was 1.7 ± 1.5 mm. When the same technique was employed to analyze the subchondral bone, the radii of curvature of the humeral heads and glenoids were 25.2 and 33.4 mm, respectively. These findings lend more importance to the articular cartilage, or more specifically the preservation of this tissue. It appears that the articular cartilage of the glenohumeral joint is a factor in the maintenance of stability in the joint. Given the inherently unstable nature of the joint with its small surface area, it is paramount to save as much cartilage as possible in order to preserve normal joint function.

Another consideration is the impact of associated coexistent disease processes in the shoulder. More importantly, focal articular lesions are often found incidentally at the time of arthroscopic evaluation of the joint for other presumptive diagnoses. This problem has been seen less frequently as a result of the improvements made in prospective diagnosis with the use of MRI techniques, particularly those employing gadolinium-enhanced arthrograms.

Several studies allude to the coexistence of other disease processes with cartilage lesions, however, especially more advanced lesions seen with osteoarthritis (8,9,10). In their study, Feeney and colleagues assessed 33 cadaveric shoulder joints and documented the incidence of rotator cuff tearing and cartilage lesions (10). Articular cartilage degeneration was almost twice as frequent in the group with rotator cuff tears as in those without tearing (10).

Another study revealed that in a series of 52 patients undergoing surgery for subacromial impingement syndrome, humeral cartilage lesions were found in 29%, of which four lesions were subtle and eleven were marked (9). In the glenoid, 15% were found to have lesions with three subtle and five marked. In essence, patients with clear surgical indications for impingement surgery may have coexistent cartilage lesions in up to one third of instances. This consideration should be taken into account at the time of preoperative discussion with the patient, as other procedures may be essential for complete treatment.

Types of Lesions

Cartilage repair response has been the focus of investigations for more than 250 years. In 1742 Hunter noted that "ulcerated cartilage is a troublesome thing . . . once destroyed it is not repaired (15). Since that time, the observations made by Hunter have been reiterated by nearly every scientific study on the topic. The lack of predictability of repair of cartilage is attributable to the many factors that often come together in a specific injury. Some of the factors include the precise injury, the age of the individual, the condition of the joint before injury, the quality, extent, and durability of the repair and the long-term function of the joint.

The types of injuries can be divided into mechanical and biologic. The mechanical types of injuries include direct trauma to the cells and matrix causing an acute disruption of the surface, or more subtle changes attributable to damage of the matrix macromolecules. This type of damage occurs with surgical disruption of the synovial membrane, infection and other inflammatory diseases, immobilization and possibly joint irrigation (15).

In cases of blunt injury, the degree of disruption is often underestimated in the acute phases. The response of articular cartilage to penetrating injury depends on the depth of injury such that injuries limited to cartilage elicit a different repair response than injuries involving cartilage and subchondral bone. Likewise, blunt trauma can have much more significant impact than is acutely appreciated as a result of the consequent cell injury and effect on the cellular matrix, as well as any injury to the subchondral supporting bone (16).

The biologic injuries include metabolic abnormalities, most commonly osteoarthritis, but also avascular necrosis and a variety of osteochondral injuries that damage the articular layer indirectly as a result of the collapse of the supporting structures. For example, MRI analysis in degenerative joint disease, osteochondritis dissecans, and avascular necrosis has shown that the subchondral region shows reactive enhanced vascularization and heightened metabolism with insufficient repair (17).

One particular disease process that deserves further mention is that of avascular necrosis because the humeral head is the second most common site of nontraumatic osteonecrosis, after the head of the femur (18). In humeral head osteonecrosis, subchondral osteolysis occurs in the superior portion. When resorption of subchondral bone is extensive, it appears that even ordinary forces transmitted across the joint will lead to subchondral fracture and humeral head collapse (18). The likelihood of this collapse and the consequent degenerative changes that would occur make this disease process one that must be addressed more expediently than other cartilage lesions.

The treatment of specific injuries is impacted by the underlying nature of the cartilage injury. The best outcomes are obviously in isolated lesions that have a clear, mechanical etiology without any underlying metabolic abnormalities. The discussion of the factors involved is beyond the scope of this chapter, but the reader is directed to the appropriate references (14,19,20).

Separate consideration should be given to osteoarthritis, as there are clear surgical indications in the treatment of the disease in the glenohumeral joint (without prosthetic replacement). The arthroscopic management of this problem, if performed in the appropriate patient, has been shown to provide significant improvement in symptomatology (11–13,21).

Diagnosis of Cartilage Lesions

Much effort has been directed at the development of imaging techniques that effectively diagnose cartilage lesions in the shoulder. The thrust of the research has employed a variety of magnetic resonance imaging techniques to delineate not only the actual lesions, but also something about their physiology. It is well established that cartilage functions as the load-bearing surface in the joints of the musculoskeletal system. Major macromolecules in cartilage are collagen Type II and proteoglycans. Although proteoglycans provide much of the compressive stiffness through electrostatic repulsion, collagen provides tensile and shear strength. Several studies have shown that the earliest stages of cartilage degeneration are primarily associated with loss of proteoglycan and minor changes in collagen structure (22). In one study, bovine articular cartilage was analyzed with a variety of MR parameters including T2 relaxation rates and spine-lattice relaxation times in the rotating frame (T1ρ) mapping method (23). The findings included a significant correlation between the changes seen on T1ρ mapping and the sequential depletion of proteoglycan. Studies like these have served to expand the base of knowledge with regards to grading of articular lesions. Although arthroscopy is the so-called gold standard at this point for final determination of the management of these lesions, it would be ideal to have a noninvasive modality that fully assesses the lesions.

In the clinical setting, it is important to be able to delineate the presence of cartilage lesions with some certainty. There are several studies available in the literature that give some guidance (7,8,24). In one study, a double blind prospective study of 15 patients with anterior shoulder instability were analyzed with respect to the efficacy of MRI versus arthroscopy in the evaluation of chondral or osteochondral lesions of the humeral head (24). MR produced 6 true positives, 5 true negatives, and 4 false negatives for an accuracy and sensitivity of 60% and 87%, respectively. Arthroscopy gave 8 true positives, 5 true negatives, and 2 false negatives, with a sensitivity of 80% and an accuracy of 87%. All lesions diagnosed with either method were regarded as positive by definition, with the result that the specificity was always 100%. The differences in diagnosis sprang from the false negatives. As a result of the variable ability to identify the cartilage lesions prospectively, it was advised that both of these methods should be employed to ensure the correct diagnosis, and hence the correct choice of treatment.

Another study has described the MRI findings of focal articular cartilage lesion of the superior humeral head in seven patients (7). This was a retrospective study to evaluate the location and incidence of these lesions. The lesions occurred along the superior surface of the posterior humeral head (medial to the expected location of a Hill-Sachs lesion), were caused by trauma, and did not seem to have a specific mechanism of injury. It was felt that they may cause clinical symptoms and may be easily overlooked on MRI because they were missed on six out of seven of those encountered.

In the largest available study, Guntern et al. (8) determined the prevalence of articular cartilage lesions in a group of patients. Arthrographic images obtained in 52 consecutive patients with a mean age of 45.8 years were retrospectively evaluated for glenohumeral cartilage lesions. Two experienced musculoskeletal radiologists who were blinded to the arthroscopy report independently analyzed the articular cartilage. Humeral and glenoidal cartilage were assessed separately and arthroscopic findings were used as the standard of reference. At arthroscopy, humeral cartilage lesions were found in 15 patients (frequency, 29%). Four lesions were subtle, and 11 were marked. Cartilage lesions of the glenoid were less frequent (eight patients; frequency, 15%): Three were subtle, and five were marked. For reader 1 and reader 2, respectively, sensitivity of MR arthrography for humeral cartilage lesions was 53% and 100%, specificity was 87% and 51%, and accuracy was 77% and 65%; sensitivity for glenoidal cartilage lesions was 75% and 75%, specificity was 66% and 63%, and accuracy was 67% and 65%. Interobserver agreement for the grading of cartilage lesions with MR arthrography was fair (humeral lesions, kappa = 0.20; glenoidal lesions, kappa = 0.27). Based on the study, it was felt that the performance of MR arthrography in the detection of glenohumeral cartilage lesions is moderate with a high degree of variability associated with the interpretation of the images.

As can be discerned by this analysis, much work needs to be done in the delineation of cartilage lesions on a prospective basis. While the use of gadolinium-enhanced arthrograms has clearly improved the ability to find these lesions, a significant proportion is not identified prospectively. Also, the biological parameters that are discernible with the use of MRI technology are important to consider. The ideal study that addresses not only the presence of a cartilage lesion, but also something about its biology or reparative capability is clearly within the grasp of modern imaging. Its implementation and refinement, however, await further studies.

■ TREATMENT ALTERNATIVES

In the past, the most common treatment for many if not most of the articular cartilage lesions that were seen in the shoulder (and other joints) was simple debridement and symptomatic management. Today's aim, however, is to restore durable hyaline cartilage through a practical and minimally invasive approach (preferably arthroscopic), that is associated with minimal morbidity perioperatively and in the long term.

There are several avenues available to accomplish the restoration of articular cartilage (1–3,25,26); however, most of the literature has been focused on knee joint abnormalities, with less attention to the other joints. The variety of techniques includes autogenous tissues, allograft tissues, and synthetic components.

In addition, simple debridement of the area of degeneration with subchondral stimulation is used on a routine basis (6). Although the use of this technique has not been explicitly studied in the literature with respect to the shoulder, the principles of stimulation of the subchondral area for creation of a fibrocartilaginous layer over the diseased area should also apply. This technique will be discussed in more detail in a later section of this chapter.

Autologous Tissues

The use of autologous tissues about the knee has been commonplace for several years, and has included the transplantation of local tissue, transfer of remote tissue, and finally the genetic production of cloned tissue from knee cartilage cells (1–3,27).

A technique that has been used in the knee is transfer of autologous tissue from other areas to reconstruct the articular cartilage; this technique has been termed mosaicplasty. Likewise in the humerus, the technique is certainly applicable. In one study, Scheibel et al. (28) have prospectively analyzed a series of autologous osteochondral plugs from the knee to the humerus in eight patients. The lesions were all Outerbridge grade IV and averaged 150mm^2. Standard radiographs, MRI, and second-look arthroscopy (in two patients) were used to assess the transplanted tissue. After a mean of 32.6 months MRI revealed good osteointegration and congruent articular cartilage in all but one patient. Second-look arthroscopy in two cases revealed good integration macroscopically with an intact articular surface. The Constant scores also increased significantly. The study certainly lends credence to the use of the procedure in the cases of limited lesions of the humeral head.

In cases where the lesion is larger or the availability of normal cartilage from another autogenous source precludes mosaicplasty, periosteal tissue has been employed (29). Basic science studies have shown that neochondrogenesis can be seen in animal models where a free autogenous periosteal graft is applied to full thickness articular cartilage lesions (30). Periosteum contains pluripotential mesenchymal stem cells with the cambium layer being responsible for many growth factors that regulate chondrocytes and cartilage development including transforming growth factor β_1, insulin-like growth factor 1 and others (31). In a limited series of patients, a tissue quite similar to articular cartilage was observed in the knee (32).

In the shoulder, a prospective series of five patients treated with an autogenous periosteal flap following microfracture of the defect has shown satisfactory short-term results (29). The technique included the use of the technique of Steadman et al. (6) where perforations into the subchondral bone at a distance of 3 to 4 mm between perforations were created. A periosteal flap harvested from the proximal humeral metaphysis (with the cambium layer facing the cartilage lesion) was then applied to the defect and sutured into place (33). The size of the defects in these patients averaged 311 mm^2 (range 225 to 400 mm). With a mean follow-up of 25.8 months, it was found that the Constant scores improved significantly from 43.4 to 81.8. Second-look arthroscopy in three patients revealed a significantly reduced cartilage lesion. Follow-up MRI revealed that the area of the chondral defect was covered with a thin layer of regenerated cartilage tissue in all patients, but there were still signs of edema in the underlying subchondral bone plate. It was felt that this is a viable technique for larger defects not amenable to treatment with osteochondral plugs. Although the findings did not show a completely normal cartilaginous surface, the authors were encouraged by the improvement in clinical symptomatology. Certainly, further follow-up is indicated in these patients before the technique can be espoused for most defects.

An additional autogenous technique that has been extensively analyzed with respect to the knee is that of autogenous chondrocyte implantation (ACI) (2,32). The technique involves the use of cells that are harvested from the articular cartilage surface, subsequently cultured in vitro, and reimplanted under a periosteal patch (2). In the shoulder, the technique has been reported in the form of a case report (34). The patient in this case sustained a lesion that, following preparation for the ACI procedure, measured 3.3 × 1.5 cm. At one year follow-up the patient demonstrated a full range of painless motion with no complaints of rest or weather change pain.

Allograft Tissues

Allograft tissues have been employed to reconstruct a variety of joint surfaces, and the humerus is certainly no different (35,36). The use of smaller focal defects, however, is not extensively described in the literature with the exception of a few case series. In one study, Gerber et al. (26) employed a large segmental humeral head allograft to reconstruct massive posterior humeral head defects (Hill-Sachs lesions) involving more than 40% of the articular surface. This treatise included four patients treated with the technique. It was found that stability was restored and maintained in each patient at an average of 68 months following the procedure. Three patients reported little or no pain and no or slight functional restrictions in activities of daily lining. One patient had mild pain and moderate-to-severe dysfunction secondary to avascular necrosis of the remaining portion of the humeral head. Although the technique appears to be worthwhile in this patient population, the use of this type of large allograft resurfacing in the more central portion of the humeral head may fare differently. The central humeral articular surface will experience significantly more mechanical stress compared to the peripheral humeral articular surface that was reconstructed with this technique.

Prosthetic Components

Obviously, the end-stage management of many of these cartilage lesions is a replacement procedure; however, in many situations the diseased portion is a limited area that is amenable to a limited replacement approach. Several devices are currently available, some experimental and some recently devised that allow for this limited resurfacing.

The currently available device is a titanium coated shaft portion with an articular bearing surface of a cobalt-chrome alloy (Arthrosurface; Franklin, MA). The device is implanted in the central articular defect either in an open or arthroscopic fashion and recreates the circumference of the humerus

(Fig 15-1). Several sizes of implants are available such that a circular defect up to 40 mm can be reconstructed. To date, there are no series of patients available that have been published in the peer-reviewed literature.

A variety of synthetic "articular cartilage-like" materials are also available. All of the devices are currently unavailable in the United States but are presently in use in some European countries and Japan. Again, the experience has been predominantly in the knee joint with an occasional series or case report in other joints such as the hip, ankle, or shoulder. The majority of the materials are hydrogels which are encapsulated and typically contain a suspension of saline with a variety of macromolecules that simulate the properties of articular cartilage (37). In a study evaluating the response of normal cartilage to the hydrogels vs. aluminum and titanium implants in a rabbit model, there were marked pathologic changes noted on the knees with the harder implants, although the knees with the hydrogel implants had none to minimal changes (38). This supports some of the well-known literature on the use of hemiprosthetics in the shoulder and knee joint where degradation of the articular surfaces has been documented with long-term follow-up of these patients (39).

■ EARLY OSTEOARTHRITIS

Separate consideration should be given to the arthroscopic management of the early osteoarthritic shoulder. The disease in young patients is a challenging clinical problem. Nonsurgical treatment options include physical therapy, therapeutic modalities, intra-articular corticosteroid injections, activity modification, and nonsteroidal anti-inflammatory medications (40). There is a substantial amount of literature to support the use of the arthroscope in these patients; however, the proper indications must be present to obtain good, predictable results. The routine use of the arthroscope for symptomatic relief of osteoarthritis is simply not substantiated in the literature.

Indications for arthroscopic debridement of shoulder osteoarthritis include young patients with early to moderate disease, preserved range of motion (>120 degree elevation, >20 degree external rotation at the side), concentric glenoid wear without evidence of subluxation, and minimal osteophyte formation (40,41).

In the athlete and young patient with osteoarthritis, arthroscopy allows recognition and treatment of coexisting pathologies in which procedures such as subacromial decompression and capsular release have proven to be of benefit. In fact, arthroscopy is the most sensitive method for diagnosing early osteoarthritis (9,42). Disorders such as rotator cuff tendinopathy, impingement syndrome, adhesive capsulitis, and biceps tendonitis often mimic osteoarthritis and are difficult to separate clinically. Through the use of arthroscopy, the proper diagnosis and specific treatment may be applied, thus maximizing the patient's opportunity for improvement (Fig 15-2).

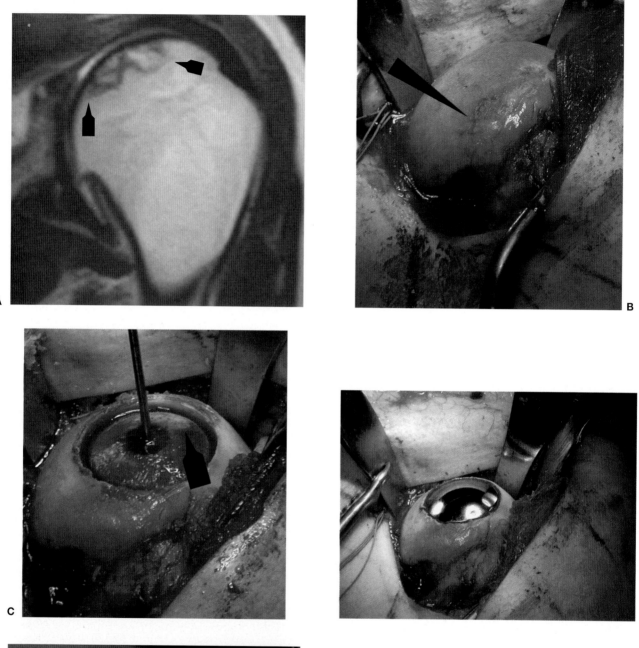

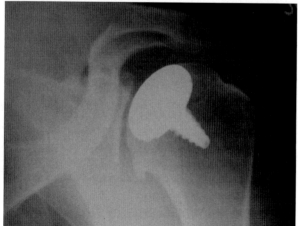

Fig 15-1. The use of a metal resurfacing device in the case of a 39-year-old patient with a history of avascular necrosis and consequent chondral damage secondary to subchondral collapse. **A:** MRI of avascular lesions (T1 weighted) depicting the area of diseased bone (*arrows*) over the superolateral head. **B:** Initial intraoperative view of chondral injury. **C:** Area of avascular bone visible (*arrowhead*) following reaming for resurfacing device. **D:** Final device implant in position (Arthrosurface). **E:** Final AP radiograph of resurfacing component in place.

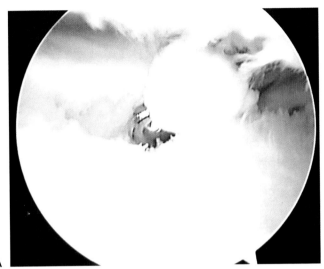
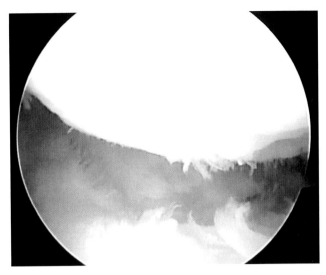

Fig 15-2. Thirty-two-year-old male with recurrent instability and now early osteoarthritic (grade A) changes radiographically. (Right shoulder viewed from posterior portal.) **A:** Loose body in anterior glenoid-labrum junction. **B:** Humeral head articular changes.

The goals of arthroscopic debridement are primarily to relieve pain and secondarily to improve function. The removal of loose tissues that cause pain and impingement helps to achieve these goals. In some situations, the microfracture technique of subchondral bone perforation can be a useful adjunct in order to induce fibrocartilage formation over areas of exposed bone **(Fig 15-3)**. Although the technique has not been specifically analyzed with respect to the shoulder, there is certainly a substantial amount of literature to support its use in the knee with studies showing that it improves symptoms, reduces defect size, and allows earlier return to activity in patients with osteochondral defects (43) **(Fig 15-4)**. It should be kept in mind, however, that the duration of relief is highly variable and the procedure is at best a temporizing one (12,13,21). It can be highly advantageous, though, in the young active patient that desires to postpone prosthetic replacement.

An important component of the decision-making process for this procedure is radiographic analysis. The proper views are critical to allow an appropriate diagnosis and these include an anteroposterior (AP) view in internal rotation, an AP view in the scapular plane with the arm in external rotation and slight abduction and an axillary view (42). The scapular AP and the axillary view are the critical ones because they are orthogonal to the plane of the joint. To improve sensitivity, the AP view may be obtained with the patient in 45 degrees of abduction while contracting the deltoid. This procedure provides joint compressive force and helps delineate joint space narrowing that can be underrepresented in standard views (41). A useful classification system that is applicable to this patient population has been devised by Walch et al. (44). A Grade A lesion shows a centralized humeral head, Grade B has posterior subluxation of the humeral head, and Grade C has a glenoid retroversion of >25 degrees. In this scheme, radiographic progression beyond a grade of A is a relative contraindication for arthroscopic debridement.

The typical arthroscopic debridement in these patients includes a thorough assessment of their motion and stability under anesthesia, as well as a thorough diagnostic arthroscopy including the subacromial space and the acromioclavicular joint (42).

An area that deserves particular mention is that of capsular release. In many of these patients, shoulder range of motion is significantly limited not only as a result of the degenerative changes, but also as a result of the capsular contractures that are often present. Certainly, part of the procedure would include a complete capsular release to improve the passive range of motion. The technique is described in other sections of this book, and the reader is directed to the appropriate references (12,42).

With regards to outcome, there are several studies in the literature that support the use of arthroscopy to improve the symptoms associated with degenerative shoulder joints (13,45–47). One study evaluated 25 patients at an average of 34 months follow-up (13). The overall results were rated as excellent in 2 patients, good in 19 patients, and unsatisfactory in 5 (20%). Two patients had complete pain relief and 18 had only occasional mild pain. Notably, of the 12 patients with marked stiffness preoperatively, 83% had improvement in range of motion. Of note in this population was the coexistence of significant intra-articular findings in 32% of the patients. This included labral tears, loose bodies, SLAP lesions, and partial cuff tears. Interestingly, there was no correlation between the radiographic grade and the clinical outcome.

Another study evaluated the results of arthroscopic debridement with or without capsular release in a group of sixty-one patients (12). At follow-up with 45 patients having a minimum of 2 years, 87% of patients indicated that

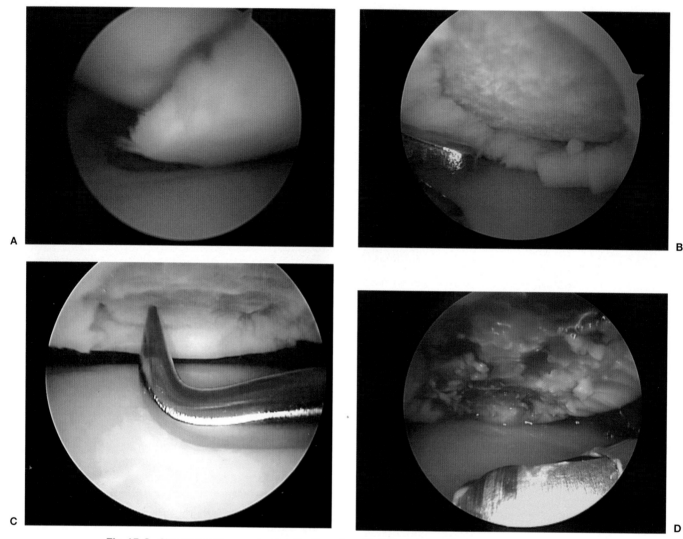

Fig 15-3. Shoulder arthroscopic visualization of cartilaginous defect treated with subchondral perforation technique (Steadman). Views are of a right shoulder, visualized from the posterior portal. **A:** Cartilaginous loose body visualized arthroscopically. **B:** Remaining defect following preliminary debridement. **C:** Arthroscopic awl employed for subchondral perforations. **D:** Final area of subchondral perforation showing good blood supply following the perforations.

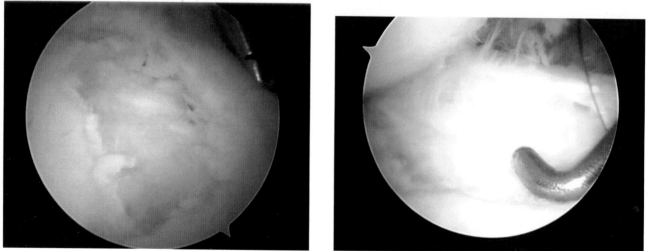

Fig 15-4. Follow-up lesions of subchondral perforation technique on the glenoid surface. **A:** Glenoid lesion at three-year follow-up showing some small, patchy areas of fibrocartilage. (Left shoulder, posterior portal view of mid-glenoid.) **B:** Glenoid lesion at two-year follow-up showing more exuberant fibrocartilage repair. (Right shoulder, posterior portal view of mid-glenoid.)

they would have the surgery again. Most patients noted the onset of pain relief within 5 weeks of surgery, and obtained a duration of pain relief of 28 months or greater. The addition of concomitant procedures, such as acromioplasty, distal clavicle resection, and labral debridement or repair did not have a negative impact on the functional results. They did note, however, that lesions greater than 2 cm appeared to be associated with a return of pain and failure of the procedure.

■ SUMMARY

Full thickness chondral defects and osteochondral defects of the shoulder can cause numerous problems for the patient such as pain, swelling, locking, and may lead to early osteoarthritis. The goals of treatment are to alleviate pain and improve function as well as delay the need for prosthetic replacement of the joint.

A variety of alternatives is available to treat these lesions; however, many limitations exist. There are several techniques that include simple debridement that clearly help in the short term, but do not change the natural course of the disease process. In most situations, the best that can be achieved with debridements and abrasions is a fibrocartilaginous covering of the articular surface with poor biomechanical characteristics (48).

The results of resurfacing the cartilage lesions, whether performed with biological tissues or synthetic materials, appear to be promising; however, there is very little large scale or long term data to support the routine use of any one technique over another.

The symptomatology associated with the early arthritic shoulder can certainly be improved with the judicious use of the arthroscope; however, appropriate patient selection is critical in this regard as significant radiographic deformities certainly do not improve with this treatment modality.

■ REFERENCES

1. Bobic V. Arthroscopic osteochondral autogenous graft transplantation in anterior cruciate reconstruction: a preliminary report. *Knee Surg Sports Traumatol Arthrosc.* 1996;3:262–262.
2. Brittberg M, Nillsson A, Petersen H, et al. Treatment of deep cartilage defects in the knee with autologous chondrocyte transplantation. *N Engl J Med.* 1994;331:889–895.
3. Hangody L, Kish G, Karpati Z. Autogenous osteochondral graft technique for replacing knee cartilage defects in dogs. *Orthopedics.* 1997;5:175–181.
4. Bert JM. Abrasion arthroplasty. *Oper Tech Orthop.* 1997;4:294–299.
5. Mitchell N, Shepard N. Resurfacing of adult rabbit articular cartilage by multiple perforation of the subchondral bone. *J Bone Joint Surg.* 1976;58A:230–233.
6. Steadman JR, Rodkey WG, Singleton SB, et al. Microfracture technique for full thickness chondral defects. *Oper Tech Orthop.* 1997;7:300–307.
7. Carroll KW, Helms CA, Speer KP. Focal articular cartilage lesions of the superior humeral head: MR imaging findings in seven patients. *Am J Roentgenol.* 2001;176:393–397.
8. Guntern DV, Pfirrmann CW, Schmid MR. Articular cartilage lesions of the glenohumeral joint: diagnostic effectiveness of MR arthrography and prevalence in patients with subacromial impingement syndrome. *Radiology.* 2002;226:165–170.
9. Ellman H, Harris E, Kay SP. Early degenerative joint disease simulating impingement syndrome: arthroscopic findings. *Arthroscopy.* 1992;8:482–487.
10. Feeney M, O'Dowd J, Kay EW, et al. Glenohumeral articular cartilage changes in rotator cuff disease. *J Shoulder Elbow Surg.* 2003; 12:20–23.
11. Bishop JY, Flatow EL. Management of glenohumeral arthritis: a role for arthroscopy? *Orthop Clin North Am.* 2003;34:559–566.
12. Cameron BD, Galatz LM, Ramsey ML, et al. Non-prosthetic management of grade IV osteochondral lesions of the glenohumeral joint. *J Shoulder Elbow Surg.* 2002;11:25–32.
13. Weinstein DM, Bucchieri JS, Pollock RG, et al. Arthroscopic debridement of the shoulder for osteoarthritis. *Arthroscopy.* 2000; 16:471–476.
14. Kelkar R, Wang VM, Flatow EL. Glenohumeral mechanics: a study of articular geometry, contact, and kinematics. *J Shoulder Elbow Surg.* 2001;10:73–84.
15. Buckwalter JD, Rosenberg L, Coutts R, et al. Articular cartilage: injury and repair. In: Woo L-Y, Buckwalter JA, eds. *Injury and repair of the musculoskeletal soft tissues.* Park Ridge, IL: American Academy of Orthopaedic Surgeons; 1988:465–537.
16. Donohue JM, Buss DD, Oegema TR, et al. The effects of indirect blunt trauma on adult canine articular cartilage. *J Bone Joint Surg.* 1983;65A:948–957.
17. Imhof H, Breitenseher M, Kainberger F, et al. Importance of subchondral bone to articular cartilage in health and disease. *Top Magn Reson Imaging.* 1999;10:180–192.
18. Nakagawa Y, Ueo T, Nakamura T. A novel surgical procedure for osteonecrosis of the humeral head: reposition of the joint surface and bone engraftment. *Arthroscopy.* 1999;15:433–438.
19. Chen FS, Frenkel SR, Di Cesare PE. Repair of articular cartilage defects: part II. treatment options. *Am J Orthop.* 1999;28:88–96.
20. Hunziker EB. Articular cartilage repair: basic science and clinical progress. A review of the current status and prospects. *Osteoarthritis Cartilage.* 2003;10:423–433.
21. Gerber A, Lehtinen JT, Warner JJP. Glenohumeral osteoarthritis in active patients. *Phys Sports Med.* 2003;31:401–410.
22. Miyauchi S, Machida A, Onaya J, et al. Alterations of proteoglycan synthesis in rabbit articular cartilage induced by intra-articular injection of papain. *Osteoarthritis Cartilage.* 1993;1: 253–262.
23. Regatte RR, Akella SVS, Bothakur A, et al. Proteoglycan depletion-induced changes in transverse relaxation maps of cartilage. *Acad Radiol.* 2002;9:1388–1394.
24. Denti M, Monteleone M, Trevisan C, et al. Magnetic resonance imaging versus arthroscopy for the investigation of the osteochondral humeral defect in anterior shoulder instability. A double blind prospective study. *Knee Surg Sports Traumatol Arthrosc.* 1995;3(3):184–186.
25. Chow JCY, Hantes ME, Houle JB, et al. Arthroscopic autogenous osteochondral transplantation for treating knee cartilage defects: a 2- to 5-year follow-up study. *Arthroscopy.* 2004;20:681–690.
26. Gerber C, Lambert SM. Allograft reconstruction of segmental defects of the humeral head for the treatment of chronic locked posterior dislocation of the shoulder. *J Bone Joint Surg.* 1996;78A: 376–382.
27. Hart R, Janecek M, Visna P, et al. Mosaicplasty for the treatment of femoral head defect after incorrect resorbable screw insertion. *Arthroscopy.* 2003;19:E80.
28. Scheibel M, Bartl C, Magosch P, et al. Osteochondral autologous transplantation for the treatment of full-thickness articular cartilage defects of the shoulder. *J Bone Joint Surg.* 2004;86B: 991–997.

29. Siebold R, Lichtenberg S, Habermeyer P. Combination of microfracture and periosteal-flap for the treatment of focal full thickness articular cartilage lesions of the shoulder: a prospective study. *Knee Surg Sports Traumatol Arthrosc.* 2003;11:183–189.

30. Carranza-Bencano A, Garcia-Paino L, Armas Padron JR, et al. Neochondrogenesis in repair of full-thickness articular cartilage defects using free autogenous periosteal grafts in the rabbit. A follow-up in six months. *Osteoarthritis Cartilage.* 2000;8:351–358.

31. O'Driscoll S, Fitzsimmons JS. The role of periosteum in cartilage repair. *Clin Orthop.* 2001;391(suppl):190–207.

32. Hominga GN, Bulstra SK, Bouwmeester PS, et al. Perichondral grafting for cartilage lesions of the knee. *J Bone Joint Surg.* 1990; 72B:1003–1007.

33. Minas T, Petersen L. Advanced techniques in autologous chondrocyte transplantation. *Clin Sports Med.* 1999;18:13–44.

34. Romeo AA, Cole BJ, Mazzocca AD, et al. Autologous chondrocyte repair of an articular defect in the humeral head. Case Report. *Arthroscopy.* 2002;18:925–929.

35. Flynn JM, Springfield DS, Mankin HJ. Osteoarticular allografts to treat distal femoral osteonecrosis. *Clin Orthop.* 1994;303:38–43.

36. Muscolo DL, Ayerza MA, Aponte Tinao LA. Distal femur osteoarticular allograft reconstruction after Grade III open fractures in pediatric patients. *J Orthop Trauma.* 2004;18:312–315.

37. Oka M, Noguchi T, Kumar P, et al. Development of an artificial articular cartilage: polyvinyl alcohol hydrogel (PVA-H). *Clin Mater.* 1990;6:361–381.

38. Oka M, Chang YS, Nakamura T, et al. Synthetic osteochondral replacement of the femoral articular surface. *J Bone Joint Surg.* 1997;79B:1003–1007.

39. Cofield RH, Frankle MA, Zuckerman JD. Humeral head replacement for glenohumeral arthritis. *Semin Arthroplasty.* 1995; 6:214–221.

40. Matthews LS, Labudde JK. Arthroscopic treatment of synovial disease. *Orthop Clin North Am.* 1993;24:101–109.

41. Iannotti JP, Naranja RJ, Warner JJP. Surgical management of shoulder arthritis in the young and active patient. In: Warner JJP, Iannotti JP, Gerber C, eds. *Complex and revision problems in shoulder surgery.* Philadelphia: Lippincott-Raven Publishers; 1997:289–302.

42. Klepps SJ, Galatz LM, Yamaguchi K. Arthroscopic treatment of osteoarthritis: Debridement and microfracture arthroplasty. In: Imhoff AB, Ticker JB, Fu FH, eds. *An atlas of shoulder arthroscopy.* London: Martin Dunitz; 2003:359–365.
(Mankin HJ. The response of articular cartilage to mechanical injury. *J Bone Joint Surg.* 1982;64A:460–466.)

43. Blevins F, Steadman JR, Rodrigo JJ, et al. Treatment of articular cartilage defects in athletes: an analysis of functional outcome and lesion appearance. *Orthopedics.* 1998;21:761–768.

44. Walch G, Boulahia A, Boileau P. Primary glenohumeral osteoarthritis: clinical and radiographic classification. *Acta Orthop Belg.* 1998;64:46–52.

45. Cofield RH. Arthroscopy of the shoulder. *Mayo Clin Proced.* 1983;58:501–508.

46. Johnson CC. The shoulder joint: an arthroscopic perspective of anatomy and pathology. *Clin Orthop.* 1987;223:113–125.

47. Ogilvie-Harris DJ, Wiley AM. Arthroscopic surgery of the shoulder. *J Bone Joint Surg.* 1986;60B:201–207.

48. Newman AP. Articular cartilage repair. Current concepts. *Am J Sports Med.* 1998;26:309–324.

PECTORALIS MAJOR TENDON RUPTURES

GEORGE K. BAL, MD, FACS, CARL J. BASAMANIA, MD

■ KEY POINTS

- The pectoralis major muscle demonstrates two distinctively different parts—the clavicular head and the sternal head.
- The clavicular head arises from the medial clavicle and upper sternum. It is supplied by the pectoral nerve off of the lateral cord and the deltoid branch of the thoraco-acromial artery.
- The sternal head arises from the sternum, upper six ribs, and the aponeurosis of the external oblique muscle. It is supplied by the medial pectoral nerve (C8-T1) off of the medial cord.
- The most common mechanism for sustaining a pectoralis muscle injury is from weight-training or athletics.
- The patient typically presents after sudden onset of pain in the shoulder. Acutely injured patients have limited shoulder range of motion; however, the more chronic injuries typically have a full range of motion. In more chronic injuries, deformity is obvious with noticeable skin retraction and loss of anterior axillary fold.
- Imaging of soft-tissue injury in the pectoralis major can be difficult. Plain x-rays can reveal bone avulsions, or loss of pectoralis shadow. Ultrasound can demonstrate intramuscular injury or loss of continuity of tendon. Hematoma is easily identified in acute injuries.
- Young, athletic patients will generally not tolerate the persistent weakness and cosmetic deformity that goes with pectoralis major ruptures; however, elderly or low-demand patients with pectoralis ruptures can be treated conservatively with success.
- The primary goal of surgical repair should be solid tendon apposition to bone.

- Postoperatively, the arm is placed in a sling. Patients are encouraged to perform limited activities of daily living as tolerated. Gentle ROM exercises begin immediately, avoiding early passive external rotation or abduction.
- Patients with acutely repaired tendon ruptures may return to full activity 4 to 6 months after repair. Elite weight lifters with chronically repaired tendon ruptures may not be able to return to pre-injury levels.

■ ANATOMY

The anatomy of the pectoralis major muscle demonstrates two distinctively different parts—the clavicular head and the sternal head **(Fig 16-1)**. We feel that when evaluating injuries to the pectoralis it is important to understand the anatomy of the pectoralis major muscle complex. Unfortunately, many of the published reports never comment on this difference, or describe it incompletely and do not distinguish if a 'complete' tear involves one or both heads of the pectoralis (1,2). Only a small number of reports specifically address the anatomy of the pectoralis and the relation of the two heads (3–5). Wolfe et al. (5) suggested the human pectoralis major to be evolved from two distinctly separate muscles in lower mammals. The sternal head of the pectoralis muscle arises from the sternum, upper six ribs, and the aponeurosis of the external oblique muscle. The sternal head is supplied by the medial pectoral nerve (C8-T1) off of the medial cord, and specific pectoral artery. The clavicular head of the pectoralis major arises from the medial clavicle, and upper sternum. The clavicular head is supplied by the lateral pectoral nerve (C5-C7) off of the lateral cord, and the deltoid branch of the thoraco-acromial artery. The sternal head primarily performs

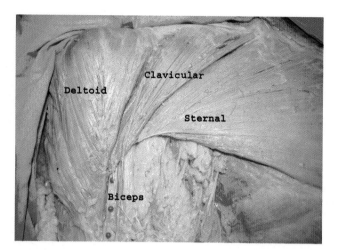

Fig 16-1. Anatomy of pectoralis major—sternal and clavicular heads.

adduction and internal rotation; the clavicular head assists with forward elevation. The two portions of the muscle form a bi-laminar tendon that inserts lateral to the long head biceps tendon. The clavicular head tendon inserts anterior and slightly distal; the sternal head folds posterior and extends superiorly. To further suggest that these are distinctly different muscles, Poland's Syndrome involves the absence of only the sternal portion of the pectoralis muscle (6), although the clavicular head is present. The primary deformity and associated weakness seen in pectoralis ruptures is related to loss of the sternal head tendon.

■ CLINICAL EVALUATION

The most common mechanism for sustaining a pectoralis muscle injury is from weight-lifting or athletics. Wolfe et al. (5) described the transition period from eccentric loading to concentric loading (bench press position) as the most stressful to the inferior muscle fibers of the pectoralis muscle. The

patient typically presents after sudden onset of pain in the shoulder. Acutely injured patients have limited shoulder range of motion; however, the more chronic injuries typically have a full range of motion. A large ecchymoses may be present on the lateral chest, but commonly extends onto the upper arm **(Fig 16-2)**. Without a careful exam, the rupture can be misdiagnosed as a biceps tendon injury (7). Acutely, it may be difficult to see a deformity in the lateral chest secondary to swelling. The classic loss of the anterior axillary fold and lateral chest border is seen in chronic injuries with either sternal head ruptures, or complete pectoralis ruptures. Often the avulsed tendon end is palpable on the chest wall. In more chronic injuries the deformity is usually obvious, with noticeable skin retraction and loss of the anterior axillary fold. Sternal head ruptures can be differentiated from complete ruptures by careful clinical exam. With forward elevation, the clavicular head of the muscle can be both palpated and visualized **(Fig 16-3)**. Resisted adduction or internal rotation will reveal the deficient sternal head **(Fig 16-4)**.

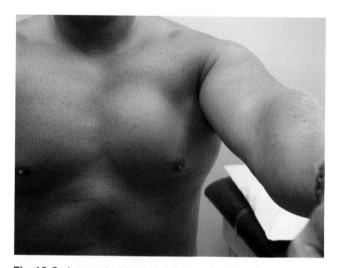

Fig 16-3. Intact clavicular head and retracted sternal head of pectoralis major. Demonstrated with resisted forward elevation.

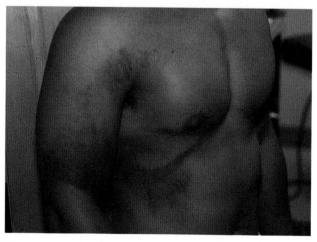

Fig 16-2. Diffuse ecchymoses from pectoralis major rupture. Note discoloration seen on distal arm and lateral chest.

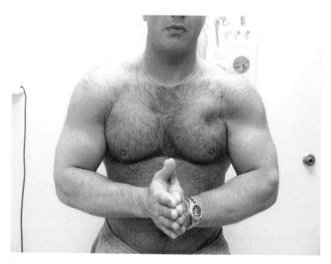

Fig 16-4. Retracted sternal head seen with resisted adduction.

■ IMAGING

Imaging of the soft tissue injury in pectoralis major ruptures can be difficult. Plain x-rays can reveal bone avulsions, or loss of the pectoralis shadow. Ultrasound exam can demonstrate intra-muscular injury or loss of continuity of the tendon (8). CT scan can outline the muscle, but has difficulty visualizing the distal soft tissue of the pectoralis. MRI has been demonstrated to reliably identify injury to the muscle and distal tendon (9) **(Fig 16-5)**. Acute injury and edema of the pectoralis muscle, however, and insertion can make identification of a complete rupture difficult (10). The hematoma is easily identified in acute injuries, but is not present in more chronic tears. It can also be difficult to differentiate a sternal head rupture versus complete injury. Incomplete tendon injuries and medial muscle ruptures are not usually amenable to repair. In our practice, we have not found MRI results to significantly affect our pre-operative planning. In general, most of the information required for surgical decision-making can be obtained from the physical exam.

■ TREATMENT OPTIONS

The past treatment of pectoralis major ruptures has been controversial. There have been studies advocating conservative treatment (9,11,12), some operative repair (8,10), and several have included both in their descriptions (5,13). More recently, most authors advocate early repair of these injuries (1,11). The pectoralis major functions to adduct, forward flex, and internally rotate the shoulder. Several studies have demonstrated significant strength deficits in conservatively treated injuries (11,13,14), with return to near or normal strength after surgical repair (4,8,9). Young, athletic patients will generally not tolerate this persistent weakness, as well as the associated cosmetic deformity; however, elderly or low-demand patients with pectoralis ruptures can be treated conservatively with success (15). The actual surgical repair technique has varied widely. There have been reports using barbed staples (3), screws and washer (4,13), suture anchors (1,16), bone trough and tunnels (2,10), and Achilles tendon allograft augmentation (17). The primary goal of surgical repair should be solid tendon apposition to bone. Although staples and screws do accomplish this, the residual hardware can raise some concerns. Sutures anchors offer an easy fixation solution, but only provide point fixation of tissue to bone. It is difficult to use anything other than simple or horizontal suture patterns with anchor fixation. Stronger, grasping suture patterns such as a Mason-Allen are much harder to accomplish with suture anchors. Our preferred surgical technique has been previously described (18), and advocates a method of direct suture repair to bone through drill holes.

The patient is placed in a supine position, with the arm supported on a hand table. We have not found the beach-chair position to be necessary. The entire upper extremity in addition to most of the thorax on the affected side is draped free. A 3–4 cm incision, at the distal end of the delto-pectoral interval, is more than adequate for exposure and repair **(Fig. 16-6)**. For sternal head ruptures, the dissection is carried medially around the intact clavicular head, not into the interval with the deltoid. With complete ruptures, no delto-pectoral interval will be present. In acute injuries, a large hematoma is frequently encountered, and the avulsed tendon easily identified. Even if retracted, minimal mobilization is needed. In more chronic injuries, a synovial tract is often present, leading medially to the retracted tendon end.

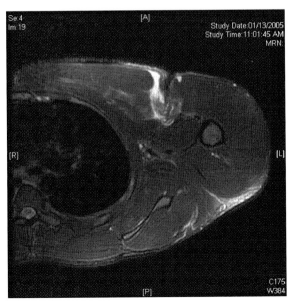

Fig 16-5. Axial image of sternal head pectoralis major rupture.

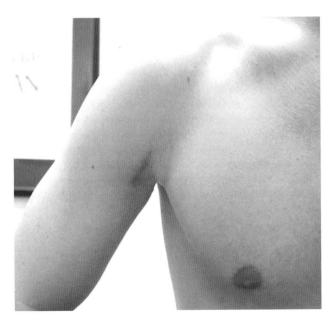

Fig 16-6. Typical incision for pectoralis repair.

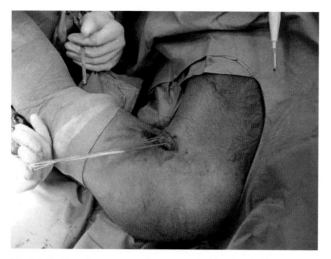

Fig 16-7. Repair sutures placed in ruptured end of tendon.

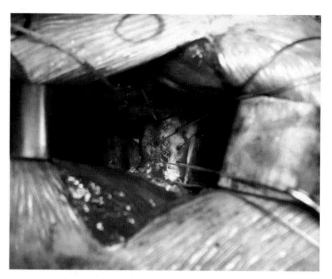

Fig 16-8. Passing sutures placed in bone tunnels.

The tendon is usually shortened and encased in scar. Aggressive scar release and mobilization is required to allow the tendon to reach the humeral insertion. Typically, the fibers of the sternal head of the pectoralis have an inferior-medial to superior-lateral obliquity. The clavicular fibers always have a superior-medial to inferior-lateral obliquity. We have seen chronic injuries that can be adequately mobilized more than 10 years after injury. It is important to feel the inferior-lateral border of the muscle when pulling tension on the tendon. A fullness and firm edge should return to the anterior axillary fold. We use 1 mm cottony Dacron (Deknatel, Fall River, MA 02720) suture in the tendon end, placing three to four sutures in a Modified Mason-Allen fashion **(Fig. 16-7)**. These sutures can be placed in the end of the muscle, for a myotendinous injury, and re-enforced as needed with soft tissue grafts or extra-cellular matrix grafts such as the Restore (DePuy, Johnson & Johnson) swine intestine submucosal graft. The insertion site of the pectoralis tendon is lateral to the bicipital groove. For sternal head injuries, the clavicular head of the muscle will have its intact insertion distal to the proposed repair site. The sternal head is brought deep and proximal to the clavicular head muscle when repaired to the insertion site. The insertion site is cleaned of any tendon remnants, and can be roughened with a curette. We have not found it necessary to create a bone trough. A Curvetek drill (Arthrotek, Ontario, CA 91761) is used to create bone tunnels at the repair site. Passing sutures are then pulled through the bone tunnels with a specific needle that matches the curve of the drill **(Fig. 16-8)**. The deep arm of each suture is passed through the bone tunnel. The arm is slightly adducted and internally rotated, and traction placed on the deep sutures. This pulls the tendon down to the bone, and the superficial sutures are tied to deep sutures **(Fig. 16-9)**. This creates a broad area of contact between the tendon and bone, with the security of tying the suture over a bone bridge. The wound is irrigated, subcutaneous tissue closed with absorbable suture, and the skin closed with running prolene suture.

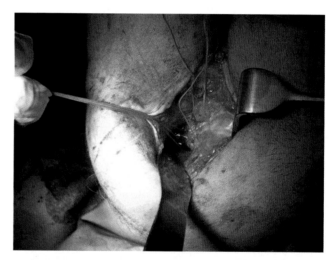

Fig 16-9. Repair sutures passed through tunnels and pectoralis tendon reduced to bone.

Postoperatively, the arm was placed in a sling. Patients were encouraged to perform limited activities of daily living as tolerated. Gentle range of motion (ROM) exercises were begun immediately, avoiding early passive external rotation or abduction. Light resistance exercises are started at six weeks, subsequent progression of strengthening, and resumption of full activity at four to six months. It has been our experience that all patients with acutely repaired tendon ruptures, less than eight weeks, have returned to full activity. The majority of patients with repairs of chronically torn pectoralis tendons have had good pain relief, cosmetic appearance **(Fig. 16-10)**, and excellent return of strength (2,5,14,19). In contrast, high-demand athletes, particularly elite weight lifters, with chronically repaired tendon ruptures have shown significant improvement, but have frequently not been able to return to pre-injury weight training levels.

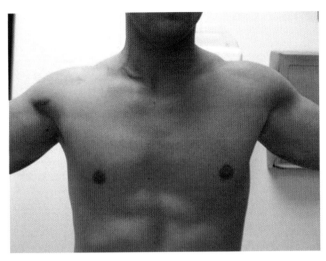

Fig 16-10. Cosmetic appearance after healed pectoralis repair.

■ REFERENCES

1. Aarimaa V, Rantanen J, Heikkila J, et al. Rupture of the pectoralis major muscle. *Am J Sports Med.* 2004;32(5):1256–1262.

2. Schepsis AA, Grafe MW, Jones HP, et al. Rupture of the pectoralis major muscle: outcome after repair of acute and chronic injuries. *Am J Sports Med.* 2000;28(1):9–15.

3. Egan TM, Hall H. Avulsion of the pectoralis major tendon in a weight lifter: repair using a barbed staple. *Can J Surg.* 1987;30:434–435.

4. Quinlan JF, Molloy M, Hurson BJ. Pectoralis major tendon ruptures, when to operate. *Br J Sports Med.* 2002;36(3): 226–228.

5. Wolfe SW, Wickiewicz TL, Cavanaugh JT. Ruptures of the pectoralis major muscle: an anatomic and clinical analysis. *Am J Sports Med.* 1992;20(5):587–593.

6. Sugiura Y. Poland's syndrome: clinico-roentgenographic study on 45 cases. *Cong Anom.* 1976;16(1):17–28.

7. Ramsey ML. Distal biceps tendon injuries: diagnosis and management. *J Am Acad Orthop Surg.* 1999;7(3):199–207.

8. Liu J, Wu JJ, Chang CY, et al. Avulsion of the pectoralis major tendon. *Am J Sports Med.* 1992;20:366–368.

9. Connell DA, Potter HG, Sherman MF, et al. Injuries of the pectoralis major muscle: evaluation with MR imaging. *Radiology.* 1999;210(3):785–791.

10. Kretzler HH, Richardson AB. Rupture of the pectoralis major muscle. *Am J Sports Med.* 1989;17(4):453–458.

11. Scott BW, Wallace WA, Barton MA. Diagnosis and assessment of the pectoralis major rupture by dynamometry. *J Bone Joint Surg Br.* 1992;74(1):111–113.

12. Zeman SC, Rosenfeld RT, Lipscomb PR. Tears of the pectoralis major muscle. *Am J Sports Med.* 1979;7:343–347.

13. McEntire JE, Hess WE, Coleman SS. Rupture of the pectoralis major muscle: a report of eleven injuries and review of fifty-six. *J Bone Joint Surg Am.* 1972;54:1040–1046.

14. Roi GS, Respezzi S, Dworzak F. Partial rupture of the pectoralis major muscle in athletes. *Int J Sports Med.* 1990;11:85–87.

15. Beloosesky Y, Grinblat J, Weiss A, et al. Pectoralis major ruptures in the elderly. Clin Orthop, 2003;413:164–169.

16. Miller MD, Johnson DL, Fu FH, et al. Rupture of the pectoralis major muscle in a collegiate football player: use of magnetic imaging in early diagnosis. *Am J Sports Med.* 1993;21:475–477.

17. Zafra M, Munoz F, Carpintero P. Chronic rupture of the pectoralis major muscle: a report of two cases. *Acta Orthop Belg.* 2005;71(1):107–110.

18. Bal GK, Basamania CJ. Pectoralis major tendon ruptures: diagnosis and treatment. *Tec Shoulder Elbow Surg.* 2005;6(3):128–134.

19. Anbari A, Kelly JD IV, Moyer RA. Delayed repair of a ruptured pectoralis major muscle. A case report. *Am J Sports Med.* 2000; 28(2):254–256.

ACUTE INJURIES: SHOULDER FRACTURES AND ACROMIOCLAVICULAR AND STERNOCLAVICULAR JOINT INJURIES

17

■ ROBERT TALAC, MD, PhD, JOEL J. SMITH, MD

■ KEY POINTS

- The most common cause of a proximal humerus fracture is a fall on outstretched hands from a standing position. Another mechanism of injury is excessive rotation while the arm is abducted.
- Although fracture of the proximal humerus significantly limits function of the upper extremity, careful neurovascular examination of the entire upper extremity should always be performed. There are three important nerves—axillary, suprascapular and musculocutanneous—in close proximity of the proximal humerus and nerve injury accompanies the majority of humerus fractures.
- The trauma series, consisting of anteroposterior (AP) view of the scapula, a lateral, Y-view of the scapula, and axillary view, is the standard initial method of evaluation for proximal humerus fracture.
- More than 80% of the proximal humerus fractures are nondisplaced and can be treated nonoperatively. The shoulder is initially immobilized in a sling at the side or in Velpaeu position. After pain has diminished and the fracture is stable (usually after 7 to 10 days), gentle pendulum exercises can be started.
- Some dislocated two-part surgical neck fractures can also be treated conservatively. They may require closed reduction in conscious sedation or general anesthesia.
- Multipart proximal humerus fractures or isolated fractures of the greater or lesser tuberosities that are displaced more than 5 mm should be treated with open reduction and internal fixation. Surgical modalities include plates, screws, intramedullary devices and their combinations.
- Clavicle fractures account for 35% of fractures about the shoulder.
- Most patients with clavicle fracture report a direct fall onto the shoulder with subsequent pain and deformity in a clavicular region.
- Most middle third clavicle fractures are treated conservatively with a sling or figure-eight dressing for 3 to 6 weeks.
- Similarly to other shoulder injuries, patients with the acromioclavicular joint injuries often report a fall or direct trauma to the shoulder. Physical exam reveals swelling and tenderness over distal clavicle associated with a deformity caused by a horizontal and/or vertical displacement of the clavicle.
- Initial radiographic confirmation and evaluation of the clavicle fracture and acromioclavicular joint injury should include AP and 45 degree cephalic tilt (apical oblique) views with patient upright which brings the clavicular image away from the thoracic cage.

The shoulder joint mobility plays a vital role in upper extremity function. It is therefore not surprising that optimal management of acute shoulder injuries remains an important issue that confronts the orthopedic profession. Modern management of shoulder injuries has become technically sophisticated. The purpose of this chapter is to provide a succinct review of current opinions and advancements in the management of proximal humerus and clavicle fractures as well as acromio- and sternoclavicular joint injuries.

■ PROXIMAL HUMERUS FRACTURES

Few areas of fracture management have been the subject of as much controversy, new information, and revisionist thinking as the management of proximal humerus fractures. Proximal humerus fractures account for 2% to 4% of all upper extremity fractures (1). They occur most often in older patients and represent complex injuries often including bony fragment displacement associated with varying degree of soft tissue injury.

■ BASIC SCIENCE

Anatomy and Biomechanics

The humerus is the largest bone of upper extremity. The proximal humerus is composed of the humeral head, the greater and lesser tuberosities, the anatomic and surgical necks of the humerus. The humeral head is the most proximal, ball-like region of the humerus that is retroverted (28 to 40 degrees) and articulates with the glenoid cavity of the scapula. The head of the humerus is significantly larger than the glenoid fossa. There is no bony structural stability to the joint. The motion of the glenohumeral joint completely relies on the balance of tension and compression of soft tissues attached to the proximal humerus and the scapula. After a fracture occurs, the pull of shoulder muscles becomes the deforming force dictating the pattern of the fracture. In addition, understanding a relationship between bony fragment position, soft tissue balancing and glenohumeral joint function is essential for successful outcome after proximal humerus injury. The greater and lesser tuberosities are close to the humeral head and they are insertion sites for the rotator cuff. Both tuberosities are separated by the intertubecular groove in which lies the tendon of the long head of the biceps muscle and the arcuate artery, a branch of the anterior circumflex humeral artery. The intertubercular groove is covered by the transverse humeral ligament. The humeral head and tuberosities are separated by a narrow region which represents the anatomic neck of the humerus. Distal to anatomic neck proximal humerus narrows connecting to humeral shaft. This area is called surgical neck and represents most vulnerable part of the proximal humerus. This area also contains the main arterial supply to the proximal humerus, anterior and posterior circumflex arteries that arise from axillary artery. Both circumflex arteries make numerous extraosseous collaterals that help to supply the most proximal areas of the proximal humerus. Despite the rich blood supply, avascular necrosis (AVN) of the humeral head is still a common sequelae of the proximal humerus fractures particularly if majority of the bony and soft tissue have been detached from the humeral head. The shoulder's innervation is derived from brachial plexus. From a clinical perspective, there are three important nerves in close proximity of the proximal humerus: These include the axillary, suprascapular, and musculocutanneous nerve.

■ CLINICAL EVALUATION

History and Physical Findings

The most common mechanism of injury for proximal humerus fracture is a fall on outstretched hands from standing. Another mechanism of injury is excessive rotation while the arm is abducted. In this situation, the proximal humerus locks against the acromion. Even minor force can cause a fracture, especially if the bone was previously weakened by osteoporosis. Inspection of the affected area often reveals significant swelling, tenderness on palpation, and obvious deformity of affected shoulder. Crepitus may be present upon motion of the fracture fragments. Although the fracture of the proximal humerus significantly limits function of the upper extremity, careful neurovascular examination of entire upper extremity should always be performed. Recently, Sommer et al. (2) reported the nerve injury in 67% of the patients with a proximal humerus fracture. The axillary nerve was involved in 58% and suprascapular nerve in 48%. All rings should be removed from the fingers. It is important to warn the patient about transient worsening of the swelling and possible development of ecchymosis within first 24 to 48 hours after injury. Although diagnosis of the fracture is made radiographically, the circumstances resulting in the injury should be elucidated and assessment for associated injuries of the neck, the clavicle, and sternoclavicular joint should be performed.

Radiographic Evaluation

Accurate radiographic evaluation of the fracture of the proximal humerus is essential for diagnosis and treatment. The trauma series **(Fig 17-1)** is still the standard initial method for evaluating proximal humeral fracture. This consists of anteroposterior (AP) view of the scapula, a lateral, Y-view of the scapula, and axillary view. This series allows evaluation of the fracture pattern in three perpendicular planes. It is not uncommon for inadequate radiographs to be done. The two most common problems include the AP view of the scapula with the arm internally rotated, and not doing an axillary view. Without an axillary view, it is almost impossible to determine the relationship between the humeral head and the glenoid. To obtain a proper AP view of the scapula, the arm should be gently externally rotated about 20 degrees. This can be easily accomplished letting the patient hold onto IV pole or the edge of the table. A similar maneuver can be used to obtain abducted axillary view. Some surgeons prefer Velpau axillary view, in which arms stay in the sling, the patient leans back, and the beam is aimed down though the shoulder (1) (Fig 17-1) .

The role of CT in the evaluation of proximal humerus fractures remains controversial. Some orthopedists order CT scan only if pattern of the fracture cannot be clearly determined. Others argue that standard radiographs are not sufficient to appreciate subtle changes in rotation and

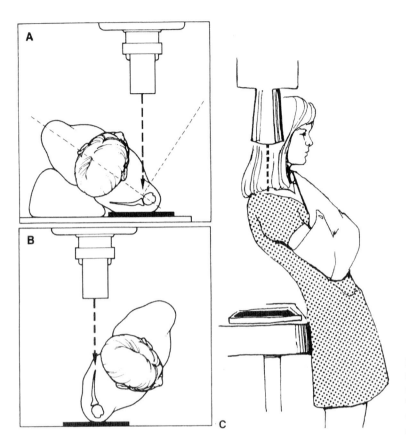

Fig 17-1. Trauma series. Trauma series consists of AP and lateral x-rays in the scapular plane as well as an axillary view. **A:** AP view in the scapular plane. **B:** Lateral view in the scapular plane. **C:** The Velpau axillary view. (Reprinted from Rockwood and Green: *Fractures in Adults,* 5th ed. Philadelphia: Saunders; 2003.)

positioning of the fragments and recommend CT scan as a part of standard radiographic evaluation of proximal humerus fractures. Moreover, CT images can be digitally manipulated to provide three-dimensional (3D) reconstruction of the fracture. Most recently, Edelson et al. (3) reported their experience with 3D-CT reconstruction of the proximal humerus fractures. They suggest that 3D-CT reconstruction provides precise information about anatomy of bony fragments that not only help to better understand fracture pattern, but may lead to improved or better surgical procedures. Magnetic resonance imaging (MRI) is rarely needed.

Decision Making Algorithms and Classification

Accurate analysis of radiographs and a reproducible classification system are desirable for the treatment of any fracture. Various classification systems have been proposed for the fractures of the proximal humerus in the past. Neer's modification of Codman's four fragments classification system **(Fig 17-2)** and AO/Orthopedic Trauma Association (OTA) system represent most commonly used schemes for classification of fractures of the proximal humerus. Both systems are based on the analysis of plain radiographs. In the Neer system, fractures are classified based on the number of segments and displacement of any of four principal fragments: humeral head, greater and lesser tuberosities, and humeral shaft. If fragments are displaced <1 cm from each other, or angulated <45 degrees, the fracture is considered minimally

displaced or one part fracture. A two-part fracture contains two fragments, and most often the fracture line runs through the surgical neck separating the shaft from the head and both tuberosities. Three-part fractures involve either the lesser or greater tuberosity fracture in conjunction with a fracture of the surgical neck. Four-part fractures have all four key components displaced from each other. AO/OTA classification is more complex and is not widely used in the United States. There is growing recognition that existing classifications schemes are inadequate in terms of interobserver reliability as well as predicting the clinical outcome (4,5). Most recently, Edelson et al. (3) reported a 3D classification for fractures of the proximal humerus based on 3D-CT reconstructions. To address inherent difficulty with presenting a 3D object on a two-dimensional (2D) printed page, they devised a fracture wheel format in which each fracture is presented in simultaneous four-quadrant views. The injury is seen from the front, side, back, and from above in one composite picture. Using this technique, they organized proximal humerus fractures into four basic types: two part fractures; three part fractures; shield fractures with their variants; and isolated fractures of the greater tuberosity. Statistical analysis of interobserver reliability demonstrated approximately twofold improvement over previous classifications (kappa 0.69). They also suggest that the experience gained from the understanding the 3D patterns of fracture provide invaluable information guiding the restitution of anatomy during the surgery.

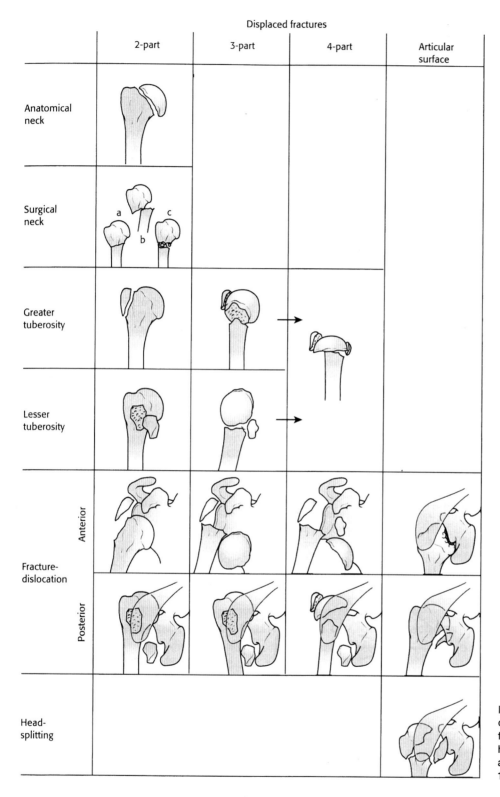

Fig 17-2. Neer's four-part classification. (Modified with permission from Neer CS. Displaced proximal humeral fractures: I. classification and evaluation. *J Bone Joint Surg.* 1970;52A:1077–1089.)

■ TREATMENT

Many treatment methods have been described through the years. In general, the choice of the treatment for a proximal humerus fracture should be based on the type of the fracture, presence of concurrent injuries, age and activity level of the patient, the presence and nature of comorbid medical conditions, and potential outcomes of specific treatment strategy.

Over 80% of the proximal humerus fractures are nondisplaced or minimally displaced and can be treated nonoperatively (1,3,6). Initially, the shoulder is immobilized in a sling at the side or in Velpaeu position. After pain is diminished and the fracture is stable (usually 7 to 10 days after injury), gentle pendulum exercises can be started. It is important to establish that the fracture is stable and moves as a unit prior to starting exercises. The exercises should be performed 3 to 4 times a day under supervision of the therapist, or at home after appropriate instruction by a physical therapist. The patient should be advised that overly aggressive exercise can lead to malunion or nonunion. Initial, immobilization and early motion have a high degree of success as documented by numerous studies (1,6).

Some dislocated two-part surgical neck fractures can also be treated conservatively. They may require closed reduction in conscious sedation or general anesthesia. In this type of injury, the shaft is usually displaced medially and anteriorly by the pull of the pectoralis major muscle, while the tuberosities remain in a neutral position. After adequate relaxation is achieved, it is possible to reduce the shaft and impact it under the head using gentle traction with flexion and adduction of the arm. Repeated and/or forceful closed reduction is not recommended. If a closed reduction is not possible, it is likely that there is an interposition of soft tissue, most commonly long head of the biceps, in the fracture site. Whenever possible, fluoroscopic C arm visualization should be employed. This allows not only visualizing the reduction, but also assessing the stability of the fracture. If the fracture is unstable, percutaneous pinning of the anterior and greater tuberosity with terminally threaded K-wires can be used to further stabilize the fracture. The greater tuberosity pins should be placed into the proximal humerus with the shoulder externally rotated and should engage the cortex at least 2 cm from most distal aspect of the humeral head. Be sure to pay close attention so that the humeral head is not penetrated (7).

Multipart proximal humerus fractures or isolated fractures of the greater or lesser tuberosities that are displaced more than 5 mm should be treated with open reduction and internal fixation. Many surgical modalities have been described in the literature. These include plates, screws, intramedullary devices, and various combinations. In general, it is important to avoid extensive exposure and soft tissue dissection because this may further compromise an already altered blood supply. As per recent literature, blade plate with interfragmentary screws or newly designed contoured proximal humerus locking compression plates seem to be most commonly used techniques for open treatment of proximal humerus fractures. The majority of orthopedists use one of the two basic surgical approaches to proximal humerus: superior deltoid approach or long deltopectoral approach. In an attempt to minimize surgical trauma to the soft tissue envelope, a new minimally invasive plating technique has been described (8). This plating technique preserves the soft tissue envelope and periosteum, maintains arterial vascularity and therefore minimizes the surgical trauma to the zone of injury. In addition, early biomechanic studies demonstrated that locking plates are less likely to fail in osteoporotic bone (9). These results

are promising, but further studies are needed to demonstrate relative merit of these new techniques.

In cases of comminuted four-part fractures, humeral head splitting injuries, or humeral head defects >40% of the articular surface, open reduction and internal fixation yields unsatisfactory results (1,6,8). Due to the high incidence of AVN, post injury early humeral head hemiarthroplasty is favored. In addition, results of late arthroplasty are inferior to those treated acutely with humeral head replacement. The studies reviewing outcomes of hemiarthroplasty for proximal humerus fractures suggest that early surgical intervention within 2 weeks of injury and accurate tuberosity reconstruction are two factors that have the greatest impact on functional outcome (10).

■ COMPLICATIONS AND SPECIAL CONSIDERATIONS

Fracture of the proximal humerus presents a therapeutic challenge. Numerous complications have been reported. Most common complications include AVN, malunion, neurovascular injury, and adhesive capsulitis (frozen shoulder) (1,2,3,6,8,10). Hardware failure, infection, and nonunion are less common.

AVN is a common complication following three- and four-part fractures. The incidence of AVN of the humeral head ranges from 21% to 75% (1). Although the exact mechanism leading to necrosis is not known, it seems that disruption of the anterior humeral circumflex artery and its branches during the injury play a critical role in development of this complication. The treatment of choice for symptomatic AVN is a humeral head arthroplasty.

Malunion is a complication occurring after inadequately closed reduction or failed open treatment. The treatment is often challenging because of excessive scarring and retraction of the fragments. Angulation or rotational malunions are treated with osteotomy and internal fixation. If malunion is associated with AVN or post-traumatic degeneration, humeral head arthroplasty or total shoulder replacement may be considered.

Neurovascular injuries occur as an associated injury during proximal humerus fracture or as a complication of surgical treatment particularly percutaneous pinning. The main trunk of the axillary nerve and posterior humeral circumflex artery is at risk during placement of the greater tuberosity pins (7). The anterior branch of the axillary nerve can be damaged during placement of the proximal lateral pin, and musculocutaneous nerve, cephalic vein, and biceps tendon can be injured during the anterior pin placement (7).

Rehabilitation is an essential part of the therapeutic plan for a proximal humerus fracture. Early range of motion exercises help prevent adhesive capsulitis (frozen shoulder) that impede adequate motion necessary for optimal function. Initial management consists of an early, staged exercise program. Patients with a frozen shoulder unresponsive to conservative treatment may be considered for arthroscopic debridement of glenohumeral joint and subacromial space and selective capsular release combined with manipulation under general anesthesia. Manipulation under general anesthesia as a stand-alone procedure has also been described and has demonstrated improvement in range of motion (11,12). Although manipulation under anesthesia was effective in terms of joint mobilization, the method can cause iatrogenic intra-articular damage such as iatrogenic superior labrum anterior-posterior lesions, partial tears of the subscapularis tendon, anterior labral detachments with a small osteochondral defect, or tears of the middle glenohumeral ligament (12).

Clavicle Fractures

Clavicle fractures account for 4% to 5% of all fractures; however, they occur in 35% fractures about the shoulder.

■ BASIC SCIENCE

Anatomy and Biomechanics

The clavicle connects the upper extremity to the axial skeleton. It extends from the manubrium of the sternum to the acromion of the scapula. In the axial plane, the clavicle assumes a gentle S-shape. The medial two-thirds of the clavicle shaft are convex anteriorly and the distal third is convex posteriorly. Both medial and lateral ends are flattened and expanded. The central part is thin and tubular. In the sagittal plane, the clavicle assumes an anteromedial to posterolateral position. It has been suggested that clavicular curvatures increase its resilience.

The functional role of the clavicle has long been debated. In reference to acute trauma, the clavicle seems to have three important biomechanical functions. It acts as a strut supporting the shoulder in such a position, which facilitates optimal range of motion of the upper extremity. Without the clavicle, contraction of muscles that cross glenohumeral joint would pull the proximal humerus towards chest instead of moving the arm. Lazarus (13) suggested that the clavicle increases the strength of the shoulder girdle movement by maintaining optimal working distance of the thoracohumeral muscles. Also, the clavicle transmits forces from the upper extremity to the axial skeleton. Hence, the fall on the shoulder may result in a clavicle fracture. The most common fracture site is a midclavicle transitional region. These account for 81% of all clavicle fractures (6). Finally, the clavicle provides attachment for muscles and ligaments that further stabilize the shoulder girdle. The attachment of the muscles and ligaments has important implications for the fracture displacement pattern. Loss of clavicle integrity secondary to the fracture leads to a characteristic displacement of its fragments. The sternocleidomastoid muscle elevates the medial fragment of the bone. The trapezius muscle is unable to hold up the lateral fragment that predictably succumbs to the weight of the arm and displaces inferiorly.

Biology

The clavicle is the first bone in the body to ossify. Intramembranous ossification begins during the 7th embryonic week. The medial clavicle physis fuses around 25 years of age. In unusual instances, the clavicle is incomplete or absent. In the former situation, the middle segment of the clavicle is absent and two ends are joined together only by a fibrous band. In latter situation, the whole clavicle is absent. This condition is known as a cleidocranial dysostosis (congenital absence of the clavicle). It is often associated with delayed ossification of the skull. It is characterized by drooping and excessive shoulder mobility (14).

■ CLINICAL EVALUATION

History and Physical Findings

Most patients with a clavicle fracture report a direct fall onto the shoulder with subsequent pain and deformity in a clavicular region. It is important to elucidate circumstances resulting in the injury that may provide sufficient clues about associated injuries (15). Because of its subcutaneous location, fractures of the clavicle do not represent a diagnostic challenge. Inspection of the affected area often reveals swelling and obvious deformity. Some patients may present with ecchymosis in the clavicular region. Skin tenting is common, but open fractures are very rare. Tenderness on palpation further reveals site of injury.

Radiographic Evaluation

As with any fracture, it is important to obtain the necessary radiographic studies to characterize the fracture appropriately. Initial radiographic confirmation and evaluation of the clavicle fracture should include AP and 45 degrees cephalic tilt (apical oblique) views with the patient upright, bringing the clavicular image away from the thoracic cage (Fig 17-3). In a case of the distal clavicle fracture, plain films should include AP clavicle, axillary and scapula Y views, as well as an AP view of the acromioclavicular joint. In these circumstances, it is not unusual to obtain a CT scan of the shoulder (with 3D reconstruction) to ensure that the correct diagnosis has been achieved and fracture adequately characterized (16).

Decision Making Algorithms and Classification

There are several classification systems for the fractures of the clavicle (13,17). Allman (17) classifies fractures of the clavicle into three groups according to the anatomic location of the injury. Group I represents middle third fractures; Group II are lateral third fractures; and Group III are medial third fractures. This system is simple, but neglects some important aspects of the fracture, such as displacement, shortening, or comminution. Neer (18) recognized the unique behavior and challenges associated with distal third clavicle fractures. He proposed to further classify Allman's Group II fractures

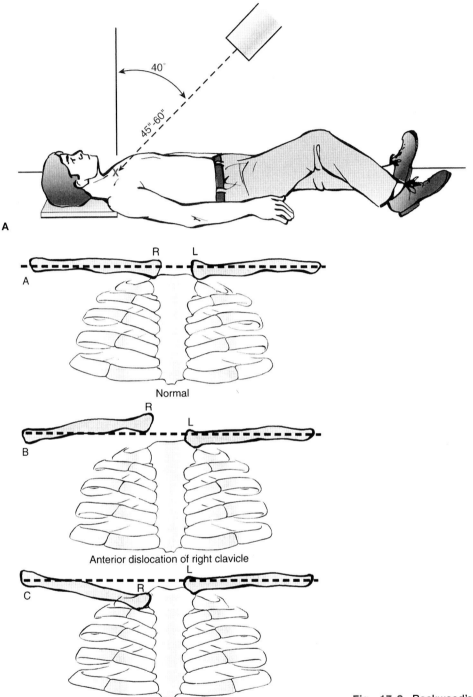

Fig 17-3. Rockwood's Serendipity view. (Reprinted from Rockwood and Green: *Fractures in Adults,* 6th edition)

into three distinct subtypes. In the Type I injury, the fracture occurs between conoid and trapezoid ligaments, or between coracoclavicular and acromioclavicular ligaments. Ligaments are not disrupted, therefore the fracture is stable with no or minimal displacement. The Neer Type II fracture represents a fracture associated with detachment of the coracoclavicular ligaments from the proximal clavicular fragment. This renders the fracture unstable and displaced. The Neer Type III fracture encompasses a distal clavicle fracture extending into the

acromioclavicular joint. Rockwood (19) further subdivides Neer Type II fractures into two subtypes: Type II A—conoid and trapezoid ligament intact and attached to distal fragment; Type IIB—conoid ligament torn. In 1990 Craig (20) combined Allman's and Neer's classification schemes and devised a new classification system (Craig's classification of clavicular fractures). Craig's classification provided more detailed anatomic and functional description of fractures of the clavicle as well as important therapeutic implications.

Naturally, any classification system is based on the premise that it covers most, if not all, of the possible fracture patterns. Unfortunately, no described system is ideal. Authors believe that for the proper treatment of a clavicular fracture, it is more important to be aware of the accurate fracture anatomy rather than to classify a fracture unreasonably and blindly follow a pre-existing classification system.

TREATMENT

The treatment of choice for a clavicle fracture should be based on the type of the fracture, presence of concurrent injuries, age and activity level of the patient, the presence and nature of comorbid medical conditions. The ultimate objective is to achieve early AP and lateral alignment and good stability of the fracture to allow rehabilitation of the limb and prevent disability.

Middle Third Clavicle Fractures

Most middle third clavicle fractures are treated conservatively with a sling or figure of eight dressing for approximately 3 to 6 weeks. Immobilization is discontinued when there are clinical signs of fracture healing (i.e., no pain or palpable fracture motion). This can be as early as 3 weeks. After there is minimal pain to palpation in the fracture site, full range of motion is begun. Shoulder stiffness is rare, but if present, physical therapy may be considered. In this case, the exercises should include forward elevation and external rotation stretches in supine position to negate the displacing effect of the gravity. Codman's pendulum exercises should be avoided because they will magnify the displacing moment of the arm weight (6,13). Most patients can resume their full activity within 1 to 3 months after injury.

Indications for open reduction and internal fixation include open fractures, neurovascular injury, fracture shortening more than 2 cm, impending skin disruption, fracture in patients with neurologic disorders such as Parkinson disease, seizures, and head injury of polytrauma that prohibits immobilization. Numerous methods of internal fixation have been described. In general, optimal internal fixation is dictated by fracture pattern. Traditionally, transverse fractures are fixed with a 3.5 mm dynamic compression (DC) plate with minimum six intact cortices on each fracture site. For an oblique fracture, the DC plate is complemented with lag screws placed across the fracture site. Plating represents rigid internal fixation that allows the patient immediate use of his/her arm for activities of daily living; however, superficial location of the clavicle with the plate makes wound closure more challenging. Authors recommend maintaining the arm in the sling for 1 to 2 weeks postoperatively, not only for comfort but to allow uneventful healing of the wound. Physical therapy is rarely needed, but if shoulder stiffness is a concern, external rotation stretches in supine position are recommended. Codman's pendulum exercises should be avoided for reasons stated previously in this chapter.

Distal Clavicle Fractures

Fractures of the distal clavicle represent a diagnostic and therapeutic challenge. Neer (18) recognized unique behavior of these fractures and recommended to treat them as a distinct entity. To date, there is a paucity of conclusive data to support one particular treatment modality. Some authors reported a good outcome with an immobilization followed by gentle range of motion exercises. Proponents of the nonoperative management recognized a relatively high rate of nonunions associated with this strategy, but emphasize that the nonunion seems to have no significant effect on functional outcome and strength. Therefore, they suggest that most Type II distal clavicle fractures can be treated nonsurgically (21,22). Others emphasize a high rate of non-unions and strongly advocate primary open reduction and internal fixation. Fixation methods described in literature include transacromial K-wires, coracoacromial screws, plates, Dacron tapes, and tension wires (22–27). Internal fixation interferes with a normal rotation of the clavicle, however, requiring hardware removal prior to full mobilization. Recently, Levi (28) described a minimally invasive technique for fixing Neer Type II distal clavicle fractures using absorbable sutures (PDS No 1). Union was achieved in all fractures with no complications. All patients demonstrated rapid return of function.

COMPLICATIONS AND SPECIAL CONSIDERATIONS

Available data demonstrates that nonoperative treatment of distal clavicle fracture is associated with a significant nonunion rate ranging from 30% to 45% (21). A more relevant issue is whether these nonunions result in clinically important symptoms or deficits.

Acromioclavicular Joint Injuries

Injuries to the acromioclavicular joint are relatively common. They account for approximately 10% of acute shoulder injuries.

BASIC SCIENCE

Anatomy and Biomechanics

The acromioclavicular joint is a small diarthrodial joint that can be palpated 2 to 3 cm medial from lateral border of the acromion. It contains an intra-articular fibrocartilageous disk. Because of an existing mismatch between the clavicle and the acromion, the stability of the acromioclavicular joint depends mostly on the joint capsule and extracapsular ligaments. Several studies suggest that the trapezoid ligament is primarily responsible for a horizontal stability, specifically posterior translation, whereas the conoid ligament mediate vertical stability, more specifically, the anterosuperior translation (29–31).

■ CLINICAL EVALUATION

History and Physical Exam

Similarly to other shoulder injuries, patients with the acromioclavicular joint injuries often report a fall or direct trauma to the shoulder. Physical exam reveals swelling and tenderness over distal clavicle associated with a deformity caused by a horizontal and/or vertical displacement of the clavicle. Shoulder motion is limited and painful, particularly with a cross-arm adduction. Thorough evaluation of the skin, vascular, and peripheral nerve structures is mandatory to rule out associated injuries.

Radiographic Evaluation

Radiographic evaluation of the acromioclavicular joint injury is identical to the evaluation of clavicle fractures. AP, axillary views, or cephalic tilt radiograph (Zanca view) provide sufficient visualization of the acromioclavicular joint **(Fig 17-4)**. They also allow comparison to the uninjuried side. In a case of suspected acromioclavicular joint injury and negative findings on initial radiographs, weighted stress views of the acromioclavicular joint may be necessary; however, these are not part of a routine initial radiographic evaluation. For patients with Type III to Type VI injuries, CT and MRI evaluation rule out concomitant injury that should

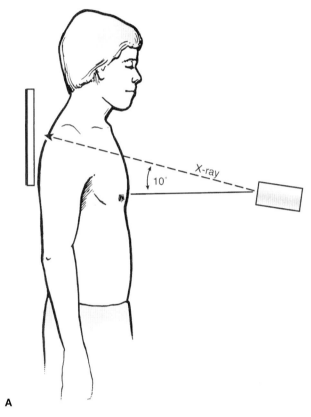

A

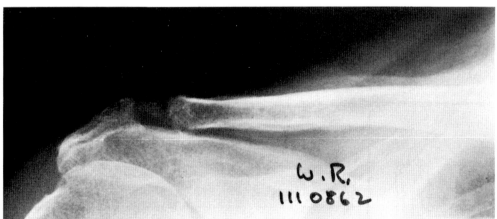

B

Fig 17-4. Zanca view of the acromioclavicular joint. **A:** Patient position. (Reprinted from Rockwood and Green: *Fractures in Adults,* 6th ed.) **B:** Radiographic Zanca view of the acromioclavicular joint. (Reprinted from Rockwood and Green: *Fractures in Adults,* 4th ed.)

be considered. CT allows for an excellent visualization of articular surfaces and joint misalignment. It is also useful for an accurate diagnosis and classification of ligamentous injury.

Decision Making Algorithms and Classification

The Rockwood classification system is widely accepted **(Fig 17-5)**. This involves dividing acromioclavicular joint injuries into 6 subtypes (32). Type I injuries represent acromioclavicular ligaments sprain. The trapezoid ligament is intact, and the clavicle remains stable. In Type II injuries, the acromioclavicular ligament is disrupted leading to AP instability. Type III injuries exhibit disruption of both the acromioclavicular and coracoacromial ligaments, resulting in vertical and horizontal instability of the distal clavicle. The deltotrapezius fascia is detached from the distal clavicle,

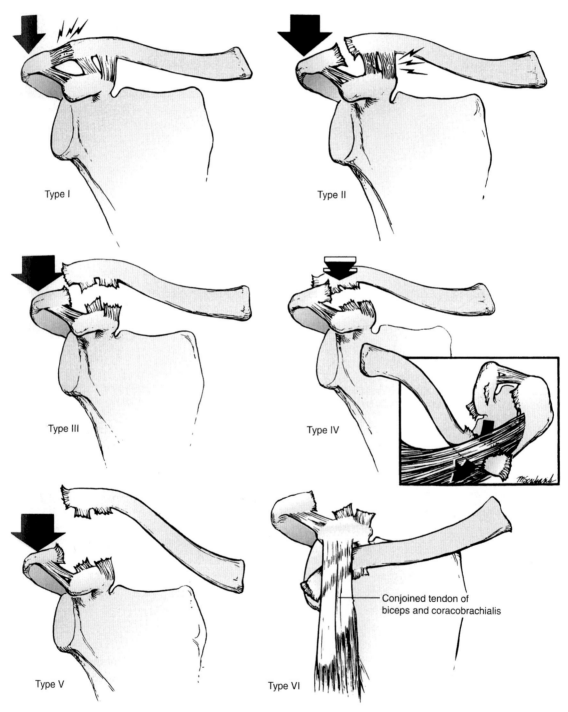

Fig 17-5. Rockwood classification of AC joint injury. (Reprinted from Rockwood and Green: *Fractures in Adults,* 6th ed.)

allowing the clavicle to displace superiorly. Type IV, V, and VI injuries exhibit significant avulsions of the deltoid and trapezius attachments, which allow more pronounced dislocation of the distal clavicle. In Type IV injuries, the distal clavicle is displaced posteriorly into the trapezius. In Type V injuries, the distal clavicle is displaced superiorly. In Type VI injuries, the distal clavicle is displaced inferiorly beneath the acromion or coracoid.

■ TREATMENT

Traditionally, Type I and Type II injuries are treated nonoperatively. Standard treatment consists of a sling and analgesics for comfort followed by a 2 to 6 week period of motion rehabilitation to control pain, regain motion, and restore strength. Most patients with Type I and Type II injuries will return to full activity within 12 weeks after injury. Controversy continues to exist in the management of Type III acromioclavicular joint injuries. Currently, most orthopedists favor nonoperative management as the initial treatment of choice (24–35). Initial management of Type III injury is identical to aforementioned treatment of Type I or Type II injuries. Patients in whom initial nonoperative treatments fail are considered for acromioclavicular joint reconstruction. Type IV, V, and VI injuries are almost always treated operatively. Most orthopedists combine distal clavicle excision with a coracoacromial ligament stabilization or reconstruction. A multitude techniques have been described. These include suture anchor and suture loop or constructs to enhance mechanical stability of coracoclavicular reconstruction (36); tendon graft reconstructions using gracilis, semitendinosus, and toe extensors (37); and coracoclavicular screw as an option for secondary stabilization of the acromioclavicular joint (38). All these techniques show early promise. Only preliminary results have been published and further clinical research is needed to define relative merit of each technique. Most recently, Phillips et al. (39) reported a meta-analysis of 24 studies evaluating the outcomes of acromioclavicular joint injury. They concluded that most patients treated conservatively will regain their strength and range of motion. In comparison to patients who underwent surgery, patients treated conservatively also experienced fewer complications. The data suggest that the only benefit of surgical intervention is decreased incidence of deformity.

■ COMPLICATIONS AND SPECIAL CONSIDERATIONS

Posttraumatic arthritis, distal clavicle osteolysis, and chronic acromioclavicular joint instability are the most common complications of nonoperative management. Complications of operative management include erosion of the coracoid or clavicle from a suture or wire and hardware failure (40,41).

Sternoclavicular Joint Injuries

Sternoclavicular joint injuries are relatively uncommon. They account for about 3% of all shoulder injuries (42). Because of a relatively low incidence, the evidence-based treatment guidelines are lacking. Treatment recommendations are based on the review of small, retrospective articles.

■ BASIC SCIENCE

Anatomy and Biomechanics

The sternoclavicular joint is a diarthrodial joint that connects the clavicle to the sternum. Because of existing mismatch between the medial clavicle and sternum, the stability of sternoclavicular joint relies mostly on surrounding ligamentous structures. These include the anterior and posterior bands of the costoclavicluar (rhomboid) ligament, the interclavicular ligament, and the capsular ligaments.

The sternoclavicular joint has limited range of motion; 0 to 30 degrees of flexion and extension and about 30 degrees of abduction (29,30). There are few biomechanical studies focusing on stability of sternoclavicular joints. Renfree and Wright (29) have suggested that the costoclavicular ligament provides stability during elevation and rotation of the clavicle. The interclavicular ligament provides suspensory function to both clavicles. The capsular ligaments seem to be the strongest of all ligamentous structures stabilizing sternoclavicular joints. Most recently, Debski et al. (30) reported results of cadaver ligament sectioning studies that provided valuable insight into the relative contribution of the anterior and posterior capsular ligaments to AP stability of the sternoclavicular ligaments. Spencer et al. (43) demonstrated that the transection of the anterior and posterior capsular ligaments result in a 25% and 41% increase in anterior translation, respectively.

Biology

As stated previously, the clavicle is the last bone to completely ossify with medial clavicular physis, closing at about 25 years of age. Sternoclavicular joint injuries in patients younger than 25 years of age are more likely physeal fractures rather than true sternoclavicular dislocations. As with other epiphyseal injuries, medial physeal separation has good remodeling capability and, therefore, closed treatment is recommended.

■ CLINICAL EVALUATION

History and Physical Findings

In the acute trauma setting, an understanding of the mechanism of the injury is essential for identification of the injury site as well as prediction of possible complications. The mechanism injury usually involves indirect trauma such as a

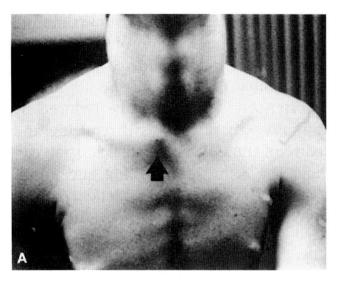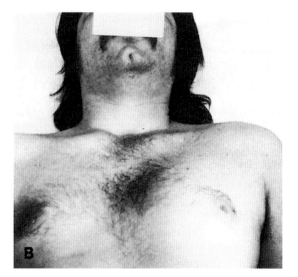

Fig 17-6. Sternocalvicular joint injury. (Reprinted from Rockwood and Green: *Fractures in Adults,* 4th ed.)

fall onto the shoulder with the arm adducted. The force applied to the shoulder is transmitted to the sternoclavicular joint via the clavicle, resulting in either an anterior or posterior dislocation. A direct mechanism has also been described with the blow to the medial clavicle resulting in posterior sternoclavicular dislocation. Patients with a sternoclavicular injury usually complain of anterior chest pain, which may radiate into the neck or chest. The diagnosis of sternoclavicular joint injury is relatively uncommon and therefore requires a high degree of clinical suspicion. After an acute shoulder trauma is encountered, sternoclavicular injury and associated complications need to be ruled out. The physical findings of acute sternoclavicular injury include tenderness to palpation over the anteromedial chest wall, soft-tissue swelling, and a characteristic prominence (anterior dislocation) **(Fig 17-6)** or depression (posterior dislocation) over the affected area. In the case of a posterior dislocation, it is imperative to rule out possible compression of anterior mediastinal structures such as esophagus, trachea, or major vessels. These are life-threatening complications that may present with dysphagia, dyspnea, and/or venous congestion of the upper extremity or face (15).

Radiographic Evaluation

The standard imaging modalities available to evaluation of sternoclavicular joint include plain radiographs, CT, and MRI. Plain x-rays have long been the standard for the initial evaluation of the trauma patient. In a case of sternoclavicular joint, plain films provide minimal information. In an attempt to obtain more accurate information about the relationship between the clavicle and sternum, a specialized "serendipity view" has been devised (Fig 17-3). These views are helpful in determining the displacement of the clavicle, but their reliability is still poor (44,45). More detailed evaluation of known or suspected abnormalities found on plain

films may be better carried out with the use of computed tomography (CT). Poor reliability of plain films, the wide availability CT, short scanning time, and excellent visualization of joint anatomy makes the CT a standard imaging modality for the evaluation of the sternoclavicular joint. Although plain films and CT are useful in the initial assessment of the sternoclavicular joint trauma, they are severely limited in their capability to detect ligamentous and other soft tissue injuries. Most recently, Siddiqui and Turner (45) reported the utility of ultrasonography in assessment of sternoclavicular joint injury. They reported that ultrasound correctly identified dislocated sternoclavicular joint in 89% of the cases. In addition, it can be used for an intraoperative monitoring of closed reduction.

Decision Making Algorithms and Classification

Classification of sternoclavicular joint injuries is based on direction of the medial clavicle displacement. In the anterior dislocations, the medial clavicle displaces anteriorly or anterosuperiorly to the sternum. In the posterior dislocations, medial clavicle displaces posteriorly or posterosuperiorly to the sternum. Because of close proximity of vital structures right behind the sternum, posterior dislocations are more concerning.

Treatment

Treatment of sternoclavicular joint injuries is dictated by the severity of the injury as well as the direction of the clavicle displacement. Mild to moderate anterior dislocations are usually treated with a period of 3 to 6 weeks immobilization in a sling or figure eight bandage followed by progressive return to activity. A complete dislocation is treated with a closed reduction followed by a period of 4 to 6 weeks immobilization with a Velpeau or figure eight bandage; however, even with successful closed reduction, there is a high rate of redislocation. Recurrent instability is not an indication for a surgical intervention unless it is associated with pain and disability. Although resection of medial clavicle can be considered to reduce the symptoms, it is imperative to preserve the costoclavicular ligaments during this procedure because its violation may lead to worsening of instability and symptoms (39). More recently, several dynamic stabilization techniques using subclavius tendon, fascia lata, sternocleidomastoid muscle, or modified Balser plate have been described (47,48). Initial results are promising, but long-term results remain to be seen.

Posterior dislocations are relatively rare. The treatment strategy is similar to those for anterior dislocations. After the posterior dislocation is identified, an attempt for closed reduction followed by immobilization may be considered. It is vital to identify posterior dislocations before attempting closed reduction. As much as 30% of posterior dislocations are associated with the injury to the mediastinal structures (i.e., trachea, esophagus or major vessels) (15). If the closed reduction is unsuccessful, or there is an associated injury to mediastinal structures, open reduction with aforementioned techniques of sternoclavicular joint stabilization is indicated. When performing these procedures, it is recommended to have a thoracic surgeon available.

■ REFERENCES

1. Flatow EL. Fractures of proximal humerus In: Bucholz RW, Heckman JD, Green DP, eds. Rockwood and Green's *Fractures in adults*, 5th ed. Philadelphia: Saunders; 2003:997–1041.
2. Visser CP, Coene LN, Brand R, et al. Nerve lesions in proximal humeral fractures. *J Shoulder Elbow Surg.* 2001;10:421–427.
3. Edelson G, Kelly I, Vigder F, et al. A three-dimensional classification of proximal humerus fractures. *J Bone Joint Surg.* 2004; 86B,413–425.
4. Brien H, Noftall F, MacMaster S, et al. Neer's classification system: a critical appraisal. *J Trauma.* 1995;38:257–260.
5. Brorson S, Bagger J, Sylvest A, et al. Improved interobserver variation after training of doctors in the Neer system. *J Bone Joint Surg Br.* 2002;84B:950–954.
6. Lyons RP, Lazarus MD. Shoulder and arm trauma: bone. In: Vaccaro AR, ed. *Orthopedic knowledge update 8.* Rosemont, IL: AAOS; 2005:267–281.
7. Rowles DJ, McGrory JE. Percutaneous pinning of the proxial part of the humerus: an anatomic study. *J Bone Joint Surg.* 2001;83A:1695–1699.
8. Gardner MJ, Griffith MH, Dines JS, et al. The extended anterolateral acromial approach allows minimally invasive access to the proximal humerus. *Clin Orthop Relat Res.* 2005;434:123–129.
9. Stoffel K, Dieter U, Stachowiak G, et al. Biomechanical testing of the LCP: how can stability in locked internal fixators be controlled? *Injury.* 2003;34(suppl 2):B11–B19.
10. Mighell MA, Kolm GP, Collinge CA, et al. Outcomes of hemiarthroplasty for fractures of the proximal humerus. *J Shoulder Elbow Surg.* 2003;12:569–577.
11. Bigliani L.U. Fractures of the proximal humerus. In: Rockwood CA, Matsen F, eds. *The shoulder.* Philadelphia: WB Saunders; 1990:278–334.
12. Placzek JD, Roubal PJ, Kulig K, et al. Theory and technique of translational manipulation for adhesive capsulitis. *Am J Orthop.* 2004;33(4):173–179.
13. Lazarus MD. Fractures of the clavicle. In: Bucholz RW, Heckman JD, Rockwood CA, Green DP, eds. Rockwood and Green's *fractures in adults.* 5th ed. Philadelphia: Saunders; 2003: 1041–1074.
14. Schmidt-Rohlfing B, Niedhart C, Schwer EH, et al. Clavicular pseudarthrosis in childhood: differential diagnosis, clinical aspects, therapy and results. *Z Orthop Ihre Grenzgeb.* 2001;139(5):447–451.
15. Torretti J, Lynch SA. Sternoclavicular joint injuries. *Curr Opin Orthop.* 2004;15:242–247.
16. Ritchie PK, McCarthy EC. Distal clavicle fractures: a current review. *Curr Opin Orthop.* 2004;15:257–260.
17. Allman FL Jr. Fractures and ligamentous injuries of the clavicle and its articulation. *J Bone Joint Surg.* 1967;49A:774–784.
18. Neer CS. Fractures of the distal third of the clavicle. *Clin Orthop.* 1968;58:43–50.
19. Rockwood CA. Fractures of the outer clavicle in children and adults. *J Bone Joint Surg.* 1982;64B:642.
20. Craig EV. Fractures of the clavicle. In: Rockwood CA Jr, Matsen F, eds. *The shoulder.* Philadelphia: Saunders; 1990:367–412.
21. Anderson K, Nuber GW, Bowen MK. Outcome of distal clavicle fractures treated nonoperatively. *J Shoulder Elbow Surg.* 1999;8:661.
22. Anderson K. Evaluation and treatment of distal clavicle fractures. *Clin Sports Med.* 2003;22:319–326.
23. Mall JW, Jacobi CA, Philipp AW, et al. Surgical treatment of fractures of the distal clavicle with polydioxanone suture tension band wiring: an alternative osteosynthesis. *J Orthop Sci.* 2002; 7:535–537.
24. Chen CH, Chen WJ, Shih CH. Surgical treatment for distal clavicle fracture with coracoclavicular ligament disruption. *J Trauma.* 2002;52:72–78.
25. Fuchs M, Losch A, Sturmer KM. Surgical treatment of fractures of the clavicle-indication, surgical technique, and results. *Zentralbl Chir.* 2002;127:479–484.
26. Wilfinger C, Hollwarth M. Lateral clavicular fractures in children and adolescents. *Unfallchirurg.* 2002;105:602–605.
27. Flinkkila T, Ristiniemi J, Hyvonen P, et al. Surgical treatment of unstable fractures of the distal clavicle: a comparative study of Kirschner wire and clavicular hook plate fixation. *Acta Orthop Scand.* 2002;73:50–53.
28. Levy O. Simple, minimally invasive surgical technique for treatment of type II fractures of the distal clavicle. *J Shoulder Elbow Surg.* 2003;12:24–28.
29. Renfree KJ, Wright TW. Anatomy and biomechanics of the acromioclavicular and sternoclavicular joints. *Clin Sports Med.* 2003;22:219–237.
30. Debski RE, Parsons IM III, Fenwick J, et al. Ligament mechanics during three degree-of-freedom motion at the acromioclavicular joint. *Ann Biomed Eng.* 2000;28:612–618.
31. Debski RE, Parsons IMT, Woo SL, et al. Effect of capsular injury on acromioclavicular joint mechanics. *J Bone Joint Surg Am.* 2001; 83A:1344–1351.
32. Bradley JP, Elkousy H. Decision making: operative versus nonoperative treatment of acromioclavicular joint injuries. *Clin Sports Med.* 2003;22:277–290.
33. Cox JS. Current method of treatment of acromioclavicular joint dislocations. *Orthopedics.* 1992;15:1041–1044.
34. McFarland EG, Blivin SJ, Doehring CB, et al. Treatment of grade III acromioclavicular separations in professional throwing athletes: results of a survey. *Am J Orthop.* 1997;26:771–774.
35. Kwon YW, Iannotti JP. Operative treatment of acromioclavicular joint injuries and results. *Clin Sports Med.* 2003;22:291–300.
36. Breslow MJ, Jazrawi LM, Bernstein AD, et al. Treatment of acromioclavicular joint separation: suture or suture anchors? *J Shoulder Elbow Surg.* 2002;11:225–229.
37. Lee SJ, Nicholas SJ, Akizuki KH, et al. Reconstruction of the coracoclavicular ligaments with tendon grafts: a comparative biomechanical study. *Am J Sports Med.* 2003;31:648–655.

38. Talbert TW, Green JR III, Mukherjee DP, et al. Bioabsorbable screw fixation in coracoclavicular ligament reconstruction. *J Long Term Eff Med Implants.* 2003;13:319–323.

39. Phillips AM, Smart C, Groom AF. Acromioclavicular dislocation: conservative or surgical therapy. *Clin Orthop.* 1998;353: 10–17.

40. Yadav V, Marya KM. Unusual migration of a wire from shoulder to neck. *Indian J Med Sci.* 2003;57:111–112.

41. Boldin C, Fankhauser F, Ratschek M, et al. Foreign-body reaction after reconstruction of complete acromioclavicular dislocation using PDS augmentation. *J Shoulder Elbow Surg.* 2004;13: 99–100.

42. Rockwood CA Jr, Wirth M. Injuries to the sternoclavicular joint. In: Bucholz RW, Heckman JD, Rockwood CA, Green DP, eds. Rockwood and Green's *Fractures in adults.* 5th ed. Philadelphia: Saunders; 2003:1245–1292.

43. Spencer EE, Kuhn JE, Huston LJ, et al. Ligamentous restraints to anterior and posterior translation of the sternoclavicular joint. *J Shoulder Elbow Surg.* 2002;11:43–47.

44. Ernberg LA, Hollis PG. Radiographic evaluation of the acromioclavicular and sternoclavicular joints. *Clin Sports Med.* 2003;22: 255–275.

45. Siddiqui AA, Turner SM. Posterior sternoclavicular joint dislocation: the value of intra-operative ultrasound. *Injury.* 2003;34:448–453.

46. Bisson LJ, Dauphin N, Marzo JM. A safe zone for resection of the medial end of the clavicle. *J Shoulder Elbow Surg.* 2003;12:592–594.

47. Franck WM, Jannasch O, Siassi M. Balser plate stabilization: an alternate therapy, for traumatic sternoclavicular instability. *J Shoulder Elbow Surg.* 2003;12:276–281.

48. Spencer EE, Kuhn JE. Biomechanical analysis of reconstructions for sternoclavicular joint instability. *J Bone Joint Surg Am.* 2004; 86:98–105.

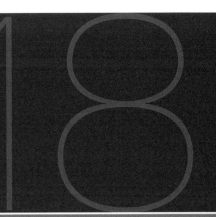

ADHESIVE CAPSULITIS

SCOTT P. FISCHER, MD, SERGE KASKA, MD

■ KEY POINTS

- True shoulder stiffness is the loss of passive range of motion in the shoulder.
- Many patients who complain of stiffness do not have true shoulder stiffness. Rather, they have pain and inflammation, and because movement results in discomfort, they guard against painful movement and appear to have lost range of motion.
- Stiffness arising out of adhesive capsulitis is a primary and idiopathic condition due to intrinsic changes within the glenohumeral joint capsule. These changes result in thickening and contracture of the capsule.
- The working definition of adhesive capsulitis is "a condition of uncertain etiology characterized by significant reduction of both active and passive shoulder motion that occurs in absence of a known intrinsic shoulder disorder."
- Adhesive capsulitis is commonly observed in patients during their fifth and sixth decades, with an incidence of 2% to 5% in this age group, and a greater frequency in women. There is an increased occurrence in patients having suffered closed head injuries, Parkinson disease, autonomic disorders of the upper extremity, and diabetes mellitus.
- Adhesive capsulitis typically progresses through three clinical phases—the initial inflammatory phase, the proliferative or "freezing" phase, and the "thawing" phase, characterized by resolution of painful contracture.
- Patients with adhesive capsulitis have a global reduction in range of motion with a marked decrease in glenohumeral translation. Examination of the opposite shoulder (if normal) is performed to identify the patient's expected range of motion.

- Evaluation is not complete without an appropriate series of plain radiographs. True glenohumeral anterior-posterior views, along with axillary, scapular outlet and acromioclavicular views, are necessary to exclude other shoulder girdle conditions.
- Nonoperative treatment commonly begins with measures to reduce pain and inflammation. The mainstay of treatment is administration of range of motion stretching exercises. Medication is also used.
- Because adhesive capsulitis is due only to a tight and thickened glenohumeral capsule, arthroscopic surgery seems ideal for treatment. The capsule is best viewed, and more directly surgically addressed, by an intra-articular approach.

It is common for patients to present to orthopaedic surgeons with complaints of shoulder stiffness. Many of these patients, although they initially appear to have limited range of motion, do not have true shoulder stiffness. Instead, they have pain and inflammation in the shoulder girdle, and because shoulder movement results in discomfort, they guard against the painful movement, only appearing to have lost range of motion. In other patients, stiffness may be confused with a decreased ability to produce active range of motion. Although these individuals are limited in the active mobility of their shoulder due to weakness, they have no joint contracture and have normal passive range of motion.

A smaller group of patients present with true shoulder stiffness—the loss of passive range of motion in the shoulder. True shoulder stiffness can be a primary condition arising independent of any other abnormality or illness (so called idiopathic stiffness), it can be a primary condition arising in conjunction with another medical condition (such as diabetes mellitus), or it can develop secondary to another condition (such as prior surgery, arthritis, or trauma). The stiffness arising out of adhesive capsulitis is a primary and idiopathic condition due to intrinsic changes within the glenohumeral joint capsule. These changes result in thickening and contracture of the capsule, which is often painful. This condition may be persistent and difficult to endure. Treatment of these patients is often challenging and their recovery may be limited as described by Simmonds (1) who wrote in 1949, "Complete recovery . . . is not my experience." DePalma (2) agreed when he wrote, "It is erroneous to believe that in all instances restoration of function is attained." Patients who develop shoulder stiffness associated with other conditions such as diabetes may appear to have adhesive capsulitis. Both of these conditions arise out of a primary capsular contracture, so they display great similarity in their presentation and development. Treatment for these patients, although similar, can be more difficult due to the additional dimension of medical illness present. In some cases, stiffness associated with another medical condition is more resistant to treatment than adhesive capsulitis. Treating patients with shoulder stiffness arising secondary to other abnormalities (such as prior surgery, arthritis, or trauma) is often challenging as well. To regain range of motion in these patients, the orthopaedist often must address not only any capsular contracture present, but he or she must also treat the primary abnormalities of intra-articular deformity or extra-articular scarring to improve the patient's function. This chapter will focus its attention mostly upon the characteristics and treatment of adhesive capsulitis.

■ HISTORICAL DESCRIPTION AND DEFINITION OF ADHESIVE CAPSULITIS

According to Cuomo (3), a medical description of true shoulder stiffness was first recorded in 1896 when Duplay introduced the term scapulohumeral periarthritis to describe this condition. He believed the initiating lesion was obliteration of the subdeltoid bursa. During subsequent years, the entity of scapulohumeral periarthritis evolved to include a myriad of pathologic shoulder conditions associated with shoulder pain and stiffness. In 1934, Codman (4) focused his attention more narrowly on true shoulder stiffness and described a clinical disorder that he termed "frozen shoulder." He captured the feelings of many physicians who diagnose and treat this condition when he described it as "a condition difficult to define, difficult to treat, and difficult to explain from the point of view of pathology." In 1945, J.S. Neviaser (5) first used the term "adhesive capsulitis," which he felt better described the pathology causing this condition. He reported the condition of the shoulder capsule as tense, markedly adherent to the humeral head and associated with decreased joint volume and

synovial fluid. The current working definition of adhesive capsulitis was formulated by a workshop committee at the 1992 symposium, "The Shoulder: A Balance of Mobility and Stability," and was subsequently published by the American Academy of Orthopaedic Surgeons in 1993 (6). They defined adhesive capsulitis as "a condition of uncertain etiology characterized by significant restriction of both active and passive shoulder motion that occurs in the absence of a known intrinsic shoulder disorder."

Anatomy and Biomechanics of the Glenohumeral Capsule

The shoulder is an inherently loose articulation permitting a wide range of motion. The glenohumeral capsule remains lax throughout mid-range motion where stability is conferred by the dynamic action of the rotator cuff and the conforming articulation of the humeral head and the glenolabral surface. The capsuloligamentous structures about the glenohumeral joint act as passive restraints when capsular tension develops at the extremes of motion and contributes to glenohumeral stability. Each portion of the joint capsule performs its primary "checkrein" responsibility at different glenohumeral positions. The rotator interval develops tension in external rotation with the arm adducted. The middle glenohumeral ligament restricts motion with the arm in external rotation in the midrange of abduction, while the anterior band of the inferior glenohumeral ligament stabilizes the glenohumeral joint in full abduction and external rotation. Tension is developed in the posterior-superior capsule with the arm adducted and internally rotated. This tension shifts posterior-inferior with abduction and internal rotation. Contracture of any given portion of the glenohumeral capsule will cause reduction in glenohumeral motion as though the end range of motion were reached prematurely. In addition, some capsular contractures cause an obligate and abnormal translation of the humeral head during motion (7). The abnormal joint mechanics associated with posterior capsular contracture have been observed to result in superior migration, which can be associated with subacromial impingent or superior labral tearing (8,9). Chronic anterior asymmetric tightness may cause posterior translation with increased posterior glenohumeral joint reaction forces resulting in posterior glenoid wear (10). Normal shoulder range of motion requires a smooth glenohumeral articulation with a surrounding capsule of normal volume and compliance, unrestricted gliding of the rotator cuff tendons under the coraco-acromial arch and under the deep surface of the deltoid muscle, and normal translation of the scapula over the chest wall. Adhesions or contracture in any of these locations may result in shoulder stiffness.

Pathophysiology of Adhesive Capsulitis

At this time there is no accepted complete understanding of the pathophysiological basis for the development of adhesive capsulitis. Harryman and Lazarus (11) credit Reidel's report in the early German literature as the first to propose that a pathologic process originating in the glenohumeral capsule was responsible for shoulder stiffness. Neviaser (5) subsequently described the histologic findings of perivascular infiltration, capsular fibrosis, and capsular thickening associated with the clinical development of adhesive capsulitis. These findings were later confirmed by Lundberg (12), who noted capsular changes including an increase in the density of collagen and a glycosaminoglycan pattern similar to that found in repair tissue. Omari and Bunker (13) studied biopsies of rotator interval tissue in patients with frozen shoulder and described a dense matrix of Type 3 collagen populated with fibroblasts and myoblasts. Some authors have hypothesized that autoimmune processes might be involved in the development of adhesive capsulitis. Studies showing reduced levels of IgA as well as an increased incidence of the immunohistocompatability antigen HLA-B27 initially suggested this relationship; however, subsequent reports have failed to establish an autoimmune etiology or identify an immunologic test to diagnose this condition. The possibility of a relationship between Dupuytrens contracture and adhesive capsulitis has intrigued investigators for many years. Many of the histologic characteristics of Dupuytrens disease have been observed in capsuloligamentous biopsies obtained from patients with adhesive capsulitis. Investigators have suggested these two conditions may share a common biochemical pathway that leads to contracture (14,15). More recently, investigations into the activity of polypeptide growth factors and matrix metalloproteinases have suggested a possible contribution to the development of adhesive capsulitis through their effects upon the activation and migration of fibroblasts and their alteration of normal collagen matrix remodeling (16).

Demographic Factors Associated with Adhesive Capsulitis

Adhesive capsulitis is commonly observed in patients during their fifth and sixth decades of life with an incidence of 2% to 5% in this age group, and a greater frequency in women than men. There is an increased occurrence in patients having suffered closed head injuries (as high as 25%), Parkinson disease (13%), autonomic disorders of the upper extremity (such as post-stroke shoulder-hand syndrome with an incidence of approximately 25%), and diabetes mellitus (with an incidence varying from 10% to 35%) (11,17–20). Prior authors have suggested an association between adhesive capsulitis and other medical disorders including thyroid disease, cardio-pulmonary disease, cervical spine degenerative disease, neoplasia in general (and more specifically in the lung), and the presence of personality disorders such as depression and anxiety disorder; however, no causal relationship has been clearly established for these entities.

Clinical History and Classification

Adhesive capsulitis is a disease that typically progresses through three clinical phases. Patients with this condition will have varying clinical complaints depending upon the phase they are experiencing at the time of interview. The initial inflammatory "painful" phase begins with a spontaneous onset of aching discomfort at rest and the development of pain with use. Pain at night that interferes with sleep commonly occurs and early limitation of motion begins to develop. The arm may be held in an adducted and internally rotated position to reduce tension in the inflamed glenohumeral capsule. Occasionally the patient attributes the onset of their problem to a trivial trauma, but more often no inciting injury can be recalled. This phase may last as long as 9 months according to Reeves (21).

The proliferative or "freezing" phase occurs next and is characterized by progressive and global loss of motion. Range of motion often becomes quite restricted during this portion of the disease process, and it is common for shoulder function to be dramatically reduced by the contracture present. Night pain usually continues, especially when lying on the involved side. Pain with the arm at rest may begin to decrease, although pain with use persists when the patient reaches the end of his or her available motion and the capsule is placed under increased tension. This phase is often described as lasting between 3 to 12 months; however, we have observed it to last significantly longer in numerous patients.

The third and final "thawing" phase is characterized by resolution of the painful contracture. The process is often slow and may be punctuated by periods where recovery seems to plateau before resuming its course of progress. Improvement may extend over a period of time ranging from 3 months to 3 years, but it can be prolonged up to 6 or 7 years. Even after the discomfort resolves and acceptable function returns, limitation in final range of motion is commonly present.

Physical Findings

The physical examination of patients with adhesive capsulitis reveals a global reduction in range of motion with a marked decrease in glenohumeral translation also present. Examination of the opposite shoulder (if normal) is performed to identify the patient's expected normal range of motion for comparison. Evaluation for limitation of pure glenohumeral motion (best measured in the supine position with the scapula immobilized) is often more demonstrative of the extent of contracture present than the measurement of total shoulder girdle range of motion (glenohumeral plus scapulothoracic motion). The latter, however, is more closely linked to the patient's clinical perception of their ability to function, so frequently both types of shoulder motion are measured and followed. Patients with adhesive capsulitis will demonstrate at least a 20% reduction in range of motion, and findings of 50% or greater loss of motion are not uncommon.

Some degree of weakness is often noted when examining for shoulder girdle strength in patients with adhesive capsulitis. The magnitude of this finding may be misleading however if the patient is experiencing an inflammatory component to their disease. When this is present, strength testing can produce substantial pain and result in a limited resistive effort. To obtain the most representative assessment of the patient's true shoulder strength, resistive strength testing should be performed within the patient's comfortable arc of motion, often testing elevation strength at approximately 30 to 45 degrees of elevation, and rotational strength with the arm at the side.

Pain is often reported to be present diffusely throughout the shoulder girdle; however tenderness with palpation is often greatest over the anterior subacromial bursa, the proximal biceps tendon, the rotator interval area and the anterior capsule. The posterior capsule, the lateral subdeltoid recess, and rotator cuff area often have less tenderness with the acromioclavicular joint often spared. Depending upon the phase of the disease process tenderness can be quite severe, so palpation is often best performed at the end of the exam to avoid patient guarding while examining for range of motion and strength.

Imaging Studies

The evaluation of a patient with adhesive capsulitis is not complete without an appropriate series of plain radiographs. True glenohumeral anterior-posterior views, along with axillary, scapular outlet and acromioclavicular views are considered necessary to exclude other shoulder girdle conditions which result in pain and stiffness. These films may often reveal osteopenia, but should not show any other definitive pathology. Additional radiographs of the neck, chest, or arm should be obtained if clinically indicated to exclude such problems as cervical radiculopathy, lung cancer, or humeral bone tumor.

Other types of advanced imaging have been used in patients with adhesive capsulitis. Magnetic resonance imaging (MRI) may demonstrate thickening of the inferior capsule, and when performed with intravenous gadolinium may reveal enhancement in the capsule or synovium (22). MRI arthrography and standard arthrography can show decreased intra-articular volume and will commonly reveal a reduction in the size of the inferior capsular recess. Additional findings can include variable distention of the biceps sheath or the subscapularis recess. Dynamic ultrasound has been shown to display a reduction in supraspinatus excursion with attempted shoulder movement (23). Radionucleide scanning has demonstrated increased uptake of technetium on "posterior views" in frozen shoulder (24), versus increased anterior uptake in subacromial conditions and uptake involving the distal upper extremity in patients with reflex sympathetic dystrophy. None of these advanced tests, however, have been shown to be diagnostic of adhesive capsulitis and often are unnecessary unless needed to exclude other diagnoses.

Approach to Treatment

A decision regarding whether and when to provide treatment for a medical condition is most often based on a complete understanding of the natural history of that disease. Unfortunately, the natural history of adhesive capsulitis is poorly understood. Although reports on this disease and its treatment have been numerous, clinical observations have varied widely with regards to the degree of disability and the duration of symptoms encountered. The response to treatment has also varied widely due to the employment of many different treatment regimens with confounding variables and conflicting results. Historically, idiopathic adhesive capsulitis has been referred to as a self-limited condition that usually resolves in 1 to 3 years regardless of treatment (19,21,25,26). Numerous studies, however, have described symptoms and disability that persist in 20% to 50% of patients for as long as 7 to 10 years (21,27). For this reason, the treatment approach of benign neglect often accepted in the past seems inappropriate, and intervention to reduce its impact upon the lives of its victims is clearly appropriate.

Nonsurgical Treatment

Nonoperative treatment commonly begins with measures to reduce shoulder pain and inflammation including topical treatments of heat, ice, transcutaneous electric stimulation, transcutaneous salves and balms, acupuncture, massage and systemic medications [nonsteriodal anti-inflammatory drug (NSAID) class medicines and oral corticosteroids]. The relative contribution to recovery that any of these treatment measures provide remains unclear and their use at this time is best individualized based upon the response each individual patient manifests during their use. Many other treatment regimens including trigger point injections, suprascapular nerve block, ultrasound, and the injection of hyaluronic acid have been studied and found to have no demonstrable long term benefit. Intra-articular injections of corticosteroid medications are often used to relieve the symptoms of painful inflammation and some believe they may alter the inflammatory process within the glenohumeral capsule. Hannafin and Chiaia (28) have observed that the use of intra-articular steroids coupled with range of motion therapy can result in a "rapid and striking improvement" if administered early in Stage 1 adhesive capsulitis and can even provide "significant improvement" during Stage 2 disease. Other investigators have found no long term improvement in outcome when these injections are used (29). The mainstay of nonoperative treatment for adhesive capsulitis is the administration of range of motion stretching therapy. This may be accomplished by the patient on their own at home; it can be administered by a physical therapist, or most commonly as a combination of both. Review of numerous articles in the orthopaedic and physical therapy literature reveal the reported success rate for formal physical therapy to average between 50% to 70% of patients. Miller et al. (19) have reported their results with a patient administered home therapy program directly supervised by the treating orthopaedist, which they call "Orthotherapy." At an average of 14 months treatment, they observed that 100% of patients were improved, having painless range of motion within 20% of normal or having no restriction during activities of daily living. Other researchers, however, have had less success with nonoperative treatment regimens. Griggs et al. (30) reported that with an average 22 months of follow-up, 50% of their patients had abnormal function, 37% continued to have pain, and 10% were not satisfied. Shaffer et al. (27) reported results after an average follow-up of 7 years and found 60% of patients had a persisting deficit in range of motion measuring between 10% to 30% of normal, 50% of their patients had continuing pain or a sense of stiffness and 11% felt they experienced continuing restriction in function.

■ OPERATIVE TREATMENT

Manipulation Under Anesthesia

Manipulation under anesthesia (MUA) has been used to treat adhesive capsulitis for many years. This treatment has commonly been described to prospective patients as "stretching the tight capsule" or "breaking up adhesions" within the shoulder joint. Arthroscopic visualization of the glenohumeral joint after this procedure, however, reveals that a MUA does not stretch a tight capsule; instead, it uniformly results in a traumatic rupture of the inferior glenohumeral capsule which extends superiorly into both the anterior and posterior capsule to varying degrees, depending on the severity of the contracture present **(Fig 18-1)**. Although incidental findings of labral tearing and rotator cuff tearing have been observed, they are not routinely encountered after this procedure. Post manipulation dislocation, fractures of the humerus or glenoid **(Fig 18-2)**, and neurologic injury to the brachial plexus have also been described. Although these types of complications are serious, and they may result in a more complicated course of

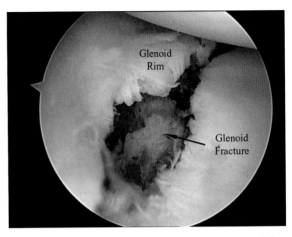

Fig 18-2. An inadvertent glenoid rim fracture resulted from a manipulation under anesthesia in this patient (photo courtesy of Benjamin D. Rubin, MD).

treatment, their occurrence is uncommon and is reported by Harryman and Lazarus (11) to be less than 1%.

The results of manipulation under anesthesia for patients with adhesive capsulitis have been reported upon by many authors with an average success rate of approximately 70% at 3 to 6 months of follow-up (11,31,32), but with variation in satisfactory outcomes ranging from as little as 30% (33) to as high as 97% (34,35). An average recurrence rate of stiffness seems to be approximately 8% (31,35). The treatment of patients with adhesive capsulitis and diabetes mellitus traditionally has seemed to be more difficult to most clinicians than the treatment of patients who have only adhesive capsulitis. This impression was confirmed by Janda and Hawkins (18) who reported in 1993 that MUA in a group of six of these patients resulted in 100% recurrence of stiffness at 8 months. Goldberg et al. (32) also found poorer outcomes with MUA in diabetic patients. Although they observed a 70% response rate to MUA in patients without diabetes, their results decreased to what they termed a "partial response" in approximately 25% of patients with shoulder stiffness who also had endured insulin-dependant diabetes mellitus for more than 10 years. Other authors, however, have offered more encouraging observations on their treatment of diabetic patients using MUA. Massoud et al. (36) found 80% acceptable results in those diabetic patients whose contracture yielded to a "gentle manipulation." (In their study protocol, those patients with more severe contractures, which would require a "forceful" MUA, received a different treatment.) Andersen et al. (31), who treated adhesive capsulitis with manipulation under anesthesia and diagnostic arthroscopic evaluation, found no difference in results for diabetic versus nondiabetic patients. Seventy-five percent of their patients returned to work after 9 weeks, and 79% had slight or no pain at both 6 and 12 months follow up. A report by Pollock et al. (37) reviewed their experience with a treatment regimen consisting of a gentle manipulation under anesthesia followed by arthroscopic

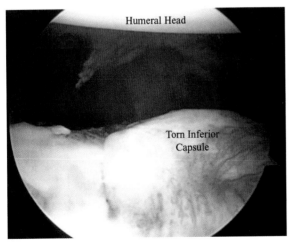

Fig 18-1. Arthroscopic visualization after manipulation under anesthesia confirms that the inferior glenohumeral capsule is completely torn by this procedure.

glenohumeral and subacromial debridement. These investigators "aggressively debrided" rotator interval synovitis, coracohumeral ligament and anterosuperior capsular tissues torn by the MUA, and bursal adhesions when present. They also occasionally used electrocautery to detach the coracohumeral ligament in those patients in whom full external rotation was not accomplished by the MUA, and in some cases performed acromioplasty and acromioclavicular joint debridement. They had excellent results in patients with idiopathic adhesive capsulitis, for whom they reported 100% success, but this approach provided only 64% success in their diabetic patients. In light of these studies, there seems to be grounds for greater optimism than Janda's initial paper suggested; however, most practitioners continue to find the management of adhesive capsulitis in patients with diabetes mellitus to be more challenging than in those without diabetes, and many remain cautious to utilize MUA to treat this group of patients.

Arthroscopic Capsular Release

Because adhesive capsulitis of the shoulder, by definition, is due only to a tight and thickened glenohumeral capsule, arthroscopic surgery seems ideal for the treatment of this problem. The capsule is best viewed, and more directly surgically addressed, by an intra-articular approach rather than an extra-articular, open surgical approach. Arthroscopy allows circumferential capsular release as needed, and post operative pain is often much less due to the absence of transmuscular surgical dissection. An important additional benefit to arthroscopic capsular release is that it can be performed without having to detach and then repair the subscapularis tendon that may be necessary with an open release. This becomes important during postoperative rehabilitation, as there is no need to limit the patient's abduction or rotation to protect against rupture of this tendon during early postsurgical range of motion.

The risks associated with arthroscopic glenohumeral capsular release include iatrogenic damage to the joint surfaces, excessive soft tissue swelling and axillary nerve injury. The safe performance of this procedure requires sufficient prior experience with shoulder arthroscopy to prevent inadvertent intra-articular injury to the joint surfaces when inserting the arthroscopic cannulae, and an appropriate amount of skill and caution to avoid injury to the labrum and the rotator cuff tendons during debridement. Lack of arthroscopic experience may also result in slower surgical progress, which invites excessive fluid extravasation and soft tissue swelling which can interfere with successful completion of the procedure. These risks, however, diminish as surgeons become more practiced with arthroscopic surgical techniques in general. The axillary nerve, due to its close proximity to the extra-articular surface of the inferior glenohumeral capsule, is at risk for injury during this and any surgical procedure involving the inferior capsule region of the shoulder joint. With open surgical approaches, the nerve can be identified,

retracted and protected prior to division of the capsule. During an arthroscopic approach, the axillary nerve most often cannot be seen through the capsule. To avoid inadvertent neural injury, a thorough understanding of its location is mandatory. In a cadaveric study, Zanotti and Kuhn (38) performed an arthroscopic circumferential capsular release using an electrocautery tip approximately 1 cm lateral to the glenoid rim while the arm was in a position of 45 degrees abduction and 20 degrees flexion. Subsequent dissection showed that in all specimens the axillary nerve lay anterior to the inferior edge of the subscapularis muscle at the level of the glenoid rim and it continued laterally and inferiorly under the subscapularis close to the inferior capsule approximately 17 mm lateral to the inferior glenoid rim. These findings indicated that a capsular incision a few millimeters lateral to the glenoid labrum should not place the nerve at risk for injury. The clinical experience of many surgeons performing arthroscopic capsular release has confirmed the safety of this approach. Some variation in the normal course of the nerve might occur, so one must always exercise caution not to penetrate or "plunge" beyond the external capsular border when incising the inferior capsule. Because patients with prior open surgery in the inferior capsular area will have postoperative scarring which may distort and displace this nerve into an abnormal location, capsular release surgery in these patients may be safer if performed with open techniques.

Clinical outcomes after arthroscopic capsular release have been gratifying, with published reports documenting 69% to 94% patient satisfaction (32,39–48). Harryman et al. (42) used this technique on 30 of their most refractory patients with glenohumeral stiffness. The average pre-operative shoulder range of motion was 41% of the uninvolved shoulder. Average postoperative range of motion at one day post surgery was 78% of normal and 93% of normal at final follow up. Pre-operatively only 6% of their patients could sleep on the involved side while postoperatively 73% could do so. In 10% of patients, they observed postoperative recurrence of refractory stiffness. Watson et al. (48) reported that their group of 73 patients experienced diminished pain at an average of 2.24 weeks with the return of motion to within 10% of the uninvolved shoulder after an average of 5.5 weeks postoperative. They noted that many patients, mostly in those operated upon during the proliferative phase of their disease and experiencing significant night pain, developed recurrence of pain at an average 4.5 weeks post-surgery, but these symptoms were adequately treated with massage or corticosteroid injection. With 12 months of postoperative follow up, they reported a recurrence rate of 11%. Ogilvie-Harris et al. (46) observed favorable results using arthroscopic capsular release to treat patients with diabetic adhesive capsulitis. They reported that 76% of these patients had no pain and full range of motion while another 12% had only mild persisting loss of function after arthroscopic release. In the patient group treated by Harryman et al. (42), approximately 47% of their patients were diabetic and they observed no difference in any outcomes when these patients were compared to the nondiabetic patients. Goldberg et al. (32) also noted no difference in outcome after arthroscopic capsular release in diabetic patients.

Open Capsular Release

Open surgical release of the glenohumeral capsule was more commonly utilized to treat patients with severe and refractory adhesive capsulitis prior to the advancement of arthroscopic techniques to treat this difficult patient population. Although the peri-operative morbidity of this open approach to treatment is now accepted to be somewhat greater than its arthroscopic counterpart, use of this technique has resulted in acceptable rates of clinical success. Open release of the contracted rotator interval tissues associated with adhesive capsulitis facilitated reduction of pain and return of motion in all patients treated by Ozaki et al. (49) and provided high rates of success for Nobuhara et al. (50). Kieras and Matsen (51) reported reduction or elimination of pain and uniform return to work after open capsular release in patients with chronic, refractory frozen shoulder. Restoration of range of motion was significantly improved, although incomplete in many cases. Omari and Bunker (13) reported good or excellent results in 80% of their most severely affected patients who were treated with open release after having failed treatment with prior MUA. Because of the good results obtained with open capsular release, but the lower degree of peri-operative morbidity and very good outcomes associated with arthroscopic capsular release, open release currently seems best reserved for patients suffering from shoulder stiffness with extracapsular abnormalities requiring treatment in addition to their contracted glenohumeral capsule. Open release also continues to have potential application to those patients who intra-operatively do not obtain adequate return of range of motion after arthroscopic release; however, in practical application, we have yet to experience this occurrence in any patients being treated for adhesive capsulitis.

Complications

The complications associated with arthroscopic capsular release surgery have included postoperative instability of the glenohumeral joint, injury to the axillary nerve, and recurrence of shoulder stiffness. Although release of the glenohumeral capsule and ligaments to treat shoulder stiffness raises the theoretical concern that postoperative instability may result, experimental cadaveric studies by Moskal et al. (52) have shown no increase in glenohumeral instability after this procedure. Postoperative instability has not been observed clinically by the authors, and very few anecdotal reports of glenohumeral instability immediately after arthroscopic release have been noted in the course of personal conversations with fellow shoulder surgeons. When this phenomenon has occurred, it has corrected shortly after surgery with the return of rotator cuff tension, and was not

present after healing at clinical follow-up. Although 3% of Pearsall et al.'s (26,47) patients reported the presence of a subjective sense of instability, no clinical instability after capsular release was observed in their series. The risk of possible injury to the axillary nerve during this procedure must be taken into account during pre-operative consultation and preparation, and careful attention to surgical technique must be observed to ensure that the capsular incision made during this procedure remains close to the labral margin and does not extend more than 5 to 10 mm lateral to the glenoid rim. It is important to note, however, that the occurrence of neural injury during this procedure has been rare, and the clinical reports reviewed have only described patients with transient nerve dysfunction, which recovered over time. Finally, the recurrence of stiffness after arthroscopic capsular release has not been common in patients with adhesive capsulitis. For some patients with more severe or more chronic pre-operative stiffness, postoperative recovery of motion may be prolonged and more difficult to maintain, but recurrence has been reported to occur in only 10% to 11% of patients (42,48).

Author's Preferred Decision Making and Treatment Algorithm

Our initial treatment for patients with adhesive capsulitis always consists of local measures and medication to reduce pain and inflammation. Most often this approach is comprised of the use of an appropriate NSAID, occasional analgesics, and the application of heat. As pain is reduced, a home stretching and range of motion program is begun under the supervision of both the attending surgeon and a physical therapist, with formal therapy visits administered as needed. During the patient's home stretching program, heat is utilized to relax the local tissues; then stretching is performed for 10 to 15 minutes. This sequence is performed at least 3 times daily. Pain is to be avoided during shoulder rehabilitation and with daily use. Intra-articular corticosteroid injections are often utilized on one or two occasions if treatment is initiated early in the course of the disease. The patient is evaluated at monthly intervals to measure their progress.

Timing

If the patient has inadequate recovery after 4 to 6 months of diligent participation in this stretching program; if their recovery plateaus during treatment, and improvement does not resume despite 6 to 8 weeks additional stretching; or if there is progressive worsening during the course of treatment, the option of surgical treatment is discussed with the patient. Those who have endured chronic adhesive capsulitis for more than 4 to 6 months prior to presenting to our office, also begin an initial course of nonoperative care. For these patients, if progress is not observed during the first 3 months of treatment, surgical care is likely to be offered.

Technique

If surgical intervention is selected, the patient is prepared for a manipulation under anesthesia and possible arthroscopic capsular release. At the time of surgery, the patient is placed under general anesthesia and a supplemental scalene block is administered for post operative analgesia. The patient's pure glenohumeral range of motion is measured and recorded. If the patient does not have significant osteoporosis, an assessment is then made regarding the resistance of the contracture to manipulation. A forceful manipulation is never performed. If the contracted capsule easily begins to yield with gentle manipulation (using only mild force), a manipulation will be performed first in forward elevation and then in horizontal cross body adduction in various positions of elevation. Next, external rotation is obtained with the arm at 90 degrees of abduction and then at several additional levels of abduction (including 120, 45 and 0 degrees). Finally, the arm is placed back into 90 degrees of abduction and manipulation for internal rotation is performed, after which the arm is lowered to the side while maintaining the arm in internal rotation. The entire manipulation is performed while loosely holding the arm above the elbow. If moderate force is required to obtain adequate release of the contracture in any plane of motion, the manipulation is discontinued and an arthroscopic capsular release is performed under the same anesthetic. This approach is used for both patients with and without diabetes mellitus.

Arthroscopic capsular release is performed in our standard position for shoulder arthroscopy, the lateral decubitus position. The arm is suspended by just enough weight to maintain a position of balanced suspension (generally 5 to 10 pounds) with the arm in approximately 45 degrees of abduction and 20 degrees of flexion. After standard skin preparation and draping, the posterior-superior cannula is carefully placed into the glenohumeral joint, taking care to do so atraumatically with regard to the articular surfaces. (The glenohumeral capsular contracture significantly reduces the intra-capsular volume, which makes insertion of an arthroscopic cannula more difficult than it is in patients without shoulder stiffness.) The arthroscope is then inserted into the cannula and a fluid pump set between 30 to 45 mmHg pressure is used to lavage and distend the joint. Often the initial view of the joint is limited to the rotator interval and the superior glenohumeral recess **(Fig 18-3)**, while an adequate view of the inferior portions of the joint cavity are obscured by the humeral head **(Fig 18-4)**. An anterior superior portal is made in the center of the rotator interval under direct visualization. A bipolar radiofrequency electrosurgical probe is used to cauterize any hypervascular synovitis present in the rotator interval and is then used to ablate the contents of the rotator interval until the coracoid process and the coraco-acromial ligament can be seen from within the joint. (Note: One must take care not to damage the lateral most portion of the coracohumeral ligament, which might destabilize the biceps tendon.) This subtotal removal of the rotator interval tissue results in a complete release of

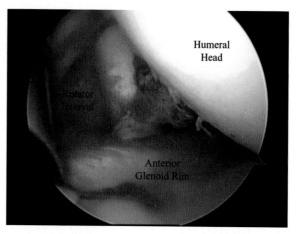

Fig 18-3. This initial view obtained upon introduction of the arthroscope into the glenohumeral joint of a patient with adhesive capsulitis demonstrates the vascular synovitis commonly observed filling the rotator interval area.

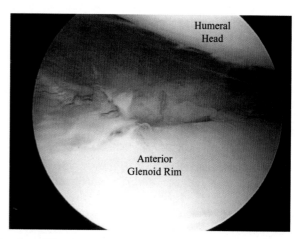

Fig 18-4. The decreased intra-articular volume associated with adhesive capsulitis severely restricts the amount of glenohumeral capsule that can be visualized upon initial introduction of the arthroscope into the shoulder joint.

the contracted coracohumeral ligament (53) that allows an increase in lateral displacement of the humeral head and increased anterior and posterior joint visualization. During the process of this capsular ablation, the thermal probe is used in its cauterizing mode to maintain hemostasis as needed. Next, the middle glenohumeral ligament and the mid-anterior capsule are released using the thermal probe at a distance of approximately 5 mm from the capsulolabral margin (where the glenohumeral capsule and subscapularis tendon are separate structures) **(Fig 18-5)**. The capsule is divided until the fleshy muscular fibers of the subscapularis can be seen **(Fig 18-6)**. The tendinous portion of the subscapularis is not divided. The anterior release is continued down to the inferior glenohumeral ligament if adequate visualization is present. Under no circumstances is any portion of the capsule divided blindly. Next, the arthroscope is transferred to the anterior portal and the thermal probe is

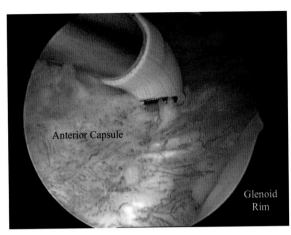

Fig 18-5. A radiofrequency electrosurgical probe is used to divide the joint capsule approximately 5 mm lateral to the glenoid labral margin.

(using whichever portal provides the best inferior capsular view), the bipolar thermal probe is reintroduced into the joint through the posterior inferior portal. The power setting for the device is adjusted to the lowest ablation setting that still divides tissue and the active surface of the probe is rotated so it faces in toward the joint cavity rather than outwards towards the capsule. Using the edge of the probe's active element the thickened capsule is slowly divided, initially with a partial thickness incision, immediately adjacent to the labral margin, keeping the probe faced toward the joint at all times **(Fig 18-7)**. Careful observation is maintained for any sign of axillary nerve stimulation such as an unexpected deltoid or teres minor muscle twitch. If there is no evidence of axillary nerve stimulation, successive layers of inferior capsule are then divided, keeping the active surface of the bipolar radiofrequency probe in full view to prevent any inadvertent penetration beyond the capsule **(Fig 18-8)**.

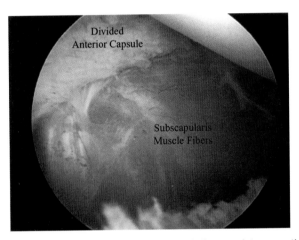

Fig 18-6. Release of the anterior capsule is complete once the fleshy muscle fibers of the subscapularis are fully visualized.

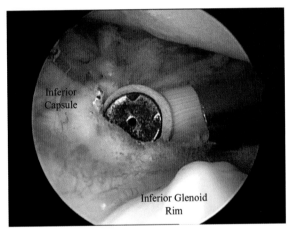

Fig 18-7. The superficial layer of the inferior capsule is released with an electrosurgical probe. To prevent inadvertent plunging through the capsule, the active tip of the device is kept in full view by rotating it in towards the joint cavity while it is being used.

inserted into the posterior cannula. It is uncommon in our experience for the superior capsule overlying the supraspinatus to require release; however, if it does, this portion of the capsule is now released by dividing it with the thermal probe 5 to 8 mm from the labral margin, taking care not to pass beyond the limits of the capsule where the suprascapular nerve might be encountered. The posterior capsule is then divided in the same fashion, at a distance of 5 to 8 mm from the labral margin, until the fleshy fibers of the posterior rotator cuff muscles are seen. This portion of the release can often be continued down into the posterior inferior recess while viewing from anterior. Next, a posterior inferior portal is made at the level of the posterior inferior corner of the glenoid (approximately the 8 o'clock position in a right shoulder). While viewing from the posterior superior portal, a blunt arthroscopic elevator can be introduced through the posterior inferior portal to sweep away the tissues on the extra-articular side of the inferior capsule; then, while viewing from either the anterior or posterior-superior portal

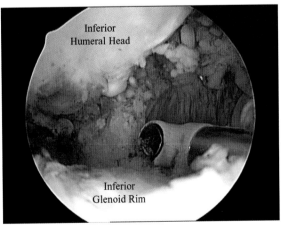

Fig 18-8. Release of the deepest layer of the inferior capsule is completed while maintaining the tip of the cutting probe in full view.

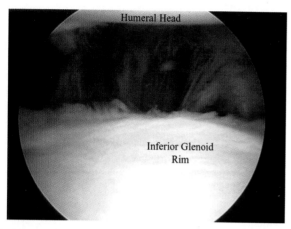

Fig 18-9. At the conclusion of this procedure, extra-articular soft tissues are easily visualized through the capsular incision confirming complete capsular release.

After all the fibers of the inferior capsule are released **(Fig 18-9)**, the arm is removed from its balanced suspension and range of motion is assessed. Full range of motion should be present at this point in the procedure. If it is not, a gentle stretching type of manipulation can be performed to release any secondary extracapsular adhesions which may have developed over time. If during the inferior capsular release, axillary nerve stimulation does occur, the release is terminated at that point in the procedure. The arm is then removed from balanced suspension and a gentle manipulation completes the inferior capsular release. If a significant limitation in motion persists, an open release can be performed (although this has not occurred in any of our cases).

If open capsular release should be indicated, it would be performed through a standard delto-pectoral approach. Careful lysis of adhesions should be performed at each successive level of the dissection to release restrictions to movement first in the subdeltoid space and the subpectoral spaces and then in the plane between the conjoined tendon and the subscapularis as well as in the subacromial space. Next, a careful release of the rotator interval tissues would be performed and range of motion evaluated. If inadequate motion persisted, then after mobilization and protection of the axillary nerve, detachment of the subscapularis from the lesser tuberosity would be performed with subsequent dissection of this muscle off of the glenohumeral capsule. A vertical capsulotomy just lateral to the glenoid margin would then be created, preserving the attachment of the labrum to the glenoid rim. Successive release of the inferior and posterior capsule would be performed until adequate motion is restored. A partial anterior capsulectomy is considered appropriate to diminish recurrent scarring. The subscapularis is then repaired either to the lesser tuberosity, if there is no significant subscapularis contracture, or to the medial end of the anterior glenohumeral capsule, if a significant subscapularis contracture is present. Routine layered closure of the wound should then be completed.

Postoperative Rehabilitation

Although the principles of shoulder rehabilitation are thoroughly reviewed in another chapter within this text, the nature of the postoperative therapeutic regimen is so intimately intertwined with the overall treatment of this condition, that a brief discussion seems necessary.

Immediately after the performance of a manipulation under anesthesia or an arthroscopic capsular release, the patient is enrolled into an aggressive program of pain control using a combination of postoperative scalene block and oral narcotic analgesics as needed. Intra-articular "pain pumps" can also be used. Continuous cold therapy is administered by a cold-water pump with a cutaneous pad for approximately 4 to 7 days. A continuous passive motion machine is utilized at home for 2 to 3 hours per session, 3 sessions a day, for 7 to 14 days. Home stretching is performed at least 3 times a day and formal physical therapy is provided each weekday for 2 weeks and then 3 times weekly until glenohumeral range of motion is satisfactory (often an additional 6 to 8 weeks). The range of motion and functional recovery is often dependant upon the patient's postoperative rehabilitation effort, with many patients recovering approximately 90% of their normal motion, at 2 or 3 months after surgery.

■ CONCLUSIONS

The clinical disorder of adhesive capsulitis is a medical problem whose etiology remains poorly understood. It produces significant morbidity in those afflicted with it and is not routinely self-limited in duration (as was previously believed). Treatment with conservative measures may achieve satisfactory subjective results, but leave the patient with persisting motion deficits and functional limitations, which they may accept and "work around." Treatment of this disorder with operative techniques is indicated for those patients with a more severe and unremitting manifestation of this disease and is often clinically successful after 2 to 3 months of postoperative rehabilitation, which significantly shortens the average duration of the recovery process for these individuals.

■ REFERENCES

1. Simmonds FA. Shoulder pain: with particular reference to the frozen shoulder. *J Bone Joint Surg Br.* 1949;31:426–432.
2. DePalma AF. Loss of scapulohumeral motion (frozen shoulder). *Ann Surg.* 1952;135:194–204.
3. Cuomo F. Diagnosis, classification, and management of the stiff shoulder. In: Ionnoti JP, Williams GR, eds. *Disorders of the shoulder: diagnosis and management.* Philadelphia: Lippincott Williams & Wilkins; 1999:397–417.
4. Codman EA. *The Shoulder.* Boston: Thomas Todd; 1934.
5. Neviasier JS. Adhesive Capsulitis of the shoulder. A study of the pathological findings in periarthritis of the shoulder. *J Bone Joint Surg Am.* 1945;27:211–222.

6. Zuckerman JD, Cuomo F. Frozen shoulder. In: Madsen FA III, Fu FH, Hawkins RJ, eds. *The shoulder: a balance of mobility and stability.* Chicago: American Academy of Orthopaedic Surgeons; 1993:253–267.

7. Poppen NK, Walker PS. Normal and abnormal motion of the shoulder. *J Bone Joint Surg Am.* 1976;58:195–201.

8. Harryman DT II, Sidles JA, Clark JM, et al. Translation of the humeral head on the glenoid with passive glenohumeral motion. *J Bone Joint Surg Am.* 1990;72:1334–1343.

9. Burkhart SB, Morgan CD, Kibler WB. Current concepts: The disabled throwing shoulder: spectrum of pathology part I: pathoanatomy and biomechanics. *Arthroscopy.* 2003;19:404–420.

10. Hawkins RJ, Angelo RL. Glenohumeral osteoarthritis: a late complication of the Putti-Platt repair. *J Bone Joint Surg Am.* 1990; 72:1193–1197.

11. Harryman DT II, Lazarus MD. The stiff shoulder. In: Rockwood CA Jr, Matsen FA III, Wirth MA, et al. *The shoulder.* 3rd ed. Philadelphia: Saunders; 2004:1121–1172.

12. Lundberg BJ. The frozen shoulder: clinical and radiographic observations: the effect of manipulation under general anesthesia: structure and glycosaminoglycan content of the joint capsule: local bone metabolism. *Acta Orthop Scand Suppl.* 1969;119:1–59.

13. Omari A, Bunker TD. Open surgical release for frozen shoulder: surgical findings and results of the release. *J Shoulder Elbow Surg.* 2001;10:353–357.

14. Smith SP, Devaraj VS, Bunker TD, The association between frozen shoulder and Dupuytren's disease. *J Shoulder Elbow Surg.* 2001;10:149–151.

15. Bunker TD. Frozen shoulder: unraveling the enigma. *Ann R Coll Surg Engl.* 1997;79:210–213.

16. Bunker TD, Reilly J, Baird KS, et al. Expression of growth factors, cytokines and matrix metalloproteinases in frozen shoulder. *J Bone Joint Surg Br.* 2000;82:768–773.

17. Balci N, Balci MK, Tuzuner S. Shoulder adhesive capsulitis and shoulder range of motion in type II diabetes mellitus: association with diabetic complications. *J Diabetes and Its Complicat.* 1999; 13:135–140.

18. Janda DH, Hawkins RJ. Shoulder manipulation in patients with adhesive capsulitis and diabetes mellitus: a clinical note. *J Shoulder Elbow Surg.* 1993;2:36–38.

19. Miller MD, Wirth MA, Rockwood CA. Thawing the frozen shoulder: the "patient" patient. *Orthopedics.* 1996;19:849–853.

20. Ogilvie-Harris DJ, Myerthall S. The diabetic frozen shoulder: arthroscopic release. *Arthroscopy.* 1997;13:1–8.

21. Reeves B. The natural history of the frozen shoulder syndrome. *Scand J Rheumatol.* 1975;4:193–196.

22. Carrillon Y, Noel E, Fantino O, et al. Magnetic resonance imaging findings in idiopathic adhesive capsulitis of the shoulder. *Rev Rhum Engl Ed.* 1999;66:201–206.

23. Ryu KN, Lee SW, Rhee YG, et al. Adhesive capsulitis of the shoulder joint: usefulness of dynamic ultrasonography. *J Ultrasound Med.* 1993;12:445–449.

24. Clunie G, Bomanji J, Ell PJ. Technetium-99m-MDP patterns in patients with painful shoulder lesions. *J Nucl Med.* 1997;38:1491–1495.

25. Grey R. The natural history of "idiopathic" frozen shoulder. *J Bone Joint Surg.* 1978;60:564.

26. Pearsall AW, Holovacs TF, Speer KP. The intra-articular component of the subscapularis tendon: anatomic and histological correlation in reference to surgical release in patients with frozen-shoulder syndrome. *Arthroscopy.* 2000;3:236–242.

27. Shaffer B, Tibone JE, Kerlan RK. Frozen shoulder. *J Bone Joint Surg Am.* 1992;74:738–740.

28. Hannafin JA, Chiaia TA. Adhesive Capsulitis. *Clin Orthop.* 2000; 372:95–109.

29. Carrette S, Moffet H, Tardif J, et al. Intaarticular corticosteroids, supervised physiotherapy or a combination of the two in the treatment of adhesive capsulitis of the shoulder. A placebo controlled trial. *Arthritis-Rheum.* 2003;48:829–838.

30. Griggs SM, Ahn A, Green A. Idiopathic adhesive capsulitis. *J Bone Joint Surg Am.* 2000;82:1398–1407.

31. Andersen NH, Sojbjerg JO, Johannsen HV, et al. Frozen shoulder: arthroscopy and manipulation under general anesthesia and early passive motion. *J Shoulder Elbow Surg.* 1998;7:218–222.

32. Goldberg BA, Scarlat MM, Harryman DT. Management of the stiff shoulder. *J Orthop Sci.* 1999;4:462–471.

33. Warner JP, Answorth A, Marks P, et al. Arthroscopic release for chronic refractory adhesive capsulitis of the shoulder. *J Bone Joint Surg.* 1996;78:1808–1816.

34. Dodenhoff RM, Levy O, Wilson A, et al. Manipulation under anesthesia for primary frozen shoulder: effect on early recovery and return to activity. *J Shoulder Elbow Surg.* 2000;9:23–26.

35. Reichmister JP, Friedman SL. Long-term functional results after manipulation of the frozen shoulder. *Maryland Med J.* 1999; 48:7–11.

36. Massoud SN, Pearse EO, Levy O, et al. Operative management of the frozen shoulder in patients with diabetes. *J Shoulder Elbow Surg.* 2002;11:609–613.

37. Pollock RG, Duralde XA, Flatow EL, et al. The use of arthroscopy in the treatment of resistant frozen shoulder. *Clin Orthop.* 1994; 304:30–36.

38. Zanotti RM, Kuhn JE. Arthroscopic capsular release for the stiff shoulder. Description of technique and anatomic considerations. *Am J Sports Med.* 1997;25:294–298.

39. Beaufils P, Prevot N, Boyer T, et al. Arthroscopic release of the glenohumeral joint in shoulder stiffness: a review of 26 cases. *Arthroscopy.* 1999;15:49–55.

40. Bennett WF. Addressing glenohumeral stiffness while treating the painful and stiff shoulder arthroscopically. *Arthroscopy.* 2000;126:142–150.

41. Berghs BM, Sole-Molins X, Bunker TD. Arthroscopic release of adhesive capsulitis. *J Shoulder Elbow Surg.* 2004;13:180–185.

42. Harryman DT II, Matsen FA III, Sidles JA. Arthroscopic management of refractory shoulder stiffness. *Arthroscopy.* 1997;13: 133–47.

43. Holloway GB, Schenk T, Williams GR, et al. Arthroscopic capsular release for the treatment of refractory postoperative or post-fracture shoulder stiffness. *J Bone Joint Surg Am.* 2001;83:1682–1687.

44. Ide J, Katsumasa T. Early and long-term results of arthroscopic treatment for shoulder stiffness. *J Shoulder Elbow Surg.* 2004;13: 174–179.

45. Nicholson GP. Arthroscopic capsular release for stiff shoulders: effect of etiology on outcomes. *Arthroscopy.* 2003;19:40–49.

46. Ogilvie-Harris DJ, Biggs DJ, Fitsialos DP, et al. The resistant frozen shoulder. Manipulation versus arthroscopic release. *Clin Orthop.* 1995;319:238–248.

47. Pearsall AW, Osbahr DC, Speer KP. An arthroscopic technique for treating patients with frozen shoulder. *Arthroscopy.* 1999;15:2–11.

48. Watson L, Dalziel R, Story I. Frozen shoulder: a 12-month clinical outcome trial. *J Shoulder Elbow Surg.* 2000;9:16–22.

49. Ozaki J, Nakagawa Y, Sakurai G, et al. Recalcitrant chronic adhesive capsulitis of the shoulder. Role of contracture of the coracohumeral ligament and rotator interval in pathogenesis and treatment. *J Bone Joint Surg.* 1989;71:1511–1515.

50. Nobuhara K, Sugiyama D, Ikeda H, et al. Contracture of the shoulder. *Clin Orthop.* 1990;254:105–110.

51. Kieras DM, Matsen FA III. Open release in the management of refractory frozen shoulder. *Orthop Trans.* 1991;15:801–802.

52. Moskal MJ, Harryman DT II, Romeo AA, et al. Glenohumeral motion after complete capsular release. *Arthroscopy.* 1999;15: 408–416.

53. Tetro AM, Bauer G, Hollstien SB, et al. Arthroscopic release of the rotator interval and the coracohumeral ligament: an anatomic study in cadavers. *Arthroscopy.* 2002;18:145–150.

ARTHROSCOPIC ROTATOR CUFF REPAIR

JAMES C. ESCH, MD, JEFFREY W. TAMBORLANE, MD

■ KEY POINTS

- The glenohumeral space and arcomiohumeral distance are carefully evaluated on the anteroposterior (AP) radiograph for arthritis, aseptic necrosis, and calcifications.
- A magnetic resonance image (MRI) provides an excellent image of a torn rotator cuff, showing the subscapularis tendon and status of the deltoid muscle. The size and shape of tendon tears can also be evaluated.
- Surgery usually provides good pain relief. Weakness, however, is slower to recover and will not recover completely if there is significant muscle atrophy.
- If the tear is irreparable, bursal tissue and spurs can be debrided but the coracoacromial arch should be preserved.
- The methods for tendon immobilization are capsular release, coracohumeral ligament releases at the rotator interval, and interval slides.
- Some surgeons recommend use of a shoulder immobilizer for 4 to 8 weeks after surgery, particularly after repairs of massive cuff tears.

Shoulder arthroscopy has improved our understanding and treatment of rotator cuff tears. It facilitates easy viewing from different angles, as opposed to open treatment, which when performed through a small incision has a limited exposure in part due to the acromion. This arthroscopic viewpoint has led to the recognition of several common rotator cuff tear patterns (1). Tear pattern recognition, suture anchors, and tissue-passing instruments enable the surgeon to mobilize and repair a torn rotator cuff to its bony footprint with consistency. Associated pathology within the shoulder joint-articular cartilage, glenoid labrum, and biceps tendon problems can also be treated. We rely on the arthroscope to repair most rotator cuff tears.

■ RADIOGRAPHY AND MAGNETIC RESONANCE IMAGING

The surgeon must carefully examine routine anteroposterior (AP), axillary, and arch radiographs. The glenohumeral space and acromiohumeral distance are carefully evaluated on the AP view for arthritis, aseptic necrosis, and calcifications. The axillary view is routinely obtained because it tells the surgeon whether an os acromion is present. The arch view shows acromion shape and thickness. Additionally, a weight-bearing "push-up" AP view, in which upward pressure is placed on the humerus, can be obtained to evaluate narrowing of the acromiohumeral space **(Fig 19-1)**.

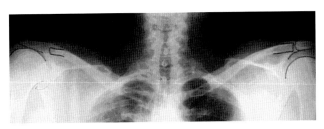

Fig 19-1. AP "Push-up" view with narrowed acromion to humeral head space on the right shoulder. (From Warner JJP, Iannotti JP, Flatow EL, eds. *Complex and Revision Problems in Shoulder Surgery*. 2nd ed. Philadelphia: Lippincott Williams & Wilkins; 2005.)

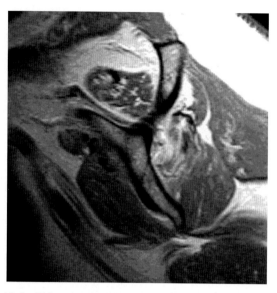

Fig 19-2. Oblique sagittal T2-weighted MRI of patient with massive rotator cuff tear shows atrophy and fatty degeneration of the supraspinatus and infraspinatus muscles. (From Mellado JM, Calmet J, Olona M, et al. Surgically repaired massive rotator cuff tears: MRI of tendon integrity, muscle fatty degeneration, and muscle atrophy correlated with intraoperative and clinical findings. *AJR.* 2005;184:1456–1463.)

Magnetic resonance imaging (MRI) imparts the best image of a torn rotator cuff, showing the subscapularis tendon and status of the deltoid muscle. The size and shape dimensions of supraspinatus and infraspinatus tendon tears are also revealed. Pre-operative evaluation of muscle atrophy is another advantage of MRI. MRI muscle evaluation can show normal muscle, partial fatty infiltration of one muscle, complete atrophy of the supraspinatus, or atrophy of the supraspinatus and infraspinatus **(Fig 19-2)**.

Smaller scanners and newer software afford excellent images in a convenient office setting. The orthopaedic surgeon should personally review the MRI scan.

■ SURGICAL OPTIONS, INDICATIONS, AND DECISION MAKING

The office radiographs and MRI complement the patient's history of symptom onset, discomfort, and loss of function. Discuss the ease or difficulty of repair with the patient as well as the extent of rehabilitation and the expected result. Surgery provides good pain relief. Weakness, however, is slower to recover and will recover incompletely if there is significant muscle atrophy. Patients with significant pain are usually unaware of any accompanying weakness. The patient should have a clear idea of the goals and problems of surgery. Despite these caveats, some patients will have unrealistic expectations for surgical correction of their symptoms. We also point out to the patient that an MRI obtained after surgery may show incomplete healing of the rotator cuff repair (1).

Small to large tears of the supraspinatus and infraspinatus tendons can be repaired by standard arthroscopic repair

techniques. Tear size and configuration dictate the specific surgical technique. Repair usually requires a combination of a margin convergence and a tendon-to-bone repair using suture anchors. The goal of margin convergence is to reduce the tension on the tendon to bone repair. Margin convergence involves suturing the anterior and posterior leaves of the tear in a sequential side-to-side manner, starting medially and proceeding laterally until the tear converges toward the bony footprint. The free edge is then attached to the footprint with suture anchors. The value of an arthroscopic rotator cuff repair is that one obtains a secure arthroscopic repair through smaller incisions, without disruption of the deltoid muscle attachment. The final repair is "decompressed" by smoothing the undersurface of the acromion.

Arthroscopic repair of a massive cuff tear is unpredictable. Surgical visualization and mobilization determine whether a massive tear is repairable, partially repairable, or irreparable. A tear is not deemed irreparable until it is evaluated at the time of arthroscopy. Many tears that appear irreparable pre-operatively can be mobilized by capsular techniques and interval slides (2), enabling a partial or complete repair of a once "irreparable" tear. These patients with massive tears usually obtain good pain relief but continue to have weakness due to atrophy of a cuff muscle (3).

If the tear is indeed irreparable, debride the bursal tissue but preserve the coracoacromial arch. Some surgeons prefer to "decompress" the undersurface of the acromion by making the underside of the acromion flat. But the insertion of the coracoacromial ligament onto the undersurface of the acromion must be preserved. If the coracoacromial ligament is removed, the humeral head may "escape" anteriorly, leading to anterosuperior shoulder instability.

Partial repair of a massive rotator cuff tear—namely, the subscapularis or infraspinatus tendons while leaving a defect in the supraspinatus tendon—may be helpful (4), improving pain and function by restoring the rotator cuff cable and force couples necessary for arm elevation (2).

■ SURGICAL TECHNIQUE

There are many different strategies that have been described regarding the management of rotator cuff tears arthroscopically. The following techniques are the authors' preferred approach to this problem.

The surgeon must balance skill versus ego in arthroscopic rotator cuff repair. He or she must be in control of the operating theater. Detailed knowledge of the proper tools for passing suture through the cuff, suture management, and knot tying techniques is essential. The skills required for the specific steps can be honed using a shoulder model.

The surgeon must have not only a favorite plan, which we will call Plan A, but also Plan B as well as Plan C. A surgeon who is learning arthroscopic rotator cuff repair can easily bail out of the arthroscopic procedure at any time and proceed to an open repair of the rotator cuff through a mini deltoid-splitting incision.

Control Bleeding

Controlling bleeding is essential for a good repair. Some tips for efficient control of bleeding include flowing fluid in through the arthroscope, controlling outflow through the shaver blades, and being aware of the nuances of an arthroscopic fluid management system.

The anesthesiologist lowers and safely monitors the systolic blood pressure in the range of 90 to 100 mmHg. Electrocautery or radiofrequency devices can be useful to stop any troublesome bleeding vessels. Nonsteroidal anti-inflammatory drugs (NSAIDs) and other drugs that can cause bleeding should be discontinued at least seven days before surgery. We recommend avoidance of NSAIDs after rotator cuff repair because they may interfere with healing of the rotator cuff tendon to the bone (5).

Patient Positioning

In our practice we place the patient in the lateral decubitus position. Turn the operating table so the anesthesiologist is at the foot **(Fig 19-3)**.

Prepare and drape the shoulder after the arm is suspended with 10 to 15 pounds of weight. Perform a glenohumeral arthroscopy in a systematic fashion using a standard posterior portal and an anterior portal through the rotator interval. Treat any cartilage and labrum pathology. Examine the rotator cuff tear and evaluate the cuff footprint.

Portal Placement

Create three portals for the rotator cuff repair. Enter the subacromial bursa from the posterior portal for initial viewing. Create the lateral portal three fingerbreadths lateral to

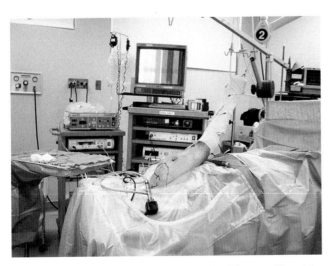

Fig 19-3. Patient positioning in lateral decubitus position. The anesthesiologist is at the foot of the table. (From Warner JJP, Iannotti JP, Flatow EL, eds. *Complex and Revision Problems in Shoulder Surgery*. 2nd ed. Philadelphia: Lippincott Williams & Wilkins; 2005.)

the acromion. Remove any bursa that interferes with visualization and debride dystrophic calcifications and irregular edges of the torn rotator cuff. Make the anterior subacromial portal by entering the bursa just lateral to the coracoacromial ligament. This enables the cannula to be easily moved and does not disrupt the coracoacromial arch. Excise bursa as necessary for visualization. Use electrocautery as necessary to control bleeding. Create additional portals as necessary. Insert suture anchors through a mini-portal off the edge of the acromion. The additional superior portal behind the acromioclavicular joint can be used for a suture-retrieving device to pass sutures through the edge of a crescent-shaped tear (6).

We prefer the lateral subacromial portal—the "50-yard line" view—for optimal viewing of the rotator cuff. Place plastic 7- to 8.5-mm cannulas in the anterior and posterior portals for use in passing tools and suture. Move the tools, suture, and arthroscope as needed. Do not lock yourself to one portal.

Preparing the Site and Beginning the Repair

Remove the bursa tissue as necessary for visualization of the cuff repair. Find a tissue plane that allows you to see the extent of the cuff tear. Free up any adhesions between the cuff or bursa and the overlying acromion. Use a shaver-blade or high-speed burr to remove any remaining rotator cuff at the greater tuberosity insertion. Gently debride the surface of the bone to provide bleeding for repair of the cuff to bone. Gently shave the edges or layers of the rotator cuff edges, but do not excise any significant pieces of the torn cuff that are mechanically sound.

Determine Tear Configuration

The next step involves determining the configuration and reparability of the cuff. Use probes or grasping forceps to assess how you are going to repair the rotator cuff. You can use grasping forceps in both hands while your assistant holds the arthroscope. You must determine first the feasibility of a repair and then, if feasible, the steps necessary to achieve it. You should be able to diagram on paper your final repair, even if you ultimately make changes as you proceed.

Rotator cuffs tear in a crescent-, L-, or U-shaped fashion. Crescent-shaped tears **(Fig 19-4)** are supraspinatus (and sometimes infraspinatus) tears that can be repaired directly to the bony footprint under minimal tension with double-loaded suture anchors placed though a mini-portal off the edge of the acromion.

The sutures can be passed though the free edge of the tear using direct suturing, penetrate and grab, or shuttle techniques. The suturing and grasping tools can be passed from the anterior, posterior, superior, or lateral portal. Create additional portals as necessary.

L-shaped tears run parallel to the anterior edge of the supraspinatus **(Fig 19-5)**, and U-shaped tears are located in

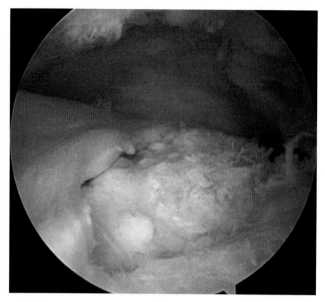

Fig 19-4. Crescent shaped rotator cuff tear. These tears can be repaired directly to bone with suture anchors under minimal tension. (From Warner JJP, Iannotti JP, Flatow EL, eds. *Complex and Revision Problems in Shoulder Surgery.* 2nd ed. Philadelphia: Lippincott Williams & Wilkins; 2005.)

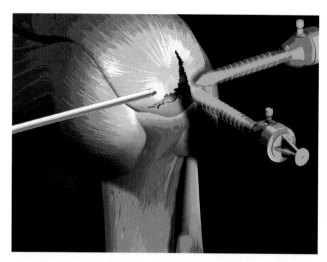

Fig 19-5. L-shaped rotator cuff tear. These tears require margin convergence sutures placed side-to-side along the anterior leaf. This will result in a crescent shaped tear, which can be repaired directly to bone. (From Warner JJP, Iannotti JP, Flatow EL, eds. *Complex and Revision Problems in Shoulder Surgery.* 2nd ed. Philadelphia: Lippincott Williams & Wilkins; 2005.)

the infraspinatus-supraspinatus interval. With L-shaped tears, the posterior leaf is more mobile then the anterior leaf (capsule in the rotator interval), whereas both leaves are mobile with U-shaped tears.

Therefore, repair L- and U-shaped tears initially by a side-to-side margin convergence using a free suture, creating in effect a small crescent-shaped tear; then attach the free edge of the tear to the bone using the suture anchor technique. Sometimes, you will need to place the sutures through

the torn cuff only *after* the suture anchors have been appropriately positioned in the bony footprint because the footprint will be covered during margin convergence and access to it will be lost. Include any layering of the torn rotator cuff into your suturing technique, just as is done in open surgery.

Suture Passage and Stitch Configuration

The author uses one of three methods for passing suture from a suture anchor through the rotator cuff. These are direct suture passage, penetrate and grab, and, suture shuttle techniques. By using these devices, the sutures can be passed as a simple, mattress or T- stitch configurations. The simple stitch requires passage of one limb of the suture through the rotator cuff and tying the suture (**Fig 19-6**). A mattress stitch is performed by passing both ends of a suture through the rotator cuff and tying the ends together (**Fig 19-7**).

The T stitch involves placement of a horizontal mattress with one of two sutures from a double loaded anchor. One

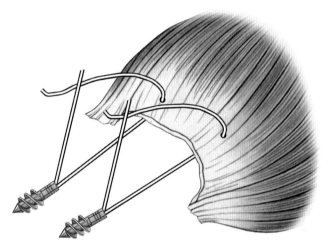

Fig 19-6. Simple stitch.

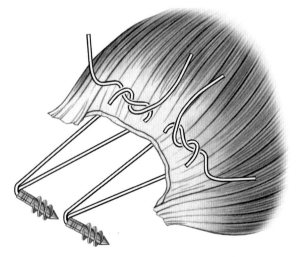

Fig 19-7. Mattress stitch.

T-Suture Steps

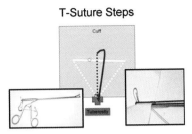

Fig 19-8. T stitch. (From Warner JJP, Iannotti JP, Flatow EL, eds. *Complex and Revision Problems in Shoulder Surgery*. 2nd ed. Philadelphia: Lippincott Williams & Wilkins; 2005.)

limb of the second suture is passed medial to the first mattress. The mattress suture is tied first, followed by the simple suture, resulting in a T formation **(Fig 19-8)**.

Mobilization Techniques for Retracted Tendons

Three methods are used for tendon mobilization. These are capsular release, coracohumeral ligament releases at the rotator interval, and interval slides.

Perform the capsular release by inserting an elevator to between the capsule and the undersurface of the rotator cuff. This maneuver reduces the tension on the final repair (7). Care must be taken to avoid damage to the suprascapular nerve motor branches to the infraspinatus which are located 2.1 +/− 0.5 cm from the posterior rim of the glenoid (8).

The coracohumeral ligament release is done by using a shaver to remove the bursa from the posterior surface of the coracoid. As the tool moves medially, the short coracohumeral ligament will be seen coursing from the posterior surface of the coracoid to the anterior edge of the supraspinatus. This is best done while viewing from laterally, using the shaver or electocautery from the anterior portal, and a grasper from the posterior portal applying tension to the supraspinatus.

The interval slide technique described by Tauro (9) **(Fig 19-9)** involves release of the rotator interval to improve cuff mobility. A double interval slide is created by releasing the supraspinatus and infraspinatus toward the scapular spine until the fat about the suprascapular nerve is seen. This is best done with anterior supraspinatus and posterior infraspinatus traction sutures while cutting from posterior with scissors or electrocautery and viewing from the lateral portal. This enables the surgeon to have a one to two centimeter strip of tendon to advance to the greater tuberosity (10). Surgeons must appreciate the locations of the anterior and posterior neurovascular structures when performing these releases to avoid serious complications.

The surgeon usually can mobilize the tendon for a complete repair to bone. If not, a partial repair of the infraspinatus can be done by mobilizing and shifting anteriorly the leading edge of the infraspinatus to a bony bed where a suture anchor is placed. Occasionally the surgeon may be unable to mobilize the cuff and call the repair irreparable.

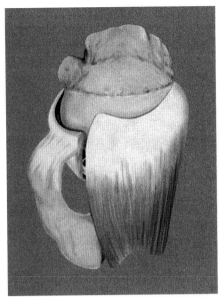

Fig 19-9. Rotator interval slide. The rotator interval is released to improve mobility of the rotator cuff. (From Tauro JC. Arthroscopic repair of large rotator cuff tears using the interval slide technique. *Arthroscopy*. 2004;20:13–21.)

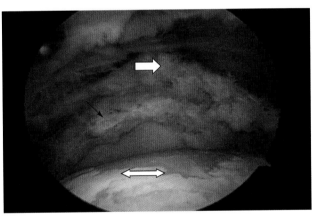

Fig 19-10. Irreparable rotator cuff tear. Biceps tenotomy was performed for pain relief. The retracted rotator cuff tissue *(top white arrow)*. The superior labrum *(thin black arrow)*. The arthritic humeral head *(double ended arrow)*. (From Warner JJP, Iannotti JP, Flatow EL, eds. *Complex and Revision Problems in Shoulder Surgery*. 2nd ed. Philadelphia: Lippincott Williams & Wilkins; 2005.)

A bursectomy may afford pain relief in these situations. We also perform a biceps tenotomy or tenodesis if the biceps tendon is diseased, due to its ability to be a potential pain generator **(Fig 19-10)**.

Margin Convergence

Figure 19-11 illustrates the initial margin convergence suture just 5 mm from the apex of the tear. This proximity prevents extension of the tear. From the posterior portal, pass a relatively straight Cuff Stitch device loaded with #2 braided polyester suture through the tear limbs from posterior to

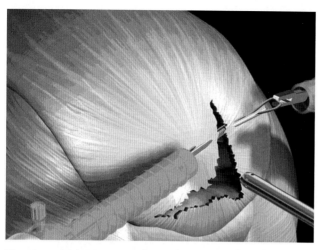

Fig 19-11. Margin convergence with a Cuff-Stitch suture passer. (From Warner JJP, Iannotti JP, Flatow EL, eds. *Complex and Revision Problems in Shoulder Surgery.* 2nd ed. Philadelphia: Lippincott Williams & Wilkins; 2005.)

anterior. Unload the suture from the anterior portal and withdraw the cuff stitch from the posterior portal. Load the knot pusher on this posterior suture limb. This is the "post" limb for your arthroscopic knot. Use a suture-grabbing device or crochet hook in the posterior portal to withdraw the anterior suture limb.

This is the "loop" strand for your arthroscopic knot. Next, tie a sliding knot. Pull on the post suture limb while guiding and manipulating the knot with the knot pusher as it brings the tissue of the torn cuff together. Secure the knot with three half-hitches, changing posts after each loop. Cut the knot. Repeat as necessary.

Subsequent margin convergence sutures are placed by grasping and moving the tissue to an optimal position without creating a large dog-ear at the repair site. We prefer a "suture-handoff" technique for accurate placement of the sutures on either side of the repair. Our preferred technique is a Cuff Stitch-to-ArthroPierce handoff.

To perform this handoff, use a straight Cuff Stitch device to pass a #2 braided suture from the anterior portal through the tear; then "hand it off" to an ArthroPierce passed through the predetermined point in the posterior limb of the tear from the posterior portal. The posterior suture strand is the post limb of the arthroscopic knot. The anterior strand is the loop limb. Tie a sliding arthroscopic knot plus three half-hitches, reversing posts. Insert as many sutures as necessary to approximate the edges of the tear. Margin convergence can also be done by placing sutures with direct suture passage or shuttle techniques.

Completing the Repair with Suture Anchors

Insert the suture anchors into bone, carefully watching them enter and remain below the surface of the bone. Use an 18-gauge needle off of the edge of the acromion to get the

correct angle for insertion of the suture anchor into the bony footprint. We prefer to insert the anchor through a cannula into the subchondral bone near the articular cartilage.

Insert one to three anchors at this time, depending on the size of the tear. Visualize the proper steps and arrangements for suture repair. Mark the sutures with hemostats. They can be left in this portal or changed as desired.

Pass the suture through the edge of the cuff in the appropriate position for repair. The "penetrate and grab" technique of passing suture is accomplished by using an ArthroPierce to penetrate through the tissue to retrieve the suture.

Pass the first suture by inserting the ArthroPierce through the posterior attachment of the infraspinatus or supraspinatus portion of the rotator cuff and retrieve one of the sutures from the most posterior anchor; pull this suture out the posterior portal. Load the knot pusher on this posterior suture limb. This is the post limb for your arthroscopic knot. Use a suture-grabbing device or crochet hook in the posterior portal to withdraw the other suture limb from the anchor. This is the loop strand for your arthroscopic knot. Tie a sliding knot and pull on the post suture limb while guiding and manipulating the knot into place as it brings the tissue of the torn cuff together. Secure the knot with three half-hitches, changing posts after each loop. Cut the knot. Repeat these simple sutures as necessary.

The author also performs the "direct" suture passage technique by utilizing the Elite-Pass (Smith and Nephew). This is accomplished by viewing from the posterior portal and removing the suture end to be passed from the lateral portal. The suture is loaded into the Elite-Pass, which then bites the desired amount of rotator cuff tissue from the lateral edge of the tear. The needle is then deployed from the Elite-Pass and the suture is passed through the tissue. The suture is then retrieved through the anterior portal by using a flat grasping device. The Elite-Pass is then removed from the lateral cannula. The suture that was just passed through the tissue is the post strand which is brought out the lateral portal and tied to the loop strand.

Tie your arthroscopic knots in the appropriate portal so they will easily slide, avoiding friction of the suture on the bone or anchor eyelet. Pay attention to the depth and orientation of the anchor and its eyelet in the bone. Do not bury the suture anchor deeper than the recommended insertion depth. This can lead to early clinical failure as the suture cuts through the bone, resulting in gap formation at the insertion zone [seen in a bovine model (11)] or as the deep anchor becomes superficial, again resulting in gap formation at the insertion zone [seen in a human cadaver model (12)] during cyclic loading. We often tie knots from the lateral portal with the arthroscope in the posterior portal. We prefer a sliding knot with three half-hitches, alternating posts. If the suture does not easily slide, tie alternating half-hitch knots with the first two or three loops on the same post. If the first simple half-hitch does not lie down easily, use a small needle holder to stabilize the first throw while the second throw is put down the cannula. Bring the needle holder through an adjacent portal or the one used for anchor insertion. This knot-stabilizing maneuver is similar to placing your finger on the ribbon when tying a bow on a package.

A "tension-band" option is available to reduce stress on repairs of large or massive tears. In this situation, we place an additional suture anchor from the greater tuberosity and pass a suture medial to the repair, through intact tendon tissue, and then tie this suture to an anchor that is placed the greater tuberosity lateral to the first row of anchors. This creates a tension band repair on the first row of sutures.

Place an anchor on the greater tuberosity from the lateral portal while viewing from posterior. Pass the sutures from this anchor out the anterior portal. Move the arthroscope back to the lateral portal. Place one suture limb through the intact supraspinatus tendon medial to the previous sutures by passing an ArthroPierce from the posterior portal proximal through the supraspinatus tendon to grasp the suture that is in the anterior portal. Pull this suture out the posterior portal. The second limb is passed in a similar retrograde fashion through the infraspinatus. Pass an ArthroPierce through the infraspinatus and grasp the suture on the greater tuberosity anchor. Tie the suture from the posterior portal. Repeat this with the second suture on the anchor.

Restore the Cuff Footprint

Apreleva et al. (13) studied the restoration of the supraspinatus footprint by four different rotator cuff repair types. By using human cadavers and a 3-D digitizer they found that single row suture anchor repairs restored only 67% of the original supraspinatus footprint while transosseous simple suture repairs restored 85% of the footprint. They concluded that restoration of the original insertion of the rotator cuff would provide larger area for healing and this could improve mechanical strength and function. Therefore, attention should be given to the capability of a procedure to restore the original tendon insertion site.

In an attempt to improve results of arthroscopic rotator cuff repairs, Burkhart (14) described a technique involving a double row of suture anchors. The technique involves use of a medial and lateral row of suture anchors which would re-establish the rotator cuff footprint. The medial suture anchors are tied with a mattress configuration and the lateral suture anchors are tied with a simple configuration. He concluded that using a double-row repair may result in greater strength and healing of rotator cuff. The authors prefer to use a double row, but this is dictated by the mobility of the tissue. For mobile tears, double-row repairs are feasible without placing tension on the repair. Retracted tears can be difficult to mobilize and single-row repairs are sometimes the only option.

Recent data suggest that the footprint restoration is clearly improved with double-row rotator cuff repair compared to single-row repairs. Results of strength testing of double-row repairs compared to single row-repairs has been variable. Some studies have illustrated significantly improved strength with double-row repairs, and others have shown no statistically significant differences (15–17).

■ POSTOPERATIVE CARE

Pain control immediately after surgery is important. Ice packs, especially for the first 3 days, and oral narcotics as needed are the mainstays of pain control. We inject 0.25% bupivacaine with epinephrine into the subacromial space, around the portals, and around the suprascapular nerve from the supraclavicular fossa portal. Healing of the rotator cuff to bone is necessary for optimal function (18). Immobilize the shoulder in a shoulder immobilizer for 4 to 8 weeks, depending on the size of the tear, except when the patients are performing physical therapy. Physical therapy consists of passive shoulder exercises, which are begun immediately, with passive supine forward elevation from 0 to 90 degrees and external rotation to 10 degrees. Active assistive motion is allowed between 6 and 8 weeks, and active motion is allowed at 8 to 12 weeks. As a rule, we tend to go slow rather than fast with these repairs. No weightlifting is allowed till 4 to 6 months after surgery.

Some patients will experience postoperative stiffness, especially with smaller tears. If this is present 12 weeks postoperatively, a Dynasplint (Dynasplint Systems, Severna Park, MD) is used for gentle home stretching.

■ RESULTS

In a review of 51 shoulders in 48 patients more than 2 years postoperatively (19), surgery had improved the pain scores in all patients, with 48 of 51 shoulders (94%) getting a satisfactory rating by the patient. Three patients with larger and massive tears reported unsatisfactory results secondary to shoulder weakness. Average time to return to work among those who were employed was 3.2 months, with an average recovery of 5.1 months. Smaller tears recovered faster than medium or large tears. Postoperative supraspinatus strength was significantly better for small and medium tears than for larger and massive tears. UCLA scores for all tears significantly improved from the preoperative average of 10.3 ($\pm$2.4) to 32.1 ($\pm$4.3) postoperatively. Small tears had an average score of 35, medium tears of 33.2, and large tears of 30. Excellent results on postoperative UCLA scores were achieved in 26 (51%) patients and good results in 17 (33%) patients. Fair results were seen in 7 shoulders (14%), and 1 shoulder (2%) had a poor result. The average overall Western Ontario Rotator Cuff (WORC) score was 86.8% ($\pm$17.1) of normal (20). Scores for smaller and medium tears were significantly better than for large or massive tears. Scores for motion, lifestyle, and physical symptoms were slightly higher than those for work and sports recreation. The only complication of this study was that 2 screws (of 75) were loose postoperatively.

One patient with a massive tear experienced superior migration of the humeral head and degenerative changes of the glenohumeral joint. One patient had symptomatic AC arthrosis at his most recent follow-up.

Metcalf (21) performed a meta-analysis that compared open and arthroscopic rotator cuff repairs. There was no significant difference in the overall results between open, arthroscopic, and mini-open techniques with regard to pain relief, range of motion, percentage of good and excellent results, satisfaction percentage, and strength. The results seem to be more dependent on the surgeon's expertise rather than repair technique (Table 19-1). The patient populations from different surgeons could not be assumed to be similar with regard to demographics, method of documentation, tear size, prior treatment, and social and medical comorbidities (22).

Warner retrospectively compared the results of 9 patients who had arthroscopic rotator cuff repairs (ARCR) versus 12 patients who had mini-open rotator cuff repairs (MOR) (23). The patients were matched for age, gender, dominance, side of injury, history of trauma, duration of symptoms, and type of rotator cuff injury. The mean follow-up for the ARCR group and the MOR group was 44 months and 55 months, respectively. They found no difference between the two groups and concluded that the choice of type of repair should be based on the surgeon and patient preferences.

Rebuzzi (24) performed a retrospective analysis of 54 shoulders in patients older than 60 years. Each patient had an arthroscopic rotator cuff repair performed by the same surgical team with average of 27 months follow-up. The mean postoperative UCLA score improved from 10.4 to 30.5. The results were comparable to those obtained from traditional open repairs. Rebuzzi believes that arthroscopic evaluation of the rotator cuff tears results in a more precise repair.

Yamaguchi reported results of 18 patients who had complete arthroscopic rotator cuff repairs of tears measuring >2 cm. The patients showed excellent clinical results despite 17 of 18 patients having recurrent tears at one year follow-up. These results deteriorated at a minimum follow-up of 2 years (25).

■ COMPLICATIONS

Complications of arthroscopic rotator cuff surgery are similar to those associated with open surgery, such as infection, stiffness, incomplete healing, loosening of an anchor, and injury to the deltoid muscle. The potential of deltoid muscle detachment is much less because the deltoid is not taken down for exposure.

TABLE 19-1 Summary of Rotator Cuff Repair Results

Author	Mean Age (y)	Mean Follow-up (mo)	% Good or Excellent	% Satisfactory	Mean ROM	% Pain Relief	Strength (out of 5)
Kersey & Esch[a] (arthroscopy)	68	53	84	94	170	92	4.8
Murray et al.[b] (arthroscopy)	58	39	96	98	170	93	4.9
Wilson et al.[c] (arthroscopy)	52	48	91	90	141	91	4.7
Burkhart et al.[d] (arthroscopy)		42	95	100	141	84	4.6
Gartsman et al.[e] (arthroscopy)	61	30	84	90	149	78	4.3
Mean arthroscopic repair[f]	56	46	90	92	147	87	4.6
Mean open repair[f]	55	58	81	89	146	78	4.2
Mean mini-open repair[f]	58	35	87	93	150	86	4.5

[a]Kersey RC, Esch JC. Arthroscopic repair of complete, isolated rotator cuff tears. Presented at the Annual Meeting of the AANA Seattle, WA; 2000.
[b]Murray TF Jr, Lajtai G, Mileski RM, et al. Arthroscopic repair of medium to large full thickness rotator cuff tears: outcome at 2- to 6-year follow-up. *J Shoulder Elbow Surg.* 2002;11:19–24.
[c]Wilson F, Hinov V, Adams G. Arthroscopic repair of full thickness tears of the rotator cuff: 2- to 14-year follow-up. *Arthroscopy.* 2002;18:136–44.
[d]Burkhart SS, Danaceau SM, Pearce CE. Arthroscopic rotator cuff repair: analysis of results by tear size and by repair technique-margin convergence versus direct tendon-to-bone repair. *Arthroscopy.* 2001;17:905–12.
[e]Gartsman GM, Khan M, Hammerman SM. Arthroscopic repair of full-thickness tears of the rotator cuff. *J Bone Joint Surg Am.* 1998;80:832–40.
[f]Metcalf MH, Savoie FH III, Smith KL, et al. Meta-analysis of the surgical repair of rotator cuff tears. A comparison of arthroscopic and open techniques. Presented at AAOS annual meeting; 2003.
From Warner JJP, Iannotti JP, Flatow EL, eds. *Complex and Revision Problems in Shoulder Surgery.* 2nd ed. Philadelphia: JB Lippincott Co; 2005.

Intraoperatively, the surgeon should know proper suture and knot management, so that the surgery proceeds in a timely fashion. Excessive operative time may lead to excessive swelling, which can make visualization and therefore repair difficult. Additionally, it can increase swelling in the area of the trachea if the patient is in the lateral position, making extubation difficult.

For certainty of placement, the anchors should be visualized going into the bone rather than being placed transtendon.

■ CONCLUSION

Short-term studies have demonstrated good results for arthroscopic rotator cuff repairs. Long-term studies are still necessary to fully evaluate outcomes of arthroscopic rotator cuff repairs. Arthroscopy offers the advantages of a minimally invasive approach, smaller incisions, easy access to the glenohumeral joint for treatment of intra-articular disease, less tissue dissection, and less potential injury to the deltoid muscle. Arthroscopy has improved our diagnostic assessment and recognition of the major tear patterns of the rotator cuff that require different repair techniques. With the development of various arthroscopic suture-passing instruments and techniques, it is now possible for the surgeon to consistently accomplish a secure repair of the rotator cuff with relative ease.

■ REFERENCES

1. Galatz LM, Ball CM, Teefey SA, et al. Complete arthroscopic repair of large and massive rotator cuff tears: correlation of functional outcome with repair integrity. Presented at AAOS annual meeting; 2002.
2. Lo I, Burkhart SS. Current concepts in arthroscopic rotator cuff repair. *Am J Sports Med.* 2003;31:308–324.
3. Cofield RH. Surgical repair of chronic rotator cuff tears. A prospective long-term study. *J Bone Joint Surg Am.* 2001;83:71.
4. Tippett JW. Partial repair of rotator cuff tears greater than five centimeters. Presented at AANA annual meeting; 1998.
5. Cohen DB, et al. Inhibitory effects of traditional NSAIDS and Cyclooxygenase-2 inhibitors on rotator cuff tendon healing. Presented at the ORS; San Francisco, CA; 2004.
6. Ciccone WJ II, Miles JW III, Cheon SJ, et al. The use of the supraclavicular fossa portal in arthroscopic rotator cuff repair. *Arthroscopy.* 2000;16:399–402.
7. Zuckerman JD, Leblanc JM, Choueka J, et al. The effect of arm position and capsular release on rotator cuff repair. A biomechanical study. *J Bone Joint Surg Br.* 1991;73:402–405.
8. Warner JP, Krushell RJ, Masquelet A, et al. Anatomy and relationships of the suprascapular nerve: anatomical constraints to mobilization of the supraspinatus and infraspinatus muscles in the management of massive rotator-cuff tears. *J Bone Joint Surg Am.* 1992;74:36–45.
9. Tauro JC. Arthroscopic repair of large rotator cuff tears using the interval slide technique. *Arthroscopy.* 2004;20:13–21.
10. Lo IK, Burkhart SS. Arthroscopic repair of massive, contracted, immobile rotator cuff tears using single and double interval slides: technique and preliminary results. *Arthroscopy.* 2004;20: 22–33.
11. Bynum CK, Lee S, Mahar A, et al. Failure mode of suture anchors as a function of insertion depth. *AJSM.* 2005;33:1–5.
12. Mahar AT, Tucker BS, Upasani VV, et al. Increasing the insertion depth of suture anchors for rotator cuff repair does not improve biomechanical stability. *J Shoulder Elbow Surg.* 2005;14(6): 626–630.
13. Apreleva M, Ozbaydar M, Fitzgibbons PG, et al. Rotator cuff tears: the effect of the reconstruction method on three-dimensional repair site area. *Arthroscopy.* 2002;18:519–26.
14. Burkhart SS, Lo IKY. Double-row arthroscopic rotator cuff repair: re-establishing the footprint of the rotator cuff. *Arthroscopy.* 2003;19(9):1035–1042.
15. Costic RS, et al. Biomechanical properties of arthroscopic roator cuff repair: Single and double row of suture anchors. Presented at the 24th Annual AANA Meeting; Vancouver, BC; 2005.
16. Ma CB, Comerford L, Wilson J, et al. Biomechanical analysis of arthroscopic rotator cuff repairs-double row versus single row. Presented at the 51st meeting of the Orthopaedic Research Society; Washington, DC; 2005.
17. Tamborlane JW, Mahar A, Esch J, et al. Strength of double row arthroscopic rotator cuff repair in bovine cadaveric humerus model. Presented at the San Diego Shoulder Course; June 2005.
18. Harryman DT II, Mack LA, Wang KY, et al. Repairs of the rotator cuff. Correlation of functional results with integrity of the cuff. *J Bone Joint Surg Am.* 1991;73:982–989.
19. Kersey RC, Esch JC. Arthroscopic repair of complete, isolated rotator cuff tears. Presented at the Annual Meeting of the AANA Seattle; WA: 2000.
20. Kirkley A, Litchfield RB, Jackowski DM, et al. The use of the impingement test as a predictor of outcome following subacromial decompression for rotator cuff tendonosis. *Arthroscopy.* 2002; 18:8–15.
21. Metcalf MH, Savoie FH III, Smith KL, et al. Meta-analysis of the surgical repair of rotator cuff tears. A comparison of arthroscopic and open techniques. Presented at AAOS annual meeting; 2003.
22. Harryman DT II, Hettrich CM, Smith K, et al. A prospective multipractice investigation of patients with full-thickness rotator cuff tears. *J Bone Joint Surg Am.* 2003;85:690–696.
23. Warner JJ, Tetreault P, Lehtinen J, et al. Arthroscopic versus mini-open rotator cuff repair: a cohort comparison study. *Arthroscopy.* 2005;21:328–32.
24. Rebuzzi E, Coletti N, Schiavetti S, et al. Arthroscopic rotator cuff repair in patients older than 60 years. *Arthroscopy.* 2005;21: 48–54.
25. Galatz LM, Ball CM, Teefey SA, et al. The outcome and repair integrity of completely arthroscopically repaired large and massive rotator cuff tears. *J Bone Joint Surg Am.* 2004; 86:219–224.

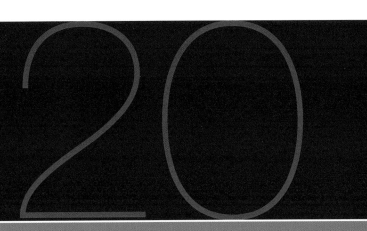

THERMAL TREATMENT, SUTURES, KNOTS, AND BONE ANCHORS

ROBERT A. PEDOWITZ, MD, PhD

■ KEY POINTS

- Arthroscopic methods for shoulder surgery offer superior visualization and open the door for complex procedures with minimal surgical morbidity, but technological advances do not necessarily guarantee better clinical results.
- The selection of a device for supplying heat to the shoulder should be driven by safety, ease, and cost-effectiveness. Depth of penetration of heat can affect risk of injury to adjacent neurologic structures and probably also plays a role in the ultimate healing and remodeling of the tissue.
- The outcome of thermal modification surgery depends upon tissue remodeling. The biological response requires either initial fibroblast viability or repopulation with viable cells and in either case, tissue vascularity is essential for ultimate biomechanical durability.
- Destruction of the capsule by thermal treatment can be extremely difficult to treat, and this condition may require tissue transfer or grafting procedures in order to reconstruct the deficient capsule.
- Axillary nerve injury is an infrequent but important complication that has been associated with thermal capsular shrinkage. The axillary nerve is vulnerable due to its proximity to the capsule in the axillary recess, and heat application should be well-controlled in this region to minimize the risk.
- The rotator cuff must be stabilized with suture material that is strong enough and lasts long enough to provide mechanical stability until adequate tissue healing is achieved.
- At a minimum, the arthroscopic surgeon must master one sliding knot and one non-sliding knot. Much of the security of arthroscopic knots is achieved by placement of

at least three reversed throws on reversed posts to back up the initial knot.

- Bio-absorbable anchors remain hard for many months or even years after surgery, making concerns about anchor migration paramount regardless of anchor material. Magnetic reasonance imaging (MRI) can be useful for radiolucent anchor localization and may help with surgical planning if a broken anchor is suspected.

Recent decades have seen tremendous advances in surgical options for shoulder disorders. Arthroscopic methods for shoulder stabilization, labral repair, biceps tendon management, and rotator cuff treatment offer superior visualization and open the door for complex procedures with minimal surgical morbidity; however, technological advances do not necessarily guarantee better clinical results. The purpose of this chapter is to review some of the recent information regarding fixation and stabilization technology for shoulder arthroscopy. This section will present basic biomechanical information that may be used by the arthroscopic surgeon for clinical application in the burgeoning field of minimally invasive shoulder surgery.

■ THERMAL TREATMENT

Thermal capsulorrhaphy went through a phase of rapid clinical adoption based upon early reports of clinical success, but subsequent clinical experience led to a marked decrease in clinical enthusiasm. This early excitement was fueled, in part, by frustration with existing surgical techniques and clinical results, the obvious ease and speed of arthroscopic application of thermal methods, and perhaps by premature commercial hype for general application of the technique. This initial enthusiasm, however, was followed by an equally rapid period of surgeon rejection, as reports of clinical failures and significant complications began to surface. At the moment, it is not clear whether thermal tissue modification will retain a specific niche in our orthopaedic armamentarium. Therefore, it makes sense to review some of the relevant basic science information regarding thermal tissue treatment.

■ BASIC SCIENCE CONSIDERATIONS

Heat can be applied in various ways to the shoulder joint, including the brutal though perhaps effective "hot poker" technique described many centuries ago. Current methods are more refined (we think); however, the basic mechanisms of thermal shrinkage are much more dependent upon the magnitude and speed of tissue temperature change than they are upon the method of inducing that change. Lasers devices and monopolar and bipolar radiofrequency probes are available for clinical application, but selection of a specific method should be driven by the safety, ease, and cost-effectiveness of the device in question. For example, the depth of penetration of heat can affect risk of injury to adjacent neurologic structures, and probably also plays a role in the ultimate healing and remodeling of the tissue because full-thickness tissue necrosis may obliterate the opportunity for revascularization and a fibroblastic response. Ciccone et al. (1) noted that human cadaveric glenohumeral capsular thickness varied from an average of 2.4 mm anteriorly to 2.8 mm in the inferior capsular pouch and to 2.2 mm posteriorly. Global shoulder capsule thickness ranged from 1.3 to 4.5 mm. Thinning of the capsule occurred from the labrum to the humerus, with a mean capsular thickness of 3.0 mm at the glenoid and 2.2 mm at the humeral insertion, and capsular thickness ranged from 2.8 to 3.2 mm in the regions in closest proximity to the axillary nerve.

Arnoczky and Aksan (2) and Gerber and Warner (3) have presented excellent reviews of the important basic science issues pertaining to tissue thermal modification. When collagenous tissue is heated, cross-links are broken and protein denaturation leads to a random, gel-like state. Upon cooling, the tissue shrinks along an axis parallel to the dominant direction of fiber orientation. Tissue shortening increases with increased temperature and time exposure to increased temperature; however, greater tissue heating is also associated with a greater loss of tissue stiffness. At tissue temperatures that are sufficient to induce collagen shortening, all cellular elements at the zone of thermal application are killed, with varying depth of necrosis based upon the magnitude and degree of thermal penetration. After thermal treatment, there is a phase of tissue fibroplasia; however,

there are no accepted opinions regarding the time frame for equilibration of mechanical properties or the ultimate degree of mechanical strength that is recovered by the treated tissues. It is also not clear whether the initial degree of shrinking has a major bearing on the long-term biologic and biomechanical status of the capsule. Associated changes in the afferent neurologic pathways may affect shoulder function after thermal treatment.

Naseef et al. (4) noted that bovine knee capsular shortening was both temperature and time dependent. No shrinkage occurred until temperature reached at least 60°C, and above that temperature, heat initiated a phase transition in the collagen triple helix leading to collagen fibril denaturation and gel formation. At or above 65°C, there was complete loss of the native fine fibrillar collagen structure and complete loss of birefringence. The loss of birefringence signifies unwinding of the collagen triple helix with loss of collagen fiber organization. The maximal observed shrinkage was about 50% of the original tissue length. Hayashi et al. (5) studied human cadaveric shoulder capsule and also found that shrinkage occurred at temperatures of 65°C and above. Shrinkage was time-dependent. Hyalinization of collagen and ultrastructural changes were observed when the tissue was subjected to temperatures of 65°C or greater (6) (Fig 20-1).

Wall et al. (7) examined the early mechanical properties of bovine tendon as a function of tissue shrinkage. They found that with greater thermal shrinkage, a higher proportion of collagen fibrils underwent a conformational change from an extended, crystalline, inextensible state to that of a contracted, random coil, extendible state. Baseline collagen packing and fiber orientation probably play a role in the amount of shrinkage that is possible. Of importance, greater tendon shrinkage was associated with a more extendible structure upon subsequent testing, and after about 15% to 20% shrinkage, extendibility may be so great that the tissue may stretch beyond its original length.

Vangsness et al. (8) found that collagen shortening in cadaveric human tendons started at a temperature just below

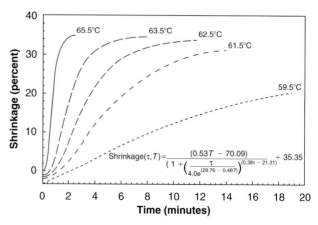

Fig 20-1. Demonstration of temperature/time dependence of tissue shrinkage.

70°C, but at temperatures greater than 80°C, the collagen physically fell apart. Histology revealed that the typical collagen striations and crimp patterns were not present in the heated tissue. Ten percent shortening of the patellar tendon was associated with a 70% loss of tensile load; however, these experiments did not address potential recovery of mechanical properties after tissue healing. In a separate study, Selecky et al. (9) used laser thermal treatment to induce 10% shortening of cadaveric glenohumeral ligaments. Early mechanical evaluation demonstrated higher ultimate strain and yield strain in the lased ligaments compared to control specimens, but no significant difference in ultimate stress, yield stress, or elastic modulus.

Several groups have examined acute changes in glenohumeral joint mechanics following thermal capsulloraphy, and it is clear that an acuter change in joint translation for a given load can be achieved by thermal treatment (10–17). It is less clear that these changes are maintained after a relevant period of biological remodeling and subsequent high-demand activity. Tibone et al. (16) found that thermal shrinkage of cadaveric anterior capsuloligamentous structures reduced anterior translation by 41% and 43% with 15 N and 20 N applied loads, respectively. Shrinkage reduced posterior translation of the shoulder by 35% and 36% with 15 N and 20 N loads, respectively.

Victoroff et al. (17) applied pancapsular radiofrequency heat to human cadaveric shoulders and noted a 37% reduction of joint volume. This amount of shrinkage was associated with significantly reduced anterior, posterior, and inferior translation at 45 degrees and 90 degrees of abduction with an applied 30 N load, with some effect of humeral rotation upon observed translation changes. Luke et al. (12) compared thermal shrinkage to standard open capsulorrhaphy, and found 30% and 50% decreases in joint volume, respectively. Karas et al. (11) found that intracapsular volume was reduced 19% by four capsulolabral tucks, compared to 33% by "paintbrush" thermal shrinkage and 41% reduction by a combination of both methods. The authors note that these acute volume reductions in a cadaveric model do not necessarily correlate with ultimate volume alterations after surgery and rehabilitation in patients.

Selecky and Tibone (14) demonstrated that thermal treatment of the rotator interval alone can significantly decrease both anterior and posterior translation with the arm abducted 30 degrees and in neutral rotation. The same author (13), however, found that arthroscopic thermal capsuloplasty of the posterior capsule alone did not significantly decrease posterior glenohumeral translation, suggesting that thermal treatment is probably not a reliable method of treatment for posterior shoulder instability.

The outcome of thermal modification surgery depends upon tissue remodeling after the thermal insult. This biological response requires either initial fibroblast viability or repopulation with viable cells and in either case, tissue vascularity is essential for ultimate biomechanical durability. Schaefer et al. (18) examined rabbit patellar tendon after laser-induced thermal shrinkage. There was a significant positive correlation between the depth of laser penetration and the percentage of tissue shrinkage. After 4 weeks, the laser treated tendon was significantly longer than the immediate post-laser length. After 8 weeks, the laser treated tendons were significantly longer than both the post-laser and the baseline, pre-laser length. At this time point, the tendons were less stiff, had an increase in cross sectional area and demonstrated fibroblastic responses that were all significantly different than the bilateral control tendon. Based upon these data, the authors recommended immobilization for a period of time following thermal shrinkage in order to prevent the collagen from "stretching out."

Schulz et al. (19) studied rabbit knee capsule up to 12 weeks after laser thermal treatment. They found decreased biomechanical properties immediately after treatment with recovery that was close to normal 12 weeks after treatment. Ultimate load, ultimate stiffness, and ultimate stress were all significantly decreased at 0 and 6 weeks post treatment but recovered by 12 weeks after thermal modification. Based upon these data, the authors recommended activity precautions particularly for the first 12 weeks after thermal tissue modification; however, these experiments were performed in rabbit knee capsule, and the pace and magnitude of biomechanical recovery may not extrapolate directly to human shoulder treatment. Lu et al. (20) compared a grid pattern (stripes of treatment separated by untouched tissue) to a paintbrush pattern (treatment of the entire surface area) to induce shrinkage in sheep knee joint capsule using a monopolar radiofrequency device, and followed the response up to 12 weeks after surgery. Although initial tissue shrinkage was similar, the grid pattern was associated with faster tissue healing and improved biomechanical recovery. These differences may be due to better preservation of cellular viability with the grid method, with associated improvement in biologic remodeling.

It is unclear from a review of the literature how much load can be tolerated by thermally modified tissue in the immediate postoperative period, and how that load changes during the healing phase. These basic questions are critical for establishment of postoperative rehabilitation protocols. Lack of optimal postoperative activity control (however that is defined), may explain some of our disappointing clinical results.

Clinical Results

Abrams (21) presented a thorough review of the important concerns related to clinical application of shoulder thermal capsulorrhaphy. Major issues include inconsistent tissue shrinkage, capsular ablation, over constraint, and neurologic complications. Anderson et al. (22) reported a 14% failure rate after thermal shoulder stabilization, with failure noted on average of 6 months after surgery. Failure was associated with multiple dislocations and prior surgery, with a tendency (inadequate statistical power) for decreased results with multidirectional instability and contact sports.

Early reports of thermal capsulorrhaphy tended to describe encouraging results. Lyons et al. (23) described a 12% unsatisfactory rate in 27 shoulders treated with laser shrinkage for multidirectional instability with a minimum follow-up of 2 years. Fitzgerald et al. (24) followed 30 of 33 consecutive multidirectional instability patients treated with radiofrequency thermal capsulorrhaphy in a military setting, with an average follow-up of 36 months. There were 3 excellent, 20 good, and 7 poor results, and 76% returned to active duty.

More recent reports tend to be more pessimistic about the clinical outcomes of thermal shrinkage. D'Alessandro et al. (25) followed 84 shoulders after thermal capsulorrhaphy performed with a monopolar radiofrequency device; most surgeries were done with the capsular "painting" technique. With an average follow-up of 38 months, the overall success rate was 63%, and the most favorable outcomes were seen in the patients with a traumatic dislocation. The worst outcomes were in patients with multidirectional instability with only a 55% success rate. Of note, these patients did well for the first year after which the clinical results declined. The most common complication was axillary nerve dysaethesias, seen in 14% of the patients. Patients who underwent open revision had a success rate of only 50% with the secondary procedure. In contrast, Savoie and Field (26) reported satisfactory results in 28 of 30 multidirectional instability patients treated with thermal capsulorrhaphy and adjunctive interval closure followed for an average of 26 months.

Levy et al. (27) noted a 36.1% failure rate at a mean follow-up of 40 months after laser capsular shrinkage, compared to a 23.7% failure rate at a mean follow-up of 23 months after shrinkage with a radiofrequency device. Noonan et al. (28) followed 59 patients after laser thermal treatment (some patients also had a suture anchor repair of a labral lesion); they observed a 4% failure rate after treatment of unidirectional instability compared to a 39% failure rate with multidirectional laxity. This report is concerning because unidirectional laxity is the best condition for treatment with current suture anchor and plication methods, whereas multidirectional laxity continues to be associated with the least predictable outcomes. In a very discouraging report, Miniaci and McBirnie (29) describe clinical failure in 9/19 instability patients treated by thermal techniques, with stiffness observed in 5 patients and neurologic symptoms noted in 4 patients.

Overhead athletes may be a specific subset of patients who may benefit from limited capsular shrinkage. Dugas and Andrews (30) reported on 170 overhead athletes treated by standard shoulder arthroscopy and debridement with addition of capsular shrinkage and a well-defined postoperative rehabilitation protocol. They noted that 81% returned to competition, and felt that, in their hands, addition of thermal capsular shrinkage resulted in about a 20% improvement in the rate of return to play. Follow-up averaged 30 months in this study. In a prior report by the same authors (31), however, heat shrinkage was not felt to improve the rate of return to

play in baseball players, although the authors thought that treatment of internal impingement with thermal capsulorrhaphy might decrease the re-injury rate after return to sports.

Another clinical situation that may be reasonable for application of thermal tissue modification involves augmentation in cases of labral repair, such as SLAP repair or Bankart repair (32–34) utilized thermal capsular treatment as an adjunct to suture anchor stabilization in 42 patients with recurrent traumatic anterior instability. Recurrent instability occurred in 3 patients (7%). Although these authors report that thermal treatment was an important adjunct, it should be emphasized that comparable results are achievable with suture anchor placation methods alone. The selection criteria for adjunctive thermal treatment are not well-defined, and use of this approach as during suture anchor stabilization is at best left to the subjective judgment of the surgeon at the time of arthroscopic evaluation of capsular laxity.

Complications

Failure of treatment is typically thought of as recurrent instability, with a subset of patients requiring a subsequent stabilization procedure. Destruction of the capsule by thermal treatment can be extremely difficult to treat, and this condition may require tissue transfer or grafting procedures to reconstruct the deficient capsule (35,36). McFarland et al. (37) did not observe a specific histologic feature that could explain capsular deficiency in 7 patients who underwent biopsy after failed thermal treatment. Denuded synovium was observed in all of these patients, and 71% had changes in the collagen including "hyalinization."

However, postoperative stiffness can also occur, and this complication may require additional surgical intervention as well (36). Gerber and Warner (3) believe that the major complication of thermal capsulorrhaphy is postoperative stiffness, with an incidence between 1% and 10% in their review.

Axillary nerve injury is an infrequent but important complication that has been associated with thermal capsular shrinkage (3,38,36). The axillary nerve is vulnerable due to its proximity to the capsule in the axillary recess, and heat application should be well-controlled in this region to minimize the risk of neurologic injury (39,40). McCarty et al. (41) noted a significant increase in temperature along the course of the axillary nerve in 11 of 15 cadaveric specimens during thermal application to the capsule; the branch to the teres minor appeared to be most vulnerable during this procedure. In a clinical follow-up study, however, shoulder proprioception returned to baseline when evaluated 6 months to 24 months after thermal treatment in twenty patients (42). These results suggest that normal neurologic function can be anticipated unless there is a catastrophic injury along the axillary nerve's ramifications.

■ SUTURES AND KNOTS

The overall strength of a repair construct, either arthroscopic or open, is defined by the "weakest link" in the chain. In the case of rotator cuff repair with suture anchors, the weak link may be the bone, anchor, eyelet, suture, knot, or rotator cuff tissue itself **(Table 20-1)**. A variety of suture materials is available for clinical application; some are resorbable, others permanent, some are monofilament and others braided. Endoscopic knot tying is technically demanding and has a relatively steep learning curve (43,44), and the

surgeon should select the appropriate knot for a given situation based upon the suture to be used, the mechanical requirements of the repair in question, and the surgeon's experience and personal preference (45). Suture materials have unique handling characteristics and knot tying behavior (46), which the surgeon must understand to create the strongest possible repair. In addition, super high strength sutures have been introduced recently and these materials have been very helpful for minimizing suture breakage during surgery. Extraordinarily high tensile load to failure does not, in and of itself, guarantee secure surgical knots (Table 20-1).

There are multiple basic science and clinical reports of suture anchor fixation for shoulder instability (47–61), and detailed clinical outcomes for these procedures will be discussed elsewhere in this book. The mechanical aspects of suture anchor stabilization tend to be more challenging with rotator cuff repair than with capsulolabral repair, due to obvious anatomic and age-related differences in bone and soft tissue quality. Although this section will focus upon issues specific to sutures and knots for arthroscopic rotator cuff repair, the principles are relevant to other surgical procedures as well.

Suture Materials

Rotator cuff repair sutures can be conveniently separated into monofilament or braided sutures and absorbable or nonabsorbable sutures **(Table 20-2)**. An advantage of monofilament suture is the relative ease of tissue passing, particularly with devices that utilize hollow needles, because the inherent stiffness of the suture facilitates "pushing" or "wheeling" the suture within the tool; however, that stiffness comes with a price in terms of knot tying, because knots don't lay

TABLE 20-1	Variables That Affect Construct Stability, Healing, and Recovery After Rotator Cuff Repair

Tissue	Anchor
Bone Quality	Geometry/Bone Interface Design
Tendon Quality	Material
Muscle Retraction	Eyelet Design
Fatty Infiltration	
Technique	**Suture**
Angle of Insertion	Size
Depth of Insertion	Material
Eyelet Orientation	Abrasion Resistance
Suture Handling	Handling Ability
Initial Loop Tension	Number of Sutures per Anchor
Initial Knot Security	Knot Configuration
Rehabilitation Protocol	**Postoperative Biology**

TABLE 20-2	Common Suture Materials for Rotator Cuff Repair[a] [1/2 life in brackets[b]]	
	Monofilament	**Braided**
Absorbable Sutures	Polyglecaprone (Monocryl) [2 wks]	Polyglycolic Acid (Dexon) [2 wks]
	Polyglyconate (Maxon) [3 wks]	Polyglactin (Vicryl) [2 wks]
	Polydioxanone (PDSII) [6 wks]	Poly(l-lactide/glycolide) (Panacryl) [~ 6 mo]
Nonabsorbable Sutures	Nylon (Dermalon, Ethilon)	Ethibond
	Polypropylene (Prolene)	Ticron
		Tevdek
		Fiberwire
		Ultra-high-molecular-weight polyethylene (ForceFiber, Ultrabraid, MaxBraid, Herculine)
Blended Suture	—	OrthoCord

[a]Trade name in parentheses.
[b]Adapted from Bourne RB, Bitar H, Andreae PR, et al. In-vivo comparison of four absorbable sutures: Vicryl, Dexon Plus, Maxon and PDS. *Can J Surg.* 1998;31(1):43–45.

down easily with monofilaments, and they have a greater tendency for knot slippage (62). In contrast, braided sutures tend to be quite pliable and are generally relatively strong compared to similar size monofilaments. The introduction of antegrade suture passing tools has made management of braided sutures a bit more convenient (these instruments grab the suture on a needle prior to tendon puncture).

Absorbable sutures are advantageous in the long term because they minimize residual knots that can cause mechanical impingement/irritation in the subacromial space. However, mechanical integrity must be maintained at least until the strength of the healing response is sufficient to withstand physiologic loads. Rapid hydrolysis can lead to an inflammatory response, which in some cases can be confused with an early postoperative infection. In the case of a rotator cuff repair, it is unlikely that the bone-tendon interface is particularly strong before 6 weeks, and it probably takes 12 weeks or more for the bone tendon junction to partially mature. Bourne et al. (63) noted significant mechanical degradation between 2 and 6 weeks after in-vivo placement with various resorbable suture materials (Table 20-2). Similar findings were noted by Greenwald et al. (64), with the important observation the PDS suture was only about 10% to 15% as strong after 6 weeks compared to time zero in-vivo. Boileau et al. (65) recently reported a 71% healing rate with arthroscopic cuff repair using predominantly PDS sutures, suggesting that sufficient early mechanical integrity was maintained for cuff healing using this resorbable suture construct. In another recent study, Boehm et al. (66) found no significant difference in clinical outcome or re-tear rate (about 20%) after cuff repair with either Ethibond or PDS suture. At this time, there is no clearly optimal suture material for rotator cuff repair. The basic principle, however, holds that we must stabilize the cuff with suture material that is strong enough and lasts long enough to provide mechanical stability until adequate tissue healing is achieved.

Obviously, sutures and knots must be at least a minimal strength to achieve sufficient security during tissue healing. Knots should be low profile and minimally bulky so to minimize the risk of mechanical impingement in the subacromial space and to minimize the inflammatory process induced by the knot itself. Babetty et al. (67) noted that addition of many throws to a suture knot added more foreign body to the wound and generated a greater amount of inflammation. This inflammatory response depended on the knot volume, suture size, and knot configuration.

Knot Types

Surgeon's knots, or square knots, are considered the standard for comparison with other knot configurations. Surgeon's knots are easy to create during open surgery, but are challenging during arthroscopic procedures because they can slip before placement of the initial back-up hitch, and after locked by that hitch, they are hard to advance. Surgeon's knots achieve mechanical equilibrium after placement of

two back-up square hitches, with little advantage to placement of further hitches (68,69) emphasized that loop security is just as important as knot security for the ultimate stability of the repair construct because loose loops give up slack with early load, thereby creating a gap at the bone-tendon interface. Loutzenheiser et al. (70) pointed out that knots perform differently for specific suture materials; therefore it is important to test knot strength for a given suture material before applying the material clinically.

Burkhart et al. (71) modeled an idealized 4 cm long rotator cuff, and thought that maximal load per suture would be about 60 N per suture (assuming a maximal supraspinatus muscle force of about 300 N and a three anchor repair/three suture repair). Adding more sutures per anchor theoretically decreases the load per suture (and increased the load on the suture anchor/bone interface). These calculations assume uniform tension (load sharing) for the sutures, which is probably not exactly achieved intra-operatively. In any event, most of the tested knot configurations with #1 polydioxanone (PDS) and #2 Ethibond failed between 35 N and 50 N, which is a range that would be of concern clinically. Reversed posts and reversed hitches were significantly more secure that stacked half hitches on a single post. It is possible to reverse the post of an arthroscopic knot by changing the tension on the limbs as the hitch is brought into the cannula (72,73); this concept allows the arthroscopic surgeon to "finesse" a flat knot during the last moment prior to cinching down the half hitch. This point is worth emphasis: **Hitches that mimic a square surgeon's knot will provide substantially better knot security than sequential half-hitches over a single post.**

Many arthroscopic knots are described and most work well as long as the surgeon adheres to the principles of knot security and loop security. Common knots include the Duncan loop, Roeder knot, Weston knot, Tennessee slider, Revo knot, and the SMC knot, to name a few **(Fig 20-2)**. At a minimum, the arthroscopic surgeon must master one sliding knot and one non-sliding knot. Much of the security of arthroscopic knots is achieved by placement of at least three reversed throws on reversed posts to back up the initial knot (74,75). This maneuver essentially locks the knot in position, and given that, it would seem that variations in initial knot selection are more relevant to discussions of loop security (i.e., the amount of slack that comes out of the initial knot with subsequent load), and the personal preference of the surgeon. Hughes et al. (76) noted that knots perform differently for different surgeons, and therefore there is no one best knot for all surgeons. Different suture materials also handle in unique ways (77–80), and surgeons should practice their knot-tying skills with various suture materials to establish what works best in their own hands.

Delimar (81) described a knot that is created by wrapping the post strand around a grasping instrument and then using the grasper to pull the non-post strand through the loops. DeBeer et al. (82) described "Nicky's" knot, which is a one-way slip knot (a "ratchet" knot) that can be pulled into the

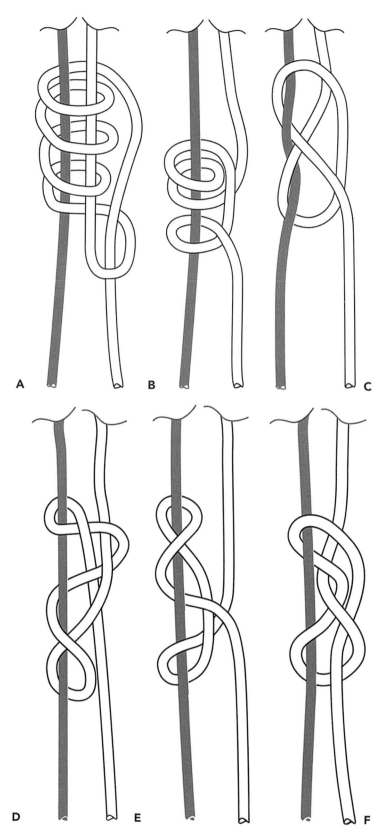

Fig 20-2. Commonly used arthroscopic knots: **(A)** Duncan loop; **(B)** Nicky's knot; **(C)** Tennessee slider; **(D)** Roeder knot; **(E)** SMC (Samsung Medical Center); **(F)** Weston knot. (Reprinted with permission from Burkhart SS, Lo KY, Brady PC. Creating a stable construct. In: *Burkhart's view of the shoulder: a cowboy's guide to advanced shoulder arthroscopy*. Philadelphia: Lippincott Williams & Wilkins; 2006:33–52).

joint but decreases the chance of the knot backing out during placement of subsequent throws. Field et al. (83) described a sliding-lockable knot that was modified from a technique for ligature of the bile duct during open cholecystectomy. Fleega and Sokkar (84) described the "Giant knot," which is a self-locking knot that they thought could be placed without a need for additional half hitches, although the authors did not provide compelling data to support that claim. Rolla and Surace (85) described the double-twist knot, which uses a loop of suture through the anchor eyelet that is used to create a complex twisted suture configuration that was stronger than the Snyder knot and the Tennessee slider.

Kim and Ha (86) described the SMC knot, which is a sliding-locking knot. Subsequently, Kim et al. (87) reported that the SMC knot was as strong as the Duncan loop and Tennessee slider, and comparable to the Revo knot (which is non-sliding). Ilahi et al. (88) found that the the SMC knot was less reliable in their hands, but noted that the Modified Revo knot was as durable as a hand tied square knot. They emphasized the importance of post switching for ultimate knot security. Lee et al. (89) noted that the French knot, which is a slight variation from the standard Duncan loop, had decreased tendency for knot slippage. They also noted that #1 PDS deformed more than #1 Ethibond prior to failure. The Tuckahoe knot was described by Wiley and Goradia (90), who thought that this locking slip knot was easy to learn and reproduce. We recently described the San Diego knot, which is a sliding-locking knot that decreases the tendency for suture slippage compared to standard arthroscopic knot configurations using ultra-high strength sutures (91,92).

Richmond (93) described an ultrasonic welding technique for polypropylene suture that eliminated the need for knot tying. The welded loops had less elongation than the knotted loops, but also lower mean loads to failure. Bonutti et al. (94) demonstrated comparable mechanical performance of an ultrasonically welded "suture seat" to fix the suture strands compared to standard knots using braided polyester suture. Recently we tested the ultrasonic weld technique in our lab using nylon suture, and have found strength and loop elongation comparable to #2 Ethibond suture (95). The in-vivo tissue performance and clinical outcomes of suture welding technology has yet to be determined.

Suture Configurations

Various suture configurations can be used to stabilize tendons during arthroscopic cuff repair. Some of these methods mimic open procedures, whereas several suture configurations have been developed specifically for arthroscopic techniques. Some techniques, such as lateral plate augmentation, are currently limited to an open approach. It hardly accomplishes much if a solid anchor, strong suture, and a good knot fail to hold the tendon because the suture rips through the tissue (96). This is a significant challenge for both open and arthroscopic techniques because the tendon is often atrophic and degenerative, which significantly compromises suture holding power.

Gerber et al. (97) examined the mechanical strength of nine different suture configurations for rotator cuff repair. They noted that simple sutures performed poorly, whereas the ultimate tensile strength was significantly increased by the modified Mason-Allen suture. This is a grasping suture that is created by three passes of the suture through the tendon, with a self-locking mechanism of the suture upon itself once tension is applied. They also noted marked strength improvement by augmentation of the laterally exiting trans-osseous sutures with a 2 mm plate. Subsequent in-vivo studies in sheep demonstrated superior results with the Mason-Allen suture and a lateral augmentation plate compared to simple trans-osseous sutures (98). Of note, strength of the bone-tendon interface was only 52% of normal at 3 months and 81% of normal at 6 months after surgery, which is relevant to clinical protocols for return to activity after rotator cuff surgery. The same research group examined an *arthroscopic* Mason-Allen technique, however, and found that this suture method did not increase the strength of repair compared to an arthroscopic mattress suture configuration (99).

We examined the mechanical characteristics of several suture anchor configurations compared to a bioabsorbable screw/washer (BioCuff Screw, Linvatec, Largo, FL) for rotator cuff repair using an immature bovine infraspinatus model (100). The bioabsorbable screw/washer performed well, but this fixation device is most suitable for open or mini-open repairs. Of note, the mattress suture performed better than simple sutures, but very early bone-tendon gap formation was observed consistently with the modified Mason-Allen stitch. This was thought to be related to the slack that was present in the complex loops of the suture within the tendon prior to cyclic load (initial suture slack may account for differences between experimental studies, referenced above). The observation emphasizes the importance of taking slack out of any grasping stitch prior to arthroscopic knot tying in order to minimize early bone-tendon gap formation with postoperative stress.

As a side note, we subsequently examined a different bioabsorbable screw-in fixation device (BioTwist, Linvatec, Largo, FL) using the same methodology used in our prior study (100); in this experiment the screw-in device failed completely very early during the cyclic load protocol (101). A key implant design difference is that the BioCuff Screw has an independent spiked washer that allows for better fixation of the cuff against bone, whereas the BioTwist is a single molded unit with a relatively small, smooth outer shelf for tissue fixation. Similar concerns regarding bioabsorbable screw fixation were voiced by Cummins et al. (102), who noted inferior clinical outcomes and biomechanical performance compared to suture anchor fixation. In contrast, Goradia et al. (103) reported essentially equivalent fixation of the rotator cuff using bioabsorbable tacks compared to suture anchor or trans-osseous fixation in cadaveric specimens. These observations serve to emphasize an important concept: **Implants should be tested using appropriate laboratory models prior to clinical application, and similar-looking implants are *not* necessarily equivalent in-vivo.**

Logically, a greater number of sutures in a cuff repair should decrease the load per suture/knot, and should improve the holding power of the construct (assuming the suture/tendon interface is the weak link). In addition, adding more points of fixation may also increase the surface contact area for tendon healing, which is the rationale for footprint restoration with a double row repair (104,105). Of course, more sutures carry some down sides in terms of the potential for devascularization and interference with the healing response, bulkiness and subsequent mechanical irritation in the subacromial space, and technical difficulty and expense of the procedure itself.

The massive cuff stitch, as described by Ma et al. (106) is created by placing an initial transverse simple loop across the tendon (this loop is tied) and then the suture from the anchor is positioned medial to that loop so that tension on the repair is borne (in part) by the initial transverse loop. This configuration was noted to be approximately four times stronger than a simple suture or horizontal mattress suture, and roughly equivalent to the load to failure of an openly placed modified Mason-Allen stitch. Scheibel and Habermeyer (107) described an arthroscopic modification of a Mason-Allen concept using both sutures from a double-loaded anchor; however, biomechanical data were not presented to demonstrate superiority of this technique.

Transosseous Fixation and Double Row Repair

It is not clear whether tendon stability and healing are better with suture anchor or bone tunnel fixation. St. Pierre et al. (108) found no histologic or mechanical differences between goat rotator cuffs that were fixed into a cancellous trough versus those fixed to the cortical surface, when the animals were followed 6 and 12 weeks after surgery. Rossouw et al. (109) noted better mechanical performance with transosseous fixation than with suture anchor fixation in cadaveric specimens. Of note, significant gap formation was noted with all repairs after a period of cyclic load (109). Lewis et al. (110) found that time zero fixation was better with bone tunnels than with suture anchors in sheep rotator cuff, however interface strength was not significantly different between 3 weeks and 12 weeks after repair. In contrast, Reed et al. (111) and Burkhart et al. (112) found better initial fixation strength with suture anchors than with bone tunnels in cadaveric models. Craft et al. (113) reported that, in general, cuff fixation strength was similar for suture anchor stabilization compared to classic transosseous suture technique.

Waltrip et al. (114) observed greater initial fixation strength with a double-layer repair technique using both suture anchors and transosseous sutures compared to a single-layer repair using either suture anchors or transosseous sutures alone. In this study, the "weak link" for all repair types was the bony attachment rather than the suture-tendon interface. On the other hand, Cummins and Murrell (96) found at revision cuff surgery that the failure mode tended to be suture pulling through tendon, as opposed to suture breakage or anchor migration in bone. So although there are good arguments for taking advantage of the stronger lateral humeral cortical bone and the vector of fixation with oblique bone tunnels, achieving this is a challenge with current arthroscopic approaches and the effect upon clinical outcome is yet to be determined.

Recently there has been more interest in achieving a double row repair construct with suture anchors alone, and at this point the data is not decisive. The contact area of double-row fixation is better than single-row fixation; however, the mechanical superiority of the double-row technique is questionable. Waltrip et al. (114) compared a double-row method (anchors and bone tunnels) to simple sutures or a modified Mason-Allen method, and found that the double row had significantly greater strength than the other groups. Demirhan et al. (115) also noted better strength with a combination of suture anchors and bone tunnel fixation compared to either method alone. We recently evaluated gap formation with cyclic load of a cuff repair performed with either single row (two anchors, four sutures), double row (four anchors, six sutures), or double row (four anchors, four sutures), and found no significant differences in mechanical characteristics between the three groups (116). Although the concept of footprint restoration is logical and appealing, we should balance our zeal for footprint coverage against the potential for overtension of the repair, especially with chronically retracted cuff tears that are not suitable for anatomic repositioning.

■ BONE ANCHORS

Suture anchors were developed about 20 years ago (117), and have become commonplace throughout orthopaedic surgery as a popular method for fixation of soft tissue to bone. These devices eliminate the anatomic and practical challenges associated with transosseous sutures (for example neurovascular anatomy on the far side) and the bulk associated with other forms of superficial fixation (such as screws, staples, and buttons). Suture anchors vary widely in terms of design, anchor and suture material composition, method of insertion, and implications in terms of subsequent treatment choices **(Table 20-3)**. Surgeons should be aware of these differences in order to select the ideal method of fixation for a given patient (113). This section will focus upon suture anchors for rotator cuff repair because this is a more challenging area of fixation than glenoid fixation for instability surgery, due to the bone quality and postoperative loads on the cuff repair construct. The biomechanics of superior labral repair likely fall between the two, due to the unusual loading characteristics of the biceps tendon/SLAP complex (118).

Barber et al. (119–123) performed a series of experimental studies looking at the fixation strength of various suture

TABLE 20-3	Relevant Issues for Selection of Suture Anchors

Anchor design
  Anchor size
 	
  Threaded/barbed/
    expandable/tack
  Specific thread design
  Partially or fully threaded
	Anchor material
	  Nonabsorbable (steel vs
	    titanium alloy)
	  Absorbable
	    Initial properties
	    Absorption characteristics

Eyelet
  Recessed or prominent
  Hard eyelet or suture
    eyelet
  Edge design
	Mechanical performance
	  Straight pullout
	  Cyclic load
	  Cortical versus cancellous
	    bone

Manufacturer suture
  selection
  Absorbable or
    nonabsorbable
  Standard or ultra
    high strength
	Revision issues
	  Retrievable or permanent
	  Bone loss/osteolysis
	  Impact on imaging (MRI)

Ergonomic issues (insertion simplicity)	Cost

MRI, magnetic resonance imaging.

anchors, and excellent reviews of this work are available in the literature. These extensive studies demonstrated differences in the pullout strength of different anchors and differences related to their placement in cortical versus cancellous bone (121). Larger diameter screw-in suture anchors are stronger than smaller anchors in cancellous bone (120,124), and newer non-screw anchors may be approaching the strength of screw-in designs (123).

Some suture anchors are designed for good purchase in cortical bone, but these anchors may not hold well in the softer cancellous bone of the humeral head (97). Tingart et al. (125) noted that the pullout strength of metallic suture anchors correlated with the bone mineral density of the proximal humerus, and recommended placement of the anchors into the proximal anterior part of the greater tuberosity in order to maximize fixation quality. Barber et al. (122, 123) concluded that newer bioabsorbable suture anchors were generally stronger than the loaded suture, and therefore the weak link should be the suture itself; however, the very recent introduction of ultra high strength sutures should temper that conclusion.

The majority of early suture anchor testing involved application of a single load to failure that was parallel to the angle of anchor insertion because this pullout force was thought to provide the worst case failure mechanism for the suture anchor (119,123). The rotator cuff is subjected to cyclic loads after surgical fixation, however, which significantly alters the mode of failure of suture anchor constructs (112,126). In addition, in-vivo loads are actually *oblique* to the angle of anchor insertion, which creates a cantilever force against the bone-anchor interface, in addition to bone-suture interactions that would be unappreciated with straight pullout studies **(Fig 20-3)**.

Burkhart (127) believes that anchor purchase is facilitated by insertion approximately 45 degrees off the vertical (the "Deadman's Angle"). Studies provide evidence in support (88) and against (128) the concept. We demonstrated recently that the depth of anchor insertion in bovine humerus had a significant effect upon the mode of construct failure because deep anchors failed by suture cutting through bone whereas proud anchors were associated with suture failure at the eyelet (129). In a separate study, anchor insertion

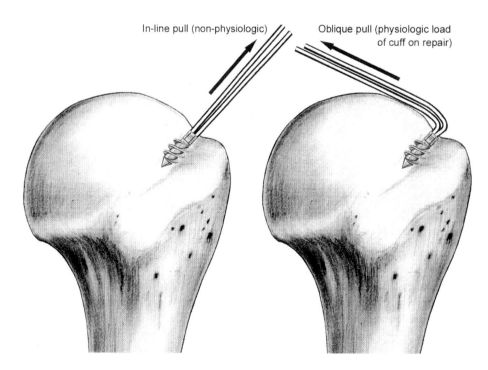

In-line pull (non-physiologic)   Oblique pull (physiologic load of cuff on repair)

Fig 20-3. Straight (in-line) pull versus oblique pull of suture relative to anchor.

depth affected construct displacement prior to failure in human cadaver bone (relatively osteoporotic material), with deep anchors rotating and translating toward the cortical surface (130). Although ultimate load was not affected by anchor depth, the observed anchor translation (on average 3 mm) would portend construct failure by early gap formation at the bone-tendon interface. Similar observations regarding early anchor migration in human osteoporotic bone are noted by other investigators as well (Steven W. Meyer, MD, New Jersey, *personal communication*, 2005). In fact, Wetzler et al. (131) demonstrated early anchor migration with cyclic load in anchors placed in cadaveric glenoids, and since glenoid bone stock is typically much better than greater tuberosity bone stock, it seems reasonable to expect more anchor displacement issues with rotator cuff repair than with instability reconstructions. These observations emphasize the importance of utilizing laboratory models that mimic the oblique, cyclic loads and the bone qualities that occur in patients who undergo rotator cuff repair. Recent studies suggest that the anchor eyelet is an important and vulnerable area for suture failure (125, 132,133). Rotation of eyelet relative to line of force affects suture fretting (132), and the line of suture load relative to anchor/eyelet also affects failure force (133). In general the failure mode differs between absorbable and nonabsorbable anchors; absorbable anchors tend to fail at the eyelet of the anchor (134), whereas nonabsorbable anchors tend to fail by anchor pullout, assuming the suture and/or tissue does not fail first. A knotless suture anchor that has a double-looped suture construct had increased failure strength compared to a standard barbed anchor (Mitek GII) in the glenoid margin (135–137); this device was intended for fixation of the labrum to the glenoid but was not designed for rotator cuff fixation (138).

Poly-L Lactic Acid (PLLA) anchors tend to be stronger than blended absorbable polymers (123), and bioabsorbable anchors can deform under static load over time (134). Failure of biodegradable screw-in anchors was noted at the eyelet compared to non-screw designs that tended to fail by bone pullout (120–124). A collagen-derived anchor was designed to hydrate after insertion, and this device was stronger 15 minutes after insertion compared to 2 minutes after insertion (139). Some authors believe that osseous integration may actually be *better* with certain absorbable polymers compare to titanium alloy suture anchors (140).

Implant absorption rates vary as a function of the specific bioabsorbable polymer, bulk, and perhaps the location of implantation (in terms of local blood flow). Some implants dissolve very quickly, for example the original Suretac (Acufex, Mansfield, MA) lost all of its fixation strength by four weeks after implantation (141–144). This loss of mechanical integrity may precede biological healing in capsulolabral and rotator cuff repairs. Bioabsorbable implants must retain strength during the critical period of tissue healing, but after healing occurs, other factors become more important, such as bone-implant reactions and the potential for implant breakage/loose body formation.

Although there are significant advantages of bioabsorbable fixation in terms of future patient management, these devices can also cause problems in terms of early material reactions (145), synovitis/osteolysis (146), and premature loss of mechanical integrity (147,148). Suture anchor failure and migration can lead to significant clinical morbidity related to damage of the articular surface, rotator cuff, the undersurface of the acromion (149–152), and can also be associated with infection (152,153). Some suture anchors are constructed from nonabsorbable radiolucent materials such as polyacetal; these anchors can perform well in vitro (154) and probably produce less tissue reaction than bioabsorbable materials. Surgeons should remember, however, that although plastic anchors may be invisible on plain radiographs, these anchors remain hard indefinitely. Migration of a plastic anchor can cause significant local tissue injury and if the anchor migrates, it can be quite challenging to localize for subsequent retrieval. Bioabsorbable anchors also remain hard for many months or even years after surgery, however, making concerns about anchor migration paramount regardless of anchor material. Magnetic resonance imaging can be useful for radiolucent anchor localization and may help with surgical planning (155) if a broken anchor is suspected.

■ REFERENCES

1. Ciccone WJ II, Hunt TJ, Lieber R, et al. Multiquadrant digital analysis of shoulder capsular thickness. *Arthroscopy.* 2000;16(5): 457–461.
2. Arnoczky SP, Aksan A. Thermal modification of connective tissues: basic science considerations and clinical implications. *J Am Acad Orthop Surg.* 2000;8:305–313.
3. Gerber A, Warner JP. Thermal capsulorrhaphy to treat shoulder instability. *Clin Orthop.* 2002;400:105–116.
4. Naseef GS, Foster TE, Trauner K, et al. The thermal properties of bovine joint capsule. *Am J Sports Med.* 1997;25(5):670–674.
5. Hayashi K, Thabit G, Massa KL, et al. The effect of thermal heating on the length and histological properties of the glenohumeral joint capsule. *Am J Sports Med.* 1997;25(1):107–112.
6. Hayashi K, Thabit G, Bogdanske JJ, et al. The effect of nonablative laser energy on the ultrastructure of joint capsular collagen. *Arthroscopy.* 1996;12(4):474–481.
7. Wall MS, Deng XH, Torzilli PA, et al. Thermal modification of collagen. *J Shoulder Elbow Surg.* 1999;8:339–344.
8. Vangsness CT, Mitchell W III, Nimni M, et al. Collagen shortening: an experimental approach with heat. *Clin Orthop.* 1997; 1(337):267–271.
9. Selecky MT, Vangsness CT, Liao WL, et al. The effects of laser-induced collagen shortening on the biomechanical properties of the inferior glenohumeral ligament complex. *Am J Sports Med.* 1999;27(2):168–172.
10. Gagey OJ, Boisrenoult P. Shoulder capsule shrinkage and consequences on shoulder movements. *Clin Orthop.* 2004;419: 218–222.
11. Karas SG, Creighton RA, DeMorat GJ. Glenohumeral volume reduction in arthroscopic shoulder reconstruction: a cadaveric analysis of suture placation and thermal capsulorrhaphy. *Arthroscopy.* 2004;20(2):179–184.
12. Luke TA, Rovner AD, Karas SG, et al. Volumetric changes in the shoulder capsular shift versus arthroscopic thermal capsular shrinkage: a cadaveric model. *J Shoulder Elbow Surg.* 2004;13:146–149.

13. Selecky MT, Tibone JE, Yang BY, et al. Glenohumeral joint translation after arthroscopic thermal capsuloplasty of the posterior capsule. *J Shoulder Elbow Surg.* 2003;12:242–246.

14. Selecky MT, Tibone JE, Yang BY, et al. Glenohumeral joint translation after arthroscopic thermal capsuloplasty of the rotator interval. *J Shoulder Elbow Surg.* 2003;12:139–143.

15. Tibone JE, McMahon PJ, Shrader TA, et al. Glenohumeral joint translation after arthroscopic, nonablative, thermal capsuloplasty with a laser. *Am J Sports Med.* 1998;26(4):495–498.

16. Tibone JE, Lee TQ, Black AD, et al. Glenohumeral translation after arthroscopic thermal capsuloplasty with a radiofrequency probe. *J Shoulder Elbow Surg.* 2000;9:514–518.

17. Victoroff BN, Deutsch A, Protomastro P, et al. The effect of radiofrequency thermal capsulorrhaphy on glenohumeral translation, rotation, and volume. *J Shoulder Elbow Surg.* 2004;13:138–145.

18. Schaefer SL, Ciarelli MJ, Arnoczky SP, et al. Tissue shrinkage with the Holmium:Yttrium aluminum garnet laser: a postoperative assessment of tissue length, stiffness, and structure. *Am J Sports Med.* 1997;25(6):841–848.

19. Schulz MM, Lee TQ, Sandusky MD, et al. The healing effects on biomechanical properties of joint capsular tissue treated with Ho:YAG laser: an in vivo rabbit study. *Arthroscopy.* 2001;17(4):342–347.

20. Lu Y, Hayashi K, Edwards RB, et al. The effect of monopolar radiofrequency treatment pattern on joint capsular healing. *Am J Sports Med.* 2000;28(5):711–719.

21. Abrams JS. Thermal capsulorrhaphy for instability of the shoulder: concerns and applications of the heat probe. *Instr Course Lect.* 2001;50:28–36.

22. Anderson K, Warren RF, Altchek DW, et al. Risk factors for early failure after thermal capsulorrhaphy. *Am J Sports Med.* 2002;30(1):103–107.

23. Lyons TR, Griffith PL, Savoie FH, et al. Laser-assisted capsulorrhaphy for multidirectional instability of the shoulder. *Arthroscopy.* 2001;17(1):25–30.

24. Fitzgerald BT, Watson BT, Lapoint JM. The use of thermal capsulorrhaphy in the treatment of multidirectional instability. *J Shoulder Elbow Surg.* 2002;11:108–113.

25. D'Alessandro DF, Bradley JP, Fleischli JE, et al. Prospective evaluation of thermal capsulorrhaphy for shoulder instability. *Am J Sports Med.* 2004;32(1):21–33.

26. Savoie FH, Field LD. Thermal versus suture treatment of symptomatic capsular laxity. *Clin Sports Med.* 2000;19(1):63–75.

27. Levy O, Wilson M, Williams H, et al. Thermal capsular shrinkage for shoulder instability: mid-term longitudinal outcome study. *J Bone Joint Surg Br.* 2001;83B:640–645.

28. Noonan TJ, Tokish JM, Briggs KK, et al. Laser-assisted thermal capsulorrhaphy. *Arthroscopy.* 2003;19(8):815–819.

29. Miniaci A, McBirnie J. Thermal capsular shrinkage for treatment of multidirectional instability of the shoulder. *J Bone Joint Surg Am.* 2003;85A(12):2283–2287.

30. Dugas JR, Andrews JR. Thermal capsular shrinkage in the throwing athlete. *Clin Sports Med.* 2002;21(4):771–776.

31. Levitz CL, Dugas J, Andrews JR. The use of arthroscopic thermal capsulorrhaphy to treat internal impingement in baseball players. *Arthroscopy.* 2001;17(6):573–577.

32. Fanton GS, Khan AM. Repair of athletic shoulder injuries: monopolar radiofrequency energy for arthroscopic treatment of shoulder instability in the athlete. *Orthop Clin North Am.* 2001;32(3):511–523.

33. Sekiya JK, Ong BC, Bradley JP. Thermal capsulorrhaphy for shoulder instability. *Instr Course Lect.* 2003;52:65–80.

34. Mishra DK, Fanton GS. Two-year outcome of arthroscopic bankart repair and electrothermal-assisted capsulorrhaphy for recurrent traumatic anterior shoulder instability. *Arthroscopy.* 2001;17(8):844–849.

35. Rath E, Richmond JC. Case report: capsular disruption as a complication of thermal alteration of the glenohumeral capsule. *Arthroscopy.* 2001;17(3):E10.

36. Wong KL, Williams GR. Complications of thermal capsulorrhaphy of the shoulder. *J Bone Joint Surg Am.* 2001;83A(Suppl 2):151–155.

37. McFarland EG, Kim TK, Banchasuek P, et al. Histologic evaluation of the shoulder capsule in normal shoulders, unstable shoulders, and after failed thermal capsulorrhaphy. *Am J Sports Med.* 2002;30(5):636–642.

38. Greis PE, Burks RT, Schickendantz MS, et al. Axillary nerve injury after thermal capsular shrinkage of the shoulder. *J Shoulder Elbow Surg.* 2001;10:231–235.

39. Gryler EC, Greis PE, Burks RT, et al. Axillary nerve temperatures during radiofrequency capsulorrhaphy of the shoulder. *Arthroscopy.* 2001;17(6):567–572.

40. Uno A, Bain GI, Mehta JA. Arthroscopic relationship of the axillary nerve to the shoulder joint capsule: an anatomic study. *J Shoulder Elbow Surg.* 1999;8:226–230.

41. McCarty EC, Warren RF, Deng XH, et al. Temperature along the axillary nerve during radiofrequency-induced thermal capsular shrinkage. *Am J Sports Med.* 2004;32(4):909–914.

42. Lephart SM, Myers JB, Bradley JP, et al. Shoulder proprioception and function following thermal capsulorrhaphy. *Arthroscopy.* 2002;18(7):770–778.

43. Young WW. Teaching surgical knot-tying skills. *Acad Med.* 1992;67(1):64.

44. Vossen C, Van Ballaer P, Shaw RW, et al. Effect of training on endoscopic intracorporeal knot tying. *Hum Reprod.* 1997;12(12):2658–2663.

45. Nottage WM, Lieurance RK. Arthroscopic knot tying techniques. *Arthroscopy.* 1999;15(5):515–521.

46. Zimmer CA, Thacker JG, Powell DM, et al. Influence of knot configuration and tying techniques on the mechanical performance of sutures. *J Emerg Med.* 1991;9:107–113.

47. Barber FA, Snyder SJ, Abrams JS, et al. Arthroscopic Bankart reconstruction with a bioabsorbable anchor. *J Shoulder Elbow Surg.* 2003;12:535–538.

48. Bhagia SM, Ali MS. Bankart operation for recurrent anterior dislocation of the shoulder using suture anchor. *Orthopedics.* 2000;23(6):589–591.

49. Cole BJ, Romeo AA. Arthroscopic shoulder stabilization with suture anchors: technique, technology, and pitfalls. *Clin Orthop.* 2001;390:17–30.

50. Dora C, Gerber C. Shoulder function after arthroscopic anterior stabilization of the glenohumeral joint using an absorbable tac. *J Shoulder Elbow Surg.* 2000;9:294–298.

51. Kandziora F, Bischof F, Herresthal J, et al. Arthroscopic labrum refixation for post-traumatic anterior shoulder instability: suture anchor versus transglenoid fixation technique. *Arthroscopy.* 2000;16(4):359–366.

52. Kartus J, Ejerhed L, Funck E, et al. Arthroscopic and open shoulder stabilization using absorbable implants: a clinical and radiographic comparison of two methods. *Knee Surg Sports Traumatol Arthrosc.* 1998;6:181–188.

53. Martin AAM, Rodriguez AH, Sebastian JJP, et al. Use of the suture anchor in modified open Bankart reconstruction. *Int Orthop.* 1998;22:312–315.

54. Norlin R. Use of Mitek anchoring for Bankart repair: a comparative, randomized, prospective study with traditional bone sutures. *J Shoulder Elbow Surg.* 1994;3:381–385.

55. Potzl W, Witt KA, Hackenberg L, et al. Results of suture anchor repair of anteroinferior shoulder instability: a prospective clinical study of 85 shoulders. *J Shoulder Elbow Surg.* 2003;12:322–326.

56. Richmond JC, Donaldson WR, Fu F, et al. Modification of the Bankart reconstruction with a suture anchor. *Am J Sports Med.* 1991;19(4):343–346.

57. Shall LM, Cawley PW. Soft tissue reconstruction in the shoulder: comparison of suture anchors, absorbable staples, and absorbable tacks. *Am J Sports Med.* 1994;22(5):715–718.

58. Silver MD, Daigneault JP. Symptomatic interarticular migration of glenoid suture anchors. *Arthroscopy.* 2000;16(1):102–105.

59. Tamai K, Higashi A, Tanabe T, et al. Recurrences after the open Bankart repair: a potential risk with use of suture anchors. *J Shoulder Elbow Surg*. 1999;8:37–41.

60. Warme WJ, Arciero RA, Savoie FH, et al. Nonabsorbable versus absorbable suture anchors for open Bankart repair. *Am J Sports Med*. 1999;27(6):742–746.

61. Wolf E. Arthroscopic capsulolabral repair using suture anchors. *Orthop Clin North Am*. 1993;24(1):59–69.

62. Mishra DK, Cannon D, Lucas DJ, et al. Elongation of arthroscopically tied knots. *Am J Sports Med*. 1997;25(1):113–117.

63. Bourne RB, Bitar H, Andreae PR, et al. In-vivo comparison of four absorbable sutures: Vicryl, Dexon Plus, Maxon and PDS. *Can J Surg*. 1998;31(1):43–45.

64. Greenwald D, Shumway S, Albear P, et al. Mechanical comparison of 10 suture materials before and after in vivo incubation. *J Surg Res*. 1994;56:372–377.

65. Boileau P, Brassart N, Watkinson DJ, et al. Arthroscopic repair of full-thickness tears of the supraspinatus: does the tendon really heal? *J Bone Joint Surg Am*. 2005;87A:1229–1240.

66. Boehm TD, Werner A, Radtke S, et al. The effect of suture materials and techniques on the outcome of repair of the rotator cuff: a prospective randomised study. *J Bone Joint Surg Br*. 2005;87(6):819–823.

67. Babetty Z, Sumer A, Altintas S, et al. Changes in knot-holding capacity of sliding knots in vivo and tissue reaction. *Arch Surg*. 1998;133:727–734.

68. Brown RP. Knotting techniques and suture materials. *Br J Surg*. 1992;79:399–400.

69. Burkhart SS, Wirth MA, Simonick M, et al. Loop security as a determinant of tissue fixation security. *Arthroscopy*. 1998;14(7):773–776.

70. Loutzenheiser TD, Harryman DT, Ziegler DW, et al. Optimizing arthroscopic knots using braided or monofilament suture. *Arthroscopy*. 1998;14(1):57–65.

71. Burkhart SS, Wirth MA, Simonick M, et al. Knot security in simple sliding knots and its relationship to rotator cuff repair: how secure must the knot be? *Arthroscopy*. 2000;16(2):202–207.

72. Chan KC, Burkhart SS. How to switch posts without rethreading when tying half-hitches. *Arthroscopy*. 1999;15(4):444–450.

73. Chan KC, Burkhart SS, Thiagarajan P, et al. Optimization of stacked half-hitch knots for arthroscopic surgery. *Arthroscopy*. 2001;17(7):752–759.

74. Loutzenheiser TD, Harryman DT, Yung SW, et al. Optimizing arthroscopic knots. *Arthroscopy*. 1995;11(2):199–206.

75. Lo IKY, Burkhart SS, Chan KC, et al. Arthroscopic knots: determining the optimal balance of loop security and knot security. *Arthroscopy*. 2004;20(5):489–502.

76. Hughes PJ, Hagan RP, Fischer AC, et al. The kinematics and kinetics of slipknots for arthroscopic Bankart repair. *Am J Sports Med*. 2001;29(6):738–745.

77. Shimi SM, Lirici M, Vander Velpen G, et al. Comparative study of the holding strength of slipknots using absorbable and nonabsorbable ligature materials. *Surg Endosc*. 1994;8:1285–1291.

78. Trimbos JB, Niggebrugge A, Trimbos R, et al. Knotting abilities of a new absorbable monofilament suture: poliglecaprone 25 (Monocryl). *Eur J Surg*. 1995;161:319–322.

79. Lieurance RK, Pflaster DS, Abbott D, et al. Failure characteristics of various arthroscopically tied knots. *Clin Orthop*. 2003;408:311–318.

80. Li X, King M, MacDonald P. Comparative study of knot performance and ease of manipulation of monofilament and braided sutures for arthroscopic applications. *Knee Surg Sports Traumatol Arthrosc*. 2004;12(5):448–452.

81. Delimar D. A secure arthroscopic knot. *Arthroscopy*. 1996;12(3):345–347.

82. De Beer JF, van Rooyen K, Boezaart AP. Nicky's Knot-a new slip knot for arthroscopic surgery. *Arthroscopy*. 1998;14(1): 109–110.

83. Field MH, Edwards TB, Savoie FH. Repair of athletic shoulder injuries. *Orthop Clin North Am*. 2001;32(3):525–526.

84. Fleega BA, Sokkar SH. The Giant Knot: a new one-way self-locking secured arthroscopic slip knot. *Arthroscopy*. 1999;15(4): 451–452.

85. Rolla PR, Surace MF. The double-twist knot: a new arthroscopic sliding knot. *Arthroscopy*. 2002;18(7):815–820.

86. Kim SH, Ha KI. The SMC Knot-a new slip knot with locking mechanism. *Arthroscopy*. 2000;16(5):563–565.

87. Kim SH, Ha KI, Kim SH, et al. Significance of the internal locking mechanism for loop security enhancement in the arthroscopic knot. *Arthroscopy*. 2001;17(8):850–855.

88. Ilahi OA, Younas SA, Alexander J, et al. Cyclic testing of arthroscopic knot security. *Arthroscopy*. 2004;20(1):62–68.

89. Lee TQ, Matsuura PA, Fogolin RP, et al. Arthroscopic suture tying: a comparison of knot types and suture materials. *Arthroscopy*. 2001;17(4):348–352.

90. Wiley WB, Goradia VK. The Tuckahoe Knot: a secure locking slip knot. *Arthroscopy*. 2004;20(5):556–559.

91. Abbi G. Espinoza L, Odell T, et al. Evaluation of 5 knots and 2 suture materials for arthroscopic rotator cuff repair: very strong sutures can still slip. *Arthroscopy*. 2006;22:38–43.

92. Mahar AT, Moezzi DM, Serra-Hsu F, et al. Comparison and performance characteristics of 3 different knots when tied with 2 suture materials used for shoulder arthroscopy. *Arthroscopy*. 2006:610–614.

93. Richmond JC. A comparison of ultrasonic suture welding and traditional knot tying. *Am J Sports Med*. 2001;29(3):297–299.

94. Bonutti PM, Cremens MJ, Gray TJ. Evaluation of a suture seat, a biodegradable suture fastener, to eliminate knot-tying in arthroscopic rotator cuff repair. *J Bone Joint Surg Am*. 2003;85A (Suppl 4):147–152.

95. Mahar A, Odell T, Thomas W, et al. A biomechanical analysis of a novel arthroscopic suture method compared to standard suture knots and materials for rotator cuff repair. Presented at the Annual Meeting of the Orthopaedic Research Society. Chicago, IL; March, 2006.

96. Cummins CA, Murrell GA. Mode of failure for rotator cuff repair with suture anchors identified at revision surgery. *J Shoulder Elbow Surg*. 2003;12(2):128–33.

97. Gerber C, Schneeberger AG, Beck M, et al. Mechanical strength of repairs of the rotator cuff. *J Bone Joint Surg Br*. 1994;76(3): 371–380.

98. Gerber C, Schneeberger AG, Perren SM, et al. Experimental rotator cuff repair. a preliminary study. *J Bone Joint Surg Am*. 1999;81(9):1281–1290.

99. Schneeberger AG, von Roll A, Kalberer F, et al. Mechanical strength of arthroscopic rotator cuff repair techniques: an in vitro study. *J Bone Joint Surg Am*. 2002;84A(12):2152–2160.

100. Petit CJ, Boswell R, Mahar A, et al. Biomechanical evaluation of a new technique for rotator cuff repair. *Am J Sports Med*. 2003; 31(6):849–853.

101. Lee S, Mahar A, Bynum K, et al. Biomechanical comparison of a bioabsorbable sutureless screw anchor versus suture anchor fixation for rotator cuff repair. *Arthroscopy*. 2005;21(1):43–47.

102. Cummins CA, Strickland S, Appleyard RC, et al. Rotator cuff repair with bioabsorbable screws: an in vivo and ex vivo investigation. *Arthroscopy*. 2003;19(3):239–248.

103. Goradia VK, Mullen DJ, Boucher HR, et al. Cyclic loading of rotator cuff repairs: a comparison of bioabsorbable tacks with metal suture anchors and transosseous sutures. *Arthroscopy*. 2001;17(4):360–364.

104. Burkhart SS, Lo IKY. Double-row arthroscopic rotator cuff repair: re-establishing the footprint of the rotator cuff. *Arthroscopy* 2003;19(9):1035–1042.

105. Millett, PJ, Mazzocca AD, Guanche CA. Mattress double anchor footprint repair: a novel, arthroscopic rotator cuff repair technique. *Arthroscopy*. 2004;20(8):875–879.

106. Ma CB, MacGillivray JD, Clabeaux J, et al. Biomechanical evaluation of arthroscopic rotator cuff stitches. *J Bone Joint Surg Am*. 2004;86A(6):1211–1216.

107. Scheibel MT, Habermeyer P. A modified Mason-Allen technique for rotator cuff repair using suture anchors. *Arthroscopy*. 2003; 19(3):330–333.

108. St. Pierre P, Olson EJ, Elliott JJ, et al. Tendon-healing to cortical bone compared with healing to a cancellous trough. *J Bone Joint Surg Am*. 1995;77A(12):1858–1866.

109. Rossouw DJ, McElroy BJ, Amis AA, et al. A biomechanical evaluation of suture anchors in repair of the rotator cuff. *J Bone Joint Surg Br*. 1997;79B:458–461.

110. Lewis CW, Schlegel TF, Hawkins RJ, et al. Comparison of tunnel suture and suture anchor methods as a function of time in a sheep model. *Biomed Sci Instrum*. 1999;35:403–408.

111. Reed SC, Glossop N, Ogilvie-Harris DJ. Full-thickness rotator cuff tears: a biomechanical comparison of suture versus bone anchor techniques. *Am J Sports Med*. 1996;24(1):46–48.

112. Burkhart SS, Pagan JLD, Wirth MA, et al. Cyclic loading of anchor-based rotator cuff repairs: confirmation of the tension overload phenomenon and comparison of suture anchor fixation with transosseous fixation. *Arthroscopy*. 1997;13(6):720–724.

113. Craft DV, Moseley JB, Cawley PW, et al. Fixation strength of rotator cuff repairs with suture anchors and the transosseous suture technique. *J Shoulder Elbow Surg*. 1996;5:32–40.

114. Waltrip RL, Zheng N, Dugas JR, et al. Rotator cuff repair. A biomechanical comparison of three techniques. *Am J Sports Med*. 2003;31(4):493–497.

115. Demirhan M, Atalar AC, Kilicoglu O. Primary fixation strength of rotator cuff repair techniques: a comparative study. *Arthroscopy*. 2003;19(6):572–576.

116. Tamborlane J, Oka R, Mahar A, et al. Strength of double row arthroscopic rotator cuff repair. Presented at the Annual Meeting of the Orthopaedic Research Society. Chicago, IL: March, 2006.

117. Goble EM, Somers WK, Clark R, et al. The development of suture anchors for use in soft tissue fixation to bone. *Am J Sports Med*. 1994;22(2):236–239.

118. DiRaimondo CA, Alexander JW, Noble PC, et al. A biomechanical comparison of repair techniques for type II SLAP lesions. *Am J Sports Med*. 2004;32(3):727–733.

119. Barber FA, Cawley P, Prudich JF. Suture anchor failure strength—an in vivo study. *Arthroscopy*. 1993;9(6):647–652.

120. Barber FA, Herbert MA, Click JN. The ultimate strength of suture anchors. *Arthroscopy*. 1995;11(1):21–28.

121. Barber FA, Feder SM, Burkhart SS, et al. The relationship of suture anchor failure and bone density to proximal humerus locations: a cadaveric study. *Arthroscopy*. 1997;13(3):340–345.

122. Barber FA, Herbert MA, Click JN. Internal fixation strength of suture anchors-update 1997. *Arthroscopy*. 1997;13(3):355–362.

123. Barber FA, Herbert MA. Suture anchors-update 1999. *Arthroscopy*. 1999;15(7):719–725.

124. Barber FA, Herbert MA, Click JN. Suture anchor strength revisited. *Arthroscopy*. 1996;12(1):32–38.

125. Tingart MJ, Apreleva M, Zurakowski D, et al. Pullout strength of suture anchors used in rotator cuff repair. *J Bone Joint Surg Am*. 2003;85A(11):2190–2198.

126. Rupp S, Georg T, Gauss C, et al. Fatigue testing of suture anchors. *Am J Sports Med*. 2002;30(2):239–247.

127. Burkhart SS. The deadman theory of suture anchors: observations along a south Texas fence line. *Arthroscopy*. 1995;11(1): 199–123.

128. Liporace FA, Bono CM, Caruso SA, et al. The mechanical effects of suture anchor insertion angle for rotator cuff repair. *Orthopedics*. 2002;25(4):399–402.

129. Bynum CK, Lee S, Mahar A, et al. Failure mode of suture anchors as a function of insertion depth. *Am J Sports Med*. 2005; 33(7):1030–4.

130. Mahar A, Tucker B, Upasani V, et al. Increasing the insertion depth of suture anchors for rotator cuff repair does not improve biomechanical stability. *Shoulder Elbow Surg*. 2005;14(6): 625–630.

131. Wetzler MJ, Bartolozzi AR, Gillespie MJ, et al. Fatigue properties of suture anchors in anterior shoulder reconstructions: Mitek GII. *Arthroscopy*. 1996;12(6):687–693.

132. Meyer DC, Nyffeler RW, Fucentese SF, et al. Failure of suture material at suture anchor eyelets. *Arthroscopy*. 2002;18(9):1013–1019.

133. Bardana DD, Burks RT, West JR, et al. The effect of suture anchor design and orientation on suture abrasion: an in vitro study. *Arthroscopy*. 2003;19(3):274–281.

134. Meyer DC, Fucentese SF, Ruffieux K, et al. Mechanical testing of absorbable suture anchors. *Arthroscopy*. 2003;19(2):188–193.

135. Thal R. A knotless suture anchor: technique for use in arthroscopic Bankart repair. *Arthroscopy*. 2001;17(2):213–218.

136. Thal R. A knotless suture anchor: design, function, and biomechanical testing. *Am J Sports Med*. 2001;29(5):646–649.

137. Thal R. Knotless suture anchor: arthroscopic repair without tying knots. *Clin Orthop*. 2001;390:42–51.

138. Yian E, Wang C, Millett PJ, et al. Arthroscopic repair of SLAP lesions with a bioknotless suture anchor. *Arthroscopy*. 2004;20(5): 547–551.

139. Stanford RE, Harrison J, Goldberg J, et al. A novel, resorbable suture anchor: pullout strength from the human cadaver greater tuberosity. *J Shoulder Elbow Surg*. 2001;10:286–291.

140. Kaab MJ, Rahn BA, Weiler A, et al. Osseous integration of poly-(L-co-D/L-Lactide) 70/30 and titanium suture anchors: an experimental study in sheep cancellous bone. *Injury*. 2002;33(Suppl 3): S-B-37–42.

141. Speer KP, Warren RF. Arthroscopic shoulder stabilization: a role for biodegradable materials. *Clin Orthop*. 1993;291:67–74.

142. Arciero RA, Taylor DC, Snyder RJ, et al. Arthroscopic bioabsorbable tack stabilization of initial anterior shoulder dislocations: a preliminary report. *Arthroscopy*. 1995;11(4):410–417.

143. Speer KP, Warren RF, Pagnani M, et al. An arthroscopic technique for anterior stabilization of the shoulder with a bioabsorbable tack. *J Bone Joint Surg Am*. 1996;78A(12):1801–1807.

144. Laurencin CT, Stephens S, Warren RF, et al. Arthroscopic Bankart repair using a degradable tack: a follow-up study using optimized indications. *Clin Orthop*. 1996;1(332):132–137.

145. Chow JCY, Gu Y. Material reaction to suture anchor. *Arthroscopy*. 2004;20(3):314–316.

146. Burkart A, Imhoff AB, Roscher E. Foreign-body reaction to the bioabsorbable Suretac device. *Arthroscopy*. 2000;16(1):91–95.

147. Demirhan M, Kilicoglu O, Akpinar S, et al. Time-dependent reduction in load to failure of wedge-type polyglyconate suture anchors. *Arthroscopy*. 2000;16(4):383–390.

148. Meyer DC, Gerber C. Failure of anterior shoulder instability repair caused by eyelet cutout of absorbable suture anchors. *Arthroscopy*. 2004;20(5):521–523.

149. Roth CA, Bartolozzi AR, Ciccotti MG, et al. Failure properties of suture anchors in the glenoid and the effects of cortical thickness. *Arthroscopy*. 1998;14(2):186–191.

150. Ekelund A. Cartilage injuries in the shoulder joint caused by migration of suture anchors or mini screw. *J Shoulder Elbow Surg*. 1998;7:537–539.

151. Rhee YG, Lee DH, Chun IH, et al. Glenohumeral arthropathy after arthroscopic anterior shoulder stabilization. *Arthroscopy*. 2004;20(4):402–406.

152. Karr TK, Schenck RC, Wirth MA, et al. Complications of metallic suture anchors in shoulder surgery: a report of 8 cases. *Arthroscopy*. 2001;17(1):31–37.

153. Ticker JB, Lippe RJ, Barkin DE, et al. Infected suture anchors in the shoulder. *Arthroscopy*. 1996;12(5):613–615.

154. Hecker AT, Hayhurst JO, Myers ER, et al. Pull-out strength of suture anchors for rotator cuff and Bankart lesion repairs. *Am J Sports Med*. 1993;21(6):874–879.

155. Magee T, Shapiro M, Hewell G, et al. Complications of rotator cuff surgery in which bioabsorbable anchors are used. *AJR*. 2003;181:1227–1231.

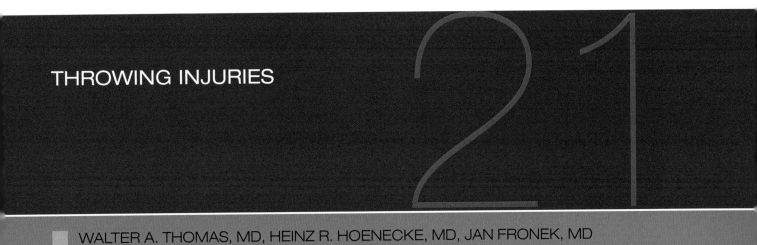

THROWING INJURIES

21

■ WALTER A. THOMAS, MD, HEINZ R. HOENECKE, MD, JAN FRONEK, MD

■ KEY POINTS

- Specific questions of an overhead athlete should include the type of throwing, level of competition, and any history of previous trauma, such as shoulder dislocation.
- Juvenile throwers are more likely to present with a physeal injury and symptoms related to laxity and associated labral tears, while older throwers tend to injure the rotator cuff.
- Sports-specific questions are helpful; for example, where in the pitching cycle symptoms are experienced; changes in throwing accuracy, velocity, or stamina; as well as changes in training regimens.
- Physical examination should include focus on general posture, position of the head and neck, and trunk, as well as on the affected arm.
- Various provocative tests are useful to help identify the source of pain in a throwing athlete. Overlap exists with the tests designed to identify biceps pathology because these may be positive in an athlete with labral pathology.
- Radiographs should include a throwers' series—an anteroposterior (AP) view in internal and external rotation, a scapular outlet view for assessment of acromion morphology, and an axillary lateral to identify bony Bankart lesions.
- Electrodiagnostic imaging may be warranted in cases where weakness is believed to be neurologic in nature. The electromyogram (EMG) can help differentiate mononeuropathies for more diffuse, widespread processes such as

radiculopathy or brachial plexopathy. The most common mononeuropathies in the throwing athlete are suprascapular and long thoracic neuopathies.
- Partial-thickness articular-sided tears of the supraspinatus and infraspinatus are well recognized in the throwing athlete. The etiology of these tears is multifactorial, but a significant component is believed to be tensile force overload during the deceleration phase in addition to the mechanical abrasion of internal impingement.
- How and when the injury occurred and what took place right before the injury is important in establishing a diagnosis when dealing with the elbow. Changes in throwing accuracy, velocity, stamina, and strength are important, as well as changes in training regimens.
- Ulnar nerve compressions may occur at various sites. Throwing athletes experience ulnar nerve irritation from traction injuries, compression from adjacent structures, or friction due to subluxation of the ulnar nerve. Complaints are typically paresthesia of the small and ring finger during or after the throwing motion.

The throwing athlete places far greater stress on his or her shoulder and elbow than the average population and consequently injuries commonly occur. The pathoanatomy and biomechanics of the throwing motion is complex and our understanding of injury mechanism and etiology continues to evolve. Specific injuries can occur in isolation and also as part of a spectrum of interrelated pathology, making a comprehensive understanding of pathoanatomy critical for rapid diagnosis and effective treatment.

■ THE THROWING MOTION

The throwing motion has been divided into six phases (Fig 21-1):

Phase I: The wind up
Phase II: Early cocking
Phase III: Late cocking
Phase IV: Acceleration
Phase V: Deceleration
Phase VI: Follow through

Phase I is the initial wind up. This represents the coiling phase in which potential energy is developed. During this phase, the center of gravity is raised and no appreciable stress is placed on the shoulder and elbow.

Phase II is early cocking. During this phase, the arm is positioned in preparation for maximal external rotation which occurs with stride initiation as the arm is positioned in 90 degrees of abduction. Early deltoid and late rotator cuff activity is show by electromyogram (EMG).

Phase III is late cocking. This phase initiates with the foot plant. It is also the point of maximal external rotation of the shoulder, approaching 170 degrees. The shoulder is positioned in abduction and external rotation, and the humeral head translates posteriorly on the glenoid. High rotator cuff activity is seen in supraspinatus, infraspinatus, and teres minor during the middle of this phase, while the subscapularis fires later coinciding with the opening of the torso. Maximal stress to the anterior restraints of the shoulder occurs and the shear forces approach 400 N, with the compensatory rotator cuff forces reaching 650 N.

Phase IV is the acceleration phase. The shoulder delivers the ball to the release point during this phase. Peak rotational velocity can approach 7,000 per second. The shoulder rapidly internally rotates and returns the humeral head to a neutral position; this occurs with minimal load to the glenohumeral joint during energy transfer.

Phase V is the deceleration phase. This is the most forceful phase of the throwing cycle. Deceleration occurs from the point of ball release. It occurs with substantial eccentric contraction of the rotator cuff to slow the arm. Posterior capsule stress is at a maximum. Joint loads are as follows: posterior shear 400 N, inferior shear 300 N, and compressive force approaching 1,000 N.

Phase VI is the follow through. This phase is a time of muscle rebalancing with stress still present in the posterior capsule. The entire throwing cycle spans approximately 2 seconds.

■ THE SHOULDER

History

An evaluation of the overhead athlete begins with a thorough history. The specific questions should address the patient's history regarding handedness, type of throwing, level of competition, and any history of previous trauma (such as previous shoulder dislocation). The age of the athlete is particularly important, because the juvenile athletes may present with a physeal injury; the younger throwers are more likely to have symptoms related to laxity and associated labral tears while the older throwers tend to injure their rotator cuff.

The history should include questions concerning the mechanism of onset, the duration of symptoms, aggravating and alleviating factors, and any previous treatments and their effectiveness. Is pain the major concern? Does the patient experience weakness or fatigue? Does the patient have a feeling of generalized looseness or tightness in his or her shoulder? Are there any episodes of catching or popping that may be indicative of labral pathology or instability? Understanding the patient's specific concern is important, as is understanding his or her short- and long-term goals. Are these goals realistic, given the patient's age, previous level of performance, severity of injury, and other medical factors?

Sport-specific questions will often be helpful. Where in the pitching cycle do they experience symptoms? Pain occurring during the cocking phase may be related to internal impingement, labral pathology, or instability (usually anterior or antero-inferior). Pain occurring during deceleration may be suggestive of cuff pathology, or posterior subluxation. Do the symptoms occur early in the game or during the later innings? What is the specific location of the symptoms? Does the patient experience a dead arm, can he or she continue throwing, and is there associated paresthesia? Does the thrower experience signs or symptoms of fatigue?

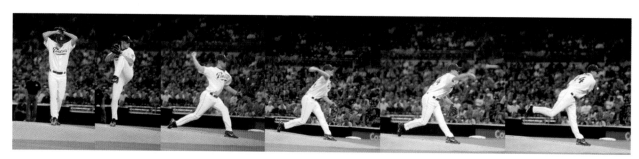

Fig 21-1. Phases of the throwing motion: I. Wind up; II. Early Cocking; III. Late Cocking; IV. Acceleration; V. Deceleration; VI. Follow through.

Physical Examination

The physical examination begins with inspection; focus should be not only on the affected arm, but also on the athlete's general posture and the position of the head, neck, and trunk. Muscle contour and balance should be observed with attention given to subtle signs of asymmetry or atrophy, which may help focus the examination. When viewing the back of the patient, the examiner can appreciate a scapular asymmetric depression, protraction, or winging of the scapula, which may be present as an isolated finding or in combination with an intra-articular problem.

Range of motion should be observed, both glenohumeral and scapulothoracic contributions. Scapulothoracic motion should be smooth and pain free; comparison with the contralateral shoulder should be noted for symmetry of position and motion; crepitus may be suggestive of inflammatory bursitis. Total rotation of the throwing shoulder should be recorded and compared with the nonthrowing shoulder. It is common for throwing athletes to have increased external rotation in abduction and decreased internal rotation in abduction in their throwing shoulder; however, the arc of total motion should be similar.

Palpation for pain is helpful to identify specific areas of injury and can distinguish between various types of pathology that can often present with similar symptoms. Specific focus should be on the muscles of the rotator cuff, long head of the biceps, conjoined tendon, anterior and posterior capsule, acromioclavicular (AC) joint, and suprascapular notch.

Strength testing of the rotator cuff muscles and the periscapular stabilizing muscles should be performed. The supraspinatus is tested with resisted forward elevation with the arms in 30 degrees of abduction with the thumbs pointed to the floor. The infraspinatus and teres minor are tested with resisted external rotation with the arms adducted at the side. The subscapularis is tested with the lift-off test or the belly press test. When weakness or muscle pain is present, the testing should be repeated with the scapula actively retracted and depressed. If strength improves or pain decreases, this represents a positive scapular retraction test consistent with scapular dyskenesis.

Laxity and translation of the glenohumeral joint should be assessed in the anterior, posterior, and inferior directions. This should be performed with the arm in both internal and external rotation and with the athlete sitting and also lying supine. Increased laxity is an expected finding in the dominant arm and is not necessarily pathologic, but laxity associated with discomfort or with reproducing the thrower's symptoms is likely to be pathologic instability.

Various provocative tests are useful to help identify the source of pain in a throwing athlete. Hawkins and Neers tests may be useful for identifying impingement. The apprehension and relocation test may be useful when they elicit discomfort or apprehension, but are less helpful when they are associated with pain. Various tests have been described for assessing labral pathology; recent reports reveal limited sensitivity and specificity with the active compression test, the anterior slide test, and the compression rotation test (1–3). Overlap exists with tests designed to identify biceps pathology because these may be positive in an athlete with labral pathology.

Ancillary Tests

Radiographs are useful in evaluating bony anatomy and include a throwers' series, an anteroposterior (AP) view in internal and external rotation (internal rotation view is helpful to assess Hill-Sachs lesions), a scapular outlet view for assessment of acromion morphology, and an axillary lateral to identify bony Bankart lesions **(Fig 21-2A)**. Additional views and MRIs may be ordered when physical examination indicates that they would be useful **(Figs 21-2B** and **C**, and **Figs 21-3–5)**.

Computed tomography (CT) scanning has limited applications, but may be useful in evaluation of glenoid bone loss. Ultrasound can be helpful for rotator cuff tendinopathy, but is of limited application because it is very operator dependent and few institutions have the experience necessary for consistent interpretation.

Magnetic resonance imaging (MRI) may be helpful in certain situations for establishing a specific diagnosis. Magnetic resonance arthrography (MRA) can also be a useful adjuvant diagnostic tool; dilute gadolinium is injected into the shoulder and gives more anatomic detail in athletes with suspected labral lesions or potentially other instability-related pathology [humeral avulsion of the glenohumeral ligament (HAGL lesion), anterior labor-ligamentous periosteal sleeve avulsion (ALPSA lesion), and glenoid labral articular disruption (GLAD lesion)].

Electrodiagnostic testing may be warranted in cases when weakness is believed to be neurologic in nature. The EMG can help differentiate mononeuropathies for more diffuse, widespread processes such as radiculopathy or brachial plexopathy. The most common mononeuropathies seen in the throwing athlete are suprascapular and long thoracic neuropathies.

The Shoulder

The Thrower's "Dead Arm"

In the overhead athletes, the "dead arm" syndrome has long been recognized as a potentially career-ending condition. Historically, the specific pathology has been poorly understood; only recently has greater insight been achieved into etiology; however, treatment remains controversial.

Athletes often complain of pain during the late cocking and acceleration phase, as the arm moves forward. The arm then "goes dead" and the athlete has loss of velocity and control; this, along with pain, prevents continued throwing and results in compromised performance. Various conditions have been observed, and debate concerning which model of pathology is most accurate is further complicated by the fact that

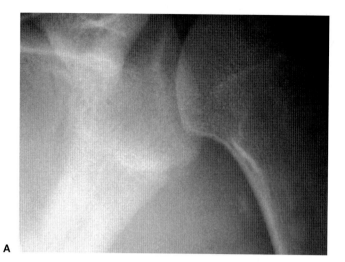

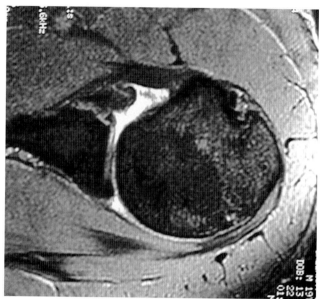

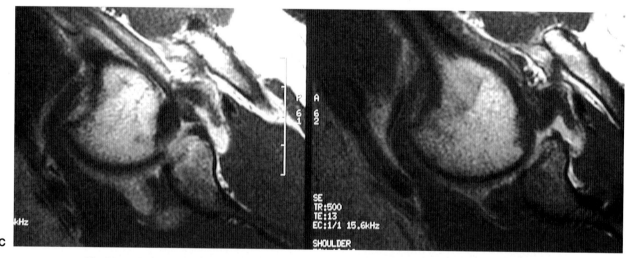

Fig 21-2. A: AP radiograph showing the periarticular bone avulsed from the anterior-inferior glenoid resulting in a Bankart lesion. **B:** MRI scan of the same patient documenting the bony Bankart defect. **C:** MRI scan obtained while the patient's arm was in the Abduction and External Rotation (ABER) position showing the bony Bankart, anteroinferior subluxation, and Hill-Sachs defect on the postero-lateral aspect of the humeral head.

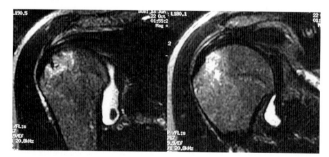

Fig 21-3. MRI after anterior dislocation of the shoulder, documenting the proximal humeral Hill-Sachs lesion with subchondral bleeding and intra-articular loose body.

these conditions may be present in asymptomatic throwing athletes, thus suggesting a spectrum of variation, often with no clear distinction from the adaptive to the pathologic changes.

Internal Impingement

Internal impingement is a topic that has been controversial and also can be very confusing. Originally described by Walch et al. (4) as naturally occurring impingement between the posterior superior rotator cuff and the glenoid rim with arm in position of abduction and external rotation. Others noted this same occurrence in asymptomatic throwing athletes.

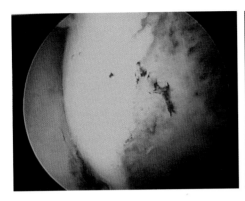
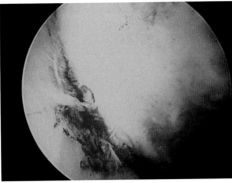

Fig 21-4. Arthroscopic view via posterior portal of the patient's right shoulder revealing the Hill-Sachs defect (A) and with external rotation, the defect is engaged with the anterior glenoid rim (B).

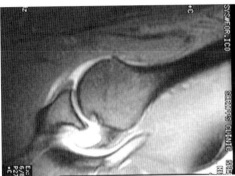
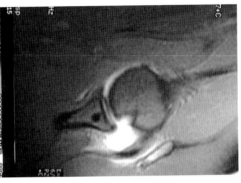

Fig 21-5. MRI study, two adjacent images demonstrate the Hill-Sachs defect seen in abduction and external rotation.

Jobe (5) later popularized the term as a pathologic condition occurring in overhead athletes leading to throwing injury. In this model, anterior capsular insufficiency was the inciting occurrence that subsequently led to further disability and the "dead arm." Loss of integrity of the capsule is a direct result of hyperangulation of the throwing arm. The symptoms are exacerbated by the loss of the posterior rollback, which leads to anterior translation and results in greater internal impingement posteriorly. If untreated, it may lead to posterior labral tears, Superior Labrum Anterior and Posterior (SLAP) lesion due to peel-back, and partial thickness articular-sided rotator cuff tears. Treatment is focused at correcting the underlying instability and treating any additional pathology. Reports of capsulolabral reconstruction have shown some success in allowing pitchers to return to their previous level of competition (6,7).

The Morgan-Burkhart model (7a, 7b) suggests that the posterior capsular contracture is the inciting occurrence in the cascade of disability and injury. Posterior capsule tightness has long been recognized as a component of the throwing shoulder (8–12); at what point this becomes pathologic has been less well delineated. As the shoulder develops progressively worsening posterior contracture, the glenohumeral contact point is shifted further posterior and superior when the shoulder is in abduction and external rotation. A relative redundancy of the anterior capsule is observed due to the tightening of the posterior capsular structures—this is what has been observed as anterior capsular stretching in the Jobe model. As the thrower attempts to reach his or her set point

for throwing, hyperangulation and hyperexternal rotation forces cause tensile overload of the rotator cuff leading to partial tears; additionally, a dynamic peel-back phenomenon generates SLAP lesion of the labrum. Glenohumeral Internal Rotation Deficit (GIRD) is defined as the loss in degrees of internal rotation as compared with the contralateral shoulder, with the arm positioned in 90 degrees of abduction and external rotation. Burkhart et al. (13) believe that symptomatic GIRD is present when the deficit is 25 degrees or greater. Treatment focuses on stretching the posterior capsule with the use of "sleeper stretches." Although the nonsurgical treatment is usually successful, those who do not respond to relative rest, stretching, and strengthening programs may be candidates for arthroscopy, debridement, and occasional posterior capsulotomy, which is often performed with treatment of other coexistent pathology.

Labral pathology is well recognized as a component of the disabled throwing shoulder. The acronym SLAP describes the location of pathology, Superior Labrum Anterior and Posterior. It was first observed by Andrews (13a) in throwing athletes and was later named by Snyder. Multiple subtypes have been described. Some believe that SLAP lesion is the most common pathologic entity associated with the throwers "dead arm" (9,13,14). If left untreated, athletes typically cannot return to throwing. Debate has existed concerning the mechanism of injury during throwing. Fleisig et al. (15) and Andrews et al. (16) proposed a deceleration mechanism of injury, as the bicep contracts to slow down the arm in follow through. This tensile load acts to pull the biceps and superior labral complex from the bone. Burkhart et al. (13) support an acceleration mechanism of injury. As the shoulder is positioned in abduction and external rotation coinciding with late cocking and acceleration, the labrum is peeled off the glenoid rim. Kuhn et al. (17) performed experimental comparison of the two mechanisms in a cadaveric model; their results support the acceleration mechanism. Treatment is dictated by the stability of the biceps/labral complex. If complex is unstable, a repair is necessary; if stable, a débridement of damaged tissue may be adequate. Surgical repair has been very successful in allowing return to throwing, some reports approaching 90% (14).

Rotator Cuff Tears

The repairs of full-thickness cuff tears has been associated with low success rate (17a). Partial-thickness articular-sided tears of the supraspinatus and infraspinatus are well recognized in the throwing athlete. The etiology of these tears is multifactorial, but a significant component is believed to be tensile force overload during the deceleration phase in addition to the mechanical abrasion of internal impingement. Various grading systems have been described. The thickness of involvement can be determined arthroscopically by direct examination and by the amount of exposed footprint at the insertion site of the tendon itself. Tears <50% thickness often only require debridement and attention to other coexistent pathology. For the few tears that are >50%, consideration may be given to repair of the tendon; this can be performed insitu or after completion of the tear to full thickness **(Figs 21-6–9)**.

Biceps Lesions

Biceps pathology is a contributing factor to shoulder pain in the overhead-throwing athlete. The function of the biceps tendon in the shoulder is controversial and treatment options

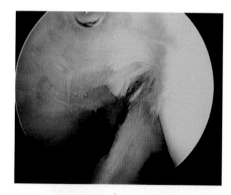
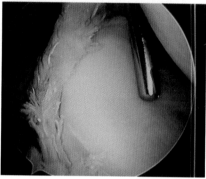

Fig 21-7. Arthroscopic views from posterior portal of the right shoulder shows the partial tear of articular surface of rotator cuff. Biceps tendon and glenoid labrum tears often seen in association with the undersurface rotator cuff tearing.

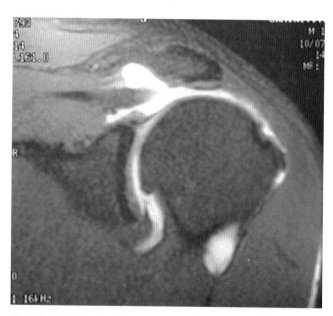

Fig 21-8. MRI arthrogram showing the massive rotator cuff tear with retraction of the tendon to the level of the glenoid.

continue to evolve. Pathology may occur at the junction with the labrum, the articular portion, directly adjacent to the transverse ligament, in the biceps groove, and distally at the musculotendinous junction. Pain with direct palpation over the proximal tendon as well as various provocative maneuvers (Speed's test—pain with resisted forward elevation of the arm

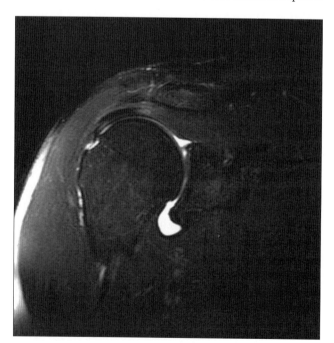

Fig 21-6. Partial-thickness rotator cuff tear.

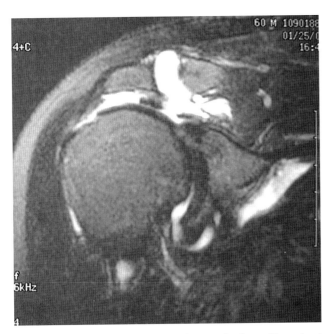

Fig 21-9. MRI arthrogram revealing the massive tear with contrast migrating into the acromioclavicular joint, creating the geyser sign.

in supination, and Yergason sign—pain with resisted forearm supination with the arm at the side and the elbow flexed 90 degrees) are helpful in identifying the biceps as a contributing factor to disability. MRI may be helpful, particularly when augmented with intra-articular contrast. Cortisone injections may also be used to help localize pathology, but injection adjacent to the tendon is often difficult and injection within the substance of the tendon may contribute to further failure. Surgical treatment options remain controversial; although the minor lesions and fraying can be debrided, the more severe lesions may require tenodesis or, in older patients, the tenotomy may offer a satisfactory solution.

Coracoid Impingement

Coracoid impingement occurs when the subscapularis tendon is compressed between the lesser tuberosity and the tip of the coracoid process. Patients will present with anterior shoulder pain and findings on exam that may mimic subacromial impingement. Pain may be elicited with passive flexion of the arm in an adducted and internally rotated position or with direct palpation over the conjoined tendon. A diagnostic and therapeutic injection in the subcoracoid space can be effective in confirming the diagnosis as well as treating the condition. A coracohumeral interval <6 mm (normally 11 mm) is helpful in confirming the diagnosis, but is not pathonomonic. If conservative measures fail to provide adequate relief, a coracoplasty may be performed; both open and arthroscopic techniques have been described.

Acromioclavicular Joint Injuries

AC joint injuries are relatively uncommon in the throwing athlete because physical contact is usually at a low to moderate

level. Less-severe injuries, grade I and II AC joint separation, are treated nonoperatively with good success. Controversy exists for the grade III lesions; randomized trials have demonstrated good results with nonoperative treatment, but despite this, some advocate early surgical reconstruction. Those who support early surgical intervention cite altered throwing mechanics and early fatigue resulting in decreased performance as reason for surgical intervention. Specific literature in throwing athletes is scant, with most recommendations reflecting personal opinion and preference. McFarland et al. (18) performed a survey of physicians of professional baseball teams; only 32 lesions had been seen by this group. In response to the theoretical treatment of a starting pitcher with a preseason grade III AC injury, 69% reported that they would treat the injury conservatively. The surgical treatment of choice in this survey was a Weaver-Dunn reconstruction with high-strength suture or graft between the clavicle and coracoid.

Bennett Lesion

A Bennett lesion is an exostosis of the posterior inferior glenoid; it is seen in throwing athletes and was first described by one of the first baseball physicians, G.E. Bennett (19). The exact cause of this lesion is not known; possible theories include traction due to the pull of the triceps tendon or possibly posterior capsule. Others have suggested that contact from the posterior superior labrum and humeral head may be responsible (19a). The location of the lesion is at the point of capsular attachment to the neck of the glenoid. It is best visualized with an axillary lateral radiograph or with the use of CT imaging.

The significance of this lesion in the throwing athlete is not well defined. Its relationship to posterior pain in the disabled throwing shoulder is also not clear. Consequently, surgical intervention to specifically address this lesion is not presently a clear indication. Labral damage and injury may occur in the presence of the Bennett lesion and in this setting the lesion may be addressed if incidental to other shoulder pathology.

Synovial Cysts

Synovial cysts can be seen with overhead athletes, but they are relatively uncommon; additionally, a lack of specific signs and symptoms make the diagnosis more challenging. They may occur in many areas around the shoulder, with symptoms typically an ill-defined ache. Occasionally, the subsequent nerve compression may occur. The suprascapular nerve can be compressed in the suprascapular notch, resulting in atrophy and weakness of both the supraspinatus and the infraspinatus, or at the spinoglenoid notch, which results in atrophy and weakness of the infraspinatus alone. The lack of specific signs and symptoms make evaluation of the posterior thorax for atrophy essential. Many lesions are discovered with use of MRI, often incidentally **(Fig 21-10)**. Nerve conduction study may also be useful in establishing a diagnosis with clinical suspicion. Normal joint extension can be confused with a synovial cyst,

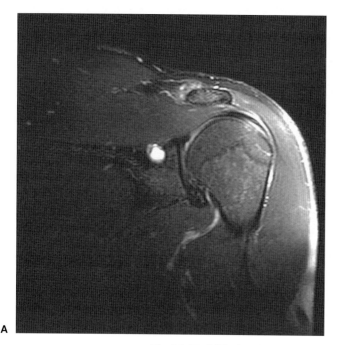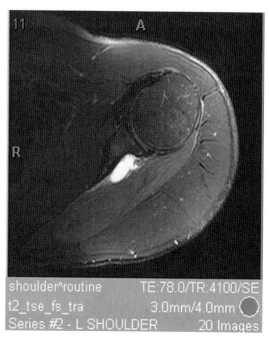

Fig 21-10. MRI of periarticular cyst **A:** Coronal view; **B:** Axial view.

as a patient with an effusion may have larger amounts of joint fluid present in a normal recess.

Treatment is nonoperative unless a clear, recent onset of nerve compression is present. Of those symptomatic patients, various surgical techniques have been described. Hawkins et al. (20) reported on aspiration of cysts with an 18% failure rate and 48% recurrence rate, with 54% reporting satisfaction with the outcome. Arthroscopy is beneficial in that the posterior and superior labrum can be assessed, because some have suggested that labral pathology may communicate with the cyst. However, not all cysts are associated with labral tears and may not be visualized arthroscopically. In addition, not all surgeons have experience with arthroscopic techniques for decompression.

Nerve Injuries
Neurological injuries may occur without the space-occupying lesions such as ganglions or cysts. Most commonly, the suprascapular and long thoracic nerves are involved. The specific etiology of injury is often unknown. When the suprascapular nerve is involved, the branch to the infraspinatus is usually injured with sparing of the branch to the supraspinatus. Volleyball players are most commonly affected in this manner, with up to 20% of professional players being affected (21). Most players will remain asymptomatic and can participate in sports without limitation, despite muscle atrophy.

Infraspinatus nerve palsy in the throwing athlete presents with symptoms that mimic tendinopathy of the shoulder with associated pain and weakness. A history will often reveal little that is helpful in establishing a diagnosis, and only with a high index of suspicion and careful inspection for atrophy and weakness can the diagnosis be made. A thorough examination is essential to ensure that no underlying neurologic condition

exists. Electromyography (EMG) can confirm the diagnosis, and MRI can be helpful to rule out a space-occupying lesion. Most patients treated nonoperatively will eventually become asymptomatic, although weakness and atrophy will persist.

Surgical intervention is reserved for those who have persistent symptoms and are not able to perform their sport. Operative intervention remains controversial, because the exact etiology of the condition is often unknown, and nerve recovery after surgery may occur in only half of those treated. The surgical technique involves decompression of the nerve and release of spinoglenoid ligament along with bony resection as needed.

Arterial and Venous Lesions
Vascular lesions of the upper extremity in throwing athletes are not common. Symptoms are vague and nonspecific initially, but progressive coolness of the hand and fingers may be suggestive. Pulses may or may not be affected, depending on the degree of the vascular compromise. Doppler ultrasound is the best initial screening test. Venogram may also be beneficial if a clot is suspected. Ultimately, venography or arteriography will identify the precise location of the lesion. Vascular consultation is recommended for assistance with medical and surgical decision making.

■ THE ELBOW

History

Information obtained during the history is usually the most important in establishing a diagnosis, including how and when the injury occurred and what took place right before the injury. Changes in throwing accuracy, velocity, stamina, and strength are important, as well as changes in training regimens. Neurologic complaints should also be noted and documented.

The Physical Examination

Observation of the elbow can provide information related to the degree of effusion present, because the capsular volume is greatest in 70 to 80 degrees of flexion and this position is most comfortable with capsular distention. Ecchymosis may be observed and serve to alert the examiner to possible fracture, tendon rupture, or capsular injury. Range of motion should be assessed both actively and passively. Any pain or crepitus should be noted during ranging and may be suggestive of loose bodies or chondral injury. Loss of elbow motion may be present in asymptomatic athletes, particularly a flexion contracture.

Palpation should be performed over all bony prominences and sites of tendon and ligament attachment. Medial epicondylar pain may be suggestive of epicondylitis or fracture or growth plate injury in the immature athlete. Proximal olecranon pain may be indicative of stress fracture. Palpation of the radial head is performed in conjunction with forearm rotation and may be suggestive of fracture, dislocation, or osteochondritis (OCD) of the capitellum. The biceps and triceps tendons should also be palpated for possible tearing or rupture. The palpation of the ulnar collateral ligament should be performed with the elbow at 60 degrees of flexion. The ligament should be evaluated along its entire course. Pain with examination may be suggestive of partial tearing to complete rupture of the ligament as well as possible concomitant injury to the flexor origin.

A complete neurovascular examination of the upper extremity should be performed. The ulnar nerve should be specifically palpated and percussion should not elicit pain or paresthesia. The nerve should also be evaluated for subluxation with range of motion or stress. Distal pulses should be noted to ensure that arterial flow is adequate.

Strength testing should be performed and comparison made with the contralateral upper extremity. Biceps and triceps muscles and pronation and supination as well as wrist flexion and extension should be performed.

Elbow stability should be assessed with the patient lying supine while the shoulder in external rotation. Valgus stress testing is performed with the elbow flexed 30 and 90 degrees in order to unlock the olecranon tip from the olecranon fossa. Recently, the moving valgus stress test may offer higher accuracy (22). Any opening of the elbow medially or reproduction of the athletes' symptoms is significant and suggestive of injury of the ulnar collateral ligament. Lateral elbow instability is significantly less common in the throwing athlete unless associated with elbow dislocation; in this setting, lateral or posteriolateral rotatory instability may be present. Valgus extension overload testing is performed with the examiner rapidly forcing the elbow into full extension from a slightly flexed position. This maneuver attempts to reproduce the pain associated with impingement of the posteromedial tip of the olecranon on the medial wall of the olecranon fossa.

Ancillary Testing

Standard radiographic analysis includes AP, lateral, and oblique views. An oblique view at 110 degrees of flexion is helpful to identify posteriomedial olecranon osteophytes. In the case of suspected medial elbow instability, stress radiographs may be taken. An increase in medial joint space opening in the symptomatic elbow is suggestive of ulnar collateral ligament injury; however, the actual amount of opening that is significant is not clearly established. CT scans or bone scans can be useful for identifying stress fractures of the olecranon.

MRI can be a useful study for evaluation of ligament injury, both complete tears and partial tears. Some evidence supports the use of CT arthrogram, with higher sensitivity for detection of partial tears compared with MRI in one series. Additionally, the MRI is useful in detection of loose bodies, osteophytes, osteochondral injuries, and nerve injuries. The MRI, with intra-articular contrast, is more valuable in the post-operative evaluation and the CT arthrogram and has greater value in the assessment of bony abnormalities.

Ulnar Collateral Ligament Injury

The anterior band of the ulnar collateral ligament (UCL) is the primary stabilizer to valgus stress during the throwing motion. The tensile stress during the acceleration phase of throwing may exceed the limit of the ligament, leading to injury and/or rupture. Athletes report pain during the acceleration phase of throwing and symptoms are often of gradual onset, though occasionally the thrower reports the rapid onset of symptoms following a single throw and inability to continue. A smaller subset of throwers reports medial elbow pain during the deceleration phase. When pain is present with the palpation of the ulnar collateral ligament or the flexor origin (may be involved with the UCL injury) or with valgus stress it is confirmatory. Stress radiographs **(Fig 21-11)** and MRI can provide additional information regarding the severity of injury.

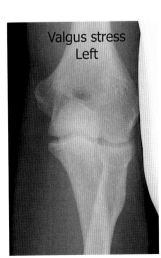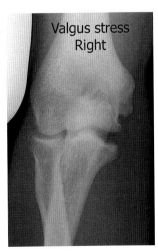

Fig 21-11. AP views with valgus stress at 30 degrees of flexion indicate markedly lax UCL of the right elbow in comparison to the left.

Nonsurgical treatment is generally limited to the non-throwing athlete and is usually successful in this lower-demand population. Attempts at nonoperative rehab in the throwing athlete have led to disappointing results (23,24), precluding return to throwing in unacceptably high numbers. For those who are treated conservatively, an initial period of rest is recommended from any throwing activities. During this time the athlete focuses on regaining range of motion, using various therapy modalities, and maintaining conditioning of the cuff and shoulder girdle musculature. As soreness and swelling resolve, strengthening of the elbow musculature may be instituted. Functional exercises may then be started followed by an interval throwing program. After the rehab program has been completed and the athlete is pain free, he or she may return to competition.

Operative treatment is usual treatment for a throwing the athlete who desires to return to throwing sports. Surgical treatment is indicated in the presence of a complete tear of the ulnar collateral ligament, or in an athlete with a partial tear that remains symptomatic despite conservative treatment. The surgical technique was first performed by Jobe et al. (25) in 1974. Prior to this time an ulnar collateral ligament tear was almost universally career ending. The original procedure (known as the "Tommy John" procedure) was performed by reconstructing the anterior band of the ulnar collateral ligament with a free palmaris longus tendon graft, which was passed through bony tunnels in the ulna and humerus in a figure-of-eight fashion and then sutured to itself. The original procedure had several modifications relating to the dissection of the flexor pronator musculature and transfer of the ulnar nerve; also, the technique for insertion of the graft into the bone was modified by Rohrbough et al. (24) with the "docking" technique, elimination of the ulnar nerve transfer in most cases and modification of the procedure to incorporate the graft into the bony tunnels with the 'docking' technique. Return to sports has been reported to be as high as 97% with current reconstruction techniques, but a rehabilitation program usually will require 8 to 18 months.

Valgus Extension Overload Syndrome with Posterior Impingement

Posterior medial osteophytes may develop in the throwing athlete as a result of valgus overload and are often symptomatic in the throwing athlete. Symptomatic athletes complain of posterior base elbow pain and will have tenderness over the proximal olecranon. Valgus stress applied to the flexed elbow causes the medial aspect of the olecranon tip to impinge on the medial wall of the olecranon fossa reproducing their symptoms. Osteophytes may subsequently generate loose body formation within the elbow joint **(Fig 21-12)**.

Treatment initially consists of active rest and conditioning of the shoulder and elbow in the absence of throwing. As symptoms progressively resolve, an interval throwing program may be initiated. When this is tolerated without symptoms, the athlete may resume competition. Those who

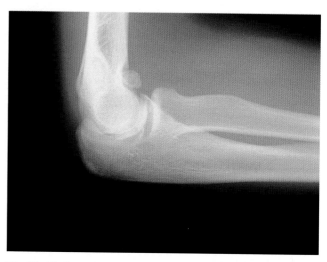

Fig 21-12. Lateral radiograph of the elbow shows intra-articular loose bodies.

have persistent symptoms despite conservative treatment may require surgical intervention. Open and arthroscopic techniques have been described. Arthroscopic debridement and osteophyte excision has been advocated in most instances, with removal of any loose bodies and debridement of any kissing lesions. Early rehabilitation is instituted, with special emphasis on regaining motion.

Ulnar Neuritis

Ulnar nerve compression may occur at various sites as the nerve passes from the arcade of Struthers, along the medial intermuscular septum, into the cubital tunnel, and past the two heads of the flexor carpi ulnaris muscle. Throwing athletes experience ulnar nerve irritation from traction injuries, compression from adjacent structures, or friction due to subluxation of the ulnar nerve. Complaints are typically paresthesias of the small and ring fingers during or after the throwing motion. Physical findings include tenderness over the ulnar nerve and/or positive Tinnel's sign. Decreased sensation in the small finger and the ring finger and decreased sensation over the dorsal ulnar aspect of the hand will rule out compression of the ulnar nerve in Guyon's canal, because the dorsal sensory branch exits the ulnar nerve proximal to the wrist. Electrophysiologic testing is useful to confirm the diagnosis. Underlying UCL ligament injury should carefully be assessed because microinstability may contribute to ulnar nerve injury.

Treatment initially consists of "active rest" with use of anti-inflammatory medication, cryotherapy, and physical therapy, followed by a gradual return to throwing. In cases of nerve subluxation, assistive devices (elbow sleeve) may be used to help prevent repeated episodes of subluxation and padding may also be used for protection. Surgical treatment is reserved for those with persistent symptoms unresponsive to conservative treatment. Surgical options include decompression in situ and submuscular transposition, but the ulnar

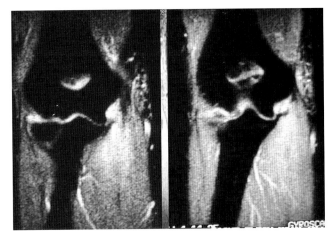

Fig 21-13. MRI showing an ulnar collateral ligament and medial flexor insertion pronator tear.

nerve subcutaneous transposition offers the best solution for the throwing athlete.

Flexor-Pronator Muscle Injury

The common flexor tendon provides dynamic support to valgus stress in the throwing elbow. Forces of contraction resist valgus stress during acceleration and aid in wrist flexion during ball release. Injury can range from mild strain to chronic tendonitis or acute muscle tears. Care should be taken to ensure that an underlying UCL injury is not misinterpreted as an isolated muscular injury, because symptoms can be confusing. Symptoms include pain over the medial elbow during late cocking and early acceleration and findings include tenderness over the muscle mass just distal to the origin. A UCL and medial flexor insertion tear can be seen in **Figure 21-13**.

Tendon injury usually responds well to a period of active rest with anti-inflammatory medication and physical therapy, followed by a gradual return to throwing. Occasional refractory cases may require corticosteroid injection; care must be taken to avoid injection into the ulnar collateral ligament. Surgical treatment is rarely necessary and should alert the health care provider to the possibility of additional underlying pathology.

Stress Fractures

Olecranon stress fractures in throwing athletes may occur as a result of repetitive tensile load from the triceps musculature or microtrauma due to olecranon impingement. Athletes report posterolateral pain and tenderness during and after throwing. Early radiographs do not reveal any bony abnormalitities and diagnosis is made with use of MRI, CT scanning, or bone scan. **Figure 21-14** is an example of the nonunion of a proximal olecranon stress fracture.

Initial treatment consists of active rest with throwing cessation and possibly uses of bone growth stimulators. Surgical treatment consists of internal fixation and is not uncommon in the competitive thrower.

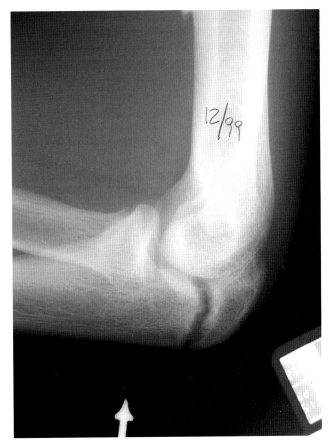

Fig 21-14. Nonunion of proximal olecranon stress fracture.

The Skeletally Immature Throwing Athlete

As juvenile sports involvement continues to increase, upper extremity injuries become more common. Injuries to the young thrower are the result of repetitive microtrauma, macrotrauma or a combination of both. Overuse injuries represent the majority of disorders of the shoulder and elbow in the young thrower. As the stress placed upon the tissues of the upper extremity exceeds the ability to recover from repetitive, cyclic loading an injury response occurs. The athlete will usually complain of pain during the throwing cycle; additionally, loss of control and a decrease in velocity may be noted.

Knowledge of the secondary ossification centers of the shoulder and elbow is essential in the evaluation and treatment of upper-extremity injuries. Additionally, range-of-motion differences and radiographic changes in the dominant versus nondominant shoulder has been described (27), as well as increased humeral head retroversion. Injuries occur most commonly to cartilage and bone in the juvenile throwers. Understanding of the age-related strength of these tissues is necessary. The level of conditioning and strength of the thrower is also useful in assessment of throwing.

Little Leaguer's Shoulder

Little Leaguer's shoulder is an injury to the proximal humeral physis in response to torsional overload. Understanding of this condition has improved recently and the pathology is similar to a stress fracture of the proximal humeral physis. The athlete will complain of pain in the region of the proximal humerus during the throwing motion; often this is the only time the shoulder will be symptomatic. Physical examination will reveal pain with palpation over the proximal humerus; this is the most common symptom, present in up to 80% in one series (28). Other presenting symptoms occur much less frequently and may include swelling or atrophy. In some instances the physical examination may be completely benign. Radiographic findings of widening of the proximal humeral physis are confirmatory; comparison radiographs may be helpful.

Treatment consists of complete rest for the initial 6 weeks. Acetaminophen may be used to treat symptoms if pain is present at rest or with activities of daily living. When the athlete is asymptomatic with activities of daily living, a scapular and rotator cuff conditioning and strengthening program may be initiated. This strengthening phase continues for an additional 6 weeks. At 3 months an interval-throwing program may be initiated and may progress to full return to competition gradually as the patient remains asymptomatic. Most athletes are able to return to competition, but should be counseled concerning proper mechanics, limited pitch count, and possibility of recurrence.

Acute Fractures

Acute fractures of the humerus may occur proximally in the physeal region and less commonly may occur in the humeral shaft.

Proximal humerus fractures are believed to be caused by rapid growth and resultant weakness of the physeal region. This injury occurs with a single throw and is associated with acute onset of pain. Further attempts at throwing are not likely because the athlete will often experience pain with simple movements of the arm. The thrower may or may not have experienced prodromal symptoms of pain. Radiographic imaging will confirm the diagnosis in most instances. Treatment is dictated by the degree of displacement, with most cases being treated conservatively, because most injuries are minimally displaced. Surgical treatment is reserved for cases of severe displacement.

Humeral shaft fractures are caused by substantial torsional stress placed on the humerus during throwing. Associated pathologic lesions in the bone should be ruled out, such as aneurysmal bone cysts, fibrous cortical defects, or malignant tumors. Treatment in most instances is functional bracing, with limitation of motion as pain dictates. Return to throwing is limited until radiographic evidence of healing is clearly visible. Return to competition is usually restricted for 6 months. Although refracture has been reported, it is relatively rare.

Medial Epicondyle Apophysitis

The medial epicondyle begins to ossify at age 5 to 7 years and is fully ossified at age 14 to 17 years, with boys experiencing ossification at the later age ranges compared with girls. Repetitive traction to the epicondyle is the inciting force

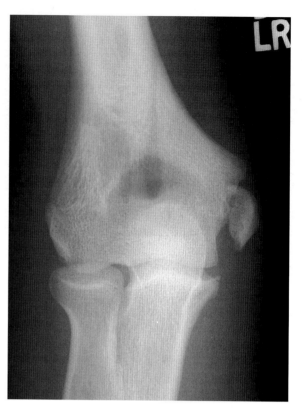

Fig 21-15. The young athlete with a medial epicondyle avulsion injury.

causing microfracture and widening of the physis and may eventually progress to avulsion or fragmentation. This occurs as a result of the ability of bone, tendon, and muscle to resist traction stress better than the apophyseal cartilage. Risk factors are directly related to the number of pitches thrown and to the pitches requiring forceful pronation or wrist flexion. Pain over the medial elbow and point tenderness over the epicondyle are characteristic. Valgus stress applied to the elbow at 25 degrees of flexion will cause pain and may reveal laxity if avulsion has occurred. Radiographs will reveal widening of the medial physis or actual displacement of the apophysis (Fig 21-15).

Treatment consists of rest until the elbow is nontender; this is usually accomplished with cessation of throwing. If pain persists, ice, massage, and acetaminophen may be used. Nonsteriodal anti-inflammatory medication should be avoided, because this has been shown to have detrimental effects on healing of bone, tendon, and muscle in laboratory animals. Surgical treatment is reserved for displacement of greater than 5 mm or if widening is demonstrated on stress testing.

Capitellar Ostechondritis Dissecans

The capitellum begins to ossify at age 1 to 2 years and is completely ossified at age 14 to 17 years (9). The highly vascularized growing bones of young throwing athletes are thought to resist compression forces poorly and may experience compression fractures with repetitive loading (10). Repetitive loading in the face of microfracture may lead to compromise in the circulation and subsequent avascular necrosis, which may then generate loose bodies. The athlete will complain of lateral elbow pain with throwing. If untreated and if throwing persists, pain may then occur at rest. The radiocapitellar joint may be painful with palpation. Radiograph will reveal osteopenia and bony changes consistent with necrosis. MRI can be used to stage the lesion or may be useful if surgical intervention is indicated. Relative rest is indicated for low-grade lesion without evidence of fluid in between the fragment and the underlying bone or displacement of the fragment. Those lesions not responding to conservative treatment may require drilling to stimulate healing. Loose bodies will need to be removed arthroscopically or open. Rehab is focused on return of motion followed by strengthening and eventually interval throwing programs prior to return to competition.

■ REFERENCES

1. O'Brien SJ, Pagnani MJ, McGlynn SR, et al. The active compression test: a new and effective test for diagnosing labral tears and acromioclavicular joint abnormality. *Am J Sports Med.* 1998;26: 610–613.
2. Liu SH, Henry MH, Nuccion SL. A prospective evaluation of a new physical examination in predicting glenoid labrum tears. *Am J Sports Med.* 1996;24:721–725.
3. Kibler WB. Sensitivity and specificity of the anterior slide test in throwing athletes with superior glenoid labrum tears. *Arthroscopy.* 1995;11:296–300.
4. Walch G, Boileau J, Noel E, et al. Impingement of the deep surface of the supraspinatus tendon on the posterior superior glenoid rim: an arthroscopic study. *J Shoulder Elbow Surg.* 1992;1:238–243.
5. Jobe CM. Posterior superior glenoid impingement: expanded spectrum. *Arthroscopy.* 1995;11:530–537.
6. Jobe FW, Giangarra CE, Kvitne RS, et al. Anterior capsulolabral reconstruction of the shoulder in athletes in overhead sports. *Am J Sports Med.* 1991;19:428–434.
7. Rubenstein DL, Jobe FW, Glousman RE, et al. Anterior capsulolabral reconstruction of the shoulder in athletes. *J Shoulder Elbow Surg.* 1992;1:229–237.
7a. Burkhart SS, Morgan CD. Technical note: The peel-back mechanism. Its role in producing and extending posterior type II SLAP lesions and it effect on SLAP repair rehabilitation. *Arthroscopy.* 1998;14:637–640.
7b. Burkhart SS, Morgan CD, Kibler WB. Shoulder injuries in overhead athletes. *Clin Sports Med.* 2000;19:125–158.
8. Kibler WB. The role of the scapula in athletic shoulder function. *Am J Sports Med.* 1998;26:325–337.
9. Morgan CD, Burkhart SS, Palmeri M, et al. Type II SLAP lesions: three subtypes, and their relationship to superior instability and rotator cuff tears. *Arthroscopy.* 1998;14:553–565.
10. Johansen RL, Callis M, Potts J, et al. A modified internal rotation stretching technique for overhead and throwing athletes. *J Orthop Sports Phys Ther.* 1995;21:216–219.
11. Kamkar A, Irrgang JL, Whitney SL. Nonoperative management of secondary shoulder impingement. *J Orthop Sports Phys Ther.* 1993;17:212–224.
12. Barber FA, Morgan CD, Burkhart SS, et al. Labrum/biceps/cuff dysfunction in throwing athlete. *Arthroscopy.* 1999;15:852–857.
13. Burkhart SS, Morgan CD, Kibler BW. The disabled throwing shoulder: spectrum of pathology Part I: pathology and biomechanics. *Arthroscopy.* 2003;19:404–420.
13a. Andrews JR, Carson W Jr, McLeod W. Glenoid labrum tears related to the long head of the biceps. *Am J Sports Med.* 1998; 16:97–100.
14. Burkhart SS, Morgan CD. SLAP lesions in the overhead athlete. *Orthop Clin North Am.* 2001;32:431–441.
15. Fleisig GS, Andrews JR, Dillman CD, et al. Kinetics of baseball pitching with implications about injury mechanisms. *Am J Sports Med.* 1995;23:233–239.
16. Andrews JR, Carson WG, McLeod WD. Glenoid labrum tears related to the long head of the biceps. *Am J Sports Med.* 1991;10: 901–911.
17. Kuhn JE, Lindholm SR, Huston LJ, et al. Failure of biceps-superior labral complex (SLAP lesion) in the throwing athlete: a biomechanical model comparing maximal cocking to early deceleration. *J Shoulder Elbow Surg.* 2000;9:463.
17a. Tibone JE, Elrod B, Jobe FW, et al. Surgical treatment of tears of the rotator cuff in athletes. *J Bone Joint Surg Am.* 1986;68: 887–891.
18. McFarland EG, Blivin SJ, Doehring CB, et al. Treatment of grade III acromioclavicular separations in professional throwing athletes: results of a survey. *Am J Orthop.* 1997;26:771–774.
19. Hawkins RJ, Piatt BE, Fritz RC, et al. Clinical evaluation and treatment of spinoglenoid notch ganglion cysts. *J Shoulder Elbow Surg.* 1993;8:551.
19a. Lombardo SJ, Jobe FW, Kerlan RK, et al. Posterior shoulder lesions in throwing athletes. *Am J Sports Med.* 1978;5:106–110.
20. Ringel SP, Treihaft M, Carry M, et al. Suprascapular neuropathy in pitchers. *Am J Sports Med.* 1990;18:80–86.
21. O'Driscoll SW, Lawton RL, Smith AM. The "moving valgus stress test" for medial collateral ligament tears of the elbow. *Am J Sports Med.* 2005;33(2):231–9.
22. Kenter K, Behr CT, Warren RF, et al. Acute elbow injuries in the National Football League. *J Shoulder Elbow Surg.* 2000;9:1–5.
23. Miller CD, Savoie FH III. Valgus extension injuries of the elbow in the throwing athlete. *J Am Acad Orthop Surg.* 1994;2: 261–269.
24. Rohrbough JT, Altcheck DW, Hyman J, et al. Medial collateral ligament reconstruction of the elbow using the docking technique. *Am J Sports Med.* 2002;30:541–548.
25. Jobe FW, Stark H, Lombardo SJ. Reconstruction of the ulnar collateral ligament in athletes. *J Bone Joint Surgery* 1986;68A: 1158–1163.
26. Mair SD, Robbe RG, Brindle KA. Physeal changes and range-of-motion differences in the dominant shoulders of skeletally immature baseball players. *J Shoulder Elbow Surg.* 2004;13: 487–491.
27. Wasserlauf BL, Paletta GA. Shoulder disorders in the skeletally immature throwing athlete. *Orthop Clin North Am.* 2003;34: 427–437.
28. Bennett GE. Elbow and shoulder dislocations of baseball players. *Am J Surg.* 1959;98:484–488.

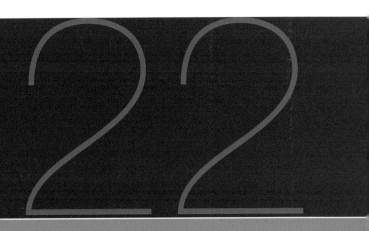

PRINCIPLES OF SHOULDER REHABILITATION

BENJAMIN D. RUBIN, MD, MS

■ KEY POINTS

- The shoulder functions in the context of a kinetic chain, a series of links and segments activated sequentially in a coordinated fashion to generate and transmit force.
- The axioscapular shoulder muscles, which attach the scapula to the thorax, include the serratus anterior, the trapezius, the rhomboids, and the levator scapulae posteriorly, and the pectoralis minor anteriorly.
- The scapulohumeral shoulder muscle group consists of supraspinatus, infraspinatus, teres minor, subscapularis, deltoid, and teres major.
- The axiohumeral muscles are the "power" muscles of the shoulder and include the pectoralis major and latissimus dorsi.
- Abnormal scapular kinematics occur as a result of alterations in anatomy, physiology, and/or biomechanics; or musculoskeletal adaptations to these aberrations.
- The goal of functional rehabilitation goes beyond resolving symptoms to regaining normal function by re-establishing normal anatomy, physiology, biomechanics, and kinematics, thus restoring the integrity of the kinetic chain.

The goal of successful shoulder rehabilitation following an injury or surgery is to establish normal function rather than to merely resolve symptoms. In order to accomplish this, restoration of the normal anatomy, physiology, and biomechanics of the shoulder, as well as correction of any associated musculoskeletal adaptations that have occurred, are necessary

to re-establish the normal kinematics. To many, the concept of evaluating and treating the shoulder in the context of the musculoskeletal system, rather than in isolation, represents a paradigm shift from the more traditional approach. This chapter will address shoulder function and dysfunction, and in that light, address the concepts and specifics of core-based functional rehabilitation of the shoulder.

■ THE SHOULDER IN THE KINETIC CHAIN

The shoulder functions in the context of a kinetic chain, which is defined as a series of links and segments activated sequentially in a coordinated fashion to generate and transmit forces to accomplish a specific function (1–3). This can easily be understood by remembering the mechanics of the childhood game "crack the whip," when a group of children holds hands in a line to try to increase the speed of the last child. The first child forms the base and whips the second child, who whips the third, thus transmitting the force and velocity, which are sequentially passed on until the final child is maximally accelerated. Each child represents a segment of the chain, and their joined hands represent links in the chain. In activities that utilize a throwing motion, (e.g., pitching or tennis), there is an open-ended kinetic chain with proximal to distal muscle activation and coordination of body segments producing interactive moments at the terminal segment (hand or racket) (4,5). In throwing, the sequence of link activation begins with the creation of a ground reaction force as a result of the foot and leg pushing against the ground. The force is increased as it is transmitted through the knees and hips through the large muscles of the legs, into the lumbopelvic region and the rest of the trunk. The proximal segments, i.e., the legs and trunk, produce roughly half the energy (51%) and force (54%) that is ultimately delivered to the distal end of the kinetic chain (6–8). The scapula and glenohumeral joint function as both a link and a segment in the kinetic chain, increasing the kinetic energy and force generated; and as a conduit to funnel and transmit these forces to the distal segments (9).

When an individual reaches, pushes, or pulls from a sitting position, there is less energy and force contribution from the legs, and the primary generator for upper-extremity motion is the initiation of trunk stabilization. Hodges has shown that before either arm or leg movement is initiated, the transverses abdominis is consistently activated first, increasing the intra-abdominal pressure in preparation of the action (10). Coordinated muscle activation sequences result in movement patterns, which create joint motions to efficiently accomplish specific tasks. These diagonal activation patterns create a "serape" effect from the knee or lumbopelvic region to the shoulder (11), act locally on one joint or harmonize several joints, provide co-contraction force couples that control joint perturbations and provide stability, and generate and transmit force. This enables the scapular stabilizing muscles to position the scapula optimally for shoulder function and for the rotator cuff to compress and position the humeral head in the glenoid fossa.

■ FUNCTIONAL SHOULDER ANATOMY

The Scapula in Shoulder Function

The scapula provides both anatomic and kinematic connections between the torso and the upper extremity. The shoulder muscles can be classified anatomically by their origins and insertions into the axioscapular, scapulohumeral, and the axiohumeral groups (12). The axioscapular muscles, which attach the scapula to the thorax, include the serratus anterior, the trapezius, the rhomboids, and the levator scapulae posteriorly, and the pectoralis minor anteriorly. These scapular stabilizing muscles position the scapula optimally for the humeral head. In the case of the serratus anterior and the trapezius, the muscles are so large and the muscle fibers course in different directions; therefore, each muscle may have multiple functions that relate to activity and arm position (13).

The scapulohumeral group consists of the supraspinatus, infraspinatus, teres minor, subscapularis, deltoid, and teres major. The rotator cuff muscles provide concavity/compression at the glenohumeral joint and fine tune humeral head rotation and depression, thus keeping the humeral head centered in the glenoid throughout the arc of upper-extremity motion. The axiohumeral muscles are the "power" muscles of the shoulder and include the pectoralis major and latissimus dorsi. The biceps and triceps comprise a special category, because they extend from the scapula to the forearm.

The shoulder is an important kinematic link between the trunk and arm, providing a stable platform for arm rotation during throwing. The shoulder includes the scapulothoracic articulation and the glenohumeral, acromioclavicular, and sternoclavicular joints, which together form two individual but paired mechanisms—one an open chain and one a closed chain (14). A closed kinetic chain, such as the one formed by the thorax, scapula, and clavicle is defined by the terminal link being fixed or immovable. The open kinetic chain mechanism, i.e., the glenohumeral joint, involves movement of the terminal link, which is the hand. Normal function requires that all four articulations participate in a simultaneous, synchronous, and coordinated manner, as well as in succession, creating what is termed scapulohumeral rhythm (15).

Every movement of the scapula involves six degrees of freedom of motion, which involves three rotations and three translations along three orthogonal axes (Fig 22-1). The medial-lateral axis is parallel to the spine of the scapula; the superior-inferior (vertical) axis is perpendicular to the transverse plane; and the anterior-posterior axis is perpendicular to the coronal plane. This six degrees of freedom motion of the scapula can be quite complex and confusing from a biomechanical perspective; therefore, for clinical purposes, the most dominant kinematic parameter for each *functional* motion is described below. The motions include anterior/posterior tilt (rotation on the sagittal plane about a medial-lateral axis—**Fig 22-2A**), internal and external rotation (rotation on the transverse plane about a vertical axis—**Fig 22-2B**), and upward and downward rotation (rotation on the coronal plane about an anterior-posterior axis—**Fig 22-2C**). Scapular translations are elevation/depression (translation along the vertical axis), abduction/adduction (translation along the medial-lateral axis), and anterior-posterior movement (translation along the anterior-posterior axis). Protraction and retraction, which are terms frequently used in the clinical setting, represent combinations of motions and translations to describe scapular movements and are dependent on the rotation of an intact clavicle about the sternoclavicular joint. Protraction, a movement frequently associated with shoulder dysfunction, involves anterior movement, anterior tilt, and upward rotation. During glenohumeral elevation, the normal scapula demonstrates a pattern of upward rotation, external rotation, and posterior tilting (16). The predominant motion is upward rotation, and to a lesser degree external rotation and posterior tilt. In addition, the scapula translates into a more superior and posterior position (16). Dynamic scapulohumeral rhythm depends on scapular motions and translations, combined with arm motion.

The scapular stabilizing muscles function as force couples to control the motions of the scapula. A force couple is formed when two forces act in opposite directions to impose rotation about an axis (17). The serratus anterior controls the movements of protraction and retraction (abduction and adduction), depending on shoulder position (18). This is counteracted by the upper and lower trapezius and the rhomboids, which act as retractors (adductors). Scapular

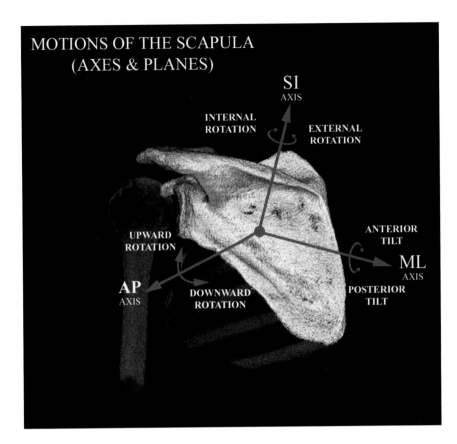

Fig 22-1. Motions of the scapula (axes and planes).

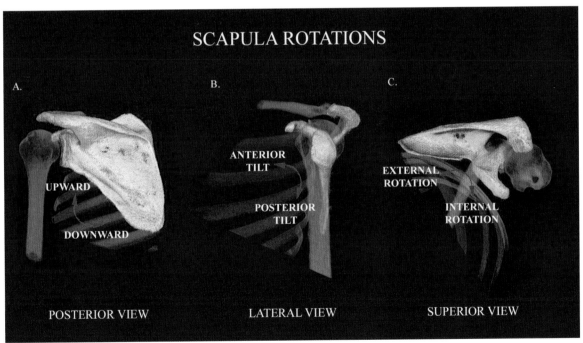

Fig 22-2. Scapula rotations.

elevation is a function of the upper trapezius, the levator scapula, and the upper serratus anterior. This is balanced by the scapular depression resulting from the function of the lower portions of the trapezius and serratus anterior (12,13,18,19).

The Scapula in Shoulder Dysfunction

Abnormal scapular kinematics occur as a result of alterations in anatomy, physiology, and/or biomechanics, or musculoskeletal adaptations to these aberrations, and can usually be classified

TABLE 22-1	Causes of Scapular Dyskinesis

1. Proximally derived scapular dyskinesis (PDSD)
   A. Neurologic
      a. Long thoracic neuropathy
      b. Spinal accessory neuropathy
      c. Dorsal scapular neuropathy
   B. Axial
      a. Postural dysfunction
      b. Scoliosis
      c. Lumbopelvic instability (weakness)
      d. Proximal kinetic chain interruption
   C. Scapulothoracic
      a. Axioscapular force couple imbalance (weakness/injury)
      b. Pectoralis minor contracture or increased tension
      c. Malunited scapula fracture
      d. Muscle avulsion
      e. Scapulothoracic bursitis
      f. Osteochondroma
      g. Muscular dystrophy
      h. Fibrous contracture

2. Distally derived scapular dyskinesis (DDSD)
   A. Glenohumeral
      a. Labral tear or detachment
      b. Instability
      c. Internal impingement
      d. Capsular laxity
      e. Biceps tendonitis/tears/pulley lesions
      f. Focal capsular restrictions (e.g., GIRD)
      g. Adhesive capsulitis
      h. Glenohumeral arthritis
      i. Fracture of glenoid or humeral head
   B. Rotator cuff
      a. Rotator cuff tears (partial or complete)
      b. Rotator cuff tendinosis/tendonitis
      c. Calcific tendonitis
      d. Primary subacromial impingement syndrome
   C. Clavicle and acromion
      a. Acromioclavicular dislocations/arthropathy/arthritis
      b. Sternoclavicular instability/arthropathy/arthritis
      c. Malunion/nonunion of clavicle
      d. Malunion/nonunion of acromion
      e. Os acromiale

as being proximally or distally derived **(Table 22-1)** (20). When the basic problem occurs proximal and posterior to the glenohumeral joint, the observed scapular dyskinesis is considered proximally derived (PDSD). When an abnormality of the glenohumeral joint, subacromial space, clavicle, acromioclavicular or sternoclavicular joints occurs, the resulting dyskinesis that is usually observed is considered distally derived (DDSD). The exception to this classification is the presence of shortening or tightness of the pectoralis minor or clavipectoral fascia, which fits best into PDSD despite its anterior position. Recently, Borstad and Ludewig (21) have documented the effect of altered pectoralis minor resting length on scapular kinematics in healthy individuals. In the context of the kinetic chain, PDSD is associated with proximal link or segment weakness or interruption, while DDSD is the result of "recoil" or "kick back" from a distal link or segment dysfunction. This

has important implications in the treatment of shoulder and upper-extremity conditions. The pattern of abnormal scapular motion is usually multi-planar and frequently changes with the plane of arm elevation, concentric or eccentric function of the scapular stabilizers, and fatigue; however, if scapular dyskinesis is observed, the sensitivity of the observation is 0.74 and the positive predictive value is 0.84 (22).

PDSD is frequently associated with postural dysfunction. The classic presentation is that of the patient who sits or stands with the head and neck in a forward position, with focal cervical lordosis (usually at C5-C6), thoracic kyphosis, and protracted scapulae (23). Lumbar lordosis with poor control of the abdominal musculature is frequently associated. Proximal kinetic chain weakness can be due to abnormalities of the lower extremities, lumbopelvic, lumbar, or thoracolumbar deficits. Lumbopelvic weakness appears to be one of the most common causes of primary scapular dyskinesis in the throwing athlete (11). Injury to either the long thoracic nerve or spinal accessory nerve causes weakness and atrophy of the serratus anterior and trapezius, respectively. Long thoracic stretch mononeuropathy is actually more common in overhead athletes than previously thought, and recently has been associated with the use of heavy backpacks by children and young adults (backpack palsy). When these muscles are compromised either from neurologic interruption or fatigue, force couple imbalances ensue, and a significant adverse cascade of events occurs **(Fig 22-3)**. Proprioception is altered, a dyssynchronous muscle firing pattern occurs, with an abnormal increase in scapular mobility (usually loss of external rotation) and subsequent increased stress on the glenohumeral joint capsule, glenoid labrum, and rotator cuff (24-28). Increased protraction has been shown to specifically increase the strain on the anterior band of the inferior glenohumeral ligament and decrease anterior translation of the humeral head (28). As indicated in the discussion above concerning the role of the scapula as a kinematic link between the trunk and the arm, optimum rotator cuff activation occurs only in the presence of a scapula that is optimally positioned for stability (27). As a result, increased intrinsic joint loads and decreased force are delivered to the terminal segment (4).

DDSD is very common. Almost all shoulder pathology is associated with alterations in the ability to position the scapula properly, usually quite early in the pathologic process (8,27,29–38). Related intra-articular pathology may include labral tears or detachments and capsular attenuation or tears (with resultant instability), focal capsular restrictions such as glenohumeral internal rotation deficit (GIRD), which is commonly seen in overhead athletes, biceps lesions, adhesive capsulitis, and glenohumeral arthritis. Rotator cuff tendonitis and tears, primary impingement syndrome, and calcific tendonitis have been observed to be associated with scapular malposition. In these cases, the pain and altered biomechanics associated with the pathology causes inhibition of the serratus anterior and lower trapezius, with the subsequent events outlined earlier. This results in the vicious cycle of scapular dysfunction and shoulder pathology summarized in Figure 22-3.

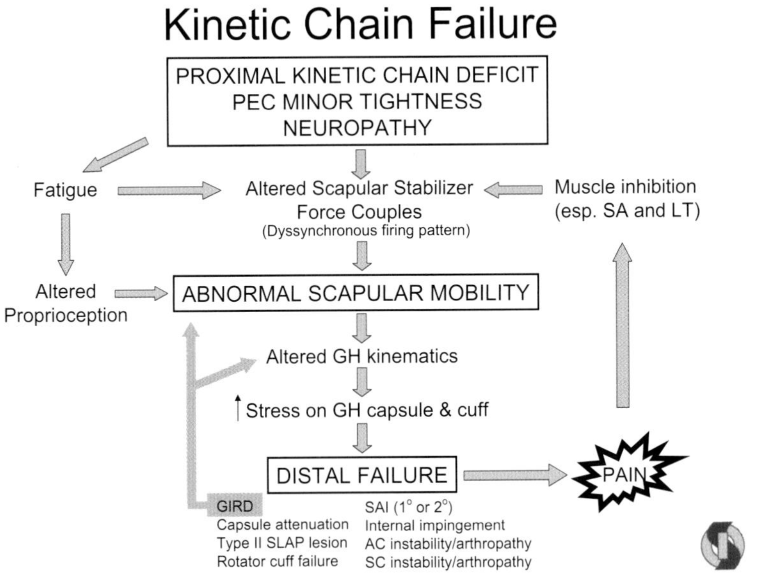

Kinetic Chain Failure

Fig 22-3. Cascade of kinetic chain failure.

Subacromial impingement syndrome has been associated with increased flexion of the thoracic spine, which results in elevation and anterior tilting of the scapula at rest, decreased upward rotation and posterior tilt of the scapula with glenohumeral elevation, decreased elevation of the glenohumeral joint, and decreased force generated at 90 degrees of scapular plane abduction (39). In addition, they have shown that with cervical spine flexion of 25 degrees, there is an increase in scapular upward rotation and a decrease in posterior tilting in healthy subjects. Recently, Meskers et al. (40) have demonstrated that the supraspinatus outlet narrows during elevation in the frontal plane from 30 to 130 degrees; however, with external rotation and movement in the horizontal plane the greater tuberosity moves away from the coracoacromial ligament. Borstad and Ludewig (41) have shown an association between subacromial impingement and anterior tilting, increased internal rotation, and decreased upward rotation of the scapula. Cools et al. (42,43) has shown that patients with subacromial impingement demonstrate a decrease in peak force for isokinetic protraction, decreased protraction/retraction ratio, and decreased EMG activity in the lower trapezius, as well as abnormal muscle recruitment in overhead athletes with delayed activation of the middle and lower trapezius.

Loss of the normal strut function of the clavicle as a result of a displaced, malunited, or ununited fracture, or higher degree acromioclavicular joint dislocation is commonly associated with dyskinetic scapular motion. The pain associated with arthrosis or arthritis of the acromioclavicular or sternoclavicular joint can also cause compromise of the periscapular muscle firing patterns.

In many cases in which shoulder symptoms are chronic, especially glenohumeral instability, GIRD, and rotator cuff tendon failure, it is difficult to determine whether the scapular dyskinesis was instrumental in causing the intra-articular and/or subacromial pathology or vice versa. Over time, there is a significant overlap due to the cyclic nature of the interaction between the segments of the kinetic chain.

Although it is not always possible to determine the primary underlying cause of abnormal scapular motion, it is important to attempt to do so, because correction of the dyskinetic pattern of motion must occur to restore normal shoulder function. This differentiation is made by clinical evaluation, selective injections and response to rehabilitation. In PDSD, surgical intervention is usually not necessary, because most patients respond to correction of posture and weaknesses in the kinetic chain. If the dyskinesis is determined to be distally derived, and the patient does not respond to functional rehabilitation techniques or specific local steroid injections, then surgical intervention is usually required to correct the underlying pathoanatomy to restore the integrity of the kinetic chain.

■ PRINCIPLES AND RATIONALE OF CORE-BASED FUNCTIONAL REHABILITATION

The goal of functional rehabilitation is not merely to resolve symptoms, but to regain normal function by re-establishing normal anatomy, physiology, biomechanics, and kinematics, thus restoring the integrity of the kinetic chain (20,44). In some cases, such as in swimmers or patients who function in a seated position, the kinetic chain is somewhat shortened. For this reason, the concept of core-based functional rehabilitation has been introduced (10,45). Based on the concepts outlined above regarding scapular function and dysfunction in the context of the kinetic chain, the rehabilitation process can be made more predictable and successful if the clinician, physical therapist, and athletic trainer adhere to certain principles and guidelines.

1 Core Stabilization. Hodges has demonstrated that before either arm or leg movement is initiated, the transverses abdominis is consistently activated first, to increase the intra-abdominal pressure and stabilize the torso for the anticipated action (10). Therefore, strengthening of the abdominal musculature and the other core muscles is done early in the rehabilitation process. We have found that the incorporation of the principles of Pilates-based exercises, including concentration, breathing, centering, control, precision, flowing motion, isolation, and routine is quite helpful in re-establishing core strength (46).

2 Postural Alignment. In order for the body to function properly, it must be in proper alignment. Upper-quarter posture depends on correct positioning of the pelvis, lumbopelvic region, cervical and thoracic spine, scapula, and shoulder. Rehabilitation exercises should be carried out with a neutral spine, appropriate pelvic position, and proper activation of trunk musculature. Shoulder protraction, excessive cervical and lumbar lordosis, and thoracic kyphosis are frequent causes of scapular dysfunction. Postural abnormalities, especially thoracic hypomobility, which is commonly seen, must be corrected early in the rehabilitation process. Exercises should be performed in the erect position as much as possible in order to replicate function.

3 Kinetic Chain. Proximal stability must be regained (or obtained) before distal mobility; otherwise, there can be an exacerbation of the distal problem, especially in subacromial impingement (see 4. Scapular Position below). Proper activation of trunk musculature and normal trunk and leg strength and flexibility will facilitate scapular position. Therefore, rehabilitation progresses from proximal to distal. When possible, correct proximal weaknesses first; then add the upper extremity. During this time, scapular and upper extremity exercises can be done in the seated position to separate the dysfunctional segments. The rehabilitation program should integrate functional movement patterns as

soon as possible. Trunk stabilization exercises (balance work) are critical to enhance return of normal function.

4 Scapular Position. Ability to position the scapula properly by retraction and depression is critical to the success of any shoulder rehabilitation program. The scapular stabilizing muscles control protraction when functioning in an eccentric mode. Patients should be taught very early in the process (preoperatively if surgery is contemplated) how to "find" their scapula and position it properly in order to enhance humeral head compression by the rotator cuff and decrease subacromial impingement due to anterior tilting of the acromion. In some cases it is helpful to use either single- or dual-channel surface biofeedback techniques to monitor muscle activity with auditory and/or visual cues. The electrodes are placed to monitor the activity of the muscles and the patient is encouraged to either facilitate (increase) or inhibit (decrease) muscle activity. We have found inhibition of the upper trapezius or latissimus dorsi and activation of the lower trapezius to be particularly beneficial in these patients. It is frequently necessary to re-establish normal length of the periscapular muscles (see 5. Range of Motion below). It is very common for the postoperative patient to develop subacromial bursitis as a result of inability to position the scapula correctly. Various taping and bracing techniques have been developed to decrease the incidence of this occurrence. These techniques do not hold the scapula in position, but rather they provide a proprioceptive link to the brain to stimulate the scapular stabilizing muscles to externally rotate and posteriorly tilt (retract and depress) the scapula, to widen the subacromial space. Recently, Walther and Werner (47) have shown that bracing improves shoulder function. This is consistent with our observations utilizing the Scapular Stabilizing System (S3) device (Alignmed, Inc.) in patients with postural dysfunction and difficulty positioning their scapulae **(Fig 22-4)**.

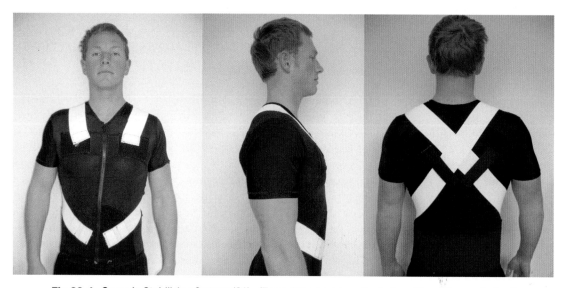

Fig 22-4. Scapula Stabilizing System (S3). (From Alignmed, Inc. Santa Ana, Ca; with permission.)

5 Range of Motion. To achieve normal scapular position, soft tissue restrictions must be addressed. Areas of particular concern in scapular dyskinesis include pectoralis minor, which causes anterior tilting; subscapularis, which causes scapular internal rotation; upper trapezius and levator scapulae, which cause elevation; infraspinatus and teres minor, which prevent normal protraction; and the posterior capsule of the glenohumeral joint. In cases where GIRD is present, the posterior inferior capsule contracture must be corrected early to restore normal glenohumeral kinematics. Postoperatively, range of motion is usually initiated in the scapular plane, but all planes must be included as the patient progresses. Specific surgical procedures must be taken into account during the period of healing.

6 Pain. *A painful joint will not progress.* During rehabilitation, pain is a sign that the wrong exercise is being done for that phase of the patient's recovery, the exercise is being done incorrectly, or the muscles are showing fatigue. Do not try to push the patient through the pain. Lack of pain is a major criterion for advancement.

7 Functional Progression. Progression is based on acquisition of function rather than time; therefore, the phases of the program are based on obtaining normal proximal control and proceeding distally. Learning speed and neuromuscular control differ among patients as a result of different learning abilities, intelligence, age, ability to focus, complicating medical issues, etc. Monitor progress by the overall trend of improvement rather than by chronological landmarks. In general, exercise progression is from general to specific, simple to complex, easy to difficult, proximal to distal, single-plane to multiple-plane, isometric stability to isometric movement, stability to mobility, controlled mobility to skill movements, controlled environment to uncontrolled environment, horizontal movements to vertical movements, and unidirectional movements to multidirectional movements (48). In addition, the patient moves from lesser to greater volume, lesser to greater intensity, and lesser to greater frequency.

8 Therapeutic Exercise. Strengthening exercises should incorporate whole-body movements whenever possible. Teach patients to isolate muscles; then train muscle groups in a coordinated, synchronous pattern to re-establish force couples, and thus functional patterns and proprioception. Muscles should be strengthened in concentric and eccentric patterns, with emphasis on control of eccentric movements.

Closed-chain exercises replicate both the physiologic and biomechanical patterns of movement. Physiologically, there is coordinated muscle firing resulting in rotator cuff muscle coactivation, reciprocal inhibition, and proprioceptive feedback. Biomechanically, there is increased joint compression with decreased shear, translational, and distractive forces on the glenohumeral joint and rotator cuff, with resultant improved control of joint movement and re-establishment of scapulohumeral rhythm. This allows the patient to increase strength and motion while protecting

healing and repaired tissue (44,49,50). Closed-chain activities for the shoulder should be primarily eccentric to slow the effects of gravity and inertia and may be used in the reverse-origin mode, for example, using the latissimus dorsi as a trunk extensor rather than as an extensor and medial rotator of the shoulder (50). Open-chain exercises, which enable movement of the terminal segments, increase the stress on the soft tissue structures; however, they are important in completing the recovery to normal function. These exercises involve concentric movement against gravity with no fixation feedback, e.g., free weight training. In general, progression is from closed-chain to open-chain exercises as healing, strength, and control are improved. Incorporation of motor patterns that include the legs and trunk should be done as soon as the patient can tolerate these activities. Sequential distal segment activation is facilitated with exercises that connect the hip and trunk with the scapula, and the scapula with the rotator cuff. Some exercises are performed in diagonal patterns to reproduce the "serape effect."

9 Quality versus Quantity. Quality is more important than quantity. Focus on control rather than the number of repetitions. Strengthening exercises should never be performed past the point of fatigue, which is frequently manifested by pain or "loss of form" in doing the exercise. In the postoperative patient, watch for elevation of the scapula as a sign of fatigue of the scapular stabilizing muscles, because this will frequently lead to subacromial bursitis, which usually inhibits functional progression.

10 Cardiovascular Training. Aerobic activity is encouraged early in the rehabilitation process to enhance blood flow and healing, as well as encouraging a feeling of control and well being for the patient. Postoperative patients can utilize a stationary bike, stair stepper, treadmill for walking, or elliptical trainer while still in a sling as long as they are comfortable and there is no impact or downward traction such as with running. Impact activities such as running are usually deferred until healing is more advanced, which is usually between 2 and 3 months postoperatively, depending on the procedure.

■ PHASES OF REHABILITATION— GOALS AND PROGRESSION CRITERIA

In the traditional approach, rehabilitation is divided into the acute, recovery, and functional phases. In the acute phase, the goals are to decrease pain and inflammation, promote healing, begin to restore range of motion, and establish more-normal scapulohumeral rhythm, scapular position, and postural and core strength. In the recovery phase, attention is directed to restoring normal range of motion, flexibility, strength, control, and endurance, and normalizing kinematics. Finally, in the functional phase, the goal is to restore work- and sport-*specific* kinematics, by re-establishing the strength, power, coordination,

TABLE 22-2	Phases of Core-based Functional Rehabilitation

1. PROXIMAL KINETIC CHAIN
   Goals
   a. Optimize postural alignment.
   b. Correct proximal kinetic chain strength and flexibility deficits.
   c. Achieve lumbo-pelvic stability and improve core strength.
   d. Improve thoracic spine mobility.
   e. Normalize upper quarter soft tissue mobility to accomplish a-d.
   Progression Criteria
   a. Normal postural alignment, thoracic spine mobility, and core stability.
   b. Normal soft tissue mobility in upper one-fourth and periscapular musculature.

2. SCAPULOTHORACIC
   Goals
   a. Normalize upper quarter soft tissue mobility.
   b. Achieve independent scapular positioning to control pain, decrease subacromial impingement, and facilitate muscle education.
   c. Strengthen scapular stabilizers and re-establish force couples to position scapula for optimal shoulder function.
   d. Restore scapulothoracic kinematics.
   Progression Criteria
   e. Functional scapular stability and mobility.

3. GLENOHUMERAL
   Goals
   a. Strengthen rotator cuff in context of kinetic chain; re-establish rotator cuff force couples for joint compression.
   b. Begin to restore normal glenohumeral motion and kinematics.
   c. Begin to restore normal upper quarter kinematics.
   Progression Criteria
   d. Full AROM in glenohumeral and scapulothoracic joints.
   e. Ability to recruit and train rotator cuff musculature without joint pain.
   f. Joint symptoms resolved or at a tolerable level.
   g. Independent in-home exercise program.

4. FUNCTION SPECIFIC
   Goals
   a. Restore function-specific glenohumeral kinematics.
   b. Restore function-specific upper quarter kinematics.
   Progression Criteria
   c. Normal activity-specific upper quarter kinematics, strength, mobility, endurance, and function.

quickness, speed, and endurance required for the desired activity of the patient (20).

This organization of phases, however, does not seem to relate as well to functional rehabilitation of the shoulder in the context of the kinetic chain as the model that we have recently developed. In our classification **(Table 22-2)**, progression is divided into the proximal kinetic chain, scapulothoracic, glenohumeral, and function-specific phases based on the concepts and principles that have been addressed earlier. Although in this scheme, there may be overlap of phases depending on strength and flexibility deficits of the patient, it is felt that this approach focuses on the return of function in a more kinematic and physiologic manner.

Table 22-3 presents a rehabilitation protocol that is based on these phases and can be used for patients with proximally or distally based scapular dyskinesis, glenohumeral instability, subacromial impingement syndrome, partial-thickness or small full-thickness rotator cuff tears, GIRD, other nonoperative disorders, and preoperative preparation. When surgical intervention is anticipated, preoperative therapy is usually performed for 4 to 6 weeks to improve scapular control preoperatively and to give the patient a head start on postoperative rehabilitation. This list of exercises and treatment options is in an approximate order of progression. By design and necessity it is incomplete, to allow for individualization of the program to meet the specific needs of an individual patient and to encourage physical therapist creativity based on the previously outlined principles. Not all exercises are appropriate for all patients.

In patients who have undergone surgery to correct a problem with instability or labral injury, the phases are divided into the protective, preparatory, progressive, and

TABLE 22-3	Nonoperative Shoulder Rehabilitation Protocol

PROXIMAL KINETIC CHAIN PHASE
1. Correct proximal kinetic chain weaknesses in lower extremity as necessary
   - Ankle, knee, hip, etc.
2. Postural correction
   - Instruction in neutral spine position
   - T roll or foam roll for thoracic mobility
3. Soft tissue releases as necessary
   - Especially pec minor, subscapularis, pec major, and lat dorsi
4. Core strengthening
   - Pelvic tilt
   - Supine alternate/double leg slides
   - Abdominal crunches
   - Supine supported marching/progression
   - Supine unsupported marching/progression
   - Exercise ball progression-foot slides
   - Sports-specific progression
5. Posterior capsule/cuff stretch
   - Side lying scapula fixed—done at 70 degrees, 90 degrees, 110 degrees elevation
   - Sleeper stretch
   - Stand against wall 90 degrees FF/elbow at 90 degrees passive horizontal add
6. Latissimus dorsi stretch
7. Prayer stretch
8. Passive pectoralis minor stretch (rolled towel or polystyrene foam roll between scapulae)
9. Passive pectoralis major stretch (doorway —> progress to corner)
10. Full kinetic chain movements—all done with scapular retraction at end
    - Grid lunges
    - Grid lunges with opposite trunk rotation dips
    - Step ups with opposite/same side hip flexion
    - Step ups with opposite/same side hip extension
    - Grid lunges with shoulder flexion
    - Grid lunges with shoulder punch
    - Step ups with shoulder flexion and opposite/same side hip flexion
    - Step ups with shoulder flexion and opposite/same side hip extension
    - Step down lunge punch/forward and to side
    - Step down lunge drop punch/forward and to side

SCAPULOTHORACIC PHASE
1. Scapular squeeze
2. Scapular clocks
3. Scapular clocks—closed chain
4. Scapular external rotation/depression-reverse corner push ups
5. Lawnmower starts
6. Isometric ball/table humeral head depression
7. Lower trapezius isometics (low rows)
8. Isometric ball/wall
9. Scapular PNF (if P.T. available)
   - Upper one-fourth pivots enables P.T. to identify specific location of weakness
10. Wall rocking
11. Weight shifting on table progression
    - Single leg balance
    - Double leg balance on bubble
    - Single leg balance on bubble
11. Weight shifting—knee to toe progression, then single arm lift
12. Single arm pull down progression
    - Single arm pull down—rotation/same side
    - Single arm pull down—hip flexion/same side
    - Single arm pull down—hip flexion/rotation same side
13. Single arm pull down progression while on bubble
14. Single arm rows progression
    - Single arm rows—rotation/same side
    - Single arm rows—bent knee/same side
    - Single arm rows—bent knee/rotation/same side

TABLE 22-3	Nonoperative Shoulder Rehabilitation Protocol—cont'd

15. Single arm rows progression while on bubble
16. Push up plus progression
17. Closed-chain perturbations
18. Prone middle/lower trap lifts
19. Wall angels (isometrics at varying degrees of elevation —> full elevation movements)
20. Scapular depressions on blocks (press up plus)
21. Prone bilateral ER with T-band (on elbows)
22. Exercise ball weight shifting—chest/hips/feet
23. Exercise ball walk outs—chest/hips/feet
24. Rowing/bilateral arms
25. Pull downs/bilateral arms
26. Iron cross with resistance band

GLENOHUMERAL PHASE
1. Cuff-specific exercises (done with scapular retraction and depression, correct axial alignment)
   - Isometrics
   - Resistance band IR/ER with good scapular position
   - IR/ER walkouts
   - Sidelying ER
   - Prone ER
   - Flexion, scaption, empty can raises
   - PNF with resistance band-standing/exercise ball
   - Closed-chain perturbations
2. Full kinetic chain coordination
   - Snatch with resistance band
   - Wall wash-standing with squat
   - Pail dumps
   - Exercise ball sitting/tubing in PNF patterns
   - Activity-specific coordinated movements without resistance
   - Progress activity-specific full kinetic chain movements from Phase I item #10 to:
     e.g., throwing technique
       swimming technique (breast, freestyle, backstroke, butterfly)
       tennis strokes (forehand —> backhand —> overhead —> serve) diving hurdle

FUNCTION-SPECIFIC PHASE (with Examples)
1. Full range of motion strengthening
   - Activity-specific strengthening progression with resistance (tubing and weights)
   - Open-chain perturbations
2. Activity-specific strength, agility, power, and endurance drills (work with coach and/or trainer)
   - Resistance band mock throwing
   - Ball bounce/wall-single/double arm
   - Sport-specific medicine ball progression
   - Tennis strokes with weights
   - Exercise ball ceiling press (diving)
   - Resistance band swimming prone on exercise ball
   - Sport-specific medicine ball work for swimmers, throwers, divers
   - Handstand sways and pushups for divers
3. Progress activity-specific full kinetic chain movements from Phase I item #10—add weight, repetitions, and plyometrics
   - Grid lunges with shoulder flexion
   - Grid lunges with shoulder punch
   - Step ups with shoulder flexion and opposite/same side hip flexion
   - Step ups with shoulder flexion and opposite/same side hip extension
   - Step down lunge punch/forward and to side
   - Step down lunge drop punch/forward and to side
   - Hurdle with jump for divers

FF, forward flexion; PNF, proprioceptive neuromuscular facilitation; P.T., physical therapy; ER, external rotation; IR, internal rotation.

TABLE 22-4	Postoperative Progression Criteria (Anterior instability, posterior instability, multidirectional instability, SLAP, or Bankart repair)

<u>Protective to Preparatory</u>
Minimal pain on range of motion and with isometric exercises
Adequate scapular control
Adequate soft tissue healing
Soft tissue restrictions cleared (improving soft tissue, thoracic spine, and GH mobility)
Understanding and performance of core stabilization exercises
Compliance with home exercise program

<u>Preparatory to Progressive</u>
Pain-free range of motion
Minimal pain with therapeutic exercise
Active elevation to 150 degrees
Normal soft tissue, thoracic spine, and GH mobility
Improved joint kinematics and control
Compliance with home exercise program

<u>Progressive to Performance</u>
Full functional range of motion and flexibility
Normal kinematics
Pain free with all exercises
Adequate scapular control for functional demands
Compliance with home exercise program
Approximately 75% strength, power, and endurance

<u>Graduation</u>
Normal upper quarter kinematics, range of motion, flexibility for specific activity or sport
Approximately 90% strength, power, and endurance
Symptom free with activity or sport-specific drills

performance phases. The goals of these phases are similar to those outlined in the classification in Table 22-2 with the protective and preparatory phases stressing proximal stability and the progressive and performance phases stressing distal mobility. In the protective phase, it is critical to the success of the program to maintain control of pain and inflammation and to educate the patient regarding postural alignment and scapular control exercises. Progression must take into account adequate time for soft tissue healing. The progression criteria following stabilization surgery are outlined in **Table 22-4**.

Rehabilitation following rotator cuff repair is controversial. Steinman (51) reported that it takes 12 weeks for the development of Sharpey fibers at the footprint of the supraspinatus following surgical repair. On this basis, many surgeons delay range of motion exercises for 4 to 6 weeks and strengthening exercises for 12 weeks. Our postoperative protocol is determined by the size of the tear, quality of repaired tissue, age and physiology of the patient, and quality of the repair. Although postoperative stiffness is a concern, passive range of motion exercises have been shown to activate the rotator cuff musculature (53) and therefore should be done only under optimal conditions. Wise et al. (52) have demonstrated that early closed chain

exercises can improve shoulder function while avoiding shear on the glenohumeral joint and excessive traction on the repaired tissue. In a majority of cases, we maintain the operated extremity in a sling for 4 to 6 weeks, permitting active assistive external rotation in adduction and gentle closed-chain active assistive elevation when the patient is comfortable enough to tolerate it. Our goal is for the patient to have approximately 90 degrees of elevation by this time. Passive elevation in the scapular plane is then allowed with a goal of 150 degrees of scaption. After this motion is achieved, open-chain eccentric rotator cuff strengthening between 90 and 150 degrees is encouraged in addition to closed-chain strengthening exercises that were initiated earlier. Wise et al. (52) have shown that based on rotator cuff activation levels, progression can be from closed to open chain, horizontal to vertical to diagonal, and from slow to fast speed.

The programs that have been outlined above allow for functional progression of range of motion, strength and kinematics; however, in the postoperative patient, it is important to protect healing tissues from adverse stress while advancing the process of rehabilitation. **Table 22-5** summarizes specific precautions that should be observed after surgical correction of pathology.

TABLE 22-5	Specific Postoperative Precautions by Procedure

Suprapinatus Repair
1. Sling is worn for 3 to 6 weeks (depending on size of tear, quality of tissue, security of repair). Ultrasling is worn at night.
2. Avoid lifting with operated arm, although it is OK to move hand to mouth.
3. Avoid reaching across the body or out to the side.
4. Avoid behind the back reaching for 6 weeks.

Subscapularis Repair
1. Sling is worn for 3 to 4 weeks. Ultrasling is worn at night.
2. Avoid lifting with operated arm, although it is OK to move hand to mouth.
3. Limit external rotation to neutral.

SLAP Repair
1. Ultrasling is worn 3 to 4 weeks.
2. Avoid lifting with the operated arm, although it is OK to move hand to mouth.
3. Limit ROM to 90 degrees for 3 to 4 weeks.
4. ROM work done with active assistance with elbow bent.
5. Avoid horizontal abduction. Avoid internal rotation in posterior slap repairs.
6. Elevation in scapular plane or forward flexion.
7. External rotation to 45 degrees done in scapular plane for 3 to 4 weeks.

Capsular Shift and Capsulolabral Reconstructions
Anterior
1. Sling is worn 3 to 4 weeks. Ultrasling at night.
2. No lifting with operated arm for 6 weeks, although it is OK to move hand to mouth.
3. No external rotation in adduction past neutral for 2 to 3 weeks, then OK to externally rotate to 45 degrees in scaption.
4. Elevation in the scapular plane or forward flexion.
5. Avoid combined abduction and external rotation; allow full ROM at 6 weeks post operatively.

Posterior
1. Ultrasling worn in gunslinger position for 6 weeks.
2. Avoid forward flexion for 3 weeks.
3. No internal rotation movements past neutral for 3 weeks.
4. Limit active motions to scapular plane, with bias toward external rotation.
5. Avoid horizontal adduction for 6 weeks.
6. Begin gentle active internal rotation in scaption at 4 weeks and reaching behind back for at least 6 weeks post operatively.

SUMMARY

Successful rehabilitation of the injured or surgically repaired shoulder should be carried out in the context of the kinetic chain in which upper-extremity function occurs. Core-based functional rehabilitation encompasses the concepts of proximal stability and core strengthening before distal mobility; exercising with proper postural alignment; correcting soft tissue restrictions early; teaching the patient to isolate muscles, then training muscle groups in a coordinated, synchronous pattern to re-establish functional patterns and proprioception; and ultimately restoring dynamic stability and normal kinematics. Following the principles that have been discussed in this chapter should allow physicians and therapists to improve the outcomes of treatment in patients with shoulder disorders.

REFERENCES

1. Feltner ME, Dapena J. Three-dimensional interactions in a two-segment kinetic chain. Part I: general model. *Int J Sport Biomech.* 1989;5:403–419.
2. Feltner ME, Dapena J. Three-dimensional interactions in a two-segment kinetic chain. Part II: application to the throwing arm in pitching. *Int J Sport Biomech.* 1989;5:420–450.
3. Dillman CJ. Proper mechanics of pitching. *Sports Med Update.* 1990;5:15–18.
4. Kibler WB. Biomechanical analysis of the shoulder during tennis activities. *Clin Sports Med.* 1995;14:79–86.
5. Putnam CA. Sequential motions of body segments in striking and throwing skills: descriptions and explanations. *J Biomech.* 1993;26:125–135.
6. Atwater AE. Movement characteristics of the overarm throw; a kinematic analysis. *Dissertation Abstracts International.* 1971;31:5819A.
7. Toyoshima C, Hoshikawa T, Miyashita M. Contribution of the body parts to throwing performance. In: Nelson RC, Morehouse CA, eds. *Biomechanics IV.* Baltimore: University Park Press; 1974: 169–174.
8. Kibler WB. The role of the scapula in athletic shoulder function. *Am J Sports Med.* 1998;26:325–337.
9. Kibler WB. Role of the scapula in the overhead throwing motion. *Contemp Ortho.* 1991;22:525–532.
10. Hodges PW. Is there a role for the transverses abdominis in lumbo-pelvic stability? *Manual Therapy.* 1999;4:74–86.
11. Young JL, Herring SA, Press JM. The influence of the spine on the shoulder in the throwing athlete. *J Back Musculoskeletal Rehab.* 1996;7:5–17.

12. Inman JT, Saunders M, Abbott L. Observations on the function of the shoulder joint. *J Bone Joint Surg.* 1944;26:1–30.
13. Happee R, Van der Helm FCT. The control of shoulder muscles during goal-directed movements: an inverse dynamic analysis. *J Biomech.* 1995;28:1179–1191.
14. Dvir Z, Berme N. The shoulder complex in elevation of the arm: a mechanism approach. *J Biomech.* 1978;11:219–225.
15. Codman EA. *The Shoulder.* Boston: Thomas Todd Co; 1934:1–64.
16. Van der Helm FCT, Pronk GM. Three-dimensional recording and description of motions of the shoulder mechanism. *J Biomech Eng.* 1995;117:27–40.
17. Kent BE. Functional anatomy of the shoulder complex. a review. *Phys Ther.* 1971;51:867–887.
18. Bagg SD, Forrest WJ. EMG study of the scapular rotators during arm abduction in the scapular plane. *Am J Phys Med.* 1986;65:111–124.
19. Bagg SD, Forrest WJ. A biomechanical analysis of scapular rotation during arm abduction in the scapular plane. *Am J Phys Med and Rehab.* 1988;67:238–245.
20. Rubin BD, Kibler WB. Fundamental principles of shoulder rehabilitation: conservative to postoperative management. *Arthroscopy.* 2002;18(9 Suppl 2):29–39.
21. Borstad JD, Ludewig PM. The effect of long versus short pectoralis minor resting length on scapular kinematics in healthy individuals. *J Orthop Sports Phys Ther.* 2005;35(4):227–238.
22. Uhl TL, Tripp B. Validation of a clinical assessment of scapular dyskinesis. A preliminary report: Paper presented at: *ASES Open Meeting*; 2003; Dana Point, CA.
23. Greenfield B, Catlin PA, Coats PW, et al. Posture in patients with shoulder overuse injuries and healthy individuals. *J Orthop Sports Phys Ther.* 1995;21:287–295.
24. Rubin BD. The basics of competitive diving and its injuries. *Clin Sports Med.* 1999;18:293–303.
25. McQuade KJ, Dawson J, Smidt GL. Scapulothoracic muscle fatigue associated with alterations in scapulohumeral rhythm kinematics during maximum resistive shoulder elevation. *J Orthop Sports Phys Ther.* 1998;28:74–80.
26. Glousman R, Jobe FW, Tibone JE. Dynamic electromyographic analysis of the throwing shoulder with glenohumeral instability. *J Bone Joint Surg.* 1988;70A:220–226.
27. Kebaetse M, McClure P, Pratt NA. Thoracic position effect on shoulder range of motion, strength, and three-dimensional scapular kinematics. *Arch Phys Med Rehabil.* 1999;80:945–950.
28. Weiser WM, Lee TQ, McMaster W, et al. Effects of simulated scapular protraction on anterior glenohumeral stability. *Am J Sports Med.* 1999;27:801–805.
29. Solem-Bertoft E, Thuomas KA, Westerberg CE. The influence of scapula retraction and protraction on the width of the subacromial space. *Clin Orthop.* 1993;296:99–103.
30. Burkhart SS, Morgan CD, Kibler WB. Shoulder injuries in the overhead athlete: the dead arm revisited. *Clin Sports Med.* 2000;19:125–159.
31. Ikeda H, "Rotator interval" lesion: II. Biomechanical study. *Nippon Ganka Gakkai Zasshi.* 1986;60:1275.
32. Nobuhara K, Ikeda H. Rotator interval lesion. *Clin Orthop.* 1987;223:44–50.
33. Ozaki J. Glenohumeral movements of involuntary inferior and multidirectional instability. *Clin Orthop.* 1989;238:107.
34. Warner JJ, Micheli LJ, Arslanian LE. Scapulothoracic motion in normal shoulders and shoulders with glenohumeral instability and impingement syndrome: a study using Moire topographical analysis. *Clin Orthop.* 1992;285:191–199.
35. Tamai K, Ogawa K. Intratendinous tear of the supraspinatus tendon exhibiting winging of the scapula: a case report. *Clin Orthop.* 1985;194:159–163.
36. Fiddian NJ, King RJ. The winged scapula. *Clin Orthop.* 1984;185:228–236.
37. Steinmann SP, Higgins DL, Sewell D. Nonparalytic winging of the scapula (poster exhibit): Paper presented at: 61st Annual Meeting of the American Academy of Orthopedic Surgeons; 1994; New Orleans, LA.
38. Kuhn JE, Plancher KD, Hawkins RJ. Scapular Winging. *J Am Acad Orthop Surg.* 1995;3:319–325.
39. Michener LA, McClure PW, Karduna AR. Anatomical and biomechanical mechanisms of subacromial impingement syndrome. *Clin Biomech.* 2003;18:369–379.
40. Meskers CG, van der Helm FCT, Rozing PM. The size of the supraspinatus outlet during elevation of the arm in the frontal and sagittal plane: a 3-D model study. *Clin Biomech.* 2002;17:257–266.
41. Borstad JD, Ludewig PM. Comparison of scapular kinematics between elevation and lowering of the arm in the scapular plane. *Clin Biomech.* 2002;17:650–659.
42. Cools AM, Witvrouw EE, Declercq GA, et al. Evaluation of isokinetic force production and associated muscle activity in the scapular rotators during a protraction-retraction movement in overhead athletes with impingement symptoms. *Br J Sports Med.* 2004;38:64–68.
43. Cools AM, Witvrouw EE, Declercq GA, et al. scapular muscle recruitment pattern: trapezius muscle latency in overhead athletes with and without impingement symptoms. *Am J Sports Med.* 2003;31:542–549.
44. Kibler WB, Livingston BP. Closed-chain rehabilitation for the upper and lower extremities. *J Am Acad Orthop Surg.* 2001;9:412–421.
45. Rubin BD. Core-based functional rehabilitation of the shoulder: Paper presented at: 17th Annual San Diego Shoulder Meeting; 2000; La Jolla, CA.
46. Muirhead M. *Total Pilates.* San Diego: Thunder Bay Press; 2003:18–19.
47. Walther M, Werner A. The subacromial impingement syndrome of the shoulder treated by conventional physical therapy, self training, and a shoulder brace: results of a prospective randomized study. *J Shoulder Elbow Surg.* 2004;13(4):417–423.
48. Kelley MJ, Clark WA. *Orthopedic Therapy of the Shoulder.* Philadelphia: JB Lippincott Co; 1994:348.
49. Uhl TL, Carver TJ. Shoulder musculature activation during upper extremity weight-bearing exercise. *J Orthop Sports Phys Ther.* 2003;33:109–117.
50. Cipriani D. Open and closed chain rehabilitation for the shoulder complex. In: Andrews JR, Wilk KE, eds. *The Athlete's Shoulder.* New York: Churchill Livingstone; 1994.
51. Sonnabend D. Paper presented at: *ASES Closed Meeting*; 2000; Austin, TX.
52. Wise MB, Uhl TL, Mattacola CG, et al. The effect of limb support on muscle activation during shoulder exercises. *J Shoulder Elbow Surg.* 2004;13:614–620.

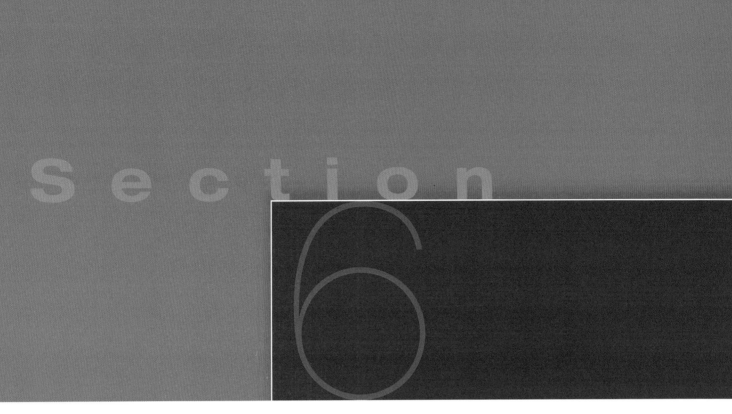
UPPER EXTREMITY

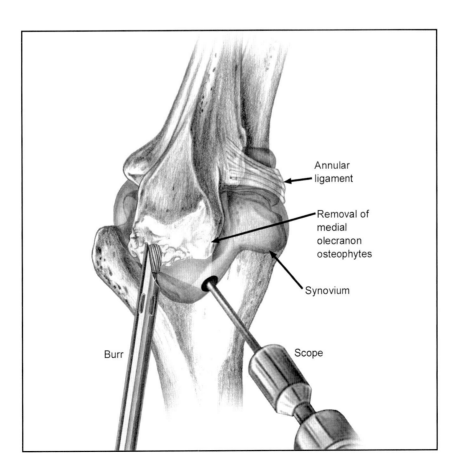

Annular ligament

Removal of medial olecranon osteophytes

Synovium

Burr

Scope

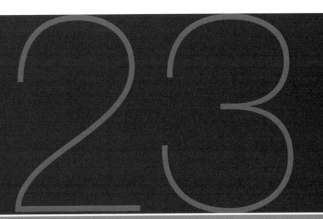

ELBOW INJURIES

RONALD M. SELBY, MD, MARC R. SAFRAN, MD, STEPHEN J. O'BRIEN, MD, PLLC

■ KEY POINTS

- The elbow joint is multifaceted and works primarily in conjunction with the shoulder to position the hand in space. It also serves as a fulcrum for the forearm lever and transmits load between the forearm and the upper arm.
- Inner elbow pain may be the result of injury to the ulnar collateral ligament (UCL). Injury to the UCL may be acute, chronically disrupted, or chronically attenuated.
- Treatment of UCL injury consists of a very structured approach that includes relative rest, anti-inflammatory measures, and physical therapy. With this conservative regimen, approximately 50% of throwing athletes are able to return to throwing.
- The elbow of the skeletally immature athlete is susceptible to two main problems—apophyseal injury and osteochondritis dissecans (OCD). The physis is the weakest link in the skeletally immature musculoskeletal system, resulting in apophysitis and avulsion injuries, rather than ligament injuries as seen in adults. Lateral elbow pain may reflect OCD, which is particularly common in young throwing athletes and gymnasts.
- Fracture or avulsion of the medial epicondylar physis can be a stress fracture or overt fracture due to repetitive valgus forces, falling, or repetitive violent forearm flexor muscle contraction in the skeletally immature athlete.
- Abnormal stresses of the triceps attachment on the olecranon apophysis can result in an injury syndrome similar to Osgood-Schlatter disease of the knee.
- The ulnar nerve is the most commonly injured nerve around the elbow.
- Acute tendon ruptures about the elbow often require surgical reattachment. They may be treated with protection,

rest, ice, compression, and elevation, along with medications (PRICEM), as long as it does not interfere with, or delay, surgical reattachment.
- Pain at the triceps insertion at the proximal olecranon is common in athletes who lift inordinate amounts of weight or participate in explosive field events such as shot put. However it is also seen in javelin throwing and baseball pitching.
- Lateral epicondylosis (tennis elbow) is arguably the most common source of elbow pain in the general population. Lateral epicondylosis, which also affects nontennis players, is a chronic, noninflammatory condition of the extensor muscles, primarily the extensor carpi radialis brevis (ECRB), due to overuse.
- Athletes participating in overhead sports such as tennis, volleyball, swimming, weightlifting, gymnastics, and especially throwing activities, subject their elbows to repetitive stresses most marked in specific phases of the activity. These athletes are vulnerable to injuries and present with a myriad of problems including tendonitis, bursitis, nerve injuries and instability. Repetitive overhead stress to the elbow can and does cause cumulative injuries to soft tissue static stabilizers, with recurrent micro injuries to the primary stabilizers including the UCLs and capsule.
- The athlete involved in throwing (baseball, javelin, water polo, football quarterback) and overhead sports (such as volleyball and tennis) is most often exposed to chronic repetitive valgus stress at the elbow.
- Although pitching a baseball places the elbow at some risk, application of the proper pitching mechanics can assist in minimizing potential risk for injury while maximizing performance.
- The elbow is the second-most commonly dislocated major joint in patients of all ages. In children under the age of

10 years, the elbow is the most commonly dislocated major joint.

■ Medial epicondylar fractures may be the result of an acute injury or repetitive overuse. Skeletally immature overhead throwing athletes may develop an injury to the medial epicondylar growth plate, because the apophysis is the weakest link in the growing musculoskeletal unit.

■ FUNCTIONAL ANATOMY

The elbow joint is formed by an articulation at the distal end of the humerus with the radius and the ulna and by an articulation of the radius with the ulna. Thus, the elbow joint is a composite of three articulations composed of a hinge (ginglymus) joint and a pivot (trochoid) joint **(Figs 23-1 and 23-2)**. Flexion and extension of the forearm in the frontal plane take place at the humeroulnar articulation, while pronation and supination occur at the articulation of the radius with the ulna (the radio-ulnar joint) **(Fig 23-3)**. The distal humerus is triangular in shape and composed of two condyles covered with a continuous layer of hyaline cartilage supporting the joint surfaces of the spool-shaped trochlea which articulates

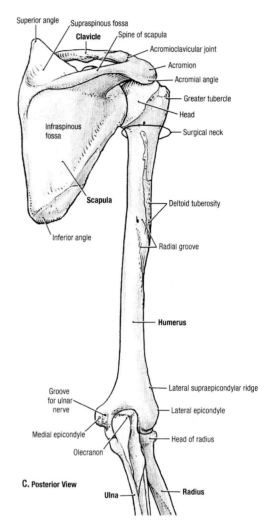

Fig 23-2. Posterior osseous anatomy. (Reprinted with permission from Agur AMR, Dally AF II. *Grant's Atlas of Anatomy.* 11th ed. Philadelphia: Lippincott Williams & Wilkins; 2005:499.)

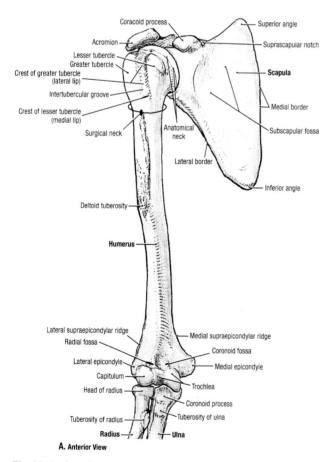

Fig 23-1. Anterior osseous anatomy. (Reprinted with permission from Agur AMR, Dally AF II. *Grant's Atlas of Anatomy.* 11th ed. Philadelphia: Lippincott Williams & Wilkins; 2005:498.)

with the reciprocally saddle-shaped trochlear notch of the proximal ulna and the rounded capitellum (Fig 23-3), which articulates with the slightly concave superior end of the radial head **(Fig 23-4)**. The capitellum is limited to the anterior and inferior surface of the distal humerus, while the trochlea is present anteriorly, inferiorly, and posteriorly. Stability of the elbow joint is largely a function of the bony congruity of the humerus, ulna, and radius, with contributions from some ligaments and muscles. In the distal humerus, the coronoid fossa anteriorly and olecranon fossa posteriorly are divided by a thin layer of bone. The proximal ulna is composed of two processes, the olecranon and the coronoid with the trochlear notch between them. The proximal radius is composed of the radial head that articulates with the capitellum, the radial neck, and a tuberosity onto which inserts the biceps tendon. The humerus is a tubular bone that articulates with the shoulder proximally and the elbow distally. Superior to the trochlea, the medial epicondyle provides the attachment for the flexor-pronator group of forearm muscles and the medial

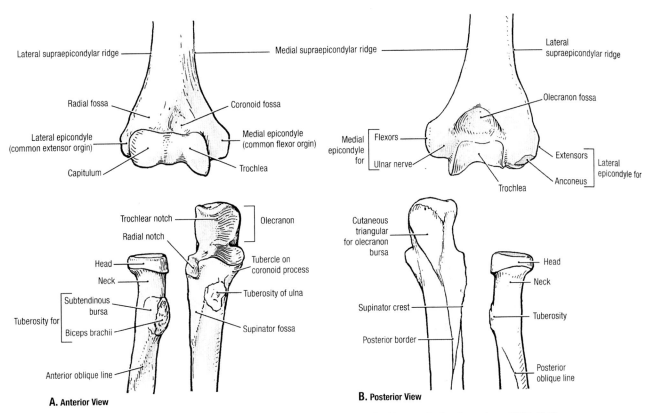

Fig 23-3. Elbow osseous articulating anatomy. (Reprinted with permission from Agur AMR, Dally AF II. *Grant's Atlas of Anatomy.* 11th ed. Philadelphia: Lippincott Williams & Wilkins; 2005:524.)

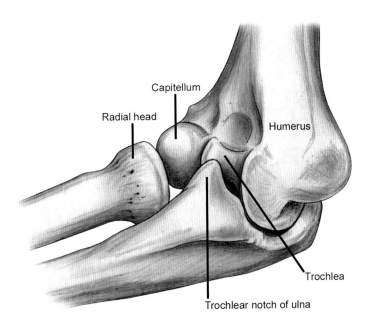

Fig 23-4. The proximal radius and ulna.

collateral ligament. Superior to the capitellum, the lateral epicondyle is not as prominent as the medial epicondyle, which serves as the site for forearm extensor and supinator muscles attachment.

Just superior to the capitellum, the radial fossa is found on the lateral humerus. This fossa accommodates the radial head in forearm flexion. The coronoid fossa is located medial to

the radial fossa in the midline of the anterior distal humerus and similarly accommodates the coronoid process in forearm flexion. The olecranon fossa up is found posteriorly, midline in the distal humerus, and provides space for the olecranon process during extension. These fossae are bordered by the robust lateral supracondylar column and a smaller medial supracondylar column.

The ulna is asymmetrical with a cylindrical cross section at the wrist changing from a triangular cross section in its midshaft to its thickened proximal section (Fig. 23-4). The greater sigmoid notch of the ulna comprises a 190-degree arc and articulates with the trochlea of the humerus. The sigmoid notch is composed of the coronoid process at its distal extent with an articular and cortical surface where the brachialis muscle and the oblique cord insert and the olecranon at its proximal extent where the triceps muscle inserts. The medial portion of the coronoid serves as the origin for the medial part of the pronator teres, flexor pollicis longus, flexor digitorum profoundus, and flexor digitorum superficialis. The anterior portion of the medial collateral ligament of the elbow inserts onto the medial aspect of the coronoid process. The lateral surface of the coronoid process is composed of a radial notch, which serves as a site for articulation with the radial head. The radial head is stabilized by the annular ligament that surrounds it and attaches to the anterior and posterior margins of the notch. From the inferior portion of the notch, a depression extends distally, which serves as the origin of the supinator muscle. The medial collateral ligament inserts onto a tuberosity at the proximal extent of this depression.

The radius has a cylindrical cross section proximally and tapers to an elliptical cross-section distally. The radial head, held securely by the annular ligament, has a proximal concavity for articulating with the capitellum. The anterior face of the radial tuberosity is covered by a bursa that protects the biceps tendon during pronation. The biceps brachii tendon attaches to the posteromedial surface of the radial tuberosity and thereby plays a role in flexion as well as supination of the forearm. The interosseous membrane is found between the medial crest of the radius and the lateral crest of the ulna.

The humeroulnar, radiohumeral, and proximal radioulnar joints are all enclosed within one synovial and fibrous capsule **(Fig 23-5)**. Elbow flexion is constrained by the trochlea articulating with the trochlear notch of the ulna. Articular cartilage covers an arch of 300 to 330 degrees on its anterior, distal, and posterior surfaces and is responsible for absorbing compressive forces (1,2). This allows for a tongue and groove, captive interface with the proximal ulna. The trochlear is not symmetrical and allows for approximately 5 degrees of internal rotation in early flexion and approximately 5 degrees of external rotation in terminal flexion. The medial lip is larger and protrudes more distally than the lateral. The two lips are partitioned by a helical groove that traverses in an anterolateral to posteromedial fashion. The capitellum of the distal humerus is spherical and covered with a thick articular cartilage. The posteromedial capitellum is marked by a prominent tubercle separating it from the lateral lip of the trochlea, where the radial head articulates through the entire range of flexion. The orientation of the articular surface of the distal humerus is rotated anteriorly about 30 degrees with respect to the longitudinal axis of the humerus. The center of the arc formed by the trochlea and capitellum is on a line that is coplanar to the anterior distal

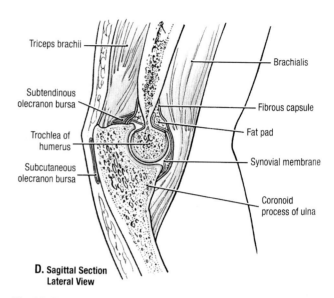

Fig 23-5. Bursae and synovium of the elbow. (Reprinted with permission from Agur AMR, Dally AF II. *Grant's Atlas of Anatomy.* 11th ed. Philadelphia: Lippincott Williams & Wilkins; 2005:524.)

cortex. Therefore, 5 to 7 degrees of internal rotation is observed at the distal humeral articular surface with respect to the midline to the humeral epicondyle. In a frontal plane there is about 6 degrees of valgus tilt of the condyles with respect to the longitudinal axis of the humerus. This articular surface accounts for more that 50% of elbow stability in extension and more than 70% of elbow stability when the elbow is flexed 90 degrees.

Articular cartilage covers the radial depression anteriorly within the radial head. This concavity has an arc of about 40 degrees (2). Additionally, 240 degrees of the outside circumference of the radial head articulates with the ulna. The lesser trochlea notch forms an arc of approximately 60 to 80 degrees delegating the remaining 160 to 180 degrees to pronation and supination (3). The head is largely covered with articular cartilage with the exception of the anterolateral one-third of the circumference of the head. This part of the radial head is devoid of subchondral bone and does not have the same structural integrity as covered areas. The head and neck of the radius form a 15-degree varus angle with the distal portion of the radius relative to the midline distally.

The trochlear notch is divided medially and laterally by a ridge that forms four quadrants. The sigmoid notch is situated approximately 30 degrees posterior to the longitudinal axis of the ulna, which corresponds to the 30-degree inferior rotation of the distal humerus. This allows for stability. Anteriorly, 1 to 6 degree rotation of the shaft lateral to the articulating surfaces contributes to the carrying angle (1). Laterally, the notch forms a 190-degree elliptical arc (3).

The congruous bony anatomy affords stability to the elbow joint. Medial (ulnar) and lateral collateral ligament complexes (LCLCs) comprise the ligaments of the elbow and provide stability in varying degrees of flexion to varus, valgus, and rotational forces. The ulnar collateral ligament

(UCL) complex is composed of the anterior oblique, posterior oblique, and transverse ligaments **(Fig 23-6)**. This is the primary stabilizer of the elbow to valgus stress. Within the UCL complex the anterior bundle is the most discrete component composed of anterior and posterior bands. These bands tighten in reciprocal fashion as flexion and extension of the elbow occurs. The posterior bundle is a thickening of the posterior capsule and defined well only with the elbow in about 90 degrees of flexion. The transverse ligament appears to contribute little to elbow stability because its fibers span the ulnar border of the trochlea notch from the coronoid process to the olecranon. The UCL originates from the anteroinferior surface of the medial epicondyle. The anterior oblique ligament (AOL) is the primary stabilizer of the elbow and resists valgus stress between 20 and 120 degrees of flexion (4–6). The AOL is composed of two bands **(Fig 23-7)**. The anterior and posterior oblique ligaments have distinct biomechanical roles. The anterior band is the primary restraint to valgus stresses at 30, 60, and 90 degrees of flexion and a co-primary restraint at 120 degrees of flexion (7). The posterior band functions as a secondary restraint to valgus stress with the elbow held at 120 degrees of flexion (7).

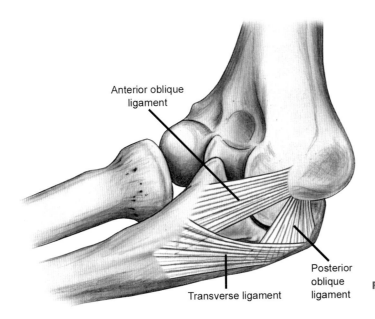

Fig 23-6. The medial ligament complex.

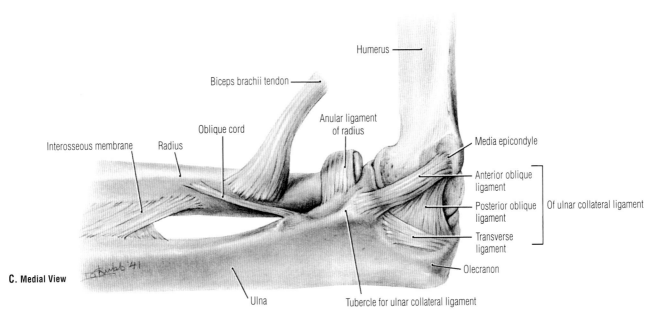

Fig 23-7. Ligaments of the medial elbow. (Reprinted with permission from Agur AMR, Dally AF II. *Grant's Atlas of Anatomy*. 11th ed. Philadelphia: Lippincott Williams & Wilkins; 2005:526.)

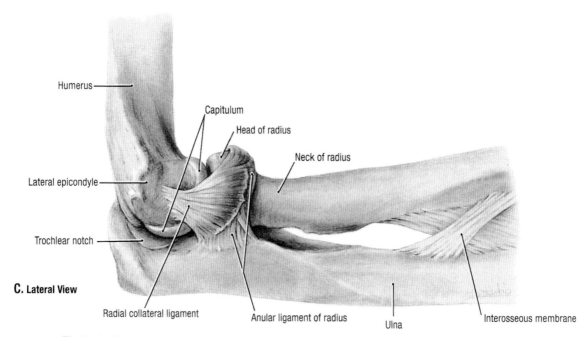

Humerus

Capitulum

Head of radius

Neck of radius

Lateral epicondyle

Trochlear notch

C. Lateral View

Radial collateral ligament

Anular ligament of radius

Ulna

Interosseous membrane

Fig 23-8. The lateral collateral ligament complex. (Reprinted with permission from Agur AMR, Dally AF II. *Grant's Atlas of Anatomy.* 11th ed. Philadelphia: Lippincott Williams & Wilkins; 2005:527.)

The LCLC encompasses the lateral collateral, lateral ulnar collateral, and annular ligaments **(Fig 23-8)**. The lateral complex consists more of a blend of poorly demarcated fan-shaped ligamentous fibers compared to the discrete bands of the medial collateral ligament complex. The function of the lateral collateral ligament is to provide an external rotation and varus stability as the elbow flexes. The LCLC effect gradually increases as the elbow flexes toward 110 degrees. The lateral collateral ligament origin is from the entire inferior surface of the lateral epicondyle. This is near the axis of rotation and subsequently remains taut throughout flexion and extension. The fibers of the lateral collateral ligaments and the lateral UCLs cannot be separated proximally. The lateral UCL is the posterior portion of the lateral collateral ligament. The annular ligament attaches to the anterior and posterior margins of the lesser sigmoid notch. It becomes taut during supination at its anterior insertion and becomes taut at the extremes of pronation at its posterior insertion. This ligament is funnel shaped and assists in stabilizing the proximal radius throughout the range of pronation and supination.

The blood supply to the elbow is composed of the vessels that comprise the collateral circulation about the elbow. This is from the superior and inferior ulnar collateral arteries on the medial side superiorly and the two ulnar recurrent arteries inferiorly **(Fig 23-9)**. Laterally, the radial recurrent and middle collateral arteries of the profunda brachii supply the joint superiorly and the radial and interosseous recurrent arteries inferiorly.

Nervous innervation to the elbow joint arises typically from all four nerves that cross the joint **(Fig 23-10)**. In general, the distribution of each nerve to the joint is overlapped by the distribution of branches from other nerves (9).

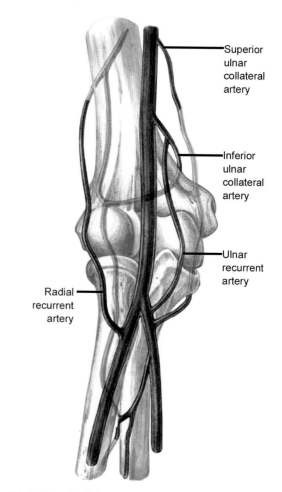

Superior ulnar collateral artery

Inferior ulnar collateral artery

Ulnar recurrent artery

Radial recurrent artery

Fig 23-9. Vessels of the upper extremity.

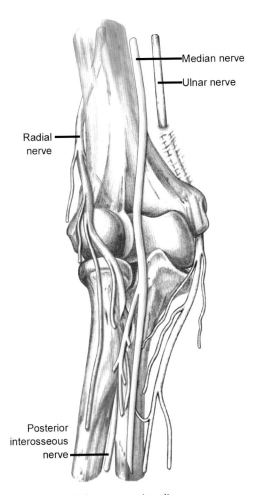

Fig 23-10. Nerves of the upper extremity.

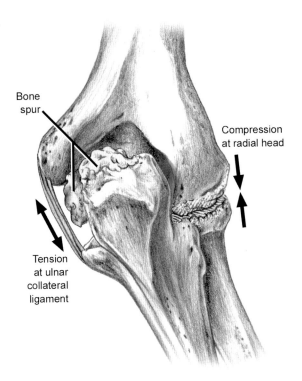

Fig 23-11. The relationship of biomechanical forces within the elbow.

■ BIOMECHANICS AND KINEMATICS

Elbow function is an inherent component of the normal use of the arm in daily activities and athletic endeavors. The elbow joint is multifaceted and works primarily in conjunction with the shoulder to position the hand in space. It also serves as a fulcrum for the forearm lever and transmits load between the forearm and the upper arm. The structural makeup of the bony articulations, ligaments, and capsule contribute to the elbow's renowned stability. As the anatomic link between the humerus and forearm, the elbow is consistently subjected to intense compressive, tensile, and shear forces **(Fig 23-11)**. Effects of the culmination of these forces can be seen in repetitive activities; this effect is magnified in the overhead athlete. Stiffness or instability of the elbow can severely compromise the function of the entire upper extremity. An understanding of the biomechanical function and kinematics of the elbow is paramount for treating physicians.

Flexion and extension about a transverse axis is permitted by the humeral trochlea serving as a pulley for the trochlear notch of the ulna. The radial head glides along the articular surface of the capitellum during flexion and extension without influencing the path of motion. Elbow flexion is limited by contact of the biceps brachii muscle and other soft tissue structures. Forearm extension is limited by the olecranon process of the ulna when it contacts the olecranon fossa of the humerus. Posteriorly the margins of the trochlea extend obliquely superiorly and laterally so that when the forearm is extended it deviates laterally rather than in line with the upper arm and thereby forms the carrying angle of the elbow.

The normal range of flexion and extension of the elbow is 135 degrees (10). Rotation as well as varus and valgus forces of the elbow are limited by the inherent bony stability as well as a significant restraint to varus and valgus forces from the collateral ligaments. The radio-ulnar joint plays a role in pronation and supination. The axis of rotation runs through the center of the radial head and styloid process of the ulna. During supination and pronation, the ulna remains fixed while the radius rotates internally during pronation or externally in supination. Supination is limited largely by ligaments between the ulna and carpal bones. Pronation is limited by soft tissues on the anterior radius and ulna. The normal range is about 80 degrees of supination and 80 degrees of pronation.

The elbow is in essence a slightly loose hinge with small amounts of varus, valgus, and rotational laxity throughout its range of motion. The center of the arc formed by the trochlea and capitellum is on a line that is coplanar to the anterior distal cortex. Therefore, 5 to 7 degrees of internal rotation is observed at the distal humeral articular surface with respect to the midline to the humeral epicondyle. In a frontal plane there is about 6 degrees of the valgus tilt of the condyles with respect to the longitudinal axis of the humerus. This articular surface accounts for more that 50% of elbow stability in extension and more than 70% of elbow stability when the elbow is flexed 90 degrees.

The range of motion of the elbow is composed of extension to about zero to 5 degrees, flexion to approximately 145 degrees, supination to 85 degrees, and pronation to about 75 degrees **(Fig 23-12)**. The normal valgus angle at the elbow (in full extension this is known as the carrying angle) is about 5 degrees in males and 10 to 15 degrees in females. Bony and soft tissue constraints contribute to the noted stability of the elbow joint. The bony structure resists valgus and varus forces and shows increased stability in extension. Static stability is also enhanced by the medial and lateral collateral ligaments and the joint capsule. This is especially noted in flexion. Dynamic stabilization is also aided by several muscles that cross the elbow joint. The primary constraint to valgus forces of the elbow is the anterior bundle of the UCL. During overhead motion, tensile forces are applied across the medial aspect of the elbow, compressive forces across the lateral aspect of the elbow, and valgus extension forces in the posterior aspect of the elbow.

The biomechanics of pitching involves coordination of the entire body with sequential activation of different body parts to culminate in maximum velocity at ball release. The motion of the arm in throwing, and this is repeatedly magnified in pitching, is rapid and violent. Elbow injuries in pitching are fairly common. The peak angular velocity during throwing has been measured to be 6,180 degrees per second for shoulder internal rotation and 4,595 degrees per second for elbow extension (11). Peak elbow acceleration has ranged from 225,000 to 500,000 degrees per second. Stresses at the elbow occur during acceleration and follow-through phases, which last approximately 15 milliseconds. During this time period the arm undergoes organized deceleration, which requires normally functioning elbow musculature to prevent the articular and ligamentous stabilizers from having to absorb all the force. The pitching motion is divided into five phases to more easily enable study of the biomechanics of the elbow during pitching. During the windup and stride phases, the elbow is not subjected to significant forces. In the arm-cocking phase, contraction of the wrist flexor pronator group generates varus torque to counter the valgus extension loading of the UCL, which is not strong enough to resist the torque by itself (12). The anconeus and triceps are also active during this phase to decrease the stress on the UCL by compressing the joint and conferring dynamic stability. During acceleration, triceps activity increases and biceps activity decreases. When the shoulder arm reaches maximum internal rotation,

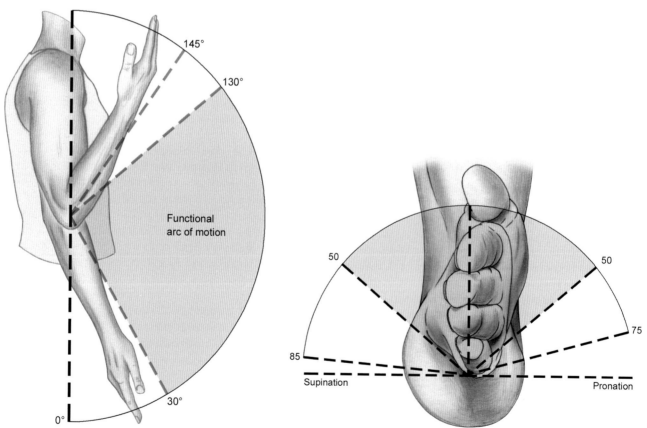

Fig 23-12. A: Normal flexion and extension of the elbow. **B:** Normal pronation and supination. The functional arc of rotation is shaded.

the deceleration phase begins with increased contraction in the biceps, triceps, reflectors, and wrist extensors to counter wrist flexion. The trunk and legs help to dissipate forces during the follow-through phase. (See Throwing Mechanics and the Elbow section.)

◼ LIGAMENT INJURY–ULNAR COLLATERAL LIGAMENT AND POSTEROLATERAL ROTATORY INSTABILITY

Ligament injuries of the elbow have been of particular interest to the sports physician with increasing amounts of research and literature being written in recent years. Due to better understanding and awareness, the diagnosis of ligament injuries is becoming more common. Particularly for the UCL, it is now understood that subtle degrees of laxity are the hallmark of injury to this ligament, thus careful examination, in addition to newer, advanced imaging techniques, help in the ability to diagnose this problem. On the lateral side, enhanced understanding of the lateral ligament complex, its role in injury and subsequent disability was brought to the forefront by O'Driscoll in the early 1990s and is now recognized as a major factor in the ligamentous stability of the elbow.

◼ ULNAR COLLATERAL LIGAMENT INJURY

Inner elbow pain may be the result of injury to the UCL. Injury to the UCL may be acute, chronically disrupted, or chronically attenuated. Waris (13) was the first to recognize and describe UCL tears, particularly isolated anterior oblique ligament disruption, in javelin throwers half a century ago. Early publications suggested that UCL tears are a rare lesion; however, with better understanding, evaluation, and imaging of the UCL, it is clear that UCL injury is not uncommon. Individuals who sustain an acute UCL rupture, note sudden onset of medial elbow pain, with or without a popping sensation, that occurred with throwing or falling. Usually the individual notes they were unable to throw after the injury and may complain of symptoms of ulnar nerve irritation.

Individuals with chronic elbow valgus instability from either complete disruption or attenuation of the UCL give a history of having pain or soreness along the inner elbow with throwing. The number one cause of UCL injuries in the throwing athlete is overuse, or repetitive microtrauma (14). The athlete gives a history of repeated bouts of inner elbow pain during and after throwing that would respond to conservative treatment. However, with the final injury, the athlete notes that he or she is unable to throw greater than 75% of maximal capacity due to this pain (14). The athlete may note, however, that there was a single "giving way" episode or sudden severe inner elbow pain, which was distinct and isolated and likely represents the final insult. The throwing athlete most commonly complains of pain at the acceleration phase of throwing and with ball release or point of impact in hitting the ball being the second-most commonly reported timing of pain (15). Due to chronicity of the instability, the athlete may have ulnar nerve irritation due to stretching of the nerve with the increased valgus laxity or symptoms of medial epicondylitis (due to attempts at muscular stabilization of the medial elbow), or symptoms of loose bodies, such as catching or locking.

On physical examination, these individuals will have point tenderness 2 cm distal to the medial epicondyle, over the UCL itself, and pain and instability with valgus stress **(Fig 23-13)**. The athlete may have pain with resisted wrist flexion, indicative of medial epicondylitis, which can co-exist with UCL injury. However, the absence of increased pain with resisted wrist flexion and the location of pain posterior to the common flexor muscle origin help differentiate this problem from flexor-pronator muscle rupture. In some cases, ecchymosis may appear at the medial joint line and

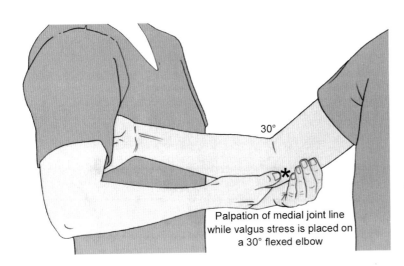

30°

Palpation of medial joint line while valgus stress is placed on a 30° flexed elbow

Fig 23-13. Valgus stress test of the elbow. The subject's hand is placed between the examiner's elbow and body while the medial joint line and UCL are palpated. A valgus stress is applied to the elbow flexed at 30 degrees, palpating the ulnar collateral ligament for tenderness, opening the medial joint line and quality of endpoint. The *asterisk* denotes the medial epicondyle.

proximal forearm 2 to 3 days after an acute injury. With a torn UCL, the medial joint gaps opens with valgus stress and the ulnar nerve is stretched. Baseball pitchers and tennis players often have long-standing fixed-flexion and valgus deformities, which are static deformities that may predispose to traction neuritis (16,17).

Examination to determine the functional integrity of the UCL is performed with the humerus stabilized and a valgus force applied to the elbow. This can be done classically with the elbow flexed 30 degrees, while holding the patient's hand between the examiner's elbow and body (Fig 23-13). The author finds this test to be a bit less useful than some of the following tests because (a) humeral rotation is poorly controlled, making examination difficult, if not confusing, and (b) the UCL is most autonomous in resisting valgus force at 70 to 90 degrees of elbow flexion (18,19). Thus, other tests utilized include the "milking maneuver," which was described by Veltri et al. (20) produces a valgus stress to the joint in greater flexion **(Fig 23-14)**. The elbow being tested is flexed beyond 90 degrees, and the opposite hand of the patient is placed under the elbow to grasp the thumb of the affected hand, thereby exerting a valgus stress on the UCL. The examiner palpates the UCL tenderness, joint line gapping, and quality of endpoint during this maneuver (20,21). This technique of examination was advocated based on the increased valgus rotation of the elbow at 90 degrees compared with 30 degrees when using the normal elbow as the control (22). Several authors prefer a modification of this technique, where the patient's elbow is flexed 70 degrees with the humerus in maximal external rotation (23). The

examiner pulls on the subject's thumb and also palpates the medial joint line with the thumb of the examiner's other hand **(Fig 23-15)**. This allows for evaluation of pain with stress testing, as well as medial joint gapping and quality of endpoint at the degree of elbow flexion deemed most important in cadaveric testing (18). As with all the above tests, medial joint gapping is usually only a few millimeters with complete, isolated UCL injuries (24).

Recently, another test has been described to identify UCL insufficiency, the Moving Valgus Stress Test described by O'Driscoll et al. (25) **(Fig 23-16)**. In this examination, the athlete's shoulder is placed in an abducted and externally rotated position. The elbow is then flexed and extended while imparting a valgus force to the elbow. For those athletes with UCL insufficiency, pain is felt at a specific and reproducible point within the arc of 80 to 120 degrees of elbow flexion. This examination reproduces the pain of throwing in the athlete, since the shearing force is applied to the attenuated UCL in a similar way as with throwing.

Though ligaments are not radiodense, radiographs still may help confirm the diagnosis or provide clues of UCL injury. A small avulsion fracture fragment may be identified radiographically, confirming the diagnosis. Secondary findings on plain films suggestive of chronic UCL insufficiency include ossification within the ligament (18%) (26), loose bodies in the posterior or lateral compartments, marginal osteophytes about the radiocapitellar or ulnohumeral articulations, or olecranon and condylar hypertrophy—this latter finding more common in throwing athletes or tennis players, and not necessarily in UCL-injured elbows. UCL injury may

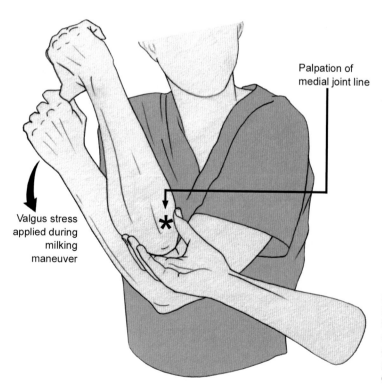

Palpation of medial joint line

Valgus stress applied during milking maneuver

Fig 23-14. Milking maneuver as described by Veltri et al. (20). The patient's contralateral extremity helps lock the shoulder of the elbow being examined. While pulling down on the thumb of the elbow being examined, a valgus stress is imparted on the elbow and the examiner palpates the medial joint line of gapping. The *asterisk* denotes the medial joint line of the elbow being examined.

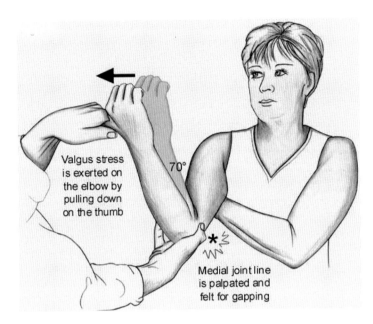

Fig 23-15. The author's modification of the milking maneuver. The patient still locks the shoulder of the upper extremity being examined by using the other arm. The examiner positions the patient's elbow at 70 degrees and pulls on the subject's thumb imparting the valgus stress while palpating the medial joint line with the other hand. This author performs the examination in this fashion because biomechanical studies on cadavers suggest that 70 degrees of elbow flexion is the best position to detect medial joint laxity to valgus stress. (From Safran MR. Injury to the ulnar collateral ligament: diagnosis and treatment. *Sports Medicine and Arthroscopy Review.* 2003;11:15–24 (figure 6, page 19).

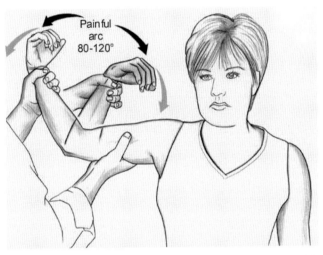

Fig 23-16. The moving valgus stress test: The patient brings his or her shoulder into abduction and external rotation. The examiner flexes and extends the patient's elbow while applying a valgus force. In the patient with a UCL injury, this should reproducibly cause pain in the arc between 80 and 120 degrees. (From Safran MR. Injury to the ulnar collateral ligament: diagnosis and treatment. *Sports Medicine and Arthroscopy Review.* 2003;11:15–24 (figure 7, page 20).

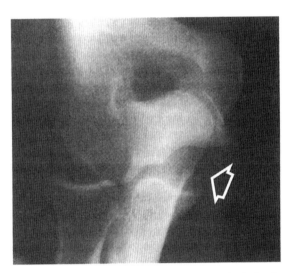

Fig 23-17. Stress radiograph showing valgus laxity indicative of rupture of the ulnar collateral ligament complex.

be confirmed with the use of stress radiographs **(Fig 23-17)**. In the acute setting, stress radiographs may be difficult due to guarding and may require anesthesia. A commercially available stress device enables evaluation of the UCL with consistent elbow flexion, rotation, and forces, resolving a problem seen with manual stress testing. This mechanical device has been reported to be 94% sensitive and 100% specific in diagnosing UCL tears, though these results have yet to be confirmed (27). Further, it should be noted that there is increased laxity of the dominant elbow to valgus stress

(nearly 0.5 mm) in uninjured, asymptomatic professional baseball pitchers when compared with their nondominant elbow (28). This is distinctly different from the general population where there is a lack of difference (up to 0.5 mm) in laxity between the dominant and nondominant elbow (29,30). Thus, there may be a continuum of elbow laxity in overhead athletes, blurring the line between asymptomatic laxity and symptomatic instability by this relatively sensitive method. Because this difference is so small, injuries to the UCL may be underestimated and misdiagnosed initially (31). Conway (32) presented his initial findings of stress radiographic findings in professional baseball pitchers and found that 2 mm of relative increased laxity and 3 mm of absolute medial joint gapping were consistent with an incompetent UCL in his series.

The gravity stress test is of historical significance to determine instability of the elbow, but is not used much anymore (33,34). The gravity stress test is performed with the patient supine and the shoulder brought into maximal external rotation with the sagittal plane of the elbow parallel to the floor **(Fig 23-18)**. There is no support under the forearm allowing the weight of the forearm, resisted only by the flexor-pronator muscle group and the UCL, to work with gravity to apply a valgus stress. A standard anteroposterior (AP) radiograph is taken, enabling assessment of medial joint gapping or displacement of a medial elbow fragment (following avulsion of the medial epicondyle). A standard arthrogram was also classically utilized, particularly in the acute injury; however, its value was lost in the chronic setting because dye leakage from the ruptured medial capsule is usually not seen in cases of chronic UCL insufficiency. On the other hand, computed tomographic (CT) arthrogram is quite sensitive and specific for acute and chronic injuries to the UCL, as reported in one study of 25 baseball players (35). The advantage of the CT arthrogram is in visualizing a partial or undersurface tear of the UCL (35,36). The role of CT arthrography must also still be confirmed and clarified. The role of magnetic resonance imaging (MRI) is more clear and can be of help in identifying torn UCL as well. MRI has been shown to be helpful in identifying UCL injury (35,37,38). The MRI visualizes the ligament directly, including acute and chronic injury, and can demonstrate secondary structures that may be injured, including the insertion of the UCL or radiocapitellar overload, by demonstrating bony edema and chondral thinning. Timmerman et al. (35) found the MRI was 57% sensitive and 100% specific. However, Thompson et al. (39) found the MRI to be positive in 79% of athletes undergoing UCL reconstruction, but "falsely" negative in 21%. The addition of intra-articular contrast to the MRI improves the ability to detect UCL injuries, while maintaining the benefit of visualization of other bony and soft tissue elbow structures. Azar et al. (40)

reported that MRI arthrography was 97% sensitive in detecting UCL injury, including partial undersurface UCL tears.

Dynamic ultrasonography has recently been studied in asymptomatic major league professional baseball players to evaluation the UCL of the elbow. Dynamic ultrasound revealed that this modality provides a rapid means for evaluating the UCL. In these baseball players, dominant UCL had a thicker anterior band, and the UCL was more likely to have hypoechoic foci and/or calcifications. Further, dynamic ultrasound demonstrated increased medial elbow laxity with valgus stress (41,42).

Timmerman and Andrews described the arthroscopic valgus stress test of the elbow and have found this to be the most sensitive and specific way to diagnose UCL disruptions in their hands. With this test, the authors arthroscopically visualize the medial compartment of the elbow while applying a valgus stress at 70 degrees. Timmerman et al. (35) noted that if the medial compartment gaps open, UCL insufficiency exists. Field and Altchek (24) confirmed in vitro that valgus stability of the elbow is best assessed in 60 to 75 degrees of elbow flexion. They found that rupture of the anterior bundle resulted in only 1 to 2 mm of medial joint gapping when viewed arthroscopically, whereas complete release of the UCL resulted in only 4 to 10 mm of medial joint opening. Thus, history and physical examination remain the mainstay for diagnosis and imaging studies may help confirm injury.

Recently, Safran et al. (43) reported their findings with a custom, noninvasive, nonradiographic stress test device. The authors developed a testing device based on in vitro studies (19) demonstrating that valgus stress testing of the elbow in 50 or 70 degrees of flexion and neutral rotation was the best position to demonstrate laxity after injury to the UCL of the elbow (19). The measurement of elbow laxity was based on angular displacement of the forearm. Then, in a comparative study of both a commercially available stress radiographic device and the noninvasive elbow tester, two groups

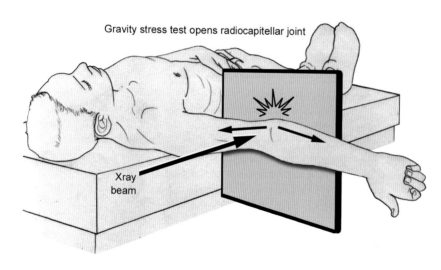

Gravity stress test opens radiocapitellar joint

Xray beam

Fig 23-18. Gravity stress test. AP radiograph of the elbow taken in the supine position while the arm hangs freely to allow the weight of the arm to apply a valgus stress to the elbow, demonstrating ulnar collateral ligament insufficiency by increased distance in the ulnohumeral joint.

of patients were evaluated (43). Seven patients had a history of isolated UCL injury treated conservatively by the senior author. These seven were able to "cope" with their UCL injury on one elbow and the other elbow was normal. The second group was 11 patients with no history of elbow injury or surgery. The noninvasive elbow testing device was able to demonstrate a side-to-side difference between the injured and noninjured elbow, whereas the radiographic stress device was unable to show a difference. Further, neither device demonstrated a side-to-side difference between the normal elbows of the controls, as one would expect.

Treatment of UCL injury consists of aggressive therapy with relative rest, anti-inflammatory measures, and physical therapy. With this conservative regimen, approximately 50% of throwing athletes are able to return to throwing (17,44). The most recent study of nonoperative treatment of 31 UCL injuries in throwing athletes demonstrated that 42% of throwing athletes were able to return to their previous level of activity at an average of 24 weeks (13 to 54 weeks) (44). Jobe prescribes two cycles of 3 months of rest from throwing and rehabilitation, and if pain occurs when throwing over 75% capacity, surgery is indicated; however, the success rate of this program in his patient population is not reported (15,45). Rettig's program includes restriction from throwing for two or more months, upper-extremity strengthening, and bracing. When the athlete is pain free, a throwing program is initiated and advanced over a period of 1 to 2 months (44).

Surgical treatment for UCL tears has evolved over the past few decades. Primary repair of the UCL when acutely injured had been advocated for years (17,34,46). Most UCL avulsion injuries were treated by surgically reattaching the ligament to bone using drill holes, whereas midsubstance tears were repaired with sutures primarily (46). Conway et al. (15) published their data of 70 athletes with acute UCL disruptions noting that 87% of UCL injuries were midsubstance, 10% were avulsions from the ulna, and only 3% were humeral avulsions. Jobe's (15,45,47) recommendation was to perform UCL reconstruction with a free tendon graft in the acute setting with the main exception being an individual undergoing surgery soon after a proximal UCL tear, with no ulnar nerve symptoms, and with the remainder of the ligament appearing normal. Currently, the most popular surgical recommendation is to perform UCL reconstruction for both acute and chronic injuries (21). Transposition of the ulnar nerve was recommended in all cases; however, there is a significant incidence of neurologic symptoms postoperatively (up to 21%), which has led to a more conservative approach (15). The techniques currently employed by most surgeons do not involve transposition of the ulnar nerve unless there is significant ulnar nerve involvement including motor weakness or significant sensory changes.

Current popular indications for UCL reconstruction are for (a) acute ruptures in overhead sports athletes, (b) significant chronic elbow instability; (c) after debridement for calcific tendinitis, if there is insufficient tissue to effect a primary repair in an overhead or throwing athlete; and

(d) multiple episodes of recurring elbow pain (with subtle instability) with throwing after periods of conservative treatment.

Current results appear better than after initial reports of UCL reconstruction. Conway et al. (15) reported the results of 56 UCL reconstructions using a palmaris longus free tendon graft and found 80% good-to-excellent results at 2 to 5 years, with 68% of the athletes returning to their previous level of competition for after more than 1 year. In that series, the authors transposed the ulnar nerve in all cases and found that 21% had postoperative ulnar neurologic symptoms, 40% were transient (all but one patient returned to previous sports activity), but 60% required a second operative procedure for the nerve (with almost half returning to previous sports activity) (15). These results have been confirmed by others (31). Jobe noted that UCL reconstruction results were not as good when there had been a previous operative procedure performed on the same elbow. In the last decade, there have been revisions in surgical technique for UCL reconstruction to make the surgery easier, more reproducible, and to reduce the incidence and risk of complications including not transposing or addressing ulnar nerve and splitting the FCU muscle mass (48), elevating flexor-pronator tendon without detaching it (31), these latter two eliminating the need to detach and reattach the flexor pronator mass with the risk of weakness and delayed avulsion of the musculotendinous unit. Other variations including fixation and tunnel techniques such as the docking procedure (49) and interference screw fixation (50) to reduce the need for multiple drill holes to reduce the risk of blow out of the bony bridge and making it easier to tension the graft. There has been a report of fixation of the graft with suture anchors onto bone as compared with tunnels (51); however, this biomechanical study is lacking clinical follow up and other studies to confirm the efficacy. Schwab et al. (52) had recommended transfer of the anterior oblique ligament anteriorly and superiorly with its bony attachment when the UCL is present but attenuated. However, this treatment is generally not recommended because the attenuated ligament is weaker due to microscopic injury, its position is not functionally isometric compared to its natural position, and elbow extension tends to be lost when using this technique, all of which is likely not acceptable to most individuals when there is a more anatomic reconstruction technique available without those risks. Synthetic ligament research has continued over the years; however, no long-term clinical data exists showing efficacy of this approach.

Repetitive valgus stress and microtrauma to the elbow may result in chronic UCL injury that occasionally heals with calcification. These calcifications are generally removed during the UCL reconstruction. It is important to note, however, that these calcifications are within the UCL. Individuals with medial elbow pain and these calcifications must be carefully examined. Care must be taken to not mistake these intraligamentous calcifications for intra-articular loose bodies. These calcifications are extra-articular, and removal of them without UCL reconstruction will result in an unstable elbow.

■ POSTEROLATERAL ROTATORY INSTABILITY

Though there were case reports years prior, posterolateral rotatory instability (PLRI) was brought to the forefront in the early 1990s by O'Driscoll (53,54). This elbow injury pattern is a rotatory instability due to injury to the lateral UCL. The mechanism of injury is a combination of axial compression, valgus stress, and supination (or external rotation) that imparts a rotational force to the elbow resulting in a spectrum of soft tissue injury (53). The initial injury is to the ulnar portion of the LCLC and progresses to capsular disruption (anterior and posterior capsule) and eventually may involve the UCL complex if the injury is severe (53–56).

Understanding the pathomechanics is the key to understanding PLRI. PLRI of the elbow results from a rotatory subluxation of the radius and ulna (which move together as a unit) relative to the distal humerus. Because the annular ligament is intact in this injury, the radio-ulnar joint maintains its normal relationship and thus the proximal radius and ulna move together in a "coupled" motion. Most give credit to Osborne and Cotterill (57) as the ones who probably were the first investigators to appreciate fully the importance of the lateral ligamentous complex in recurrent instability and describe the findings of PLRI. While much of the initial literature by O'Driscoll (53,54) and the laboratory at the Mayo Clinic reported the results of biomechanical studies demonstrating that the primary stabilizer to PLRI is the lateral ulnar collateral ligament (LUCL) (53–56,58), much of the recent literature suggests that the injury may not be to the LUCL alone. It was reported that the radial collateral ligament and capsule serve as secondary restraints. However, clinically it is known that elbow dislocations and injury to the LCLC occurs proximally. And it is after this injury that the PLRI most commonly manifests. Subsequent research by other investigators has suggested that isolated injury to the LUCL alone may not be enough to produce PLRI (18,59,60). Some suggest that the complex works in a "Y" configuration and that a proximal injury, near the epicondyle, as seen clinically, can and does produce PLRI (61).

The diagnosis of PLRI is much more elusive than other ligament injuries, including the UCL, and requires a careful history and physical examination. The physician must be diligent and maintain a high degree of suspicion in patients with vague reports of elbow discomfort. It is frequently reported in patients with PLRI that they have painful clicking, snapping, clunking, locking, dislocating, or giving way. Position of the hand during maneuvers that elicit these symptoms is critical, because the symptoms are often produced when the patient extends his or her elbow, with the forearm supinated (53). An example would be using their hands to get out of a chair with their forearms maximally supinated.

Standard, preliminary physical examination of the elbow generally is unremarkable with regard to strength, range of motion, and tenderness. The diagnosis requires a provocative test of stability described by O'Driscoll et al. (53) and termed the lateral pivot-shift test of the elbow **(Figs 23-19 and 23-20A)**. The pivot shift test is performed with the patient supine and the examiner standing above the patient's head. The extremity being tested is brought above the patient's head into forward elevation, and the shoulder is placed in full external rotation to stabilize the humerus for the test. The patient's forearm is held in maximal supination, with one hand grasping the wrist distally. A valgus force is applied with the examiner's other hand as the elbow is slowly flexed from a starting position of full extension. The combination of supination and valgus results in an axial joint compression, which produces a posterolateral rotatory subluxation of the combined radius and ulna relative to the humerus. In the unanesthetized patient, this maneuver reproduces the sensation of instability and often elicits apprehension or guarding. Usually, the subluxation is maximized as the elbow reaches 40 degrees flexion and further flexion results in a sudden clunk as a result of joint reduction. Dimpling of the skin proximal to the radial head (posterolateral elbow) can be seen with PLRI in degrees of extension before the reduction **(Fig 23-20B)**. The clunk of reduction in PLRI is generally only felt by the examiner in a patient under general anesthesia or occasionally following an intra-articular injection of anesthetic. If a patient does display apprehension or guarding during the pivot-shift maneuver in the office, then we usually recommend confirmation of posterolateral instability with an examination under anesthesia (Fig 23-20A). Lateral stress radiographic studies or fluoroscopy during the pivot maneuver demonstrates posterolateral radial head dislocation with widening of the ulnohumeral joint (due to the

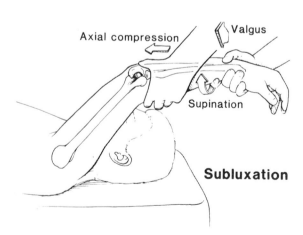

Fig 23-19. Schematic representation of the lateral pivot-shift test of the elbow for posterolateral rotatory instability. (From O'Driscoll SW, Bell DF, Morrey BF. Posterolateral rotatory instability of the elbow. *J Bone Joint Surg Am.* 1991;73:440–446; with permission.)

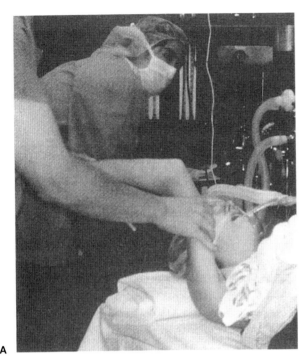
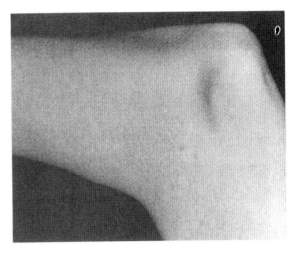

A   B

Fig 23-20A and B. Examination under anesthesia of a patient with PLRI. A: Performing the lateral pivot shift test. B: Demonstration of the posterolateral prominence of the radial head with dimpling of the skin, consistent with PLRI. (From Safran MR, Caldwell GL, Fu FH. Chronic instability of the elbow. In: Peimer CA, ed. *Surgery of the hand and upper extremity.* New York: McGraw-Hill; 1996:478; with permission.)

subluxation of the ulna out of the trochlear groove) and may be helpful for confirmation and documentation of the pathomechanics.

Plain radiographs are usually unremarkable unless there is a bony avulsion off the lateral epicondyle. Stress radiographs can often show the posterolateral subluxation if the patient is relaxed and allows application of the forces necessary. Lateral stress radiographs show that the ulna is rotated off the distal humerus (slight gapping of the ulnohumeral joint with otherwise maintained relationship) while the radial head is rotated with the ulna so that the radial head rests posterior to the capitellum **(Fig 23-21)**. The normal radio-ulnar relationship differentiates PLRI from radial head subluxation or dislocation in which the radial head is displaced but the ulnohumeral joint is entirely normal. While arthrography has not been shown to be of benefit in aiding the diagnosis, advances in MRI have allowed good visualization of the LCLC and can be helpful in confirming the diagnosis in some cases. However, since this is a dynamic problem, and the ligament may be stretched but intact, the sensitivity and specificity of MRIs for PLRI is less than one would like; however, studies are still forthcoming.

No nonoperative treatment regimens have been reported to be successful in the management of PLRI (62). For PLRI that markedly interferes with the patient's daily function, one can consider activity modification and a hinged brace with forearm pronation and an extension block, although few patients are content with this option and most require surgical intervention.

Surgical treatment of PLRI involves reattaching the avulsed LCLC or reconstructing the LUCL with a free tendon graft to the lateral epicondyle, similar to reconstruction of the medial UCL. Because the annular ligament is intact in these patients, radio-ulnar dislocation does not occur, and surgery on this ligament is not indicated (62). If the condition is diagnosed acutely, primary repair of the lateral UCL may be performed, and this is usually an avulsion from the humerus and can be repaired back to the bone (63) **(Fig 23-22)**. Modifications of the technique originally described by O'Driscoll include making the distal connecting tunnels perpendicular to the isometric point to the lateral epicondyle as well as using the interference screw technique. Results for these latter techniques are lacking, but in general, surgical reconstruction of the LUCL has been excellent (64). Osborne and Cotterill (57) reported excellent results in eight patients with transosseous repair and Nestor et al. (64) reported excellent results in three patients. Ligamentous reconstruction results have been mixed. O'Driscoll and Morrey reported a 90% success rate in restoring stability in the absence of arthritis or radial head fracture. 60% resulted in excellent results while 40% continued to have pain or some loss of motion.

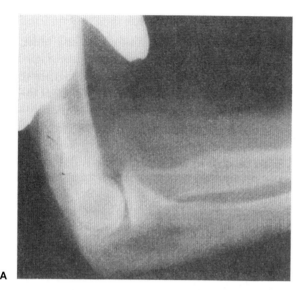
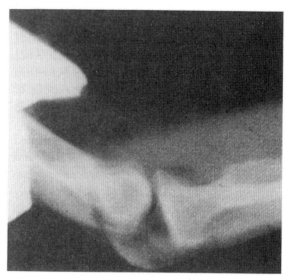

Fig 23-21A and B. Lateral radiographs of a cadaver elbow after sectioning of the LUCL. **A:** Without stress at approximately 90 degrees of flexion. **B:** Radiograph with axial compression, valgus stress, and supination (lateral pivot-shift test) at 45 degrees of elbow flexion resulting in posterolateral subluxation. Note that the ulnohumeral articulation is not concentric, while the radial head is posteriorly subluxated in **(B)**. This is contrasted with isolated radial head subluxation, in which the radial head is subluxated, yet the ulnohumeral articulation is normal. (From Safran MR, Caldwell GL, Fu FH. Chronic instability of the elbow. In: Peimer CA, ed. *Surgery of the hand and upper extremity.* New York: McGraw-Hill; 1996:479; with permission.)

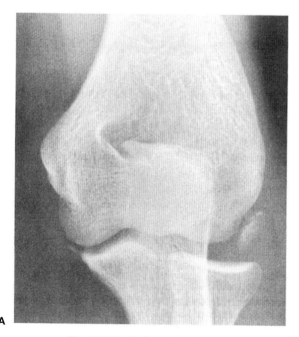
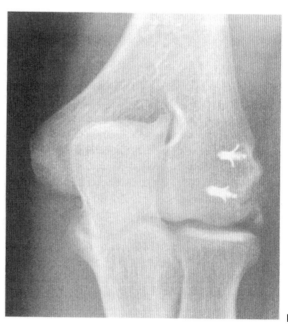

Fig 23-22. Radiograph of a snowboarder who fell on his outstretched hand. **A:** Acute PLRI was diagnosed, suggested radiographically by this lateral condyle avulsion fracture. **B:** The lateral ligament complex was repaired acutely with suture anchors. This radiograph shows the elbow 6 months after primary repair for PLRI.

■ PEDIATRIC INJURIES— OSTEOCHONDRITIS DISSECANS/AVULSION

The elbow of the skeletally immature athlete is susceptible to two main problems: apophyseal injury and osteochondritis dissecans (OCD). The physis is the weakest link in the skeletally immature musculoskeletal system, resulting in apophysitis and avulsion injuries, rather than ligament injuries as seen in adults. OCD is also common in young athletes, particularly throwing athletes. The term "Little Leaguer's Elbow" has been applied to both medial- and lateral-sided injuries (generally medial epicondylar apophyseal injury and OCD of the capitellum) and thus has very little usefulness and is avoided in this chapter.

Medial Epicondylar Physeal Injury

Fracture or avulsion of the medial epicondylar physis can be a stress fracture or overt fracture due to repeated valgus forces, falling, or repetitive violent forearm flexor muscle contraction in the skeletally immature athlete. Throwing results in a repetitive valgus stress and can result in accelerated growth of the medial epicondylar apophysis, which can be followed by separation and eventual fragmentation if the body does not have the opportunity to recover and heal from the repetitive forces (65,66) **(Fig 23-23)**. Pediatric athletes with medial epicondylar apophysitis complain of pain with throwing while also noting their throwing accuracy, speed, and distance are reduced. On examination, the patient has point tenderness over the medial epicondyle. Frequently, these pediatric athletes have an elbow flexion contracture of more than 15 degrees based on muscular and capsular tightness. Radiographs demonstrate that the medial epicondylar apophysis can be widened and occasionally fragmented. This is as compared with the contralateral elbow, which should always be obtained when evaluating an injured elbow in the skeletally immature patient with elbow pain due to the complexity and various ages of closure of the multiple different physes about the elbow **(Fig 23-24)**. Care should be taken, since this finding may be normal in throwing athletes (34). The treatment of the stress fracture or inflamed apophysis is rest from throwing for 4 to 6 weeks, along with the

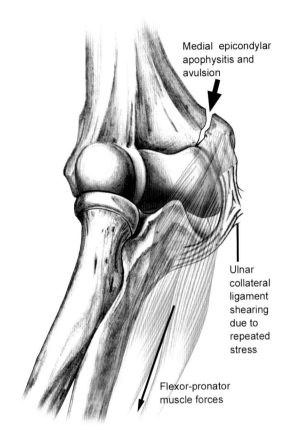

Fig 23-23. Medial epicondylar apophysitis and avulsion occur due to repeated stress from the ulnar collateral ligament (*arrow*) and flexor-pronator muscle forces.

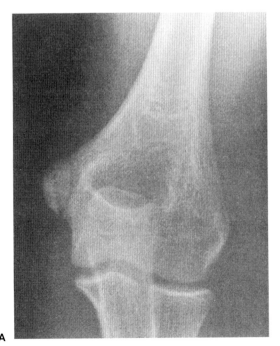 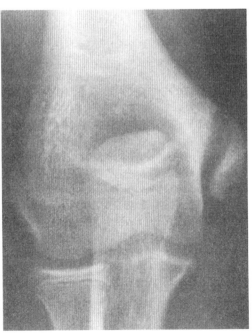

Fig 23-24. Thirteen-year-old baseball pitcher with medial elbow pain. **A:** Left (normal) elbow. **B:** Right, throwing elbow showing widening of the medial epicondyle physis.

application of ice (take care to protect the ulnar nerve from ice injury by placing a wet towel between the ice and the medial elbow). NSAIDs may also be used to reduce pain and the acute inflammation. After the symptoms subside, a rehabilitation program is instituted consisting of stretching to eliminate the flexion contracture, strengthening of the muscles that cross the elbow, and then transitioning to a gradual throwing program.

Continued stress to the elbow with apophysitis may result in progression to a complete fracture or separation of the medial epicondyle. The avulsion fracture of the medial epicondyle, however, may occur without any preceding symptoms of medial elbow pain and is usually due to a single, more severe, valgus force or violent muscle contraction. Medial epicondylar apophyseal fracture can have two distinct patterns, as described by Woods (67) and Woods et al. (68). A Woods Type 1 fracture occurs in the younger child and is characterized radiographically by a large fragment, involving the entire epicondyle that is often displaced and rotated anteriorly and distally, and may even become entrapped in the joint. A Woods Type 2 fracture occurs in the adolescent and is radiographically notable for medial epicondylar fragmentation with a small fracture fragment. In this type of injury, the flexor-pronator muscle is essentially avulsed; however, the anterior oblique ligament of the UCL complex is usually intact. Treatment of this entity, however, depends on elbow stability (Fig 23-18).

The treatment of these injuries where the elbow is stable and epicondyle is nondisplaced is rest for 2 to 3 weeks, with return to throwing by 6 weeks after attaining full motion. Unstable elbows are treated by open reduction and internal fixation, using wires, pins, or screws. If, however, the medial epicondyle is displaced more than 1 cm, then surgery should be performed to anatomically reduce the fragment and internally fix it with pins or screw(s) (69,70) **(Fig 23-25)**. It should be noted that displacement of 1 cm as an indication for surgery is somewhat arbitrary, and it is easy to see how malunion of this fracture could lead to functional medial ligamentous laxity, which would be expected to be symptomatic in a throwing athlete. Therefore, we recommend aggressive management, including open reduction and internal fixation, to obtain adequate fracture reduction. In nonthrowing pediatric athletes or for the nondominant elbow, some authors recommend surgery only if the fragment is displaced 2 cm or more.

Occasionally, elbow dislocation is complicated by avulsion of the medial epicondyle fragment, which may become entrapped within the elbow joint. Closed manipulation of the elbow by applying valgus stress and wrist extension can free the fragment from within the joint, enabling the child to avoid open surgery. As an adjunct, air can be injected into the lateral joint, which may help to move the incarcerated fragment out of the joint, helping to avoid open reduction (69,71). Minimally displaced medial epicondyle avulsion injuries and apophysitis (widening of the growth plate without fracture or displacement) can usually be managed without surgery. If surgery is required to manage this problem, UCL evaluation is also performed and the ligament is repaired as needed.

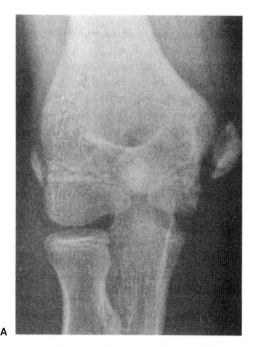 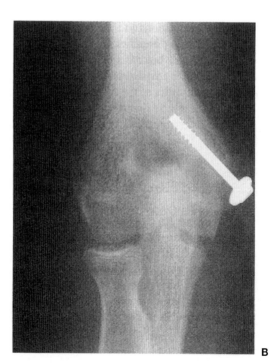

A

B

Fig 23-25. Medial epicondylar avulsion fracture. **A:** Displaced medial epicondyle fracture. **B:** Fracture fixed with internal fixation.

Olecranon Apophysitis

Abnormal stresses of the triceps attachment on the olecranon apophysis can result in an injury syndrome similar to Osgood-Schlatter disease of the knee. An intrinsic overload from repeated triceps pull can lead to inflammation and separation of the olecranon secondary ossification center (72). This injury may also be due to valgus extension overload and has been reported in a baseball pitcher (73,74). Generally, those afflicted are adolescents. Typical complaints are those of pain on resisted elbow extension and tenderness over the olecranon. Radiographs demonstrate widening of the olecranon apophysis, and should be confirmed by comparison with radiographs of the contralateral elbow.

When the apophysis is widened, but not separated or avulsed, initial treatment is rest from the offending activity, gentle range-of-motion and flexibility exercises, eventually progressing to strengthening exercises. Ice and NSAIDs are useful if acute inflammation is present. If the child is in severe pain, a short period of immobilization in a splint or brace may be beneficial. In the situation where there is separation of the secondary growth center or adolescents have persistent pain despite conservative management due to lack of fusion of the physis, internal fixation is recommended. Surgical intervention to promote fusion of the apophysis may require internal fixation with a screw in addition to bone grafting, due to the high incidence of fibrous union when bone grafting is not used (75,76). Left untreated, apophysitis of the olecranon may result in an incompletely fused olecranon apophysis, which may later fracture as a result of direct trauma when older (73–75,77,78). It is generally recommended that unfused olecranon physis fractures in adults be treated with open reduction, internal fixation, and primary bone grafting, though recent case series have been presented calling into question the need for bone grafting (75).

Osteochondritis Dissecans

OCD is a focal lesion of the lateral elbow that occurs most frequently in young throwers and gymnasts. Although OCD can occur in throwers and nonthrowers, in the dominant and nondominant elbows, and in the capitellum, radial head, or both, it tends to occur in the capitellum of the dominant arm in throwers and gymnasts 10 to 15 years of age (79,80–85). The exact etiology of OCD remains a mystery. A current leading hypothesis of the etiology of OCD is that it is a result of vascular insufficiency due to repetitive trauma or microfracture in a genetically predisposed adolescent. The capitellar blood supply is tenuous, with end-arterioles terminating at the subchondral plate (86). The current leading pathogenesis theory proposes that compression at the radiocapitellar joint produces arterial injury at the subchondral plate resulting in bone death (34). As noted in the section on throwing injuries, the radiocapitellar joint functions as a secondary restraint to the valgus stresses associated with throwing resulting in compression of this joint (Figs 23-26 and 23-27). OCD can be a disabling problem.

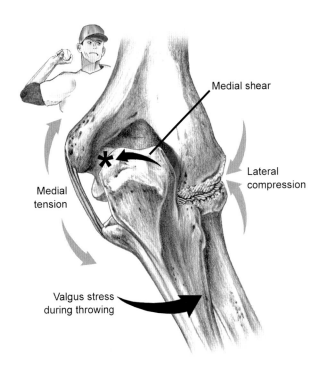

Fig 23-26. The effects of valgus elbow forces during throwing as viewed posteriorly. There are tensile forces medially, compressive forces laterally, and compressive and shear forces within the olecranon fossa.

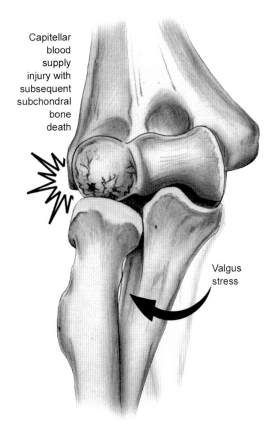

Fig 23-27. Schematic representation of radiocapitellar compression associated with valgus force and ulnar collateral ligament laxity thought to result in OCD of the capitellum or radial head.

There is a debate as to whether OCD is a distinctly different entity from Panner disease; however, it should be clear that these diagnoses have different prognoses and treatments. The difference between the two problems focuses on age and degree of involvement of the capitellar secondary ossification center. Panner disease occurs in the young child, usually 7 to 12 years of age, and is characterized by a focal, localized lesion of the subchondral bone and its overlying articular cartilage (anterior central capitellum) (86). In comparison, OCD occurs in the older child, 13 to 16 years of age, and is characterized as a focal lesion in the capitellum demarcated by a rarefied zone, with or without loose bodies (34).

The skeletally immature athlete often gives a history of insidious onset of lateral elbow pain and reduced throwing effectiveness and distance. The child may have a flexion contracture of more than 15 degrees on examination. A provocative test, which may reproduce symptoms and suggest the diagnosis, known as the "active radiocapitellar compression test," consists of forearm pronation and supination with the elbow in full extension resulting in pain if OCD is present. Early in the process, radiographs may be normal, although with time, islands of subchondral bone demarcated by a rarified zone can be seen, and with even more time, loose bodies may be generated **(Fig 23-28)**. MRI, computed tomography (CT), and ultrasound have all been found to be helpful in defining the extent of the lesion. The critical factor in determining treatment is the status of the overlying cartilage. The diagnosis is usually made by MRI, MR arthrogram, arthro-CT scan, ultrasound, or arthroscopy if plain films do not show free fragments to help detect early OCD lesions and to assess the integrity of the overlying articular cartilage (87). If the overlying articular cartilage is intact, treatment is relative rest and occasionally splinting, followed by range-of-motion

and then strengthening exercises. Some have also advocated an unloading type of elbow brace. Symptoms generally subside with rest alone; however, throwing is contraindicated because the healing process may lag behind symptomology and tends to be slow. The athlete is restricted from throwing and other heavy activities until there is radiographic evidence of healing. Bennett and Tullos (34) have suggested that fragmentation is likely if pain and flexion contracture persist for more than 6 weeks. If the overlying articular cartilage is not intact at the time of surgery, some recommended excising the fragment regardless of size. They note the patient will have a functional elbow; however, the patient should be discouraged from throwing or performing heavy labor. The current recommended management for elbows where the articular cartilage is not intact is to reattach and internally fix large fragments with screws, wires, or biodegradable pins after drilling the bed to enhance vascularity, similar to the procedure described by Indelicato et al. (88). Smaller fragments, on the other hand, are usually just removed. The surgeon usually attempts to fix the larger fragments to help reduce articular surface incongruity and potentially degenerative changes, while smaller fragments, if removed, would have less impact on contact stresses.

If the large fragment has been chronically detached, the fragments may have continued to grow, and/or become incarcerated within the joint, resulting in multiple smaller fragments or in a fragment that is rounded and hypertrophied, and in either scenario, reattachment may not be possible. In these situations, the bony fragment(s) is removed and the crater is cleared of the fibrous tissue and roughened to attempt to stimulate fibrocartilaginous growth. Yamamoto has also recommended filling the defect, particularly if it involves the lateral columnar wall, with an autogenous osteochondral graft from the knee (88a). There have been several reports of excellent short-term results of arthroscopic debridement of loose articular cartilage flaps and loose bodies removal for OCD (89,99). However, studies have also shown that the late sequelae of OCD after removal of loose bodies include deformity of the capitellum and radial head, arthritis, loss of motion, pain, and often residual disability (91,92).

Radial Neck Physeal Fracture

Fracture of the radial neck at the physis may be the result of a fall on an outstretched hand or due to valgus stresses at the elbow with attenuation or insufficiency of the UCL resulting in increased compressive forces to the radiocapitellar joint. This injury tends to be acute due to a sudden force to the radiocapitellar joint in the skeletally immature athlete. These children complain of lateral elbow pain and reduced forearm rotation. On examination, these kids have tenderness over the radial head and concomitant loss of supination and pronation. Radiographs reveal a fat pad sign is present, and the fracture may be identified if displaced or with stress films. The treatment for nondisplaced fractures is rest for 4 to 6 weeks, until the fracture is healed. Displaced fractures

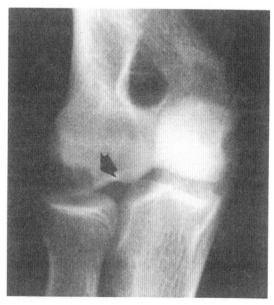

Fig 23-28. Osteochondritis dissecans of the capitellum *(arrow)*.

are treated with closed versus open reduction, which is based on the degree of angular displacement.

■ NERVE: CUBITAL TUNNEL, PRONATOR SYNDROME, ANTERIOR INTEROSSEOUS

The ulnar nerve is the most commonly injured around the elbow. This is likely due to the tight path it follows, which changes its dimensions with elbow flexion and extension, its subcutaneous location, and the considerable excursion required of it to accommodate the full motion of not only the elbow but also the shoulder. The ulnar nerve may be injured by traction, direct trauma, friction, or compression. Compression, either alone or in combination with the other causes, can produce cubital tunnel syndrome. Interneuron pressure increases six times over resting levels when the elbow is flexed, wrist extended, and shoulder abducted. With full elbow flexion the confines of the cubital tunnel become restrictive and the retinaculum becomes taut and compresses the nerve **(Fig 23-29)**. Beginning proximally to distally, the most common sites of ulnar nerve compression are the arcade of Struthers, medial intramuscular septum, medial epicondyle, cubital tunnel, and deep flexor pronator aponeurosis. Other causes of ulnar nerve compression that are less common include cubitus valgus and cubitus varus, which are sometimes associated with snapping triceps syndrome, a subluxing medial head of the triceps.

Injury to the ulnar nerve can result in significant long-term morbidity. The relatively high incidence of ulnar neuropathy is likely related to its posteromedial location in the elbow with its path through a confined space and the necessity for generous excursion to accommodate motion of the elbow and shoulder **(Fig 23-30)**. The ulnar nerve is a terminal branch of the medial cord of the brachial plexus. Through the upper two-thirds of the arm it travels along the anterior aspect of the medial intramuscular septum

near the median nerve and brachial artery. At the distal third of the arm, the ulnar nerve pierces the intramuscular septum and passes under the anteromedial margin of the triceps to the medial epicondyle. There it passes through the cubital tunnel where the retinaculum joining the medial epicondyle to the olecranon encloses the tunnel configuration **(Fig 23-31)**. The floor of the tunnel is the joint capsule and posterior band of the ulnar collateral ligament. Cubital tunnel retinaculum can display considerable anatomic variation. This is also known as the arcuate ligament. It may be muscular, known as the anconeus epitrochlearis, or fibrous and tight or alternately absent. Distal to the cubital tunnel, the nerve passes between the ulnar and humeral heads of the pronator teres. There are no clinically significant branches from the ulnar nerve to the upper arm. A sensory branch to the elbow joint is the first noted branch and usually arises proximal to the medial epicondyle. Occasionally, a branch to the FCU arises proximal to the cubital tunnel and courses in intimate relationship with the ulnar nerve itself in the cubital tunnel. Distally, in the cubital tunnel, the ulnar nerve distributes two to three branches to the FCU. The medial brachial cutaneous and antebrachial cutaneous nerves both pass through the posteromedial arm and medial epicondyle.

Pronator syndrome involves the median nerve at the level of the elbow and is painful. As a cause of median nerve compressive neuropathy, it is a distant second to carpal tunnel syndrome. The median nerve originates from branches from the medial and lateral cords that pass through the upper arm next to the brachial artery. It contains contributions from the sixth through the eighth cervical roots and the first thoracic nerve root of the brachial plexus.

The median nerve crosses the elbow joint medial to the brachial artery. It passes distally under the lacertus fibrosis and then penetrates the pronator teres. Considerable anatomic variation can be noted as the nerve traverses the pronator teres. Entrapment of the median nerve around the elbow may occur at various anatomic sites.

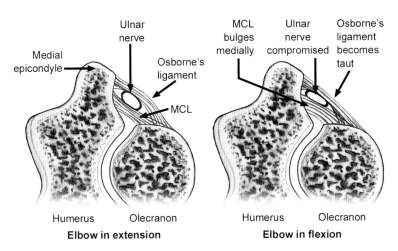

Fig 23-29. Anatomy of the cubital tunnel in elbow extension and flexion.

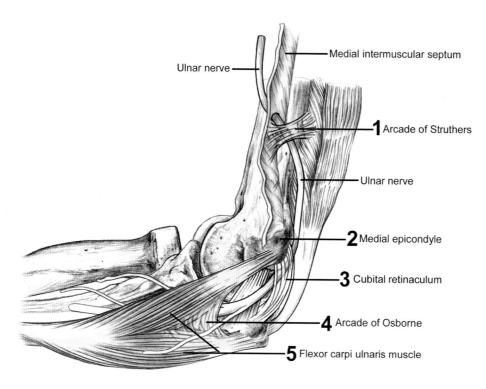

Medial intermuscular septum

Ulnar nerve

1 Arcade of Struthers

Ulnar nerve

2 Medial epicondyle

3 Cubital retinaculum

4 Arcade of Osborne

5 Flexor carpi ulnaris muscle

Fig 23-30. Sites of potential ulnar nerve compression and the causes of compression at each site. In Site 1, compression is caused by the Arcade of Struthers, medial intermuscular septum, hypertrophy of the medial head of the triceps, and snapping of the medial head of the triceps. In Site 2, compression is caused by valgus deformity of the bone. In Site 3, compression is caused by lesions within the epicondylar groove, conditions outside the groove, and subluxation or dislocation of the nerve. In Site 4, compression is caused by thickened Osborne's ligament. In Site 5 (exit of ulnar nerve from flexor carpi), compression is caused by deep flexor-pronator aponeurosis.

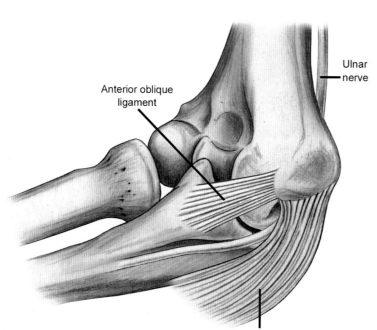

Ulnar nerve

Anterior oblique ligament

Fascial sheath continuous with flexor pronator fascia

Fig 23-31. Cubital tunnel retinaculum.

A supracondylar process when present and ligament of Struthers may cause compression of the median nerve just proximal to the elbow and is a possible cause of pronator syndrome. The causes are compressive. The possible compressive structures beginning proximally include the ligament of Struthers, lacertus fibrosis, fibrous band of the pronator teres, and the fibrous band in the flexor digitorum superficialis. Pronator syndrome presents as a dull ache and pain in the proximal anterior forearm just distal to the antecubital fossa and may radiate distally to the volar wrist. Rarely will it radiate proximally. Dysesthesias in the radial three and one-half digits and weakness and clumsiness may also be noted. Pronator syndrome usually occurs in the fifth decade of life and is four times more common in women than men. The history may involve a direct blow to the forearm, repetitive trauma, or, more commonly, no known cause. Physical findings include a positive Tinel sign over the nerve at the elbow, reproduction of symptoms with resisted pronation (or less commonly with supination), a positive median nerve compression test at the elbow that reproduces the symptoms, or tenderness over the proximal edge of the pronator teres. Initial conservative treatment of the pronator syndrome is rest, modified activities, nonsteroidal anti-inflammatory medication, and splintering. The majority will respond to conservative management. In recalcitrant cases surgery may be indicated.

With anterior interosseous syndrome, a deep unremitting pain in the proximal forearm usually precedes the symptoms that define the syndrome. The patient may complain of loss of dexterity or weakness of pinch. Clinically, loss of the function of the flexor pollicis longus and flexor digitorum profundus to the index and middle fingers with weakness of the pronator quadratus is noted. No tenderness over the proximal forearm is usually noted and sensibility is unaffected. The thumb and index finger assume a classic position during pinch in anterior interosseous syndrome. The index finger extends at the distal interphalangeal joint with compensatory increased flexion of the proximal interphalangeal joint. The thumb hyperextends at the interphalangeal joint and demonstrates increased flexion at the metacarpophalangeal joint. Conservative measures for treating anterior interosseous nerve syndrome include rest, activity modification, protective immobilization, holding the elbow in flexion, forearm in slight pronation and wrist in slight flexion, cryotherapy, nonsteroidal anti-inflammatory medication later followed by physical therapy and rehabilitation.

TENDINOPATHIES EPICONDYLITIS, DISTAL BICEPS, TRICEPS

Tendinopathy and epicondylopathy are the more appropriate terms for pain and injuries of the tendons about the elbow. Unfortunately, the nomenclature of tendonitis and epicondylitis has been used for many years, and while the concepts of lack of inflammatory changes within these injured tendons has been readily accepted, changing the names have been slow in general usage. Nonetheless, this section will discuss the etiology, presentation, evaluation, and treatment of injuries to the distal biceps, triceps, medial, and lateral musculotendinous structures. In general, treatment for these tendinopathies (not acute tendon ruptures) is the same initially. Initial management can be summed up in the acronym PRICEMM: P, protection: protect the area that is injured from further injury; R, rest: rest from the offending activity and further overuse; I, ice: ice the area after activity and if it reduces the pain; caution should be taken, however, when icing medial epicondylitis to not injure the ulnar nerve; C, compression: mild compression may help reduce the pain and swelling, especially if symptoms are acute; E, elevation: elevate the injured extremity, especially if the injury is acute; M, modalities: frequently, tendinopathies will respond to physical therapy, including the use of modalities such as iontophoresis or phonphoresis; M, medications: ironically or

possibly counterintuitively, anti-inflammatories may be of benefit, including nonsteroidal and/or injectible or oral steroids—to reduce the pain to enable appropriate rehabilitation, and other medications may also be of benefit in this setting.

Acute tendon ruptures, which often require surgical reattachment, may be treated with protection, rest, ice, compression, and elevation, along with medications (PRICEM), as long as it does not interfere with, or delay, surgical reattachment.

DISTAL BICEPS TENDINOPATHY

Distal biceps tendinopathy is an uncommon problem. Tendinopathy of the distal biceps occurs in association with repetitive pull-ups and elbow flexion, hyperextension, or repeated forceful supination. Occasionally, biceps tendinopathy may be the result of a violent or excessive elbow extension against a forceful contraction (extrinsic overload). However, generally, this is considered an overuse syndrome. It is generally thought that the bicipital tuberosity of the radius may produce friction and inflammation of the biceps tendon, resulting in pain in the antecubital fossa. Physical examination is notable for elbow pain with resisted supination or elbow flexion, frequently with reduced strength attributable to the pain. Treatment is based on the aforementioned PRICEMM protocol. This includes resting from weight lifting, throwing, or climbing activities (all associated with this injury). Treatment should also focus on early range of motion, because patients are more comfortable with their elbow flexed and, left unchecked, this may result in a flexion contracture. Typically, improvement is slow and steady, and surgical intervention is rarely warranted.

DISTAL BICEPS TENDON RUPTURE

Rupture of the distal biceps tendon is an uncommon injury, representing only 3% of all biceps ruptures (93). The incidence of complete distal biceps tendon avulsion injuries is 1.2 per 100,000 in the general population (94). The vast majority of distal biceps tendon avulsion injuries are complete, although partial tears have been reported (95–97). Untreated significant partial distal biceps tears may progress to become complete ruptures (95). The common mechanism of injury is a sudden, forceful overload, with the elbow near 90 degrees of flexion (98,99). Although the rupture tends to occur as an acute event, there is usually preexisting degenerative change within the tendon. The source of this preexisting degenerative change is felt to be as a result of friction and erosion of the tendon from repetitive rubbing against the bicipital tuberosity, although hypovascularity within areas of the distal portion of the tendon may also predispose the tendon to chronic degenerative change and ultimate rupture (98,100). Despite the existence of degenerative change within the tendon insertion, most patients have had no prior symptoms related to the elbow or biceps tendon (98). Examination of the elbow in a patient with an acute distal biceps tendon avulsion reveals localized pain and tenderness at the bicipital tuberosity, proximal displacement of the distal biceps tendon with a bulge in the distal arm, inability to palpate the taut tendon within the antecubital fossa, and marked weakness of forearm supination and elbow flexion (often associated with increased pain). The pain and tenderness identified after the acute rupture quickly subside, but a dull ache may persist for weeks. Ecchymosis is usually present in the antecubital fossa, and sometimes above and below the elbow, 48 to 72 hours after the injury.

Treatment for partial tears of the distal biceps begins with PRICEMM. Additionally, splinting or bracing may be used initially until pain and inflammation subside. This is followed by a range of motion, stretching, and strengthening program. If symptoms persist, surgical exploration with debridement or detachment with reinsertion of the tendon into the radial tuberosity may be indicated (95,97).

Current treatment of complete ruptures has traditionally been primary repair of the tendon into the bicipital tuberosity. The most popular technique for many years has been the two-incision Boyd-Anderson technique (101,102). This technique allows for reinsertion of the biceps tendon to restore power, while reducing the risk of radial nerve injury seen with the single anterior incision approach. Currently, there is increased enthusiasm again for the single-incision surgical technique using suture anchors or endobutton to help reduce the morbidity of two incisions and hasten the surgical time, while reducing the risk of nerve injury (103). Biomechanical studies, however, suggest that transosseous sutures fail at a significantly higher load than suture anchors and that the anchors may protrude from the bone (104). Further, these approaches with suture anchors reattach the biceps tendon onto the bone, while the two-incision technique (and the endobutton one-incision technique) reinserts the tendon into the medullary cavity of the radius. Anchor protrusion out of the tuberosity during cyclic loading has been seen in the lab and clinically, and this may potentially result in a gap at the repair site and interfere with forearm rotation (105). There are no published large series evaluating the results of a single-incision technique using suture anchors, the recently discussed endobutton (105), or comparing the results with other surgical techniques in the treatment of distal biceps ruptures. Nonsurgical management of distal biceps tendon ruptures has been found to result in strength deficits of 30% in flexion and 40% in supination, whereas immediate repair results in near-normal strength (106). Nonoperative treatment of distal biceps tendon avulsions frequently results in weakness, fatigue, pain, and disability, particularly with supination activities (99,107). Subjective results of surgical reattachment of the distal biceps have been reported to be good to excellent in up to 98% of patients (108). A meta-analysis of the treatment of distal biceps tendon avulsion injuries revealed 90% good to excellent results with anatomic repair and reinsertion at 3 years, as compared with only 60% good-to-excellent results at the same time period for nonanatomic surgical repair, and only 14% for patients treated nonoperatively (109). In general, it is recommended that distal biceps tendon reattachment be performed acutely, although excellent results have been obtained after anatomic reinsertion 3 years after injury (109). The key to delayed surgery is the status of the lacertus fibrosis. If the lacertus fibrosis is intact, the tendon will retract to the level just proximal to the antecubital fossa. The amount of muscle shortening is not very significant and delayed repair is easily attainable. However, if the lacertus is ruptured, the tendon may "slingshot" into the arm, significant muscle shortening may occur, along with scarring within the arm, and delayed primary reattachment may be difficult.

■ MEDIAL EPICONDYLOSIS (GOLFER'S ELBOW)

Medial epicondylosis is a tendinosis of the flexor-pronator muscle group. Medial epicondylosis primarily involves the tendons of the pronator teres and flexor carpi radialis (FCR) muscles, and occasionally the flexor carpi ulnaris (FCU) (110, 111). These muscle-tendon units are susceptible to inflammation and injury as a result of repetitive valgus stress, resulting in overload from both extrinsic and intrinsic forces. The flexor-pronator muscles are subjected to significant extrinsic forces. Because the muscles span two or more joints, they are exposed to increased stretching in addition to valgus forces at the elbow and intrinsic forces from muscular contraction.

Medial epicondylosis is a much less common entity when compared to its lateral counterpart, tennis elbow, 1/7 to 1/20 (110,112). Medial epicondylosis, like lateral epicondylosis, seems to have a peak incidence in the fourth and fifth decades of life (110,111). Sports that are more commonly associated with medial epicondylosis are golf, tennis, and baseball (predominantly pitchers). In golf, medial epicondylosis is caused by repeatedly hitting behind the ball (called hitting it fat), imparting large amounts of stress to the medial structures. Advanced tennis players who forcibly extend their wrist while striking the ball on overheads and serves are at risk for this injury. Baseball pitchers are susceptible to this problem while compensating for a lax or injured UCL or from repetitive use resisting the valgus forces of throwing.

Patients with medial epicondylosis may occasionally note swelling of the medial elbow. The most consistent complaint from those athletes suffering from medial epicondylosis is inner elbow pain that is worse with throwing, serving, or hitting a forehand. These individuals are tender over the medial epicondyle, particularly slightly distal, anterior, and lateral to the epicondyle, and have increased pain with resisted wrist flexion or pronation, as well as with passive wrist extension. It has been found that nearly 60% of athletes with medial epicondylosis have associated ulnar nerve symptoms (111,113–115).

Treatment is conservative, again using the PRICEMM program. Recalcitrant cases may require a local corticosteroid injection at the site of maximal tenderness, which provides pain relief in the short term, allowing for adequate rehabilitation (116). However, when injecting the area for medial epicondylosis, care must be taken to not inject into the tendon or ulnar nerve owing to the risk of tendon rupture or nerve damage. After the symptoms have resolved with relative rest, ice, anti-inflammatory medications, and modalities, a systematic regimen of strengthening exercises is initiated. As strength improves, a counterforce brace may be applied and sports resumed. It is often prudent to recommend the patient to seek professional advice to improve the biomechanics of the desired sport. It is important to stress to the patient the treatment is relative rest and the exercise program, not an injection or medications. Most patients (85%–90%) respond to nonsurgical treatment (110–112, 114,117,118). If symptoms persist after at least 10 weeks of the appropriate conservative management program, then surgical treatment may be necessary. Surgery consists of releasing the flexor-pronator origin, excising the granulation tissue, roughening or decorticating the medial epicondylar bone to stimulate bleeding, and reconstructing the medial musculotendinous unit, thus restoring a good vascular bed to induce healing (111,119). Alternatively, the flexor-pronator muscle group may be split in line with the fibers, allowing exposure to excise the granulation tissue, decorticate the bone, and close the muscle split. This latter approach reduces the risk associated with detachment-reattachment and post-operative protection of a muscle tendon group, but may not allow complete identification and resection of the granulation tissue. When operating for medial epicondylosis, care must be taken to not damage the UCL during surgery, because this ligament is adherent to the flexor pronator muscle group, and, in fact, serves as a partial origin of one of the muscles. There are not as many series published on the surgical results of medial epicondylosis; however, the results with surgical treatment reveal 97% subjectively good to excellent results and 86% of patients without limitation in elbow use at an average 7 years of follow-up (118). It should be noted, however, that the results are not as good when there is associated ulnar neuropathy (114). As one may expect, surgical release of the flexor-pronator muscle origin alone, without repair or reconstruction, does not provide as good results. In fact, in one report of 38 patients, only 69% of patients reported good to excellent results for medial release when the injury was not associated with ulnar nerve symptomology and significantly worse when associated with ulnar nerve symptoms and an ulnar nerve release needed to also be performed (115). Some surgeons recommend exploration of the UCL at the time of medial epicondylosis surgery if the patient is a throwing athlete and clinical examination is suggestive of elbow instability.

■ FLEXOR-PRONATOR MUSCLE GROUP DISRUPTION

Avulsion of the flexor-pronator muscle group from the medial epicondyle is more common than avulsion of the extensor muscle group, even though epicondylosis is more common on the lateral side. The mechanism of this uncommon injury is often forceful extension of the elbow and pronation of the forearm, although it may occur with forceful valgus stress. Norwood found that the flexor-pronator muscle group ruptured in all four of his patients with acute tears of the UCL, whereas Conway et al. (15) found a 13% incidence of flexor-pronator muscle rupture near its origin on the medial epicondyle in patients undergoing surgery for UCL injury (46). The patient will often relay a history of sudden onset of pain along the medial epicondyle, although pain may be insidious with partial ruptures. Examination reveals tenderness at, or slightly distal to the medial epicondylar origin of the muscle and pain that is worse with wrist flexion. A complete rupture or avulsion is usually associated with wrist flexion weakness. A palpable defect in the tendon may be felt just distal to the medial epicondyle, while a bulge may be felt in the proximal forearm. Radiographs (including stress radiographs) are usually normal, although some calcific deposits may be identified within the tendon. Surgical reattachment is the recommended treatment because the common flexor origin is an important stabilizer for the medial elbow. However, repair can be difficult and rarely restores competitive function.

■ TRICEPS TENDINOPATHY

Pain of the triceps insertion at the proximal olecranon is common in athletes who lift inordinate amounts of weight or in explosive field events such as shot put, although it is also seen in javelin throwing and baseball pitching. The cause of triceps tendinopathy is intrinsic muscle overload of the triceps associated with the sudden snap of elbow extension. Patients with this problem complain of pain at the tip of the olecranon that is aggravated by throwing. On examination, the point of maximal tenderness is just proximal to the attachment of the triceps on the olecranon, or exactly at the triceps insertion. The posterior elbow pain is accentuated by resisted active elbow extension or with complete passive flexion with shoulder flexion (resulting in a stretching of the triceps musculotendinous complex). Triceps tendinopathy may be an acute or chronic problem. In the chronic setting, radiographs frequently will reveal calcific deposits within the tendon. However, usually, radiographs are normal. Treatment again is conservative utilizing the PRICEMM protocol. It is important not to inject steroids into the tendon in any circumstance due to the significant risk of tendon rupture and its consequences. If the symptoms do not respond to this conservative program, and particularly if calcific deposits are present, surgery may be warranted to explore the tendon, excise intratendinous and extratendinous degeneration and granulation tissue, remove the calcification, and primarily to repair the tendon (120).

■ TRICEPS TENDON RUPTURE

The triceps tendon is the least common of all tendon ruptures in the body and, fortunately, is a very uncommon cause of pain in the posterior elbow (106). This tendon may be ruptured or avulsed due to a decelerating counterforce during active extension of the elbow or a direct blow. Systemic and local corticosteroid injections have been implicated as etiologic factors for triceps tendon rupture, which is why these injections are contraindicated for the triceps tendon (121). Patients with triceps tendon rupture cannot actively extend their elbow against gravity and have a palpable defect in the tendon proximal to the olecranon. Radiographs frequently show a fleck of bone (up to 80% of cases) **(Fig 23-32)**. This is usually an avulsion injury, although there are reports of tears at the musculotendinous junction (106,122–125). Triceps tendon avulsions should be treated as soon as possible with a direct repair through drill holes in the olecranon, with or without fascial or tendon augmentation (106,126). The results are universally good with surgical repair.

■ LATERAL EPICONDYLOSIS (TENNIS ELBOW)

Lateral epicondylosis is arguably the most common source of elbow pain in the general population. As noted earlier, it occurs seven to twenty times more frequently than medial

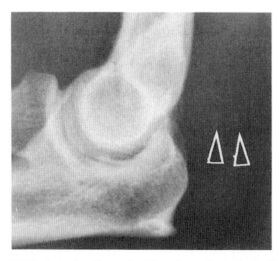

Fig 23-32. Lateral radiograph of the elbow of a patient with an acute triceps rupture sustained while weight lifting. The triceps tendon ruptured during eccentric contraction while bench pressing. The arrowheads point to two flecks of bone, which is consistent with avulsion of the triceps tendon.

epicondylosis (110,112). Though it was initially reported more than 100 years ago in a tennis player (127), it has since been described in association with many other athletic and nonathletic endeavors, with most clinicians noting a predominance of nontennis players having tennis elbow. Lateral epicondylosis is a chronic, noninflammatory condition of the extensor muscles, primarily the extensor carpi radialis brevis (ECRB), due to overuse (from both intensity and duration). The pathology has been described as angiofibroblastic proliferation, appearance of vascular ingrowth into a degenerative area, provoked by repetitive trauma (128).

It has been shown that there is a prevalence of tennis elbow of approximately 50% of club tennis players older than 30 years of age (128). Half of these players noted minor symptoms lasting less than 6 months, whereas the other half had significant symptoms that lasted an average of 2.5 years. Lateral epicondylosis tends to occur in recreational tennis players 35 to 50 years of age (average 41 years) playing three to four times per week, who are inadequately conditioned and often use poor technique. Several factors are associated with tennis elbow: heavier, stiffer, more tightly strung rackets; incorrect grip size; metal rackets; inexperienced players; and bad backhand technique (128–132). Increased racquet vibration, typically initiated by off-center hitting (miss hits—correlating with poor mechanics), is another factor felt to produce this injury. High-level tennis players who warm up, use good technique, and are well conditioned rarely develop tennis elbow. Individuals who use a one-handed backhand technique are at higher risk of developing lateral epicondylosis when compared with those who use two hands. This is believed to be the result of better mechanics in using body rotation to swing at the ball when using two hands.

Individuals with lateral epicondylosis complain of dull lateral elbow pain that started with an insidious onset, beginning gradually after vigorous activity and progressing to pain with activity. Frequently, the patient notes pain with normal daily activities, such as turning a doorknob, lifting a milk carton, opening a jar, or typing on a computer. Night pain is not common, usually appearing in patients with chronic epicondylosis. On physical examination, pain may be elicited with passive wrist flexion and with active resisted wrist extension or resisted supination. Frequently, there is tenderness 1 to 2 cm distal to the lateral epicondyle. Grasping or pinching with the wrist extended (the "coffee cup" test) usually reproduces pain at the point of maximal tenderness (112). Radiographs are frequently normal, although it has been reported that 22% of patients have evidence of a spur at the lateral epicondyle or calcification of the common extensor tendon (117). Calcification of the extensor tendon is believed to be secondary to the chronic repetitive tension forces placed on the musculotendinous origin. Surgical pathology reveals that the ECRB is the tendon involved as the source of injury and pain; however, the anterior extensor digitorum communis (EDC), the underside of the extensor digitorum radialis longus (EDRL), and rarely, the origin of the extensor carpi ulnaris (ECU) may be involved too.

Initial treatment again is PRICEMM, which often is quite successful. Wrist extension splints have been advocated by some to rest the wrist extensor muscles as well during the acute and subacute phases. The key to treating patients with this problem is making them aware that this is an overuse syndrome. Additionally, recognition that other factors, such as using proper technique, reducing tension on the strings of racquets, using a cushioned synthetic grip, conditioning, and using the counterforce brace may all be helpful, though scientific proof is lacking. Counterforce bracing has been found to be useful treating patients with tennis elbow (133,134). Many theories have been put forth to explain the mechanism of success for counterforce bracing **(Table 23-1)**. The overlying theme is the brace works by causing a change in the sequence and direction of muscle contraction, which short circuits muscle forces by shortening the effective length of the muscle and reducing pull at the lateral epicondylar origin. If this conservative program is not effective, injection of lidocaine (Xylocaine) and corticosteroids just below the ECRB may be beneficial for short-term use (135–139). It is important to realize that repeated injections of corticosteroids may result in tendon compromise and complications. After the symptoms subside following the injection, a comprehensive rehabilitation program is again initiated, emphasizing strength and flexibility of the forearm flexors and extensors. The patient should be reminded that the exercises and proper mechanics are important for prevention of recurrence. It should also be emphasized that the medications and injections are only temporizing factors to reduce the symptoms to allow them to do the exercises, and not the definitive treatment. The patient should be encouraged to seek professional instruction to eliminate biomechanical errors in stroke production. Typical errors seen in tennis include (a) improper weight transfer (hitting off the back foot), (b) hitting with the leading elbow during the backhand, and (c) excessive pronation of the forearm during the serve or the overhead. In golf, lateral epicondylosis is associated with "hooker's grip," which is an attempt to close the club face by over-pronating the hand.

TABLE 23-1   Counterforce Bracing

Theories of function:
1. Inhibit maximal contraction of wrist and finger flexor and extensors
2. Constrain full muscle expansion, reducing intrinsic muscle force to sensitive or vulnerable areas
3. Limit stress absorbed by the joint protected
4. Reduce activity of forearm muscles reducing the overload forces to the muscle
5. Partially fix the muscle to the underlying forearm bone and soft tissue, creating a new muscle origin that shortens the length of the muscle pull, slightly changing the direction of force and bypassing the inflamed and injured portion of the muscle that is proximal to the strap

---

If conservative treatment fails to return the athlete to usual activities after an adequate attempt at the conservative PRICEMM program, which occurs in 4% to 12% (110,137, 140,141) most surgeons recommend surgical intervention (117). Some authors also recommend surgery for recurrence following successful resolution by conservative means (142), although most clinicians recommend another trial of conservative treatment before proceeding with surgery. There have been many described surgical procedures at the elbow and wrist in the treatment of lateral epicondylosis (117,137, 143–149). The authors prefer removal of the granulation tissue and decortication of the lateral epicondyle (119). Basically, the common extensor hood is elevated carefully, and the underlying granulation tissue is excised. The epicondyle is drilled or burred to bleeding bone to create a good vascular bed, and the extensor hood is repaired (119). Care is taken to not injure the lateral ligamentous complex because cases of PLRI have been reported following surgery for lateral epicondylosis.

Lateral epicondylosis can also be treated arthroscopically. Baker and Cummings (150) first reported capsular rents or holes in patients with lateral epicondylosis noted at the time of arthroscopy. This has been confirmed by these authors and others, bringing the pathogenesis into further question. Arthroscopic release for lateral epicondylosis has been shown to result in improvement in 93.3% of patients, with 71% having good to excellent results in patients followed for at least 6 months (150). Subsequent studies have confirmed the success and safety of this procedure (149,151–153).

Most studies find good success with open surgical treatment, averaging 85% returned to full activities without pain, 12% improved but still had some pain with vigorous activities, and 3% showed no improvement (137,141,154). Revision surgery using the open approach described above has also been successful in 83% of patients (155). It has been reported that the most common cause of failure of surgery for lateral epicondylosis was incomplete excision of the degenerative tissue (155).

Another approach is percutaneous release of the common extensor origin—supinator origin, which can be performed in the office or operating room. Proponents of this procedure prefer this technique because the surgical results are similar to other, more complicated procedures with less-invasive means. In a retrospective study in 1982, Baumgard and Schwartz (156) described his results of percutaneous release of the common extensors as an office procedure. The lateral epicondyle release included 37 lateral releases (3 bilateral and 3 re-operations) followed for a mean of 35 months. They reported 91.4% excellent results and 8.6% unsatisfactory results at 3-year follow up. There have been other case series of percutaneous releases all with similar results (157,158).

Some have recommended multiple repeated steroid injections as an alternative to surgical treatment. Most clinicians and authors recommend a maximum of three injections into this area per year (129); however, others believe that more than this is not a problem for lateral epicondylosis.

The philosophy behind this repeated injection approach is that the consequence of more than three injections per year is degeneration of the tendon and subsequent rupture (159). The goal of several different surgical approaches for this problem is just to release the tendon; the end result is the same without the risk of surgery or the time away from sports. The repeated injection approach does, however, put the other normal surrounding tissues at risk for degeneration from the steroids (160), and as such is not generally recommended.

Savoie et al. (161) compared the results of percutaneous, open, and arthroscopic techniques in the surgical management of lateral epicondylosis and found no difference between the techniques with regard to outcome or complications. A recent evidence-based review and meta-analysis (149) also was unable to conclude which surgical approach is superior. Although multiple studies show comparable results without looking intra-articularly, the incidence in more recent studies suggest that the rate of concomitant intra-articular pathology varies and in some cases is as high as 18% to 69% (151,161, 162). Because of this latter revelation, and with the lack of proven superiority of one technique over the other, at least one author prefers to treat lateral epicondylosis arthroscopically to identify and treat the concomitant intra-articular pathology, because this may be the cause of "failed lateral epicondylosis surgery" in some cases.

■ EXTENSOR-SUPINATOR MUSCULAR DISRUPTION

Common extensor musculotendinous origin disruption or avulsion, without previous cortisone injection, is an uncommon injury (110). Patients who do have lateral musculotendinous avulsion describe severe acute lateral elbow pain, often associated with a pop or snap. On examination, weakness of wrist extension and forearm supination can be detected. Surgery to reattach the extensor origin is indicated if weakness persists after the pain subsides and if all or a major part of the extensor tendon origin is ruptured.

■ OVERUSE INJURIES

Athletes participating in overhead sports such as tennis, volleyball, swimming, weightlifting, gymnastics, and especially throwing, subject their elbows to repetitive stresses most marked in specific phases of the activity. These athletes are vulnerable to injuries and present with a myriad of problems including tendonitis, bursitis, nerve injuries, and instability. Repetitive overhead stress to the elbow can and does cause cumulative injuries to soft tissue static stabilizers, with recurrent micro injuries to the primary stabilizers including the UCLs and capsule. The spectrum of valgus overload extension syndrome points to the stresses then being picked up by

the secondary stabilizers including bony injuries such as wear and osteophytes of the olecranon.

A frequent cause of lost playing time and lost training time, particularly in overhead athletes, is overuse injuries. Athletes beginning the season are exposed to sudden increases in the intensity and volume of overhead throwing and consequently stress on the elbow. Another common expression of this mechanism is the Little League pitcher who is not compliant with pitch count or innings pitched by playing on multiple teams in different leagues. Often, as the best pitcher on the team, these young athletes are asked to do the bulk of the pitching and are happy to comply. This is combined with a trend towards a "year-round season" and specialization to a single sport at an earlier age. A much-repeated scenario is well-meaning parents who encourage or even insist that the child keep pitching and perhaps "work his way through whatever elbow pain may be present." This in an effort to maintain prospects for future advancement in sports or perhaps college.

Another common scenario of overuse problems related to pitching, and particular to the elbow, is seen in the valgus extension overload syndrome. Senior pitchers or, less commonly, more-mature tennis players experience repetitive overuse with gradual failure of the UCL. This is very common as successful players continue for many years and start to see a rather sudden decline in their abilities very late in their careers. This has been only recently recognized and will bring more diligence to evaluations of the ulnar side of the elbow. The human elbow presents an anatomic risk factor inherently for overuse injuries in overhead sports best exemplified by pitching a baseball. Intuitively it was not designed to perform this activity at this level for such an extended period of time.

Treatment of soft tissue overuse injuries involves review of training technique and errors, modification of perpetuating activity, cryotherapy, anti-inflammatory medications and other modalities, and a stretching and strengthening program along with a gradual monitored return to the activity. If patients do not respond readily to this program, a judicious re-evaluation of shoulder pathology should be undertaken.

Throwing Injuries and Posterior Compartment Elbow Injuries

This section begins with a review of the functional anatomy of the elbow as it relates to throwing, then throwing mechanics, and completing with pathomechanics and injury. Most of the injuries associated with throwing are discussed in other sections within this chapter with the exception of posterior compartment injuries, such as valgus extension overload and olecranon stress injury, which will be covered here.

Functional Anatomy

The athlete involved in throwing (such as baseball, javelin, water polo, football quarterback) and overhead sports (such as volleyball and tennis) is most often exposed to chronic repetitive valgus stress at the elbow. While bony articulation resists these stresses with the elbow flexed less than 20 degrees (including the olecranon within the olecranon fossa, or posterior compartment) or greater than 120 degrees (20,79, 163), the UCL complex valgus stress is the primary restraint in the ranges of motion between 20 and 120 degrees of elbow flexion (20,79,163–165). The anterior band of the anterior oblique ligament is felt to be the critical portion of the UCL complex resisting forces imparted by throwing sports, and it is this part of the ligament complex that is usually injured as a result of throwing. The radiocapitellar joint is a secondary stabilizer to valgus stress (30%) and thus, when the UCL is injured, there is an even greater load on the lateral elbow joint (166). This is important because, occasionally, an athlete may present with lateral elbow pain when the primary problem is UCL injury.

The soft tissues also contribute dynamic stability through muscular forces. The flexor-pronator muscle group originates as a common tendon from the medial epicondyle and is an important dynamic stabilizer to the medial elbow. Specifically, the FCU lays directly over the UCL and is believed to be the primary dynamic contributor to valgus stability, while the flexor digitorum superficialis, which originates in part from the UCL, may also support valgus stability in greater degrees of extension (167,168). Additionally, the wedge shape of the bony olecranon central ridge within the trochlea provides some stability to varus-valgus stress with the contribution of joint compression from muscular forces across the elbow (from all the muscles that cross the joint and are contracting during activity) in a concavity compression mechanism, similar to that described in the shoulder.

Throwing Mechanics and the Elbow

Understanding the mechanics involved in overhand sports can help in understanding injury pathomechanics and patterns in the throwing athlete. While other overhand sports have been studied, most research involves analysis of the baseball throw, particularly baseball pitching. It has been shown that, although pitching a baseball is an inherently destructive or injurious force to the elbow, application of the proper pitching mechanics can assist in minimizing potential risk for injury while maximizing performance. To simplify analysis of pitching, the motion is commonly divided into six phases: wind-up, stride, cocking, acceleration, deceleration, and follow-through (169), though the cocking and acceleration phases are also sometimes subdivided. Following is a description of the elbow biomechanics during each phase of pitching.

Wind-Up

The wind-up phase begins with initiation of leg movement and ends when the pitcher's forward knee has reached its maximum height. During this phase, the pitcher is attempting to balance his weight over his rear leg, preparing for forward motion toward the plate with weight on the forward leg. The elbow is flexed throughout this phase, though there are minimal elbow kinetics and muscle action present during this phase (169–171).

Stride

The stride phase begins at the end of the wind-up phase when the forward leg begins to descend toward the ground, the ball leaves the glove, and the two arms separate from each other. The stride phase ends when the forward foot contacts the pitching mound. In the beginning and middle periods of this phase the elbow is extended. From the middle to the end of this phase the elbow becomes flexed. At foot contact with the mound, the elbow is positioned in approximately 80 to 100 degrees of flexion (169,171).

Cocking

The cocking phase begins when the forward foot has initial contact with the mound and ends when the throwing shoulder reaches maximum external rotation—just before the ball starts in forward motion. After forward foot contact, the pelvis and upper trunk begin to rotate to face the batter. As this pelvic and trunk rotation occurs, elbow torques and joint forces are generated. A low-to-moderate flexion torque of 0 Nm to 32 Nm is produced at the elbow throughout this phase (172). The upper trunk and pelvis rotate forward as the throwing shoulder externally rotates, rotating the arm and ball backward, producing a large valgus torque onto the upper arm at the elbow. This occurs in the last 25% of the cocking phase, and is sometimes referred to as the late cocking phase. To resist the valgus torque, the upper arm generates a varus torque of up to 64 ± 12 Nm onto the forearm shortly before maximum external rotation of the shoulder in baseball players (172) and more than 60 Nm with the tennis serve (173,174). Due to significant valgus torque imparted upon the elbow during this phase, large tensile forces are produced on the medial aspect of the elbow. The flexor-pronator mass helps dynamically stabilize the medial elbow from these distraction forces. However, the repetitive nature of valgus loading on the elbow with pitching at this instance in the throwing mechanics is most often associated with a possible injury to the UCL. Morrey and An (175) demonstrated that the UCL contributes approximately 54% of the resistance to valgus stress with the elbow in the flexed position. If this were the case, it has been shown that the strength of the UCL is only 32 Nm in cadaveric specimens (176), and thus, the UCL would be injured with every throw. However, the Morrey and An study was done on cadaveric specimens, where the contribution of dynamic muscular stabilization could not be accounted for. The UCL likely combines with dynamic muscular stabilizers and quite possibly long arm rotation to reduce the stress and to resist this valgus loading (177). As noted above, muscular contraction may reduce the stress seen on the UCL by the concavity compression effect (169). The study by Morrey and An also showed that a third of the resistance to valgus loading is provided by bony articulation. As noted in the section on OCD, compressive force on the radiocapitellar joint to resist valgus can lead to OCD and radiocapitellar degeneration.

Some investigators divide this phase into the early and late cocking phase. The early cocking phase is the first 75% of cocking, that essentially is where the ball moves back by active arm motion. The late cocking phase, the last 25% of the phase, is where the body momentum of the pitcher is moving forward and the ball moves backwards as the shoulder moves into greater external rotation passively. It is this late cocking phase where the forces are greatest on the elbow.

Acceleration

The acceleration phase is the shortest phase of the pitching motion, but one of the most intense for the elbow and shoulder (178). This phase begins at maximal shoulder external rotation (the initiation of forward ball motion) and ends at ball release. Sometimes this phase is also subdivided into early and late phases. The early acceleration phase is the first 25% where the greatest forces are generated, the initiation of forward ball motion, and the last 75%, the late acceleration phase. During the acceleration phase, the elbow extends as the trunk continues to rotate. The maximum elbow extension velocity has been recorded at 2,100 to 2,700 degrees per second at approximately halfway through the acceleration phase in baseball (169,179) and 1,300 degrees per second in tennis (174). The maximum elbow angular velocity is not statistically different when comparing the fastball, curveball, and slider pitches. However, the angular velocity is significantly less during the change-up pitch (180). Elbow extension is too rapid to be attributed to the elbow extensors. Most of the elbow extension velocity is the result of the summation of more proximal parts, the premise for the kinetic chain. It is the rotary actions of the other parts of the body (e.g., leg, thigh, hips, trunk, back, and shoulder) than to the action of the triceps. In support of this concept, a differential nerve block was used to paralyze the triceps in a baseball pitcher who was then able to throw a ball at more than 80% of the speed attained before triceps were paralyzed (181). Using computer simulation, Ahn (182) reinforced the concept of the kinetic chain, concluding that velocity of the ball at release was primarily generated by the lower extremities, hips, and trunk.

During the acceleration phase, significant amounts of varus torque are generated in order to resist the valgus torque and forces accelerating the arm forward. Valgus torque as the elbow is being extended can result in impingement of the olecranon against the trochlear groove and the olecranon fossa, resulting in valgus extension overload (below) (183). As the elbow extends and the upper trunk continues to rotate, a maximum elbow proximal force of 800 N to 1,000 N is produced by ball release to resist the distraction forces after ball release (172). The elbow flexors (biceps, brachioradialis, and brachialis) add compressive joint stability by contracting throughout this phase while also eccentrically contracting to control the rate of elbow extension.

Deceleration

The deceleration phase begins at ball release and ends when the shoulder reaches maximum internal rotation. The body helps decelerate the rapidly moving arm and dissipate the energy through the shoulder and elbow. During this phase, there is an elbow flexion torque produced by the elbow flexors of approximately 10 Nm to 35 Nm to decelerate elbow extension (169,170,172,184). Elbow extension ends approximately 20 degrees before full extension (169,171). To prevent elbow distraction after ball release, the large proximal compression-contraction forces are generated (172). Thus the elbow flexors resist the distraction forces in addition to decelerating elbow extension before the olecranon impingement (169). This proximal force is greatest when the pitcher is throwing a fastball or a slider pitch (185). It should also be noted that the proximal forces of the elbow flexors are increased with increasing skill level (186).

Follow-through

The final phase of the baseball pitch is the follow-through. This phase begins when the shoulder reaches maximum internal rotation and ends when the pitcher reaches a balanced fielding position. Motion of the larger body parts, such as the trunk and lower extremities, continue to help dissipate energy in the throwing arm during this phase (178). During follow-through, the elbow flexes into a comfortable position as the trunk rotates forward and the arm moves across the body (171).

Pathophysiology of the Thrower's Elbow

As described above, valgus stress as a result of throwing produces tensile or distraction forces to the medial elbow. The chronic tensile stress is initiated by the repetitious high-velocity nature of overhead sports and often predisposes the elbow to overuse syndromes (172). As described earlier, many sports activities require similar motion and mechanics: rapid forceful extension of the elbow, frequently accompanied by valgus stress and pronation of the supinated forearm (187). The normal valgus carrying angle of the elbow may predispose the medial aspect of the elbow to valgus overuse injuries, which, as noted above, may be increased in baseball and tennis players.

The forces at the elbow due to recurring valgus stress result in (a) traction of the medial-sided structures of the elbow **(Fig 23-33)**, (b) compression of the lateral side of the elbow, and (c) medially directed posterior shear and compression of the posteromedial olecranon **(Fig 23-34)**. The medial traction forces may result in tensile injury to the soft tissues of the medial elbow, including the UCL, ulnar nerve, and the components of the flexor-pronator musculotendinous complex. The exception to this is the immature athlete, where the physis (medial epicondylar apophysis) is the weakest link in the adolescent musculoskeletal system and thus is most susceptible to injury. The bony tissues of the lateral elbow (radiocapitellar joint) are subjected to repetitious

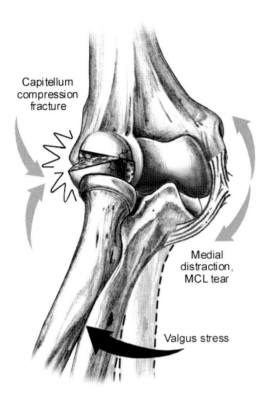

Fig 23-33. Valgus stress to the elbow imparts a tensile force to the medial elbow, resulting in injury to the ulnar collateral ligament. Other medial structures, such as the flexor-pronator muscles, can be injured due to repeated eccentric contraction and while attempting to provide dynamic stability to the medial elbow. The ulnar nerve is susceptible to injury due to these tensile forces as well as compression within a narrowed cubital tunnel, secondary to the scarring within the ligament and osteophytes. With continued valgus stress, the radiocapitellar joint is compressed, which may result in chondromalacia, osteophyte formation, and, eventually, loose bodies. (From Safran MR. Injury to the ulnar collateral ligament: diagnosis and treatment. *Sports Medicine and Arthroscopy Review.* 2003;11:15–24 (figure 2, page 17).

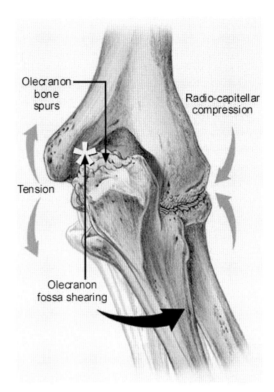

Fig 23-34. Posteriorly, the olecranon is subjected to medial shearing forces with valgus stress, which may be accentuated by increased valgus laxity, resulting in valgus extension overload, with osteophyte formation and loose bodies. (From Safran MR. Injury to the ulnar collateral ligament: diagnosis and treatment. *Sports Medicine and Arthroscopy Review.* 2003;11:15–24 (figure 3, page 17).

compressive forces, which is accentuated when there is UCL laxity.

Effects on Medial Elbow

The medial elbow structures are primarily susceptible to injury due to the valgus forces that are associated with repetitive throwing, because these soft tissues are susceptible to tensile forces. As noted on the section on the UCL, the UCL is particularly at risk for injury due to repetitive tensile (valgus) overload as seen with overhead throwing sports and valgus stress with throwing-type mechanics. When the UCL is injured, the tensile forces will then be imparted to other structures of the medial elbow, including the flexor-pronator musculotendinous unit and the ulnar nerve.

As noted earlier, the primary *dynamic* stabilizer to valgus stress is the flexor-pronator muscle mass, particularly the FCU and flexor digitorum superficialis (168,188). With repetitive valgus stress as a result of throwing, these

muscles may fatigue, imparting increasing stress to the UCL, producing microtraumatic ligamentous injury resulting in stretching of the ligament (Fig 23-33). Also, as previously noted, the UCL is the most important *static* stabilizer to valgus stress to the elbow in the arc between 30 and 120 degrees elbow flexion, greater than the range of motion needed from the elbow during throwing (22,164,172). As a result, the UCL is particularly at risk for injury, including microtears or frank tears, from excessive repetitive valgus force during throwing and overhead sports, depending on the magnitude of force and rate of loading of the ligament.

Further, fatigue of the medial muscles may result in inflammation and injury to the musculotendinous unit of the medial elbow (189). This may result in medial epicondylitis in adults and medial epicondylar apophysitis or avulsion in the skeletally immature thrower (189,190). An athlete may be even more susceptible to these problems if there is concomitant laxity of the UCL due to repeated injury resulting in increased dependence on these dynamic stabilizers. Further, there are reports of flexor-pronator muscle avulsion injuries associated with UCL tears, demonstrating the similar function of these structures (191,192). Chronic traction injury to the UCL may result in thickening of the ligament and/or traction osteophytes at its insertion on the ulna. Chronic UCL laxity may also result in shear forces at the posteromedial elbow that may produce osteophytes and loose bodies in the posterior compartment of the elbow, which will be discussed in more detail below.

Pressure within the ulnar nerve has been found to be elevated to three times more than normal with the elbow flexed at 90 degrees and the wrist extended, the position of late cocking and early acceleration (193,194). The intraneural pressure elevation is felt to be the result of physiologic stretching of the nerve combined with compression by the FCU aponeurosis (195). With further elbow flexion, wrist extension, and shoulder abduction, which can occur with throwing, this pressure can be elevated to as much as six times the resting normal intraneural pressure (194,195). Further, ulnar nerve has been shown to elongate an average 4.7 mm with elbow flexion and can be displaced by more than 7 mm by the medial head of the triceps (196). As a result, the cubital tunnel narrows 40% to 55% with elbow flexion, resulting in compression of the ulnar nerve (193, 196). The cubital tunnel may be encroached further by a variety of associated pathologies commonly seen in overhead athletes resulting in further compression of the ulnar nerve.

Traction neuritis may be made worse by the valgus forces associated with throwing activities. With an incompetent or lax UCL, the medial joint widens with valgus stress, imparting a tensile stress to the nerve as it is stretched beyond its normal elongation. It is not uncommon for professional baseball and tennis players to have fixed elbow flexion and valgus deformities—static malalignments that further predispose them to ulnar nerve problems. The end result of excessive traction is fibrosis from direct injury and possibly ischemia of the nerve due to prolonged or repeated elevation of pressures and stretching injury (197).

Effects on the Lateral Elbow

As introduced above, valgus stress to an elbow with an attenuated UCL may result in compression of the bony structures of the lateral elbow functioning as a secondary stabilizer. In the adult, valgus stresses in the setting of a lax UCL may result in a radiocapitellar overload syndrome (Fig 23-33). This is manifest by repetitive compressive forces to the radiocapitellar joint that result in radial head abutment against the capitellum. This chronic, repetitive compressive force may result in chondromalacia of the radiocapitellar joint surfaces, followed by cartilage and then bony degeneration. Persistent radiocapitellar compression may eventually result in osteochondral fracture and the production of loose bodies within the joint. In the skeletally immature athlete, it is proposed that this may be clinically manifest as OCD of the capitellum, possibly as a result of interruption of the subchondral blood flow due to repeated compressive forces, discussed in more detail in the pediatric elbow section.

Effects on the Posterior Elbow

Throwing forces may also result in posterior elbow pain as the olecranon is repeatedly and forcefully driven into the olecranon fossa. Typically a valgus stress causes shearing of the posterior compartment resulting in the olecranon impinging against the medial wall of the olecranon fossa. Ahmad et al. (198) has demonstrated that UCL injury results in contact alterations in the posterior compartment that leads to osteophyte formation. The results of this study suggest that osteophyte formation may result from subtle UCL injury, or increased valgus laxity, due to increased shear forces to the posteromedial elbow (Fig 23-34). Amplifying this posterior impingement is the bony hypertrophy of the distal humerus and proximal ulna that is commonly seen in those athletes involved in sports such as tennis and baseball (199,200). Hypertrophy of the distal humerus decreases the size of the olecranon fossa, making less olecranon translation necessary to result in bony impingement. Additionally, proximal ulna hypertrophy also decreases the free space between the olecranon fossa and the olecranon, allowing for impingement to occur with lesser degrees of medial laxity and posterior shearing. To add to this situation, the fixed valgus deformity often seen in throwing athletes who have played for many years also positions the medial olecranon closer to the medial wall of the olecranon fossa. Thus, less translational motion (and thus UCL laxity) is needed before the olecranon contacts the distal humerus resulting in posterior impingement and valgus extension overload.

The repeated large extension velocities may result in impaction of the olecranon tip within the fossa, further compounding the problem. The intra-articular tip of the olecranon causes localized inflammation when impacted within the fossa. With repetitive impaction, chondromalacia and osteophyte formation can occur. With persistent impingement and shear forces, these osteophytes may break off and become loose bodies within the joint (183). Loose bodies may cause mechanical symptoms, such as blocking flexion or extension, or may produce a synovitic reaction resulting in an effusion and stiff elbow. These forces may also result in other olecranon injury, including stress reaction, stress fracture, or apophyseal injury in the skeletally immature ball player (201–204).

Valgus Extension Overload Syndrome

The valgus extension overload syndrome is a common final pathway for posterior elbow problems that result from excessive valgus and hyperextension forces (Fig 23-26). Athletes who participate in racquet sports, baseball, or throw javelin are more susceptible to this problem because the olecranon is repeatedly and forcefully driven into the olecranon fossa. In addition, there is the valgus stress of throwing that causes the olecranon to shear and impinge against the medial wall of the olecranon fossa. This situation is made worse when there is concomitant laxity of the UCL (198).

The tip of the olecranon, which is intra-articular, causes local inflammation and, if it persists, eventually chondromalacia and osteophyte formation occur, as noted above. With continued impingement, these osteophytes can break off from the olecranon and become loose bodies within the elbow (205) **(Fig 23-35)**. Loose bodies may cause intermittent locking with a mechanical block to flexion or extension or may produce a synovitis, resulting in an effusion and stiff elbow. As mentioned earlier, professional baseball pitchers and tennis players have increased valgus angulation of the elbow as well as hypertrophy of the distal humerus resulting in narrowing of the olecranon fossa. Such morphologic changes, in addition to the valgus force of throwing, predispose pitchers to impingement of the olecranon process on the medial wall of the olecranon fossa (16).

Individuals with valgus extension overload complain of posterior elbow pain, sometimes with a clicking or grating sensation. When loose bodies develop, individuals often complain of catching or locking and that they need to manipulate the elbow to release or unlock it. They may also note that their pain occurs with full extension—either passive or active—which can be demonstrated on physical examination. Further, this posterior elbow pain can be accentuated by applying a valgus stress upon an extended elbow. Examination may also demonstrate tenderness posteriorly along the margins of the olecranon, although it is rare to palpate loose bodies within the elbow. Radiographs may reveal calcification at the olecranon tip, which frequently is confused with triceps tendinitis. An arthrogram or tomogram can be helpful in distinguishing between the two conditions and may reveal the loose bodies. Radiographs may also reveal osteophytes or enlargement of the olecranon, or both **(Fig 23-36)**. A modified cubital tunnel view may help demonstrate posteromedial olecranon osteophytes. When there is any question, a CT scan can show osteophytes and a CT arthrogram is very sensitive at demonstrating small loose bodies within the elbow.

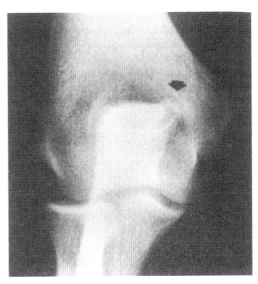

Fig 23-36. Radiograph showing a posterior medial spur *(arrow)* associated with valgus extension overload.

Treatment for early phases of this syndrome, particularly if there are no loose bodies, include NSAIDs and strengthening of the flexor-pronator muscle group to reduce inflammation and symptoms and to protect the joint. However, when posteromedial osteophytes are present, physical therapy is usually not effective (205). Arthroscopy can be used to determine whether osteophytes or loose bodies are present and can be used to shave down the osteophytes and remove the loose bodies (206). Arthrotomy traditionally has been used with good results (17,88,205,207,208). Yet, current results with the arthroscope in the elbow are quite good, with low complication rates (28,89,209–211), while allowing for earlier and more aggressive rehabilitation and earlier return to sport, making this the preferred treatment for loose bodies and osteophytes **(Fig 23-37)**.

Removal of the osteophytes and removal of the loose bodies do not treat a frequent underlying cause of the loose bodies—attenuation of the UCL (28). As a result, there is a high reoperation rate (41%) if just removal of the loose bodies or osteophyte is undertaken (28). In fact, this study showed 25% of the professional baseball players who underwent olecranon debridement for valgus extension overload eventually required UCL reconstruction (28).

A recent biomechanical study suggests olecranon resection subjects the UCL to greater strain and places the UCL at increased risk for injury (212). Kamineni et al. (213) also showed the strain in the AOL is increased with increasing posteromedial olecranon resection beyond 3 mm. Thus, based on clinical and basic science studies, we advocate careful evaluation of the UCL in patients presenting with valgus extension overload. We feel consideration should be given to UCL reconstruction in combination with posterior debridement in these patients who fail nonoperative treatment and have combined posteromedial impingement and UCL injury. Further, based on these studies, we feel posterior debridement

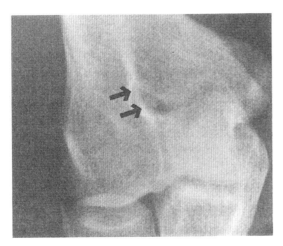

Fig 23-35. Radiograph demonstrating loose bodies in the posterior compartment *(arrows)* of the elbow in a baseball pitcher who reported intermittent locking of the elbow.

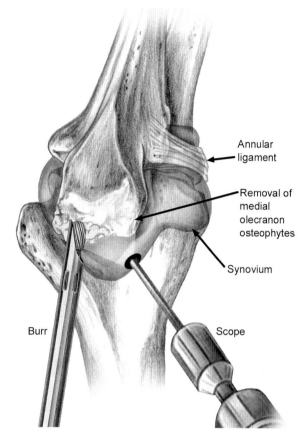

Annular ligament

Removal of medial olecranon osteophytes

Synovium

Burr

Scope

Fig 23-37. Schematic representation of arthroscopic burring of olecranon osteophytes.

should be limited to removal of the osteophytes only, leaving normal olecranon intact.

Osteophyte removal also does not prevent recurrence, but because it often takes years to redevelop osteophytes and loose bodies, many authors consider this an acceptable treatment.

Olecranon Stress Fracture

An uncommon cause of pain in the throwing athlete is a stress fracture of the olecranon. Stress fractures of the olecranon may occur through the growth plate or the persistence of the olecranon apophysis (discussed earlier). In skeletally mature athletes, this fracture usually occurs distally and is oblique, but may occur at the tip (214–216). The mechanisms of this injury are the result of intrinsic forces from the triceps or as a result of shear forces from valgus extension overload. Athletes with an olecranon stress fracture may have pain at rest during or after throwing. The pain usually is insidious in onset and increases with an increased amount and intensity of throwing. Most frequently it is the result of the repetitive sudden snap of full extension in the deceleration phase. Healing of the midolecranon stress fracture is slow with a high risk of nonunion (76). If symptoms persist despite an adequate trial of rest, NSAIDs, and modalities, surgery is usually necessary. Surgical options

include excision of the tip fragment if it is quite distal (214) or internally fixing the olecranon if the fragment is large (76,215).

◼ RADIOCAPITELLAR OVERLOAD SYNDROME, ARTHROFIBROSIS

Olecranon bursitis is more common in athletes involved in contact sports than in throwing athletes. Two bursae near the olecranon have clinical significance. One found between the attachment of the triceps to the olecranon and the skin is the more superficial and is inflamed much more often. The deeper bursa lies between the tendon of the triceps muscle and the posterior ligament of the elbow and the olecranon. The superficial bursa is frequently distended with fluid when inflamed. The fluid tends to recur after aspiration. The clinician should be suspicious for an associated crystalline deposition disease such as gout. Palpable fibrotic or synovial nodules may be felt to move within this bursa and it is frequently painful to direct pressure even when not extended. The superficial bursa may easily be excised when indicated but recurrences are frequent unless careful technique is observed.

Radiocapitellar overload syndrome encompasses radiocapitellar chondromalacia, degeneration, osteochondral fracture fragmentation, and loose bodies. In the throwing elbow of the senior skeletally mature longtime athlete, lateral compression follows the development of posteromedial impingement and UCL injury. It is a late finding in valgus extension overload syndrome. The increased load transmission across the radiocapitellar joint leads to chondromalacia of the articular surfaces, which advances to more severe degeneration and, perhaps, osteochondritis dissicans. The development of pathological findings in this compartment in general occurs near the end of a pitching career. Compared to the conservative treatment of skeletally immature athletes with osteochondritis dissicans, skeletally mature athletes with osteochondral lesion are sometimes treated early with arthroscopic debridement before loose bodies are generated. Debridement of the articular defects, chondroplasty, and microfracture technique is sometimes employed to stimulate a fibrocartilaginous healing response. As these patients often present with significant flexion contractures, these may also be released arthroscopically at the time of surgery. This is followed by an aggressive range-of-motion physical therapy program immediately after surgery.

PLRI is another common cause of lateral elbow pain. Pain referral to the LCLC is infrequent because lateral structures are rarely stressed in athletic activities. Subtle PLRI may cause elbow pain. An incompetent LUCL possibly caused by a previous injury may be the cause of this pain. The patients present complaining of painful clicking, clunking, locking, or snapping when the forearm and supinated in the extension half of the arc of motion. The physical examination is only remarkable for a positive lateral pivot shift or posterolateral rotatory apprehension test.

Fibrosis can occur to the synovial tissues lining the lateral side of the elbow joint from repetitive injuries. A synovial plica band can be a normal finding in the lateral gutter of many people. The repetitive compression in the radiocapitellar joint, however, can lead to synovial hypertrophy and plica band fibrosis. At arthroscopy the extent of the pathology and the robustness of this band must be examined. An associated radial head or capitellar chondromalacia is often seen in association with a pathological plica. In their absence, other more common diagnoses should be looked for. When treating arthroscopically with debridement, care must be taken not to reset the normal annular ligament, which could lead to instability.

■ FRACTURES AND DISLOCATIONS

The elbow is the most commonly injured joint in children, with dislocations accounting for 6% to 8% of elbow injuries (54,217). Following shoulder dislocations, the elbow is the second most commonly dislocated major joint in patients of all ages. In children under the age of 10 years, the elbow is the most commonly dislocated major joint (218). About one-half of all elbow dislocations occur in patients under the age of 20, with a peak incidence between the ages of 13 and 14 (219–221). In most reports, the etiology most commonly listed as the cause is sports. Typically, it is the nondominant extremity that is most commonly dislocated, as a result of a fall on the outstretched hand (219–222). Thus, sports where there is the risk of a fall, especially a violent fall, are the more common sports where the athlete is at increased risk of an elbow dislocation. These sports include cycling, gymnastics, football, and wrestling (223).

Classification of elbow dislocation is based on the displacement of the radius and ulna, which usually move together when the elbow is dislocated. This includes posterior (straight, posterolateral, or posteromedial), anterior, medial, and lateral. A divergent dislocation occurs when the proximal radio-ulnar joint is disrupted, and is divided into anterior, posterior, or mediolateral (224–227). The vast majority of elbow dislocations are posterior or posterolateral (80%–90% of all dislocations) (219–222). Isolated radial head dislocations are rare.

As previously stated, a fall on an outstretched hand is the typical history given by a patient sustaining a posterior elbow dislocation. It has been proposed that there are two main pathophysiologic mechanisms involved: (a) The olecranon levers on the olecranon fossa as the elbow hyperextends until the coronoid process slips posteriorly, while a varus or valgus stress can create a posteromedial or posterolateral dislocation; or (b) the arm is slightly flexed with the lateral sloping surface of the trochlea acting as a cam, converting the vertical force to lateral rotation and valgus stress, which ruptures the medial collateral ligament or avulses the medial epicondyle, allowing the ulna to slip laterally and come to lie posteriorly or posterolaterally (223). Alternatively, a currently popular thought is that a varus rotational force results in lateral collateral ligament or lateral condyle or epicondyle avulsion injury resulting in injury to the LCL and extending anteriorly and posteriorly, resulting in dislocation.

The less common anterior elbow dislocation is often reported to be the result of a direct blow to the olecranon with the elbow flexed.

In children, elbow dislocations are associated with fractures in up to 50% of cases, especially fractures of the radial head and neck, and the medial or lateral epicondyle (228). With posterior elbow dislocations, significant injury to the soft tissues must also occur, including tearing of the anterior capsule, usually from the ulna, while the posterior capsule may be stripped off proximally along the distal humerus.

With elbow dislocations, the medial or lateral collateral ligaments are usually ruptured (57,229). In children, the medial epicondyle apophysis may be avulsed instead of direct ligament injury. There is a spectrum of positioning of the apophysis after dislocation. The avulsed fragment may be nondisplaced, displaced a few millimeters, or can even come to lie within the joint (see medial epicondylar fracture) **(Figs 23-38** and **23-39)**. Associated medial epicondyle fractures in the scenario of elbow dislocation varies from 0% (222) to 30% (219–222). Although current research suggests that the lateral collateral ligament is the essential lesion for elbow dislocation, the lateral epicondyle fracture is less frequently seen in elbow dislocations in children.

In association with elbow dislocations, it is not uncommon to also identify injury to wrist flexor or extensor musculotendinous origins. In the setting of a medial epicondyle fracture or avulsion, the flexor origin usually remains attached to the fracture fragment and acts as a displacing force. Five to 10% of elbow dislocations are associated with radial head or neck fractures (230).

The force of elbow dislocation can uncommonly result in tearing of the brachial artery. In some situations, a tear in the brachial artery can be treated nonoperatively due to excellent collateral flow. However, it has been shown that the collateral vessels about the elbow are usually injured with elbow dislocation as well; thus it is strongly recommended to repair the brachial artery when it is torn during an elbow dislocation (231). Although these injuries have been reported, they are rare; no cases were noted in the West Point series nor in my own personal experience with athletics-induced elbow dislocations (222).

Posterior or posteromedial dislocations may also result in traction injury to the ulnar nerve. In children, there have been reports of median nerve entrapment within the joint. Median nerve entrapment has been classified into three types: (a) displacement posteriorly to the humerus and passes through the joint, (b) an entrapment occurs between fracture surfaces, and (c) there is a kinking nerve in the elbow joint (232). Again, fortunately, these are also uncommon injuries, with Protzman's series (222) reporting no cases of residual neurologic deficits.

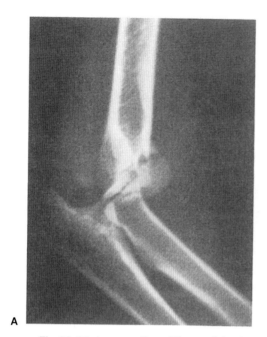
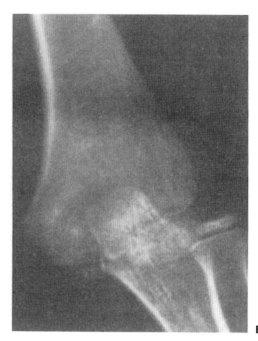

Fig 23-38. Incarceration of the medial epicondyle in the joint prevented closed reduction of this elbow dislocation. (From Safran MR, Salyers S, Fu FH. Elbow dislocations. In: Reider B, ed. *Sports medicine—the school age athlete.* 2nd ed. Philadelphia: WB Saunders; 1996:242; with permission.)

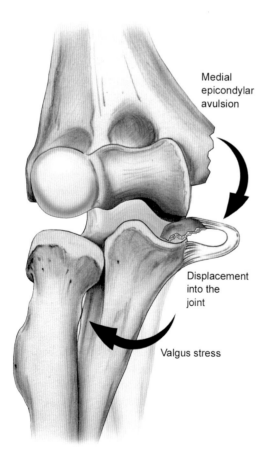

Medial epicondylar avulsion

Displacement into the joint

Valgus stress

Fig 23-39. Schematic representation of medial epicondylar avulsion with displacement into the joint.

The diagnosis of posterior elbow dislocation is easy, especially when the patient is seen soon after the injury (223). The general position is that of the extremity held in flexion and the forearm appearing shortened. The olecranon is prominent posteriorly. The individual is usually in significant pain. There is fullness in antecubital fossa as noted on palpation, while the olecranon and the radial head are felt and noted to be prominent posteriorly. Proximal to the olecranon, a palpable indentation in the triceps is noted. Manual flexion and extension of the elbow in a short arc while palpating for crepitus can help rule out a fracture.

Delayed evaluation of the elbow is hampered by significant swelling—at that point there is difficulty in differentiating this injury from a supracondylar fracture, lateral condylar fracture, and, in the young child, transcondylar fracture. Excessive manipulation in this scenario is unnecessary, because radiographic confirmation of the diagnosis is easy and reliable.

A key part of the elbow examination, before sending the patient for radiographic evaluation, is a careful neurovascular examination. This takes only a few moments, can be performed without undue stress, and helps avoid important delay while also being important from a medicolegal standpoint.

The radiographic series includes a standard AP and lateral radiograph, while special views or arthrography may additionally be performed if your clinical suspicions are not confirmed with routine radiographs (233). When an arterial injury is suspected, an arteriogram or digital subtraction studies should be performed.

Interpretation of radiographs in the setting of a posterior, posterolateral, or divergent elbow dislocation is not difficult **(Fig 23-40)**. However, the rare medial or lateral dislocation can be overlooked on casual reading of the radiograph, but, fortunately, the physical findings are not subtle. Radiographic evaluation is critical in the evaluation of the elbow dislocation to help identify associated fractures. The radial head and neck, coronoid, and medial and lateral epicondyles all are frequently injured in the setting of elbow dislocation and must be carefully examined. All views are repeated and reevaluated after reduction, because fractures may be identified that were not seen in the prereduction films.

The clinician must be aware that spontaneous reduction of a dislocated elbow is common, especially in children. Often, the only evidence of a spontaneously reduced elbow dislocation is a history of a fall, while examination reveals a swollen, boggy elbow with no obvious radiographic injury. However, radiographs must be carefully reviewed because they may reveal signs of a previous dislocation, including an avulsed coronoid fragment.

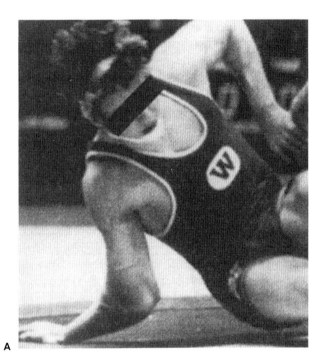

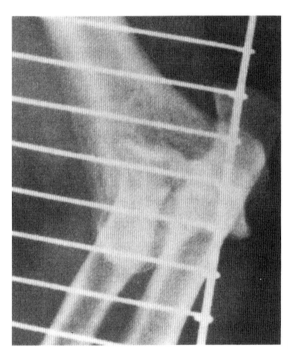

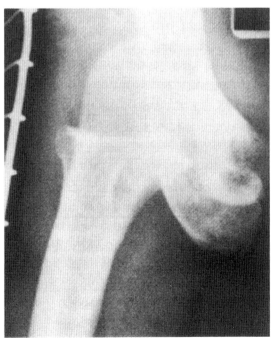

Fig 23-40. A: A newspaper photographer caught this wrestler in the process of sustaining a posterior dislocation of the elbow. **B/C:** A severely displaced posterior dislocation of the elbow of another wrestler. (From Safran MR, Salyers S, Fu FH. Elbow dislocations. In: Reider B, ed. Sports *medicine—the school age athlete*. 2nd ed. Philadelphia: WB Saunders; 1996:239; with permission.)

"All methods of reduction are directed toward sufficiently overcoming the muscle forces so that the coronoid process and radial head can slip from posterior to anterior past the distal end of the humerus" (234). In order to achieve reduction and overcome muscular forces, adequate anesthesia is needed in the form of general anesthetic, regional block, local joint injection, and/or sedation. If one is confident of the diagnosis at the time of injury, a single attempt at gentle reduction may be attempted on the playing field before muscle spasms become pronounced if the clinician is also experienced with the technique of reduction. However, caution is advised that one needs to be sure of the diagnosis of dislocation, because this can lead to disaster if the injury is a supracondylar fracture rather than an elbow dislocation. Reduction within 6 hours of the time of injury is usually preferred to help reduce the periarticular edema and postreduction stiffness.

After adequate anesthesia and relaxation is obtained, closed reduction using gentle force usually can be obtained. It is important to first correct medial or lateral displacement prior to reducing the posterior displacement.

It is absolutely critical to take the elbow through a full range of motion following reduction because there should be no grinding, mechanical block, or spongy feel with motion. If these problems occur, further evaluation is necessary to rule out intra-articular entrapment of the median nerve or the medial epicondyle. Further, the postreduction examination should include assessment of varus and valgus stability. The degree of varus-valgus laxity helps determine how aggressive postreduction rehabilitation can be.

After reduction, it is also important to perform careful and complete postreduction radiographic and neurovascular evaluations. After postreduction evaluation is complete, a long arm plaster splint with adequate padding is applied with the elbow flexed 90 degrees or an elbow brace may alternatively be applied within the stable range of motion. Hospitalization may be considered if there is pronounced elbow swelling, a questionable vascular examination, concern about a compartment syndrome, or if the patient is unreliable. Otherwise, instructing the parent how to observe the

circulatory status is sufficient. Ice and elevation are recommended after reduction, taking care not to cause thermal injury to the ulnar nerve. Some recommend joint aspiration to assist in resolving the hematoma, improving joint motion after reduction, and decreasing pain.

Protzman's (222) series at West Point contains a population very similar to that seen in a sports medicine practice because all the cadets are required to participate in sports. Protzman astutely noted that decreasing the period of postreduction immobilization resulted in a decreased loss of motion and a decreased disability, which we have also found in our patients (235). An individual with a posterior or posterolateral dislocation without an associated fracture can start hand, wrist, and shoulder motion the day of injury. Flexion can begin 3 or 4 days after reduction, and the splint can usually be discarded in 7 to 10 days. If not already fitted for a brace, 1 week after the reduction, the splint can be removed and the patient fitted for a hinged elbow brace. At this point, gentle active flexion and extension ranges of motions are encouraged. It should be noted that forced passive motion or manipulation has no place in elbow dislocation treatment due to the risk of loss of elbow motion and increased risk of heterotopic ossification. Using this protocol, recurrent dislocation is uncommon. Three weeks after reduction, elbow stability will determine the course of therapy or bracing. Gentle strengthening exercises usually can begin 3 to 5 weeks after the injury and may be progressed as pain allows.

Treatment must be altered if there is an associated fracture or gross instability. A single axis elbow orthosis has traditionally been recommended to allow early motion in elbows that are unstable to varus or valgus stress **(Fig 23-41)**. However, there is an increasing interest in primary repair or reconstruction of the collateral ligaments to provide elbow stability to allow for early range of motion. The currently recommended approach is to repair the LCLC. If the elbow is stable with just the LCL repaired, the skin is closed and the patient immobilized to allow wound healing and then started with physical therapy. If the elbow is still unstable,

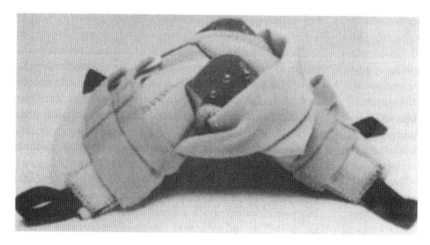

Fig 23-41. Single-axis orthosis used for patients with elbow instability. (From Safran MR, Salyers S, Fu FH. Elbow dislocations. In: Reider B, ed. *Sports medicine—the school age athlete,* 2nd ed. Philadelphia: WB Saunders; 1996:241; with permission.)

then the UCL is repaired. This usually provides elbow stability, provided there is no associated fracture. If there is an associated coronoid fracture, this must be fixed, especially in cases of Type II or III coronoid fracture, due to the high risk of recurrence associated with this fracture. If the radial head is fractured, this must be repaired or replaced to provide stability.

Currently, the indications for open treatment of elbow dislocations are (a) open injury, (b) vascular injury, (c) fracture management, (d) median nerve entrapment, and (e) inability to obtain reduction (a situation that is quite rare). It has been noted that there is up to a 10% rate of failure of closed reduction of traumatic elbow dislocations. Josefsson et al. (236) performed a prospective randomized study of surgical versus nonsurgical management of elbow dislocation in 30 consecutive patients and found no advantage of operative treatment. However, Norwood et al. (46) and Durig et al. (237) found surgery beneficial for those with elbow dislocation. DeLee et al. (238) concluded that "the incidence of recurrent dislocation is not sufficiently high nor the results of treatment by closed reduction sufficiently poor to warrant primary operative repair in pure elbow dislocations."

If an associated fracture of the radial head or neck is noted, these should be treated in the routine fashion. Coronoid fractures should be managed as discussed below because these are critical to the success of elbow stability. Osteochondral fractures and chondral flaps can occur in association of elbow dislocations and should be looked for in the evaluation of the patient with elbow dislocation (239). If surgery is undertaken and the joint is opened for any reason, inspection should be carried out to look for intra-articular osteochondral or chondral fragments associated with the dislocation or the reduction.

The most common complication of elbow dislocation is loss of extension, and, as such, patients should be counseled that 5 to 10 degrees' loss of extension is to be expected. Fortunately, this amount of motion loss infrequently causes symptoms. Institution of early range of motion helps prevent this problem. Heterotopic ossification within the ligaments is a common radiographic finding, yet it is associated with few symptoms and appears to be less common in children. Myositis ossificans can lead to significant loss of motion, but it is a rare complication, particularly if the dislocation is not associated with a fracture (221). If myositis ossificans occurs and limits the individual's function, then excision after the inflammatory phase is complete may be recommended. This can be confirmed by a "cold" technetium bone scan. Prevention of recurrence after excision using oral diphosphonates (240,241), irradiation (242–245), or oral NSAIDS (246,247) is recommended.

Recurrent dislocation is a rare phenomenon. In the West Point series, no recurrent dislocations were identified in the active cadet population when treated with a minimum of postreduction immobilization (222), as has been seen in other studies as well (219–222,229,235).

Josefsson et al. (229) followed 52 patients 24 years after elbow dislocation. In this series, there were no patients with elbow redislocations, persistent neurologic symptoms, or symptoms of instability. However, there were eight patients with evidence of abnormal valgus laxity, but these patients were asymptomatic. However, in a more recent study by Eygendaal et al. (248), long-term follow up of patients with elbow dislocation, those with greater valgus laxity at final follow up have a poorer functional and radiographic result compared to those with less laxity.

Comparing adults with children, adult dislocators had an average loss of extension of 12 degrees at follow up, whereas juvenile dislocators lost an average of only 4 degrees of elbow extension. There was essentially no loss of elbow pronation, supination, or flexion. There were some mild radiographic findings of osteoarthritis, but the only associated symptom was a mild increase in extension loss. Other large series reflect the above-mentioned findings (219–222, 229,230,235).

The individual with an elbow dislocation often can return to noncontact sports 2 to 3 weeks after reduction (223). Contact sports require at least twice as long for return, and the throwing athlete may not return for considerably longer. The long-term prognosis, however, is for most of these athletes to return to their sport with little disability.

Coronoid Fractures

The coronoid process forms a significant portion of the articular surface of the proximal ulna. It appears that this process is critical in the stability of the elbow by functioning as an osseous buttress as well as serving a role as an important attachment site for muscles and ligaments about the elbow. Fractures of the coronoid may occur in approximately 2% to 15% of acute elbow dislocations (219,230,239). Nonunion of fractures of the coronoid may result in chronic, recurrent elbow dislocations.

In 1989, Reagan and Morrey (249) described a classification system of coronoid fractures based on lateral radiographs, CT scans, or tomograms. They classified three types of coronoid fractures: Type I—avulsion of the tip of the coronoid process, Type II—fracture involving less than 50% of the process, and Type III—fracture involving greater than 50% of the process (Fig 23-42). Coronoid fractures may also be described in relation to the degree of comminution and the presence of associated dislocation of the elbow. Anatomic studies have revealed the patho-anatomy correlated with the classification of coronoid fractures. The Type I coronoid fracture is actually a fracture of the tip of the coronoid. This tip fragment is intra-articular and has no soft tissue attachment. The Type II coronoid fracture fragment is attached only to the anterior capsule. A Type III coronoid fracture fragment includes the attachment of the brachialis, capsule, and anterior band of the UCL (250). An attempt must be made at the time of patient presentation to assess the extent of injury to the soft tissues, because radiographs show only the bony injury.

The coronoid appears to play an important role in elbow stability (239,249,251–255). The incidence of acute elbow

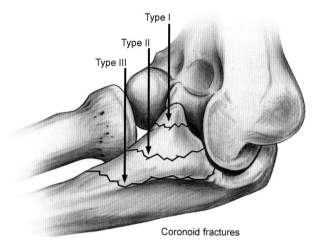

Fig 23-42. Schematic representation of the classification of coronoid fractures.

dislocation with associated coronoid fractures is reported to be 14% with Type I fractures, 56% with Type II coronoid fractures, and 80% with Type III (249). Thus, greater extent of fracture involvement of the coronoid seems to be associated with instability of the elbow due to loss of at least half of the anterior wall of the elbow joint (61).

Evaluation of a patient with an elbow dislocation includes careful clinical assessment of the elbow and careful assessment of lateral radiographs to determine involvement of the UCL, radial head, and coronoid. The combination of injuries to these three structures has been termed the terrible triad (256). The terrible triad reveals the significance of ligamentous and osseous contributions to elbow stability.

Untreated, recurrent dislocations of the elbow due to nonunion of large coronoid fractures may result in destruction of the distal humeral articular surface, chronic dislocation, arthritic pain, painful subluxation, weakness, and instability.

Fortunately, this difficult scenario may be avoided by early identification and treatment of the coronoid fracture with good radiographs. Being just the tip of the coronoid, Type I fractures are not frequently associated with recurrent instability due to its minimal amount of the coronoid involved. As such, those with Type I coronoid fractures are treated as one would treat an elbow dislocation without fracture—early mobilization (21). The treatment of elbow dislocations associated with a Type II coronoid fracture is based on the stability of the elbow. If the elbow is stable after reduction in the setting of a Type II coronoid fracture, management is early motion (21). However, a Type II fracture associated with an unstable fracture or a Type III fracture should be treated with open reduction and internal fixation (21). A comminuted Type III or unstable Type II fracture may also require the application of an external fixation distraction device (21). Nonunion may occur if the fracture is not recognized and treated, resulting in chronic instability. A displaced fragment that blocks full elbow motion should be treated with fracture fixation or excision of the fragment, depending on the size and comminution of the fragment.

Nonoperative treatment includes triceps strengthening and a hinged elbow brace. Due to the fact that the elbow is more stable in pronation, a hinged elbow brace in pronation with an extension block may provide limited stability. However, fulltime brace wear is usually not satisfactory to the patient. Furthermore, brace treatment for the unstable elbow is unlikely to provide a satisfactory functional result.

Olecranon Fracture

The olecranon functions as the final link in transmitting force from the triceps mechanism to enable elbow extension. Fractures of the olecranon usually involve an intra-articular component; therefore, olecranon fractures often combine joint effusions with loss of active elbow extension. Ulnar neuropathy may accompany this injury; thus, initial evaluation should include a good neurologic examination. Currently, no accepted classification of olecranon fractures exists that is considered useful to predict the outcome or guide in the management of these injuries.

Management of nondisplaced olecranon fractures begins with cast immobilization at 40 degrees of elbow flexion for 2 weeks. After this, patients must be able to demonstrate the ability to actively extend the elbow against gravity. At the end of 2 weeks, active motion may begin; however, full flexion is discouraged until 6 weeks. Weekly radiographs for the first 4 weeks are necessary to confirm that the fracture has not displaced.

Fractures with more than 2 mm of articular displacement are treated surgically. Noncomminuted, displaced olecranon fractures in an elbow that is stable to ligament testing is usually fixed with the tension band wire technique. Tension band wiring of stable olecranon fractures allows for early active range of motion. Stable elbows with comminuted olecranon fractures are usually treated with open reduction and internal fixation with reconstruction plates and screws. Fractures associated with ligament instability are usually treated with open reduction and internal fixation (tension band technique or plates and screws) in addition to ligament repair or reconstruction to provide stability. External fixation is occasionally recommended in this situation as well, the key being early range of motion of a stabilized elbow.

On some occasions, excision of the fracture fragment and reattachment of the triceps may be recommended in the treatment of olecranon fractures (257). However, this option is rarely recommended in the athlete because it has been shown that serial excision of the olecranon (25%, 50%, 75%, 100%) is associated with a near-linear decrease in ulnohumeral stability in extension and flexion (258).

Radial Head

Radial head fractures occur in 5% of all fractures and a third of all elbow fractures (259,260). The mechanism of injury of radial head fractures generally is a fall onto an outstretched hand, which transmits force to the elbow. This injury can also occur in conjunction with elbow dislocations. Fractures of the radial head and neck may be associated with injuries of the distal radio-ulnar joint, interosseous membrane, and nerve injuries. The Mason classification of radial head fractures is a useful guideline for management of the fractures (261). A Mason Type 1 fracture is a nondisplaced fracture involving less than 25% of the radial head. Type 2 fractures of the radial head are marginally displaced, including angulation, impaction, or depression fractures, although the degree of displacement is not defined. Mason Type 3 fractures involve the entire radial head and are comminuted. Mason Type 4 injuries are any radial head fracture associated with ulnohumeral dislocation.

Treatment of Mason Type 1 fractures is nonoperative and includes splint support and early range-of-motion exercises. Early range of motion may be facilitated by joint aspiration and introduction of a long-acting anesthetic. Use of a simple sling as needed and motion as tolerated by the patient is the preferred mobilization regimen. Some degree of limitation of elbow motion is to be expected, with a loss of extension of up to 10 degrees being common (262).

Many reliable options are available in the management of Mason Type 2 fractures, including (a) splinting and early range of motion, (b) open reduction and internal fixation, and (c) excision of the radial head. The final outcome for Mason Type 2 fractures is the same regardless of the method undertaken. Surgery is often necessary if the fracture is displaced more than 2 mm; however, many surgeons treat these fractures nonoperatively because late resection of the radial head has a similar outcome to early excision (263). One potential complication is that of myositis ossificans. Surgical intervention, including open reduction and internal fixation, should be carried out within the first 48 hours or radial head excision may be carried out 3 to 4 weeks following injury, because surgery between 2 days and 3 weeks is associated with a higher risk of myositis ossificans. Open reduction and internal fixation is best achieved when at least 50% of the radial head remains intact to provide a stable internal fixation platform. However, it should be noted that open reduction and internal fixation can be a demanding procedure that requires meticulous technique and special instrumentation.

Excision of the radial head in Type 3 fractures is usually required, although if possible, open reduction and internal fixation should be undertaken. Prior to excision, the integrity of the interosseous ligament and distal radioulnar joint must be confirmed on clinical examination and wrist radiographs, as injury to these structures during radial head excision can lead to wrist pain and dysfunction. Currently, the direct lateral approach is recommended to reduce risk to the LUCL over the previously favored anconeus approach.

A Mason Type 4 fracture associated with an elbow dislocation is a complex problem, and as such there is controversy regarding the management of this injury. If the radial head is comminuted, excision could be considered, but again, evaluation of the interosseous ligament and DRUJ is important in decision making. However, in general, if open reduction and internal fixation is feasible, the radial head should be retained. Radial head replacement should be considered if ORIF is not possible, and is mandatory if there is associated interosseous ligament and/or DRUJ injury and the head is not repairable. Generally, the prognosis for return to sports at the same level of activity following a Mason Type 4 injury is poor (264).

Particular attention needs to be paid to those individuals with a radial head fracture and associated wrist pain or distal radio-ulnar joint pain, particularly for Mason Type 2, 3, or 4 radial head fractures. Attempts should be made to maintain the length of the radius during healing of the soft tissues, particularly the interosseous membrane in this setting, because removal of the radial head in this setting may result in proximal migration of the radius and degenerative change at the wrist. Thus, internal fixation should be attempted if possible. If fixed and if the bone does not heal or a malunion or arthritis develops, the radial head may be excised later with satisfactory results. However, if open reduction and internal fixation is not feasible, radial head replacement is the treatment of choice. Radial head replacement generally consists of a metallic radial head implant; however, there still may be a place for temporary placement of a Silastic (Dow-Corning Wright, Arlington, TN) implant. Prosthetic radial head implant functions as a spacer while the interosseous membrane heals and may prevent long-term distal radio-ulnar joint dysfunction and pain. Removal of the Silastic implant after 2 to 3 months is recommended because this allows for interosseous membrane healing while preventing the complications of long-term Silastic implantation. Permanent Silastic implants have been associated with synovitis and osteolysis, and thus are not recommended. Currently, metal radial head implants are preferred, because these require only one surgery and are not associated with the complications of Silastic.

Surgery of radial head fractures may require additional procedures, including ulnar collateral or radial collateral ligament repair and/or open reduction of ulnohumeral dislocation.

Distal Humerus Fracture

Distal humerus fractures are severe injuries that, fortunately, are uncommon in athletes. These are usually high-energy injuries that are the result of either a direct injury or a fall on an outstretched hand. These fractures may be intra-articular or extra-articular. Nondisplaced extra-articular and intra-articular fractures may be treated nonoperatively. Displaced intra-articular fractures are most frequently treated by open reduction and internal fixation with plates and screws. Other alternative treatment methods include traction, limited open reduction and internal fixation, external fixation, and arthroplasty. Risks associated with these injuries include a high incidence of elbow stiffness (after this injury and any treatment), as well as fixation failure, malunion, nonunion, infection, and ulnar nerve injury.

Supracondylar Humerus Fracture

Supracondylar humerus fractures are the second most common fracture encountered in the pediatric age group (265). There are two types of supracondylar humerus fractures: extension and flexion. The extension type fracture is usually produced by an extension mechanism (i.e., fall onto outstretched hand) in which the distal fragment is pulled proximally and posteriorly, usually by the pull of the triceps (Fig 23-19). The flexion type of supracondylar humerus fracture is much less common and is often the result of a direct injury to the back of the elbow. Clinically, it is important to distinguish supracondylar humerus fractures from simple elbow dislocations. Clinically, those with supracondylar fractures maintain the normal triangular anatomic relationship between the medial and lateral epicondyle and the olecranon process, which is not the case in elbow dislocations.

Treatment of displaced supracondylar humerus fractures in the pediatric age group is fraught with potential problems. Treatment of these fractures is based on the neurovascular status of the affected extremity and the ability to maintain fracture reduction. Generally, gentle closed reduction (using skin traction, gentle manipulation, or skeletal traction through the olecranon) followed by cast immobilization is adequate. If the reduction of the fracture cannot be maintained closed or if neurovascular compromise is present, percutaneous or open surgical treatment may be indicated. Risks of this injury and surgery include compartment syndrome, brachial artery laceration or thrombosis, loss of motion, cubitus varus, and risks of surgery, including pin tract infections and nerve injury.

Medial Epicondyle Fracture

Medial epicondylar fractures may be the result of an acute injury or repetitive overuse. Skeletally immature overhead throwing athletes may develop an injury to the medial epicondylar growth plate, because the apophysis is the weakest link in the growing musculoskeletal unit. The spectrum of injuries to the medial epicondylar apophysis includes widening of the growth plate to frank fracture and separation of the apophysis from the distal humerus. (See Pediatric Injuries section.)

■ REFERENCES

1. Shiba R, Sorbie C, Siu DW, et al. Geometry of the humeroulnar joint. *J Orthrop Res.* 1988;6(6):897–906.
2. Steindler A. *Kinesiology of the Human Body under Normal and Pathological Conditions.* Baltimore: Charles C Thomas Publisher; 1955.
3. Bass RL, Stern PJ. Elbow and forearm anatomy and surgical approaches. *Hand Clin.* 1994;10(3):343–356.
4. Morrey BF, Tanaka S, An KN. Valgus stability of the elbow: a definition of primary and secondary restraints. *Clin Orthop.* 1991;265:187–195.
5. Schwab GH, Bennett JD, Woods GW, et al. Biomechanics of elbow instability: the role of the medial collateral ligament. *Clin Orthop.* 1980;146:42–52.
6. Sojbjerg JO, Ovesen J, Nielsen S. Experimental elbow instability after transection of the medial collateral ligament. *Clin Orthop.* 1987;218:186–190.
7. Callaway GH, Field LD, Dens XH, et al. Biomechanical evaluation of the medial collateral ligament of the elbow. *J Bone Joint Surg Am.* 1997;79(8):1223–1231.
8. Conway JE, Jobe FW, Glousman RE, et al. Medial instability of the elbow in throwing athletes: treatment by repair or reconstruction of the ulnar collateral ligament. *J Bone Joint Surg Am.* 1992;74(1): 67–83.
9. Gardner, E. *Anat Rec.* 1 0f 2:161, 1948.
10. Behr CT, Altchek DW. The elbow. *Clin Sports Med.* 1997; 16(4):681–704.
11. Pappas AM, Zawacki RM, Sullivan TJ. Biomechanics of baseball pitching: a preliminary report. *Am J Sports Med.* 1985;13: 216–222.
12. Werner SL, Fleisig GS, Dillman CJ, et al. Biomechanics of the elbow during baseball pitching. *J Orthop Sports Phys Ther.* 1993; 17(6):274–278.
13. Waris W. Elbow injuries in javelin throwers. *Acta Chir Scand.* 1946;93:563.
14. Kvitne RS, Jobe FW. Ligamentous and posterior compartment injuries. In: Jobe FW, ed. *Operative techniques in upper extremity sports injuries.* St Louis: Mosby; 1996:411–430.
15. Conway JE, Jobe FW, Glousman RE, et al. Medial instability of the elbow in throwing athletes: treatment by repair or reconstruction of the ulnar collateral ligament. *J Bone Joint Surg Am.* 1992; 74:67–83.
16. King JW, Brelsford HJ, Tullos HS. Analysis of the pitching arm of the professional baseball pitcher. *Clin Orthop.* 1969;67:116.
17. Barnes DA, Tullos HS. An analysis of 100 symptomatic baseball players. *Am J Sports Med.* 1978;6:62–67.
18. Safran MR, Baillargeon, D. Soft tissue stabilizers of the elbow. *J Shoulder Elbow Surg.* 2005;14(1)(suppl):179S–185S.
19. Safran MR, McGarry MH, Shin S, et al. Effects of elbow flexion and forearm rotation on valgus laxity of the elbow. *J Bone Joint Surg Am.* 2005;87:2065–2074.
20. Veltri DM, O'Brien SJ, Field LD, et al. The milking maneuver— a new test to evaluate the MCL of the elbow in the throwing athlete: Paper presented at: 10th Open Meeting of the American Shoulder and Elbow Surgeons Specialty Day; New Orleans, LA; 1994.
21. Safran MR, Caldwell GL III, Fu FH. Chronic instability of the elbow. In: Peimer CA, ed. *Surgery of the hand and upper extremity.* New York: McGraw-Hill; 1996:467–490.
22. Callaway GH, Field LD, Deng XH, et al. Biomechanical evaluation of the medial collateral ligament of the elbow. *J Bone Joint Surg Am.* 1997;79:1223–1231.
23. Safran MR. Injury to the ulnar collateral ligament: diagnosis and treatment. *Sports Medicine and Arthroscopy Review.* 2003;11:15–24.
24. Field LD, Altchek DW. Evaluation of the arthroscopic valgus instability test of the elbow. *Am J Sports Med.* 1996;24:177–181.
25. O'Driscoll SW, Lawton RL, Smith AM. The "moving valgus stress test" for medial collateral ligament tears of the elbow. *Am J Sports Med.* 2005;33(2):231–239.
26. Pappas AM. Elbow problems associated with baseball during childhood and adolescence. *Clin Orthop.* 1982;164:30–41.
27. Goitz HT, Rijke AM, Andrews JP, et al. Evaluation of elbow medial collateral ligament injury in the throwing athlete: Paper presented at: 61st Annual Meeting of the American Academy of Orthopaedic Surgeons; New Orleans, LA; 1994.
28. Ellenbecker TS, Mattalino AJ, Elam EA, et al. Medial elbow joint laxity in professional baseball pitchers: a bilateral comparison using stress radiography. *Am J Sports Med.* 1998;26:420–424.

29. Lee GA, Katz SD, Lazarus MD. Elbow valgus stress radiography in an uninjured population. *Am J Sports Med.* 1998;26:425–427.

30. Rijke AM, Goitz HT, McCue FC. Stress radiography of the medial elbow ligaments. *Radiology.* 1994;191:213–216.

31. Andrews JR, Timmerman LA. Outcome of elbow surgery in professional baseball players. *Am J Sports Med.* 1995;23:407–413.

32. Conway JE. Secondary effects of ulnar collateral ligament injury—clinical, radiographic and arthroscopic perspective. Instruction course presented at: 25th Annual Meeting of the American Orthopaedic Society for Sports Medicine; Traverse City, MI; June 21, 1999.

33. Safran MR. Elbow injuries in athletes. *Clin Orthop.* 1995;310:257–277.

34. Bennett JB, Tullos HS. Ligamentous and articular injuries in the athlete. In: Morrey BF, ed. *The elbow and its disorders.* Philadelphia: WB Saunders; 1985:502–522.

35. Timmerman LA, Schwartz ML, Andrews JR. Preoperative evaluation of the ulnar collateral ligament by magnetic resonance imaging and computed tomography arthrography: evaluation in 25 baseball players with surgical confirmation. *Am J Sports Med.* 1994;22:26–31.

36. Timmerman LA, Andrews JR. Undersurface tear of the ulnar collateral ligament in baseball players: a newly recognized lesion. *Am J Sports Med.* 1994;22:33–36.

37. Jobe FW, Kvitne RS. Elbow instability in the athlete. *Instr Course Lect.* 1991;40:17–23.

38. Mirowitz SA, London SL. Ulnar collateral ligament injury in baseball pitchers: MR imaging evaluation. *Radiology.* 1992;185:573.

39. Thompson WH, Jobe FW, Yocum LA, et al. Ulnar collateral ligament reconstruction in athletes: muscle splitting approach without transposition of the ulnar nerve. *J Shoulder Elbow Surg.* 2001;10:152–157.

40. Azar FM, Andrews JR, Wilk KE, et al. Operative treatment of ulnar collateral ligament injuries of the elbow in athletes. *Am J Sports Med.* 2000;28:16–23.

41. Nazarian LN, McShane JM, Ciccotti MG, et al. Dynamic US of the anterior band of the ulnar collateral ligament of the elbow in asymptomatic major league baseball pitchers. *Radiology.* 2003;227:149–154.

42. Sasaki J, Takahara M, Ogino T, et al. Ultrasonographic assessment of the ulnar collateral ligament and medial elbow laxity in college baseball players. *J Bone Joint Surg Am.* 2002;84A:525–531.

43. Safran MR, Greene H, Lee TQ. Comparison of elbow valgus laxity using radiographic and non-radiographic objective measurements. Paper presented at the 73rd Annual Meeting of the American Academy of Orthopaedic Surgeons; Chicago, IL; March 22, 2006.

44. Rettig AC, Sherrill C, Snead DS, et al. Non-operative treatment of ulnar collateral ligament injuries of the elbow in the throwing athlete. *Am J Sports Med.* 2001;29:15–17.

45. Jobe FW. Medial collateral ligament reconstruction. Paper presented at the Shoulder and Elbow in Sports AAOS Meeting; Beverly Hills, CA; October 1992.

46. Norwood LA, Shook JA, Andrews JR. Acute medial elbow ruptures. *Am J Sports Med.* 1981;9:16–19.

47. Jobe FW, Stark H, Lombardo SJ. Reconstruction of the ulnar collateral ligament in athletes. *J Bone Joint Surg Am.* 1986;68:1158–1163.

48. Smith GR, Altchek DW, Pagnani MJ, et al. A muscle-splitting approach to the ulnar collateral ligament of the elbow: neuroanatomy and operative technique. *Am J Sports Med.* 1996;24:575–580.

49. Rohrbough JT, Altchek DW, Hyman J, et al. Medial collateral ligament reconstruction of the elbow using the docking technique. *Am J Sports Med.* 2002;30:541–548.

50. Ahmad CD, Lee TQ, elAttrache NS. Biomechanical evaluation of a new ulnar collateral ligament reconstruction technique with interference screws fixation. *Am J Sports Med.* 2003;31:332–337.

51. Hechtman KS, Tjin-A-Tsoi EW, Zvijac JE, et al. Biomechanics of a less invasive procedure for reconstruction of the ulnar collateral ligament of the elbow. *Am J Sports Med.* 1998;26:620–624.

52. Schwab GH, Bennett JB, Woods GW, et al. The biomechanics of elbow stability: the role of the medial collateral ligament. *Clin Orthop.* 1980;46:42–52.

53. O'Driscoll SW, Bell DF, Morrey BE. Posterolateral rotatory instability of the elbow. *J Bone Joint Surg Am.* 1991;73:440–446.

54. O'Driscoll SW, Morrey BF, Korinek SL, et al. Elbow subluxation and dislocation: a spectrum of instability. *Clin Orthop.* 1992;280:86–197.

55. O'Driscoll SW. Classification and spectrum of elbow instability: recurrent instability. In: Morrey BF, ed. *The elbow and its disorders.* 2nd ed. Philadelphia: WB Saunders; 1993:453–463.

56. O'Driscoll SW, Morrey BF, Korinek SL, et al. The pathoanatomy and kinematics of posterolateral rotatory instability (pivot shift) of the elbow. *Transactions of the Orthopaedic Research Society.* 1990;15:6.

57. Osborne G, Cotterill P. Recurrent dislocation of the elbow. *J Bone Joint Surg Br.* 1966;48B:340–346.

58. Olsen BS, Sojbjerg JO, Nielsen KK, et al. Posterolateral elbow joint instability: the basic kinematics. *J Shoulder Elbow Surg.* 1998;7:19–29.

59. Olsen BS, Sojbjerg JO, Dalstra M, et al. Kinematics of the lateral ligamentous constraints of the elbow joint. *J Shoulder Elbow Surg.* 1996;5:333–341.

60. Dunning CE, Zarzour ZDS, Patterson SD, et al. Ligamentous stabilizers against posterolateral rotatory instability of the elbow. *J. Bone Joint Surg.* 2001;83A:1823–1828.

61. Seki A, Olsen BS, Jensen SL, et al. Functional anatomy of the lateral collateral ligament complex of the elbow: configuration of Y and its role. *J Shoulder and Elbow Surg.* 2002;11:53–59.

62. Morrey BF, O'Driscoll SW. Lateral collateral ligament injury. In: Morrey BF, ed. *The elbow and its disorders.* 2nd ed. Philadelphia: WB Saunders; 1993:573–580.

63. Imatani J, Hashizume H, Ogura T, et al. Acute posterolateral rotatory subluxation of the elbow joint. A case report. *Am J Sports Med.* 1997;25:77–80.

64. Nestor BJ, O'Driscoll SW, Morrey BF. Ligamentous reconstruction for posterolateral rotatory instability of the elbow. *J Bone Joint Surg Am.* 1992;74:1235–1241.

65. Adams JE. Injury to the throwing arm: a study of traumatic changes in the elbow joints of boy baseball players. *Calif Med.* 1965;102:127.

66. Brodgon BG, Crow NE. Little leaguer's elbow. *AJR Am J Roentgenol.* 1960;8:671.

67. Woods GW. Elbow instability and medial epicondyle fractures. *Am J Sports Med.* 1977;5:23.

68. Woods GW, Tullos HS, King JW. The throwing arm: elbow injuries. *Am J Sports Med.* 1973;1(suppl):4.

69. Fowles JV, Slimane N, Kassab M. Elbow dislocation with avulsion of the medial humeral epicondyle. *J Bone Joint Surg Br.* 1990;72:102–104.

70. Wilkins KE. Fractures of the medial epicondyle in children. *Instruct Course Lect.* 1991;40:3–10.

71. Masse B. Technique de reduction des luxations du conde avec fracture ou interposition de l'epitrochlee. *Revue Prat.* 1955;5:1038.

72. Micheli LJ. The traction apophyses. *Clin Sports Med.* 1987;6:389.

73. Torg JS, Moyer RA. Non-union of a stress fracture through the olecranon epiphyseal plate observed in adolescent baseball pitcher. a case report. *J Bone Joint Surg Am.* 1977;59:264–265.

74. Pavlov H, Torg JS, Jacobs B, et al. Nonunion of olecranon epiphysis: two cases in adolescent baseball pitchers. *AJR Am J Roentgenol.* 1981;136:819–820.

75. Kovach J, Baker BE, Mosher JE. Fracture separation of the olecranon ossification center in adults. *Am J Sports Med.* 1985;13:105–111.

76. Orava S, Hulkko A. Delayed unions and non-unions of stress fractures in athletes. *Am J Sports Med.* 1988;16:378–382.

77. Lowery WD Jr, Kurzweil PR, Forman SK, et al. Persistence of the olecranon physis: a cause of "Little League Elbow." *J Shoulder Elbow Surg.* 1995;4:143–147.

78. Skak SV. Fracture of the olecranon through a persistent physis in an adult. A case report. *J Bone Joint Surg Am.* 1993;75:272–275.

79. Tullos HS, Schwab GH, Bennett JB, et al. Factors influencing elbow stability. *Instr Course Lect.* 1982;8:185–199.

80. Aronen JG. Problems of the upper extremity in gymnastics. *Clin Sports Med.* 1985;4:61–71.

81. Ellman H. Unusual affections of the preadolescent elbow. *J Bone Joint Surg Am.* 1967;49:203.

82. Fixsen JA, Maffulli N. Bilateral intra-articular loose bodies of the elbow in an adolescent BMX rider. *Injury.* 1989;20:363–364.

83. Gugenheim JJ, Stanley RF, Woods GW, et al. Little league survey: the Houston study. *Am J Sports Med.* 1976;4:189.

84. Hang VS, Lippert FG, Spolek GA, et al. Biomechanical study of the pitching elbow. *Int Orthop.* 1979;3:217.

85. Pintore E, Maffulli N. Osteochondritis dissecans of the lateral humeral condyle in a table tennis player. *Med Sci Sports Exer.* 1991;23:889–891.

86. Panner HJ. A peculiar affection of the capitulum humeri resembling Calve-Perthes disease of the hip. *Acta Radial.* 1928;10:234.

87. Takahara M, Shundo M, Kondo M, et al. Early detection of osteochondritis dissecans of the capitellum in young baseball players: report of three cases. *J Bone Joint Surg Am.* 1998;80:892–897.

88. Indelicato PA, Jobe FW, Kerlan RK, et al. Correctable elbow lesions in professional baseball players. *Am J Sports Med.* 1979;7:72.

88a. Yamamoto Y, Ishibashi Y, Tsuda E, et al. Osteochondral autograft transplantation for osteochondritis dissecans of the elbow in juvenile baseball players: minimum two-year followup. *Am J Sports Med.* 2006;34:714–720.

89. O'Driscoll SW. Arthroscopy of the elbow. *J Bone Joint Surg Am.* 1992;74:84–94.

90. Baumgarten TE, Andrews JR, Satterwhite YE. The arthroscopic classification and treatment of osteochondritis dissecans of the capitellum. *Am J Sports Med.* 1998;26:520–523.

91. Bauer M, Jansson K, Josefsson PO, et al. Osteochondritis dissecans of the elbow. *Clin Orthop.* 1992;284:156–160.

92. Ruch DS, Cory JW, Poehling GG. The arthroscopic management of osteochondritis dissecans of the adolescent elbow. *Arthroscopy.* 1998;14:797–803.

93. Gilcreest EL. The common syndrome of rupture, dislocation and elongation at the long head of the biceps brachii: an analysis of one hundred cases. *Surg Gynecol Obstet.* 1934;58:322.

94. Safran MR, Graham S. *Distal biceps tendon ruptures: incidence of disruption, demographics and other observations.* Submitted for publication, 2001.

95. Bourne MH, Morrey BE. Partial rupture of the distal biceps tendon. *Clin Orthop.* 1991;271:143–148.

96. Nielsen K. Partial rupture of the distal biceps brachii tendon. *Acta Orthop Scand.* 1987;58:287.

97. Rokito AS, McLaughlin JA, Gallagher MA, et al. Partial rupture of the distal biceps tendon. *J Shoulder Elbow Surg.* 1996;5:73–75.

98. Davis WM, Yassine Z. An etiological factor in tear of the distal tendon of the biceps brachii. A report of two cases. *J Bone Joint Surg Am.* 1956;38:1365–1368.

99. Morrey BF, Askew LJ, An KN, et al. Rupture of the distal tendon of the biceps brachii: a biomechanical study. *J Bone Joint Surg Am.* 1985;67:418–421.

100. Seiler JG III, Parker LM, Chamberland PDC, et al. The distal biceps tendon. Two potential mechanisms involved in its rupture: arterial supply and mechanical impingement. *J Shoulder Elbow Surg.* 1995;4:149–156.

101. Boyd HB, Anderson LD. A method for reinsertion of the distal biceps brachii tendon. *J Bone Joint Surg.* 1961;43:1041.

102. Safran MR. Management of acute distal biceps brachii tendon ruptures: single versus two incision technique. *Oper Tech Orthop.* 1995;5:248–253.

103. Lintner S, Fischer T. Repair of the distal biceps tendon using suture anchors and an anterior approach. *Clin Orthop.* 1996;322:116–119.

104. Berlet GC, Johnson JA, Milne AD, et al. Distal biceps brachii tendon repair. An in vitro biomechanical study of tendon reattachment. *Am J Sports Med.* 1998;26:428–432.

105. Bain TI, Prem H, Heptinstall RJ, et al. Repair of distal biceps tendon rupture: a new technique using the endobutton. *J Shoulder Elbow Surg.* 2000;9(2):120–126.

106. Morrey BF. Tendon injuries about the elbow. In: Morrey BF, ed. *The elbow and its disorders.* Philadelphia: WB Saunders; 1985:452–463.

107. Baker BD, Bierwagen D. Rupture of the distal tendon of the biceps brachii. Operative versus nonoperative treatment. *J Bone Joint Surg Am.* 1985;67:414–417.

108. Dobbie RP. Avulsion of the lower biceps brachii tendon. Analysis of fifty-one previously reported cases. *Am J Surg.* 1941;51:661.

109. Rantanen J, Orava S. Rupture of the distal biceps tendon. A report of 19 patients treated with anatomic reinsertion, and a meta-analysis of 147 cases found in the literature. *Am J Sports Med.* 1999;27:128–132.

110. Leach RE, Miller JK. Lateral and medial epicondylitis of the elbow. *Clin Sports Med.* 1987;6:259–272.

111. Ollivierre CO, Nirschl RP, Pettrone FA. Resection and repair for medial tennis elbow. A prospective analysis. *Am J Sports Med.* 1995;23:214–221.

112. Coonrad RW. Tendonopathies at the elbow. *Instruct Course Lect.* 1991;40:25–32.

113. Nirschl RP. Prevention and treatment of elbow and shoulder injuries in the tennis player. *Clin Sports Med.* 1988;7:289.

114. Gabel GT, Morrey BF. Operative treatment of medial epicondylitis. Influence of concomitant ulnar neuropathy at the elbow. *J Bone Joint Surg Am.* 1995;77:1065–1069.

115. Kurvers H, Verhaar J. The results of operative treatment of medial epicondylitis. *J Bone Joint Surg Am.* 1995;77:1374–1379.

116. Stahl S, Kaufman T. The efficacy of an injection of steroids for medial epicondylitis. A prospective study of sixty elbows. *J Bone Joint Surg Am.* 1997;79:1648–1652.

117. Nirschl RP. Muscle and tendon trauma: tennis elbow. In: Morrey BF, ed. *The elbow and its disorders.* Philadelphia: WB Saunders; 1985:481–496.

118. Vangsness CT Jr, Jobe FW. Surgical treatment of medial epicondylitis: results in 35 elbows. *J Bone Joint Surg Br.* 1991;73:409–411.

119. Safran MR. Elbow tendinopathy—surgical repair of the epicondylitides. In: Craig EV, ed. *Clinical orthopaedics.* Philadelphia: Lippincott Williams & Wilkins; 1999:274–284.

120. Dobyns JH. Musculotendinous problems at the elbow. In: Evarts CM, ed. *Surgery of the musculoskeletal system.* 2nd ed. New York: Churchill-Livingstone; 1990:1661–1681.

121. Sollender JL, Rayan GM, Barden GA. Triceps tendon rupture in weight lifters. *J Shoulder Elbow Surg.* 1998;7:151–153.

122. Farrar EL, III, Lippert FG, III. Avulsion of the triceps tendon. *Clin Orthop.* 1981;161:242.

123. Gilcreest EL. Ruptures of muscles and tendons. *JAMA.* 1925;84:1819.

124. Montgomery AH. Two cases of muscle injury. *Surg Clin Chic.* 1920;4:871.

125. Tarsney FE. Rupture and avulsion of the triceps. *Clin Orthop.* 1972;83:177.

126. Bennett BS. Triceps tendon rupture. Case report and a method of repair. *J Bone Joint Surg Am.* 1962;44:741–744.

127. Runge E. Zur genese und behandlung des schreibekrampfes. *Berl Klin Wnschr.* 1873;10:245.

128. Nirschl RP. Tennis elbow. *Orthop Clin North Am.* 1973;4:787.

129. Nirschl RP, Sobel J. Conservative treatment of tennis elbow. *Phys Sports Med.* 1981;9:42.

130. Gerberich SG, Preist JD. Treatment for lateral epicondylitis: variables related to recovery. *Br J Sports Med.* 1985;19:224.

131. Hang Y, Peng S. An epidemiologic study of upper extremity injury in tennis players. *J Formos Med Assoc.* 1984;83:307.

132. Kelley JD, Lombardo SJ, Pink M, et al. Electromyographic and cinematographic analysis of elbow function in tennis players with lateral epicondylitis. *Am J Sports Med.* 1994;22:359–363.

133. Froimson AI. Treatment of tennis elbow with forearm support band. *J Bone Joint Surg Am.* 1971;53:183.

134. Ilfeld FW, Field SM. Treatment of tennis elbow: use of a special brace. *JAMA.* 1966;195:67.

135. Day BH, Govindasamy N, Patnaik R. Corticosteroid injections in the treatment of tennis elbow. *Practitioner.* 1978;220:459–462.

136. Dijs H, Mortier G, Driessens M, et al. A retrospective study of the conservative treatment of tennis elbow. *Acta Belgica Med Phys.* 1990;13:73–77.

137. Nirschl RP, Pettrone E. Tennis elbow. The surgical treatment of lateral epicondylitis. *J Bone Joint Surg Am.* 1979;61:832.

138. Solveborn SA, Buch F, Mallmin H, et al. Cortisone injection with anesthetic additives for radial epicondyalgia (tennis elbow). *Clin Orthop.* 1995;316:99–105.

139. Verhaar JAN, Walenkamp GHI, van Mameren H, et al. Local corticosteroid injection versus Cyriax-type physiotherapy for tennis elbow. *J Bone Joint Surg Br.* 1996;78:128–132.

140. Boyd HB, McLeod AC Jr. Tennis elbow. *J Bone Joint Surg Am.* 1973;55:1183–1187.

141. Coonrad RW, Hooper WR. Tennis elbow. Its course, natural history, conservative and surgical management. *J Bone Joint Surg Am.* 1973;55:1177.

142. Dreyfuss U, Kessler I. Snapping elbow due to dislocation of the medial head of the triceps. *J Bone Joint Surg Br.* 1978;60:56.

143. Bosworth DH. The role of the orbicular ligament in tennis elbow. *J Bone Joint Surg Am.* 1955;37:527.

144. Cyriax JH. The pathology and treatment of tennis elbow. *J Bone Joint Surg.* 1936;18:921–940.

145. Garden RS. Tennis elbow. *J Bone Joint Surg Br.* 1961;43:100.

146. Goldie I. Epicondylitis lateralis humeri (epicondylagia or tennis elbow). A pathogenetical study. *Acta Chir Scand.* 1964;339(Suppl):1–119.

147. Hohmann G. Das wesen und die behandlung des sogenannten tennissellenbogens. *Munch Med Whenschr.* 1933;80:250.

148. Kaplan EB. Treatment of tennis elbow (epicondylitis) by denervation. *J Bone Joint Surg Am.* 1959;41:147.

149. Lo MY, Safran MR. Surgical Treatment of Lateral Epicondylitis: A Systematic Review. Accepted for publication in Clinical Orthopaedics and Related Research; 2006.

150. Baker CL Jr, Cummings PD. Arthroscopic management of miscellaneous elbow disorders. *Oper Tech Sports Med.* 1998;6:16–21.

151. Owens BD, Murphy KP, Kuklo TR. Arthroscopic release for lateral epicondylitis. *Arthroscopy.* 2001;17(6):582–587.

152. Kuklo TR, Taylor KF, Murphy KP, et al. Arthroscopic release for lateral epicondylitis: a cadaveric model. *Arthroscopy.* 1999;15(3):259–264.

153. Smith AM, Castle JA, Ruch DS. Arthroscopic resection of the common extensor origin: anatomic considerations. *J Shoulder Elbow Surg.* 2003;12(4):375–379.

154. Kvitne RS. Epicondylitis. Paper presented at the Shoulder and Elbow in Sports AAOS Meeting; Beverly Hills, CA; October, 1992.

155. Organ SW, Nirschl RP, Kraushaar BS, et al. Salvage surgery for lateral tennis elbow. *Am J Sports Med.* 1997;25:746–750.

156. Baumgard SH, Schwartz DR. Percutaneous release of the epicondylar muscles for humeral epicondylitis. *Am J Sports Med.* 1982;10(4):233–236.

157. Yerger B, Turner T. Percutaneous extensor tenotomy for lateral epicondylitis. An office procedure. *Orthopaedics.* 1985;10:1261–1263.

158. Powell SG, Burke AL. Surgical and therapeutic management of tennis elbow: an update. *J Hand Ther.* 1991;4:64–68.

159. Balasubramaniam P, Prathap K. The effect of injection of hydrocortisone into rabbit calcaneal tendons. *J Bone Joint Surg Br.* 1972; 54:729.

160. Unverferth LJ, Olix ML. The effect of local steroid injection on tendon. *J Sports Med.* 1973;1:31.

161. Savoie FH, Szabo SJ, Field LD. Lateral epicondylitis: an evaluation of three methods of operative treatment. Paper presented at the American Shoulder and Elbow Surgeons 21st Meeting; Washington D.C. Edited; 2005.

162. Baker CL Jr, Murphy KP, Gottlob CA, et al. Arthroscopic classification and treatment of lateral epicondylitis: two-year clinical results. *J Shoulder Elbow Surg.* 2000;9(6):475–482.

163. Fuss FK. The ulnar collateral ligament of the human elbow joint. Anatomy, function and biomechanics. *J Anat.* 1991;175: 203–212.

164. Safran MR, McGarry MH, Shin, S, et al. Effects of elbow flexion and forearm rotation on valgus laxity of the elbow. *J Bone Joint Surg Am.* 2005;87A:2065–2074.

165. Safran MR, Baillargeon D. Soft tissue stabilizers of the elbow. *J Shoulder Elbow Surg.* 2005;14(1)(suppl):179S–185S.

166. Morrey BF, Tanaka S, An KN. Valgus stability of the elbow. A definition of primary and secondary constraints. *Clin Orthop.* 1991;265:187–195.

167. Davidson PA, Pink M, Perry J, et al. Functional anatomy of the flexor pronator muscle group in relation to the medial collateral ligament of the elbow. *Am J Sports Med.* 1995;23:245–250.

168. Park MC, Ahmad CS. Dynamic contributions of the flexor-pronator mass to elbow valgus stability. *J Bone Joint Surg.* 2004; 86A:2268–2274.

169. Werner SL, Fleisig GS, Dillman CJ, et al. Biomechanics of the elbow during baseball pitching. *J Orthop Sports Phys Ther.* 1993; 17:274–278.

170. Sisto DJ, Jobe FW, Moynes DR. An electromyographic analysis of the elbow in pitching. *Am J Sports Med.* 1987;15:260–263.

171. Feltner M, Dapena J. Dynamics of the shoulder and elbow joints of the throwing arm during the baseball pitch. *Int J Sport Biomech.* 1986;2:235–259.

172. Fleisig GS, Dillman CJ, Escamilla RF, et al. Kinetics of baseball pitching with implications about injury mechanisms. *Am J Sports Med.* 1995;23:233–239.

173. Elliott B, Fleisig G, Nicholls R, et al. Technique effects on upper limb loading in the tennis serve. *J Sci Med Sport.* 2003;6:76–87.

174. Fleisig G, Nicholls R, Elliott B, et al. Kinematics used by world class tennis players to produce high-velocity serves. *Sports Biomech.* 2003;2:51–64.

175. Morrey BF, An KN. Articular and ligamentous contributions to the stability of the elbow joint. *Am J. Sports Med.* 1983;11(5): 315–319.

176. Dillman CJ, Smutz P, Werner S. Valgus extension overload in baseball pitching. *Med Sci Sports Exerc.* 1991;23:355.

177. Marshall RN, Elliott BC. Long-axis rotation: the missing link in proximal-to-distal segmental sequencing. *J Sports Sci.* 2000;18(4): 247–254.

178. Fleisig GS, Escamilla RF, Andrews JR. Biomechanics of throwing. *Ath Inj and Rehab.* 1996;17:332–353.

179. Escamilla RF, Fleisig GS, Zheng N, et al. Kinematic comparisons of 1996 Olympic baseball pitchers. *J Sports Sci.* 2001;19:665–676.

180. Escamilla RF, Fleisig GS, Barrentine SW, et al. Kinematic comparisons of throwing different types of baseball pitches. *J Appl Biomech.* 1998;14:1–23.

181. Roberts TW. Cinematography in biomechanical investigation. Selected topics in biomechanics. In: CIC symposium on biomechanics. Chicago, The Athletic Institute, 1971:41–50.

182. Ahn BH. *A model of the human upper extremity and its application to a baseball pitching motion* [Dissertation]. East Lansing, MI: Michigan State University; 1991.

183. Wilson FD. Valgus extension overload in the pitching elbow. *Am J Sports Med.* 1983;11:83–88.

184. DiGiovine NM, Jobe FW, Pink M, et al. An electromyographic analysis of the upper extremity in pitching. *J Shoulder Elbow Surg.* 1992;1:15–25.

185. Escamilla RF, Fleisig GS, Alexander E, et al. A kinematic and kinetic comparison while throwing different types of baseball pitches. *Med Sci Sports Exer.* 1994;26:S175.

186. Fleisig GS, Barrentine SW, Zheng N, et al. Kinematic and kinetic comparison of baseball pitching among various levels of development. *J Biomech.* 1999;32:1371–1375.

187. Loftice J, Fleisig GS, Zheng N, et al. Biomechanics of the elbow in sports. *Clin Sports Med.* 2004;23:519–530.

188. Davidson PA, Pink M, Perry J, et al. Functional anatomy of the flexor pronator muscle group in relation to the medial collateral ligament of the elbow. *Am J Sports Med.* 1995;23:245–250.

189. Ciccotti MC, Schwartz MA, Ciccotti MG. Diagnosis and treatment of medial epicondylitis of the elbow. *Clin Sports Med.* 2004; 23:693–706.

190. Safran MR. Elbow injuries in athletes. *Clin Orthop.* 1995;310: 257–277.

191. Conway JE, Jobe FW, Glousman RE, et al. Medial instability of the elbow in throwing athletes. Treatment by repair or reconstruction of the ulnar collateral ligament. *J Bone Joint Surg Am.* 1992; 74(1):67–83.

192. Norwood LA, Shook JA, Andrews JR. Acute medial elbow ruptures. *Am J Sports Med.* 1981;9:16–19.

193. Gelberman RH, Yamaguchi K, Hollstien SB, et al. Changes in interstitial pressure and cross-sectional area of the cubital tunnel and of the ulnar nerve with flexion of the elbow. *J Bone Joint Surg Am.* 1998;80A:492–501.

194. Pechan J, Julis I. The pressure measurement in the ulnar nerve. A contribution to the pathophysiology of the cubital tunnel syndrome. *J Biomechanics.* 1975;8:75.

195. MacNichol MF. Extraneural pressure affecting the ulnar nerve at the elbow. *Hand.* 1982;14:5–11.

196. Apfelberg DB, Larson SJ. Dynamic anatomy of the ulnar nerve at the elbow. *Plast Reconstr Surg.* 1973;51:76–81.

197. Jobe FW, Fanton GS. Nerve injuries. In: Morrey BF, ed. *The elbow and its disorders.* Philadelphia: WB Saunders; 1985:497–501.

198. Ahmad CS, Park MC, El Attrache NS. Elbow medial ulnar collateral ligament insufficiency alters posteromedial olecranon contact. *Am J Sports Med.* 2004;32:1607–1612.

199. Jones HH, Priest JD, Hayes WC, et al. Humeral hypertrophy in response to exercise. *J Bone Joint Surg Am.* 1977;59A:204–208.

200. Krahl H, Michaelis U, Pieper H-G, et al. Stimulation of bone growth through sports. A radiologic investigation of the upper extremities in professional tennis players. *Am J Sports Med.* 1994; 22:751–757.

201. Suzuki K, Minami A, Suenaga N, et al. Oblique stress fracture of the olecranon in baseball pitchers. *J Shoulder Elbow Surg.* 1997;6: 491–494.

202. Schickendantz MS, Ho CP, Koh J. Stress injury of the proximal ulna in professional baseball players. *Am J Sports Med.* 2002;30: 737–741.

203. Miller JE. Javelin thrower's elbow. *J Bone Joint Surg Br.* 1960;42B: 788–792.

204. Ahmad CS, El Attrache NS. Valgus extension overload syndrome and stress injury of the olecranon. *Clin Sports Med.* 2004;23: 665–676.

205. Wilson FD, Andrews JR, Blackburn TA, et al. Valgus extension overload in the pitching elbow. *Am J Sports Med.* 1983;11:83–88.

206. Andrews JR. Bony injuries about the elbow in the throwing athlete. *Instr Course Lect.* 1985;34:323–331.

207. Baratz RL, Bryan WJ. Open proximal olecranonectomy for treatment of posterior impingement in baseball pitchers. Transactions of the 25th Annual Meeting of the American Orthopaedic Society for Sports Medicine; Traverse City, Michigan; June 21, 1999:450.

208. DeHaven KE, Evarts CM. Throwing injuries of the elbow of athletes. *Orthop Clin North Am.* 1973;4:801–808.

209. Andrews JR, St Pierre RK, Carson WG Jr. Arthroscopy of the elbow. *Clin Sports Med.* 1986;5:653–662.

210. Faulkner JR, Jackson RW. Arthroscopy of the elbow. *J Bone Joint Surg Br.* 1980;62B:130.

211. Kvitne RS. Arthroscopy of the elbow. Paper presented at the Shoulder and Elbow in Sports AAOS Meeting; Beverly Hills, CA; October, 1992.

212. Kamineni S, Hirahara H, Pomianowski S, et al. Partial posteromedial olecranon resection: a kinematic study. *J Bone Joint Surg Am.* 2003;85A:1005–1011.

213. Kamineni S, El Attrache NS, O'Driscoll SW, et al. Medial collateral ligament strain with partial posteromedial olecranon resection. A biomechanical study. *J Bone Joint Surg.* 2004;86A: 2424–2430.

214. Miller JE. Javelin thrower's elbow. *J Bone Joint Surg Br.* 1960; 42:788–792.

215. Suzuki K, Minami A, Suenaga N, et al. Oblique stress fracture of the olecranon in baseball pitchers. *J Shoulder Elbow Surg.* 1997; 6:491–494.

216. Tullos HS, Erwin WD, Woods GW, et al. Unusual lesions of the pitching arm. *Clin Orthop.* 1972;88:169–183.

217. Blount WP. *Fractures in Children.* Baltimore: Williams & Wilkins; 1955.

218. Letts M. Dislocations of the child's elbow. In: Morrey BF, ed. *The elbow and its disorders.* 2nd ed. Philadelphia: WB Saunders; 1993:288–315.

219. Linscheid RL, Wheeler DK. Elbow dislocations. *JAMA.* 1965; 194:1171–1176.

220. Nevaiser JS, Wickstrom JK. Dislocation of the elbow: a retrospective study of 115 patients. *South Med J.* 1977;70:172–173.

221. Roberts PH. Dislocation of the elbow. *Br J Surg.* 1969;56: 806–815.

222. Protzman RR. Dislocation of the elbow joint. *J Bone Joint Surg Am.* 1978;60:539–541.

223. Safran MR, Salyers S, Fu FH. Elbow dislocations. In: Reider B, ed. *Sports medicine—the school age athlete.* 2nd ed. Philadelphia: WB Saunders; 1996:235–246.

224. DeLee JC. Transverse divergent dislocation of the elbow in a child. *J Bone Joint Surg Am.* 1981;63:322.

225. Holbrook JL, Green NE. Divergent pediatric elbow dislocation. A case report. *Clin Orthop.* 1988;234:72–74.

226. McAuliffe TB, Williams D. Transverse divergent dislocation of the elbow. *Injury.* 1988;19:279.

227. Sovio OM, Tredwell SJ. Divergent dislocation of the elbow in a child. *J Pediatr Orthop.* 1986;6:96–97.

228. Beaty JH. Fractures and dislocations about the elbow in children. *Instr Course Lect.* 1992;16:373–384.

229. Josefsson PO, Johnell O, Gentz CE. Long-term sequelae of simple dislocation of the elbow. *J Bone Joint Surg Am.* 1984;66: 927–930.

230. Linscheid RL, O'Driscoll SW. Elbow Dislocations. In: Morrey BF, ed. *The elbow and its disorders.* 2nd ed. Philadelphia: WB Saunders; 1993:441–452.

231. Louis DS, Ricciardi JE, Spengler DM. Arterial injury: a complication of posterior elbow dislocation. *J Bone Joint Surg Am.* 1974; 56:1631–1636.

232. Hassman GC, Brunn F, Neer CS. Recurrent dislocation of the elbow. *J Bone Joint Surg Am.* 1975;57:1080–1084.

233. Greenspan A, Norman A. The radial head, capitellum view. Useful technique in elbow trauma. *AJR Am J Roentgenol.* 1982;128:1186–1188.

234. Wilkins KE. Fractures and dislocations of the elbow region. In: Rockwood CA, Wilkins KE, King RE, eds. *Fractures in children.* Vol 3. Philadelphia: JB Lippincott; 1984:363–575.

235. Mehloff TL, Noble PC, Bennett JB, et al. Simple dislocation of the elbow in the adult. *J Bone Joint Surg Am.* 1988;70:244–249.

236. Josefsson PO, Gentz CF, Johnell O, et al. Surgical versus nonsurgical treatment of ligamentous injuries following dislocation of the elbow joint. A prospective randomized study. *J Bone Joint Surg Am.* 1987;69:605–608.

237. Durig M, Muller W, Ruedi TP, et al. The operative treatment of elbow dislocation in the adult. *J Bone Joint Surg Am.* 1979;61:239–244.

238. DeLee JC, Green DP, Wilkins KE. Fractures and dislocations of the elbow. In: Rockwood CA, Green DP, eds. *Fractures in adults.* Vol 1. Philadelphia: JB Lippincott Co; 1984:559–652.

239. Selesnick FH, Dolitsky B, Haskell SS. Fracture of the coronoid process requiring open reduction with internal fixation. *J Bone Joint Surg Am.* 1984;66:1304–1305.

240. Finerman GAM, Krengel WF, Lowell JD, et al. Role of diphosphonate (EHDP) in the prevention of heterotopic ossification after total hip arthroplasty: a preliminary report. In: *The Hip.* Proceedings of the Fifth Open Scientific Meeting of the Hip Society. St. Louis: CV Mosby; 1977:222–234.

241. Thomas BJ, Amstutz HC. Results of the administration of diphosphonate for the prevention of heterotopic ossification after total hip arthroplasty. *J Bone Joint Surg Am.* 1985;67:400–403.

242. Ayers DC, Evarts CM, Parkinson JR. The prevention of heterotopic ossification in high-risk patients by low-dose radiation after total hip arthroplasty. *J Bone Joint Surg Am.* 1986;68:1423–1430.

243. Ayers DC, Pellegrini VD, Evarts CM. Prevention of heterotopic ossification in high-risk patients by radiation therapy. *Clin Orthop Rel Res.* 1991;263:87–93.

244. Bosse MJ, Poka A, Reinert CM, et al. Heterotopic ossification as a complication of acetabular fracture. *J Bone Joint Surg Am.* 1988;70:1231–1237.

245. McAuliffe JA, Wolfson AH. Early excision of heterotopic ossification about the elbow followed by radiation therapy. *J Bone Joint Surg Am.* 1997;79:749–755.

246. McLaren AC. Prophylaxis with indomethacin for heterotopic bone after open reduction of fractures of the acetabulum. *J Bone Joint Surg Am.* 1990;72A:245–247.

247. Schmidt SA, Kjaersgaard-Andersen P, Pedersen NW, et al. The use of indomethacin to prevent the formation of heterotopic bone after total hip replacement. A randomized, double-blind clinical trial. *J Bone Joint Surg Am.* 1988;70:834–838.

248. Eygendaal D, Verdegaal SH, Obermann WR, et al. Posterolateral dislocation of the elbow joint. Relationship to medial instability. *J Bone Joint Surg Am.* 2000;82:555–560.

249. Regan WD, Morrey BE. Fractures of the coronoid of the ulna. *J Bone Joint Surg Am.* 1989;71:1348–1354.

250. Cage DJ, Callaghan JJ, Botte MJ, et al. Coronoid process and its soft tissue attachments with radiographic correlation. Paper presented at the 61st Annual Meeting of the American Academy of Orthopaedic Surgeons; New Orleans, LA; 1994.

251. Josefsson PO, Gentz CF, Johnell O, et al. Dislocations of the elbow and intra-articular fractures. *Clin Orthop.* 1989;246:126–130.

252. Kapel O. Operation for habitual dislocation of the elbow. *J Bone Joint Surg Am.* 1956;33:707.

253. King T. Recurrent dislocation of the elbow. *J Bone Joint Surg Br.* 1953;35B:50–54.

254. Reichenheim PP. Transplantation of the biceps tendon as a treatment for recurrent dislocation of the elbow. *Br J Surg.* 1947;35:201–204.

255. Stone JE. Recurrent dislocation of the elbow. Proceedings of the East Anglican Orthopaedic Club. *J Bone Joint Surg Br.* 1955;37:733.

256. Hotchkiss RN, Green DP. Fractures and dislocations of the elbow. In: Rockwood CA, Green DP, Bucholz RW, eds. *Rockwood and Green's Fractures in Adults.* 3rd ed. New York: JB Lippincott Co; 1991:739–841.

257. McKeever FM, Buck RM. Fracture of the olecranon process of the ulna. *JAMA.* 1947;135:1.

258. An KN, Morrey BE. Biomechanics of the elbow. In: Morrey BF, ed. *The elbow and its disorders.* Philadelphia: WB Saunders; 1985:43–61.

259. Conn J, Wade PA. Injuries of the elbow: a ten-year review. *J Trauma.* 1961;1:248.

260. Johnston GW. A follow-up of one hundred cases of fracture of the head of the radius with a review of the literature. *Ulster Med.* J1962;31:51.

261. Mason JA. Some observations on fractures of the head of the radius with a review of one hundred cases. *Br J Surg.* 1954;42:123.

262. Mason JA, Shutkin NM. Immediate active motion in the treatment of fractures of the head and neck of the radius. *Surg Gynecol Obstet.* 1943;76:731.

263. Broberg MA, Morrey BE. Results of delayed excision of the radial head after fracture. *J Bone Joint Surg Am.* 1986;68A:669–674.

264. Bennett, JB. Acute injuries to the elbow. In Nicholas JA, Hershman EB, eds. *The upper extremity in sports medicine.* 2nd ed. St. Louis: Mosby; 1995:301–316.

265. Hanlon CR, Estes WL. Fractures in childhood: a statistical analysis. *Am J Surg.* 1954;87:312–323.

■ SUGGESTED READING

1. Alcid JG, Ahmad CS, Lee TQ. Elbow anatomy and structural biomechanics. *Clin Sports Med.* 2004;23:503–517.

2. Smith AM, Castle JA, Ruch DS. Arthroscopic resection of the common extensor origin: anatomic considerations. *J Shoulder Elbow Surg.* 2003;12:375–379.

3. Wang AA, Mara M, Hutchinson DT. The proximal ulna: an anatomic study with relevance to olecranon osteotomy and fracture fixation. *J Shoulder Elbow Surg.* 2003;12:293–296.

4. Duggal N, Dunning CE, Johnson JA. The flat spot of the proximal ulna: a useful anatomic landmark in total elbow arthroplasty. *J Shoulder Elbow Surg.* 2004;13:206–207.

5. Seki A, Olsen BS, Jensen SL, et al. Functional anatomy of the lateral collateral ligament complex of the elbow: configuration of Y and its role. *J Shoulder Elbow Surg.* 2002;11:53–59.

6. Paraskevas G, Papadopoulos A, Papaziogas B, et al. Study of the carrying angle of the human elbow joint in full extension: a morphometric analysis. *Surg Radiol Anat.* 2004;26:19–23.

7. Prasad A, Robertson DD, Sharma GB, et al. Elbow: the trochleogingylomoid joint. *Seminars In Musculoskeletal Radiology.* 2003;7:19–25.

8. Ward SI, Teefey SA, Paletta GA, et al. Sonography of the medial collateral ligament of the elbow: a study of cadavers and healthy adult male volunteers. *AJR Am J Roentgenol.* 2003;180:389–394.

9. Cohen MS, Bruno RJ. The collateral ligaments of the elbow: anatomy and clinical correlation. *Clin Orthop.* 2001;383:123–130.

10. Beckett KS, McConnell P, Lagopoulos M, et al. Variations in the normal anatomy of the collateral ligaments of the human elbow joint. *J Anat.* 2000;197:507–511.

11. Berg EE, DeHoll D. The lateral elbow ligaments. A correlative radiographic study. *Am J Sports Med.* 1999;27:796–800.

12. Imatani J, Ogura T, Morito Y, et al. Anatomic and histologic studies of lateral collateral ligament complex of the elbow joint. *J Shoulder Elbow Surg.* 1999;8:625–627.

13. Miyasaka KC. Anatomy of the elbow. *Orthop Clin North Am.* 1999;30:1–13.
14. Ochi N, Ogura T, Hashizume H, et al. Anatomic relation between the medial collateral ligament of the elbow and the humero-ulnar joint axis. *J Shoulder Elbow Surg.* 1999;8:6–10.
15. Hannouche D, Bégué T. Functional anatomy of the lateral collateral ligament complex of the elbow. *Surg Radiol Anat.* 1999;21:187–191.
16. Yamaguchi K, Sweet FA, Bindra R, et al. The extraosseous and intraosseous arterial anatomy of the adult elbow. *J Bone Joint Surg Am.* 1997;79:1653–1662.
17. Steinberg BD, Plancher KD. Clinical anatomy of the wrist and elbow. *Clin Sports Med.* 1995;14:299–313.
18. Field LD, Altchek DW, Warren RF, et al. Arthroscopic anatomy of the lateral elbow: a comparison of three portals. *Arthroscopy.* 1994;10:602–607.
19. Bass RL, Stern PJ. Elbow and forearm anatomy and surgical approaches. *Hand Clin.* 1994;10:343–356.
20. Closkey RF, Goode JR, Kirschenbaum D, et al. The role of the coronoid process in elbow stability. A biomechanical analysis of axial loading. *J Bone Joint Surg Am.* 2000;82A:1749–1753.
21. Schneeberger AG, Sadowski MM, Jacob HAC. Coronoid process and radial head as posterolateral rotatory stabilizers of the elbow. *J Bone Joint Surg Am.* 2004;86A:975–982.
22. Deutch SR, Jensen SL, Olsen BS, et al. Elbow joint stability in relation to forced external rotation: an experimental study of the osseous constraint. *J Shoulder Elbow Surg.* 2003;12:287–292.
23. Callaway GH, Field LD, Deng XH, et al. Biomechanical evaluation of the medial collateral ligament of the elbow. *J Bone Joint Surg Am.* 1997;79:1223–1231.
24. Olsen BS, Vaesel MT, Søjbjerg JO, et al. Lateral collateral ligament of the elbow joint: anatomy and kinematics. *J Shoulder Elbow Surg.* 1996;5:103–112.
25. Mullen DJ, Goradia VK, Parks BG, et al. A biomechanical study of stability of the elbow to valgus stress before and after reconstruction of the medial collateral ligament. *J Shoulder Elbow Surg.* 2002;11:259–264.
26. Posner MA. Compressive ulnar neuropathies at the elbow: I. Etiology and diagnosis. *J Am Acad Orthop Surg.* 1998;6:282–288.
27. Amadio PC. Anatomical basis for a technique of ulnar nerve transposition. *Surg Radiol Anat.* 1986;8:155–161.
28. Spinner M, Kaplan EB. The relationship of the almoner to the medial intramuscular septum in the arm and its clinical significance. *Hand.* 1976;8:239–242.
29. Gelberman RH, Yamaguchi K, Hollstien SB, et al. Changes in interstitial pressure and cross-sectional area of the cubital tunnel and of the ulnar nerve with flexion of the elbow. An experimental study in human cadavera. *J Bone Joint Surg Am.* 1998;80:492–501.
30. Wright TW, Glowczewskie F Jr, Cowin D, et al. Ulnar nerve excursion and strain at the elbow and wrist associated with upper extremity motion. *J Hand Surg Am.* 2001;26:655–662.
31. Posner MA. Compressive neuropathies of the ulnar nerve at the elbow and wrist. *Instr Course Lect.* 2000;49:305–317.
32. Golovchinsky V. Ulnar-to-median anastomosis and its role in the diagnosis of lesions of the median nerve at the elbow and the wrist. *Electromyogr Clin Neurophysiol.* 1990;30:31–34.
33. Kelly EW, Morrey BF, O'Driscoll SW. Complications of elbow arthroscopy. *J Bone Joint Surg Am.* 2001;83A:25–34.
34. Cain E, Lyle Jr, Dugas JR, et al. Elbow injuries in throwing athletes: a current concepts review. *Am J Sports Med.* 2003;31:621–635.
35. Nazarian LN, McShane JM, Ciccotti MG, et al. Dynamic US of the anterior band of the ulnar collateral ligament of the elbow in asymptomatic major league baseball pitchers. *Radiology.* 2003;227:149–154.
36. David TS. Medial elbow pain in the throwing athlete. *Orthopedics.* 2003;26:94–103; quiz 104–105.
37. Chen FS, Rokito AS, Jobe FW. Medial elbow problems in the overhead-throwing athlete. *J Am Acad Orthop Surg.* 2001;9:99–113.
38. Chumbley EM, O'Connor FG, Nirschl RP. Evaluation of overuse elbow injuries. *Am Fam Physician.* 2000;61:691–700.
39. Maloney MD, Mohr KJ, El Attrache NS. Elbow injuries in the throwing athlete. Difficult diagnoses and surgical complications. *Clin Sports Med.* 1999;18:795–809.
40. Breck LW, Higinbotham NL. Patellar and olecranon bursitis: with the report of an improved operative procedure. *Milit Surg.* 1946;98:396.
41. Stell IM. Management of acute bursitis: outcome study of a structured approach. *J R Soc Med.* 1999;92:516–521.
42. Stewart NJ, Manzanares JB, Morrey BF. Surgical treatment of aseptic olecranon bursitis. *J Shoulder Elbow Surg.* 1997;6:49–54.
43. Caldwell GL Jr, Safran MR. Elbow problems in the athlete. *Orthop Clin North Am.* 1995;26:465–485.
44. Chen J, Alk D, Eventov I, et al. Development of the olecranon bursa. An anatomic cadaver study. *Acta Orthopaedica Scandinavica.* 1987;58:408–409.
45. Ogilvie-Harris DJ, Gilbart M. Endoscopic bursal resection: the olecranon bursa and prepatellar bursa. *Arthroscopy.* 2000;16:249–253.

INJURIES OF THE WRIST AND HAND

24

ETHAN R. WIESLER, MD, JIAN SHEN, MD, ANASTASIOS PAPADONIKOLAKIS, MD

■ KEY POINTS

- Wrist ligaments are classified as either extrinsic or intrinsic. Extrinsic ligaments connect the forearm bones with the carpus. Intrinsic ligaments originate and insert within the carpus. Extrinsic ligaments are stiffer but have a lower ultimate yield point than the intrinsic ligaments.
- There are two main carpal instability patterns: static and dynamic. Static instability is present at rest and can be diagnosed on routine anteroposterior (AP) and lateral radiographs. Dynamic instability requires certain maneuvers to occur with stress; motion fluoroscopy is often required for diagnosis.
- Scapholunate (S-L) instability is the most common form of carpal instability. Two ligaments out of interosseous S-L ligament, the dorsal S-L ligament and the volar radioscapholunate ligament, must be disrupted for dissociation to occur.
- Injuries to the ligaments and other supporting structures in the thumb offer results in joint instability.
- The periscaphoid area is the site of 95% of all wrist degenerative diseases. Scapholunate advanced collapse (SLAC) of the wrist is the most common pattern of degenerative arthritis in the wrist.
- The extrinsic flexors of the finger consist of the flexor digitorum profundus (FDP) and the flexor digitorum superficialis (FDS). The FDP originates from the proximal ulna and interossesus membrane; and then divides into two muscle groups in the forearm, the most radial part supplying the index finger and the ulnar part supplying the middle, ring, and little fingers. The FDS has two heads: the radial head originates from the proximal shaft of the radius and the humeral ulnar head originates from the medial epicondyle of the humerus and the coronoid process of the ulna.
- The most common complication following flexor tendon surgery is the formation of adhesions, which may occur in spite of appropriate therapy and a compliant patient. Tenolysis should be considered when active flexion is restricted despite a normal passive range of motion, in a wound that has reached soft-tissue equilibrium (usually more than 3 months since repair).
- Fractures of the distal radius are the most common of all skeletal injuries. These fractions, which are the most frequent type of bone injury in the upper extremity, occur in athletes of all ages. Distal radius injuries in the athlete typically occur secondary to high energy and are encounted most often in impact sports, but they can occur in any activity where falling onto an outstretched hand is possible.
- Carpal scaphoid fractures are the most common and yet problematic fractures of the wrists of athletes. The pattern of scaphoid fractures depends on the force and position of the wrist. The most common mechanism of scaphoid fractures is a fall on an outstretched hand with the wrist in extension and the forearm in pronation.
- Fracture of the hamate usually occurs at the hook and is most common in stick- or racquet-handling sports, such as golf, baseball, or tennis. The hook of the hamate is the site of origin for the hypothenar muscles, pisohamate ligaments, and the distal attachment of the transverse ligament.
- Fractures of the thumb metacarpal occur most frequently at the base and are subdivided into intra-articular and extra-articular types. Extra-articular fractures occur in transverse and oblique fracture patterns and can be managed without surgery.

- Most metacarpal fractures occur in adolescents and young adults from sports or industrial accidents. Fractures of the metacarpals and phalanges comprise approximately 10% of all fractures and 30% to 40% of all hand fractures.
- Phalangeal fractures are a common injury affecting all age groups and they are among the most common in all sports. Most phalangeal fractures are caused by direct blows and result in transverse fractures. Distal phalanx fractures are most often caused by crushing forces that lead to comminuted fracture patterns and are frequently accompanied by nailbed lacerations.
- Ganglion cyst is the most common soft-tissue lesion of the hand and wrist. Ganglions have been reported at almost every joint in the hand and wrist. The most common location is the dorsum of the wrist. Cyst lining is usually a bland, fibrous, relatively acellular membrane with compressed collagen fibers.
- Nerve injuries in athletes are usually the result of chronic overuse or overload, although they may result from acute compression. Chronic overuse injuries are mainly dependent on the sport and biomechanical loading related to the activity. Fractures, compartment syndromes, or blunt trauma may result in acute compression nerve syndromes.

While many sports injuries occur to the lower extremity, the use of the upper extremity for many sports places the wrist and hand in an extremely vulnerable position. Knowledge of both basic science of the structures at risk, and common injuries and their treatment will be outlined in this chapter.

■ WRIST LIGAMENTS

There are multiple anatomic variations in ligament shape and size (1) **(Fig 24-1)**. This explains the existence of so many different descriptions of carpal ligaments in the orthopedic literature (2,3). Wrist ligaments are classified as either extrinsic or intrinsic (4). Extrinsic ligaments connect the forearm bones with the carpus. Intrinsic ligaments originate and insert within the carpus. The existing literature indicates that the extrinsic ligaments are stiffer but have lower ultimate yield point than the intrinsic ligaments (5). The extrinsic ligaments usually rupture mid-substance but the intrinsic ligaments appear to more typically avulse from their osseous origins and insertions than rupture (6).

Extrinsic Ligaments

Superficial Extrinsic Radiocarpal Ligaments: The most lateral superficial ligaments are the radioscaphoid (RS), radiocapitate (RC), and long radiolunate (long RL) ligament (7). The dorsal extrinsic radiocarpal ligamentous complex is formed by the dorsal radiotriquetral (RTq) ligament.
Superficial Extrinsic Ulnocarpal Ligaments: The ulnocapitate (UC) ligament, which inserts into the neck of the capitate (8), forms this complex.

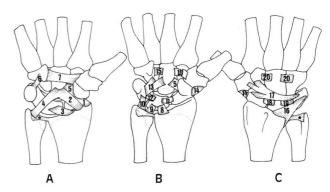

Fig 24-1. Schematic representation of the most consistently present wrist ligaments. These drawings do not aim to replicate the exact shape and dimensions of the actual ligaments, nor their frequent anatomic variations. **A:** Palmar superficial ligaments: *(1)* radioscaphoid, *(2)* radiocapitate, *(3)* long radiolunate, *(4)* lunocapitate, *(5)* scaphocapitate, *(6)* pisohamate, and *(7)* flexor retinaculum or transverse carpal ligament. **B:** Palmar deep ligaments: *(8)* short radiolunate; *(9)* ulnolunate; *(10)* ulnotriquetral; *(11)* palmar scapholunate; *(12)* palmar lunotriquetral; *(13)* triquetral-hamate-capitate, also known as the ulnar limb of the arcuate ligament; *(14)* dorsolateral scaphotrapezial; and *(15)* palmar transverse interosseous ligaments of the distal row. **C:** Dorsal ligaments: *(16)* radiotriquetral; *(17)* triquetrum-scaphoid-trapezium-trapezoid, also known as the dorsal intercarpal ligament; *(18)* dorsal scapholunate; *(19)* dorsal lunotriquetral; and *(20)* dorsal transverse interosseous ligaments of the distal row.

Deep Extrinsic Radiocarpal Ligaments: This complex is made up of the short radiolunate (short RL) ligament and the radioscapholunate ligament.
Deep Extrinsic Ulnocarpal Ligaments: The ulnotriquetral (UTq) and the ulnolunate (UL) form this complex.

Intrinsic Ligaments

These ligaments connect the bones of the proximal and distal carpal bones or link the two rows to each other.
S-L Interosseous Ligaments: Is formed by three distinct structures: two SL ligaments (palmar and dorsal) and the proximal fibrocartilaginous membrane.
Lunotriquetral Interosseous Ligaments: Two interosseous ligaments (palmar and dorsal) formed by stout transverse fibers connecting the palmar and dorsal aspects of the two bones (9).
Distal Carpal Row Interosseous Ligaments: These ligaments connect transversely the distal carpal row bones and they are classified into dorsal, palmar, or deep intra-articular (10).
1-Dorsal Intercarpal Ligament: It arises from the dorsal ridge of the triquetrum and fans out to insert on the dorsal rim of the scaphoid, the trapezium, and the trapezoid bones (11).
2-Palmar Intercarpal Ligaments: Medially, the triquetral-hamate-capitate (TqHC) ligamentous complex. And laterally, the anteromedial scaphocapitate (SC) ligament and the dorsolateral scaphotrapeziotrapezoid (STT) ligament (12) form this complex.

Neither true radial nor ulnar collateral ligaments of the wrist exist.

Carpal Instability

Carpal instability is defined as the inability to bear physiologic loads without losing the normal carpal alignment (13). There are two main carpal instability patterns: static and dynamic. Static instability is present at rest and can be diagnosed on routine AP and lateral radiographs. Dynamic instability requires certain maneuvers to occur with stress, and motion fluoroscopy is often required for diagnosis. Larsen et al. (14) has classified wrist instability into acute (<1 week, maximum primary healing potential), subacute (1 to 6 weeks, some healing potential), and chronic (>6 weeks, little primary healing potential). Most instability patterns can be identified on the lateral radiograph. In the normal wrist in the neutral position, the axes of the radius, the lunate, and the capitate co-align. Dorsal intercalary segmental instability (DISI) is present when the lunate lies palmar to the capitate but is flexed dorsally **(Fig 24-2)**. Volar intercalary segmental instability (VISI) is present if the lunate lies dorsal to the capitate and is palmar flexed **(Fig 24-2)**. Either of these collapsed patterns can be associated with carpal instabilities.

Scapholunate Instability

Scapholunate (S-L) instability is the most common form of carpal instability. Diagnosis can be challenging due to the subtle findings in this entity. Three ligaments are involved in this condition: the interosseous S-L ligament, the dorsal S-L ligament, and the volar radioscapholunate ligament. Two of the three ligaments must be disrupted for dissociation to occur. It is generally thought that the volar radioscapholunate ligament must be disrupted before complete subluxation can occur (15). The mechanism of injury usually involves a fall or direct blow that causes hyperextension of the wrist. Pain, swelling, and tenderness are noted over the dorsoradial aspect of the wrist. Watson and Hempton (16) described a diagnostic test in which the examiner stabilizes the scaphoid by placing his or her thumb over the volar pole of the scaphoid while the wrist is held in ulnar deviation. When the wrist is brought into radial deviation, pain is produced as the force is transmitted to the injured S-L ligaments **(Fig 24-3)**.

Radiograph Findings. An AP view in full supination may demonstrate widening of the S-L interval. A gap of more than 2 mm is abnormal and should be compared to the contralateral side, provided it is uninjured. The scaphoid will be shortened and a ring sign may be present, which presents the cortical projection of the distal pole of the scaphoid in its more flexed position **(Fig 24-4)**. On the lateral radiograph, a S-L angle of more than 70 degrees (normal range from 30 to 60 degrees) is also suggestive of S-L dissociation **(Fig 24-5)**. Bone scans, arthrography, and, more recently, magnetic resonance imaging (MRI) can be helpful in localizing the area of injury (17).

Management. Injuries diagnosed within 3 weeks are considered acute (18). Cast immobilization with the wrist in full supination, mild dorsiflexion, and ulnar deviation is recommended (19). Closed reduction and cast immobilization for 6 to 10 weeks may allow healing. In complete tears, it is

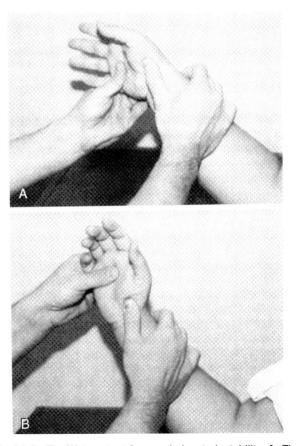

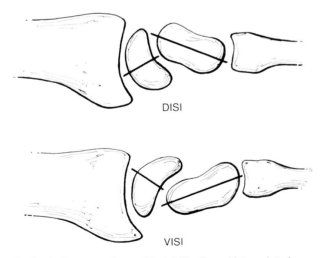

Fig 24-2. Patterns of carpal instability. Dorsal intercalated segmental instability (*DISI*) is present when the lunate lies volar to the capitate but is flexed dorsally. Volar intercalated segmental instability (*VISI*) is present if the lunate lies dorsal to the capitate and is flexed volarly.

Fig 24-3. The Watson test for scapholunate instability. **A:** The scaphoid is stabilized with the thumb over the volar pole. **B:** When the hand is brought from ulnar to radial deviation, pain results.

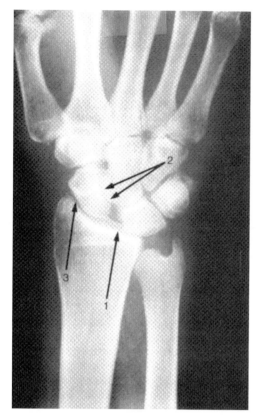

Fig 24-4. Radiographic findings of scapholunate dissociation.

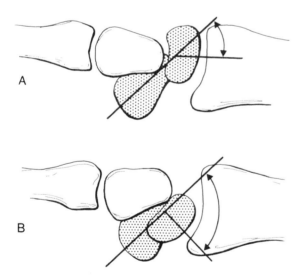

Fig 24-5. The normal scapholunate angle **A:** is 30 to 60 degrees. A scapholunate angle of more than 70 degrees **B:** suggests scapholunate dissociation. (Redrawn from Green DP. *Operative Hand Surgery.* 2nd ed. New York: Churchill Livingstone; 1988.)

difficult to obtain a satisfactory reduction by closed means.

Closed reduction and percutaneous pinning in which the wrist is maintained in dorsiflexion to reduce the proximal pole of the scaphoid while the S-L joint is pinned may be successful. A Kirschner wire (K-wire) is passed percutaneously through the snuffbox and across the S-L joint. The wrist should then be gently palmar-flexed to approximate the volar ligaments. A K-wire is then passed across the scaphoid into the capitate for final stabilization. The wires can be removed after 6 to 8 weeks. A protective splint is used for another 4 weeks. Open reduction internal fixation (ORIF) of the S-L joint through a dorsal approach with direct repair of the ligament can be successful, especially if done in the acute period (20). Newer techniques based on improved understanding of carpal kinematics are being developed, but in all cases outcomes are proportional to the severity of injury and the early recognition of the injury pattern. Other treatment options for acute open repair of the injured S-L ligament, with direct repair or ligamentous reconstruction, is generally indicated.

Chronic instability is defined as an injury that has lasted longer than 3 months. There is no reliable procedure for treatment of chronic injuries. Some use a dorsal capsulodesis technique in which the dorsal capsule acts as a check rein to prevent palmar rotation of the distal pole of the scaphoid (21). Others have used various tendon grafts to reconstruct the S-L ligament or the radioscapholunate ligament (15,22).

A variety of intercarpal arthrodeses have been proposed. In S-L joint arthrodesis, it is difficult to attain successful fusion. There is currently no accepted means to achieve successful SL fusion, due to the high stresses imparted to this joint; nonunion rates are unacceptably high in the reported literature. The capitate can be included in the S-L arthrodesis to increase success rate in attaining solid fusion. This, however, is at the cost of loss of wrist motion (23), primarily palmar flexion. Triscaphe (trapezium-trapezoid-scaphoid, S-T-T) fusion (16) is a demanding technique; however, it prevents subluxation of the proximal pole. Although bony S-L arthrodesis may not occur, a fibrous union does occur to prevent capitate migration. Including the capitate in the fusion increases the chances of obtaining a bony fusion but results in restriction of motion. The scapho-trapezial-trapezoid arthrodesis described by Peterson and Lipscomb (24) may increase the stress on other joints, especially the RS joint.

It is the authors' opinion that acute repair of the S-L ligament should be performed within the first 3 months. This may be done with tissue augmentation from the extensor or flexor tendons, or with a capsulodesis. After 3 months, especially in the case of significant static carpal instability, other options such as, but not limited to, those mentioned above should be performed to prevent the 9 to 12 year gradual progression to SLAC.

Medial (Ulnar) Carpal Instability
With medial (ulnar) carpal instability, patients present with wrist pain and often have a painful click, which may be audible or palpable. Often the patient does not recall a specific injury episode.

Triquetrohamate Instability

Triquetrohamate dissociation is the most common ulnar instability. The patients usually have a characteristic "clunk," which maybe audible and/or palpable as produced by active motion. This clunk represents the triquetrum suddenly snapping back and forth over the lunate articulation with ulnar and radial deviation. Physical examination may elicit tenderness over the triquetrum. Plain radiographs are usually not helpful. Fluoroscopy is useful and sufficiently demonstrates abnormal motion (25). The lunate can be seen to snap suddenly when the triquetrum reduces on the lunate.

Lunotriquetral Instability

With lunotriquetral instability, patients may or may not have a wrist click on examination. For diagnostic purpose, a ballottement test **(Fig 24-6)** has been described (9) in which the lunate is stabilized by one hand while the other hand shifts the triquetrum in a palmar and dorsal direction. This reproduces the same pain that the patient is experiencing. Plain radiographs are not helpful. Fluoroscopy is usually normal.

Treatment includes a trial of conservative measures consisting of immobilization in a cast or a splint and an anti-inflammatory medication. From our own experience, local steroid injection into the joint can be helpful. Athletes who are mostly symptomatic during game activity can be fitted with a splint to correct triquetrohamate instability (26). This splint reduces the VISI sag of the proximal row by pushing dorsally on the pisiform. Surgery can be considered in those who fail conservative treatment. The triquetrohamate and lunotriquetral joints are first inspected, and then the wrist is stressed by axial compression and side deviation to confirm the location of the instability. The triquetrum is then reduced and fixed internally by inserting K-wires across the involved joint. The joint space is filled with cancellous bone graft to maintain the joint space. The wrist is then immobilized for 6 to 8 weeks in a short-arm cast, after which the pins are removed and a rehabilitation program is started. This joint has had more success than the S-L joint in arthrodesis in the literature. Consideration for arthroscopic debridement in mild cases with partial limited intercarpal (L-T) tears should be the first step in treatment; L-T fusion is an option in advanced cases of ligamentous instability.

Thumb Metacarpophalangeal Joint Instability

The human thumb plays a central role in almost all hand functions. Injuries to the ligaments and other supporting structures in the thumb often result in instability.

The most common thumb metacarpophalangeal (MCP) joint dislocation is dorsal dislocation **(Fig 24-7)**. The mechanism is usually a hyperextension injury. The condition of the volar plate will determine if a dislocation is easily reducible or if it will require open reduction.

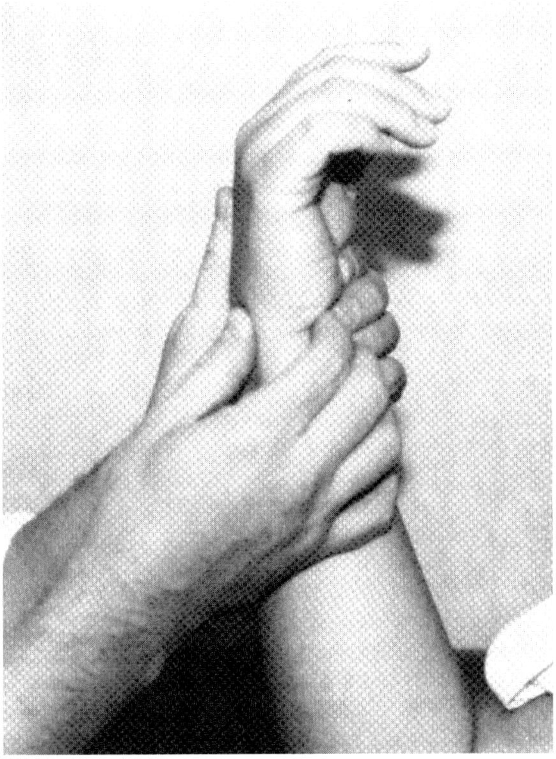

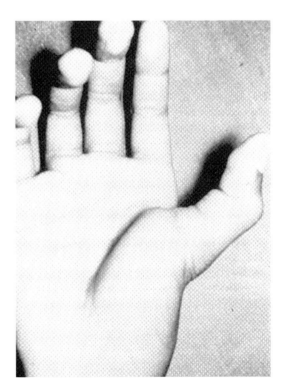

Fig 24-6. The ballottement test described by Reagan et al. The lunate is stabilized by one hand while the triquetrum is shifted in a palmar and dorsal direction with the examiner's opposite hand. (From Reagan DS, Linscheid RL, Dobyns JH. Lunotriquetral sprains. *J Hand Surg Am*. 1984;9A(4):502–514; with permission)

Fig 24-7. Clinical image of a dorsal metacarpophalangeal joint dislocation of the thumb. Most often the result of a hyperextension force, dorsal dislocations are far more common than their volar counterparts.

Volar dislocation of the thumb MCP joint is encountered in practice. However, it represents a global instability pattern resulting from extensive tearing of the dorsal capsule and the extensor pollicis brevis (EPB) tendon (27). The simple dislocation or subluxation is the most striking with regard to physical findings because the proximal phalanx assumes a posture of almost 90° to the metacarpal axis. This is relatively easy to reduce, with sufficient anesthesia and reversal of the responsible mechanism.

In complex dislocation, the position of the proximal phalanx is almost parallel to the metacarpal. The finding of skin dimpling over the volar MCP suggests complex dislocation. In complex dislocation, the surgeon should initially attempt a closed reduction. This would include insufflating the joint with anesthetic agent to essentially float out the volar plate. The procedure should include hyperextension combined with an attempt to coapt the dorsal rim of the proximal phalanx and the dorsal aspect of the articular surface of the metacarpal head, then dragging the base of the proximal phalanx over the articular surface of the metacarpal head in an attempt to push the volar plate out of the joint. This approach will result in successful closed reduction in a reasonable number of these somewhat rare injuries.

After closed reduction of either simple or complex dislocation is attained, the physician should check lateral stability to evaluate the integrity of the collateral ligaments. Anteroposterior (AP) translation, extension, and flexion should be checked while the thumb is still anesthetized. If surgical reduction is elected, digital nerves, which are more central and subcutaneous in the thumb MCP dislocations, are at significant risk in the volar approach. Recovery of almost normal stability and motion is expected. After surgery, thumb spica splinting, including the interphalangeal (IP) joint, is advisable to allow healing of the dorsal or volar skin incision and the underlying tissues. It is reasonable to allow protected return to play at 3 weeks.

Collateral Ligament Injuries of the Thumb Metacarpophalangeal Joint

Injury to the ulnar collateral ligament is more common than that of the radial counterpart (28). The proper collateral ligaments are the main stabilizers of the thumb MCP joint to valgus and varus stress and are the most important structures to repair to restore stability to the destabilized thumb MCP joint. The accessory collateral ligaments and the EPB tendon contribute static stability. Repair of these structures is critical in restoring stability when they are significantly compromised. Volar subluxation as seen on lateral radiograph of the thumb is twice as common in radial collateral ligament injuries as ulnar collateral injuries. In general, radial collateral ligament injuries are less prone to need acute or delayed repair or reconstruction.

Radial Collateral Ligament Injuries

In radial collateral ligament injuries, tenderness, deviation to ulnar-directed stress, and asymmetry of skin findings in contralateral comparison are the basic tenants of the diagnosis.

However, incomplete ligament injury can be converted to a complete injury by vigorous examination.

The treatment of the radial collateral ligament is determined by the competence of the remaining ligament. Anatomy on the radial side of the joint does not include any soft tissue structures that routinely interfere with direct opposition of the torn ends of the ligament as opposed to the ulnar side (Stener lesion). In radial collateral ligament injuries, nonoperative treatment has a greater chance of success.

For complete tears, open treatment is still advocated. Reattachment of the avulsed ligament back to (usually) the proximal phalanx through pullout wire or suture anchor is performed. The joint is typically held after soft tissue repair with a single percutaneous pin for the first 4 weeks, followed by protected mobilization. Protection in a cast for 4 to 6 weeks is standard.

Ulnar Collateral Ligament Injuries

Gamekeeper's thumb, or skier's thumb, is one of the most common injuries in sports medicine and hand surgery. Palpation of the ulnar side of the MCP joint immediately after the injury may reveal a swelling that represents the distal edge of the displaced ulnar collateral ligament, the Stener lesion, which represents an avulsion of the UCL with proximal migration volar to the thumb adductor musculature (29) **(Fig 24-8)**. The stress examination, under local anesthesia, is the most critical physical examination maneuver.

Examination should be performed by applying radially directed stress with the MCP joint in both neutral and 30-degree flexed posture. The flexed position isolates the UCL stabilization effect from that of the other ulnar-sided restraints. When compared to the other thumb, relative deviation compared with the contralateral side of greater than 10 to 15 degrees usually indicates complete tear.

The quality of the end point is an important indicator of ligament integrity. Radiographs should be used for all patients to detect the presence and extent of bony injury.

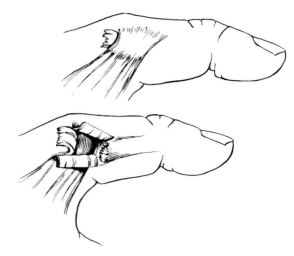

Fig 24-8. Stener lesion.

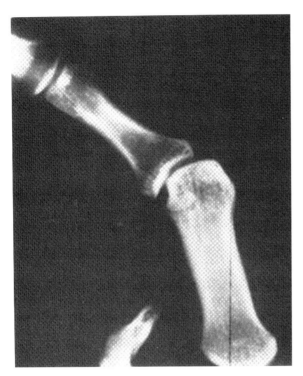

Fig 24-9. Stress radiographs of ulnar collateral ligament injuries of the thumb are indicated if complete rupture is not obvious on clinical examination.

Radiographs should be performed prior to vigorous examination. Arthrography has been employed in several studies to determine the extent of MCP injury and the presence of a Stener lesion (30). The combination of palpation, stress examination, and fluoroscopic evaluation **(Fig 24-9)** remain the primary tools for diagnosis of these injuries.

Treatment. Partial tears treatment: 2 to 6 weeks of immobilization in a forearm-based thumb spica with the IP joint included, followed by hand-based orthosis that allows wrist motion up to the fourth week to be followed by taping for an additional 2 to 4 weeks.

Complete tears treatment: anatomic repair is the rule (31). Because the Stener lesion is present in up to half of the suspected complete tears, open treatment is indicated. The primary repair is believed to yield superior results to late reconstruction and is thought to be possible up to 1 year post injury, after which an allograft reconstruction (using palmaris longus tendon) should be considered. Finding volar subluxation related to an ulnar-sided injury is an indication for open repair because it indicates severe tissue compromise

Technique of Repair of the Thumb MCP Ulnar Collateral Ligament. If the diagnosis is complete tear of the UCL, then surgical repair is indicated. A "lazy-S-shaped" incision is used that courses from the ulnar mid-axial line across the dorsum of the MCP joint and then proximally along the radial border of the metacarpal. Branches of the superficial radial nerve lying in the deep subcutaneous layer should be

identified and protected. The proximal edge of the adductor aponeurosis is identified. A longitudinal incision is made in the adductor aponeurosis parallel and approximately 2 to 3 mm volar to the ulnar border of the extensor pollicis longus (EPL). The aponeurosisis reflected volarly to expose the ulnar aspect of the MCP joint, including the volar base of the proximal phalanx.

Tears in the middle two-thirds of the ligament can be re-approximated with interrupted figure-of-eight sutures using nonabsorbable suture material like 3-0 or 4-0 nylon. The ligament, however, is usually avulsed distally and can be approximated to the distal stump or into the bone defect from which it was detached with pull-out suture technique or a bone anchor. Secure fixation of the ligament to bone can be achieved by pull-out suture technique after scarifying the bone at the site of reattachment. A monofilament synthetic suture such as 3-0 Prolene, nylon, or stainless steel wire is placed in the proximal stump of the UCL with a modified Kessler technique. Keith needles are drilled across the base of the proximal phalanx to exit percutaneously on the radial side. The ends of the suture in the UCL stump are threaded through the eye of the Keith needles, which are then pulled through the proximal phalanx. The ligament is pulled up to the shallow trough previously made in the ulnar base of the phalanx and the ends of suture then tied over a button. An important technical point here is that the ligament repair needs to be performed such that the ligament is reinserted volar to the axis of rotation of the joint, so as not to cause undue tension to the repair and ultimately limit joint flexion.

If a fragment of bone accompanies the avulsed ligament, the repair technique is based on the size of the fragment. If the fragment is less than 15% of the articular surface, it can be excised and the ligament inserted directly into the defect with a pull-out suture. If the fragment is larger than 15% of the articular surface, it is reduced anatomically into the defect with a pull-out suture. A suture is placed between the distal volar portion of the repaired ligament and the volar plate to secure this three-dimensional complex. Repair of the dorsal ulnar capsule is performed to prevent volar subluxation of the joint. Radial stress is applied to the joint to test the stability of the repair. The thumb is immobilized in a thumb spica cast with the IP joint left free to move, which is encouraged to prevent adhesions of the extensor mechanism during healing time. Cast immobilization is continued for approximately 4 weeks, after which a hand-based orthosis is used to immobilize the MCP joint. Splint protection is discontinued 2 weeks later. Unrestricted use is not recommended for at least 3 months following surgery.

■ FINGER DISLOCATIONS

Metacarpophalangeal Joint

The MCP joint is a condyloid joint that allows greater freedom of movement than the interphalangeal joint. The collateral ligaments, volar plate, joint capsule, deep transverse intermetacarpal ligament, and tendons all play a role in the stability of the MCP joint.

The safe position of the MCP joint is fully flexed because the proper collateral ligaments are at their greatest length and thus will not contract. Dislocations or subluxation of the MCP joint is relatively uncommon.

Lateral Plane Injury: Full-blown lateral injury is rare, but strains of the ligaments and small avulsion or impaction fractures are commonly seen.

Spontaneous reduction with reasonable stability is the rule for these injuries. Splinting and gradual liberation to play with appropriate buddy taping is the typical modality of treatment.

Dorsal Metacarpophalangeal Dislocations

The term *simple* dislocation has historically referred to an MCP joint that is in 70- to 90-degree of extension; however, the proximal phalanx is still in articular contact with the metacarpal head.

Complex dislocation, as described previously in the thumb section, denotes axial, dorsally translated, arrangement between the metacarpal and the proximal phalanx. As described previously in the thumb section, an attempt at closed reduction under adequate anesthesia should be made in all MCP dislocations. The reduction technique entails hyperextension at the MCP joint, enabling the *dorsal* margin of the proximal phalanx to contact the dorsal margin of the metacarpal head. The phalanx may be translated proximally or distally to "capture" the volar plate. The phalanx is then pushed across the metacarpal articular surface, with care to maintain the dorsal rim contact as long as possible to cause the volar plate to "pop" out of the joint and back into position. Postreduction radiographs are a must. Brief splinting for 3 to 5 days in the functional or safe position is followed by a buddy taping regimen to prevent hyperextension and allow motion. If closed reduction is unsuccessful, immediate open reduction is warranted. The common surgical approach to dorsal MCP dislocation is dorsal.

Volar Metacarpophalangeal Joint Dislocations

Volar MCP dislocation is extremely rare (32). The tissue that almost always causes difficulty in achieving closed reduction is likely a combination of the collateral ligament, the volar plate, the MCP capsule, and possibly the extensor mechanism. To reduce a volar MCP dislocation, the steps in reduction of a dorsal dislocation can simply be reversed. Failed closed reduction necessitates immediate open reduction through a volar approach to remove the interposed tissue. After reduction and brief splinting, motion is encouraged.

Proximal Interphalangeal Joint Dislocation

The proximal interphalangeal (PIP) joint dislocation is very common in all sports. The collateral ligaments along with the volar plate provide the most resistance to stress forces in lateral deviation. Secondary restraints include the joint capsule, flexor tendon sheath, and parts of the extensor apparatus. PIP dislocations are classified as dorsal and volar based on the direction of the distal segment.

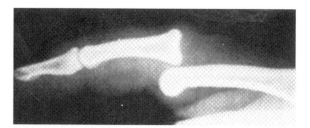

Fig 24-10. Dorsal dislocation is by far the most common type of dislocation of the PIP joint.

Dorsal Proximal Interphalangeal Dislocations

The dorsal PIP dislocation is the most common PIP dislocation (**Fig 24-10**). Hyperextension of the middle phalanx is the usual mechanism. This entity can be either pure soft tissue or combined soft tissue and bone injury. Reduction is usually performed under digital block anesthesia. After reduction has been attained, while the patient's finger is still anesthetized, it is important to test the range of motion through which the PIP remains stable and to observe the quality of the end points. The majority of these injuries will resume a concentric reduction and will have immediate stability in all directions but the extremes of hyperextension forces. The hallmark of closed treatment of these injuries is dorsal extension block splinting.

Volar Proximal Interphalangeal Dislocations

Volar dislocations are rare (33) (**Fig 24-11**). This is usually sustained when an extended digit is forcibly flexed at the PIP joint. The determining factors of treatment are the ability to achieve and maintain closed reduction and the extent of extensor mechanism disruption. Stable closed reduction should be kept in a position of PIP extension for a period of 4 to 6 weeks. Joint pinning can be used instead when there is difficulty in maintaining the extended posture in a splint. Formal open reduction is necessary when the lateral band of the extensor mechanism is blocking reduction. Primary repair of the rent between the lateral band and the central

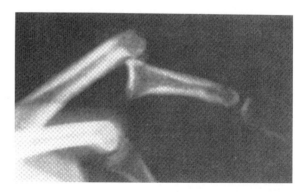

Fig 24-11. Volar dislocation of the PIP joint is a relatively uncommon injury. It should be obvious from this radiograph that the central slip must be torn for this injury to occur; therefore, these patients should be treated in the same manner as those with a boutonnière injury.

tendon is advocated to avoid the development of a traumatic boutonnière deformity. Pinning after open repair is recommended. Early motion in volar dislocations is discouraged because the injured extensor must be allowed to heal.

Distal Interphalangeal Dislocations

Dislocation of the distal interphalangeal (DIP) joint is often seen in contact sports. The great majority of these dislocations are dorsal dislocations. After reduction, immediate stability is the rule. These injuries are commonly treated in a DIP extension splint, which keeps the DIP in a full extension or slightly hyperextended position for 6 weeks. DIP pinning can be used instead if DIP cannot be maintained in a splint, mostly due to patient's occupation. Joint pinning is performed after open reduction for 4 weeks, while the PIP joint is left free for movement.

Distal Radioulnar Joint Anatomy

The anatomy of the distal radioulnar joint (DRUJ) is complex. The DRUJ articulation is trochoid. The marginal ligaments of the triangular fibrocartilage (TFC) are important in load transference from the carpus to the ulna and in the stability of the DRUJ.

The joint is most stable in the extremes of rotation, where the compressive forces between the radius and the ulna are resisted by the reciprocal tensile forces developed within the opposite TFC marginal ligament (34,35). Clinical stability is obviously related to many factors.

Ulnocarpal Ligaments. TFC and ulnocarpal ligaments constitute the triangular fibrocartilage complex (TFCC). The ulnocarpal ligaments are the combined volar UL and UTq ligaments. These ligaments originate at the base of the styloid, in tandem with the apical attachment of the TFC and insert volarly on the lunate and triquetrum.

Other Stabilizing Factors. The TFC and ulnocarpal ligaments make up the TFCC. Stability of the radioulnar-carpal unit is further influenced by the conformation of the sigmoid notch and the interosseous membrane (36), the extensor retinaculum, and the forces of the ECU and the pronator quadratus, and also by the dorsal carpal ligament complex. The DRUJ capsule is uniformly thin and cannot be thought of to offer stability in the usual sense.

Acute Joint Instability. *Triangular Fibrocartilage Complex Disruption with Distal Radioulnar Joint: Instability Associated with Fractures or Dislocations.* When the TFCC and DRUJ disruption is associated with radial or ulnar fractures or other dislocations, accurate closed reduction of the dislocation and associated fracture, followed by appropriate cast immobilization in mid-rotation with slight ulnar deviation and palmar flexion will often solve the problem. Alternative fracture management should be considered rather than accepting abnormal joint positioning. Ligament repair (DRUJ and TFCC) should be strongly considered when

open reduction of the fracture is required and DRUJ disruption is evident.

The Essex-Lopresti Lesion (Radial Head Fracture with Injury to the Interosseous Membrane and Triangular Fibrocartilage Complex). DRUJ disruption associated with a displaced radial head fracture and proximal migration of the radius is termed the Essex-Lopresti fracture (37,38). The injury is complex, with sequential forces disrupting the DRUJ ligaments, interosseous membrane, and radiocapitellar articular surface. A high index of suspicion should occur in any patient with a displaced radial head fracture or acute DRUJ displacement. Posteroterior (PA) and lateral comparison views of both forearms, including the elbow and wrist, should be followed by comparison computed tomography (CT) scans of the DRUJ if any suspicion of this injury persists on plain films. If the forearm is to be opened for associated fractures, one should look at the interosseous membrane with a tendency toward repair or reconstruction. Acute large-fragment radial head fractures should be fixed in addition to reduction, repair, and pinning of the DRUJ (39). Acute, comminuted radial head fractures should be excised with replacement by radial head prostheses and the DRUJ reduced, repaired, and pinned. Fortunately, this combination of injuries is rare, and forearm longitudinal instability, though rare, is often missed. Early surgical address of associated injuries in this entity is critical in order to avoid late and often nonsalvageable forearm pathology.

Isolated Triangular Fibrocartilage Complex Disruption with Dislocation or Instability of the Distal Radioulnar Joint. Isolated DRUJ dislocations will respond to cast immobilization for 6 weeks if an accurate closed reduction can be obtained. If the ulna is palmar relative to the radius, pronation will reduce the dislocation. If the ulna is dorsal, supination will usually reduce the joint (40). It has been recommended that a long arm cast be used with the forearm in full supination for ulna dorsal and in full pronation for ulna volar. Most acute closed DRUJ disruptions can be satisfactorily handled by a careful nonoperative approach as described above.

The joint should be opened and reduced and the TFCC repaired only if the dislocation is locked or the reduction is incongruous. If instability persists after cast treatment and reasonable rehabilitation, the problem may be satisfactorily solved by operative intervention.

Management of Chronic Joint Instability. Stabilization by primary repair of the TFCC is recommended if possible. Although this approach should be considered first, problems such as contracture or loss of tissue may demand a reconstructive approach. There is no single optimal operation, but the following have received some support.

Triangular Fibrocartilage Complex Reconstruction or Substitution. The Bunnell-Boyes procedure (41) is innovative and anatomic insofar as reconstruction of DRUJ instability **(Fig 24-12)**.

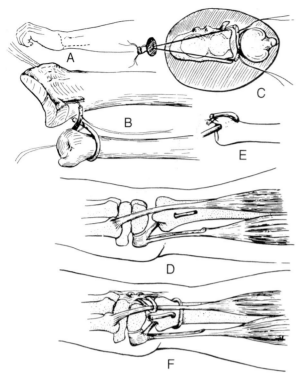

Fig 24-12. Boyes/Bunnell reconstruction of the distal radioulnar articulation. (From Boyes JH. Surgical repair of joints. In: *Bunnell's surgery of the hand*. 5th ed. Philadelphia: JB Lipincott Co; 1970:94–313; with permission.)

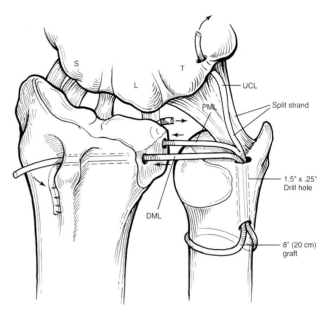

Fig 24-13. A proposed method of augmentation or reconstruction of the ulnotriquetral (UTq) and dorsal and palmar radioulnar marginal ligaments of the triangular fibro-cartilage (TFC). The donor graft material may be palmaris longus, plantaris, or toe extensor. The unique aspect of the technique is the graft loop around the neck of the ulna and then passage of the two (three) ends through an oblique drill hole exiting at the fovea—the natural insertion point of the TFC. This provides a strong ulnar anchor where needed. The remaining anchor points are to the radius through dorsal and palmar exposure and to the triquetrum as shown.

The procedure uses distally based portion of the FCU harvested proximally and stripped distally to the pisiform attachment. The new ligament is stabilized distally by weaving it through the remaining volar capsule. This new ligament is then passed through a drill hole in the styloid area and exits in the apex of the ulnar articular surface. The repair is completed with imbrication of the dorsal capsule. Others have used a reconstructive approach as illustrated in Figure 24-13. A palmaris or plantaris graft is harvested and doubled on itself. The two ends are looped around the neck of the ulna and passed distally through an oblique one-quarter-inch drill hole in the ulna. The hole begins proximally at the neck of the ulnar articular prominence and exits in the fovea at the TFC's normal anatomic attachment site. The two ends are then used to reinforce or replace deficient portions of the dorsal and/or palmar marginal ligament or ulnocarpal ligaments. Many techniques have been described to accomplish the same extrinsic stability of the disrupted DRUJ. No single technique has been deemed superior, due to the absence of controlled trials in the literature.

Substitution. Radioulnar tether procedures are the historical approach to substitution (42,43). Johnson (44) has proposed advancement of the pronator quadratus from its normal insertion on the ulna to a more lateral and dorsal insertion. He postulated that this might increase radioulnar joint stability.

Osteotomy. This is included in several procedural approaches to disorders of the DRUJ. The types of osteotomy vary, but it is used to correct abnormal rotation, angulation, or length discrepancies between the two forearm bones (45). Osteotomies should be considered only when there is demonstrable maintenance of the articular cartilage of the DRUJ. A CT scan of the DRUJ is a critical step in assessing the congruence and anatomy of the joint, as well as providing insight as to the quality of the cartilage. In the absence of joint cartilage, arthrodesis, arthroplasty, or excision should be considered. Algorithms have been developed to assist in the decision-making process.

Osteotomy of the Distal Radius. Osteotomy of the distal radius should be considered when correction of malunion or deformity of the distal radius is needed. The surgical technique usually requires a buttress plate and the addition of a bone graft.

If the original injury or insult involved the sigmoid notch, one must presume that this DRUJ surface is abnormal. An osteotomy done proximal to this level might not correct the sigmoid irregularity but instead change its angular relationship to the distal ulnar articular surface. If the deformity is the result of an injury not involving the notch, one might expect a well-done osteotomy to be highly beneficial if radial length, tilt, and inclination are well corrected.

Osteotomy of the Ulna. Performed to correct problems with ulnar shortening, rotation, or angulation. A variety of procedures have been utilized including ulnar head excision (46), hemiresection interposition arthroplasty with shortening (47,48), and ulnar recession and fusion of the ulnar head to the radius with restoration of forearm motion through creating a proximal pseudo-arthrosis (Sauve-Kapandji procedure) (49,50).

■ HAND AND WRIST ARTICULAR CARTILAGE

Articular cartilage is composed of hyaline cartilage that covers articulating surfaces. It is composed of

A Chondrocytes (5%)
B Extracellular matrix (95%)
1 Water (75%)
2 Collagen (mainly Type 2) (5%)
3 Proteoglycans (20%)
4 Enzymes
5 Growth Factors (PDGF, Platelet-derive growth factor; TGF beta, Transforming growth factor; FGF, Fibroblast growth factor; IGF-1, Insulin-like growth factor 1)
6 Lipids
7 Adhesives (fibronectin, chondronectin)

Articular cartilage zones **(Fig 24-14)** (superficial to deep) are:

1 Surface
2 Superficial Tangential Zone: Collagen fibers (Type 2) orientated tangential to surface. This layer has the greatest ability to resist shear stresses.
3 Transitional/Middle Zone: This is the transition between the shearing forces of surface layer to compression forces in the cartilage layer. In this layer collagen is arranged obliquely. This layer is composed almost entirely of proteoglycans.
4 Radial/Deep Zone: Here the collagen fibers are attached radially (vertical) into the tidemark. This layer distributes loads and resists compression.
5 Calcified Zone: This layer contains the Tidemark Layer (basophilic line that straddles the boundary between calcified and uncalcified cartilage). This layer contains Type 10 collagen.

Chondrocytes (5% wet weight): Chondroblasts, which are derived from mesenchymal cells, become trapped in lacunae and develop into chondrocytes. Chondrocytes are important in the control of matrix turnover through production of collagen, proteoglycans, and enzymes for cartilage metabolism.

Organic Matrix: Proteoglycans (PG): 10% to 15% of wet weight. They are produced by chondrocytes and secreted into the matrix. These are responsible for the compressive strength of

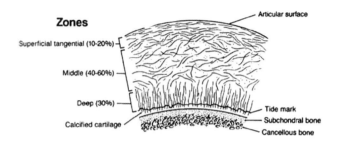

Fig 24-14. Articular cartilage zones.

cartilage and serve to trap and hold water to regulate matrix hydration and bind growth factors. Proteoglycans look like test tube brush with keratan and chondroitin sulphate chains (glycosaminoglycans, GAGs) bound to a protein core molecule monomer **(Fig 24-15)**. The monomer is attached via a link protein to hyaluronic acid. GAGs include: chondriotin-4-suphate (decreases with age), chondriotin-6-sulphate (increases with age), and keratan sulphate (increases with age). GAGs are bound to a protein core by sugar bonds to form a proteoglycan aggregen molecule. Link proteins stabilize aggregen molecules to hyaluronic acid to form a proteoglycan aggregate **(Fig 24-16)**. The aggregated proteoglycans and water are strongly electronegative. This generates a resistance to compressive force and contributes to the elasticity of cartilage. Hyaluronic acid is the major aggregating factor.

Collagen: Mainly Type 2. Other Types = 5, 6, 9, and 11. Type 9 lies on the surface of Type 2, acting as interfibrillary glue. Type 10 is associated with calcification of cartilage. Disruption

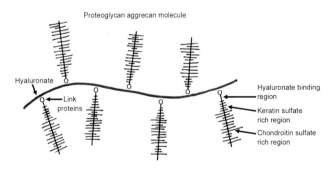

Fig 24-15. Proteoglycan aggregate molecule.

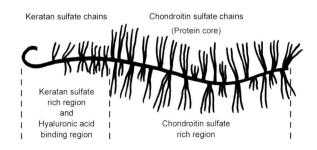

Fig 24-16. Link proteins stabilize aggregen molecules to hyaluronic acid to form a proteoglycan aggregate.

of the collagen network is a key factor in the development of OA. Collagen forms the cartilaginous framework and is responsible for the tensile strength of cartilage.

Water: 75% of wet weight. Allows for deformation of the surface by shifting in and out in response to stress. Increased water content causes an increase in the permeability, decreased strength, and decreased Young's modulus (less stiff). Water content increases in osteoarthritis.

Articular Cartilage Function: 1- Decreases friction in joints. 2- Load distribution in joints.

Articular Cartilage Nutrition: Mature articular cartilage is avascular, aneural, and alymphatic. Chondrocytes receive nutrition and oxygen via diffusion from synovial fluid through the cartilage matrix.

Articular Cartilage Biomechanics: Creep occurs when a viscoelastic tissue, like cartilage, is subjected to a constant load. Stress relaxation occurs with constant deformation. In contrast to bone, articular cartilage tends to stiffen with increasing strain.

Changes with Aging: With aging, cartilage becomes hypocellular and has decreased elasticity. Chondrocytes increase in size, increase their lysosomal enzymes, and cartilage becomes hypocellular (cells stop reproducing). Proteoglycans decrease in mass and size due to a decrease in the length of chondroitin sulfate chains and change in proportion. Keratin sulfate increases and hyaluronic acid decreases. Water content decreases with aging (increases in OA) and protein content increases due to a decrease in the ratio of carbohydrates to protein. Much of hyaline cartilage of the body ultimately calcifies with aging. When calcification occurs, chondrocytes die and matrix disintegrates. The superficial zones do not calcify, except in pathologic states such as pseudogout.

Healing of Articular Cartilage

Deep Lacerations: Extend below the tidemark and heal with *fibrocartilage*. Blunt trauma may cause osteoarthritic changes.

Superficial Lacerations: Above the tidemark. Chondrocytes proliferate but do not heal. Immobilization leads to atrophy while continuous passive motion is beneficial to healing.

Degenerative Joint Disease of the Hand: Osteoarthritis of the hand preferentially involves the DIP joint and the carpometacarpal (CMC) joint of the thumb. The PIP joint is affected less commonly. A multitude of hypotheses have been suggested for factors involved in osteoarthritis. Alterations in cartilage metabolism, trauma, infection, joint laxity, diet, hormonal changes, gout, calcium pyrophosphate

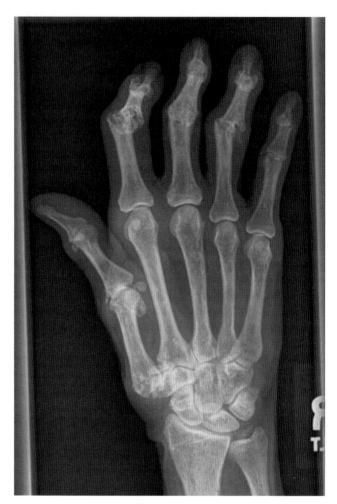

Fig 24-17. Advanced OA with PIP and DIP involvement.

deposition, microfractures, and immunologic factors have all been implicated in the etiology of osteoarthritis. Genetic factors play a role in some forms of osteoarthritis. The arthritic PIP joint demonstrates fusiform joint swelling. With progression of the condition, marginal osteophytes (Bouchard nodes) become evident with progressive lateral deviation of the digits **(Fig 24-17)**.

Pain, stiffness, diminished strength, and angular deformities are the most common complaints. Early in the degenerative process, the patient complains of pain aggravated by activities. Often, in time, pain decreases but the deformity remains. Radiologic findings include severe joint destruction, subchondral sclerosis, and osteophyte formation. The differential diagnosis usually includes inflammatory arthritides, including rheumatoid arthritis. Periarticular osteopenia and involvement of the MCP joint characteristic of rheumatoid arthritis are usually absent in erosive osteoarthritis. Nonoperative treatment of patients with PIP joint arthritis is directed toward relieving pain, reducing swelling, and protecting the joint from further deterioration. During episodes of inflammatory response, rest rather than increased activity is indicated by using a removable resting splint of a thermoplastic material to immobilize the PIP joint in full extension. Coban elastic bandage is used to wrap the finger in a circumferential manner from the fingertip to the web space of the digits in order to diminish morning swelling, and it can be used in association with the immobilization splint. Occasional injections of intraarticular glucocorticoids into the PIP joint may provide pain relief and decrease the inflammatory process. However, the authors are reluctant to prescribe this modality of treatment on a routine basis. More recently, multiple nonsteroidal antiinflammatory drugs (NSAIDs) have emerged with preeminent efficacy. Adverse effects include upper gastrointestinal intolerance, ulceration, platelet dysfunction, and renal dysfunction. NSAIDs should not be considered in the presence of recent or active peptic ulcer or upper gastrointestinal bleeding and should be used with caution in older patients (>70 years) or in patients with a history of asthma.

Surgical Therapy

Operative treatment is indicated for the PIP joint when medical management has failed to relieve the pain, when the digit deformity is interfering with hand function, or when a significant restriction of motion limits the activities of daily living. When choosing the method of surgical treatment for a painful arthritic PIP joint, consider the clinical role of the PIP joint in the patient's particular activities.

Flatt (51) noted that the PIP joint has the greatest degree of movement and functional adaptations of the hand. He has found loss of movement to be a frequent complaint, especially in the third, fourth, and fifth digits.

Stability is equally important, especially in the radial digits involved during pinching activities, in which the index finger must withstand forceful contact with the thumb, especially in the lateral or key pinch. Patients with impaired index fingers pinch with the middle finger when possible, so stability of the middle finger becomes more important when the index finger is affected also. Relatively few surgical options exist for the painful arthritic PIP joint. Most surgeries are arthroplasties or arthrodeses. There has also been limited success with joint denervation when other techniques are either not indicated or not desired by the physician or patient.

Arthroplasty

A Swanson silicone interpositional arthroplasty (52) of the PIP joint through a dorsal approach has been recommended. However, a volar surgical approach is advocated by many because it minimizes the risk of extensor lag, avoids interference with the extensor tendons, preserving the central slip, allows for more prompt active range of motion in the postoperative period, and eliminates the risk of central slip rupture with a resultant boutonniere deformity or a flexion contracture deformity.

The volar approach also has better cosmetic and functional results. This approach provides an excellent exposure, which is critical given the importance of the technique with this type of procedure. However, with the volar approach, the risk of creating a swan-neck deformity exists.

One potential shortcoming of the silicone implant is if the collateral ligaments are compromised, implantation of the device in the index or long finger PIP joint may affect lateral pinch stability. In contrast, most surface resurfacing implants preserve collateral ligaments.

Many surgeons favor a dorsal approach, with longitudinal splitting of the extensor tendon or through a distally based flap of the central slip, as described by Chamay in 1988 (53). The Chamay approach is the favored approach for surface replacement arthroplasty (SRA). Various nonsilicone implant arthroplasties are either available for use or under investigation. They include the Saffar, the Digitos, the DJO3A, the Mathy, the Ascension, and the Avanta PIP SRA.

An alternative treatment for PIP joint osteoarthritis is arthrodesis of the joint in a functional position. This option continues to be the best surgical treatment for the painful unstable PIP joint in the index or long finger, which is usually subjected to lateral stress during pinching activities. Arthrodesis offers stability, durability, and little need for further procedures. It is the procedure of choice for the index finger. However, depending upon the patient's needs, arthrodesis may impair or even be incompatible with satisfactory function. On the ulnar aspect of the hand, preservation of mobility at the level of the PIP joint is important, especially to obtain functional ability to grasp small objects. Arthrodesis of the PIP joint is indicated mainly for the index and middle fingers in patients who are young or active or when a significant loss of bone has occurred.

Surgical Methods

Arthroplasty. In the volar approach, a radial- or ulnarbased Bruner incision is made, with the apex at the PIP joint flexion crease. After the skin flap is elevated, the Grayson ligaments are completely released from their origin, exposing the neurovascular bundle. The bundle is retracted, exposing the Cleland ligaments dorsally. These also are released.

The proximal and interphalangeal transverse digital arteries, which consistently are present as communicating branches from the digital arteries, are cauterized and transected, allowing full mobilization of the neurovascular structures. The flexor tendon sheath is released by dividing the origin of the first and second cruciform pulleys and the third annular pulley at the volar plate. The volar plate is fully exposed and is released proximally and along its lateral margins from the accessory collateral ligaments, which are seen upon release of the transverse retinacular ligament from the volar capsule and tendon sheath. The collateral ligaments are then released proximally and the joint is opened by hyperextension. The flexor tendons retract to one side, and the neurovascular bundles are displaced dorsally. Both articular surfaces are completely exposed in this manner. The medullary cavities of the bone are reamed in order to accommodate the proper size of implant. After the implant is inserted in place, it is essential that full range of motion exists and the implant is stable.

Resurfacing prosthetic procedures, with or without bone cement, have been designed for the replacement of this joint. Limited experience with this design has shown promise for future consideration as an alternative treatment. The exposure for most SRAs spares the collateral ligaments; therefore, these joint replacements are an option for the index and long fingers.

Arthrodesis. The preferred position for arthrodesis of the PIP joints is 30 to 40 degrees for the index and the middle finger, 50 degrees for the ring finger, and 55 degrees for the small finger.

Several different arthrodesis techniques for the PIP joint are based on the type of fixation used. The appropriate finger position varies for the radial to the ulnar fingers and with the assessment of the patient's particular needs. K-wires, interosseous wiring, tension band wiring, and screw fixation have been used to achieve a solid nonpainful arthrodesis. The rate of nonunion is reported to be at 0% to 10%.

Postoperative Care: Primary wound healing is the first goal of postoperative care. Elevation is important to prevent swelling. Active motion of the PIP joint usually begins on the third to seventh day, as the swelling subsides. A Coban elastic bandage helps to control swelling.

Following arthrodesis surgery, the PIP joint is protected in a dorsal and volar Orthoplast splint for approximately 4 to 6 weeks. Motion of the MCP and DIP joints is allowed shortly after surgery.

A hand therapist evaluates the patient to ensure adequate splinting, joint protection, and assistive devices to carry out activities of daily living. Patients with silicone implant arthroplasties are monitored indefinitely for signs of fracture. Patients who have undergone SRAs are likewise monitored indefinitely for signs of loosening.

Patients who have undergone arthrodeses are monitored radiographically for signs of bony union. Hardware removal may become necessary but is not recommended until a year after surgery.

■ CARPAL DEGENERATIVE JOINT DISEASE

The periscaphoid area is the site of 95% of all wrist degenerative diseases. SLAC of the wrist is the most common pattern of degenerative arthritis in the wrist. Watson and Ballet (54) coined the term SLAC wrist in 1984. The hallmark of the disorder is scaphoid or S-L ligament injury with collapse on the radial side of the wrist. It is most common in the dominant wrist. A SLAC wrist pattern is the result of many radial-sided wrist pathologies. Most common is S-L dissociation with rotatory subluxation of the scaphoid. Scaphoid nonunion advanced collapse (SNAC) is another common cause **(Fig 24-18)**. Other etiologies include Preiser disease (avascular necrosis of the scaphoid), midcarpal instability, intra-articular fractures involving the RS or capitate-lunate

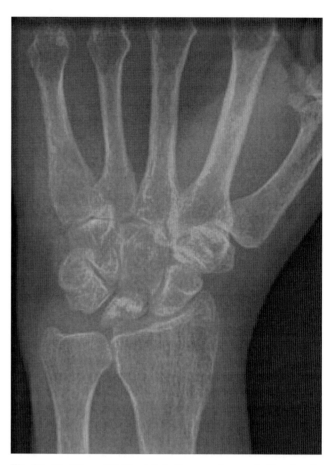

Fig 24-18. Stage 3B Kienböck disease demonstrating lunate collapse and scaphoid rotation.

joints, Kienböck disease, primary degenerative arthritis with attenuation of the S-L ligament and S-L dissociation, capitolunate degeneration, and inflammatory arthritis, such as seen in the crystalline deposition disorders of gout and calcium pyrophosphate dihydrate deposition disease (CPPD).

Pathophysiology and Staging

The distal radius has two articular fossae for the scaphoid and lunate. The scaphoid fossa is elliptical or ovoid. It narrows towards the radial styloid in a dorsal-volar plane. Thus, the scaphoid proximal articular surface is shaped like a spoon. The lunate fossa is spherical. Injury of the scaphoid or its supportive ligaments can cause radial-sided collapse with flexion of the scaphoid, thus resulting in incongruency of the RS joint.

Thus, narrowing of the RS joint first begins at the radial styloid aspect (Stage 1A). Radiographic changes appear as a sharp elongation on the radial styloid. As the disease progresses, the rest of the RS joint is destroyed (Stage 1B). In Stage 1B, the entire scaphoid fossa is involved. Complete collapse of RS joint alters the normal load-bearing ability of the capitolunate joint. This results in a radial or dorsal radial position of the capitate. Shear stress destroys cartilage in the capitolunate joint leading to the most advanced stage,

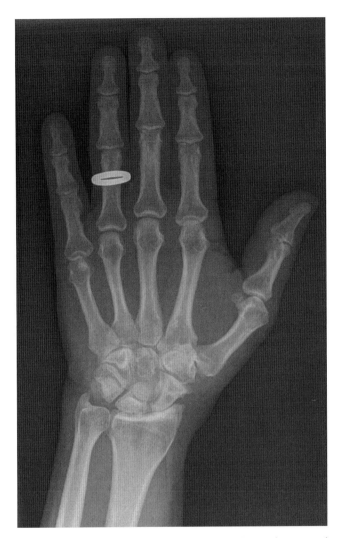

Fig 24-19. Stage II SNAC wrist, with RS narrowing and preserved capitolunate and radiolunate joints.

midcarpal SLAC (Stage 2). In Stage 2 **(Fig 24-19)**, the capitolunate joint is additionally narrowed and sclerotic. As the arthritic pattern thus progresses, it shifts from the scaphoid fossa of the radius to the midcarpal capitate articulation.

At all stages of SLAC wrist, the radiolunate joint is least involved because of its spherical shape. The lunate is congruently loaded in every position and, thus, highly resistant to degenerative changes. This sparing of the lunate fossa provides a basis for some of the motion-preserving procedures to treat SLAC wrist.

Long-standing and untreated SLAC wrist can lead to a painful wrist at rest and during use, deterioration of range of motion (ROM), and decreased grip strength. The radiographic SLAC appearance does not always correlate with the patient's symptoms.

Clinical Presentation and Evaluation

A history of wrist injury, scaphoid fracture, carpal tunnel decompression, or carpal ganglion excision may be present.

Many patients with SLAC wrist have minimal symptoms and may present because of a secondary problem, such as carpal tunnel syndrome (CTS). Patients may have a variable duration history of wrist pain during activity. Patients relate their symptoms to increased activity and overuse. Post activity pain may be present. Patients may have modified their activities, depending on the severity of symptoms. Many patients have used NSAIDs for pain relief.

Wrist edema may be present, and patients may have pain with motion, especially when loading the wrist in an extended position. Limited wrist ROM is typical, and an average wrist flexion/extension arc of 80 to 90 degrees has been reported. Direct palpation of the S-L joint or radiocarpal joint generally elicits pain. Pain with resistance against active finger extension while the wrist is held in passive flexion is common. A scaphoid shift test also elicits pain.

Plain wrist radiographs [posteroanterior (PA), lateral, and oblique] are usually sufficient to make the diagnosis and permit staging. They can reveal joint narrowing, sclerosis, osteophytes, cysts, S-L dislocation, and carpal collapse. Early changes at the RS articulation can appear as an elongated radial styloid process. The scaphoid may assume a vertical position with a cortical ring sign. In SLAC secondary to S-L dissociation, increased distance between the scaphoid and lunate as well as lunate ulnar translocation will be obvious. A lateral view can show an increase in the S-L angle with a dorsiflexion of the lunate [dorsal intercalated segment instability (DISI) deformity]. As the disease progresses, the whole RS joint becomes narrowed. In subtle cases, PA and lateral wrist CT can reveal these joint changes. For imaging of the skeletal morphology or occult fracture, CT is most useful. If avascularity is a concern, then magnetic resonance imaging is the best imaging modality.

Nagle (55) recommends staging wrist arthroscopy for articular surface evaluation since lunate fossa changes may be present in advanced cases of SLAC wrist but may not be appreciated on plain radiographs. Since scaphoid resection and ulnar column fusion in the presence of lunate fossa degenerative changes are contraindicated, an accurate assessment of the radiolunate joint is critical for correct surgical planning. When necessary, staging arthroscopy is performed as part of the definitive procedure.

Management

Nonoperative
Mild symptomatic SLAC can often be managed nonoperatively with periodic steroid injections, splinting, and NSAIDs. If the grip strength registers more than 80% that of the uninvolved wrist and the condition is not significantly impairing, then living with the condition is a valid option.

Operative Management: SLAC Reconstruction (Limited Wrist Fusion)
A SLAC reconstruction involves scaphoid excision and arthrodesis of the capitate, lunate, hamate, and triquetrum

(four-corner). Two parallel dorsal transverse incisions, a lazy S, or a central longitudinal incision over the distal radio-carpal joint and styloid process is made. The extensor retinaculum is incised through the third dorsal compartment. The terminal branch of the posterior interosseous nerve (PIN) in the floor of the fourth extensor compartment can be sacrificed as an adjunctive pain relief measure. The wrist capsule is opened over the capitolunate joint. The scaphoid is resected in piecemeal fashion. Articular cartilage and subchondral bone are removed from the capitate, lunate, hamate, and triquetrum. Care should be taken to maintain the anatomic relationship of the intercarpal intervals. Cancellous bone is harvested from the distal radius, the proximal ulna, or the iliac crest.

Lunate DISI should be corrected, and five percutaneous K-wires are used. Two wires are placed through the capitate into the lunate, one each through the hamate and triquetrum into the lunate, and a fifth wire through the triquetrum into capitate. Cancellous bone graft is packed between the interstices of the four bones.

A long arm splint is placed after the procedure. After a week, the splint is replaced with a long arm cast, which is maintained for 3 weeks. Then, a short arm cast is placed and maintained for an additional 2 to 4 weeks. The cast and wires are removed when fusion is evident on radiographs.

Alternative methods for this four-quadrant fusion, such as the use of intercalary screws and a dorsal carpal plate, are made especially for this fusion. It remains to be seen whether the increased cost of such devices results in improved outcomes. More solid fixation does enable the use of a short arm cast and an earlier initiation of wrist ROM therapy. Patients with evidence of advanced radiocarpal arthritic changes are not candidates for this limited arthrodesis, and pre-operative discussion should include other options, such as devervation, total wrist arthrodesis, or wrist arthroplasty.

Proximal Row Carpectomy. PRC requires resection of the proximal row of wrist bones to enable articulation of the capitate within the lunate fossa. For a successful procedure, both the proximal capitate articular surface and the lunate fossa should ideally be free of pathology (56). The procedure is usually effective only when the disease is restricted to the RS joint; satisfactory capitate head articular surface and lunate fossa congruity must be confirmed. PRC provides the best motion but may be associated with painful narrowing of the RC joint. It is not indicated for Stage 2 SLAC wrist. It may serve as a salvage procedure for Stages 1A and 1B when limited wrist fusion is not indicated. Failure of PRC requires conversion to wrist arthrodesis.

A dorsal longitudinal or transverse incision is used. The extensor tendons are retracted. A longitudinal capsulotomy is extended radially and ulnarly. The capitate is identified and its articular surface is inspected. In the presence of capitate degenerative changes, the procedure should not be performed. If both proximal capitate articular surface and lunate fossa are free of pathology, the scaphoid, lunate, and

triquetrum are excised. Both radioscaphocapitate and long RL ligaments are preserved. Wrist collapse follows, with placement of the capitate head in the lunate fossa along with radial deviation of the wrist. If impingement between the radial styloid and the trapezium is present, a limited radial styloidectomy is performed. Following the procedure, the wrist is splinted for 4 weeks. Early active digital flexion and extension are recommended. ROM exercises start 4 weeks after the procedure. Strengthening exercises and heavy lifting may begin 3 months after the procedure.

Total Wrist Arthrodsis. Total wrist fusion diminishes pain, but wrist function is sacrificed. Patients may have functional limitations interfering with lifestyle, but current literature supports the fact that this procedure is compatible with most activities and job duties.

Using a central, dorsal, longitudinal incision, the extensor retinaculum is incised. The incision is carried down to bone surface from middle finger metacarpal to distal radius, raising capsular and periosteal flaps. Articular cartilage and subchondral bone are resected from the RS, RL, lunocapitate, scaphocapitate, and middle finger CMC joints. The radioulnar joint should not be entered unless distal ulna resection is planned. The radial metaphysis is generally used for the necessary cancellous bone graft and more distal harvest is not required.

Bone grafts are placed in the radiocarpal, midcarpal, and CMC fusion sites, and a wrist fusion plate is applied. The fusion plate is secured with screws at the middle finger metacarpal, the capitate, and the radius. Periosteal and capsular flaps are reapproximated. A short arm splint is applied until fusion can be seen on radiographs. Fusion is usually evident in 8 weeks.

Total Wrist Arthroplasty. Total wrist arthroplasty is an alternative to diffuse arthrosis of the wrist, especially in rheumatoid arthritis and if bilateral disease is present. With bilateral disease, a combination of a total wrist arthroplasty and a contralateral total wrist fusion is an option. Numerous implants have been used; however, major complications of implant loosening and wear of the components are common. In general, indications are in the lower-demand patient, especially with contralateral disease or prior arthrodesis. Newer implants and techniques have improved survivability of this prosthesis.

■ THUMB BASAL DEGENERATIVE JOINT DISEASE

A common area of hand involvement in osteoarthritis is the CMC joint of the thumb. This is the joint that most commonly requires surgery in the osteoarthritic hand. Patients present with increasing pain at the base of the thumb. The joint space between the first metacarpal and trapezium narrows with loss of articular cartilage. Rotary motions of the joint are particularly painful. With a gradual lateral subluxation of the joint, typically the thumb develops a "shoulder" or a prominence at its base. The patient has increasing difficulty applying pressure with the thumb, making any activity requiring pinch painful. A simple activity such as opening a car door becomes difficult and painful. Secondary deformities include adduction of the metacarpal and MCP hyperextension; these can cause further limitation in function, especially in activities involving grasp.

Resting and splinting are frequently helpful in relieving pain and certainly should be tried before surgery is contemplated. Many of these patients respond to a conservative approach with relief of pain that is long-lasting in spite of advanced radiographic findings. When conservative treatment fails to relieve pain, arthroplasty affords an excellent solution. Three surgical approaches have been successful. The simplest procedure is osteotomy of the first metacarpal, which can provide satisfactory pain relief in 80% of patients (57). In another procedure, resection arthroplasty, the trapezium is removed and replaced by autogenous soft tissue, such as joint capsule or tendon. In the third approach, the trapezium is replaced by a prosthesis (58).

Resection arthroplasty gives predictable relief of pain but with some loss of pinch power and some residual proximal migration of the metacarpal. The advantages of this technique are the simplicity of surgical procedure and the consistency of satisfactory results. Other resection techniques may use a tendon sling to prevent proximal migration or to preserve the proximal half of the trapezium (59).

Trapezium replacement arthroplasties can also be used to maintain space and thumb alignment. Results with this technique, mainly using the silicone rubber trapezium prosthesis, were initially encouraging. However, this approach is surgically more demanding, and longer followup has shown increasingly frequent reports of prosthetic erosion or breakage or "Silastic synovitis" and deterioration of results (60). Thus, in most cases, complete trapezial resection with autogenous tissue interposition, with or without ligamentous reconstruction, is the procedure of choice (61).

CMC joint fusion can be successful in restoring stability and relieving pain in these patients but should be used only in patients who have localized CMC joint involvement and in whom MCP flexion is maintained. CMC joint fusion is currently advised only in traumatic arthritis in the young patient. This procedure requires 10 to 12 weeks of postoperative casting and has become less frequently used since the introduction of successful arthroplasties.

■ FLEXOR TENDON INJURIES

Flexor Tendon Anatomy

Tendons are vital structures connecting muscles to bones. The extrinsic flexors of the finger consist of the flexor digitorum profundus (FDP) and the flexor digitorum superficialis (FDS). The FDP originates from the proximal ulna and the interosseous membrane. In the forearm, it divides into two muscle groups, the most radial part supplying the index finger and the ulnar part supplying the middle, ring, and little fingers. The FDP and the flexor pollicis longus (FPL) form the deep compartment of the volar forearm, and they travel through the floor of the carpal tunnel. The FDP tendon passes through the bifurcation of the FDS before inserting into the proximal palmar base of the distal phalanx. The innervation of the FDP of the index and occasionally middle finger, and the FPL, is by the anterior interosseous branch of the median nerve (AIN), whereas the profundus of the ring and little fingers is innervated by the ulnar nerve. The FDP provides digital flexion at both the proximal and DIP joints.

The FDS has two heads: the radial head originates from the proximal shaft of the radius and the humeral ulnar head originates from the medial epicondyle of the humerus and the coronoid process of the ulna. As the FDS tendons pass through the carpal tunnel, the tendons of the middle and ring finger are more superficial and central than those of the index and little fingers. In the proximal aspect of the finger, the FDS tendon bifurcates around the FDP at the beginning of the A2 pulley. The FDS tendon slips then reunites distally at Camper chiasm, with approximately half of the fibers staying on the ipsilateral side and half crossing to the contralateral side of the finger. The tendon then inserts via radial and ulnar slips into the proximal metaphysis of the middle phalanx. The entire FDS muscle is innervated by the median nerve. The primary function of FDS is digital flexion at the PIP joints.

The FPL has two heads: the radial head originates from the proximal radius and interosseous membrane, and an accessory head originates from the coronoid process of the ulna and from the medial epicondyle of the humerus. In the palm, the FPL tendon transverses between the abductor pollicis longus (APL) and the flexor pollicis brevis (FPB). The FPL inserts into the proximal base of the distal phalanx and is innervated by the AIN. The FPL flexes both the interphalangeal and MCP joints of the thumb.

Tendons need to glide smoothly and are enclosed by synovium. The synovium also provides a source of nutrition to the tendon. It does so by producing a lubrication similar to that present in joints. This bathes the tendon and is thought to contribute to the metabolic requirements of the tendon. The other source of nutrition comes from the tendon's own blood supply **(Fig 24-20)**.

The tenosynovial sheath of the FPL is continuous with the radial bursa and the tenosynovial sheath to the little finger is continuous with the ulnar digital bursa. In some patients, these two bursae communicate, allowing a so-called "horseshoe abscess" to spread between the thumb and the little finger if the flexor tendon sheath of either digit is infected.

Biomechanics of Flexor Tendons

As the flexor tendons pass distal to the metacarpal neck, they enter the fibro-osseous tunnel, or digital flexor sheath.

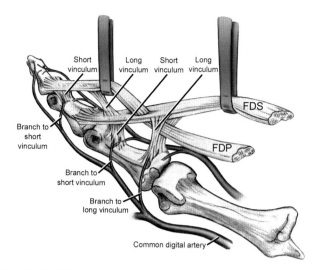

Short vinculum   Long vinculum   Short vinculum   Long vinculum

FDS

Branch to short vinculum

FDP

Branch to short vinculum

Branch to long vinculum

Common digital artery

Fig 24-20. Blood supply to flexor tendons. The direct vascular supply to the flexor tendons in the digits comes from vincula. Each tendon is supplied by two vincula. The vinculum longus superficialis and vinculum brevis superficialis supply the FDS. The vinculum longus profundus and vinculum brevis profundus supply the FDP. The vinculae are remnants of mesotenon and provide the blood supply and nutrition to the flexor tendons. The vincular system is supplied by the transverse communicating branches of the common digital artery.

The digital flexor sheath extends distally to the proximal aspect of the distal phalanx. The tendinous sheath consists of annular pulleys, which provide mechanical stability, and cruciate pulleys, which provide flexibility **(Fig 24-21)**. The first, third, and fifth annular pulleys (A1, A3, and A5) are located over the MCP, PIP, and DIP joints, respectively, while the second and fourth annular pulleys (A2 and A4) are situated over the middle portion of the proximal and middle phalanges. The moment arm, excursion, and joint rotation produced by the flexor tendons are governed by the constraint of the pulley system. The A2 and A4 pulleys are the most biomechanically important in maintaining the mechanical advantages of the flexor tendons, loss of either may diminish digital motion and power and lead to flexion contractures of interphalangeal joints (62,63).

As much as 9 cm of flexor tendon excursion may be required to produce composite wrist and digital flexion, while approximately 2.5 cm is required for full digital flexion with the wrist stabilized at neutral. The greater the distance a tendon is from the axis of joint rotation, the greater the moment arm and the less motion a given muscle contraction will generate at that joint. Conversely, a shorter moment arm will result in more joint rotation from the same tendon excursion (64).

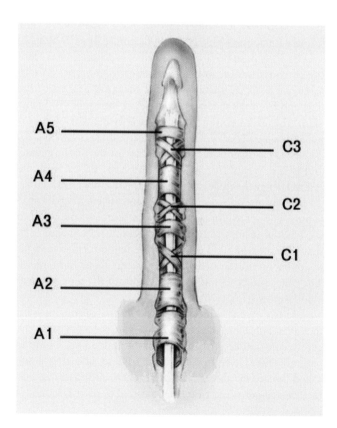

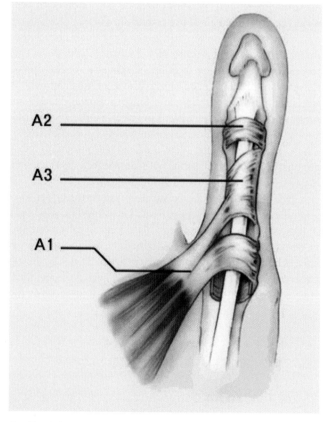

Fig 24-21. A: Digital flexor sheath. The sturdy annular *(A1-A5)* pulleys are important biomechanically in keeping the tendons closely applied to the phalanges. The thin and pliable cruciate pulleys *(C1-C3)* collapse to allow full digital flexion. **B:** Thumb: oblique pulley over proximal phalanx.

Biology of Flexor Tendon Healing

Restoration of normal hand function following tendon injury requires reestablishment not only of the continuity of the tendon fibers, but also of the gliding mechanism between the tendon and its surrounding structures. Research on the biology of tendon healing has provided a basic understanding of the processes by which tendons heal after laceration or other injuries. This healing process has three sequential phases: inflammatory, fibroblastic, and remodeling. During the inflammatory phase, inflammatory cells from the surrounding tissues migrate to the injury site. These cells phagocytize necrotic tissue and clot. During the fibroblastic phase, fibroblasts proliferate about the injury site and synthesize collagen and other components of the extracellular matrix. Finally, during the remodeling phase, newly produced collagen fibers become organized longitudinally along the axis of the tendon. Fibroblasts are the main cells in fibrotic healing reactions and are responsible for collagen deposition and the formation of scar. Two mechanisms of tendon healing have been proposed. The first is an extrinsic mechanism, whereby fibroblasts and inflammatory cells from the periphery invade the healing site to promote repair of the injured tendon. The second mechanism is the so-called intrinsic mechanism, whereby fibroblasts and inflammatory cells from within the tendon and epitenon invade the healing site. It is likely that the healing response observed clinically is a combination of extrinsic and intrinsic mechanisms (65,66). The extrinsic mechanism appears to be active earlier in the healing sequence, while the intrinsic mechanism is delayed (67).

A series of experiments have been performed recently that have demonstrated the positive effects of loading on the resultant repair strength and stiffness using a flexor tendon system. It is shown in the chicken tendon repair model, a tendon that is subjected to early active motion does not experience the decrease in repair strength in the early phase of tendon healing (68).

Zones of Flexor Tendon Injury

The anatomical relationships of the flexor tendons usually are discussed in terms of zones (Fig 24-22). The five flexor tendon zones are modifications of Verdan's original work, which based zone boundaries on anatomic factors that influenced prognosis following flexor tendon repair. The zones are numbered from distal to proximal (69):

- Zone I consists of the profundus tendon only and is bounded proximally by the insertion of the superficialis tendons and distally by the insertion of the profundus tendon into the distal phalanx.
- Zone II is also known as "no man's land," indicating the frequent occurrence of restrictive adhesion bands around lacerations in this area. Proximal to Zone II, the superficialis tendons lie superficial to the profundus tendons. Within Zone II and at the level of the proximal third of the proximal phalanx, the superficialis tendons split into two slips. These slips then divide around the profundus tendon and reunite on the dorsal aspect of the profundus, inserting into the distal end of the middle phalanx. This split of the superficialis tendon is known as Camper chiasma.
- Zone III extends from the distal edge of the carpal ligament to the proximal edge of the A1 pulley. Within Zone III, the lumbrical muscles originate from the profundus tendons. The distal palmar crease superficially marks the termination of Zone III and the beginning of Zone II.
- Zone IV includes the carpal tunnel and its contents (i.e., the nine digital flexors and the median nerve).
- Zone V extends from the origin of the flexor tendons at their respective muscle bellies to the proximal edge of the carpal tunnel.
- Thumb TI extends from the FPL insertion to A2 pulley.
- Thumb TII extends from Zone I to distal part A1 pulley. FPL tendon lacerations often retract into the thenar area or wrist; unlike the other fingers, the FPL often lacks a vinculum and does not have a lumbrical, and therefore the tendon is free to retract.
- Thumb TIII extends from Zone II to carpal tunnel. Most times, injuries also involve damage to thenar muscles and the recurrent motor branch of median nerve.

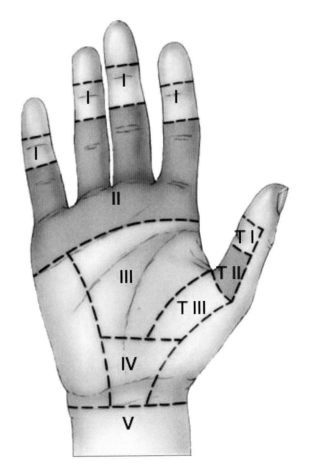

Fig 24-22. Zones of flexor tendon injury.

Clinical Evaluation of Flexor Tendon Injury

The time since injury as well as the mechanisms of injury should be noted in the history. The mechanism of injury generally includes lacerations, crush injuries, avulsions, burns, and deep abrasions. Usually, the position of the hand at the time of injury determines the tendon retraction: flexed fingers—distal tendon retracts; extended fingers—proximal tendon retracts. The resting posture of the fingers should be observed. Disruption of the normal cascade of increasing flexion in the relaxed fingers as one moves from the index finger to the little finger should arouse suspicion of tendon disruption. Tendon integrity may also be evaluated by taking advantage of the normal tenodesis positioning of the digits, which occurs as the wrist is passively brought through a range of motion and the motion of the fingers is observed. As the wrist is dorsiflexed, the digital extensors relax and the finger flexors become taught, passively flexing the fingers in the normal cascade pattern. When the muscles of the proximal forearm are squeezed, the fingers normally flex involuntarily.

Isolated testing of the superficialis and profundus tendon is employed to determine the integrity of each tendon. It is important to know that the FDS of the little finger is not independent of ring finger in some individuals, either because of cross-connections between the two tendons or because of congenital absence of the tendon. The strength of flexion should be noted as each of the tendons is tested. If the patient is able to flex the finger but experiences pain with flexion and is unable to generate full power against resistance, a partial flexor tendon injury should be suspected.

To differentiate the index finger FDP, the patient is told to pinch and pull a sheet of paper with each hand using the index fingers. If the superficialis tendon is injured, the distal IP joint will hyperflex, and the proximal IP joint will hyperextend. The finger with an intact superficialis tendon will allow hyperextension of the distal IP joint so that the maximal pulp of the finger stays in contact with the paper.

Diagnostic Imaging

Ultrasound for evaluation of soft tissue injuries has been used with success in orthopedics and sports medicine. Sonography can be used for focused assessment of the soft tissues including tendons and may be useful especially when performing a dynamic examination such as assessment for subtle tendon tears. The normal appearance of a tendon by ultrasound is hyperechoic with a fibrillar echotexture (70). Specific injuries including full and partial tears, tendonitis, and sprains have unique findings. High-frequency transducers allow assessment of the tendon architecture. A focal tendon tear may be well defined and appear anechoic or hypoechoic, with cortical irregularity. Tendonitis may present with enhanced echogenicity.

MRI has been shown to be highly sensitive in detecting tendon injuries. MRI of the hand and wrist tendons has greatly benefited from the use of dedicated surface coils, which allow fine depiction of the intricate anatomy of these structures, owing to high spatial resolution images as well as superb soft tissue contrast. Wrist and hand MRI is obtained in the axial, sagittal, and coronal planes. The axial and sagittal planes provide most of the information necessary to assess the tendons at the wrist and hand. The axial images are optimal for evaluating tendon morphology, longitudinal splits, tendon sheath fluid, and adjacent soft tissues such as overlying retinacula. The sagittal images are most useful for depicting abnormalities of the finger flexor and extensor tendons (71).

Treatment of Flexor Tendon Injuries

Functional outcomes are equivalent if the repair is done the day of injury (primary repair) or within the first 7 to 10 days after the injury (delayed primary repair). Because trauma to the flexor tendon sheath will create adverse scarring, the tendon ends must be gently retrieved, and tendons should not be grasped along their tenosynovial surfaces. The A2 and A4 pulleys should be preserved, if possible. A maximal of one centimeter may be débrided from the tendons before compromising digital extension. A core suture of either 3-0 or 4-0 braided synthetic material is secured to coapt tendon ends. The flexor tendon repair is strengthened by employing four to six strands of suture across the repair site rather than two. A running 6-0 epitendinous suture completes the tendon repair. The role of flexor tendon sheath repair remains controversial.

For Zone I injury, the tendon may be directly repaired if the distal stump is large enough, or it may be reinserted to bone. Care must be taken not to advance the tendon more than one centimeter, due to the possible cause of a quadriga hand, especially with overadvancement of the FDP repair.

For Zone II injuries, care must be taken to preserve the vincular blood supply. When both the FDS and FDP tendons are divided, it is preferable to repair both tendons because greater digital independence of motion may be achieved with a lower risk of tendon rupture during the rehabilitation period. Repair of the FDS tendon as well as the FDP tendon also diminishes the likelihood of PIP joint hyperextension deformity.

In Zone IV, the area beneath the transverse carpal ligament, a step-cut release and repair of the transverse carpal ligament should be performed to prevent flexor tendon bowstringing. Thumb TI and TII injuries are handled similarly to those of analogous finger zones. For thumb Zone TIII injuries, it is difficult to access the FPL tendon as it passes through the thenar musculature. Options for treatment of injuries at this level include either primary tendon grafting or step-cut lengthening of the tendon in the forearm, so that the repair is distal to the obscuring thenar muscles.

Immobilization of the finger after tendon repair is appropriate only in very young or otherwise uncooperative patients. The wrist should be immobilized at approximately 30 degrees of flexion, the MCP joints at approximately 45 degrees of flexion, and the interphalangeal joints at 0 to 15 degrees of flexion. A program of passive range-of-motion exercises should be initiated under the supervision of a certified hand therapist. This will decrease the adhesions at the repair site and enhance intrinsic tendon healing. Passive range-of-motion can be done either through rubber band splinting to passively flex the finger or by having the patient passively move the finger. At 4 to 6 weeks following surgery, active flexion and extension exercises are allowed as splinting is discontinued. At 6 to 8 weeks, passive extension exercise and isolated blocking is encouraged. After 8 weeks, flexion against resistance may begin.

When a four- or six-strand repair is performed, active assisted motion is begun within the first 2 weeks. In this program, the wrist is extended and the fingers are passively flexed. The patient is then asked to actively flex the fingers to hold this position. With four- and six-strand techniques for flexor tendon repair, active motion can begin earlier than with a two-strand repair. In properly motivated and compliant patients, an active hold program could begin within the first week after surgery. The hand therapist passively brings the hand into flexion and the patient is asked to maintain the position. Results for this surgical and postoperative program appear superior. The modified Duran protocol of flexor tendon rehabilitation, as supervised by a certified hand therapist, is a critical component of the post-operative care.

Partial Flexor Tendon Injuries

Basic research work has shown that the strength of the tendon is maintained even when the tendon has sustained a significant laceration. It has been shown that transverse lacerations of up to 70% would have sufficient residual strength to enable treatment by debridement. Further, it is reported that tendon repair may have an adverse effect on the mechanical properties of the repair site for smaller lacerations (72).

Clinical investigators have reported that some partial lacerations may be complicated by entrapment of the tendon within the digital sheath, triggering the tendon beneath the adjacent annular pulley and tendon rupture. To avoid the commonly reported complications of partial tendon laceration, Strickland has recommended repair of lacerations greater than 50% of the tendon and debridement of the edges for lacerations that are less than 50% of the tendon, and all cases should be evaluated for satisfactory intra-operative range of motion and tendon excursion (73).

Flexor Tendon Reconstruction

Direct repair of the flexor tendon is not possible if there is loss of the tendon substance, long-standing myostatic contracture, or unresolved soft-tissue defects. If FDS tendon is present with a full active range of PIP joint motion, arthrodesis or tenodesis of the DIP joint, creating a "superficialis finger," may be used. If the patient requires active motion at the DIP joint, tendon grafting can be done. Primary tendon grafting may be performed when there is satisfactory skin coverage,

full passive range of MCP and interphalangeal joint motion, an intact annular pulley system, minimal scarring in the sheath, adequate digit circulation, and at least one intact digital nerve. Possible donor tendons include the palmaris longus, plantaris, or toe extensor tendons.

Primary tendon repair is contraindicated if the fibro-osseous sheath is extensively scarred or if critical pulleys are absent. Restoration of flexion in such cases will require a staged tendon reconstruction. In the first stage, the tendon remnants are excised from the sheath and joint contractures are released. The A2 and A4 pulleys are reconstructed using either a flexor tendon remnant or a strip of the wrist extensor retinaculum. A silicone rod (Hunter) similar in size to the anticipated tendon graft is secured to the distal phalanx and passed within the tendon sheath. Early passive range-of-motion stimulates the development of a pseudosheath surrounding the silicone tendon rod. The second stage of the reconstruction occurs at least 3 months after the initial procedure, because full digital passive range-of-motion and soft tissue equilibrium must be achieved before the start of second stage. The silicone tendon rod is replaced with a tendon graft. The donor tendon is secured to the distal phalanx and to the donor motor in a manner similar to primary tendon grafting.

Recent studies have shown that tendons derived from intrasynovial sources are superior to extrasynovial tendons for the purpose of grafting into the synovial space. Intrasynovial donor tendons heal and incorporate into the recipient tendon using minimal adhesion formation, whereas extrasynovial tendons are associated with significant peritendinous adhesion formation (74).

Flexor Tendon Avulsion Injuries

The avulsion of the profundus tendon from the distal phalanx (Jersey Finger) occurs when the digit is forcibly extended while attempting to flex at the DIP joint. Seventy-five percent of FDP avulsion injuries involve the ring finger. Such injuries commonly occur in football or rugby, when the athlete grabs an opponent's jersey and a finger is involuntarily extended as the opponent attempts to elude tackle. The player presents with the loss of the normal cascade of the fingers and the inability to flex the DIP joint actively. It is not uncommon for this injury to be missed initially and go untreated. There is no classic diagnostic deformity, and the pathognomonic sign of loss of active flexion at the DIP joint may be dismissed because of swelling and pain. Radiographs are often negative, and pain, swelling, and ecchymosis are not always present. It is therefore important to specifically test for active flexion of the DIP joint. It is also important to localize precisely the area of maximum tenderness to try to identify the distal end of the retracted tendon. Factors that can alter the prognosis include: time from injury to treatment, the level to which the tendon retracts, the presence and size of bony avulsion, and the remaining blood supply of the tendon (75).

Avulsion injuries that are promptly recognized are best treated by anatomic repair. Recent work using a clinically relevant animal model concluded that the tendon–to-bone repair is slow. During the first 6 weeks following repair, a significant increase in the repair site strength did not occur. Repair methods that employ suture anchors to insert the tendon into cancellous bone troughs may provide the best opportunity for more rapid tendon repair. Missed or neglected profundus avulsion injuries, if symptomatic, may be treated by primary or staged tendon reconstruction or distal phalangeal joint arthrodesis.

Complications of Flexor Tendon Repair

The most common complication following flexor tendon surgery is formation of adhesions, which may occur in spite of an appropriate therapy program and compliant patient. Tenolysis should be considered when active flexion is restricted despite a normal passive range of motion in a wound that has reached soft-tissue equilibrium (usually more than 3 months since repair). Active range-of-motion therapy should begin within the first 24 hours after tenolysis surgery.

The second major postoperative complication of flexor tendon repair is rupture of the repair. When the rupture is immediately diagnosed, repair should be done a second time, because success rate approaches those of uncomplicated primary repair. If the rupture is not promptly diagnosed, the ruptured tendon ends must be resected, and either tendon grafting or staged tendon reconstruction will be done to restore active flexion.

If staged reconstruction has failed, arthrodesis or amputation of the digit may be considered, especially when neurovascular compromise occurs.

Trigger Finger (Stenosing Tenosynovitis)

Trigger digits, or stenosing tenosynovitis of the digits, are one of the most common causes of hand pain and dysfunction. Although stenosing tenosynovitis of the digital flexors is usually secondary to degenerative changes in the A-1 pulley and flexor tendons, direct pressure on the distal palm and metatarsophalangeal flexion crease from a racquet, golf club, or bat can cause acute inflammation and produce "trigger

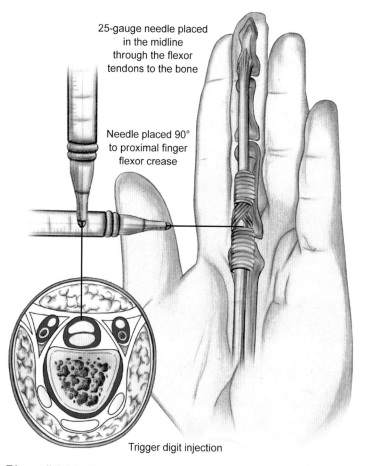

25-gauge needle placed in the midline through the flexor tendons to the bone

Needle placed 90° to proximal finger flexor crease

Trigger digit injection

Fig 24-23. Trigger digit injection. Trigger digit injection for finger is placed 90 degrees to flexor sheath at level of proximal finger flexor crease. (For thumb, place 1 cm proximal to interphalangeal flexion crease.) The 25-gauge needle is placed in the midline through the flexor tendon sheath; the needle is adjusted to avoid intratendinous injection.

finger" in the athlete. The athlete complains of pain in the flexor aspect of the digit and can experience catching or even locking. Passive extension may be required to unlock the digit or the patient may be unable to fully flex the finger. Multiple digit involvement is not uncommon nor is bilateral involvement. Chronic cases of locked trigger digits may result in fixed joint contractures. Trigger digit in children is very rare (affecting 0.05% of children) and is a separate entity from adult trigger digit. Involvement of digits other than the thumb is rare.

Clinical examination often reveals a noticeable catching of the digit during active extension from a flexed position. Tenderness is often present on the palmar aspect of the MP joint. The flexor sheath should also be palpated for a discrete nodule or diffuse tenosynovitis. Most proposed classification systems divide trigger digits to one of five grades, based on physical exam findings.

Trigger digits occur due to a size mismatch between the digital retinacular sheath and its contents, the flexor tendons and synovial sheath. Anatomically, the first annular pulley (A1) is the usual site of obstruction in trigger fingers. Preservation of the second annular pulleys (A2) in the fingers, and the oblique pulleys in the thumb, is important to prevent bowstringing of the flexor tendons, which results in decreased tendon excursion and ultimately decreased active IP joint flexion. The digital arteries are volar to the digital nerves in the palm but become dorsal to the digital nerves in the fingers. Both structures lie in close proximity to the flexor sheath, paralleling the sheath on both its radial and ulnar borders. The neurovascular bundles are at risk for injury during surgery. The radial neurovascular bundle to the thumb is the most at risk because it passes obliquely across the thenar eminence from ulnar to radial and lies just deep to the dermis at the MP joint crease.

Most primary trigger digits in adults can be successfully treated nonoperatively, including activity modification, splinting, ice, massage, NSAIDS, and corticosteroid injections. Corticosteroid injection without splinting is recommended as the initial treatment for symptomatic primary trigger digits, with success rate of 40% to 90% **(Fig 24-23)**. Patients with multiple digit involvement, symptoms lasting longer than 6 months, or diabetes mellitus respond less favorably to corticosteroid injections. Intratendinous injection should be avoided.

Surgical treatment may be indicated for nodular trigger digits that are unresponsive to a series of two corticosteroid injections or trigger digits that are locked, involve multiple digits, are due to diffuse stenosing tenosynovitis, or are of long duration (greater than 6 months). Open release of the A1 pulley is the standard surgical treatment for trigger digits. The A2 pulley in the proximal region of the proximal phalanx should be preserved. The procedure is best done under local anesthesia so that the patient may actively flex and extend the digit following A1 pulley release. A1 pulley release is not recommended in patients with rheumatoid arthritis because of the risk of exacerbating ulnar drift of the digits. Instead, flexor tenosynovectomy is performed to eliminate the cause of triggering.

In one study, triggering is eliminated with no complications in approximately 90% of patients undergoing A1 pulley release. Complications generally occur in less than 5% of patients and include scar tenderness, mild PIP flexion contractures, neurovascular bundle injuries, ulnar drift of the digit, and tendon bowstringing. Percutaneous A1 pulley release has been proposed as an alternative technique and has been reported successful in approximately 93% of patients treated (76). But some authors recommend not performing percutaneous release in the thumb and the index finger because the neurovascular bundle may be at increased risk.

■ EXTENSOR TENDON INJURIES

Extensor Tendon Anatomy

The extrinsic extensor tendons are divided into superficial and deep groups based on their position in the forearm. The superficial group is composed of the extensor carpi radialis longus and brevis (ECRL and ECRB), the extensor digitorum communis (EDC), extensor digiti minimi (EDM), and extensor carpi ulnaris (ECU). The deep group consists of the APL, EPB, and extensor indicis proprius (EIP). All the above muscles are innervated by the deep branch of the radial nerve, the PIN.

The extrinsic extensors run through six different fibro-osseous retinacular compartments at the wrist level **(Table 24-1)**.

The first compartment is the most radial and contains the APL and the EPB. The APL inserts at the base of thumb metacarpal and radially abducts the thumb, whereas the EPB inserts on the dorsum of the proximal aspect of the proximal phalanx of the thumb and actively extends the MCP joint of the thumb.

TABLE 24-1	Extrinsic Extensor Compartments	
Compartment	**Tendons**	**Anatomy Notes**
1.	EPB, APL	Both in separate synovial sheaths
2.	ECRL, ECRB	Radial to Lister tubercle
3.	EPL	Ulnar to Lister tubercle
4.	EDC, EIP	Common synovial sheath
5.	EDM	Double tendon, over DRUJ
6.	ECU	Lies over distal ulna

EPB, extensor pollicis brevis; APL, abductor pollicis longus; ECRL, extensor carpi radialis longus; ECRB, extensor carpi radialis brevis; EPL, extensor pollicis longus; EDC, extensor digitorum communis; EIP, extensor indicis proprius; EDM, extensor digiti minimi; ECU, extensor carpi ulnaris.

The second extensor compartment contains the ECRL and the ECRB. The ECRL, inserting on the index metacarpal, dorsiflexes and radially deviates the wrist, and the ECRB, inserting into the base of the middle metacarpal, provides balanced wrist dorsiflexion.

The third compartment contains the EPL, which runs longitudinally down the forearm through the third compartment and turns abruptly radial-ward about Lister's tubercle, a dorsal prominence on the distal radius. Inserting

on the distal phalanx, the EPL provides forceful extension of the thumb interphalangeal joint.

The fourth extensor compartment contains the EIP and the EDC, while the fifth compartment contains the EDM. These three muscles each have a role in digital extension at the MCP, PIP, and DIP joints of the fingers. The principal bony insertion of the extrinsic digital extensors is on the dorsal proximal aspect of the middle phalanx. MCP joint extension is provided by extrinsic extensor force transmitted

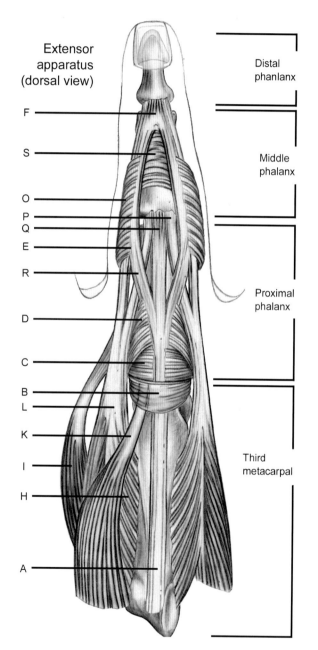

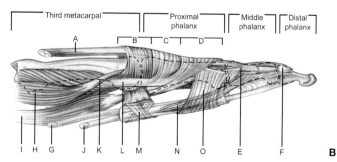

Fig 24-24. Anatomy of the extensor apparatus of the finger. **A:** Dorsal. **B:** Lateral *(A)* EDC tendon, *(B)* sagittal bands, *(C)* transverse fibers of the interossei, *(D)* oblique fibers of the interossei, *(E)* lateral conjoined tendon, *(F)* terminal tendon, *(G)* FDP tendon, *(H)* interosseous muscle (2nd dorsal), *(I)* lumbrical muscle, *(J)* FDS tendon, *(K)* medial tendon, superficial head of 2nd dorsal interosseous, *(L)* lateral tendon of deep head of 2nd dorsal interosseous, *(M)* fibrous flexor pulley, *(N)* oblique retinacular ligament, *(O)* transverse retinacular ligament, *(P)* medial interosseous band, *(Q)* central slip of the common extensor, *(R)* lateral slip of the common extensor, *(S)* triangular ligament

through the sagittal bands. DIP joint extension is achieved through the conjoined lateral bands that are composed of tendinous slips from the extrinsic and intrinsic tendons. The EIP inserts on the index finger ulnarly to the EDC. The EDC inserts on the index, middle, ring, and, in some cases, little fingers. The EDM tendon inserts on the little finger ulnar ward to the EDC insertion.

The ECU tendon runs through the sixth compartment and inserts at the base of the little finger metacarpal. It provides wrist extension and ulnar deviation.

The intrinsic muscles of the hand are intricately connected to the extensor mechanism. The lumbricals arise from the tendon of the FDP and are innervated by the median (for the index and long fingers) and the ulnar (for the ring and small fingers) nerves. There are three palmar and four dorsal interosseous muscles. The palmar interossei adduct the fingers and the dorsal interossei abduct the fingers. All the intrinsic muscles course palmar to the axis of the MCP joint and dorsal to the axis of the PIP joint, therefore acting to extend the proximal and DIP joints while flexing the MCP joints.

The extensor tendons on the dorsum of the hand are interconnected by the juncturae tendinum: narrow connective tissue bands proximal to the MCP joint that extend between the EDC tendons as well as to the EDM, although rarely to the EIP. The juncturae tendinum pass distally and obliquely between the ulnar three EDC tendons and are primarily responsible for grouped extension. Laceration of the juncturae may cause snapping and subluxation of the EDC tendon over the MCP joint. Conversely, laceration of the extensor tendon may be masked by an intact juncturae because of the bridging between tendons.

At the level of metacarpophalangeal joint (MCPJ), the sagittal bands centralize the extensor tendon and connect to the volar plate of the MCPJ and to the periosteum of the proximal phalanx. The sagittal bands act as a support sling for the MCPJ and aid the EDC tendon with joint extension. Distal to the MCPJ, the extrinsic and intrinsic tendons blend into a thin sheet of complex fibers called the dorsal apparatus. The continuation of the extrinsic extensor tendon is the central slip, inserting into the base of the middle phalanx.

Biomechanics of Extensor Tendons

The extensor tendons have much fewer excursions than the flexor tendons and therefore even minimal shortening results in a significant decrease in joint motion **(Fig 24-24)**. The EDC has an average excursion of 50 mm, as compared to the FDP (excursion of 70 mm). It has been shown that 6 mm of shortening in the extensor tendon produces an 18 degree decrease in motion at both the MCP and the PIP joints (77).

The dorsal apparatus is frequently referred to as the extensor mechanism. Through dorsal hood attachments, the extrinsic extensor muscles extend the MCPJ, the intrinsic muscles flex the MCPJ, and both the intrinsic and extrinsic muscles extend the proximal and DIP joints.

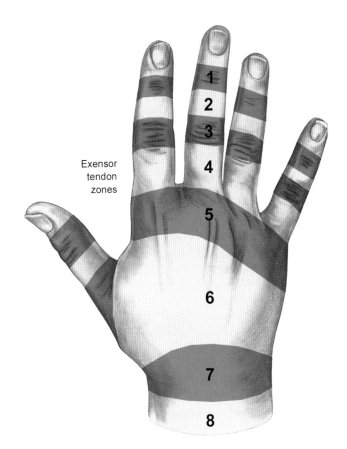

Exensor tendon zones

Fig 24-25. The eight extensor tendon zones.

Extension of the MCPJ is achieved through the action of the extrinsic extensor tendons pulling through the sagittal band sling mechanism, which lift up the proximal phalanx. Flexion of the MCPJ is achieved both by the tendinous insertion of the intrinsics on the proximal phalanx and by a similar sling effect with oblique fibers of the intrinsic mechanism blending into the hood and converging at the level of the central slip to create a sling, which flexes the MCPJ. Extension of the PIP joint is achieved through the action of the central slip, which is the bony insertion of the extrinsic digital extensors on the middle phalanx. In addition, the intrinsic muscles contribute to PIP joint extension through medial slips from the lateral band, which run centrally to insert on the proximal dorsal aspect of the middle phalanx as part of the central slip.

DIP joint extension is achieved through both intrinsic and extrinsic forces pulling through the radial and ulnar conjoined lateral bands, which merge to form the terminal tendon insertion. The intrinsic contribution to the conjoined lateral band is through its insertion into the lateral band. The extrinsic contribution to DIP joint extension occurs through lateral slip fibers that diverge from the central slip over the dorsum of the proximal phalanx and join the lateral band to form the conjoined lateral band. The conjoined lateral bands from the radial and ulnar side converge distally as the terminal tendon inserting on the distal phalanx.

The Eight Extensor Tendon Zones. The extensor mechanism is often divided into eight zones for the evaluation and treatment of extensor tendon injuries (**Fig 24-25**). The odd-numbered zones are located over joints and the even-numbered zones are over bones. Zone VIII, the most proximal zone, contains the musculotendinous junction of the extrinsic extensors in the forearm. Zone VII lies over the carpus and includes the area of the extensor retinaculum where the tendons are within the tenosynovial sheaths. The dorsum of the hand contains both the extensor tendons and the juncturae tendinum and is considered Zone VI. The level of the MCP joints is Zone V, where the extensor tendon is held in place by the sagittal bands. Zone III is over the PIP joints and zone I is over the DIP joints. The thumb is numbered differently owing to its differing number of phalanges: TI is over the interphalangeal joint, TIII is over the MCP joint, and TV is over the radiocarpal joint.

The vascular supply to the extensor apparatus varies depending on the zone. In Zone I through Zone VI, nutrition is through perfusion through the paratenon. In Zone VII, nutrition is through diffusion from the synovium. In Zone VIII, small arterial branches from the surrounding fascia provide vascularity.

Clinical Evaluation and Imaging of Extensor Tendon Injury

A careful evaluation of the injured hand, including neurovascular examination and flexor tendon function, is very important in treatment of extensor tendon injuries. Appropriate radiographs should be obtained to assess bony involvement. Of note, MR imaging shows in detail the musculotendinous and retinacular structures of the extensor apparatus. In the different extensor zones, MR imaging findings are similar to those seen macroscopically in anatomic sections (78).

The wound should be thoroughly inspected and attention given to possible violation of the joint capsule. Injuries that involve substantial loss of bone or overlying soft tissue should be treated first with adequate irrigation and debridement. Skeletal stabilization and skin coverage are priorities.

Lacerations in Zones V through VIII may affect MCP joint extension. Evaluation should be performed with the wrist in neutral extension and the PIP joints in full extension to eliminate the contributions from the intrinsic muscles on joint extension. The patient should be asked to fully extend each finger at the MCP joint against gentle resistance. A complete laceration of the extensor tendon usually manifests as incomplete MCP extension.

Injuries proximal to the juncturae tendinum in Zone VI require special attention, because a finger may extend fully even if the tendon is fully lacerated. While holding all other fingers flexed at the MCP joint and blocking the pull of the juncturae tendinum, the patient is asked to extend each finger individually against gentle resistance.

Treatment of Extensor Tendon Lacerations

Various techniques have been described for repair of an extensor tendon laceration. It is important to know that the extensor tendons have fewer excursions than the flexor tendons and even minimal shortening will result in significant decrease in motion.

The ideal suture technique would generate minimal shortening and maximal tensile strength with a high load to failure. Most suture techniques are considerably weaker than those achieved when similar techniques are used on flexor tendons. Of the commonly used repair techniques for extensor tendons, the modified Kessler or modified Bunnell techniques have been shown to produce the strongest results with minimal gapping and least amount of loss-of-motion. For lacerations in Zone I through VI, nonabsorbable 4-0 or 5-0 sutures provide adequate strength to the repair. The lateral bands should be repaired separately with 5-0 or 6-0 nonabsorbable sutures, if they have been damaged. In Zones VI and VII, 4-0 sutures provide adequate strength. In Zone VIII, repair is best accomplished with 3-0 sutures. Of note, small tapered needles in Zones VI and VII should be used to prevent shredding of the thin, flat tendon (79).

Rehabilitation of Extensor Tendon Injuries

Static splinting has a long history with well-documented results following extensor tendon repairs in the various zones. However, immobilized tendons lose strength over time and aggressive rehabilitation following prolonged immobilization can further attenuate the repair. Recently, attention has been turned to early active motion using dynamic splinting to improve results. Controlled early motion has been shown to increase tensile strength of tendons and improve gliding properties.

Dynamic extension splinting allows several millimeters of extensor gliding without placing stress across the repair site. This splinting technique has improved outcomes in repairs in the proximal extensor zones (80). The splint is applied dorsally 3 to 5 days after injury and the wrist is held in 30 degrees of extension with the MCP joints in 10 to 15 degrees of flexion. The IP joints are held in full extension by rubber bands attached to slings.

For Zones III and IV injuries, static splinting of the involved digit is used for 4 to 6 weeks after repair, followed by active range-of-motion for 2 weeks until passive motion can be started.

Complications of Extensor Tendon Injuries

In addition to extensor tendon injuries, complex injuries to the dorsum of the hand are complicated with skin loss, nerve injuries, and multiple fractures. Soft tissue management and skeletal stabilization are very important for an optimal functional outcome. Tendon injuries are commonly complicated by adhesion formation with secondary loss of motion in both extension and flexion. Treatment should begin with aggressive hand therapy regime and may require tenolysis or capsulotomies. Immediate postoperative active motion is necessary to prevent recurrent adhesion formation.

Mallet Finger (Zone I Injuries)

Disruption of the extensor tendon over the DIP joint results in the classic "mallet finger" deformity. Mallet finger is also referred to as "baseball finger" and "drop finger." It is most commonly seen in softball, baseball, basketball, and football players. This injury is usually caused by a direct blow to the tip of the extended finger, which forces the distal phalanx into flexion. A mallet finger can also result from a direct blow to the dorsum of the DIP joint or secondary to a hyperextension force at this joint. There is disruption of the extensor mechanism over the dorsum of the DIP joint. The resultant deformity is caused by unopposed flexion of the distal phalanx. Clinically, the athlete has pain and swelling on the dorsum of the DIP joint with lack of active extension at this joint.

The mallet deformity can be caused by disruption of the terminal extensor mechanism through its substance or associated with an avulsed bony fragment (the "bony mallet"). It is believed that the degree of flexion present during disruption of the extensor tendon will determine whether or not there is an associated bony avulsion. If the tear is through the substance of the tendon, the radiograph is normal except for a flexion deformity at the DIP joint.

Four types of mallet finger injuries have been described: Type I: closed, with or without avulsion fractures; Type II, laceration at or proximal to the DIP joint with loss of tendon continuity; Type III, deep abrasion with loss of skin, subcutaneous soft tissue, and tendon substance; Type IVa, transepiphyseal plate fracture in children; Type IVb, hyperextension injury with fracture of the articular surface of 20% to 50%; Type IVc: fracture of the articular surface greater than 50% with palmar subluxation of the distal phalanx.

The treatment for a mallet finger deformity depends on the patient's age, mechanism of injury, associated fractures, and the chronicity of the injury (81). Closed acute mallet fingers are best treated by continuous splinting in extension for at least 6 weeks (82). Active PIP joint motion should be maintained during splinting to avoid a swan neck deformity **(Fig 24-26)**. The patient may be gradually weaned from splinting after 6 to 8 weeks of continuous treatment. If deformity recurs at this point, full-time splinting should be restarted. After the initial period of continuous treatment, nighttime splinting should continue for at least 6 more weeks. Care should be taken to avoid complications such as skin necrosis. Dorsal splints that hold the DIP joint in slight hyperextension may be more effective.

Type II mallet finger deformity should be repaired with a simple figure-of-eight suture through the tendon only or incorporating the tendon and skin in the same suture (dermatotenodesis). Type III injuries usually require soft tissue coverage and primary grafting or late reconstruction. Type IVa usually is a Salter-Harris Type II injury and should be managed with closed reduction and splinting. Type IVb injuries heal well with closed treatment for articular surface remodeling. Type IVc injuries with palmar subluxation of the distal phalanx are usually treated with ORIF with a K-wire and possibly using a pullout suture with a button.

Chronic mallet finger injuries that are up to 12 weeks old and are still flexible may respond to conservative treatment with full-time splinting. Failure of response to splinting is an indication for advancement of the terminal tendon to bone with an associated dermodesis and a transarticular K-wire. If the deformity is rigid, arthrodesis may be a better treatment choice. A swan neck deformity occurs with chronic mallet finger deformity resulting in hyperextension of the PIP joint as the central extensor tendon retracts and the lateral bands subluxate dorsally. Treatment includes ligament reconstruction using the spiral oblique retinacular ligament or a superficialis tenodesis, or conservative treatment with long-term splinting.

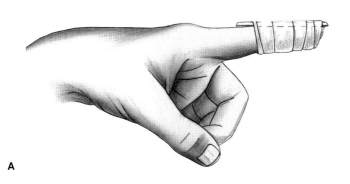

A

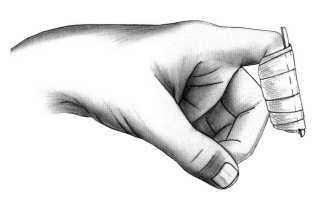

B

Fig 24-26. DIP splinting for "mallet finger" deformity.

DeQuervain Syndrome

DeQuervain's syndrome is stenosing tenosynovitis of the first dorsal compartment of the wrist, which contains the APL and EPB tendons. It is the most common tendinitis of the wrist in athletes. Sports most commonly associated with DeQuervain's syndrome include golf, racquet sports (especially racquetball, badminton, and squash), and fishing.

Patients usually present with radial-sided wrist pain exacerbated by thumb movements, especially thumb abduction and/or extension. Pain may radiate distally or proximally along the course of the APL and EPB tendons. Localized swelling and tenderness may be present over the first dorsal compartment, 1 to 2 cm proximal to the radial styloid process. Symptoms are usually present for weeks to months by the time of presentation. On physical examination, tenderness over the first dorsal compartment is present, and a positive Finkelstein test is pathognomic for the diagnosis. This test is performed by flexing the thumb into the palm and passively deviating the wrist ulnarly, thus causing maximum stretch to the APL and EPB tendons. In chronic cases, thickening of the fibrous sheath and occasionally a ganglion cyst can be present. Thumb CMC joint, radiocarpal, and intercarpal arthritis can be distinguished from DeQuervain syndrome based on radiographs, although the conditions may co-exist.

The anatomy of the first dorsal compartment of the wrist is highly variable. Failure to recognize these anatomic variations could lead to treatment failure in DeQuervain syndrome. The EPB tendon is rounder and smaller than the APL and absent in approximately 5% of individuals. The APL usually has two or more tendon slips and may insert onto the trapezium, volar carpal ligament, opponens pollicis, or abductor pollicis brevis, in addition to the consistent insertion onto the base of the first metacarpal. In up to 34% of cadaveric specimens, the first dorsal compartment is subdivided by a septum into two separate fibro-osseous tunnels, with the EPB tendon in the ulnar tunnel and the APL tendon slips in the radial tunnel. A higher incidence of subdivided first dorsal compartments is reported in patients with DeQuervain syndrome, suggesting that separate fibro-osseous tunnels may predispose to developing DeQuervain syndrome (83). The deep branch of the radial artery passes through the anatomic snuff-box distal to the radial styloid process and just deep to the first and second dorsal compartments, and need not be exposed during first dorsal compartment release. Several branches of the superficial radial nerve lie within the subcutaneous fat overlying the first dorsal compartment and should be preserved during surgical approaches.

Treatment options of DeQuervain syndrome depend on the stage at presentation, and include splinting, corticosteroid injections, and various techniques of surgical release of the first dorsal compartment. Splinting alone may be beneficial for acute symptomatic relief but has shown an approximately 70% failure rate. Corticosteroid injections into the first dorsal compartment are a moderately effective nonoperative treatment option. Single injections into the first dorsal compartment sheath are successful in alleviating symptoms in 62% of patients and two injections are successful in 80% of patients. Complications of corticosteroid injections include depigmentation, fat necrosis, and subcutaneous atrophy. Furthermore, corticosteroid injections in diabetic patients may be less desirable and less successful.

For surgical approaches for DeQuervain syndrome, care must be taken to protect and avoid excessive dissection of the superficial radial nerve and its branches. Symptoms secondary to superficial radial nerve injury may be far more severe than those due to DeQuervain syndrome alone. In a septated first dorsal compartment, complete release of both fibro-osseous tunnels is recommended. Most authors agree that sheath excision is unnecessary and could predispose the patient to symptomatic volar tendon subluxation. Volar subluxation of the APL and EPB tendons can be treated with a retinacular sling or a lip of brachioradialis tendon. Ninety percent of patients can be expected to have satisfactory outcomes following surgical release of the first dorsal compartment for DeQuervain syndrome (84).

■ DISTAL RADIAL FRACTURE

Fractures of the distal radius are among the most common of all skeletal injuries. These fractures are the most frequent type of bone injury in the upper extremity; they occur in athletes of all ages, from preadolescent to the elderly (85). Distal radius fractures are more common in the adolescent athlete than in the adult. Distal radius injuries in the athlete typically occur secondary to high energy and they are encountered most often in the impact sports such as football, basketball, snow boarding, rollerblading, and soccer; in the racquet and stick sports such as baseball, tennis, hockey, golf, skiing, and racquetball; and in the apparatus or external contact sports such as gymnastics, rock climbing, and weight lifting. Distal radius fractures can occur, however, in any athletic activities where falling onto the outstretched hand is possible, such as horseback riding and cycling.

Anatomy

The wrist is an extremely complex joint. The distal end of the radius is the anatomic foundation of the wrist joint. Both stability and mobility are dependent on the design and interaction of the radius with its carpal and ulnar articulations. Beginning 2 to 3 cm proximal to the radiocarpal joint at the metaphyseal flare, the distal radius is unique to transmit axial load and provide mobility. The distal articular surface is biconcave and triangular in shape. The apex of the triangle points to the radial styloid process, and the base of the triangle forms the sigmoid notch, which articulates with the distal end of the ulna. The articular surface of the distal radius is separated into two distinct facets, and they articulate individually with the scaphoid and lunate. These facets are concave in both the AP and the radioulnar directions. The articular surface slopes in an ulnar and palmar direction, so the carpus has a natural tendency to slide in this direction. This tendency is resisted by the intracapsular and interosseous carpal ligaments.

The sigmoid notch is semicylindrical and oriented parallel to the ulnar head. This articulation plays an important role in the functional anatomy of the hand and wrist, as the radius and hand rotate about the fixed ulna. It has been shown in cadaveric studies that this rotation of the radius about the ulna is also accompanied by a relative volar translation of the ulna with forearm supination and a relative dorsal translation with forearm pronation.

The TFC arises from the ulnar aspect of the lunate facet of the radius and extends on to the base of the ulnar styloid process to function as another important stabilizer of the distal radial ulnar joint.

Biomechanics

Axial compressive loads pass through the carpus mostly to the radius, and, to a much lesser degree, the ulnar head. Approximately 46% of the contact force across the carpus is transmitted through the lunate fossa and 43% through the scaphoid fossa, and only 11% through the ulnar side of the wrist (86). A cadaveric study has shown that the load through the ulna increased from 21% to 67% as the angulation of the distal radial fragment from 10 degrees of palmar tilt to 45 degrees of dorsal tilt (87). Loss of palmar tilt has also been associated with a pattern of midcarpal instability, most commonly seen in younger patients. In a clinical series of patients with fracture malunions that result in a dorsal collapse alignment of the carpus, dynamic instability developed resulting in pain and decreased grip

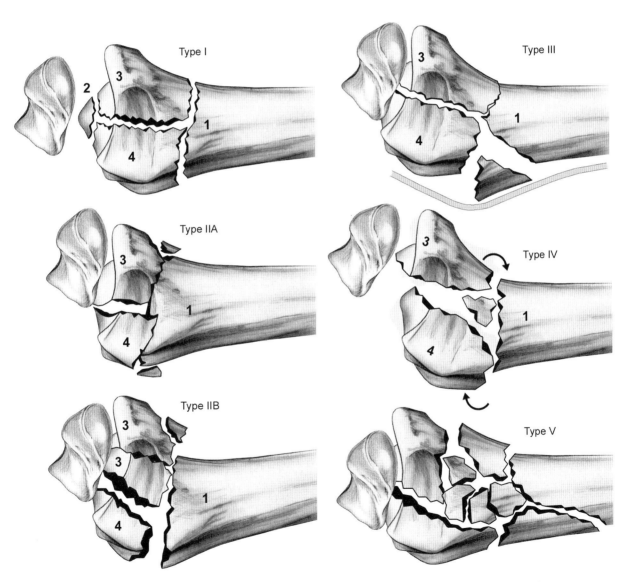

Fig 24-27. The Melone Distal Radius Fracture Classification. This classification incorporates the underlying pattern of fracture with four relatively constant readily identifiable components: *(1)* metaphyseal or shaft, *(2)* radial styloid, *(3)* dorsal medial, and *(4)* palmar medial fragments. Fractures Type I to Type V demonstrate progressive instability as well as comminution.

strength. It has also been shown that of all radial deformities, radial shortening has the greatest influence on DRUJ function, which is manifested as limited rotation of the forearm and impingement of the ulna.

Rikli et al. (88) divided the distal metaphyseal and articular regions into three columns: a medial column comprising the distal ulna, the TFC, and the DRUJ, an intermediate column including the medial part of the distal radius with its lunate fossa and sigmoid notch, and a lateral column comprising the scaphoid fossa and the radial styloid process.

Classifications

There are many classification systems for describing distal radius fractures. The more commonly used systems are the Frykman, Fernandez, Melone, and the A.O. The Melone classification is particularly helpful in recognizing and treating intra-articular distal radius fractures **(Fig 24-27)**. He observed that the components of the radiocarpal articular surface appeared to fall into four basic parts: radial shaft, radial styloid, dorsal medial fragment, and palmar medial fragment. He defines the medial fragments of the lunate facet and their strong ligamentous attachments with the proximal carpal bones as the "medial complex." The extent and direction of displacement of the fragments formed the basis of this classification as well as the prognostic view of the fracture reducibility and stability. The progression of the classification is from nondisplaced stable configuration to a pattern of displacement, comminution, and instability (89).

The AO system is the most detailed classification system to date and is organized in order of increasing severity of the bony and articular lesions. This classification divides these fractures into extra-articular (Type A), partial articular (Type B), and complete articular (Type C). Each type can be further divided into three main groups. These, in turn, can be further subdivided to reflect the morphologic complexity, difficulty of treatment, and prognosis (90).

One component of distal radius fractures that has not been the subject of extensive classification is injury to the DRUJ. Three basic types of DRUJ lesions have been established: Type I, stable lesions, the DRUJ is clinically stable and the radiographs show the radioulnar joint to be congruous. The primary stabilizers of the DRUJ, including the TFCC and capsular ligaments, are intact. These lesions include avulsion of the tip of the ulnar styloid and a stable fracture of the ulnar neck. Type II, unstable lesion, the DRUJ is subluxated or dislocated. There is either a massive substance tear of the TFCC or an avulsion fracture of the base of ulnar styloid. Type III, potentially unstable lesions, and they reflect skeletal disruption of the distal radioulnar articular surfaces of the sigmoid notch (four-part fracture of the distal radius) or the ulnar head.

Clinical Evaluation and Diagnosis

A complete history and physical examination is critical to the appropriate care of patients with distal radius fractures.

The diagnosis is typically obvious in most patients with wrist fractures. The wrist is displaced dorsally with associated ecchymosis and tenderness over the fracture site. Detailed neurovascular examination with special attention to the function of the median nerve is indicated.

The diagnosis is confirmed by radiographs. The standard views for examination of the distal radius include a PA, a true lateral, and an oblique view. Especially, oblique views are useful in degree, if any, of intra-articular involvement. In addition, a "facet" lateral view, done by tilting the beam 20 degrees distal to proximal to simulate normal radial inclination, gives a better assessment of the subchondral articular surface and the degree of dorsal angulation.

The role of advanced imaging techniques such as arthrography, CT, and arthroscopy continues to be explored. The diagnostic role of arthroscopy is reinforced with a study of 50 patients who sustained displaced distal radius fractures. All patients but one were found to have a ligamentous injury in the wrist (91).

Treatment of Distal Radius Fractures

There are four principles in the treatment of distal radius fractures: restoration of articular congruity and axial alignment, maintenance of reduction, achievement of bony union, and restoration of hand and wrist function. Several excellent treatment algorithms can be used to assist the orthopedist in the decision-making process. However, there is currently no consensus regarding the treatment of unstable distal radial fractures, which are defined by the presence of metaphyseal comminution, intra-articular extensions, shearing fractures, radiocarpal fracture-dislocations, or reduction that cannot be maintained with a cast (92).

Nonoperative Treatment

Extra-articular, nondisplaced fractures and displaced, stable, reducible fractures are managed best with cast or splint immobilization and early therapy. In general, closed treatment of distal radius fractures requires weekly vigilance. By definition, progressive displacement after reduction implies failure to appreciate initial instability and warrants modification.

Operative Treatment

Displaced, stable fractures are treated best with closed reduction under anesthesia and percutaneous pin fixation.

External fixation is a commonly utilized method for fixation of unstable distal radius fractures. A fixator is typically indicated for a fracture that demonstrates significant comminution in both the volar and dorsal cortical surfaces of the radius. Several recent studies have reported the difficulty in achieving and maintaining volar tilt with an external fixator alone. To achieve improved stability, the fracture should be augmented with one or two trans-styloid K-wires and one or two dorsal-to-volar wires.

Internal fixation with a dorsal plate for dorsally comminuted fractures is a viable option for unstable extra-articular fractures with extensive comminution. However, this technique may be complicated by interference with the extensor tendon system. To address this issue, several newer low-profile plate systems with countersunk screw heads have been developed for dorsal fixation.

Volar plating is a relatively new concept in treating extra-articular distal radius fractures (93). This technique employs a fixed angle plate with traditional blade plate "tongs" or a number of screws or smooth pegs that lock into threaded screw holes in the plate to provide a shelf, or cantilever, on which the subchondral bone rests. A plate on the volar surface is attractive because of the ease of the operative approach and the abundant soft tissue sleeve to protect digital and wrist tendons.

Intra-articular distal radius fractures still present the greatest challenge. Even nondisplaced, stable intra-articular fractures can be associated with serious ligamentous or TFCC injuries, as discussed above. Certainly, the displaced and unstable intra-articular fractures will require some modality of surgical treatment. Closed reduction under anesthesia with percutaneous pinning (94), pins and plaster, external fixation (95) limited open reduction, ORIF including plate fixation (96), and small implant "fragment-specific" fixation (97), supplemental bone grafting, and arthroscopically assisted reduction and internal fixation (98) are all viable treatment options.

Rehabilitation

In general, there is currently no consensus regarding whether or not a true benefit exists to physical therapy in the management of distal radius fractures. Investigation is needed to identify which patients and which treatments are best suited for physical therapy after high-energy distal radius fractures.

It is important to maintain the athlete in good physical condition through combined vigorous training while the wrist fracture is protected by cast, external fixator, or splint.

If the fracture is stable and the acute symptoms of the injury have resolved, the athlete could return to competition in a custom-molded silicone wrist splint. It must be emphasized, however, that unrestrained activity before stable distal radius fracture union is an unacceptable risk that could lead to serious complications.

■ SCAPHOID FRACTURES

Carpal scaphoid fractures are the most common and yet the most problematic fractures in the wrists of athletes. Although the true incidence is unknown because many people remain asymptomatic throughout life, it is reported to account for approximately 70% of all carpal fractures and is most prevalent in the 15- to 30-year-old population (99).

Anatomy

Scaphoid means "boat" in Greek. The scaphoid bone has an irregular shape, and it has a concave curvature in both the palmar and ulnar direction. It is tilted both palmarly and radially 45 degrees. Approximately 80% of the scaphoid surface is covered by articular cartilage. It is well documented that dorsal vessels supply 70% to 80% of vascularity, the majority of which enters at the dorsal ridge of the scaphoid **(Fig 24-28)**. Intra-osseous blood flow is retrograde, leaving the proximal pole with a tenuous blood supply (100). The vascular anatomy explains the slower healing time (up to 10 months), increased risk of osteonecrosis (up to 60%), and nonunion in proximal pole fractures (101).

The synchronous motion of the carpal bones during wrist motion depends on the rotation of the scaphoid. Many ligaments, both intrinsic and extrinsic, attach to the scaphoid. Intrinsic ligaments connect carpal bones while extrinsic

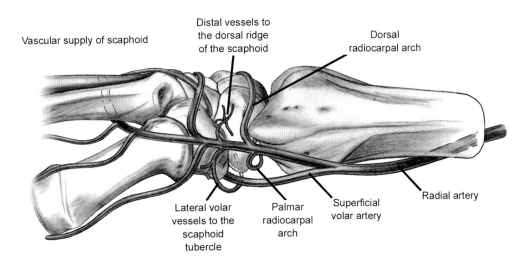

Fig 24-28. The vascular supply of the scaphoid arises from dorsal branches of the radial artery, which perforate the distal third of the dorsal cortex of the scaphoid.

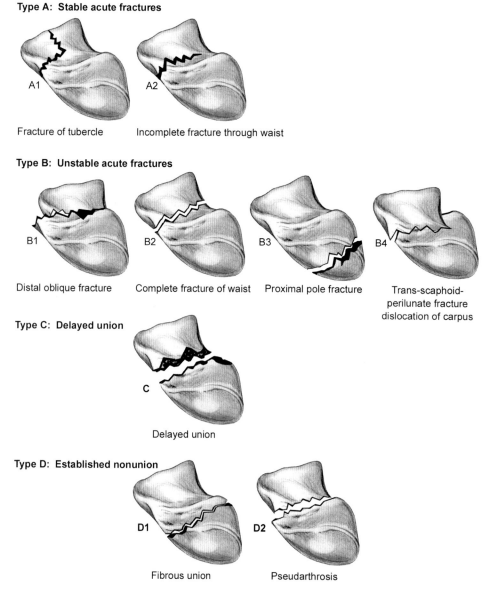

Type A: Stable acute fractures

A1 — Fracture of tubercle

A2 — Incomplete fracture through waist

Type B: Unstable acute fractures

B1 — Distal oblique fracture

B2 — Complete fracture of waist

B3 — Proximal pole fracture

B4 — Trans-scaphoid-perilunate fracture dislocation of carpus

Type C: Delayed union

C — Delayed union

Type D: Established nonunion

D1 — Fibrous union

D2 — Pseudarthrosis

Fig 24-29. Herbert classification of scaphoid fractures.

ligaments cross the radiocarpal joint. As the wrist is radially deviated, the scaphoid flexes. If the S-L ligaments are intact, the lunate is also slightly flexed. As the wrist is ulnarly deviated, the scaphoid extends. The average S-L angle is 45 degrees (range: 30 to 60 degrees) with the distal scaphoid tilted palmarly. In displaced fractures, a "humpback" deformity of the scaphoid can occur. If left untreated, the S-L angle can be greater than 60 degrees. This in turn can develop into midcarpal arthritis or scaphoid nonunion.

Biomechanics of Scaphoid Fractures

The pattern of scaphoid fractures depends on the force and position of the wrist. The most common mechanism of

scaphoid fractures is a fall on an outstretched hand with the wrist in extension and the forearm in pronation. A cadaveric study reproduced scaphoid fracture in the laboratory in wrists in more than 90 degrees of dorsiflexion and more than 10 degrees of radial deviation and with more than 400 kg of force (102).

Classification

Commonly, scaphoid fractures are described as distal pole or tuberosity, waist, and proximal pole. Most fractures of the scaphoid (75%) involve the waist. Approximately 20% involve the proximal pole, with the remaining 5% being distal or tuberosity fractures. A detailed classification by Herbert separating scaphoid fractures by stability and whether the fracture is acute or chronic can be seen in **Figure 24-29.** Recently, a new system has divided scaphoid fractures into two groups: stable and unstable. Stable fractures include occult, incomplete, and complete nondisplaced fractures, while unstable fractures include complete displaced, comminuted, dislocated, and those associated with other injuries (103). Most acute fractures in the athlete are waist and minimally displaced.

Clinical Evaluation and Diagnosis

Any contact-sport athlete who has radial wrist pain should be considered to have a scaphoid fracture until proven otherwise. Physical examination in the acute setting usually reveals tenderness in the "anatomic snuffbox," and this finding alone should be enough to justify immobilization until a definite diagnosis is made. Other physical findings include decreased range of motion, swelling, and pain with dorsiflexion.

Routine radiographs should include a posteroanterior, lateral, and oblique view in 45 degrees to 60 degrees of pronation, and a scaphoid or "clenched fist" view, which is a posteroanterior view in slight ulnar deviation. Some fractures can be seen initially on plain radiographs. However, many fractures are not evident on plain radiographs until resorption at the fracture site occurs. The S-L interval must also be carefully examined for any widening.

Occult fractures can be detected with other imaging studies including MRI, bone scan, or CT. MRI has been shown to be more sensitive and specific than bone scintigraphy. Gadolinium-enhanced MRI is the most useful modality for evaluating vascularity to the scaphoid (104). MRI is also very useful in detecting avascular necrosis of the scaphoid.

Treatment of Scaphoid Fractures

Treatment of acute scaphoid fracture in the athlete depends on location and stability of the fracture, sport, and desires of the athlete. Treatment options include: cast with no sports participation until healed, cast treatment plus use of a playing cast/splint in sports where applicable, percutaneous fixation or internal fixation of the fracture with return to sport as symptoms permit.

Nonoperative Treatment. Nondisplaced stable scaphoid fractures can achieve union in the majority of cases when treated with adequate cast immobilization (105). The average healing time in these cases is 8 to 10 weeks. Application of a Muenster-type or long arm spica cast for 4 weeks, followed by a short arm cast, is the typical method of treatment. If serial radiographs taken monthly demonstrate no progress toward union after 3 to 4 months, consideration can be given to internal fixation with bone grafting.

Fractures initially determined to be nondisplaced can displace over time. Many surgeons now recommend internal fixation of nondisplaced waist and proximal pole fractures.

Operative Treatment. Percutaneous fixation may be used for minimally displaced or nondisplaced scaphoid fractures and has proven to be successful in healing (106). Advantages of this technique include preservation of vital ligaments in the wrist, decreased risk of vessel injury, less postoperative pain, and faster return to pre-injury activity.

Displaced scaphoid fractures require internal fixation. Open reduction with internal fixation improves the ability for the scaphoid to be anatomically reduced and improves the chances of healing. In addition, wrist motion can begin earlier and even return to pre-injury activities. The two most common approaches to the scaphoid are the dorsal and volar approaches. The volar approach is ideal for waist and distal third fractures (107), while the dorsal approach is preferred for proximal pole scaphoid fractures (108).

Bone graft use should be liberal in acute comminuted scaphoid fractures. Autograft can be taken very easily from the distal radius through the dorsal approach. Iliac crest bone graft or allograft can be utilized too.

The key to either approach is anatomic reduction and rigid fixation. K-wires can be used as joysticks or derotational devices to achieve anatomic reduction. Solid and cannulated screws are available for fixation. These screws have differential pitch allowing for compression at the fracture site. Most are self-tapping and can be countersunk below the articular surface.

Scaphoid Nonunions

Scaphoid fractures with delayed union or nonunion are frequently seen in athletes because the initial injury is often ignored. Often, the patient can remain symptom free for a long period of time. When wrist pain does present, there is frequently evidence of carpal arthrosis. If left untreated, scaphoid nonunions lead to predictable patterns of wrist arthrosis similar to S-L dissociation. Scaphoid nonunions occur most often with proximal pole and waist fractures. Nonunions can cause scaphoid deformity and collapse, avascular necrosis, and carpal collapse making treatment difficult.

The goals of surgery for a scaphoid nonunion include not only union but also restoring alignment. The standard procedure consists of an iliac crest bone graft. More recently, vascularized bone graft from the distal radius has been shown to result in accelerated healing (109). Poor prognostic factors in scaphoid union include: smoking, proximal pole, chronicity, and unstable fixation.

■ HAMATE FRACTURES

Fracture of the hamate usually occurs at the hook, and the diagnosis is commonly missed. Hamate injuries are most common in stick- or racquet-handling sports such as golf, baseball, or tennis. The nondominant hand usually is affected in golf and baseball players, whereas the dominant hand is involved in tennis and racquetball players.

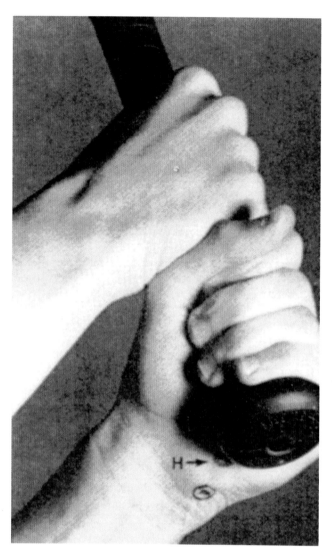

Fig 24-30. Location of the hook of the hamate relative to a bat handle.

pression of the handle against the protruding hook is the primary cause of fracture **(Fig 24-30)**. Another mechanism involves indirect avulsion through forceful pull of the flexor carpi ulnaris and avulsion through the pisohamate ligament.

Hamate body fractures may result from severe wrist fracture dislocations, direct blows to the ulnar head, AP crush injury, or transcarpal CMC dislocation resulting in a dorsal coronal fracture with posterior subluxation of the fourth or fifth metacarpal. CT scan is necessary to establish this diagnosis.

Because of the hamate's proximity to neurovascular and tendinous structures, fracture of the hamate may lead to ulnar nerve compression in the Guyon canal, CTS, and finger flexor tendon rupture, especially if nonunion occurs.

Classifications of Hamate Fractures

Hamate hook fractures can be further subdivided based on anatomic location of the fractures: tip avulsions, waist fractures, and base fractures. Hamate body fractures can be subdivided into proximal pole, medial tuberosity, sagittal, and dorsal coronal fractures.

Clinical Evaluation and Diagnosis

Fractures of the hook of the hamate occur frequently, but usually present late as chronic pain at the base of the hypothenar eminence, ulnar nerve paresthesias into the ring and small fingers, and weakness in grip strength. Patients are usually tender to palpation over the hamate hook, located approximately 2 cm distal and radial to the pisiform.

The hamate hook can be visualized with a radiograph taken with the wrist in slight supination and full radial deviation, or by carpal tunnel views. Alternatively, CT scans and MRI may assist with the diagnosis.

Anatomy

The hook of the hamate protrudes from the base of the hamate into the hypothenar eminence. The hook of the hamate is the site of origin for the hypothenar muscles (flexor digiti minimi, opponens digiti minimi), pisohamate ligaments, and the distal attachment of the transverse ligament. The hook of the hamate acts as an important pulley for the ring and small finger flexors, especially in ulnar deviation. Its nonunion or irregularity may lead to attritional rupture of the flexors as they pass the hamate hook. The vascular supply is most tenuous at the waist of the hamate hook because of a dual vascular supply to the tip and base of the hook with a watershed region at the waist.

Biomechanics of Hamate Fractures

The hook of hamate is at risk for fracture in any athlete who actively swings a racquet, club, or a bat. Direct com-

Treatment

Hamate hook fractures are treated based on location and displacement. Nondisplaced fractures, regardless of the location, are treated with immobilization. The wrist is cast in slight radial deviation to minimize the deforming force of the ulnar finger flexors. Displaced tip avulsion fractures may be treated with excision of the fragment if it remains symptomatic after 4 to 6 weeks of immobilization. It is currently controversial regarding the treatment of displaced hook waist or base fractures. Traditional treatment is excision of symptomatic fractures. Recently, interest has turned toward preservation of the hook and ORIF through a palmar approach (110).

Rehabilitation

Athletes with fractures treated nonoperatively may return to play immediately. The wrist is protected in a semi-rigid cast.

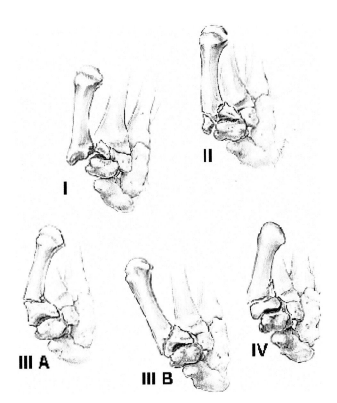

Fig 24-31. Thumb MC fracture classifications.

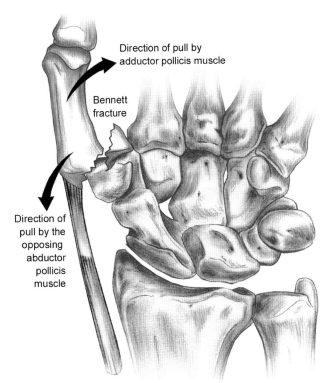

Direction of pull by adductor pollicis muscle

Bennett fracture

Direction of pull by the opposing abductor pollicis muscle

Fig 24-32. In Bennett fracture, first metacarpal shaft is displaced by divergent pull of muscles.

Athletes with surgically treated fractures are usually restricted from active participation in sports until after 4 to 6 weeks of mobilization. Protective splint is continued for approximately 3 months or until the wrist has normal strength and range of motion.

■ THUMB METACARPAL FRACTURES

Anatomy

The base of the thumb metacarpal articulates with the trapezium in the form of a saddle joint, and this allows the thumb metacarpal a wide range of motion. Thumb opposition is its most important function, and this motion can occur because of the ability of the thumb metacarpal to move in abduction as well as pronation at the thumb CMC joint. The stability of the thumb CMC joint is due to the stout surrounding ligamentous complex. In a recent study, 16 ligaments were identified (111); the dorsoradial and deep anterior oblique ligaments play the most substantial role in stabilizing the thumb CMC joint.

Classification

Fractures of the thumb metacarpal occur most frequently at the base and are subdivided into intra-articular and extra-articular types **(Fig 23-31)**. Extra-articular fractures occur in transverse and oblique fracture patterns. It is important to distinguish the intra-articular fractures [Type I (Bennett)

+II (Rolando)] from the extra-articular (III + IV) fractures, because the extra-articular fractures can be managed adequately with nonoperative management. Rolando fracture is analogous to the pilon fracture of the distal tibia and appears to be secondary to a significant axial load that splits and crushes the articular surface. In addition to the volar lip fracture, there is also a large dorsal fragment. All comminuted metacarpal base fractures are commonly referred to in this category.

Biomechanics

Large loads are impacted to the thumb CMC joint. Axial and bending loads are applied to the joint during pinch and grasp. The trapezium is unstable due to its anatomic location at the radial aspect of the wrist and its bony structure. The basal articulation of the trapezium with the mobile scaphoid also contributes to its potential for instability.

The mechanism of injury of thumb metacarpal base fracture is an axially directed force through the metacarpal shaft. In Bennett and Rolando fractures, the strong deep anterior oblique ligament remains intact and prevents displacement of the volar fragment. However, the dorsal fragment and metacarpal are displaced radially and dorsally by the pull of the APL and the adductor pollicis longus **(Fig 24-32)**.

Clinical Evaluation and Diagnosis

An accurate evaluation of the injury depends on adequate radiographic examination. Obtain standard postero-anterior,

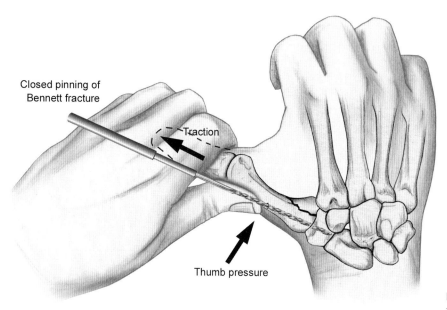

Closed pinning of Bennett fracture

Traction

Thumb pressure

Fig 24-33. Closed pinning of Bennett fracture.

lateral, and oblique radiographs in patients with suspected fractures or dislocations of the thumb. Traction radiography may be used to assess the degree of comminution in certain fractures (e.g., Bennett, Rolando, comminuted metacarpal base fractures).

A true lateral of the CMC joint must be obtained. It can be done by placing the palmar surface of the hand flat on the imaging plate, and the hand and wrist approximately 20 to 30 degrees pronated. The imaging beam is then directed obliquely at 15 degrees in a distal to proximal direction centered over the trapeziometacarpal joint. A "broken V sign" may be present on the lateral radiograph, indicating disruption of the normal V that is formed by the radial aspect of the trapeziometacarpal articulation. This may indicate undetected CMC joint subluxation. In addition, CT studies may help define the degree of comminution within a fracture as well as suspected impaction of the articular surface.

Treatment of Thumb Metacarpal Fractures

Nonoperative

Extra-articular fractures can usually be managed with closed reduction. The reduction maneuver includes traction, downward pressure at the fracture, and pronation of the distal fragment. If the reduction is stable, the fracture may be managed in a thumb spica cast for 4 weeks. Angulation of up to 30 degrees is acceptable due to the mobility of the thumb CMC joint.

For Bennett fractures, if a stable reduction can be achieved and maintained with less than 1 mm displacement, the thumb spica cast immobilization is effective treatment. However, it is important to note that the strong pull of the APL frequently leads to displacement, necessitating open reduction and internal fixation or closed reduction with percutaneous pinning. More than 1 mm of articular incongruity

or persistent CMC joint subluxation after closed reduction indicates the need for surgical treatment.

Operative Treatment

Generally, closed reduction and percutaneous K-wire fixation is successful treatment for Bennett fractures **(Fig 24-33)**. Two 0.045-inch K-wires are drilled through the dorsal radial thumb metacarpal base into the reduced volar ulnar fragment. If the fragment is very small, reduction may be maintained by placing the K-wire from the thumb metacarpal into the trapezium or the index metacarpal. Recently, arthroscopic-assisted reduction has been introduced as an adjunct to percutaneous pinning to allow direct visualization of the articular reduction.

If adequate reduction cannot be achieved utilizing this percutaneous technique, open reduction and internal fixation with K-wires or Herbert screws is performed. Of note, external fixation may be necessary in the presence of associated soft tissue injury and loss.

Treatment of Rolando fractures requires both restoration of length and articular congruity. These fractures are difficult to manage and may be destined to develop posttraumatic arthritis and instability despite surgical intervention. Various open surgical techniques have been described including the use of multiple K-wires, tension bands, and plates.

Complications

Generally, complications for Bennett and Rolando fractures include post-traumatic arthritis, first web space contracture, and those that are associated with hardware use. In a study comparing open and closed reduction of Bennett fractures, osteoarthritis was found to correlate with the quality of reduction of the fracture, but had developed in all cases even after exact reduction (112).

■ METACARPAL FRACTURES

Most metacarpal fractures occur in adolescents and young adults from sports or industrial accidents. Fracture of the metacarpals and phalanges comprises approximately 10% of all fractures. Metacarpal fractures account for 30% to 40% of all hand fractures. Fractures of the fifth metacarpal neck alone account for 10% of all fractures in the hand.

Anatomy

The metacarpals are long, tubular bones with an intrinsic longitudinal arch and a collective transverse arch. The bones are concave on their palmar surface and are joined proximally and distally by ligamentous attachments. The index and middle metacarpals are fixed rigidly at their bases, while the fourth and fifth fingers are capable of 15 and 25 degrees of motion at their respective CMC joints. The cam-shape of the metacarpal heads leads to relaxation of the collateral ligaments in extension, permitting adduction and abduction of the finger. With flexion of the MCP joints the collateral ligaments become taut, stabilizing the finger for power pinch and grip. The metacarpal shafts are the origin for the dorsal and palmar interossei muscles. These muscles are important deforming forces in metacarpal shaft fractures, leading to apex dorsal angulation. The volar plate is a cartilaginous ligament on the palmar aspect of each MCP joint. Volar plates are interconnected via the deep transverse intermetacarpal ligaments, which provide additional volar stability.

Metacarpal Base Fractures

Metacarpal base fractures and dislocations of the CMC joint commonly result from a fall or other stress on the hand with the wrist flexed. The index, middle, and ring metacarpals are rigidly fixed. Extensive force is necessary to fracture and displace these metacarpals.

Fractures of the metacarpal base can be associated with carpal fractures. Requiring considerable force, these fracture dislocations can separate the hand similar to LisFranc fracture dislocations. The longitudinal force may split the arch and lead to its collapse. Special imaging including Brewerton views or CT scans may reveal unsuspected fractures or dislocations.

Impaction fractures of the metacarpal bases that are not significantly displaced can be treated with splinting, followed by early mobilization.

CMC fracture dislocations usually are unstable. These fractures are easy to reduce but difficult to maintain due to deforming forces. Although historically these fractures were treated with closed reduction and immobilization, frequently with good results, current literature supports closed reduction and pin fixation because closed management leads to residual pain and weakness of grip.

Open reduction with pin fixation is often required with multiple CMC joint injuries, especially when there is a large hamate fracture or the dislocation is irreducible. Fracture-dislocations of the metacarpal in which the dorsal portion of the hamate is fractured and displaced should also be treated with ORIF. Care should be taken to ensure anatomic reduction of the hamate to preserve the CMC joint surface of the mobile lateral digits.

Metacarpal Shaft Fractures

Metacarpal shaft fractures tend to angulate apex dorsal with the head displaced palmarly due to the deforming pull of the interossei muscles. The more proximal the fracture, the greater the deformity and less angulation that is acceptable. Small amounts of angulation (<15 degrees are acceptable in the second and third metacarpals due to their limited CMC motion). The fourth and fifth finger metacarpals are much more mobile and angulation of 40 degrees can be accepted.

Usually the diagnosis of metacarpal shaft fractures is easily made with swelling, pain, and deformity noted at the fracture site, although swelling may mask the deformity. AP, lateral, and oblique radiographs readily demonstrate the fracture and displacement.

Most injuries to the metacarpal shaft can be managed nonoperatively. Management usually consists of sedation or local anesthesia followed by closed reduction of the fracture or dislocation. A forearm-based splint is then applied, which is held by a loose compressive wrap.

With the improvement in surgical implants, management of metacarpal shaft fractures has become more aggressive. Shaft fractures should be approached with a variety of surgical techniques to fit individual fracture patterns. Transverse patterns may enable the use of plates, intramedullary nails, or stacked pins. Long spiral or oblique fracture patterns may be fixed with multiple lag screws. Comminuted fractures may need bone graft with plating or external fixation.

Metacarpal Neck Fractures

The typical "boxer's fracture" is a misnomer, because true boxers are more likely to fracture their index and middle metacarpals than their fifth metacarpal.

Metacarpal neck fractures usually can be managed closed without operative intervention. Although the degree of angulation acceptable is variable and contested in the literature, high degrees of angulation can be accepted with little or no functional deficits in fractures of the neck, especially in the fourth and fifth digits. However, fixation should be strongly considered in unstable patterns.

Metacarpal Head Fractures

Fractures of the metacarpal head are rare injuries. Pain, swelling, and loss of motion often accompanied by soft tissue trauma are the key clinical signs of injury to the MCP joint. Crepitus may be present with motion in intra-articular injuries.

Nondisplaced fractures can be managed with splinting for 2 to 3 weeks, followed by gentle motion. Noncomminuted fractures with greater than 25% of the articular surface involved and/or greater than 1 mm of articular displacement should be treated with open reduction and internal fixation.

Comminuted metacarpal head fractures present a major problem. K-wire and cerclage wire fixation often fail. Multiple fine wires placed through drill holes made with a Keith or Bunnell needle as a drill bit may provide better reduction and greater stability of important small bone fragments. Plate and screw fixation with condylar plates is bulky, and anatomic fixation is difficult. Satisfactory results can be obtained with immobilization of the MCP joint in 70 degrees of flexion for 2 weeks, followed by aggressive therapy (113).

PHALANGEAL FRACTURES

Phalangeal fractures are a common injury affecting all age groups and they are among the most common in all sports, especially in ball-playing athletes. Most phalangeal fractures are caused by direct blows and result in transverse fractures. Distal phalanx fractures are most often caused by crushing forces that lead to comminuted fracture patterns and are frequently accompanied by nailbed lacerations.

Anatomy

The phalanges do not contain muscle bellies, and motor function is accomplished only by the flexor and extensor tendons. The thenar muscles consist of three intrinsic muscles including the abductor pollicis brevis, the FPB, and the opponens pollicis. All three intrinsic thenar muscles are supplied by the recurrent branch of the median nerve. The adductor pollicis adducts the thumb and is supplied by the deep branch of the ulnar nerve. The hypothenar muscles include the following: The abductor digiti minimi abducts the fifth digit and flexes its proximal phalanx. The flexor digiti minimi is deeper and also flexes the proximal phalanx of the fifth digit. The opponens digiti minimi opposes the fifth digit. The hypothenar muscles also are supplied by the deep branch of the ulnar nerve.

The lumbricals are four muscles that arise from the tendons of FDP. Their tendons insert into the radial side of each of the proximal phalanges of the fingers and into the dorsal hood. They flex the MCP joints and extend the interphalangeal joints. The first and second lumbricals are supplied by the median nerve, and the third and fourth lumbricals are supplied by the ulnar nerve.

The palmar and dorsal interossei arise from the metacarpals. The palmar interossei insert into the proximal phalanx and the expansion of the EDC. The palmar interossei are adductor muscles. Dorsal interossei are abductors and insert into the proximal phalanges and the dorsal digital hood. The interosseous muscles are all supplied by the deep branch of the ulnar nerve.

Clinical Evaluation and Diagnosis

The signs of injury are usually obvious: swelling, tenderness, ecchymosis, deformity, and/or skin abrasions. Usually three x-ray views (PA, lateral, and oblique) of the injured hand must be obtained with the imaging beam centered over the metacarpal phalangeal joint of the long finger to screen for trauma. PA and lateral views of the injured digit centered on the PIP joint should be obtained when a particular digit is of concern. Evaluation for subtle joint subluxation must be made on true lateral views of the DIP or PIP joints. In addition, stress views can be obtained with a digital block.

Treatment

Nonoperative

The goal in treatment of every phalangeal fracture is to obtain union with normal alignment and complete active range of motion. Most hand fractures can be treated by closed, nonoperative methods. The preferred position of immobilization of the hand is the intrinsic plus or safe position—the wrist in 30 degrees of extension, MP joints in 90 degrees of flexion, and the IP joints in full extension. MP joint flexion maintains the collateral ligaments in maximum stretch, whereas extension of the PIP joints will prevent volar plate contractures. Several muscles that act as deforming forces on the fracture originate in the forearm; thus it is advised to immobilize the wrist as well as the fingers, using a mid-forearm-based splint or cast. Immobilization should always include at least one joint proximal and distal to the fracture.

Operative

When phalangeal fractures are reducible but unstable, supplemental percutaneous pinning may be required. K-wires can be passed across the fracture and affix adjacent cortices or pass intramedullary and act as internal splints. Of note is that periarticular pins may limit joint motion by obstructing collateral ligament glide over the condyles.

Open reduction may be required for severe comminution or bone loss and can provide a bridging or spanning function across unstable segments. Fixation techniques include interfragmentary screws, intraosseous wiring, plating, and intramedullary devices.

External fixation of phalangeal fractures is uncommon and is reserved for severe open injuries with associated soft-tissue or bone loss.

LUNATE AVASCULAR NECROSIS

The lunate is the most common carpal bone affected by avascular necrosis (**Kienböck Disease**). The etiology of avascular necrosis is generally uncertain and is most likely multifactorial. At times, a traumatic event or heavy use can be clearly identified as a precipitating factor, but often this condition presents as a challenging idiopathic situation, particularly in young adults.

Kienböck disease must be considered in young adults presenting with wrist pain; there may be tenderness over the lunate and decreased range of motion (particularly in extension). On occasion, symptoms of CTS have been noted.

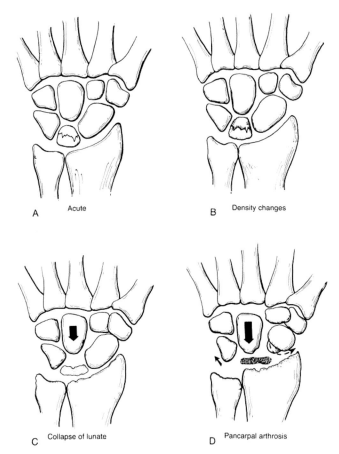

Fig 24-34. Modified Stahl classification of Kienböck disease. **A:** Stage I: Normal-appearing lunate with a compression fracture demonstrated by a radiolucent line. **B:** Stage II: Sclerosis of the lunate. **C:** Stage III: Collapse of the lunate. **D:** Stage IV: Pancarpal arthrodesis (including subchondral cyst formation, sclerosis, and articular cartilage narrowing). (From Lichtman DM, Alexander AH, Mack GR, et al. Kienbock's disease—Update on silicone replacement arthroplasty. *J Hand Surg Am.* 1982;7:343–347; with permission.)

Classification

The classification of Kienböck disease was first described by Stahl in 1947 based on the radiographic changes, and since modified by subsequent authors, is very helpful in guiding treatment **(Fig 24-34)**.

Imaging

Routine radiographs in the early stages may reveal no changes in the lunate, but the ulnar–minus variant may be noted. Tomography is sometimes helpful to demonstrate early lunate changes. Bone scans may demonstrate increased local uptake of contrast material. MRI studies provide useful information with decreased signal intensity in both the T1 and T2 weighted images. In addition, transient edema involving a portion of the lunate can be appreciated with MRI studies. Intraosseous ganglion cysts are usually clearly delineated on T2 weighted images.

Treatment

The above-described radiographic staging system is very helpful in guiding the treatment of Kienböck disease. Stage I patients may improve with immobilization and activity modification.

Before collapse of the lunate in Stage III, leveling and unloading procedures, including radial shortening osteotomies, capitate shortening, and scaphoid trapezium trapezoid arthrodesis, are based on the theory that relieving stress on the lunate allows healing.

Advances in understanding the vascular anatomy of the distal radius have led to increased use of vascularized bone grafts for treatment of Kienböck disease (114).

For advanced stage of Kienböck disease with arthritic changes, salvage procedures can be considered. Proximal row carpectomy remains a reasonable option for patients interested in preserving motion.

■ BENIGN TUMORS OF THE HAND

Ganglion Cysts

Ganglion cyst is the most common soft-tissue lesion of the hand and wrist, representing approximately 33% to 69% of all hand tumors. Ganglions have been reported at almost every joint in the hand and wrist. The most common location is the dorsum of the wrist (originating from the scapho-lunate ligaments). Other joints of origin include the scaphotrapezial joint of the wrist, the PIP joint, and DIP joint. Cyst lining is usually a bland, fibrous, relatively acellular membrane with compressed collagen fibers. Cyst content is highly viscous mucin, composed of hyaluronic acid, glucosamine, albumin, and globulin. The exact pathogenesis of ganglion cysts still remains unclear.

Patients usually present with mildly tender or nontender soft-tissue mass, which may vary in size. The mass typically transilluminates. In some patients, concomitant carpal instability may contribute to wrist symptoms. Vascular evaluation (the Allen test) is recommended for volar ganglions due to the possibility of radial artery aneurysm. Radiographic assessment is usually normal. MRI is useful to identify occult ganglion cysts as a source of local symptoms.

Recent series have reported improved success rates using various aspiration techniques. However, recurrence rate can be as high as 40%. The most definite treatment is open surgical excision. The key to the surgery is the identification and removal of the ganglion stalk with tracing of the stalk to the joint capsule. Recently, arthroscopic ganglion removal is gaining popularity for dorsal wrist ganglions. Recurrence following surgical excision is approximately 5% (115).

Giant Cell Tumor of Tendon Sheath

The giant cell tumor of tendon sheath (GCT) is the second most common tumor of the hand. It is also referred to as nodular synovitis or fibrous xanthoma. This slow-growing, painless lesion usually presents along the volar hand and digits. In contrast to ganglion cysts, GCTs do not transilluminate. A soft tissue shadow may be identified on plain radiographs. MRI is useful for both diagnosis and assessment of local tissue infiltration, including osseous erosion. Treatment is surgical marginal excision and curettage/bone graft for osseous erosion. Recurrence is notable in these lesions with reports as high as 50% (116).

Epidermal Inclusion Cyst

Epidermal inclusion cysts are among the most common soft-tissue lesions of the hand. They are caused by the result of traumatic implantation of epithelial cells from the skin surface into the underlying soft-tissue or bone. The resulting well-circumscribed, firm growth of epithelial cells is usually painless. The most common location of this lesion is the finger tip. On x-ray, osseous involvement is often identified as a well-demarcated lytic lesion with or without cortical penetration. Marginal surgical excision is curative. Intraosseous lesions require curettage with or without bone grafting.

Lipoma

Lipomas are common, slow-growing, benign fatty tumors of the hand, usually subcutaneous or intramuscular. Lipomas are often not tender and do not transilluminate. When present in the carpal tunnel or Guyon canal, neurologic symptoms may arise. X-ray radiographs may demonstrate a soft tissue mass. MRI is useful to evaluate signal characteristics with surrounding fat. If signal characteristics remain uncertain, then incisional biopsy may be indicated for deeper lesions. Generally, marginal excision is curative.

Vascular Tumors

Glomus Tumor

Usually subungual, the lesion is an arteriovenous shunt formed from neoplastic proliferation of the smooth muscle cells. Classic triad symptoms include intermittent severe pain, point tenderness, and cold intolerance. Localized subungual bluish discoloration with or without nail ridging may be present. The tumor is most effectively treated by surgical excision.

Pyogenic Granuloma

Pyogenic granulomas are considered to be disorders of angiogenesis, but the exact etiology is still unknown. Patients often present with a friable polypoid purple-red lesion. Cauterization with silver nitrate applicators is a mainstay of treatment. Recurrent lesions or those refractory to silver nitrate treatment may require marginal excision.

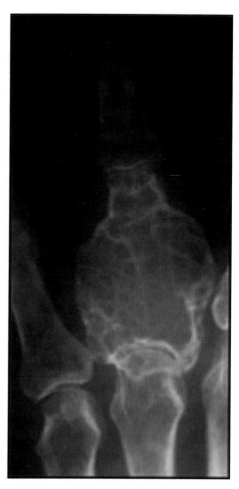

Fig 24-35. Aneurysmal bone cyst in the hand. (From Seiler JG, ed. *Crucial elements in hand surgery*. Rosemont, IL: American Association for Surgery of the Hand; 2004 with permission.)

Hemangioma

Hemangioma is a true neoplasm with a biphasic growth curve: rapid proliferation during infancy with elevation and reddening of the overlying skin, followed by a phase of involution, usually at the age of 5 to 7 years, which leaves an area of mild skin depigmentation and fibrous thickening. In adults, symptomatic hemangiomas of the hand are removed by marginal excision. More diffuse lesions are prone to recurrence.

Nerve Tumors

Schwannoma/Neurilemoma

This lesion is the most common benign nerve tumor of the upper extremity. It arises from the Schwann cell and usually presents in adults, characterized by a slow-growing, well-circumscribed, eccentric lesion on the peripheral nerve. MRI is useful to delineate the lesion; however, distinguishing it from neurofibroma or malignant nerve sheath tumors is difficult. Treatment is surgically "shelling out" the lesion from the nerve. Recurrence and malignant transformation are rare.

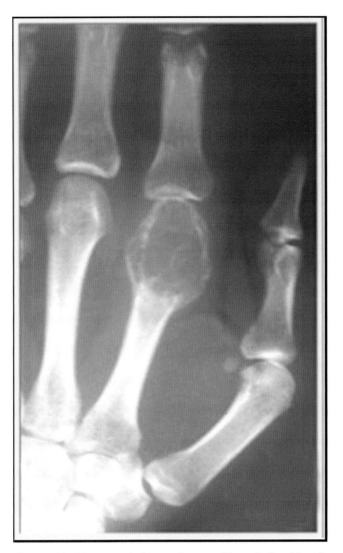

Fig 24-36. Metacarpal giant cell tumor (From Seiler JG, ed. *Crucial elements in hand surgery*. Rosemont, IL: American Association for Surgery of the Hand; 2004; with permission.)

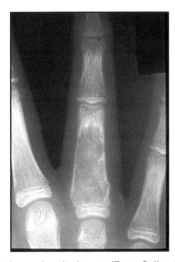

Fig 24-37. Phalangeal endochroma (From Seiler JG, ed. *Crucial elements in hand surgery*. Rosemont, IL: American Association for Surgery of the Hand; 2004; with permission.)

Neurofibroma

In contrast to the schwannoma, the neurofibroma arises in nerve fascicles making excision more difficult. Clinical presentation may include a palpable mass and nerve dysfunction. Surgical excision requires transection of nerve fascicles that enter/exit the lesion.

Aneurysmal Bone Cyst

Aneurysmal bone cyst only rarely occurs in the hand **(Fig 24-35)**. Lesions are most often seen in the phalanges or metacarpals. Mild swelling is often present; lesion may or may not be painful. Radiographs usually demonstrate an expansile cystic mass. MRI or CT are useful to assess for cortical destruction or soft tissue mass which may suggest other causes. Curettage and bone grafting are mainstays of treatment if there is adequate bone stock; whereas wide resection may be necessary if there is inadequate bone stock. Recurrence rate can be as high as 60%.

Giant Cell Tumor of Bone

Giant cell tumor of the bones of the hand is very uncommon. Distal radius is the third most common site in body of presentation of giant cell tumor of bone. However, lesions in the hand and wrist present a higher risk of local recurrence following treatment and a higher risk for metastasis compared with lesions elsewhere in the body. Patients usually present with complaints of pain and swelling. Radiographs usually demonstrate a lytic lesion without distinct borders (in contrast to aneurysmal bone cysts) **(Fig 24-36)**. Chest x-ray and bone scan are indicated to evaluate for possible pulmonary metastasis and/or synchronous lesions.

For contained lesions, curettage, adjuvant treatment, and bone grafting of metacarpal or phalangeal lesions is acceptable. Metacarpal or phalangeal lesions with cortical destruction or soft-tissue extension are effectively treated with amputation or wide en-bloc resection and reconstruction. Distal carpal row lesions are treated with wide excision and

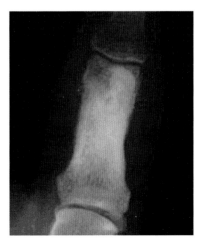

Fig 24-38. Osteoid osteoma.

L-T arthrodesis, while proximal carpal row lesions may be treated with proximal row carpectomy.

Enchondroma

Enchondroma is a benign cartilaginous lesion. It is the most common bone tumor that arises in the hand (accounts for approximately 90% of osseous tumors in the hand), and it is most commonly seen as an incidental finding. On radiographs, it is usually presented as a well-defined, central intramedullary lytic lesion with a thin, sclerotic border; intralesional/matrix calcification may be present **(Fig 24-37)**.

Small, asymptomatic enchondromas may be observed, and larger or symptomatic lesions should be biopsied and surgically treated (resection with curettage and bone grafting). Pathologic fractures may be treated acutely or after fracture healing. Local recurrence is approximately 5%.

Osteoid Osteoma

Osteoid osteoma is a benign osseous lesion presenting in the second to third decade of life, often presented as a dull ache that may be relieved with anti-inflammatories. Classic radiographic findings are of reactive sclerosis surrounding a lucency area **(Fig 24-38)**. Surgical excision with curettage of the nidus with or without bone grafting, or by en-bloc resection, is the treatment for lesions in the hand.

■ MALIGNANT TUMORS OF THE HAND

Soft Tissue Sarcomas

In general, soft tissue sarcomas are very rare in hand/upper extremity, with approximately 5,000 new cases per year in the United States of which 15% affect the upper limb. They often present as a slowly enlarging, painless mass which may have undergone recent growth. They may present with neurogenic symptoms, and less commonly, mass may be painful or may involve skin ulceration. Soft tissue sarcomas in the upper extremity most commonly metastasize to the lungs and regional lymph nodes. The most common soft tissue sarcoma of the hand is the squamous cell carcinoma, often seen to arise on the dorsum of the hand.

Clinical exam should assess for location, size, depth, and mobility of the mass. Regional lymph nodes should be evaluated. Local mass effect on surrounding neurovascular or musculotendinous structures should be considered. X-ray radiographs (osseous involvement, soft-tissue calcification) and an MRI (tissue pathology) can be done for diagnosis and preoperative planning.

For staging purpose, small, isolated lesions which may be removed with a margin of normal tissue may be considered for excisional biopsy. Larger lesions, particularly those adjacent to major nerves, vessels, or within tendinous compartments,

incisional biopsy should be considered. Following tissue diagnosis, a CT scan of the chest and axilla is usually done to assist in tumor staging. Tumor staging is based on tumor grade, size, and metastasis.

In general, surgical planning is crucial to the success of both tumor resection and limb reconstruction. Treatments for soft tissue sarcomas include wide tumor excision with a normal tissue cuff of 2 to 3 cm. Amputation may be considered when normal margins cannot be obtained, or when neurovascular structures cannot be excluded from resection margins. Digital, ray, or multiple-ray amputations may provide the best outcome for patients with sarcomas involving the digits. A below-elbow amputation is considered for those lesions involving the carpal canal. In addition, postresection treatment with radiation therapy or chemotherapy is often indicated for lesions of more than 5 cm in size. Re-excision versus amputation should be considered for patients with positive tumor margins at primary excision.

Malignant Bone Tumors

Chondrosarcoma

Chondrosarcoma is a malignant tumor of cartilage and the most common malignant primary bone tumor arising in the hand. Nonetheless, it remains rare. Proximal phalanx and metacarpals are the most common sites in hand, and it usually presents as a slowly growing, firm mass which is often painful. Typically, radiographs demonstrate a poorly demarcated lesion with cortical expansion and erosion, and tumor extension into the soft tissues. There are areas of lysis and focal or stippled calcification. Incisional biopsy and chest CT scan (to evaluate for pulmonary metastasis) may be done for staging. Wide en-bloc resection or digital/ray amputation is recommended for chondrosarcoma of the hand. Adjuvant chemotherapy or radiation therapy plays little role in treatment. Risk of metastasis from primary hand lesions is approximately 10%.

Osteogenic Sarcoma

Osteogenic sarcoma is a highly malignant tumor that produces neoplastic osteoid. It only rarely occurs in the hand, and usually presents as a firm, rapidly enlarging, and painful mass. Radiographs demonstrate an expansile, sclerotic lesion with malignant bone formation or a lytic pattern of bone destruction and soft-tissue mass. MRI is useful to evaluate the soft-tissue component of the lesion and to detect "skip" lesions within bone. Incisional biopsy may be performed to establish the diagnosis. Treatment for hand lesion is wide en-bloc excision or amputation. Neoadjuvant chemotherapy may improve surgical tissue margins. Long-term survival is not well known for primary hand lesions, although the prognosis in general is poor.

Ewing Sarcoma

Ewing sarcoma is a malignant primary bone tumor occurring in childhood, with most cases diagnosed before the age of 20 years. It only rarely occurs in the hand; metacarpals and phalanges are most common sites. It often presents with pain, swelling, erythema, and fever, which mimics infection. X-ray radiographs often demonstrate a permeative, poorly demarcated lesion; may be lytic or lytic/sclerotic. MRI is useful to assess extent of bone and soft tissue involvement. Treatment for lesion in the hand is wide en-bloc excision or amputation. Patients require systemic chemotherapy due to the high risk of metastasis. There are several reported cases of patients with hand lesion treated with only chemotherapy and external beam radiation with success. It should be noted that local recurrence is usually associated with systemic metastasis and poor prognosis.

Metastatic Carcinoma

In general, metastasis to the hand is uncommon, and it only occurs in less than 0.3% of cancer patients. Bronchogenic carcinoma is most common primary (approximately 50% of all cases), and other sources include renal, esophageal, breast, colon, prostate, thyroid, and bone. It usually presents with localized pain, swelling, and erythema. Radiographs typically demonstrate destructive or lytic lesions. However, sclerotic lesions have been reported with metastatic prostate carcinoma. Systemic staging should include evaluation for metastatic disease or for assessment of an unknown primary tumor source. Chest and abdominal CT scans and bone scan are often indicated. Treatment of metastatic lesions should emphasize pain relief, maintenance of function, and prevention of pathologic fractures.

■ NERVE

The nerve injuries in athletes are usually the result of chronic overuse or overload, although they may result from acute compression. Chronic overuse injuries are mainly dependent on the sport and the biomechanical loading related to the activity; however, general population causes also apply to athletes. Fractures, compartment syndromes, or blunt trauma may result in acute compression nerve syndromes. Nevertheless, muscular hypertrophies and chronic inflammatory lesions can contribute to the development of compression syndromes and nerve irritation. In addition, nerve compression may be the result of anatomic causes like anomalous muscles or ligaments and congenital anomalies.

The biomechanics of the sport and training program are of particular interest to the clinician because they are helpful in the establishment of a diagnosis and understanding of the mechanism of the disease. Repetitive motion, such as in throwing athletes, or multiple joint loading like the repetitive movements of gymnastics are significant factors related to the mechanism and severity of the wrist or hand injury.

According to Sunderland (117) the nerve injuries are classified in five degrees:

Sunderland Classification of Nerve Injury

1 degree	*Neuropraxic*—nerve is not functioning.
2 degrees	*Axonotmesis*—total interruption of the axons. Wallerian degeneration occurs distal to site of compression. Supporting stroma is intact.
3 degrees	Like grade II. Axonal disintegration and Wallerian degeneration. Perineurium is intact. Internal damage to the bundles. Endoneurial tubes are distorted.
4 degrees	*Neurotomesis*—Neuroma in continuity, mass of scar within epineural sheath.
5 degrees	Loss of continuity. Nerve is pulled apart or severed.

Metabolic conduction block can be considered the mildest type of nerve dysfunction. It is usually the result of compression. The mechanism of disturbance in nerve conduction is related to the decreased local energy supply. For example, when the peroneal nerve is compressed by one leg crossed over the knee of the opposite side there is a transient blockade of the blood flow to the nerve that results in reversible conduction disturbance. In general, 6 to 8 hours of ischemia can be considered a time limit before permanent impairment of nerve function occurs.

The median, ulnar, or digital nerves may be involved in athletic hand or wrist injuries.

Pathophysiology of Nerve Compression

Nerve compression affects several neural, fibrous, and vascular structures. However, the clinical results of compression are mainly defined by the (a) *duration* and (b) *magnitude* of the increased pressure to the nerve. The connective tissue of the nerve protects the axon from immediate damage during the early stage of the compressive phenomena. However, if the energy of trauma is increased, then a significant tissue reaction in the superficial layers of the nerve (epineurium) will be produced, which is associated with decreased microvascular blood flow, edema, and finally *intraneural fibrosis*. Interestingly, the compressive phenomena due to fibrosis may lead to disturbance of parts of the neuron proximal and distal to the site of compression. The nerve cell body may also be affected, while surrounding cells may also be involved in the compression syndrome.

At significant levels of energy, trauma to the nerve may have direct effect on the function of the nerve fibers. Damage of the myelin sheath or axonal disintegration can be the result. The patients usually report sensory and motor deficits due to conduction abnormalities, which are associated with acute or chronic compressive phenomena.

Nerve compression can be noted at several anatomical sites. Anatomic tunnels or muscles can be the sites of compression.

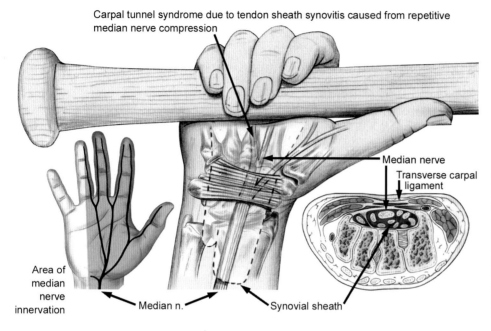

Carpal tunnel syndrome due to tendon sheath synovitis caused from repetitive median nerve compression

Median nerve

Transverse carpal ligament

Area of median nerve innervation

Median n.

Synovial sheath

Fig 24-39. Carpal tunnel syndrome may be associated with racquet sports and is usually due to hypertriphic synovitis. Fractures of the hook of the hamate characteristically occur in the hand that grips the butt end of the racquet. Ulnar nerve compression neuropathy has been reported in association with fractures of the hook of the hamate.

Congenital abnormalities, chronic inflammation, muscle hypertrophy, and high intratunnel pressures can result in compression.

The surgical intervention produces a progressive restoration of nerve function. Immediate relief is associated with restoration of microvascular circulation to the nerve. Relief that is achieved over days is related to edema reduction. Over the period of weeks, repair to the myelin occurs. Unfortunately, regeneration of nerve fibers occurs over the period of months or years.

Median Nerve

Anatomy

- Brachial plexus: C5, C6, C7, C8, T1
- Condensation of lateral and medial cords of brachial plexus
- Travels lateral to brachial artery in arm, but crosses medial to artery in antecubital fossa
- There are no branches before elbow; however, it is between two heads of pronator teres at the elbow. Five to 6 cm distal to elbow gives off anterior interosseous branch
- The palmar cutaneous branch (sensory to thenar skin) arises 5 cm proximal to wrist joint and overlies flexor retinaculum
- Enters carpal tunnel between PL and FCR
- Recurrent motor branch to thenar muscles arises at distal end of carpal tunnel
- Motor
    —Supplies pronator teres, flexor carpi radialis, palmaris longus, FDS, radial two lumbricals, opponens pollicis, abductor pollicis, FPB

    —Anterior interosseous branch supplies FPL, radial half of FDP, and pronator quadratus
- Sensation
- Radial 3 1/2 digits
- Autonomous zone is located in the tip of index finger

Classification of Injury/Disease

CTS is the most common nerve injury seen in athletes (118). It may be related to wrist/distal radius fractures, dislocation of the carpus, or repetitive use especially in gripping athletes (119) **(Fig 24-39)**. Muscle hypertrophy can be related to CTS, which is usually seen in weight lifters because of hypertrophy of the lumbricals (120). Except for compression due to space-occupying lesions, high intracarpal tunnel pressures may also be involved in median nerve compression, especially in athletes in which the activity is related to repetitive wrist flexion and extension (121,122). In neutral wrist position, the average intracarpal tunnel pressure is 2.5 mmHg, in 90 degrees of palmar flexion is 94 mmHg, and in 90 degrees of extension is 110 mmHg. Furthermore, repetitive digital flexion may cause tenosynovitis of the digital flexors, which can result in compression of the medial nerve.

Anatomic factors may be involved in females in which the incidence of CTS is increased. According to Armstrong and Chaffin (123), smaller canal size in the female is associated with a two to ten times greater incidence of CTS in women. Overall, vascular insufficiency is implicated as a primary pathologic process.

Evaluation

Patients may present with the classical symptoms of CTS, which include pain at the wrist or hand that may be radiated to the forearm, elbow, shoulder, and not very often to the cervical spine. Numbness in the radial three digits is also a hallmark clinical complaint. Although it is rare, it is important to evaluate the cervical spine for evidence of nerve compression as a possible etiology for the cause of upper-extremity pain, especially if there is evidence of multiple crush injuries. The pain and paresthesias are frequent complaints and affect the radial 3 1/2 digits.

During physical evaluation, a positive Phalen test is more sensitive than a Tinel sign. However, it is important to highlight that the Phalen test and Tinel sign are not always diagnostic and their presence may not be constant. Sensibility testing can delineate abnormal results in the middle finger, while motor weakness is not frequent and mainly localized in the thenar eminence. Weakness of the abductor pollicis brevis is frequent and the thenar eminence can be atrophied. Laboratory evaluation includes electromyography and nerve conduction studies. Neurophysiologic tests have a sensitivity of approximately 85% to 90% (124). Tests are considered positive when sensory conduction prolongation is above 3.5 ms or distal motor latency is above 4.0 ms.

Management

Nonoperative. Splinting of the wrist in a neutral position, especially during the nighttime, and rest must be the initial management. It is important to identify positions during athletic activity that may worsen the symptoms. In such cases, modification of the technique can be of benefit. Young patients may present with CTS due to significant tenosynovitis of the digital flexors. However, routine flexor tenosynovectomy along with carpal tunnel release is not of particular benefit when compared to isolated carpal tunnel release (125). Corticosteroid injection is often helpful in treatment and diagnosis of patients with continuous symptoms or symptoms that persist with splinting. Alternatively, infiltration with lidocaine is beneficial in relieving symptoms; however, local infiltration with morphine before carpal tunnel release does not have an analgesic benefit (126). The use of morphine was associated with increased pain intra-operatively and 1 day postoperatively as well as with a high prevalence of postoperative complications.

Operative. For patients with atrophy or evidence of ongoing denervation, treatment should consist of surgical intervention via release of the transverse carpal ligament. It is unusual that surgical intervention is required because, most commonly, EMG are usually normal in the athlete (127). On the other hand, in cases of acute CTS due to wrist fractures or carpal dislocations, prompt surgical intervention is paramount.

Carpal tunnel release can be performed either with an open or an arthroscopic procedure. Arthroscopic procedures are two- or one-portal techniques. Currently, there is a debate about the optimal treatment. According to Chow, contraindications to endoscopic carpal tunnel release include (a) the patient requires neurolysis, tenosynovectomy, Z-plasty of the transverse carpal ligament, or decompression of the Guyon canal; (b) the surgeon suspects a space-occupying lesion or other severe abnormality of the muscles, tendons, or vessels in

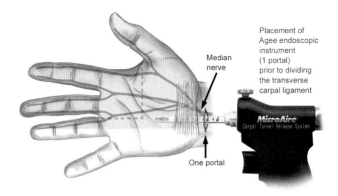

Fig 24-40. One-portal technique (Agee technique).

the carpal tunnel; and (c) the patient has localized infection or severe hand edema, or the vascular status of the upper extremities is tenuous. Fischer and Hastings add contraindications to the use of endoscopic technique as follows: (a) revision surgery for unresolved or recurrent CTS; (b) anatomical variation in the median nerve, suggested by clinical findings of wasting in the abductor pollicis brevis without significant median sensory changes; and (c) previous tendon surgery or flexor injury that would cause scarring in the carpal tunnel, preventing the safe placement of the instruments for endoscopic carpal tunnel release.

Although both procedures are highly effective in relieving symptoms, there are prospective randomized studies (128,129) in which arthroscopic procedures are safe and relief of symptoms is achieved more quickly. This is of particular interest to the athletes. Scar sensitivity during the 3-month post-operative period is less significant in patients treated with endoscopic release in comparison to patients treated with the open technique.

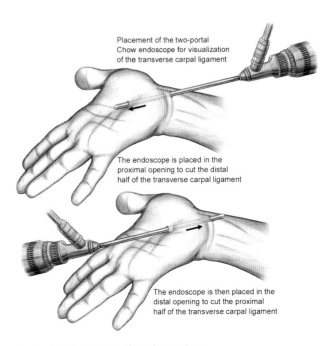

Fig 24-41. Two-portal (Chow) technique.

Nevertheless, at 1 year after surgery the scar tenderness is equally mild in both groups (128). Persistent weakness and pain in the thenar are considered limitations of the open techniques; however, the probability of complications in patients treated endoscopically and the risk of recurrence due to incomplete distal release cannot be overlooked (130).

In a multicenter study involving 169 wrists, the two-portal technique resulted in only four complications (131): one partial transection of the superficial palmar arch, one digital-nerve contusion, one ulnar-nerve neuropraxia, and one wound hematoma. Chow and Hantes (132) reported after reviewing 2,402 patients treated during a 13-year period that the two-portal Chow technique resulted in an overall complication rate of 1.1% 48.

Technique: A. Endoscopic release.

One-portal technique (Agee technique). **(Fig 24-40)** In the one-incision (Agee) technique, the blade assembly and viewing device are inserted into the carpal canal anterograde through the proximal incision. The safe zone for blade elevation is a triangle defined by the ulnar half of distal edge of transverse carpal ligament (TCL), ulnar border of the median nerve, and the superficial palmar arch. With the wrist in extension, the device is advanced to the distal edge of the TCL. Video picture, ballottement, and translumination confirm the position. When correctly positioned, the cutting blade is elevated, and the device is withdrawn, cutting the distal half of the ligament. The device then is reinserted to inspect ligament division, and additional passes then are made to complete the division of the remaining proximal portions of the ligament.

Two-portal technique (Chow technique). **(Fig 24-41)** In the two-incision (Chow) technique, the patient is placed supine with the wrist placed on a hand table and extended. The first incision for the entry portal is essentially the same that is being used for the Agee technique (Fig 24-40). The second incision for the exit portal is made transversely in the palm on a line bisecting the angle formed by lines drawn along the distal border of the fully abducted thumb and the third web space. Blunt dissection is performed in the palm to identify the superficial palmar arch, the common digital nerves, and the distal edge of the TCL. Following the axis of the forearm, a blunt curved instrument is inserted into the carpal canal through the proximal incision to free soft tissues from the undersurface of the TCL.

Open carpal tunnel release. (128) A line is drawn from the apex of the interdigital fold between the thumb and index finger, toward the ulnar side of the hand and parallel to the proximal palmar crease, and passing 4.0 mm to 5.0 mm distal to the pisiform bone (Kaplan oblique). The incision is made 2 mm ulnar to the thenar crease, just distal to the Kaplan oblique line (a line drawn), and extended 3.0 cm to 4.0 cm proximally toward the distal wrist crease. The superficial palmar fascia, transverse carpal ligament, and antebrachial fascia are divided under loupe magnification. The tourniquet is deflated after the wound is closed with monofilament sutures.

■ ULNAR NERVE COMPRESSION

Anatomy

- C7, C8, T1 from medial and lateral cords of brachial plexus
- Passes through intermuscular septum in mid-arm
- Behind medial epicondyle
- Between two heads of flexor carpi ulnaris

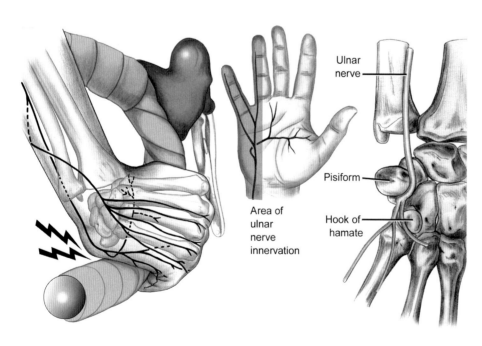

Ulnar nerve

Area of ulnar nerve innervation

Pisiform

Hook of hamate

Fig 24-42. Ulnar nerve compression syndrome.

- Lies anterior to FDP
- Gives off dorsal cutaneous branch 5 cm proximal to wrist
- At wrist lies between FDS and flexor carpi ulnaris
- Through Guyon canal at wrist (between pisiform and hook of hamate), medial to ulnar artery
- Motor branch winds around hook of hamate
- Sensory—ulnar 1 1/2 digits both sides; autonomous zone is located at the tip of little finger

Classification

Ulnar nerve compression syndromes are related to the anatomic location of the nerve. The nerve can be compressed in the Guyon canal when edema and inflammation is present, which are frequently seen in racquet sports because of its superficial location (119,133) **(Fig 24-42)**. Other causes of compression may include (134,135,136,137):

- Fractured hook of hamate or pisiform, which is usually seen in sports that require a forceful grip
- Instability of the pisiform
- Pisotriquetral arthritis
- Tumors—ganglion, lipoma
- Ulnar artery true or false aneurysms related to repeated blows to the ulnar artery in the Guyon canal.

Furthermore, push-up palmar palsy may be related to exercise on a hard surface without hand protective measures (138).

In bicycle riders, compressive ulnar neuropathies are very common. They usually result from continued compressive forces to the hypothenar eminence during supporting of the body weight, or from repetitive hyperextension of the wrist (139,140).

Additionally, inflammation may be the etiology, which is usually seen in the entity of racquet player's pisiform (141). In these patients, the inflammatory process is related to pisotriquetral degenerative lesions causing ulnar neuropathy (139). Masses may also be involved in the pathogenesis, like a neuroma that can be developed in the dorsal sensory branch. Neuromas are the result of adherence to the extensor tendon to the small finger (142).

According to Shea and McClain classification (143), the ulnar nerve compression syndrome is divided into three types: Type I, which is proximal to the Guyon canal, Type II, which is distal to Guyon, and Type III, which is proximal to the Guyon canal and involves the dorsal sensory branch of the ulnar nerve.

Evaluation

Patients usually present with pain and paresthesias of the small and medial one-half of the ring fingers. A positive Tinel sign with radiation to the small finger and the ulnar side of the ring finger can be found. It must be pointed out that testing of the motor function of the ulnar nerve should include measuring the grip strength. Additionally, the Froment sign may be positive (inability of the adductor pollicis brevis to produce a key pinch when FPL is activated with thumb interphalangeal joint flexion). Hypothenar and interossei atrophy can be present. Dorsal sensory branch irritation symptoms can be present with pain over the dorsal ulnar wrist, tenderness, and a positive Tinel sign. It is important to clinically localize the lesion by differentiation of motor and/or sensory findings. The deep branch of ulnar–to-median nerve anastomosis (Riche-Cannieu anastomosis) can account for unusual clinical findings (142).

Radiographs are not required on a routine basis. However, a CT scan of the wrist or a carpal tunnel view should be ordered in patients with pain around the hamate. The pain in these cases can be related to a hook of the hamate fracture (144,145).

Tumors or ganglions are usually delineated with MRI. A thorough vascular examination is necessary to differentiate vascular from neurologic pathology. In cases of ulnar artery thrombosis, the Allen test and angiography are crucial in making the diagnosis (146). Patients have normal nerve conduction velocity and EMG results and rarely show delayed motor latency from wrist to 1st dorsal interosseous (147).

Management

- Nonoperative (splinting, avoidance of repetitive trauma, NSAIDs)
- Operative (decompression of motor and sensory branches, +/− excision of pisiform/hook of hamate)

Resting, splinting, and NSAIDs may provide symptomatic relief. Conservative treatment must be accompanied by avoidance of offending activities. EMG and nerve conduction studies can be done serially to document progression or improvement. Failure of conservative care and denervation can be considered indications for surgery. Furthermore, nonunions of the hook of the hamate, ulnar artery thrombosis, ganglions, and tumors require operative treatment.

Surgical techniques consist of decompression of motor and sensory branches depending on the location of the compression. Excision of the hook of the hamate is indicated for nonunion. Vascular reconstruction consists of excision of the aneurysm with primary vascular repair. Intercalary vascular grafting is often necessary, depending on the size of the lesion.

■ DIGITAL NERVE COMPRESSION

Classification of Injury/Disease

Compression of the digital nerves is usually the result of repetitive impact seen most commonly in racquet sports, throwing pitchers, and bowling. Ulnovolar neuroma of the thumb has been described as "bowler's thumb" (148).

Bowler's thumb is a rare disorder related to repetitive trauma to the thumb characterized by perineural fibrosis of the ulnar digital nerve of the thumb (149). Symptoms include paresthesias and numbness associated with a painful mass. Interestingly, people who have not developed callus in the area of repeated use of the thumb are more susceptible to the development of the disease (149). These injuries occur in the common digital nerve to the long and ring fingers. However, the motor nerve to the first dorsal interossei can also be involved (150,139). Pitchers may present with severe digital ulcers that must be treated with surgical decompression at the lumbrical canal and at the Cleland ligament (151).

Pain, hypo/hyperesthesias, or paresthesias are usually found during physical examination. Furthermore, palpable masses can be present with a Tinel sign and an abnormal two-point discrimination sensibility testing. In the differential diagnosis (a) ganglia and tumors, (b) vascular thrombosis, and (c) tenosynovitis must be included.

Evaluation

Histopathology may be helpful in cases where hyperplastic neuromas are difficult to differentiate from neoplastic lesions.

Management

Nonoperative

Apart from preventive measures, which are considered the most important method of protection, conservative treatment should be initially applied. Modification of the technique or even discontinuance of the athletic activity may be helpful. In cases where preventive measures do not result in improvement, immobilization after infiltration of a corticosteroid is indicated.

Operative

Surgical decompression, neurolysis, and transposition are often effective in the treatment of bowler's thumb. Excision is not recommended. For Pacinian tumors, the terminal lesions can be excised (152).

■ VESSEL

Wrist and/or hand vascular disorders are usually seen in sports that require absorption of energy by the hand. These disorders are rare and are usually seen in baseball catchers, handball players, golfers, tennis players, weight lifters, volleyball players, and athletes who participate in sports that involve repetitive impact to the hand. These athletes have a higher incidence of vascular disorders and trauma to the hand from catching in comparison to other athletes. The mechanism of vascular lesion is usually related to repetitive

impact to the superficial vascular structures. However, aneurysms of the subclavian/axillary artery and its branches are at risk to embolize distally to the peripheral vessels and produce ischemic phenomena.

Anatomy

The blood supply to the hand is derived from the ulnar and radial arteries, which form the superficial and deep palmar arterial arches by anastomosis. Sometimes the median artery provides a significant contribution to the hand's vascular supply. The ulnar artery supplies the superficial palmar arch, while the deep palmar arch is mainly a branch of the radial artery. In the majority of individuals, both radial and ulnar arteries contribute to the blood supply of the hand. However, in 20% of individuals a reduction in blood flow to the digits may be related to loss of contribution of one of the main arteries. The superficial palmar arch supplies common digital arteries, which are divided into the radial and ulnar proper digital arteries. The side of the ulnar artery and nerve lesions is usually the Guyon canal. Neurovascular injuries are usually located distal to the pisiform because of inadequate protection at this level. Repetitive trauma at this site can result in neurovascular syndromes (145).

Classification of Injury/Disease

Hypothenar Hammer Syndrome

Initially, HHS was described in patients who take repetitive force or impact in their hands due to hammering activities. In 1934, Von Rosen described the disease in a 23-year-old factory workser. Today, HHS is considered a frequent disorder in air hammer operators; however, athletes are also susceptible to the development of HHS. Athletes that use the palms of their hands during athletic activities can develop the syndrome (karate and judo, baseball and handball). The vascular disorder seen in HHS may be similar to Raynaud phenomenon and is related to damage to the ulnar artery in or distal to the Guyon canal. Nevertheless, the vulnerable portion of the ulnar artery is located over the hamate bone, which may result in thrombosis, irregularity, and true or false aneurysm formation. In true aneurysms, all layers of the vessel wall are involved. On the contrary, false aneurysm involves laceration of the vessel wall with formation of hematoma, which is encapsulated.

Ischemic phenomena are the result of decreased blood flow due to thrombosis, aneurysms, or vasospasm. The mechanism is usually related to minor repetitive blunt trauma to the hand (153,154,155). Mild repetitive trauma usually results in reversible distal ulnar or digital arterial ischemia; however, the prolonged and repetitive arterial spasm may lead to the development of vessel occlusion.

Patients with HHS usually present with pain in the palm associated with coldness of the digits. Catching a ball or vibration may worsen the pain; however, in severe cases the pain can be constant and not related to activity. In such cases digital ulceration may be present (156). The pain can radiate to the forearm, which can make the diagnosis difficult. Symptoms may also include heaviness, coolness, and blanching of the arm and/or hand.

Evaluation. Physical examination includes both sensory/ motor evaluation for compression of the ulnar nerve and damage of the ulnar artery. It is important to differentiate the possibility of HHS from Raynaud phenomenon in athletes because HHS can be cured. Color and temperature changes occur more diffusely in HHS than in Raynaud phenomenon, while absence of the triphasic color change, which is usually seen in Raynaud phenomenon, may lead to suspicion and diagnosis of HHS.

Compressive neuropathy of the ulnar nerve can be evaluated with the Tinel sign, while the Allen test is very important for the delineation of ischemia related to ulnar artery patency. Compressing both the ulnar and radial arteries while the patient makes a fist reproduces the Allen test. One of the arteries is released after relaxation of the fist. The hand will "blush" within 5 seconds if the vessel in normal. In case of ischemia, the "blush" will be either absent or delayed. A similar test may be performed on the digital vessels. Auscultation proximal along the vessels of the upper extremity is important in differential diagnosis and should not be overlooked because the cause of HHS may be distal embolization. Bruits or thrills located proximally in the infraclavicular and supraclavicular fossae should be further evaluated and a chest radiograph should be ordered in case it is suspected that a cervical rib may exist.

Adjunctive tests may include use of the cold testing, Doppler scanner or B-mode ultrasonography, photo plethysmography, and digital thermistors. The initial phase of a radionuclide scan is valuable in providing information about the vascular supply. While these tests may be helpful in making the diagnosis, if a vascular injury is suspected based on clinical examination and presentation, angiogram or magnetic resonance angiography (MRA) is the test of choice, especially when surgical repair is considered (154). The use of nitroglycerin or papaverine can be useful to distinguish spasm from chronic occlusion in these cases.

Management. Conservative treatment consists of rest and use of pads. Furthermore, the use of vasolytic and sympatholytic drugs may be beneficial. Surgical intervention is required when conservative treatment has no result. Establishment of a patent artery is performed through excision of the aneurysm or thrombosal segment and reconstruction either with direct anastomosis or vein interposition grafting (154,157).

Digital Ischemia
Evaluation. Trauma to the hand from catching can lead to decreased digital vessel perfusion, which has been described mainly in baseball players. In a study involving 36 otherwise

healthy baseball players, it was found that gloves used by professional catchers do not adequately protect the hand from microvascular trauma (158).

However, there are some reports in the literature in which increased padding of the glove can decrease the symptoms of digital ischemia (154,159,160).

Primary ischemic phenomena to these athletes may be related to repetitive trauma to the digital arteries or lumbrical enlargement or entrapment by the Cleland ligaments in the throwing hands of baseball pitchers (151,161). Secondary ischemia may be the result of arterial embolization from proximal arterial injury.

Patients usually present with ischemic symptoms like coolness or numbness of the involved digit, which is frequently the index finger of the catching hand. Cyanosis, paleness, and, in severe cases, digital ulceration may be present. Diagnosis may be established with the digital Allen test, although noninvasive tests, such as thermography, digital ultrasonography, and photo plethysmography, are usually diagnostic. It should be pointed out that the gold standard of diagnosis is the delineation with the use of arteriography.

Management. Conservative treatment includes extra padding of the glove in baseball catchers, rest, and sympatholytic drugs. Surgical intervention is indicated if the conservative treatment fails. During the surgical procedures the digital vessels are examined for evidence of pressure due to hypertrophy or ligamentous entrapment.

■ REFERENCES

1. Berger RA, Garcia-Elias M. General anatomy of the wrist. In: An KN, Berger RA, Cooney WP, eds. *Biomechanics of the wrist joint.* New York: Springer-Verlag; 1991:1–22.
2. Bonnel F, Allieu Y. The radioulnocarpal and midcarpal joints: anatomical organization and biomechanical basis. *Ann Chir Main.* 1984;3:287–296.
3. Cooney WP, Garcia-Elias M, Dobyns JH, et al. Anatomy and mechanics of carpal instability. *Surg Rounds Orthop.* 1989;3:15–24.
4. Jobe FW, Pink MM. Shoulder pain in golf. *Clin J Sports Med.* 1996;15:55–63.
5. Johnston RB, Seiler JG, Miller EJ, et al. The intrinsic and extrinsic ligaments of the wrist: a correlation of collagen typing and histologic appearance. *J Hand Surg Br.* 1995;20B(6):750–754.
6. Linscheid RL, Dobyns JH. Treatment of scapholunate dissociation. *Hand Clin.* 1992;8(4):645–652.
7. Siegel DP, Gelberman RH. Radial styloidectomy: an anatomical study with special reference to radiocarpal intracapsular ligamentous morphology. *J Hand Surg Am.* 1991;16A(1):40–44.
8. Hogikyan JV, Louis DS. Embryologic development and variations in the anatomy of the ulnocarpal ligamentous complex. *J Hand Surg Am.* 1992;17:719–723.
9. Reagan DS, Linscheid RL, Dobyns JH. Lunotriquetral sprains. *J Hand Surg Am.* 1984;9A(4):502–514.
10. Garcia-Elias M, An KN, Cooney WP, et al. Transverse stability of the carpus. *J Orthop Res.* 1989;7(5):738–743.
11. Mizuseki T, Ikuta Y. The dorsal carpal ligaments: their anatomy and function. *J Hand Surg Br.* 1989;14B(1):91–98.
12. Masquelet AC, Strube F, Nordin JY. The isolated scapho-trapezio-trapezoid ligament. *J Hand Surg Br.* 1993;18B(6):730–735.

13. Kauer JMG. The mechanism of the carpal joint. *Clin Orthop*. 1986;202:16–26.

14. Larsen CF, Amadio PC, Gilula LA, et al. Analysis of carpal instability: description of the scheme. *J Hand Surg Am*. 1995;20(5):757–764.

15. Taleisnik J. Wrist: anatomy, function, and injury. *Instr Course Lect*. 1978;27:61–87.

16. Watson HK, Hempton RF. Limited wrist arthrodeses I. The triscaphoid joint. *J Hand Surg Am*. 1980;5(4):320–327.

17. Hudson RM, Caragol WJ, Faye JJ. Isolated rotary subluxation of the carpal navicular. *AJR Am J Roentgenol*. 1976;126(3):601–611.

18. Blaine ES. Lunate osteomalacia. *JAMA*. 1931;96:492.

19. King RJ. Scapholunate diastasis associated with a Barton fracture treated by manipulation, or Terry-Thomas and the wine waiter. *J R Soc Med*. 1983;76(5):421–423.

20. O'Brien ET. Acute fractures and dislocations of the carpus. *Orthop Clin North Am*. 1984;15:237–258.

21. Blatt G. Capsulodesis in reconstructive hand surgery: dorsal capsulodesis for the unstable scaphoid and volar capsulodesis following excision of the distal ulna. *Hand Clin*. 1987;3:81–102.

22. Dobyns JH, Linscheid RL, Chao EYS, et al. Traumatic instability of the wrist. *Instr Course Lect*. 1975;24:182–199.

23. Green DP, ed. *Operative Hand Surgery*. 2nd ed. New York: Churchill Livingstone; 1988.

24. Aldridge JM III, Mallon WJ. Hook of the hamate fractures in competitive golfers: results of treatment by excision of the fractured hook of the hamate. *Orthopedics*. 2003;26(7):717–719.

25. Alexander CE, Lichtman DM. Ulnar carpal instabilities. *Orthop Clin North Am*. 1984;15(2):307–320.

26. Lichtman DM, Alexander AH, eds. *The Wrist and Its Disorders*. Philadelphia: WB Saunders; 2004.

27. Moneim MS. Volar dislocation of the metacarpophalangeal joint: pathologic anatomy and report of two cases. *Clin Orthop*. 1983;176:186–189.

28. Durham HW, Khuri S, Kim MH. Acute and late radial collateral ligament injuries of the thumb metacarpophalangeal joint. *J Hand Surg Am*. 1993;18A(2):232–237.

29. Stener B. Displacement of the ruptured ulnar collateral ligament of the metacarpophalangeal joint. *J Bone Joint Surg Br*. 1962;44B:8769–79.

30. Engel J, Ganel A, Ditzian R, et al. Arthrography as a method of diagnosing tear of the ulnar collateral ligament of the metacarpophalangeal joint of the thumb. *J Trauma*. 1979;19(2):106–109.

31. Green DP, Strickland JW. The hand. In: DeLee JC, Drez Jr D, eds. *Orthopaedic sports medicine*. 1st ed. Philadelphia: WB Saunders; 1994:945–1017.

32. Renshaw TS, Louis DS. Complex volar dislocation of the metacarpophalangeal joint: a case report. *J Trauma*. 1973;13(2):1086–1088.

33. Meyn MA Jr. Irreducible volar dislocation of the proximointerphalangeal joint. *Clin Orthop*. 1981;158:215–218.

34. Ekenstam F. *The distal radioulnar joint: an anatomical, experimental, and clinical study* [Dissertation from the Faculty of Medicine]. *Acta Univ Abstr Uppsala*. 1984;505:1–55.

35. Hagert CG. Functional aspects on the distal radioulnar joint [abstract]. *J Hand Surg*. 1979;4A:585(abst).

36. Tolat AR, Stanley JR, Trail IA. A cadaver study of the anatomy and stability of the distal radioulnar joint in the coronal and transverse planes. *J Hand Surg Br*. 1996;21B(5):587–594.

37. Hergenroeder PT, Gelberman RH. Distal radioulnar joint subluxation secondary to excision of the radial head. *Orthopedics*. 1980;3:649–650.

38. Hotchkiss RN, An KN, Sowa DT, et al. An anatomic and mechanical study of the interosseous membrane of the forearm: pathomechanics of proximal migration of the radius. *J Hand Surg Am*. 1989;14A(2 Pt 1):256–261.

39. Geel CW, Palmer AK. Radial head fractures and their effect on the distal radioulnar joint. *Clin Orthop*. 1992;275:79–83.

40. Heiple KG, Freehafer AA, Van't Hof A. Isolated traumatic dislocation of the distal end of the ulna or distal radio-ulnar joint. *J Bone Joint Surg Am*. 1962;44A:1387–1394.

41. Boyes JH. Surgical repair of joints. In: *Bunnell's surgery of the hand*. 5th ed. Philadelphia: JB Lippincott Co; 1970:94–313.

42. Liebolt FL. Surgical fusion of the wrist joint. *Surg Gynecol Obstet*. 1938;66:1008–1023.

43. Lowman CL. The use of fascia lata in the repair of disability at the wrist. *J Bone Joint Surg*. 1930;12:400–402.

44. Johnson RK. Stabilization of the distal ulna by transfer of the pronator quadratus origin. *Clin Orthop*. 1992;275:130–132.

45. Biyani A, Mehara A, Bhan S. Morphological variations of the ulnar styloid process. *J Hand Surg Br*. 1990;15B(3):352–354.

46. Darrach W. Anterior dislocation of the head of the ulna. *Ann Surg*. 1912;56:802–803.

47. Bowers WH. The distal radioulnar joint. In: Green DP, ed. *Operative hand surgery*. 3rd ed. New York: Churchill Livingstone; 1993:973–1019.

48. Fernandez DL. Radial osteotomy and Bowers arthroplasty for mal-united fractures of the distal end of the radius. *J Bone Joint Surg*. 1988;70A(10):1538–1551.

49. Millroy D, Coleman S, Ivers R. The Suave-Kapandji operation. *J Hand Surg*. 1992;17B(4):411–414.

50. Miinami A, Suzuki K, Suenaga N, et al. The Suave-Kapandji procedure for osteoarthritis of the distal radioulnar joint. *J Hand Surg*. 1995;20A(4):602–608.

51. Flatt AE. *The Care of the Rheumatoid Hand*. 2nd ed. St Louis: CV Mosby; 1983.

52. Swanson AB. Flexible implant for replacement of arthritic or destroyed joints in the hand: inter-clinic information bulletin. Ref Type: Generic. New York: New York University; 1966:16–19.

53. Chamay A. A distally based dorsal and triangular tendinous flap for direct access to the proximal interphalangeal joint. *Ann Chir Main*. 1988;7(2):179–189.

54. Watson HK, Ballet FL. The SLAC wrist: scapholunate advanced collapse pattern of degenerative arthritis. *J Hand Surg Am*. 1984;9A(3):358–365.

55. Nagle DJ. Arthroscopy. In: Russell RC, ed. *Hand surgery*. St Louis: Mosby; 2000.

56. Imbriglia JE, Broudy AS, Hagberg WC, et al. Proximal row carpectomy: clinical evaluation. *J Hand Surg Am*. 1990;15A(3):426–430.

57. Hobby JL, Lyall HA, Meggitt BF. First metacarpal osteotomy for trapeziometacarpal osteoarthritis. *J Bone Joint Surg Br*. 1998;80B(3):508–512.

58. Simmons B, Smith G. The hand and wrist. In: Kelley WN, Harris ED Jr, Rudy S, et al., eds. *Textbook of rheumatology*. Philadelphia: WB Saunders; 1997:1647.

59. Damen A, VanderLei B, Robinson PH. Carpometacarpal arthritis of the thumb. *J Hand Surg Am*. 1996;21A(5):807–812.

60. Sollerman C, Herrlin K, Abrahamsson S, et al. Silastic replacement of the trapezium for arthrosis—a twelve year follow-up study. *J Hand Surg Br*. 2004;14B(4):426–429.

61. Muermans S, Coenen L. Interpositional arthroplasty with Gore-Tex, Marlex or tendon for osteoarthritis of the trapeziometacarpal joint. *J Hand Surg Br*. 1998;23B(1):64–68.

62. Lin GT, Amadio P, An KN, et al. Functional anatomy of the human digital flexor pulley system. *J Hand Surg Am*. 1989;14A(6):949–956.

63. Zissimos AG, Szabo RM, Yinger KE, et al. Biomechanics of the thumb flexor pulley system. *J Hand Surg Am*. 1994;19A(3):475–479.

64. Idler RS. Anatomy and biomechanics of the digital flexor tendons. *Hand Clin*. 1985;1(1):3–12.

65. Gelberman RH, Vandeberg JS, Manske PR, et al. The early stages of flexor tendon healing: a morphologic study of the first fourteen days. *J Hand Surg Am.* 1985;10(6 Pt 1):776–784.

66. Gelberman RH, Manske PR, Akeson WH, et al. Flexor tendon repair. *J Orthop Res.* 1986;4(1):119–128.

67. Khan U, Kakar S, Akali A, et al. Modulation of the formation of adhesions during the healing of injured tendons. *J Bone Joint Surg Br.* 2000;82B(7):1054–1058.

68. Aoki M, Kubota H, Pruitt DL, et al. Biomechanical and histologic characteristics of canine flexor tendon repair using early postoperative mobilization. *J Hand Surg Am.* 1997;22A(1): 107–114.

69. Scheffler P, Uder M, Gross J, et al. Dissection of the proximal subclavian artery with consecutive thrombosis and embolic occlusion of the hand arteries after playing golf. *Am J Sports Med.* 2003;31(1):137–140.

70. Jacobson JA. Ultrasound in sports medicine. *Radiol Clin North Am.* 2002;40(2):363–386.

71. Bencardino JT. MR imaging of tendon lesions of the hand and wrist. *Magn Reson Imaging Clin N Am.* 2004;12(2):333–347.

72. Amadio PC, An KN, Couvreur P, et al. The effect of suture technique on adhesion formation after flexor tendon repair for partial lacerations in a canine model. *J Trauma.* 2002;51(5): 917–921.

73. Strickland JW. Flexor tendon injuries: I. Foundations for treatment. *J Am Acad Orthop Surg.* 1995;3(1):44–54.

74. Gelberman RH, Leversedge F, Seiler JG, et al. Flexor tendon grafting to the hand: an assessment of the intrasynovial donor tendon. *J Hand Surg.* 2000;25A(4):721–730.

75. Leddy JP. Avulsions of the flexor digitorum profundus. *Hand Clin.* 1985;1(1):77–83.

76. Pope DF, Wolfe SW. Safety and efficacy of percutaneous trigger finger release. *J Hand Surg Am.* 1995;20A(2):280–283.

77. vonSchroeder HP, Botte MJ. Functional anatomy of the extensor tendons of the digits. *Hand Clin.* 1997;13(1):51–62.

78. Clavero JA. Extensor mechanism of the fingers: MR imaging-anatomic correlation. *Radiographics.* 2003;23(3):593–611.

79. Newport ML. Extensor tendon injuries in the hand. *J Am Acad Orthop Surg.* 2004;5(2):59–66.

80. Chester DL, Beale S, Beveridge L, et al. A prospective, controlled, randomized trial comparing early active extension with passive extension using a dynamic splint in the rehabilitation of repaired extensor tendons. *J Hand Surg Br.* 2002;27B(3): 283–288.

81. Doyle JR. Extensor tendons-acute injuries. In: Green DP, Hotchkiss RN, Pederson WC, eds. *Operative hand surgery.* 4th ed. New York: Churchill Livingstone; 1999:1950–1987.

82. Garberman SF, Diao E, Peimer CA. Mallet finger: results of early versus delayed closed treatment. *J Hand Surg Am.* 1994;19A(5): 850–852.

83. Jackson WT, Viegas SF, Coon TM, et al. Anatomical variations in the first extensor compartment of the wrist. *J Bone Joint Surg.* 1986;68A(6):923–926.

84. Harvey FJ, Harvey PM, Horsley MW. DeQuervain's disease: surgical or nonsurgical treatment. *J Hand Surg Am.* 1990;15A(1):83–87.

85. Rettig ME, Dassa GL, Raskin KB, et al. Wrist fractures in the athlete: distal radius and carpal fractures. *Clin J Sports Med.* 1998;17(3):469–489.

86. Linscheid RL. Biomechanics of the distal radioulnar joint. *Clin Orthop.* 1992;275:46–55.

87. Short WH, Palmer AK, Werner FW, et al. A biomechanical study of distal radial fractures. *J Hand Surg Am.* 1987;12A:529–534.

88. Rikli DA, Regazzoni P. Fractures of the distal end of the radius treated by internal fixation and early function. *J Bone Joint Surg Br.* 2004;78B:588–592.

89. Melone CPJ. Distal radius fractures: patterns of articular fragmentation. *Orthop Clin North Am.* 1993;24:239–253.

90. Kreder HJ, Hanel DP, McKee M, et al. Consistency of AO fracture classification for the distal radius. *J Bone Joint Surg Br.* 1996;78B:726–731.

91. Lindau T, Arner M, Hagberg L. Intraarticular lesions in distal fractures of the radius in young adults: a descriptive arthroscopic study in 50 patients. *J Hand Surg Br.* 2004;22B:638–643.

92. Fernandez DL, Jupiter JB. *Fractures of the distal radius.* New York: Springer-Verlag; 2002.

93. Orbay JL, Fernandez DL. Volar fixed-angle plate fixation for unstable distal radius fractures in the elderly patient. *J Hand Surg Am.* 2004;29A:96–102.

94. Walton NP, Brammar TJ, Hutchinson J, et al. Treatment of unstable distal radial fractures by intrafocal, intramedullary K-wires. *Injury.* 2001;32:383–389.

95. Krishnan J, Chipchase LS, Slavotinek J. Intraarticular fractures of the distal radius treated with metaphyseal external fixation. Early clinical results. *J Hand Surg Br.* 1998;23(3):396–399.

96. Kamano M, Honda Y, Kazuki K, et al. Palmar plating for dorsally displaced fractures of the distal radius. *Clin Orthop.* 2002;397: 403–408.

97. Dodds SD, Cornelissen S, Jossan S, et al. A biomechanical comparison of fragment-specific fixation and augmented external fixation for intra-articular distal radius fractures. *J Hand Surg* Am. 2002;27A:953–964.

98. Doi K, Hattori Y, Otsuka K, et al. Intra-articular fractures of the distal aspect of the radius: arthroscopically assisted reduction compared with open reduction and internal fixation. *J Bone Joint Surg Am.* 1999;81A(8):1093–1110.

99. Rettig AC, Patel DV. Epidemiology of elbow, forearm, and wrist injuries in the athlete. *Clin J Sport Med.* 1995;14(2):289–297.

100. Panagis JS, Gelberman RH, Taleisnik J, et al. The arterial anatomy of the human carpus: part II: the intraosseous vascularity. *J Hand Surg Am.* 1983;8A(4):375–382.

101. Burge P. Closed cast treatment of scaphoid fractures. *Hand Clin.* 2001;17(4):541–552.

102. Weber ER, Chao EY. An experimental approach to the mechanism of scaphoid waist fractures. *J Hand Surg Am.* 1978;3A(2): 142–148.

103. Jupiter JB, Shin AY, Trumble TE, et al. Traumatic and reconstructive problems of the scaphoid. *Instr Course Lect.* 2001;50: 105–122.

104. Cerezal L, Abascal F, Canga A, et al. Usefulness of gadolinium-enhanced MR imaging in the evaluation of the vascularity of scaphoid nonunions. *AM J Am J Roentgenol.* 2000;174(1): 141–149.

105. Kozin SH. Incidence, mechanism, and natural history of scaphoid fractures. *Hand Clin.* 2001;17(4):515–524.

106. Yip HS, Wu WC, Chang RY, et al. Percutaneous cannulated screw fixation of acute scaphoid waist fracture. *J Hand Surg Br.* 2002;27B(1):42–46.

107. Herbert TJ. Open volar repair of acute scaphoid fractures. *Hand Clin.* 2001;17(4):601–610.

108. Raskin KB, Parisi D, Baker J, et al. Dorsal open repair of proximal pole scaphoid fractures. *Hand Clin.* 2001;17:601–610.

109. Steinmann SP, Bishop AT, Berger RA. Use of the 1,2 intercompartmental supraretinacular artery as a vascularized pedicle bone graft for difficult scaphoid nonunion. *J Hand Surg Am.* 2002;27A(3): 391–401.

110. Walsh JJ, Bishop AT. Diagnosis and management of hamate hook fractures. *Hand Clin.* 2000;16(3):397–403.

111. Bettinger PC, Linscheid RL, Berger RA, et al. An anatomic study of the stabilizing ligaments of the trapezium and trapeziometacarpal joint. *J Hand Surg Am.* 1999;24A(4):786–798.

112. Timmenga EJ, Blokhuis TJ, Maas M, et al. Long-term evaluation of Bennett's fracture. *J Hand Surg Br.* 1994;19B(3):373–377.

113. Light TR, Bednar MS. Management of intra-articular fractures of the metacarpophalangeal joint. *Hand Clin.* 1994;10(2): 303–314.

114. Shin AY, Bishop AT. Vascularized bone grafts for scaphoid nonunions and Kienbock's disease. *Orthop Clin North Am.* 2001;32(3):263–277.

115. Thornburg LE. Ganglions of the hand and wrist. *J Am Acad Orthop Surg.* 1999;7(4):231–238.

116. Al-Qattan MM. Giant cell tumours of tendon sheath: classification and recurrence rate. *J Hand Surg Br.* 2001;26B(1):72–75.

117. Sunderland S. A classification of peripheral nerve injuries producing loss of function. *Brain.* 1951;74(4):491–516.

118. Nuber GW, Assenmacher J, Bowen MK. Neurovascular problems in the forearm, wrist, and hand. *Clin J Sport Med.* 1998; 17(3):585–610.

119. Aulicino PL. Neurovascular injuries of the hands of athletes. *Hand Clin.* 1990;6(3):455–466.

120. Mosher JF. Current concepts in the diagnosis and treatment of hand and wrist injuries in sports. *Med Sci Sports Exerc.* 1985;17(1):48–55.

121. Gelberman RH, Hergenroeder PT, Hargens AR, et al. The carpal tunnel syndrome: a study of carpal canal pressures. *J Bone Joint Surg.* 1981;63A(3):380–383.

122. Szabo RM, Gelberman RH. The pathophysiology of nerve entrapment syndromes. *J Hand Surg Am.* 1987;12A(5, Part 2):880–884.

123. Armstrong TJ, Chaffin DB. Some biomechanical aspects of the carpal tunnel. *J Biomech.* 1979;12(7):567–570.

124. Louis DS, Hankin FM. Symptomatic relief following carpal tunnel decompression with normal electroneuromyographic studies (RETRACTED). *Orthopedics.* 1988;11(4):532.

125. Shum C, Parisien M, Strauch RJ, et al. The role of flexor tenosynovectomy in the operative treatment of carpal tunnel syndrome. *J Bone Joint Surg Am.* 2002;84A(2):221–225.

126. Stahl S, Ben-David B, Moscona RA. The effect of local infiltration with morphine before carpal tunnel release. *J Bone Joint Surg Am.* 1997;79A(4):551–554.

127. Fulcher SM, Kiefhaber TR, Stern PJ. Upper-extremity tendinitis and overuse syndromes in the athlete. *Clin J Sport Med.* 1998;17(3):433–448.

128. Trumble TE, Diao E, Abrams RA, et al. Single-portal endoscopic carpal tunnel release compared with open release: a prospective randomized trial. *J Bone Joint Surg Am.* 2002;84A(7): 1107–1115.

129. Brown RA, Gelberman RH, Seiler JGI, et al. Carpal tunnel release: a prospective randomized assessment of open and endoscopic methods. *J Bone Joint Surg Am.* 1993;75A(9): 1265–1275.

130. Papageorgiou CD, Georgoulis AD, Makris CA, et al. Difficulties and early results of the endoscopic carpal tunnel release using the modified Chow technique. *Knee Surg Sports Traumatol Arthrosc.* 1998;17:987–995.

131. Brown LG, Wright JG. Endoscopic compared with open carpal tunnel release. *J Bone Joint Surg.* 2003;85A:964.

132. Chow JC, Hantes ME. Endoscopic carpal tunnel release: thirteen years' experience with the Chow technique. *J Hand Surg Am.* 2002;27A(6):1011–1018.

133. Kulund DN, McCue FCI, Rockwell DA, et al. Tennis injuries: prevention and treatment: a review. *Am J Sports Med.* 1979;7(4): 249–253.

134. Cabrera JM, McCue FCI. Nonosseous athletic injuries of the elbow, forearm, and hand. *Clin J Sport Med.* 1986;5(4):681–700.

135. Carter PR, Eaton RG, Littler JW. Ununited fracture of the hook of the hamate. *J Bone Joint Surg Am.* 1977;59A(5):583–588.

136. McCue FCI, Baugher WH, Kulund DN, et al. Hand and wrist injuries in the athlete. *Am J Sports Med.* 1979;7(5):275–286.

137. Torisu T. Fracture of the hook of the hamate. *Clin Orthop.* 1972; 83:91–94.

138. Walker FO, Troost BT. Push-up palmar [Letter]. *JAMA.* 1988;259(1):45–46.

139. Rettig AC. Neurovascular injuries of the wrists and hands of athletes. *Clin J Sport Med.* 1990;9(2):389–417.

140. Wilmarth MA, Nelson SG. Distal sensory latencies of the ulnar nerve in long distance bicyclists: pilot study. *J Orthop Sports Phys Ther.* 1988;9(11):370.

141. Helal B. Racquet player's pisiform. *Hand.* 1978;10(1):87–90.

142. Weinstein SM, Herring SA. Nerve problems and compartment syndromes in the hand, wrist, and forearm. *Clin Sports.* 1992; 11(1):161–188.

143. Shea JD, McClain EJ. Ulnar nerve compression syndromes at and below the wrist. *J Bone Joint Surg Am.* 1969;51A(6):1095–1103.

144. Hoyt CS. Ulnar neuropathy in bicycle riders [Letter]. *Arch Intern Med.* 1976;33(5):372.

145. Colemann SS, Anson BJ. Arterial patterns in the hand based upon a study of 650 specimens. *Hand Clin.* 1961;8(2):359–367.

146. Converse TA. Cyclist's palsy [Letter]. *N Engl J Med.* 1979; 301(25):1397–1398.

147. Jackson DL. Electrodiagnostic studies of medial and ulnar nerves in cyclists. *Physician in Sports Medicine.* 1989;17(9):137.

148. Dunham W, Haines G, Spring JM. Bowler's thumb: ulnovolar neuroma of the thumb. *Clin Orthop.* 1972;83:99–101.

149. Minkow FV, Bassett FHI. Bowler's thumb. *Clin Orthop.* 1972;83: 115–117.

150. Goodman CE. Unusual nerve injuries in recreational activities. *Am J Sports Med.* 1983;11(4):224–227.

151. Itoh Y, Wakano K, Takeda T, et al. Circulatory disturbances in the throwing hand of baseball pitchers. *Am J Sports Med.* 1987;15(3):264–269.

152. Dobyns JH. Digital nerve compression. *Hand Clin.* 1992;8(2): 359–367.

153. Conn J, Bergan JJ, Bell JL. Hypothenar hammer syndrome: posttraumatic digital ischemia. *Surgery.* 1970;68:1122–1128.

154. Nuber GW, McCarthy WJ, Yao JS, et al. Arterial abnormalities of the hand in athletes. *Am J Sports Med.* 1990;18:520–523.

155. Porubsky GL, Brown SI, Urbaniak JR. Ulnar artery thrombosis: a sports-related injury. *Am J Sports Med.* 1986;14(170):175.

156. Lowery CW, Chandwick RO, Waltman EN. Digital vessel trauma from repetitive impact in baseball catchers. *J Hand Surg Am.* 1976;1:236–238.

157. DeMonaco D, Fritsche E, Rigoni G, et al. Hypothenar hammer syndrome: retrospective study of nine cases. *J Hand Surg Br.* 1999;24B(6):731–734.

158. Ginn TA, Smith AM, Snyder J, et al. Vascular changes of the hand in professional baseball players: digital ischemia in catchers. American Academy of Orthopaedic Surgeons; 2004.

159. Sugawara M, Ogino T, Minami A, et al. Digital ischemia in baseball players. *Am J Sports Med.* 1986;14:329–334.

160. Buckout BC, Warner MA. Digital perfusion of handball players. *Am J Sports Med.* 1980;8:206–207.

161. Dugas JR, Weiland AJ. Vascular pathology in the throwing athlete. *Hand Clin.* 2000;16(3):477–485.

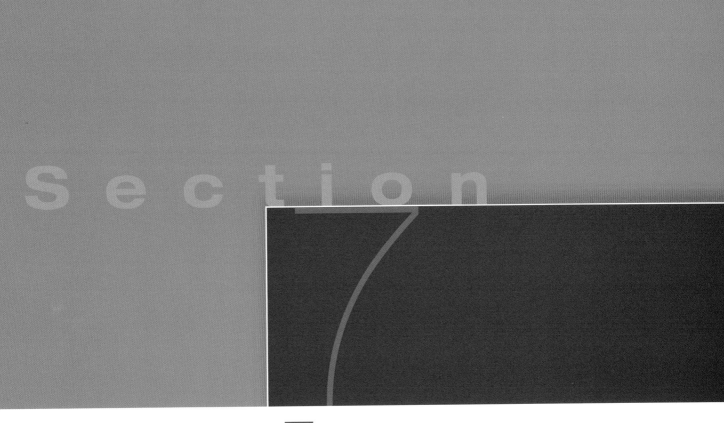

HIP AND THIGH

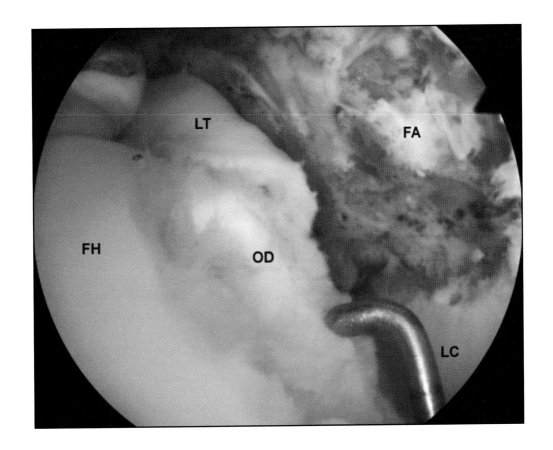

ANATOMY AND KINEMATICS OF THE HIP

MARK R. HUTCHINSON, MD, JOHN HUNG, MD, J.W. THOMAS BYRD, MD

■ KEY POINTS

- Normal range of motion of the hip is measured from a neutral or anatomic position of erect posture with the toes pointed forward.
- The presence of labral tears is directly associated with degenerative changes in adjacent articular cartilage.
- Labral tear location should be described as anterior, superior, or posterior and, if possible, peripheral or central. Tears may also be described as longitudinal, radial, or flap tears.
- The muscles crossing the hip joint are some of the most powerful in the body. Twenty-two muscles cross the hip joint and provide motor power for functional range of motion, balance, and gait.
- Both supine and lateral positions in arthroscopy require some element of traction along the femur to open the joint space; therefore, both have a risk of pudendal nerve palsy due to excessive traction against a perineal post.

■ ANATOMY AND KINEMATICS OF THE HIP

The hip joint is an important link in the kinetic chain connecting the lower extremity to the core. It must have the structural integrity to assume the loads of body weight not only through static stance but also through a myriad of dynamic activities such as walking, climbing, running, and jumping. The hip must also be both flexible and powerful. Normal range of motion is measured from a neutral or anatomic position of erect posture with the toes pointed forward. From this position, the normal hip can flex 120 to 130 degrees, extend 15 to 30 degrees, adduct 25 to 30 degrees,

abduct 30 to 50 degrees, externally rotate 40 to 60 degrees, and internally rotate 30 to 40 degrees. Extremes of motion are limited by bony anatomy, ligamentous and capsular restraints, and active motor tension. Coordinated motor power of the muscles that cross the joint is essential for balance, normal gait, and transferring energy up the kinetic chain. Indeed, the muscles crossing the hip joint are some of the most powerful in the body.

The purpose of this chapter is to review the anatomy of the hip as it relates to orthopaedic sports medicine and arthroscopy. Anatomy is the foundation of diagnosis, physical examination, and successful surgical intervention. This chapter will cover in sequence superficial anatomic landmarks; bony anatomy including facets of the pelvis, acetabulum, and proximal femur; capsule, labrum, and ligamentous structure; muscle tendon units that cross the hip joint and power motion; associated bursae including the trochanteric bursa and iliopsoas bursa; and neurovascular structures that supply the anatomic structures about the hip and are at risk during surgical and arthroscopic approaches **(Fig 25-1)**. The final section will be dedicated to the unique perspective of anatomy from an arthroscopic point of view.

Superficial Anatomic Landmarks

Superficial bony landmarks assist in the examination of the hip to specifically identify pathology and to guide safe surgical approaches and portal placement. The anterior and posterior surfaces of the pelvis are an obvious delineation between anterior and posterior structures. Laterally, the border can be palpated from the border of the iliac crest, the anterior superior iliac spine, and the greater trochanter. Medially, the delineation between anterior and posterior

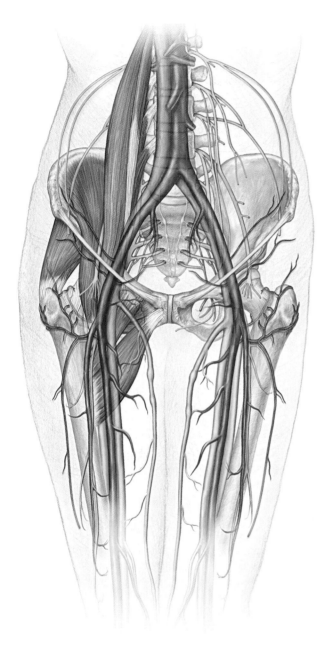

Fig 25-1. Anterior perspective of the hip demonstrates the relationship of bone structure, muscles, nerves, arteries, and veins about the hip.

structures extend distally from the symphysis pubis along the palpable superficial adductor, the gracilis.

Additional superficial anatomic landmarks anteriorly include the hip flexion crease, the palpable inguinal ligament (creating the roof of the femoral triangle), and the femoral artery (palpated by pulse) **(Fig 25-2)**. The obvious superficial anatomic landmark laterally is the greater trochanter, which serves as the insertion point of the hip abductors and defines the site of trochanteric bursitis when present. The anterior edge of the tensor fascia lata can frequently be palpated with internal and external rotation of the hip as it passes over the greater trochanter. Posteriorly, important palpable landmarks

include the spinous processes of the lumbo-sacral spine, the posterior superior iliac spine, the sacroiliac joints, the ischium serving as insertion of the hamstring musculature, and the sciatic notch, which can relatively be assessed as a soft spot medial and superior to the ischium deep to the gluteal musculature.

Bone Anatomy/Osteology

The pelvis is a complex structure composed of bony and ligamentous constructs. There are two inominate bones connected at the pubis symphysis, in addition to their interconnections with the sacrum. The inominate bones are composed of three components: ilium, ischium, and pubis. These bones converge to form the acetabulum, which articulates with the femoral head to comprise the hip joint **(Fig 25-3)**. The bony pelvis is maintained structurally by dense ligamentous structures. The formation of the sacroiliac joint is one of excellent stability due to the expanse of the articular surfaces as well as the broad extensive ligamentous structures that make up the sacroiliac joint. The ligaments that provide the structural stability include the interosseus sacroiliac ligaments, posterior sacroiliac ligaments, anterior sacroiliac ligaments, and the sacrotuberous, sacrospinous ligaments. Posteriorly, the construct of the ligaments act in the same way suspension bridges function. The posterior superior iliac spines act as the pillars, the interosseus ligaments serving as the suspensory bars, and the sacrum acts as the bridge.

The acetabulum is described as an incomplete hemisphere and serves as the socket for this classic diarthrodial, ball and socket joint. The articular surface is shaped like a horseshoe surrounding the nonarticular cotyloid fossa **(Figs 25-4** and **25-5)**. The socket is supported by the anterior and posterior columns of bone oriented in an inverted Y-shape. The posterior column is composed of the ischium, the ischiala spine, the posterior half of the acetabulum, and the dense bone of the sciatic notch. The anterior column is composed of the anterior iliac crest, the anterior iliac spines, the anterior half of the acetabulum, and the pubis. The inferior aspect of the acetabulum (the lower two limbs of the horseshoe) is connected by the transverse ligament, which plays an important role in maintaining joint congruity and accepting transfer loads across the joint.

The acetabulum is obliquely oriented in the coronal plane 45 degrees to the floor and is usually anterior-faced (anteverted) at about 15 degrees. The anteversion is directly affected by the amount of pelvic tilt or rotation in the sagittal plane. With increased pelvic tilt the relative anteversion increases and with loss of pelvic tilt the acetabulum can actually face posteriorly. With neutral pelvic alignment, anteversion ranges from 5 to 20 degrees in men and 10 to 24 degrees in women (1–3).

The weight-bearing surface of the acetabulum is the dome or roof. This portion supports the femur during normal standing. This dome can be defined as the area encompassed by a 45-degree arc with a central axis through the

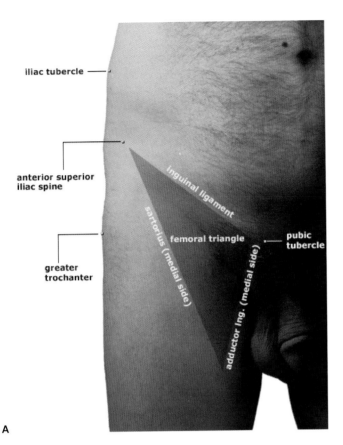

A

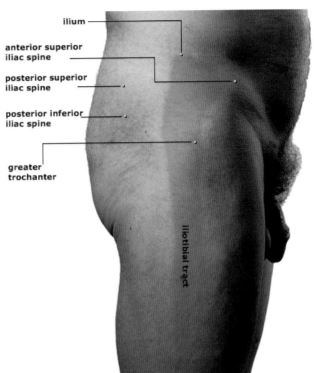

B

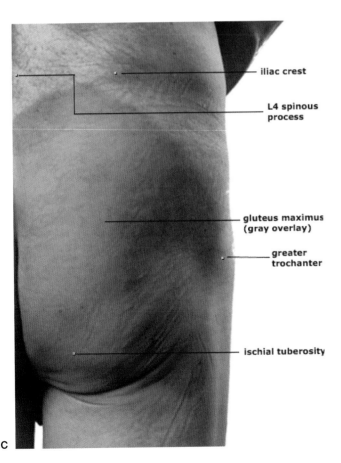

C

Fig 25-2. Superficial anatomic landmarks are important guides to diagnosis and surgical approaches of the hip. The anterior view (A) demonstrates the anterior superior iliac spine, the inguinal ligament, the symphysis pubis, and the sartorius, which defines the femoral triangle. The lateral view (B) demonstrates the greater trochanter, the iliotibial tract, the iliac crest, the anterior superior iliac spine, the posterior superior iliac spine, and the posterior inferior iliac spine. The posterior view (C) demonstrates the iliac crest, the lumbar spinous processes, the ischial tuberosity, and gluteus maximus muscle. (Courtesy of Dartmouth Medical School, Board of Trustees, Hanover, New Hampshire, 03755. Joseph Mehliing photographer. www.Dartmouth.edu/anatomy/hip/http.)

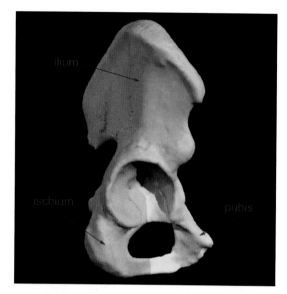

Fig 25-3. Lateral view of the pelvis demonstrates the developmental contributions to the acetabulum from the ischium, ileum, and pubis. (Courtesy of Primal Pictures 2000, Interactive Hip, Tennyson House, 159 Great Portland Street, London, England, W1W 5PA.)

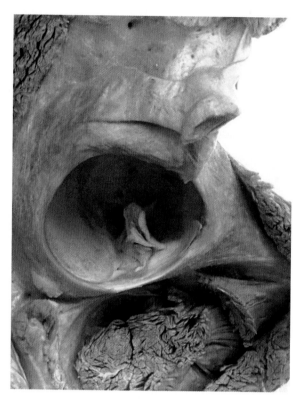

Fig 25-5. Lateral view of acetabulum in a cadaver specimen. (Courtesy of Primal Pictures 2000, Interactive Hip, Tennyson House, 159 Great Portland Street, London, England, W1W 5PA.)

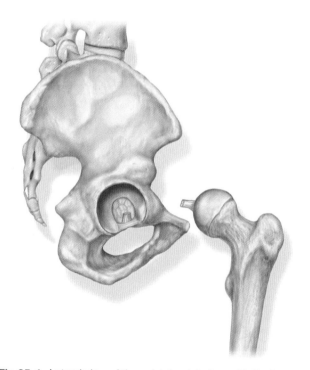

Fig 25-4. Lateral view of the pelvis/acetabulum with the femoral head removed demonstrates the relationship of the labrum, transverse ligament, ligamentus mucosum, acetabulum and femoral head. (Courtesy of Anatomic Chart Company.)

and superiorly on the articular surface and serves as the insertion of the ligamentum teres (Fig 25-4). The femoral neck is anteverted between 8 to 14 degrees in relation to the femoral condyles. This angle is determined by the femoral neck and the transcondylar axis of the knee. The femoral neck shaft angle averages 127 to 135 degrees (with angles >135 degrees known as coxa valga, and angles <120 degrees knows as coxa vara). The effect of this femoral offset or overhanging head and neck is to lateralize the hip abductors, which increases their potential torque and reduces the overall force necessary to balance the pelvis. The base of the femoral neck broadens into the lesser and greater trochanters, which serve as strong sites for hip abductor and adductor motor attachments.

Capsule, Ligaments, and Labrum

The articular capsule of the hip joint is a strong, dense, fibrous capsule. Proximally, it is attached to the edge of the acetabulum, just peripheral to the labrum. It is attached distally to the neck of the femur. Anteriorly, it inserts along the intertrochanteric line and posteriorly, just proximal to the intertrochanteric crest. The capsule blends with a number of intrinsic ligaments, which serve to provide static stability to the hip joint on extremes of motion as well as maintain joint fluid in an enclosed space for lubrication.

superior pole of the acetabulum. This area must be intact for adequate support in weight bearing through the acetabulum.

The femoral head is a spherical structure that serves as the ball of the ball and socket joint and is predominantly covered by articular hyaline cartilage. A fovea sits centrally

The capsular ligaments include the iliofemoral ligament, pubofemoral ligament, and ischiofemoral ligament **(Figs 25-6 and 25-7)**. These capsular ligaments thicken the capsule and make it challenging at times to penetrate when placing arthroscopic portals.

The iliofemoral ligament, also known as the Y ligament of Bigelow, originates from the anterior inferior iliac spine and the acetabular rim distally to the intertrochanteric line of the femur. This ligament is Y-shaped and becomes taut in extension of the hip. This ligament serves an important role in hip biomechanics to prevent hyperextension and maintain an erect posture in the standing position. The pubofemoral ligament originates from the pubic portion of the acetabular rim and blends with the iliofemoral ligament. It serves to provide strength to the inferior and anterior aspect of the hip joint. It becomes tight into abduction and extension. The ischiofemoral ligament originates from the ischial acetabular rim and inserts to the superior lateral femoral neck along the medial aspect of the greater trochanter. It also becomes taut into hip extension, again, preventing hyperextension of the hip joint.

The ligamentum teres is an intra-articular ligament originating from the acetabular notch (with extension to the transverse acetabular ligament) inserting into the fovea of the femoral head. Within this ligament, there exists a foveal artery originating from the obturator artery. The artery is viable in children but may not play a significant role of arterial supply to the femoral head in adults. This ligament is contained within a sleeve of synovial membrane but rupture with hip dislocation usually leads to violation of both. A torn ligamentum teres may catch within the articular surface of the joint and be an intra-articular source of a snapping hip.

The labrum is composed of fibro-elastic cartilage with interlacing network of collagen fibers, proteoglycans, glycoproteins, and cellular elements. Scanning electron microscopy revealed three distinct layers in the acetabular labrum: (a) the articular surface covered by a meshwork of thin fibrils; (b) beneath the superficial layer a layer of lamella-like collagen fibrils; and (c) the deepest layer of collagen fibrils oriented in a circular manner to absorb hoop stresses. The vascular supply reaches only the peripheral third of the labrum (4,5).

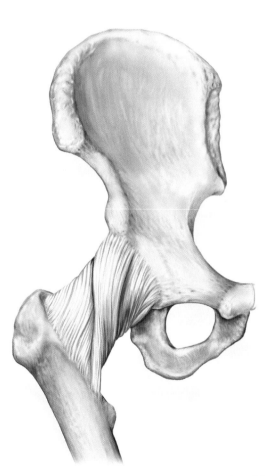

Fig 25-6. Anterior view of the capsuligament complex of the hip demonstrates the Y ligament of Bigelow, the iliofemoral ligament, and the pubofemoral ligament. (Courtesy of Anatomic Chart Company.)

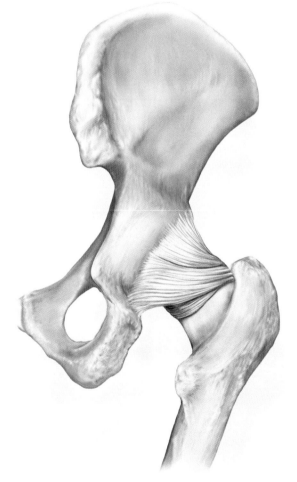

Fig 25-7. Posterior view of the capsuloligamentous complex of the hip demonstrates the ischiofemoral ligament. (Courtesy of Anatomic Chart Company.)

The role of the labrum is still not completely understood, but there is a number of proposed theories. An important role is likely in providing increased joint stability. By increasing the depth of the socket, the labrum assists in structurally maintaining the humeral head in the socket. In addition, the labrum provides a seal to the joint, thereby providing stability utilizing ambient and intra-articular pressures to keep the joint reduced. Hydrostatic fluid pressure with the intra-articular space is greater with an intact labrum than without which may enhance joint lubrication (6).

The labrum probably plays a significant role in load transmission across the hip **(Fig 25-8)**. A number of studies have revealed that the presence of labral tears is directly associated with degenerative changes in adjacent articular cartilage (7,8). Nonetheless, the direct relationship with labral injury and increased cartilage degeneration may not be so clear because another study revealed increased degeneration only when both the labrum and the transverse acetabular ligaments were resected (5,9). Tear location should be described as anterior, superior, or posterior and, if possible, peripheral or central. Tears may also be described as longitudinal, radial, or flap tears **(Fig 25-9)**. The majority of the tears involve the anterior labrum. This is true for sports-related injures, which are commonly torsional, occult tears with no specific mechanism, and in patients with degenerative joint disease or hip dysplasia. Isolated posterior labral tears typically occur with posterior hip dislocations or occasionally in dysplastic hips. Complex and severe injuries may involve the anterior, superior, and posterior labrum; therefore, thorough examination is always necessary (10,11). Degenerative tears may be associated with intra-articular degeneration and appear as friable tissue with complex tear patterns. Acute tears, radial flap, and longitudinal peripheral tears, may have sharper borders. Longitudinal peripheral tears have the potential for repair if identified early. Labral pathology associated with dysplastic hips may present with hypertrophy or degenerative tearing.

Motor and Neurovascular Anatomy

The hip joint is a very dynamic joint with 3 degrees of freedom including abduction/adduction, flexion/extension, and internal/external rotation. The hip allows very little anterior-posterior, mediolateral, or proximodistal translation. Twenty-two muscles cross the hip joint and provide motor power for functional range of motion, balance, and gait. **Table 25-1** lists each muscle categorized by function including its origin, insertion, and nerve supply. All five flexors are innervated by the femoral nerve (iliacus, psoas, pectineus, rectus, and sartorius). All four adductors are innervated by the obturator nerve: adductor magnus (with some contribution from sciatic), adductor brevis, adductor longus, and gracilis. Four of the seven external rotators have self-named nerves (gluteus maximus, priformis, obturator internus, and obturator externus.). The remaining external rotators are innervated by the obturator nerve (superior and inferior gamellus and quadrator femoris). The three abductors (gluteus medius, gluteus minimus, and tensor fascia lata) are all innervated by the superior gluteal nerve.

Innervation to the lower extremity is accomplished by a network of terminal nerve roots from the spinal cord, the lumbosacral plexus. The spinal levels that incorporate this plexus originate from the ventral rami of T12 to S4. These lie posterior to the psoa muscle and are further differentiated into anterior and posterior divisions. The anterior division includes obturator nerve (also sometimes the accessory obturator nerve), the tibial component of the sciatic nerve, nerve to the quadratus femoris, nerve to obturator internus, pudendal nerve, coccygeus nerve, and levator ani nerve. The posterior division includes lateral femoral cutaneous nerve, femoral nerve, the peroneal component of the sciatic nerve, superior gluteal nerve, inferior gluteal nerve, piriformis, and posterior femoral cutaneous nerve. All important nerves about the hip leave the pelvis by way of the sciatic foramen. The pudendal and obturator internus nerves leave via the greater sciatic notch and then re-enter via the lesser sciatic notch. Within the sciatic notch, the superior gluteal nerve and artery lie above the piriformis and all other structures lie below it. When exiting the pelvis and entering the thigh, the great vessels lie beneath the inguinal ligament in the femoral triangle. These structures can be at risk in open and arthroscopic approaches to the hip joint.

The blood supply to the lower extremity and pelvis comes from the two iliac arteries that serve as the terminal end of the abdominal aorta (Fig 25-1). The iliac vessels diverge into internal and external components with the internal iliac supplying the internal pelvic structures, acetabulum, and musculature, and the external iliac becoming the femoral artery at the level of the inguinal ligament. The internal iliac artery gives off branches to the obturator, superior gluteal, inferior gluteal, and internal pudendal arteries. The obturator

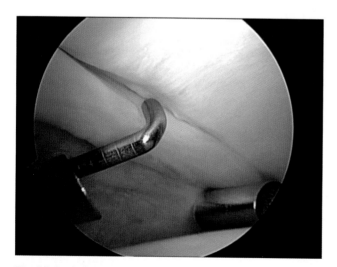

Fig 25-8. Arthroscopic view of a normal labral variant. The labrum may be continuous with the bony acetabulum or have a small sublabral recess making it look similar to a meniscus. (Courtesy of J.W. Thomas Byrd MD.)

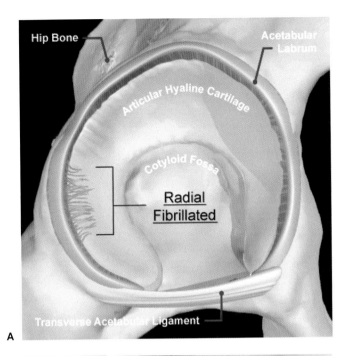

A

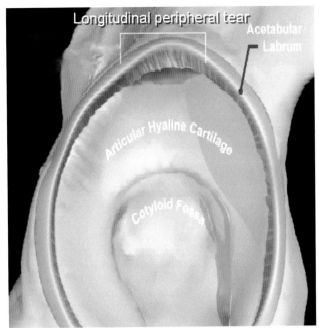

B

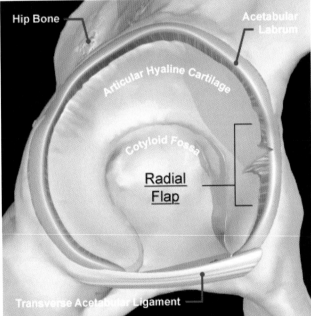

C

Fig 25-9. Representative illustrations of the lateral view of the acetabulum demonstrate posterior radial fraying (A), peripheral superior longitudinal (B), and anterior flap tears (C) of the labrum. (Courtesy of Primal Pictures 2000, Interactive Hip, Tennyson House, 159 Great Portland Street, London, England, W1W 5PA.)

is notably at risk with over-penetrance of acetabular screws placed in the anterior inferior quadrant during total hip arthoplasty. The external iliac is at risk of injury with over-penetrated screws in the anterior superior quadrant of the acetabulum.

The femoral artery can be easily palpated just distal to the inguinal ligament in the anterior-medial aspect of the groin. It is at risk of injury during anterior approaches to the hip and acetabulum via arthroscopic or open surgical procedures. A commonly used acronym to remember the relationship between neurovascular structures at this level is "NAVEL," with the "Nerve being lateral followed sequentially by the artery vein, empty space, and lymphatics as one proceeds medially." The femoral artery then branches into the superficial femoral artery and the profundus femorus artery (Fig 25-10). The superficial femoral artery travels medially and becomes the popliteal artery in the mid to distal thigh and in turn is the terminal blood supply to the leg, ankle, and foot. The profundus femorus artery supplies a majority of structures in the thigh.

TABLE 25-1

Muscle	Origin	Insertion	Innervation	Spinal level/segment
Adductors				
Adductor Magnus	Inf pubic ramus/ischial tuberosity	Linea aspera/ adductor tubercle	Obturator (Posterior) Sciatic (Tibial)	L2-4
Adductor Brevis	Inf pubic ramus	Linea aspera/ pectineal line	Obturator (Posterior)	L2-4
Adductor Longus	Anterior pubic ramus	Linea aspera	Obturator (Anterior)	L2-4
Gracilis	Inf Symphysis/ pubic arch	Proximal medial tibia	Obturator (Anterior)	L2-4
Flexors				
Iliacus	Iliac fossa	Lesser trochanter	Femoral	L2-4
Psoas	Transverse process L1-L5	Lesser trochanter	Femoral	L2-4
Pectineus	Pectineal line of pubis bone	Pectineal line of femur	Femoral	L2-4
Rectus Femoris	AIIS/Ant acetabular rim	Patella/tibial tubercle	Femoral	L2-4
Sartorius	ASIS	Proximal medial tibia	Femoral	L2-4
Abductors				
Gluteus Medius	Ilium (between Post/ Ant gluteal lines	Greater trochanter	Superior Gluteal	L4-S1
Gluteus Minimus	Ilium (between Ant/ Inf gluteal lines	Greater trochanter	Superior Gluteal	L4-S1
Tensor fasciae Latae	Anterior iliac crest	IT band (Gerdy's turbercle)	Superior Gluteal	L4-S1
External Rotators				
Gluteus Maximus	Ilium along crest post to post gluteal line	IT band/Posterior femur	Inferior Gluteal	L5-S2
Piriformis	Ant Sacrum, through sciatic notch	Proximal greater trochanter (piriformis fossa)	Piriformis	S1-S2
Obturator Internus	Ischiopubic rami/ obturator membrane	Medial greater trochanter	Obturator internus	L5-S2
Obturator Externus	Ischiopubic rami/ obturator membrane	Medial greater trochanter	Obturator	L2-4
Superior Gemellus	Ischial spine	Medial greater trochanter	Obturator internus	L5-S2
Inferior Gemellus	Ischial tuberosity	Medial greater trochanter	Obturator femoris	L4-S1
Quadratus Femoris	Ischial tuberosity	Quadrate line of femur	Obturator femoris	L4-S1
Extensors				
Gluteus Maximus	as above			
Biceps femoris	Med ischial tub (long), linea aspera/lat IM septum (short)	Fibular head/ lateral tibia	Tibial (long), Peroneal (short)	L5-S2
Semitendinosus	Distal medial ischial tuberosity	Ant tibial crest	Tibial	L5-S2
Semimembranosus	Proximal lateral ischial tuberosity	Posterior/medial tibia, posterior caspule, medial meniscus, popliteus, popliteal ligament	Tibial	L5-S2

The primary blood supply to the femoral head and neck of the femur comes from the medial femoral circumflex, which is a branch off the deep femoral artery (the profunda femoris). The medial femoral circumflex wraps around the iliopsoas tendon passing between the iliopsoas and pectineus muscles then to the medial and posterior aspect of the femoral neck. It is at risk of injury with posterior hip dislocations and posterior approaches to the hip. The femoral head receives blood supply from an anastomosis of three sets of arteries: (a) the medial circumflex and, to a lesser extent,

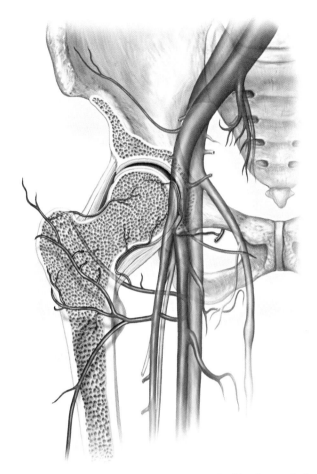

Fig 25-10. Cross-sectional illustration of the hip demonstrates the vascular supply to the femoral head via branches from the profunda femoris artery. (Courtesy of Anatomic Chart Company.)

olecronon bursa of the elbow, which serve as cushions between the skin and bony prominences, or the subacromial bursa of the shoulder, which reduces friction between the rotator cuff muscles and the acromion. There are a number of potential bursa about the hip, including the obturator externus bursa (12) and the piriformis bursa, but the most common that lead to pathologic problems are the trochanteric bursa and the iliopsoas bursa.

The trochanteric bursa is a large bursa that sits between the fascia lata and the greater trochanter of the femur on the lateral aspect of the hip. A series of cadaveric dissections revealed this bursa to be immediately superficial to the common attachment of the gluteus medius, minimus, and vastus lateralis onto the greater trochanter and in almost a third of the cases a superficial bursa was noted reflected by the gluteus maximus muscle (13). In two of 16 cases, branches of the inferior gluteal nerve were visualized innervating the bursa. It is important to be aware of the potential variations and proximity of the inferior gluteal nerve proximally or sciatic nerve posteriorly when considering addressing chronic treo-chanteric bursitis arthroscopically.

The iliopsoas bursa has been described as the largest bursa in the body and lies between the iliopsoas tendon and the lesser trochanter and may extend beneath the iliopsoas tendon as it passes over the brim of the pelvis **(Fig 25-11)**. It communicates with the joint space (via a gap between the

the lateral circumflex femoral artery, (b) terminal branches of the medullary artery from the shaft of the femur, and (c) the artery of the ligamentum teres from the posterior division of the obturator artery (from the internal iliac artery). The retinacular arteries traverse from the circumflex vessels along the femoral neck into the femoral head. The specific contribution of each source to total femoral head blood supply is age dependent. From birth to 4 years, the medial and lateral circumflex are most important and the ligamentum teres is more likely to be viable. From 4 years to adult, the posterior superior retinacular vessels from the medial femoral cirmcumflex are most important. In the adult, the lateral epiphyseal artery from the medial femoral circumflex plays an important role. Each of these vessels may be at risk with femoral neck fractures, hip dislocations, surgical approaches, or arthroscopy that proceeds from the hip capsule down the femoral neck.

Anatomy of Bursae about the Hip

Bursae are fluid-filled sacs that serve as cushions or pads between structures that produce friction between each other. Examples include the prepatellar bursa of the knee or the

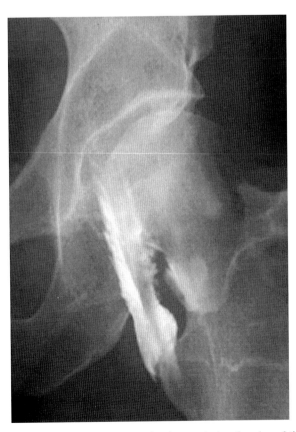

Fig 25-11. Iliopsoas bursography demonstrates the size of the bursa and can be helpful in making the diagnosis of snapping hip secondary to the iliopsoas tendon. (Courtesy of Martin Lazarus MD.)

iliofemoral and pubofemoral ligaments) in about 15% of normal hips and up to 30% to 40% of patients with intra-articular diseases such as osteoarthritis, rheumatoid arthritis, infection, calcium pyrophosphate deposition disease, and idiopathic synovial chondromatosis. Iliopsoas bursal imaging has been proposed as a simple, rapid, and reproducible method to evaluate abnormal iliopsoas tendon motion in patients with a snapping hip (14).

Hip Joint Kinematics and Biomechanics

Kinematic measurements in the hip joint are generally described in terms of joint rotation. The translational component of this joint is relatively small and difficult to quantify. These motions are typically flexion-extension, internal-external rotation, and abduction-adduction.

Clinically, normal flexion range of motion is about 135 degrees with normal extension about 40 degrees. However, if the pelvis is stabilized to neutral and not allowed to rotate, true hip flexion is slightly less at about 120 degrees with extension of 10 degrees. Internal and external rotation occurs along a longitudinal axis extending from the femoral head to the intercondylar region of the distal femur. The total arc of motion is approximately 50 degrees, being slightly greater in external rotation (about 35 degrees) compared to internal rotation (about 15 degrees). Normal hip abduction is approximately 45 degrees and normal hip adduction is about 25 degrees. Naturally, these ranges can vary depending on anatomic variants of femoral version, anatomic variants of the acetabulum, or pathology within or about the hip joint.

Biomechanics is a dynamic science evaluating the effect of forces and loads across an anatomic structure. Of all the species in the animal kingdom, only birds and man habitually use a bipedal gait. When standing, the center of gravity is centered between the two hips and equal force is exerted across both hips. The compressive force is about one-third body weight when standing on both legs (15,16). In single leg stance, the center of gravity moves away from the stance limb (the non-supported limb is now calculated as part of the body mass) and requires abductor muscle activity to avoid dropping the contralateral pelvis (a positive Trendelenberg sign). Those abductors include upper fibers of the gluteus medius, the tensor fascia lata, the gluteus medius and minimus, the piriformis, and the obturator internus. Due to active muscle compression and increased loads, the compressive force across the hip joint increases to four times body weight in the single leg stance phase of gait. These forces can be reduced through weight loss or the use of a walking stick.

In normal stance, when the hips are viewed in the sagittal plane, the center of gravity should pass directly through the centers of the femoral heads implying that minimal muscle forces necessary to maintain an erect position. If the upper body is leaned slightly posteriorly, the hip is slightly extended and the center of gravity will fall posterior to the centers of the femoral heads. Stability is provided primarily by the static restraints of the anterior capsule or more specifically the Y ligament of Bigelow. If the Y ligament is damaged or lax, the patient may have difficulty maintaining an erect posture because the anterior motor power is not as powerful as the posterior motor power (gluteals) to maintain the upright position.

The anatomic design of the acetabulum plays a valuable role in accepting/transferring the forces across the hip joint. The intact acetabulum has been described as an inverted horseshoe in which the superior, anterior, and posterior articular surface wraps around the femoral head. As load is applied across the joint, the horseshoe expands slightly to accept the load, allowing a more congruous seating of the femoral head (16,17). The expansion is resisted by both the rigid bony structure and the transverse ligament that connects both limbs of the inferior horseshoe and closes the acetabular socket.

Arthroscopic Anatomy: A Different Perspective

Open surgical procedures and classic dissections provide a direct outside in assessment of anatomic structures. We are able to understand the common relationships between structures and we know which structures are supplied by which artery and nerve to try to find a safe plane to approach the deeper anatomy by moving the more superficial anatomy aside. This retraction and removal of superficial structures carries the risk of distorting anatomy or altering the functional performance of these structures. Arthroscopy provides a different perspective by looking inside out rather than outside in. It allows the examiner to evaluate the structures inside a joint while minimizing dissection of superficial structures and the inherent morbidity of doing so. Naturally, safely performing arthroscopy requires a keen knowledge of normal anatomy to optimally place portals and avoid neurovascular structures (18). In addition, the new perspective achieved looking from inside out may vary on the perspective of the examiner (i.e., which portal you are viewing through and which way your scope is oriented). This section will briefly review the relevant anatomy of portal placements, anatomic advantages or disadvantages of the lateral or supine position, and the arthroscopic normal anatomy through anterior, anterior-lateral, and posterior portals.

Debate continues regarding the ideal patient position in which to perform hip arthroscopy: supine or lateral. Each has its advantages and disadvantages. What is likely more important is an intricate knowledge of anatomy to allow for safe portal placements and to avoid complications in either position. Both positions require some element of traction along the femur to open the joint space; therefore, both have a risk of pudendal nerve palsy due to excessive traction against a perineal post. The lateral position introduces some potential risk of injury to the downside limbs if not carefully monitored or padded; for example, the downside fibula head should be well padded or sit on a pillow to avoid injury to the peroneal nerve and the downside upper extremity should be protected with an axillary roll to avoid injury to the axillary nerve. Proponents of the lateral position have argued a reduced risk of injury to the sciatic nerve, because gravity helps to displace the neurovascular structures medially in this position. In either case, the fundamentals are the same, identify neurovascular structures at risk and avoid them (19–21).

Arthroscopic portal placements are made using superficial anatomic landmarks with the goal of minimizing risk of adjacent neurovascular structures **(Fig 25-12)**. The primary landmark for portal placement when the patient is placed in the lateral or supine positions is the greater trochanter. Subtle variations exist between arthroscopists, but most will use an anterior-lateral portal as a starting portal because it is the farthest away from major neurovascular structures. (This has been described as the anterior paratrochanteric portal by some arthroscopists who prefer the lateral position.) This portal is placed at the level of the tip of the greater trochanter and about 1 to 2 cm anterior to it. Flouroscopic assistance enables appropriate aim into the joint itself. The primary structure at risk is the lateral femoral cutaneous nerve; therefore, a skin stab wound with blunt dilation is preferred over a sharp portal placement down to the capsule. The femoral

artery and nerve may also be at risk if the arthroscopist aims anterior to the acetabular socket. The superior gluteal nerve lies an average 4.4 cm from the portal. The anterior lateral portal enables visualization of the anterior femoral head, anterior labrum, and anterior synovium **(Fig 25-13)**. It is used as the arthroscopic portal when working tools are used in the anterior or posterolateral portals.

An accessory portal used more commonly in the lateral position is the proximal trochanteric portal. This portal is located directly cephalad to the tip of the trochanter and equidistant between the anterior and posterior margins. The cannula must penetrate the gluteus medius and minimus on its way to the capsule. The advantage of this portal is that it can enable visualization to both the anterior and posterior labral tissue. The disadvantage is that there may not be significant distance between this and the working portals, making it difficult to handle both the arthroscope and instruments in a limited space.

The posterolateral or posterior paratrochanteric portal is a mirror image of the anterolateral portal at the level of the tip of the greater trochanter but 2 to 3 cm posterior to it. The cannula should penetrate the capsule anterior to the piriformis tendon and posterior to the gluteus minimus tendon. The key structure at risk is the sciatic nerve. The portal

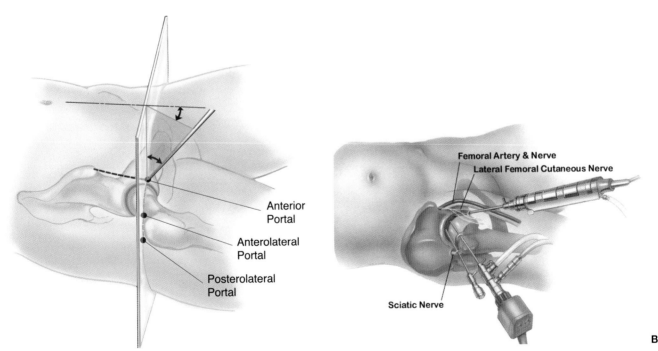

A

B

Fig 25-12. Portal placements are made in line with a plane that cuts sagitally through the pelvis at the level of the acetabulum. The anterior portal coincides with the intersection of that plane with a vertical line dropped from the anterior superior iliac spine. The anterolateral and posterolateral portals are positioned just superior to the trochanter at its anterior and posterior borders. [(A) Courtesy of J.W. Thomas Byrd MD and Smith & Nephew Endoscopy, Andover, Massachusetts.] The sciatic nerve is at risk with the posterior portal and the lateral femoral cutaneous nerve, femoral nerve, and femoral artery are in proximity to the anterior portal. [(B) Courtesy of J.W. Thomas Byrd MD.]

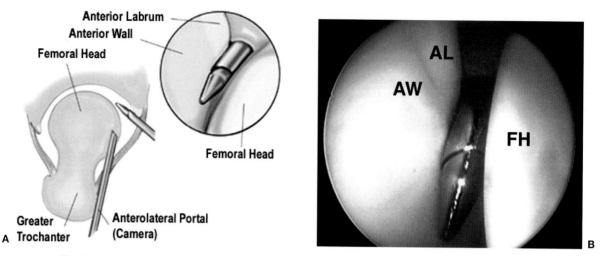

Fig 25-13. Arthroscopic placement of the anterolateral portal **(A)** allows visualization of the anterior wall *(AW)*, anterior labrum *(AL)*, and femoral head *(FH)* articular surface. [**(A)** courtesy of Smith & Nephew Endoscopy, Andover, Massachusetts; **(B)** courtesy of J.W. Thomas Byrd MD.]

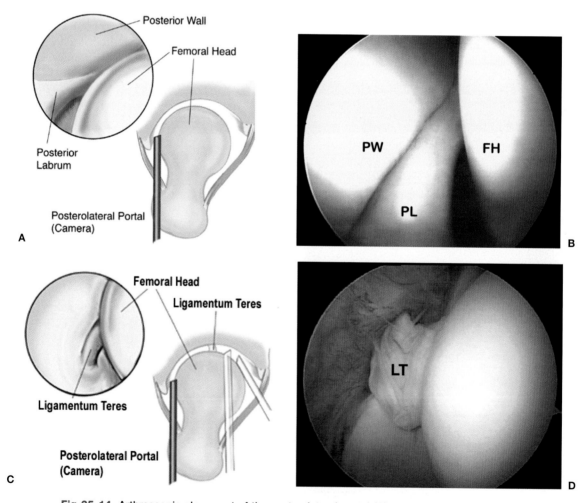

Fig 25-14. Arthroscopic placement of the posterolateral portal **(A)** enables visualization of the posterior wall *(PW)*, posterior labrum *(PL)*, and posterior aspect of the femoral head *(FH)* when directed posteriorly **(B)** and enables visualization of the femoral head and ligamentus teres when directed central into the acetabulum **(C,D)**. [**(A)** and **(C)** courtesy of Smith & Nephew Endoscopy, Andover, Massachusetts; arthroscopic photos **(B)** and **(D)** courtesy of J.W. Thomas Byrd MD.]

lies closest to the sciatic nerve at the level of the capsule with the distance average 2.9 cm. The average distance from the superior gluteal nerve is 4.4 cm. Proponents of the lateral position feel that the muscles and neurovascular structures tend to fall medially and therefore reduce the risk of injury in that position. Attention should be given to maintaining a neutral or slightly internally rotated position of the femur. With external rotation, the trochanter tends to block access to the posterior capsule, forcing the arthroscopist to slip posteriorly, risking the sciatic nerve. Neutral or slight internal rotation can minimize this risk. True posterior portals are rarely placed due to the proximity of the sciatic nerve. Nonetheless, some authors have proposed a mini-incision posterior with retraction of the nerve as a safe way to approach from even more posteriorly than a posterolateral portal will allow. The posterolateral portal enables visualization of the posterior labrum, posterior wall, and posterior aspect of the femoral head **(Fig 25-14)**.

Various anatomic landmarks have been used to most safely place a direct anterior portal. Clearly, it must begin lateral to the palpable femoral pulse. The most common guidelines using superficial landmarks guiding portal placement is the intersection between a vertical line dropped from the anterior superior iliac spine and a horizontal line drawn from the tip of the greater trochanter. The angle of the portal is about 45 degrees medially and 30 to 45 degrees proximally into the anterior superior aspect of the acetabulum. This tract will penetrate the belly of the sartorius and rectus muscles before it enters the capsule. The most common structure at risk is the lateral femoral cutaneous nerve; however, great care should be made to avoid beginning too medially where the femoral nerve and artery could be at risk. Average distance to the femoral nerve is 3.2 cm and to the femoral artery is 3.7 cm. The anterior portal enables visualization of the anterior femoral head and neck, the superior retinacular fold, and the ligamentum teres **(Fig 25-15)**.

By flexing the hip joint and redirecting the cannulas to the periphery along the femoral neck, it is possible to inspect the intracapsular anatomy of the hip that is not within the acetabular socket itself. From this distal perspective, one

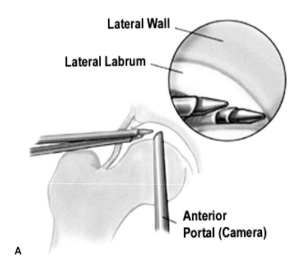

A

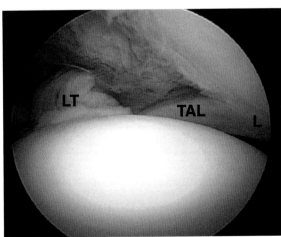

C

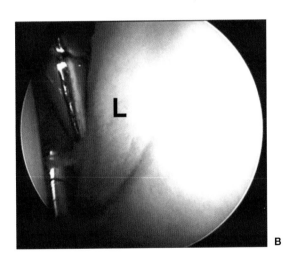

B

Fig 25-15. Arthroscopic placement of the anterior portal **(A)** enables visualization of the lateral aspect of the labrum and its relationship to the lateral portals **(B)**. Directing the scope inferiorly and medially enables visualization of the ligamentum teres *(LT)* and transverse acetabular ligament *(TAL)* **(C)**. [**(A)** courtesy of Smith & Nephew Endoscopy, Andover, Massachusetts; arthroscopic photos **(B)** and **(C)** courtesy of J.W. Thomas Byrd MD.]

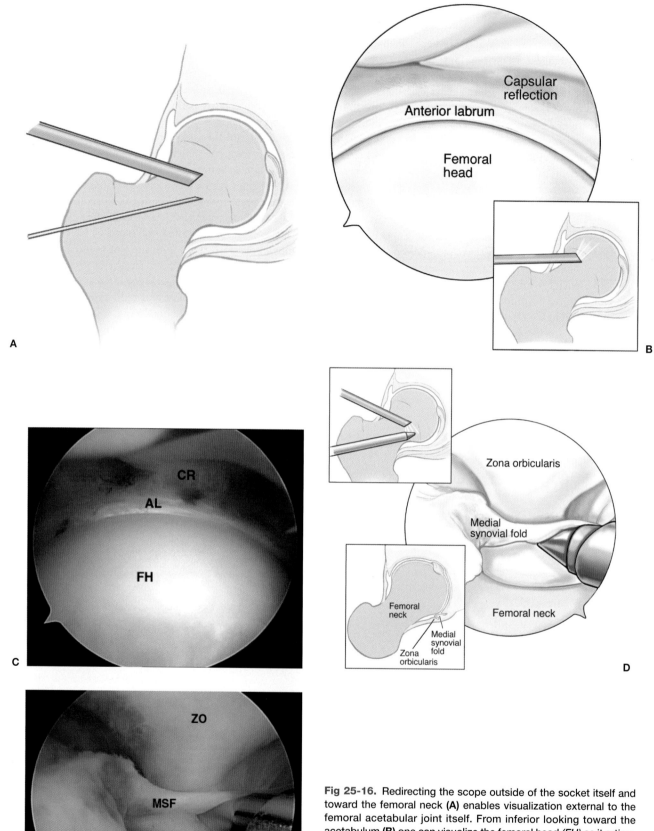

Fig 25-16. Redirecting the scope outside of the socket itself and toward the femoral neck **(A)** enables visualization external to the femoral acetabular joint itself. From inferior looking toward the acetabulum **(B)** one can visualize the femoral head *(FH)* as it articulates in the socket while visualizing the outer periphery of the anterior labrum *(AL)* and capsular reflection *(CR)* **(C)**. When the scope is directed toward the base of the neck, one can visualize the femoral neck *(FN)*, medial synovial fold *(MSF)*, and zona orbicularis *(ZO)* **(D)** and **(E)**. [Art renderings **(A,B,D)** courtesy of Smith & Nephew Endoscopy, Andover, Massachusetts; arthroscopic photos **(C,E)** courtesy of J.W. Thomas Byrd MD.]

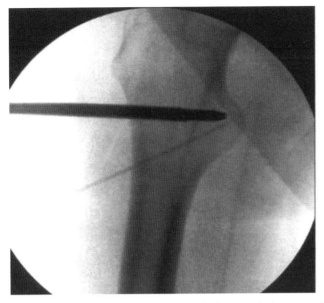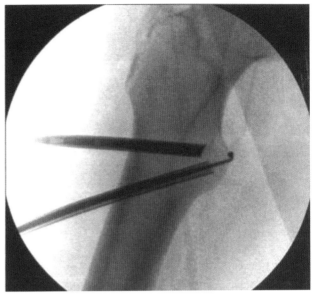

Fig 25-17. Fluoroscopic images during an endoscopic-assisted release of the psoas tendon. Arthroscopic treatment of the painful internal snapping hip: Results of a new endoscopic technique and imaging protocol. (From Flanum ME, Keene JS, Blankenbaker DG, et al. Arthroscopic treatment of the painful internal snapping hip: results of a new endoscopic technique and imaging protocol: Paper presented at: Annual Meeting of the American Orthopaedic Society for Sports Medicine; July 2005; Keystone, CO; with permission.)

can visualize the femoral head, the medial synovial fold, the femoral neck, the anterior capsule, the anterior and free edge of the zono orbicularis, the anterior synovial fold, the base of the labrum, the posterior capsule, the perilabral sulcus, and the reflection of the capsule at the intertrochanteric crest **(Fig 25-16)**. Some authors have exited the capsule to treat pathology including endoscopically assisted release of the psoas tendon from the base of the lesser trochanter **(Fig 25-17)**.

In conclusion, a thorough understanding of the anatomy about the hip is necessary for optimal diagnosis, focused treatment, and safe and optimal performance of open and arthroscopic treatment portal placement. This anatomic overview of the hip should serve as an introduction to the subsequent focused chapters on the hip in this text dedicated to practical orthopaedic sports medicine and arthroscopy.

■ REFERENCES

1. McKibbin B. Anatomical factors of the hip joint in the newborn. *J Bone Joint Surg Br.* 1970;52:148.
2. Sienbenrock KA, Schoeniger R, Ganz R. Anterior femoroacetabular impingement due to acetabular retroversion. *J Bone Joint Surg Am.* 2003;85A(2):278–286.
3. Tonnis D, Heineck A. Current concepts review—acetabular and femoral anteversion: relationship with osteoarthritis of the hip. *J Bone Joint Surg Am.* 1999;81:1747–1770.
4. Peterson W, Peterson F, Tillman B. Structure and vascularization of the acetabular labrum with regard to pathogenesis and healing of labral lesions. *Arch Orthop Trauma Surg.* 2003; 123(6):283–288.
5. Dameron TB Jr. Bucket-handle tear of acetabular labrum accompanying posterior dislocation of the hip. *J Bone Joint Surg Am.* 1959;41A:131–134.
6. Ferguson SJ, Bryant JT, Ganz R, et al. An in vitro investigation of the acetabular labral seal in hip joint mechanics. *J Biomech.* 2003; 36:171–178.
7. McCarthy JC, Noble PC, Schuck MR, et al. The watershed labral lesion; its relationship to early arthritis of the hip. *J Arthroplasty.* 2001;16(8):81–87.
8. Mozzari HH, Clark JM, Jacob HA, et al. Effects of removal of acetabular labrum in a sheep model. *Osteoarthr Cartil.* 2004; 12(5):419–430.
9. Konrath GA, Hames AJ, Olsen JA, et al. The role of the acetabular labrum and transverse ligament in load transmission in the hip. *J Bone Joint Surg Am.* 1998;80(12):1781–1788.
10. Lage LA, Patel JV, Villar RN. The acetabular labral tear: an arthroscopic classification. *Arthroscopy.* 1996;12(3):269–272.
11. McCarthy J, Noble P, Aluisio FV, et al. Anatomy, pathologic features, and treatment of acetabular labral tears. *Clin Orthop Rel Res.* 2003;406:38–47.
12. Robinson P, White LM, Agur A, et al. Obturator externus bursa: anatomic origin and MR imaging features of pathologic involvement. *Radiology.* 2003;228:230–234.
13. Dunn T, Heller, CA, McCarthy SW, et al. Anatomical study of the trochanteric bursa. *Clin Anat.* 2003;16(3):233–240.
14. Vaccaro JP, Sauser DD, Beals RK. Iliopsoas bursa imaging: efficacy in depicting abnormal iliopsoas tendon motion in patients with internal snapping hip syndrome. *Radiology.* 1995; 197:853–856.
15. Pauwels F. *Biomechanics of the Locomotor Apparatus.* New York: Springer-Verlag; 1980:1–228.
16. Radin EL. Biomechanics of the Human Hip. *Clin Orthop.* 1980; 152:28.

17. Lhe F, Eckstein F, Sauer T, et al. Structure, strain, and function of the transverse acetabular ligament. *Acta Anat (Basel)*. 1996; 157(4):315–323.
18. Byrd JWT, Pappas JN, Pedley MJ. Hip arthroscopy: an anatomic study of portal placement and relationship to the extra-articular structures. *Arthroscopy*. 1995;11(4):418–423.
19. Bohannon MJ, McCarthy JC, O'Donnell J, et al. Hip arthroscopy: surgical approach, positioning, and distraction. *Clin Orthop Rel Res*. 2003;406:29–37.
20. McCarthy JC, Lee J. Hip arthroscopy: indications, outcomes, and complications. *J Bone Joint Surg Am*. 2005;87A(5):1137–45.
21. Clarke MT, Arora A, Villar RN. Hip arthroscopy: complications in 1054 cases. *Clinical Orthopaedics and Related Research* 2003; 406:84–88.

■ SUGGESTED READINGS

1. Byrd JWT, ed. *Operative Hip Arthroscopy*. New York: Thieme Medical Publishers; 1998.
2. Byrd JWT. Diagnostic and operative arthroscopy of the hip. In: Andrews JR, Timmerman LA, eds. *Diagnostic and operative arthroscopy*. Philadelphia: WB Saunders; 1997:207–220.
3. Byrd JWT, Pappas JN, Pedley MJ. Hip arthroscopy: an anatomic study of portal placement and relationship to the extra-articular structures. *Arthroscopy*. 1995;11(4):418–423.
4. Grant JCB. *An Atlas of Anatomy*. Baltimore: Williams & Wilkins; 1943:126–153.
5. Johnson L. Hip joint. In: Johnson L, ed. *Diagnostic and surgical arthroscopy*. 3rd ed. St. Louis: Mosby; 1986:1491–1519.
6. Kim SJ, Choi NH, Kim HJ. Operative hip arthroscopy. Clinical *Orthopaedics and Related Research*. 1998;353:156–65.
7. Moore KL. *Clinically Oriented Anatomy*. 3rd ed. Philadelphia: Williams & Wilkins; 1992:243–294, 373–497.

HIP ARTHROSCOPY

26

■ MICHAEL H. DIENST, MD

■ KEY POINTS

- Various anatomical features make placement of portals and movement of the arthroscope and instruments within the hip more difficult than in other joints.
- The central compartment (CC) of the hip, made up of the lunate cartilage, acetabular fossa, ligamentum teres and the loaded articular surface of the femoral head, can be visualized almost exclusively with traction.
- The peripheral compartment (PC) can be better seen without traction. The PC consists of the unloaded cartilage of the femoral head, the femoral neck with the medial, anterior, and posterolateral synovial folds and the articular capsule with the intrinsic ligaments, including the zona orbicularis.
- The key to an accurate and complete diagnosis of lesions within the hip joint is a systematic approach to viewing. A methodical sequence of examination should be developed, progressing from one part of the joint cavity to another.
- Evaluation should exclude spinal, abdominal-inguinal, neurologic, and rheumatologic diagnoses before the patient is considered for a diagnostic hip scope.
- For contouring of the femoral head in CAM-type of impingement, the arthroscope is introduced via the anterolateral or distal anterolateral portal, the shaver and burr are placed via the anterior portal. Usually, trimming of the femoral head starts at the insertion of the medial synovial fold medially and extends up to the lateral synovial fold laterally.

The need for less invasive, joint preserving, operative techniques has led to a massive improvement of minimally invasive procedures not only of the knee and shoulder, but also of arthroscopic surgery of the hip joint. For the past ten years,

many surgeons have been contributing to the development and improvement of innovative techniques of hip arthroscopy. With its increasing frequency has grown the knowledge of the normal hip anatomy with the ability to differentiate between anatomic variations and pathologic conditions of the hip joint. Moreover, hip arthroscopy has left its limited function as a diagnostic tool and resection operation such as removal of loose bodies and resection of the acetabular labrum or ligamentum teres. It has made the step to become a reconstructive procedure in the treatment of femoroacetabular impingement, repair of a torn acetabular labrum and for treatment of cartilage defects.

Based on the classification of the arthroscopic compartments of the hip joint, the following report presents the current diagnostic and operative technique of hip arthroscopy of both compartments with and without traction. A systematic mapping of the normal arthroscopic anatomy is included followed by a summary of indications, contraindications, and complications.

■ ARTHROSCOPIC COMPARTMENTS OF THE HIP JOINT

Placement of portals and maneuverability of the arthroscope and instruments within the hip joint is more difficult than in other joints. This is related to various anatomical features: a thick soft tissue mantle, close proximity of two major neurovascular bundles, a strong articular capsule, a relatively small intraarticular volume, permanent contact of the articular surfaces, and the sealing of the deep, central part of the joint by the acetabular labrum. Thus, if no traction is applied to the hip, only a small film of synovial fluid separates the articular surface of the femoral head from the lunate carti- lage and acetabular labrum ("artificial space").

The anatomy of the acetabular labrum must be consid- ered before accessing the hip joint. The labrum seals the joint space between the lunate cartilage and the femoral head (1–3). To overcome the vacuum force and passive resis- tance of the soft tissues, traction is needed to separate the head from the socket, to elevate the labrum from the head and to allow the arthroscope and other instruments access to the narrow "artificial space" between the weight-bearing car- tilage of the femoral head and acetabulum. However, if trac- tion is applied, the joint capsule is tensioned and the joint space peripheral to the acetabular labrum decreases. Thus, in order to maintain the space of the peripheral hip joint cavity for better visibility and maneuverability during arthroscopy, traction should be avoided.

In consequence, Dorfmann and Boyer (4,5) divided the hip arthroscopically into 2 compartments separated by the labrum. The first is the central compartment (CC) compris- ing the lunate cartilage, the acetabular fossa, the ligamentum teres, and the loaded articular surface of the femoral head. This part of the joint can be visualized almost exclusively with traction. The second is the peripheral compartment (PC) consisting of the unloaded cartilage of the femoral head, the femoral neck with the medial, anterior, and posterolateral synovial folds (Weitbrecht's ligaments) and the articular cap- sule with its intrinsic ligaments including the zona orbicularis. This area can be better seen without traction (6).

Positioning

Hip arthroscopy, with and without traction, can be performed in the lateral (7,8) or supine position (6,9,10). Some authors claim that there are advantages to the lateral position, includ- ing better access to the posterolateral area (11,12), and better application of traction in line with the femoral neck (13). However, this author's studies in fresh cadaveric hip joints showed no significant differences in distraction of the hip between the supine and the lateral position (14). From the author's experience, the decision whether to use the supine or lateral position appears to be more a matter of individual training and habit of use. Because of the almost exclusive use of the anterolateral and anterior portals during hip arthroscopy without traction, the author prefers the supine position (5,6,15,16). The author usually combines the tech- nique with traction and without traction. If distraction of the CC is not sufficient, only the PC is operated without traction. The combination of both techniques is important to allow a complete diagnostic arthroscopic examination of the hip.

Hip Arthroscopy With Traction

In the supine position, the patient is pulled distally onto the counterpost, so that the medial side of the thigh presses against the post. This is important not only to avoid pressure to the perineum and pudendal nerve, but also to increase the cantilever effect of the post on subsequent adduction of the

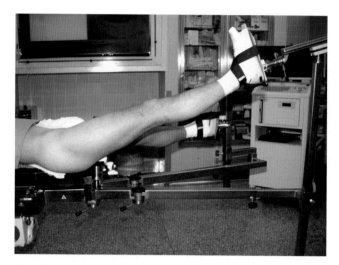

Fig 26-1. Supine position for hip arthroscopy with traction. (Courtesy of Michael Dienst, MD.)

leg (3). Both feet and ankles are well padded and fixed tightly into the traction boots. The ipsilateral hip is slightly flexed to 10 to 20 degrees for relaxation of the strong anterior parts of the hip joint capsule, and tensioned by lengthening of the extension bar. The leg is adducted to about 0 to 10 degrees of abduction in order to increase the distraction force vector by a cantilever effect of the counterpost (3) **(Fig 26-1)**. The first AP radiograph is taken with the image intensifier. The hip is then distracted by pulling with the traction module until the joint vacuum is broken. Another radiograph is taken to assess distraction of the hip joint **(Fig 26-2)**. Traction is released until the hip is scrubbed and draped and portals to the CC are established. Sometimes distraction may be moderate only. In these cases, better separation can often be achieved once the vacuum seal is broken with the spinal needle. However, if adequate distraction cannot be achieved with a combination of traction, distension, and proper joint positioning, the surgeon needs to be prepared to abandon arthroscopy of the CC. Under these circumstances, he can still perform arthroscopy of the PC without traction.

Hip Arthroscopy Without Traction

Traction is released; the foot is taken out of the traction boot and covered with a sterile hood. The traction bar and the counterpost are removed, and the leg rest extension is reat- tached to the extension table. The hip can be flexed, rotated and ab-/adducted to the desired position **(Fig 26-3)**. Cadaver experiments and in vivo experience (17) have shown that free draping and a good range of movement is important to relax parts of the capsule and increase the intra-articular vol- ume of the area that is inspected (18).

Distraction and Distension

For arthroscopy of the CC, sufficient joint distraction is necessary: More space will improve the intra-articular maneuverability of the arthroscope and additional instruments

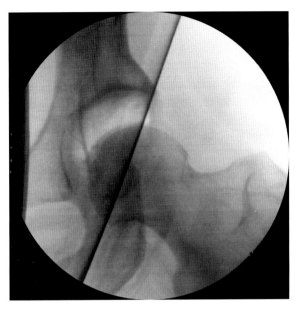

Fig 26-2. Preoperative AP radiographs after application of traction with breakage of the joint seal. (Courtesy of Michael Dienst, MD.)

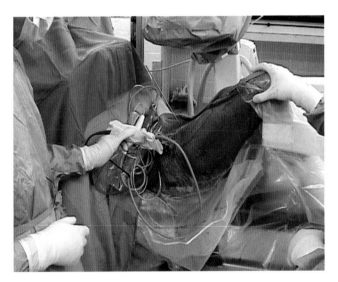

Fig 26-3. Supine position for hip arthroscopy without traction. (Courtesy of Michael Dienst, MD.)

and may reduce the risk of intra-articular complications, such as damage to the acetabular labrum and articular cartilage. On the other hand, high traction forces can cause nerve and soft tissue injuries around the hip, at the perineum, and the ankle (10,12,19–21).

Little is known on the direct effect of tension of the femoral and sciatic nerve during hip arthroscopies. To my knowledge, only temporary sensory and motor deficits of the femoral and sciatic nerve were reported. Griffin and Villar (21) identified in their retrospective analysis of 640 consecutive hip arthroscopies: 3 patients with temporary sciatic nerve palsy; and one patient with temporary femoral nerve palsy. All deficits recovered within the first few hours postoperatively.

There is consensus not to exceed traction time over 2 hours. In addition, flexion over 20 degrees should be avoided to not increase tension to the sciatic nerve. This author's studies have shown that creep of the periarticular structures reduces the need for force to maintain distraction (22). Thus traction should be reduced as soon as the hip has been distended and the portals have been established.

The effect of distension has already been studied. In-vivo and cadaver studies have shown that the breakage of the joint vacuum leads to a significant increase of distraction (3,23). Distraction can be improved by additional distension up to 81% in vivo (23). Thus, the joint should be distended with a spinal needle before the first portal is established.

■ ACCESS TO THE HIP JOINT-PORTALS

A complete diagnostic round trip and access to damaged structures can be achieved only with precise portal placement. In addition, potential complications of portal placement, mainly to the CC, have to be considered. The space between the acetabular labrum and the cartilage of the femoral head is small, so both structures are at risk for direct lesions from scuffing to deep cartilage defects or labral tears. Neurovascular structures are close, but usually not at risk, if distinct lines are not crossed. So, the surgeon should take his time especially for this part of the procedure.

From my experience, fluoroscopy is mandatory for safe portal placement at least for the first portal to each compartment. Further access of additional portals can be controlled via the arthroscope and triangulation. Special guides may be of further help (24). Beneficial is the use of cannulated trokars, or dilating instruments, for introduction of the sheaths and flexible working cannulas.

Central Compartment

Different portals are currently being used. Some surgeons prefer a 2-portal technique, others a 3-portal technique for arthroscopy of the CC. From our experience a 2-portal technique may be sufficient in hips with very good distraction. However, usually a 3-portal access to the hip is required for a complete inspection and access to different structures **(Fig 26-4)**.

The following paragraphs describe the "classic" technique for portal placement to the CC. However, the author has established a new technique, which he has been increasingly using over the past year. This technique is presented afterward.

Anterolateral and Lateral Portal

With respect to neurovascular structures both the anterolateral and lateral portal are most centrally in the safe zone for arthroscopy (25). For placement of the anterolateral portal, the skin is incised about 2 cm anterior to the anterosuperior ca. 4-6 cm — Anterior Portal

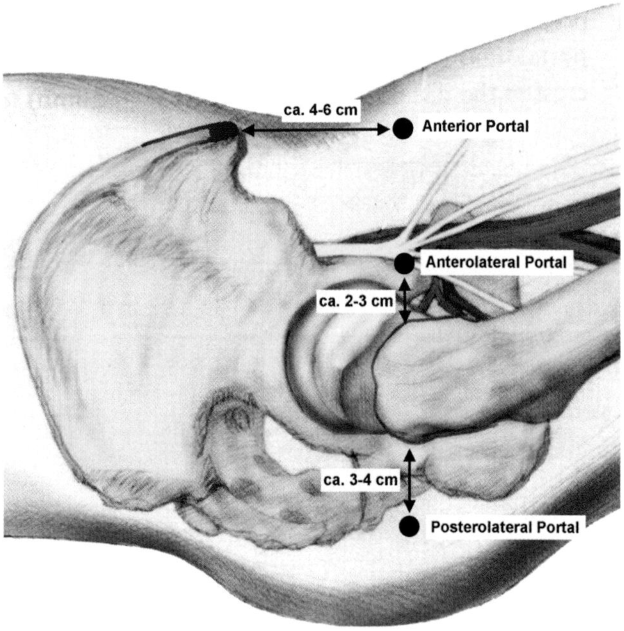

Anterolateral Portal

ca. 2-3 cm

ca. 3-4 cm — Posterolateral Portal

Fig 26-4. Portals to the CC of the hip. (Courtesy of Michael Dienst, MD.)

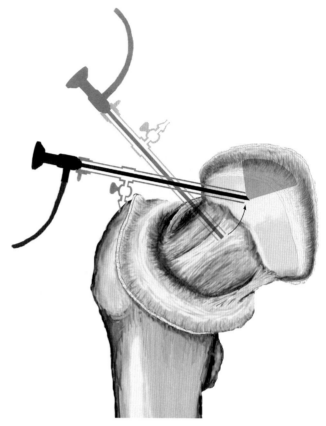

Fig 26-5. Position of the arthroscope for inspection of the peripheral anterior head area for subsequent placement of the anterior portal to the CC. (Courtesy of Michael Dienst, MD.)

edge of the greater trochanter. The needle is directed about 10 to 20 degrees cranially and 20 to 30 degrees posteriorly. It penetrates the gluteus medius and/or the tensor fasciae latae before entering the joint. The lateral portal may be used alternatively to the anterolateral portal. It lies just proximal to the tip of the greater trochanter. Anterior and posterolateral portal placement can be controlled arthroscopically as soon as the arthroscope is introduced via the anterolateral portal.

Posterolateral Portal

The skin is incised about 3 cm posterior to the posterosuperior edge of the greater trochanter at the same height as the anterolateral portal. The needle is directed about 10 degrees cranially, and 30 degrees anteriorly, penetrating the gluteus maximus, medius, and minimus, and the capsule close to the posterior horn of the labrum. Here, the distance to the sciatic nerve was measured with a minimum of 2 cm (25).

Anterior Portal

The skin incision for this portal is 4 to 6 cm distally to the anterior superior iliac spine. The needle is directed about 30 degrees medially, and 30 to 45 degrees cranially. On its way into the joint it penetrates the muscle belly of the sartorius and the rectus femoris, before entering the joint (25). If the entry point for the anterior portal is not placed further medially, the minimum distance to the femoral nerve has been measured as 2.7 cm in cadavers (25).

Since 2003, the author has used a "new" technique for the first access to the CC (26). Under fluoroscopy, the arthroscope is introduced via the anterolateral portal to the anterior neck area of the PC, in the standard technique using a needle, guidewire, and cannulated trocars. The 30 degree

arthroscope is advanced over the head-neck-transition, into the anterior head area, and changed to the 70 degree arthroscope, to visualize the junction of the anterior labrum and anterior femoral head cartilage (Fig 26-5). The anterior portal to the CC can be placed under arthroscopic control. Entry site and direction of the needle are the same as described before. The tip of the needle with a guide wire can be maneuvered precisely between the labrum and the femoral head cartilage (Fig 26-6). As soon as the anterior portal is placed to the CC, further portal placement can be controlled via the 70 degree arthroscope with less risk of injury to the labrum and cartilage.

When all 3 portals are established, the diagnostic round trip and operative treatment, in case of pathologic changes of the CC, can be initiated.

Peripheral Compartment

From Dorfmann and Boyer's (5), and my experience (6,27), a comprehensive overview can be obtained from the anterolateral portal only. Because the soft tissue mantle is relatively thin and the position of the portal is near the lateral cortex of the femoral neck, maneuverability of the arthroscope is sufficient for moving the arthroscope into the medial recess, gliding over the anterior surface of the femoral head to the

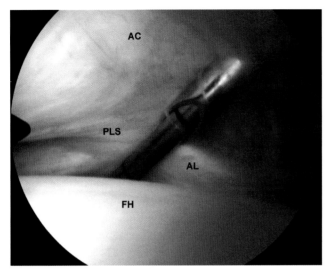

Fig 26-6. Arthroscopic control from the PC of anterior portal placement to the CC femoral head *(FH)*, anterior labrum *(AL)*, perilabral recess *(PR)*, anterior capsule *(AC)*. (Courtesy of Michael Dienst, MD.)

lateral recess, and frequently passing the lateral cortex of the femoral neck for inspection of the posterior recess (6). With the need for better access to the lateral and posterolateral neck and head area for therapy, or CAM-type of femoro-acetabular impingement, a 3 portal technique for the PC has recently been established **(Fig 26-7).**

The position and direction of the anterolateral portal (PC) is different to the anterolateral portal to the CC. The incision lies more proximally and anteriorly. Usually the perfect spot for the skin incision can be found by palpating a soft spot, one third of the distance of a line drawn from the anterior superior iliac spine to the tip of the greater trochanter. Here, one can

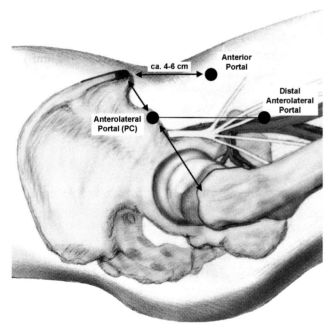

Fig 26-7. Portals to the PC. (Courtesy of Michael Dienst, MD.)

feel the anterior margin of the gluteus medius. The needle thus penetrates only the tensor fasciae latae on its way to the joint capsule. Under fluoroscopy, the needle is directed perpendicular to the femoral neck axis to the anterolateral transition from the femoral head to the femoral neck.

Anterior portal (PC)

Using the same skin incision of the anterior portal to the CC, the needle is directed more inferiorly and not so far medially aiming to the anterior junction of the femoral head and neck.

Distal anterolateral portal (PC)

Especially in order to improve viewing of the anterolateral and lateral head and neck areas during recontouring of the femoral head in impingement surgery, placement of another anterolateral portal further distally, is beneficial. The portal incision lies at the junction of a vertical line drawn from the anterolateral portal (PC) with the superior border of the femoral neck. The needle is directed to the anterior neck area.

■ DIAGNOSTIC ROUND AND ANATOMY

Similar to the knee joint, the key to an accurate and complete diagnosis of lesions within the hip joint is a systematic approach to viewing. A methodical sequence of examination should be developed, progressing from one part of the joint cavity to another and systematically carrying out this sequence in every hip.

Central Compartment

For a complete inspection of the CC all 3 portals are used. No matter from which portal the 30 degree arthroscope allows inspection of the acetabular fossa and central parts of the lunate cartilage only. For viewing of the peripheral parts of the lunate cartilage, the acetabular labrum, perilabral recess, and the more circumferential aspects of the femoral head, the use of the 70 degree arthroscope is mandatory **(Fig 26-8)**. From each portal, different areas within the CC can be inspected. Both lenses are brought into all 3 portals scanning the complete CC.

Peripheral Compartment

For arthroscopic examination, the PC of the hip can be divided routinely into the following areas: anterior neck area, medial neck area, medial head area, anterior head area, lateral head area, lateral neck area, and posterior area, **(Fig 26-9)**.

■ INDICATIONS

Hip arthroscopy has made the step from a diagnostic and removing/resecting tool to a reconstruction procedure. The

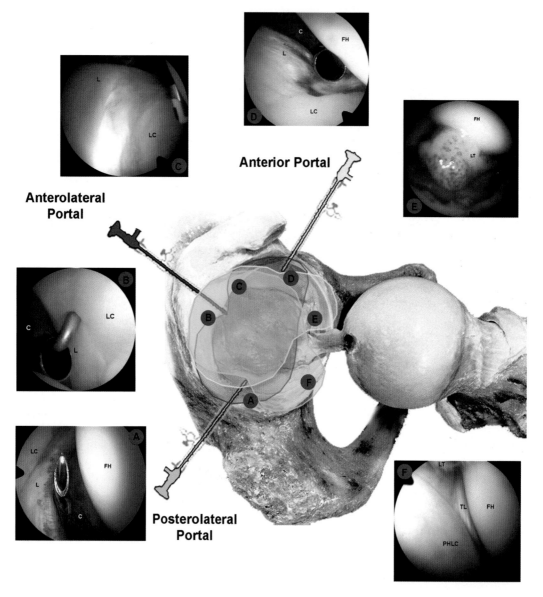

Fig 26-8A–F. Inspection areas of the 70° arthroscopes from the anterior, anterolateral, and posterolateral portal to the CC. No matter which portal is used, the 30° arthroscope allows inspection of the central parts of this compartment only (intersection of the marked areas). The 70° arthroscope is mandatory for viewing the more peripheral parts (colored areas corresponding to portals). Femoral head *(FH)*, lig. teres *(LT)*, acetabular fossa *(FA)*, lunate cartilage *(LC)*, articular capsule *(C)*, posterior horn of the lunate cartilage *(PHLC)*, transverse ligament *(TL)*. (Courtesy of Michael Dienst, MD.)

following paragraphs summarize classic indications such as unclear hip pain, loose bodies, and labral tears, and more recent indications such as unstable, longitudinal labral tears for labral repair and femoroacetabular impingement for recontouring of the femoral head and cartilage defects.

Unclear Hip Pain

With respect to the limited sensitivity and specificity of preoperative radiologic methods for intra-articular hip joint lesions, indicating hip arthroscopy for patients with "unclear

hip pain" is not uncommon (10,11,28–33). However, preoperative evaluation should exclude spinal, abdominal-inguinal, neurologic, and rheumatologic diagnoses before the patient is considered for a hip scope. In addition, radiologic imaging of intra-articular loose bodies, and labral and cartilage lesions has improved since the advent of computed tomography (CT) and magnetic resonance arthrograms (MRA) (17,34–36). Intra-articular application of radiopaque material and air (double contrast CT) or Gadolinium MRA enhances the contrast between intra-articular structures. Relief of pain with a local anesthetic is another strong indicator that the hip is the

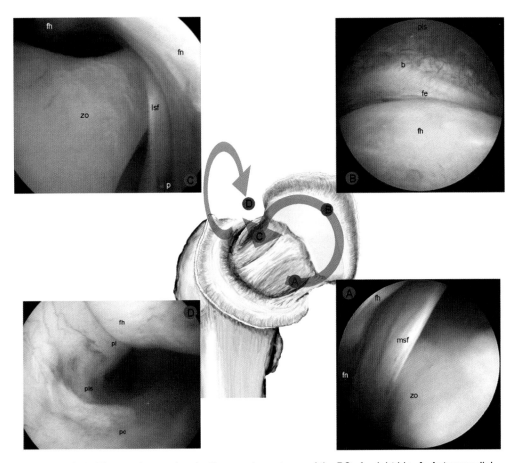

Fig 26-9A–D. Diagnostic round and arthroscopic anatomy of the PC of a right hip. **A:** Anteromedial neck area with the medial synovial fold *(msf)*, femoral head *(fh)*, femoral neck *(fn)* and anteromedial capsule with the zona orbicularis *(zo)*. **B:** Anterior head area with the cartilage of the femoral head *(fh)*, free edge of the labrum *(fe)* and base of the labrum *(b)*, and perilabral sulcus *(pls)*. **C:** Lateral neck area with the lateral margin of the femoral neck *(fn)* and head *(fh)*, lateral synovial fold *(lsf)* building a small subplical pouch (p) and zona orbicularis *(zo)*. **D:** Posterior area with the posterior surface of the femoral head *(fh)*, posterior labrum *(pl)*, perilabral sulcus *(pls)*, and thin posterior capsule *(pc)*. (Courtesy of Michael Dienst, MD.)

source of pain. Since preoperative evaluation has been improving by these techniques, "unclear hip pain" has become more and more rare.

If the etiology remains unclear, a complete diagnostic inspection of the hip joint is mandatory. Especially in this situation, it is important to combine the traction with the nontraction technique. Loose bodies can be easily missed if only the CC is scanned. Synovial diseases such as a chondromatosis or an inflammatory synovitis typically manifest first in the hip joint periphery.

Loose Bodies

Radiologic evidence of loose bodies may be the classical indication for hip arthroscopy (8,13,24,30,31,37–41). Loose bodies prefer to accumulate within the acetabular fossa **(Fig 26-10 A**, **B** and **C)** and in the peripheral recesses **(Fig 26-11A** and **B)**. This is important in assessing preoperative

radiographs, CT or magnetic resonance imaging (MRI) and also for operative planning (5,6). The fossa, medial neck area, the perilabral recesses, and the recess underneath the transverse ligament especially need to be scanned. The technique of removal depends on the size and consistency of the loose bodies. In case of small loose bodies, they may be easily washed or sucked out via an additional portal cannula. The removal of bigger loose bodies especially with a bony core within the acetabular fossa is more demanding. They may need to be chopped up with a strong forceps. In these cases, it is very helpful to place a larger cannula from posterolateral. The cannula cannot be brought into the joint, but can be placed directly outside the articular capsule. For the PC, bigger cannulas can be brought directly into the joint. Inspection and removal of loose bodies in the posterior area of the PC of the hip is more demanding. As indicated before, it may be difficult to pass the lateral femoral neck and bring the 70 degree scope

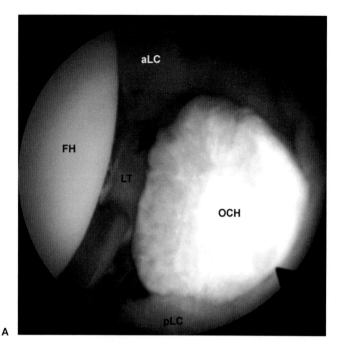

A

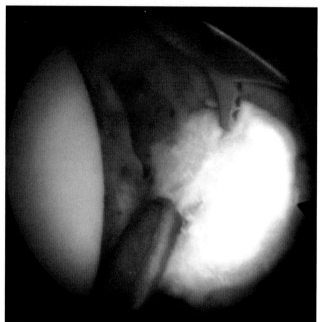

B

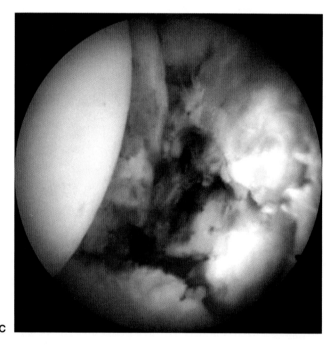

C

Fig 26-10A and B. Big osteochondroma *(OCH)* of the acetabular fossa viewed from the anterolateral portal **(A)**, femoral head *(FH)*, anterior lunate cartilage *(aLC)*, posterior lunate cartilage *(pLC)*, lig. teres *(LT)*. Removal of the osteochondroma from posterolateral, the osteochondroma is fixed with forces introduced from the anterior portal **(B)**. Acetabular fossa after removal of the osteochondroma **(C)**. (Courtesy of Michael Dienst, MD.)

into the posterior area, particularly if visibility is decreased by synovitis or the joint is tight. Sometimes, rotation of the hip, manual ballotement or intra-articular suction can bring loose bodies from the posterior area into the visible anterior or medial areas (15).

Synovial Diseases

If the hip joint is under distraction, the synovium (pulvinar) of the acetabular fossa can be seen. The anterolateral portal is ideal for inspection, whereas operative therapy such as biopsies, removal hof the pulvinar and removal of

chondromas are done via the anterior and posterolateral portal (Fig 26-10A, B, and C). With traction, only small parts of the synovial lining of the medial, anterior, and lateral capsule are visible. From my and other authors' experience, this part of the synovium can best be seen without traction (5,6). As indicated before, chondromas prefer to accumulate in the medial neck area, the perilabral recesses, and the recess underneath the transverse ligament (Fig 26-11A and B). Here, cannulas can be easily placed via another anterolateral or anterior portal for synovial biopsies [reactive or specific synovitis, pigmented villonodular synovitis (PVNS)], synovectomies, and

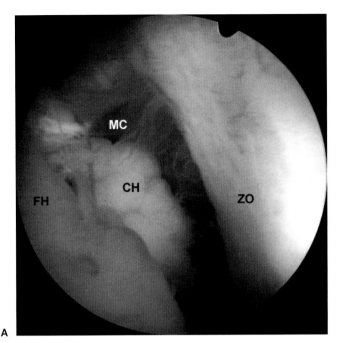

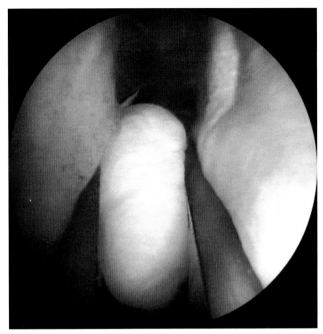

Fig 26-11A and B. View of a chondroma *(CH)* of the medial head area in synovial chondromatosis via the anterolateral portal to the PC without traction **A:** femoral head *(FH)*, medial articular capsule *(MC)*, zona orbicularis *(ZO)*. **B:** Removal of the chondroma with a forceps introduced via the distal anterolateral portal. (Courtesy of Michael Dienst, MD.)

removal of chondromas (5,42,43) **(Fig 26-12)**. In addition, other pathologic conditions such as cysts of the labrum, anterior capsule, and variations of the anatomy such as

Fig 26-12. Diffuse pigmented villonodular synovitis (PNVS) of the right hip joint. View from the anterolateral portal without traction to the medial neck area. Femoral head *(FH)* and neck *(FN)*, anteromedial capsule *(AMC)*. (Courtesy of Michael Dienst, MD.)

communications with the iliopectineal bursa have to be ruled out. Particularly in patients with rheumatoid arthritis, an iliopectineal cyst has to be considered as a source of a painful hip. Depending on the size of the cyst, arthroscopic decompression may be performed.

Labral Lesions

Tears of the acetabular labrum must not be confused with normal variations of the anatomy such as the sublabral recess. Most series report that the majority of labral tears are located anteriorly and anterolaterally (44,45). The morphology of labral tears has been classified by Lage et al. (45) into radial flap tears, radial fibrillated labra, longitudinal peripheral tears, and the unstable labrum.

Tears are usually located at the articular side of the base of the labrum, directly at the junction of the labrum to the articular cartilage of the lunate cartilage (Fig 26-13A and B). Thus, it appears mandatory to use traction to check the articular side of the labrum and to treat them properly. Frequently, the tears come along with concomitant lesions of the articular cartilage, especially with femoroacetabular impingement (46). So, removal of the bump of the femoral head with the nontraction technique alone is not sufficient. Not only in these cases, I scope the CC first to take care of labral and cartilage lesions. Afterwards, traction is released and the recontouring of the femoral head is performed. In general, the surgeon should debride all torn tissue and leave as much healthy substance intact as possible.

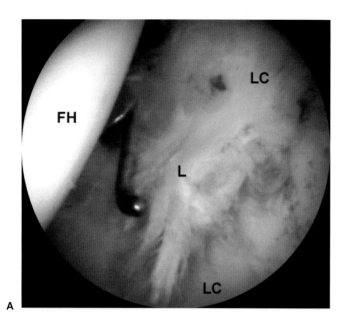 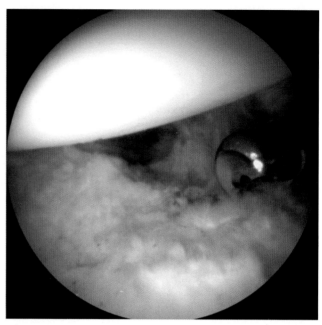

Fig 26-13A and B. Degenerative radial flap tear of the acetabular labrum *(L)* with underlying lesions of the lunate cartilage *(LC)* before **(A)** and after resection **(B)**. Femoral head *(FH)*, lateral capsule *(LC)*. (Courtesy of Michael Dienst, MD.)

Sometimes labral lesion can be seen from the periphery without traction, especially if the labrum is altered and lifted up from the femoral head. In these cases, an instrument can be passed underneath the labrum for partial resection or trimming. With the nontraction technique, the labrum has to be checked for labral cysts, which are better accessible from the peripheral side. A typical location of a labral cyst is the anterior labrum close to the iliopsoas tendon. Here, the differential diagnosis should include an iliopectineal, capsular cyst.

For the past few years, surgeons have gained first experience with labral repairs. From my experience, the indications are rare. Only unstable longitudinal tears of the base of the labrum and the unstable labrum should be indicated for a repair. It has been shown—similar to the meniscus—that only the base of the acetabular labrum has sufficient vascularity to heal (47). In these cases, the labrum can be sutured back to the rim with anchors, which is a technically demanding procedure. Particularly the angle of insertion of the anchor has to be controlled—similar to a Bankart repair of the shoulder—in order not to skive into the cartilage of the socket. Alternatively, the labrum may be fixed to the articular capsule, which is however not as anatomic as the fixation to the acetabular rim.

The prognosis of trimming and repair of the labrum is mostly depending on the status of the articular cartilage (45,48,49). As indicated before, concomitant cartilage defects are frequent. Smaller cartilage flaps should be removed; in case of circumscribed full thickness tears, microfracturing of the subchondral bone appears beneficial. However, if a larger area of the bony socket is uncovered,

arthroscopy should be limited to resect unstable parts of the labrum and cartilage.

Chondral Lesions

A review of the literature reveals that a considerable number of hip arthroscopies (HA) are performed for traumatic and nontraumatic (osteoarthritis, osteochondritis dissecans) chondral lesions. In osteoarthritis, associated lesions such as loose bodies, labral lesions, and synovitis can be frequently found pre- and intraoperatively (16). If arthritis is not advanced, arthroscopic treatment is beneficial for treatment of these findings (31,50). However, in severe osteoarthritis and a long history of symptoms, improvement is for only short time and probably related to the washout and distraction of the joint. In these cases, frequently the hip cannot be distracted adequately because of significant capsular fibrosis and thickening, leading to a high risk of labral or cartilage injury during portal placement and operative treatment. Hip arthroscopy may be limited to the PC of the joint, but probably better not indicated.

In trauma and osteochondritis dissecans, successful treatment of cartilage injuries by hip arthroscopy is usually of much higher success **(Fig 26-14A and B)**. Cartilage flaps and chondral fragments are frequently not seen on MRI, and the correct diagnosis with extent of the cartilage lesion is often only shown by the arthroscope (51). Unstable cartilage flaps can be trimmed, and chondral and osteochondral fragments as in stage 3 and 4 osteochondritis dissecans lesions removed. Cartilage defects can be treated with microfracture tools, which can be a technically demanding step depending on

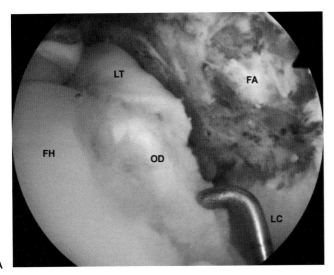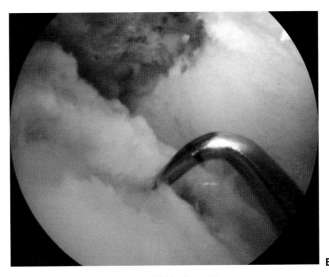

Fig 26-14A and B. View from the anterior portal of an osteochondritis dissecans *(OD)* lesion of the anterosuperior femoral head *(FH)*. The osteochondral fragment is loose **(A)** thus subsequently removed and the bed microfractured **(B)**. Acetabular fossa *(FA)*, lunate cartilage *(LC)*, ligamentum teres *(LT)*. (Courtesy of Michael Dienst, MD.)

the location of the lesion and the extent of subchondral sclerosis. If distraction is sufficient, an extra long microfracture awl can be used to pick the subchondral bone (Fig 26-14B). Depending on the angle, a 90 degree awl may be necessary. Here, the awl cannot be tapped; it needs to be turned for breakage of the sclerosis. If the sclerosis is hard, abrasion with a burr may be necessary first or exclusively. Depending on the trauma, cartilage injuries are found at the femoral head superiorly and at the periphery of the lunate cartilage close to the base of the labrum. From my experience, osteochondritis dissecans lesions are found typically at the femoral head, at its anterior to superior curvature. Probing of the lesion is essential to decide whether to drill the lesion only or to remove the osteochondral fragment with subsequent microfracture or arthroscopic or open refixation.

Rupture of the Ligamentum Teres

From my own experience and reports of the past years (52,53), arthroscopic resection of traumatic and nontraumatic ruptures of the ligamentum teres has excellent results. Especially after trauma, and in patients with deformities of the proximal femur, such as in dysplasia, slipped epiphysis, and Perthes' disease, a ruptured ligamentum teres has to be taken into consideration in cases of unclear hip pain. Even by MRA, lesions of the ligamentum teres are very difficult to be identified. The ligamentum can be torn from its insertion at the femoral head with or without an avulsion fragment, at its midsubstance, or even stripped off its origin from the bottom of the acetabular fossa. On conventional MRI, an osteochondral fragment within the acetabular fossa, chondral fragments in the joint, an effusion and thickening of the

pulvinar may be indirect indicators of a tear of the ligamentum. On MRA, absence of the ligamentum, or an unusual course through the fossa may be found. Resection of the ligament is done via the anterior and posterolateral portal **(Fig 26-15A** and **B)**. The distal part of the ligament at its insertion at the femoral head and the anterior part of the synovium of the fossa in case of reactive synovitis is removed with a curved shaver or bowed electrothermic device via the anterior portal, the proximal part with the synovium of the base of the fossa via the posterolateral portal. Concomitant lesions such as cartilage injury must not be overlooked.

Femoracetabular Impingement

This entity has been added to hip pathology within the past decade by Ganz et al. from Berne, Switzerland (54). The first promising results of open treatment of this condition of the hip joint have recently been reported (55). However, the approach for open treatment is considerably invasive, the greater trochanter needs to be osteotomized, and the ligamentum teres removed for dislocation of the femoral head for inspection and treatment of concomitant labral and cartilage pathology. Thus, in the meantime, arthroscopic techniques for the treatment of femoroacetabular impingement are being developed. I started with the first cases of mild to moderate femoroacetabular impingement in 2003, still performing open dislocations for impingement cases with more severe loss of head-neck offset and Pincer-type of impingement. My and other authors' early results are very promising.

I usually start with arthroscopy, with traction of the CC first, in order to treat the concomitant lesions of the acetabular labrum and lunate cartilage. They are always found at a different extent from anterior to lateral and can best be treated

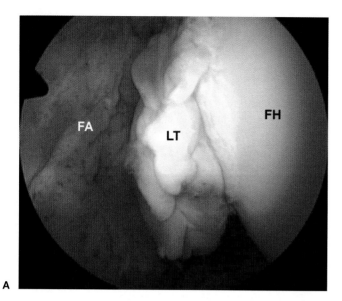

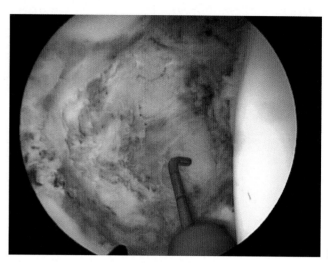

A

B

Fig 26-15A and B. Degenerative tear of the Lig. teres before **(A)** and after resection and synovectomy within the acetabular fossa **(B)**. View from the anterolateral portal to the acetabular fossa *(FA)* with severe synovitis, to the lig. teres *(LT)* and femoral head *(FH)*. (Courtesy of Michael Dienst, MD.)

via the anterior and anterolateral portal. In mild impingement, softening of the lunate cartilage directly beneath the base of the labrum is seen. In more severe cases, the base of the labrum is torn and possibly elevated from the acetabular rim, and significant cartilage flaps with full thickness defects of the lunate cartilage can be found. Here, the unstable fragments need to be removed possibly in combination with a microfracturing of the subchondral bone. The labrum needs to be trimmed or repaired. From my experience, the hip needs to be distracted to check for these lesions and to treat them. Hip arthroscopy without traction for recontouring of the femoral head only is insufficient and a possible reason of failures.

For recontouring of the femoral head in CAM-type of impingement, the arthroscope is introduced via the anterolateral or distal anterolateral portal, and the shaver and burr are placed via the anterior portal. Usually, trimming of the femoral head starts at the insertion of the medial synovial fold medially and extends up to the lateral synovial fold laterally **(Fig 26-16A, B** and **C)**. These two structures are very important landmarks for orientation. Moreover, the lateral synovial fold marks the entry point of the vessel of the medial circumflex artery, which is very important for vascular supply of the femoral head. It must not be injured. In order to remove an adequate part of the head-neck-cartilage and -bone, flexion of the hip must be controlled regularly. Usually, the transition from the good cartilage to the altered cartilage of the bump can be seen. Part of the joint capsule needs to be released mainly anterolaterally and laterally for inspection and access to the lateral head-neck-junction. Impingement must be checked before and after trimming of the bump; thus the hip must be flexed over 90 degrees and

rotated in- and outward in order to see the stress of the head-neck-junction to the anterior and anterolateral labrum and acetabular rim.

The more experience I gained, the more severe CAM-type of impingement has been indicated for arthroscopic surgery. However, in patients with a severe loss of offset extending laterally, I am still performing open hip dislocations. In these cases, the arthroscopic treatment is technically demanding and very time consuming. In Pincer-type of impingement, the decision whether to treat the patient arthroscopically or open is made individually. Detachment of the labrum from medial to posterolateral, resection of the prominent acetabular rim, and reattachment of the labrum on such a long distance is arthroscopically a very challenging procedure. I still do these cases open. However, if the labrum is worn or calcified, resection of the labrum in combination with a trimming of the acetabular rim can be done arthroscopically.

Septic Arthritis

Arthroscopic treatment of a septic arthritis of the hip joint should include a debridement of detritus and necrotic tissue, a lavage with at least 3 to 4 L irrigation fluid, placement of a drain into the femoral neck area, and antibiotic treatment for at least 7 days (56–59). The combination of traction with the nontraction technique is important to have access to the complete joint. During traction, the labrum and the zona orbicularis hinder flow of the irrigation fluid to and back from the peripheral recesses. Direct access to the peripheral areas without traction eases direct inspection, washing and debridement of necrotic tissues

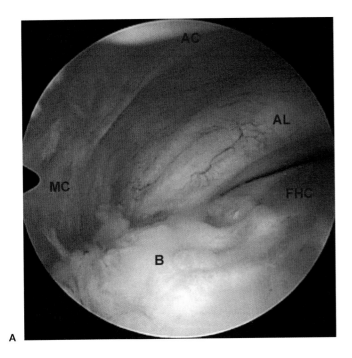

A

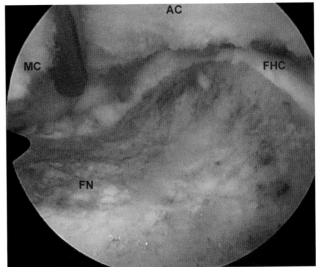

B

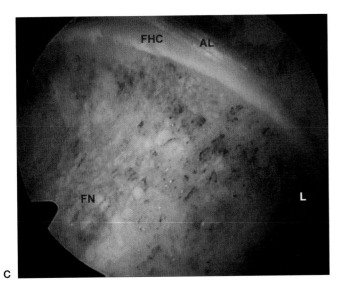

C

Fig 26-16A, B and C. Anterior femoroacetabular impingement of the left hip. View of the anterior head and neck area at 60 degrees of flexion **(A)** bump **(B),** anterior femoral head cartilage *(FHC)*, anterior labrum *(AL)*, anterior *(AC)* and medial capsule *(MC)*. Status post bump resection: anterior **(B)** and anterolateral **(C)** head and neck area with the anterior femoral neck *(FN)*, femoral head cartilage *(FHC)*, anterior labrum *(AL)*, anterior *(AC)* and medial capsule *(MC)*, lateral area *(L)*. (Courtesy of Michael Dienst, MD.)

and detritus. In addition, placement of a drain can easily be performed.

Other Indications

Hip arthroscopy may be used for the treatment of associated pathology in avascular necrosis, Perthes' disease, and complications in total hip arthroplasty. In avascular necrosis, arthroscopy may be used for staging, trimming of unstable cartilage flaps, or to control the correct position of core decompression and drilling (8,40,60,61). In Perthes' disease, arthroscopy may be indicated for loose bodies, debridement of the lateral calcification, or for dilation of the articular capsule in loss of motion (40,62–67). After total hip arthro-

plasties, hip arthroscopy may be useful for the removal of pieces of cement or wires or impinging parts of the articular capsule (60,68–70).

■ CONTRAINDICATIONS

Hip arthroscopy in a recent acetabular fracture has been reported with a risk of leakage of irrigation fluid into the retroperitoneal space and the abdomen (71,72). In patients with advanced osteoarthritis of the hip, the benefit of an arthroscopic debridement is small. In addition, access to the hip may be hindered by insufficient distraction of the femoral head caused by fibrosis and thickening of the articular capsule or femoral head osteophytes.

■ COMPLICATIONS

Extra-articular complications are rare. Byrd (71) reported in a meta-analysis of 1491 cases a complication rate of 1.34%. Griffin and Villar (21) described in their own series of 640 consecutive cases a similar complication rate of 1.6%. Both authors show that the rate of complications significantly decreases with the experience of the surgeon.

However, from the analysis of various reports, it has to be stated that intra-articular complications have not been reported. From my own experience and communication with many other surgeons, intra-articular complications are frequent in the beginning. Iatrogenic scuffing of the articular cartilage especially of the femoral head and tearing of the acetabular labrum is usually not documented. These and other complications can only be minimized if beginners spend time with experienced hip arthroscopists and use a cadaver course to gain first experience with the procedure. Newer techniques such portal placement to the CC controlled by arthroscopic inspection from the PC are tools to reduce the scope trauma.

The possibility of complications during HA without traction is small. Since no traction is used, the perineum and pudendal nerve are not at risk. Instruments do not have to pass between labrum and cartilage of the femoral head, thus tearing the labrum and scuffing the load-bearing cartilage of the femoral head is unlikely. The zone of portal placement is very safe, if only anterolateral portals are used. Byrd et al. (25) showed that the superior gluteal nerve is the only structure with significance relative to the anterolateral portal and has been shown to be at least 3.2 cm from the portal. If the portal is placed further medially and proximally the lateral femorocutaneous nerve comes more at risk. To avoid direct cutting of one of the branches of the superficial nerve, skin incisions must be made superficially. Dilators and portal sheath should be introduced stepwise using blunt instruments. Forceful lever movements in the presence of portal sheaths should be avoided. Skin sutures must be placed superficially (27). If paresthesias of the lateral femorocutaneous nerve occur, those are usually transient and regress within a few days. After perforation of the articular capsule, scuffing of the articular cartilage of the anterior part of the femoral head and the anterior synovial fold covering the anterior femoral neck is possible (6). As for HA with traction, unnecessary perforations of the articular capsule must be avoided. Leakage of fluid into the periarticular soft tissues can cause an increasing narrowing of the joint cavity. The shaft, particularly of the 70 degree arthroscope, should remain inside the joint and not come too close to the capsule, since the optic of the 70 degree arthroscope exceeds the shaft more than that of the 30 degree arthroscope. This carries the danger of direct fluid leaking from the sheath into the periarticular soft

tissues. For this reason, we recommend that shafts and portal sheaths be used that are not fenestrated. In particular, after sliding out of the joint, the irrigation pressure should be kept as low as possible (27).

■ REFERENCES

1. Wingstrand H, Wingstrand A, Krantz P. Intracapsular and atmospheric pressure in the dynamics and stability of the hip. A biomechanical study. Acta *Orthop Scand*. 1990;61:231–235.
2. Weber W, Weber E.Über die Mechanik der menschlichen Gehwerkzeuge nebst der Beschreibung eines Versuches über das Herausfallen des Schenkelkopfes aus der Pfanne im luftverdünnten Raum. *Ann Phys Chem*. 1837;40:1–13.
3. Dienst M, Seil R, Gödde S, et al. Effects of traction, distension and joint position on distraction of the hip joint: an experimental study in cadavers. *Arthroscopy*. 2002;18:865–871.
4. Dorfmann H, Boyer T. Hip arthroscopy utilizing the supine position. *Arthroscopy*. 1996;12:264–267.
5. Dorfmann H, Boyer T. Arthroscopy of the hip: 12 years of experience. *Arthroscopy*. 1999;15:67–72.
6. Dienst M, Goedde S, Seil R, et al. Hip arthroscopy without traction: in vivo anatomy of the peripheral hip joint cavity. *Arthroscopy*. 2001;17:924–931.
7. Hawkins RB. Arthroscopy of the hip. *Clin Orthop*. 1989;249:44–47.
8. Glick JM, Sampson TG, Behr JT, et al. Hip arthroscopy by the lateral approach. *Arthroscopy*. 1987;3:4–12.
9. Suzuki S, Awaya G, Okada Y, et al. Arthroscopic diagnosis of ruptured acetabular labrum. *Acta Orthop Scand*. 1986;57:513–515.
10. Byrd JWT. Hip arthroscopy utilizing the supine position. *Arthroscopy*. 1994;10:275–280.
11. Funke E, Munzinger U. Zur Indikation und Technik der Hüftarthroskopie: Möglichkeiten und Grenzen. *Schweiz Rundschau Med (PRAXIS)*. 1994;83:154–157.
12. Funke EL, Munzinger U. Complications in hip arthroscopy. *Arthroscopy*. 1996;12:156–159.
13. Norman-Taylor FH, Villar RN. Arthroscopic surgery of the hip: Current status. *Knee Surg Sports Traumatol Arthroscopy*. 1994;2:255–258.
14. Dienst M, Romain S, Brang M, et al. Effects of supine and lateral position, joint position, distension and traction for distraction of the hip in arthroscopy. An experimental study in cadavers. ISAKOS, Montreux, Switzerland, 2001.
15. Klapper RC, Silver DM. Hip arthroscopy without traction. *Contemp Orthop*. 1989;18:687–693.
16. Dienst M, Seil R, Gödde S, et al. Hüftarthroskopie bei radiologisch beginnender bis mäßiggradiger Koxarthrose. Diagnostische und therapeutische Wertgkeit. *Orthopäde*. 1999;28:812–818.
17. Personal Communication with H. Dorfmann und T. Boyer, Paris, France. 1998.
18. Dvorak M, Duncan CP, Day B. Arthroscopic anatomy of the hip. *Arthroscopy*. 1990;6:264–273.
19. Eriksson E, Arvidsson I, Arvidsson H. Diagnostic and operative arthroscopy of the hip. *Orthopedics*. 1986;9:169–176.
20. Glick J.M. Complications of hip arthroscopy by the lateral approach. In: Sherman OH, Minkoff J, eds. Arthroscopic surgery. Baltimore: Williams & Wilkins; 1990:193.
21. Griffin DR, Villar RN. Complications of arthroscopy of the hip. *J Bone Joint Surg Br*. 1999;81:604–606.
22. Dienst M, Grün U, Köhler C, et al. Improvement of hip joint distraction by distension and release of the Zona orbicularis and iliofemoral ligament: An investigation in cadaveric hip joints. Arthroscopy Association of North America, Phoenix; 2003.

23. Byrd JWT, Chern KY. Traction versus distension for distraction of the joint during hip arthroscopy. *Arthroscopy*. 1997;13:346–349.
24. Villar RN. Hip arthroscopy. Review. *B J Hosp Med*. 1992;47:763–766.
25. Byrd JWT, Pappas JN, Pedley MJ. Hip arthroscopy: an anatomic study of portal placement and relationship to the extra-articular structures. *Arthroscopy*. 1995;11:418–423.
26. Dienst M, Kohn D. Safe arthroscopic access to the central compartment of the hip. *Arthroscopy*. 2005;21:1510–1514.
27. Dienst M, Goedde S, Seil R, et al. Diagnostic arthroscopy of the hip joint. *Orthop Traumatol*. 2002;10:1–14.
28. Nishii T, Nakanishi K, Sugano M, et al. Acetabular labral tears: contrast-enhanced MR imaging under continuous leg traction. *Skeletal Radiol*. 1996;25:349–356.
29. Ikeda T, Awaya G, Suzuki S, et al. Torn acetabular labrum in young patients. Arthroscopic diagnosis and managment. *J Bone Joint Surg Br*. 1988;70B:13–16.
30. Villar RN. Arthroscopy. *BMJ*. 1994;308:51–53.
31. McCarthy JC, Busconi B. The role of hip arthroscopy in the diagnosis and treatment of hip disease. *CJS*. 1995;38(suppl):S13–S17.
32. Byrd JWT. Labral lesions: an elusive source of hip pain. Case reports and literature review. *Arthroscopy*. 1996;12:603–612.
33. Baber YF, Robinson AHN, Villar RN. Is diagnostic arthroscopy of the hip worthwhile? A prospective review of 328 adults investigated for hip pain. *J Bone Joint Surg Br*. 1999;81:600–603.
34. Czerny C, Hofmann S, Neuhold A, et al. Lesions of the acetabular labrum: accuracy of MR imaging and MR arthrography in detection and staging. *Radiology*. 1996;200:225–230.
35. Urban M, Hofmann S, Tschauner C, et al. MR-Arthrographie bei der Labrumläsion des Hüftgelenks. Technik und Stellenwert. *Orthopäde*. 1998;27:691–698.
36. Personal communication with J.W. Thomas Byrd, Nashville, U.S.A.; 2000.
37. Ide T, Akamatsu N, Nakajima I. Arthroscopic surgery of the hip joint. *Arthroscopy*. 1991;7:204–211.
38. Gondolph-Zink B. Aktueller Stand der diagnostischen und operativen Hüftarthroskopie. *Orthopäde*. 1992;21:249–256.
39. Goldman A, Minkoff J, Price A, et al. A posterior arthroscopic approach to bullet extraction from the hip. *J Trauma*. 1987;27:1294–1300.
40. Schindler A, Lechevallier JJC, Rao NS, et al. Diagnostic and therapeutic arthroscopy of the hip in children and adolescents: evaluation of results. *J Ped Orthop*. 1995;15:317–321.
41. Klapper R., Dorfmann H, Boyer T. Hip arthroscopy without traction. In: Byrd JWT, ed. *Operative hip arthroscopy*. New York: Thieme; 1998:139.
42. Okada Y, Awaya G, Ikeda T, et al. Arthroscopic surgery for synovial chondromatosis of the hip. *J Bone Joint Surg*. 1989;71B:198–199.
43. Janssens X, Van Meirhaeghe J, Verdonk R, et al. Diagnostic arthroscopy of the hip joint in pigmented villonodular synovitis. Case report. *Arthroscopy*. 1987;3:283–287.
44. Fitzgerald RH Jr. Acetabular labrum tears. Diagnosis and treatment. *Clin Orthop*. 1995;311:60–68.
45. Lage LA, Patel JV, Villar RN. The acetabular labral tear: an arthroscopic classification. *Arthroscopy*. 1996;12:269–272.
46. Leunig M, Podeszwa D, Beck M, et al. Magnetic resonance arthrography of labral disorders in hips dysplasia and impingement. *Clin Orthop*. 2004;204:74–80.
47. Schuck M, Noble P, McCarthy JC. The healing potential of lesions of the acetabular labrum. *Trans ORS*. 2000.
48. Sampson TG, Farjo LA. Hip arthroscopy by the lateral approach: technique and selected cases. In: Byrd JWT, ed. *Operative hip arthroscopy*. New York: Thieme; 1998:105.
49. Kelly BT, Williams RJ, Philippon MJ. Hip arthroscopy: current indications, treatment options, and management issues. *Am J Sports Med*. 2003;31:1020–1037.
50. Villar RN. Arthroscopic debridement of the hip: a minimally invasive approach to osteoarthritis. *J Bone Joint Surg Br*. 1991;73B (supp II):170–171.
51. Byrd JWT. Lateral impact injury. A source of occult hip pathology. *Clin Sports Med*. 2001;20:801–816.
52. Gray AJR, Villar RN. The ligamentum teres of the hip: an arthroscopic classification of its pathology. *Arthroscopy*. 1997;13:575–578.
53. Rao J, Zhou YX, Villar RN. Injury to the ligamentum teres. Mechanism, findings, and results of treatment. *Clin Sports Med*. 2001;20:791–800.
54. Ganz R, Parvizi J, Beck M, et al. Femoroacetabular impingement: a cause for osteoarthritis of the hip. *Clin Orthop*. 2003;417:112–120.
55. Beck M, Leunig M, Parvizi J, et al. Anterior femoroacetabular impingement: part II. Midterm results of surgical treatment. *Clin Orthop*. 2004;418:67–73.
56. Bould M, Edwards D, Villar RN. Arthroscopic diagnosis and treatment of septic arthritis of the hip joint. Case report. *Arthroscopy*. 1993;9:707–708.
57. Blitzer CM. Arthroscopic management of septic arthritis of the hip. *Arthroscopy*. 1993;9:414–416.
58. Chung WK, Slater GL, Bates EH. Treatment of septic arthritis of the hip by arthroscopic lavage. *J Ped Orthop*. 1993;13:444–446.
59. Carls J, Kohn D. Arthroskopische Therapie der eitrigen Koxitis. *Arthroskopie*. 1996;9:274–277.
60. Byrd JWT. Arthroscopy of select hip lesions. In: Byrd JWT, ed. *Operative hip arthroscopy*. New York: Thieme; 1998:153.
61. Ruch DS, Satterfield W. The use of arthroscopy to document accurate position of core decompression of the hip. *Arthroscopy*. 1998;14:617–619.
62. Suzuki S, Kasahara Y, Seto Y, et al. Arthroscopy in 19 children with Perthes' disease. Pathologic changes of the synovium and the joint surface. *Acta Orthop Scand*. 1994;65:581–584.
63. Gross RH. Arthroscopy in hip disorders in children. *Orthop Rev*. 1977;6:43–49.
64. Kuklo TR, Mackenzie WG, Keeler KA. Hip arthroscopy in Legg-Calve-Perthes disease. Case Report. *Arthroscopy*. 1999;15:88–92.
65. Bowen JR, Kumar VP, Joyce JJ, et al. Osteochondritis dissecans following Perthes' disease. Arthroscopic-operative treatment. *Clin Orthop*. 1986;209:49–56.
66. Lechevallier J, Bowen JR. Arthroscopic treatment of the late sequelae of Legg-Calve-Perthes disease. *J Bone Joint Surg* 1993;75B(suppl 2):160–161.
67. Majewski M. Arthroscopic mobilisation of the hip joint in children and adolescents by distension and bump resection. 18th annual meeting of the Association of Germanspeaking Arthroscopists (AGA), Saarbruecken; 2001.
68. Shifrin LZ, Reis AN. Arthroscopy of a dislocated hip replacement: a case report. *Clin Orthop*. 1980;146:213–214.
69. Vakili F, Salvati EA, Warren RF. Entrapped foreign body within the acetabular cup in total hip replacement. *Clin Orthop*. 1980;150:159–162.
70. Nordt W, Giangarra CE, Levy M, et al. Arthroscopic removal of entrapped debris following dislocation of a total hip arthroplasty. *Arthroscopy*. 1987;3:196–198.
71. Byrd JWT. Complications associated with hip arthroscopy. In: Byrd JWT, ed. *Operative hip arthroscopy*. New York: Thieme; 1998:171.
72. Bartlett CS, DiFelice GS, Buly R, et al. Cardiac arrest as a result of intraabdomial extravasation of fluid during arthroscopic removal of a loose body from the hip joint of a patient with an acetabular fracture. *J Orthop Trauma*. 1998;12:294–300.

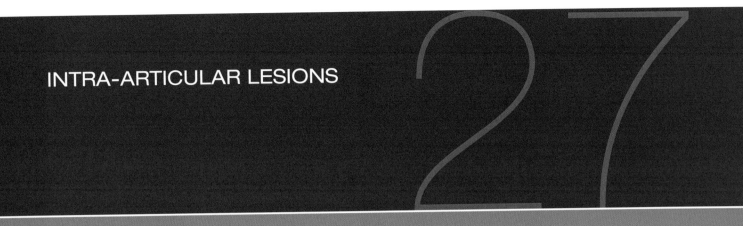

INTRA-ARTICULAR LESIONS

AARON A. BARE, MD, CARLOS A. GUANCHE, MD

■ KEY POINTS

- When a pathologic process alters the function of the homeostatic chemical and mechanical forces within the hip joint, articular cartilage breakdown can occur and joint deterioration may follow.
- Disruption of the articular surface dynamics usually responds best to surgical debridement, repair, or removal of the offending lesion or lesions.
- Arthroscopy offers a minimally invasive solution compared to traditional open techniques.
- Open exposure of the joint remains an option for conditions not amenable to arthroscopic technique, such as fixation of large osteochondral lesions.
- Loose bodies within the joint can cause pain and may mimic the snapping hip phenomenon.
- A disruption of the acetabular labrum alters the biomechanical properties of the hip. The forces acting on the hip in the setting of a torn labrum often cause pain during sports participation. Patients with labral tears often present with mechanical symptoms, such as buckling, clicking, catching, or locking.
- The most commonly reported cause of a traumatic labral tear is an externally applied force to a hyperextended and externally rotated hip. However, a specific inciting event often is not identified, and the patient presents for evaluation after failed attempts to management of groin pulls, muscle strains, or hip contusions.
- Femoroacetabular impingement is a structural abnormality of the femoral neck which can lead to chronic hip pain and subsequent acetabular labral degenerative tears. The repetitive microtrauma from the femoral neck abutting

against the labrum produces degenerative labral lesions in the anterior-superior quadrant.
- Impingement often occurs in extreme ranges of motion. While in flexed position, patients exhibit a decrease in both internal rotation and adduction, often accompanied by pain.
- Osteonecrosis can cause severe pain and disability in young patients. It occurs most commonly between the third and fifth decades of life. Osteonecrosis can be the result of trauma that disrupts the blood supply of the femoral head. *Non*traumatic risk factors include: corticosteroid use, heavy alcohol consumption, sickle cell disease, Gaucher and Caisson disease, and hypercoaguable states.
- Instability of the native hip is much less common than shoulder instability, but can cause a significant amount of disability. The labrum provides a great deal of stability at extremes of motion, particularly flexion. With a torn or absent labrum, a great deal of force is transmitted through the capsule.
- Traumatic dislocations of the hip can lead to capsular redundancy and clinical hip laxity.
- Hip instability has been recognized in sports with repetitive hip rotation with axial loading, such as golf, figure skating, football, gymnastics, ballet, and baseball. A common injury pattern for athletes is labral degeneration combined with subtle rotational hip instability. This has been successfully treated with labral debridement and thermal capsulorrhaphy.
- Rheumatoid arthritis is a common inflammatory arthritis that can affect the hip. Arthroscopic synovectomy has been used as a treatment aimed to improve symptoms and slow progression of the disease.

■ Patients with underlying chronic conditions, such as osteonecrosis or connective tissue disorders, may benefit from a diagnostic and therapeutic arthroscopy, when mechanical symptoms are present.

Approximately 2.5% of all sports related injuries are located in the hip region, and this figure increases to 5% to 9% of high school athletes (1). Painful hips in the young and middle-aged patients impose a diagnostic challenge. With improved imaging modalities and an increasing capacity to treat intra-articular pathology, more diagnoses and treatments are available than a decade ago. Arthroscopic treatment of intra-articular and extra-articular lesions of the hip continues to expand, with recent advances providing an invaluable diagnostic as well as treatment vehicle for hip pathology. As a result, our awareness of many hip problems has increased. We now have more definitive answers for the active patient without radiographic evidence of degenerative joint disease and less commonly must formulate vague diagnoses such as generalized hip sprains, strains, or tendonitis.

The hip joint often functions without problems for 7 or 8 decades under normal physiologic loads, which include loads of up to five times body weight. When a pathologic process alters the function of the homeostatic chemical and mechanical forces within the joint, articular cartilage breakdown can occur and joint deterioration may follow. Unfortunately, a large percentage of patients are not evaluated or diagnosed until the process affecting the joint is established. Once bony changes have occurred, the process of joint deterioration becomes progressive and usually irreversible. While aging defines a large portion of patients with hip degenerative joint disease, younger patients with intra-articular disruptions have acute symptoms and are at risk of developing a chronic disability. Improved imaging modalities and arthroscopic techniques have introduced the ability to identify and treat intra-articular pathology in hopes of preventing the degenerative cascade.

The majority of intra-articular pathology does not respond well to conservative treatment. Disruption of the articular surface dynamics usually responds best to surgical debridement, repair, or removal of the offending lesion or lesions. Treatment of intra-articular lesions can be performed either open or arthroscopically. Arthroscopy, however, offers a minimally invasive solution compared to the traditional open techniques. It spares extensive surgical dissection and violation of the hip capsule. While the range of pathology amenable to arthroscopic treatment in the hip continues to expand, open exposure of the joint remains an option for conditions not amenable to arthroscopic techniques such as fixation of large osteochondral lesions. The goal of surgical treatment of intra-articular lesions is to restore near normal intra-articular anatomy and biomechanical forces. Inferior arthroscopic results, therefore, should not be accepted from inexperienced surgeons.

Burman (2) first introduced arthroscopic surgery of the hip in 1931. While procedures for the shoulder and knee flourished in the 1980s, hip arthroscopy received relatively little attention. Within the last 10 years, a variety of studies have documented the success of treating a wide range of intra-articular pathology of the hip. Current indications for intra-articular hip arthroscopy include removal of loose bodies, treatment of acetabular labral tears, avascular necrosis (AVN), synovial and connective tissue disorders, chondral lesions, and the treatment of impingement.

■ LOOSE BODIES

Loose bodies within the joint can cause pain and may mimic the snapping hip phenomenon. Anterior groin pain, episodes of clicking or locking, buckling, giving way, and persistent pain during activity suggest an intra-articular loose body. McCarthy and Busconi (3) showed that loose bodies within the hip, whether ossified or not, correlated with locking episodes and inguinal pain.

In cases of traumatic injury or dislocation, suspicion should be high for loose bodies to explain hip symptoms. Besides hip trauma, other diseases known to be associated with loose bodies include Perthes disease, osteochondritis dissecans, AVN, synovial chondromatosis, and osteoarthritis. When identified by computed tomography (CT) scanning during closed treatment of an acetabular fracture or a hip dislocation, Keene and Villar (4) advocate early arthroscopic retrieval of traumatic loose bone fragments from the joint to eliminate additional insult to the articular surface.

Radiographs often identify loose bodies, but noncalcified lesions may not appear on standard radiographs. CT scans are highly sensitive for detection of suspected loose bodies and are more sensitive than magnetic resonance imaging (MRI) (5). Loose bodies may occur as an isolated lesion following trauma or may present with many intra-articular lesions as seen in synovial chondromatosis.

Although arthrotomy remains the gold standard for direct observation and removal of intra-articular and extra-articular objects or loose bodies, the morbidity of an open approach and hip dislocation is significant. Hip arthroscopy offers an excellent method for removal of the lesions. McCarthy and Busconi (3) reported that radiographs did not visualize 67% of loose bodies in the hip. When persistent symptoms of locking or catching are present, further work-up for loose bodies should be performed. A CT scan is the imaging modality of choice to pursue, followed by a diagnostic or therapeutic hip arthroscopy **(Fig 27-1)**. A history of trauma followed by mechanical symptoms suggests either an articular loose body, chondral injury, or a labral injury. While CT scans best evaluate loose bodies, an MRI offers the best imaging modality for labral injures, therefore occasionally both studies are required for the diagnosis.

Osteoarthritic changes in the hip can be caused by intra-articular bone and chondral fragments or from a step-off at the articular surface. Osteoarthritis has been documented to

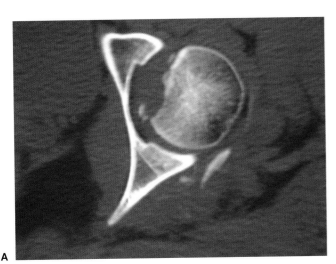
A

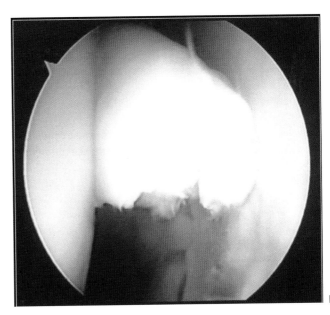
B

Fig 27-1. A: Axial CT illustrates loose bodies within the hip joint along with a humeral head defect following a posterior hip dislocation. **B:** Arthroscopy of the joint allows for loose body removal.

occur at a rate of approximately 25% to 55% following all native hip dislocations at a follow-up of 10 years, with simple dislocations having a better prognosis (6). Upadhyay et al. (7) reported osteoarthritic changes at 5 years following traumatic posterior dislocation of the hip. Yamamoto et al. (6) evaluated 11 hips arthroscopically after major hip trauma. In seven cases, small osteochondral or chondral fragments visualized arthroscopically were not seen on radiographs or CT scans. Even though the patient series was small, because over half of the patients had free fragments documented on arthroscopy, there is a broadening indication for diagnostic arthroscopy and lavage following hip trauma.

The presence of a loose body within the articulating surfaces of any joint theoretically will result in destruction of the hyaline cartilage, and ultimately result in premature arthritic degeneration. The significance of a symptomatic loose body in the hip should not be understated, and the treatment, arthroscopically or open, should not be delayed. When hip disease or a pathologic condition results in loose body formation, symptomatic improvement can be expected after arthroscopic removal, but the effect on the future of the joint remains dependent on the natural history of the underlying condition. The minimally invasive nature and low morbidity associated with hip arthroscopy make the procedure ideal for establishing an early preventive strategy to treat symptomatic patients with loose bodies in the hip.

■ LABRAL TEARS

The acetabular labrum is a rim of triangular fibrocartilage that attaches to the base of the acetabular rim. It surrounds the perimeter of the acetabulum and is absent inferiorly where the transverse ligament resides. The labrum provides structural resistance to lateral motion of the femoral head within the acetabulum, enhances joint stability, and preserves joint congruity (8). Similar to the meniscus, it also functions to distribute synovial fluid and provides proprioceptive feedback (9).

A disruption of the acetabular labrum alters the biomechanical properties of the joint. The forces acting on the hip in the setting of a torn labrum often cause pain during sports participation in athletes. Altenberg (10) in 1977 was the first to describe tearing of the acetabular labrum as a source of hip pain. Patients with labral tears often present with mechanical symptoms, such as buckling, clicking, catching, or locking. Athletes may present with subtle findings, including dull, activity-induced, positional pain that fails to respond to rest. The most commonly reported cause of a traumatic labral tear is an externally applied force to a hyperextended and externally rotated hip (11). However, a specific inciting event often is not identified and the patient presents for evaluation after failed attempts at conservative management for groin pulls, muscle strains, or hip contusions.

The mechanism of labral tearing can be either traumatic and acute, or chronic and degenerative. Hip impingement chronically loads the anterosuperior labrum and leads to degenerative tears in that region of the acetabulum. The location of labral tears has varied based on different regions. North American series have reported that the vast majority of tears are located anteriorly and acute tears result from sudden pivoting or twisting motions (12). In contrast, in Asian populations, tears are found more frequently posteriorly and are associated with hyperflexion or squatting (11).

Lage et al. (13) have described an arthroscopic classification of labral tears. Labral tears were divided into four groups: radial flap tears, radial fibrillated tears, longitudinal peripheral tears, and mobile tears. Radial flaps were the most common, followed by radial fibrillated, longitudinal peripheral and mobile tears. They also classified degenerative tears based on location and the extent of the tear. Stage I degenerative tears are localized to one segment of an anatomic region, anterior or posterior. Stage II tears involve an entire anatomic region, and stage III tears are diffuse and involve more than one region. They found that the extent of the degenerative tear correlated to the degree of degenerative changes within the joint. The degree or increasing stage of degenerative labral tears correlated with erosive changes of the acetabulum or femoral head. The articular lesions are most often located adjacent to the labral tear, often at the labrochondral junction.

Labral tears secondary to trauma generally are isolated to one quadrant depending on the direction and extent of the trauma. For instance, patients with a known posterior subluxation or dislocations most frequently have posterior labral tears. If a bone fragment is avulsed as a result of a dislocation, the labral injury most often occurs on the capsular or peripheral region of the labrum and may be amenable to an arthroscopic repair (14). Patients with minor trauma often have anterior and more central tears, located in the same region as those for impingement and those seen in athletes.

Idiopathic tears are often seen in the athletic population. Chronic, repetitive loading of the hip can subject the labrum to tensile and compressive forces and lead to tearing (Fig 27-2). Often, no specific recognizable injury is reported. The majority of patients participate in sports requiring repetitive pivoting or twisting, such as football, soccer, basketball, or ballet. It has been theorized that recurrent torsional maneuvers subject the anterior portion of the articular-labral junction to recurrent microtrauma and eventual mechanical attrition (14). McCarthy et al. (14) performed arthroscopic labral debridement on 13 hips in ten competitive athletes with mechanical symptoms stemming from labral tears. All hips had anterior labral tears, with two hips having additional posterior tears. Twelve of thirteen patients had successful results following arthroscopy and returned to competitive activities. Of note, four of the twelve hips had associated chondral lesions requiring debridement. Stated in their conclusion, "hip arthroscopy is the new gold standard for treating the elite athlete with intractable hip pain with mechanical symptoms."

Radiographs are often unremarkable when evaluating for a labral tear. Specific attention should be given to the superior neck, looking for subtle irregularities in the femoral head-neck offset and decreased neck concavity compared to the contralateral side, which would suggest impingement.

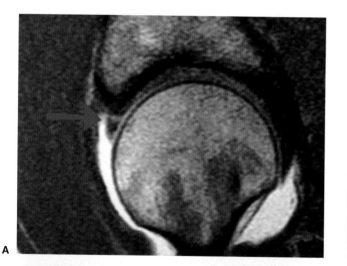

A

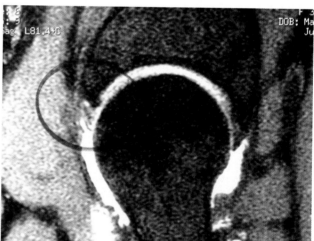

B

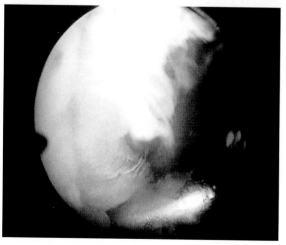

C

Fig 27-2. A T1 **(A)** (*arrow*) and a T2 **(B)** (*circle*) MRI sagittal oblique illustrate a degenerative labral lesion in the anterosuperior quadrant. Arthroscopy **(C)** reveals the degenerative lesion.

Contrast enhanced MRI arthrography is more sensitive than standard MRI at detecting intra-articular lesions of the hip (15). Czerny et al. (15) compared conventional MRI with MR arthrography in the diagnosis of labral lesions. They reported a sensitivity and accuracy of 80% and 65% for conventional MRI compared with 95% and 88% with MR arthrography. However, hip MR arthrograms are not without frequent misinterpretation. Byrd and Jones (16) found an 8% false-negative rate and a 20% false-positive interpretation of MR arthrograms for all types of intra-articular pathology of the hip. While MR arthrograms offer a diagnostic advantage over conventional MRI for labral tears and other intra-articular pathology, their reported false-positive rate dictates cautious interpretation. Newer MR imaging modalities such as fast spin echo have improved the imaging capability of articular cartilage and may obviate the need for intra-articular gadolinium in the future (5).

Not only should imaging studies be interpreted with caution but physical exam findings are often inconsistent. Farjo et al. (17) did not find specific exam findings to correlate with labral injuries. However, Fitzgerald (18) found the Thomas test correlated with surgical pathology. Bilateral hip flexion, followed by abduction and extension of the involved hip with a palpable or audible click along with pain defines a positive Thomas test. Another available test, similar to the Thomas test, is the McCarthy test: Both hips are flexed; the affected hip is then extended, first in external rotation, then in internal rotation. Hip extension in internal rotation will stress the anterior labrum, and extension with external rotation will elicit posterior pathology.

MRI may confirm the diagnosis, but the decision to proceed with operative intervention should be heavily weighted on refractory, mechanical symptoms. The majority of labral tears are treated by debridement; however some tears are amenable to arthroscopic repair. Petersen et al. (19) studied blood supply to the labrum and found blood vessels enter the labrum from the adjacent joint capsule. Vascularity was detected in the peripheral one-third of the labrum and the inner two-thirds of the labrum are avascular, similar to the meniscus. Thus, peripheral tears have healing potential and repairs should be considered **(Fig 27-3)**. Peripheral tears, however, are a rarity. McCarthy et al. (14) reported 436 consecutive hip arthroscopies performed over 6 years and treated 261 labral tears, all of which were located at the articular junction.

For articular or centrally based as well as degenerative tears, the goal of arthroscopic debridement is to relieve pain and mechanical symptoms while preserving healthy, intact portions of the labrum. Kelly et al. (20) reviewed the results of more the 500 acetabular debridements and found nearly 90% good to excellent results at short-term follow-up. Farjo et al. (17) reported good to excellent results for debrided acetabular tears without concomitant arthritis and only 21% good or excellent results for patients with articular cartilage damage discovered intra-operative. McCarthy et al. (14) published good to excellent results for debridement of labral

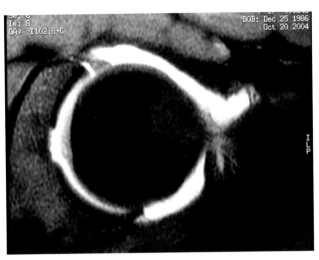

Fig 27-3. An anterior peripheral labral tear is seen on this T2 axial MRI.

lesions without articular cartilage involvement and less than 40% good to excellent results for patients with associated articular cartilage lesions. Therefore, patient outcomes are significantly more favorable after operative treatment for labral lesions without concomitant degenerative joint disease.

Whether acetabular labral tears lead to degenerative joint disease has yet to be determined. McCarthy et al. (21) reported that labral tears might contribute to the progression of degenerative disease of the hip. They found an association between the progression of labral lesions and the progression of anterior acetabular articular cartilage lesions. The frequency and severity of acetabular articular degeneration was statistically significantly higher in patients with labral lesions than those without. This association, however, does not offer a definitive causal relationship. Currently, arthroscopic findings have supported the theory that labral disruptions and degenerative joint disease are linked as part of a continuum. Labral tears, idiopathic, traumatic, or degenerative in nature, can progress to articular cartilage delamination adjacent to the labral lesions and slowly progress to more global labral and articular destruction. Therefore, treatment of patients with mechanical symptoms with underlying labral pathology will not only alleviate symptoms but may prevent the development of degenerative cartilage lesions.

■ IMPINGEMENT

Femoral neck impingement against the acetabular labrum or femoroacetabular impingement has been described as a structural abnormality of the femoral neck which can lead to chronic hip pain and subsequent acetabular labral degenerative tears. The repetitive microtrauma from the femoral neck abutting against the labrum produces degenerative labral lesions in the anterior-superior quadrant of the labrum. This mechanical impingement is believed to originate from either a "pistol grip" deformity of the femoral neck or a retroverted acetabulum.

A "pistol grip" femoral neck is a neck with a decreased femoral head-neck offset on the superior or anterolateral neck. A decreased offset of the anterolateral head-neck junction causes a reduction in joint clearance and can lead to repetitive contact between the femoral neck and the acetabular rim. Several recent studies (21–23) have shown an association between labral tears and osteoarthritis as well as labral tears in the setting of impingement. Therefore, a specific subset of patients may be predisposed to the development of labral lesions and osteoarthritis based on an altered morphology of the anterolateral femoral neck. Evidence to support this theory remains circumstantial, but treatment of symptoms by attempting to correct the structural abnormality often allows patients to return to normal activities.

Impingement often occurs in extreme ranges of motion. Abutment from the superior neck occurs in flexion, often with a variable degree of adduction and internal rotation. The repetitive trauma not only damages the labrum, but can create adjacent chondral injuries. Beck et al. (24) noted all patients treated operatively for impingement had labral lesions in the anterosuperior quadrant and that labral and cartilage lesions correlated with an absent anterolateral offset of the head-neck junction.

The etiology of the abnormal neck morphology is not completely understood. The pistol grip deformity has been attributed as a form of mild or subclinical slipped capital epiphysis (25). *Non*spherical heads with a wide neck have also been described as the result of a growth disturbance of the proximal femur (26). Recently, Siebenrock et al. (27) reported an increase in the lateral epiphyseal extension in patients with decreased head-neck offset and a larger extension of the epiphysis onto the neck in the anterosuperior quadrant. They showed that an increased physeal extension into the cranial hemisphere of the femoral head neck is associated with a decreased head-neck offset. This suggests that a growth abnormality of the capital physis is a possible cause of the development of a decreased head-neck offset in patients with anterolateral impingement. Overall, several theories exist to explain the femoroacetabular impingement phenomenon but the inciting event has not been agreed upon.

Currently, evidence suggests that femoroacetabular impingement may play a role in the cascade of hip osteoarthritis in some patients: those with structural proximal femoral head-neck abnormalities (21–24,28). This entity usually appears in younger and more physically active adults and can be physically debilitating. Subsequent labral and chondral lesions have been linked to repetitive microtrauma caused by the pistol grip deformity of the femoral neck (29). The operative management of these lesions offers two benefits. First, for symptomatic patients: who fail conservative treatment, the removal of the structural abnormality will provide significant pain relief. Because labral and chondral lesions are seen more frequently in early osteoarthritic hips, early recognition and treatment of this entity may curb or halt the unfortunate progression to osteoarthritis in these younger patients.

The typical patient is a middle-aged, athletic individual complaining of groin pain with activity. This often occurs during activities requiring hip flexion. Sporting activities may cause symptoms, but often-simple acts like walking may aggravate the situation. Symptoms range from mild to severe and are often intermittent in presentation. The groin pain can become activity limiting, especially for athletes. Patients often have been seen by multiple physicians and have been given a wide range of diagnoses, such as a sports hernia, tendonitis, or synovitis.

Patients often exhibit a decrease in both internal rotation and adduction while in a flexed position, often accompanied by pain. The impingement test, done by passively flexing the adducted hip and gradually internally rotating, will often elicit groin pain. This moves the proximal and anterior part of the femoral neck into contact with the rim of the acetabulum (29). Leunig et al. (30) have shown that positive impingement tests correlate with labral tears on MR arthrograms, corresponding to the location of impingement. A complete examination to rule out other sources of hip pain such as bursitis, nerve entrapments, and referred pain will help ascertain the diagnosis.

Although many patients will have been previously told that their hip radiographs are normal, subtle abnormalities may be present and should be suspected. An anteroposterior (AP) pelvis allows a gross comparison of both proximal femurs, with particular attention given to head-neck offset **(Fig 27-4)**. The contour of the anterolateral neck should be compared to the unaffected side. A normal superior neck will have a distinctive concave appearance, with the concave contour takeoff at the head-neck junction through the neck-greater trochanter junction. A cross table lateral radiograph is essential in addition to the AP radiograph. A properly taken cross-table radiograph will illustrate the appearance of the femoral neck, allowing for an additional view of the anterolateral neck **(Fig 27-5)**. MR arthrography detects labral pathology in addition to an assessment of the femoral head, neck, and acetabulum **(Fig 27-6)**.

Hip impingement can be a difficult entity to diagnose and treat. We feel that conservative treatment should be attempted for all patients with the understanding that a structural abnormality often does not improve with conservative treatment, especially in the younger, active patient group. When conservative modalities fail, the location of the pathology dictates the treatment plan. Impingement secondary to variations in proximal femoral anatomy is often amenable to arthroscopic debridement. With a normal head-neck offset, repetitive impingement will not occur and subsequent labral and chondral damage may be obviated.

While open techniques have been the traditional approach to address a retroverted acetabulum or altered morphology of the femoral neck, arthroscopy has recently been introduced as a method of treating hip impingement secondary to structural abnormalities of the anterolateral neck. The peripheral

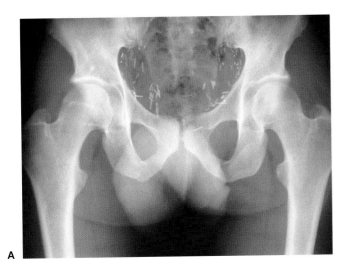

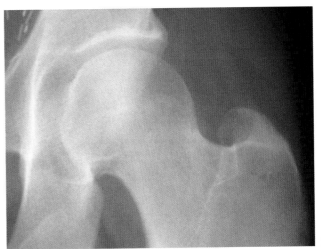

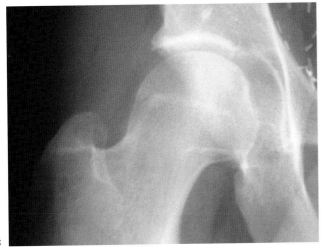

Fig 27-4. A: An AP pelvis XR offers a comparison of the morphology of both femoral necks. The asymptomatic hip **(B)** has a normal superior neck contour with a normal head-neck offset. The affected hip **(C)** has a near vertical superior neck slope with a loss of the normal head-neck offset.

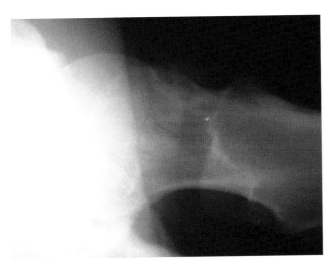

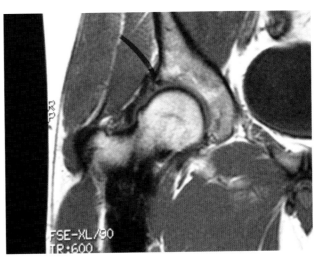

Fig 27-5. A cross table lateral XR illustrates the abnormal head-neck junction.

Fig 27-6. An MRI confirms the abnormal morphology of the femoral neck as well as a degenerative tear of antero-superior labrum.

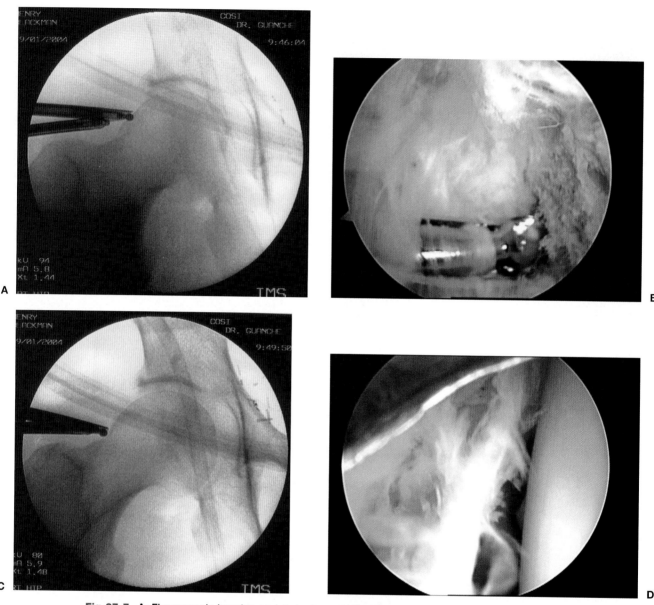

Fig 27-7. A: Fluoroscopic imaging assists in documenting the correct positioning for debridement. **B:** Debridement of the prominent with a burr. **C:** Fluoroscopic documentation of the femoral neck after completion of the debridement. **D:** Intra-compartmental visualization of the degenerative labral lesion.

compartment or extracapsular compartment is entered and the neck is debrided with the help of fluoroscopy. After the anterolateral femoral neck has been contoured, the central or intra-articular region is explored and concomitant labral and chondral pathology is addressed **(Fig 27-7)**.

■ CHONDRAL LESIONS

Articular surface lesions create an irregular contour of the joint surface and lead to abnormal intra-articular forces with motion and weight bearing, predisposing the patient to the development of progressive degenerative disease. Chondral injuries are found following trauma and have been associated

with degenerative labral lesions as well as with early arthritic hips. McCarthy et al. (21) reported 74% of patients with a torn labrum had some degree of articular surface damage. In 80% of these patients, the labral and articular lesions occurred in the same quadrant. They also found an association between labral tears, the severity of articular injury, and age. The frequency and severity of cartilage lesions increased with age, and 24% of chondral injuries were observed arthroscopically in patients less than 30 years of age compared to 81% of patients with chondral lesions in patients older than 60 years of age.

Arthroscopic debridement of chondral flaps can be performed through a standard arthroscopic approach. Chondral flaps are debrided and associated labral pathology is treated as well. Full thickness chondral defects, more often associated with trauma, can be treated with microfracture or acute repair of large full-thickness acute lesions. Arthroscopic microfracture as well as internal fixation of large lesions can be challenging and an open approach should be considered if the desired results cannot be achieved through the arthroscope.

◼ LIGAMENTUM TERES

The ligamentum teres is a triangular shaped ligament, arising from the posteroinferior region of the cotyloid fossa, inserting on the base of the femoral head. It provides blood supply to the femoral head in children. Its function in adults remains unclear. Gray and Villar (31) suggest that the ligamentum teres injury causing symptoms without a history of traumatic hip dislocation may be more common than previously reported. Byrd and Jones (16) reported that rupture of the ligament was the third most commonly encountered pathology during hip arthroscopy. The ligament becomes taut in flexion, adduction, and external rotation. This has been a proposed mechanism for traumatic rupture (31).

Gray and Villar (31) reported twenty injuries to the ligamentum teres observed among 472 consecutive hip arthroscopies. They discovered three distinct patterns of ligament injury: complete rupture, partial tears, and degenerative ligaments, which were associated with degenerative changes of the hip **(Fig 27-8)**. Complete ruptures were associated with trauma, and labral or chondral injuries were often present. Partial tears often occurred without associated pathology and presented as hip pain of unknown etiology prior to arthroscopy. The degenerative ligament all had articular changes on both the femoral and acetabular surfaces. All patients presented with groin or thigh pain and most complained of a limp or clicking sensation with weight bearing. They were unable to elicit any specific exam finding path

gnomonic for ligament tears and reported the imaging studies did not aid in the diagnosis **(Fig 27-9)**.

Byrd and Jones (32) reported 41 lesions of the ligamentum teres among 271 consecutive hip scopes: 23 injuries were traumatic, including 12 complete and 11 partial ruptures; 18 ligaments were found to be hypertrophic or degenerative. Of the patients with traumatic injuries, 80% complained of mechanical symptoms, 15 resulted from major trauma, and 8 from twisting injuries. Preoperative diagnosis was made on imaging studies in only 2 of 23 cases. Eight lesions were isolated findings during arthroscopy, and 15 hips had additional pathology discovered during arthroscopy. All patients improved with arthroscopic debridement, with an average preoperative hip score of 47, and postoperative score of 90 with more than a 1-year follow-up **(Fig 27-10)**.

Overall, ligamentum teres ruptures respond well to arthroscopic debridement. Ligamentum teres disruption has been known to occur with hip dislocations, and its occurrence following minor trauma, and twisting injuries has just recently been appreciated. Twisting injuries often result in labral tears, so the clinician should consider ligamentum teres disruption as a potential source of pain after twisting injuries. The diagnosis of ligament tears remains elusive to imaging technology and an index of suspicion should be maintained in the presence of mechanical symptoms and a history of trauma or twisting injury. Debridement of a complete or partial rupture has not been shown to produce detrimental effects on hip stability; however the complete function of the ligament has not been fully elucidated.

◼ OSTEONECROSIS

Osteonecrosis can cause severe pain and disability in young patients, occurring most commonly between the third and fifth decades of life (32). Approximately 10,000 to 20,000 of

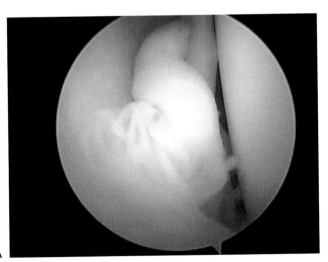
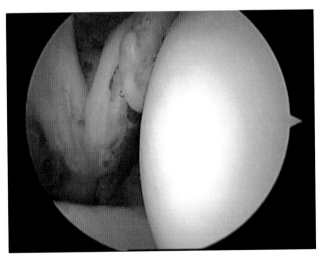

Fig 27-8. A: Arthroscopy confirms a complete ligamentum rupture. **B:** A partial ligamentum tear with surrounding synovial inflammation.

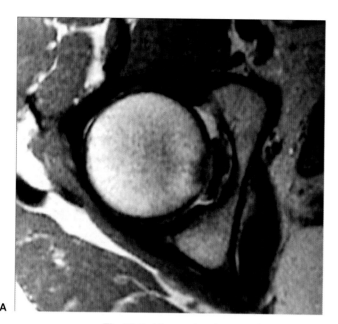

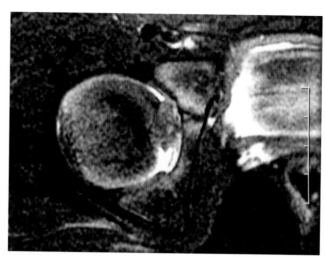

A

B

Fig 27-9. Ligamentum tears are best visualized on axial MRI images. T1 image **(A)** shows ligamentous discontinuity (*arrow*) and a T2 image **(B)** often reveals corresponding fluid within the fovea.

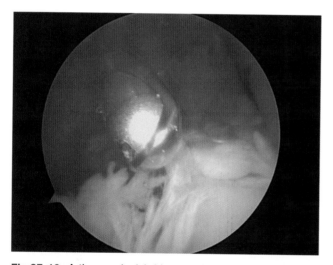

Fig 27-10. Arthroscopic debridement of the torn ligament.

new cases of hip osteonecrosis are reported each year in the United States (34). It has been estimated that up to 10% of total hip arthroplasties are performed because of AVN (35). It can be the result of trauma that disrupts the blood supply of the femoral head. Other nontraumatic risk factors include corticosteroid use, heavy alcohol consumption, sickle cell disease, Gaucher and Caisson disease as well as hypercoaguable states. However, the etiology of a large percentage of patients is idiopathic. Without treatment, AVN often progresses to articular collapse and degenerative joint disease. Prior to femoral head collapse, joint preserving procedures such as core decompression, vascularized fibular grafts and osteotomies attempt to obviate the problem by stimulating the vascular supply to the involved area of the femoral head.

While the traditional joint preserving procedures attempt to alter the intrinsic composition of the diseased subchondral bone, intra-articular changes do occur, most often in the form of chondromalacia, chondral flaps, and loose bodies. Arthroscopic evaluation of the joint offers the ability to treat intra-articular pathology and improve mechanical symptoms. Prior to subchondral collapse, some patients complain of mechanical symptoms such as locking, buckling, and clicking (33). O'Leary et al. (36) reported the results of hip arthroscopy for treatment of 37 cases of hip AVN. They found that outcomes were most favorable for patients with mechanical symptoms without articular collapse. As would be expected, patients with degenerative changes and no mechanical symptoms had the worst outcome. Of patients with stage Ficat III or IV, only 34% had significant pain relief following arthroscopy **(Table 27-1)**.

Patients with stage III (crescent sign with or without collapse) or stage IV (collapse with involvement of the acetabular cartilage) are best treated with either a total hip arthroplasty, hemiarthroplasty, or resurfacing arthroplasty. Resurfacing

TABLE 27-1	**Ficat Classification of Femoral Head Avascular Necrosis**

Ficat Classification

I – Precollapse: Radiographs normal, clinical exam positive

II – Precollapse: Diffuse porosis, sclerosis, cysts

III – Collapse: Broken contour of the femoral head, joint space maintained

IV – Collapse: Flattened contour, joint space collapse

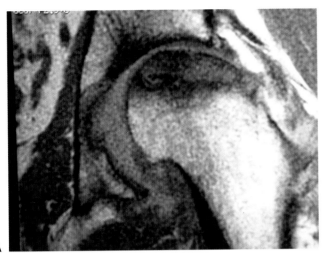
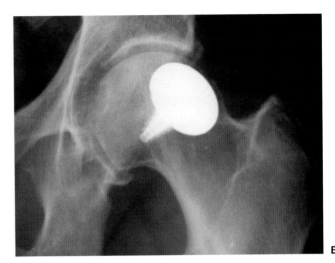

Fig 27-11. A: Femoral head AVN with involvement of a large portion of the femoral head. **B:** Resurfacing arthroplasty of the femoral head.

arthroplasty of the femoral head **(Fig 27-11)** preserves bone stock and only removes the diseased portion of the head while not compromising future conversion to a total hip arthroplasty. It is indicated for Ficat stage III or early stage IV disease. Mont et al. (35) showed that resurfacing arthroplasty had a survival rate of 90% at 10 years, nearly identical to the total hip arthroplasty group. While survival rates are good, patient outcomes are less predictable with good to excellent results at early follow-up reported between 60% to 80% (35). Stage IV Ficat is best treated with a total hip arthroplasty.

In general, the goal in treating AVN of the hip is to improve patients' symptoms and give them the best opportunity to prevent subchondral collapse and degeneration, which often occurs at a young age. Patients without subchondral collapse (Ficat stage I or II and some stage III) and those complaining of pain associated with mechanical symptoms often will improve with hip arthroscopy and debridement. Arthroscopic debridement can be performed in conjunction with joint sparing procedures such as a core decompression or a vascularized fibular graft (33). After the femoral head has shown signs of collapse, the patient is best served by a prosthetic implant, either a total hip arthroplasty or a hemi-resurfacing implant.

Arthroscopy may also have a role for the evaluation and treatment of osteochondritis dissecans (OCD) and Perthes disease (20). Treatment parameters parallel those for osteonecrosis. OCD prevalence in the hip is estimated to be much less than the knee (37). Sporadic case reports have reported OCD in the hip in young patients (38). Perthes, more common than OCD of the hip, is often monitored conservatively, focusing attention on preserving range of motion with frequent follow-ups. Conservative treatment often is successful in treating the condition. However, if young patients with either OCD or Perthes develop symptomatic mechanical symptoms, consideration should be given to arthroscopic evaluation of the joint surfaces. Chondral flaps or

loose bodies can be treated with limited morbidity to the patient.

■ CAPSULAR LAXITY

Instability of the native hip is much less common than shoulder instability, but its presence can cause a significant amount of disability (20). The hip relies less on the surrounding soft tissues for stability because it has a significant amount of inherent osseous stability. The labrum provides a great deal of stability at extremes of motion, especially flexion. With a torn or absent labrum, a great deal of force is transmitted through the capsule (20).

Hip instability can be difficult to diagnose. Patients often are performing a motion of pelvic rotation and external rotation of the hip to elicit symptoms (39). Motions such as swinging a golf club or throwing a football often precipitate symptoms in active patients (20). The cause of instability may be traumatic or atraumatic. Atraumatic patients are often able to voluntary sublux or nearly dislocate the affected hip and may exhibit generalized ligamentous laxity **(Fig 27-12)**. Some young patients may have an undiagnosed connective tissue disorder causing the ligamentous laxity (i.e., Ehlers-Danlos, Marfans, or Down syndromes). Bellabarba et al. (40) linked a group of atraumatic patients with idiopathic hip instability to subclinical capsular laxity from mild residual acetabular dysplasia.

Traumatic dislocations of the native hip can lead to capsular redundancy and clinical hip laxity. Liebenberg and Dommisse (41) described the development of capsular redundancy after recurrent posterior dislocation of the hip. They suggest that the presence of subclinical hip instability in these patients may result from a damaged capsulolabral complex. The labrum may be torn and may not function as it did prior to the injury. The normal contribution of labrum to

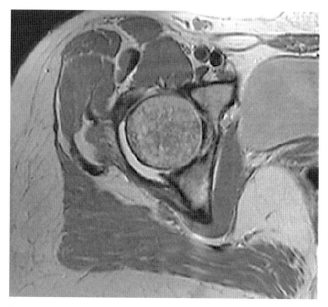

Fig 27-12. MRI with contrast illustrates a redundant posterior capsule with disproportionate amount of contrast posteriorly (*arrow*).

instability requires the hip to rely more on the redundant hip capsule, thus stressing an already lax capsule, which results in further instability.

High level athletes are also subject to hip instability. It has been recognized in sports requiring repetitive hip rotation with axial loading such as golf, figure skating, football, gymnastics, ballet, and baseball. A common injury pattern in athletes is of labral degeneration combined with subtle rotational hip instability. This has been successfully treated by labral debridement and thermal capsulorrhaphy (20). Early results of this procedure have yielded very positive results with 82% return to pre-injury level of athletic competition (39).

Philippon (39) has described the role of arthroscopic thermal capsulorrhaphy for hip instability. Early results have been promising but long term results are necessary to make a conclusion about its effectiveness. Capsular suture plication of the hip arthroscopically in the future will allow us to treat the hip capsule in a similar manner as we treat the shoulder capsule. Improved arthroscopic techniques and equipment as well as experience will make this procedure possible.

■ SYNOVIAL PLICAE

In the knee, diagnosis and treatment of plica syndrome are well described (42–44). Other joints, including the elbow, tibiotalar joint and hip are also known to have synovial plicae that may become symptomatic, but few cases have been reported. Currently, six cases of symptomatic hip plica have been reported in the literature (45–47). Hip plicae have been described in cadavers (48) and have been discovered in patients either through diagnostic arthroscopy (46), or during arthrography (47). Plicae are present as unusually large folds that are vulnerable to impingement between the articular.

Repeated minor entrapments of a plica or one traumatic episode of entrapment can cause pain.

Patients may have a palpable click during the examination with passive motion. One case reported by the senior author found flexion, abduction, and external rotation created pain as well as a click and this corresponded to a plica along the anteromedial aspect of the femoral neck (45). Plain films and nonenhanced MRI are likely to be reported as normal. Often, a gadolinium-enhanced MRI arthrography is obtained with the suspicion of a labral tear **(Fig 27-13)**. MRI can reveal an elongated ligamentous-like structure extending from the region of the femoral head-neck to a region of the hip capsule. Chondromalacia, if present, suggests repeated impingement from the plica on the articular surface has taken place.

Although plica syndrome of the hip seems to be rare, its true incidence may be underestimated. The presence of a symptomatically impinged hip plica should be considered in the differential diagnosis of recalcitrant hip pain. Suspicion of a hip plica that has failed conservative treatment should be treated with diagnostic arthroscopy, debridement of the plica, and thorough evaluation of the articular surfaces, looking in particular for associated chondromalacia from chronic plica impingement.

■ DEGENERATIVE JOINT DISEASE

Hip arthroscopy has a limited role in the treatment of osteoarthritis. The best indications are for patients with mechanical symptoms such that degenerative disease may improve with arthroscopic evaluation and debridement.

Santori and Villar (49) reported a series of 234 consecutive hip arthroscopies, of which 66% had normal radiographs. Of these patients, more than 30% had evidence of early degenerative changes documented during the diagnostic arthroscopic examination. Therefore, osteoarthritis of the hip can present clinically prior to development of radiographic changes, with those complaining of mechanical symptoms responding most favorably to arthroscopic debridement.

■ SYNOVIAL AND CONNECTIVE TISSUE DISORDERS

Advances in hip arthroscopy have improved the treatment of synovial-based disorders. These include synovial chondromatosis, osteochondromatosis, pigmented villonodular synovitis (PVNS), and inflammatory arthropathies such as rheumatoid arthritis. Also, other conditions that result in acute and chronic synovitis of the hip such as hemosideric deposits from hemophilia as well as deposits from chondrocalcinosis may benefit from arthroscopic treatment. Indications for early treatment of progressive synovial diseases may curb the progression of articular destruction.

Synovial chondromatosis, or intrasynovial cartilage metaplasia, can form multiple or extracapsular loose bodies. More

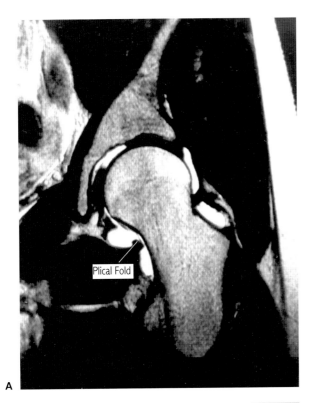

A

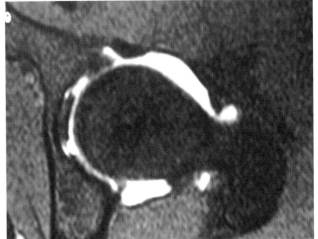

B

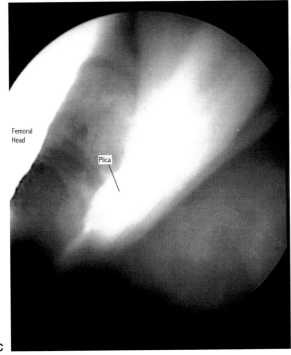

C

Fig 27-13. **A:** A sagittal MRI reveals a synovial plicae along the inferior neck. This is also visualized on the axial MRI (*arrow*) **(B)** as well during arthroscopy **(C)**. **(A,C:** from Atlihan D, Jones DC, and Guanche, CA. Arthroscopic treatment of a symptomatic hip plica. *Clin Orthop.* 2003;411:174–177; with permission).

cases have been reported for the knee, shoulder and elbow, but hip involvement is not uncommon (50). Symptoms include the onset of dull, aching pain, catching or locking, and often-mild restriction of motion. Periarticular loose bodies are seen on radiographs less than 50% of the time as the lesions are often not calcified (51).

The best imaging modality is an MR arthrogram with gadolinium enhancement. Multiple filling defects within the joint suggest synovial chondromatosis. Conservative treatment of multiple intra-articular lesions can lead to articular erosions and hip subluxation. The standard of treatment includes removal of the loose bodies, while the role of concomitant synovectomy is controversial. While some authors recommend only removal of loose bodies (12,52), others support concomitant partial or complete synovectomy (50,53). No large series of hip synovial chondromatosis exist and the role of synovectomy has not been defined. If arthroscopic treatment is chosen, surgeons are limited to a partial synovectomy as complete synovectomy is technically extremely demanding.

Both arthroscopic (54) and open procedures have been described for removal of hip lesions. Limited disease often is more amenable to arthroscopic treatment, while extensive disease may require a formal open approach. Lesions also may be present in the extra-articular peripheral compartment and this compartment should be inspected independent of what operative procedure is performed. Recurrence does occur following removal of the lesions and estimates can best be extrapolated from the knee and shoulder experiences. Recurrence rates have been reported between 7% and 23% (50,55). The senior author recommends arthroscopy debridement and partial synovectomy for all lesions amenable to arthroscopic treatment and formal open debridement and complete synovectomy for recurrences, with a complete evaluation of the joint, paying particular attention to the peripheral compartment.

■ RHEUMATOID ARTHRITIS

Rheumatoid arthritis is a common inflammatory arthritis that can affect the hip. Traditional treatment modalities consisted of medical management with anti-inflammatory medications, disease modifying agents as well as immunosuppressive medications. The role of an orthopedic surgeon was relegated to patients with degenerative hips. Recently, arthroscopic synovectomy has been used as a treatment adjunct aimed to improve symptoms and slow disease progression. It is not a curative procedure and there has been no concrete evidence to suggest that synovectomy retards the bony destruction or the disease process (56). However, Holgersson et al. (57) showed that arthroscopic intervention can benefit patients early in the disease process with minimal degenerative changes. In their series, arthroscopy provided better information about the articular surface in addition to debulking of the synovial membrane and improving patient symptoms.

Arthroscopic synovectomy may be most useful for patients with minimally erosive stages of the disease when synovitis is not controlled by conservative suppressive modalities. As previously mentioned, a disparity exists between arthroscopically diagnosed degenerative changes and radiographic changes (57). In symptomatic hips without degenerative changes on radiographs, articular changes may be present during the diagnostic exam and this may help future decisions regarding treatment.

■ CHONDROCALCINOSIS

Calcium pyrophosphate deposition disease is a crystalline arthropathy that can affect the hip. While the cause is unknown, it results from increased calcium or inorganic phosphate in hyaline or fibrocartilage that precipitates to form crystals. Chondrocalcinosis is the descriptive term used to denote the presence of crystals in cartilage, and it often is not observed radiographically in the hip. The deposition of crystals can lead to acute, as well as chronic synovitis. While it has been postulated that chronic synovitis from calcium pyrophosphate deposition disease plays a role in the initiation of hip degenerative joint disease (58), this has yet to be proven. However the same authors (59) showed that the presence of chondrocalcinosis in the hip at the time of arthroplasty was found to be significantly higher in patients with rapidly destructive hips when compared to patients with osteoarthritis presenting in the 7th or 8th decade.

Currently, it is unknown whether lavage, synovectomy, or arthroscopic, or open crystal debulking will help symptoms or prevent articular degeneration. In patients with chronic or severe symptoms, diagnostic arthroscopy, synovial debulking, and lavage may provide clinical relief, but the literature has yet to confirm this observation.

■ PIGMENTED VILLONODULAR SYNOVITIS

PVNS is a non-neoplastic proliferative disorder that most commonly occurs in the knee, but hip involvement has been reported (60,61). It can affect any synovial lined structures including bursa, tendons, and intra-articular compartments. It typically presents in younger patients, with an average age within the 4th or 5th decade, without gender predilection. It should be considered in the differential diagnosis of this age group in patients with hip pain.

While similar to chondrocalcinosis, the pathogenesis remains unknown. It has been attributed to a chronic inflammatory response, or a benign but locally aggressive growth of fibrohistiocytic origin. Long-standing PVNS of the hip often results in hip degeneration (60). Treatment includes debulking of the lesion, synovectomy, and possible chemical or radio nuclear adjunctive therapy. Hips with degenerative arthritis are treated with a total hip arthroplasty. As these lesions present in the middle-age population, early diagnosis and treatment may prevent a younger patient from requiring a total hip arthroplasty.

Hip arthroscopy can provide tissue for pathologic identification and allow evaluation of the joint surfaces and the ability to perform a partial synovectomy. As a complete synovectomy is difficult to perform, adjunctive chemical synoviothesis in addition to partial synovectomy offers the most minimally invasive treatment option. This treatment regimen is most successful for patients with no or very limited degenerative joint disease. If the lesion recurs, as is common for PVNS (60), more aggressive open complete synovectomy can be attempted. Total hip arthroplasty, a concern for young patients, is the treatment of choice for PVNS presenting as, or progressing to diffuse, advanced degenerative disease.

■ COMPLICATIONS

Whether an open or arthroscopic procedure is chosen to treat intra-articular pathology, knowledge of the surrounding neurovascular structures is crucial to prevent iatrogenic injury. Accurate portal placement during arthroscopy will usually prevent iatrogenic injury to the neurovascular structures. Complications from traction and fluid management can also occur during arthroscopy and these complications should be realized by the arthroscopist.

Sampson reviewed 530 consecutive hip arthroscopies and published a total complication rate of 5.5% with 5.0% described as transient and 0.5% as permanent. The most common complication was secondary to traction and this caused temporary neuropraxias of the peroneal, femoral, sciatic, and lateral femoral cutaneous nerves. Most neuropraxias resolved within three days. Iatrogenic injuries to the femoral head from the instruments were also reported. No major nerve and vessel injuries were encountered but were mentioned as a potential problem. Extra-articular arthroscopy caused a few cases of excessive fluid extravasation, with some cases requiring a paracentesis for fluid removal and one case requiring an exploratory laparotomy. Rodeo et al. (63) reported similar complications and also identified direct injury to cutaneous nerves such as the lateral femoral cutaneous as well as injuries to the foot, scrotum, or perineum from inadequate padding of the traction apparatus. New traction apparatuses will eliminate the need for the standard fracture table for traction **(Fig 27-14)**.

■ CONCLUSION

The indications for arthroscopic management of intra-articular lesions continue to expand and hip arthroscopy is gradually replacing the open approach as the preferred treatment modality. Until the last decade, the hip was thought to be arthroscopically inaccessible because of anatomical and technical constraints. As our experience with hip arthroscopy advances, our ability to diagnose and treat these lesions successfully with a minimally invasive procedure greatly benefits patients. Many patients are young, and avoiding an open approach with the complications associated with dislocation, certainly helps decrease morbidity. With the recent improvement in hip arthroscopy, the majority of intra-articular procedures can be performed safely, effectively and in an outpatient setting.

Selecting the correct patient for an operative procedure and understanding the limitations of the currently available imaging studies is important for providing the patient with an appropriate diagnosis and treatment plan. Imaging, even MR arthrography, has less success in identifying the correct pathology or lack there-of, than MR arthrography of the knee or shoulder. Patients with underlying chronic conditions, such as osteonecrosis or connective tissue disorders may benefit from a diagnostic and therapeutic arthroscopy when mechanical symptoms are present. Labral pathology is the most common pathology treated arthroscopically. Most lesions are degenerative and require debridement and assessment of the chondral surfaces. Labral repairs should be attempted for acute peripheral lesions. The entity of hip impingement should alert the clinician to routinely look for altered femoral neck morphology on radiographs. Early treatment of this abnormality may provide great benefits to patients. The future of hip arthroscopy for intra-articular lesion is bright and the future will likely see the advancement of challenging procedures such as labral repairs, capsular plications and impingement, as well as outcome studies for these procedures.

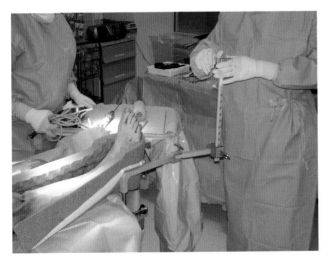

Fig 27-14. A sterile leg traction apparatus allows the surgeon to manipulate the leg during the procedure.

■ REFERENCES

1. DeAngelis NA, Busconi BD. Assessment and differential diagnosis of the painful hip. *Clin Orthop.* 2003;406(1):11–18.
2. Burman M. Arthroscopy or the direct visualization of joints. *J Bone Joint Surg.* 1931;4:669–695.
3. McCarthy JC, Busconi B. The role of hip arthroscopy in the diagnosis and treatment of hip disease. *Orthopedics.* 1995;18: 753–756.
4. Keene GS, Villar RN. Arthroscopic anatomy of the hip: an in vivo study. *Arthroscopy.* 1994;10:392–399.
5. Potter HG, Linklater JM, Allen AA, et al. Magnetic resonance imaging of articular cartilage of the knee. An evaluation with use of fast-spin-echo imaging. *J Bone Joint Surg.* 1998;80A:1276–1288.
6. Yamamoto Y, Ide T, Ono T, et al. Usefulness of arthroscopic surgery in hip trauma cases. *Arthroscopy.* 2003;19(3):269–273.
7. Upadhyay SS, Moulton A, Srikrishnamurthy K. An analysis of the late effects of traumatic posterior dislocation of the hip without fracture. *J Bone Joint Surg Br.* 1983;65:150–152.
8. Ferguson SJ, Bryant JT, Ganz R, et al. An in vitro investigation of the acetabular labral seal in hip joint mechanics. *J Biomech.* 2003;36:171–178.
9. Kim YT, Azuma H. The nerve endings of the acetabular labrum. *Clin Orthop.* 1995;320:176–181.
10. Altenberg AR. Acetabular labrum tears: a cause of hip pain and degenerative arthritis. *South Med J.* 1977;70:174–175.

11. Mason JB. Acetabular labral tears in the athlete. *Clin Sports Med.* 2001;20:779–790.
12. Dorfmann H, Boyer T. Arthroscopy of the hip: 12 years of experience. *Arthroscopy.* 1999;15:67–72.
13. Lage LA, Patel JV, Villar RN. The acetabular labral tear: an arthroscopic classification. *Arthroscopy.* 1996;12:269–272.
14. McCarthy J, Noble P, Aluisio FV, et al. Anatomy, pathologic features, and treatment of acetabular labral tears. *Clin Orthop.* 2003; 406:38–47.
15. Czerny C, Hofmann S, Urban M, et al. MR arthrography of the adult acetabular capsular-labral complex: Correlation with surgery and anatomy. *AJR Am J Roent.* 1999;173:345–349.
16. Byrd JWT, Jones KS. Traumatic rupture of the ligamentum teres as a source of hip pain. *Arthroscopy.* 2004;20(4):385–391.
17. Farjo LA, Glick JM, Sampson TG. Hip arthroscopy for acetabular labral tears. *Arthroscopy.* 1999;15(2):132–137.
18. Fitzgerald RH Jr. Acetabular labrum tears. Diagnosis and treatment. *Clin Orthop.* 1995;311:60–68.
19. Petersen W, Petersen F, Tillman B. Structure and vascularization of the acetabular labrum with regard to the pathogenesis and healing of labral lesions. *Arch Orthop Trauma Surg.* 2003;123(6): 282–288.
20. Kelly BT, Williams RJ, Philippon MJ. Hip arthroscopy: current indications, treatment options, and management issues. *Am J Sports Med.* 2003;31(6):1020–1037.
21. McCarthy JC, Noble PC, Schuck MR, et al. The role of labral lesions to development of early hip disease. *Clin Orthop.* 2001; 393:25–37.
22. Ganz R, Parvizi J, Beck M, et al. Femoroacetabular impingement: a cause for early osteoarthritis of the hip. *Clin Orthop.* 2003;417: 112–120.
23. Ito K, Minka M, Leunig, et al. Femoroacetabular impingement and the cam-effect. *J Bone Joint Surg.* 2001;83B(2):171–176.
24. Beck M, Leunig M, Parvizi J, et al. Anterior femoroacetabular impingement: Part II: midterm results of surgical treatment. *Clin Orthop.* 2004;418:67–73.
25. Goodman DA, Feighan JE, Smith A, et al. Subclinical slipped capital femoral epiphysis. *J Bone Joint Surg.* 1997;79A:1489–1497.
26. Morgan JD, Sommerville EW. Normal and abnormal growth at the upper end of the femur. *J Bone Joint Surg.* 1960;42B:810–824.
27. Siebenrock KA, Wahab KHA, Werlen S, et al. Abnormal extension of the femoral head epiphysis as a cause of cam impingement. *Clin Orthop.* 2004;418:54–60.
28. Lavigne M, Parvizi J, Beck M, et al. Anterior femoroacetabular impingement: Part I: technique of joint preserving surgery. *Clin Orthop.* 2004;413:61–66.
29. Klaue K, Durnin C, Ganz R. The acetabular rim syndrome. *J Bone Joint Surg.* 1991;73B(3):423–429.
30. Leunig M, Werlen S, Ungersbock A, et al. Evaluation of the acetabular labrum by MR arthrography. *J Bone Joint Surg.* 1997; 79B:230–234.
31. Gray AJR, Villar RN. The ligamentum teres of the hip: an arthroscopic classification of its pathology. *Arthroscopy.* 1997;13: 575–578.
32. Byrd JWT, Jones KS. Traumatic rupture of the ligamentum teres as a source of hip pain. *Arthroscopy.* 2004;20(4):385–391.
33. McCarthy J, Barsoum W, Puri L, et al. The role of hip arthroscopy in the elite athlete. *Clin Orthop.* 2003;406:71–74.
34. Etienne G, Mont MA, Ragland PS. The diagnosis and treatment of Nontraumatic Osteonecrosis of the Femoral Head. *Ins Course Lectures.* 2004;53:67–85.
35. Mont MA, Rajadhyaksha AD, Hungerford DS. Outcomes of limited femoral resurfacing arthroplasty compared with total hip arthroplasty for osteonecrosis of the femoral head. *Clin Orthop.* 2001;386:85–92.
36. O'Leary JA, Berend K, Vail TP. The relationship between diagnosis and outcome in arthroscopy of the hip. *Arthroscopy.* 2001; 17(2):181–188.
37. Linden B, Jonsson K, Redlund-Johnell I. Osteochondritis dissecans of the hip. *Acta Radiol.* 2003 Jan;44(1):67–71.
38. Rowe SM, Yoon TR, Jung ST, et al. Free osteochondral fragment caught in the acetabular fossa in the osteochondritis dissecans after Legg-Calve-Perthes'—disease-report of 2 cases. *Acta Orthop Scand.* 2003;74(1):107–10.
39. Philippon MJ. The role of arthroscopic thermal capsulorrhaphy in the hip. *Clin Sports Med.* 2001;20:817–819.
40. Bellabarba C, Sheinkop MB, Kuo KN. Idiopathic hip instability. An unrecognized cause of coax Saltans in the adult. *Clin Orthop.* 1998;355:261–271.
41. Liebenberg F, Dommisse GF. Recurrent post-traumatic dislocation of the hip. *J Bone Joint Surg.* 1969;51B:632–637.
42. Dorchak JD, Barrack RL, Kneisl JS, et al. Arthroscopic treatment of symptomatic synovial plica of the knee: Long-term follow-up. *Am J Sports Med.* 1991;19:503–507.
43. Dupont JY. Synovial plicae of the knee: Controversies and review. *Clin Sports Med.* 1997;16:87–122.
44. Johnson DP, Eastwood DM, Witherow PJ. Symptomatic synovial plicae of the knee. *J Bone Joint Surg.* 1993;75A:1485–1496.
45. Atlihan D, Jones DC, Guanche CA. Arthroscopic treatment of a symptomatic hip plica. *Clin Orthop.* 2003;411:174–177.
46. Frich LH, Lauritzen J, Juhl M. Arthroscopy in diagnosis and treatment of hip disorders. *Orthopedics.* 1989;12:389–392.
47. Hélénon CH, Bergevin H, Aubert JD, et al. Plication of hip synovia at upper border femoral neck. *J Radiol.* 1996;67:737–740.
48. Fu Z, Peng M, Peng Q. Anatomical study of the synovial plicae of the hip joint. *Clin Anat.* 1997;10:235–238.
49. Santori N, Villar RN. Arthroscopic findings in the initial stages of hip osteoarthritis. *Orthopedics.* 1999;22:405–409.
50. Maurice H, Crone M, Watt I. Synovial chondromatosis. *J Bone Joint Surg.* 1988;70B:807–811.
51. Wilson WJ, Parr TJ. Synovial chondromatosis. *Orthopedics.* 1988; 11:1179–1183.
52. Shpitzer T, Ganel A, Engelberg S. Surgery for synovial chondromatosis: 26 cases followed up for 6 years. *Acta Orthop Scand.* 1990; 61:567–569.
53. Murphy F, Dahlin D, Sullivan C. Articular synovial chondromatosis. *J Bone Joint Surg.* 1962;44A:77–86.
54. Okada Y, Awaya G, Ikeda T, et al. Arthroscopic surgery for synovial chondromatosis of the hip. *J Bone Joint Surg.* 1989;71B:198–199.
55. Ogilvie-Harris DJ, Weisleder L. Arthroscopic synovectomy of the knee: Is it helpful? *Arthroscopy.* 1995;11:91–95.
56. Ochi T, Iwase R, Kimura T, et al. Effect of early synovectomy on the course of rheumatoid arthritis. *J Rheumatol.* 1991;18: 1794–1798.
57. Holgersson S, Brattstrom H, Mogensen B, et al. Arthroscopy of the hip in juvenile chronic arthritis. *J Pediatr Orthop.* 1981;1:273–278.
58. Menkes CJ, Simon F, Delrieu F, et al. Destructive arthropathy in chondrocalcinosis articularis. *Arthritis Rheum.* 1976;19(3):329–348.
59. Menkes CJ, Decraemere W, Postel M, et al. Chondrocalcinosis and rapid destruction of the hip. *J Rheumatol.* 1985;12:130–133.
60. Goldman AB, DiCarlo EF. Pigmented villonodular synovitis: diagnosis and differential diagnosis. *Radiol Clin North Am.* 1988; 26:1327–1347.
61. Cotton A, Flipo RM, Chastanet P, et al. Pigmented villonodular synovitis of the hip: Review of radiographic features in 58 patients. *Skeletal Radiol.* 1995;24:1–6.
62. Sampson TG. Complications of hip arthroscopy. *Clin Sports Med.* 2001;20:831–835.
63. Rodeo SA, Forster RA, Weiland AJ. Neurological complications due to arthroscopy. *J Bone Joint Surg.* 1993;75A:917–926.

■ SUGGESTED READING

1. Byrd JWT. Indications and contraindications. In: Byrd JWT, ed. *Operative hip arthroscopy.* New York: Thieme; 1998:69–82.

2. Byrd JWT. Complications associated with hip arthroscopy. In: Byrd JWT, ed. *Operative hip arthroscopy*. New York: Thieme; 1998:171–176.

3. Byrd JWT. Hip arthroscopy in athletes. *Instructional Course Lectures*. 2003;52:701–709.

4. Byrd JWT. Hip arthroscopy: patient assessment and indications. *Instructional Course Lectures*. 2003;52:411–719.

5. McCarthy JC. Hip Arthroscopy: When it is and when it is not indicated. *Instructional Course Lectures*. 2004;53:615–621.

6. Monllau JC, Solano A, Leon A, et al. Tomographic study of the arthroscopic approaches to the hip joint. *Arthroscopy*. 2003;19(4): 368–372.

7. Sampson TG, Glick JM. Indications and surgical treatment of hip pathology. In: McGinty J, Caspari R, Jackson R, et al., eds. *Operative arthroscopy*. 2nd ed. New York: Raven Press; 1995: 1067–1078.

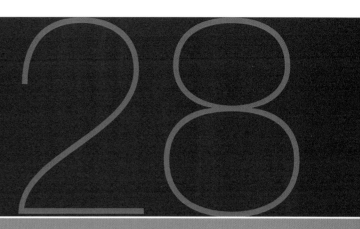

HIP MORPHOLOGY AND RELATED PATHOLOGY

■ J.W. THOMAS BYRD, MD

■ KEY POINTS

- Development dysplasia of the hip (DDH) is a morphological condition that makes the hip vulnerable to an intra-articular lesion that may then cause pain.
- Dysplasia is an etiologic factor in the development of various painful intra-articular lesions, which may be amenable to arthroscopic intervention.
- Patients must be assessed for the presence of dysplastic disease of the hip. Whereas arthroscopic debridement may result in significant symptomatic improvement, it may not seriously influence the long-term outlook.
- Radiographic evidence of dysplasia is not a contraindication to arthroscopy or necessarily an indicator of poor outcome. Results are more dictated by pathology.
- Femoroacetabular impingement (FAI) occurs in the native hip and is believed to be a precursor to the development of osteoarthritis. It has been grouped into pincer type and cam type. Pincer type is attributed to a bony lip of the anterior acetabulum. Cam type is associated with bony abnormalities of the anterior and lateral femoral head/neck junction.

In the past sports-related injuries of the hip joint have gone mostly unrecognized and untreated. Arthroscopy has been instrumental in identifying the nature and extent of numerous intra-articular lesions. In a study of athletes undergoing arthroscopy, in 60% of the cases, the hip was not recognized as the source of symptoms at the time of initial treatment and were managed for an average of 7 months, before the hip was considered as a potential contributing source. Most commonly, these were erroneously diagnosed as a musculotendinous strain.

The arthroscopic anatomy has been defined including normally occurring anatomic variations. Numerous pathological lesions have been identified with efforts at both grading and staging the pathology. Armed with a preliminary understanding of this intra-articular pathology, efforts have focused on interpreting the causative pathomechanics. An appreciation for these pathomechanics is essential to reliably altering the natural history of these processes and perhaps advocating early intervention as a preventative measure.

The correlation of hip morphology and hip disease is not a recent concept. Congenital dislocation of the hip (CDH) more recently referenced as dysplastic disease of the hip (DDH), left untreated, and has long been known to result in early joint deterioration and disability. Femoroacetabular impingement (FAI) is a more recent concept felt to be a causative factor in many cases of osteoarthritis. Osteoarthritis is not so much a specific diagnosis, but simply a common final pathway for a variety of conditions culminating in the osteoarthritic process. In general, dysplasia and impingement are considered to exist on two ends of a spectrum: dysplasia associated with a shallow acetabulum and instability, and impingement associated with over coverage of the acetabulum or insufficient clearance for the proximal femur. However, it is also recognized that in some cases dysplasia and impingement may coexist in the same joint.

■ DYSPLASIA

Developmental DDH is not a cause of hip pain. It is simply a morphological condition that makes the hip vulnerable to an intra-articular lesion that may then become symptomatic.

The three most likely structures to be involved include the acetabular labrum, articular surface, and ligamentum teres.

Accompanying a shallow bony acetabulum, the labrum may be enlarged assuming a more important role as a weight-bearing surface as well as added responsibility for joint stability. This hypertrophic labrum is thus exposed to greater joint reaction forces and may be at increased risk for developing symptomatic tearing (1–3). Inversion of the acetabular labrum is also known to occur in association with dysplasia, being entrapped within the joint and again being a source of painful tearing (4–5).

The reduced area of the acetabular articular surface results in increased contact forces (6–7). This can result in early development of degenerative wear and may make the articular cartilage more vulnerable to acute fragmentation (8–11).

Lastly, elongation or hypertrophy of the ligamentum teres accompanies lateral subluxation of the femoral head within the acetabulum (12–13). Entrapment of this ligament can be a source of significant mechanical hip pain, whether from its redundant nature or partial degenerate rupture.

Thus, dysplasia is well recognized as an etiologic factor in the development of various painful intra-articular lesions, which may be amenable to arthroscopic intervention. In fact, in a study by this author, which is the only published report on outcomes of arthroscopy in a dysplastic population, the results were comparable to those previously published in a general population (14). However, there are several caveats, which need to be fully appreciated.

It is important to assess patients carefully for the presence of dysplastic disease of the hip. While arthroscopic debridement may result in significant symptomatic improvement, it may not seriously influence the long-term outlook. Especially for young individuals, arthroscopy should not be used solely for symptomatic improvement when long-term issues need to be addressed. Specifically, patients who are candidates for osteotomy to improve the joint mechanics and weight distribution must be carefully assessed.

As noted, the enlarged labrum accompanying a shallow acetabulum may carry greater weight-bearing responsibility as well as provide a buttress to superolateral subluxation of the femoral head. It is unlikely that simple debridement of the deteriorated portion of the labrum will accentuate this subluxation potential, but great care must be taken in the debridement procedure, especially avoiding an overly zealous resection.

Similarly, indiscriminate debridement of the ligamentum teres should be avoided. The vessel of the ligamentum teres remains patent and contributes to the blood supply of the femoral head in a significant percentage of adults. Arbitrary debridement could unnecessarily place the femoral head at risk for avascular necrosis. However, it seems unlikely that debridement of the ruptured portion should present a problem, and has produced very gratifying symptomatic results.

In summary, radiographic evidence of dysplasia is not a contraindication to arthroscopy, nor is it necessarily an indicator of poor outcome. Results are more dictated by the nature of the pathology. Nonetheless, it is prudent to view arthroscopy as but one tool in the complement of resources necessary in the assessment and management of patients with developmental DDH.

Case Examples

Case 1

A 14 year old female was referred with a 4 month history of painful locking and catching of her right hip. This first occurred while simply raising her leg to step over a railing. Her symptoms had since been unremitting. Her history was remarkable for dysplastic disease of both hips since birth. These were initially treated with closed reduction, but she had subsequently undergone multiple osteotomies of the proximal femur and pelvis. Most recently, she was being evaluated for an acetabular procedure to improve the coverage of her femoral head, when she developed incapacitating mechanical right hip symptoms. Radiographs revealed changes consistent with her underlying disease and previous surgical procedures as well as slight lateral joint space loss on the right compared to the left **(Fig 28-1A)**.

Based on her symptoms and exam findings, arthroscopy was recommended as a method to assess the extent of intra-articular damage that may be contributing to her symptoms and to see if this could be addressed. She was found to have an unstable inverted labrum **(Fig 28-1B)**. This was debrided in a cautious fashion **(Fig 28-1C)**. Care was taken to excise the entrapped portion contributing to her symptoms, while preserving as much of the remaining labrum as possible, to avoid potentially destabilizing the joint. Additionally, there was grade IV articular loss of the acetabulum. The unstable fragments were debrided, creating a stable edge of surrounding cartilage **(Fig 28-1D)**. Microfracture of the lesion was performed to stimulate a fibrocartilaginous healing response **(Fig 28-1E)**. Occluding the inflow, confirmed vascular access through the perforations **(Fig 28-1F)**. Postoperatively, she was maintained on a strict protected weight-bearing status for 2 months emphasizing range of motion. She was then able to resume normal light daily activities with resolution of her mechanical hip pain.

Case 2

A 16 year old male presented with a 9 month history of pain and locking of his left hip. This first occurred while playing football as a freshman in high school. He had received no previous specific treatment, but was known to have a developmental abnormality of his hip since early childhood. Radiographs revealed evidence of a separate bone fragment within the femoral head **(Fig 28-2A)**, which was further substantiated by a computed tomography (CT) scan **(Fig 28-2B)**.

With his mechanical symptoms and imaging evidence of a loose fragment, arthroscopy was recommended. The fragment was actually found to be fixed within the femoral head, but there was a grade IV unstable articular fragment over this area, which was debrided **(Fig 28-2C,D and E)**. Postoperatively, he had resolution of his mechanical pain and catching.

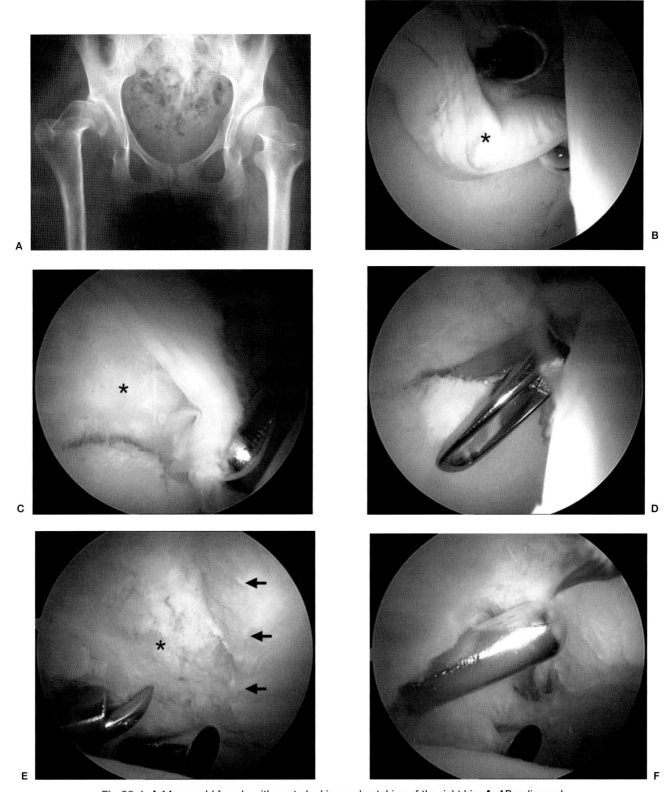

Fig 28-1. A 14 year old female with acute locking and catching of the right hip. **A:** AP radiograph demonstrates evidence of residual DDH of both hips and changes consistent with multiple previous osteotomies. There is slight lateral joint space narrowing of the right hip compared to the left. **B:** Arthroscopic view from the anterolateral portal demonstrates an unstable entrapped anterior labrum (*asterisk*). **C:** Debridement of the unstable portion of the labrum is begun, revealing extensive exposed subchondral bone (*asterisk*) with full thickness articular loss. **D:** Debridement of unstable articular fragments is performed with a basket. **E:** Now viewing from the anterior portal, a stable articular edge has been achieved (*arrows*) and microfracture is begun through the subchondral surface (*asterisk*) that still has a thin covering of fibrous tissue. **F:** With suction through the shaver, bleeding confirms vascular access through the areas of perforation.

493

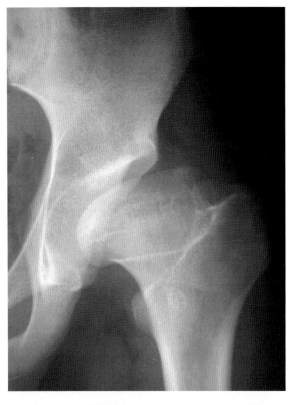

A

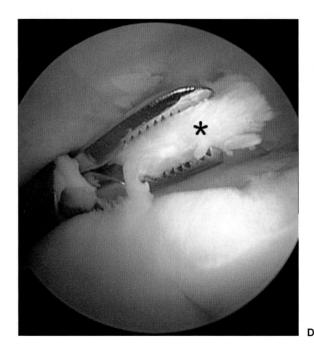

D

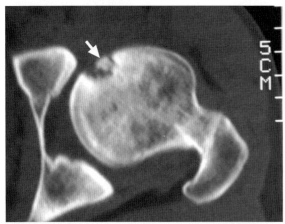

B

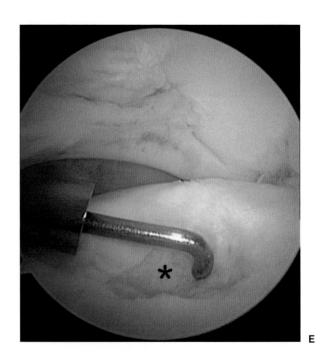

E

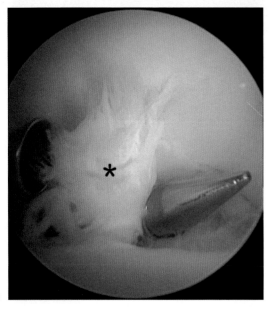

C

Fig 28-2. A 16 year old male with pain and locking of the left hip from playing football. **A:** AP radiograph demonstrates congenital deformity of the joint with a 10 degree CE angle. **B:** CT scan demonstrates evidence of a bone fragment within the femoral head (*arrow*). **C:** Arthroscopic view from the posterolateral portal demonstrates an unstable full-thickness articular flap (*asterisk*). **D:** Now viewing from the anterolateral portal, the fragment (*asterisk*) is excised. **E:** A stable edge is created around the crater (*asterisk*) with no loose bone fragment.

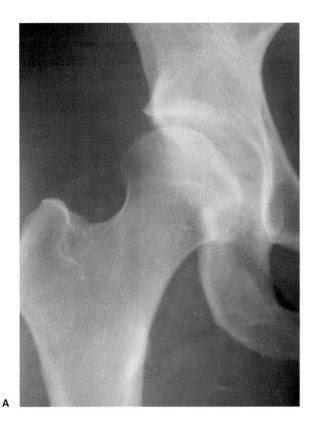

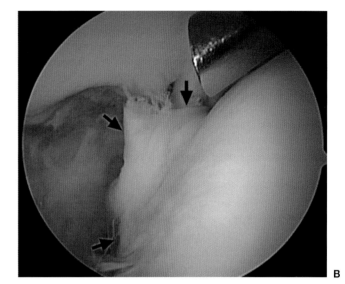

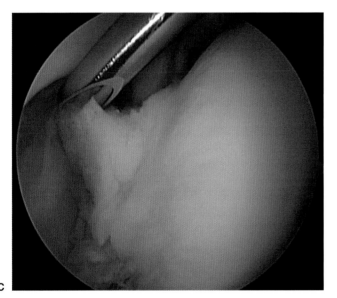

Fig 28-3. A 37 year old female with recalcitrant right hip pain. A: AP radiograph demonstrates moderate dysplasia with an 18 degree CE angle. B: Arthroscopy reveals a hypertrophic ligamentum teres (*arrows*). C: The degenerated hypertrophic portion of the ligament is debrided.

Case 3

A 37 year old female presented with a 4 year history of progressively worsening right hip pain. There was no history of injury or precipitating event, she simply began experiencing discomfort that had worsened over recent months. Twisting maneuvers were especially painful. Her examination findings suggested that her hip joint was the source of her pain. Radiographs revealed evidence of modest underlying dysplasia, but were otherwise unremarkable (Fig 28-3A). An

MRI was also unremarkable. She then underwent 6 months of continued activity restriction as well as various trials of oral anti-inflammatory medications, and physical therapy without improvement. She obtained pronounced temporary alleviation of her symptoms from a fluoroscopically guided intra-articular injection of anesthetic.

Based on her clinical circumstances, arthroscopy was offered as the next step in her management. She was found to have a hypertrophic ligamentum teres with an accompanying degenerate rupture, which was debrided **(Fig 28-3B,C)**. Postoperatively she demonstrated pronounced symptomatic improvement and was able to resume fitness exercises.

■ FEMOROACETABULAR IMPINGEMENT

Impingement of the hip is not an entirely new concept. Open chilectomy of the femoral head has long been proposed as a salvage procedure for painful restricted motion associated with the late sequela of childhood disorders including Legg-Calve-Perthes disease and slipped capital femoral epiphysis (15,16).

The concept of FAI has been proposed by Ganz and numerous co-authors from the Berne group (17–20). This was first recognized as an iatrogenic process associated with overcorrection of periacetabular osteotomy (PAO) performed for dysplasia (17). Since then, FAI has been recognized to occur in the native hip and is felt to be a precursor to the subsequent development of osteoarthritis (18). It has also been subgrouped into a pincer type and a cam type. The impingement test has been described where pain is elicited by forced flexion combined with adduction and internal rotation of the hip (18). However, we have found this examination maneuver to be nonspecific and painful in association with a variety of joint pathology (21).

Pincer impingement is attributed to a bony lip of the anterior acetabulum. With flexion of the hip, the labrum becomes entrapped between the acetabular lip and the anterior neck of the femur. The principal lesion is labral deterioration with some secondary articular breakdown. Assessment of pincer impingement necessitates a properly centered AP radiograph of the pelvis, including both hips. A poorly centered film will result in either over- or underestimating the amount of impingement. The cross-over sign is indicative of overcoverage of the anterior acetabulum, while the posterior wall sign reflects the presence of acetabular retroversion.

Pincer impingement may be due to simple bony build-up of the anterior acetabular rim, or associated with more complex acetabular retroversion. Rarely, the retroversion is severe enough to warrant correction with PAO. Technically, this is more challenging than PAO for dysplasia because of the risk of destabilizing the joint. More commonly, the anterior acetabulum is simply recontoured ("acetabuloplasty") to eliminate the impingement.

Acetabuloplasty has traditionally been performed via a surgical dislocation of the hip, as described by Beck et al (20). Our experience has been that this acetabular impingement can be readily addressed with arthroscopic methods and this has been substantiated by other reports as well (22–24). There are three arthroscopic hallmarks of this process. First, is the presence of anterior and anterolateral labral pathology. It is the labral tearing that causes symptoms, presenting the patient for treatment. Second, there is more difficulty establishing the anterior portal than would be expected, even with adequate joint distraction.

The impinging lip may hinder access, making this technically more challenging. Third, as the damaged labrum is debrided, it becomes evident that there is a lip of bone overhanging this portion of the labrum. Normally, there should be only the capsulolabral reflection peripheral to the labrum.

It is a relatively simple process to excise the impinging bone. As the damaged labrum is removed, this exposes the impinging lip, which is then excised with a burr. Technically, this is analogous to taking down a distal tibial spur impinging on the anterior aspect of the ankle joint.

Cam impingement is associated with bony abnormalities of the anterior and lateral femoral head/neck junction. Bony prominence in this area results in a nonspherical femoral head. A cam effect occurs with flexion, as this nonspherical head is forced into the acetabulum. The resultant pathology is selective articular breakdown with lesser degrees of associated labral tearing. The articular surface is essentially peeled away from its articulolabral junction by this bony prominence as it pushes up inside the joint.

Cam impingement is most clearly associated with childhood disorders including slipped capital femoral epiphysis and Perthes disease. Both of these are conditions that leave the hip with an abnormal bony prominence of the anterior and lateral femoral head/neck junction. The "pistol-grip deformity" is another developmental condition that can lead to cam impingement. Less clear are bony "bumps" which are acquired in adulthood and are often described as impingement lesions. It is often uncertain whether these bumps are a cause, or a consequence, of osteoarthritis. Pincer impingement and cam impingement can occur separately or together. When one sees acquired bony buildup on the femoral head, look closely for acetabular impingement that may secondarily precipitate the "kissing lesion" to occur on the femoral side.

Cam impingement is easier to diagnose with AP and lateral radiographs of the proximal femur. However, these radiographic abnormalities are often observed in patients with no hip symptoms, and in these cases the significance of the findings is less certain. It is postulated that FAI is a cause of secondary osteoarthritis. Successful results have been reported in the surgical management of this condition. It seems reasonable that addressing these lesions may improve the long-term outlook, but there is no data to state that this truly alters the natural course of this process. Nonetheless, it seems prudent that, in the presence of persistent symptoms, and earlier intervention may be preferable to letting the process go unchecked for an indefinite period of time.

CT, with 3D reconstructions, can be especially helpful for mapping the bony morphology in preparation for surgery. Cam impingement is often more extensive than suggested by 2D radiography. An overhanging acetabular lip may also be better discerned. This assists the surgeon in planning the extent of bony resection and recontouring to be done.

Recontouring of the proximal femur is most thoroughly accomplished with open surgical dislocation of the hip. Visualization is excellent for assessing the bony lesion and intraoperative freedom of motion assures the adequacy of the chondro osteoplasty. Arthroscopy has the advantage of significantly less morbidity, but is technically demanding. Cam impingement is assessed and addressed from the peripheral compartment. Visualizing the entirety of the lesion to be resected is more difficult and necessitates careful arthroscopic mapping of its dimensions prior to beginning resection. This lessens the risk of either inadequate or excessive resection. Intraoperative freedom of motion is also more restricted with arthroscopy, again challenging the surgeon to assure the completeness of the procedure. The low morbidity associated with the arthroscopic technique seems to outweigh the technical challenges imposed, but should only be undertaken by surgeons after having gained considerable experience in hip arthroscopy for less complex pathology.

Case Examples

Case 4

A 20 year old male military recruit was referred with a one year history of mechanical right hip pain following an injury sustained while assisting another 300 pound recruit over a wall. An AP radiograph demonstrated evidence of pincer impingement with a positive cross over sign **(Fig 28-4A)**. An MRI showed pathology of the anterior labrum. Arthroscopy

revealed the tear with anterior acetabular impingement **(Fig 28-4B,C)**. The damaged portion of the labrum was resected, exposing the impinging bone, which was excised **(Fig 28-4D,E and F)**. The post operative radiograph illustrates correction of the cross-over sign **(Fig 28-4G)**.

Case 5

A 20 year old male hockey player was referred with a 4 year history of worsening right hip pain. Radiographs demonstrated evidence of cam impingement **(Fig 28-5A and B)** and an MRI was unremarkable. The extent of the bony lesion was further defined by a 3D CT scan **(Fig 28-5C)**. Arthroscopy of the intra-articular compartment revealed articular damage indicative of cam impingement **(Fig 28-5D)**. The bony lesion was then identified and excised from the peripheral compartment **(Fig 28-5E and F)**. A post operative CT scan illustrates the extent of bony resection **(Fig 28-5G)**.

Case 6

A 38 year old female presented with a 3 year history of progressively worsening right hip pain and restricted motion. Radiographs revealed osteophyte formation around the femoral head reflecting cam impingement **(Fig 28-6A and B)**. A 3D CT scan further defined the cam lesion, but also

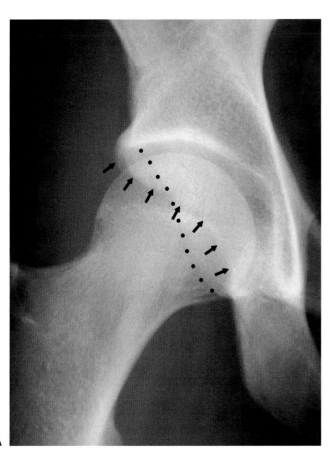

A

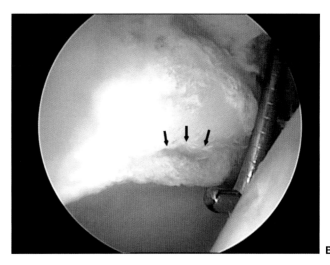

B

Fig 28–4. A 20 year old male with persistent hip pain following an acute injury. **A:** AP radiograph demonstrates a positive cross-over sign indicative of pincer impingement. Superiorly the anterior wall (*arrows*) lies lateral to the posterior wall (*dotted line*), reflecting anterior acetabular impingement. Inferiorly it lies medial to the posterior wall, creating the cross-over sign. **B:** Viewing from the anterolateral portal, tearing of the anterior labrum is identified (*arrows*). The probe is introduced from the anterior portal. **C:** Retracting the torn portion of the labrum exposes the overhanging bony impingement (*). **D:** The damaged labrum has been resected, exposing the impinging lesion (*). **E:** Acetabuloplasty is performed excising the bony impingement. **F:** The arthroscope has been switched to the anterior portal, completing the acetabuloplasty with the burr in the anterolateral portal. The healthy lateral labrum (*) demarcates the limit of the bony resection. **G:** Postoperative AP radiograph illustrates correction of the cross-over sign.

Fig 28-4. (*continued*)

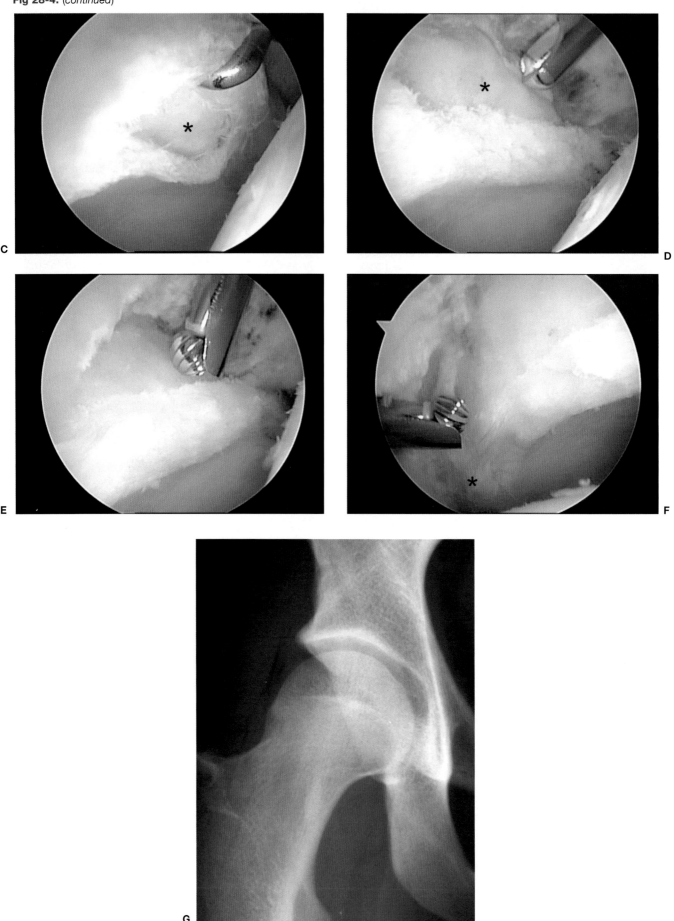

C

D

E

F

G

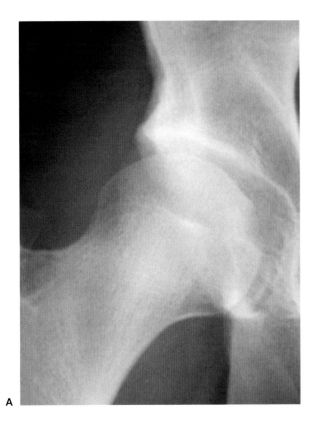
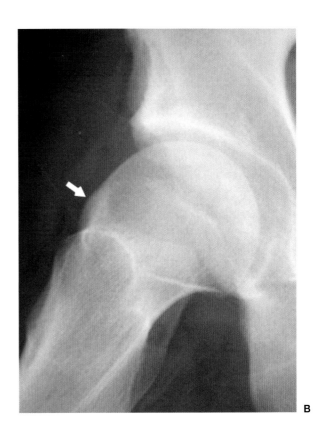

A

B

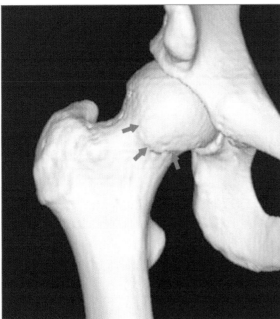
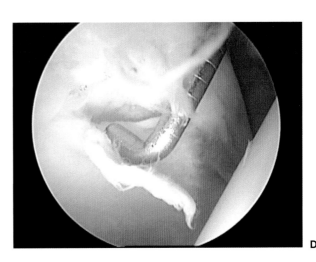

C

D

Fig 28-5. A 20 year old hockey player with a four year history of right hip pain. **A:** AP radiograph is unremarkable. **B:** Frog lateral radiograph demonstrates a morphological variant with bony build up at the anterior femoral head/neck junction (*arrow*) characteristic of cam impingement. **C:** A 3D CT scan further defines the extent of the bony lesion (*arrows*). **D:** Viewing from the anterolateral portal, the probe introduced anteriorly displaces an area of articular delamination from the anterolateral acetabulum characteristic of the peel back phenomenon created by the bony lesion shearing the articular surface during hip flexion. **E:** Viewing from the peripheral compartment the bony lesion is identified (***) immediately below the free edge of the acetabular labrum (*L*). **F:** The lesion has been excised, recreating the normal **concave** relationship of the femoral head/neck junction immediately adjacent to the articular surface (*arrows*). Posteriorly, resection is limited to the mid portion of the lateral neck to avoid compromising blood supply to the femoral head from the lateral retinacular vessels. **G:** Post operative 3D CT scan illustrates the extent of bony resection.

Fig 28-5. (*continued*)

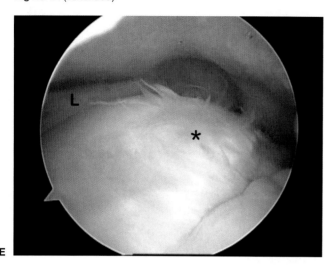

E

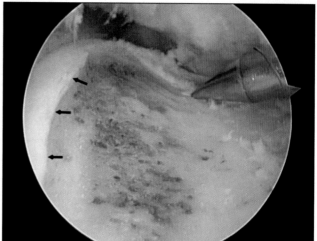

F

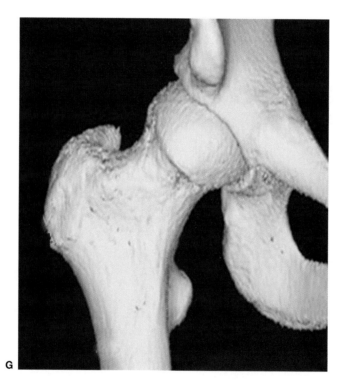

G

revealed pincer impingement as the primary cause resulting in secondary bony build up on the femoral head as a "kissing" lesion **(Fig 28-6C)**. At arthroscopy the central articular surfaces of the joint were still healthy **(Fig 28-6D)**.

The pincer **(Fig 28-6E)** and cam **(Fig 28-6F)** lesions were excised. A post operative CT scan illustrates the extent of resection at both the acetabulum and femoral head **(Fig 28-6G)**.

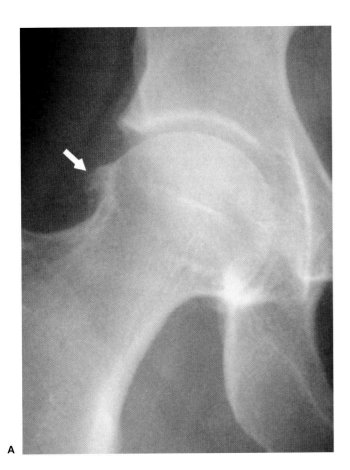

A

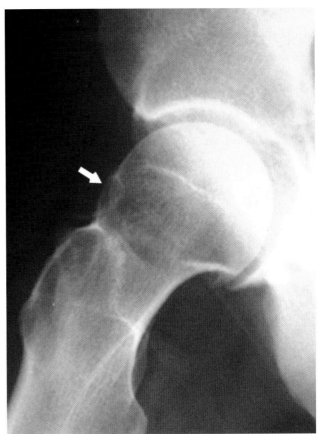

B

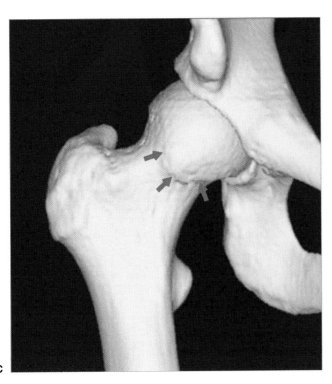

C

Fig 28-6. A 38 year old female with progressive pain and loss of motion of the right hip. **A:** AP radiograph demonstrates acquired bony build up/osteophyte formation on the lateral femoral head (*arrow*). **B:** A frog lateral radiograph further defines the bony build up on the anterior femoral head (*arrow*). **C:** A 3D CT scan further defines the femoral head osteophyte (*asterisk*) and the anterior acetabular lesion (*arrows*). **D:** Arthroscopy of the central weight bearing surface of the joint demonstrates good articular preservation of both the acetabulum (*A*) and femoral head (*FH*) with some reactive synovitis within the fossa (S). **E:** The anterior acetabular osteophyte is excised. **F:** Viewing peripherally, the femoral head has been recontoured showing the edge of the femoral articular surface (*white arrows*) and the labrum (*black arrows*). **G:** A post operative 3D CT scan demonstrates the extent of bony recontouring of both the acetabulum and femoral head.

Fig 28-6. (*continued*)

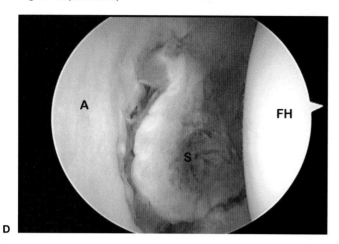

D

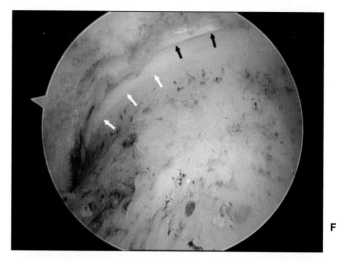

F

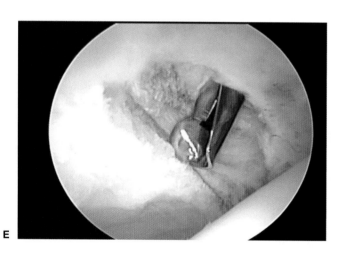

E

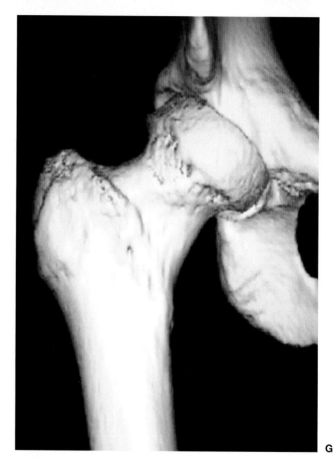

G

■ REFERENCES

1. Dorell JH, Catterall A. The torn acetabular labrum. *J Bone Joint Surg.* 1986;68B(3):400–403.
2. Klaue K, Durnin CW, Ganz R. The acetabular rim syndrome. *J Bone Joint Surg.* 1991;73B:423–429.
3. Nishina T, Saito S, Ohzono K, et al. Chiari pelvic osteotomy for osteoarthritis: the influence of the torn and detached acetabular labrum. *J Bone Joint Surg.* 1990;72B(5):765–769.
4. Byrd, JWT. Labral lesions: an elusive source of hip pain: case reports and review of the literature. *Arthroscopy.* 1996;12(5) 603–612.
5. Byrd JWT, Jones KS. Inverted acetabular labrum and secondary osteoarthritis: radiographic diagnosis and arthroscopic treatment. *Arthroscopy.* 2000;16(4):417.
6. Hadley NA, Brown TD, Weinstein SL. The effect of contact pressure elevations and aspetic necrosis on the long term outcome of congenital hip dislocation. *J Orthop Rev.* 1990;8(4):504–513.
7. Maxian TA, Brown TD, Weinstein SL. Chronic stress tolerance levels for human articular cartilage: two nonuniform contact models

applied to long term follow up of CDH. *J Biomech*. 1995;28:159–166.

8. Cooperman DR, Wallensten R, Stulberg SD. Acetabular dysplasia in the adult. *Clin Orthop*. 1983;175:79–85.

9. Malvitz TA, Weinstein SL. Closed reduction for congenital dysplasia of the hip. Functional and radiographic results after an average of thirty years. *J Bone Joint Surg*. 1994;76A:1777–1792.

10. Nishii T, Sugano N, Tanaka H, et al. Articular cartilage abnormalities in dysplastic hips without joint space narrowing. *Clin Orthop*. 2001;383:183–190.

11. Noguchi Y, Miura H, Takasugi S, et al. Cartilage and labrum degenerative in the dysplastic hip generally originates in the anterosuperior weight-bearing area: an arthroscopic observation. *Arthroscopy*. 1999;15:496–506.

12. Michaels G, Matles AL. The role of the ligamentum teres in congenital dislocation of the hip. *Clin Orthop*. 1970;71:199–201.

13. Ippolito E, Ishii Y, Ponseti IV. Histologic, histochemical, and ultrastructural studies of the hip joint capsule and ligamentum teres in congenital dislocation of the hip. *Clin Orthop*. 1980;146:246–258.

14. Byrd JWT, Jones KS. Hip arthroscopy in the presence of dysplasia, *Arthroscopy*. 2003;19(10):1055–1060.

15. Garceau, GJ. Surgical treatment of coxa plana. *J Bone Joint Surg*. 1964;46B:779.

16. Heyman, CH, Herndon CH, Strong JM. Slipped femoral epiphysis with severe displacement: a conservative operative treatment. *J Bone Joint Surg*. 1957;39A:293.

17. Myers SR, Eijer H, Ganz R. Anterior femoroacetabular impingement after periacetabular osteotomy. *Clin Orthop*. 1999;363: 93–99.

18. Ganz R, Parvizi J, Beck M, et al. Femoroacetabular impingement: a cause for osteoarthritis of the hip. *Clin Orthop*. 2003;417:112–120.

19. Lavigne M, Parvizi J, Beck M, et al. Anterior femoroacetabular impingement: part I. Techniques of joint preserving surgery. *Clin Orthop*. 2004;418:61–66.

20. Beck M, Leunig M, Parvizi J, et al. Anterior femoroacetabular impingement: part II. Midterm results of surgical treatment. *Clin Orthop*. 2004;418:67–73.

21. Byrd JWT. Physical examination. In: Byrd JWT, ed. *Operative hip arthroscopy*. 2nd ed. New York: Springer; 2005:36–50.

22. Byrd JWT. Hip arthroscopy: evolving frontiers: op tech in orthop. In: Beaule PE, Garbuz DS, eds. *Special Issue: Novel Techniques in Hip Surgery*. 2004;14(2):58–67.

23. Sampson TG. Arthroscopic treatment of femoroacetabular impingement. *Tech Orthop*. 2005;20(1):56–62.

24. Bare AA, Guanche CA. Hip impingement: the role of arthroscopy. *Orthopedics*. 2005;28(3):266–273.

EXTRA-ARTICULAR LESIONS

AARON A. BARE, MD, CARLOS A. GUANCHE, MD

■ KEY POINTS

- The anatomic and biomechanical considerations involved with these injuries include some of the more complex areas of the musculoskeletal system with a large overlap between the intra-abdominal contents and the pelvic musculature. The immature skeleton can add significant levels of complexity and broaden the differential diagnosis.

- The body's center of gravity is located within the pelvis, immediately anterior to the second sacral vertebra. Loads that are generated or transferred through this area are important in virtually every athletic endeavor.

- The incidence of groin pain accounts for only approximately 5% of patient injuries, but is responsible for a large proportion of time loss from competition.

- Athletic pubalgia may be the more appropriate term than sports hernia in many cases because an actual hernia is not seen.

- The physical examination for a possible sports hernia includes a thorough assessment of the pelvic musculature and plain radiographs to assure no significant bony pathology is present.

- The most common athletic injuries about the hip and groin are muscle strains. In an adolescent athlete, the same eccentric mechanism leading to a muscle strain may cause an apophyseal avulsion.

- There appears to be a predisposition for the development of stress fractures in females with rates as high as four to ten times that of males. Amenorrhea appears to be especially prevalent in endurance athletes with notable decreases in bone mineral density as compared to those menstruating normally. The important principle is that a menstrual and dietary history should always be included in the diagnosis and treatment of the female athlete with potential stress fracture.

- Avulsion fractures are most commonly seen in athletes between the ages of 14 and 17 years of age with males more commonly affected.

- Avulsion fractures often occur during athletic competition. The mechanism of injury is a powerful muscle contraction that takes place during sprinting, while playing soccer or football, or in sports that require jumping. The clinical presentation is usually localized swelling, tenderness, and limitation of motion of the hip, secondary to pain.

- Osteitis pubis is an unusual injury that occurs more commonly in long-distance runners. The mechanism of injury appears to be overtraining of the rectus abdominis and adductor muscles.

- Pudendal neuropathy can cause groin pain and numbness, often exacerbated in the seated position and relieved by standing or lying supine.

- Obturator nerve entrapment can cause groin pain in athletes. The cause of the nerve entrapment is uncertain. Repetitive kicking, side-to-side movements, and twisting are common motions which correlate with the problem.

- Referred pain from lower lumbar and sacral nerves frequently cause gluteal or posterior thigh symptoms. Facet joint and erector spinae muscle abnormalities may also refer pain.

- Groin and hip symptoms have a large overlap with many disciplines of medicine from the orthopaedic surgeon to the neurologist, the general surgeon, gynecologist, and endocrinologist. It is important to maintain this perspective and to seek appropriate consultations.

Orthopedic injuries about the hip and groin occur at a low frequency relative to injuries distal to the hip. Epidemiological studies have shown that injuries to the hip region comprise approximately 5% to 9% of the injuries in high school athletes (1). The incidence of hip pathology appears to be expanded as a result of an increased fund of knowledge in this area. This has occurred as a result of the improved imaging modalities as well as the implementation of hip arthroscopy.

The anatomic and biomechanical considerations involved with these injuries include some of the more complex areas of the musculoskeletal system with a very large overlap between the intra-abdominal contents and the pelvic musculature. This makes the management of these injuries very challenging. Also, the immature skeleton can add significant levels of complexity and broaden the differential diagnosis.

In addition to the complex anatomic considerations involved, the hip joint can see loads of up to eight times body weight, with even larger loads present during vigorous athletic competition (2). It appears that the structures about the hip are uniquely adapted to transfer such forces. The body center of gravity is located within the pelvis immediately anterior to the second sacral vertebra. This becomes increasingly important when one realizes that loads that are generated or transferred through this area are important in virtually every athletic endeavor (3).

Imaging modalities are now available that can help clinicians diagnose more accurately. They may provide indirect diagnostic and prognostic information. In addition, an important aspect of many hip and pelvic injuries is that of rehabilitation. The importance of trunk stability rehabilitation is being increasingly recognized and plays a part in many common injuries (4).

Finally, as a result of the large anatomic overlap between several disciplines, several different medical and surgical specialties may be involved in the treatment of a patient with many of these injuries.

This chapter will delineate many common hip injuries. These can be broken down into several components, namely soft tissue injuries, bony injuries, and nerve injuries. Many of the soft tissue injuries are particularly troublesome to the average sports medicine physician as the result of the large overlap with general surgical problems including those of hernias. In addition, there are several bursae around the pelvis and hip which can cause a significant amount of symptomatology and, in some cases, are misdiagnosed as a result of their unusual presentation.

Bony problems can be separated into a variety of injuries. Stress fractures can have a very insidious onset. Osteitis pubis is another poorly understood condition that can impact athletes and whose treatment is simple; however, the diagnosis is often not made until much later in the course. Neural injuries likewise are unusual in presentation. The most common injuries are meralgia paresthetica, obturator nerve entrapment, and sciatica.

■ SOFT TISSUE INJURIES

Sports Hernias

While the incidence of groin pain accounts for only approximately 5% of patient injuries, it is responsible for a very large proportion of time loss from competition (5,6). The sports hernia, also known as the hockey hernia, has become a more common injury in athletes participating in sports requiring repetitive twisting and turning such as ice hockey, tennis, field hockey, soccer, and American football. The incidence in several high level athletic groups has been documented to be significantly increased over the last decade (7). Although it is true that the increased frequency of this diagnosis may be partly attributable to the heightened awareness of trainers and physicians, there is also the notion that the increasingly rigorous off season conditioning programs that concentrate on strengthening the lower extremities, but neglect the abdominal and pelvic musculature cause a significant imbalance, and may contribute to this problem. In addition, various theories regarding contractures of the hip flexor and adductor muscles are developing as a result of this preferential strengthening of one muscle group over another. One study has attempted to document radiographically a lack of hip extension when pelvic tilt is controlled (8). In this study, 25 professional hockey players and 25 age-matched controls were evaluated using the Thomas test and an electrical circuit device to determine pelvic tilt motion. The results demonstrated that the players had a reduced maximum hip extension in comparison with age-matched controls. The authors theorized that hockey players demonstrated a decreased extensibility of the iliopsoas musculature.

In making the diagnosis of a sports hernia, the more appropriate term may be that of athletic pubalgia since in many cases an actual hernia is not seen (9). Although the definite pathophysiology behind the development of this problem has not been implicated in overuse syndrome, in most of the athletes involved, a series of hip abduction/adduction and flexion/extension maneuvers with the resultant pelvic motion may produce a shearing force across the pubic symphysis leading to stress in the inguinal wall musculature perpendicular to the fibers of the muscle. In these cases a chronic pull from the adductor musculature against a fixed lower extremity can cause significant shear forces across the hemipelvis with subsequent attenuation or tearing of the transversalis fascia or the conjoined tendon (10). In some studies there have also been changes noted at the rectus abdominis muscle insertion (9), while in some situations, avulsions of part of the internal oblique muscle fibers at the pubic tubercle have also been documented (11). One additional theory suggests that entrapment of the genital branches of the ilioinguinal or genital femoral nerves may be the source of pain in some patients (12).

In, summary, it is apparent that the variety of abnormalities that have been reported leading to the diagnosis of sports hernias are a clear indication for the need to further delineate this area through research. In order to understand the treatment, however, it is best to think of these problems as a relative incompetence of the abdominal wall musculature in the absence of a clinically detectable hernia bulge **(Fig 29-1).**

Although the diagnosis of a sports hernia is made in many patients retrospectively or after eliminating the more common injuries noted about the pelvis, it is important to know the common presenting symptoms. Often, there is an insidious onset of unilateral groin pain, although some present with bilateral symptoms. Many are evaluated for a common inguinal hernia that is not typically seen and are then further misdiagnosed. In some cases, an acute tearing sensation is felt by the patient, making a diagnosis somewhat more straightforward. In many cases pain usually occurs only during exercise. It does not typically become exacerbated with coughing or sneezing as is often seen in an inguinal hernia.

By definition, no clinically detectable hernia will be present during examination. The need for a thorough examination by an experienced examiner with an understanding of the anatomy cannot be over-emphasized. The physical examination includes a thorough assessment of the pelvic musculature and plain radiographs to assure no significant bony pathology is present. Tenderness is commonly seen over the conjoined tendon, pubic tubercle, and the mid inguinal region (13). In some cases, a tender internal inguinal ring is noted. While the diagnosis of an inguinal hernia is not typically missed as a result of the significant radiation into the groin, this needs to be assessed to assure that it is not a more common inguinal hernia. The most common clinical findings have been pain with resisted leg adduction in 88%, while only 22% had pubic tenderness (9). Commonly positive findings include pain with a resisted sit-up and pain reproduction with a valsalva maneuver.

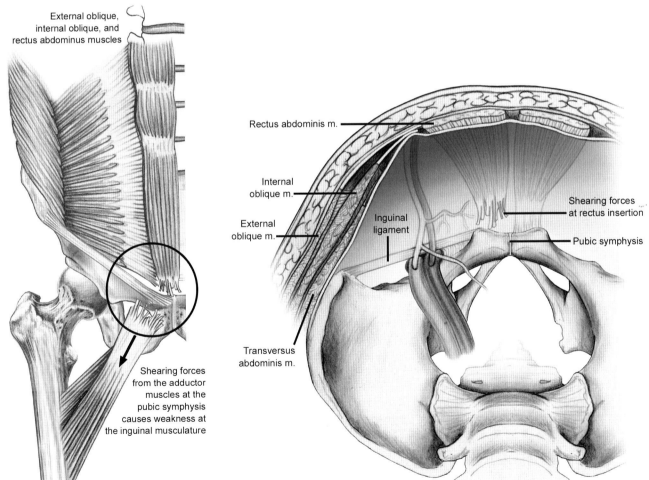

Fig 29-1. Diagrammatic representation of the typical pathology encountered in a sports hernia as compared to the more common inguinal hernias. **A:** Extra-abdominal view. **B:** Intra-abdominal view.

Imaging modalities are typically employed including plain radiographs in order to evaluate for the possibility of either a different or coexisting pathology. Most commonly, there is a significant overlap with osteitis pubis as well as chronic adductor musculature irritation. In addition, herniography may be used as a treatment to evaluate the area and has had some support in the recent literature (14,15). In a study by Hamlin and Kahn (14) 333 consecutive herniographic studies were performed (14). An equivocal physical examination was the most common reason for requesting a herniogram. In 56 of the 57 patients who came to operation, the herniogram and the physical examination were concordant.

In a study by Sutcliffe et al. (15) a prospective study of 112 patients undergoing herniorrhaphy were evaluated over a 5-year period. In this study 30 hernias were diagnosed with one false positive and one false-negative examination, thus giving herniography a sensitivity of 96.6% and a specificity of 98.4%. There were no complications noted with the herniographic procedures.

Magnetic resonance imaging (MRI) has also been employed in these difficult patients (16). In one study, the MRI findings of athletic pubalgia were delineated in 32 athletes studied with T1 weighted and T2 weighted as well as STIR images. The abnormalities found included pubic symphysis abnormalities, abdominal wall defects, and musculature abnormalities including rectus abdominis, pectineus, and adductor muscle groups. The authors felt that pubalgia, although a complex process and frequently multifactorial, could be delineated with MRI. More importantly it was felt that MRI could alter the surgical approach.

More invasive delineations of the hernias have been undertaken through endoscopic means. In these situations, the treatment is considered both diagnostic and curative in the same sitting. In one study, 18 patients were prospectively evaluated with undiagnosed chronic groin pain (17). Radiography, bone scintigraphy, and ultrasound were all performed pre-operatively without a definitive diagnosis. The patients underwent transabdominal or extraperitoneal diagnostic endoscopy. The pathology found by endoscopy included 9 inguinal hernias, 4 femoral hernias, a preperitoneal lipoma, and an obturator hernia. In 17 patients, a mesh was placed preperitoneally, with 93% of the patients returning to full activities within three months of surgery.

The treatment of sports hernias can be nonoperative, in some cases However, it should be noted that approximately 8 to 12 weeks of a concerted effort with respect to pelvic musculature strengthening is necessary (9). A well delineated conservative protocol has been developed, consisting of four phases over a 6 week period (18). In the first phase, massage and stretching are employed over the involved musculature with a focus on "trigger points." During weeks 3 and 4, a period of strengthening is instituted. In this period, areas of core strengthening are addressed as well as proprioceptive stabilization of the pelvis. The fifth week begins with a more functional return including rotational and lateral drills. The final phase returns the patient to sports-specific activities and a gradual return to competition.

The operative treatment of sports hernia has been documented both through endoscopic and open methods (5,11,19,20). The classic study by Gilmore (5) documented a pentad of surgical findings: a torn external oblique aponeurosis, a torn conjoined tendon, conjoined tendon torn from the pubic tubercle, dehiscence between the torn conjoined tendon and the inguinal ligament and the absence of a frank hernia. He described a six-layer closure of the inguinal floor. Based on his early description of the problem, the eponym of Gilmore's groin is often ascribed to this pathology.

Hackney (10) has reported that 15 patients (87%) returned to full sports activities with an open repair technique. Meyers et al. (9) reported a success rate of 97% in 157 patients undergoing an open rectus abdominis reattachment as well as recession of the adductor muscle in approximately 25%. In their series 44% of the patients had bilateral procedures. Based on this study, it is important to assess the area of the adductor musculature and to document any significant pain in that area. Should there be a fair amount of muscle pain noted on clinical examination pre-operatively, then adductor muscle release or recession combined with the herniorrhaphy may be required. It is important to note, however, that simple adductor tenotomy has shown poor results in patients with chronic groin pain (21).

Laparoscopic techniques have also been described. In one study, 15 professional athletes were treated for sports hernia by a single surgeon (22). Laparoscopic hernia repairs were performed using an extraperitoneal approach. Athletes presented with symptoms lasting several months to several years. Long-term follow-up was obtained by phone to assess overall patient satisfaction, efficacy of surgery, and effect on athletic performance. Nearly all (87%) of the athletes were able to return to full, unrestricted athletic activity in 4 weeks or less. Overall long-term satisfaction was high. Long-term follow-up revealed no adverse sequelae or recurrence of symptoms at a median of 46 months.

Muscle Strains

The most common injuries about the hip and groin resulting from athletic competition are muscle strains. Most commonly these occur in biarticular muscles undergoing an eccentric contraction. Most often the injury occurs at the myotendinous junction, but may also be seen in the muscle belly (23,24). In addition to the strain injuries, it is important to realize that in an adolescent athlete, the same eccentric mechanism leading to a muscle strain may cause an apophyseal avulsion (25).

The commonly injured muscles are the sartorius, rectus, iliopsoas, and adductor muscles. In the clinical examination, it is important to assess the pelvic musculature and to specifically check for the function of all of the above-mentioned muscles. With respect to adductor testing, it is important to resist adduction and to delineate whether the muscular origin or perhaps the muscle belly is tender. By the same token, forced hip flexion should assess for palpable pain or a muscle defect along the rectus muscle belly and toward its origin, as well as over the sartorius muscle belly and toward its origin at the anterosuperior iliac spine.

Rectus femoris muscle injuries commonly result in palpable swelling and tenderness along the anterior thigh approximately 10 cm below the anterosuperior iliac spine. These injuries result from explosive hip flexion maneuvers such as sprinting or kicking, but can occur from eccentric overload such as with hip extension. It is important to delineate whether there is possible knee extension weakness or hip flexion weakness. A rupture or strain of the iliopsoas muscle can also occur during resisted hip flexion or passive hyperextension such as in an eccentric overload (26). Psoas strength can be measured with resisted hip external rotation. This can mimic intra-articular pathology as a result of its course over the hip capsule (Fig 29-2). An important clinically associated injury in patients with a psoas strain is that significant swelling is possible along the muscle belly, leading to acute femoral nerve palsy. Objective weakness in any of these large muscles may be difficult to ascertain. In many cases the diagnosis is made presumptively.

Bony avulsions should be ruled out via radiographic analysis including an anteroposterior (AP) pelvic radiograph, as well as oblique images in questionable cases. Most commonly MRI is useful in order to delineate the intramuscular component of the injury as well as to serve as a prognostic factor in the injury (27). In one study 14 professional athletes with a hamstring injury were analyzed (27). The injuries were categorized according to the muscle group involved, the percentage of cross sectional area affected and the location of T1 and T2 signal intensity. In their analysis, a longer interval of convalescence was seen in injuries with complete transection, those with greater than 50% of the cross sectional area of the muscle being involved, those with ganglion-like fluid collections with long T1 and T2 signal intensities, and those with hemorrhage-like signal intensity both on short T1 and T2. In addition, distal myotendinous junction tears and deep muscular tears also had significantly increased convalescence.

The initial treatment of muscle strains involves control of hemorrhage and edema with compressive wrapping, icing, and rest. Gentle range of motion should be instituted rather quickly. The use of nonsteroidal anti-inflammatory medications (NSAIDs) is somewhat controversial. NSAIDs appear to have a paradoxical effect on the healing of muscle injuries with early signs of improvement and subsequently impairment in functional capacity and histology (28). Following establishment of full range of motion in the acute phase, strengthening becomes the focus. It is important to assess the patient on a regular basis and to assure that return to full activity occurs only after the athlete is pain free. Recurrences may be more severe and require longer rehabilitation, if a re-injury occurs during the acute phases (7).

Bursitis

Bursitis most commonly is seen about the greater trochanter. There are several other areas, however, that not infrequently present with acute inflammation in the bursae. In some cases, a variety of bursitis can cause the so-called "snapping hip," which will be discussed later. The other areas that are anatomically related to the hip and can present with symptoms attributable to the bursae, include the lesser trochanteric, or psoas bursa, and occasionally the bursa about the ischial tuberosity (Fig 29-3).

The inciting factors in bursitis appear to be related to overuse. Most commonly, trochanteric bursitis is attributable to the wider pelvis seen in women, a prominent trochanter, or in runners who adduct beyond the midline (Fig 29-4). In addition, running on banked surfaces may cause an uneven pelvis and abnormal stress at the trochanter, precipitating inflammation.

The diagnosis of trochanteric bursitis is one that presents significant difficulty in some cases. Often there is diffuse pain in the hip, thigh, and leg with occasional proximal and distal radiation. The presentation can be similar to acute low back conditions. It is not unusual for the tenderness in the region of the greater trochanter, buttock, or lateral thigh to mimic the symptoms of lumbar nerve root compression. Despite these known features, the diagnosis is often missed. In one study, the prevalence of trochanteric bursitis in patients referred to a tertiary care orthopedic spine referral center for the evaluation of low back pain was assessed retrospectively in 247 consecutive

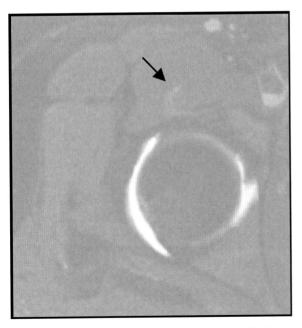

Fig 29-2. 30 year old karate teacher with an acute hip hyperextension injury presentation with weakness of the extremity and subjective locking of the joint. MRI (T1 weighted) depicting a muscle belly injury of the psoas.

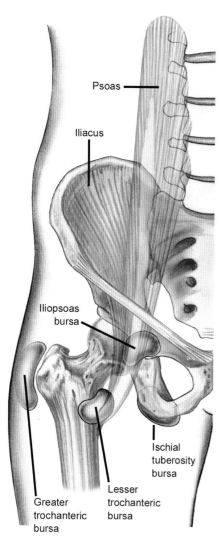

Fig 29-3. Diagrammatic representation of the commonly pathologic bursae about the hip and pelvis.

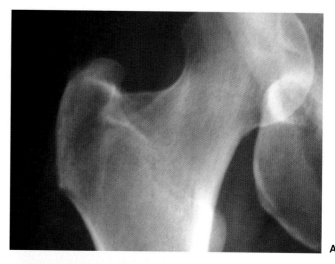

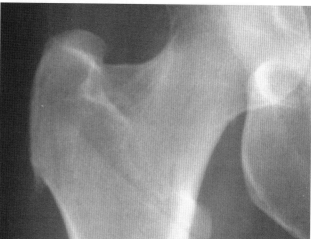

Fig 29-4. Greater trochanteric spur in an active 28 year old person, refractory to conservative measures including corticosteroid injections and physical therapy. **A:** AP radiograph with inferior greater trochanteric osteophytes. **B:** AP radiograph following endoscopic resection.

patients (29). The diagnosis of bursitis was made based on history and physical examination and was confirmed by response to anesthetic corticosteroid injection. It was found that the prevalence of bursitis was 20.2% (51 of 252) in the population. 62.7% (32 of 51) of the patients had previously been evaluated by an orthopedist or neurosurgeon and one patient had undergone two lumbar decompressions without clinical improvement.

Psoas bursitis can also be a difficult problem to diagnose. The findings are frequently diffuse and a percentage of the patients will complain of snapping about the hip. The clinical maneuvers that will elicit pain in these patients include resisted flexion and abduction of the hip, followed by resisted extension and adduction. This exacerbates the pain by compressing the tendon of the iliopsoas over the bursa.

The treatment of most bursitis includes rest, stretching of the involved tendons, and NSAIDs. In refractory cases, a corticosteroid injection is certainly acceptable and these are often repeated in many cases. The delivery of corticosteroid

in the case of psoas bursitis, however, must be made with the use of radiographic localization. In refractory cases, surgical excision of the either the trochanteric bursa or the iliopsoas bursa can be undertaken (30). Recently, the arthroscopic management of trochanteric bursitis has been discussed in the literature and is becoming more commonplace (31) **(Fig 29-5).**

Snapping Hip

Coxa saltans or "snapping hip" is typically seen in patients with an audible snapping, usually with flexion and extension of the hip during exercise or with normal activities. It is often accompanied by pain. The causes can be classified into three broad categories: external, internal, and intra-articular. The final type, which can be caused by loose bodies or labral tears, will not be discussed in this section. The external type is most commonly caused by the iliotibial band, but can also involve the gluteus maximus tendon. The internal type

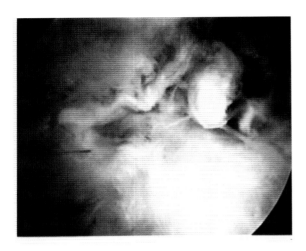

Fig 29-5. Endoscopic view of psoas tendon. The lesser tuberosity is identified fluoroscopically and then palpated with the arthroscopic cannula for localization of the appropriate area.

involves the musculotendinous iliopsoas as it moves over structures located behind it, the most common being the femoral head (32).

In the external snapping, the iliotibial band slides over the greater trochanter, where there is a thickening of the posterior part of the tract (32). The band lies posterior to the trochanter, when the hip is in extension and snaps forward with flexion. The two attachments of the iliotibial band proximally are to the tensor fascia femoris anteriorly and the gluteus maximus posteriorly. Because the iliotibial tract remains taut throughout motion of the hip, not only does it act as a tension band on the lateral thigh, but also any small anatomic change can cause snapping over the trochanter (33). In some cases, the snapping can also cause an irritation of the overlying trochanteric bursa.

The internal form of snapping is most often attributed to the confluence of the iliacus and psoas muscles through a groove between the iliopectineal eminence and the anterior inferior iliac spine (34). It appears that the musculotendinous junction occurs at the level of this groove and remains within the groove throughout hip motion. However, with rotation, the tendon translates across the femoral head while fixed in the groove, thus causing the snapping. Some anatomic variants have been described in this area including osteophytes on the lesser trochanter and anomalous tendon slips (34).

The other area of concern with respect to internal snapping is the psoas bursa itself. The musculotendinous part of the iliopsoas muscle is anterior to the bursa and the capsule is posterior. In about 15% of cases the bursa communicates with the hip joint, such that any effusion within that joint may affect the space available for the tendon, thus exacerbating snapping (34).

The history provided by most patients with snapping is fairly straightforward and does not present a clinical challenge. However, the identification of the snapping can be difficult to isolate in some cases, especially in the internal and intra-articular types. It is most important to delineate what activities exacerbate the symptomatology to isolate the problem.

The physical examination of patients with suspected internal snapping should include examining the patient in a supine position and having him or her demonstrate the snapping with active leg motion. Most commonly, simple flexion and extension of the hip can reproduce the symptoms. In order to make the symptoms more prominent, the hip should be abducted with flexion and adducted with extension. The snapping can often be eliminated or significantly lessened by applying pressure over the iliopsoas tendon at the level of the femoral head (33).

The external type likewise is reproduced with hip flexion and extension, although the patient typically can reproduce the snap more effectively while in a standing position. Much like the internal type, the snapping can be decreased, or eliminated altogether by applying manual pressure over the greater trochanter. Unlike internal snapping, which is typically painless, the external type of snapping is often accompanied by pain secondary to trochanteric bursitis (35).

Imaging of the symptomatic snapping hip can be difficult. In cases of the external variety, the diagnosis is typically not difficult to make and simple radiographs are usually sufficient to rule out coexistent pathology. In cases of intra-articular snapping, MRI can be effective, especially if an arthrogram is performed. The imaging study of choice in the delineation of internal snapping, however, has not been well established. Radiographs are typically nondiagnostic. MRI can be used to delineate the anatomy, however the images are obviously static and often do not lead to a conclusive diagnosis.

The two dynamic studies that have been commented on the most in the literature are the use of ultrasound and iliopsoas bursography (36). With bursography, the psoas tendon is usually seen as a filling defect adjacent to the opacified psoas bursa. The hip can then be moved through a full range of motion while imaging. A sudden jerking of the iliopsoas tendon is diagnostic of the snapping (36).

The vast majority of snapping hips are asymptomatic from the perspective of pain. In most cases, the snapping is a curiosity that has been present for long periods of time (35). In the occasional patient, some new activity may exacerbate the problem and simple avoidance may be curative. In some acute exacerbations, a corticosteroid injection may be useful for alleviation of the symptoms.

In the rare patient with external snapping that does not respond to conservative measures, the treatment of choice is excision of the trochanteric bursa along with either Z-plasty or elliptical excision of the iliotibial band over the prominence of the greater trochanter (35,37).

Painful internal snapping is also treated in a conservative fashion with occasional use of corticosteroids. In those patients that fail these measures, consideration should be given to lengthening of the iliopsoas tendon performed either in an open or arthroscopic fashion (33,38) **(Fig 29-6)**. Although the lengthening procedures do relieve much of the

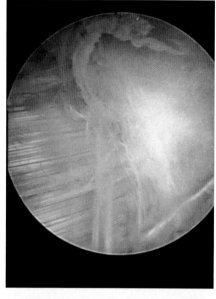

A

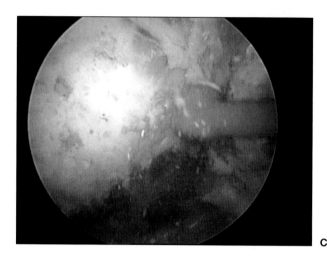

C

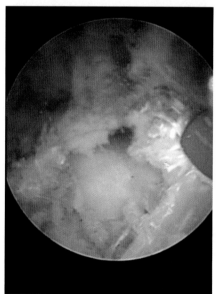

B

Fig 29-6. Endoscopic trochanteric bursectomy (Left hip with patient in lateral decubitus position and leg to the left). **A:** View of iliotibial band prior to debridement. **B:** View of partially debrided band about the central trochanteric area. **C:** View of final debridement. Note the visible vastus lateralis fibers to the left and the gluteus maximus fibers to the right and above.

pain symptomatology, it is not unusual for patients to still note a fair amount of snapping over the area of the tendon.

Stress Fractures

Although stress fractures were described initially in military recruits and were clinically seen in these populations for many years, the incidence in the average civilian population has certainly exploded (39). This larger incidence is reflective of the increased athletic participation level of the average person, especially as it relates to women participants (40).

It is important, to begin with, to delineate the difference between a stress fracture in a normal, healthy individual and that of a metabolically abnormal person. To this end the distinction to be made is to classify these types of fractures into two different groups. The first is a fatigue fracture that occurs in normal bone, when subjected to abnormal forces (such as the military recruit or marathon runner). The second subgroup is an insufficiency fracture, where a fracture of abnormal bone subjected to normal forces occurs. This is typically seen in the elderly as well as other metabolically deficient persons, and will not be discussed in this chapter.

The most important principle in the diagnosis of a stress fracture is the clear association between the level or running (or other high-impact activity), and the likelihood of a fracture. This has been described as a dose-response relationship between the amount of training and the likelihood of injury (41). The common denominator for all stress fractures is a change in the frequency, intensity, or duration of an activity to which the bone is unaccustomed. As a general rule of thumb, increases in training distance should not exceed 10% per week in order to avoid undue stress in the bony architecture (3).

There also appears to be a predisposition for the development of stress fractures in females with rates as high as four to ten times higher than that of males (41). Amenorrhea appears to be especially prevalent in endurance athletes with notable decreases in bone mineral density as compared to those normally menstruating (42). Taking this into consideration there may be a subset of patients that do not fit into the above-mentioned populations of stress and fatigue fractures. The important principle is that a menstrual and dietary history should always be included in the treatment of the female athlete with a potential stress fracture (40).

The factors in the development of these fractures are poorly understood. There are theories that implicate the repetitive muscle forces that occur across weight bearing joints as being the major factor (43). Others, however, take a differing view and attribute the injuries to a repetitive sub maximal stress being applied to the bone with a frequency that exceeds the inherent capacity of the bone to heal. Along these lines, Baker et al. (44) have concluded that muscle fatigue leads to abnormal gait patterns, altered stress distribution and ultimately excessive forces to the underlying bone.

In one study rabbit tibiae were studied in order to determine their adaptive capability. Continued excessive stress weakened by accelerated osteoclastic resorption due to circulatory disturbances within the Haversian system was hypothesized as the underlying cause of injuries going on to complete fractures (45). Most of the bones, however, remodeled appropriately and did not go on to fracture. On the basis of this study, it appears that fatigue fractures result from the failure of a bone to react quickly enough and with sufficient adaptive response to counter a repetitive sub maximal load that occurs at an unaccustomed frequency.

The characteristic clinical presentation of a stress fracture depends, to some extent, on the area of the femur that is involved. The most confusing and dangerous are those of the femoral neck. The typical presentation of these injuries is activity related groin pain that is relieved by rest, which brings to mind a rather large differential diagnosis (39). In the more distal fractures, the pain may be more diffuse and typically is associated with more significant antalgia on presentation. Strenuous activity may intensify the pain to prohibit further athletic activity. Femoral shaft stress fractures, can present with symptoms that include anterior thigh pain, increasing with activity (46). In some cases, the patient presents with a complete fracture after having had minimal prodromal symptomatology.

Physical examination will occasionally reveal tenderness to palpation, but obviously depends on the level of the fracture. In general, the neck fractures would be difficult to palpate and the pain is more diffuse. Limitation of the extremes of range of motion is often the only clinically obvious finding (47). The other maneuvers that are typically employed with respect to hip pathology are useful in at least isolating the area of pathology. These maneuvers include log rolling of the extremity as well as a resisted (or active) straight leg raise. Other maneuvers that can be employed include percussion of the heel; however this type of exam has not shown a high correlation with the present pathology (47).

It is important to realize that a stress fracture can occur anywhere in the pelvis and femur, including the iliac wings (48,49) **(Fig 29-7)**. The pubic stress fractures can present with diffuse hamstring spasm and adductor tightness and are not typically as dangerous with respect to likely displacement requiring surgical intervention. Likewise, iliac wing

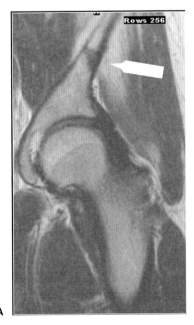
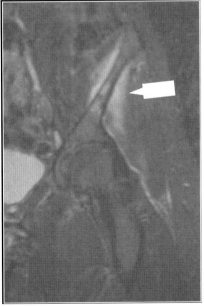

Fig 29–7. Iliac wing stress fracture in a 32-year-old healthy woman following completion of a marathon. A: T1 coronal view of area of fracture in supraacetabular region. B: T2 coronal view depicting the significant soft tissue injury associated with the fracture.

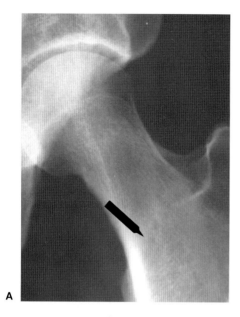

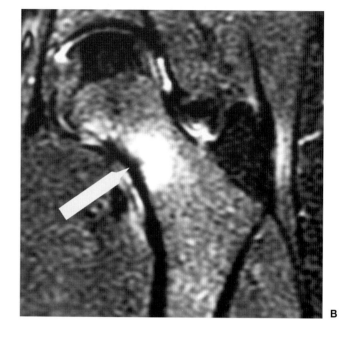

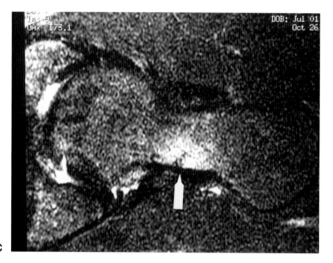

Fig 29–8. Stress fracture of the femoral neck in a 34-year female police officer following a marathon. **A:** AP radiograph with subtle fracture line (*arrowhead*). **B:** T2 coronal view with area of bony reactive tissue (*arrowhead*). **C:** Axial view (T2 weighted) with the posterior neck fracture line visible.

stress fractures can present with acute symptomatology, but are unlikely to cause significant residual, once they heal (48).

As a result of the variety of areas of stress fractures that can present with hip or groin pain, any imaging modality chosen should be carefully evaluated for its potential to delineate the cause of the problem as completely as possible. In many, if not most situations, radiographs are normal at least in the first 2 to 4 weeks. There is a suggestion in the literature that up to 55% of stress fractures may never have positive radiographic findings (40). Radiographs are typically good for the depiction of late changes such as cortical thickening or periosteal bone formation. Nonetheless, the standard of care would include AP pelvis view with a lateral view of the involved leg.

The use of bone scintigraphy has become commonplace in the diagnosis of stress fractures. The changes that accompany a stress fracture can be noted within 24 hours after the onset of pain in most healthy individuals (50). However, in

the older athlete and in patients with significant medical problems, the findings may lag for as much as 72 hours (51). In the young patient, therefore, the use of bone scintigraphy with technetium 99 m methylene diphosphonate will yield a sensitivity of 93% to 100% and a specificity of 76% to 95%, as compared with plain radiographs in the diagnosis of a stress fracture (52). In addition, the study serves as a broad screening device for the rest of the pelvis and femur should the diagnosis not be a femoral neck stress fracture.

More recently, the use of MRI has become more commonplace in the evaluation of these injuries. The characteristic findings of fatigue or insufficiency fractures on MRI imaging include a decreased signal on T1-weighted images, and increased signal on T2-weighted images as well as short-tau inversion recovery (STIR) sequences (53) **(Fig 29–8).** Although somewhat controversial, the findings are believed to represent edema secondary to microscopic trabecular fractures (40).

The use of MRI in these injuries has been studied by Shin and Gillingham (40). In most of the studies, MRI has been found to be superior as compared to radiographs, and more importantly as compared to bone scintigraphy. The reason for the superiority has been the ability of MRI to delineate not only the acute findings of the stress fracture within the bone, but also to help assess the soft tissues about the area of injury. In addition, the findings of edema and trabecular changes occur immediately, as opposed to some of the metabolic events that need to take place before scintigraphy is positive (51). The use of MRI may therefore supplant bone scintigraphy as the procedure of choice in the diagnosis of stress fractures.

The most important stress fracture to consider about the hip is that of the femoral neck. While the others are obviously important as well, the femoral neck fractures present a challenge with respect to diagnosis as well as treatment. For that reason the classification of these fractures will be discussed to some extent in this chapter, since it is important to be familiar with the more dangerous variants.

The most accepted and modern classification is that developed by Fullerton and Snowdy (47). They analyzed 54 femoral neck fatigue fractures in soldiers with both plain radiography and bone scintigraphy. They divided the fractures into three types which they felt added significant prognostic significance.

The first type is the compression-side fracture. This type most commonly demonstrated as sclerosis on the compression side of the neck. The diagnosis was also made in some cases on positive scintigraphy, only on that side of the neck. This is a stable type that can be treated with non weight-bearing for 6 weeks, followed by a gradual progression to increased activities.

The second type is the tension-side fracture that typically shows callus or overt tension-side cortical disruption. There is a spectrum of pathology noted with this type of fracture from the above-mentioned periosteal changes on the tension side to tension-side uptake on bone scintigraphy without obvious radiographic changes. Finally, there are displaced fractures of the femoral neck, which are surgical emergencies.

The treatment of the compression type fracture is mostly nonoperative with strict non weight-bearing recommended for a period of 6 weeks, before allowing gradual progression to increasing activity. A caveat of the nonoperative treatment is that weekly radiographs should be obtained to assure that no significant progression of the fracture line occurs or that displacement is not seen. The determination for surgical intervention is reserved for those fractures showing a fatigue line greater than or equal to 50% of the width of the femoral neck (40). In these cases, percutaneous fixation with large cannulated screws is the technique of choice.

The tension type of fracture should be surgically addressed with cannulated screw fixation and treated as a relative emergency (39,47). There is literature to support the nonoperative treatment of these fractures, which involves at least three weeks of bed rest (54). However, given the significant morbidity associated with a displaced fracture and the problems associated with prolonged bed rest, the modern treatment of these fractures is surgical intervention. The potential lifelong disability associated with a displaced fracture with the possible development of either a malunion or avascular necrosis far outweighs the surgical risk (40).

The treatment of the displaced fracture is obviously a surgical emergency (39,47). Expeditious, open reduction, and internal fixation is required to prevent further complications. Despite aggressive management, the prognosis in young patients is poor with a prolonged period of non weight-bearing and the potential to develop avascular necrosis in about 25% of cases up to 18 months after the fracture (53).

■ AVULSION FRACTURES

Avulsion fractures are most commonly seen in athletes between the ages of 14 and 17 years of age, with males more commonly affected than females. The mechanism of injury is usually a sudden, intense muscular contraction or an excessive amount of muscle stretch, across an open physis. External trauma is rarely involved. A similar overload injury in adults would result in a muscle strain. However, an avulsion fracture without external trauma in adults should raise suspicion for a pathologic fracture, especially for avulsions of the lesser trochanter (55). The avulsions most frequently occur at the anterior superior iliac spine from the sartorius, the ischium from the hamstrings, the lesser trochanter from the iliopsoas, the anterior inferior spine from the rectus, as well as the iliac crest from the abdominal muscles.

These injuries often occur during athletic participation. A powerful muscle contraction takes place during participation in sports such as sprinters, soccer, and football players, as well as sports that require jumping. The clinical presentation is usually localized swelling, tenderness, and limitation of motion of the hip secondary to pain. The pain is often described as severe following the injury on the playing or practice field. Resisted contraction or stretch of the involved muscle usually reproduces the pain. Radiographs of the hip and pelvis confirm the diagnosis. Multiple views, including inlet and outlet views of the pelvis may be required to define the extent of displacement of the lesion. The index of suspicion should remain high if the clinical exam and history suggest an avulsion in spite of normal radiographs, because secondary ossification centers may not have formed yet in children.

Conservative treatment, including rest, ice, and positioning the limb to lessen the stretch on the affected muscle will often improve the patient's symptoms and lessen the risk of further displacement of the apophysis. Metzmaker and Pappas (55) introduced a five-stage rehabilitation program to treat avulsion fractures around the hip and pelvis. The first phase includes rest and positioning the limb to relax the offending muscle group along with pain management. Next, as the pain subsides, excursion of the muscle group is gradually increased. When the patient has achieved full, active range of motion, resisted range of motion activities are instituted. When the patient achieves 50% of anticipated strength, he or she begins

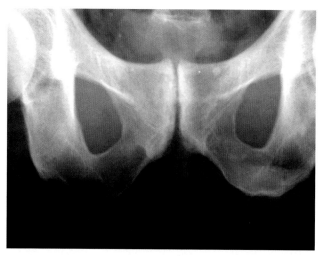

Fig 29-9. Osteitis pubis in a 28 year old recreational soccer player. Player had a long history of diffuse groin pain for one year.

to integrate the use of the injured muscle group with other muscle in the pelvis. They showed that at this stage, the athlete is most at risk of re-injury, if full strength and function is not obtained prior to returning to full participation. Therefore, full participation is guided by achieving full strength and integration of the injured muscle group.

Rarely will avulsion fractures lead to chronic pain and disability. Fortunately, the periosteum and surrounding fascia often limit severe displacement. Greater amounts of displacement can lead to the development of a fibrous nonunion. Persistent, chronic pain has been suggested as an indication for surgical intervention (56). However, early open reduction and internal fixation has been advocated only when there is significant displacement of a fragment (57). Overall, definitive guidelines for operative management of avulsion fractures are unclear, as it is very uncommon for one to become severely displaced or lead to a long-term disability.

Osteitis Pubis

Osteitis pubis is an unusual injury that occurs more commonly in long-distance runners, but has been described in a variety of athletic activities. The mechanism of injury appears to be overtraining of the rectus abdominis and adductor muscles. The patient often complains of tenderness directly over the symphysis pubis. Radiographs are initially negative but sclerosis on one or both sides of the pubis may be present several weeks after onset of symptoms **(Fig 29-9)**. Bone scans, however, are positive in the symphysis early and can be used, if the diagnosis is in question and the need for a definitive diagnosis is important, such as for high level athletes. Rest, heat, and conditioning exercises that do not cause pain are recommended (58).

Iliac apophysitis presents as iliac crest tenderness to palpation with associated muscular contraction usually seen in adolescent long-distance runners. Patients do not report a specific inciting event or trauma and a history often reveals a recent or current intensive training regimen. Radiographs

are unremarkable. The etiology seems to be traction apophysitis similar in nature to Osgood-Schlatters disease. Treatment consists of rest with ice and anti-inflammatories for 4 to 6 weeks (59).

Nerve Entrapment

Piriformis Syndrome

Piriformis syndrome has been a controversial diagnosis since it was introduced. Yeoman in 1928, first linked the piriformis muscle to sciatica and considered sacroiliac joint degeneration as the cause. However, Robinson in the 1940s is credited with naming the syndrome. The theory linking the SI joint to piriformis syndrome has been refuted (60) and piriformis syndrome currently consists of primary and secondary causes. Primary piriformis syndrome includes all pathology intrinsic to the muscle, such as myofascial pain, pyomyositis, and myositis ossificans. Secondary piriformis syndrome results from external influences on the nerve, such as a mass effect (61).

The typical patient with piriformis syndrome complains of buttock pain with or without radiation to the ipsilateral posterior thigh that sometimes extends below the knee to the calf, resembling sciatica. Buttock pain may be reproduced with activity, such as hip adduction and internal rotation that stretches the muscle. However, the most common complaint is sitting intolerance (60). Symptoms are often exacerbated by activity of the hip rotators or prolonged sitting on hard surfaces. Benson and Schutzer (65) reported sitting intolerance in all 14 patients whom they had treated surgically with all 14 patients having immediate and long-lasting pain relief.

Trauma or a fall involving the gluteal region is common. Pregnancy also has been implicated as a possible risk factor. Because of the proximity of the piriformis muscle to the lateral pelvic wall, patients may complain of dyspareunia or pain with bowel movements. These symptoms can often be relieved initially by externally rotating the leg.

The primary goal when diagnosing piriformis syndrome is to rule out all potential sources of intraspinal pathology. On gross inspection, the patient may hold the leg in an externally rotated position while lying supine. This is called the piriformis sign. Buttock tenderness over the greater sciatic foramen is present in almost all patients. Specific piriformis tests are based on either active contraction of the muscle in resistance or by passive stretching of the muscle. The Pace test, an active contraction test, elicits pain with resisted abduction of a flexed thigh. The Freiberg test, a passive stretch test, causes pain with internal rotation during thigh extension. The FADIR test, producing pain with flexion, adduction, and internal rotation is another passive stretch test.

Radiographic and other imaging studies are usually not helpful with the diagnosis. An MRI can evaluate for a mass effect. Neurophysiologic testing provides more consistent and reliable results. Results affect the peroneal division of the sciatic nerve that supplies the hamstrings, but the tibial nerve innervations are spared. Positive nerve conduction studies demonstrate delayed F waves and H reflexes. Hughes et al. (62) feel that piriformis syndrome should be diagnosed electrodiagnostically prior to operative intervention.

Most patients with piriformis syndrome respond successfully to conservative treatment. Nonsteroidal anti-inflammatories, analgesics, and muscle relaxants reduce pain and inflammation. Ultrasound treatment was effective in reducing pain in a small series (62). Physical therapy consisting of stretching with hip internal rotation with adduction and flexion has also been advocated (63,64).

Diagnostic and therapeutic injections with anesthetics and corticosteroids can be attempted for those patients that fail conservative treatment. Operative release is performed via a limited posterior approach. The tendon is released off the femur, a neurolysis is performed, and any obstructing lesions are also removed (61). Patients ambulate with crutches and progress to full weight-bearing by 5 to 10 days after surgery (63). The two largest series, both with less than twenty patients, reported satisfactory results, and both

authors suggest proper patient selection as an important factor for a good outcome (63,65).

Pudenal Nerve Compression

Pudendal neuropathy can cause groin pain and numbness, often exacerbated in the seated position and relieved by standing or lying supine. Symptoms can also involve the perineal region as well as pain in the genital region.

Pudendal nerve compression is thought to occur at two different locations based on cadaveric studies (66). The junction of the sacrotuberous and sacrospinous ligaments as well as the pudendal canal can impinge the nerve. Also, the dorsal branch of the pudendal nerve can be compressed between the symphysis pubis and a bicycle seat. Therefore, this condition is seen frequently in competitive cyclists. The nerve compression causes a temporary ischemia and pain follows. Scrotal anesthesia suggests compression of the genital branch of the genitofemoral nerve. This may occur in tandem with pudendal ischemia, especially in cyclists.

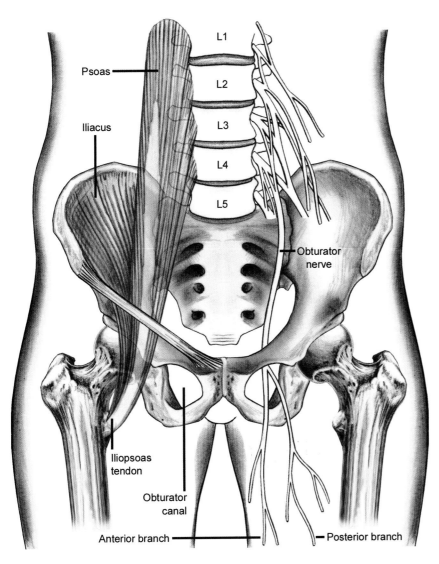

Fig 29-10. Nerve course and cutaneous distribution of the obturator nerve through the pelvis and leg.

The diagnosis is often made based on the patient's history. Pain exacerbated with prolonged sitting was the most reproducible finding. Electrodiagnostic testing, using an intrarectal technique has been reported (66). Thoumas et al. (67) have described Pudendal nerve blocks for diagnostic and therapeutic purposes. With an average of 2.2 injections, more than 65% of patients reported relief at more than one-year follow-up (67).

For cyclists, activity and equipment modification can resolve the problem. Specifically, making sure the bicycle seat does not tilt upward and adding padding to bicycle pants can help resolve the symptoms. Other patients that fail extensive conservative treatment may be candidates for an operative release. Robert et al. (66) achieved a 67% good to excellent results with surgical release.

Obturator Nerve Compression

Obturator nerve entrapment is a recently described cause of groin pain in athletes. The cause of the nerve entrapment is uncertain; however myofascial compression exacerbated during exercise is the current theory (68). Repetitive kicking, side-to-side movements, and twisting are common motions, which correlate with the problem. Patients usually report a pattern of exercise induced groin pain over the adductor region, which radiates along the medial thigh. A common complaint is that of a poorly localized deep ache centered on the adductor origin at the pubic tubercle. The pain will often subside with rest and recur when exercise resumes. In addition, many patients also will complain of paresthesias in the cutaneous distribution of the obturator nerve **(Fig 29–10)**.

Findings on clinical exam are often unremarkable as symptoms are usually not present in an office setting. Occasionally, subtle adductor weakness or pain induced by perineal muscle stretch (passive hip external rotation and abduction while standing) or resisted hip internal rotation may be present.

Similar to pudendal entrapment, standard-imaging modalities often do not aid in the diagnosis. Needle electromyography demonstrates denervation of the adductor muscles. A post-exercise anesthetic block will relieve the pain, as well as relieve pain from previous provocative stretches (68,69).

Conservative treatment should be attempted, and this includes anti-inflammatories, rest, massage, ultrasound, and discontinuation of activity. Failed measures warrant obturator nerve neurolysis. Bradshaw et al. (69) report universally good results for all 32 patients treated with internal neurolysis and reported all patients resumed athletic participation, symptom free within 3 to 6 weeks.

Meralgia Paresthetica

Meralgia paresthetica describes compression or injury to the lateral femoral cutaneous nerve (LFCN) and produces symptoms of pain, numbness, tingling, and paresthesias in the anterolateral thigh.

The nerve has a highly varied anatomical course and passes either above, through, or below the inguinal ligament from the pelvis to the lateral thigh. Meralgia paresthetica often occurs spontaneously, but can result from iatrogenic injury such as from autogenous bone grafting from the anterior superior iliac spine, the ilioinguinal approach to the pelvis or from local trauma. Irritation of the nerve usually occurs near the inguinal ligament.

Patients describe numbness, tingling, pain, burning, and decreased sensitivity to pain, touch, and temperature in the distribution of the LFCN. Direct palpation often exacerbates symptoms. Standing may worsen and sitting may decrease the severity of the symptoms. Hip extension during walking will put stretch on the nerve and aggravate symptoms. Patients are often seen massaging the region to attempt to alleviate the discomfort. The clinical exam is usually sufficient for the diagnosis, but electrodiagnostic testing can be performed for difficult clinical presentations. Radiographs should be obtained to rule out bone pathology and an MRI can be ordered, if a lesion causing a mass effect is suspected.

Conservative treatment for idiopathic entities consist of anti-inflammatories and making the patient aware of any lifestyles changes that may have initiated the symptoms such as weight gain or tight clothing. Anesthetic injections with corticosteroids may be beneficial to decrease inflammation. The injection should be performed 1 cm medial to the anterior superior iliac spine. The results of the injections have been variable (70). In general, conservative treatment for meralgia paresthetica has yielded excellent results. Kalangu (71) reported that approximately two-thirds of their patients were improved with conservative treatment at 2 years from the initial evaluation. Williams and Trzil (72) published a 91% success rate for nonoperative management of their patients.

Surgical intervention should be considered when symptoms reach an unacceptable level. Three surgical options are available: neurolysis of the constricting tissue, neurolysis and transposition of the LFCN, and transection with excision of a portion of the LFCN. Macnicol and Thompson reported a 44% success rate for neurolysis at more than 5 years of follow-up (73). Nahabedian and Dellon (74) documented complete relief in 18 of 23 patients treated with neurolysis. There has not been a large series of neurolysis with medial transposition of the nerve, but Keegan described two patients with good results (71). Williams and Trzil (72) reported success in 23 of 24 patients treated with nerve transection after conservative treatment had failed. This procedure leaves patients with permanent anterolateral thigh anesthesia, but other symptoms are alleviated. Van Eerten et al. (75) compared the results of decompression and neurolysis to those of transaction, and reported better long-term results for transaction. Grossman et al. (76) recommend neurolysis with decompression as the initial procedure and nerve transection if neurolysis fails.

Lateral femoral cutaneous iatrogenic injuries such as from iliac crest bone grafts or ilioinguinal approaches to the pelvis usually do not require additional procedures. Occasionally patients are left with permanent numbness over the anterolateral thigh, but symptoms often improve to a certain degree with time. It is important to inform patients of the possibility of this injury prior to performing the procedure.

Other Sources of Groin Pain

Referred pain from lower lumber and sacral nerves, frequently cause gluteal or posterior thigh symptoms. Facet joint and erector spinae muscle abnormalities may also be refer pain to this distribution. The upper lumbar nerves (L1-3) travel anteriorly and may be the source of groin or thigh pain. The femoral nerve stretch test can cause groin and anterior thigh pain. A thorough physical examination and neurological assessment may be sufficient to identify spinal abnormalities.

Slipped capital femoral epiphysis is a disorder of adolescence that may be precipitated during sports participation. It occurs most commonly in African American males or obese children and can be associated with hormonal imbalances such as hypothyroidism. Patients will often have hip or groin pain, or symptoms may be referred to the knee. Internal rotation is limited because the femoral neck is externally rotated and positioned anterior to the femoral neck. Many of these patients will require percutaneous stabilization.

SUMMARY

Despite the fact that the hip and pelvis are designed to withstand significant amounts of stress on weight-bearing and with higher-level activities, a significant amount of injuries can and do occur. With the advent of arthroscopic surgery of the hip, a large body of knowledge has begun to develop that delineates that pathophysiology of many poorly understood problems. With increasing education a lot of the unknown issues will be clearly delineated in the next few years. However, the biggest factor in preventing the advancement of many of these problems is lack of understanding of the clinical overlap of many of these problems and the history and physical examination maneuvers that can help decipher the individual problems.

One thing that should be reiterated with regard to these injuries is that there is a large overlap with many disciplines of medicine from the orthopaedic surgeon to the neurologist, the general surgeon, gynecologists, and endocrinologists. It is important to maintain this perspective with these injuries and to seek appropriate consultations when necessary.

■ REFERENCES

1. DeLee JC, Farney WC. Incidence of injury in Texas high school football. *Am J Sports Med.* 1992;20:575–580.
2. Crowninshield RD, Johnston RC, Andrews JG, et al. A biomechanical investigation of the human hip. *J Biomech.* 1978;11:75–85.
3. Anderson K, Strickland SM, Warren RF. Hip and groin injuries in athletes. *Am J Sports Med.* 2001;29:521–533.
4. Holmich P, Uhrskou P, Ulnits L, et al. Effectiveness of active physical training as treatment for long-standing adductor-related groin pain in athletes: randomized trial. *Lancet.* 1999;353:439–443.
5. Gilmore J. Groin pain in the soccer athlete: fact, fiction, and treatment. *Clin Sports Med.* 1998;17:787–793.
6. Renstrom P. Swedish research in sports traumatology. *Clin Orthop.* 1984;191:144–158.
7. Emery CA, Meeuwise WH, Powell JW. Groin and abdominal strain injuries in the National Hockey League. *Clin J Sport Med.* 1999; 9:151–156.
8. Tyler T, Zook L, Brittis D, et al. A new pelvic tilt detection device; roentgenographic validation and application to assessment of hip motion in professional ice hockey players. *J Orthop Sports Phys Ther.* 1996;24:303–308.
9. Meyers WC, Foley DP, Garrett WE, et al. Management of severe lower abdominal or inguinal pain in high-performance athletes. *Am J Sports Med.* 2000;28:2–8.
10. Hackney RG. The sports hernia: A cause of chronic groin pain. *Br J Sports Med.* 1993;27:58–62.
11. Taylor DC, Meyers WC, Moylan JA, et al. Abdominal musculature abnormalities as a cause of groin pain in athletes. Inguinal hernias and pubalgia. *Am J Sports Med.* 1991;19:239–242.
12. Akita K, Niga S, Yamato Y, et al. Anatomic basis of chronic groin pain with special reference to sports hernia. *Surg Radiol Anat.* 1999; 21:1–5.
13. Schuricht A, Haut E, Wetzler M. Surgical options in the treatment of sports hernia. *Oper Tech Sports Med.* 2002;10:224–227.
14. Hamlin JA, Kahn AM. Herniography: a review of 333 herniograms. *Am Surg.* 1998;64:965–969.
15. Sutcliffe JR, Taylor OM, Ambrose NS, et al. The use, value and safety of herniography. *Clin Radiol.* 1999;54:468–472.
16. Albers SL, Spritzer CE, Garrett WE Jr, et al. MR findings in athletes with pubalgia. *Skeletal Radiol.* 2000;30:270–277.
17. Kluin J, den Hoed PT, van Linschote R, et al. Endoscopic evaluation and treatment of groin pain in the athlete. *Am J Sports Med.* 2004;32:944–949.
18. Larson CM, Lohnes JH. Surgical management of athletic pubalgia. *Oper Tech Sports Med.* 2002;10:228–232.
19. Azurin DJ, Go LS, Schuricht A, et al. Endoscopic preperitoneal herniorrhaphy in professional athletes with groin pain. *J Laparoendosc Adv Surg Tech A.* 1997;7:7–12.
20. Ingoldby CJ. Laparoscopic and conventional repair of groin disruption in sportsmen. *Br J Surg.* 1997;84:213–215.
21. Akermark C, Johansson C. Tenotomy of the adductor longus tendon in the treatment of chronic groin pain in athletes. *Am J Sports Med.* 1992;20:640–643.
22. Srinivasan A, Schuricht A. Long-term follow-up of laparoscopic preperitoneal hernia repair in professional athletes. *J Laparoendosc Adv Surg Tech.* 2002;12:101–110.
23. Garrett WE Jr. Muscle strains injuries. *Am J Sports Med.* 1996; 24S:S2–S8.
24. Garrett WE Jr, Nikolau PK, Ribbeck BM, et al. The effect of muscle architecture on the biomechanical failure properties of skeletal muscle under passive extension. *Am J Sports Med.* 1988; 16:7–12.
25. Giacomini S, Di Gennaro GL, Donzelli O. Fracture of the lesser trochanter. *Chir organi Mov.* 2002;87:255–258.
26. Mozes M, Papa MZ, Zweig A, et al. Iliopsoas injury in soccer players. *Br J Sports Med.* 1985;91:168–170.
27. Pomeranz SJ, Heidt RS Jr. MR imaging in the prognostication of hamstring injury. *Radiology.* 1993;189:897–900.
28. Prisk V, Huard J. Muscle injuries and repair: the role of prostaglandins and inflammation. *Histol Histopathol.* 2003;18:1243–1256.
29. Tortolani PJ, Carbone JJ, Quartararo LG. Greater trochanteric pain syndrome in patients referred to orthopedic spine specialists. *Spine J.* 2002;2:251–254.
30. Janzen DL, Partidge E, Logan PM, et al. The snapping hip: clinical and imaging findings in transient subluxation of the iliopsoas tendon. *Can Asso Radiol J.* 1997;47:202–208.
31. Fox JL. The role of arthroscopic bursectomy in the treatment of trochanteric bursitis. *Arthroscopy.* 2002;18:E34.
32. Jacobson T, Allen WC. Surgical correction of the snapping iliopsoas tendon. *Am J Sports Med.* 1990;18:470–474.

33. Allen WC, Cope R. Coxa Saltans: the snapping hip revisited. *J Am Acad Orthop Surg.* 1995;3:303–308.

34. Schaberg JE, Harper MC, Allen WC. The snapping hip syndrome. *Am J Sports Med.* 1984;12:361–365.

35. Zoltan DJ, Clancy WG Jr, Keene JS. A new operative approach to snapping hip and refractory trochanteric bursitis in athletes. *Am J Sports Med.* 1986; 14:201–204.

36. Harper MC, Schaberg JE, Allen WC. Primary iliopsoas bursography in the diagnosis of disorders of the hip. *Clin Orthop.* 1987;221: 238–241.

37. Brignall CG, Stainsby GD. The snapping hip: treatment by Z-plasty. *J Bone Joint Surg.* 1991;73B:253–254.

38. Byrd JWT. Hip arthroscopy: Evolving frontiers. *Op Tech Orthop.* 2004;14:58–67.

39. Blickenstaff LD, Morris JM. Fatigue fracture of the femoral neck. *J Bone Joint Surg.* 1966;48A:1031–1047.

40. Shin AY, Gillingham BL. Fatigue fractures of the femoral neck in athletes. *J Am Acad Orthop Surg.* 1997;5:293–302.

41. Jones BH, Harris JM, Vinh TN, et al. Exercise-induced stress fractures and stress reactions of bone: Epidemiology, etiology, and classification. *Exerc Sport Sci Rev.* 1989;17:379–422.

42. Drinkwater BL, Nilson K, Chestnut CH III, et al. Bone mineral content of amenorrheic and eumenorrheic athletes. *N Engl J Med.* 1984;311:277–281.

43. Stanitiski CL, McMaster JH, Scranton PE. On the nature of stress fractures. *Am J Sports Med.* 1978;6:391–396.

44. Baker J, Frankel VH, Burstein A. Fatigue fractures: Biomechanical considerations(abstract). *J Bone Joint Surg.* 1972;54A:1345–1346.

45. Li GP, Zhang SD, Chen G, et al. Radiographic and histologic analyses of stress fracture in rabbit tibias. *Am J Sports Med.* 1985;13: 285–294.

46. McBryde AM Jr. Stress fractures in runners. *Clin Sports Med.* 1985;4:737–752.

47. Fullerton LR Jr, Snowdy HA. Femoral neck stress fractures. *Am J Sports Med.* 1988;16:365–377.

48. Atlihan D, Quick DC, Guanche CA. Stress fracture of the iliac bone in a young female runner. *Orthopedics.* 2003;26:729–730.

49. Iwamoto J, Takeda T. Stress fractures in athletes: review of 196 cases. *J Orthop Sci.* 2003;8:273–278.

50. Greany RB, Gerber FH, Laughlin RL, et al. Distribution and natural history of stress fractures in U.S. Marine recruits. *Radiology.* 1983;146:339–346.

51. Guanche CA, Kozin SH, Levy AS, et al. The use of MRI in the diagnosis of occult hip fractures in the elderly: a preliminary review. *Orthopedics.*1994;17:327–330.

52. Prather JL, Nusynowitz ML, Snowdy HA, et al. Scintigraphic findings in stress fractures. *J Bone Joint Surg.* 1977;59A:869–874.

53. Aro H, Dahlstrom S. Conservative management of distraction-type stress fractures of the femoral neck. *J Bone Joint Surg.* 1986; 68B: 65–67.

54. Lee CH, Huang GS, Chao KH, et al. Surgical treatment of displaced stress fractures of the femoral neck in military recruits: a report of 42 cases. *Arch Orthop Trauma Surg.* 2003;123:527–533.

55. Metzmaker JN, Pappas AM. Avulsion fractures of the pelvis. *Am J Sports Med.* 1985;13:349–358.

56. Schlonsky J, Olix ML. Functional disability following avulsion fracture of the ischial epiphysis. *J Bone Joint Surg.* 1972;54A: 641–644.

57. Canale TS, King RE. Pelvic and hip fractures. In: Rockwood CA, Wilkins KE, King RE, eds. *Fractures in children.* Philadelphia: JB Lippincott; 1984.

58. Koch R, Jackson D. Pubic symphysitis in runners. *Am J Sports Med.* 1981;9:62–70.

59. Clancy WG, Foltz AS. Iliac apophysitis in stress fractures in adolescent runners. *Am J Sports Med.* 1976;4:214–218.

60. Papadopoulos EC, Khan SN. Piriformis syndrome and low back pain: a new classification and review of the literature. *Orthop Clin North Am.* 2004;35:1–10.

61. Foster MR. Piriformis syndrome. *Orthopedics.* 25(8):821–825.

62. Hughes SS, Goldstein MN, Hicks DG, et al. Extrapelvic compression of the sciatic nerve. *J Bone Joint Surg Am.* 1992;74: 1553–1559.

63. Hallin RP. Sciatic pain and the piriformis muscle. *Postgrad Med.* 1983;74:69–72.

64. Parziale JR, Hidgins TH, Fishman LM. The piriformis syndrome. *Am J Orthop.* 1996;25:819–823.

65. Benson ER, Schutzer SF. Posttraumatic piriformis syndrome: diagnosis and results of operative treatment. *J Bone Joint Surg.* 1999;81A:941–949.

66. Robert R, Prat-Pradal D, Labatt JJ, et al. Anatomic basis of chronic perineal pain: Role of the pudendal nerve. *Surg Radiol Anat.* 1998; 20:93–98.

67. Thoumas D, Leroi AM, Mauillon J, et al. Pudendal neuralgia: CT-guided pudendal nerve block technique. *Abdom Imaging.* 1999;24: 309–312.

68. Bradshaw C, McCrory P. Obturator nerve entrapment. *Clin J Sport Med.* 1997;7(3):217–219.

69. Bradshaw C, McCrory P, Bell S, et al. Obturator nerve entrapment: a cause of groin pain in athletes. *Am J Sports Med.* 1997; 25(3):402–408.

70. Edelson R, Stevens P. Meralgia paresthetica in children. *J Bone Joint Surg.* 1994;76:993–999.

71. Kalangu KK. Meralgia paresthetica: a report on two cases treated surgically. *Cent Afr J Med.* 1995;41:227–230.

72. Williams PH, Trzil KP. Management of meralgia paresthetica. *J Neurosurg.* 1991;74:76–80.

73. Macnicol MF, Thompson WJ. Idiopathic meralgia paresthetica. *Clin Orthop.* 1990;254:270–274.

74. Nahabedian MY, Dellon AL. Meralgia paresthetica: etiology, diagnosis, and outcome of surgical decompression. *Ann Plast Surg.* 1995; 35:590–594.

75. Van Eerten PV, Polder TW, Broere CAJ. Operative treatment of meralgia paresthetica: transection versus neurolysis. *Neurosurgery.* 1995;37:63–65.

76. Grossman MG, Ducey SA, Nadler SS, et al. Meralgia paresthetica: diagnosis and treatment. *J Am Acad Orthop Surg.* 2001;9: 336–344.

SNAPPING HIP SYNDROME

30

■ J.W. THOMAS BYRD, MD

■ KEY POINTS

- External coxa saltans is snapping due to the tensor fascia lata and iliotibial band flipping back and forth across the greater trochanter.
- Internal coxa saltans is snapping caused by the iliopsoas tendon.
- Intra-articular coxa saltans refers to a variety of intra-articular lesions that can cause painful clicking or popping within the joint.
- Coxa vara and reduced bi-iliac width have been proposed as predisposing anatomic factors of external coxa soltans.
- Symptomatic cases of external coxa saltans are most commonly associated with repetitive activities, but may occur following trauma.
- Snapping of the iliotibial band usually can be demonstrated by the patient better than it can be produced by passive examination.
- Radiographs and further investigative studies are rarely of benefit except to assess for other associated disorders.
- Surgical intervention rarely is necessary. Published results of a variety of surgical techniques to address recalcitrant snapping of the iliotibial band range from poor to excellent.
- Snapping of the iliopsoas tendon can be difficult to differentiate from and may co-exist with intra-articular pathology.
- Certain activities, such as ballet, have a tendency to develop snapping of the iliopsoas tendon as an overuse phenomenon.
- Endoscopic release of the iliopsoas tendon seems to represent an excellent alternative to traditional open techniques for recalcitrant cases.

- When treatment is necessary, most patients will respond to a proper conservative strategy.

"Coxa saltans" is a popular term to describe snapping syndromes around the hip, with an external, internal, and intra-articular type described (1). External coxa saltans is snapping due to the tensor fascia lata and iliotibial band flipping back and forth across the greater trochanter. Internal coxa saltans refers to snapping caused by the iliopsoas tendon. Intra-articular coxa saltans is a nonspecific term for a variety of intra-articular lesions that can cause painful clicking or popping emanating from within the joint.

■ ILIOTIBIAL BAND

Snapping of the iliotibial band is visually evident. The patient will describe a sense that the hip is subluxing or dislocating but radiographs show that the hip remains concentrically reduced despite the outward appearance.

Etiology and Pathomechanics

The snapping occurs as the iliotibial band flips back and forth across the greater trochanter (Fig 30-1). This is often attributed to a thickening of the posterior part of the iliotibial tract or anterior border of the gluteus maximus (1,2). Coxa vara and reduced bi-iliac width have been proposed as predisposing anatomic factors (3,4). Tightness of the iliotibial band may also be an exacerbating feature. This condition has classically been described in the downside leg of runners training on a sloped surface, such as a roadside (5). Some patients can demonstrate this phenomenon as an incidental asymptomatic maneuver. Symptomatic cases are most commonly associated

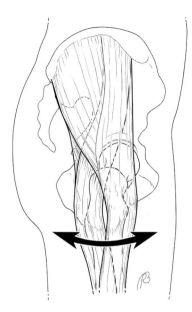

Fig 30-1. As the iliotibial band snaps back and forth across the greater trochanter, the tendinous portion may flip across the trochanter with flexion and extension, or the trochanter may move back and forth underneath the stationary tendon with internal and external rotation.

with repetitive activities, but the snapping may occur following trauma. It has also been reported as a postsurgical iatrogenic process (6,7).

Assessment

The snapping or subluxation sensation described by the patient is a dynamic process that they can usually demonstrate better than it can be produced by passive examination. The symptoms and findings are located laterally and the patient can usually produce this best while standing. The snap can be palpated over the greater trochanter and applying pressure to this point may block the snap from occurring. The Ober test evaluates for associated tightness of the iliotibial band.

The diagnosis is usually clinically evident. Radiographs and further investigative studies are rarely of benefit except to assess for other associated disorders. Ultrasonography may help to substantiate the diagnosis, but is rarely necessary. Magnetic resonance imaging (MRI) may demonstrate evidence of trochanteric bursitis or inflammation within the abductor mechanism.

Treatment

Once the diagnosis is established, most will respond to conservative measures. These include modification of activities to avoid offending factors, oral anti-inflammatory medication, therapeutic modalities, and a gentle stretching and conditioning program directed specifically at the iliotibial

band. Corticosteroid injection in the trochanteric bursa does not resolve the snapping, but may alleviate the symptoms so other measures can be effective.

The published results of surgical intervention for recalcitrant snapping of the iliotibial band range from poor to excellent. Various techniques have been described, but it is generally accepted that the common goal, regardless of the method, is to eliminate the snapping by some type of relaxing procedure of the iliotibial band. The success of the operation may be less dependent on the exact technique as much as careful patient selection. In fact, the published results of the same operation among two different military populations ranged from "less than optimal" to "excellent and predictable" (8,9).

It is important to remember that snapping of the iliotibial band is usually a dynamic process, better demonstrated by the patient than observed by passive examination, and there may be a deliberate or voluntary component to this snapping phenomenon. Thus, the surgeon must carefully evaluate that patient's motivation and emotional stability. The patient is causing no harm by living with the condition but, if they have exhausted all efforts at conservative treatment, then surgical intervention is an appropriate final step for select recalcitrant cases. The patient must be aware that, while the results of surgery may be successful at eliminating the snapping, there is a risk that they may still experience similar or different pain or dysfunction. For correctly diagnosed cases that do not respond to surgical intervention, it is unlikely that there is a reliable subsequent salvage procedure.

Most recent published literature has been based on the Z-plasty technique popularized by Brignall and Stainsby in 1991 (10) **(Fig 30-2)**. They reported eight hips in six patients, mean age 19 years, all with resolution of the snapping and excellent pain relief. Three hips in two patients experienced occasional aching, and one patient underwent a second, more extensive Z-plasty in order to achieve a successful outcome. Faraj et al. (11) in 2001, reported on 11 hips in 10 patients, mean age 17.3 years. All experienced resolution of pain and snapping, although three patients developed painful scars requiring desensitization treatment for 2 to 6 months. In 2002, Kim et al. (8) reported on three active duty soldiers with a successful result in only one case. Conversely, a report by Proventure et al. (9) in 2004 included eight hips in seven active duty military personnel with six of the seven returning to full military duties. One underwent subsequent surgical intervention and was eventually medically discharged from the service. Of note, this study excluded an unknown number of patients who had other concomitant diagnoses, prior fracture, childhood hip pathology, or had undergone previous surgical procedures.

In 1986, Zoltan et al. (12) described seven athletic individuals treated with excision of an ellipsoid-shaped segment of the iliotibial band over the greater trochanter **(Fig 30-3)**. All experienced resolution of the snapping, were able to return to sports activities, and considered themselves significantly

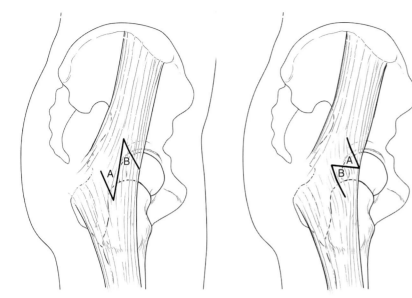

Fig 30-2. Illustration of the incision and transposition Z-plasty technique originally described by Brignall and Stainsby. (From Brignall CG, Stainsby GD. The snapping hip, treatment by Z-plasty. *J Bone Joint Surg Br.* 1991;73:253–254; with permission.)

improved, although only three were asymptomatic. One patient underwent a subsequent revision procedure with further excision of the iliotibial band in order to achieve a successful outcome.

The largest single series was published by Larsen and Johansen (4) in 1986 with 31 hips in 24 patients who underwent resection of the posterior half of the iliotibial tract at

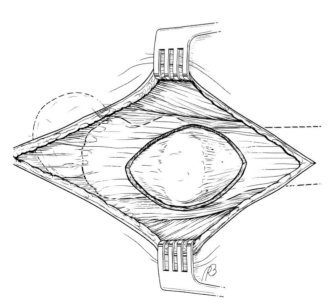

Fig 30-3. Ellipsoid-shaped segment excision of the iliotibial band over the greater trochanter described by Zoltan et al. (From Zoltan DJ, Clancy WG Jr, Keens JS. A new operative approach to snapping hip and refractory trochanteric bursitis in athletes. *Am J Sports Med.* 1986;14(3):201–204; with permission.)

its insertion with the gluteus maximus. The details of this study were brief, but they reported that 22 (71%) were pain-free, six (19%) had persistent snapping without pain, three (10%) had persistent snapping with pain, and there were no major complications. Two of the three with pain underwent revision surgery with good results.

In 1979, Brooker (13) described a cruciate incision of the iliotibial band over the greater trochanter as a successful method of management for severe trochanteric bursitis. William Allen from Missouri (*personal communication*, 1995) has proposed a modification of the cruciate incision in the management of the snapping iliotibial band. This is a method that these authors have employed which includes an 8 to 10 cm longitudinal incision just posterior to the midpoint of the greater trochanter in the thickest portion of the iliotibial band along with two pairs of 1 to 1.5 cm transverse incisions (6) **(Fig 30-4)**. Limited experience in five cases has resulted in complete resolution of the snapping, excellent patient satisfaction, and no complications. The advantage of this technique is that it is simple, it accomplishes the desired effect, it minimizes violation of the iliotibial band, and there are no repair lines that must be counted upon to heal. This also facilitates a liberal, although structured, postoperative rehabilitation program. Crutches are used only for comfort as the gait pattern is normalized, typically in 10 to 14 days. Gentle stretching and flexibility is emphasized, although aggressive stretching is not necessary.

Recent experience has begun to emerge on the role of trochanteric bursoscopy (14,15). A natural progression of this may be toward endoscopic release of the iliotibial band. The concern is either inadequate or excessive resection. Currently, the open method still seems to be better suited for quantitating the extent of tendinous release.

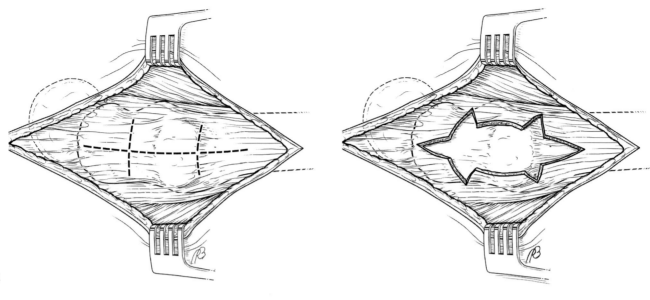

A

B

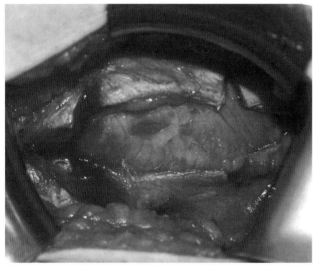

C

Fig 30-4. Approach used by this author includes an 8 to 10 cm longitudinal incision, posterior to the mid-point of the greater trochanter with two pairs of 1 to 1.5 cm transverse incisions. This relaxes the iliotibial band, eliminating the snapping, without creating any suture repair lines that would necessitate prolonged convalescence. **A:** Illustration of incision pattern. **B:** Illustration of relaxing response to incision. **C:** Appearance at surgery.

■ ILIOPSOAS TENDON

Snapping of the iliopsoas tendon can be difficult to differentiate from intra-articular pathology and the two may co-exist (16,17). It is also estimated that snapping of the iliopsoas tendon is an asymptomatic incidental observation in at least 5% of an active population (16).

Etiology and Pathomechanics

Certain activities, such as ballet, have a predilection for developing this process as an insidious overuse phenomenon (3). Snapping may occur as a consequence of injury, but the structural change that precipitates the snapping is elusive. It is well accepted that the snapping phenomenon occurs as the iliopsoas tendon subluxes from lateral to medial while the hip is brought from a flexed, abducted, externally rotated position into extension with internal rotation **(Fig 30-5)**. It is less clear which structure is responsible for impeding the translation of the iliopsoas, thus creating the snapping phenomenon (18,19). This issue has some importance as authors have proposed various surgical techniques based on which structure seems to be most responsible for the snapping (20,21). The most popular theories are that the tendon snaps back and forth across the anterior aspect of the femoral head and capsule, or that it lodges across the pectineal eminence at the anterior brim of the pelvis (20,22). A less commonly proposed concept is that it can snap across an exostosis of the lesser trochanter.

Assessment

Characteristically, the patient will describe a painful clicking sensation emanating from deep within the anterior groin. Usually, this is audible, but sometimes it may occur more as

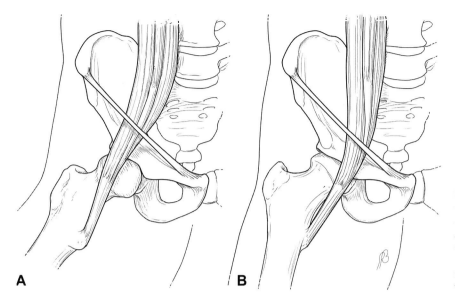

Fig 30-5. Illustration of the iliopsoas tendon flipping back and forth across the anterior hip and pectineal eminence. **A:** With flexion of the hip, the iliopsoas tendon lies lateral to the center of the femoral head. **B:** With extension of the hip, the iliopsoas shifts medial to the center of the femoral head.

a sensation experienced by the patient rather than what the examiner can objectively observe. The most specific examination maneuver is performed with the patient lying supine, bringing the hip from a flexed, abducted, externally rotated position down into extension with internal rotation, producing the associated pop (1). Applying pressure over the anterior joint may block the tendon from snapping and assist in confirming the diagnosis. Some patients may also describe an element of aching rising from the flank, buttock, or sacroiliac region attributed to irritation of the iliacus and psoas muscle origins.

Radiographs are an integral part of the assessment, but there are no findings specific for involvement of the iliopsoas tendon. Similarly, MRI findings are rarely specific for involvement of the iliopsoas, but may reveal indirect evidence if there is inflammation within the surrounding iliopsoas bursa **(Fig 30-6)**. Iliopsoas bursography can be quite specific for snapping of the iliopsoas tendon when the tendon is visualized under fluoroscopy flipping back and forth in concert with the patient's snapping sensation (24,25) **(Fig 30-7)**. Problems with this technique include that it requires that the patient be able to produce the snapping while lying supine on the fluoroscopy table, and the fluoroscopy imaging unit may block the patient's ability to produce the snap in a position where it can be visualized. Concomitant injection of bupivicaine may have some diagnostic value and injecting corticosteroid may potentially have some therapeutic benefit. Ultrasonography may also be quite good at visualizing the dynamic motion of the iliopsoas tendon (26). The advantages are that it is noninvasive and can easily allow comparison with the uninvolved hip. It does require a high resolution ultrasound unit and an experienced ultrasonographer.

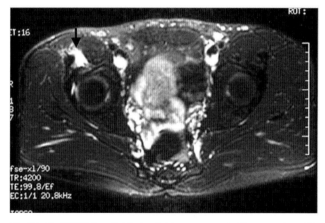

Fig 30-6. MRI T-1 weighted axial image reveals iliopsoas bursitis characterized by high-signal fluid (*arrow*) surrounding the right iliopsoas tendon (Courtesy of J.W. Thomas Byrd, MD.)

Treatment

Once the diagnosis has been established, the treatment for most people is little more than assurance that this is a normal variant and that the snapping is not indicative of future problems. For symptomatic cases, standard conservative methods include identifying and modifying offending activities and a gentle stretching and flexibility program to reduce tension in the iliopsoas, while incorporating a core stabilization program. Oral anti-inflammatory medications are routinely employed and a corticosteroid injection in the iliopsoas bursa may be tried, although this is rarely curative. When a patient fails conservative measures, careful attention should be given to assess for influencing motivational and emotional factors.

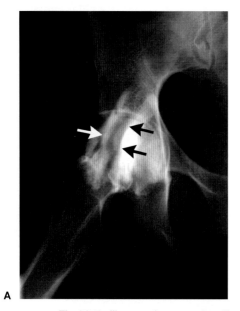

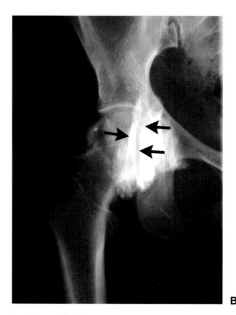

Fig 30–7. Iliopsoas bursography silhouettes the iliopsoas tendon (*arrows*) with contrast. **A:** In flexion, the iliopsoas tendon lies lateral to the femoral head. **B:** In extension, the iliopsoas tendon moves medial. (Courtesy of J.W. Thomas Byrd, MD.)

Surgery consists of relaxation of the iliopsoas to eliminate the snapping. This is accomplished by partial or complete release of its tendinous portion. Various open techniques have been described, mostly influenced by the authors' interpretation of the principal location of the snapping.

Surgery to address snapping of the iliopsoas tendon has been most influenced by Allen et al. (1,22,23). They felt the tendon most commonly snapped across the anterior femoral head and capsule and described an anterior approach to address the tendon at this level. They initially used a vertical incision but then switched to a much more cosmetic transverse incision **(Fig 30-8)**. They release the posteromedial tendinous portion of the iliopsoas, leaving the anterior muscular portion intact, effectively producing a lengthening of the musculotendinous unit. Their cohort consisted of 20 hips in 18 patients (22). Seventy percent had complete resolution of snapping, 25% had partial resolution and, overall, 85% were subjectively improved. Complications included 50% with reduced skin sensation, 15% with subjective weakness, and 10% underwent re-operation.

Gruen et al. (20) hypothesized that the tendon was most taut over the pelvic brim and proposed fractional lengthening of the iliopsoas tendon at this location. They described an ilioinguinal approach used in 11 patients **(Fig 30-9)**. They reported 100% resolution of snapping with overall 83% patient satisfaction. Complications included 45% subjective weakness and one patient who underwent multiple re-operations.

Dobbs et al. (21) hypothesized that fractional lengthening of the tendon over the iliopectineal eminence might lead to less postoperative loss of hip flexion strength. They described a modified iliofemoral approach used in 11 hips of 9 adolescent children **(Fig 30-10)**. All were satisfied with the results of the procedure, and none had detectable loss of flexion strength; however, one patient developed recurrent snapping and two experienced an area of decreased skin sensation. They acknowledged that, although the approach was extensive, it did provide excellent visualization, which is important because they emphasized the extreme caution necessary to correctly identify the tendon from the femoral nerve, which lies in close proximity at this level.

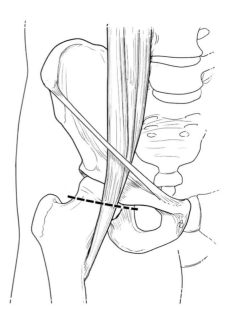

Fig 30-8. Anterior approach for iliopsoas release described by Allen and Cope utilizing a cosmetic transverse incision. (From Allen WC, Cope R. Coxa saltans: the snapping hip revisited. *J Am Acad Orthop Surg.* 1995;3(5):303–308; with permission.)

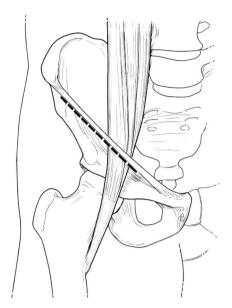

Fig 30-9. Ilioinguinal approach for release of the iliopsoas over the pelvic brim described by Gruen, et al.

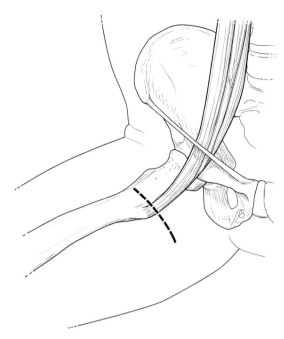

Fig 30-11. Medial approach for release of the iliopsoas from its insertion on the lesser trochanter: described by Taylor and Clarke.

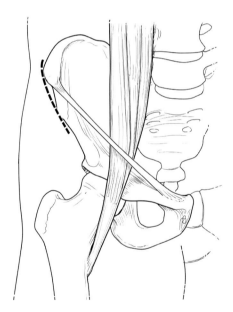

Fig 30-10. Modified iliofemoral approach for release of the iliopsoas over the iliopectineal eminence described by Dobbs, et al.

Taylor and Clark (27) advocated a medial approach, citing cosmesis and avoidance of sensory deficits associated with the anterior approach as its principal advantages **(Fig 30-11)**. They reported on 16 hips in 14 patients where the tendinous portion of the iliopsoas was released from the lesser trochanter, leaving its muscular portion in tact. All patients were subjectively improved with 57% experiencing complete resolution of the snapping and 36% partial resolution.

Fourteen percent experienced persistent weakness of hip flexion above 90 degrees.

Recently, these authors have gained experience with an endoscopic method of releasing the tendinous portion of the iliopsoas at the lesser trochanter (16,28). Among the open techniques, this most closely simulates the method described by Taylor and Clark (27).

The hypothesis is that the solution to snapping of the iliopsoas tendon centers on relaxation of the musculotendinous structure. Successful results have been reported with relaxation at various levels. Thus, the principal feature is to develop a technique that reliably allows relaxation of the iliopsoas with the least amount of morbidity. In this regard, these authors have found the endoscopic method to satisfy this criterion. Also, it has been recognized that snapping of the iliopsoas tendon can occur in association with intra-articular pathology. Thus, the endoscopic method accommodates simultaneous arthroscopic assessment of the joint.

Endoscopic release of the iliopsoas tendon is a continuation of routine hip arthroscopy as previously described using a standard supine technique on a fracture table (29,30). After completing arthroscopy of the hip, the instruments are removed and the traction released. The hip is flexed 15 to 20 degrees, which slightly relaxes the iliopsoas tendon, and the hip is externally rotated. This brings the lesser trochanter more anterior for access to the endoscopic portals.

A portal is established distal to the standard anterolateral hip portal at the level of the lesser trochanter using fluoroscopic guidance. An ancillary portal is then established for instrumentation **(Fig 30-12A)**. The iliopsoas bursa is the largest bursa in the body. Adhesions within the bursa can be cleared, providing excellent visualization of the iliopsoas tendon.

The tendinous portion of the iliopsoas is then transected directly adjacent to its insertion on the lesser trochanter, using either an arthroscopic bovie or other thermal device **(Fig 30-12B)**. As the tendon is released, it will retract 1 to 2 cm, exposing its muscular remnants which are preserved.

Postoperatively, the patient is maintained on crutches for approximately 2 weeks until their gait pattern is normalized. Aggressive hip flexion strengthening is avoided for the first 6 weeks but otherwise the patient follows a normal post-arthroscopy protocol.

Preliminary experience in nine cases with at least 1 year follow up has been quite good (16). There was 100% resolution of the snapping and patient satisfaction, with no complications. No patient has experienced subjective weakness; however these authors have been cautious to select only patients with severe recalcitrant symptoms and it is likely that their improved function due to pain relief may have overshadowed any residual strength deficit. Also five of these nine cases (56%) had associated intra-articular pathology addressed at the time of releasing the iliopsoas tendon. This is similar to the experience of Ilizaliturri, et al. who found associated intra-articular pathology in four of seven cases (57%) who underwent successful endoscopic release of the iliopsoas tendon (17). It is postulated that failure to address this intra-articular pathology in conjunction with open procedures could be a factor in poorer outcomes.

For recalcitrant cases, endoscopic release of the iliopsoas tendon seems to represent an excellent alternative to traditional open techniques. It is an outpatient procedure that allows concomitant assessment for hip joint pathology and

excellent cosmesis. The results are at least comparable to those reported for open methods, with minimal morbidity. However, few patients require surgery for snapping of the iliopsoas tendon, regardless of whether it is performed open or endoscopic. When the surgeon is certain of the diagnosis, the patient must still demonstrate convincing evidence that he or she is an appropriate candidate for the procedure. They must acknowledge that they would not be deterred by the chance of residual weakness. This is especially important for athletes where weakness could be an inhibiting factor to resuming their competitive career.

Conclusions

Snapping hip, or coxa saltans, most clearly encompasses two distinct entities, the external type due to the iliotibial band and the internal type due to the iliopsoas tendon (1). With an understanding of the anatomy, etiology, and pathomechanics, the characteristic history and examination findings will usually lead the clinician to the correct diagnosis. Further investigative studies may occasionally assist in substantiating this.

An intra-articular type of coxa saltans has also been proposed (1). This term is less clear as it encompasses numerous intra-articular lesions that can cause symptoms. It may be a challenge to distinguish whether the source of the patient's symptoms is entirely extra-articular, or whether there may be an intra-articular component. It is not uncommon that patients may present with an element of both. The treatment strategy for hip joint pain may vary sharply from the symptomatic management employed for the extra-articular disorders.

The prevalence of asymptomatic snapping hips in the normal population is unknown. Similarly, the incidence of

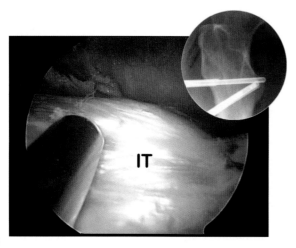

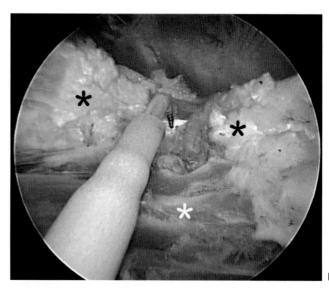

Fig 30-12. A: The arthroscope and shaver are positioned within the iliopsoas bursa directly over the lesser trochanter, identifying the fibers of the iliopsoas tendon (*IT*) at its insertion. **B:** An electrocautery device is used to transect the tendinous portion of the iliopsoas *(black asterisks)* revealing the underlying muscular portion (*white asterisk*) which is preserved. (Courtesy of J.W. Thomas Byrd, MD.)

symptomatic cases is not well-defined. However, it is clear that when treatment is necessary, most will respond to a properly constructed conservative strategy. It is rare that surgical intervention is necessary. Various techniques have been described with moderate success. The ultimate goal is the least invasive procedure with the lowest potential complications that accomplishes the desired effect of correcting the painful snapping. Certainly it is important to select an operation that adequately addresses the structural problem but, perhaps more important to this success is selecting the appropriate patient. This is only partly determined by the anatomic lesion and perhaps more so by the patient's motivation and expectations of what the procedure may accomplish.

■ REFERENCES

1. Allen WC, Cope R. Coxa saltans: the snapping hip revisited. *J Am Acad Orthop Surg*. 1995;3(5):303–308.
2. Brignall CG, Brown RM, Stainsby GD. Fibrosis of the gluteus maximus as a cause of snapping hip. *J Bone Joint Surg Am*. 1993;75(6):909–910.
3. Reid DC. Prevention of hip and knee injuries in ballet dancers. *Sports Med*. 1988;6(5):295–307.
4. Larsen E, Johnasen J. Snapping hip. *Acta Orthop Scand*. 1986;57:168–170.
5. Clancy WG. Runners' injuries part two: evaluation and treatment of specific injuries. *Am J Sports Med*. 1980;8:287–289.
6. Byrd JWT. Snapping hip. *Oper Tech Sports Med*. 2005;13(1):46–54.
7. Larsen E, Gebuhr P. Snapping hip after total hip replacement. *J Bone Joint Surg Am*. 1988;70:919–920.
8. Kim DH, Baechler MF, Berkowitz MJ, et al. Coxa saltans externa treated with Z-plasty of the iliotibial tract in a military population. *Military Medicine*. 2002;167:172–173.
9. Provencher MT, Hofmeister EP, Muldoon MP. The surgical treatment of external coxa saltans (the snapping hip) by Z-plasty of the iliotibial band. *Am J Sports Med*. 2004;32(2):470–476.
10. Brignall CG, Stainsby GD. The snapping hip, treatment by Z-plasty. *J Bone Joint Surg Br*. 1991;73:253–254.
11. Faraj AA, Moulton A, Sirivastava VM. Snapping iliotibial band, report of ten cases and review of the literature. *Acta Orthopaedica Belgica*. 2001;67(1):19–23.
12. Zoltan DJ, Clancy WG Jr, Keens JS. A new operative approach to snapping hip and refractory trochanteric bursitis in athletes. *Am J Sports Med*. 1986;14(3):201–204.
13. Brooker AF Jr. The surgical approach to refractory trochanteric bursitis. *Johns Hopkins Medical Journal*. 1979;145:98–100.
14. Bradley DM, Dillingham MF. Bursoscopy of the trochanteric bursa. *Arthroscopy*. 1998;14(8):884–887.
15. Fox JL. The role of arthroscopic bursectomy in the treatment of trochanteric bursitis. *Arthroscopy*. 2002;18(7):E34.
16. Byrd JWT. Evaluation and management of snapping iliopsoas tendon. *Tech Orthop*. 2005;20:45–51.
17. Ilizaliturri VM, Chaidez PA, Valero FS, et al. Arthroscopic release of the "snapping ilio-psoas tendon" (SS-90). *Arthroscopy*. 2004;20:41–42
18. Tatu L, Parratte B, Vuillier F, et al. Descriptive anatomy of the femoral portion of the iliopsoas muscle. Anatomical basis of anterior snapping of the hip. *Surg Radiol Anat*. 2001;23:371–374.
19. Lyons JC, Peterson LFA. The snapping iliopsoas tendon. *Mayo Clin Proc*. 1984;59:327–329.
20. Gruen GS, Scioscia TN, Lowenstein JE. The surgical treatment of internal snapping hip. *Am J Sports Med*. 2002;30(4):607–613.
21. Dobbs MB, Gordon JE, Luhmann SJ, et al. Surgical correction of the snapping iliopsoas tendon in adolescents. *J Bone Joint Surg Am*. 2002;84(3):420–424.
22. Jacobson T, Allen WC. Surgical correction of the snapping iliopsoas tendon. *Am J Sports Med*. 1990;18(5):470–474.
23. Schaberg JE, Harper MC, Allen WC. The snapping hip syndrome. *Am J Sports Med*. 1984;12(5):361–365.
24. Harper MC, Schaberg JE, Allen WC. Primary iliopsoas bursography in the diagnosis of disorders of the hip. *Clin Orthop*. 1987;221:238–241.
25. Vaccaro JP, Sauser DD, Beals RK. Iliopsoas bursa imaging: efficacy in depicting abnormal iliopsoas tendon motion in patients with internal snapping hip syndrome. *Radiology*. 1995;197:853–856.
26. Pelsser V, Cardinal E, Hobden R, et al. Extraarticular snapping hip: sonographic findings. *AJR Am J Roentgenol*. 2001;176:67–73.
27. Taylor GR, Clarke NMP. Surgical release of the "snapping iliopsoas tendon." *J Bone Joint Surg*. 1995;77(6):881–883.
28. Byrd JWT. Hip arthroscopy: evolving frontiers: Op Tech in Orthop. Special issue: Novel Techniques in Hip Surgery, Beaule PE, Garbuz DS (eds), 14(2):58–67;2004.
29. Byrd JWT. Hip arthroscopy: the supine position. *Instr Course Lect*. 2003;52:721–730.
30. Byrd JWT. Hip Arthroscopy. *J Am Acad Orthop Surg*. Publication pending.

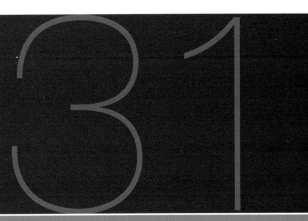

OCCULT GROIN INJURIES: ATHLETIC PUBALGIA, SPORTS HERNIA, AND OSTEITIS PUBIS

MICHAEL B. GERHARDT, MD, JOHN A. BROWN, MD, ERIC GIZA, MD

■ KEY POINTS

- Although most disorders of the groin in athletes are the result of injury, the broad differential diagnosis includes traumatic and atraumatic etiologies.
- The groin involves the musculoskeletal, gastrointestinal, and genitourinary systems, as well as a complex array of intertwining neurovascular structures. Groin pain can be the primary complaint in disorders involving any of these systems.
- The most challenging cases involve presentation after weeks or months of symptoms or when pain persists despite rest and attempts at rehabilitation.
- An occult groin injury is a painful, symptomatic injury isolated to the groin or pelvis region in which no clinically obvious signs are present upon exam.
- Classic hernias are straightforward in that the physical exam often confirms the diagnosis and allows for early detection. Many other groin disorders can be diagnosed by clinical exam with the assistance of various imaging studies. Magnetic resonance imaging (MRI) is a useful tool to rule out serious issues in the differential diagnosis.
- There is sometimes overlap between the three major categories of occult groin injuries—athletic pubalgia, sports hernia, and osteitis pubis.
- Sports hernias may stem from an athletically induced tear during an episode of aggressive hip abduction and extension, such as occurs with lateral cutting in a football running back or the aggressive kick in soccer. The result is an incompetent abdominal wall, usually localized to the posterior inguinal canal, where the transversalis fascia resides.

- The athletic pubalgia/sports hernia occurs most frequently in professional, high performance pivoting athletes.
- Athletic pubalgia and sports hernias occur almost exclusively in males. Women who present with a clinical history consistent with either syndrome should be scrutinized carefully. All other sources of potential pathology and rehabilitation should be exhausted before attempting a surgical solution.
- Caution should also be exercised when considering treatment of athletic pubalgia or sports hernia in nonathletes.
- A significant number of patients improve with a forced period of rest. If the injury recurs upon return to the playing field, a more aggressive approach should begin.

Disorders of the groin and pelvis are a significant diagnostic challenge for the sports medicine specialist. While most disorders of the groin in athletes occur as a result of injury, the broad differential diagnosis includes traumatic and atraumatic etiologies. Several confounding clinical variables exist in this part of the body making it a difficult area to accurately assess. The groin involves a crossroads of multiple systems, including the musculoskeletal, gastrointestinal, and genitourinary systems, as well as a complex array of intertwining neurovascular structures. Groin pain can be the primary chief complaint in disorders involving each of these systems. Thorough evaluation is essential in order to hone in on the correct diagnosis.

Unfortunately this is not always an easy task because the pathoanatomy of groin injuries remains poorly understood.

For example an athlete with a complaint of chronic deep groin pain may have a stress injury of the hip or pelvis, an intrarticular hip injury such as a superior acetabular labral tear (SALT lesion), a classic inguinal hernia, an upper lumbar spine disorder, or an occult groin injury. Other less common diagnostic entities such as genitourinary infections or tumors must also be kept in mind. The clinical complexity of these disorders may lead to delay in diagnosis, which is frustrating for patients and clinicians alike. Therefore it is important to have a sound general knowledge base of the various disorders causing groin pain, and to be familiar with the basic diagnostic and treatment algorithms.

The most challenging cases involve presentation after weeks or months of symptoms or when pain persists despite rest and attempted rehabilitation. Some cases present very subtle clinical signs on physical examination. We classify these disorders as occult groin injuries, and they will be the focus of this chapter (Table 31-1). Other differential diagnoses will be listed, but will be covered in detail elsewhere in the textbook.

In general, we prefer to classify these disorders into three major groups: (a) occult groin injuries, and (b) classic hernias, (c) other diagnostic entities (Fig 31-1). An occult groin injury is defined as a painful, symptomatic injury isolated to the groin or pelvis region in which no clinically obvious signs are present upon exam. This is in contradistinction to a typical groin injury, such as a classic inguinal hernia in which groin pain is accompanied by hard clinical signs, such as a reducible or possibly irreducible bowel loop demonstrable by digital exam. Classic hernias are fairly straightforward in that the physical exam often confirms the diagnosis and allows for early detection and treatment. Many other groin disorders, which we classify as other diagnostic entities, can usually be diagnosed by clinical exam with the assistance of various imaging studies, e.g., a soft tissue tumor or an avascular necrosis of the hip.

At this point, we do not have a well accepted classification system for occult groin injuries, and the published nomenclature is confusing and conflicting. We prefer to consider three major categories of occult groin injuries: (a) *Athletic Pubalgia,* (b) *Sports Hernia, and* (c) *Osteitis Pubis.* It is sometimes impossible to separate these clinical entities, as overlap exists between the three groups (Fig 31-2). However, this classification system is useful as a framework for clinical evaluation and may help guide appropriate clinical management.

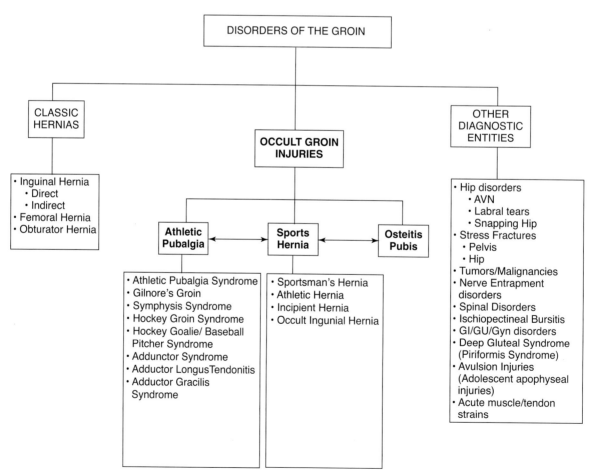

Fig 31-1. Disorders of the groin.

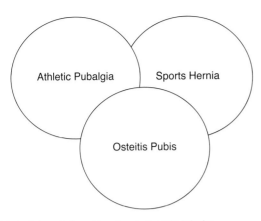

Fig 31-2. Interrelationship of occult groin injuries.

■ ATHLETIC PUBALGIA AND SPORTS HERNIA

Athletic pubalgia and sports hernia are debilitating groin pain syndromes that have become major focal points in the diagnosis and treatment of the professional athlete. The concept of a debilitating focal groin injury was first described by Gilmore in 1980 as a "groin disruption" (1,2). To date there has been no real consensus on the classification of the syndromes. A variety of terms has been used to describe groin pain syndromes, including Gilmore's groin, symphysis syndrome, hockey groin syndrome, adductor gracilis syndrome, occult inguinal hernia, sportsman's hernia, and incipient hernia (2-9) **(Table 31-1)**.

From a conceptual basis, athletic pubalgia is based on a biomechanical model, and sports hernia is best considered from an anatomical perspective. Both syndromes are associated with a significant loss of playing time and can be career ending. However, current treatment strategies can facilitate return to an elite level of play (2,4-7,9-16).

Athletic pubalgia is defined as an injury to the rectus abdominis insertion on the pubic symphysis, often accompanied by injury to the conjoined tendon insertion and the adductor longus attachment to the pelvis (7) **(Fig 31-3)**. We believe the hallmark feature of this disorder is subtle pelvic instability. The sports hernia is defined as an injury of the transversalis fascia leading eventually to incompetency of the posterior inguinal wall (11,15,17) **(Fig 31-4)**.

Anatomy

The pathoanatomy of athletic pubalgia and sports hernia is complex. The zone of injury includes the medial extent of the inguinal canal with the transversalis fascia posterior, the tendinous rectus abdominis and conjoined tendon anterior, and the bony pubic symphysis medial. The adductor tendons and their attachment along the anterior pelvis define the distal extent of the zone of injury (2,7). The various nerves of the inguinal region are involved commonly, which may explain the typical cutaneous pain distribution to the scrotum (ilioinguinal nerve), ipsilateral and contralateral inguinal area (genitofemoral nerve), and medial thigh (obturator nerve) (18). Fon (17) describes the "sportsman's hernia" and proposes the cause as an incipient hernia based on the findings of a posterior bulge found in 80% to 85% of the operations. He considers this analogous to a classic inguinal hernia, where the absence of striated muscle at the posterior inguinal wall and the passage of the spermatic cord predispose the abdominal wall to weakness. In the "sportsman's hernia" an anatomically thin transversalis fascia forms this part of the posterior wall, and is prone to injury. Similarly, Joesting (14) defines the "sportsman's hernia" as an actual tear in the transversalis fascia in the posterior inguinal wall. The tear is located between the internal inguinal ring and the pubic tubercle, typically 3-5cm in length. Lynch and Renstrom (19) also localize the pathology to the posterior inguinal wall.

Susmallian (16) describes the entity of "sportsman's hernia" as a result of a tear of the structures around the internal

TABLE 31-1	Common Features of Occult Groin Injuries		
Type	**Clinical Features**	**Pathological Features**	**Treatment**
Sports Hernia	■ Inguinal pain ■ Lower abdominal pain	■ Posterior inguinal wall deficiency ■ Thinning/tearing of transversalis fascia	■ Conservative ■ Surgery (refractory cases only) ■ Laparoscopic vs. Open
Athletic Pubalgia	■ Inguinal pain ■ Lower abdominal pain ■ +/−Adductor pain	■ Tearing of abdominal muscle attachment to pelvis ■ Tearing of conjoined tendon ■ Adductor microtearing ■ Subtle pelvic instability/anterior pelvic tilt	■ Conservative ■ Surgery (if refractory) ■ Open pelvic floor repair
Osteitis Pubis	■ Peri-symphyseal pain ■ Groin pain ■ +/−Adductor pain	■ Peri-symphyseal inflammation	■ Conservative ■ Cortisone injection ■ Surgery (refractory cases only) ■ Curettage vs. arthrodesis

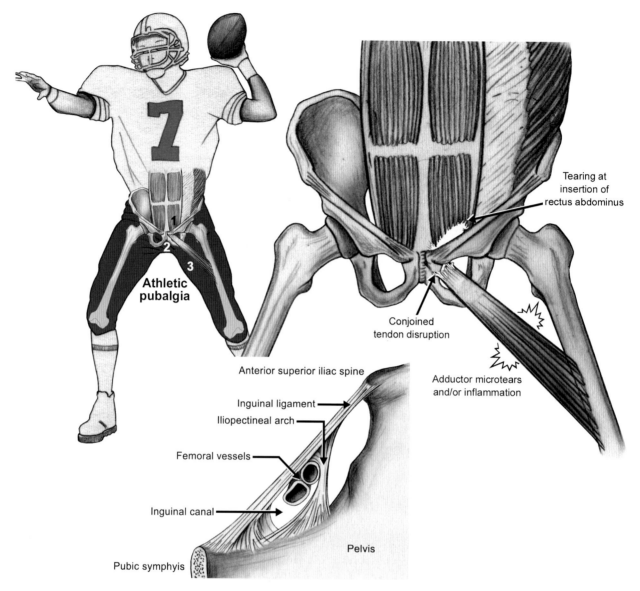

Fig 31-3. Proposed mechanism of injury in *athletic pubalgia*. Primary sites of involvement include: **(A)** tearing at the insertion of the rectus abdominis (*arrow*); **(B)** conjoined tendon disruption (*arrow*); **(C)** adductor microtears and/or inflammation (*arrow*).

inguinal ring and the subsequent progressive weakness of the posterior wall. Kluin et al. (15) also define the term sports hernia as a weakness of the posterior inguinal wall resulting in an occult medial hernia. Genitsaris et al. (11) echoed this sentiment and under endoscopic visualization defined a defect in the posterior wall in Hesselbach's triangle without forming a true hernia. Srinivasan and Schuricht (9) state the cause, in general, to be incompetent abdominal wall musculature. In his series, he subjectively noted the presence of an occult hernia in all cases. In a thorough review of the literature, Mora and Byrd (8) define the cause as a nonpalpable, small hernia with microscopic tearing of the internal oblique muscle attachments. Leblanc and Leblanc (20) state that the entity is a spectrum of injuries, principally involving the conjoined tendon, inguinal ligament, transversalis fascia, internal oblique muscle, and external oblique aponeurosis.

Although more broadly defined, several authors describe a constellation of injuries around the groin that can also fall under the auspices of sports hernia. Macleod and Gibbon (21) define the groin pathology in terms of pain generators. They describe four general contributors to the groin pain:

1 Adductor or rectus abdominis musculotendinous strains or tendoperiosteal enthesopathies
2 Osteitis pubis
3 Disruption of the inguinal canal with tearing of the superficial ring and thinning of the posterior wall
4 Nerve entrapment of the ilioinguinal, genitofemoral, and/or obturator nerve

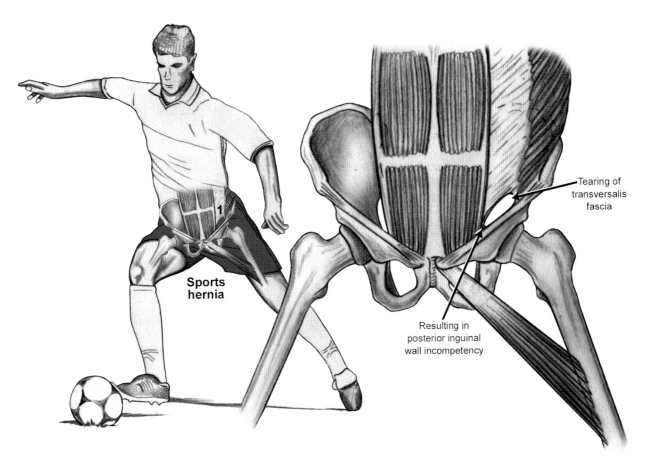

Tearing of
transversalis
fascia

Sports
hernia

Resulting in
posterior inguinal
wall incompetency

Fig 31–4. Proposed mechanism of injury in *sports hernia*. Primarily involves injury to the transversalis fascia, resulting in eventual incompetency of posterior inguinal wall (*arrow*).

Similarly, Anderson (3) describes three possible sources of pain:

1 Abnormalities at the insertion of the rectus abdominis muscle
2 Avulsion of part of the internal oblique muscle fibers at the pubic tubercle
3 Abnormality in the external oblique muscle and aponeurosis

Some authors focus upon the effects of soft tissue injury and the biomechanics of the pelvis, without specific focus upon a structural hernia. This is what we broadly define as athletic pubalgia. Again, this is to serve as a generic term under which several clinical syndromes can be subclassified.

"Gilmore's groin" is an entity that falls under the athletic pubalgia category. Gilmore describes variability in the intraoperative findings, but the main features include a torn external oblique aponeurosis, tearing of the conjoined tendon and avulsion from the pubic tubercle, and a dehiscence between the conjoined tendon and inguinal ligament. He reports no evidence of an actual hernia (1,2,6).

Martens et al. (22), in 1987, were the first to actually describe the concept of associated abdominal muscle and adductor injuries, as they described a specific entity composed of adductor tendinitis and musculus rectus abdominis tendonopathy. Subsequent articles introduced the term pubalgia, later to be amended to the term athletic pubalgia, upon which we base our current classification system (23). These are thought to involve microscopic tears or avulsions of the internal oblique muscle in the area commonly referred to as the conjoined tendon.

Meyers et al. (7,24) refined this definition of athletic pubalgia as injury to the rectus abdominis tendinous insertion onto the pubic symphysis with associated adductor longus related pain. They emphasize that no true hernia is present. In general, Meyers defined the injury localized to the flexion-adduction apparatus of the lower abdomen and hip, and theorized that pelvic instability secondarily occurs as a result of imbalance between the rectus and adductor muscles. Other authors agree, as evidenced by Biedert's claim (5) that pelvic instability plays a major role in the etiology of occult groin injuries. He uses the phrase "symphysis syndrome" as a means to describe the combination of weak groin, abnormalities of the rectus abdominis at its small attachment area on the pubis, and chronic adductor pain from overuse. In his proposed model, the symphysis pubis represents the center of the different local or referred pains.

The end result of these injuries is an imbalance of the pelvic anterior stabilizing musculature, with the strong adductors overpowering the torn rectus muscles anteriorly, allowing for subtle anterior tilt of the pelvis (7). This anterior tilt leads to further abnormalities in the biokinetic chain, which ultimately causes more pain around the anterior groin, resulting in the athlete's inability to compete at a high level.

Holmich (25) focuses on the adductor component of the groin pain and correlates the pathophysiology with the poor blood supply at the tendon/bone interface combined with local muscular imbalance. A traumatic event or multiple microtraumas result in injury and pain in the adductor region, which is richly innervated with nociceptive fibers. Ashby (4) localizes the origin of pain to be at the medial insertion of the inguinal ligament onto the pubic symphysis; essentially an enthesopathy of the inguinal ligament.

Athletic pubalgia and sports hernia have also been described in terms of sport specific syndromes. Meyers et al. (24) describe the Hockey goalie/Baseball pitcher syndrome in which there is a localized infolding of the adductor muscle fibers between the torn fibers of the epimysium. Pain is related to the muscle entrapment that occurs. Leblanc and Leblanc (20) describe an associated entity, a subset of sports hernia, called Hockey player's syndrome or slap shot gut. Anatomically, this may represent a tear in the external oblique aponeurosis associated with inguinal nerve entrapment. Irshad et al. (26) describe the "hockey groin syndrome." All patients were reported to have tearing of the external oblique aponeurosis with branches of the ilioinguinal nerve emanating from the tear. He considers the entrapment of the nerve as the causative agent in the persistent pain.

A potential source of pain in these syndromes includes the cutaneous nerves that pass through the inguinal region. Akita et al. (18) performed a study in which they examined the cutaneous branches of the inguinal region in 54 halves of 27 male adult cadavers. The ilioinguinal nerve and cutaneous branches were present in 49 of 54 and genitofemoral cutaneous branches were present in 19 of 54. The cutaneous branches of the ilioinguinal nerve wind around the spermatic cord and also are distributed to the skin of the dorsal surface of the scrotum. The ilioinguinal nerve and the genital branch of the genitofemoral nerve probably play important roles in chronic pain associated with occult groin injuries. Pain resolution after "sports herniorraphies" may indeed be due to nerve decompression during the surgical procedure.

Biomechanics

The biomechanics of the pelvis are not completely understood. Sports hernias may stem from an athletically induced tear during an episode of aggressive hip abduction and extension, such as occurs with lateral cutting in a football running back or the aggressive kick in soccer (9,11,15,16). The results are an incompetent abdominal wall, usually localized to the

posterior inguinal canal, where the transversalis fascia resides. This theory does not address the adductor symptoms that frequently accompany inguinal pain.

Pelvic pathomechanics can be a useful conceptual basis of athletic pubalgia. Proponents consider the initial injury event, the subsequent propagation of pain, the eventual chronicity, and the final disability as a continuum related to changes in the biomechanics of the pelvis, localized to the region of the pubic symphysis (2,5,7,22-24). The initial insult occurs at the tendinous attachments that stabilize the pelvis.

With this theory, the pubic symphysis is considered a single large joint. Along the superior edge of the symphysis are the attachments of the rectus abdominis, external oblique, internal oblique, and transversus abdominis. Along the inferior edge are the attachments for the adductor group, namely the adductor longus, pectineus, and gracilis. The theoretical mechanism of injury seems to be an overuse syndrome due to repetitive hip hyperextension and truncal rotational movements leading to wear and tear and eventual failure (acute or acute on chronic) of the abdominal musculotendinous attachments to the pelvis (6).

More specifically, hip adduction/abduction and flexion/extension with the resultant pelvic motion produces a shearing force across the pubic symphysis leading to stress on the inguinal wall musculature. In combination, pull from the adductor musculature against a fixed lower extremity causes shear forces across the hemipelvis (3). Once the injury has progressed to the point of pelvic microinstability, the rectus attachment is incompetent and allows the pelvis to tilt anteriorly. Theoretically, the anterior tilt and the unopposed adductor muscle group results in increased pressure in the adductor compartment, possibly creating an "adductor compartment syndrome" with resulting adductor pain (7). With time, the failure of the support mechanism on one side of the pubis creates an overuse type scenario for the contralateral rectus and adductor group, resulting in the same problem on the opposite side. It is emphasized that the problem is not related to a classical inguinal hernia mechanism.

Clinical Evaluation

History

The athletic pubalgia/sports hernia occurs most frequently in professional, high performance pivoting athletes. In the United States, NFL football players and NHL hockey players are most commonly affected (7,24), while in Europe professional soccer players are at highest risk (2,11). It may occur in recreational athletes; however, treatment of this group is much less predictable (7,14).

These syndromes occur almost exclusively in males (7,15). Women who present with a clinical history consistent with athletic pubalgia or sports hernia should be scrutinized carefully. Routine laparoscopic evaluation is recommended for females being worked up for an occult groin injury (7). In one study, 17 of 20 females, who were suspected of having athletic pubalgia underwent diagnostic laparoscopy, and all but one of these women were found to have another cause for the pain, with endometriosis being the most common diagnosis (7).

Typically, these athletes present with a long standing history of lower abdominal pain with exertion. Though the pain may be insidious, often the athlete recalls a specific injury event (2,9,14,24). The pain is localized to the inguinal region, just medial to the external inguinal ring, near the insertion of the rectus abdominis on the pubic tubercle. It usually is unilateral, but can present bilaterally (6,13,24). Pain may be localized to the tendon and insertional region of the adductor longus. Radiation of the pain into the scrotum, laterally in the upper thigh, or to the opposite groin can also be present (8,18). The pain is aggravated by sudden movements such as running, lateral cutting, kicking, shooting a slap shot, pushing off with ice skates, and other activities that involve torso rotation and abdominal stress during intense physical activity. Pain is usually absent or minimal at rest. A common early symptom is that the athlete will have pain getting out of bed in the morning (2). The syndrome is often refractory to conservative management (2,9,24).

Physical Findings

The first goal of the physical exam is to first rule out a classic hernia. After that, the work up of athletic pubalgia or sports hernia is fairly straightforward. The exam is surprisingly consistent (2,3,5,20,24), and in fact, in one study it was shown that the majority of tests for pain, strength, and flexibility of the adductor, iliopsoas, and abdominal muscles are reproducible (27).

Gross observation is important to document any evidence of mass, bruising, or other soft tissue lesions of the groin. Testicular masses must be ruled out. The inguinal canal is examined next and is best done supine with the hip slightly flexed and externally rotated. Examination of the unaffected side should be performed first to establish a baseline (2,6,14). The tip of the 5th digit is inserted through the scrotum into the external inguinal ring to a depth of approximately 2 to 3 cm. In the sports hernia, there may be slight enlargement of the inguinal ring along with tenderness of the posterior wall of the canal. Sometimes a subtle defect can be appreciated in the transversalis fascia as it makes up the posterior wall (2,14). A cough impulse may be evident as well. These findings are not consistently found in athletic pubalgia.

In athletic pubalgia, adductor tenderness is quite common. Maximal points of tenderness in the adductor region are located along the adductor tendons near the pubis with the patient in full passive abduction (5,7,24). Provocative maneuvers such as sit-ups, resisted hip adduction, and Valsalva will oftentimes reproduce the symptoms. Diffuse tenderness over the pubic tubercle and the peripubic region is common. Clinical exam of the hip joint is usually normal with supple range of motion and normal gait.

Imaging

Imaging is particularly important for ruling out other forms of pathology in the differential diagnosis of athletic pubalgia and sports hernia. Most of the important diagnoses listed as "other diagnostic entities" will be evident with imaging studies.

Magnetic Resonance Imaging. MRI is a useful tool to help rule out serious diagnoses in the differential diagnosis, however, only 9% of the scans show discrete musculotendinous injury in the region of concern (7). More recently, an MRI study of athletes with surgically confirmed athletic pubalgia reported that the authors were able to identify several common findings (28):

1 Increased signal within one or both pubic bones
2 Attenuation or asymmetry of the abdominal wall musculofascial layers
3 Increased signal within one or more of the groin muscles

Attenuation of the abdominal wall musculofascial layers was seen most often (27 of 30 patients). MRI can assist in creating a more precise preoperative plan, in particular, whether to do unilateral or bilateral repair.

Overdeck recommends the use of MRI as the modality of choice. STIR and T2-weighted sequences are recommended (29). Close scrutiny should be applied to the abdominal wall, groin, symphysis, pelvic viscera, scrotum, proximal femur, inguinal region, sacroiliac joints, and hip. Robinson also recommends the use of intravenous gadolinium enhanced MR. He demonstrated that in patients with chronic adductor complaints, the extent of the abnormal MRI signal at the adductor longus insertion correlated with the athlete's current symptoms (30).

Currently, absence of MRI findings should not dissuade one from surgical intervention as long as the clinical signs and symptoms are consistent. In fact, the majority of patients do not have positive MRI findings suggestive of rectus or inguinal canal disruption. However, as knowledge of the pathoanatomy improves, associated MRI findings are likely to be better-delineated.

Ultrasound. Orchard et al. (31) looked at a group of Australian Rules Football players with clinically evident sports hernia. They determined that dynamic ultrasound examination was able to detect inguinal canal posterior wall insufficiency in young males with no clinical signs of hernia, and thought this modality could improve decision making for associated hernia repair. Many groin specialists in Europe, including Dr. Urlike Muschaweck from Germany, consider ultrasound as the diagnostic modality of choice for evaluating occult groin injuries.

In experienced hands, ultrasound may help visualize a weak, bulging posterior wall. As technology and clinical acceptance evolve, ultrasound may become the modality of choice in identifying pathology in the inguinal region for those presenting with unresolved chronic groin pain.

Conventional Radiography/Computed Tomography/Bone Scan.
Plain radiographs should be completed as the first line of imaging. In athletic pubalgia and sports hernia, this exam will be nondiagnostic except to rule out other causes of the pain or in cases of associated osteitis pubis. If there is any question of a bony abnormality, computed tomography (CT) scan should be obtained as it has proven superior to plain film radiography for its demonstration of the extent of both osseus and soft-tissue injury (29). Bone scan may also be used, again, mainly to rule out other causes of the pain.

Herniography.
Some authors advocate herniography to rule out occult hernias (32-34). It is performed by injecting contrast material into the peritoneal cavity followed by fluoroscopy to visualize the path of the dye. Any extraperitoneal extravasation is consistent with an occult hernia (32-34). However it is not a risk-free procedure. Complication rates of 5% to 6%, including bowel perforation and peritonitis have been reported (15,17,32).

The current literature remains mixed in regard to the indications for this study. Leander et al. (34) compared the use of MR and herniography and concluded that herniography should be the primary diagnostic tool for diagnosing hernias. Kesek et al. (33) reviewed a group of 51 athletes all with unexplained groin pain who underwent herniography as part of the workup. A quarter of these athletes were found to have a hernia. They concluded that herniography should be included as part of the diagnostic workup. Gwanmesia et al. (32) report the results of 43 herniograms for occult groin pain with a true positive rate of 90.5% and a true negative rate of 100% and conclude that herniography is an effective tool in the workup of occult groin pain. Some believe that herniography is associated with unreasonable risks (4%-6%) such as bradyarythmias, peritonitis, and small bowel and bladder injection (15,32). The risk/benefit ratio has to be carefully considered in regard to how the results of the test will change treatment decisions for a particular patient. Other less invasive tests such as MRI or ultrasound may provide similar information without posing risk to the patient.

Decision Making Algorithm and Classification

A treatment algorithm has been developed for sports hernias and athletic pubalgia **(Fig 31-5)**. Nonoperative treatment is initiated first, since a significant number of patients improve with a forced period of rest. During this initial phase, the basic work up includes plain radiographs and/or CT to rule out any acute bony injury.

Upon return to the playing field, if the injury recurs then a more aggressive work-up should begin. Imaging studies, as outlined in the previous section, may be obtained to confirm the diagnosis and to rule out other pathoetiologies. MRI, ultrasound (US), and (perhaps) herniography can also be useful for pre-operative planning. Failure of conservative treatment may justify surgical intervention.

The management of adductor pain can be challenging. Isolated adductor pain is treated with typical conservative measures such rest, ice, anti-inflammatories, and physical therapy for stretching and muscle balance. The most commonly involved tendon is that of the adductor longus. Treatment of adductor pain in the face of athletic pubalgia can be quite difficult. The literature is largely empiric as described by Meyers et al. (7); however other authors present similar findings (2,5).

Adductor pain with minimal to no pubalgic type pain is treated conservatively. If the adductor pain persists, despite conservative treatment, adductor release in conjunction with an open pelvic floor repair should be performed. The adductor symptoms are considered a consequence of pelvic microinstability and therefore both need to be addressed. Adductor pain with pubalgia symptoms is also initially treated conservatively. If, after conservative treatment the pubalgic pain and adductor pain persists, then a pelvic floor repair and adductor release is performed. If the pubalgic pain persists, but the adductor pain completely disappears, then the adductor can be left alone. The threshold for releasing the adductors has significantly decreased and in most cases, if any adductor pain remains, the adductor is released. This seems to avoid a second operation for adductor release in the future **(Fig 31-6)**. The concept of adductor release still remains highly controversial.

Surgical Treatment

If pelvic instability is suspected then an open procedure that reconstitutes the pelvic attachment of the abdominal musculature should be performed. Meyers et al. (7) describe a modified Bassini herniorrhaphy pelvic floor repair. Of 157 high level athletes who underwent the repair, 152 (97%) returned to their previous level of play after this type of procedure. In addition, the study included 12 athletes who had undergone previous hernia type repairs for "occult hernia." These athletes continued to have a clinical picture of athletic pubalgia. Following the pelvic floor repair, 11 of 12 of these athletes had complete relief of their symptoms with return to their desired levels of athletic performance.

Joesting (14) describes repair of the transversalis fascia with mesh augmentation. He argues against the laparoscopic technique because it fails to address the true pathology. In 40 patients, 36 returned to full, pain-free activity. Irshad et al. (26) report on the results of 22 NHL hockey players with debilitating groin pain, who underwent open operative exploration. All patients were reported to have tearing of the external oblique aponeurosis with branches of the ilioinguinal nerve emanating from the tear. Treatment consisted of reinforcement of the external oblique aponeurosis with mesh

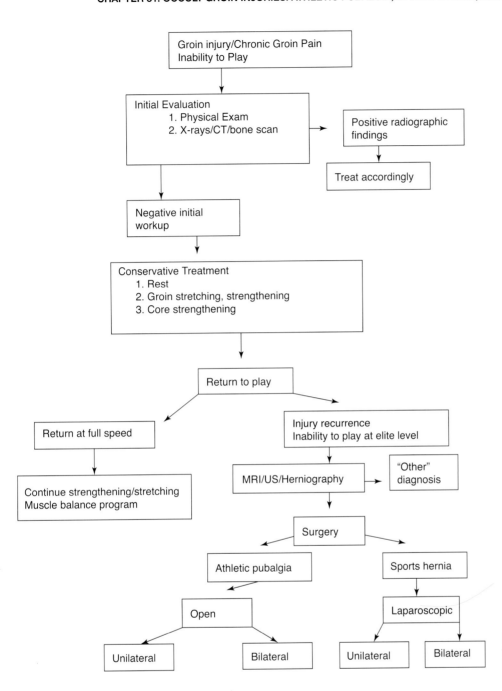

Fig 31-5. Treatment algorithm for athletic pubalgia and sports hernia.

and ablation of the ilioinguinal nerve. All 22 were able to return to hockey with 19 of 22 resuming their career.

Gilmore describes open restoration of the anatomy with meticulous repair of the affected structures without mesh. Exploration is carried out through a 6 cm incision. The principles of the repair include reconstitution of the posterior inguinal wall, repair of the rectus abdominis and external oblique, and reattachment of the conjoined tendon to the pubic tubercle (1,2,6). In his report of 915 cases, 887 (97%) were successful (1,2).

Brannigan et al. (6) prospectively evaluated 85 patients undergoing 100 groin repairs for "Gilmore's groin hernia": Ninety-six percent returned to competitive sports within 15 weeks. Beidert et al. (5) describe 24 patients with symphysis

syndrome, 20 of which had adductor pain. 20 patients underwent spreading of the lateral border of the rectus sheath together with an epimysial adductor release. Return to full sport occurred at 10 to 12 weeks, with 96% of athletes returning to their previous level of sport.

In patients with the diagnosis of sports hernia, the surgical repair focuses on the deficiency of the posterior wall of the inguinal canal. Both laparoscopic and open procedures have been successful, however the recent literature reflects a trend toward laparoscopic intervention. Debate regarding unilateral verses bilateral repair is ongoing, without current consensus. The arguments for prophylactic repair of the unaffected side include prevention of contralateral symptoms, balanced reinforcement, and a single surgical procedure

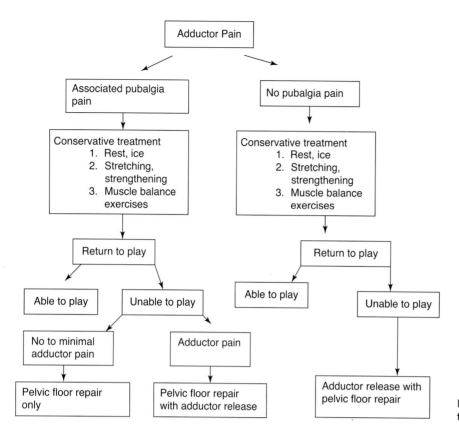

Fig 31-6. Treatment algorithm for adductor symptoms.

(9,11,16,20). Opponents of bilateral repair cite the inherent risks of surgery and the routine performance of potentially unnecessary surgery.

Genitsaris (11) reports on bilateral laparoscopic repair in 131 professional athletes. All patients returned to activity in 1 week with the majority back to full sport in 2 to 3 weeks. Mean follow up was 5 years with one reported failure, successfully treated laparoscopically with mesh. Kluin et al. (15) advocate endoscopic evaluation and repair in athletes as well. They report a 93% return to activity within 3 months. The only failure in this group was a female. In Srinivasan and Schuricht's (9) series of 15 professional athletes repaired laparoscopically with mesh, all resumed unrestricted athletic activity in 2 to 8 weeks. Interestingly, they indirectly address the biomechanical issue by stating that it is "theoretically possible that this reinforcement contributes to the structural integrity of the groin in those athletes, who have an associated musculoskeletal problem."

Complications and Special Considerations

In a review of the literature regarding athletic pubalgia and sports hernia, no serious surgical complications were reported. Minor complications included superficial wound infections, hematoma, and peri-incisional numbness. Failures in recognition of a neoplastic disorder such as a seminoma, or serious gynecologic condition such as endometriosis, would be far more devastating than the clinician's failure to precisely recognize an occult groin injury.

Concomitant adductor pathology is a common finding in athletic pubalgia. Some surgeons advocate adductor release in this situation. This approach should minimize the chance of incomplete pain relief and potentially the need for additional subsequent surgery. However, adductor release remains controversial and further research is needed to determine if this procedure is truly indicated. Certain authors argue against adductor release and report excellent results and quicker return to play with a "minimal repair" technique as advocated by Muschaweck (34a).

Another dilemma involves surgery on the asymptomatic side. In Meyers et al. (7) review of 157 athletes, five (out of 86) patients, who had unilateral repairs returned for contralateral symptoms. Three of these five patients were subsequently repaired and did well. Two patients had tolerable symptoms, which did not require an operation. In Gilmore's (2) series of 915 cases, 10% returned with contralateral symptoms. Meyers et al. (24) now routinely use MRI specifically to assist with the decision.

Those surgeons that perform laparoscopic repair have the option of applying the mesh reinforcement to both inguinal regions. Some, regardless of the laparoscopic findings, perform bilateral mesh reinforcement, citing the need for a balanced repair (11,16). Currently, there is no definitive test or investigation to predict whether an athlete who undergoes a unilateral repair will subsequently require a repair on the contralateral side.

A red flag should be raised when a female presents with groin pain. All other sources of potential pathology need to be investigated and rehabilitation exhausted before turning to a surgical solution (7,15). Similarly, caution should be exercised when considering treatment for athletic pubalgia or sports hernia in nonathletes. Both Meyers et al. (7) and Joesting (14) have demonstrated significantly less satisfactory results in nonathletes, though the explanation is not entirely clear.

OSTEITIS PUBIS

Basic Science—Anatomy

The symphysis pubis is composed of opposed hyaline cartilage covered pubic bones with an intervening fibrocartilage disc. The articulation is supported superiorly by the suprapubic ligament and inferiorly by the arcuate ligament (35). The thickest portion of the fibrous joint is superior and anterior (36). Remodeling of the symphysis is usually complete by age 26. The adult symphysis is about 3 mm wide with sclerosis at the joint margins, with continued narrowing and sclerotic change throughout adult life, and eventual osteoarthritic degeneration (35).

There are numerous muscle attachments about the symphysis, including the rectus and abdominal musculature superiorly, and the adductors and gracilis inferiorly. The blood supply of the bones arise from a periosteal plexus and involve valveless venous outflow from the pudendal plexus (35). The innervation involves both sympathetic (L1, L2) and parasympathetic (S2-4) supply. The sympathetic fibers respond to ischemic pain and can induce muscle spasm, while the parasympathetic fibers respond to mechanical stimuli and can create referred pain to the groin, thigh, and perineum (35).

Pathoetiology

Mobility about the symphysis is generally less than 2 mm; however, both laboratory and clinical studies have identified increased mobility associated with pregnancy (37,38). Shear forces are greatest during mid-stance, when the unsupported pelvis begins to drop (39). Osteitis pubis is probably caused by repetitive microtrauma across the symphysis leading to periosteal inflammation, osseous resorption, or osteolysis along the symphyseal margin of the inferior pubic ramus (40,41). It has also been postulated that following an initial muscle strain, a cycle of events is created, which is then exacerbated by further activity (42). Spinelli first described the condition in athletes in 1932 (43). Inciting activities include unilateral leg support, cutting, sudden acceleration-deceleration, and multi-directional cutting from sports such as soccer, rugby, ice hockey, and football (35,41,44-46). Osteitis pubis accounted for 3% to 5% of all injuries of a professional Mexican soccer club over a 10 year period. It was also found that a higher percentage of midfield players, who perform more multidirectional cutting than other players,

suffered from the condition (45). Excessive firing of the rectus abdominus or adductors, or imbalance between these muscles can lead to inflammation across the joint (35,41-43). This muscle imbalance between the abdominal muscles and the adductors can lead to anterior pelvic tilt as described in athletic pubalgia. Sacroiliac abnormalities can be present, and instability of one or both joints can contribute to excessive forces across the symphysis (35,41,47,48).

Though the etiology of osteitis pubis in athletes is typically mechanical, the condition was originally described as an infectious complication of urologic suprapubic surgery (44,49). Infection of the symphysis has also been described in gynecologic surgery, intravenous drug users, and after herniorraphy, with pseudomonas aeruginosa the most common pathogen (35,44). Depending on the severity of the infection, there can be destruction of the periosteum and hyaline cartilage, with subsequent osteomyelitis of the pubic bones (35).

Coventry and Mitchell (50) reported on the histology of symphysis in seven cases of noninfectious osteitis pubis (35). They found moderate lymphocytes, plasma cells, and an inflammatory reaction along with marrow fibrosis, hyaline cartilage degeneration, and bone resorption.

Clinical Evaluation

History

The typical presenting complaint is the insidious onset of anterior pubic pain, adductor pain, or lower abdominal pain that is exacerbated by activity (43). The symptoms are often consistent with several pathologic conditions about the groin, and the variability of the presenting complaints can contribute to diagnostic delay (39,42). Patients commonly describe pain, when standing on one leg, while dressing (41). Fricker et al. (35) reported on 59 cases of osteitis pubis and found that the range of symptom onset was from 1 month to 5 years, with an average of 14.8 months in women and 9.3 months in men. A thorough history is important to exclude genitourinary related causes, obstetric related issues, and seronegative arthropathies.

Physical Findings

The most common physical sign is tenderness of the symphysis pubis. Fricker et al. (35) found pubic tenderness in 70% of male patients, adductor longus tenderness in 42%, and impairment of hip range of motion in 24%. There is often pain with resisted adduction and active abdominal muscle contracture. We have found that loading of the symphysis with external compression of the pelvis often elicits pain. The patient is placed in a lateral position on the exam table with the symphysis pubis oriented perpendicular to the floor. One hand is placed anterior to the pubis to prevent forward leaning and the other hand applies a downward pressure on the exposed iliac crest. Examination of the sacroiliac joints, lumbar spine, inguinal region, and hip are also important to exclude other causes of symptoms, and laboratory work up for infection or inflammatory arthropathy should be performed, if indicated.

Imaging

Radiographic evaluation of osteitis pubis begins with routine films of the pelvis. Visualization of articular surface irregularity, erosion, sclerosis, and osteophyte formation is often possible **(Fig 31-7)**. Flamingo views of the pelvis can demonstrate symphyseal joint laxity or disruption, defined by widening of more than 7 mm or greater than 2 mm of malalignment of the upper margins of the superior pubic rami (40).

Fricker et al. (35) found that the severity of sclerosis on radiography did not reliably match symptoms and signs. For cases where exam and history are consistent with osteitis pubis, but plain radiographs are equivocal, scintography with Tc99 is useful to confirm the diagnosis. A positive scan will reveal focal accumulation of radionucleotide at or adjacent to the symphysis pubis (40). MRI may demonstrate abnormal signal at the pubic symphysis and/or symphyseal disc extrusion (40). Both CT and MRI can be helpful to identify concomitant lesions of the sacroiliac joint or pubic rami, such as stress fractures. In a retrospective review of MRI and plain radiographs, Major and Helms (48) demonstrated that 6 out of 11 patients with combined complaints of pubic pain and sciatic pain or low back pain, had secondary lesions of the sacroiliac joint.

Classification

Two types of osteitis pubis exist, infectious and traumatic. As discussed above, infectious is often secondary to direct inoculation after a surgical procedure in the vicinity of the pubis symphysis. Traumatic osteitis pubis was separated into four stages by Rodriguez et al. (45) in a retrospective cohort of 44 players:

Stage 1 included unilateral symptoms that subsided after warm-up and returns after training,
Stage 2 involved bilateral symptoms,
Stage 3 players were unable to continue playing,
Stage 4 players had pain and difficulty with activities of daily living.

Debate exists regarding whether osteitis pubis represents a unique disorder, or if it is part of a larger syndrome. Our impression is that it can be both. In our experience, patients can present with isolated pain at the symphysis and positive focal imaging studies. Other patients have pain in the adductor region, inguinal pain, and lower abdominal discomfort. Several authors have described osteitis pubis in addition to a larger syndrome such as athletic pubalgia or sports hernia (2,17,27,51).

Treatment

Nonoperative

Nonoperative treatment of osteitis pubis is usually effective. The first phase of recovery involves rest from all physical activity, the use of ice, ultrasound stimulation, and oral anti-inflammatory medications (35,39,41–43,45,50,52). Oral corticosteroids have also been used with some benefit; however, the risks of this treatment make it a second line treatment option (35,42,44). Phonophoresis with 10% hydrocortisone or topical ketoprofen can also be useful (42).

After reduction of acute pain and inflammation, a second phase of stretching and strengthening should be initiated to reduce the forces across the pelvis. Both Batt et al. (42) and Williams et al. (41) recommend stretching of all muscle groups; however, the hip flexors and external rotator muscles should be emphasized as they are the least flexible. The third phase involves a gradual return to exercise starting with low impact activities that will not stress the pubic symphysis, such as rowing and freestyle swimming. Sim et al. (53) outlined a helpful swimming rehabilitation activity, which includes the use of a flotation jacket with the legs tied together to prevent torque across the pelvis. The fourth and final phase includes a progression to biking, jogging, running, cutting, and ultimately high level sporting activities.

Recurrence has been reported to be as high as 25%, with only 25% of athletes returning to their previous level of competition; therefore, an immediate and aggressive approach to nonoperative treatment is necessary (42). Batt et al. (42) found an average of 3 to 6 months for full return to play, while Fricker et al. (35) report a range of 3 weeks to 48 months. Rodriguez et al. (45) showed that the time to symptom remission was dependent upon the stage of the condition. Stage 1 and 2 took 3.8 and 6.7 weeks, respectively, while stage 3 took 10 weeks.

Another conservative treatment modality includes corticosteroid injection into the symphysis. Holt et al. (43) recommend injection of 4 mg dexamethasone, 1 ml 1% lidocaine, and 1 ml of 0.25% bupivicaine in athletes that do

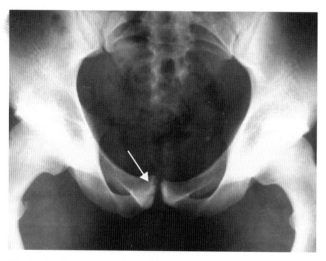

Fig 31-7. Twenty-two year old male soccer player with 6 month complaint of groin pain. Note the unilateral resorption and fragmentation of the pubic symphysis (*arrow*).

not respond to simpler treatment modalities. In their series, seven of eight college level athletes returned to their prior level of play, and three of eight returned within 3 weeks. O'Connell et al. (40) also advocate early injection of the symphysis with 14 of 16 athletes returning to sport after 48 hours; however, only five of 16 remained completely pain free at 6 month follow-up.

Reports of other alternative treatment modalities have been reported with varying degrees of success. Maksymowych et al. (49) described the use of intravenous pamidronate infusions (two injections per month for 3 to 6 months) for refractory osteitis pubis. A total of three patients (two with idiopathic osteitis pubis and one with spondyloarthropathy), who failed conservative treatment were symptom free at 6 month follow-up, and two of three patients had negative uptake on repeat bone scan.

Operative

Up to 90% of cases will respond to nonoperative care, and operative treatment should be reserved for refractory cases and recurrences only (35) **(Fig 31-8)**. Absolute indications for surgical treatment of the symphysis pubis include acute infection or excessive widening of the symphysis with sacroiliac joint disruption. Surgical options include wedge resection, curettage, and bone grafting with rigid fixation (50). Mullhall et al. (52) reported on two soccer players who returned to professional sport six months after open curettage and methylprednisolone injection. Williams reported on 13 professional rugby players with at least 13 months of

failed conservative treatment and found that all players were pain free at an average of 52.4 months after bone grafting and arthrodesis (41).

There is no current consensus on the ideal operative treatment. Rigid plate fixation has been advocated for athletes with refractory osteitis pubis; however, the long term biomechanical effects are unknown at this time. The question remains as to the effects anterior arthrodesis will have on the posterior pelvic ring, specifically the SI joint. Until this issue is resolved, the indication for arthrodesis should be reserved for those refractory patients who demonstrate large osteophytes, gross instability, and complete loss of joint space. Conversely, potential problems could arise from surgical curettage of the symphysis as the possibility of increased anterior instability arises. Curettage has been shown to provide relief in elite athletes, but care should be taken to minimize dissection such that the surrounding stabilizing ligaments are not disrupted.

Conclusions and Future Directions

There is some evidence that muscular imbalance, which may be present in disorders such as osteitis pubis and athletic pubalgia, can be affected by a conditioning program. Hölmich et al. (54) investigated athletes with a mean of 40 weeks of groin pain into an active physical rehabilitation group and a physiotherapy only group. The active physical training consisted of a gradual abdominal and adductor strengthening program and the physiotherapy group underwent rest, stretching, and

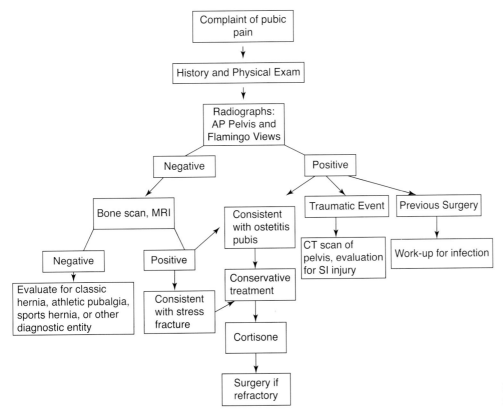

Fig 31-8. Ostetitis pubis treatment algorithm.

modalities. They found that 23 of 29 athletes in the active group and four of 30 athletes in the control group returned to sport after 8 to 12 weeks.

Prevention programs can have a significant impact on sporting injuries. Tyler et al. (55) found that an adductor strengthening program may be effective in the prevention of adductor strains in professional ice hockey players. Thirty-three of 58 who were identified as "at risk" on the basis of preseason hip adductor strength and participated in an intervention program, which consisted of 6 weeks of exercises aimed at functional strengthening of the adductor muscles. They found that there were three adductor strains in the two seasons subsequent to the intervention, compared with 11 in the previous two seasons (55). Similarly, a groin injury prevention program in Major League Soccer teams has been implemented in the United States and our preliminary results appear to be promising. It is our belief that these types of sport specific prevention programs will be the key to minimizing the number of missed playing hours due to groin injuries. Further research is needed to determine the precise etiology, biomechanics, and pathophysiology of occult groin injuries.

■ REFERENCES

1. Gilmore J. Gilmore's groin—ten years experience of groin disruption. *Sports Med Soft Tissue Trauma.* 1992;3.
2. Gilmore J. Groin pain in the soccer athlete: fact, fiction, and treatment. *Clin Sports Med.* 1998;17:787–793.
3. Anderson K, Strickland SM, Warren R. Hip and groin injuries in athletes. *Am J Sports Med.* 2001;29:521–533.
4. Ashby E. Chronic obscure groin pain is commonly caused by enthesopathy: 'tennis elbow' of the groin. *Br J Surg.* 1994;81:1632–1634.
5. Biedert RM, Warnke K, Meyer S. Symphysis syndrome in athletes: surgical treatment for chronic lower abdominal, groin, and adductor pain in athletes. *Clin J Sports Med.* 2003;13:278–284.
6. Brannigan AE, Kerin MJ, McEntee GP. Gilmore's groin repair in athletes. *J Orthop Sports Phys Ther.* 2000;30:329–332.
7. Meyers WC, Foley DP, Garrett WE, et al. Management of severe lower abdominal or inguinal pain in high-performance athletes. PAIN (Performing Athletes with Abdominal or Inguinal Neuromuscular Pain Study Group). *Am J Sports Med.* 2000;28:2–8.
8. Mora SA MB, Byrd T. Hip and groin injuries. In: JG G, ed. *Orthopaedic knowledge update 3, sports medicine. Vol. 3.* Rosemont, IL: American Academy of Orthopaedic Surgeons; 2004:143–144.
9. Srinivasan A, Schuricht A. Long-term follow-up of laparoscopic preperitoneal hernia repair in professional athletes. *J Laparoendosc Adv Surg Tech.* 2002;12:101–106.
10. Ekberg O, Persson NH, Abrahamsson PA, et al. Longstanding groin pain in athletes. A multidisciplinary approach. *Sports Med.* 1988;6:56–61.
11. Genitsaris M, Goulimaris I, Sikas N. Laparoscopic Repair of Groin Pain in Athletes. *Am J Sports Med.* 2004;32:1238–1242.
12. Holmich P. Groin pain in 207 consecutive athletes — a prospective clinical approach. *Scand J Med Sci Sports.* 1998;8:332.
13. Ingoldby C. Laprascopic and conventional repair of groin disruption in sportsmen. *Br J Surg.* 1997;84:213–215.
14. Joesting DR. Diagnosis and treatment of sportsman's hernia. *Curr Sports Med Rep.* 2002;1:121–124.
15. Kluin J, den Hoed PT, van Linschoten R, et al. Endoscopic evaluation and treatment of groin pain in the athlete. *Am J Sports Med.* 2004;32:944–949.
16. Susmallian S, Ezri T, Elis M, et al. Laparoscopic repair of "sportsman's hernia" in soccer players as treatment of chronic inguinal pain. *Med Sci Monit.* 2004;10:CR52–CR54.
17. Fon L, Spence R. Sportsman's hernia. *Br J Sports Med.* 2000;87:545–552.
18. Akita K, Niga S, Yamato Y, et al. Anatomic basis of chronic groin pain with special reference to sports hernia. *Surg Radiol Anat.* 1999;21:1–5.
19. Lynch SA, Renstrom PA. Groin injuries in sport: treatment strategies. *Sports Med.* 1999;28:137–144
20. LeBlanc KE, LeBlanc KA. Groin pain in athletes. *Hernia.* 2003;7:68–71.
21. McLeod D, Gibbon W. The sportsmans' groin. *Br J Surg.* 1999;86:849–850.
22. Martens M, Hansen L, Mulier J. Adductor tendinitis and musculus rectus abdominis tendopathy. *Am J Sports Med.* 1987;15:353–356.
23. Taylor DC, Meyers WC, Moylan JA, et al. Abdominal musculature abnormalities as a cause of groin pain in athletes. Inguinal hernias and pubalgia [Comment]. *Am J Sports Med.* 1991;19:239–242.
24. Meyers W, Lanfranco A, Castellanos A. Surgical management of chronic lower abdominal and groin pain in high-performance athletes. *Curr Sports Med Rep.* 2002;1:301–305.
25. Holmich P. Adductor-related groin pain in athletes. *Sports Med Arth Rev.* 1997;5:285–291.
26. Irshad K, Feldman LS, Lavoie C, et al. Operative management of "hockey groin syndrome": 12 years of experience in National Hockey League players. Discussion 64–6 [See comment]. *Surgery.* 2001;130:759–764.
27. Holmich P, Holmich L, Berg A. Clinical examination of athletes with groin pain: an intraoberserver and interobserver reliability study. *Br J Sports Med.* 2004;38:446–451.
28. Albers SL, Spritzer CE, Garrett WE Jr., et al. MR findings in athletes with pubalgia. *Skeletal Radiol.* 2001;30:270–277.
29. Overdeck KH, Palmer WE. Imaging of hip and groin injuries in athletes. *Semin Musculoskelet Radiol.* 2004;8:41–55.
30. Robinson P, Barron DA, Parsons W, et al. Adductor-related groin pain in athletes: correlation of MR imaging with clinical findings. *Skeletal Radiol.* 2004;33:451–457.
31. Orchard JW, Read JW, Neophyton J, et al. Groin pain associated with ultrasound finding of inguinal canal posterior wall deficiency in Australian Rules footballers. *Br J Sports Med.* 1998;32: 134–139.
32. Gwanmesia II, Walsh S, Bury R, et al. Unexplained groin pain: safety and reliability of herniography for the diagnosis of occult hernias. *Postgrad Med J.* 2001;77:250–251.
33. Kesek P, Ekberg O, Westlin N. Herniographic findings in athletes with unclear groin pain. *Physician Sports Med.* 1998;26:78–103.
34. Leander P, Ekberg O, Sjoberg S, et al. MR imaging following herniography in patients with unclear groin pain. *Eur Radiol.* 2000;10:1691–1696.
34a. Muschaweck U. Hernia surgery in soccer players—a minimal repair technique presentation. Major League Soccer SIMS meeting, 2005.
35. Fricker P, Taunton J, Ammann W. Osteitis pubis in athletes. *Sports Med.* 1991;12:266–279.
36. Keller J, Browner B. Fractures of the pelvic ring. In: Browner B, Jupiter A, Levine A, et al., eds. *Skeletal trauma. Vol. 1.* Philadelphia: WB Saunders; 1998:1117–1180.
37. Samuel CS, Butkus A, Coghlan JP, et al. The effect of relaxin on collagen metabolism in the nonpregnant rat pubic symphysis: the influence of estrogen and progesterone in regulating relaxin activity. *Endocrinology.* 1996;137:3884–3890.
38. Heckman J, Sassard R. Musculoskeletal considerations in pregnancy. *J Bone Joint Surg Am.* 1994;76A:1720–1730.

39. Langeland R, Carangelo R. Injuries to the thigh and groin. In: Garrett WE, Speer KP, Kirkendall DT, eds. *Principles and practice of orthopaedic sports medicine.* Philadelphia: Lippincott Williams & Wilkens; 2000:583–22.
40. O'Connell MJ, Powell T, McCaffrey NM, et al. Symphyseal cleft injection in the diagnosis and treatment of osteitis pubis in athletes. *AJR Am J Roentgenol.* 2002;179:955–959.
41. Williams P, Thomas D, Downes E. Osteitis pubis and instability of the pubic symphysis. *Am J Sports Med.* 2000;28:350–355.
42. Batt ME, McShane JM, Dillingham MF. Osteitis pubis in collegiate football players. *Med Sci Sports Exerc.* 1995;27:629–633.
43. Holt MA, Keene JS, Graf BK, et al. Treatment of osteitis pubis in athletes. Results of corticosteroid injections. *Am J Sports Med.* 1995;23:601–606.
44. Andrews SK, Carek PJ. Osteitis pubis: a diagnosis for the family physician. *J Am Board Fam Pract.* 1998;11:291–295.
45. Rodriguez C, Miguel A, Lima H. Osteitis pubis syndrome in the professional soccer athlete: a case report. *J Athl Train.* 2001;36:437–440.
46. Amendola A, Wolcott M. Bony injuries around the hip. *Sports Med Arth Rev.* 2002;10:163–167.
47. Harris N, Murray R. Lesions of the symphysis in athletes. *BMJ.* 1974;4:211.
48. Major NM, Helms CA. Pelvic stress injuries: the relationship between osteitis pubis (symphysis pubis stress injury) and sacroiliac abnormalities in athletes. *Skeletal Radiol.* 1997;26:711–717.
49. Maksymowych WP, Aaron SL, Russell AS. Treatment of refractory symphysitis pubis with intravenous pamidronate. *J Rheumatol.* 2001;28:2754–2757.
50. Coventry M, Mitchell W. Osteitis pubis: observations based on a study of 45 patients. *JAMA.* 1961;178:898–905.
51. Lovell G. The diagnosis of chronic groin pain in athletes: a review of 189 cases. *Aust J Sci Med Sport.* 1995;27:76–79.
52. Mulhall KJ, McKenna J, Walsh A, et al. Osteitis pubis in professional soccer players: a report of outcome with symphyseal curettage in cases refractory to conservative management. *Clin J Sport Med.* 2002;12:179–181.
53. Sim F, Rock M, Scott S. Pelvis and hip injuries in athletes: anatomy and function. In: Nichols J, Hershman E, eds. *The lower extremity and spine in sports medicine.* Vol. 2. St. Louis: Mosby; 2001: 1025–1265.
54. Holmich P, Uhrskou P, Ulnits L. Effectiveness of active physical training for long-standing adductor-related groin pain in athletes. *Lancet.* 1999;353:439–443.
55. Tyler T, Nicholas S, Campbell R, et al. The effectiveness of a preseason exercise program to prevent adductor muscle strains in professional ice hockey players. *Am J Sports Med.* 2002;30:680–683.

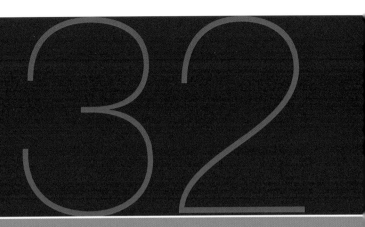

SPORTS RELATED BONY LESIONS OF THE HIP: FRACTURES, STRESS FRACTURES, AVULSION, AVN, DISLOCATION, AND SUBLUXATION

CARLOS A.M. HIGUERA, MD, JOSHUA M. POLSTER, MD,
WAEL K. BARSOUM, MD, VIKTOR E. KREBS, MD

■ KEY POINTS

- Sports related hip injuries are most common in activities that require acceleration-deceleration, side-to-side movement, jumping, kicking, quick directional changes, repetitive twisting, endurance running, and cyclical impact loading.
- In athletes, the distinction between an injury, event, and overuse is important in the comprehensive history.
- A normal function of the hip joint is requisite for successful sports performance, and is based on the anatomic bony architecture that provides the foundation for movement and inherent mechanical stability. Deviations in bony anatomy can result in biomechanical alterations that amplify force transmission, affect the strength and movement-generating capacity of the muscles, and can increase susceptibility to injury and early degeneration.
- Plain radiographs of the hip and pelvis remain the standard for initial evaluation of sports injuries.
- Advanced diagnostic imaging such as magnetic resonance imaging (MRI), computed tomography (CT) scans, and radionuclide scans are useful adjuncts when occult injuries and pathology warrant further assessment.
- Stress fractures are more common in females and result from overuse and overload injuries sustained during endurance in running, jumping, and dance.
- Injuries and lesions of the axial skeleton in the hip joint region, especially those encountered by athletes, are all activity limiting and also have the potential for devastating outcomes. Most bony injuries require an extended recovery and rehabilitation.

Sports related hip injuries are relatively uncommon, occurring in only 2% to 5% of athletes (1). These injuries are most common in sports and activities that require rapid acceleration-deceleration, side-to-side movement, jumping, kicking, quick directional changes, repetitive twisting, endurance running, and cyclical impact loading. There have been reports in the literature describing hip injuries in football, basketball, rugby, soccer, hockey, skiing, martial arts, running, dance, and track and field (2–13). Contact sports have the most highly reported incidence of severe skeletal injury to the hip region (4,8,10). In the acute injury the diagnosis can be relatively straightforward, but in the more chronic and subtle injuries the diagnosis can remain undefined in approximately 30% of cases. This difficulty arises from the complex anatomy of the hip joint, its deep anatomic location, and a high frequency of coexisting injuries that can obscure a hip problem (3). The differential diagnosis for hip and groin pain is extensive (Table 32-1), and should be defined by the clinical setting, as most of the etiologies have subtle or no radiographic evidence of abnormality.

A comprehensive history is critical, and in athletes, the distinction between an injury, event, or overuse is important. Most bony lesions of the hip joint fall into the emergent category, and should be approached with a high index of suspicion. Initially, considering the patient's diagnosis from deep to superficial is an effective strategy, as critical problems that require prompt treatment usually involve the axial skeleton. The most emergent orthopaedic and nonorthopaedic causes of hip and groin pain should be the focus of the initial assessment (Table 32-2), as failure to diagnose these conditions

TABLE 32-1	Differential Diagnosis of Hip and Groin Pain in Athletes

Infection
Slipped capital femoral epiphysis (SCFE)
Femoral neck fracture
Acetabular labral tears
Avascular necrosis (AVN)
Osteoarthritis
Iliopsoas abscess
Pelvic inflammatory disease
Loose bodies
Synovitis (transient)
Stress fracture
Hip subluxation
Appendicitis
Herniated lumbar disk
Adductor strain
Athletic pubalgia
Nerve entrapments
Piriformis syndrome
Snapping hip
Iliopsoas tendonitis
Iliotibial band syndrome
Osteitis pubis/Gracilis syndrome
Contusion
Avulsion fracture
"Sports hernia"
Transient osteoporosis

TABLE 32-2	Emergent Causes of Hip and Groin Pain

Orthopaedic	Nonorthopaedic
Infection	Appendicitis
SCFE	Abscess
Legg-Calve-Perthes	- Retroperitoneal
Dislocation/Subluxation	- Iliopsoas
AVN	Bowel obstruction
Femoral neck fracture/	Carcinoma
Stress fracture	-Testicular
Tumors	-Rectal

SCFE, slipped capital femoral epiphysis; AVN, Avascular Necrosis.

can result in a potentially devastating situation for the patient/athlete.

The age of the athlete should be considered, primarily in the assessment of hip pain, as the nature of the injuries, tendencies, and pathologies differ with the age. The growth of organized sports and practice schedules for children has increased the number of injuries seen by physicians treating the pediatric age group. Fortunately these young athletes are most likely to sustain only musculotendinous sprains and contusions in the hip and groin region. Skeletal injuries are less frequent in this population, and when present are typically apophyseal avulsions and stress fractures that rarely require treatment beyond conservative rest, icing, anti-inflammatory medications, and physical therapy (14). In the adolescent and young adult athlete, more significant sports related hip injuries are being reported (14,15). This trend may be related to a societal impetus for progressive levels of competition, sport specialization, and unremitting practice that exceeds the repair and regenerative capabilities of the immature and growing musculoskeletal system. Sports injuries to the hip and groin region have been noted in 5% to 9% of high school athletes, a higher percentage than that of the overall population of athletes (9). Another level and type of sports related injury has also emerged in adults and mature athletes, and is associated with the effects of tissue aging, systemic disease, and joint degeneration (3,14).

The goal in all age groups of athletes with hip related injuries is to first understand the types of injuries that occur, make the diagnosis, and rapidly treat the problem so the participants may return to their sport with a pain-free hip. Another objective is to identify any underlying bony abnormalities that increase the susceptibility to injury, and counsel them to modify activities and sport to avoid irreparable damage, when subjected to the high demands and hip joint stresses.

Ultimately, the patient and surgeon share a common goal: a painless hip that is strong enough and mobile enough to allow normal function and activity. The use of thorough history and comprehensive physical exam when evaluating hip injuries will establish the working foundation for successful and safe sports participation.

■ BASIC SCIENCE

Hip Joint Anatomy and the Biology of Development

The hip joint is classified as an enarthrosis, or ball and socket joint. The slightly incongruous articulation occurs between the acetabulum, which is less than a hemisphere, and the femoral head, which is normally about two-thirds of a sphere. It is a complex joint and allows rotational movement in three anatomic planes: sagittal, coronal, and transverse. The capsule, which is reinforced by the iliofemoral, pubofemoral, and ischiofemoral ligaments, contains and stabilizes the joint, protecting it from the extremes of motion. The capsule tightens in extension, providing maximum passive stability, and loosens in flexion. In flexion, the 27 separate musculotendinous units that cross the hip joint work both individually and in groups to provide positional dynamic stability. These muscles are unique in their large volume and length, spanning the hip and knee joint both anteriorly and posteriorly, and allowing the hip joint to generate large forces through an extremely broad range of motion between 240 to 300 degrees **(Table 32-3)**.

TABLE 32-3	Normal Hip Joint Range of Motion

Flexion - 130 degrees
Extension - 15 to 30 degrees
Abduction - 40 to 60 degrees (increased in flexion)
Adduction - 30 degrees
Internal Rotation - 70 degrees (increased in extension)
External Rotation - 90 degrees (increased in extension)

Total Motion 240 to 300 degrees

Understanding the normal and abnormal growth and development of the bony hip joint in relation to its muscular, ligamentous, and capsular support is paramount in comprehending the injuries and pathologic conditions that can affect it. Both the acetabulum and proximal femur develop from multiple primary ossification centers, and their final shape is influenced by a dynamic interaction between the developing bone, joint position, and its response to internally and externally transmitted forces (15,16). The physeal growth sections of the iliac, pubic, and ischial portions of the acetabulum join centrally through a common epiphysis, the triradiate cartilage. This common epiphysis is responsible for relatively spherical expansion of the acetabulum during growth, and simultaneously accommodates uninterrupted congruency with the femoral head as it enlarges. In addition to growth of the head, complex structural dynamics occur during development of the proximal femur, which includes elongation and anteversion of the femoral neck, differentiation of the extra-capsular greater and lesser trochanteric apophyses, and transition of the neck-shaft angle (17). Hip joint structural maturation occurs from before birth to approximately age 16 to 18, when the majority of the physeal growth plates have closed. Critical time frames include; formation of acetabular morphology by age 8 to 9, structural quiescence from 9 to 12, rapid growth of the capital femoral epiphysis from age 13 to 15, and closure of the triradiate cartilage and femoral epiphysis by age 16 (16,18). These time frames are important, as they correspond to the types of hip injuries that can occur in the growing athlete.

Applied Biomechanics

The normal function of the hip joint is requisite for successful sports performance, and is based on the anatomic bony architecture that provides the foundation for movement and inherent mechanical stability. The prime function of the hip joint is to act as a fulcrum to provide a mechanical advantage to the muscles moving the leg, stabilizing the pelvis, and holding the body upright. The biomechanical study of hip kinematics and kinetics describes this relationship and defines how the joint interacts with the surrounding soft tissues and environment to generate motion and accommodate the static and dynamic forces that are generated and absorbed. The explanation of joint reactive forces and gait analysis is beyond the scope of this chapter, but should be reviewed by the physician evaluating and treating hip injuries and disorders. Awareness of the normal or "ideal" biomechanical configuration can be helpful in assessing radiographs, providing clues to the mechanism of injury, making a difficult diagnosis, and planning surgical correction.

Deviations in the bony anatomy of the hip can result in biomechanical alterations that amplify force transmission, affect the strength and moment-generating capacity of the muscles, and can increase susceptibility to injury and early degeneration (19). Developmental dysphasia of the hip (DDH) is the most frequently encountered example, and describes a variety of structural problems and malformations that can also result in increased susceptibility to instability, subluxation, and/or dislocation of the joint (20). In the athletic population, the less severely affected joints are typically diagnosed after an injury, and should be evaluated for variations in acetabular position/joint center location, femoral neck anteversion angle, head-neck angle, neck length, and resultant leg length discrepancy.

Clinical Evaluation of Bony Hip Lesions

History

The history and chief complaint are critical in the initial assessment of an athlete with a hip injury, and the information gathered allows the physician to formulate a provisional diagnosis, focus the physical exam, and direct the most appropriate diagnostic testing. Considering the entire patient without isolating the hip injury is of paramount importance. Other historical information that is necessary includes a general medical history, account of previously treated musculoskeletal conditions, family history, and a social history. Autonomous treatments, modalities, compensations, and responses should also be noted. For some bony hip lesions the consequences of a delayed diagnosis and treatment can be significant, and may be the difference between life-long disability and a normally functioning joint.

Groin and/or thigh pain are a typical consequence of hip joint capsule or sensorial inflammation. The possibility of infection should always be considered in a patient with the acute onset of groin and thigh pain, especially when it is constant and unremitting accompanied by fevers, chills, and malaise. Bony hip lesions can present similarly with an acute limp or inability to bear weight, but also can result in more chronic situations with vague nonlocalized pain and/or limited motion, which impairs functional ability. The pain characteristics should be investigated, noting the location, severity, and frequency. A team physician is in a unique position to do this because in many cases they are present to witness the incident and/or receive the patient exiting the field of play. This real-time history and exposure can make the diagnosis straightforward. In situations where the injury is not witnessed, the patient's account and description of the events surrounding the problem become more important.

Aspects of the history in this athletic population that can influence a prompt diagnosis and expedient treatment include: a) the age of the patient, b) injury acuity, c) description and mechanism of the injury event, and d) potential for overuse. These historical aspects will be detailed for each of the bony hip lesions discussed in this chapter.

Physical Exam

The physical examination begins the moment a physician encounters the injured athlete, on the field or in the office. The exam differs for the acute and more chronic injury, and should be guided by the patient's level of pain and guarding. Active and passive motion is significant in this triaxial joint, varies considerably between individuals, and should be measured side to side for relative equivalence. In the acute hip injury, when motion is restricted, palpation of the bony and soft tissue landmarks for pain and asymmetry is most important. Fractures and dislocations result in abnormalities that should be quickly recognized, and should increase the level of urgency to acquire appropriate diagnostic tests and prepare for expedient treatment. In the patient with a subacute or chronic hip problem, the exam follows basic principles. A general musculoskeletal exam including an assessment of gait, posture, physical maturity, muscular symmetry, and body habitus should be done before focusing on the injured hip. Specific exam maneuvers and findings will be presented in this chapter as they relate to the bony lesions and injuries presented.

Imaging

Plain radiographs of the hip and pelvis remain the standard for initial evaluation of sports injuries. Routine radiographic evaluation of a painful hip joint should include the anteroposterior (AP) view of the pelvis and dedicated AP and frog lateral views of the symptomatic hip (21). The information derived either establishes a diagnosis of the primary disorder or screens for other differential pathology, directing acquisition of advanced imaging techniques. In the acute injury setting detection of fracture is paramount, and involves systematic inspection of bony landmarks; iliopubic line–anterior column, ilioischial line–posterior column, obturator rings, anterior acetabular rim, posterior acetabular rim, and medial acetabular wall (radiographic tear drop). Slight variation and malalignment should be scrutinized for symmetry, as they may represent fractures that are not immediately obvious. When clinical presentation does not coincide with the radiographic findings, advanced studies should be considered.

Advanced diagnostic imaging such as magnetic resonance imaging (MRI), computed tomography (CT) scans, and radionuclide scans are useful adjuncts important when occult injuries and pathology warrant further assessment. MRI imaging with or without intra-articular contrast has been considered the second line of evaluation by many because of its high sensitivity and specificity for the wide range of bony, intra-articular, and soft tissue problems that can occur in the

hip region (21–23). In situations where no radiographic abnormalities are visible, MRI imaging has become an indispensable technique with the capability to differentiate the most frequent diagnoses responsible for the painful hip.

■ HIP FRACTURES

Hip fractures, and fracture-dislocations are extremely uncommon in sports. When they do occur, they are associated with direct trauma encountered during contact and high-speed sports such as football, rugby, snow/cross-country skiing, cycling, and all forms of motor sports/racing (3). The injury is more common in the mature athlete, and the incidence may be directly related to increased age, and osteopenic bones. These high-energy and often violent injuries have the potential to damage the blood supply to the proximal femur and femoral head, and even when treated appropriately have a possible higher risk for a compromised long-term prognosis and poor outcome (24,25). Stress and avulsion hip fractures are fortunately the most common type encountered in sports, and occur in a younger age group, and carry a much better prognosis (14).

The hip fractures may be divided into the following categories, based on the anatomical configuration of the joint: femoral head fractures, femoral neck fractures, intertrochanteric hip fractures, subtrochanteric fractures, and acetabular fractures. The majority of reported cases refer only to fractures of the femoral neck or proximal portion of the femoral shaft (26). Regardless of the configuration and etiology, traumatic displaced and nondisplaced fractures of the hip are best treated surgically with open reduction and internal fixation (27). In athletes, these are season-ending injuries, with the potential to be career ending and disabling.

Clinical and Radiographic Evaluation

Patients with suspected hip fractures should always go through the trauma initial assessment (Advance Trauma Life Support). Special attention should be placed on the ipsilateral upper extremity to rule out possible associated injuries. At the same time, careful evaluation of the lower extremity should be performed to identify other injuries. A neurovascular assessment needs to be done as soon as possible. When a life-threatening condition is identified, it should be managed first. The patient should be transported as soon as possible to a facility that can perform definitive evaluation and treatment.

During the physical exam, pain and deformity around the hip joint are the hallmarks for a fracture, which usually present as shortening with deformation in flexion and rotation, depending on the fracture pattern. The athlete is disabled with severe groin pain and an inability to bear weight on the affected limb. When a hip fracture is suspected, AP and lateral radiographs should be performed and will usually reveal the fracture pattern. However, occult or stress fractures of the femoral neck may require additional imaging to establish the diagnosis. MRI is the most commonly used diagnostic test after radiographs, and helps to identify the location and verticality of the fracture (23,28). When the hip pain has been present for several days, a bone scan may be useful to identify stress fractures and pathologic fractures associated with tumors and/or infections.

Treatment

Selection of the appropriate treatment is based on the fracture pattern, patient age, associated injuries, and medical comorbidities.

Femoral head fractures should undergo emergent closed reduction with a posterior CT scan evaluation to determine displacement (25). These fractures are treated based on fragment location, size, displacement, and stability. When the displacement is minimal, the fracture can be treated nonsurgically with limitation of weight-bearing and daily activities, if the patient is reliable. If significant displacement is present, open reduction and internal fixation should be performed expediently within 6 hours of the injury, with titanium screws. When associated with acetabular fractures, usually located on the posterior wall, a concomitant internal fixation of the acetabulum is performed.

Femoral neck fractures are treated based on the Garden classification (29), as nondisplaced (stage I and II) and displaced (stage III and IV), because prognosis is also grouped in this manner. The Orthopaedic Trauma Association classification is also broadly used. Nondisplaced fractures are treated with internal fixation using multiple parallel cannulated cancellous screws, near the cortex of the femoral neck avoiding varus, shortening and external rotation displacement. Nonsurgical treatment is reserved for very friable patients. Displaced fractures should be treated emergently to avoid necrosis of the femoral head (10,24,25). If closed reduction is adequate, internal fixation should be performed based on the verticality pattern. If closed reduction cannot be performed, open reduction is indicated. Radiographic examination of the contralateral hip may guide the anatomical angle orientation of the femoral neck. In older patients, a hemiarthroplasty or total hip arthroplasty are recommended depending upon the degree of degenerative arthritis in the acetabulum (30).

The equivalent of the femoral neck fracture in the adolescent athlete is a slipped capital femoral epiphysis (SCFE). These injuries can occur up until the growth plates are closed, and are most commonly seen in 11 to 14 year old males who are overweight and growing rapidly (15,31). SCFE commonly presents as a limp, groin pain, limited passive internal rotation of the hip, and/or isolated medial knee pain. The onset can be associated with acute trauma or chronic overuse, but does not require these mechanisms for establishment of the diagnosis. In either acute or chronic situations, the diagnosis is critical, and should top the differential list in this age group. If the diagnosis is suspected the athlete should be immediately placed on crutches nonweight

bearing, sent for bilateral hip radiographs, and referred to an orthopaedic surgeon. The standard treatment for these lesions is surgical pinning in situ for stabilization. Up to 40% of cases have been reported bilaterally, and long-term monitoring of both hips is indicated in any patient with a confirmed diagnosis (15,31). Delayed treatment may result in slip progression, and increases the incidence of subsequent avascular necrosis (AVN).

Intertrochanteric hip fractures are described and treated based on the number of fragments and stability pattern. The correct device selection and adequate reduction are the most important variables in the management of this type of fracture. A sliding hip screw is the most commonly used device for this treatment, except in the case of reverse obliquity pattern, in which a 95 degree angle device such as dynamic condylar screw or a condylar blade plate is recommended (32). Another option is the use of intramedullary devices (33). Prosthetic replacement for salvage of failed internal fixation has shown excellent results (34). This type of treatment for acute fractures should be reserved for pathologic fractures, poor bone stock limiting internal fixation, and contralateral severe joint degeneration/fracture that may preclude rehabilitation (34).

When fractures are in the area below the lesser trochanter to the proximal aspect of the femoral isthmus, these are considered as subtrochanteric fractures. Different classifications are based on the location relative to the lesser trochanter and the presence of the fracture line extension into the piriformis fossa. Different fixation devices have been described, including the sliding hip screw, dynamic condylar screw, angled blade plate for proximal fractures, and interlocking cephalomedullary nailing for distal fractures (35). In case of comminution, these areas should be bridged and stable proximal and distal fixation should be obtained maintaining correct length, alignment and rotation using plating techniques. However, intramedullary nailing is the most commonly used method for fixation in this type of fractures (36).

In the pediatric population, acute traumatic hip fractures are approached in a different manner, frequently using the Delbet's classification (37) that includes:

I Transepiphyseal fractures of the femoral head
II Transcervical fractures
III Cervicotrochanteric fractures
IV Intertrochanteric fractures

In transepiphyseal fractures the results are generally poor (38). Only closed reduction and application of spica cast, as well as fixation with pins across the growth plate following reduction have been described (37). For minimally displaced transcervical fractures, treatment with closed reduction and internal fixation with small-diameter, smooth pins, in addition to spica cast has been recommended (37). Cervico trochanteric fractures in children are similar to that of adults, and are treated in the same fashion as femoral neck fractures in adults. The surgeon should be cautious, when applying the fixation devices since the cancellous trabeculae on the pediatric neck are different from those in the adult. The cancellous trabeculae are not oriented along the lines of stress, which may cause distraction during fixation (39). Intertrochanteric fractures are easier to treat due to a more stable pattern, and can be treated with a spica cast (39).

Complications

Nonunion rates of femoral neck fractures are reported as <10%. Rates of posttraumatic osteonecrosis are 10% for nondisplaced fractures and 25% for displaced fractures (25).

Special consideration should be taken in young athletes due to the bone growth pattern that may be affected by the configuration of the hip fracture. Any interruption of the vascular supply may injure the growth plate at the proximal femur, which may cause premature closure of the physis resulting in varus deformity of the femoral head and neck. Additionally, in trans epiphyseal fractures in children, some series described rates of AVN close to 100%. In transcervical fractures, the rates are 15% to 50% depending upon the amount of displacement. In cervico trochanteric fractures the rates of AVN are between 30% to 40% (37).

■ HIP STRESS FRACTURES

Stress fractures are most common in the lower extremities in the athletes and are seen at all levels of training and competition. There is a predilection for females, which may be mediated by hormonal mechanisms (11,40). These types of fractures are typically overuse and overload injuries sustained during endurance running, jumping, and dance (41). The mechanism involves microfractures sustained during repetitive and cyclical impact loading that overwhelm the body and bone's ability to remodel and heal. Once a certain threshold is past, the fractures become symptomatic. Structural and chemical metabolic imbalances can alter this threshold. These fractures can occur in normal bone exposed to persistent abnormal stress, or in abnormal bone exposed to normal stress (12,31). Anything that interferes with bone remodeling, i.e., medications, nutritional deficiencies, and hormonal disturbances, can predispose an athlete to stress fractures under normal conditions. Altered bony anatomy and pathology can also be responsible and should not be overlooked (42,43).

In the hip, stress fractures can occur on both the femoral and pelvic sides of the joint. On the pelvic side, fractures occur in the medial wall and roof of the acetabulum, and in the pubic rami. These types of stress fractures should alert the physician to metabolic or structural abnormalities, as most occur due to bone insufficiency. These fractures are uncommon in young athletes, and can usually be treated symptomatically, when identified. On the femoral side, stress fractures can occur in the femoral head and neck, and depending on the configuration may have much more significant consequences, when diagnosis and treatment is delayed (5,44).

The history and clinical presentation for all stress fractures in the hip region involve the vague onset of groin and anterior thigh pain that is initially bothersome and later becomes unremitting and activity limiting. There is usually no history of trauma. Important antecedent events that should raise the level of suspicion for stress fracture include a recent increase or change in a training or practice program, footwear or training surface, and episodes of extreme muscle fatigue (14,45). When the pubic rami are affected, patients are tender to direct palpation. The physical examination is relatively nonspecific when the proximal femur and acetabulum are involved, and the only finding may be slight limitation of internal rotation in flexion. These findings can occur in numerous less consequential injuries, so frequent consecutive exams should be performed if a stress fracture is suspected. Single leg hopping is a provocative maneuver that can also help identify the problem, but it is should be done cautiously. Further diagnostic testing should be considered if the pain pattern persists after a 3 to 4 week period of relative rest.

Plain radiographs should be obtained in all patients with unremitting hip pain, despite the fact that they will likely be normal in patients with stress fractures two to four weeks after the onset of symptoms (7). The plain radiographs should be evaluated for unsuspected abnormalities, and are also useful later in the treatment process to assess healing. When plain radiographs are normal and the index of suspicion remains high for pathology because of continued or increased symptoms, advanced imaging is indicated. There is controversy as to the best modality for evaluation bone scintigraphy or MRI. Both tests have a sensitivity approaching 100% for stress fracture, but bone-scan lacks specificity and when positive is typically followed by an MRI. MRI including the proximal femur and pelvis has become our initial preference after plain films in the athlete, because the scans are readily available, identify stress fractures, localize and quantify the lesions, define the peri-articular soft-tissue, and can identify other pathology.

Femoral neck stress fractures carry the most significant consequences when diagnosis and treatment are delayed. They are more common in the skeletally mature athlete, but do occur in younger patients (7). The significance of the fracture depends on its location and extent, and if it is associated with any cortical irregularity or displacement. If displacement is present, treatment is expedient surgical reduction and fixation with cannulated titanium screws. Nondisplaced femoral neck stress fractures are assessed and treated based on a classification that combines location and biomechanical stability, lateral "tension-side" or medial "compression-side" fractures. Lateral tension-side fractures are inherently unstable, and are best treated with operative fixation (44). Compression-side fractures are biomechanically stable (Fig 32-1), and have been treated successfully with rest, limited weight bearing, and activity restriction in dependable patients (44). Unfortunately, these stable

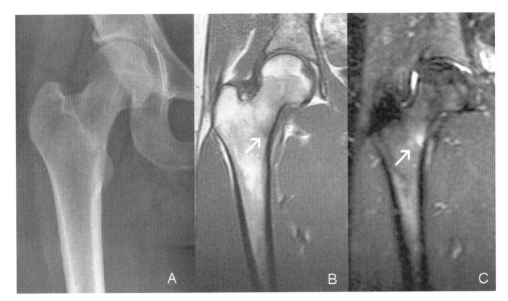

Fig 32-1. A medial "compression-side" fracture of the right femoral neck. AP radiograph of the proximal femur demonstrates a subtle area of trabecular condensation in the medial femoral neck consistent with stress fracture just above the lesser trochanter **(A)**. T1-weighted coronal MR image depicts a zone of decreased signal intensity perpendicular to the cortex in the medial femoral neck **(B)**. A coronal STIR image **(C)** highlights the stress fracture as a zone of marked brightening/edema (*arrow*) on the compression side of the femoral neck.

fractures can go on to nonunion, and additional classification, based on radiographic/MRI findings, is recommended. Compression-side fractures with a visible fatigue line ≥50% of the width of the femoral neck should be treated operatively with screws. Those being treated nonoperatively should be followed with bi-weekly serial radiographs, and if delayed healing or fracture progression is noted, internal fixation is recommended (44).

Fatigue fractures of the subchondral femoral head have also been reported, and are important to consider and recognize because it can be misdiagnosed as AVN, and treated inappropriately (12). This is a rare condition in athletes, and is more likely to occur in individuals with poor bone quality. In the healthy athlete with no risk factors for AVN, the hip MRI should be evaluated closely by a musculoskeletal radiologist alerted to the possible diagnosis. In a hip with a subchondral fatigue fracture, the signal changes and bone marrow edema patterns differ. In cases without evidence for collapse, successful treatment involves limited weight-bearing and rest. When collapse is evident, bone grafting has been successful (12).

The complications associated with delayed diagnosis of hip joint related stress fractures can be devastating and extremely disabling for a healthy, athletic individual. Elite athletes seldom return to their prior level of function or sport (5). When these lesions displace, the outcome has been globally dismal, and reported complications associated with surgical fixation include infection, malalignment, leg-length discrepancy, nonunion, and AVN (44). It is therefore imperative that the physician caring for the athlete develops a high index of suspicion for hip stress fractures, understands the natural history of the process, and becomes comfortable either fully assessing and treating the problem or expediently referring the patient. In all cases, treatment should include careful evaluation and modification of the anatomic, metabolic, and environmental factors that contributed to the injury.

■ AVULSION FRACTURES

Avulsion fractures are the most common type of fracture encountered by the sports practitioner, especially in young male athletes (3). This type of fractures is seen more often in football and soccer players, sprinters, and jumpers (14). When the skeletal system is immature, a sudden violent muscular contraction or an excessive amount of sustained muscle action across an open apophysis may cause an avulsion fracture. Separation occurs in the cartilaginous area between the apophysis and the bone. Occasionally, they may be the result of chronic overuse apophysitis, similar to the Osgood-Schlatter's syndrome in the knee. Different types of avulsion fractures around the hip joint have been described, and the most common are avulsion of the lesser trochanter, avulsion of the anterior superior iliac spine (ASIS), anterior inferior iliac spine (AIIS), and ischial apophysis.

Clinical Evaluation

Generally, when the avulsion fracture is in the pelvis, there is localized pain and edema after an extreme effort. Often, there is no history of external trauma. They are often mistaken for muscle or tendon injuries. Plain radiographs (AP pelvis, AP and lateral of the compromised hip) are useful to confirm diagnosis. When the suspected fracture is present in children, it is necessary to obtain contralateral side radiographs for comparison and evaluation of the skeletal maturity. If the fracture is not shown clearly in the radiographs, but suspicion is high, then further imaging should be obtained. A computer tomography is helpful when the amount of displacement is minimal (23).

Avulsion of the Lesser Trochanter

Approximately 85% of the avulsion fractures of the lesser trochanter occur in patients under 20 years of age (46). This injury results from a sudden contracture of the iliopsoas muscle and presents with sudden onset of severe anteromedial hip pain mainly while running (47). At the physical exam, resisted hip flexion exacerbates the pain. Most of the time, plain radiographs reveal the avulsed fragment of the lesser trochanter (47).

Avulsion of the Anterior Superior Iliac Spine

This injury occurs when there is an over pull of the sartorius muscle during activities that involve extension of the hip and flexion of the knee, like running and jumping (48). The patient presents with localized pain, tenderness exacerbated by flexion or abduction and mild edema. The diagnosis is confirmed with plain radiographs. Sometimes, the fascia lata and the inguinal ligament prevent significant displacement, and a CT scan may be helpful to confirm the diagnosis.

Avulsion of the Anterior Inferior Iliac Spine

This is less common than the ASIS due to earlier ossification and less exposure to stress during running. This type of fracture occurs with vigorous contraction of the straight head of the rectus femoris muscle, a muscle action that occurs with distance ball kicking seen in soccer or football (14). In the course of physical exam, active flexion of the hip reproduces the pain. Plain radiographs show distal displacement of a fragment of the AIIS.

Avulsion of the Ischial Apophysis

This type of fracture may happen in patients up to age 25, when the ischial apophysis unites with the bony skeleton, one of the last to fuse (48). Avulsion is caused by maximum hamstring contraction with the pelvis fixed in flexion and the knee in extension (47). This mechanism of injury may be seen in gymnastics and hurdling. The patient usually presents with sudden onset of pain at the ischial tuberosity with tenderness to palpation, discomfort when sitting and occasionally an antalgic gait. Physical exam reveals pain when the knee is extended and the hip is flexed, the classic hamstring stretch

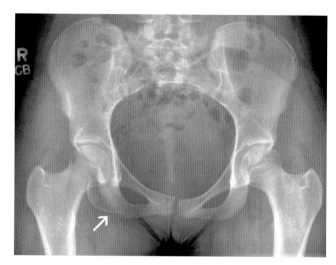

Fig 32-2. AP radiograph of the pelvis demonstrates an acute displaced avulsion fracture of the right ischial tuberosity (*arrow*) in a skeletally immature female athlete.

position. Plain radiographs show a displaced fragment of the ischial tuberosity **(Fig 32-2)**. Displacement of this fragment is rarely significant because of the robust sacrotuberous ligament.

Treatment

The treatment of avulsion fractures depends on the type of fracture and amount of displacement. Most avulsion fractures of the pelvis and hip can be treated nonoperatively, with initial bed rest, ice, and analgesics (47,49–51). Open reduction and internal fixation have been advocated by some when the displacement is significant enough to create a functional disability in competitive athletes (50). The implementation of a rehabilitation program is key in the treatment of these fractures, with increased excursion an early goal can be achieved through gentle active and passive range of motion exercises (49). Progressive resistance exercise is started when 75% of the range of motion is achieved. Once the involved muscles have regained 50% of their anticipated strength the resistance exercise can be stopped. Before returning to competitive sports integration of muscle function should be attained through stretching and strengthening exercises combined with pattern motions (49).

Complications

After conservative treatment, the development of hypertrophic callus has been described (14). Additionally, nonunion and chronic pain may cause functional disability and may require surgical intervention remote to the injury (14).

■ AVASCULAR NECROSIS OF THE FEMORAL HEAD

AVN or osteonecrosis of the femoral head as a direct result of sports participation or training without significant prior injury has not been described. Often the diagnosis is made incidentally, when an athlete is being evaluated for another problem, because more than one-third of the cases are idiopathic. AVN is more common in males, typically affects patients in their 30s and 40s, and is bilateral in 50% of the cases (52). It usually presents with pain in the groin region, exacerbated with activity and ambulation, but may also be asymptomatic in early stages. It should be suspected in athletes with recurrent groin pain, especially in individuals with risk factors such as steroid use, smoking, alcohol abuse, and hypercoagulable states. Special attention should be taken in the athlete with recurrent groin pain after trauma, as the reported incidence of traumatic AVN is 10% (53). Femoral head osteonecrosis is the result of altered blood supply, which causes bone necrosis, subcortical fractures, and finally collapse of the hip joint. It has been reported after hip subluxation, dislocation, and femoral neck fractures, which can all cause traumatic disruption of the vasculature (29). In the young athlete under age 12 experiencing continued groin pain and limping, Legg-Cálve-Perthes Syndrome is a variant of AVN that should be considered. In this condition, the growing femoral head loses its blood supply and a portion of the femoral head dies, causing a flattening of the weight-bearing surface of the femoral head that has a characteristic radiographic appearance.

Clinical and Radiographic Evaluation

Osteonecrosis of the femoral head should be always considered as a possible cause of persistent hip or groin pain in young, high-level athletes, because the institution of the appropriate treatment may help to prevent later degenerative sequelae. The onset of hip pain may coincide temporally with a traumatic injury. These patients generally have normal findings on radiographs at presentation (54). However, if the symptoms persist, a further diagnostic imaging with MRI is required.

Classification and treatment of AVN are based on symptoms, radiographs, and MRI findings (55). Stage 0 is when asymptomatic patients have osteonecrotic findings in MRI. Stage I is when symptomatic patients have positive MRI findings without abnormality in plain radiographs. In stage II, radiographs show sclerotic bone in the femoral head without subchondral bone collapse and in stage III subchondral bone collapse is evident (crescent sign). In stage IV, there is collapse of the femoral head with secondary degenerative changes of the hip joint. When >30% of the femoral head is involved the prognosis is considered to be poor (56).

Treatment

Treatment of these lesions depends on the stage of AVN at the time of diagnosis. The initial stages (0 to II) are best treated conservatively. Wang et al. (57) compared the use of noninvasive treatment with extracorporeal shock waves to core decompression and bone grafting in young patients

with early-stage osteonecrosis, and concluded that the former appeared to be more effective than the latter.

Joint preserving-measures such as core decompression and vascularized fibular graft have been described. Core decompression involves drilling multiple holes through the avascular portion of the femoral head under fluoroscopic guidance. Vascularized bone grafting involves the use of a vascularized fibular graft with microsurgical anastomosis to local blood vessels. The vascularized graft is harvested from the mid-shaft fibula, which is then inserted through a drill hole into the avascular zone of the femoral head. In a study done by Kim et al. (58), vascularized fibular grafting was associated with better clinical results and was more effective than nonvascularized fibular grafting for the prevention of collapse of the femoral head in a population with stage II or higher AVN lesions. The results of vascularized grafting were best when the procedure was used to treat precollapse lesions.

In more advanced stages (III and IV), hemi-resurfacing arthroplasty may be considered in the younger athlete. In middle-aged and older patients, total hip arthroplasty is the treatment of choice. Recently, bone grafting of the femoral head by elevating the articular cartilage flap (trapdoor approach) has been described for patients with stage II and III AVN, and may be an excellent alternative to arthroplasty in the younger patient (56).

■ DISLOCATION AND SUBLUXATION

Hip dislocation is a high-energy traumatic injury, and is an absolute orthopaedic emergency. The injury is most commonly seen in motor vehicle accidents and motor sports. In nonvehicle based sports the incidence of hip dislocation is rare, but the injury has been reported in football, rugby, hockey, gymnastics, skiing, and snowboarding (8,10,59–61). Although hip dislocation in contact sports is usually isolated and not associated with other visceral injuries, a screening trauma evaluation should always be performed. The age of the patient is an important consideration when dislocation is suspected because the injury may occur in lower energy situations, but has the same consequences (62). Traumatic hip subluxation follows the same injury pattern as dislocation, and is essentially the same injury with the same implications, but occurs in lower energy circumstances. The transient nature of these injuries and lack of deformity may result in under-diagnosis, and for this reason subluxation may ultimately be more significant than dislocation, because they are not evaluated and treated with the same level of urgency (8). The hip subluxation/dislocation continuum is associated with a very high incidence of long-term complications and disability, when the diagnosis and treatment are delayed (25,63,64).

Hip dislocation and subluxation can occur in anterior and posterior directions. Classification systems reference this directionality, which is based on the underlying biomechanics of the joint and capsule. The patient's bony morphology and capsular compliance also influence susceptibility; dysplastic hips with shallow acetabuli, patients with connective tissue disorders, and young patients with cartilaginous pliability and ligamentous laxity are at increased risk for dislocation or subluxation. The hip is in its most stable configuration in full extension, with the capsule and ligaments twisted tight and the articular surfaces compressed. In flexion the ligaments are lax and stability depends on articular congruence, which is optimized in abduction and external rotation, and least congruent in adduction. These biomechanical concepts are supported clinically by the fact that posterior dislocations are by far the most common, and account for up to 90% of all hip dislocations (25). The extent of bony damage is also dependent on the position of the leg when axial force is transmitted. When the leg is neutral or adducted, a simple dislocation without fracture occurs, but when the leg is abducted, a posterior wall acetabular and femoral head fracture is likely because increased force is required to overcome the congruence of the articular surfaces. Conversely, anterior dislocations are rare, accounting for 10% to 18% of hip dislocations, as would be predicted by the biomechanics (25). In sports, anterior dislocations have only been reported in snowboarding (60). Anterior dislocations occur in superior and inferior directions, the later being more common because the hip is in a relaxed capsule position of flexion.

Dislocations and subluxations typically present acutely during sports competition, and are caused by falls on a flexed knee with the hip adducted and flexed, but also can occur with direct blows to the hip region and knee in the same position (8). Dislocations are obvious and extremely painful, the affected leg is typically in a flexed and internally or externally rotated position, and a leg length discrepancy may be evident. Subluxations occur from the same mechanism, but spontaneous relocation can occur and the leg length discrepancy is not present. In both situations joint movement is actively and passively limited by pain. The athlete is not capable of standing when a dislocation has occurred, and should not be encouraged to stand if a subluxation is suspected. There are advocates for attempting gentle closed reduction immediately when these injuries are witnessed on the field, while the trauma literature supports reduction under anesthesia or sedation to avoid further damage to the femoral head or acetabular rim caused by muscle spasm and involuntary resistance (10,65).

When a hip dislocation or subluxation is suspected, plain radiographs with oblique views should be obtained emergently. In the case of dislocation, the patient should be taken to the operating room within 6 to 12 hours of the injury for attempted reduction under anesthesia, with the orthopaedic surgeon prepared to open the hip if a stable reduction cannot be achieved (63,65). The need for repeated attempts at relocation increases the complication rate (65). After a closed reduction and in cases of suspected subluxation with joint asymmetry on plain films and/or evidence of a posterior rim fracture, an MRI and/or CT scan should be obtained to

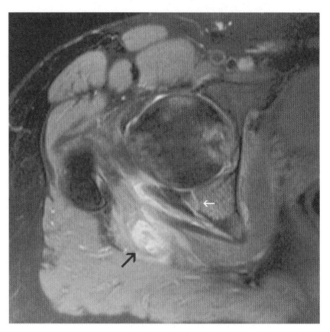

Fig 32-3. Axial T2 fat-saturation MRI performed after closed reduction of a traumatic right hip dislocation. The scan reveals a concentric reduction, a nondisplaced posterior acetabular lip fracture (*white arrow*), and significant posterior capsular disruption and tissue edema (*black arrow*).

assess congruency, hemarthrosis, and to exclude associated femoral head or acetabular fractures **(Fig 32-3)**. When fractures are found, open concentric reduction of the joint and fixation of substantial bony rim or head fragments should be performed. In cases of subluxation, aspiration of a hemarthrosis has been shown to effectively decompress the joint and decrease the likelihood of AVN and chondrolysis (8). Postreduction stability should be assessed, as it will determine the postoperative treatment. After definitive reduction and decompression have been confirmed, postoperative motion and weight-bearing are based on the postreduction stability of the joint. Unstable joints are treated in skeletal traction for 4 to 6 weeks, and then progressed like stable joints and subluxations that are treated with touch down weight-bearing, crutches, and progressive motion for 6 weeks before the joint is loaded. MRI is repeated at 6 weeks to evaluate for signs of osteonecrosis with further surveillance based on the results (66).

Complications and the prognosis for a hip joint that has dislocated are related to the severity of the dislocation, the presence of associated fracture, and the timing of the reduction in relation to the injury (25,63,64). Femoral artery and nerve injury can occur, but are not common; in contrast sciatic nerve injuries are relatively common, with an incidence approaching 10% in posterior dislocations (67). Osteonecrosis of the femoral head is the most serious and disabling consequence. In simple dislocations, the rate of osteonecrosis is about 10%, which is similar in adults and children. In fracture dislocations, the rate of osteonecrosis can approach 50%. In cases of subluxation, the true rate of osteonecrosis cannot be determined. In the series reported by Mooreman et al. (8), 2 out of 8 patients developed osteonecrosis, suggesting a rate of 25%. Posttraumatic hip degeneration is the most significant and common complication that occurs after hip dislocation, and has been shown to increase in situations where concentric reduction is not achieved, the time delay to reduction is greater than 12 hours, hemarthrosis are not evacuated, and in patients that develop osteonecrosis (8,25,63,64).

■ CONCLUSIONS AND FUTURE DIRECTIONS

Injuries and lesions of the axial skeleton in the hip joint region, especially those encountered in the athletic population, are all activity limiting and also have the potential for devastating outcomes. Most bony injuries have an extended recovery and rehabilitation. Frustration from all involved—athlete, parents, and coaches—will likely be directed at the medical team. Understanding the bony pathology responsible for these hip injuries, the mechanisms, and clinical presentation is critical for the physician to appropriately care for the athlete and safely return them to their sport. When any bony injury to the hip is suspected, every athlete should be placed on crutches nonweight bearing, plain radiographs should be obtained without delay, and advanced radiography should be considered if the symptoms and exam do not correlate. The most important aspect to understand is that the majority of these bony injuries require prompt diagnosis and treatment to avoid lifelong pain and disability, a consequence that will always be significantly greater than missing any sporting event, season, scholarship, or career.

■ REFERENCES

1. Morelli V, Smith V. Groin injuries in athletes. *Am Fam Physician.* 2001;64:1405–1414.
2. Beck T, Messmer P, Regazzoni P. Unilateral apophyseal fracture of the superior anterior iliac crest—a case report. *Swiss Surg.* 2003;9:31–34.
3. Boyd KT, Peirce NS, Batt ME. Common hip injuries in sport. *Sports Med.* 1997;24:273–288.
4. Giza E, Mithofer K, Matthews H, et al. Hip fracture-dislocation in football: a report of two cases and review of the literature. *Br J Sports Med.* 2004;38:E17.
5. Johansson C, Ekenman I, Tornkvist H, et al. Stress fractures of the femoral neck in athletes. The consequence of a delay in diagnosis. *Am J Sports Med.* 1990;18:524–528.
6. LeBlanc KE, LeBlanc KA. Groin pain in athletes. *Hernia.* 2003;7:68–71.
7. Lehman RA, Jr, Shah SA. Tension-sided femoral neck stress fracture in a skeletally immature patient. A case report. *J Bone Joint Surg Am.* 2004;86A:1292–1295.
8. Moorman CT III, Warren RF, Hershman EB, et al. Traumatic posterior hip subluxation in American football. *J Bone Joint Surg Am.* 2003;85A:1190–1196.
9. Morelli V, Espinoza L. Groin injuries and groin pain in athletes: part 2. *Prim Care.* 2005;32:185–200.
10. Pallia CS, Scott RE, Chao DJ. Traumatic hip dislocation in athletes. *Curr Sports Med Rep.* 2002;1:338–345.
11. Paluska SA. An overview of hip injuries in running. *Sports Med.* 2005;35:991–1014.
12. Song WS, Yoo JJ, Koo KH, et al. Subchondral fatigue fracture of the femoral head in military recruits. *J Bone Joint Surg Am.* 2004;86A:1917–1924.
13. Weaver CJ, Major NM, Garrett WE, et al. Femoral head osteochondral lesions in painful hips of athletes: MR imaging findings. *AJR Am J Roentgenol.* 2002;178:973–977.
14. Waters PM, Millis MB. Hip and pelvic injuries in the young athlete. *Clin Sports Med.* 1988;7:513–526.
15. Adkins SB III, Figler RA. Hip pain in athletes. *Am Fam Physician.* 2000;61:2109–2118.
16. Bullough P, Goodfellow J, Greenwald AS, et al. Incongruent surfaces in the human hip joint. *Nature.* 1968;217:1290.
17. Ponseti IV. Growth and development of the acetabulum in the normal child. Anatomical, histological, and roentgenographic studies. *J Bone Joint Surg Am.* 1978;60:575–585.
18. Bombelli R, Santore RF, Poss R. Mechanics of the normal and osteoarthritic hip. A new perspective. *Clin Orthop Relat Res.* 1984;69–78.
19. Reikeras O, Bjerkreim I, Kolbenstvedt A. Anteversion of the acetabulum and femoral neck in normals and in patients with osteoarthritis of the hip. *Acta Orthop Scand.* 1983;54:18–23.
20. Delp SL, Maloney W. Effects of hip center location on the moment-generating capacity of the muscles. *J Biomech.* 1993;26: 485–499.
21. Bencardino JT, Kassarjian A, Palmer WE. Magnetic resonance imaging of the hip: sports-related injuries. *Top Magn Reson Imaging.* 2003;14:145–160.
22. De Paulis F, Cacchio A, Michelini O, et al. Sports injuries in the pelvis and hip: diagnostic imaging. *Eur J Radiol.* 1998;27(suppl 1):S49–S59.
23. Overdeck KH, Palmer WE. Imaging of hip and groin injuries in athletes. *Semin Musculoskelet Radiol.* 2004;8:41–55.
24. Ogden JA. Changing patterns of proximal femoral vascularity. *J Bone Joint Surg Am.* 1974;56:941–950.
25. Sahin V, Karakas ES, Aksu S, et al. Traumatic dislocation and fracture-dislocation of the hip: a long-term follow-up study. *J Trauma.* 2003;54:520–529.
26. Bartonicek J. Pauwels' classification of femoral neck fractures: correct interpretation of the original. *J Orthop Trauma.* 2001;15: 358–360.
27. Lu-Yao GL, Keller RB, Littenberg B, et al. Outcomes after displaced fractures of the femoral neck. A meta-analysis of one hundred and six published reports. *J Bone Joint Surg Am.* 1994;76:15–25.
28. Boutin RD, Newman JS. MR imaging of sports-related hip disorders. *Magn Reson Imaging Clin N Am.* 2003;11:255–281.
29. Garden RS. Malreduction and avascular necrosis in subcapital fractures of the femur. *J Bone Joint Surg Br.* 1971;53:183–197.
30. Bhandari M, Devereaux PJ, Swiontkowski MF, et al. Internal fixation compared with arthroplasty for displaced fractures of the femoral neck. A meta-analysis. *J Bone Joint Surg Am.* 2003;85A: 1673–1681.
31. O'Kane JW. Anterior hip pain. *Am Fam Physician.* 1999;60: 1687–1696.
32. Haidukewych GJ, Israel TA, Berry DJ. Reverse obliquity fractures of the intertrochanteric region of the femur. *J Bone Joint Surg Am.* 2001;83A:643–650.
33. Adams CI, Robinson CM, Court-Brown CM, et al. Prospective randomized controlled trial of an intramedullary nail versus dynamic screw and plate for intertrochanteric fractures of the femur. *J Orthop Trauma.* 2001;15:394–400.

34. Haidukewych GJ, Berry DJ. Hip arthroplasty for salvage of failed treatment of intertrochanteric hip fractures. *J Bone Joint Surg Am.* 2003;85A:899–904.

35. Vaidya SV, Dholakia DB, Chatterjee A. The use of a dynamic condylar screw and biological reduction techniques for subtrochanteric femur fracture. *Injury.* 2003;34:123–128.

36. Wiss DA, Brien WW. Subtrochanteric fractures of the femur. Results of treatment by interlocking nailing. *Clin Orthop Relat Res.* 1992;283:231–236.

37. Pape HC, Krettek C, Friedrich A, et al. Long-term outcome in children with fractures of the proximal femur after high-energy trauma. *J Trauma.* 1999;46:58–64.

38. Ratliff AH. Fractures of the neck of the femur in children. *J Bone Joint Surg Br.* 1962;44B:528–542.

39. Canale ST, Bourland WL. Fracture of the neck and intertrochanteric region of the femur in children. *J Bone Joint Surg Am.* 1977;59:431–443.

40. Brukner P, Bennell K. Stress fractures in female athletes. Diagnosis, management and rehabilitation. *Sports Med.* 1997;24: 419–429.

41. Reeder MT, Dick BH, Atkins JK, et al. Stress fractures. Current concepts of diagnosis and treatment. *Sports Med.* 1996;22:198–212.

42. Annan IH, Buxton RA. Bilateral stress fractures of the femoral neck associated with abnormal anatomy—a case report. *Injury.* 1986;17:164–166.

43. Voss L, DaSilva M, Trafton PG. Bilateral femoral neck stress fractures in an amenorrheic athlete. *Am J Orthop.* 1997;26:789–792.

44. Shin AY, Gillingham BL. Fatigue Fractures of the femoral neck in athletes. *J Am Acad Orthop Surg.* 1997;5:293–302.

45. Davies SJ, Walker G. Problems in the early recognition of hip dysplasia. *J Bone Joint Surg Br.* 1984;66:479–484.

46. DeLee J. Fractures and dislocations of the hip. In: *Fractures in adults.* In: Rockwood CA Jr, Wilkins DE, King RE, eds. *Fractures in children.* Philadelphia, PA: JB Lippincott Co; 1984.

47. Gross ML, Nasser S, Finerman, GA. Hip and pelvis. In: DeLee JC, Drez D Jr, eds. *Orthopaedic sports medicine.* Philadelphia, PA: WB Saunders; 1994.

48. Canale ST, King RE. Pelvic and hip fractures. In: Rockwood CA Jr, Wilkins DE, King RE, eds. *Fractures in children.* Philadelphia, PA: JB Lippincott Co; 1984.

49. Metzmaker JN, Pappas AM. Avulsion fractures of the pelvis. *Am J Sports Med.* 1985;13:349–358.

50. Moeller JL. Pelvic and hip apophyseal avulsion injuries in young athletes. *Curr Sports Med Rep.* 2003;2:110–115.

51. Soyuncu Y, Gur S. Avulsion injuries of the pelvis in adolescents. *Acta Orthop Traumatol Turc.* 2004;38(suppl 1):88–92.

52. Mont MA, Jones LC, Sotereanos DG, et al. Understanding and treating osteonecrosis of the femoral head. *Instr Course Lect.* 2000;49:169–185.

53. Vingard E, Alfredsson L, Goldie I, et al. Sports and osteoarthrosis of the hip. An epidemiologic study. *Am J Sports Med.* 1993;21:195–200.

54. Hernigou P, Poignard A, Nogier A, et al. Fate of very small asymptomatic stage-I osteonecrotic lesions of the hip. *J Bone Joint Surg Am.* 2004;86A:2589–2593.

55. Mitchell DG, Steinberg ME, Dalinka MK, et al. Magnetic resonance imaging of the ischemic hip. Alterations within the osteonecrotic, viable, and reactive zones. *Clin Orthop Relat Res* 1989;244:60–77.

56. Parvizi JP, Purtill JJ. Hip, pelvic reconstruction, and arthroplasty. In: Vaccaro AR, ed. *Orthopaedic knowledge update 8.* Rosemont, IL: American Academy of Orthopaedic Surgeons; 2005.

57. Wang CJ, Wang FS, Huang CC, et al. Treatment for osteonecrosis of the femoral head: comparison of extracorporeal shock waves with core decompression and bone-grafting. *J Bone Joint Surg Am.* 2005;87:2380–2387.

58. Kim SY, Kim YG, Kim PT, et al. Vascularized compared with nonvascularized fibular grafts for large osteonecrotic lesions of the femoral head. *J Bone Joint Surg Am.* 2005;87:2012–2018.

59. Byrd JW, Jones KS. Traumatic rupture of the ligamentum teres as a source of hip pain. *Arthroscopy.* 2004;20:385–391.

60. Matsumoto K, Sumi H, Sumi Y, et al. An analysis of hip dislocations among snowboarders and skiers: a 10-year prospective study from 1992 to 2002. *J Trauma.* 2003;55:946–948.

61. Mitchell JC, Giannoudis PV, Millner PA, et al. A rare fracture-dislocation of the hip in a gymnast and review of the literature. *Br J Sports Med.* 1999;33:283–284.

62. Price CT, Pyevich MT, Knapp DR, et al. Traumatic hip dislocation with spontaneous incomplete reduction: a diagnostic trap. *J Orthop Trauma.* 2002;16:730–735.

63. Dreinhofer KE, Schwarzkopf SR, Haas NP, et al. Isolated traumatic dislocation of the hip. Long-term results in 50 patients. *J Bone Joint Surg Br.* 1994;76:6–12.

64. Tornetta P III, Mostafavi HR. Hip dislocation: current treatment regimens. *J Am Acad Orthop Surg.* 1997;5:27–36.

65. Yang EC, Cornwall R. Initial treatment of traumatic hip dislocations in the adult. *Clin Orthop Relat Res.* 2000;377:24–31.

66. Poggi JJ, Callaghan JJ, Spritzer CE, et al. Changes on magnetic resonance images after traumatic hip dislocation. *Clin Orthop Relat Res.* 1995;319:249–259.

67. Barquet A. Traumatic anterior dislocation of the hip in childhood. *Injury.* 1982;13:435–440.

KNEE

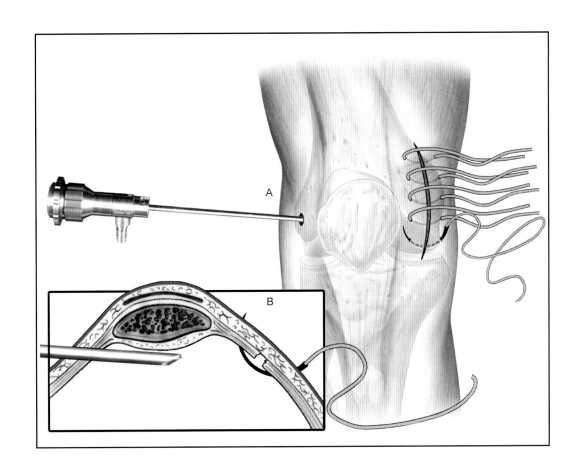

BASIC SCIENCE OF THE KNEE

DONALD H. JOHNSON, MD, FRCS, PAUL JOHNSON, MD,
ALI ALSUWAIDI, MD, FRCSI, FRCSC

■ KEY POINTS

- The knee joint is considered to be three separate compartments, the patellofemoral, the medial, and the lateral compartments.
- The knee has no inherent bony stability, but depends upon the ligaments to provide stability.
- The patellofemoral joint consists of the patella, the trochlea, and the stabilizing quadriceps mechanism.
- The condyles of the femur articulate with the condyles of the tibia but are asymmetrical and appear to have no inherent stability.
- The anterior cruciate ligament (ACL) is a two-bundle ligament with a small isometric attachment to the tibia and femur. The tension in the two bundles varies with knee flexion; the anteriomedial is tight in flexion and the posterolateral tight in extension.
- The posterior cruciate ligament (PCL) is also a two-bundle ligament with a small central isometric point on the femur.
- The pes anserinus muscles (sartorius, gracilis, and semi-membranous muscles) are flexors and internal rotators of the knee, which act as dynamic stabilizers.
- The medial and lateral meniscus are concentric lamellae that serve to deepen the contact of the tibia and provide stability to the femur.
- Articular cartilage is a thin layer of specialized connective tissue lining the articulations of diarthrodial joints.
- Age, mobilization, pregnancy and the post-partum state, and medications all are factors affecting the biomechanical properties of tendons and ligaments.
- The function of the articular cartilage is significant as the knee joint reaction force at the tibiofemoral joint is about

three times body weight in walking. The joint reaction forces are absorbed by the menisci along with the articular cartilage in the normal biomechanics of the knee.
- Soft tissue can be divided into dense, loose, and adipose subtypes depending on the histological appearance.
- Soft-tissue healing is a structured process that takes place over a specific period of time in a very coordinated way. Different tissues have different repair capacities for a variety of environmental and genetic factors.
- In the multi-ligament injury, reconstruction of the ACL may impart stability to the injured medial collateral ligament (MCL) and allow it to heal in a satisfactory manner without the need for primary repair.

■ ANATOMY

This description of anatomy of the knee will be presented with an emphasis on the practical surgical approach to each structure. The knee joint is considered to be three separate compartments, the patellofemoral, the medial, and the lateral compartments. The knee has no inherent bony stability, but depends upon the ligaments to provide stability.

Bone

The Patellofemoral Joint

The patellofemoral joint consists of the patella, the trochlea, and the stabilizing quadriceps mechanism **(Fig 33-1)**. In the normal situation, the trochlea provides stability to the patella, but with dysplasia of the lateral facet of the trochlea, and muscular imbalance, lateral instability of the patella occurs. The patella has seven facets, the three lateral: superior, medial,

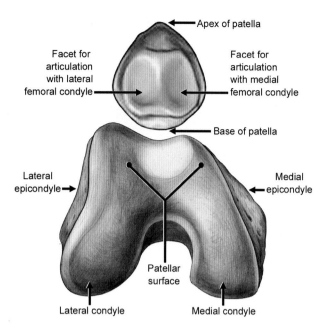

Fig 33-1. The patella articulation with the trochlea of the femur.

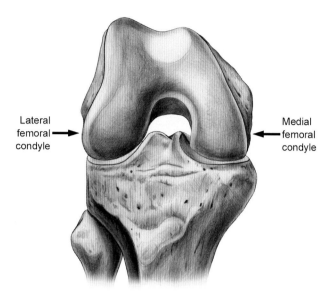

Fig 33-2. The medial and lateral femoral condyles.

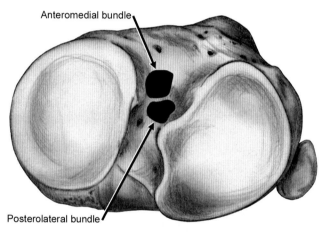

Fig 33-3. The attachment site of the ACL on the tibia.

and inferior, the three medial: superior, medial, and inferior. The medial odd facet has no articulation with the trochlea. The degree of contact between the patella and trochlea varies with knee flexion. The distal portion of the patella articulates in extension, and with increasing flexion the patella is drawn into the trochlea groove. In full flexion, the proximal patella articulates with the femur.

The patellar tendon joins the patella to the anterior tibia, and is of variable length, but averages about 5 cm. The ratio of length of the patella tendon to the length of the patella determines the position of the patella in the femoral groove. An excessively long tendon results in patella alta, with the patella lying above the trochlea in extension.

The quadriceps tendon attaches to the superior aspect of the patella. The medial patella femoral ligament stabilizes the patella on the medial side. This ligament attaches to the femur at the epicondyle, and to the patella just above the midportion. The lateral retinaculum has several thickened bands, forming the lateral stabilizing structures.

The Tibiofemoral Joint

The condyles of the femur articulate with the condyles of the tibia, but are asymmetrical and appear to have no inherent stability (Fig 33-2). The larger medial femoral condyle is round, and the lateral condyle is longer, and wider at contact with the tibia. The medial tibial plateau is flat, but the lateral tibial plateau is convex. Both tibial plateaus have a posterior inclination of 10 degrees. The meniscus provides increased stability by deepening the concavity of the tibia. The intercondylar notch of the femur is occupied by the anterior and posterior cruciate ligaments (PCLs). On full flexion of the knee there is a posterior translation of the tibial on the femur through a combination of gliding and rolling of the femur.

The Anterior Cruciate Ligament

The anterior cruciate ligament (ACL) is a two-bundle ligament with a small isometric attachment to the tibia and femur (Fig 33-3). The cross sectional area of the ACL is approximately 35 mm^2 and the average length is 25 mm. The tension in the two bundles varies with knee flexion; the anteromedial is tight in flexion and the posterolateral tight in extension. The tibial insertion is an oval attachment between the two spines of the tibia (Fig 33-4). The insertion sites are larger in cross sectional area than the midportion of the ligament. The insertion site on the femur is also oval in the posterior aspect of the medial wall of the lateral femoral condyle at the 1 to 3 o'clock position in the left knee, and 9 to 11 o'clock position in the right knee (Fig 33-5).

The Posterior Cruciate Ligament

The PCL is also a two-bundle ligament with a small central isometric point on the femur (Fig 33-6). The PCL has an average intra-articular length of 4 cm, and the cross sectional

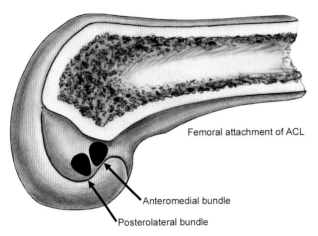

Fig 33-4. The attachment site of the ACL on the femur.

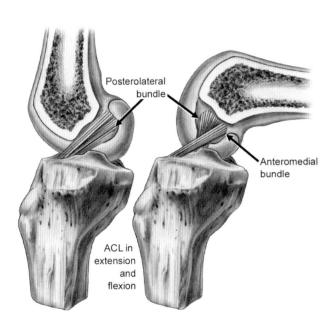

Fig 33-5. The two bundles of the ACL.

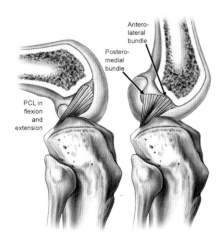

Fig 33-6. The two bundles of the PCL.

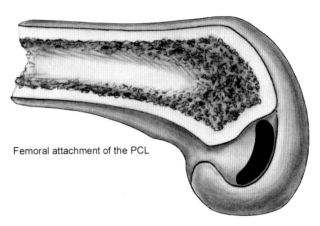

Fig 33-7. The femoral attachment of the PCL.

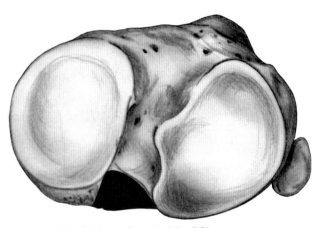

Fig 33-8. The tibial attachment of the PCL.

area is smaller in the middle compared to the femoral attachment site. The two bundles vary in tension with knee flexion, the anterolateral is tight in flexion and the posteromedial is tight in extension. The PCL insertion on the femur is a board insertion from the top of the intercondylar notch at the edge of the articular surface extending approximately 3 cm inferior **(Fig 33-7)**. The insertion of the PCL on the tibia is slightly lateral, and 1 to 2 cm below the joint line **(Fig 33-8)**.

The Meniscal Femoral Ligaments
The meniscofemoral ligaments are present in most knees, but their true function is unknown. The meniscofemoral ligaments comprise up to one third the cross sectional area of the total PCL volume. The anterior meniscofemoral ligament of Humphrey crosses obliquely the distal aspect of the PCL when the knee is flexed **(Fig 33-9)**.

The ligament of Humphrey attaches to the femur in front of the PCL, and is superficial when viewed in the flexed knee. It is attached to the femur immediately adjacent to the articular cartilage, in the 2 to 3 o'clock position, in a right knee. The distal attachment is to the posterior horn of the lateral meniscus. When the PCL is viewed arthroscopically, the anterior meniscofemoral ligament may be

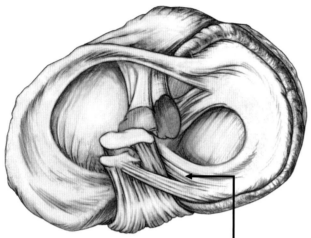

Anterior meniscofemoral ligament of Humphrey

Fig 33-9. The anterior meniscofemoral ligament of Humphrey.

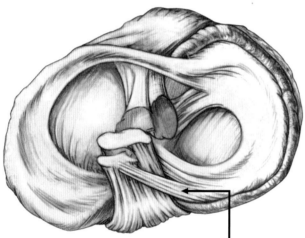

Posterior meniscofemoral ligament of Wrisberg

Fig 33-10. The posterior meniscofemoral ligament of Wrisberg.

identified by the oblique orientation of its fibers, in contrast to the vertical orientation of the PCL fibers.

The posterior meniscofemoral ligament of Wrisberg runs from the medial side wall of the femoral notch to the posterior horn of the lateral meniscus **(Fig 33-10)**. The femoral attachment is proximal to the posteromedial fibers of the PCL, and so, it is superficial to the PCL when viewed from the posterior aspect. It is on the posterior/superior aspect of the surface of the PCL. In order to make a positive identification of the posterior meniscofemoral ligament, it should be noted that it attaches directly to the posterior horn of the lateral meniscus, whereas the oblique posterior fibers of the PCL pass down to the posterior rim of the tibial plateau. The two meniscofemoral ligaments form a sling around the PCL.

The Medial Collateral Ligament

The medial supporting structures of the knee are divided into static and dynamic stabilizers. The pes anserinus muscles (sartorius, gracilis, and semimembranosus muscles)

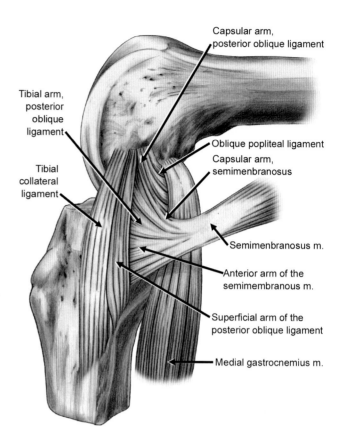

Fig 33-11. The MCL, and the attachment sites.

are flexors and internal rotators of the knee, which act as dynamic stabilizers. The semimembranosus is a stabilizer of the posteromedial corner, having insertions which provide capsular reinforcement along tibial and popliteal insertion. In addition, the vastus medialis obliquitous attaches to the adductor tubercle, and is associated with the tibial attachment of the MCL.

The static stabilizer is the capsuloligamentous complex. The MCL is a broad ligament (10 to 12 cm in length) that attaches to the medial femoral epicondyle and to the medial aspect of the tibia under the pes anserinus muscles, 4 cm below the joint line. The anterior fibers of the ligament tighten during knee flexion. The capsular tissue is reinforced by the vastus medialis anteriorly. In its middle one third of the capsule consists of meniscofemoral, meniscocapsular, and meniscotibial portions that lie under the deep MCL. Hughston and Eilers (1) have described the posterior portion of the capsule as the posterior oblique ligament (POL). This complex, which is tense in extension and loose in flexion, forms a sling around the posterior aspect of the medial femoral condyle and becomes confluent with the posterior capsule of the knee **(Fig 33-11)**.

The Posterolateal Corner

The lateral side of the knee is composed of the iliotibial band, the lateral collateral ligament (LCL), the fabellofibular ligament, the arcuate ligament, the popliteus tendon, the popliteal-fibular ligament and the capsule **(Fig 33-12)**.

The iliotibial band is the most superficial and inserts on Gerdy's tubercle. The LCL runs from the lateral epicondyle of the femur to the head of the fibula, and blends with the insertion of the biceps tendon.

The fabellofibular ligament is between the lateral ligament and the arcuate ligament. The arcuate ligament is a variable condensation of the posterior capsule. The popliteus tendon originates from the popliteus muscle on the back of the tibia, and wraps around the posterior aspect to insert just anterior to the epicondyle of the femur **(Fig 33-13)**. The popliteal-fibular ligament connects the tendon to the posterior aspect of the head of the fibula. The popliteus tendon arises below the LCL in a small sulcus on the lateral femoral condyle, passes under the LCL, descends into the popliteus hiatus, then passes under the arcuate ligament, and becomes extra-articular before finally joining its muscle belly.

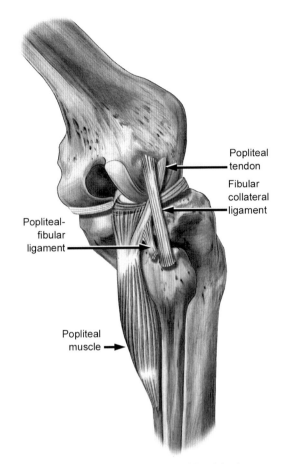

Fig 33-12. The structures of the lateral side of the knee.

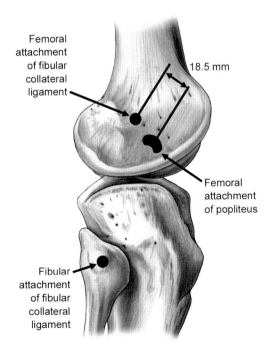

Fig 33-13. The attachment sites of the LCL and popliteus on the femur and tibia.

■ THE POSTERIOR ANATOMY OF THE KNEE

The neurovascular structures, popliteal artery and vein, and popliteal nerve lie between the heads of the gastrocnemius muscle **(Fig 33-14)**. The artery is slightly lateral, and lies directly behind the posterior horn attachment of the lateral meniscus. The nerve and artery can be retracted laterally with the medial head of the gastrocnemius to approach the PCL and the posterior aspect of the joint.

Meniscus

The medial and lateral meniscus are concentric lamellae that serve to deepen the tibial contact of the tibia, and provide stability to the femur **(Fig 33-15)**.

The peripheral border of the meniscus is thick and wedge shaped with attachments to the capsule. The medial meniscus is 3.5 cm in length and is thicker posteriorly than anteriorly **(Fig 33-16)**. It is attached to the posterior aspect of the tibia. The anterior attachment is variable, and in some cases, has no bony attachment. The transverse ligament is a variable structure that connects the anterior medial to the anterior lateral meniscus. There is less anterior to posterior motion of the medial meniscus on range of motion of the knee.

The composition of the meniscus is: 75% water, 20% collagen (Type I 90%, Type II, III, V, VI 3%), proteoglycans, noncollagenous proteins, lipids, and 2% cells (fibrochondrocytes, fibroblasts, mast cells, myofibroblasts). The collagen ultra-structure of the meniscus is composed of fine random fibers-A, the main bundle of circumferential fibers-B, and small radial fibers-C to reinforce the structure **(Fig 33-17)**.

The outer one third of the meniscus is vascular, and thus has more potential to heal. This vascularity persists into adulthood **(Fig 33-18)**. The lateral meniscus is larger, and has more motion as the knee flexes. The lateral meniscus is attached posterior to the tibia and to the meniscal femoral

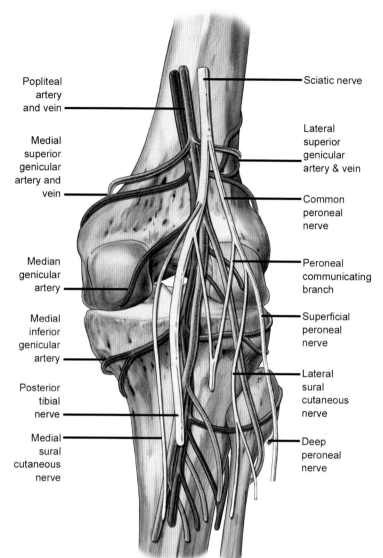

Popliteal artery and vein

Medial superior genicular artery and vein

Median genicular artery

Medial inferior genicular artery

Posterior tibial nerve

Medial sural cutaneous nerve

Sciatic nerve

Lateral superior genicular artery & vein

Common peroneal nerve

Peroneal communicating branch

Superficial peroneal nerve

Lateral sural cutaneous nerve

Deep peroneal nerve

Fig 33-14. The neurovascular anatomy of the posterior aspect of the knee.

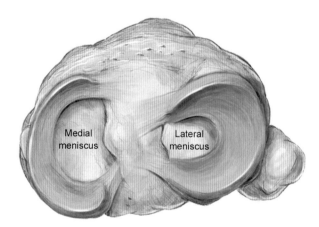

Medial meniscus

Lateral meniscus

Fig 33-15. The medial and lateral meniscus.

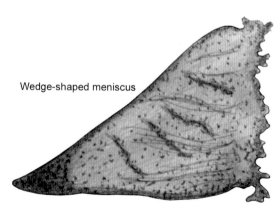

Wedge-shaped meniscus

Fig 33-16. The wedge shaped meniscus.

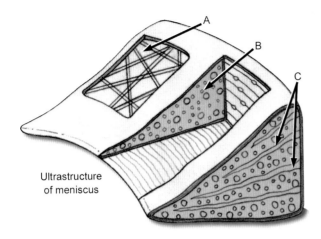

Fig 33-17. The ultrastructure of the meniscus fibers.

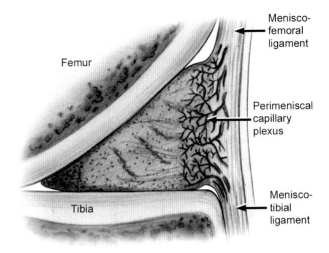

Fig 33-18. The vascular anatomy of the meniscus.

ligaments. On the lateral aspect, the popliteus tendon leaves an open hiatus in the attachment of the meniscus.

■ ANATOMY OF THE ARTICULAR CARTILAGE

Articular cartilage is a thin layer of specialized connective tissue lining the articulations of diarthrodial joints. Properties which are unique to this tissue enable an almost frictionless joint movement and afford protection to the underlying bone from excessive load and trauma by dissipating the forces produced during movement.

The structural organization of articular cartilage can be divided into four major zones: superficial, middle, deep, and calcified zones **(Fig 33-19)**. Each zone is distinctly structured with cells and extracellular matrix (ECM) organized in specific patterns. The cells, known as chondrocytes, make up 1% to 2% of the total weight of the articular cartilage. On

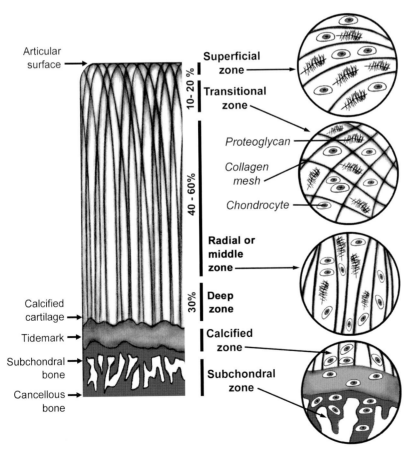

Fig 33-19. The four zones of the articular cartilage.

the other hand, the ECM, which makes up the rest of the cartilage, is generally composed of Type II collagen, glycoaminosglycans, and proteoglycans.

■ BIOMECHANICS OF TENDONS AND LIGAMENTS

Tendons and ligaments are tissues with unique biomechanical properties. Tendons have adequate strength to sustain the high tensile forces during muscle contraction, yet have adequate compliance to angulate around bone surfaces and move underneath retinacula to vary the direction of muscle tension. Ligaments are supple, permitting natural movements of bones to which they attach, yet are strong in providing resistance to external forces to a joint.

The function of tendons is to attach muscle to bone and produce joint motion via the transfer of forces from muscular tensile forces to bone. Tendons also permit the muscle belly to be at an ideal distance from the joint it acts on to prevent an excessive muscle length between origin and insertion.

The role of the ligaments and joint capsules is to increase the mechanical stability of the knee joint, guide normal kinematics or joint motions, and to prevent excessive joint motion, which may damage articular cartilage and menisci. These structures play an integral role in knee joint motion even though they are passive (i.e., they do not actively produce joint motion).

Tendons and ligaments are primarily composed of collagen, a fibrous protein, giving them great strength and flexibility. Ligaments are poorly vascularized and generally have 75% collagen composition somewhat less than tendons (2). The orientations of the parallel collagen fibers help determine the biomechanical behavior of the individual knee ligaments. Collagen fibrils in the joint capsule are less parallel than ligaments, resulting in increased compliance, but decreased resistance to linear forces. Since the biochemical composition of tendons and ligaments of humans are identical to some other species such as rabbits and dogs, a significant amount of research on tissue biomechanics has been applied from these animal studies.

■ BIOMECHANICS OF KNEE LIGAMENTS

In the knee, the ligaments are the most important static stabilizer of the joint. The knee ligaments' role is to stabilize the knee, prevent abnormal kinematics, and any abnormal displacements that may damage the articular cartilage. There are four zones pertaining to the insertion of ligaments into bone (this also applies to tendons).

Zone 1: End of ligament.
Zone 2: Collagen fibers intermesh with fibrocartilage.

Zone 3: Fibrocartilage becomes gradually mineralized.
Zone 4: Cortical bone.

This transformation zone permits a gradual increase in the stiffness of the ligaments, thus decreasing the concentration of stress at the attachment of ligament/tendon to bone. In the knee, this reduces the chance of failure of the ligaments.

Stress/Strain Curves

Load/Elongation or commonly noted as "Stress/Strain" curves allow for analysis of the biomechanics of ligaments and tendons (Fig 33-20). The tissue is subject to a constant rate of deformation and the force required to rupture the ligament is plotted versus the amount of lengthening of the tissue in question. The relationship between stress and strain of tissues can be quantified with the modulus of elasticity. The modulus of elasticity for tendons and ligaments has been calculated in several research investigations (3,4). This value is based on the linear relationship between the stress or load and the elongation or strain of the tissue in question. The stress therefore, is proportional to the strain:

$$E = \sigma/\epsilon$$

Where E = the modulus of elasticity

σ = load/stress
ϵ = elongation or strain

This modulus of elasticity can be calculated for any point on the stress/strain curve and will increase as the slope of the stress/strain curve increases as the tendon or ligament is placed under stress.

Region 1 is the "primary" or "toe" region. The tissue lengthens with a relatively small increase in load/stress. This is due to the wavy collagen fibers progressively straightening out. Thus the slope of the graph or stiffness increases gradually during this part of the curve.

Region 2 is the secondary or "linear" region where the fibers straighten out and the stiffness has become constant.

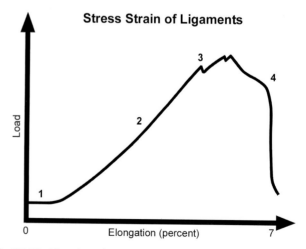

Fig 33-20. The stress/strain curve of ligaments.

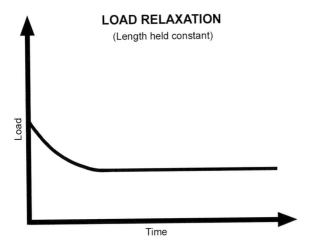

Fig 33-21. The load relaxation curve.

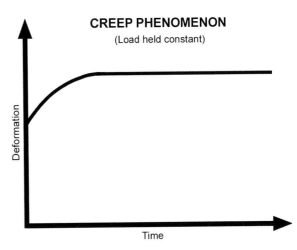

Fig 33-22. The creep curve.

This is the elastic region and deformation of the tissues begins and is proportional to the load or stress at this point.

Region 3 typifies the sequential failure of fiber bundles as the maximum load has been reached before failure begins. Small dips or drops in force occur as the collagen fibers begin to fail.

Region 4 is ultimate failure and there is a low resistance to elongation after this point as there is a steep drop in the load/stress.

Besides these elastic properties, under stress ligaments and tendons exhibit viscoelastic, or rate dependent behavior. Therefore, as the loading rate on a tendon or ligament increases, the stiffness of the tissue will increase, thus storing more energy (area under the stress/strain curve) prior to failure, and undergoing more elongation prior to failure. This would be illustrated by a steeper slope (stiffness) on the stress/strain curve prior to ultimate failure of the tissue. Stress/relaxation occurs if a tendon or ligament is held at a constant length (strain) by a load (stress), and the stress required to maintain that strain decreases **(Fig 33-21)**. This decreases rapidly during the first 6 to 8 hours of loading and then more slowly over the next few months.

Concept of Creep

Creep occurs if a tendon is held by a constant load (stress) **(Fig 33-22)**. With time, the length or strain of the tendon will increase. This strain rapidly increases initially, but then increases more slowly with time. One application of this phenomenon is the use of plaster casts or braces to correct deformity such as in scoliosis or clubfoot.

Knowledge of the viscoelastic properties of ligaments has clinical importance in knee surgery, since these properties are integral to proper ligament function. The amount of stress relaxation of a ligament is important as applied to the ACL replacement graft during reconstructive surgery. The graft is placed under an initial elongation, or tensioning, prior to fixation to host bone. The amount of tension that remains in the graft over time is an essential factor in the graft's function as a stabilizer of the knee joint.

Factors Affecting the Biomechanical Properties of Tendons and Ligaments

1 Age: The amount of collagen crosslinking increases until the age of 20 which increases the tensile strength of tendons and ligaments (5).

2 Mobilization: Tendons and ligaments, similar to bone, remodel as a response to mechanical stress. As they are subjected to stress, they become stronger and stiffer and vice versa (6).

3 Pregnancy and the post-partum state: There is an increased laxity of tendons and ligaments in the third trimester of pregnancy. This is caused by hormonal changes during pregnancy including increased estradiol levels. These levels later return to normal during the post-partum state. Increase laxity of the ACL with the KT-1000 arthometer has been correlated with increased estradiol levels during the late stages of pregnancy. As estradiol levels returned to baseline in the post-partum state ACL laxity decreased (7). Thus, the increased ligament laxity from hormonal changes potentially increases knee joint instability during pregnancy.

4 Medications: The effect of nonsteroidal anti-inflammatories (NSAIDs) on ligament healing remains controversial. Nonselective (COX-1 and COX-2 inhibitors) NSAIDs such as indomethacin have been shown to improve ligament healing strength in animals by up to 40% (8). This is explained by the increase in cross-linking of collagen molecules in ligaments. More recently research has demonstrated that COX-2 inhibitors (celecoxib) inhibit ligament healing in rats (9).

The fluoroquinolone class of antibiotics has increased significantly due to their effectiveness and versatility. However cases of tendonitis and Achilles tendon rupture have been documented in the literature most commonly with ciprofloxacin (10). Other anatomic sites for tendonopathy include the patellar, quadriceps, and rotator cuff tendons. The etiology for this tendonopathy includes a decreased collagen and fibroblast synthesis (11).

■ BIOMECHANICS OF ARTICULAR CARTILAGE

Articular cartilage is a specialized avascular tissue designed to handle the demands of the joint environment over a person's lifetime. It has two principal functions in the knee joint: first to act as a shock-absorber by distributing joint loads over a wide surface area; and second to provide a near frictionless environment for opposing joint surfaces allowing efficient movement.

To simplify the biomechanical behavior of articular cartilage it can be classified into an organic solid phase and an inorganic fluid phase. The two principal components of articular cartilage are chondrocytes and the ECM. Chondrocytes, or the cellular component of articular cartilage, comprise less than 10% of the tissue's volume (12). Despite this relatively low proportion of volume, they produce, secrete, and maintain the organic component of the extracellular component, the matrix. Collagen fibrils and proteoglycans form the organic matrix. The remainder is composed of water, inorganic salts, glycoproteins, and lipids. Collagen fibrils and proteoglycans are structural components resisting the internal forces produced by the load-bearing articular cartilage.

Collagen in articular cartilage has a heterogenous composition composed of three distinct structural layers. Through studies using electron microscopy, Mow and Lai (13) proposed a structural arrangement for the collagen network in articular cartilage (Fig 33-19).

In the superficial tangential zone, the collagen fibers are tightly woven into sheets parallel to the articular surface. This collagen-rich superficial layer provides the joint cartilage with a protective, wear-resistant skin.

In the middle zone, the randomly oriented fibers are less densely packed in a matrix of proteoglycans and water. In the deep zone, the collagen fibrils are larger and radially oriented which enter into the calcified cartilage and anchor the tissue to the underlying bone. Similar to bone, articular cartilage is anisotropic; that is, its biomechanical properties vary with the direction of loading. This arrangement is significant from a biomechanical standpoint as it distributes stress more uniformly across the load-bearing areas of the joint articular cartilage (14). Articular cartilage being viscoelastic demonstrates both properties of creep and stress-relaxation. Creep in articular cartilage occurs due to exudation of the interstitial fluid. As cartilage is compressed, initially a rapid deformation occurs since interstitial fluid exudation begins. Deformation decreases gradually as fluid

flow ceases and the compressive forces within the solid matrix alone are equal to the applied force in the joint. Thus deformation equilibrium is achieved and no fluid flows.

In the knee joint, the function of articular cartilage is significant, as the joint reaction force at the tibiofemoral joint is about three times body weight in walking (14a). The joint reaction forces are absorbed by the menisci along with the articular cartilage in the normal biomechanics of the knee. Studies using force transducers at the tibiofemoral joint have demonstrated that the lateral and medial menisci absorb at least 50% of the compressive load transmitted on the tibiofemoral joint between 0 and 90 degrees of flexion (14b). The role of the normal menisci in absorbing tibiofemoral compressive forces is increased with knee flexion. Nearly all of the tibiofemoral compressive load is absorbed by the posterior horns of the menisci in knee flexion past 75 degrees as found in research by Seedhom and Hargreaves (15). Perhaps more significantly, additional findings included the decreased transmission of forces through the tibiofemoral joint in partial meniscectomy as opposed to total meniscectomy **(Fig 33-23)**.

The medial meniscus also has a biomechanical relationship with the anterior cruciate replacement graft. In research by Papageorgeou et al. (15a) the in situ forces in the anterior cruciate replacement graft in cadaveric knees increased between 33% and 50% after medial meniscectomy. Thus total meniscectomy in the knee joint will increase the tibiofemoral compressive forces compared to a partial meniscectomy. Total meniscectomy will also significantly increase forces in the ACL replacement graft illustrating the integral biomechanical role of the menisci in the knee joint.

Articular cartilage plays a significant role in the biomechanics of the patellofemoral joint. With its low compressive stiffness and coefficient of friction, it is integral in transmitting the relatively high quadriceps force across the distal femur to the tibia via the patella. These patellofemoral compressive forces have been estimated at a peak 4,250 N or 5.6 times normalized body weight during running (16). Thus articular cartilage is designed to handle significant loads at the patellofemoral joint via a well-designed patellofemoral contact area. However if the patellofemoral contact area is decreased, and the cartilage is subject to an abnormally high patellofemoral joint reaction force (PFJR), articular cartilage is at a higher risk of defects and possibly

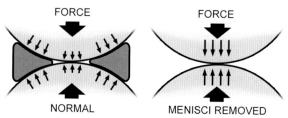

Fig 33-23. The increased stress on the articular cartilage with meniscectomy.

osteoarthritis. An example of these forces is in the use of deep squatting exercise in strength training. Although the joint contact area is increased, the joint reaction force is much greater with knee flexion toward 90 degrees. At 90 degrees of knee flexion, the joint reaction force is approximately 2.5 to 3 times body weight. Thus, activities such as deep squatting should be avoided in individuals with patellofemoral joint derangement since high forces working on the patellofemoral joint could cause pain and further joint degeneration.

Articular cartilage also works in concert with tensile forces of the ligaments in the knee to restrain knee motion. An example of this would be the ACL and tibial femoral contact areas. If a rotational torque is applied to the lower leg, the ACL would not be able to resist the relative rotation of the tibia with respect to the femur. The ligament would rotate about its tibial and femoral insertion sites. However, the internal rotation causes the femoral condyles to translate posteriorly along the tibial spine, creating compressive forces at the tibial-femoral contact regions at the articular cartilage surfaces. This tibiofemoral articular compression will combine with the tensile forces in the ACL to resist an internal rotation force at the knee joint.

Besides evenly distributing forces in the knee joint, articular cartilage decreases frictional forces to miniscule levels in the knee joint. This is due to a high level of lubrication of the articular cartilage surfaces. Both boundary lubrication and squeeze-film lubrication occur. In boundary lubrication, the lubricant synovial fluid reacts chemically with the articular cartilage forming a layer to be formed enabling the two opposing surfaces to move in a frictionless fashion. Boundary lubrication is more prevalent when the knee joint is under high loading forces. It is postulated that squeeze film lubrication occurs in less severe loading conditions. The bearing surfaces are separated by a fluid film created by external pressure. An example of this is hydrostatic lubrication where the joint fluid is pumped between the articulating surfaces. Articular cartilage is both a pump and a reservoir. Joint loading pressurizes the articular cartilage and drives the fluid out toward the surface via microscopic pores. The cartilage then expands as the knee joint is unloaded and the fluid is resorbed.

During compressive movement of the knee joint such as the stance phase in walking, fluid is squeezed out from the articular cartilage at the area of contact until the peak stress has occurred when the fluid starts to resorb. In contrast, during prolonged standing, the fluid film will gradually disappear, resulting in only boundary lubricant protecting the joint surfaces.

Thus articular cartilage in the knee joint is biomechanically complex and its unique structure helps the knee act as a shock absorber and perform repetitive motion at a relatively low amount of friction. However, anatomic alterations in articular cartilage and menisci in the knee joint will significantly change biomechanics in the knee and possibly lead to long-term morbidity.

■ SOFT TISSUE HEALING

Historical Background

Management of soft tissue injuries went through an evolution over the centuries but the greatest advances in the understanding of the process of healing took place over the past few centuries.

Hippocrates, a Roman physician, first studied the healing wound and recommended diet, rest, and cleanliness as essential factors in healing. During the middle ages little progress took place until the 16th century when a French surgeon, Paré, realized while treating soldiers that infection was not a normal process in wound healing. John Hunter in the 18th century was first to describe symptoms of inflammation. His interest was mainly in the mechanism that led to healing. Louis Pasteur, discovered bacteria and contributed more to the prevention of infection. Joseph Lister advocated the use of carbolic acid antiseptics as a method of sterilization besides boiling, and at that time aseptic surgery was born. Carrel used crushed animal tissue to enhance tissue healing. Advances in the field of biochemistry led to better understanding of mediators responsible for tissue healing. Elrich was responsible for understanding of immuno-chemical principles of wound healing and the recognition of the role of growth factors in the process of tissue repair. Howes at the beginning of the 20th century studied tensile strength of healing in soft tissue and concluded that different patterns of healing exists in different soft tissues.

Normal Connective Tissue

Biochemistry

Articular cartilage is composed of a large number of unique glycoproteins that interact in complex ways within a fluid medium. Major components of connective tissue are water, collagen, proteoglycans, elastin, and other smaller but important substances.

Water

Water constitutes approximately 70% of dense connective tissue. It is evenly distributed and functions mainly as a medium for transport of ions, cells, and other substances.

Collagen

Collagen is the most prevalent protein in all connective tissue. It comprises a triple helical chain of amino acid, which aggregates in extra cellular space. Currently there are 13 recognized collagen types. Type I, II, IV, V, and XI are mainly involved in fiber synthesis. Collagen Types I and III are found mainly in fiber of tissues such as skin, tendons, and ligaments. Types II and XI are mainly found in hyaline cartilage. Collagen fibers are stabilized by intermolecular cross links. Collagenases are responsible for degradation of collagen and they are normally inhibited by metal chelators which reduces calcium and zinc needed for their activity.

Proteoglycans

The proteoglycans are a subclass of glycol proteins with high content of carbohydrate. Glycosaminoglycan (GAG) chain comprises the major functional element, and normally attaches to core protein in proteoglycans. It functions as "cement" in both intracellular and extracellular interfaces. It has a water binding property which contributes to the visco-elastic behavior of soft tissue.

Elastin

Elastin is a highly insoluble protein found in scar tissue as well as normal tissue in varying quantities. It is responsible for elasticity through hydrophobic interactions. It is composed of two types of fibers, namely amorphous elastic and elastic fiber microfibril. Growth factor plays a role in regulation of this component.

Adhesive Proteins

Adhesive proteins function as cell adhesion ligands in soft connective tissue, modulating mechanical and load transmission between cells and EC matrix. Fibronectin, laminin, vitronectin, and thrombospodin have collagen or fibrin specific binding domains, which function to attach cells to collagen matrix.

Morphology

Soft tissue can be divided into dense, loose, and adipose subtypes depending on the histological appearance.

Dense Connective Tissue Organs

Dense connective tissue organs include ligament, tendon, and joint capsule, which are of particular interest to surgeons. These are characterized by densely arranged collagen fibers.

Ligaments

Ligaments appear microscopically as dense white cords. These are made mainly of collagen Type I in densely packed arrangements with scattered ligament cells (fibro cytes). It has a uniform microvascularity originating from insertion site. Mechanoreceptors, proprioceptors, and nociceptors are present in ligaments. Ligament collagen has a characteristic crimp pattern.

Tendons

Tendons are strong bands of dense connective tissue that connect muscles to bones. Microscopically they have a fibrillar texture and may resemble ligament. Microscopically there are differences in collagen crimp, cellularity, and cell shape between ligaments and tendons. Tendons are less metabolically active with a lesser content of reducible collagen cross-links, and Type III collagen as compared to ligaments.

Cartilage

This is classified into three subgroups: hyaline, fibro cartilage, and elastic cartilage based on the morphological characteristics of their extracellular matrix.

Hyaline Cartilage

Hyaline cartilage constitutes the layer covering articular surface and most of the epiphyseal growth plate. It is rich in fibro collagen (Type II) and large proteoglycans and aggrecan.

Fibro Cartilage

It contains a coarse collagen fiber and is mainly found in joint meniscus, labrae, cartilaginous sesamoids, and tendon insertions. The articulation of collagen fiber bundles differs in the above structures and gives its characteristic appearance.

Elastic Cartilage

Elastic cartilage is similar to Hyaline cartilage but contains elastic bundles (elastin) scattered through the matrix. This provides a tissues that is stiff yet elastic. It is found in the Larnyx and Pinna of the ear.

■ PHASES IN SOFT TISSUE HEALING

Soft tissue healing is a structured process that takes place over a specific period of time in a very coordinated way. Different tissues have different repair capacities for a variety of environmental and genetic factors. Healing often is divided into three and occasionally four phases in an organized process that is spread over months to years. It starts with clot formation followed by inflammation, proliferation, and finally remodeling.

The healing process of the MCL has been thoroughly examined by Frank. The process contains an inflammation phase (72 hours), a repair and regeneration phase (six weeks), and a remodelling phase (approximately one year). Forty weeks after trans-section in rabbit MCLs, the repair tissue was shown to be composed of Type III collagen scar tissue, and it was found to be more lax and mechanically inferior to a native ligament in a sham operation group. The maximum tensile strength regained is approximately 70%. Canine studies by Frank et al. (17,18) support the concept of increased MCL strength with surgical repair, and for improved strength and results with early range of motion and nonoperative treatment.

Hemorrhage and Clot Formation Phase

Depending on the clotting potential, local pressure, temperature, and vascularity of the tissue, a clot may or may not form. Microscopically, this process leads to formation of fibrin mass with activation of platelets, and intrinsic coagulation pathways with release of active molecules such as Growth Factors (GFs) and peptides, which contribute to inflammatory process.

Inflammatory Phase

During this phase there is local release of inflammatory factors. Macroscopically this phase is characterized by redness, swelling, and warmth. At the microscopic level there is marked presence of inflammatory cells including polymorphs, lymphocytes, and macrophages. These cells are attracted to the injury site through the process of chemotaxis. Initially polymorphs appear, but are soon replaced by monocytes and macrophage cells, which play significant roles in phagocytosis of necrotic tissue along with release of prostaglandins (PG), cytokines, tumor necrosis factor (TNF) and GFs.

Proliferative Phase

At the gross level this phase is undistinguished from the inflammatory phase, but microscopically it is characterized by the presence of fibroblasts spindle-shaped cells, which produce matrix along with new vessel formation. The presence of GF and cytokines constitute the catalyst for differentiation and growth in a complex environment with some inhibiting cells, while others promote cell proliferation. The effect of GF/cytokines is mediated through receptors present on target cells. The above mentioned process at this phase may differ in various types of soft tissues, because of variables such as endogenous cells, blood supply, innervation, and extent of inflammation and presence of inhibitory factors. Recent research has shown that Transforming Growth Factor Beta 1 (TGF-BI) and IGF-II regulate messenger ribonucleic acid (mRNA), which increases the synthesis of collagen and have proteinase inhibitor expression. IGF-II is present at a high level during fetal development, but is minimally expressed in adult cells. The findings that scar tissue is very responsive to IGF-II may have important clinical application.

Remodeling

This stage is manifested with shrinkage of scar tissue, while microscopically there is a decrease in fibroblasts with organization of new matrix, a process that may take months to years. In order to achieve scar maturation, removal of fibrin, fibronectin, and proteoglycans is needed. This process needs a fine balance between matrix removal by proteinases and secretion of matrix molecules. The level of plasminogen activator may reflect the initial activity with formation of scar tissue and the subsequent decline with maturation.

Role of Angiogenesis in Soft Tissue Healing

Formation of new vascular network in acutely injured tissue is an essential and critical step toward tissue healing. It starts within 24 hours after injury. In response to stimulus the endothelial cells secrete proteolytic enzyme, which degrades vascular basement membrane. The migration of endothelial cells toward angiogenic stimulus occurs within 48 hours. Capillary buds form in the granulating wounds. Those buds eventually become branching networks of new vessels. Angiogenesis is a complex multifactorial process occurring in response to local tissues factors following injury and it is influenced by local and systemic factors. Local factors may have a direct or indirect effect on endothelial cells. Direct acting angiogenic agents include TNF-x, TGF-x, and Fibroblast Growth Factor (FGF). Indirect acting agents include TGF-B. Oxygen tension is considered a critical factor in angiogenesis. Inhibition of angiogenesis is an important step in limiting the proliferation of new vascular networks. Both vascular smooth muscle cells and vascular pericytes have shown inhibitory effects on endothelial cell proliferation in vitro (17).

Factors that Influence Tissue Healing

Frank et al. (19) has outlined the process that optimizes soft tissue repair. Seeding wounds with embryonic stem cells, bridging gaps with cell-derived "engineered tissues," addition of exogenous hyaluronic acid, and modification of wounds to either enhance the growth factors, which have been implicated in regeneration (e.g., TGF-B3), or block those implicated in scar formation (e.g., TGF-B1) have all shown promise.

Age

There is considerable evidence that age at time of injury affects healing, but the mechanism remains unclear. Studies in fetal healing show a dramatic difference where the type of tissue is regenerated rather than scar tissue. Fetal healing features rapid healing, no scarring or acute inflammation, minimal fibroblasts proliferation in matrix rich in hyaluronic acid, and no excessive collagen formation.

Systemic Factors

Patient nutritional and metabolic status may affect the process of soft tissue healing. It has been shown in the past delayed wound healing is common in malnourished patients.

Dietary Factors

Protein deficiency may impair wound healing and decrease resistance to inflammation. Carbohydrate imbalance in a poorly controlled diabetic can seriously impair wound healing. This occurs through a defective process of inflammation and proliferation. In addition, wound infections are common in those patients. Essential fatty acids are needed for wound healing. Deficiency of some water-soluble vitamins (i.e., Vitamin C) will affect collagen formation and resistance to infection. Fat-soluble Vitamin A appears to play a significant role in collagen synthesis. Some trace elements deficiencies such as zinc may slow the response to healing.

Biochemical Factors

Local factors such as recent injury play an important role in the rate and quality of tissue healing in that area. Recent clinical observation regarding arthrofibrosis suggests that acute surgery represents an acute re-injury pattern and predisposes to excessive scar formation and poor results. Growth factors play a pivotal role in early healing process. Attempts at modulating their effects have not yet resulted, in encouraging results.

Biomechanical Factors

Canine studies showed that ligament healing is faster and stronger with unrestricted joint motion rather than immobilization in stable joints. Other studies showed the benefit of immobilization in better collagen orientation. At this time the relation between mechanical load and healing behavior in soft tissue remains tissue specific. Recent data have also suggested that cell morphology in ligament cell scar can be influenced by a mechanical load leading to selective differentiation of pluri-potent cells.

Future Methods to Improve Soft Tissue Healing

Angiogenic response in ligament injury and pattern of revascularization in healed ligament remains unclear. Further studies to enhance the knowledge of angiogenesis in healing ligament are needed. A better understanding of the role of GFs on soft tissue healing at a cellular level is needed in order to use exogenous GFs to alter biological process. Tissue response to locating stimuli has shown in animal studies to have a beneficial effect in the early stages of healing, but the frequency and response in different types of soft tissue is not yet established.

In summary, soft tissue healing follows a complex pattern of events, which remained poorly understood until recently. Opportunity may exist in the future for manipulation of soft tissue and in particular, ligament healing through further research in this area.

Laboratory Research

In the past, a controversy existed with regard to the best treatment of soft tissue injuries around the knee, particularly the MCL. Due to the accessibility and healing properties of this ligament many researchers made it a primary model for scientific experiment. Researchers have noted from an earlier work, differences in the healing of ACL (intra-articular ligament), as compared to MCL (extra-articular ligament). ACL mid substance tears showed poor healing ability, while the MCL consistently healed with good results. Many factors were attributed to the poor healing of the ACL, including the bathing of ruptured ends with synovial fluid, pattern of blood supply, and the structural and cellular difference. Biomechanical factors may play a significant role as the

ACL has multidirectional demands with regard to stability of the knee, while the MCL receives protection from intact secondary stabilizers and come under significantly less loads than the ACL (20–23).

Frank et al. (24) showed that divided MCL in rabbits healed satisfactory without immobilization or surgical repair. The repair was characterized by the formation of a "scar" rather than true ligament generation. He noticed that healed MCL was mechanically inferior to normal ligament at 40 weeks. He also showed in a long-term study in an animal model that the histological and morphologic appearance of the healed ligaments differs from the intact ligament with regard to having a smaller fiber diameter, and a poorer alignment of collagen fibers (24).

Earlier animal studies by Frank et al. (25) reported differences in the number, type, and cross linkage of collagen fibers at an earlier stage of the healing process. Greater proportion of collagen Type III was present early, but replaced by collagen Type I at a later stage, and the normal ratio returned to normal by 1 year. Cross linkage remained poor at 45% of normal values. The decrease in the collagen diameter, mass, and cross linkage resulted in the inferior biomechanical properties of the healed MCL (26).

Woo et al. (27), reported excellent results with mobilization following an MCL injury in a canine study. They treated three groups of surgically transected MCL with different methods including no repair with cage/farm activity, repair with 3 weeks of immobilization, and repair with 6 weeks of immobilization. They showed that within 12 weeks the no repair mobilized group had varus-valgus laxity and structural properties approaching that of controls. Load to failure in groups 1, 2, and 3 were 98%, 92%, and 54% of the respective controls; however, tensile strength values were only 49%, 43%, and 36% respectively. They concluded that conservative treatment with early mobilization rather than surgical repair, or prolonged immobilization, is the treatment of choice in isolated MCL injuries (25).

Burroughs and Dahners (28) demonstrated in a rat experiment with two groups of stable and unstable knees that the knees healed with excessive laxity in the unstable group while more strenuous exercise did not show beneficial results over the moderate excursive in the stable group. They reiterated the importance of secondary stabilizers on the healing of injured ligaments. Gijssen et al. (29) in a recent study reported that stiffness of 3, 6, or 9 weeks of healed murine MCL was not significantly different from the unoperated control.

Weiss et al. (30), reporting on the tensile strength of the healing MCL, found that the biomechanical properties of the healing ligament remained inferior to controls up to 1 year. Stiffness returned to near normal, while ultimate load was significantly lower than control. Mechanical properties were inferior despite the larger cross-sectional area of the healing mid substance MCL as compared to the intact control.

Simulated combined ACL/MCL injuries in animal models have been reported. Some studies on rabbits suggested that conservative treatment of MCL injury with mobilization and reconstruction of the ACL results in a satisfactory healing of the MCL (31). Other researchers have reported good outcomes from reconstructing both ligaments in terms of valgus laxity and structural properties in the short term with no difference at 1 year.

It has to be emphasized that there are limitation with regard to animal studies, including differences in animal size, ligament loading pattern, rehabilitation methods, and the use of exclusively young animals. Therefore, caution should be exercised before the application of these results directly into clinical practice. The information provided offers an understanding of the basic principles and processes that occur in the healing of ligament.

Clinical Application

Primary Repair versus No Repair
Based on scientific evidence primary repair of completely torn extra-articular ligament may produce smaller scar with some improvement in structural strength, but has no major benefits with regard to mechanical properties. Furthermore, repair did not show significant improved laxity, strength, or stiffness in a healed MCL in the ACL deficient knee.

In the multi-ligament injury, reconstruction of the ACL may impart stability to the injured MCL and allow it to heal in a satisfactory manner without the need for primary repair.

Isolated complete ACL (intra-articular ligament) injury showed poor healing potential, when transected at mid substance due to several factors mentioned previously, but primary repair has yielded unsatisfactory outcome based on clinical practice. Reconstruction with either hamstring or bone patellar tendon has been the treatment of choice for ACL tears with excellent results. Different patterns of ACL injuries including intra-substance tears and avulsion of the femoral attachment may show some healing with either elongated lax ACL, or abnormal attachment to the PCL respectively. Both may lead to dysfunctional ACL biomechanics necessitating reconstruction at a later date.

Movement versus Immobilization
Extensive research on the effects of immobilization in animal models has shown deleterious effects of prolonged immobilization on both the joints and the quality of the healed ligament. It causes the immobilized healing ligament to be less stiff and significantly weaker than the mobilized healing ligament.

Early mobilization under low stresses in a stable joint has clear benefits in the healing of injured ligaments. It improves strength and stiffness with minimal effect on the scar mass. It stimulates the synthesis of collagen and matrix remodeling.

It seems that early rather than late motion would provide those beneficial effects in ligament healing.

Effect of Early Return to Sports
Ligament injuries are common in the athletic population. The stresses on early return to sports have increased in recent times in a more competitive and demanding environment.

Previous clinical reports by Indelicato (20) and Reider et al. (32) have shown that 2 to 4 months may be required before the athlete returns to sports.

Woo (27) has shown in animal models that a mobilized healing ligament regained much of its structural properties including load at failure and varus–valgus laxity by 12 weeks, although recovery of its mechanical strength was only 49% at the same time.

Based on the above studies and other literature reports it is safe to assume that sufficient strength in the rehabilitated healing ligament has been achieved by twelve weeks to allow gradual return of sports.

■ REFERENCES

1. Hughston JC, Eilers AF. The role of the posterior oblique ligament in repairs of acute medial (collateral) ligament tears of the knee. *J Bone Joint Surg Am.* 1973;55(5):923–940.
2. Amiel D, Frank C, Harwood F, et al. Tendons and ligaments: a morphological and biochemical comparison. *J Orthop Res.* 1984; 1(3):257–265.
3. Fung YC. Elasticity of soft tissues in simple elongation. *Am J Physiol.* 1967;213:1532.
4. Viidik A. Elasticity and tensile strength of the anterior cruciate ligament in rabbits as influenced by training. *Acta Physiol Scand.* 1968;74(3):372–380.
5. Vogel H. Influence of maturation and age on mechanical and biochemical parameters of connective tissue on various organs in the rat. *Connect Tissue Res.* 1978;6:161.
6. Noyes FR. Functional properties of knee ligaments and alterations induced by immobilization: a correlative biomechanical and histological study in primates. *Clin Orthop.* 1977;(123):210–242.
7. Charlton WP, Coslett-Charlton LM, Ciccotti MG. Correlation of estradiol in pregnancy and anterior cruciate ligament laxity. *Clin Orthop.* 2001;387:165–170.
8. Dahners LE, Banes AJ, Burridge KW. The relationship of actin to ligament contraction. *Clin Orthop.* 1986;210:246–251.
9. Elder CL, Dahners LE, Weinhold PS. A cyclooxygenase-2 inhibitor impairs ligament healing in the rat. *Am J Sports Med.* 2001;29(6):801–805.
10. Lee WT, Collins JF. Ciprofloxacin associated bilateral achilles tendon rupture. *Aust N Z J Med.* 1992;22(5):500.
11. Williams RJ III, Attia E, Wickiewicz TL, et al. The effect of ciprofloxacin on tendon, paratenon, and capsular fibroblast metabolism. *Am J Sports Med.* 2000;28:364–369.
12. Muir H. The chemistry of the ground substance of joint cartilage. In: Solokoff L, ed. *The joints and synovial fluid.* New York: Academic Press;1980:27–94.
13. Mow VC, Lai WM. Some surface characteristics of articular cartilage. I. A scanning electron microscopy study and a theoretical model for the dynamic interaction of synovial fluid and articular cartilage. *J Biomech.* 1974;7(5):449–456.
14. Askew MJ, Mow VC. The biomechanical function of the collagen ultrastructure of articular cartilage. *J Biomech Eng.* 1978; 100:105.
14a. Morrison JB. The mechanics of the knee joint in relation to normal walking. *J Biomech.* 1970;3:51–61.
14b. Shrive NG, O'Conner JJ, Goodfellow JW. Load bearing in the knee joint. *Clin Orthop.* 1978;131:279.

15. Seedhom BB, Hargeaves DJ. Transmission of load in the knee joint with special reference to the role of the menisci. *Eng Med.* 1979;8:220–228.

15a. Papageorgeou C, Gil J, Kanamori A, et al. The biomechanical interdependence between the anterior cruciate replacement graft and the medial meniscus. *Am J Sports Med.* 2001;29:226–231.

16. Flynn TW, Soutas-Little RW. Patellofemoral joint compressive forces in forward and backward running. *J Orthop Sports Phys Ther.* 1995;21(5):277–282.

17. Frank CB, Bray RC, Hart DA, et al. Soft tissue healing. In: Fu F, Harner CD, Vince KG, eds. *Knee surgery.* Baltimore: Williams and Wilkins; 1994:189–229.

18. Frank C, Schar N, Dittrich D. Natural history of healing in the repaired medial collateral ligament. *J Orthop Res.* 1983;1(2):179–188.

19. Frank CS, Hiraoka N, Nakamura H, et al. Optimisation of the biology of soft tissue repair. cruciate ligament injury: an inter disciplinary study in rabbits. *J Orthop Res.* 1996;14:223–227.

20. Indelicato PA. Isolated medial collateral ligament injuries in the knee. *J Am Acad Orthop Surg.* 1995;3:9–14.

21. Johnson RJ, Beynnon BD, Nichols CE, et al. The treatment of injuries of the anterior cruciate ligament. *J Bone Joint Surg Am.* 1992;74:140–151.

22. Nickerson DA, Joshi R, Williams S, et al. Synovial fluid stimulates the proliferation of rabbit ligament: fibroblasts in vitro. *Clin Orthop.* 1992;274:294–299.

23. Woo SLY, Young EP, Ohland KJ, et al. The effects of transection of the anterior cruciate ligament on healing of the medial collateral ligament: a biomechanical study of the knee in dogs. *J Bone Joint Surg Am.* 1990;72:382–392.

24. Frank C, McDonald D, Shrive N. Collagen fibril diameters in the rabbit medial collateral ligament scar: a longer term assessment. *Connect Tissue Res.* 1997;36:261–269.

25. Frank C, Woo SLY, Amiel D, et al. Medial collateral ligament healing: a multidisciplinary assessment in rabbits. *Am J Sports Med.* 1983;11:379–389.

26. Frank C, McDonald D, Wilson J, et al. Rabbit medial collateral ligament scar weakness is associated with decreased collagen pyridinoline crosslink density. *J Orthop Res.* 1995;13:157–165.

27. Woo SL, Inoue M, McGurk-Burleson E, et al. Treatment of the medial collateral ligament injury. II: Structure and function of canine knees in response to differing treatment regimens. *Am J Sports Med.* 1987;15(1):22–29.

28. Burroughs P, Dahners LE. The effect of enforced exercise on the healing of ligament injuries. *Am J Sports Med.* 1990;18(4):376–378.

29. Gijssen Y, Sierevelt IN, Kooloos JG, et al. Stiffness of the healing medial collateral ligament of the mouse. *Connect Tissue Res.* 2004;45(3):190–195.

30. Weiss JA, Woo SLY, Ohland KJ, et al. Evaluation of a new injury model to study medial collateral ligament healing: primary repair versus nonoperative treatment. *J Orthop Res.* 1991;9:516–528.

31. Yamaji T, Levine RE, Woo SLY, et al. Medial collateral ligament healing one year after a concurrent medial collateral ligament and anterior. *J Sci Med Sport.* 1999;2(3):190–210.

32. Reider B, Sathy MR, Talkington J, et al. Treatment of isolated medial collateral ligament injuries in athletes with early functional rehabilitation: a five-year follow-up study. *Am J Sports Med.* 1994;22:470–477.

THE ANTERIOR CRUCIATE LIGAMENT

34

ANTERIOR CRUCIATE RECONSTRUCTION

34.1

ANDREW PICKLE, MD, AARON CAMPBELL, MD, DONALD H. JOHNSON, MD, FRCS

■ KEY POINTS

- The most common mechanism of anterior cruciate injury is a twisting or deceleration that may be accompanied by hyperextension and/or internal rotation forces on the knee.
- Unrecognized malalignment can be a reason for failure of ACL reconstructions.
- X-rays should be ordered in all cases to rule out associated fractures and to identify degenerative changes in middle-age patients pre-operatively.
- Reconstructive surgery is generally considered the standard treatment for athletes, who want to return to sports that involve pivoting.
- In younger patients, reconstructive surgery is necessary to prevent further damage to the knee, and minimize degenerative changes.
- An aggressive post-op rehabilitation program can diminish the problem of lack of full knee extension commonly associated with patellar tendon grafts. Therefore, if the surgeon is unable to control the post-op physiotherapy program to ensure full extension, the hamstrings may be a better graft choice.
- The ideal candidate for reconstruction with a patellar tendon graft is the young athlete competing in pivotal activities at the elite level, because of the importance of the commitment to an intensive rehabilitation program.
- Unlike hamstring grafts, which can be of variable diameter, the patellar tendon offers a graft of consistent size and shape.
- Errors in tunnel placement, tensioning, and fixation are more likely to result in a poor outcome than the choice of which graft to use.
- Patients are placed in a Continuous Passive Motion (CPM) machine prior to leaving the OR.
- Physical therapy is begun within 4 or 5 days of surgery, and patients are seen 5 to 7 days post-op to review surgical findings and postoperative rehabilitation.
- The goal for the first 2 weeks post-op is to minimize swelling, allow wound healing, and begin range of motion exercises.

577

After 3 months, light sports (cross-country skiing, curling, or golf) may be allowed, if there is full range of motion, no effusion, negative Lachman, and return to 90% strength.

Anterior cruciate ligament (ACL) injuries are very common in today's active population. Over the years, ACL reconstruction has evolved dramatically, from primary repair to extra-articular procedures, and finally intra-articular, single incision techniques. There are estimated to be over 100,000 ACL reconstructions performed in the United States annually. Once considered a career ending injury, ACL reconstruction is now an outpatient procedure with better than 90% successful outcome.

■ CLINICAL EVALUATION

History

The most common mechanism of injury is a noncontact twisting or deceleration injury. This may also have hyperextension and/or internal rotation forces on the knee. The patients often feel a "pop," followed by pain and swelling, and they are unable to continue playing. In the chronic situation the patients have symptoms of knee instability with pivoting, jumping, or lateral motions. The patients complain that the knee gives way, and it feels like the bones are coming apart. ACL ruptures can also occur with combined ligament injuries such as knee dislocations.

Physical Exam

The examination begins with observation of the patient's body habitus, gait, and alignment. Unrecognized malalignment can be a reason for failure of ACL reconstructions. An example of this would be a varus knee alignment, associated with posterolateral laxity, and a thrust when walking. A general examination of the knee is performed, including inspection, palpation, range of motion, neurovascular examination, and special tests for ligaments and menisci.

Lachman Test

This is the hallmark test to assess ACL injury **(Fig 34.1-1)**. The test is performed with the knee flexed at 30 degrees, and the hamstrings relaxed. The examiner assesses the amount of anterior translation and the presence or absence of an endpoint compared to the opposite knee.

The Lachman test can be graded as follows:

■ Grade 1+ has 0 to 5 mm displacement with a firm end point,

■ Grade 2+ has 5 to 10 mm displacement with no end point,
■ Grade 3+ has greater than 10 mm displacement.

In the acute situation, the dropped leg Lachman test is performed by letting the thigh rest on the edge of the bed, and the leg is dropped over the side with 30 degrees of knee flexion **(Fig 34.1-2)**. The hamstring muscles are relaxed in this position, and an assessment of the anterior translation can be made even in the acute situation.

Pivot Shift Test

This test is performed by the examiner supporting the patient's leg in extension. One hand then applies an axial load, and valgus force as the knee is slowly flexed **(Fig 34.1-3)**.

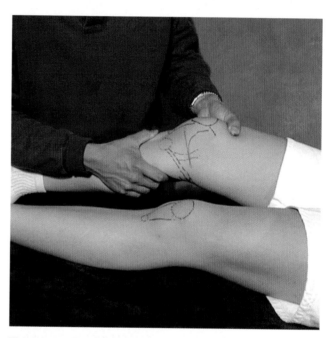

Fig. 34.1-1. The Lachman Test.

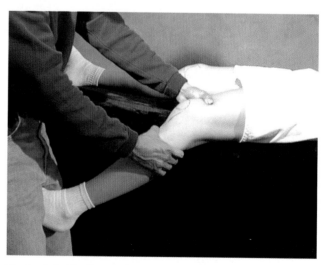

Fig 34.1-2. The Dropped leg Lachman Test.

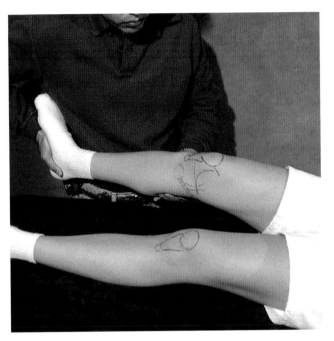

Fig 34.1-3. The Pivot Shift Test.

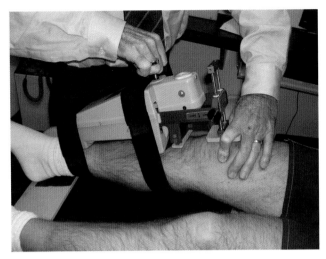

Fig 34.1-4. KT-1000 Arthrometer.

If the ACL is deficient, the tibia will sublux anteriorly in extension, and will reduce with flexion. The anatomic shape of the lateral femoral condyle is thought to be responsible for the snap or clunk that is felt with reduction (1). It can be accentuated with applying external rotation to the tibia with the maneuver.

The pivot shift test can be graded as follows:

- 1+ is a pivot glide
- 2+ is a pivot shift
- 3+ is a gross pivot shift with the feeling that the condyles will dislocate.

Anterior Drawer Test

Although the posterior drawer test is very useful for posterior cruciate ligament injuries, the anterior drawer test has limited use in ACL injuries. It is performed with the patient's knee flexed 90 degrees and stabilized by the examiner sitting on the foot, while applying an anterior directed force to the proximal tibia. The amount of anterior translation of the tibia under the femur is compared to the opposite leg.

Special tests for other ligament injuries, such as the dial test for posterolateral laxity, will not be covered here, but are very important to avoid missing associated injuries.

■ IMAGING

Plain Radiographs

These should be ordered in all cases to rule out associated fractures. They can be used to assess the growth plates and

avulsion fractures in adolescents. The Segond fracture is a lateral capsule avulsion from tibia, and is pathognomonic for ACL injury. As well, degenerative changes in middle age patients can be identified pre-operatively.

MRI

This is generally not required for routine ACL injuries. However, MRI is useful to assess associated meniscal pathology, and newer fast spin technology has improved cartilage imaging.

■ INSTRUMENTED LIGAMENT TESTING

KT-1000 Arthrometer

This is a very useful tool to give objective measurements of the amount of anterior translation of the tibia (Fig 34.1-4). The arthrometer can be used pre-operatively, intra-operatively, and post-operatively. It has been validated and generally a side-to-side difference of over 3 mm is considered pathologic, and over 5 mm difference indicates a complete tear (2,3).

■ TREATMENT

The patient who has sustained an ACL injury has three treatment choices: avoid pivoting sports, resume modified activities with a brace, or undergo ACL reconstruction.

Reconstructive surgery for torn ACLs is generally considered the standard of care for patients who want to return to pivoting sports. There are two main reasons for this: First, the natural history of an ACL deficient knee is associated with a high incidence of complex meniscal tears, chondral injuries, and late degenerative changes (4,5); second, ACL reconstruction has become a relatively routine outpatient procedure with a greater than 90% success rate (6).

Nonoperative

The initial treatment of all ACL injuries includes splinting, crutches, and early range of motion exercises. Range of motion must be re-established for optimal outcome with either operative or nonoperative treatment.

The role of functional braces is controversial. They have been shown to decrease anterior translation at low loads, but not at physiologic loads. Braces may however contribute some proprioceptive feedback, but the significance is unknown (7). A difficult scenario exists when an athlete tears one's ACL early in the season and wants to complete the season with a brace. Shelton et al. (8) followed 43 athletes, prospectively, who elected to complete the season in a brace, and found that 70% were able to complete the season, 61% experienced instability in the brace, and 62% of the athletes had associated meniscal/chondral injuries at the time of their ACL reconstruction. Generally, if patients elect for nonoperative treatment, they should be aware of the natural history, and avoid pivoting activities.

Operative

The operative management of ACL tears has evolved significantly over the years. Primary repair has been abandoned due to high failure rates (9). The extra-articular procedures such as the Macintosh and Ellison had poor long-term results, and thus have fallen out of favor. Amis and Scammell (10) have shown in the lab that the addition of an extra-articular procedure did not improve the biomechanics over an intra-articular procedure alone. For most surgeons, the standard of care would be the arthroscopically aided intra-articular reconstruction.

The indications for ACL reconstruction include active patients that experience symptoms of instability with pivoting sports. Patients who complain of instability with activities of daily living most likely have additional pathology such as a meniscal tear. In younger patients, reconstructive surgery is necessary to prevent further damage to the knee, and minimize degenerative changes (11). In older patients the treatment is more individualized to meet their physical demands.

There are several issues to consider in ACL reconstruction including the choice of graft, tunnel placement, choice of fixation, pain control, and post-op rehabilitation. The choices of graft include autogenous bone-patellar tendon-bone, hamstring, and quadriceps grafts. The same tissues are all available in all grafts.

Successful outcomes have been achieved with all graft types. The meta-analysis by Yunes et al. (12) showed better stability, but more anterior knee pain with the patellar tendon graft. There was more laxity with the hamstrings graft, but less harvest site morbidity. At International Society of

Arthroscopy, Knee Surgery, and Orthopaedic Sports Medicine, (ISAKOS) in 2003, Cohen showed that at a 15 year follow-up, 75% of patients had evidence of patellofemoral osteoarthritis with patellar tendon reconstructions. Inability of the patients to regain full extension was implicated as the reason for this finding. Shelbourne and Nitz (13) have advocated an aggressive post-op rehabilitation program, which has diminished the problem of lack of full knee extension commonly associated with patellar tendon grafts. Therefore, if the surgeon is unable to control the post-op physiotherapy program to ensure full extension, then the hamstrings may be a better graft choice.

Quadrupled hamstring grafts have been found to be stronger (i.e., higher ultimate load to failure) than patellar tendon grafts, and twice as strong as native ACLs (14). The main issue with hamstring grafts remains the method of graft fixation (15,16). With improved fixation devices and graft tensioning this problem should be minimized.

■ TECHNIQUE OF ANTERIOR CRUCIATE LIGAMENT RECONSTRUCTION WITH SEMITENDINOSUS

The following are the steps in ACL reconstruction with the four bundle hamstring graft at our institution:

- Examination under anesthesia (EUA) and Documentation
- Graft Harvest and Preparation
- Diagnostic Arthroscopy and Meniscal Repair
- Meniscectomy
- Stump Debridement and Notchplasty
- Tibial Tunnel Preparation
- Femoral Tunnel Preparation
- Graft Passage and Fixation
- Final Inspection and Measurement

Examination Under Anesthesia and Documentation

After appropriate anesthesia, a femoral nerve block and preoperative antibiotics are given. An examination under anesthesia is performed to confirm the diagnosis and check for other pathology. The collateral ligaments, the PCL, and posterior lateral corner are examined. Lachman, pivot shift, as well as, a KT-1000 arthrometer side to side difference are done to evaluate the ACL. The indication to proceed with a standard ACL reconstruction is a manual maximum difference of greater than 5 mm, and positive pivot shift. The leg is prepped and draped in the standard fashion, and the tourniquet is inflated.

Graft Harvest and Preparation

Harvesting of the hamstring grafts usually occurs first. There is some controversy in whether the diagnostic arthroscopy of the knee should be done before the graft

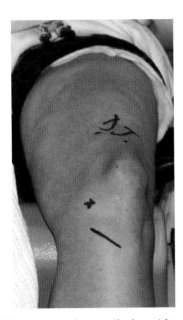

Fig 34.1-5. Skin incision to harvest the hamstring graft.

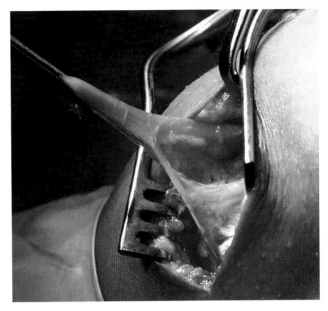

Fig 34.1-6. The bands from the tendon to the gastronemius.

harvest. If the patient has a positive pivot shift test, and KT-1000 values greater than 5 mm side to side, then the ACL is not functional, and a reconstruction will have to be performed. The leg is placed in the figure of four position, and the hamstring tendons can often be palpable approximately 5 cm below the medial joint line. An oblique 3 cm incision is made about 1 cm medial to the tibial tubercle and approximately 5 cm below the joint line (Fig 34.1-5). Dissection is made through the skin and subcutaneous fat until the sartorius fascia is identified. The gracilis and semitendinosus tendons can now be seen and felt just below the fascia. The tendons are picked up with a Kocher, and using scissors, the fascia is opened above the tendons, and the pes anserine bursa identified. The tendons are detached from the tibia by sharp dissection using a knife. This corner is lifted up to visualize the underlying medial collateral ligament. Kochers are placed on both tendon ends, and the conjoined tendon divided. The tendon ends can now be pulled into the wound to expose the adhering bands, which attach inferiorly and medially to the gastrocnemius. Avoid twisting the tendons as it changes the orientation of the bands, making them harder to find and subsequently cut (Fig 34.1-6). Pulling on the free end and watching for any dimpling in the calf is a useful check to be sure the tendon is free. It is very important to identify and cut these all the fascial bands to the gastrocnemius to prevent premature amputation of the grafts with the tendon stripper. The closed loop tendon stripper is then used to harvest the grafts by keeping distal tension on the grafts, and passing the stripper in the direction of the tendons. The tendons will be cut off by the stripper at their musculotendinus junction. The tendons are then taken to the back table to be prepared.

The tendons are prepared on the graft preparation workstation. Using a periosteal elevator, the muscle is removed, and the tendons are cut to 22 cm in length. Using No. 2 nonabsorbable

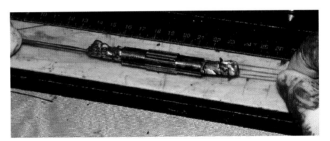

Fig 34.1-7. Sizing the graft.

braided suture, the four ends are individually stitched in a whip stitch fashion for about 4 cm. The two tendons are folded over a No. 5 braided suture, to form a quadruple graft. Their diameter is measured to the nearest 0.5 mm (Fig 34.1-7). The tendons can be kept in a moist sponge, or pretensioned at 15 N until the tunnels are prepared.

A complete diagnostic arthroscopy is performed next in a standard fashion. Any associated pathology is identified and treated. The remaining ACL stump is removed with a mechanical shaver until the footprint is seen well. A minimal notchplasty is performed to ensure there will be no graft impingement and the back wall of the femoral notch is well seen and felt with a hook. Care must be taken to ensure the true back wall is visualized and not just residents' ridge (Fig 34.1-8).

The tunnels are prepared next. The tibial tunnel is prepared using a tibial guide (Fig 34.1-9) that is inserted through the anteromedial portal and directs a K-wire 7 mm anterior to the PCL in the midline (Fig 34.1-10). The K-wire is started on the anteromedial tibia in the harvest site incision approximately halfway between the tubercle and the posterior tibia. This will allow the transtibial drilling of the femur at the 10 and 2 o'clock positions, and avoid placing the graft too vertical in the notch. After appropriate guide wire placement,

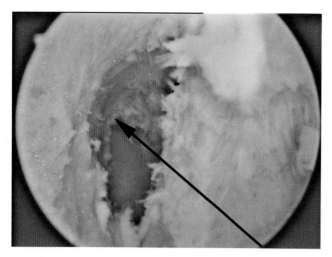

Fig 34.1-8. The completed notchplasty.

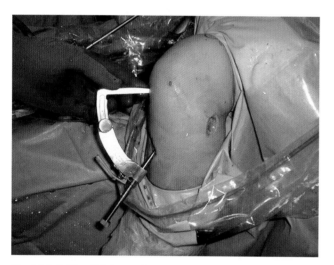

Fig 34.1-9. The tibial tunnel guide.

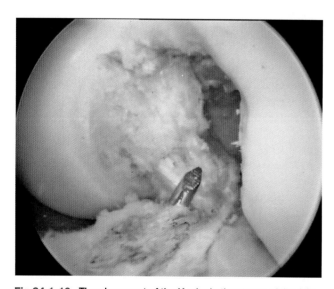

Fig 34.1-10. The placement of the K-wire in the stump of the ACL.

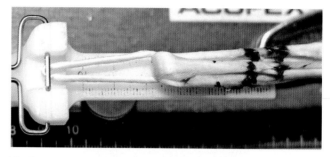

Fig 34.1-11. The closed loop endobutton attached to the four bundle graft.

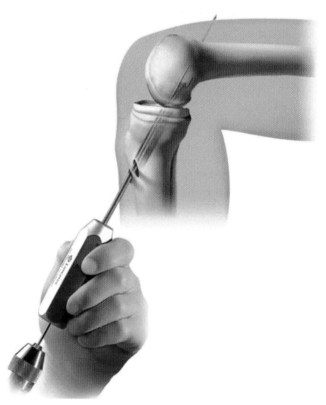

Fig 34.1-12. The Bullseye femoral aiming guide.

the tibial tunnel is first drilled with a 6 mm cannulated drill, and then dilated to the diameter of the harvested graft. The leg can be extended with the dilator in place to verify that there will be no anterior graft impingement.

The closed loop EndoButton (Smith & Nephew, Andover, MA) is the choice of femoral fixation at our institution (Fig 34.1-11). A Bullseye femoral aiming guide is placed into the notch and hooked over the back wall (Fig 34.1-12). The guide can be passed through the tibial tunnel or through a low anteromedial portal. It is important to position the guide at the 10 o'clock position for right knees and 2 o'clock position for left knees. The endobutton 4.5 mm cannulated drill is used next, to drill through both cortices, and the length of the femoral tunnel is measured with a depth gauge. After calculating the desired length of tunnel to hold the graft and allow for flipping the endobutton (5 mm), the tunnel is drilled to the

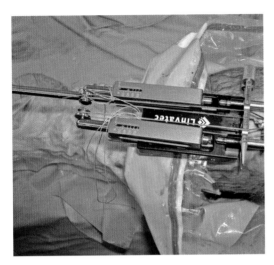

Fig 34.1-13. The Linvatec graft tensioner.

diameter of the harvested graft. The closed loop endobutton is attached to the quadrupled graft and the length of the femoral tunnel is marked on the graft. One No. 2 suture is placed in one eye of the endobutton and two No. 5 sutures are placed in the other eye. These will be used to pull the graft through the tunnels and allow flipping of the endobutton on the anterior femoral cortex. The graft is passed into the femoral tunnel from distal to proximal. After the endobutton is secured on the femur by flipping the button, the graft is tensioned distally.

In order to achieve appropriate ACL graft tension intraoperatively, we have been using the Linvatec SE Graft Tensioner (Fig 34.1-13). Small guide pins are attached at the entrance of the tibial tunnel, and the semitendinosus graft ends are marked to distinguish them from the gracilis ends. The knee is taken through a range of motion and impingement is assessed. The tensioner is now attached to the guide pins on the tibia, and the semitendinosus graft is tensioned to 50 N, and the gracilis is tensioned to 30 N, to attain an overall 80 N of tension in the graft. Again the knee is cycled several times, and the tensioner adjusted. The tensioner is left in place, keeping the tendons separated and under appropriate tension while a BioScrew XtraLok (Linvatec, Largo, FL) corticocancellous screw is placed in the middle of the four bundles of graft. Finally, the tensioner is removed, the grafts ends are cut, and the wounds are closed and dressed. An immediate post-op KT-1000 manual maximum measurement is taken and recorded.

Post-operatively, the patients are discharged home with crutches, an extension knee splint, a continuous passive motion machine, and a Cyrocuff cold therapy unit.

Anterior Cruciate Ligament Reconstruction with the Patellar Tendon Graft

Initially described by Jones in 1960, and later popularized by Erickson in the 1970s, the patellar tendon graft remains a popular graft choice for surgeons and is considered by many

to be the gold standard. The problems with postoperative stiffness have been greatly diminished as a result of more aggressive rehabilitation protocols, such those advocated by Shelbourne. Contra lateral graft harvest has also been described in order to facilitate rehabilitation and early return to sports. The popularity of this graft amongst members of the American Academy of Orthopedic Surgeons was demonstrated by a survey conducted in 2003, in which 80% of respondents preferred the use of a patellar tendon graft.

Advantages to Patellar Tendon Grafts

Several advantages of the patellar tendon graft, which serve to enhance its popularity. Unlike hamstring grafts, which can be of variable diameter, the patellar tendon offers a graft of consistent shape and size. Graft harvest is done with relative ease, and little preparation is required to make the graft ready to implant. Bone plugs at the ends of the graft allow for secure initial fixation and early bone to bone healing, which is more conducive to an aggressive rehabilitation program and early return to sport at an elite or professional level. Finally, as Shelbourne has demonstrated, contra lateral limb graft harvest can also be undertaken in an attempt to further enhance postoperative recovery.

Indications for the Patellar Tendon Graft

The ideal candidate for ACL reconstruction with a patellar tendon graft is the young athlete competing in aggressive pivotal activities at the elite or professional level. Commitment to an intensive rehabilitation program is essential for a good outcome. Thus, while there is no strict age limit for this graft, it is generally better suited to young athletes, who often have more time to commit to rehabilitation, and competitive individuals, who are highly motivated to commit to the postoperative physiotherapy required for good outcome. The patellar tendon graft is favored by 80% of the ACL study group members, and 99% of NFL team physicians.

Concerns with Patellar Tendon Autografts

Despite its popularity, the patellar tendon graft is not without its disadvantages. The graft harvest necessitates exposing and then disturbing the normal extensor mechanism. Thus the majority of problems involved the components of the extensor mechanism as well as the incision required for the exposure.

The topic of patellofemoral pain, after anterior cruciate reconstruction with the patellar tendon is graft, is controversial. The problem is confounded by the fact that older rehabilitation programs immobilized the knee and restricted early motion. The incidence of patellofemoral problems appears to have lessened with more aggressive postoperative physiotherapy and patellar mobilization exercises. However, anterior knee pain and difficulty kneeling are common complaints after patellar tendon harvest. This may be, at least in part, due to injury to the infrapatellar branch of the saphenous nerve. Harvest through two transverse incisions rather than a single longitudinal incision has been proposed in order to help minimize the risk of nerve injury and resultant anterior knee pain.

The defect left in the patellar tendon after removing its central third is also a concern for the orthopedic surgeon. If the defect is closed too tight, the patella may become entrapped producing patellar baja, and potential patellofemoral pain and crepitus. On the other hand, if the defect is not closed, it may persist, resulting in a weaker tendon susceptible to rupture.

Being able to perform the postop physiotherapy is crucial to a good outcome after anterior cruciate reconstruction. Both patellar tendonitis and quadriceps weakness are common after patellar tendon harvest, making compliance with rehabilitation a problem for some patients. For this reason, many surgeons consider an alternative graft in patients who are not highly motivated or will not be followed closely by a therapist postoperatively.

Patellar fracture may also occur as a result of harvesting the patellar bone plug. This may occur either intraoperatively or in the postoperative period. It generally mandates open reduction and internal fixation, if appropriate rehabilitation is to be carried out. Removing the patellar bone plug in a manner, which does not produce stress risers (see method of harvest), can greatly reduce the risk of fracture.

Contraindications to Patellar Tendon Graft Harvest

While there are no absolute contraindications to primary harvest of the patellar tendon in a mature patient, one should consider the previously discussed concerns prior to choosing it as the source of graft material for ACL reconstruction. As postoperative anterior knee pain remains a concern, it seems to make sense to avoid using patellar tendon grafts in patients with a history of patellofemoral pain, patellar tendonitis, or chondromalacia in order to prevent exacerbating a previous condition. Although, Shelbourne and Nitz (13) has reported that a bony ossicle within the tendon from Osgoode-Schlatters disease is not a contraindication to use of the patellar tendon, because the ossicle usually lies within a bone tunnel, such cases should be considered on an individual basis.

The patient with a narrow patellar tendon (less than 25 mm) also deserves careful consideration. Harvesting 10 mm from such tendon leaves it susceptible to rupture in the postoperative period. To reduce this risk, one should either reduce the graft width (i.e., 8 to 9 mm), or chose an alternative source of graft.

Summary

Successful ACL surgery requires a number of factors including careful patient selection, surgical technique, and

postoperative rehabilitation. While there has been much debate about graft selection, comparative studies have shown the outcome is almost the same regardless of graft choice. Errors in tunnel placement, tensioning, and fixation are more likely to result in a poor outcome, than is the choice of graft. One must remember that with any graft, meticulous surgical technique is still required to obtain an optimal result.

■ SURGICAL TECHNIQUE OF ANTERIOR CRUCIATE LIGAMENT RECONSTRUCTION WITH THE PATELLAR TENDON GRAFT

Graft Harvest and Preparation

The first step in patellar tendon graft harvest is to carefully plan the skin incisions. Preferably the skin incision, or incisions for harvest incorporate the exposure needed for the tibial tunnel in order to avoid unnecessary incisions. A longitudinal incision 8 to 10 cm long and biased 1 cm medially allows for easy exposure and harvest, while allowing the tibial tunnel to be drilled through the same incisions. As one becomes more proficient with the harvest, the incision can be shortened in order to improve cosmesis. Alternatively, two short transverse incisions may be used instead of the single longitudinal incision **(Fig 34.1-14)**. This technique has been shown to lessen the risk of injury to the infrapatellar branch of the saphenous nerve, and improve the patients' ability to kneel comfortably after the tendon harvest. Despite its merits, this method provides less exposure of the bone tendon complex, than the longitudinal incision, and thus is more technically demanding.

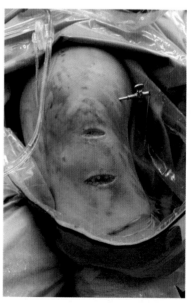

Fig 34.1-14. The two incisions for the patellar tendon harvest.

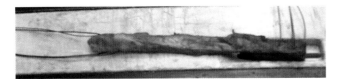

Fig 34.1-15. The patellar tendon graft.

After exposing the tendon, a double bladed knife is used to mark the central 10 mm of the tendon (picture). The bone plugs on the patella (10 x 25 mm), and tibia (10 x 35 mm) should also be marked at this time. Using a boat shaped graft minimizes the risk of stress fracture. A 2 mm (1/16 inch) drill bit is then used to drill two holes in each bone plug. It is generally easier to perform this step prior to removing the bone plug.

With the bone plugs marked and predrilled, a micro-oscillating saw is used to make the necessary cuts. Careful attention should be paid to the patella to avoid creating stress risers that can cause fractures. The initial 4 to 5 mm cut should be perpendicular to the cortex. The saw should then be angled to at 60 degrees and the cut continued to 8 to 10 mm. A deep V cut as well as a transverse proximal cut should be avoided as both create stress risers. Upon completion of the cuts, the graft is carefully freed with a 1 cm osteotome. The base of the bone plug should be flat and its proximal end tapered to minimize the risk of fracture and allow easy passage (Fig 34.1-15).

Once free, the graft is transferred to a back table and prepared for implantation. Care must be taken to avoid dropping the graft. Nonabsorbable sutures are placed through the holes previously drilled in the bone plugs. Two number five Ticron sutures are used for the femoral (patellar) plug, and two number two sutures are used for the tibia. Excess fat should be removed and rough edges trimmed with scissors. Next, the bone plugs should be tailored with a small rongeur and checked with an appropriate sizing tube (9 mm femur, 10 mm tibia) so they pass easily through the tunnels. Finally, the bone tendon junction on the femoral plug should be marked so it can easily be distinguished arthroscopically as the graft is passed through the knee. The graft is now ready to implant.

Notch Preparation

The diagnostic arthroscopy and meniscal work should be completed prior to the notch and tunnel preparation. The technique is essentially the same as for hamstring grafts.

The soft tissue is removed from the medial aspect of the lateral femoral condyle using a curette and 5.5 mm resector. Emphasis should be placed on "opening" up the roof and anterolateral corner of the notch. This allows more light to reach the back of the knee and improves visualization as one works in the posterior aspect of the notch closer to the neurovascular structures. The degree of notchplasty required is quite variable depending on the amount of notch stenosis. In the very narrow A-shaped notch, an oval burr may be used to remove bone. Oval burrs are preferred as they do not jump around as much as round burrs and are easier to control.

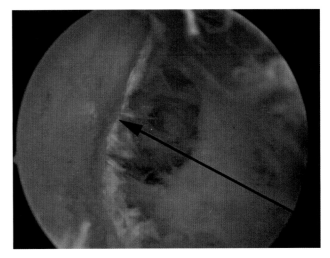

Fig 34.1-16. The completed notchplasty.

By carefully working posterior, the back of the notch can be viewed. Remember, the most common technical error in ACL reconstruction is placing the femoral tunnel too anterior. Therefore, it is critical to clearly visualize the overlying fringe of capsule and probe the drop off of the femoral condyle (Fig 34.1-16). The fringe of capsule is not present on residents ridge and together with feeling the drop off allows for accurate determination of the over the top position. Once the over the top position has been identified a mark is made with a burr or awl, 7 mm in from the drop off (assuming a 10 mm tunnel) at the eleven or one o'clock position. A visual check can be used to see that the tunnel is aimed for the intended 10 oval target area on the anterior lateral aspect of the thigh.

Tibial Tunnel

After the notch is prepared, the tunnels are drilled. Generally the tibial side is drilled first, and the femoral tunnel referenced off the tibial tunnel. However, if a transtibial technique is being used, great care must be taken to correctly orient the tibial tunnel, in order to allow for proper placement of the femoral tunnel (Fig 34.1-17). The guide positions the tunnel approximately 5 cm distal to the joint line at the anterior margin of the medial collateral ligament. Using the guide, a K-wire is then positioned in the footprint of the ACL, just anterior to the leading edge of the PCL. The guide should then be removed and the position rechecked in extension to check for possible impingement.

After confirming correct positioning of the K wire, a cannulated drill is then used to drill the tibial tunnel. Then remove any debris from around the intra articular portion of the tunnel. A 3 mm posterior wall should exist between the posterior wall of the tunnel and the PCL. Also remove any soft tissue from the tunnel entrance to facilitate passage of the femoral guide and later the graft.

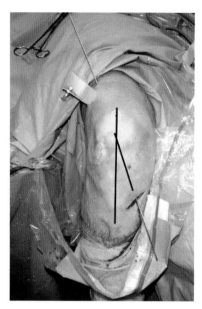

Fig 34.1-17. The correct angle for drilling the tibial tunnel.

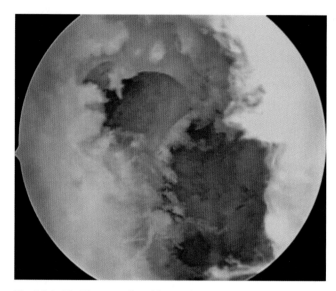

Fig 34.1-18. The completed femoral tunnel with 1 to 2 mm of posterior wall.

Femoral Tunnel

The femoral tunnel is now referenced off the tibial tunnel using the offset femoral guide. The guide is passed through the tibial tunnel and hooked behind the lateral femoral condyle. The knee is flexed to 90 degrees and a long guide wire introduced through the guide. The starting position for the guide wire should closely approximate the position marked during the notch preparation (11 or 1 o'clock). By rotating the guide slightly, the guide wire may also be positioned more obliquely (10:30 or 1:30), if so desired. With the wire in place, a 10 mm reamer is the used to drill the tunnel. A 5 mm footprint should be drilled first and the position checked to avoid drilling out the posterior wall. With this step complete, the tunnel may then be completed to a depth of 30 mm to accommodate the 25 mm bone plug. The completed femoral tunnel should have a 1 to 2 mm of posterior wall **(Fig 34.1-18)**.

After the tunnel has been drilled, the guide and wire are removed from the knee. The notcher is then introduced through the anterior medial portal and the entrance of the tunnel notched. This should be done at the starting point of the fixation screw on the superiolateral portion of the tunnel. Failure to perform this step may lead to difficulty in starting the screw or screw breakage, especially in patients with hard bone.

With notching complete, a two-pin passer is then passed through the tibia and positioned eccentrically anterior in the femoral tunnel. Again the surgeon should aim for the target zone on the anterior and lateral aspect of the thigh. The pin should be drilled through the cortex and out through the skin. A Kocher clamp is used to keep it in place. The guide wire for the femoral fixation screw is then introduced through the medial portal and into the anterior channel of the pin passer to ensure screw fixation anterior to the graft.

It should be held in place with a hemostat next to the skin on the thigh. A second guide wire is then placed anteriorly in the tibial tunnel to be used later for the tibial fixation screw.

Graft Passage

The eyelet of the two pin passer is used to pull the number five leader sutures through the knee. A Kocher is then used to pull the graft into the joint. The cancellous surfaces should be anterior. During passing, the graft should be viewed through the arthroscope. Occasionally it may be necessary to manipulate the femoral bone with a grasper or hook to facilitate its entrance into the tunnel. The graft is then pulled into the femoral tunnel until the previously marked bone tendon interface is at the tunnel entrance. Tension is then applied to the sutures at both ends of the graft and the positioning checked through a range of motion.

Graft Fixation

The two pin passer ensures that the guide wire for the fixation screw passes directly up the anterior aspect of the femoral tunnel and avoids kinking of the guide wire when the screw is inserted. Screw insertion should be performed with the knee flexed to 120 degrees to minimize damaging the graft and ensure the screw is inserted in the direction of the tunnel. As the screw advances, there should be an audible squeak and the surgeon should feel a good purchase in the bone tunnel. If the screw does not advance, the starting point should be tapped. A properly positioned screw should be against the cancellous bone and parallel to the tunnel, with the head of the screw at the tunnel entrance in order to achieve fixation at the cortex.

With the femoral fixation complete, tension is applied to the sutures on the tibial side and knee cycled repeatedly from complete flexion to complete extension. This cycling removes the "play" from the graft and can be done by simply pulling on the sutures or by using a mechanical tensioning device. This process also checks that the femoral fixation is adequate. Currently most authors recommend 80 N of tension. With continuous tension applied, the graft is then secured distally using a tibial fixation screw over the anteriorly positioned guide wire. The screw should not be countersunk, but instead should remain at the tibial cortex in order to provide maximal fixation.

Graft Inspection

After fixation, a final inspection of the graft should be undertaken. Using the arthroscope, the graft is inspected throughout a range of motion to check for possible impingement or abrasion. Tension is assessed with a hook and by performing a Lachman test, while watching the motion of the tibial spines with the arthroscope. KT measurements may also be performed at this point. Once the surgeon is satisfied that the knee is stable and fixation is secure, the leader sutures may be cut and the wounds irrigated and closed.

Postoperative Care

After wound closure sterile dressings are applied along with a cryocuff. Patients are placed in a CPM machine prior to leaving the OR. After a few hours in hospital the patients are discharged home with an extension splint and crutches. Physical therapy is begun within four or five days of surgery and patients are seen in clinic 5 to 7 days post-op to review the surgical findings and postoperative rehabilitation.

Rehabilitation

Rehabilitation for the patient begins before the surgery. Preoperatively, the patient should have a full understanding of the operative procedure and the post-operative rehabilitation. Ideally, the patient should have no effusion, full range of motion, and good strength pre-operatively. The injured knee should look like the normal uninjured knee. Physiotherapy should start 5 to 7 days post-op. The goal for the first 2 weeks post-op is to minimize swelling, allow wound healing, and begin range of motion exercises. This is done primarily with passive exercises and isometrics. Weeks 2 to 12 focus on gaining further range of motion, and strength with closed chain kinetic exercises. After 3 months, light sports may be allowed (e.g., cross-country skiing, curling, or golf) if there is full range of motion, no effusion, negative Lachman, and greater than 90% strength. Vigorous pivoting exercises are avoided until 6 months post-op, and only if the patient has full range of motion, is stable, has no effusion, and has achieved 90% strength of the opposite leg. If the patient owns an ACL brace, it is advised that they continue to use it for pivoting sports for the first year post-operatively. The patient will usually discontinue the use of

the brace when he has regained confidence in the knee, and perhaps proprioception.

Pain Management and Outpatient Anterior Cruciate Ligament Reconstruction

There are only a very few things that have been learned over the past decade about ACL reconstruction. First of all, mark the site that you are going to operate on, to avoid wrong side surgery. This should be done outside of the OR with the patient awake. The choice of graft is probably immaterial. The most important factor in a satisfactory stability outcome is to put the tunnels in the correct position, and fix the graft adequately. But, from a patient's perspective, the biggest improvement is in pain management. This is an important aspect nowadays, as all ACL reconstruction is done as an outpatient.

This is the list of pain management modalities that are currently used for outpatient anesthesia in ACL reconstruction:

- Pre-emptive multi-modal analgesia
- Oral nonsteroidal anti-inflammatory drug (NSAID) preop
- Intra-articular injection of sensocaine and morphine
- Incisional injection of sensocaine
- Femoral nerve block
- Tourniquet
- Post op NSAID
- Cryotherapy
- Continuous passive motion
- Accelerated rehab

Multimodal Analgesia

Multimodal or balanced analgesia (17) means to make use of multiple modalities to augment the anesthesia. In our protocol it refers to the oral NSAID, the femoral nerve block, and the incisional and intra-articular injection of sensocaine and morphine.

The femoral nerve block is done with the patient awake and sedated. The nerve stimulator is used to locate the nerve. This is one of the safest blocks that can be performed. We have done over 4,000 ACL reconstructions with this block. Even though physicians with varying degrees of skill have performed the block, I have not seen a significant problem or complication as a result of the femoral nerve block.

The portals, incision, and the joint are injected with sensocaine and morphine before the leg is prepped and draped. Turner and Chalkiadis (18) have demonstrated the benefit of infiltrating the incisional site with local anaesthetic. Numerous authors have shown the efficacy of the joint injection with marcaine/sensocaine and/or morphine (19–26).

We have been performing the nerve block, intra-articular injection, and NSAID pre-emptively since 1999, when we found that this improved the Visual Analog Scale (VAS) score in the recovery room (27). The long-term improvement in the pain score was not as dramatic as we had expected due to the nature of the hamstring reconstruction that we were studying. There seems to be much less morbidity from the hamstring harvest from the ipislateral knee, compared to the patellar tendon harvest from the ipislateral knee. We have been convinced of the effectiveness of the femoral nerve block, since our first study in 1987 (28). The femoral nerve block had been described by Ringrose and Cross (29) in 1984 for postoperative pain relief after open knee surgery. A poster presentation at the AAOS meeting by Thomas et al. (30) also found improved VAS scores when the block was done at the beginning of the case. In 1993, Allen et al. (31) found that the intra-articular injection of marcaine and morphine improved in the post-op VAS scores. Shelbourne et al. (32) has also emphasized the importance of pre-emptive analgesia. He uses IV Ketorlac and a local injection of the wound with marcaine pre-op. Immediately post-op in the OR, the CPM machine and cryocuff are applied. The Cox-2 inhibitors are started on the morning of surgery.

Tourniquet

We felt that the tourniquet may be a factor in increasing the pain post-op. In a study (33) to compare tourniquet versus no tourniquet, we found no difference in cases that only took under 1 hour. Tourniquet pain may be more of a factor with longer cases.

Post-op Nonsteroidal Anti-inflammatory Drugs and Cox-2 Inhibitors

Since McGuire et al. (34) pointed out to us the advantages of IV ketolorac, we have been using Toradol, both pre-op and post-op, but have switched to Cox-2 inhibitors. We have not done any randomized study of this, but have the impression that there are fewer GI complaints with Celebrex as compared to the Toradol. Reuben et al. (35) has shown that the NSAID, given 1 hour before surgery, augments the effect of the blocks. The preferred regime now should be the Celebrex taken on the morning of surgery with sips of water.

Cryotherapy and Continuous Passive Motion

We have been extremely happy with cryotherapy over the past decade. Some patients like the cold pack so much that they find it difficult to wean themselves off the device. The efficacy of cryotherapy has been documented by Cohn et al. (36), Shelbourne (37), and Barber et al. (38). Shelbourne (37) was one of the early proponents of the Cryocuff. In the 1994 study he showed less narcotic use with the use of the pneumatic cryocuff. This group also showed an improvement over the application of ice packs. This may be due to both the compression, and the use of the Cryocuff, while ambulatory. Barber et al. (38) found less Vicodin use, and

better VAS scores with the cryotherapy group. Barber (39) has also shown in a clinical trial that the cryotherapy is superior to crushed ice to cool the knee.

There have been several studies to examine the efficacy of the continuous passive motion after ACL reconstruction (40–46). The consensus seems to be that the range of motion is not significantly improved, but there is less swelling. Richmond et al. (44) examined the use of the CPM, and found that the use for 4 days post-op was as effective as 14 days. In summary, the main use of the CPM is to keep the knee elevated post-op, and consequently this reduces the pain and swelling.

Complications and Special Considerations

There are well known complications from ACL reconstructions, which the surgeon must advise their patients about. As with any operative procedure, bleeding, infection, deep venous thrombophlebitis, and neurovascular problems can occur. Prophylactic antibiotics generally keep infection rates under 1%. Be cautious when using posterior portals, because they are more prone to becoming infected. Neurovascular complications are also rare. The infrapatellar branch of the saphenous nerve can be damaged with hamstring harvest. The popliteal artery can be damaged with meniscal repairs, and the peroneal nerve with lateral meniscal repairs. Arthrofibrosisa is a well known complication arising from operating on an acutely injured and inflamed knee. It presents as a global stiffness that can be very frustrating to the patient, and requires extensive physiotherapy to regain range of motion. In severe cases arthroscopic arthrolysis, and medial and lateral retinacular releases, may be required. Anterior knee pain is more common after bone-patellar tendon-bone grafts, and has been attributed to increased patellofemoral contact forces arising from loss of extension and decreased patellar mobility. Shelbourne et al. (47) advocates regaining the patients' normal extension or hyper-extension post-operatively to minimize this complication.

Some complications the surgeon may encounter include:

- Dropped graft: What does the surgeon do if the graft is contaminated? There are a few options. The surgeon could harvest a new graft from the ipislateral knee, i.e., harvest a bone-patellar tendon-bone, if a hamstring graft was dropped. Or, a graft could be obtained from the contralateral knee, if one was not available in the ipislateral knee. If allografts are available in the hospital, these also could be considered. Finally, the surgeon may want to cleanse the graft and re-use it. The literature is sparse on this procedure, however Molina et al. (48) performed a study and found that standard 4% chlorhexidine gluconate solution was better than an antibiotic solution of neomycin + polymyxin B, or a 10% Providone-iodone solution. Whatever decision is made the surgeon should inform the patient to avoid difficulties later.

- Infected ACL grafts: What is the appropriate treatment of septic arthritis following ACL reconstruction? After urgent irrigation, debridement, and appropriate antibiotics, the surgeon must decide what is to be done with the graft and hardware. Matava et al. (49) conducted a survey of the "experts" entitled Septic Arthritis of The Knee Following ACL Reconstruction: Results of a Survey of Sports Medicine Fellowship Directors, and found that 95% of the surgeons surveyed would recommend retention of the graft at the time of first irrigation and debridement. However, only 39% would retain the graft if the infection persisted. McAllister et al. (50) reported the outcomes of patients with septic arthritis following ACL reconstruction, and found that although the patients' knees were stable they generally had lower functional scores.

- Adolescents with open physes: The number of immature athletes that are experiencing ACL injuries is rising. There are three main issues. First is whether to brace the athlete until skeletal maturity, or surgically reconstruct the ACL. The danger of waiting until maturity is the increased risk of meniscal damage. Millett has published that a delay increases the incidence of meniscal tears (51). The second issue is whether to perform an extra-articular reconstruction to avoid the growth plates or an intra-articular reconstruction that cross the epiphyseal plate. The extra-articular reconstruction is nonanatomic, and has been shown to have poor results. Numerous authors have reported minimal physeal damage, with small transphyseal tunnels filled with soft tissue grafts. The literature supports the use of these tunnels with endoscopic femoral tunnel placement (52–54). The third issue concerns which graft to use. Simonian et al. (55) presented an overview of ACL reconstruction in the skeletally immature patient, reviewed the existing literature, and made the following points:

- Post-pubertal patients who are nearing skeletal maturity should be treated as adults. Treat partial tears conservatively, especially if stable. Drill holes as small as possible. Centrally placed tunnels are less likely to cause angular deformity with growth. Only soft-tissue grafts should traverse the physis. Bone blocks or fixation devices that traverse the physis are more likely to cause growth arrest. Extra-articular procedures that require extensive dissection or fixation devices near the physis may be more damaging than transphyseal tunnels. A careful follow-up plan must be in place to monitor the growth and plan for intervention if premature physeal closure occurs. This follow up plan should include long standing x-rays yearly to assess growth and deformity.

- Based on this knowledge, Simonian recommends using the hamstring tendons through a central tibial tunnel, and a normal endoscopic femoral tunnel. Proximal femoral fixation is accomplished with an endobutton, and distally with sutures tied over a post.

OUTCOMES

ACL reconstruction has become a very successful operation with most authors reporting 90% success (56–63). Several prospective clinical trials performed comparing bone-patellar tendon-bone and hamstring grafts have demonstrated no significant difference in outcome scores (22–24,58,62,64). However, Pinczewski et al. (61) compared their results of patellar tendon, versus hamstring grafts at 5 years, and found that 18% of patients with the patellar tendon grafts had evidence of degenerative changes on their x-rays, versus only 4% of the patients with hamstring grafts (25). As well, Shaieb et al. (62) found that 42% of their patients with patellar tendon grafts had anterior knee pain at 2 years post-op, compared to 20% with hamstring grafts.

Yunes et al. (12) performed a meta-analysis on four studies that compared patellar tendon to hamstring grafts, and found that patients with patellar tendons had a greater chance to return to pre-injury level of activity. Freedman et al. (63) also performed a meta-analysis on 34 papers to compare the outcomes with patellar tendon versus hamstring graft. They found an overall failure rate of 1.9% with patellar tendons, versus 4.9% with hamstrings. 79% of patients with patellar tendons had less than 3 mm side-to-side difference at final follow-up, versus 74% of patients with hamstring tendons. However, the incidence of anterior knee pain was higher in the patellar tendon patients, than the hamstring graft patients, 17% versus 11.5%. Both graft options have proven track records, and the choice of graft should be based on patient characteristics. For example, if the patient is an elite athlete that needs to return to high level of performance as soon as possible, then the patellar tendon graft may be more suitable. It can heal more quickly with bone-to-bone healing, and the chance of returning to pre-injury level of activity is greater.

However, the patient must be made aware of potential anterior knee pain. For more recreational athletes, the hamstring grafts, which restore stability with minimal morbidity, seem an ideal choice.

FUTURE DIRECTIONS

ACL reconstruction will continue to evolve as it has for the past 30 years. Improving soft tissue fixation devices and intra-operative tensioning devices will likely continue to improve outcomes. The development of computer-assisted navigation may help tunnel placement, especially for those who do not perform a large number of reconstructions. A continued interest in preventive medicine and teaching high risk individuals proper training, and landing techniques should help decrease the incidence of ACL tears in the future. The use of biodegradable collagen stents implanted with growth factors may eventually replace the autogenous graft. The harvest of the graft will be looked on as a barbaric procedure in the future.

■ REVISION ANTERIOR CRUCIATE LIGAMENT SURGERY

In most cases after proper evaluation and preparation, the revision case is usually not much more difficult than a primary reconstruction. It is estimated that there are 100,000 ACL reconstructions done in the United States per year (65). At a conservative estimate of 10% failure that means that there are about 10,000 potential revisions per year. The type of failures has changed over the past 15 years. In the past, the common cause of failure was lack of range of motion with persistent pain. Now, re-rupture associated with return to sports seems to be the most frequent failure mode. The most common cause of the early re-rupture of the graft is a technical failure.

There are several types of failure:

- The stiff painful knee
- The knee with osteoarthritis of the patellofemoral or medial compartments
- The knee with persistent anterior knee pain preventing return to sports
- The knee with residual laxity
- The traumatic re-rupture

The Stiff Painful Knee

The painful knee that lacks motion can be a challenge to manage. Lack of extension may be due to a cyclops of scar tissue anteriorly. This can be diagnosed with an MRI. On the other hand the patella that has become bound down is a clinical diagnosis with lack of patella mobility compared to the opposite side and loss of flexion. This is a more difficult problem, and if unable to regain motion with therapy, then this has to be dealt with by medial and lateral arthroscopic retinacular releases. The results of global stiffness, or arthrofibrosis is poor, with a lower return to sport after treatment (66).

Arthritis

The ACL deficient knee with either arthritis of the patellofemoral joint or medial compartment may have to undergo osteotomy to correct the malalignment. If the medial compartment wear indicates grade 2 or grade 3 Outerbrige chondral damage and there is minimal varus, it is recommended to do an ACL reconstruction with hamstrings or an allograft. If the wear is grade 4 and there is a deficiency of both the ACL and meniscus, then an osteotomy should be done. The osteotomy may be done first and followed with a staged ligament reconstruction. In some instances both procedures may be done simultaneously, but now a more conservative approach is to stage the procedures.

Arthritis of the patellofemoral joint is a more difficult problem, but the same approach would follow as with the medial compartment. In early stages, do the ACL reconstruction, and

in advanced degenerative changes, focus initially on the patellofemoral joint and perform a tibial tubercle osteotomy. Many patients who have had an osteotomy are not too quick to volunteer to have a secondary procedure, so this may be the only chance you have to correct their problem.

Persistent Anterior Knee Pain

One of the most problematic clinical situations is the anterior knee pain that follows ACL reconstruction. Is this pain from the patellofemoral joint, the bound down patella, the cyclops lesion, patella tendonitis, or medial compartment osteoarthritis? The clinical examination supplemented by standing weight bearing flexion x-ray, bone scans, and MRI are necessary to pinpoint the exact cause of the pain. In some rare cases of anterior knee pain after patellar tendon reconstruction the patella tendon is bound to the front of the tibia and a release of this space as described by Steadman et al. (68) may be required.

Residual Laxity

The knee that gives away due to residual laxity is the most common cause of failure. If the failure occurs within the first year, it is probably due to a technical error. The anterior femoral tunnel is cited as the cause of most failures. If the tunnel is placed well anterior, it is easy to drill another new tunnel behind the previous tunnel. If the tunnel is only slightly anterior, the over the top position with a trough created with a rasp can be used. This latter technique is very infrequently used. If the second tunnel is drilled and breaks into the old tunnel it may be necessary to fill the defect with a large bioabsorbable screw or a bone graft.

Causes of recurrent laxity:

- Traumatic re-rupture
- Technical failures
- Early return to sports
- Aggressive rehab
- Biologic failure of incorporation of the graft

Traumatic Ruptures

As Shelbourne has pointed out, these rarely occur until a year, when the quads are rehabilitated and strong. This represents about 1% to 2% of the failures.

Technical Failures

Tunnel Placement

Anterior Femoral Tunnel. This is generally the easiest problem to revise. The new tunnel can usually be drilled behind the existing tunnel, and the only difficulty encountered may be drilling around the existing hardware. When the tunnel is clearly anterior, it is easy to drill a new tunnel

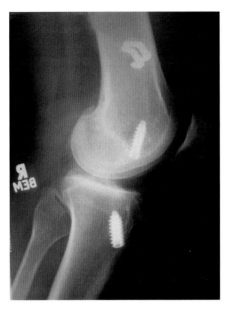

Fig 34.1-19. The incorrect anterior femoral tunnel placement.

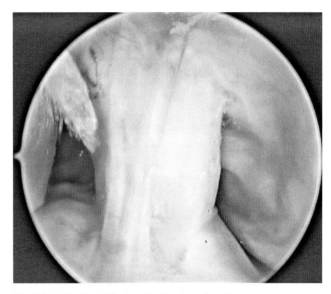

Fig 34.1-20. The failed vertically placed graft.

posterior to the existing hardware **(Fig 34.1-19)**. The guide wire can be passed by the staple on the lateral cortex without problems. None of the hardware needs to be removed, avoiding a second incision laterally. A tibialis allograft can be used with an endobutton on the femoral side and a Corticocancellous Extrlok screw on the tibial side.

Anterior Tibial Tunnel. The anterior tibial tunnel was a common mistake made in the past resulting in graft impingement anteriorly. The second tunnel is drilled behind the old tunnel. If there is considerable tunnel enlargement, a bone plug may have to be used to fill the gap anteriorly.

Vertical Graft. The vertical graft is the result of drilling the femoral tunnel through the tibial tunnel and not making the tibial tunnel oblique **(Fig 34.1-20)**. This may be avoided by using the two incision technique, or by drilling through the anteromedial portal to create the femoral tunnel low in the notch at 10 and 2 o'clock positions. In most situations, a suitable oblique graft can be done by moving the entrance of the tibial tunnel on the exterior of the tibia next to the medial collateral ligament. If the Bullseye femoral guide does not allow you to reach the 10 and 2 positions, then the femoral tunnel must be drilled through the anteromedial portal.

Inappropriate Graft Choice—Synthetic

In the past, synthetic grafts seemed initially to hold great promise. But over time the GoreTex, Leeds-Keho, and then LARS all showed unacceptable failure rates. Dandy et al. (67) reported a 40% failure of the Leeds-Kehoe synthetic ACL graft. Steadman et al. (68) and Fukubayashi and Ikeda (69) have reported the difficulties in revising the large bony defects associated with the Gore-Tex ligament. At the present time there is no place for the use of synthetic grafts for the routine primary ACL reconstruction. It may well be that

at some point in the future there will be a biodegradable stent with growth factors infused. These synthetic grafts would be available off the shelf and re-enforce the existing ligament.

Inadequate Fixation

The initial reluctance to use the hamstring graft was due to the poor results due to an inadequate fixation of the soft tissue graft. The authors initially thought that the problem was on the femoral side with interference screws. In a randomized clinical trial comparing endobutton with screws, there was no difference in the mechanical KT results in 2 years of follow-up. The tibial fixation was changed from placing the screw up to the proximal end of the tunnel to leaving it distal at the cortex. Amis has shown that the pullout strength is twice as good with cortical fixation. The initial results of our randomized clinical trial of the comparison of the corticocancellous screw and intrafix shows a trend to better mechanical results with the screw.

Posterior Wall Blowout

This was a problem on the femoral side when using the interference screw and patellar tendon grafts. Now with the use of endobutton and soft tissue grafts, as well as drilling the tunnel with the knee flexed at 90 degrees, this is not a significant problem.

Divergent Screws

If the screws are placed at more than 15 degrees of divergence within the tunnel, the pullout strength is significantly reduced. With the use of flexible guide wires there should not be a problem with divergent interference fit screws.

Osteopenic Bone

With osteopenic bone a secondary back up may be necessary. The question is how do you decide if the bone is osteopenic?

Should all the middle-aged patients undergoing ACL reconstruction have a bone mineral density study? The recent article in the *American Journal of Sports Medicine (AJSM)* by Jarvinen (Jarvinen, 2004 3197) shows that the insertion torque of the screw is not a good predictor of either the ultimate pullout or cyclic load strength.

Lack of Secondary Back Up on Tibia

This is still a problem in deciding how to do a secondary fixation. Most patients do not like the hardware on the front of their tibia, and so most surgeons are reluctant to use staple or screw posts except when clearly necessary. This may be necessary in revision cases of tunnel enlargement.

Inadequate Tensioning

There may have been many patients who have left the OR loose. This may be due to the lack of taking the play out of the construct, not seating the endobutton flush on the femur, or not seating the cross pins into the soft tissue graft. The recommended tension should be set at 80 N.

Missed Associated Ligament Laxities, Especially the Posterolateral Corner

This cause is commonly quoted as a cause for failure of the ACL reconstruction. In reality, this is very uncommon. Furthermore, how much laxity of the posterolateral corner is acceptable, before considering doing a formal reconstruction? This same principle applies to the medial side. When is the laxity sufficient to warrant reconstruction? This is still a controversial decision and the indications are very soft.

Biologic Failure of the Graft

This is a relatively uncommon cause of graft failure, but it is a real entity. Occasionally, there may be no evidence of graft in the notch **(Fig 34.1-21)**. Corsetti and Jackson (70) have discussed the causes of biological failure of the autogenous graft. Biologic factors include cellular repopulation, matrix remodeling, the ultimate small diameter collagen fibril orientation, the final cross sectional area of the graft, a favorable vascularization, and not overloading the graft during the remodeling process.

Clinical Assessment

The clinical assessment of a failure of ACL reconstruction should consist of the following:

- History and physical examination.
- Plain x-ray to assess tunnel position, tunnel enlargement, location of metal hardware, and axial alignment.
- Lateral x-ray in full extension to asses the anterior impingement of the tibial tunnel.
- MRI to assess anterior soft tissue impingement and position of the graft in the notch. Is the graft too vertical or too anterior?
- CT scan for tunnel enlargement in cases of synthetic grafts.

Assessment of Hardware

It may be necessary to stage the procedure to avoid large defects from previous hardware or from tunnel expansion due to bioabsorbable screws (71). The initial procedure is to bone graft the defects. Fluoroscopy may have to be used to locate the metal. If you use the endobutton, a small 4.5 mm drill bit is all that has to be passed by the residual metal in the femur. With this technique it is sometimes possible to leave hardware in the femur **(Fig 34.1-22)**. The x-rays will often demonstrate the anterior screw placement for the femoral and tibial tunnels.

Alignment Evaluation

In cases of failure it is important to evaluate the axial alignment of the extremity. The standing flexion views may

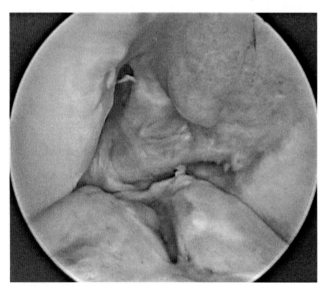

Fig 34.1-21. The absence of any graft in the notch.

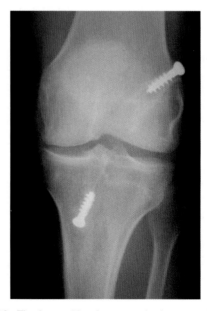

Fig 34.1-22. The femoral hardware can be by-passed using the small endobutton drill bit.

demonstrate narrowing of the medial or lateral joint space, but this has to be further assessed with a long-standing view to measure the degree of varus or valgus of the knee. If there is a significant varus deformity with narrowing of the medial joint space, then consideration should be given to high tibial open wedge osteotomy. In a review article by Noyes and Barber-Westin (72) 90% of their revision cases had associated injuries, and 16% required a high tibial osteotomy to correct varus malalignment.

Choice of Graft

There are now several choices of graft that should be discussed with the patient. The results from allograft and autogenous graft are equal in the long-term. If the patient prefers autogenous tissue there is the patellar tendon, quadriceps tendon, and hamstring tendon to choose from. The results of autogenous graft reconstruction have been reported by Noyes and Barber-Westin to be superior to the allograft (72).

■ **Autogenous Graft**
- Harvest a different graft from same knee.
- Harvest the same graft from the same site.
- Harvest the same graft from the opposite knee.

■ **Allograft has Several Common Options**
- Tibialis tendon
- Achilles tendon
- Bone tendon bone

Colosimo et al. (73) and O'Shea and Shelbourne (74) have reported a small series of revision patellar tendon grafts from the same site with good short term results. Shelbourne and O'Shea's (75) preference for revision is to use the patellar tendon from the opposite knee and have reported good results with this technique. Recently they have been using the opposite knee for primary reconstructions, so the opposite knee requires a re-harvest.

The author's preference for a routine revision is the tibialis allograft. In situations of large tunnel expansions, an Achilles tendon allograft may be preferable to fill the tunnels. Most surgeons feel that avoidance of another graft harvest is in the best interest of the patient. Vorlat et al. (76) have reported good results of revision using tendon allografts. Taking the graft from the opposite knee is a good option for the hamstring graft, but some patients don't want their normal knee violated. Perhaps in the very hyperlax patient using an allograft with hopefully better collagen than theirs may be the best alternative. If allografts are used, then a detailed explanation of the potential risks of infection and disease transmission should be outlined to the patient (77).

Indelli et al. (78) have reported good results with the Achilles tendon allograft in athletes who wish to return to play early. Sun et al. (79) have reported that the results of allograft are the same as allograft for ACL reconstruction including revision procedures.

Is there any place for electrothermal shrinking of grafts? There have been several reports of good short term results of moderate degrees of thermal shrinking of elongated grafts (80). It is important to determine if the grafts have been placed in the correct position and that the cause of elongation is not improper tunnel placement.

■ TECHNICAL TIPS

One should be well prepared for ACL revision surgery by doing a complete physical examination, x-ray work up, and arthroscopic examination. Have an allograft available as back up, even if autogenous tissue is the first choice.

If you are drilling the femoral tunnel through the tibial tunnel, create the tibial tunnel oblique in order to make a low femoral tunnel. If necessary, drill the femoral tunnel through the anteromedial portal, or in rare instances use the rear-entry two incision technique (81). Most second femoral tunnels can be drilled behind the original tunnel. The endobutton is a good soft tissue femoral fixation device for the double tibialis allograft.

■ SUMMARY AND PEARLS

The reported results are not as good as for a primary ACL reconstruction, due to the associated injuries to meniscus and articular cartilage (72,82).

The abnormally lax patient should have an allograft rather than another autograft.

The patients should be counseled to have realistic expectations after their revision surgery (83).

■ REFERENCES

1. Matsumoto H. Mechanism of the pivot shift. *J Bone Joint Surg Br.*, 1990;72(5):816–821.
2. Daniel D. Principles of knee ligament surgery. In: Akeson WH, Daniel DM, O'Connor JJ, eds. *Knee ligaments: structure, function, injury, and repair.* New York: Raven Press; 1990.
3. Bach BR Jr, Warren RF, Flynn WM, et al. Arthrometric evaluation of knees that have a torn anterior cruciate ligament. *J Bone Joint Surg Am.* 1990;72(9):1299–1306.
4. Gillquist J, Messner K. Anterior cruciate ligament reconstruction and the long-term incidence of gonarthrosis. *Sports Med.* 1999;27(3):143–156.
5. Neyret P, Donell ST, Dejour H. Results of partial meniscectomy related to the state of the anterior cruciate ligament. Review at 20 to 35 years. *J Bone Joint Surg Br.* 1993;75(1):36–40.
6. Shelbourne KD, Gray T. Results of anterior cruciate ligament reconstruction based on meniscus and articular cartilage status at the time of surgery. Five- to fifteen- year evaluations. *Am J Sports Med.* 2000;28(4):446–452.
7. Cawley PW, France EP, Paulos LE. The current state of functional knee bracing research. A review of the literature. *Am J Sports Med.* 1991;19:226–233.

8. Shelton WR, Barrett GR, Dukes A. Early season anterior cruciate ligament tears. A treatment dilemma. *Am J Sports Med.* 1997;25(5):656–658.

9. Lobenhoffer P, Tscherne H. [Rupture of the anterior cruciate ligament. Current status of treatment]. *Unfallchirurg.* 1993;96(3):150–168.

10. Amis AA, Scammell BE. Biomechanics of intra-articular and extra-articular reconstruction of the anterior cruciate ligament. *J Bone Joint Surg Br.* 1993;75(5):812–817.

11. Millett PJ, Willis AA, Warren RF. Associated injuries in pediatric and adolescent anterior cruciate ligament tears: does a delay in treatment increase the risk of meniscal tear? *Arthroscopy.* 2002;18(9):955–959.

12. Yunes M, Richmond JC, Engels EA, et al. Patellar versus hamstring tendons in anterior cruciate ligament reconstruction: A meta-analysis. *Arthroscopy.* 2001;17(3):248–257.

13. Shelbourne KD, Nitz P. Accelerated rehabilitation after anterior cruciate ligament reconstruction. *Am J Sports Med.* 1990;18:292–299.

14. Howell SM, Hull ML. Aggressive rehabilitation using hamstring tendons: graft construct, tibial tunnel placement, fixation properties, and clinical outcome. *Am J Knee Surg.* 1998;11(2):120–127.

15. Kousa P, Jarvinen TLN, Vihavainen M, et al. The fixation strength of six hamstring tendon graft fixation devices in anterior cruciate ligament reconstruction. Part II: tibial site. *Am J Sports Med.* 2003;31(2):182–188.

16. Kousa P, Jarvinen TLN, Vihavainen M, et al. The fixation strength of six hamstring tendon graft fixation devices in anterior cruciate ligament reconstruction. Part I: femoral site. *Am J Sports Med.* 2003;31(2):174–181.

17. Kehlet H, Dahl JB. The value of "multimodal" or 'balanced analgesia' in postoperative pain treatment. *Anesth Analg.* 1993;77:1048–1056.

18. Turner GA, Chalkiadis G. Comparison of peroperative with postoperative lignocaine infiltration on postoperative analgesic requirements. *Br J Anaesth.* 1994;72:541–543.

19. Joshi GP, McCarroll SM, McSwiney M. Effects of Intraarticular morphine on analgesic requirements after anterior cruciate ligament surgery. *Reg Anesth.* 1993;18:254–257.

20. Reuben SS, Steinberg RB, Cohen MA, et al. Intraarticular morphine in the multimodal analgesic management of postoperative pain after ambulatory anterior cruciate ligament repair. *Anesth Analg.* 1998;86(2):374–378.

21. Stein C, Comisel K, Haimerl E, et al. Analgesic effect of intraarticular morphine after arthroscopic knee surgery. *N Engl J Med.* 1991;325:1123–1126.

22. Heard SO, Edwards WT, Ferrari D, et al. Analgesic effect of intra-articular bupivacaine or morphine after arthroscopic knee surgery. A randomized prospective double blind study. *Anesth Analg.* 1992;72:822–826.

23. Denti M, Randelli P, Bigoni M, et al. Pre and postoperative intra-articular analgesia or arthroscopic assisted anterior cruciate ligament reconstruction. A double blind randomized prospective study. *Knee Surg Sports Traumatol Arthrosc.* 1997;5:206–212.

24. Kalso E, Tramer K, Carroll D, et al. Pain relief from intra-articular morphine after knee surgery. *Pain.* 1997;71:127–134.

25. Tetzlaff JE, Dilger JA, Abate J, et al. Preoperative intra-articular morphine and bupivacaine for pain control after outpatient anterior cruciate ligament reconstruction. *Reg Anesth Pain Med.* 1999;24:220–224.

26. Reuben SS, Sklar J, El-Mansouri M. The preemptive analgesic effect of intraarticular bupivacaine and morphine after ambulatory arthroscopic knee surgery. *Anesth Analg.* 2001;92(4):923–926.

27. Rosaeg OP, Krepski B, Cicutti N, et al. Effect of pre-emptive multi-modal analgesia for arthroscopic knee ligament repair. *Reg Anesth Pain Med.* 2001;26(2):125–130.

28. Tierney E, Lewis G, Hurtig MB, et al. Femoral nerve block with bupivicaine 0.25% for post operative analgesia after open knee surgery. *Can J. Anaesth.* 1987;34:455–458.

29. Ringrose NH, Cross MJ. Femoral nerve block in knee joint surgery. *Am J Sports Med.* 1984;12:398–402.

30. Thomas B, B.A., Levy M. *A Prospective Randomized Trial of Femoral Nerve Blocks Before and After Anterior Cruciate Ligament Reconstruction.* in *AAOS.* Dallas, 2002.

31. Allen GC, St Armand MA, Lui ACP, et al. Postarthroscopy analgesia with intraarticular bupivacaine/morphine. A randomized clinical trial. *Anesthesiology.* 1993;79:475–480.

32. Shelbourne KD, Liotta FJ, Goodloe SL. Preemptive pain management program for anterior cruciate ligament reconstruction. *Am J Knee Surg.* 1998;11(2):116–119.

33. Hooper J, Rosaeg OP, Krepski B, et al. Tourniquet inflation during arthroscopic knee ligament surgery does not increase postoperative pain. *Can J Anaesth.* 1999;46(10):925–929.

34. McGuire DA, Sanders K, Hendricks SD. Comparison of ketorolac and opioid analgesics in postoperative ACL reconstruction outpatient pain control. *Arthroscopy.* 1993;9(6):653–661.

35. Reuben SS, Sklar J, El-Mansouri M. The preemptive analgesic effect of rofecoxib after ambulatory arthroscopic knee surgery. *Anesth Analg.* 2002;94(1):55–59, table of contents.

36. Cohn BT, Draeger RI, Jackson DW. The effects of cold therapy in the postoperative management of pain in patients undergoing anterior cruciate ligament reconstruction. *Am J Sports Med.* 1989;17(3):344–349.

37. Shelbourne KD. Post-operative cryotherapy for the knee in ACL reconstructive surgery. *Orthopedics International Edition.* 1994;2(2).

38. Barber FA, McGuire D, Click S. Continuous-flow cold therapy for outpatient anterior cruciate ligament reconstruction. *Arthroscopy.* 1998;14(2):130–135.

39. Barber FA. A comparison of crushed ice and continuous flow cold therapy. *Am J Knee Surg.* 2000;13(2):97–101, discussion 102.

40. Casscells SW. Is continuous passive motion useful following cruciate ligament reconstruction? *Arthroscopy.* 1991;7(1):38.

41. Engstrom B, Sperber A, Wredmark T. Continuous passive motion in rehabilitation after anterior cruciate ligament reconstruction. *Knee Surg Sports Traumatol Arthrosc.* 1995;3(1):18–20.

42. Gaspar L, et al. Therapeutic value of continuous passive motion after anterior cruciate replacement. *Acta Chir Hung.* 1997;36(1–4):104–105.

43. McCarthy MR, Yates, CK, Anderson MA, et al. The effects of immediate continuous passive motion on pain during the inflammatory phase of soft tissue healing following anterior cruciate ligament reconstruction. *J Orthop Sports Phys Ther.* 1993;17(2):96–101.

44. Richmond JR, Gladstone J, MacGillivray J. Continuous passive motion after arthroscopically assisted anterior cruciate ligament reconstruction: comparison of short- versus long-term use. *Arthroscopy.* 1991;7(1):256.

45. Rosen MA, Jackson DW, Atwell EA. The efficacy of continuous passive motion in the rehabilitation of anterior cruciate ligament reconstructions. *Am J Sports Med.* 1992;20(2):122–127.

46. Witherow GE, Bollen SR, Pinczewski LA. The use of continuous passive motion after arthroscopically assisted anterior cruciate ligament reconstruction: help or hindrance? *Knee Surg Sports Traumatol Arthrosc.* 1993;1(2):68–70.

47. Shelbourne KD, Trumper RV. Preventing anterior knee pain after anterior cruciate ligament reconstruction. *Am J Sports Med.* 1997;25(1):41–47.

48. Molina ME, Nonweiller DE, Evans JA, et al. Contaminated anterior cruciate ligament grafts: the efficacy of 3 sterilization agents. *Arthroscopy.* 2000;16(4):373–378.

49. Matava MJ, Evans TA, Wright RW, et al. Septic arthritis of the knee following anterior cruciate ligament reconstruction: results of a survey of sports medicine fellowship directors. *Arthroscopy.* 1998;14(7):717–725.

50. McAllister DR, Parker RD, Cooper AE, et al. Outcomes of postoperative septic arthritis after anterior cruciate ligament reconstruction. *Am J Sports Med.* 1999;27(5):562–570.

51. Millett PJ, Willis AA, Warren RF. Associated injuries in pediatric and adolescent anterior cruciate ligament tears: does a delay in treatment increase the risk of meniscal tear? *Arthroscopy.* 2002;18(9):955–959.

52. Stadelmaier DM, Arnoczky SP, Dodds J, et al. The effect of drilling and soft tissue grafting across open growth plates. A histologic study. *Am J Sports Med.* 1995; 23(4):431–435.

53. Shelbourne KD, Patel DV, McCarroll JR. Management of anterior cruciate ligament injuries in skeletally immature adolescents. *Knee Surg Sports Traumatol Arthrosc.* 1996;4(2):68–74.

54. Aronowitz ER, Ganley TJ, Goode JR, et al. Anterior cruciate ligament reconstruction in adolescents with open physes. *Am J Sports Med.* 2000;28(2):168–175.

55. Simonian PT, Metcalf MH, Larson RV. Anterior cruciate ligament injuries in the skeletally immature patient. *Am J Orthop.* 1999;28(11):624–628.

56. Gobbi A, Tuy B, Mahajan S, et al. Quadrupled bone-semitendinosus anterior cruciate ligament reconstruction: a clinical investigation in a group of athletes. *Arthroscopy.* 2003;19(7): 691–699.

57. Goradia VK, Grana WA. A comparison of outcomes at 2 to 6 years after acute and chronic anterior cruciate ligament reconstructions using hamstring tendon grafts. *Arthroscopy.* 2001;17(4): 383–392.

58. Aune AK, Holm I, Risberg MA, et al. Four-strand hamstring tendon autograft compared with patellar tendon-bone autograft for anterior cruciate ligament reconstruction. A randomized study with two-year follow-up. *Am J Sports Med.* 2001;29(6):722–728.

59. Ejerhed L, Kartus J, Sernert N, et al. Patellar tendon or semitendinosus tendon autografts for anterior cruciate ligament reconstruction? A prospective randomized study with a two-year follow-up. *Am J Sports Med.* 2003;31(1):19–25.

60. Jansson KA, Linko E, Sandelin J, et al. A prospective randomized study of patellar versus hamstring tendon autografts for anterior cruciate ligament reconstruction. *Am J Sports Med.* 2003;31(1): 12–18.

61. Pinczewski LA, Deehan DJ, Salmon LJ, et al. A five-year comparison of patellar tendon versus four-strand hamstring tendon autograft for arthroscopic reconstruction of the anterior cruciate ligament. *Am J Sports Med.* 2002;30(4):523–536.

62. Shaieb MD, Kan DM, Chang SK, et al. A prospective randomized comparison of patellar tendon versus semitendinosus and gracilis tendon autografts for anterior cruciate ligament reconstruction. *Am J Sports Med.* 2002;30(2):214–220.

63. Freedman KB, D'Amato MJ, Nedeff DD, et al. Arthroscopic anterior cruciate ligament reconstruction: a metaanalysis comparing patellar tendon and hamstring tendon autografts. *Am J Sports Med.* 2003;31(1):2–11.

64. Ejerhed LK, Kartus J, Sernert N, et al. Patellar tendon or semitendinosus tendon autografts for anterior cruciate ligament reconstruction? A prospective randomized study with a two-year follow-up. *Am J Sports Med.* 2003;31(1):19–25.

65. Bach BR Jr. Revision anterior cruciate ligament surgery. *Arthroscopy.* 2003;19(suppl 1):14–29.

66. Mayr HO, Weig TG, Plitz W. Arthrofibrosis following ACL reconstruction-reasons and outcome. *Arch Orthop Trauma Surg.* 2004;124(8):518–522.

67. Dandy DJ, Gray AJ. Anterior cruciate ligament reconstruction with the Leeds-Keio prosthesis plus extra-articular tenodesis. Results after six years. *J Bone Joint Surg Br.* 1994;76(2):193–197.

68. Steadman JR, Seemann MD, Hutton KS. Revision ligament reconstruction of failed prosthetic anterior cruciate ligaments. *Instr Course Lect.* 1995;44:417–429.

69. Fukubayashi T, Ikeda K. Follow-up study of Gore-Tex artificial ligament—special emphasis on tunnel osteolysis. *J Long Term Eff Med Implants.* 2000;10(4):267–277.

70. Corsetti JR, Jackson DW. Failure of anterior cruciate ligament reconstruction: the biologic basis. *Clin Orthop.* 1996;325:42–49.

71. Martinek V, Friederich NF. Tibial and pretibial cyst formation after anterior cruciate ligament reconstruction with bioabsorbable interference screw fixation. *Arthroscopy.* 1999;15(3): 317–320.

72. Noyes FR, Barber-Westin SD. Revision anterior cruciate surgery with use of bone-patellar tendon-bone autogenous grafts. *J Bone Joint Surg Am.* 2001;83A(8)1131–1143.

73. Colosimo AJ, Heidt RS Jr, Traub JA, et al. Revision anterior cruciate ligament reconstruction with a reharvested ipsilateral patellar tendon. *Am J Sports Med.* 2001;29(6):746–750.

74. O'Shea JJ, Shelbourne KD. Anterior cruciate ligament reconstruction with a reharvested bone-patellar tendon-bone graft. *Am J Sports Med.* 2002;30(2):208–213.

75. Shelbourne KD, O'Shea JJ. Revision anterior cruciate ligament reconstruction using the contralateral bone-patellar tendon-bone graft. *Instr Course Lect.* 2002;51:343–346.

76. Vorlat PV, Verdonk R, Arnauw G. Long-term results of tendon allografts for anterior cruciate ligament replacement in revision surgery and in cases of combined complex injuries. *Knee Surg Sports Traumatol Arthrosc.* 1999;7(5):318–322.

77. Strickland SM, MacGillivray JD, Warren RF. Anterior cruciate ligament reconstruction with allograft tendons. *Orthop Clin North Am.* 2003;34(1):41–47.

78. Indelli PF, Dillingham MF, Fanton GS, et al. Anterior cruciate ligament reconstruction using cryopreserved allografts. *Clin Orthop.* 2004;(420):268–275.

79. Sun KT, Xu JW, Liu Q, et al. [A prospective study of the anterior cruciate ligament reconstruction: allograft versus autograft]. *Zhonghua Wai Ke Za Zhi.* 2004;42(16):989–992.

80. Spahn G, Shindler S. Tightening elongated ACL grafts by application of bipolar electromagnetic energy (ligament shrinkage). *Knee Surg Sports Traumatol Arthrosc.* 2002;10(2):66–72.

81. Gill TJ, Steadman JR. Anterior cruciate ligament reconstruction the two-incision technique. *Orthop Clin North Am.* 2002;33(4): 727–735, vii.

82. Harilainen A, Sandelin J. Revision anterior cruciate ligament surgery. A review of the literature and results of our own revisions. *Scand J Med Sci Sports.* 2001;11(3):163–169.

83. Getelman MH, Friedman MJ. Revision anterior cruciate ligament reconstruction surgery. *J Am Acad Orthop Surg.* 1999;7(3): 189–198.

■ SELECTED READINGS

1. Bach BR Jr. Revision anterior cruciate ligament surgery. *Arthroscopy.* 2003;19(suppl 1):14–29.

2. Mayr HO, Weig TG, Plitz W. Arthrofibrosis following ACL reconstruction-reasons and outcome. *Arch Orthop Trauma Surg.* 2004;124:518–522.

3. Dandy DJ, Gray AJ. Anterior cruciate ligament reconstruction with the Leeds-Keio prosthesis plus extra-articular tenodesis. Results after six years. *J Bone Joint Surg Br.* 1994;76(2):193–197.

4. Steadman JR, Seeman MD, Hutton KS. Revision ligament reconstruction of failed prosthetic anterior cruciate ligaments. *Instr Course Lect.* 1995;44:417–429.

5. Fukubayashi T, Ikeda K. Follow-up study of Gore-Tex artificial ligament—special emphasis on tunnel osteolysis. *J Long Term Eff Med Implants.* (YEAR);10(4): 267–277.

6. Corsetti JR, Jackson DW. Failure of anterior cruciate ligament reconstruction: the biologic basis. *Clin Orthop.* 1996;325:42–49.

7. Martinek V, Friederich NF. Tibial and pretibial cyst formation after anterior cruciate ligament reconstruction with bioabsorbable interference screw fixation. *Arthroscopy.* 1999;15(3): 317–320.

8. Noyes FR, Barber-Westin SD. Revision anterior cruciate surgery with use of bone-patellar tendon-bone autogenous grafts. *J Bone Joint Surg Am.* 2001;83A(8):1131–1143.

9. Colosimo AJ, Heidt RS Jr., Traub JA, et al. Revision anterior cruciate ligament reconstruction with a reharvested ipsilateral patellar tendon. *Am J Sports Med.* 2001;29(6):746–750.

10. O'Shea JJ, Shelbourne KD. Anterior cruciate ligament reconstruction with a reharvested bone-patellar tendon-bone graft. *Am J Sports Med.* 2002;30(2):208–213.

11. Shelbourne KD, O'Shea JJ. Revision anterior cruciate ligament reconstruction using the contralateral bone-patellar tendon-bone graft. *Instr Course Lect.* 2002;51: 343–346.

12. Vorlat P, Verdonk R, Arnauw G. Long-term results of tendon allografts for anterior cruciate ligament replacement in revision surgery and in cases of combined complex injuries. *Knee Surg Sports Traumatol Arthrosc.* 1999;7(5):318–322.

13. Strickland SM, MacGillivray JD, Warren RF. Anterior cruciate ligament reconstruction with allograft tendons. *Orthop Clin North Am.* 2003;34(1):41–47.

14. Indelli PF, Dillingham MF, Fanton GS, et al. Anterior cruciate ligament reconstruction using cryopreserved allografts. *Clin Orthop.* 2004;(420):268–275.

15. Sun KT, Xu JW, Liu Q, et al. [A prospective study of the anterior cruciate ligament reconstruction: allograft versus autograft]. *Zhonghua Wai Ke Za Zhi.* 2004;42(16):989–992.

16. Spahn G, Shindler S. Tightening elongated ACL grafts by application of bipolar electromagnetic energy (ligament shrinkage). *Knee Surg Sports Traumatol Arthrosc.* 2002;10(2):66–72.

17. Gill TJ, Steadman JR. Anterior cruciate ligament reconstruction the two-incision technique. *Orthop Clin North Am.* 2002;33(4): 727–735, vii.

18. Harilainen A, Sandelin J. Revision anterior cruciate ligament surgery. A review of the literature and results of our own revisions. *Scand J Med Sci Sports.* 2001;11(3): 163–169.

19. Getelman MH, Friedman MJ. Revision anterior cruciate ligament reconstruction surgery. *J Am Acad Orthop Surg.* 1999;7(3): 189–198.

POSTERIOR MINI-INCISION ACLR HAMSTRING HARVEST

■ CHADWICK PRODROMOS, MD

■ KEY POINTS

- Using the traditional anterior approach to perform the hamstring harvest for anterior cruciate ligament reconstruction (ACLR) can be a difficult task, particularly in large or obese patients.
- If the intertendinous cross connections are not completely divided prior to tendon stripping, the tendons can be cut too short to use necessitating a switch to autologous bone-tendon-bone (BTB) or a previously ordered allograft which is kept in reserve.
- The posterior approach to the hamstring harvest brings these intertendinous cross connections, especially the accessory semitendinosus, into plain view of the surgeon, where they can be easily sectioned under direct vision prior to tendon stripping.
- Additional benefits of the posterior approach are that it allows easier identification of the semitendinosus and gracilis tendons, improved cosmesis and reduced harvest time.

The hamstring harvest is generally acknowledged to be the most difficult part of hamstring anterior cruciate ligament reconstruction (ACLR) (1). It has traditionally been carried out through a 4 to 5 cm anterior approach. While surgeons performing large numbers of hamstring harvests become technically proficient using this traditional anterior approach, there are many surgeons who perform limited numbers of ACLRs [or who have recently switched from bone-tendon-bone (BTB) to hamstring] for whom the harvest can be daunting. Even the very best surgeons (2) acknowledge that the harvest is challenging in large and obese patients.

While it is seldom reported, it is not uncommon for the graft to be cut too short to use in clinical practice. This occurs when surgeons fail to cut tendinous cross connections prior to harvesting the tendon with the tendon stripper. The tendon stripper will then occasionally amputate the tendon itself at the point of the cross connection (rather than sectioning the cross connection), rendering the tendon too short to use. Because the cross connections often will be sectioned by the tendon stripper even if the surgeon does not cut them first, the surgeon may be lulled into a false sense of security that he doesn't need to go to the additional trouble to visualize them and cut them before harvesting. However if this shortcut is taken a tendon will eventually be cut too short to use, necessitating a switch to autologous BTB or a previously ordered allograft kept in reserve for this eventuality.

The primary difficulty lies in visualizing these posteromedial tendinous cross attachments from the traditional anteromedial approach. These cross tendons, especially the accessory semitendinosus (ST), are not described in standard anatomy texts and may be unknown to some surgeons. The references describing the accessory ST (3–5) should be read by any surgeon planning to perform hamstring ACLR. It must also be realized that these cross connections are variably present, particularly regarding the gracilis (Gr), and the tendons must be adequately visualized to a distance of roughly ten centimeters from their insertion to make sure that all such cross connections are satisfactorily found and sectioned. While these cross connections can certainly be found from the anterior approach, they lie far enough posterior to the traditional anterior incision to render the process challenging in many patients—especially large patients. Attempts to blindly cut them can result in accidentally cutting the tendon itself or the saphenous nerve. However good visualization from the traditional anterior approach may require enlargement of the incision to a degree greater than the surgeon had led the patient to believe would be used. Strong retraction can also damage the saphenous nerve, and this process can be quite time consuming.

Even if the cross connections are satisfactorily cut the tendon stripper can still occasionally become entangled in the semimembranosus sling more proximally during harvesting, cutting the tendon short at this level. Particularly in large patients, the surgeon's index finger is usually not long enough to reach this area from the traditional anteromedial approach to free the tendon stripper.

Another problem with the traditional anterior approach is that the initial differentiation of the three pes tendons by this approach can be difficult. There are no reliable landmarks for finding the tendons anteriorly before making the incision (videos showing identification of the individual tendons by external tendon palpation always show patients with extremely low body fat). The traditional anteromedial approach puts the incision over the general area of the pes insertion. However at this point all three tendons are conjoined. Differentiation of the ST and Gr (or sartorius) therefore necessitates dissecting backward to identify the tendons proximal to their conjoined insertion where they are separate structures and then returning forward.

The posterior mini-incision approach to the harvest described below greatly facilitates the harvest primarily because it obeys a basic surgical principle that the traditional anteromedial principle violates, namely to put the incision where the dissection needs to be.

The posterior approach thus has four important advantages relative to the traditional anterior approach.

1 The posteromedial accessory semitendinosus and other cross connections are easier to see and section, thus preventing the tendon from being harvested too short to use.

2 The tendons are easier to identify as separate structures posteriorly.

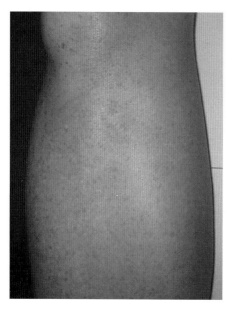

Fig 34.2-1. Picture of anterior mini-incision. Appearance of anterior mini-incision after healing.

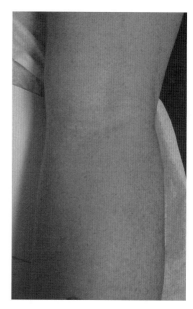

Fig 34.2-2. Picture of posterior mini-incision. Appearance of posterior mini-incision after healing.

3 The semimembranosus sling is readily accessible to allow freeing from the tendon stripper if it should get caught at this point.

4 After the tendons are first identified posteriorly, it is a simple matter to slide an index finger under the ST and find its exact anterior insertion site. By tenting the skin in this location the anterior incision can be made quite small **(Fig 34.2-1)**, one inch or less in size, and each tendon is already positively identified from the posterior incision. The cosmetic benefit of having only this one visible tiny incision (the posterior incision is both very small and hidden from view) is significant in the minds of patients – especially females—as shown by our questionnaires results (5). The posterior incision is in Langer's lines as well as the flexion crease and in most cases becomes quite inconspicuous after healing **(Fig 34.2-2)**.

■ SURGICAL TECHNIQUE

The Posterior Incision

The affected lower extremity is put on the table, flexed 30 degrees and externally rotated at the hip. A soft spot is always present in the depth of the popliteal fossa just to the medial side of the midline. In lean patients the ST can be palpated in this area. In large patients the ST cannot be palpated. But it is important to note that palpation of the ST is not important and I do not palpate or attempt to palpate it before making the incision. The tendon is always there. A 2.5 cm transverse skin incision should be made, centered over the junction of the medial and middle thirds of the popliteal fossa in this soft spot **(Fig 34.2-3)**. Longer incisions may be used and will still heal with excellent cosmetic results since the incision is within Langer's lines within the popliteal flexion creases and

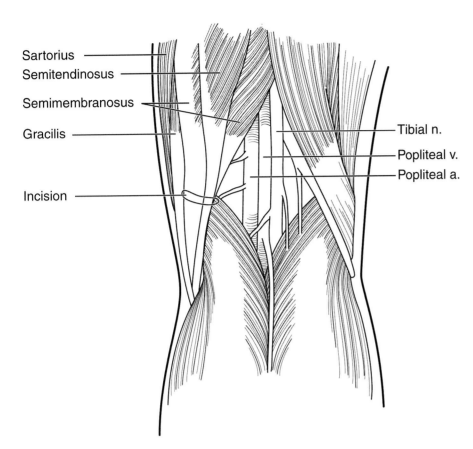

Sartorius
Semitendinosus
Semimembranosus
Gracilis
Incision

Tibial n.
Popliteal v.
Popliteal a.

Fig 34.2-3. Location of posterior mini-incision.

also within the shadow of the popliteal fossa during gait. The use of a longer incision allows the surgeon to eliminate any learning curve. The subcutaneous tissue should be carefully incised with a Metzenbaum scissors. An index finger should then bluntly dissect into this space. The leg is flexed and extended during this time until a tendinous structure is found. Most of the time it will be the ST, occasionally the Gr. The ST is generally in the middle of the incision under the subcutaneous fat. The Gr is generally at its medial border more closely adherent to the skin. The index finger is then slid under the tendon around to its anterior insertion at the pes anserinus. If the tendon is the most distal tendon felt at the pes it is the ST; if there is a tendon distal to it then it is the Gr. Rather than using blind palpation to identify the tendon in the manner just described, some surgeons may be prefer to use Senne rakes in the incision to directly visualize the tendon. Once found, a right angle clamp is passed under the tendon and a quarter of an inch penrose drain is placed around the tendon(s) and clamped.

The Anterior Incision

The surgeon should use an index finger under the insertion of the ST to tent the skin near its insertion. The skin can then be incised **(Fig 34.2-4)** just anterior to the posteromedial border of the tibia extending proximalward from the ST for a distance of about 2.5 cm. The short end of an army-navy retractor exposes the insertion and the superficial fascia should be carefully incised in a line parallel to the ST to avoid accidentally cutting it. The ST can be tented with an index finger inserted in the

posterior incision to aid in its identification. Then a right angle clamp is used to pass a quarter of an inch penrose drain passed around the tendon and clamped.

Incising the Accessory Semitendinosus

An open section tendon stripper is then fit onto the tendon and passed proximalward until tension is felt. This tension will be the accessory ST. It will occur just before the head of the stripper emerges out the posterior incision **(Figs 34.2-5)**. At this point the stripper should be firmly but gently inched proximalward while senne rakes pulls the medial edge of the posterior mini-incision over the head of the tendon stripper. The accessory ST will be located on the superior surface of the neck of the tendon stripper. It can then easily be sectioned with either a 15 blade or a Metzenbaum scissors **(Figs 34.2-6)**. The tendon stripper will then pass freely proximalward.

Stripping the Tendon

The surgeon should then put his index finger under the ST at its insertion in the anterior incision and pull it taut. The knee can be further flexed to facilitate this. This step is very important and will enable the surgeon to routinely obtain lengths of 30 cm or longer from the ST. The tendon stripper is then further advanced proximalward with a gentle rotatory motion. If firm resistance is felt the surgeon should insert an index finger in the posterior incision to dilate the track the stripper is taking. The stripper then should be advanced further until a loss

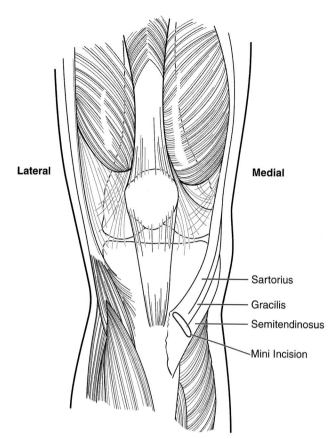

Fig 34.2-4. Location of anterior mini-incision.

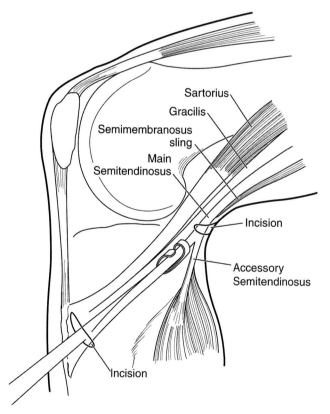

Fig 34.2-5. Tendon stripper on ST, about to deliver accessory ST into posterior incision.

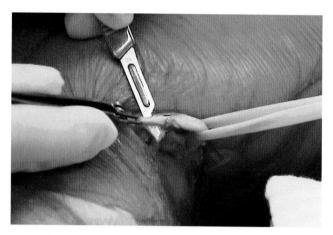

Fig 34.2-6. Sectioning the accessory ST.

of resistance is felt by the surgeon's index finger under the ST insertion. The avulsed tendon can then be delivered out the anterior incision. This procedure can be repeated for the Gr tendon. The Gr can be identified in either the posterior or anterior incision and harvested in a similar manner.

Removing the Insertion

Removal of the tendinous insertion site at the pes provides at least another cm of length of tough tendinous/periosteal tissue. It should be dissected sharply off the tibial surface.

Graft Preparation

The graft can then be given to the assistant on the back table for cleaning and preparation. We put taut whipstitches of number 5 braided nonabsorbable suture in the graft ends which are later tied around a tibial cortical screw-post. We use endobutton fixation on the femur. However the surgeon may use whatever fixation system he prefers.

■ RESULTS

Our results using this approach have been previously reported (6). We have had no complications of any kind and no tendons cut short over a period of nearly 13 years. Our cadaver studies showed that the nearest neurovascular structure, the popliteal artery, was always safely at least 2.9 cm away. The cosmesis is unsurpassed but is a side benefit. The primary advantage is the elimination of premature graft amputation. And harvest time is also reduced. I used the traditional approach for 6 years before devising this method and have found it greatly preferable. A complete technique DVD is available from our center at 847-699-6810 or research@ismoc.net. Its use is increasing worldwide as more surgeons have begun using hamstring tendons.

■ REFERENCES

1. Williams III RJ, Hyman J, Petrigliano F, et al. Anterior cruciate ligament reconstruction with a four-strand hamstring tendon autograft. *J Bone Joint Surg Am.* 2004;86A:225–232.
2. Howell SM. Short-term results ibialis Allograft vs. DLSTG. Presented at 2005 Annual Meeting of the Arthroscopy Association of North America.
3. Ferrari JD, Ferrari DA. The semitendinosus: anatomic considerations in tendon harvesting. *Orthop Rev.* 1991;20:1085–1088.
4. Pagnani MJ, Warner JJ, O'Brien SJ, et al. Anatomic considerations in harvesting the semitendinosus and gracilis tendons and a technique of harvest. *Am J Sports Med.* 1993;21:565–571.
5. Prodromos CC, Han YS, Keller BL, et al. Posterior mini-incision technique for hamstring anterior cruciate ligament reconstruction graft harvest. *Arthroscopy.* 2005;21:130–137.
6. Prodromos CC, Han YS, Keller BL, et al. Stability results of hamstring anterior cruciate ligament reconstruction at two- to eight-year follow-up. *Arthroscopy.* 2005;21:138–146.

ANATOMIC DOUBLE BUNDLE ANTERIOR CRUCIATE LIGAMENT RECONSTRUCTION

34.3

STEVEN B. COHEN, MD, JAMES STARMAN, MD, FREDDIE H. FU, MD

KEY POINTS

- The anterior cruciate ligament (ACL) is composed of two major bundles. The posterolateral (PL) bundle is posterior and lateral on the tibial footprint and the anteromedial (AM) bundle is anterior and medial on the tibial footprint.
- The posterolateral bundle originates more distally and anteriorly relative to the AM bundle on the wall of the intercondylar notch.
- When the knee is extended, the PL bundle is under tension and the AM bundle is moderately lax. With knee flexion, the AM bundle tightens and the PL bundle becomes lax.
- Patients who are having recurrent instability or giving way episodes or who are unable to return to activities of daily living or sport are appropriate for anatomic double bundle ACL reconstruction.
- ACL injury typically is the result of an acute pivoting episode, which is most commonly noncontact.
- Before ACL reconstruction, it is important to determine and address any associated injuries involving the meniscus and chondral surfaces.
- Radiographs include weight-bearing anteroposterior (AP) 30-degree flexion, lateral, and sunrise views. Magnetic resonance imaging is essential for assessing both bundles of the ACL, other ligamentous structures, menisci, chondral surfaces, and bone bruises.
- Patients wear a hinged knee brace postoperatively for 6 weeks. Continuous passive motion is started immediately after surgery. Noncutting and nontwisting sports are allowed after 12 weeks.

- No long-term study results are yet available on anatomic double bundle ACL reconstruction. Further studies are needed to show the apparent potential for reconstruction with separate AM and PL bundles to better recreate normal anatomy and biomechanics of the knee than with single bundle ACL reconstruction.

HISTORICAL PERSPECTIVE

Complete anterior cruciate ligament (ACL) ruptures can lead to recurrent knee instability, meniscal tears, and articular cartilage degeneration. Traditionally, reconstruction of the ACL has been performed using a single-bundle reconstruction technique that attempts to recreate the anteromedial bundle (AM) of the normal ACL. Review of the literature suggests that the success rates of single-bundle ACL reconstruction vary between 69% and 95%. A potential explanation for unsatisfactory results of the conventional single-bundle reconstructions may be that simply reconstructing the AM bundle does not restore the complex function of the intact ACL.

To fully understand the principles of ACL reconstruction, it is important to understand the complex anatomy of the ACL, which is composed of two major bundles. These specific bundles are named relative to their relationship on the tibial footprint; the PL bundle is posterior and lateral on the tibial footprint and the AM bundle is anterior and medial on the tibial footprint. However, the PL bundle originates more distally and anteriorly relative to the AM bundle on the wall of the intercondylar notch. When the knee is extended, the PL bundle is under tension and the AM bundle is moderately lax. With knee flexion, the AM bundle tightens and the PL bundle becomes lax. Additionally, with internal and external rotation of the tibia at 90 degrees of flexion, the PL bundle tightens.

Biomechanical studies have shown that ACL single-bundle reconstruction using either patellar tendon or quadrupled hamstring autograft is successful in limiting anterior tibial translation but is insufficient in controlling a combined rotatory load of internal and valgus torque (1). In addition, Loh et al. (2) showed that the 2 or 10 o'clock femoral tunnel position of a single-bundle ACL reconstruction improved rotatory stability when compared with the 1 or 11 o'clock position. However, neither the 10 o'clock nor the 11 o'clock tunnel position could restore the kinematics and the in situ forces of the intact knee.

Traditional techniques in ACL surgery that simply reconstruct the AM bundle do not fully address the anatomic insertion sites and the biomechanical complexity of the intact ACL. Therefore, we have begun to perform the arthroscopic technique for anatomic double-bundle ACL reconstruction that reconstructs both the AM and the PL bundle through separate anatomically based tunnels with either autogenous semitendinosus and gracilis or tibialis anterior allograft.

■ INDICATIONS AND CONTRAINDICATIONS

The indications for anatomic double bundle ACL reconstruction are similar to those for traditional single bundle reconstruction. Patients who are having recurrent instability or giving way episodes or who are unable to return to activities of daily living or sport are appropriate for surgical reconstruction. In addition, patients with complaints of instability and a single bundle or "partial" tear may benefit from single bundle augmentation or double bundle reconstruction in the event the remaining bundle is incompetent. The double bundle reconstruction has been especially useful in the revision setting, particularly when the previous femoral tunnel placement has been in the traditional "over the top" position which is too high in the femoral notch. This allows anatomic placement of the two femoral tunnels without interfering with the previous tunnel.

We have not found a contraindication to the procedure in the skeletally mature patient. The height of the patient or size of the knee has not been a factor when performing the surgery.

■ PREOPERATIVE PLANNING

A thorough history and physical examination are required prior to surgical reconstruction. Typically there is a history of an acute pivoting episode associated with an injury, most commonly noncontact. In a chronic setting, the patient complaints are generally related to knee instability or repeated giving way. Specific examination abnormalities consist of Lachman, anterior drawer, and pivot shift. It is important to determine any associated injuries involving the meniscus and chondral surfaces. A KT-1000 exam is used to determine side-to-side antero-posterior (AP) translational difference. Radiographs include weight-bearing AP 30-degree flexion, lateral, and sunrise views. Magnetic resonance imaging is essential for assessing both bundles of the ACL, other ligamentous structures, menisci, chondral surfaces, and bone bruises. Patient education is also critical prior to ACL reconstruction.

■ SURGICAL TECHNIQUE

The patient is identified in the preoperative holding area and the surgeon marks the correct limb. The procedure can be performed with general or spinal anesthesia according to the preference of the patient and the anesthesiologist. In the operating room, the patient is positioned supine on the operating table and the nonoperative leg is placed in a well-leg holder in the abducted lithotomy position. A pneumatic tourniquet is applied around the upper thigh of the operative leg, the operative limb is exsanguinated by elevation for 3 minutes, and the tourniquet is insufflated to 300 to 350 mm Hg depending on the patient size. The limb is positioned in an arthroscopic leg holder and the operative leg is prepared and draped (Fig 34.3-1). The portals used for this procedure are slightly different from standard arthroscopy portals. The anterolateral portal is placed more superior at the level of the inferior pole of the patella just lateral to the patella tendon. The anteromedial portal is placed just below the inferior pole of the patella approximately 1 cm lateral to the medial edge of the patella tendon (intratendinous portal). Finally an accessory inferior medial portal is established using direct visualization with an 18-gauge spinal needle, which is inserted medially and distally to the inferomedial portal just above the meniscus (Fig 34.3-2). This is done for better access of the lateral wall of the intercondylar notch when placing the femoral PL tunnel and femoral AM tunnel if transtibial tunnel location placement is unacceptable. Importantly, the arthroscope is placed in the anteromedial portal during femoral tunnel placement for better

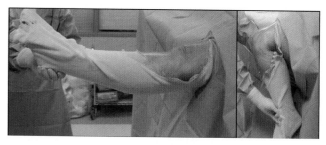

Fig 34.3-1. Leg positioning. It is essential to allow for a full range of motion between extension and 120 degrees flexion.

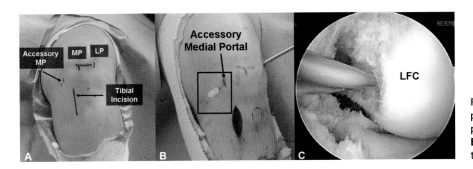

Fig 34.3-2. **A:** Arthroscopic portal placement. MP, medial portal; LP, lateral portal; AM, accessory medial portal. **B, C:** Accessory medial portal visualization with 18-gauge needle.

visualization of the intercondylar notch, while the camera is maintained in the anterolateral portal for tibial tunnel placement.

Any associated meniscal or chondral lesions are addressed prior to the ACL reconstruction. The torn ACL is carefully dissected using a thermal device to determine the injury pattern **(Fig 34.3-3)** and with special attention to the anatomic footprints of the two ACL bundles on the lateral wall of the intercondylar notch and on the tibial insertion **(Fig 34.3-4)**. The tibial footprints are left intact because of their proprioceptive and vascular contributions. The PL femoral tunnel is the first tunnel to be drilled, using the accessory anteromedial portal. A 3/32 Steinman pin is inserted through the portal and the tip of the guidewire is placed on the femoral footprint

of the PL bundle on the lateral wall of the intercondylar notch **(Fig 34.3-5)**. It is important to note that the femoral footprint of the ACL changes with the position of knee flexion. When the knee is positioned at 90 degrees of flexion, the PL and AM bundles' orientation on the femur is horizontal and in full extension, the orientation is vertical (AM bundle superior to PL bundle). Once the tip of the guidewire is placed in the correct anatomic position, the knee is flexed to 120 degrees and the guidewire is manually tapped into the femur. Hyperflexion while placing the PL femoral tunnel is performed to avoid injury to the peroneal nerve when passing a beath pin. The femoral PL tunnel is drilled with a 7 mm acorn drill that is inserted over the guidewire taking care to avoid injury to the medial femoral

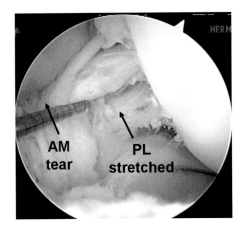

Fig 34.3-3. Arthroscopic rupture pattern of the AM and PL bundle. This case demonstrates a midsubstance AM bundle tear and a stretched-out PL bundle.

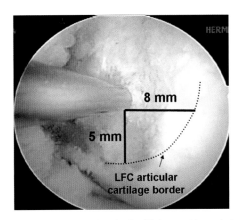

Fig 34.3-5. Anatomical landmarks for PL femoral tunnel placement.

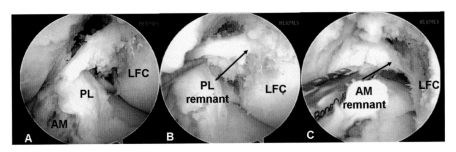

Fig 34.3-4. Marked insertion sites of the AM and PL bundle. **A:** Tibial footprints. **B:** PL Femoral insertion. **C:** AM Femoral insertion. LFC, lateral femoral condyle.

condyle articular cartilage. The PL tunnel is drilled to a depth of 25 mm to 30 mm (Fig 34.3-6). Then the far cortex is breached with a 4.5-mm EndoButton drill (Smith & Nephew, Andover, MA), and the depth gauge is used to measure the distance to the far cortex.

To establish the two tibial tunnels, a 4-cm skin incision is made over the anteromedial surface of the tibia at the level of the tibial tubercle. First the PL tunnel is drilled. An Accufex (Smith & Nephew) ACL tibial tunnel tip drill guide set to 55 degrees is placed intra-articularly on the tibial footprint of the PL bundle which was previously marked using the thermal device (Fig 34.3-7). On the tibial cortex, the tibial drill starts just anterior to the superficial medial collateral ligament fibers. A 3.2-mm guidewire is then passed into the stump of the PL tibial footprint. Next, the

AM tibial tunnel is drilled with the tibial drill guide set at 45 degrees, and the tip of the drill guide is placed on the tibial footprint of the AM tunnel (Fig 34.3-8A). The starting point of the AM tunnel on the tibial cortex is more anterior, central, and proximal than the starting point of the PL tunnel (Fig 34.3-8B). The 3.2-mm guidewire is passed into the stump of the AM tibial footprint and the placement of both guidewires is assessed for satisfactory position (Fig 34.3-9). The tibial tunnels are then over drilled with 7 mm and 8 mm compaction drill reamers for the PL and AM tunnels respectively. Finally, the femoral AM tunnel is the last tunnel to be drilled. A transtibial technique is most commonly used in a similar fashion that a femoral tunnel for ACL single-bundle reconstruction is performed. A guidewire is passed through the AM tibial tunnel and the tip of the guidewire is placed on the femoral footprint of the AM bundle, which was previously marked with a thermal device. If the position of the location of the guidewire tip is unacceptable, the accessory medial portal is used for placement of the femoral AM tunnel (Fig 34.3-10). After the guidewire is inserted in the desired position, an 8 mm acorn drill is inserted over the guidewire and the AM femoral tunnel is drilled to a depth of 35 mm to 40 mm (Fig 34.3-11). The far cortex of the AM femoral tunnel is breached with a 4.5-mm EndoButton drill (Smith & Nephew), and the depth gauge is used to measure the distance to the far cortex. During the arthroscopic procedure, the ACL grafts are prepared on the back table.

We prefer the use of two separate tibialis anterior or tibialis posterior tendon allografts. These grafts are usually 24 cm to 30 cm in length, and we fold each tendon graft to obtain 12 cm to 15 cm double-stranded grafts (Fig 34.3-12). The AM tendon double-stranded graft is typically 8 mm and

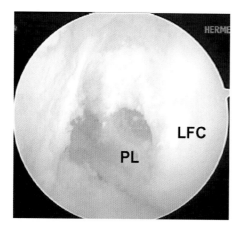

Fig 34.3-6. PL femoral tunnel.

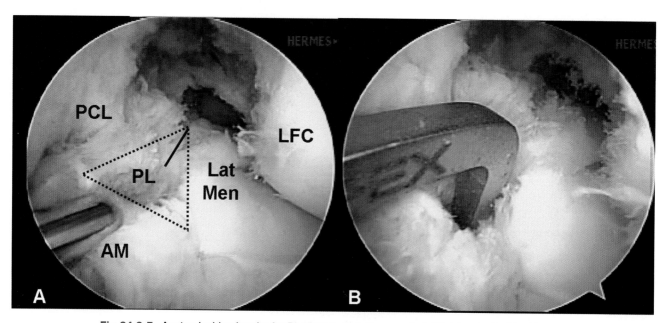

Fig 34.3-7. Anatomical landmarks for PL tibial tunnel placement. **A:** PL triangle. **B:** PL tibial pin placement with drill guide set at 55 degrees. PCL, Posterior cruciate ligament; Lat men, lateral meniscus.

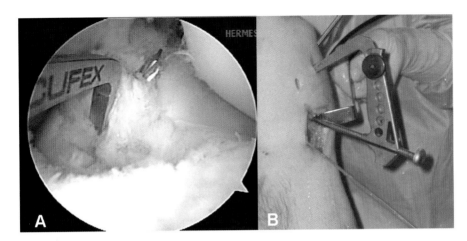

Fig 34.3-8. AM tibial pin placement. **A:** Drill guide placed in the anatomic footprint of the AM bundle. **B:** Drill guide set at 45 degrees for AM pin.

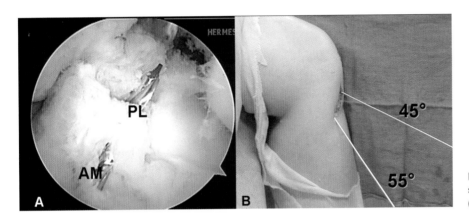

Fig 34.3-9. Tibial guide pins. **A:** Arthroscopic view. **B:** External view of AM pin (45 degrees) and PL pin (55 degrees).

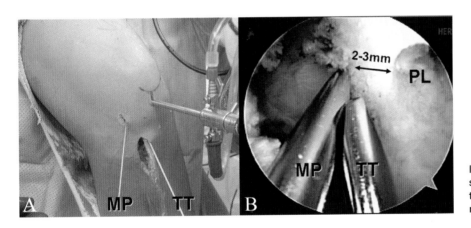

Fig 34.3-10. External **(A)** and arthroscopic **(B)** view of options for AM femoral tunnel placement. TT, transtibial; MP, medial portal approach.

the PL double-stranded graft is 7 mm. The ends of the tendon grafts are sutured using a whipstitch with number 2 Ticron sutures. Each graft is looped around an EndoButton CL (Smith & Nephew). The length of the endobutton loop is chosen according to the measured length of the femoral tunnels. The PL bundle graft is passed first with the use of a Beath pin with a long looped suture attached to the eyelet is passed through the accessory anteromedial portal and out the PL femoral tunnel and lateral aspect of the tight. Once again hyperflexion of the knee is performed to protect the peroneal nerve. The looped suture is visualized within the

joint and retrieved with an arthroscopic suture grasper through the PL tibial tunnel. The graft is passed and the endobutton is flipped in a standard fashion to establish femoral fixation of the PL bundle graft **(Fig 34.3-13)**. Next, the AM bundle graft is passed using the transtibial technique and out the anterior-lateral thigh with a Beath pin loaded with a looped suture. If the transtibial technique is not used for the AM femoral tunnel then the graft is passed in a similar fashion to the PL bundle graft. The endobutton is flipped in a standard fashion to establish femoral fixation of the AM bundle graft **(Fig 34.3-14)**. Preconditioning of the

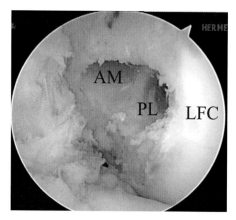

Fig 34.3-11. AM femoral tunnel.

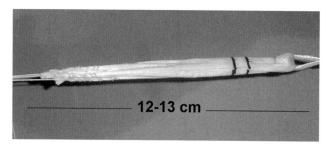

Fig 34.3-12. Doubled over tibialis anterior allograft, with "whip stitch" at left. Endobutton CL attached at right. Graft diameter for PL is 7 mm, for AM is 8 mm.

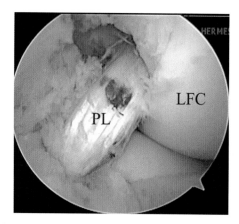

Fig 34.3-13. PL graft in situ.

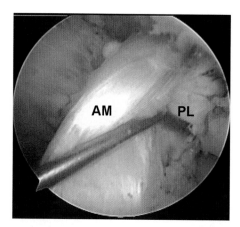

Fig 34.3-14. AM and PL grafts in situ. AM retracted to show PL position.

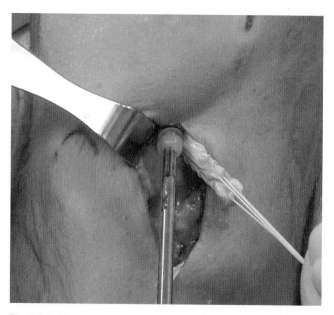

Fig 34.3-15. Bioscrew placement for primary graft fixation. PL tensioned at full extension, AM tensioned at 60 degrees flexion.

grafts is performed by flexing and extending the knee through a range of motion from 0 to 120 degrees approximately twenty to thirty times. On the tibial side, we prefer the use of a bioabsorbable interference screw fixation combined with a staple fixation for each graft **(Fig 34.3-15)**. The PL bundle graft is tensioned and fixed at full extension, and the AM bundle graft is tensioned and fixed at 60 degrees of flexion. After the fixation is complete, the knee is tested for

stability and full range of motion. The wounds are closed in a standard fashion and locked in full extension in a hinged knee brace with a Cryocuff (Aircast, Summit, NJ) placed under the brace.

■ POSTOPERATIVE MANAGEMENT

Our postoperative rehabilitation follows the same standard protocol that we have used for patients undergoing ACL single-bundle reconstruction using soft tissue grafts. Postoperatively, the patients wear a hinged knee brace for 6 weeks. For the first week, the brace is locked in extension. Continuous passive motion is started immediately after surgery from 0 to 45 degrees of flexion and increased by

10 degrees per day. The patients use crutches for four weeks postoperatively. From the first postoperative day, the patients are allowed full weight bearing as tolerated. Noncutting and nontwisting sports such as swimming, biking, and running in a straight line are allowed at 12 weeks after surgery. Return to full activity level is usually allowed at 6 months postoperatively.

■ COMPLICATIONS

Traditional complications for ACL surgery for single bundle reconstruction include graft failure, hardware complications, and infection. In our series, we have had three graft failures, all occurring after returning to sport. Two were sustained during contact injuries while playing collegiate football. The third occurred in a noncompliant patient 3 months after reconstruction when she returned to playing high school basketball without a brace. Four patients have undergone staple removal for symptomatic hardware.

There are several potential complications associated with double bundle ACL reconstruction when compared to single bundle reconstruction. Many of the issues discussed regarding double bundle reconstruction revolve around risk of femoral condyle fracture, graft impingement, incorrect tunnel placement, tunnel enlargement, and difficulty with revision surgery. Currently, after 186 double bundle ACL reconstructions, we have had no fractures, no radiographic signs of femoral condylar avascular necrosis, or tunnel widening.

Biomechanical and computer modeling studies by Bell et al. (3) have been performed comparing single and double femoral tunnels and the risk of femoral condyle fracture. Results of these studies have shown that fracture risk increased significantly for single tunnel versus the native condyle, but no significant increase in fracture risk for one versus two tunnels. Range of motion studies are currently ongoing but preliminary results have shown earlier return to full extension and symmetric flexion to the contralateral knee by three months after surgery. Proper tunnel location is achieved by marking the anatomic sites for each bundle prior to ACL debridement. Additionally, prospective studies are ongoing measuring for radiographic tunnel enlargement. Thus far, no significant tunnel enlargement has been found; however follow-up has been short term. Finally, revision surgery has not been compromised in the two patients in our cohort who have undergone repeat ACL surgery following traumatic re-tear after double bundle reconstruction.

■ RESULTS

There are no current long-term studies on the results of anatomic double bundle ACL reconstruction. However, there are several short-term studies and multiple prospective studies currently ongoing in Japan, France, Italy, and the United States on the clinical results of double bundle ACL reconstruction.

Muneta et al. (4) reported on 54 patients at 2 years after double bundle ACL reconstruction using autogenous hamstring and found a trend toward improved anterior stability compared with single-bundle technique. Zaricznyj (5) found 86% good or excellent results at 3.6 years follow-up in 14 patients after using doubled hamstring autograft for ACL reconstruction with one femoral and two tibial tunnels. Rotational stability was achieved in each patient as demonstrated by a negative pivot shift.

In a case series with 57 consecutive patients, Yasuda et al. (6) demonstrated that anatomic ACL double-bundle reconstruction appears to be a safe technique with satisfactory outcomes. They evaluated the functional outcomes at 24 to 36 months follow up and compared their results with historic data on ACL single-bundle reconstruction. Patients undergoing anatomic ACL double-bundle reconstruction trended toward better AP knee stability, as measured by the KT-2000, compared with the single-bundle group.

In a prospective, randomized clinical trial including 108 patients, Adachi et al. (7) compared the outcomes of anatomic ACL double-bundle reconstruction with the ACL single-bundle technique at an average follow up of 32 months. Their outcome measures included the AP knee stability, as measured by the KT-2000, and the joint position sense of the knee. These authors did not find any difference between the ACL double-bundle and the ACL single-bundle group.

■ CONCLUSION

Reconstruction of the ACL with separate AM and PL bundles recreates normal anatomy and has greater potential to restore the normal biomechanics of the knee compared with single bundle ACL reconstruction. Future studies are needed to show distinct advantages of improved stability, improved range of motion, higher rate of return to sport, and decreased degenerative changes of double bundle reconstruction compared with single bundle ACL surgery.

■ REFERENCES

1. Woo SL, Kanamori A, Zeminski J, et al. The effectiveness of reconstruction of the anterior cruciate ligament with hamstrings and patellar tendon: a cadaveric study comparing anterior tibial and rotational loads. *J Bone Joint Surg Am*. 2002;84:907–914.
2. Loh JC, Fukuda Y, Tsuda E, et al. Knee stability and graft function following anterior cruciate ligament reconstruction: Comparison between 11 o'clock and 10 o'clock femoral tunnel placement. *Arthroscopy*. 2003;19:297–304.
3. Bell KM, Egan M, Fu FH, et al. Femoral fracture risk analysis of single- and double-bundle ACL reconstruction. 52nd Annual Meeting of the Orthopaedic Research Society (ORS), Chicago, IL: March 19-22; 2006.

4. Muneta T, Sekiya I, Yagishita K, et al. Two-bundle reconstruction of the anterior cruciate ligament using semitendinosus tendon with endobuttons: operative technique and preliminary results. *Arthroscopy*. 1999;15:618–624.

5. Zaricznyj B. Reconstruction of the anterior cruciate ligament of the knee using a doubled tendon graft. *Clin Orthop Relat Res*. 1987;220:162–175.

6. Yasuda K, Kondo E, Ichiyama H, et al. Anatomic reconstruction of the anteromedial and posterolateral bundles of the anterior cruciate ligament using hamstring tendon grafts. *Arthroscopy*. 2004;20:1015–1025.

7. Adachi N, Ochi M, Uchio Y, et al. Reconstruction of the anterior cruciate ligament. Single- versus double-bundle multi-stranded hamstring tendons. *J Bone Joint Surg Br*. 2004;86:515–520.

LIGAMENT INJURY
AND PAIN
MANAGEMENT

34.4

■ R. LANCE SNYDER, MD, ERIC C. MCCARTY, MD

■ KEY POINTS

- Bleeding, swelling, inflammation, pain, and impaired function follow a ligament injury. Multiple nerves around knee ligaments can lead to considerable pain.
- Because side effects can be an issue, various methods are used to control pain after injury and after surgery.
- When narcotics are used for postoperative patients, they are often given in a combination of methods, including orally, intramuscularly, intravenously, or by intra-articular infusion. Controlled release oral narcotics may be more effective than immediate release narcotics.
- Preoperative anesthesia can interrupt the pain cycle before it begins.
- In theory, intra-articular pain infusion pumps have the advantage of administering analgesia directly to the site of the injury, but studies question whether the advantage is only theoretical.
- A femoral nerve block is typically not recommended for patients who are going to have hamstring autograft anterior cruciate ligament (ACL) reconstruction.

When an injury to a ligament occurs, a series of cascading events is set in motion. These events include a course of bleeding, swelling, inflammation, pain, and ultimately impaired function. The physician's role is to minimize this course and thus speed healing.

The cruciate ligaments are supplied by the middle geniculate artery. Rupture of this artery may be responsible for the ensuing hemarthrosis that occurs after injury to the anterior cruciate ligament. In addition, swelling and inflammation result from the release of mediators on the surface of damaged cells. Some of these mediators are prostoglandins which aid in

the degradation of cellular debris. These prostoglandins are in turn linked to the pain associated with ligamentous injury.

The knee ligaments are also richly innervated. The posterior articular nerve arises from the tibial nerve to supply the cruciates. The posterior articular nerve forms a plexus that also receives branches from the obturator and saphenous nerves. Thus multiple nerves innervate the knee ligaments. The lateral ligaments are innervated by the lateral articular nerve, a branch of the common peroneal nerve. The infrapatellar branch of the saphenous nerve innervates the anterior medial ligaments, including the patellar tendon (1,2). Free nerve endings, responsible for pain as well as mechanoreceptors responsible for proprioception, have been found in the cruciate ligaments (3,4). When ruptured, the knee ligaments can produce considerable pain and joint instability.

Pain begins after injury on the athletic field and continues after surgery. There are several methods used to control pain in the injured knee, including narcotics, anesthetic agents, nonsteroidal anti-inflammatory agents (NSAIDs), and modalities such as cold therapy, electrical stimulation, and continuous passive motion. The rationale supporting each of these methods is variable and often controversial. Many methods are also associated with significant side effects. The purpose of this chapter is to summarize the rationale, advantages, and disadvantages of common methods used to control pain in the injured and postoperative knee.

■ NARCOTICS

Narcotics block opiod receptors which are responsible for conducting pain to the central nervous system. These narcotics may be given to the patient orally, intramuscularly, intravenously, or by intra-articular infusion. Narcotics are associated with complications such as nausea, vomiting, pruritis, sedation, respiratory depression, confusion, hypotension, urinary retention, and addiction. The best route is not known, and frequently a combination of methods is used in the postoperative patient.

Oral Narcotics

Oral narcotics have to be broken down by the digestive tract. They differ in activation time and in the blood concentration. Controlled release oral narcotics may be more effective than immediate release narcotics, particularly in the immediate postoperative period. Reuben et al. (5) compared controlled release to immediate release oxycodone in patients undergoing ACL reconstruction. Less pain and vomiting, better sedation scores, and greater satisfaction were reported in patients receiving controlled release oxycodone. Popp et al. (6) found fewer side effects with a regimen of oral oxycodone and ketorolac versus morphine in patients undergoing ACL reconstruction. The morphine was delivered by a patient controlled analgesia device (PCA). According to visual analog scores, the pain control was identical between methods. Intra-articular morphine could theoretically block pain receptor sites in the knee thus providing a direct relief from painful surgery.

Meperidine should be used with caution in the elderly because one of its metabolites, normeperidine, is toxic to the central nervous system. This drug also has anticholinergic side effects.

Intra-articular Narcotics

Intra-articular morphine has been used extensively to aid in postoperative pain control. It theoretically blocks pain receptor sites in the knee and thus provides direct relief from painful surgery. It has been found to provide analgesia in arthroscopic knee surgery as well as patients undergoing ACL reconstruction (7). A needle is typically placed within the knee joint preoperatively or postoperatively. The mu-receptors of opoids have been found on articular cartilage, which is a possible explanation for the benefit of intra-articular morphine (8). Lawrence et al. (9) performed a study on biopsied synovium. They found evidence for the presence of opoid binding receptor sites in this tissue.

In a canine study inflamed articular cells were found to have increased opoid binding sites (10). This upregulation of opoid receptors on inflamed tissues likely validates the use of intra-articular opoid usage in postoperative patients. Brandsson et al. (11) compared intra-articular morphine to a placebo in patients undergoing ACL reconstruction. In a double blinded placebo controlled study the authors showed that the group of patients receiving morphine had lower pain scores than those in the placebo groups.

Karlsson et al. (12) found that a combination of bupivicaine and morphine given in an intra-articular fashion reduced pain scores after ACL reconstruction. In a previous study, authors had similar conclusions when patients undergoing ACL reconstruction received intra-articular morphine (13). In a multimodal study these results were somewhat refuted. Reuben et al. (14) looked at patients undergoing ACL reconstruction who received a placebo, bupivicaine, and/or morphine. Patients receiving bupivicaine had prolonged analgesia and decreased postoperative analgesia requirements. The addition of intra-articular morpine did not provide added benefit to these patients.

Tourniquet release may have an effect on the benefit of intra-articular morphine. In a study looking at the time to deflation of the tourniquet Whitford et al. (15) showed that when the tourniquet was maintained for 10 minutes after injection, pain scores were lower compared to a group of patients who had immediate release of their tourniquet. Another study looked at the concentration of the medicine delivered into the knee. The authors found no difference in pain relief when different concentrations of bupivicaine were delivered to the knee in an intra-articular fashion.

■ ANESTHESIA

Preemptive Anesthesia

Preoperative anesthesia has the theoretical benefit of interrupting the pain cycle before it begins. A study looking at preemptive intra-articular morphine showed lower analgesic usage and greater duration of analgesia in patients undergoing arthroscopic knee surgery (16). McCarty et al. (17) performed a prospective randomized double blind study comparing a preoperative injection of morphine (5 mg) to a placebo. Sixty-two patients underwent arthroscopically assisted ACL reconstruction using the central third of the patella as an autograft. There was no significant difference between the two groups in their Visual Analog Scale (VAS) scores or their postoperative narcotic requirements. Hoher et al. (18) found a reduction in VAS scores in patients receiving a preoperative intra-articular injection of bupivacaine on the day after their ACL reconstruction surgery. Tetzlaff et al. (19) found a reduction in the need for postoperative opoid usage in a group of patients who received a preoperative intra-articular injection of bupivacaine and morphine.

A study looking at patients undergoing ACL reconstruction did not show a great benefit for the use of preemptive intra-articular analgesia. In this study 30 patients were placed into three groups: one group had a preoperative placebo, one group had a preoperative injection with bupivicaine, and a third group had an injection with bupivicaine and morphine. Postoperative pain was significantly greater in the placebo group. However this difference became less apparent with time and after one hour there was no significant difference. Another finding of the study was that patients in the third group used significantly less narcotic than the other groups; the authors recommended the use of preemptive analgesia (20). Based on the available literature, an intra-articular injection of bupivacaine and morphine should be carried out prior to ligament reconstruction.

Intra-articular Anesthesia

An intra-articular infusion of analgesia medication may be given as a bolus. This is given as a one time injection either before or after the procedure. This one time injection has the theoretical benefit of a lower chance for infection versus the prolonged placement of the catheter for the infusion pump. The medication typically used is bupivicaine. This medicine has a longer half life than lidocaine and thus provides longer analgesia. The one time bolus may be given preoperatively or postoperatively. Studies have validated the use of a one time bolus of bupivacaine but have not shown a benefit of a preoperative over a postoperative injection.

Intra-articular pain infusion pumps using anesthetic have the theoretical advantages of administering analgesia directly to the site of injury. However, this theoretical advantage may be only theoretical. Alford and Fadale (21) did an excellent prospective, randomized, placebo-controlled, double-blinded study examining the use of a bupivacaine infusion pump in patients undergoing ACL reconstruction. One group had infusion with normal saline and a second group had infusion with bupivacaine. There was no significant difference in the median pain rating between the two groups, though the maximum pain rating was better in the bupivacaine group. Narcotic usage was lower in both groups when compared with a group that did not have an infusion catheter. There was also no difference in the ability to progress with therapy between the two groups. The authors felt the catheter may have provided a psychological difference and thus the reason for lower narcotic usage.

A study done by Chew et al. (21a) examined infusion into the infrapatellar fat pad in patients undergoing ACL reconstruction using autograft central third of the patellar tendon. Opioid usage was decreased compared to historic controls in the bupivacaine group. The authors felt the fat pad infusion provided significant enhancement of pain relief after surgery. Dauri et al. (22) compared epidural analgesia, continuous femoral nerve blocks, and intra-articular infusion in patients undergoing ACL reconstruction. The patients receiving an intra-articular infusion required more ketorolac to help them cope with the pain and their pain as measured by the VAS was higher. Potential side effects of intra-articular anesthesia include the risk of infection.

Femoral Nerve Blocks

Femoral nerve blocks are a method of anesthetizing the lower limb. They have the advantage of delivering analgesia in a safe and effective way without the side effects of narcotics. They are particularly useful in the acute postoperative period, but their long term benefit has not been proven. The femoral sheath is infiltrated with an anesthetic agent which blocks the femoral nerve. There is some controversy as to whether the obturator and lateral femoral cutaneous nerves are blocked as well (23). Potential side effects include incomplete anesthesia, hematoma, and infection.

Preoperative femoral nerve blocks may aid in the amount of anesthesia during the operative procedure. Postoperative blocks probably aid in the initial pain after surgery but do not aid in the rehab after surgery. Edkin et al. (24) retrospectively reviewed their charts in 161 patients undergoing outpatient ACL reconstruction using patellar tendon autograft. Ninety-eight percent of patients surveyed found femoral nerve blocks to be beneficial in helping to control the post surgical pain. Williams et al. (25) found a 2.5 fold reduction in unplanned hospital admissions in patients undergoing ACL reconstruction using patellar tendon autograft and femoral nerve block versus a control group. Several other studies have documented the effectiveness of femoral nerve blocks in this patient population as well (26–28). Another study in patients undergoing ACL reconstruction found femoral nerve blocks with bupivacaine 0.5% found lower pain scores and lower narcotic usage compared to a placebo group however there was no difference in time to discharge between the two groups (29).

Femoral nerve blocks have been found to deliver superior analgesia to intra-articular ropivicaine infusion as well. Iskandar et al. (30) looked at patients undergoing ACL reconstruction. They found that the intra-articular group had higher VAS scores and narcotic use was lower in the femoral nerve block group. Analgesia duration was longer in the femoral nerve block group as well. The type of analgesia administered in the intra-articular injection may have an effect as well. A study looking at intra-articular bupivicaine versus femoral nerve block using bupivicaine found no difference in postoperative VAS scores (31). These two studies seem to contradict each other and more work should be done in this area.

The type of graft used in ACL reconstruction may affect the ability of a femoral nerve block to deliver pain relief. One study looked at femoral nerve blocks (Bupivacaine 0.25%) in patients undergoing ACL reconstruction using hamstring autograft. There was no significant difference in VAS scores or short form questionnaires between placebo and femoral nerve block groups. There was also no significant difference in narcotic usage. This study suggest that femoral nerve blocks may be of benefit for patella tendon autograft surgery but not hamstring autograft ACL reconstruction (32) **(Fig 34.4-1)**.

Epidural

An epidural is another means by which anesthesia can be achieved. In this technique a catheter is placed in the space

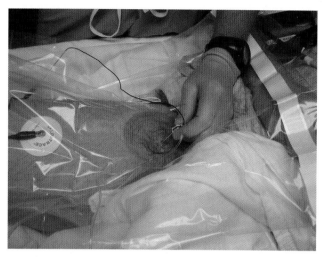

Fig 34.4-1. Femoral nerve block.

above the thecal sac and a continuous infusion of anesthetic solution is delivered. It has been used with success in other orthopedic procedures as well as ligament reconstruction (33). Several complications with this procedure have been, reported, including dural leaks, infection, hematoma, and nerve damage. A case of compartment syndrome in the leg has also been reported as being missed secondary to the anesthesia provided by the epidural. A problem with this technique is that the patient must be monitored in the hospital and most patients are discharged on the same day making this technique unnecessary and inefficient.

Spinal

A spinal block is another means to deliver anesthesia. The location differs from an epidural in that the agent is delivered into the subarachnoid space. The anesthetic, typically bupivicaine, is mixed with dextrose to render it heavier than cerebrospinal fluid and thus controllable with patient positioning. Benefits of this type of anesthesia include less need for analgesia in the Postoperative Anesthesia Care Unit (PACU). Risks of the procedure include nerve damage, infection, postoperative urinary retension, and a prolonged stay in the recovery room until the block has worn off.

■ ANALGESICS

Tramadol

Tramadol is a centrally acting analgesic. It is not a narcotic but can decrease the feeling of pain like one. It is given in an oral fashion and works by blocking Mu-opioid receptors and inhibiting the reuptake of norepinephrine and serotonin. It has fewer side effects than most narcotics including addiction and respiratory depression but can cause nausea and vomiting (34). Tramadol can be used as an adjunct to other drugs in the postoperative period.

Non Steroidal Anti-Inflammatory Drugs

Anti-inflammatory agents such as aspirin and ibuprofen work on the cellular level to stop the production of prostaglandins by blocking the enzyme cyclooxygenase. This inhibition results in decreased swelling and analgesia. Several studies have validated the use of nonsteroidal anti-inflammatory drugs (NSAIDS) to reduce pain after injury and surgery (35). NSAIDS can be toxic to the kidneys and liver. They also can result in gastrointestinal ulceration. Diclofenac is an oral NSAID. In a study on patients undergoing knee arthroscopy Diclofenac appeared to have an effect on reducing pain VAS scores (36). Ketorolac is a NSAID that be given parenterally or in an oral form. Barber and Gladu (37) analyzed the effectiveness of parenteral ketorolac compared to hydrocodone with acetomenophen in patients undergoing outpatient anterior cruciate ligament reconstruction using the central third of the patellar tendon. The study was randomized, double-blinded, and multi-centered. Patients were placed into two groups. Both groups received a loading dose of parental ketorolac. Then patients were given two doses of an unknown. The patients given two doses of ketorlac showed lower categegorical pain intensity than those who took hydrocodone and acetomenophen. McGuire et al. (38) compared ketorolac and patient controlled anesthesia with morphine or meperidine in patients undergoing ACL reconstruction. The ketorolac group had better pain scores. Based on the cost and side effects, the author's conclusion was that ketorolac was a better agent for pain control.

Newer NSAIDS have been developed that selectively block the COX-2 receptors that are responsible for inflammation. They do not interfere with cytoprotective COX-1 receptor sites and therefore should not have gastrointestinal side effects. Their effectiveness with other types of orthopedic procedures has been documented (39). In summary, NSAIDS probably have a role preoperatively in the oral form to reduce pain. They also have a role in the acute postoperative period in the I.V. form of ketorolac. They may also be used in the oral form for the longer period of postoperative ligament reconstruction. Their side effects are serious and they must be used with caution.

Acetominophen

Acetominophen is an analgesic which differs from NSAIDS in its method of action and its effect. It acts to decrease relative pain by elevating the pain threshold and affecting the hypothalamus to cause antipyresis.

It does not affect inflammation and therefore has a theoretical benefit over NSAIDS when it comes to allowing bony ingrowth to occur as in the case of ACL reconstruction using the central third of the patellar tendon. Acetaminophen works well and has been shown to reduce pain in the injured athlete. In an animal study by Rahusen et al. (40) acetomenophen had similar effects on damaged muscle compared to a Cox-2 anti-inflammatory agent. Their conclusions suggested that the lower risk and cost of acetaminophen may cause it to be a more attractive drug than some of the NSAIDs. Hepatic toxicity can occur with overdosage and anyphylaxis has been reported with this medication.

MODALITIES

Cold Therapy

The method by which cold therapy works is poorly understood. Cold therapy reduces inflammation and causes vasoconstriction. The vasoconstriction produced does not stop acute swelling but may decrease the enlargement of a hematoma. Enzymatic degradation is decreased by cold therapy as well. Decreased enzyme activity along with decreased nerve function probably help to reduce overall pain. The main side effect of cold therapy is that of frost bite damage to the skin. Cold therapy has been found to be beneficial for patients undergoing ligament reconstruction. Barber et al. (41) performed a randomized prospective study using cold therapy. They found decreased narcotic use and lower VAS scores for the cold therapy group versus the control group. Brandsson et al. (42) found that patients receiving an external cooling device as well as a postoperative intra-articular injection of bupivacaine had lower pain scores than control patients undergoing ACL reconstruction. However, some authors have found the use of cold therapy to be of no benefit (43).

Ice alone may have benefit over cold compressive devices. Warren et al. (44) compared ice to cryotherapy. They found that ice was able to lower temperature in the knee more than a cold compression device but the VAS was reduced more with the cold compressive device (44). Cold therapy in some form is recommended both pre- and postoperatively based on the literature.

Electrical Stimulation

Electrical stimulation is thought to drive electrically charged particles through the soft tissue. Its benefit is somewhat controversial and has not been proven to definitively help with the recovery after ligament injury. Electrical stimulation has been shown to reduce edema and this reduction could theoretically aid in advancement in rehab and return to play. There is no literature regarding electrical stimulation and its ability to aid in the rehabilitation of ligament injuries.

Continuous Passive Motion

Continuous passive motion (CPM) has potential benefit in terms of improving motion and reducing pain. In a randomized study McCarthy et al. (45) found decreased narcotic usage and decreased perceived pain in the CPM versus control group. This study was small (only thirty patients) and not blinded. Other authors have not found the same benefits from the use of a CPM and its use is controversial.

■ CONCLUSIONS AND PERSONAL EXPERIENCE

Outpatient surgery to reconstruct damaged ligaments has become commonplace in today's society. It has been determined to be safe for the patient (46). Of concern is our patients' pain and our ability to control that pain so that their recovery is as quick and as comfortable as possible. For injuries to the medial collateral ligament, posterior cruciate ligament, and lateral collateral ligament the treatment is often nonsurgical. These ligaments are typically treated with bracing, ice, and physical therapy. An anti-inflammatory has been shown to not be harmful. This medication is typically coupled with a mild narcotic in the acute period.

The anterior cruciate ligament often must be surgically reconstructed. We typically use a multimodal approach in this situation. In the preoperative holding area patients are given the option of a femoral nerve block at our institution. We typically do not recommend a block if the patients are going to have hamstring autograft ACL reconstruction. The patients are given prescription for postoperative pain management as well. We give the patient an anti-inflammatory, such as naproxen 500 mg, to decrease swelling and inflammation. The patient is also given an immediate release narcotic such as hydrocodone 5 mg as well as a controlled release narcotic for the acute period only. Oxycontin is typically used in this acute period. We do not use a pre-operative injection of narcotic but bupvicaine 0.25% is injected into the portal sites as well as intra-articularly in this period.

During the case an attempt is made to not use a tourniquet. After the case is over we will inject morphine in an intra-articular fashion. We use about 5 cc of this solution. A cold compressive device is then wrapped around the leg and is placed in a knee immobilizer. I.V. narcotics are given in the recovery room. Morphine is the drug of choice at our institution because of its relatively few side effects and adequate pain relief. Physical therapy is begun the day after surgery to prevent stiffness. We feel that this multimodal approach is the best way to delver safe and effective pain relief to our patients (Table 34.4-1).

TABLE 34.4-1		Summary of Methods Used to Control Pain				
		Advantages	**Disadvantages**	**Intra-Op Pain Relief***	**Post-Op Pain Relief***	**Recommended Use**
Oral Narcotics		Outpatient	Strength	N/A	+	First 6 weeks
I.V. Narcotics		Strength	Inpatient	N/A	+ +	PACU, ms typically
I.A. Narcotics		Ease	■ Infection ■ One time	+	+ +	5 mg Duramorph
I.A. Anesthesia	Infusion	N/A	■ Toxicity ■ Infections	N/A	+ − + +	N/A
	Single bolus	Ease	Toxicity	Minimal	+ − + +	Recommended w/ Duramorph postoperative
Femoral Nerve Block	Pre-Op	■ One time ■ Less anesthesia required	■ Infection ■ Nerve damage	+ + +	+ + +	On BTB only
	Post-Op		■ Infection ■ Nerve damage	N/A	+ + +	On BTB only
Epidural		Greater pain relief	■ Infection ■ Inpatient ■ Dural leak	+ + + +	+ + + +	N/A
NSAIDS	I.V.	No addiction	■ Ulcer ■ Kidney ■ Inpatient ■ Ulcer	+	+ +	Ketorolac Postoperative
	P.O.	Self-regulated	■ Kidney ■ Strength	N/A	+	Naprosyn for ten days
Acetaminophen		Self-regulated	Liver toxicity	N/A	+	In combo with oral narcotic
CPM		No addiction	Cost	N/A	N/A	N/A

*Degree of pain relief indicated by "+".

■ REFERENCES

1. Kennedy JC, Alexander IJ, Hayes KC. Nerve supply of the human knee and its functional importance. *Am J Sports Med.* 1982;10(6):329–335.
2. Kennedy JC, Weinberg HW, Wilson AS. The anatomy and function of the anterior cruciate ligament. As determined by clinical and morphological studies. *J Bone Joint Surg Am.* 1974;56(2): 223–235.
3. Schutte MJ, Dabezies EJ, Zimny ML. Neural anatomy of the human anterior cruciate ligament. *J Bone Joint Surg Am.* 1987; 69(2):243–247.
4. Katonis PG, Assimakopoulos AP, Agapitos MV. Mechanoreceptors in the posterior cruciate ligament. Histologic study on cadaver knees. *Acta Orthop Scand.* 1991;62(3):276–278.
5. Reuben SS, Connelly NR, Maciolek H. Postoperative analgesia with controlled-release oxycodone for outpatient anterior cruciate ligament surgery. *Anesth Analg.* 1999;88(6):1286–1291.
6. Popp JE, Sanko WA, Sinha AK, et al. A comparison of ketorolac tromethamine/oxycodone versus patient-controlled analgesia with morphine in anterior cruciate ligament reconstruction patient. *Arthroscopy.* 1998;14(8):816–819.
7. Gupta A, Bodin L, Holmstrom B, et al. A systematic review of the peripheral analgesic effects of intraarticular morphine. *Anesth Analg.* 2001;93(3):761–770.
8. Elvenes J, et al. Expression of functional mu-opioid receptors in human osteoarthritic cartilage and chondrocytes. *Biochem Biophys Res Commun.* 2003;311(1):202–207.
9. Lawrence AJ, Joshi GP, Michalkiewicz A, et al. Evidence for analgesia mediated by peripheral opioid receptors in inflamed synovial tissue. *Eur J Clin Pharmacol.* 1992;43(4):351–355.
10. Keates HL, Cramond T, Smith MT. Intraarticular and periarticular opioid binding in inflamed tissue in experimental canine arthritis. *Anesth Analg.* 1999;89(2):409–415.
11. Brandsson S, Karlsson J, Morberg P, et al. Intraarticular morphine after arthroscopic ACL reconstruction: a double-blind placebo-controlled study of 40 patients. *Acta Orthop Scand.* 2000;71(3):280–285.
12. Karlsson J, Rydgren B, Eriksson B, et al. Postoperative analgesic effects of intra-articular bupivacaine and morphine after arthroscopic cruciate ligament surgery. *Knee Surg Sports Traumatol Arthrosc.* 1995;3(1):55–59.
13. Joshi GP, McCarroll SM, O'Brien TM, et al. Effects of intraarticular morphine on analgesic requirements after anterior cruciate ligament repair. *Reg Anesth.* 1993;18(4):254–257.
14. Reuben SS, Steinberg RB, Cohen MA, et al. Intraarticular morphine in the multimodal analgesic management of postoperative pain after ambulatory anterior cruciate ligament repair. *Anesth Analg.* 1998;86(2):374–378.

15. Whitford A, Healy M, Joshi GP, et al. The effect of tourniquet release time on the analgesic efficacy of intraarticular morphine after arthroscopic knee surgery. *Anesth Analg*. 1997;84(4):791–793.

16. Reuben SS, Sklar J, El-Mansouri M. The preemptive analgesic effect of intraarticular bupivacaine and morphine after ambulatory arthroscopic knee surgery. *Anesth Analg*. 2001;92(4):923–926.

17. McCarty EC, Spindler KP, Tingstad E, et al. Does intraarticular morphine improve pain control with femoral nerve block after anterior cruciate ligament reconstruction? *Am J Sports Med*. 2001;29(3):327–332.

18. Hoher J, Kersten D, Bouillon B, et al. Local and intra-articular infiltration of bupivacaine before surgery: effect on postoperative pain after anterior cruciate ligament reconstruction. *Arthroscopy*. 1997;13(2):210–217.

19. Tetzlaff JE, Dilger JA, Abate J, et al. Preoperative intra-articular morphine and bupivacaine for pain control after outpatient arthroscopic anterior cruciate ligament reconstruction. *Reg Anesth Pain Med*. 1999;24(3):220–224.

20. Gatt CJ Jr, Parker RD, Tetzlaff JE, et al. Preemptive analgesia: its role and efficacy in anterior cruciate ligament reconstruction. *Am J Sports Med*. 1998;26(4):524–529.

21. Alford JW, Fadale PD. Evaluation of postoperative bupivacaine infusion for pain management after anterior cruciate ligament reconstruction. *Arthroscopy*. 2003;19(8):855–861.

21a. Chew HF, Evans NA, Stanish WD. Patient-controlled bupivacaine infusion into the infrapatellar fat pad after anterior cruciate ligament reconstruction. *Arthroscopy*. 2003;19(5):500–505.

22. Dauri M, Polzoni M, Fabbi E, et al. Comparison of epidural, continuous femoral block and intraarticular analgesia after anterior cruciate ligament reconstruction. *Acta Anaesthesiol Scand*. 2003;47(1):20–25.

23. Edkin BS, Spindler KP, Flanagan JF. Femoral nerve block as an alternative to parenteral narcotics for pain control after anterior cruciate ligament reconstruction. *Arthroscopy*. 1995;11(4):404–409.

24. Edkin BS, McCarty EC, Spindler KP, et al. Analgesia with femoral nerve block for anterior cruciate ligament reconstruction. *Clin Orthop*. 1999;369:289–295.

25. Williams BA, Kentor ML, Williams JP, et al. Femoral-sciatic nerve blocks for complex outpatient knee surgery are associated with less postoperative pain before same-day discharge: a review of 1,200 consecutive cases from the period 1996-1999. *Anesthesiology*. 2003;98(5):1206–1213.

26. Mulroy MF, Larkin KL, Batra MS, et al. Femoral nerve block with 0.25% or 0.5% bupivacaine improves postoperative analgesia following outpatient arthroscopic anterior cruciate ligament repair. *Reg Anesth Pain Med*. 2001;26(1):24–29.

27. Ng HP, Cheong KF, Lim A, et al. Intraoperative single-shot "3-in-1" femoral nerve block with ropivacaine 0.25%, ropivacaine 0.5% or bupivacaine 0.25% provides comparable 48-hr analgesia after unilateral total knee replacement. *Can J Anaesth*. 2001; 48(11):1102–1108.

28. Tierney E, Lewis G, Hurtig JB, et al. Femoral nerve block with bupivacaine 0.25 per cent for postoperative analgesia after open knee surgery. *Can J Anaesth*. 1987;34(5):455–458.

29. Peng P, Claxton A, Chung F, et al. Femoral nerve block and ketorolac in patients undergoing anterior cruciate ligament reconstruction. *Can J Anaesth*. 1999;46(10):919–924.

30. Iskandar H, Benard A, Ruel-Raymond J, et al. Femoral block provides superior analgesia compared with intra-articular ropivacaine after anterior cruciate ligament reconstruction. *Reg Anesth Pain Med.*, 2003;28(1):29–32.

31. Mehdi SA, Dalton DJN, Sivarajan V, et al. BTB ACL reconstruction: femoral nerve block has no advantage over intraarticular local anaesthetic infiltration. *Knee Surg Sports Traumatol Arthrosc*. 2004;12(3):180–183.

32. Frost S, Crossfield S, Kirkley A, et al. The efficacy of femoral nerve block in pain reduction for outpatient hamstring anterior cruciate ligament reconstruction: a double-blind, prospective, randomized trial. *Arthroscopy*. 2000;16(3):243–248.

33. Loper KA, Ready LB. Epidural morphine after anterior cruciate ligament repair: a comparison with patient-controlled intravenous morphine. *Anesth Analg*. 1989;68(3):350–352.

34. Raffa RB, Friderichs E, Reimann W, et al. Opioid and nonopioid components independently contribute to the mechanism of action of tramadol, an atypical opioid analgesic. *J Pharmacol Exp Ther*. 1992;(260):275–285.

35. Power I, Barratt S. Analgesic agents for the postoperative period. Nonopioids. *Surg Clin North Am*. 1999;79(2):275–295.

36. Rautoma P, Santanen U, Avela R, et al. Diclofenac premedication but not intraarticular ropivacaine alleviates pain following daycase knee arthroscopy. *Can J Anaesth*. 2000;47(3):220–224.

37. Barber FA, Gladu DE. Comparison of oral ketorolac and hydrocodone for pain relief after anterior cruciate ligament reconstruction. *Arthroscopy*. 1998;14(6):605–612.

38. McGuire DA, Sanders K, Hendricks SD. Comparison of ketorolac and opioid analgesics in postoperative ACL reconstruction outpatient pain control. *Arthroscopy*. 1993;9(6):653–661.

39. Reuben SS, Fingeroth R, Krushell R, et al. Evaluation of the safety and efficacy of the perioperative administration of rofecoxib for total knee arthroplasty. *J Arthroplasty*. 2002;17(1):26–31.

40. Rahusen FT, Weinhold PS, Almekinders LC. Nonsteroidal anti-inflammatory drugs and acetaminophen in the treatment of an acute muscle injury. *Am J Sports Med*. 2004;32(8):1856–1859.

41. Barber FA, McGuire DA, Click S. Continuous-flow cold therapy for outpatient anterior cruciate ligament reconstruction. *Arthroscopy*. 1998;14(2):130–135.

42. Brandsson S, Rydgren B, Hedner T, et al. Postoperative analgesic effects of an external cooling system and intra-articular bupivacaine/morphine after arthroscopic cruciate ligament surgery. *Knee Surg Sports Traumatol Arthrosc*. 1996;4(4):200–205.

43. Dervin GF, Taylor DE, Keene GC. Effects of cold and compression dressings on early postoperative outcomes for the arthroscopic anterior cruciate ligament reconstruction patient. *J Orthop Sports Phys Ther*. 1998;27(6):403–406.

44. Warren TA, McCarty EC, Richardson AL, et al. Intra-articular knee temperature changes: ice versus cryotherapy device. *Am J Sports Med*. 2004;32(2):441–445.

45. McCarthy MR, Yates CK, Anderson MA, et al. The effects of immediate continuous passive motion on pain during the inflammatory phase of soft tissue healing following anterior cruciate ligament reconstruction. *J Orthop Sports Phys Ther*. 1993;17(2):96–101.

46. Kao JT, Giangarra C, Singer G, et al. A comparison of outpatient and inpatient anterior cruciate ligament reconstruction surgery. *Arthroscopy*. 1995;11(2):151–156.

MEDIAL COLLATERAL LIGAMENT

■ DONALD H. JOHNSON, MD, FRCS

■ KEY POINTS

- The medial collateral ligament (MCL) is a broad ligament that attaches to the medial femoral epicondyle and to the medial aspect of the tibia under the pes anserinus muscles, 4 cm below the joint line. The anterior fibers of the ligament tighten during knee flexion.
- The MCL is the primary restraint against valgus stress, which in turn is the primary cause of injury to the ligament. This stress is common in contact sports such as football, hockey, and wrestling. MCL injury is the most common ligament injury to the knee.
- The clinical examination of the MCL involves stressing the knee with a valgus force. The knee should be examined both in 30 degrees of flexion and in full extension.
- Most injuries of the MCL are partial isolated injuries and can be treated conservatively.
- Operative repair is only considered in Grade 3 MCL injuries. Grade 3 injuries, which are often associated with injuries to the anterior cruciate ligament (ACL) and posterior cruciate ligament (PCL), involve instability both in 30 degrees of flexion and in extension.
- When warranted, medial repair is performed after a diagnostic arthroscopy with attention to conservative use of a fluid pump, for fear of fluid extravasation through the ruptured medial capsule.
- The reconstructed knee must be protected postoperatively against valgus stress, but range of motion is allowed to prevent stiffness and to stimulate healing of the ligament.

The medial supporting structures of the knee are divided into static and dynamic stabilizers. The pes anserinus muscles (sartorius, gracilis, and semimembranosus muscles) are flexors and internal rotators of the knee, which act as dynamic stabilizers. The semimembranosus is a stabilizer of the posteromedial corner, having insertions, which provide capsular reinforcement along tibial and popliteal insertion. In addition, the vastus medialis obliquitous attaches to the adductor tubercle and is associated with the tibial attachment of the medial collateral ligament (MCL).

The static stabilizer is the capsuloligamentous complex. The MCL is a broad ligament (10 to 12 cm in length) that attaches to the medial femoral epicondyle and to the medial aspect of the tibia under the pes anserinus muscles, 4 cm below the joint line. The anterior fibers of the ligament tighten during knee flexion. The capsular tissue is reinforced by the vastus medialis anteriorly. In its middle third, the capsule consists of meniscofemoral, meniscocapsular, and meniscotibial portions that lie under the deep MCL. Hughston and Eilers (1) have described the posterior portion of the capsule as the posterior oblique ligament (POL). This complex, which is tense in extension and loose in flexion, forms a sling around the posterior aspect of the medial femoral condyle and becomes confluent with the posterior capsule of the knee.

The MCL is the primary restraint against valgus stress. At 25 degrees of knee flexion this structure provides 78% of the restraining force against valgus injury. With extension, it provides a decreasing role, providing 57% of the restraining force at five degrees. In knee extension, the anterior cruciate ligament (ACL) and the posteromedial corner (POL, medial meniscus, and the semimembranosus) increase their contribution to valgus restraint. Some authors have suggested that the ACL is much more significant in providing valgus restraint (2).

Hughston (1) suggested that the MCL and ACL act synergistically. When the tibia is displaced anteriorly, the ACL becomes taut and restricts additional anterior displacement; however, the femur's posterior translation is also impeded by the conformity of the medial meniscus and its attachment to the POL. Similarly, both the ACL and medial capsuloligamentous complex check valgus instability.

The healing process of the MCL has been thoroughly examined by Frank et al. (2a). The process contains an inflammation phase (72 hours), a repair and regeneration phase (six weeks), and a remodelling phase (approximately one year). Forty weeks after trans-section in rabbit medial collateral ligaments, the repair tissue was shown to be composed of Type III collagen scar tissue, and it was found to be more lax and mechanically inferior to a native ligament in a sham operation group. The maximum tensile strength regained is approximately 70%. Canine studies can be found to support the concept of increased MCL strength with surgical repair, and for improved strength and results with early range of motion and nonoperative treatment.

■ MECHANISM OF INJURY

The MCL is injured primarily by a valgus stress to the knee. This is a common mechanism of stress in many contact sports such as football, hockey, and wrestling; therefore, the MCL injury is one of the most common ligament injury seen in the knee.

Clinical Evaluation: History and Physical Exam

The patient gives a history of a blow to the outside of the knee, followed by pain, swelling, and limitation of motion.

The clinical examination of the MCL involves stressing the knee with a valgus force. The knee should be examined both in 30 degrees of flexion and full extension. The degree of injury can be divided into three groups. The first degree injury presents with local tenderness, pain on valgus stress, but minimal detectable laxity of less than 5 mm. Grade 2 injuries have local tenderness, pain on valgus stress, and 5 to 10 mm of laxity with an end point. Grade 3 injuries have 10 mm of laxity, and no end point on valgus stress in full extension. The Grade 3 injury usually is associated with an injury to either the ACL or posterior cruciate ligament (PCL).

Imaging

Plain x-rays are usually required to rule out an associated lateral tibial plateau fracture. Stress radiography using the Telos (Austin Associates, Fallston MD) device can quantify and compare the laxity to the opposite normal knee. MRI evaluation can determine the site and degree of injury to the ligament, as well as evaluate other associated injuries (3).

Treatment

Most injuries to the MCL are partial isolated injuries, and can be treated conservatively. The early literature suggested that MCL injuries should be treated operatively (4); however, Indelicato (5) advocated conservative treatment for all tears of the MCL. Similarly, a concept to repair only the MCL and leave the cruciate ligament injury in the recreational athlete has fallen out of favor. It is important to diagnose any associated injuries to the cruciate ligaments because early surgical intervention may necessary.

The conservative care of the isolated MCL injury should be protection against valgus stress using a brace that allows motion of the knee, but protects against a valgus stress. Prolonged immobilization, such as a long leg cast, has been shown to have a deleterious effect on the healing of the medial ligament (2).

Treatment of the Combined Medial Collateral Ligament Injury

In distinction from the isolated ACL injury, there is less information published on the treatment of combined ligament injuries in the MCL and ACL or PCL.

Operative repair is only considered in the Grade 3 MCL injury that is unstable both in 30 degrees of flexion and in extension. Shelbourne and Carr (6) has advocated conservative treatment of the MCL for the combined injuries. They feel that the MCL and the PCL have potential to heal, as long as they are protected. They also suggest that the MCL should be allowed to heal, and a late reconstruction done for the cruciates only if necessary. This approach avoids the stiffness that may be associated with doing an open MCL repair combined with a anterior cruciate ligament reconstruction. The patient would rather have a knee with some residual laxity compared to a stiff painful knee that may result from overly aggressive surgery.

Surgical Technique of Repair of the Medial Aspect of the Knee

When warranted, medial repair is performed after a diagnostic arthroscopy with attention to conservative use of a fluid pump, for fear of fluid extravasation though the ruptured medial capsule. To avoid extravasation of the fluid into the posterior compartment, the medial incision should be made before the arthroscopy to allow the fluid to leak out through the wound. Waiting for 7 to 10 days after injury will allow the capsule to heal sufficiently to prevent significant extravasation of fluid during arthroscopy. After the diagnostic arthroscopy, meniscal tears may be treated, and the reconstruction of the cruciate may be carried out.

When the decision has been made to repair the medial structures, a medial utility incision is made, avoiding injury to the saphenous vein and nerve. The retinaculum is opened in line with the skin incision, and the MCL examined. If an avulsion of the ligament from the tibia or femur is identified, the ligament can be repaired with suture anchors. Care should be taken to prevent over-tightening of the anterior band of the MCL, which could limit its excursion, and thus, knee motion. After this repair has been completed, the POL can be reattached to the tibia or femur with suture anchors or drill holes. Finally, the vastus medialis muscle insertion should be examined, as it is often disrupted. If this is the case, it can be reattached to the adductor tubercle to reinforce the anterior capsuloligamentous structures. In the acute setting, augmentation of the repair is not routinely required.

The knee is then placed in a knee immobiliser, and started on early range of motion. The patient is permitted to weight bear in an extension splint. Early transfer to a hinged orthosis will allow full range of motion with protection of the MCL repair. Full range of motion is usually possible by 8 to 10 weeks post operatively. The patient then continues with an ACL rehabilitation protocol. During the rehabilitation phase, care should be taken to prevent unprotected weight bearing, which might allow the knee to drift into valgus, resulting in residual valgus instability. Attention is directed toward early range of motion to prevent knee stiffness. Both knee stiffness and the formation of heterotopic bone are complications of acute MCL repair.

Decision Making: The Medial Collateral Ligament Repair

Isolated injury to the MCL is generally believed to heal without operative intervention, and without residual symptoms. Instability following isolated injury to the ACL may impair a patient from participation in pivotal activities, and thus many authors recommend ACL reconstruction for those who regularly participate in those activities (7); however, the management of a combined anterior cruciate and MCL injury is more controversial.

The primary restraint to anterior displacement of the knee is the anterior cruciate ligament. The primary restraint to valgus instability is the MCL, with the cruciate ligaments acting as a secondary restraint; therefore, sectioning of both structures results in both anterior and valgus instability. Further, it has been suggested that the increased valgus instability, which results from anterior cruciate ligament laxity, may result in poorer quality healing of the MCL and residual instability.

Sullivan et al. (8) has shown that after sectioning the superficial MCL in cadavers, there was 3 mm of opening at 30 degrees, and with complete sectioning, there was 7 mm. Hughston and Eilers (1) reported the results of operative repair of the MCL for instability greater than 10 mm. As a result of this review, they recommended nonoperative treatment of mild/moderate instability, and operative repair for severe instability. Jokl et al. (9) evaluated 28 patients who had been managed nonoperatively for combined tears of the

ACL and MCL. Twenty patients had good or excellent results with normal or nearly normal function and no limitation.

Some authors believe that combined injuries are best treated with operative intervention and repair of all of the damaged structures. Fetto and Marshall (10) compared operative (repair of both ACL and MCL) and nonoperative (repair of ACL alone) treatments of the MCL in combined ACL/MCL injuries. Seventy-nine percent of the nonoperative group had unsatisfactory outcomes with pain and instability.

Authors such as Shelbourne and Porter (11) believe that combined injuries are best treated with operative reconstruction of the ACL and nonoperative treatment of the MCL. These authors believe that the MCL can be treated nonoperatively, regardless of severity, and that it will heal and provide functional stability to the knee. These authors have reported good results with retrospective reviews of patient cohorts treated in this manner. In addition, MCL injuries torn near the femoral condyle or proximal to the joint line can result in knee stiffness. Therefore, they believe that it is important to restore a full active and passive range of motion before agreeing to undertake ACL reconstruction. In fact, in low demand patients the stability conferred by a healed MCL in association with some knee stiffness may provide adequate knee function for activities of daily living without ACL reconstruction.

Some authors, however, argue that reconstruction of the ACL is required to allow proper healing of the MCL. If this were true, the ACL reconstruction would need to occur within one to two weeks of the injury to allow healing of the MCL. Some reports have emphasized few problems with early ACL reconstruction; others have suggested that ACL surgery during this period may result in an increased rate of post-operative knee stiffness (12). As a consequence, it is necessary to balance the advantages gained by early repair of the ACL against the potential morbidity that might be associated with early reconstruction.

Hillard-Sembell et al. (7) used radiographs to document valgus instability in 24 patients who had a repair of an isolated tear of the MCL and in 41 patients who had a combined ligament injury. The increased medial opening of the injured knee on a valgus stress radiography compared to the normal knee was at least 3 mm on reconstructed knees in seven patients (29%) with isolated MCL repairs and in five patients (12%) with combined ACL/MCL injuries. In Ballmer's review, 3 mm of increased laxity was detected in 12 of 20 patients (60%) who had been managed nonoperatively (13). Ballmer also reviewed 14 patients with combined ACL/MCL reconstruction noting that 12 were stable and two patients had 3 to 5 mm of valgus laxity (17%). Peterson's group compared the results of early and delayed operative management of the ACL in combined ACL/MCL injuries (14). His group suggested that there was no functional improvement in outcome and an increased rate of complications associated with early ACL reconstruction.

Hillard-Sembell (7) reviewed 66 patients with combined injuries of the ACL and Grade II to III injuries to the MCL (33% of which occurred during snow skiing). Eleven patients had ACL and MCL reconstructions, 33 had reconstruction of the ACL alone, and 22 were managed nonoperatively. Operative indications for the MCL included a Grade III MCL injury (before 1987) and an indication for an ACL reconstruction. Patients with a grade II MCL injury were managed nonoperatively for that ligament.

Hillard-Sembell (7) showed that in 8 of 60 (13%) patients, there was persistent valgus instability (greater than 2.5 mm) according to stress-radiography at final follow-up (seven with a Grade III injury and one with a Grade II injury). Combined reconstruction of both ligaments did not alter the preponderance valgus laxity. In addition, they suggested that isolated ACL reconstruction in the presence of an MCL injury did not alter the natural history of the ACL reconstruction when the repair was performed within the first 90 days of injury.

This group identified four patients who required knee manipulation (two with ACL/MCL reconstructions, one with ACL reconstruction, and one with nonoperative management). Residual flexion deficits were greatest in the group with combined ACL/MCL reconstruction (mean 6 degrees, range 0 to 20), intermediate for ACL reconstruction alone (mean 2 degrees, range 0 to 15), and least for the nonoperative group (0 degrees), p < 0.01. This study was done in a period of conservative post-operative rehabilitation. The results may have been improved with current aggressive ACL rehabilitation protocols.

For the Grade III MCL injury associated with a complete tear of the ACL, there is evidence to support early operative management of both structures. Operative treatment of both ligaments is recommended only when gross knee extension instability exists that can't be controlled by bracing. In less significant cases of MCL injury, the consensus is that the benefits of combined reconstruction outweigh the risks of knee stiffness and morbidity associated with early surgical reconstruction. The conventional wisdom is to perform isolated ACL reconstruction after the nonoperative management of the MCL, and when knee motion and strength have been restored.

Chronic Medial Collateral Ligament Laxity

This scenario of chronic MCL laxity associated with either an ACL or PCL injury is one of the most difficult to surgically reconstruct. If one reconstructs only the cruciate ligament, the medial ligament laxity will eventually cause the cruciate reconstruction to fail. Lab studies have also confirmed the synergistic stabilizing effect of the MCL on the ACL reconstruction (2,15). There have been several procedures recommended to reconstruct the medial complex.

The procedure of advancement of the MCL attachment on the femoral condyle has evolved into a recession of the epicondyle, and fixation with a staple. Recession is preferred to advancement to maintain the isometricity of the ligament. The posterior capsule and POL are then plicated to the posterior aspect of the tightened ligament. If the medial ligament is very thin and attenuated, this may be reconstructed using an Achilles tendon allograft. The bone block is fixed into a trough on the epicondyle of the femur and the tendon sutured along the anterior edge of the MCL. The posterior portion of the tendon is fanned out and sutured to the posterior capsule. In this fashion the wedge shape of the MCL may be reconstructed. For minor degrees of laxity, a plication of the ligament may be done using a locking suture on the anterior and posterior bands of the ligament. The posterior capsule and POL are then sutured to the posterior limb of this shortened ligament.

Post-operatively the reconstruction must be protected against valgus stress, but range of motion is allowed to prevent stiffness and to stimulate healing of the ligament.

■ REFERENCES

1. Hughston JC, Eilers AF. The role of the posterior oblique ligament in repairs of acute medial (collateral) ligament tears of the knee. *J Bone Joint Surg Am.* 1973;55(5): p.923–940.
2. Inoue M, McGurk-Burleson E, Hollis JM, et al. Treatment of the medial collateral ligament injury. I: The importance of anterior cruciate ligament on the varus-valgus knee laxity. *Am J Sports Med.* 1987;15(1):15–21.
2a. Frank C, Shrive N, Hiraoka H, et al. Optimisation of the biology of soft tissue repair. *J Sci Med Sport.* 1999;2:190–210.
3. Nakamura N, Horibe S, Toritsuka Y, et al. Acute Grade III medial collateral ligament injury of the knee associated with anterior cruciate ligament tear. The usefulness of magnetic resonance imaging in determining a treatment regimen. *Am J Sports Med.* 2003;31(2):261–267.
4. Oster A, Okholm K, Hulgaard J. Operative treatment of rupture on the medial collateral ligament of knee. *Acta Orthop Scand.* 1971;42(5):439.
5. Indelicato PA, Hermansdorfer J, Huegel M. Nonoperative management of complete tears of the medial collateral ligament of the knee in intercollegiate football players. *Clin Orthop.* 1990;(256): 174–177.
6. Shelbourne KD, Carr DR. Combined anterior and posterior cruciate and medial collateral ligament injury: nonsurgical and delayed surgical treatment. *Instr Course Lect.* 2003;52:413–418.
7. Hillard-Sembell D, Daniel DM, Stone ML, et al. Combined injuries of the anterior cruciate and medial collateral ligaments of the knee. Effect of treatment on stability and function of the joint. *J Bone Joint Surg Am.* 1996;78(2):169–176.
8. Sullivan DL, Levy IM, Sheskier S, et al. Medical restraints to anterior-posterior motion of the knee. *J Bone Joint Surg Am.* 1984;66(6):930–936.
9. Jokl P, Kaplan N, Stovell P, et al. Non-operative treatment of severe injuries to the medial and anterior cruciate ligaments of the knee. *J Bone Joint Surg Am.* 1984;66(5):741–744.
10. Fetto JF, Marshall J L. Medial collateral ligament injuries of the knee: a rationale for treatment. *Clin Orthop.* 1978;(132):206–218.
11. Shelbourne KD, Porter DA. Anterior cruciate ligament-medial collateral ligament injury: nonoperative management of medial collateral ligament tears with anterior cruciate ligament reconstruction. A preliminary report. *Am J Sports Med.* 1992;20(3):283–286.

12. Mohtadi NG, Webster-Bogaert S, Fowler PJ. Limitation of motion following anterior cruciate ligament reconstruction. A case-control study. *Am J Sports Med*. 1991;19(6):620–624, discussion 624–625.
13. Ballmer PM, Ballmer FT, Jakob RP. Reconstruction of the anterior cruciate ligament alone in the treatment of a combined instability with complete rupture of the medial collateral ligament. A prospective study. *Arch Orthop Trauma Surg*. 1991;110(3):139–141.
14. Petersen W, Laprell H. Combined injuries of the medial collateral ligament and the anterior cruciate ligament. Early ACL reconstruction versus late ACL reconstruction. *Arch Orthop Trauma Surg*. 1999;119(5–6):258–262.
15. Ichiba A, Nakajima M, Fujita A, et al. The effect of medial collateral ligament insufficiency on the reconstructed anterior cruciate ligament: a study in the rabbit. *Acta Orthop Scand*. 2003;74(2):196–200.

THE POSTERIOR CRUCIATE LIGAMENT

36

POSTERIOR CRUCIATE LIGAMENT AND POSTEROLATERAL RECONSTRUCTION

36.1

GREGORY C. FANELLI, MD

■ KEY POINTS

- The posterior cruciate ligament (PCL) is integral to knee joint stability and is the primary restraint to posterior tibial translation at all flexion angles greater than 30 degrees.
- The PCL consists of two major inseparable bundles. The anterior bundle makes up the bulk of the ligament, and is tight in flexion and lax in extension. The posterior bundle is much thinner, and these fibers are tight in extension and lax in flexion.
- PCL injury occurs more frequently in trauma patients than injured athletes.
- Isolated PCL tears most often result from a direct blow to the proximal tibia, causing a posteriorly directed force.
- Patients with chronic PCL/posterolateral instability present with a functionally unstable knee. Symptoms will include hyperextension instability, posterior lateral knee pain, and different degrees of a varus thrust when ambulating.

- Graft choices for posterolateral reconstruction include free graft procedures, split biceps tendon transfer, biceps tendon transfer, and capsular advancement procedures.
- Indications for surgical treatment of acute PCL injuries include insertion site avulsions, tibial step off decreased 5 mm or greater, and PCL tears combined with other structural injuries.
- Indications for surgical treatment of chronic PCL injuries are when an isolated PCT tear becomes symptomatic or when progressive functional instability develops.
- Post-operatively, the knee is kept locked in a long leg brace in full extension for 6 weeks, with non-weight bearing using crutches. Progressive range of motion occurs during weeks 4 through 6. Progressive weight bearing begins after 6 weeks and crutches are discontinued after 10 weeks.

Much has been learned and written about the anterior cruciate ligament (ACL). Interest in the posterior cruciate ligament (PCL) is increasing, and more articles are appearing

625

the literature. The natural history of PCL tears has not been well defined. The general consensus has been that isolated PCL tears do well when treated nonoperatively, and multiple ligament injuries about the knee should be surgically stabilized (1–3).

The benign natural history of the isolated PCL tear has been recently challenged (4–6). Trickey (6), in 1980, calling the PCL the central pivot point of the knee, recommended early surgical treatment of all PCL tears.

Dandy and Pusey (4) studied 20 patients treated conservatively for a mean interval of 7.2 years, and found that 14 continued to have pain while walking, whereas nine had episodes of giving way.

Keller et al. (5) studied 40 patients with isolated PCL tears treated nonoperatively. At an average follow up interval of 6 years from the time of injury, 90% continued to experience pain, and 65% noted that their activity level was limited despite excellent muscle strength. Additionally, 65% of patients had radiographic evidence of degenerative changes that increases in severity as the time interval from injury increased. This supports Trickey's earlier recommendation that PCL tears should be treated early surgically (6).

The purpose of this chapter is to review the anatomy and biomechanics of the PCL and posterolateral corner, describe our surgical technique, present our results of PCL-posterolateral reconstruction, and to briefly discuss rehabilitation following PCL surgery.

■ POSTERIOR CRUCIATE LIGAMENT ANATOMY AND BIOMECHANICS

The PCL has been considered by some to be the strongest knee ligament (7). More recent studies indicate that the ACL and PCL are of approximately equal strength (8–10). The PCL is the primary restraint to posterior tibial translation at the knee, and plays an integral part in knee joint stability.

The PCL is named because of its posterior insertion on the tibia (11,12). PCL fibers are more vertically aligned than those of the oblique ACL fibers. The PCL originates on the posterior lateral aspect of the medial femoral condyle where its attachment is in the form of a segment of a circle. The tibial attachment of the PCL is situated in a depression between the two tibial plateaus. This attachment in the PCL fossa extends for a few millimeters below the tibial articular surface (13).

Synovial tissue reflected from the posterior capsule covers the ligament on its medial, lateral, and anterior surfaces. Distally, the posterior portion of the PCL blends with the posterior capsule and periosteum. Strictly anatomically speaking, the PCL is extra-articular while lying within its own synovial sheath (12).

Girgis et al. (13) found in cadaver and fresh knee dissections that the PCL averaged 38 mm in length and 13 mm in width, whereas the ACL averaged 38 mm in length and 11 mm in width.

The PCL has been shown to consist of two major inseparable bundles. The anterior bundle makes up the bulk of the ligament and is tight in flexion and lax in extension. The posterior bundle is much thinner, and these fibers are tight in extension and lax in flexion. In reality, there is a gradually changing pattern of fiber tension going from anterior to posterior as the knee is extended (11–14). Recent studies suggest that the PCL consists of four fiber regions: anterior, central, posterior longitudinal and posterior oblique. These fiber regions are based on fiber orientation and osseous attachment sites with the anterior and central groups comprising approximately 85% of the PCL bulk (15).

The fiber regions should not be confused with the meniscofemoral ligaments, which are distinct and separate structures. In approximately 70% of knees, an accessory meniscofemoral ligament is present (13,16). The anterior meniscofemoral ligament of Humphry lies anterior to the PCL, arising from the posterior horn of the lateral meniscus and inserting on the femur with the PCL. It is approximately one third the diameter of the PCL. The posterior meniscofemoral ligament of Wrisberg arises as a continuation of the posterior horn of the lateral meniscus and is closely associated with the PCL. It has been measured to be up to one half the diameter of the PCL (16). There are no attachments between the PCL and the medial meniscus.

The majority of the blood supply to the PCL stems from the middle genicular artery, a branch of the popliteal artery (17). The middle genicular artery also supplies the synovial sheath which itself is a major contributor of nourishment to the PCL (18,19). Capsular vessels also supply the base of the PCL via branches from the popliteal and inferior genicular arteries (19). Katonis et al. (20) observed three types of nerve endings in the PCL in a histologic study (20). They observed Ruffini corpuscles (Type I, pressure receptors), Vater-Pacini corpuscles (Type II, velocity receptors), and free nerve endings (Type IV, pain receptors). They further postulated that damage to the PCL not only creates a mechanical disturbance, but a central neurologic one as well. This is most likely secondary to lack of feedback mechanisms.

The PCL is the primary restraint to posterior tibial translation at all flexion angles >30 degrees (21,22). It provides 95% of the total restraining force for the straight posterior drawer (21). Gollehon et al. (22) found in a biomechanical study of cadaveric knees that isolated sectioning of the PCL did not affect varus or external rotation of the tibia at any position of knee flexion. As expected, isolated sectioning of the PCL increased posterior tibial translation with a posteriorly directed force at all angles of flexion (maximum at 90 degrees). Sectioning of the lateral collateral ligament and the posterolateral complex, leaving the PCL intact, resulted in small but significant increases in posterior translation at all angles of flexion (maximal at 30 degrees).

As the knee progresses from flexion to extension, the tibia externally rotates relative to the femur. This has been traditionally called the "screw home" mechanism of the knee. Possible hypotheses of this mechanism include bony anatomy and relative lengths of the cruciates (23). Van Dommelen and Fowler (12) suggested that the PCL plays an important role in the screw home mechanism because of variable region tautness at different flexion angles.

Covey and Sapega (24) have conducted a biomechanical study of cadavers to determine the effects of normal knee joint motion and loading on end to end fiber length behavior of the four fiber regions. They found obvious differences in tautness of the region when comparing passive joint motion with simulated quadriceps force. This data may help in determining optimum graft placement and post PCL reconstruction rehabilitation programs.

■ POSTEROLATERAL CORNER ANATOMY AND BIOMECHANICS

The posterior lateral corner consists of the lateral collateral ligament, the acucuate ligament, the popliteus tendon, the popliteofibular ligament, the short lateral ligament, the fabellofibular ligament, and the posterior lateral capsule. The fibular attachment of the popliteus tendon, the popliteofibular ligament, is a common supporting structure of the posterolateral corner of the knee. This structure reinforces the posterolateral capsule. Its oblique anatomical orientation indicates that it may act as a static restraint to varus and external rotation movements (25).

The posterolateral corner structures serve to resist varus stress, posterior tibial translation near full extension, and external rotation of the tibia relative to the femur. Sectioning of the posterolateral corner structures results in small increases in posterior tibial translation, but major increases in varus rotation and external tibial rotation (25).

■ INCIDENCE OF PCL/POSTEROLATERAL CORNER INJURIES

The incidence of PCL injuries has been reported to be in the range of 1% to 40% of acute knee injuries (2,26–31). This appears to be patient population dependent, and PCL injury occurs more frequently in trauma patients than athletic injury patients (28,29). We have reported the incidence of PCL injuries in acute knee injuries from our tertiary care regional trauma center (32). We have shown a 38% incidence of PCL tears in acute knee injuries from our center. The two most frequent combined PCL injuries were ACL/PCL (45.9%), and PCL/posterolateral corner injuries (41.2%). PCL/posterolateral corner injuries are the second most frequently encountered multiple ligament injuries of the knee involving the PCL (2,28,29,32).

■ MECHANISM OF INJURY

PCL and posterolateral corner tears may result from a variety of injuries. Isolated PCL tears most likely result from a direct blow to the proximal tibia, causing a posteriorly directed force. This occurs with the so-called dashboard knee in motor vehicle accidents, or when the proximal tibia contacts an immovable object. A fall on a flexed knee with the foot in plantar flexion may also induce an isolated PCL tear (13). Forced flexion plus internal rotation has also been reported to cause isolated PCL tears (33). Hyperextension, forced varus, forced tibial external rotation have been associated with PCL/posterolateral corner injuries (28,29,32). The most frequent PCL/posterolateral corner injury mechanism seen in our clinic is a direct blow to the proximal medial tibia causing forced posterolateral tibial translation.

Clinical Presentation

Patients with PCL/posterolateral instability in the chronic situation will present with a functionally unstable knee. Symptoms will include hyperextension instability, posterior lateral knee pain, and different degrees of a varus thrust when ambulating. Depending on the degree of instability, peroneal nerve symptoms may also be present (25). Physical examination features of an isolated PCL instability include the following:

■ Abnormal posterior laxity less than 5 to 10 mm (tibial step-off is still palpable)
■ No abnormal varus
■ Abnormal external rotation of the tibia on the femur <10 degrees compared to the uninvolved side tested with the knee at 30 and 90 degrees of flexion

Physical examination features of combined PCL/posterolateral instability include the following:

■ Abnormal posterior laxity >5 to 10 mm; tibial step-off is flat or negative
■ Abnormal varus rotation at 30 degrees of knee flexion (variable)
■ Abnormal external rotation thigh foot angle of greater than 10 degrees compared to the normal lower extremity tested at 30 and 90 degrees of knee flexion
■ Positive external rotation recurvatum test (variable)
■ Positive posterolateral drawer test
■ Positive reversed pivot shift test (variable)

Treatment

The surgical treatment principles for PCL-posterolateral instability are to correct the abnormal motion by addressing all the injured ligaments (34–49). PCL reconstruction is performed as an arthroscopically assisted procedure using the surgeons' autograft, or allograft tissue of choice. We believe that the success for posterolateral reconstruction consists in creating a strong "posterolateral post" of autograft or allograft tissue to recreate the function of the popliteofibular ligament. In acute cases, we perform a direct repair of all injured posterolateral structures, and augment this repair with a "posterolateral post" of soft tissue to reinforce the primary repair. Chronic posterolateral instability is addressed by capsular repair if possible, and by reconstructing the function of all the injured posterolateral and lateral structures. Graft choices for the posterolateral reconstruction include free graft procedures, split biceps tendon transfer, biceps tendon transfer, and capsular advancement procedures. Certain cases of chronic PCL/posterolateral instability may require high tibial valgus osteotomy to correct bony varus deformity prior to ligament reconstruction. Failure to correct the bony varus deformity exposes the ligament reconstruction to high tensile loads increasing the risk of ligament reconstruction failure (25).

Surgical Indications

Our indications for surgical treatment of acute PCL injuries include insertion site avulsions, tibial step off decreased 5 mm or greater, and PCL tears combined with other structural injuries. Our indications for surgical treatment of chronic PCL injuries are when an isolated PCL tear becomes symptomatic or when progressive functional instability develops.

Surgical Timing

Surgical timing of acute PCL/posterior lateral corner injuries depends upon the grade of the lateral side injury (A, B, or C), and/or presence or absence of a bony avulsion of the lateral ligament complex. Our preferred timing for PCL/posterior lateral corner tears is to allow capsular sealing to occur over 2 to 3 weeks, followed by arthroscopic PCL reconstruction, and posterior lateral corner primary repair/reconstruction. The use of strong graft material in the posterior lateral corner independently, or to augment primary repair, is essential for the success of this procedure. Cases of bony avulsion or fibular head avulsion are repaired acutely, and arthroscopic PCL reconstruction is performed 2 to 6 weeks later.

Surgical Technique

The single bundle/single femoral tunnel trans tibial tunnel PCL reconstruction is an anatomic reconstruction of the anterolateral bundle of the PCL. The anterolateral bundle tightens in flexion, and this reconstruction reproduces that biomechanical function. Although the SB/SFT TTT PCL reconstruction does not reproduce the broad anatomic

insertion site of the normal PCL, there are certain factors that lead to success with this surgical technique:

1 Identify and treat all pathology (especially posterolateral instability).
2 Accurate tunnel placement.
3 Anatomic graft insertion sites.
4 Strong graft material.
5 Minimize graft bending.
6 Final tensioning at 70 to 90 degrees of knee flexion.
7 Graft tensioning.
   a. Arthrotek mechanical tensioning device.
8 Primary and back-up fixation.
9 Appropriate rehabilitation program.

■ PATIENT POSITIONING AND INITIAL SET UP

The patient is positioned on the operating table in the supine position, and the surgical and non-surgical knees are examined under general anesthesia. A tourniquet is applied to the operative extremity, and the surgical leg prepped and draped in a sterile fashion. Allograft tissue is prepared prior to beginning the surgical procedure, and autograft tissue is harvested prior to beginning the arthroscopic portion of the procedure. The arthroscopic instruments are inserted with the inflow through the superior lateral patellar portal, the arthroscope in the inferior lateral patellar portal, and the instruments in the inferior medial patellar portal. The portals are interchanged as necessary. The joint is thoroughly evaluated arthroscopically, and the PCL evaluated using the three zone arthroscopic technique (5). The PCL tear is identified, and the residual stump of the PCL is debrided with hand tools and the synovial shaver.

Initial Incision

An extra capsular posteromedial safety incision approximately 1.5 to 2.0 cm long is created (**Fig 36.1-1**). The crural fascia is incised longitudinally, taking precautions to protect the neurovascular structures. The interval is developed between the medial head of the gastrocnemius muscle and the posterior capsule of the knee joint, which is anterior. The surgeon's gloved finger is able to have the neurovascular structures posterior to the finger, and the posterior aspect of the joint capsule anterior to the surgeon's finger. This technique enables the surgeon to monitor surgical instruments such as the over the top Arthrotek PCL instruments (Arthrotek Inc., Warsaw, Indiana), and the Arthrotek Fanelli PCL/ACL drill guide (Arthrotek Inc., Warsaw, Indiana) as they are positioned in the posterior aspect of the knee. The surgeon's finger in the posteromedial safety incision also confirms accurate placement of the guide wire prior to tibial tunnel drilling in the medial-lateral and proximal-distal directions (**Fig 36.1-2**).

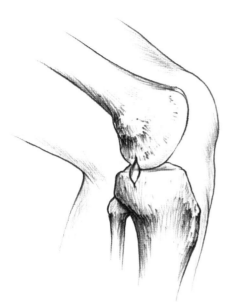

Fig 36.1-1. Posteromedial extra-articular extracapsular safety incision. (From Arthrotek, Inc. Warsaw, Indiana; with permission.)

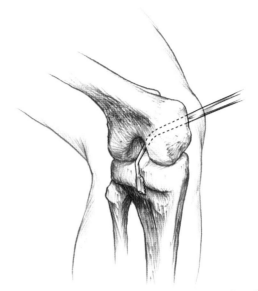

Fig 36.1-3. Posterior capsular elevation using the Arthrotek PCL instruments. (From Arthrotek, Inc. Warsaw, Indiana; with permission.)

Drill Guide Positioning

The arm of the Arthrotek Fanelli PCL-ACL Drill Guide (Arthrotek Inc., Warsaw, Indiana) is inserted into the knee through the inferior medial patellar portal and positioned in the PCL fossa on the posterior tibia **(Fig 36.1-4)**. The bullet portion of the drill guide contacts the anterior medial aspect of the proximal tibia approximately one centimeter below the tibial tubercle, at a point midway between the tibial crest anteriorly and the posterior medial border of the tibia. This drill guide positioning creates a tibial tunnel that is relatively vertically oriented, and has its posterior exit point in the inferior and lateral aspect of the PCL tibial anatomic insertion site. This positioning creates an angle of graft orientation such that the graft will turn two very smooth 45-degree angles on the posterior aspect of the tibia eliminating the "killer turn" of 90 degree graft angle bending **(Fig 36.1-5)**.

The tip of the guide in the posterior aspect of the tibia is confirmed with the surgeon's finger through the extracapsular posteromedial safety incision. Intraoperative AP and lateral x-ray may also be used, as well as arthroscopic visualization to confirm drill guide and guide pin placement. A blunt spade tipped guide wire is drilled from anterior to posterior and may be visualized with the arthroscope, in addition to being palpated with the finger in the posteromedial safety incision. We consider the finger in the posteromedial safety incision the most important step for accuracy and safety.

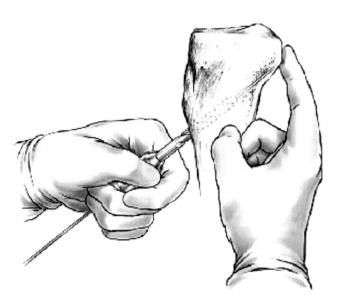

Fig 36.1-2. The surgeon is able to palpate the posterior aspect of the tibia through the extracapsular extra-articular posteromedial safety incision. This enables the surgeon to accurately position guide wires, create the tibial tunnel, and to protect the neurovascular structures. (From Arthrotek, Inc. Warsaw, Indiana; with permission.)

Elevating the Posterior Capsule

The curved over the top Arthrotek PCL instruments (Arthrotek Inc., Warsaw, Indiana) are used to carefully lyse adhesions in the posterior aspect of the knee, and to elevate the posterior knee joint capsule away from the tibial ridge on the posterior aspect of the tibia. This capsular elevation enhances correct drill guide and tibial tunnel placement **(Fig 36.1-3)**.

Tibial Tunnel Drilling

The appropriately sized standard cannulated reamer is used to create the tibial tunnel. The closed curved PCL curette may be positioned to cup the tip of the guide wire **(Fig 36.1-6)**. The arthroscopic, when positioned in the posteromedial portal, visualizes the guide wire being captured by the curette,

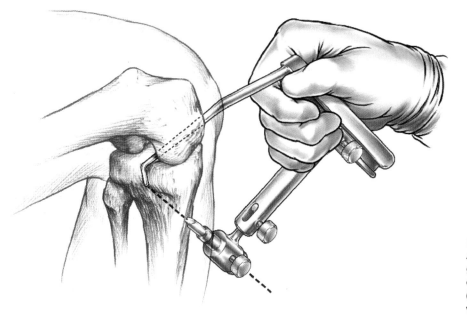

Fig 36.1-4. Arthrotek Fanelli PCL-ACL drill guide positioned to place guide wire in preparation for creation of the Transtibial PCL tibial tunnel. (From Arthrotek, Inc. Warsaw, Indiana; with permission.)

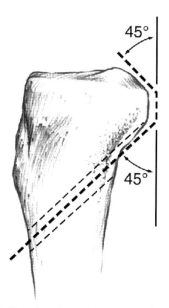

Fig 36.1-5. Drawing demonstrating the desired turning angles the PCL graft will make after the creation of the tibial tunnel. (From Arthrotek, Inc. Warsaw, Indiana; with permission.)

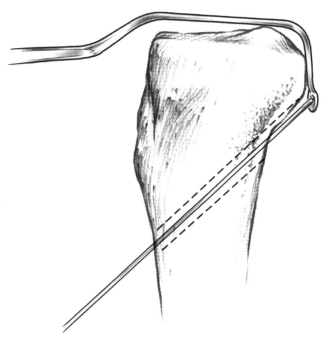

Fig 36.1-6. The Arthrotek PCL closed curette may be used to cap the guide wire during tibial tunnel drilling. (From Arthrotek, Inc. Warsaw, Indiana; with permission.)

and protecting the neurovascular structures in addition to the surgeon's finger in the posteromedial safety incision. The surgeon's finger in the posteromedial safety incision is monitoring the position of the guide wire. The standard cannulated drill is advanced to the posterior cortex of the tibia. The drill chuck is then disengaged from the drill, and completion of the tibial tunnel reaming is performed by hand. This gives an additional margin of safety for completion of the tibial tunnel. The tunnel edges are chamfered and rasped with the Arthrotek Fanelli PCL/ACL system rasp (Arthrotek Inc., Warsaw, Indiana) **(Fig 36.1-7)**.

The Femoral Tunnel

The Arthrotek Fanelli PCL-ACL Drill Guide is positioned to create the femoral tunnel **(Fig 36.1-8)**. The arm of the guide is introduced into the knee through the inferior medial patellar portal and is positioned such that the guide wire will exit through the center of the stump of the anterolateral bundle of the PCL. The blunt spade tipped guide wire is drilled through the guide, and just as it begins to emerge through the center of the stump of the anterolateral

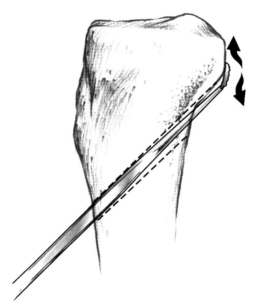

Fig 36.1-7. The tunnel edges are chamfered after drilling to smooth any rough edges. (From Arthrotek, Inc. Warsaw, Indiana; with permission.)

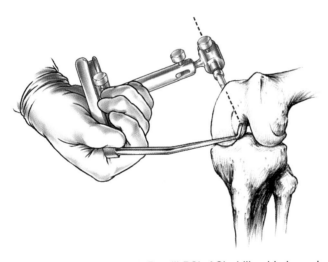

Fig 36.1-8. The Arthrotek Fanelli PCL-ACL drill guide is positioned to drill the guide wire from outside in. The guide wire begins at a point half way between the medial femoral epicondyle and the medial femoral condyle trochlea articular margin, approximately two to three centimeters proximal to the medial femoral condyle distal articular margin and exits through the center of the stump of the anterolateral bundle of the posterior cruciate ligament stump. (From Arthrotek, Inc. Warsaw, Indiana; with permission.)

bundle of the PCL, the drill guide is disengaged. The accuracy of the guide wire position is confirmed arthroscopically by probing and direct visualization. Care must be taken to ensure the patellofemoral joint has not been violated by arthroscopically examining the patellofemoral joint prior to drilling the femoral tunnel.

The appropriately sized standard cannulated reamer is used to create the femoral tunnel. A curette is used to cap the tip of the guide so there is no inadvertent advancement

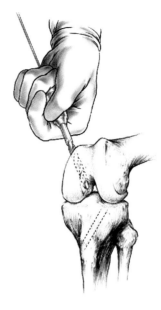

Fig 36.1-9. Completion of femoral tunnel reaming by hand for an additional margin of safety. (From Arthrotek, Inc. Warsaw, Indiana; with permission.)

of the guide wire causing damage to the articular surface, the ACL, or other intra-articular structures. As the reamer is about to penetrate the wall of the intercondylar notch, it is disengaged from the drill, and the final femoral tunnel reaming is completed by hand for an additional margin of safety **(Fig 36.1-9)**. The reaming debris is evacuated with a synovial shaver to minimize fat pad inflammatory response with subsequent risk of arthrofibrosis. The tunnel edges are chamfered and rasped. The PCL femoral tunnel may also be created from inside out through a low anterolateral portal depending upon the surgeons' preference.

Tunnel Preparation and Graft Passage

The Arthrotek Magellan suture-passing device (Arthrotek, Inc., Warsaw, Indiana, USA) is introduced through the tibial tunnel and into the knee joint and is retrieved through the femoral tunnel with an arthroscopic grasping tool **(Fig 36.1-10)**. A 7.9 mm Gortex Smoother (W.L. Gore, Inc., Flagstaff, AZ) flexible rasp may be used, and when used is attached to the Magellan suture-passing device, and the Gortex Smoother is pulled into the femoral tunnel, into the joint, and into and out the tibial tunnel opening. The tunnel edges are chamfered and rasped at 0, 30, 60, and 90 degrees of knee flexion. Care must be taken to avoid excessive pressure using the Gortex Smoother, because the tunnel configuration could be altered or the bone destroyed. The traction sutures of the graft material are attached to the loop of the flexible rasp, and the PCL graft material is pulled into position.

Graft Tensioning and Fixation

Fixation of the PCL substitute is accomplished with primary and backup fixation on both the femoral and tibial sides. Our preferred graft source for PCL reconstruction is the Achilles tendon allograft with or without the calcaneal

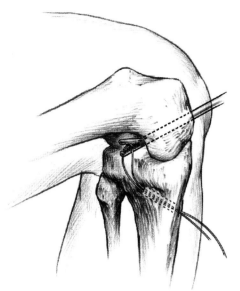

Fig 36.1-10. Retrieval of suture passing wire. (From Arthrotek, Inc. Warsaw, Indiana; with permission.)

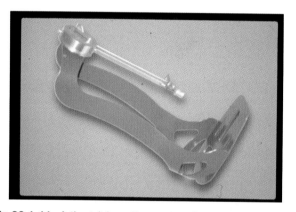

Fig 36.1-11. Arthrotek knee ligament graft tensioning boot. This mechanical tensioning device uses a ratcheted torque wrench device to assist the surgeon during graft tensioning. (From Arthrotek, Inc. Warsaw, Indiana; with permission.)

bone plug. Femoral fixation is accomplished with press fit fixation of a wedge shaped calcaneal bone plug and aperture opening fixation using the Arthrotek Gentle Thread bioabsorbable interference screw (Arthrotek Inc., Warsaw, Indiana), or with primary aperture opening fixation using the Arthrotek Gentle Thread bioabsorbable interference screw (Arthrotek Inc., Warsaw, Indiana), and back up fixation with an Arthrotek ligament fixation button (Arthrotek Inc., Warsaw, Indiana), or screw and spiked ligament washer, or screw and post assembly when no calcaneal bone plug is present. The Arthrotek Tensioning Boot (Arthrotek Inc., Warsaw, Indiana) is applied to the traction sutures of the graft material on its distal end, set for 20 pounds, and the knee cycled through full flexion-extension cycles for graft pre-tensioning and settling **(Fig 36.1-11)**. The knee is placed in approximately 70 degrees of knee flexion, and tibial fixation of the Achilles tendon allograft is achieved with primary aperture opening fixation using the Arthrotek

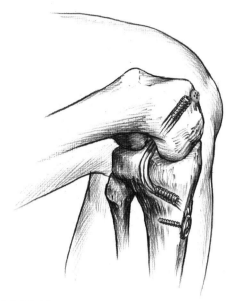

Fig 36.1-12. Final graft fixation using primary and back-up fixation. (From Arthrotek, Inc. Warsaw, Indiana; with permission.)

Gentle Thread bioabsorbable interference screw (Arthrotek Inc., Warsaw, Indiana), and back up fixation with an Arthrotek ligament fixation button, or screw and post, or screw and spiked ligament washer assembly **(Fig 36.1-12)**.

■ POSTEROLATERAL RECONSTRUCTION: SPLIT BICEPS TENDON TECHNIQUE

A technique for posterolateral reconstruction is the split biceps tendon transfer to the lateral femoral epicondyle **(Fig 36.1-13A)**. The requirements for this procedure include an intact proximal tibiofibular joint, the posterolateral capsular attachments to the common biceps tendon should be intact, and the biceps femoris tendon insertion into the fibular head must be intact. This technique recreates the function of the popliteofibular ligament and lateral collateral ligament, tightens the posterolateral capsule, and provides a post of strong autogenous tissue to reinforce the posterolateral corner.

A lateral hockey stick incision is made. The peroneal nerve is dissected free and protected throughout the procedure. The long head and common biceps femoris tendon is isolated, and the anterior two third is separated from the short head muscle. The tendon is detached proximal and left attached distally to its anatomic insertion site on the fibular head. The strip of biceps tendon should be 12 to 14 cm long. The iliotibial band is incised in line with its fibers, and the fibular collateral ligament and popliteus tendons are exposed. A drill hole is made 1 cm anterior to the fibular collateral ligament femoral insertion. A longitudinal incision is made in the lateral capsule just posterior to the fibular collateral ligament. The split biceps tendon is passed medial to the iliotibial band, and secured to the lateral femoral epicondylar region with a screw

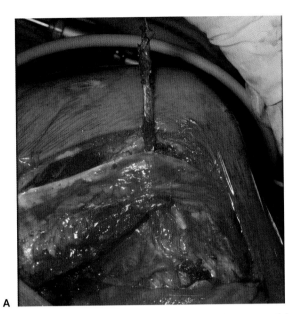
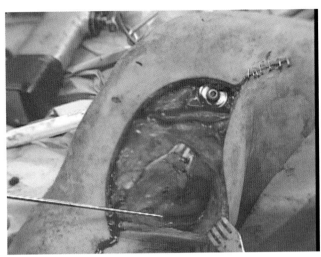

A

B

Fig 36.1-13. Surgical technique for posterolateral and lateral reconstruction are the split biceps tendon transfer **(A)** or the allograft or autograft figure of eight reconstruction **(B)** combined with posterolateral capsular shift and primary repair of injured structures as indicated. These complex surgical procedures reproduce the function of the popliteofibular ligament and the lateral collateral ligament and eliminate posterolateral capsular redundancy. The split biceps tendon transfer utilizes anatomic insertion sites and preserves the dynamic function of the long head and common biceps femoris tendon. (From Fanelli GC, Orcutt DR, Edson CJ. Current concepts. The multiple ligament injured knee: evaluation, treatment, and results. *Arthroscopy.* 2005;21(4):471–486.)

and spiked ligament washer at the above mentioned point. The residual tail of the transferred split biceps tendon is passed medial to the iliotibial band and secured to the fibular head. The posterolateral capsule that had been previously incised is then shifted and sewn into the strut of transferred biceps tendon to eliminate posterolateral capsular redundancy.

■ POSTEROLATERAL RECONSTRUCTION: FREE GRAFT TECHNIQUE

Posterolateral reconstruction with the free graft figure of eight technique utilizes semitentinosus autograft or allograft, Achilles tendon allograft, or other soft tissue allograft material. A curvilinear incision is made in the lateral aspect of the knee extending from the lateral femoral epicondyle to the interval between Gerdy's tubercle and the fibular head. The fibular head is exposed and a tunnel is created in an anterior to posterior direction at the area of maximal fibular diameter. The tunnel is created by passing a guide pin followed by a cannulated drill usually 7 mm in diameter. The peroneal nerve is protected during tunnel creation and throughout the procedure. The free tendon graft is then passed through the fibular head drill hole. An incision is then made in the iliotibial band in line with the fibers directly overlying the lateral femoral epicondyle. The graft material is passed medial to the iliotibial band, and the limbs

of the graft are crossed to form a figure of eight. A drill hole is made 1 cm anterior to the fibular collateral ligament femoral insertion. A longitudinal incision is made in the lateral capsule just posterior to the fibular collateral ligament. The graft material is passed medial to the iliotibial band, and secured to the lateral femoral epicondylar region with a screw and spiked ligament washer at the above mentioned point. The posterolateral capsule that had been previously incised is then shifted and sewn into the strut of figure of eight graft tissue material to eliminate posterolateral capsular redundancy. The anterior and posterior limbs of the figure of eight graft material are sewn to each other to reinforce and tighten the construct (Fig 36.1-13B). The iliotibial band incision is closed. The procedures described are intended to eliminate posterolateral and varus rotational instability.

■ POSTOPERATIVE REHABILITATION AND RETURN TO STRENUOUS ACTIVITY RECOMMENDATIONS

The knee is kept locked in a long leg brace in full extension for 6 weeks, with nonweight bearing using crutches. Progressive range of motion occurs during weeks 4 through 6. The brace is unlocked at the end of 6 weeks, and progressive weight bearing at 25% body weight per week during postoperative weeks 7 through 10. The crutches are discontinued at the end of postoperative week number 10. Progressive closed kinetic chain strength training and continued motion exercises are performed. Return to sports and heavy labor occurs after the sixth to ninth postoperative month, when sufficient strength, range of motion, and proprioceptive skills have returned.

RESULTS

Our 2- to 10-year results of combined PCL-posterolateral reconstruction have been previously published (48). This study presented the 2 to 10 year (24 to 120 month) results of 41 chronic arthroscopically assisted combined PCL/posterolateral reconstructions evaluated pre- and postoperatively using Lysholm, Tegner, and Hospital for Special Surgery knee ligament rating scales, KT 1000 arthrometer testing, stress radiography, and physical examination.

This study population included 31 males, 10 females, 24 left, and 17 right chronic PCL/posterolateral knee injuries with functional instability. The knees were assessed pre- and postoperatively with arthrometer testing, three different knee ligament rating scales, stress radiography, and physical examination. PCL reconstructions were performed using the arthroscopically assisted single femoral tunnel-single bundle transtibial tunnel PCL reconstruction technique using fresh frozen Achilles tendon allografts in all 41 cases. In all 41 cases, posterolateral instability reconstruction was performed with combined biceps femoris tendon tenodesis and posterolateral capsular shift procedures. The paired t-test and power analysis were the statistical tests used. Ninety-five percent confidence intervals were used throughout the analysis.

Postoperative physical exam revealed normal posterior drawer/tibial step off in 29 out of 41 (70%) of knees for the overall group, and 11 out of 12 (91.7%) normal posterior drawer and tibial step off in the knees tensioned with the Arthrotek tensioning boot. Posterolateral stability was restored to normal in 11 out of 41 (27%) knees, and tighter than the normal knee in 29 out of 41 (71%) knees evaluated with the external rotation thigh foot angle test. Thirty degrees varus stress testing was normal in 40 out of 41 (97%) knees, and grade 1 laxity in 1 out of 41 (3%) knees. Postoperative KT 1000 arthrometer testing mean side-to-side difference measurements were 1.80 mm (PCL screen), 2.11 mm (corrected posterior), and 0.63 mm (corrected anterior) measurements. This is a statistically significant improvement from preoperative status for the PCL screen and the corrected posterior measurements (p = 0.001). The postoperative stress radiographic mean side-to-side difference measurement measured at 90 degrees of knee flexion, and 32 pounds of posterior directed force applied to the proximal tibia using the Telos device was 2.26 mm. This is a statistically significant improvement from preoperative measurements (p = 0.001). Postoperative Lysholm, Tegner, and Hospital for Special Surgery knee ligament rating scale

mean values were 91.7, 4.92, and 88.7, respectively, demonstrating a statistically significant improvement from preoperative status (p = 0.001).

Conclusions drawn from this study were that chronic combined PCL/posterolateral instabilities could be successfully treated with arthroscopic PCL reconstruction using fresh frozen Achilles tendon allograft combined with posterolateral corner reconstruction using biceps tendon transfer combined with posterolateral capsular shift procedure. Statistically significant improvement is noted (p = 0.001) from the preoperative condition at 2- to 10-year follow-up using objective parameters of knee ligament rating scales, arthrometer testing, stress radiography, and physical examination. In the knees tensioned with the Arthrotek mechanical tensioning boot (Arthrotek Inc., Warsaw, Indiana), 91.7% of these knees achieved a normal posterior drawer and tibial step off postoperatively.

CONCLUSIONS

The arthroscopically assisted single bundle transtibial PCL reconstruction technique is a reproducible surgical procedure. There are documented results demonstrating statistically significant improvements from preoperative to postoperative status evaluated by physical examination, knee ligament rating scales, arthrometer measurements, and stress radiography. Factors contributing to the success of this surgical technique include identification and treatment of all pathology (especially posterolateral instability), accurate tunnel placement, placement of strong graft material at anatomic graft insertion sites, minimizing graft bending, performing final graft tensioning at 70 to 90 degrees of knee flexion using the Arthrotek graft tensioning boot, utilizing primary and back up fixation, and the appropriate postoperative rehabilitation program. In the knees tensioned with the Arthrotek mechanical tensioning boot, 91.7% of these knees achieved a normal posterior drawer and tibial step off postoperatively.

FUTURE DIRECTIONS

We have now converted to performing the double bundle, double femoral tunnel PCL reconstruction surgical technique since there is convincing basic science data supporting the efficacy of this procedure (50). This double bundle, double femoral tunnel technique more closely approximates the anatomic insertion site of the native PCL and should theoretically provide improved results. Our early clinical results are encouraging; however, there are no long-term clinical results available as of this writing.

Another area of interest is the incorporation of autologous platlette rich fibrin matrix into the grafts used in the cruciate and collateral ligament reconstructive procedures. There are several studies indicating favorable effects on the ligament graft tissue and the clinical results (51–53). We have demonstrated favorable initial clinical results with respect to graft incorporation, wound healing, and early stability; however, there is no long-term follow-up as of this writing.

■ REFERENCES

1. Parolie JM, Bergfeld JA. Long term results of nonoperative treatment of isolated posterior cruciate ligament injuries in the athlete. *Am J Sports Med*. 1986;14:35–38.
2. Fanelli GC. PCL tears-who needs surgery? Presented at the AANA Annual Meeting, Palm Dessert, CA, 1993.
3. Torg JS, Barton JM. Natural history of the posterior cruciate deficient knee. *Clin Orthop*. 1989;246:208–216.
4. Dandy DJ, Pusey RJ. The long term results of unrepaired tears of the posterior cruciate ligament. *J Bone Joint Surg Br*. 1982;64:92–94.
5. Keller PM, Shelbourne KD, McCarroll JR, et al. Nonoperatively treated isolated posterior cruciate ligament injuries. *Am J Sports Med*. 1993;12:132–136.
6. Trickey EL. Injuries to the posterior cruciate ligament. *Clin Orthop*. 1980;147:76–81. Johnson JC, Back BR. Current concepts review, posterior cruciate ligament. *Am J Knee Surg*. 1990; 3:143–153.
7. Carlin GJ. Personal communication. University of Pittsburgh biomechanics laboratory, Pittsburgh, PA: March 1994.
8. Prietto MP, Bain JR, Stonebrook SN, et al. Tensile strength of the human posterior cruciate ligament. Presented at the 34th Annual Meeting. Atlanta, Georgia: Orthopaedic Research Society; February 1–4, 1988.
9. Woo SL, Hollis JM, Adams DJ, et al. Tensile properties of the human femur-anterior cruciate ligament-tibia complex. *Am J Sports Med*. 1991;19:217–225.
10. Cooper DE, Warren RF, Warner JJ. The posterior cruciate ligament and posterolateral structures of the knee: anatomy, functions, and patterns of injury. *Instr Course Lect*. 1991; 40:249–270.
11. Van Dommelen BA, Fowler PJ. Anatomy of the posterior cruciate ligament, a review. *Am J Sports Med*. 1989;17:24–29.
12. Girgis FG, Marshall JL, Al Monajem ARS. The cruciate ligaments of the knee joint: anatomical, functional, and experimental analysis. *Clin Orthop*. 1975;106:216–231.
13. Kennedy JC, Grainger RW. The posterior cruciate ligament. *J Trauma*. 1967;367–377.
14. Covey DC, Sapega AA, Sherman GM, et al. Testing for "isometry" during posterior cruciate ligament reconstruction. *Trans Orthop Res Soc*. 1992;17:665.
15. Heller L, Langman J. The menisco-femoral ligaments of the human knee. *J Bone Joint Surg Br*. 1964;46:307–313.
16. Vladimirov B. Arterial sources of blood supply of the knee joint in man. *Acta Med*. 1968;47:1–10.
17. Arnoczky SP, Rubin RM, Marshall JL. Microvasculature of the cruciate ligaments and its response to injury. *J Bone Joint Surg Am*. 1979;61:1221–1229.
18. Scapinelli R. Studies of the vasculature of the human knee joint. *Acta Anat*. 1968;70:305–331.
19. Katonis PG, Assimakopoulos AP, Agapitos MV, et al. Mechanoreceptors in the posterior cruciate ligament. *Acta Orthop Scand*. 1991;62:276–278.
20. Butler DL, Noyes FR, Grood ES. Ligamentous restraints to anterior-posterior drawer in the human knee. *J Bone Joint Surg Am*. 1980;62:259–270.
21. Gollehon DL, Torzilli PA, Warren RF. The role of the posterolateral and cruciate ligaments in the stability of the human knee. *J Bone Joint Surg Am*. 1987;69:233–242.
22. Brantigan OC, Voshell AF. The mechanics of the ligaments and menisci of the knee joint. *J Bone Joint Surg*. 1941; 23:44–66.
23. Covey DC, Sapega AA. Posterior cruciate ligament fiber length behavior under varied joint motion and loading conditions. Presented at the AAOS Annual meeting, New Orleans, LA, 1994. Veltri DM, Warren RF. Posterolateral instability of the knee. *J Bone Joint Surg*. 1994;76A:460–472.
24. Clancy WG, Shelbourne KD, Zoellner GB, et al. Treatment of knee joint instability secondary to rupture of the posterior cruciate ligament. Report of a new procedure. *J Bone Joint Surg*. 1983;65A:310–322.
25. Degenhardt TC, Hughston JC. Chronic posterior cruciate instability: nonoperative management. *Orthop Trans*. 1981;5:486–487.
26. Fanelli GC. PCL injuries in trauma patients. *Arthroscopy*. 1993;9:291–294.
27. Fanelli GC, Edson CJ. PCL injuries in acute traumatic hemarthrosis of the knee. Presented at the AAOS Annual Meeting, New Orleans, LA, 1994.
28. O'Donoghue DH. An analysis of end results of surgical treatment of major injuries to the ligaments of the knee. *J Bone Joint Surg*. 1955;37A:1–13.
29. Parolie JM, Bergfeld JA. Long term results of non operative treatment of isolated posterior cruciate ligament injuries in the athlete. *Am J Sports Med*. 1986;14:35–38.
30. Fanelli GC, Edson CJ. PCL injuries in trauma patients. Part II. *Arthroscopy*. 1995;11:526–529.
31. Stanish WO, Rubinovich M, Armason T, et al. Posterior cruciate ligament tears in wrestlers. *Can J Appl Sports Sci*. 1986; 4:173–177.
32. Malek MM, Fanelli GC. Technique of arthroscopically PCL reconstruction. *Orthopaedics*. 1993;16(9):961–966.
33. Fanelli GC, Giannotti BF, Edson CJ. Current concepts review. The posterior cruciate ligament: arthroscopic evaluation and treatment. *Arthroscopy*. 1994;10(6):673–688.
34. Fanelli GC, Giannotti BF, Edson CJ. Arthroscopically assisted PCL/posterior lateral complex reconstruction. *Arthroscopy*. 1996;12(5).
35. Fanelli GC, Monahan TJ. Complications of posterior cruciate ligament reconstruction. *Sports Med Arthrosc Rev*. 1999; 7(4):296–302.
36. Fanelli GC. Point counter point. Arthroscopic posterior cruciate ligament reconstruction: single bundle/single femoral tunnel. *Arthroscopy*. 2000; 6(7):725–731.
37. Fanelli GC, Monahan TJ. Complications in posterior cruciate ligament and posterolateral complex surgery. *Oper Tech Sports Med*. 2001;9(2):96–99.
38. Fanelli GC, Edson CJ. Arthroscopically assisted combined ACL/PCL reconstruction. 2–10 year follow-up. *Arthroscopy*. 2002;18(7):703–714.
39. Fanelli GC, Edson CJ. Management of posterior cruciate ligament and posterolateral instability of the knee. In: Chow J, ed. *Advanced arthroplasty*. New York: Springer-Verlag; 2001.
40. Fanelli GC, Monahan TJ. Complications and pitfalls in posterior cruciate ligament reconstruction. In: Malek M, Fanelli GC, Johnson D, et al. eds. *Knee surgery: complications, pitfalls, and salvage*. New York: Springer-Verlag; 2001.
41. Fanelli GC. Arthroscopic evaluation of the PCL. In: Fanelli GC, ed. *Posterior cruciate ligament injuries. A guide to practical management*. New York: Springer-Verlag; 2001.
42. Fanelli GC. Arthroscopic PCL reconstruction: transtibial technique. In: Fanelli GC, ed. *Posterior cruciate ligament injuries. A guide to practical management*. New York: Springer-Verlag; 2001.
43. Fanelli GC. Complications in PCL surgery. In:. In: Fanelli GC, ed. *Posterior cruciate ligament injuries. A guide to practical management*. New York: Springer-Verlag; 2001.

44. Miller MD, Cooper DE, Fanelli GC, et al. Posterior cruciate ligament: current concepts. In: Beaty JH, ed. *American academy of orthopaedic surgeons instructional course lectures. Volume 51.* Rosemont, Illinois: 2002;347–351.

45. Fanelli GC. Arthrotek PCL Reconstruction Surgical Technique Guide. Fanelli PCL-ACL Drill Guide System. Arthrotek, Inc. Warsaw, Indiana. 1998.

46. Fanelli GC, Edson CJ. Combined posterior cruciate ligament—posterolateral reconstruction with Achilles tendon allograft and biceps femoris tendon tenodesis: 2–10 year follow-up. *Arthroscopy.* April-May, 2004.

47. Fanelli GC, Giannotti BF, Edson CJ. Arthroscopically assisted combined anterior and posterior cruciate ligament reconstruction. *Arthroscopy.* 1996;12(1):5–14.

48. Harner CD, Janaushek MA, Kanamori A, et al. Biomechanical analysis of a double bundle posterior cruciate ligament reconstruction. *Am J Sports Med.* 2000;28:144–151.

49. Yasuda K, Tomita F, Yamazaki S, et al. The effect of growth factors on biomechanical properties of the bone patellar tendon bone graft after anterior cruciate ligament reconstruction. *Am J Sports Med.* 2004;4:870–880.

50. Weiler A, Forster C, Hunt P, et al. The influence of locally applied platelet derived growth factor BB on free tendon graft remodeling after anterior cruciate ligament reconstruction. *Am J Sports Med.* 2004;4:881–891.

51. Sanchez M, Azofra J, Aizpurua B, et al. Application of growth factor rich autologous plasma in arthroscopic surgery. *Cuadernos de Arthroscopia.* 2003;10:12–19.

POSTERIOR CRUCIATE LIGAMENT RECONSTRUCTION WITH THE POSTERIOR INLAY GRAFT

36.2

DONALD H. JOHNSON, MD, FRCS

■ KEY POINTS

- The results of posterior cruciate ligament (PCL) reconstruction may be inconsistent due to the difficulty in reproducing the complex double bundle anatomy. It may also be due to the bending angle of the transtibial graft around the back of the tibia, the "killer tunnel angle."
- The indication for a posterior inlay graft is a symptomatic PCL deficient knee.
- A contra-indication to the posterior inlay is a previous vascular repair.
- The posterior tibia is approached with a posteromedial incision along the border of the tibia.
- The bone block is fixed to the back of the tibia first, followed by tensioning and fixation in flexion of the anterolateral bundle. The posteromedial bundle is tensioned and fixed near complete knee extension. The knee is cycled through a full range of motion to ensure that there is no restriction of motion.
- Postoperative rehab is slow. The patient is braced in extension, with a pad under the calf to push the tibia forward.

The surgical outcome of posterior cruciate ligament (PCL) reconstruction has been somewhat inconsistent, and this may be due to a number of factors that include:

- The PCL is a double bundle ligament. The single femoral tunnel may not reproduce the anatomy as well as the double femoral tunnel.
- The reconstructed graft has the continuous posterior effect of gravity that may lead to loosening in the postoperative period.

- The results may not be optimum due to the technique of transtibial tunnel reconstruction. The posterior inlay may reduce the bending angle around the posterior aspect of the tibia, and thus reduce the thinning and attenuation of the graft.
- Due to the harvest site morbidity, the use of autogenous grafts may not be as optimum as using a larger allograft.

The posterior inlay was initially described by Berg (1) in 1995. The original technique used a patellar tendon graft, and screwed a bone block to the posterior aspect of the tibia. The purported advantage of the posterior inlay was to reduce the killer tunnel angle around the back of the tibia. It was felt that with continued range of motion of the knee the graft would be thinned as it emerged from the tibial tunnel. The posterior inlay technique avoided this stress point.

■ BASIC SCIENCE

There is basic laboratory science to support the use of the posterior inlay graft. Bergfeld et al. (2) has shown that with cyclic loading the graft in the transtibial tunnel procedure is thinned and attenuated around the tibia leading to graft failure. Markolf et al. (3) compared the inlay and transtibial tunnel and concluded that the inlay technique of PCL replacement was superior to the tunnel technique with respect to graft failure, graft thinning, and permanent increase in graft length.

In another study Markoff et al. (4) showed that if the bone block of the graft is put in the very proximal end of the tibial tunnel, there is little difference compared to the posterior inlay graft. Mannor et al. (5) and Harner et al. (6) have studied the two bundle reconstruction in the lab and felt that this technique improves the kinematics. Margheritini (7) studied the kinematics and has shown that there is very little difference between the posterior inlay and the transtibial tunnel techniques.

Indications

The indication for a posterior inlay graft is for any symptomatic chronic unstable PCL deficient knee. In general, most reconstructions are done for knees that are more than 10 mm of posterior displacement and have multiple ligament laxities. A revision case that has hardware in the proximal tibia is also an indication for the posterior inlay technique. A contra-indication to the posteromedial approach of the tibial inlay is a previous vascular repair.

Graft Choice

In North America, the most common choice of graft is the achilles tendon allograft. There are numerous other options for autogenous grafts, the ipsilateral patellar tendon graft, and the quadriceps tendon graft with patellar bone plug. The same grafts may be also harvested from the opposite knee.

■ THE STEPS OF THE SURGICAL TECHNIQUE

Graft Harvest and Preparation

The autogenous patellar tendon or quadriceps tendon with a bone plug is harvested from the same or the opposite knee. The bone plug must be at least 1.5 cm in width and 3 cm in length to accept a screw without breaking.

Diagnostic Arthroscopy

The knee is arthroscoped to document the state of the articular surface and meniscus. The ACL and PCL are probed and assessed. If there is any meniscal or chondral pathology, it is dealt with at this time. The PCL is debrided from the femoral condyle leaving a footprint to guide the placement of the tunnels. The posteromedial portal is created to insert a shaver and remove the ligament on the back of the tibia. Some of the preparation of the trough on the tibia can also be done with a burr through this portal.

Femoral Tunnel

The femoral tunnel can be created with an ACL guide from outside in or from inside out. The tip of the ACL guide is placed in the center of the anterolateral bundle and a K-wire drilled from outside in. A 1.5 cm skin incision is made to accept the 10 mm drill bit. The tunnel is drilled from outside in. In the other technique, a K-wire is introduced from the far low anterolateral portal. The K-wire is placed in the center of the anterolateral bundle, the knee is flexed to 120 degrees, and is drilled through to the outside. The tunnel is then drilled from outside in with the appropriate size drill bit. A folded-over AO wire is introduced down the femoral tunnel from outside in and pushed to the back of the joint. If indicated, a second femoral tunnel for the posteromedial bundle may be drilled just inferior to the anterolateral tunnel.

Posteromedial Incision

The posteromedial incision is created longitudinally along the posteriomedial aspect of the tibia. Burks Schaffer (8) described this approach in 1990. The incision is along the posteromedial border of the tibia. The medial head of the gastrocnemius is identified and retracted medially. This retracts the neurovascular bundle laterally and protects them from injury. The PCL attachment site on the back of the tibia is identified by palpating the trough between the two eminences on each side of the PCL attachment site. This trough can be increased in size with an osteotome or a burr. It must be deep and large enough to accommodate the bone plug of the graft. A large posterior arthrotomy is created to pass the graft. The folded-over AO wire is found in the back of the joint and pulled out through the incision.

Graft Passage

The femoral soft tissue end of the graft is attached with leader sutures to the AO wire. The leader sutures are pulled with the wire into the femoral tunnel. The soft tissue end of the graft is pulled into the femoral tunnel (either single or double bundle).

Graft Fixation and Tensioning

The bone block is fixed to the back of the tibia with one or two small fragment screws. Bicortical fixation of the screws is ideal. If the bone block is small, only one screw is used. The soft tissue end of the graft is pulled firmly into the femoral tunnel and the knee placed through several cycles of knee motion. The knee is set at 90 degrees of flexion, and a screw placed from outside in is used to fix the soft tissue in the femoral tunnel. An anterior drawer force is applied to the tibia as the graft is fixed in the femoral tunnel. Secondary fixation can be done by placing a staple into the end of the soft tissue graft on the cortical surface of the femur. The posteromedial bundle is fixed close to full knee extension. The knee is cycled through a full range of motion to ensure that there is no restriction in motion. The wounds are closed, and an extension splint with a posterior pad is applied to the calf.

■ REHABILITATION

Postoperatively the rehab is much slower after PCL reconstruction. The patient is braced in extension, with a pad under the calf to push the tibia forward. Prone lying range of motion exercises only are allowed for the first few weeks. After healing of the graft gradual range of motion exercises are instituted. After 3 months more vigorous strength training may resume. The knee is braced for at least 6 months if any concomitant collateral ligament reconstruction is done.

■ RESULTS

Cooper and Stewart (9) have presented and published satisfactory results of the single bundle posterior inlay graft. The technique was a single bundle patellar tendon allograft in 44 patients that were followed for 2 to 10 years. Telos stress radiography with 25 kg posterior load applied at 90 degrees of flexion demonstrated average side-to-side difference of 4.11 mm (−2 to 10 mm).

The latest twist to try to improve the outcome of PCL reconstruction is the posterior inlay graft with two femoral bundles. Stannard et al. (10) have published a series of good results using this double femoral bundle technique. In that series 30 PCL reconstructions were followed up, and 77% had no detectable residual laxity. Noyes et al. (11) have described using the quadriceps tendon graft with a double-bundle posterior inlay technique to reconstruct the PCL.

■ REFERENCES

1. Berg EE. Posterior cruciate ligament tibial inlay reconstruction. *Arthroscopy*. 1995;11(1):69–76.
2. Bergfeld JA, McAllister DR, Parker RD, et al. A biomechanical comparison of posterior cruciate ligament reconstruction techniques. *Am J Sports Med*. 2001;29(2):129–136.
3. Markolf KL, Zemanovic JR, McAllister DR. Cyclic loading of posterior cruciate ligament replacements fixed with tibial tunnel and tibial inlay methods. *J Bone Joint Surg Am*. 2002;84A(4):518–524.
4. Markolf K, Davies M, Zoric B, et al. Effects of bone block position and orientation within the tibial tunnel for posterior cruciate ligament graft reconstructions: a cyclic loading study of bone-patellar tendon-bone allografts. *Am J Sports Med*. 2003;31(5):673–679.
5. Mannor DA, Shearn J T, Grood ES, et al. Two-bundle posterior cruciate ligament reconstruction. An in vitro analysis of graft placement and tension. *Am J Sports Med*. 2000;28(6):833–845.
6. Harner CD, Janaushek MA, Kanamori A, et al. Biomechanical analysis of a double-bundle posterior cruciate ligament reconstruction. *Am J Sports Med*. 2000;28(2):144–151.
7. Margheritini FM, Rihn CS, Stabile JA, et al. Biomechanical comparison of tibial inlay versus transtibial techniques for posterior cruciate ligament reconstruction: analysis of knee kinematics and graft in situ forces. *Am J Sports Med*. 2004;32(3):587–593.
8. Burks RT, Schaffer JJ. A simplified approach to the tibial attachment of the posterior cruciate ligament. *Clin Orthop*. 1990;254:216–219.
9. Cooper DE, Stewart D. Posterior cruciate ligament reconstruction using single-bundle patella tendon graft with tibial inlay fixation: 2- to 10-year follow-up. *Am J Sports Med*. 2004;32(2):346–360.
10. Stannard JP, Riley RS, Sheils T, et al. Anatomic reconstruction of the posterior cruciate ligament after multiligament knee injuries. A combination of the tibial-inlay and two-femoral-tunnel techniques. *Am J Sports Med*. 2003;31(2):196–202.
11. Noyes FR, Medvecky MJ, Bhargava M. Arthroscopically assisted quadriceps double-bundle tibial inlay posterior cruciate ligament reconstruction: An analysis of techniques and a safe operative approach to the popliteal fossa. *Arthroscopy*. 2003;19(8):894–905.

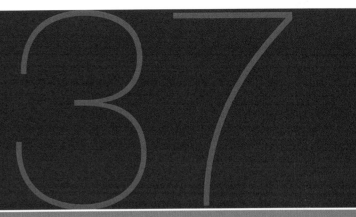

THE ACL PCL INJURED (DISLOCATED) KNEE

GREGORY C. FANELLI, MD, DANIEL R. ORCUTT, MD, JUSTIN D. HARRIS, MD, DAVID ZIJERDI, MD, CRAIG J. EDSON, MHS, PT, ATC

■ KEY POINTS

- Multiple ligament injuries to the knee occur most often after a significant force is applied, resulting in a knee dislocation.
- Knee dislocations may be easily missed at initial presentation because they often spontaneously reduce.
- When the posterior lateral corner is injured, it can be repaired, but often needs augmentation with autograft or allograft tissue.
- Each knee dislocation needs to be described using a combination of classification systems. The classification systems are: direction of the dislocation of the tibia, whether it is an open or closed injury, and whether it was a high-energy or low-energy event.
- Anterior dislocations are thought to be the most common of knee dislocations. Posterior dislocations are the next-most common.
- The typical mechanism of injury is a violent force on the proximal tibia or knee. The direction that the force is applied will determine the ultimate position of the dislocation and which ligaments are damaged.
- All four major knee ligaments, as well as the posteromedial and posterolateral corners, can be compromised in the dislocated knee. Vascular and neurologic injuries are also common, making a detailed assessment of these structures imperative.
- In frank or suspected knee dislocations, the presence of pulses does not rule out an arterial injury. Any signs of compromised vascularity following a dislocated knee warrant evaluation with an arteriogram.
- A thorough history, including the mechanism and position of the limb at the time of injury, may provide clues to the possible ligaments involved.

- Gross knee swelling with normal radiographs may indicate a spontaneously reduced knee dislocation.
- Prior to any manipulation, anteroposterior (AP) and lateral radiographs of the affected extremity should be obtained to confirm the direction of the dislocation, which will aid in planning the reduction maneuver.
- Following the acute management of the dislocated knee, a magnetic resonance image (MRI) of the affected knee may be obtained to confirm and aid in planning the reconstruction of compromised ligamentous structures.
- Critically ill patients, sedentary elderly people, and patients with grossly contaminated wounds and/or significant soft tissue injuries may require nonoperative management. The most basic method of nonoperative management is a long leg or cylinder cast.
- Acute medial collateral ligament (MCL) tears, when combined with anterior cruciate ligament (ACL)/posterior cruciate ligament (PCL) tears, may in certain cases be treated with bracing.
- The techniques of arthroscopic assisted ACL/PCL reconstruction have become popular because of several advancements in the last decade.

A multiple ligament injured knee most often occurs after a significant force is applied to the knee resulting in a knee dislocation. The knee may have spontaneously reduced and may not demonstrate radiographic evidence of a dislocation at initial presentation. As these injuries typically involve a high-energy mechanism, the physician evaluating the patient must have a high index of suspicion for additional trauma, especially involving the contralateral lower extremity. Neurovascular injuries commonly occur in the multi-ligament injured knee and a detailed assessment of these structures is imperative.

The incidence of knee dislocation is difficult to quantify. Knee dislocations may be easily missed, especially if one has spontaneously reduced. Numerous retrospective studies have attempted to evaluate the true incidence (46,57,69). Estimates indicate that approximately 0.01% or less of all hospital admissions are attributable to knee dislocations.

Evaluation beyond the initial trauma work-up commonly includes examination under anesthesia, magnetic resonance imaging, and arthroscopy. Combining these tools can give valuable information on the injury complex as well as assisting in formulating a treatment plan.

Historically, immobilization was the treatment of choice for multiligament injuries to the knee. More recently, outcome studies comparing nonoperative management versus operative repair/reconstruction have suggested an improved outcome with surgical management.

When the anterior cruciate ligament (ACL) and posterior cruciate ligament (PCL) are disrupted in the adult population it is usually in the midsubstance of the ligament and therefore reconstruction is performed. When the posterior lateral corner has been injured, it can be repaired but often needs augmentation with autograft or allograft tissue. When the medial collateral ligament (MCL) is disrupted, the treatment is usually nonoperative, allowing it to heal in a brace prior to reconstruction of the other damaged ligaments.

Surgical timing is dependent on several factors including the specific ligaments injured, the presence or absence of neurovascular injuries, the ability to keep the knee reduced by external means, and the overall health of the individual.

■ ANATOMY AND BIOMECHANICS OF THE KNEE

Several anatomic features, both static and dynamic, contribute to knee stability. Static stabilizers include the bony articulations, menisci, and ligaments. Dynamic stabilizers include the musculature that crosses the knee joint. The articulation of the tibiofemoral joint is maintained in part by the bony anatomy of the femoral condyles and tibial plateau as well as the menisci, which increase contact area between the tibia and femur. The most significant ligamentous stabilizers are the anterior and posterior cruciate ligaments, the medial and lateral collateral ligaments, and the posteromedial and posterolateral corners. The capsular ligaments of the knee are aponeurotic extensions of the thigh and leg musculature that terminate on the menisci. They function to activate motion of the joint and impart stability as ligament tension is modulated by the attached musculature (22).

The medial aspect of the knee can be conceptualized in terms of three layers and three longitudinal divisions (77,79). The first and most superficial layer is the sartorius and its fascia. Next is the tibial collateral ligament.

The third and deepest layer consists of the medial capsular ligament. The gracilis and semitendinosis muscles run between the two superficial layers. The medial aspect of the knee is divided longitudinally into thirds. The anterior third consists of the medial retinacular ligament of the extensor aponeurosis, which has only meniscal and tibial attachments. The middle third contains the medial mid-third capsular ligament and the tibial collateral ligament superficially. The posterior third contains the termination of the semimembranosis tendon, which consists of the posterior oblique ligament and the origin of the oblique popliteal ligament. Each ligament can be divided into meniscofemoral and meniscotibial components in the coronal plane.

The lateral aspect of the knee can also be divided into layers (79). The deepest layer is the lateral capsule which divides into two laminae just posterior to the overlying iliotibial tract. The laminae encompass the lateral collateral, fabellofibular, and arcuate ligaments. The second layer consists of the quadriceps retinaculum and the two patellofemoral ligaments posteriorly. The most superficial layer consists of the iliotibial tract and the superficial portion of the biceps and its expansion. The peroneal nerve lies deep to the iliotibial tract, just posterior to the biceps tendon (40).

In the popliteal fossa, the popliteal artery and vein are separated from the posterior capsule by a layer of fat. The artery is tethered proximally by the adductor hiatus and distally by the soleus arch where it bifurcates into anterior and posterior tibial arteries. Genicular arteries give rise to the collateral circulation around the joint. The close proximity of the popliteal artery to the joint as well as its immobility makes it especially susceptible to injury with dislocations of the knee joint (54). The tibial and common peroneal nerve run superficial to the artery and are less vulnerable to injury when the knee is dislocated.

To assess the structural integrity of the ligamentous structures, the function of each must be well understood. The ACL functions to prevent anterior translation of the tibia relative to the femur, limits rotation of the tibia when the knee is in extension, and limits varus and valgus stress when the lateral collateral ligament (LCL) or MCL are injured (10,83). The PCL is located near the center of rotation of the knee. It functions as the primary static stabilizer of the knee and the primary restraint against posterior translation of the tibia. The MCL and LCL function to prevent valgus and varus stresses respectively when the knee is flexed to 30 degrees. A secondary function of both is to limit anterior or posterior translation and rotation of the tibia (22). The posterolateral corner functions to resist posterolateral rotation as well as posterior tibial translation relative to the femur. The posteromedial corner functions to resist posteromedial tibial translation relative to the femur and valgus stress at the knee. A thorough clinical exam is necessary to evaluate each of these structures in the multiple ligament injured knee (19,20,21).

■ CLASSIFICATION OF KNEE DISLOCATIONS

There are several ways to classify knee dislocations: a) the direction of dislocation of the tibia; b) the presence of an open or closed injury; or c) the amount of energy required for the dislocation (high-energy vs. low-energy). Each classification system provides valuable information on the type of injury, its risk of neurovascular complication, and its risk of infection. Each knee dislocation needs to be described using a combination of these classification systems.

One common way is to describe the direction of displacement of the tibia in relation to the distal femur. This gives a combination of possible dislocations including anterior, posterior, medial, lateral, and rotational. Rotational dislocations include anteromedial, anterolateral, posteromedial, and posterolateral. Anterior dislocations are thought to be the most common, representing 31% to 70% of all knee dislocations (25,33). Posterior dislocations are the next most frequent at 25% (25,33). Rotational dislocations occur in 3% to 5% (25,33). Many knee dislocations spontaneously reduce. A high index of suspicion must exist if multiple ligaments are injured that a knee dislocation is likely to have occurred.

Open dislocations occur in 19% to 35% of all knee dislocations and have a poorer prognosis (46,69). Open dislocations also limit surgical management because it may make arthroscopic surgery difficult.

Another method to classify knee dislocations is to differentiate between high- and low-energy mechanisms. Low-energy mechanisms include nonmotorized sports injuries. These injuries have a lower incidence of neurovascular injury (67). Higher energy mechanisms include motor vehicle collisions and falls from height.

A classification system has been created by Schenck (63) that describes the injury pattern, as well as any associated neurovascular injury **(Table 37-1)**. This classification system may be helpful in planning surgical treatment and for predicting functional outcome.

TABLE 37-1	Classification of Injury Patterns
Classification	**Injury Descriptor**
KDI	Intact PCL with variable injury to collateral ligaments
KDII	Both cruciate ligaments disrupted completely with collaterals intact
KDIII	Both cruciate ligaments disrupted completely with one collateral ligament distrupted
KDIV	Both cruciate ligaments and collateral ligaments disrupted
KDV	Dislocation with periarticular fracture

Regardless of the mechanism or position of the tibia, prompt reduction is needed. If after reduction, there is an asymmetrical vascular exam between the two lower extremities urgent vascular studies should be obtained.

■ INJURY MECHANISMS

The typical mechanism of injury is a violent force on the proximal tibia or knee. The direction that the force is applied will determine the ultimate position of the dislocation as well as the ligaments injured. Hyperextension results in anterior dislocation. Kennedy (42) has described the sequence of events in a cadaveric model. The posterior capsule fails first. The ACL and PCL as well as the popliteal artery then fail at approximately 50 degrees of hyperextension (29,43). Kennedy's is the only published experimental study that has investigated mechanism of injury for knee dislocations.

A posteriorly directed force on the proximal tibia, typical of a dashboard injury, is thought to result in a posterior knee dislocation. Varus and valgus stresses result in lateral and medial dislocations, respectively. A combination of forces in the anterior-posterior plane and in the medial-lateral plane will likely produce a rotational type dislocation.

The posterolateral dislocation is thought to arise from flexed nonweight bearing knee with a rapid abduction and internal rotation moment (57).

■ ASSOCIATED INJURIES

Several anatomic structures are at risk for injury in the dislocated knee. Patients can present with varying combinations of ligamentous involvement. All four major knee ligaments as well as the posteromedial and posterolateral corners can be compromised. Additionally, vascular and neurologic injuries are common. Furthermore, bony avulsion injuries, fractures of the distal femur or tibial plateau, and ipsilateral tibial or femoral shaft fractures are often seen with concomitant knee dislocations.

Numerous reports exist in the literature citing knee dislocations in which less than three of the major knee ligaments were torn (9,13,43,47,68,69); however, this appears to be the exception rather than the rule. If a dislocation occurs solely in the sagittal plane, it would not be uncommon to find macroscopic continuity of both collateral ligaments, but several authors propose that frank dislocations invariably result in rupture of at least three of the four major knee ligaments. Sisto and Warren (69) found that all knees in their series treated operatively had three or more ligaments compromised. In a series by Frassica et al. (25), all patients were found to have disruption of the ACL, PCL, and MCL at time of surgery. In Fanelli's study, 19 of 20 patients had bicruciate disruption coupled with injury to a variable third component, either the MCL or the posterolateral corner (20). A meticulous ligamentous examination is essential in order to fully evaluate the extent of the injury.

Cruciate injuries in knee dislocations typically fall into one of two patterns: either bony avulsions or midsubstance tears. These often exist in multiple combinations with other soft tissue and ligamentous injuries. Bony avulsion or peel-off injuries are often amenable to surgical reattachment and avoid need for reconstruction of the involved cruciate. Avulsion injuries are more likely to occur in high-energy knee dislocations. Midsubstance tears of the cruciates occur commonly with knee dislocations. Results of primary repair of midsubstance tears are far inferior to that of surgical reconstruction.

In addition to cruciate rupture, injury to the soft tissues, collateral ligaments, joint capsule, and supporting tendinous structures are common in knee dislocations. These structures also frequently require operative attention. Again, a careful physical and surgical evaluation is crucial to identify injury to the MCL, LCL, menisci, and tendons of the iliotibial band, the biceps femoris, the popliteus, and the quadriceps mechanism. All open injuries require thorough debridement, pulsatile irrigation, and bony stabilization.

The incidence of vascular compromise in knee dislocation has historically been estimated to be about 32% (33). Other studies have documented rates anywhere from 16% to 64% (37,46). The more recent literature confirms the significant incidence of arterial injury (2,25,66,70) reaffirming the need for a complete vascular evaluation. The popliteal artery has very limited mobility secondary to the tethered nature of the vessel at the adductor hiatus and the entrance through the gastrocnemius-soleus arch. This tethering makes it extremely vulnerable to injury in cases of blunt trauma to the knee. Two major types of injury mechanisms are described. One involves a stretching of the artery, often seen with hyperextension, which results in extensive intimal damage. This is more common in anterior dislocations. Posterior dislocations, however, typically result in a direct contusion of the vessel by the posterior aspect of the tibial plateau and are more likely to produce complete rupture of the artery (33). As the popliteal artery is an end-artery to the leg, with minimal collateral circulation provided by the geniculate system, any compromise to the point of prolonged obstruction often leads to ischemia and eventual amputation. Furthermore, the popliteal vein is responsible for the majority of the venous outflow from the knee. Injury to this structure also compromises the viability of the lower limb.

It is important to note that in the case of frank knee dislocations and suspected dislocations, the presence of pulses does not rule out an arterial injury. Serial vascular examinations are essential as intimal flaps may often present as delayed thrombus formation. Additionally, the absence of pulses implies an arterial injury and cannot be attributed to vascular spasm. Failure to recognize an arterial injury can lead to disastrous outcomes.

Nerve injury is also quite common following dislocation of the knee. A reasonable estimate of the documented incidence is anywhere from 20% to 30% (39,43,47,69,70,74).

The majority of nerve injuries involve the peroneal nerve, but reports of tibial nerve compromise have been reported (81). Nerve palsies have been described in all types of knee dislocations, but a common theme is association with injury to the lateral ligamentous complex. The peroneal and tibial nerves are not as tightly tethered as the popliteal artery and are thus less prone to injury. A stretch neuropraxia is the most common mechanism of injury, which often extends well proximal to the fibula. Occasionally, complete nerve transection occurs. Recovery of nerve function is unpredictable with most series reporting no recovery in more than 50% of injuries, though Sisto and Warren (69) reported spontaneous complete recovery in two of two patients with an incomplete peroneal nerve palsy (46,70,72,73). Nerve injury must be differentiated from stocking paresthesias that may be indicative of a developing compartment syndrome as opposed to a simple neuropraxia.

Osseous integrity is also often times compromised in knee dislocations. Reports have indicated that the incidence of bony injury may be as high as 60% (47). Avulsion fractures of ligamentous and tendinous attachments are frequently seen in knee dislocations (Segond fractures, fibular head avulsion fractures, cruciate avulsions) but should be considered ligamentous injuries, unlike major fractures as are seen in true fracture-dislocations of the knee.

Moore (49) coined the term "fracture-dislocation" to distinguish between tibial plateau fractures and purely ligamentous knee dislocations because of different treatment protocols. Tibial plateau fractures require bony stabilization, whereas pure knee dislocations necessitate ligamentous reconstruction. Fracture-dislocations of the knee are a combination of the two, adding an element of complexity to their treatment. Similar to pure knee dislocations, these are typically high-energy injuries that can result in marked joint instability and are associated with a high risk of soft-tissue and neurovascular compromise. It is also important to differentiate between these three entities as outcomes correlate directly with the underlying injury. Tibial plateau fractures have the best prognosis and pure dislocations have the worst prognosis with fracture-dislocations lying somewhere in between.

■ INITIAL EVALUATION OF THE MULTIPLE LIGAMENT INJURED KNEE

General Considerations

Evaluation of the knee with multiple ligament involvement involves a systematic approach in order to accurately identify all potential injuries. A comprehensive physical examination supplemented by appropriate ancillary studies allows the physician to formulate a treatment plan.

A knee dislocation represents the most dramatic example of the multiple ligament injured knee. Obvious deformity may be present, and a grossly dislocated knee is unlikely to escape diagnosis. However, dislocations that have spontaneously reduced may present more subtly. Complete disruption of two or more knee ligaments should alert the clinician to the possibility of a spontaneously reduced knee dislocation (80). Without proper evaluation and treatment, considerable adverse sequelae and morbidity may result.

Physical Examination

A thorough history, including mechanism and position of the limb at the time of injury may provide clues to the possible ligamentous involvement. Injuries may be classified as low- or high-velocity based on the history. Any manipulation of the limb prior to the patient's arrival in the emergency department as well as the resting position and alignment of the injured extremity need to be recognized. Inspection of the skin for abrasions, ecchymosis, swelling, and open wounds provides clues for possible underlying pathology. Gross knee swelling with normal radiographs may indicate a spontaneously-reduced knee dislocation. Dimpling of the skin may indicate an irreducible posterolateral dislocation. This type of dislocation involves buttonholing of the medial femoral condyle through the medial joint capsule. A high incidence of skin necrosis following attempted closed reduction mandates open reduction (36).

The most essential aspect of the initial evaluation of an acutely injured knee is a detailed neurovascular examination. Prior to any attempted closed reduction, both motor and sensory findings in the superficial peroneal, the deep peroneal, and the tibial nerve distributions must be documented. A thorough vascular examination includes checking pulses, capillary refill, skin color, and skin temperature. The presence of active hemorrhage, an expanding hematoma, or a bruit over the popliteal artery are all also signs of vascular injury. These must all be carefully evaluated both prior to and after a closed reduction is performed. Serial neurovascular checks are mandatory in all patients that have or are suspected of having a knee dislocation.

Laxity testing for evaluating ligament injury is often limited in the conscious patient because of significant pain with the examination. A stabilized Lachman test in which the examiner's thigh is placed under the injured knee allows for relatively pain-free evaluation of both anterior and posterior endpoints. Gross laxity in full extension during application of a varus or valgus stress implies disruption of the collateral ligament, one or more of the cruciate ligaments, and associated capsular injury. A more detailed ligamentous examination typically requires conscious sedation or general anesthesia.

Imaging Studies

Prior to any manipulation, anteroposterior (AP) and lateral radiographs of the affected extremity should be obtained to confirm the direction of the dislocation, which will aid in planning the reduction maneuver. Plain films also afford the opportunity to evaluate for associated osseous injuries, identifying both joint surface fractures as well as bony avulsions.

Radiographs are also necessary to verify reduction. Additionally, tibiofemoral widening on AP knee films may be the only radiographic sign of a spontaneously reduced knee dislocation.

Arteriography plays an important role in the imaging of the dislocated knee. All knee dislocations raise suspicion of potential vascular injury. Any signs of compromised vascularity following a dislocated knee warrants evaluation with an arteriogram. It is the gold-standard for assessment of intimal injury.

After the acute management of the dislocated knee, magnetic resonance imaging (MRI) of the affected knee may be obtained to confirm and aid in planning the reconstruction of compromised ligamentous structures. Because of its superior soft tissue contrast and direct multiplanar acquistion, MRI has become the primary tool used to evaluate the soft tissues of the knee. Improvements in technology now enable a complete examination in less than 20 minutes, inclusive of ligaments, menisci, and articular cartilage. Numerous studies verify the high sensitivities and accuracy of MRI in diagnosing both ligamentous and meniscal lesions (48). In addition, abnormalities of the peroneal nerve can often be evaluated on MRI (56).

Magnetic resonance angiography of the popliteal fossa is now becoming considered as a method to evaluate for possible vascular injury following knee dislocation. At some institutions it is used in the acute setting, as an alternative to invasive formal arteriography. In addition to being less invasive, it avoids the potential for contrast reactions and arterial punctures. Numerous studies document the utility of MRA in other settings (8,26), but its utility in the assessment of vascular injury following knee dislocation has not been cited in the literature. As further studies involving more high-risk patients commence and technology continues to evolve, MRA may supplant arteriography as the first-line vascular study in this patient population.

Vascular Injuries

A full spectrum of vascular injuries can be encountered in the multiple ligament injured knee. The mechanism of arterial injury varies with the type of dislocation. As stated before, anterior dislocations typically produce a traction injury to the artery, resulting in an intimal tear. On the contrary, vascular injuries associated with posterior dislocations are frequently complete arterial tears (33). Green and Allen (32) reported a higher likelihood of vascular injury with posterior dislocations than with anterior dislocations, 44% to 39% respectively. Numerous other studies have stated the opposite (68).

Regardless of the direction of the dislocation, vascular injury should always be suspected and evaluated. Delay in diagnosis of major arterial injuries represents a significant contributor to high amputation rates. Prompt and accurate diagnosis of vascular trauma is essential in its successful management.

The diagnosis of vascular injury is a clinical one. A detailed history and physical are essential. A history of ischemia (pain, paresthesias, paralysis, pallor, and diminished limb temperature) should be pursued. Physical exam includes assessment of the pulses by palpation, Doppler, and ankle-brachial indices when pulse status is questionable. Distal perfusion as well as motor and neurologic function must also be evaluated. These variables must be reassessed on a frequent, scheduled basis to evaluate for changes in the immediate period following closed reduction. Any abnormalities or asymmetry are concerning and should be investigated further.

Difficulty ensuring vascularity clinicially has always been well documented in numerous reports of knee dislocations (33,36,37,39,43,47). It is well known that the presence of pulses does not eliminate the possibility of vascular compromise. Misdiagnosis of vascularity and subsequent delay in arterial repair based on palpable peripheral pulses and/or capillary refill have been documented (39). As a result, many authors recommend liberal or mandatory angiographic studies in cases of knee dislocations (1,6,12,45). Arguments for this approach have emphasized the risks of missed arterial injury including muscle ischemia and limb amputation. Others note that normal pulses, Doppler signals, and capillary refill after initial closed reduction do not rule out a vascular injury that progresses over time causing late vascular compromise (43).

More recently, several authors have proposed studying only those patients who present with diminished or absent pulses on physical examination and closely observing those patients with normal pulses (14,41,42,49). The issue of total reliance on physical examination versus routine arteriography is quite controversial. A recent prospective study used arteriography to evaluate only those patients with hard signs of potential vascular injury. Patients with normal pulses were followed clinically with serial physical examinations. They reported a 94% positive predictive value for vascular injury in those patients with hard clinical signs. A 100% negative predictive value was reported for those patients that had a negative clinical examination for vascular compromise (49). The authors concluded that arteriography is unnecessary when physical examination is negative but may avert negative vascular exploration when physical examination is positive.

Duplex ultrasonography has also been proposed as a safer, cheaper, and less invasive method of evaluating the popliteal vasculature. Results have been favorable showing a 98% accuracy of detecting extremity vascular trauma (11). Advocates state that ultrasonography offers yet another safeguard against missing a potentially disastrous injury (27). Opponents argue that ultrasounds are operator dependent, cannot account for distorted anatomy surrounding the knee following dislocation, and present an intrinsic delay as a technician must be present to complete the study (49).

Less controversy exists regarding management of patients with hard signs of limb ischemia. Arteriography is not indicated in cases with an obviously ischemic limb, as there is a danger in delaying vascular repair. Many authors contend that arteriographic studies supply little additional information as the location of the lesion is invariably within the popliteal space (33). Arteriography may be useful if more than one level of injury exists. This can often be accomplished with an intraoperative angiogram prior to vascular exploration. Emergent vascular reconstruction with a reverse saphenous vein graft is the treatment of choice for an ischemic limb following a knee dislocation.

Patients in whom angiography is absolutely indicated are those whose pulses are abnormal or asymmetric but there is no evidence of limb ischemia and those that have developed a change in their vascular status following serial examinations.

Nerve Injuries

A high incidence of nerve injury exists following knee dislocation. Little consensus has been reached regarding management of these lesions.

Multiple anatomic factors contribute to the propensity of peroneal nerve injury during knee dislocation. There is only 0.5 cm of excursion of the peroneal nerve at the fibular head during knee motion (7). Additionally, there is a significantly smaller ratio of epineural tissue to axonal tissue in this nerve compared to other peripheral nerves making it prone to stretch injuries (35).

During knee reconstruction, exploration of the peroneal nerve usually reveals that it is in continuity; however, rupture has been reported (7,64,82). A widespread zone of injury is typically encountered, which correlates with the poor results that have been documented following observation of complete nerve palsies (46,70,72,73).

The evaluation of a potential nerve injury begins with a detailed history and physical examination. Paresthesias, sensory changes, and motor function all must be documented. As stated before, common peroneal nerve injury is the most common nerve injury seen after dislocation of the knee, followed by tibial nerve injury. Sequential neurologic evaluation over the first 48 hours, and repeat evaluations one and two weeks after injury, is imperative, as motor grades are often acutely reduced after dislocation secondary to pain alone. In addition, delayed neurologic compromise may develop from swelling, hematoma, or direct compression from a splint or a cast.

Needle electromyography (EMG) can offer useful information about the status of the motor axons in the peroneal nerve. EMG changes that indicate axon disruption include fibrillation potentials, positive sharp waves, and absence of activity on voluntary effort or proximal nerve stimulation. Typically, these changes may not appear for 2 to 3 weeks following injury, so EMG is of limited use prior to this time. Absence of signs of denervation in a paralyzed muscle after 3 weeks indicates a neuropraxic lesion, and any identifiable voluntary motor unit axon potentials exclude nerve rupture. Serial EMGs are also helpful following recovery.

Three options exist for operative intervention of peroneal nerve palsies. These include neurolysis alone, primary repair, or neuroma excision with nerve grafting. A recent study proposed the following treatment algorithm. Observation is the treatment of choice for all incomplete peroneal nerve palsies. One should expect a high likelihood of complete recovery. If nerve rupture is identified at the time of ligamentous reconstruction, nerve reconstruction should be considered approximately 3 months after the original operation. Acute repairs should be avoided, unless a primary repair can be performed under no tension.

If at exploration the nerve appears to be normal, electrical studies should be obtained as a baseline anywhere from 4 to 6 weeks following the injury. If no contraction exists in the tibialis anterior at 3 months, electrophysiologic testing should be repeated and neurolysis or nerve reconstruction entertained. The chance for success falls off dramatically between 9 and 12 months following the original neurologic insult (30).

■ TREATMENT

Nonsurgical

Indications

Nonsurgical treatment of the dislocated knee is important historically as well as an important option today when circumstances dictate. Historically knee dislocations were reduced and treated in a cylinder cast. In the 1960s and 1970s there were studies supporting both nonoperative treatment as well as operative repair of the torn structures, but there was no clear consensus (2,43,46,47,58,69,70,73). More recently, with improved surgical techniques including arthroscopically assisted ligament reconstruction, and increased understanding of the ligamentous anatomy and biomechanics around the knee there has been evidence supporting surgical reconstruction (19,66). These studies demonstrate improved ligamentous stability of the knee as well as improved function postoperatively.

Multiligament knee injuries in specific circumstances warrant nonoperative treatment. Critically ill patients unable to tolerate a surgical procedure and patients with grossly contaminated wounds and/or significant soft tissue injuries around the prospective surgical site may be candidates for nonoperative management. Also in the elderly sedentary person it may be best to treat the knee dislocation nonoperatively (67).

Methods

The most basic method of nonoperative management is a long leg or cylinder cast. A long leg knee brace locked in extension may also be used. The brace may be especially helpful if there are significant wounds about the knee that a cast would conceal. The knee brace is often helpful in the setting of a critically ill patient. The brace allows easy access and evaluation of the injured extremity. If the cast or brace does not afford enough stability to maintain the knee in a reduced position, a knee spanning external fixator may be necessary **(Fig 37-1)**. The external fixator also provides better access to soft tissue injuries if it can be positioned away from contaminated wounds. Regardless of the type of nonsurgical management, frequent radiographs should be obtained to verify continued reduction of the knee.

Surgical Treatment

Knee dislocations were initially managed conservatively with a cylinder cast for several months (51,73). Early reports by Kennedy (42) and Meyers et al. (46) reported reasonable outcomes for nonoperatively treated knee dislocations; however, there was suggestion that the surgically stabilized

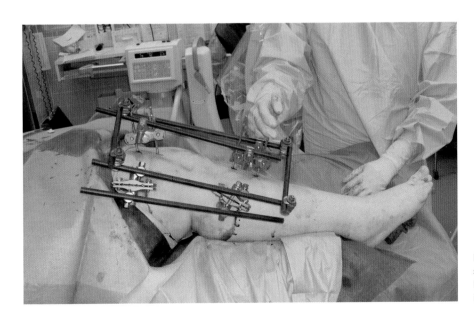

Fig 37-1. External fixation is used to stabilize the reduction in an ACL, PCL, lateral side injured knee dislocation that is grossly unstable.

dislocated knee would fare better in the long term. A recent report by Almekinders and Logan (2) compared surgically stabilized knees with conservative treatment and concluded that conservative treatment was comparable to surgical treatment. Despite similar outcomes, the conservatively treated knees were grossly unstable compared to surgically stabilized knees. Their study was retrospective from 1963 to 1988 and the typical surgical treatment during this period was in most cases open direct repair of the ligaments. Sisto and Warren (69) found similar results comparing four conservatively treated knees to 16 direct suture repair of torn ligaments. Frassica et al. (25) also evaluated early (within 5 days of injury) direct repair (with or without augmentation) of torn ligamentous structures in 13 of 17 patients. They concluded better results were obtained with early versus late direct repair of torn ligaments. This study supports surgical management of the dislocated knee and introduces the idea that long term benefits exist from a ligamentously stable knee.

Within the last decade, the technique of arthroscopic assisted ACL/PCL reconstruction has become popular. Several advancements have made these techniques possible: a) better procurement, sterilization, and storage of allograft tissue; b) improved arthroscopic surgical instrumentation; c) better graft fixation methods; d) improved surgical technique; and e) improved understanding of the ligamentous anatomy and biomechanics of the knee. Few reports of combined ACL/PCL reconstruction are available in the literature, but surgical reconstruction appears to afford at least the same results, if not better, than direct repair of the ligaments. Shapiro and Freedman (65) reconstructed seven ACL/PCL injuries with primarily allograft Achilles tendon or bone-patellar tendon-bone. They found that three patients had excellent results, three good results, and one had fair results. Furthermore, average KT-1000 was +3.3 mm side-to-side difference, with very little varus/valgus instability or significant posterior laxity. All seven of their patients were able to return to school or the workplace.

Fanelli et al. (19) reported on 20 ACL/PCL arthroscopic assisted ligament reconstructions. In their study group, there was one ACL/PCL tear, ten ACL/PCL/posterior lateral corner tears, seven ACL/PCL/MCL tears and two ACL/PCL/MCL/posterior lateral corner tears. Achilles tendon allografts and bone-patellar tendon-bone autografts were used in PCL reconstructions, auto and allograft bone-patellar tendon-bone was used in ACL reconstruction. An additional component, not previously mentioned with any consistency in the literature, was the addressing of the associated MCL or posterior lateral corner injury. It is imperative to address these injuries as well, or the results of ACL/PCL reconstruction alone will be less than optimal.

Postoperatively, significant improvement was found utilizing the Lysholm, Tegner, and Hospital for Special Surgery knee ligament rating scales, and the KT-1000 arthrometer. Overall postoperatively, 75% of patients had a normal Lachman test, 85% no longer displayed a pivot shift, 45% restored a normal posterior drawer test, and 55% displayed Grade I posterior laxity. All 20 knees were deemed functionally stable and all patients returned to desired levels of activity. These authors concluded that results of reconstruction are reproducible and that appropriate reconstruction will produce a stable knee.

Noyes and Barber-Westin (51) evaluated surgically reconstructed ACL/PCL tears (all had additional MCL or LCL/PCL reconstruction) at an average of 4.8 years. Seven of these knees were acute knee dislocations and four were chronically unstable knees secondary to knee dislocations. At follow-up, five of the seven acute knee injures had returned to pre-injury level of activity. Three of the four chronic knee injuries were asymptomatic with activities of daily living. Arthrometric measurements at 20 degrees showed less than 3 mm of side-to-side difference with anterior to posterior translation in 10 of the 11 knees; at 70 degrees, there were 9 knees that had less than 3 mm side-to-side difference in anterior-posterior translation. These authors concluded that simultaneous bicruciate ligament reconstruction is warranted to restore function to the knee.

Fanelli Sports Injury Clinic Experience

Our practice is at a tertiary care regional trauma center. There is a 38% incidence of PCL tears in acute knee injuries, with 45% of these PCL injured knees being combined ACL/PCL tears (17,24). Careful assessment, evaluation, and treatment of vascular injuries is essential in these acute multiple ligament injured knees. There is an 11% incidence of vascular injury associated with these acute multiple ligament injured knees at our center (23).

Our preferred approach to combined ACL/PCL injuries is an arthroscopic ACL/PCL reconstruction using the transtibial technique, with collateral/capsular ligament surgery as indicated. Not all cases are amenable to the arthroscopic approach and the operating surgeon must assess each case individually. Surgical timing is dependent upon vascular status, reduction stability, skin condition, systemic injuries, open versus closed knee injury, meniscus and articular surface injuries, other orthopaedic injuries, and the collateral/capsular ligaments involved.

Surgical Timing

Some ACL/PCL/MCL injuries can be treated with brace treatment of the medial collateral ligament followed by arthroscopic combined ACL/PCL reconstruction in 4 to 6 weeks after healing of the MCL. Other cases may require repair or reconstruction of the medial structures and must be assessed on an individual basis.

Combined ACL/PCL/posterolateral injuries should be surgically addressed as early as is safely possible. ACL/PCL/ posterolateral repair-reconstruction performed between 2 and 3 weeks post-injury allows healing of capsular tissues to permit an arthroscopic approach, and still permits primary repair of injured posterolateral structures.

Open multiple ligament knee injuries/dislocations may require staged procedures. The collateral/capsular structures are repaired after thorough irrigation and debridement, and the combined ACL/PCL reconstruction is performed at a later date after wound healing has occurred. Care must be taken in all cases of delayed reconstruction that the tibiofemoral joint reduction is maintained.

The surgical timing guidelines outlined above should be considered in the context of the individual patient. Many patients with multiple ligament injuries of the knee are severely-injured multiple trauma patients with multisystem injuries. Modifiers to the ideal timing protocols outlined above include the vascular status of the involved extremity, reduction stability, skin condition, open or closed injury, and other orthopaedic and systemic injuries. These additional considerations may cause the knee ligament surgery to be performed earlier or later than desired. We have previously reported excellent results with delayed reconstruction in the multiple ligament injured knee (19,20).

Graft Selection

The ideal graft material should be strong, provide secure fixation, easy to pass, readily available, and have low donor site morbidity. The available options in the United States are autograft and allograft sources. Our preferred graft for the posterior cruciate ligament is the Achilles tendon allograft because of its large cross sectional area and strength, absence of donor site morbidity, and easy passage with secure fixation. We prefer Achilles tendon allograft or other allograft for the ACL reconstruction. The preferred graft material for the posterolateral corner is a split biceps tendon transfer, or free autograft or allograft tissue when the biceps tendon is not available (18). Cases requiring medial collateral ligament and posteromedial corner surgery may have primary repair, reconstruction, or a combination of both. Our preferred method for MCL and posteromedial reconstructions is a posteromedial capsular advancement with autograft or allograft supplementation as needed.

Surgical Approach

Our preferred surgical approach is a single stage arthroscopic combined ACL/PCL reconstruction using the transtibial technique with collateral/capsular ligament surgery as indicated. The posterolateral corner is repaired, and then augmented with a split biceps tendon transfer, biceps tendon transfer, semitendinosus free graft, or allograft tissue. Acute medial injuries not amenable to brace treatment undergo primary repair, and posteromedial capsular shift, and/or allograft reconstruction as indicated. The operating surgeon must be prepared to convert to a dry arthroscopic procedure, or open procedure if fluid extravasation becomes a problem.

Surgical Technique

The principles of reconstruction in the multiple ligament injured knee are to identify and treat all pathology, accurate tunnel placement, anatomic graft insertion sites, utilize strong graft material, secure graft fixation, and a deliberate postoperative rehabilitation program. The patient is positioned supine on the operating room table. The surgical leg hangs over the side of the operating table, and the well leg is supported by the fully extended operating table. A lateral post is used for control of the surgical leg. We do not use a leg holder. The surgery is done under tourniquet control unless prior arterial or venous repair contraindicates the use of a tourniquet. Fluid inflow is by gravity. We do not use an athroscopic fluid pump.

Allograft tissue is prepared, and arthroscopic instruments are placed with the inflow in the superior lateral portal, arthroscope in the inferior lateral patellar portal, and instruments in the inferior medial patellar portal. An accessory extracapsular extra-articular posteromedial safety incision is used to protect the neurovascular structures and to confirm the accuracy of tibial tunnel placement **(Fig 37-2)**.

The notchplasty is performed first and consists of ACL and PCL stump debridement, bone removal, and contouring of the medial wall of the lateral femoral condyle and the intercondylar roof. This allows visualization of the over the top position and prevents ACL graft impingement throughout the full range of motion. Specially curved Arthrotek PCL instruments are used to elevate the capsule from the posterior aspect of the tibia **(Fig 37-3)**.

The PCL tibial and femoral tunnels are created with the help of the Arthrotek Fanelli PCL/ACL drill guide **(Fig 37-4)**. The transtibial PCL tunnel is positioned from the anteromedial aspect of the proximal tibial one cm below the tibial tubercle to exit in the inferior lateral aspect

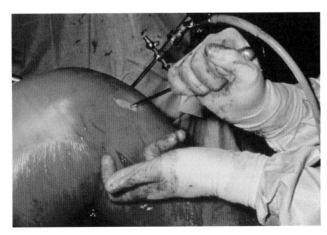

Fig 37-2. One to two centimeter extra capsular posterior medial safety incision allows the surgeon's finger to protect the neurovascular structures and confirm the position of instruments on the posterior aspect of the proximal tibia. (From Fanelli GC, Giannotti BF, Edson CJ. Current concepts review. The posterior cruciate ligament arthroscopic evaluation and treatment. *Arthroscopy.* 1994;10(6):673–688; with permission.)

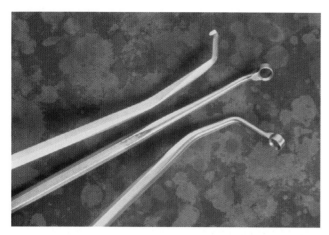

Fig 37-3. Specially curved PCL reconstruction instruments used to elevate the capsule from the posterior aspect of the tibial ridge during PCL reconstruction. Posterior capsular elevation is critical in transtibial PCL reconstruction because it facilitates accurate PCL tibial tunnel placement and subsequent graft passage. (Photograph courtesy of Arthrotek, Inc., Warsaw, Indiana. Used with permission.)

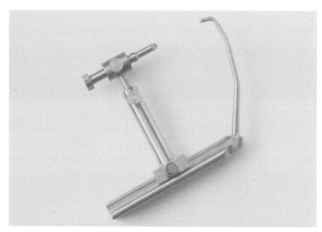

Fig 37-4. The Arthrotek Fanelli PCL/ACL drill guide system is used to precisely create both the PCL femoral and tibial tunnels and the ACL single incision technique and double incision technique tunnels. The drill guide is positioned for the PCL tibial tunnel so that a guide wire enters the anteromedial aspect of the proximal tibia approximately 1 cm below the tibial tubercle at a point midway between the posteromedial border of the tibia and the tibial crest anteriorly. The guide wire exits in the inferior lateral aspect of the PCL tibial anatomic insertion site. The guide is positioned for the PCL femoral tunnel so the guide wire enters the medial aspect of the medial femoral condyle midway between the medial femoral condyle articular margin and the medial epicondyle, 2 cm proximal to the medial femoral condyle distal articular surface (*joint line*). The guide wire exits through the center of the stump of the anterolateral bundle of the posterior cruciate ligament. The drill guide is positioned for the single incision endoscopic ACL technique so that the guide wire enters the anteromedial surface of the proximal tibia approximately 1 cm proximal to the tibial tubercle at a point midway between the posteromedial border of the tibia and the tibial crest anteriorly. The guide wire exits through the center of the stump of the tibial ACL insertion. (Photograph courtesy of Arthrotek, Inc., Warsaw, Indiana. Used with permission.)

of the PCL anatomic insertion site. The PCL femoral tunnel originates externally between the medial femoral epicondyle and the medial femoral condylar articular surface to emerge through the center of the stump of the anterolateral bundle of the posterior cruciate ligament. The PCL graft is positioned and anchored on the femoral side followed by PCL graft tensioning and tibial fixation.

The ACL tunnels are created using the single incision technique. The tibial tunnel begins externally at a point 1 cm proximal to the tibial tubercle on the anteromedial surface of the proximal tibia to emerge through the center of the stump if the ACL tibial footprint. The femoral tunnel is positioned next to the over the top position on the medial wall of the lateral femoral condyle near the ACL anatomic insertion site. The tunnel is created to leave a 1 to 2 mm posterior cortical wall so interference fixation can be used. The ACL graft is positioned and anchored on the femoral side followed by ACL graft tensioning and tibial fixation (**Fig 37-5**).

A technique for posterolateral reconstruction is the split biceps tendon transfer to the lateral femoral epicondyle (**Fig 37-6A**). The requirements for this procedure include an intact proximal tibiofibular joint, the posterolateral capsular attachments to the common biceps tendon should be intact, and the biceps femoris tendon insertion into the fibular head must be intact. This technique recreates the function of the popliteofibular ligament and lateral collateral ligament, tightens the posterolateral capsule, and provides a post of strong autogenous tissue to reinforce the posterolateral corner.

A lateral hockey stick incision is made. The peroneal nerve is dissected free and protected throughout the procedure.

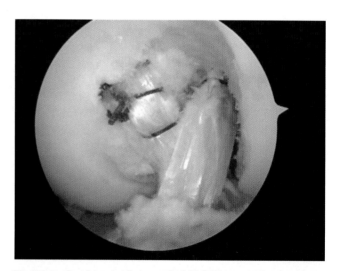

Fig 37-5. Combined arthroscopic ACL/PCL reconstruction using Achilles tendon allograft. The tunnels are precisely created to reproduce the anatomic insertion sites of the anterolateral bundle of the posterior cruciate ligament and the anatomic insertion sites of the anterior cruciate ligament. Correct and accurate tunnel placement is essential for successful combined ACL/PCL reconstructions. The Achilles tendon allograft is preferred because of its large cross sectional area, strength, and absence of donor site morbidity.

The long head and common biceps femoris tendon is isolated, and the anterior two-thirds is separated from the short head muscle. The tendon is detached proximal and left attached distally to its anatomic insertion site on the fibular head. The strip of biceps tendon should be 12 to 14 cm long. The iliotibial band is incised in line with its fibers, and the fibular collateral ligament and popliteus tendons are exposed. A drill hole is made 1 cm anterior to the fibular collateral ligament femoral insertion. A longitudinal incision is made in the lateral capsule just posterior to the fibular collateral ligament. The split biceps tendon is passed medial to the iliotibial band and secured to the lateral femoral epicondylar region with a screw and spiked ligament washer at the above mentioned point. The residual tail of the transferred split biceps tendon is passed medial to the iliotibial band and secured to the fibular head. The posterolateral capsule that had been previously incised is then shifted and sewn into the strut of transferred biceps tendon to eliminate posterolateral capsular redundancy.

Posterolateral reconstruction with the free graft figure of eight technique utilizes semitendinosus autograft or allograft, Achilles tendon allograft, or other soft tissue allograft material. A curvilinear incision is made in the lateral aspect of the knee extending from the lateral femoral epicondyle to the interval between Gerdy's tubercle and the fibular head. The fibular head is exposed and a tunnel is created in an anterior to posterior direction at the area of maximal fibular diameter. The tunnel is created by passing a guide pin followed by a cannulated drill usually 7 mm in diameter. The peroneal nerve is protected during tunnel creation and throughout the procedure. The free tendon graft is then passed through the fibular head drill hole. An incision is then made in the iliotibial band in line with the fibers directly overlying the lateral femoral epicondyle. The graft material is passed medial to the iliotibial band, and the limbs of the graft are crossed to form a figure of eight. A drill hole is made 1 cm anterior to the fibular collateral ligament femoral insertion. A longitudinal incision is made in the lateral capsule just posterior to the fibular collateral ligament. The graft material is passed medial to the iliotibial band and secured to the lateral femoral epicondylar region with a screw and spiked ligament washer at the above mentioned point. The posterolateral capsule that had been previously incised is then shifted and sewn into the strut of figure of eight graft tissue material to eliminate posterolateral capsular redundancy. The anterior and posterior limbs of the figure of eight graft material are sewn to each other to reinforce and tighten the construct **(Fig 37-6B)**. The iliotibial band incision is closed. The procedures described are intended to eliminate posterolateral and varus rotational instability.

Posteromedial and medial reconstructions are performed through a medial hockey stick incision **(Fig 37-7)**. Care is taken to maintain adequate skin bridges between incisions. The superficial medial collateral ligament is exposed, and a longitudinal incision is made just posterior to the posterior border of the MCL. Care is taken not to damage the medial meniscus during the capsular incision. The interval between the posteromedial capsule and medial meniscus is developed. The posteromedial capsule is shifted anterosuperiorly. The medial meniscus is repaired to the new capsular position, and the shifted capsule is sewn into the medial collateral ligament. When superficial MCL reconstruction is indicated,

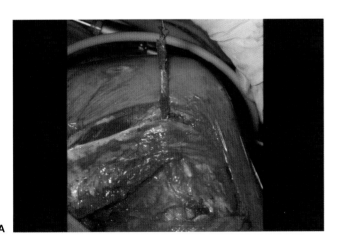
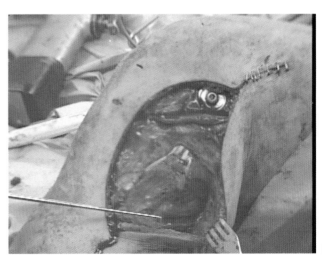

A   B

Fig 37-6. Surgical technique for posterolateral and lateral reconstruction are the split biceps tendon transfer **(A)** or the allograft or autograft figure of eight reconstruction **(B)** combined with posterolateral capsular shift and primary repair of injured structures as indicated. These complex surgical procedures reproduce the function of the popliteofibular ligament and the lateral collateral ligament and eliminate posterolateral capsular redundancy. The split biceps tendon transfer utilizes anatomic insertion sites and preserves the dynamic function of the long head and common biceps femoris tendon. (From Fanelli GC, Orcutt DR, Edson CJ. Current concepts. The multiple ligament injured knee: evaluation, treatment, and results. *Arthroscopy.* 2005;21(4):471–486; with permission.)

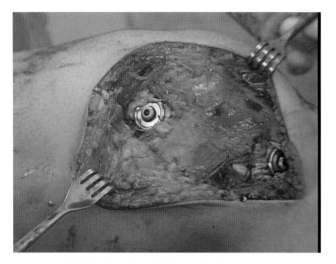

Fig 37-7. Severe medial side injuries are successfully treated with primary repair using suture anchor technique, combined with MCL reconstruction using allograft tissue combined with postero-medial capsular shift procedure. The Achilles tendon allograft's broad anatomy can anatomically reconstruct the superficial medial collateral ligament. The Achilles tendon allograft is secured to the anatomic insertion sites of the superficial MCL using screws and spiked ligament washers. The posteromedial capsule can then be secured to the allograft tissue to eliminate posteromedial capsular laxity. This technique will address all components of the medial side instability. (From Fanelli GC, Orcutt DR, Edson CJ. Current concepts. The multiple ligament injured knee: evaluation, treatment, and results. *Arthroscopy.* 2005;21(4):471–486; with permission.)

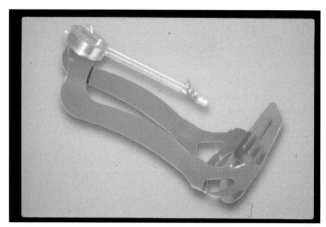

Fig 37-8. The Arthrotek knee ligament-tensioning boot is used to precisely tension PCL and ACL grafts. During PCL reconstruction, the tensioning device is attached to the tibial end of the graft and the torque wrench ratchet set to 20 pounds. This restores the anatomic tibial step off. The knee is cycled through full flexion-extension cycles, and with the knee at approximately 70 degrees of flexion, final PCL tibial fixation is achieved with an Arthrotek Gentle Thread bioabsorbable interference screw, and screw and spiked ligament washer for back up fixation. The tensioning device is applied to the ACL graft, set to 20 pounds, and the graft is tensioned with the knee in 70 degrees of flexion. Final ACL fixation is achieved with Arthrotek Gentle Thread bioabsorbable interference screws, and spiked ligament washer or ligament fixation button back up fixation. The mechanical tensioning boot assures consistent graft tensioning and eliminates graft advancement during interference screw insertion. It also restores the anatomic tibial step off during PCL graft tensioning, and applies a posterior drawer force during ACL graft tensioning. (Photograph courtesy of Arthrotek, Inc., Warsaw, Indiana. Used with permission.)

this is performed allograft tissue or semitendinosus autograft. This graft material is attached at the anatomic insertion sites of the superficial medial collateral ligament on the femur and tibia. The posteromedial capsular advancement is performed and sewn into the newly reconstructed MCL.

Graft Tensioning and Fixation

The posterior cruciate ligament is reconstructed first followed by the anterior cruciate followed by the posterolateral complex and/or medial side. The Arthrotek tensioning boot is used for tensioning the anterior and posterior cruciate ligament reconstructions **(Fig 37-8)**. Tension is placed on the PCL graft distally, and the knee is cycled through a full range of motion cycles to allow pretensioning and settling of the graft. The knee is placed in 70 degrees to 90 degrees of flexion, the Arthrotek tensioning boot is tensioned to 20 pounds to restore the normal tibial step-off, and fixation is achieved on the tibial side of the PCL graft with a screw and spiked ligament washer and Arthrotek Gentle Thread bioabsorable interference screw (Arthrotek Inc., Warsaw, Indiana). The knee is maintained at 70 degrees to 90 degrees of flexion, the Arthrotek tensioning boot is tensioned to 20 pounds with tension on the ACL graft, and final fixation is achieved of the ACL graft with an Arthrotek Gentle Thread bioabsorable interference screw and Arthrotek ligament fixation button or spiked ligament washer back-up fixation. The knee

is then placed in 30 degrees of flexion, the tibia internally rotated, slight valgus force applied to the knee, and final tensioning and fixation of the posterolateral corner is achieved. Reconstruction and tensioning of the MCL and posteromedial corner are performed after the ACP, PCL, and PLC reconstructions and are done in 30 degrees of knee flexion **(Fig 37-9)**.

Technical Hints

The posteromedial safety incision protects the neurovascular structures, confirms accurate tibial tunnel placement, and allows the surgical procedure to be done at an accelerated pace. The single incision ACL reconstruction technique prevents lateral cortex crowding and eliminates multiple through and through drill holes in the distal femur reducing stress riser effect. It is important to be aware of the two tibial tunnel directions, and to have a 1 cm bone bridge between the PCL and ACL tibial tunnels **(Fig 37-10)**. This will reduce the possibility of fracture. We have found it useful to use primary and back-up fixation. Primary fixation is with resorbable interference screws, and back-up fixation is performed with a screw and spiked ligament washer or Arthrotek ligament fixation button. Secure fixation is critical to the success of this surgical procedure.

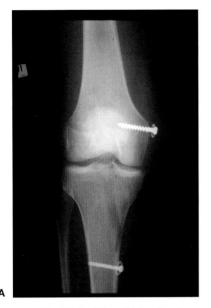
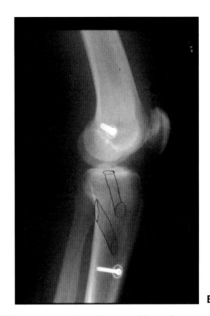

A   B

Fig 37-9. AP and lateral radiographs after combined ACL/PCL reconstruction. Note position of tibial tunnel on lateral x-ray placing the PCL graft at the anatomic PCL insertion site.

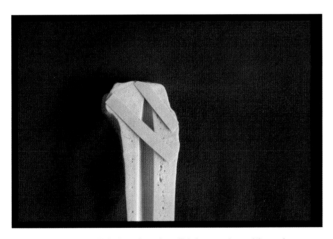

Fig 37-10. A model showing the tibial tunnel positions for combined ACL/PCL reconstructions. It is essential to have an adequate bone bridge between the two tunnels. (From Fanelli GC, Giannotti BF, Edson CJ. Current concepts review. The posterior cruciate ligament arthroscopic evaluation and treatment. *Arthroscopy*. 1994; 10(6):673–688; with permission.)

Post Operative Rehabilitation

The knee remains in full extension and a nonweight bearing status is maintained for 6 weeks. Progressive range of motion occurs after post-op week 3. The brace is unlocked at the end of 3 weeks and the crutches are discontinued after progression to full weight bearing has been achieved. Progressive closed kinetic chain strength training, and continued motion exercises are performed. The brace is discontinued after the tenth week. Return to sports and heavy labor occurs after the ninth post-operative month when sufficient strength, proprioceptive skills, and range of motion has returned. It should be noted that a loss of 10 degree to 15 degree of terminal flexion might be expected in these complex knee ligament

reconstructions. This does not cause a functional problem for these patients and is not a cause for alarm.

Complications

Potential complications in treatment of the multiple ligament injured knee include failure to recognize and treat vascular injuries (both arterial and venous), iatrogenic neurovascular injury at the time of reconstruction, iatrogenic tibial plateau fractures at the time of reconstruction, failure to recognize and treat all components of the instability, postoperative medial femoral condyle osteonecrosis, knee motion loss, and post-operative anterior knee pain.

Results

We have previously published the results of our arthroscopically assisted combined ACL/PCL and PCL/posterolateral complex reconstructions using the reconstructive technique described in this chapter (19,20,21). Our most recently published 2 to 10 year results of combined ACL-PCL reconstructions are presented here (15).

This study presented the 2 to 10 year (24 to 120 month) results of 35 arthroscopically assisted combined ACL/PCL reconstructions evaluated pre- and postoperatively using Lysholm, Tegner, and Hospital for Special Surgery knee ligament rating scales, KT 1000 arthrometer testing, stress radiography, and physical examination.

This study population included 26 males, 9 females, 19 acute, and 16 chronic knee injuries. Ligament injuries included 19 ACL/PCL/posterolateral instabilities, 9 ACL/PCL/MCL instabilities, 6 ACL/PCL/posterolateral/MCL instabilities, and 1 ACL/PCL instability. All knees had Grade III preoperative ACL/PCL laxity, and were assessed pre- and postoperatively with arthrometer testing, three different knee ligament rating scales, stress radiography, and physical examination. Arthroscopically assisted combined ACL/PCL reconstructions were performed using the single incision endoscopic ACL technique and the single femoral tunnel-single bundle transtibial tunnel PCL technique. PCLs were reconstructed with allograft Achilles tendon (26), autograft BTB (7), and autograft semitendinosus/gracilis (2). ACLs were reconstructed with autograft BTB (16), allograft BTB (12), Achilles tendon allograft (6), and autograft semitendinosus/gracilis (1). MCL injuries were treated with bracing or open reconstruction. Posterolateral instability was treated with biceps femoris tendon transfer, with or without primary repair, and posterolateral capsular shift procedures as indicated. No Arthrotek graft tensioning boot was used in this series of patients.

Postoperative physical examination results revealed normal posterior drawer/tibial step off in 16 of 35 (46%) of knees. Normal Lackman and pivot shift tests in 33/35 (94%) of knees. Posterolateral stability was restored to normal in 6 of 25 (24%) of knees, and tighter than the normal knee in 19 of 25 (76%) of knees evaluated with the external rotation thigh foot angle test. Thirty degree varus stress testing was normal in 22 of 25 (88%) of knees, and Grade 1 laxity in 3 of 25 (12%) of knees. Thirty degree valgus stress testing was normal in 7 of 7 (100%) of surgically treated MCL tears, and normal in 7 of 8 (87.5%) of brace treated knees. Postoperative KT 1000 arthrometer testing mean side-to-side difference measurements were 2.7 mm (PCL screen), 2.6 mm (corrected posterior), and 1.0 mm (corrected anterior) measurements, a statistically significant improvement from preoperative status ($p = 0.001$). Postoperative stress radiographic side-to-side difference measurements measured at 90 degree of knee flexion and 32 pounds of posteriorly-directed proximal force were 0 to 3 mm in 11 of 21 (52.3%), 4 to 5 mm in 5 of 21 (23.8%), and 6 to 10 mm in 4 of 21 (19%) of knees. Postoperative Lysholm, Tegner, and HSS knee ligament rating scale mean values were 91.2, 5.3, and 86.8 respectively demonstrating a statistically significant improvement from preoperative status ($p = 0.001$). No Arthrotek graft tensioning boot was used in this series of patients.

The conclusions drawn from the study were that combined ACL/PCL instabilities could be successfully treated with arthroscopic reconstruction and the appropriate collateral ligament surgery. Statistically significant improvement was noted from the preoperative condition at 2 to 10 year follow-up using objective parameters of knee ligament rating scales, arthrometer testing, stress radiography, and physical examination. Postoperatively, these knees are not normal, but they are functionally stable. Continuing technical improvements will most likely improve future results.

Results with the Arthrotek Graft Tensioning Boot

New data as of this writing presents the 2 year follow up results of 15 arthroscopic assisted ACL PCL reconstructions using the Arthrotek graft tensioning boot. This study group consists of 11 chronic and 4 acute injuries. These injury patterns included six ACL PCL PLC injuries, four ACL PCL MCL injuries, and five ACL PCL PLC MCL injuries. The Arthrotek tensioning boot was used during the procedures as in the surgical technique previously described. The PCL results for this study group demonstrated a normal posterior drawer and tibial step off in 13 of 15 knees (86.6%). The study group demonstrates the efficacy of using a mechanical graft-tensioning device (Arthrotek graft tensioning boot) in PCL reconstruction.

■ CONCLUSIONS/SUMMARY

Multiple ligament injuries of the knee are complex injuries requiring a systematic approach to evaluation and treatment. Gentle reduction and documentation and treatment of vascular injuries are primary concerns in the acute dislocated/multiple ligament injured knee. Arthroscopically assisted combined ACL/PCL reconstruction with appropriate collateral ligament surgery is a reproducible procedure. Knee stability is improved postoperatively when evaluated with knee ligament rating scales, arthrometer testing, and stress radiographic analysis. Acute MCL tears when combined with ACL/PCL tears may in certain cases be treated with bracing. Posterolateral corner injuries combined with ACL/PCL tears are best treated with primary repair as indicated combined with reconstruction using a post of strong autograft (split biceps tendon, biceps tendon, semitendinosis), or allograft tissue. Surgical timing depends upon the ligaments injured, the vascular status of the extremity, reduction stability, and the overall health of the patient. We prefer the use of allograft tissue for reconstruction in these cases because of the strength of these large grafts, and the absence of donor site morbidity.

■ FUTURE DIRECTIONS

We have now converted to performing the double bundle double femoral tunnel posterior cruciate ligament reconstruction surgical technique since there is convincing basic science data supporting the efficacy of this procedure. This double bundle double femoral tunnel technique more closely approximates the anatomic insertion site of the native PCL and should theoretically provide improved results. Our early clinical results are encouraging; however, there are no long-term clinical results available as of this writing.

Another area of interest is the incorporation of autologous platlette rich fibrin matrix into the grafts used in the cruciate and collateral ligament reconstructive procedures. There are several studies indicating favorable effects on the ligament graft tissue and the clinical results. We have demonstrated favorable initial clinical results with respect to graft incorporation, wound healing, and early stability, however, there is no long-term follow-up as of this writing

■ REFERENCES

1. Alberty RE, Goodfried G, Boyden AM. Popliteal artery injury with fractural dislocation of the knee. *Am J Surg*. 1981;142:36.

2. Almekinders LC, Logan TC. Results following treatment of traumatic dislocation of the knee. *Clin Orthop Rel Res*. 1991;284:203-207.

3. Applebaum R, Yellin AE, Weaver FA, et al. Role of routine arteriography in blunt lower-extremity trauma. *Am J Surg*. 1990;160:221–225.

4. Ashworth EM, Dalsing MC, Glover JL, et al. Lower extremity vascular trauma: a comprehensive, aggressive approach. *J Trauma*. 1988;28:329.

5. Athanasian EA, Wickiewicz TL, Warren RF. Osteonecrosis of the femoral condyle after arthroscopic reconstruction of a cruciate ligament. *J Bone Joint Surg*. 1995;77(9):1418–1422.

6. Barnes CJ, Pietrobon R, Higgins LD. Does the pulse examination in patients with traumatic knee dislocation predict a surgical arterial injury? A meta-analysis. *J Trauma*. 2002;53:1109–1114.

7. Berry H, Richardson PM. Common peroneal nerve palsy: a clinical electrophysiological review. *J Neurol Neurosurg Psychiatry*. 1976;39:1162–1171.

8. Bok APL, Peter JC. Carotid and vertebral artery occlusion after blunt cervical injury: the role of MR angiography in early diagnosis. *J Trauma*. 1996;40:968–972.

9. Bratt HD, Newman AP. Complete dislocation of the knee without disruption of both cruciate ligaments. *J Trauma*. 1993;34(3):383–389.

10. Butler DL, Noyes FR, Good ES. Ligamentous restraints to anterior-posterior drawer in the human knee. A biomechanical study. *J Bone Joint Surg*. 1980;62A:259–270.

11. Bynoe RP, Miles WS, Bell RM, et al. Noninvasive diagnosis of vascular trauma by duplex ultrasonography. *J Vasc Surg*. 1991;14:346–352.

12. Cone JC. Vascular injury associated with fracture-dislocations of the lower extremity. *Clin Orthop*. 1989;243:30–35.

13. Cooper DE, Speer KP, Wickiewicz TL, et al. Complete knee dislocation without posterior cruciate ligament disruption. *Clin Orthop*. 1992;284:228–233.

14. Dennis JW, Jaggar C, Butcher L, et al. Reassessing the role of arteriograms in the management of posterior knee dislocations. *J Trauma*. 1993;35:692–697.

15. Fanelli GC, Edson CJ. Arthroscopically assisted combined ACL/PCL reconstruction. Two to ten year follow-up. *Arthroscopy*. 2002;18(7):703–714.

16. Fanelli GC, Edson CJ. Arthroscopically assisted combined PCL-posterolateral reconstruction. Two to ten year follow-up. *Arthroscopy*. 2004.

17. Fanelli GC, Edson CJ. PCL injuries in trauma patients, part II. *Arthroscopy*. 1995;11:526–529.

18. Fanelli GC, Feldmann DD. The use of allograft tissue in knee ligament reconstruction. In: Parisien JS, ed. *Current techniques in arthroscopy*. 3rd ed. New York: Thieme; 1998.

19. Fanelli GC, Gianotti BF, Edson CJ. Arthroscopically assisted combined anterior and posterior cruciate ligament reconstruction. *Arthroscopy*. 1996;12(1):5–14.

20. Fanelli GC, Gianotti BF, Edson CJ. Arthroscopically assisted combined posterior cruciate ligament/posterior lateral complex reconstruction. *Arthroscopy*. 1996;12(5):521–530.

21. Fanelli GC, Gianotti BF, Edson CJ. The posterior cruciate ligament arthroscopic evaluation and treatment. *Arthroscopy*. 1994;10(6):673–688.

22. Fanelli, GC. Combined ACL/PCL/medial/lateral side injuries of the knee. In: Fanelli GC, ed. *The multiple ligament injured knee. A practical guide to management*. New York: Springer-Verlag; 2004.

23. Fanelli, GC. Arthroscopic combined ACL/PCL reconstruction. In: Fanelli GC, ed. *Posterior cruciate ligament injuries. A guide to practical management*. New York: Springer-Verlag; 2001.

24. Fanelli GC. PCL injuries in trauma patients. *Arthroscopy*. 1993;9:291–294.

25. Frassica FJ, Sim FH, Staheli JW, et al. Dislocation of the knee. *Clin Orthop*. 1991;263:200–205.

26. Friedman D, Flanders A, Thomas C, et al. Vertebral artery injury after acute cervical spine trauma: rate of occurrence as detected by MR angiography and assessment of clinical consequences. *AJR Am J Roentgenol*. 1995;164:443–447.

27. Gable DR, Allen JW, Richardson JD. Blunt popliteal artery injury: is physical examination alone enough for evaluation. *J Trauma*. 1997;43:541–544.

28. Ghalambor N, Vangsness CT. Traumatic dislocation of the knee: a review of the literature. *Bull Hosp Jt Dis*. 1995;54(1):19–24.

29. Girgis FG, Marshall JL, Monajem A. The cruciate ligaments of the knee joint. *Clin Orthop*. 1975;106:216–231.

30. Goitz RJ, Tomaino MM. Management of peroneal nerve injuries associated with knee dislocations. *Am J Orthop*. 2003;32:14–16.

31. Gollehon DL, Torzilli PA, Warren RF. The role of the posterior lateral corner and cruciate ligaments in the stability of the human knee. A biomechanical study. *J Bone Joint Surg*. 1987;69A:233–242. 1987.

32. Green A, Allen BL. Vascular injuries associated with dislocation of the knee. *J Bone Joint Surg*. 1977;59A:236–239.

33. Grimley RP, Ashton F, Slaney G, et al. Popliteal aterial injuries associated with civil knee trauma. *Injury*. 1981;13:1–6.

34. Haftek J. Stretch injury of peripheral nerve. *J Bone Joint Surg Br*. 1970;52:354–365.

35. Hill JA, Rana NA. Complications of posterolateral dislocation of the knee: case report and literature review. *Clin Orthop*. 1981;154:212–215.

36. Hoover NW. Injuries of the popliteal artery associated with fractures and dislocations. *Surg Clin North Am*. 1961;41:1099–1112.

37. Irgang JJ, Harner CD. Loss of motion following knee ligament reconstruction. *Sports Med*. 1995;19(2):150–159.

38. Jones RE, Smith EC, Bone GE. Vascular and orthopedic complications of knee dislocation. *Surg Gynecol Obstet*. 1979;149:554–558.

39. Kaplan EB. The Iliotibial tract. clinical and morphological significance. *J Bone Joint Surg*. 1958;40A:817–832.

40. Kaufman SL, Martin LG. Arterial injuries associated with complete dislocation of the knee. *Radiology*. 1992;184:153–155.

41. Kendall RW, Taylor DC, Salvian AJ, et al. The role of arteriography in assessing vascular injuries associated with dislocations of the knee. *J Trauma*. 1993;35:875–878.

42. Kennedy JC. Complete dislocation of the knee joint. *J Bone Joint Surg*. 1963;45A:889–904.

43. Malizos KN, Xenakis T, Mavrodontidis AN, et al. Knee dislocations and their management. *Acta Orthop Scand*. 1997:68(suppl 275):80–83.

44. McCoy GF, Hannon DG, Barr RJ, et al. Vascular injury associated with low-velocity dislocations of the knee. *J Bone Joint Surg*. 1987;69B:285–287.

45. Meyers MH, Harvey JP Jr. Traumatic dislocation of the knee joint: a study of eighteen cases. *J Bone Joint Surg*. 1971;53A:16–29.

46. Meyers MH, Moore TM, Harvey JP Jr. Traumatic dislocations of the knee joint. *J Bone Joint Surg*. 1975;57A:430–433.

47. Mink JH, Levy T, Crues JV. Tears of the anterior cruciate ligament and menisci of the knee: MR imaging evaluation. *Radiology*. 1988;167:769–774.

48. Miranda, FE, Dennis JW, Veldenz HC, et al. Confirmation of the safety and accuracy of physical examination in the evaluation

of knee dislocation for injury of the popliteal artery: a prospective study. *J Trauma*. 2002;52:247–252.

49. Moore TM. Fracture-dislocation of the knee. *Clin Orthop*. 1981;156:450–453.

50. Myles JW. Seven cases of traumatic dislocation of the knee. *Proc R Soc Med*. 1967;60:279.

51. Noyes FR, Barber-Westin SD. Reconstruction of the anterior and posterior cruciate ligaments after knee dislocation. *Am J Sports Med*. 1997;25(6):769.

52. O'Donnell TF Jr, Brewster DC, Darling RC, et al. Arterial injuries associated with fractures and/or dislocations of the knee. *J Trauma*. 1977;17:775–784.

53. Ottolenghi CE. Vascular complications in injuries about the knee joint. *Clin Orthop*. 1982;165:148–156.

54. Paulos LE, Winorowski DC, Beck CL. Rehabilitation following knee surgery Recommendations. *Sports Med*. 1991;111(4): 257–275.

55. Potter HG, Weinstein M, Allen AA. Magnetic resonance imaging of the multiple-ligament injured knee. *J Orthop Trauma*. 2002;16:330–339.

56. Quinlan AG, Sharrard WJW. Postero-lateral dislocation of the knee with capsular interposition. *J Bone Joint Surg*. 1958;40B:660–663.

57. Reckling FW, Peltier LF. Acute knee dislocations and their complications. *J Trauma*. 1969;9:181–191.

58. Rich NM, Hobson RW, Collins GJ, et al. The effect of acute popliteal venous interruption. *Ann Surg*. 1976;183:365–368.

59. Rich NM, Hobson RW, Wright CB. Repair of lower extremity venous trauma: a more aggressive approach required. *J Trauma*., 1974;14:639.

60. Roman PD, Hopson CN, Zenni EJ Jr. Traumatic dislocation of the knee: a report of 30 cases and literature review. *Orthop Rev*. 1987;16:917–924.

61. Savage R. Popliteal artery injury associated with knee dislocation: improved outlook? *Am Surg*. 1980;46:627–632.

62. Schenck RC Jr. The dislocated knee. American Academy of Orthopaedic Surgeons *Instr Course Lect*. 1994;43:127–136.

63. Seddon H. *Surgical Disorders of the Peripheral Nerves*. Edinburgh, Scotland: Churchill Livingstone; 1972.

64. Seebacher JR, Inglis AE, Marshall DV, et al. The structure of the posterolateral aspect of the knee. *J Bone Joint Surg*. 1982;64A(4): 536–541.

65. Shapiro MS, Freedman EL. Allograft reconstruction of the anterior and posterior cruciate ligaments after traumatic knee dislocation. *Am J Sports Med*. 1995;23(5):580–587.

66. Shelbourne KD, Porter DA, Clingman JA, et al. Low-velocity knee dislocation. *Orthop Rev*. 1991;20:995–1004.

67. Shelbourne KD, Pritchard J, Rettig AC, et al. Knee dislocations with intact PCL. *Orthop Rev*. 1992;21(5):607–608, 610–611.

68. Shields L, Mital M, Cave EF. Complete dislocation of the knee: experience at the Massachusetts General Hospital. *J Trauma*. 1969;9:192–215.

69. Sisto DJ, Warren RF. Complete knee dislocation: a follow-up study of operative treatment. *Clin Orthop*. 1985;198:94–101.

70. Sterling JC, Meyers MC, Calvo RD. Allograft failure in cruciate ligament reconstruction. *Am J Sports Med*. 1995;23(2):173–178.

71. Taft T, Almekinders L. The dislocated knee. In: Fu F, Harner C, Vince K, eds. *Knee surgery*. Baltimore: Williams & Wilkins; 1994:837–858.

72. Taylor AR, Arden GP, Rainey HA. Traumatic dislocation of the knee: a report of forty-three cases with special reference to conservative treatment. *J Bone Joint Surg*. 1972;54B:96–102.

73. Thomsen PB, Rud B, Jensen UH. Stability and motion after traumatic dislocation of the knee. *Acta Orthop Scand*. 1984;55: 278–283.

74. Trieman GS, Yellin AE, Weaver FA, et al. Evaluation of the patient with a knee dislocation: the case for selective arteriography. *Arch Surg*. 1992;127(9):1056–1063.

75. VanDommelen BA, Fowler PJ. Anatomy of the posterior cruciate ligament. A review. *Am J Sports Med*. 1989;17:24–29.

76. Voshell AF. Anatomy of the knee joint. Instructional Course Lectures. The American Academy of Orthopaedic Surgeons Ann Arbor, J.W. Edwards. 1956;Vol 13:247–264.

77. Wand JS. A physical sign denoting irreducibility of a dislocated knee. *J Bone Joint Surg*. 1989;71B:862.

78. Warren LF, Marshall DVM. The supporting structures and layers on the medial side of the knee. *J Bone Joint Surg*. 1979;61A(1): 56–62.

79. Wascher DC, Dvirnak PC, Decoster TA. Knee dislocation. Initial assessment and implications for treatment. *J Orthop Trauma*. 1997;11:525–529.

80. Welling RE, Kakkasseril J, Cranley JJ. Complete dislocations of the knee with popliteal vascular injury. *J Trauma*. 1981;21: 450–453.

81. White J. The results of traction injuries to the common peroneal nerve. *J Bone Joint Surg*. 1968;50B:346–350.

82. Wilson SA, Vigorita VJ, Scott WN. Anatomy. In: Scott WN, ed. *The knee*. St. Louis, Missouri: Mosby Books; 1994.

83. Wright DG, Covey DC, Born CT, et al. Open dislocation of the knee. *J Orthop Trauma*. 1995;9(2):135–140.

38

THE MENISCUS

MONIKA VOLESKY, MD, DONALD H. JOHNSON, MD, FRCS

■ KEY POINTS

- The importance of preserving the meniscus to protect the articular cartilage has been recognized over the past 2 decades. The original concept of the meniscus as a vestigial functionless structure has evolved to one of weight bearing, lubrication, stability, and nutrition of the articular surface.

- The clinical presentation of a meniscal tear is pain and swelling following a twisting injury. The signs are joint-line tenderness, an effusion, and limited motion.

- In the chronic situation, a McMurray test may be elicited to reproduce the loose meniscal fragment being trapped between the condyles. Imaging with plain x-rays is done to rule out fractures, loose bodies, or osteoarthritis. The magnetic resonance imaging (MRI) plays a valuable role in demonstrating a meniscal tear.

- The indications for meniscal repair depend upon the chronicity of the tear, the size and appearance of the tear, location or zone of the tear, medial or lateral tears, and whether or not an anterior cruciate ligament reconstruction will be done at the same time.

- The acute treatment of meniscal tears is conservative with protected weight bearing, modified activity, ice application, and anti-inflammatory medication. Treatment is aimed at reducing the effusion and increasing the range of motion.

- Operative treatment is indicated when a meniscal tear has been diagnosed and there is no improvement in the patient's symptoms. Some stable tears may be treated with abrasion and trephination alone. Degenerative tears are usually treated by excision of the unstable fragments of the meniscus.

- There are numerous methods for meniscal repair, inside-out sutures, outside-in sutures, rigid meniscal fixators, and fixators that are embedded leaving only a suture on the surface of the meniscus. Most authors consider meniscal suture to be the standard for repair. Inside-out suture repair should be done with a separate outside incision to retrieve the suture needles and avoid neurovascular complication.

- The use of rigid meniscal fixators for an all-inside technique has become popular due to ease of use and reduced operative time; however, there are more potential complications, including injury to the articular surface, neurovascular injury, migration of the devices, inflammatory reaction to the implant, and failure of the repair.

- The rehabilitation of the repair has been controversial in the past. Most authors restrict weight bearing flexion exercise for 6 weeks after a meniscal repair.

- Outcome of meniscal repair in the short term has been reported to be satisfactory with 80% to 90% success. The results of both fixators and sutures seem to deteriorate over time. This may be due to the incomplete healing of the tears that are reported as successes in the short-term, but will fail in the long-term in this active athletic group.

- The future holds improvement in the healing of the tears by augmenting the repair with growth factors. Meniscal transplantation with either collagen scaffolds or allograft tissue may also prove to be chondroprotective in the long-term.

The last 2 decades have called attention to the importance of preserving the meniscus to protect the articular surfaces of the knee. This evolution has been stimulated by the customary use of arthroscopy and the ongoing research on the natural history, basic science, and biomechanics of meniscal injury (1). Annandale (2) first reported meniscal repair in

1885, contradicting the conventional wisdom of the time, which thought menisci to be functionless remains of muscle origins (3). A rejuvenated interest in meniscal repair began when Ikeuchi (4) performed the first arthroscopic repair in Japan and published his findings in 1979.

Our understanding of meniscal function has evolved from the described "functionless" structure to the view that they are, indeed, crucial components of the normal biomechanics and functioning of the knee. Laboratory investigations have shown that the menisci participate in many important functions, including tibio-femoral load transmission, shock absorption, lubrication, and passive stabilization of the knee joint (5–7). Removal of meniscal tissue increases local contact stresses across the articular cartilage proportional to the amount removed. It is well accepted that total and even partial meniscectomy gradually results in radiographic Fairbank (8) changes and symptomatic degenerative changes in the knee (9–15). In fact, it is clear that the menisci are essential components of the normal knee, and that techniques intended to preserve the menisci are desirable. As evidence accumulates from both animal and clinical studies of the frequent development of degenerative changes following meniscectomy, surgeons have become increasingly aggressive in their efforts to conserve as much meniscal tissue as possible (5).

Injuries to the knee menisci are common and operations to treat them are among the most frequent procedures performed by orthopaedic surgeons (16). Although it was first described over a century ago by Annandale (2), meniscal repair has only regained popularity in the last 20 years. A variety of techniques for repair have been devised and there remains no common consensus among experts with respect to which treatment of meniscal lesions is best (17). The techniques of meniscal repair have evolved over time from an open suture meniscal repair to a number of arthroscopic techniques using diverse implants. Many of these devices have facilitated meniscal repair, making it more appealing to the arthroscopic knee surgeon. More difficult, however, is understanding the intricacies of all the devices available on the market, including their composition, indications for use, methods of insertion, as well as the advantages and drawbacks of each particular implant.

■ REGENERATIVE CAPACITY OF THE MENISCUS

Cabaud et al. (18) canine and rhesus experiments with meniscal laceration and repair showed that certain meniscal tears, particularly those involving the vascular periphery, can heal and may be repaired rather than resected. Later canine experiments confirmed that the vascular healing response originates from the peripheral synovial tissues (19). Classification of meniscal vascular anatomy is based on anatomic studies that depict a peripheral vascular zone, including a synovial fringe that extends a short distance over both the femoral and tibial surfaces of the menisci, but does not contribute any vessels to the meniscal stroma (20). The "red," or vascular,

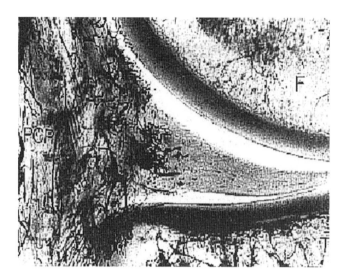

Fig 38-1. The vascular anatomy of the meniscus.

portion of the meniscus refers to the peripheral 10% to 25% of the lateral meniscus and the peripheral 10% to 30% of the medial meniscus, which is penetrated by vessels originating in the perimeniscal capsular and synovial capillary plexus (19). The central portion of the meniscus is relatively avascular, or "white," while the watershed area between them is referred to as the "red-white" zone (21) **(Fig 38-1)**.

The reparative process of the meniscus involves a coalescence of blood from the peripheral vascular zone adjacent to the meniscal tear and formation of a fibrin clot. Undifferentiated mesenchymal cells accumulate in the clot forming a cellular fibrovascular scar, which maintains the tear edges in a reduced position. The inflammatory reaction proceeds with ongoing invasion of cells from the "synovial fringe" and the fibrovascular scar tissue. This inflammatory cascade ultimately results in angiogenesis in the premeniscal capillary plexus allowing vessels to proliferate through the repair tissue.

Animal studies have shown that when a radial tear extends into the synovium, it can heal spontaneously by fibrovascular scar in approximately 10 weeks (19). In rabbit medial menisci, the mean scar strength 6 weeks after repair was 19% (no treatment), 26% (suture repair), and 42.5% (fibrin glue) of the value measured in the equivalent region of the intact contralateral controls (22). This inherent healing ability of the meniscus is the foundation on which clinical initiatives of meniscal repair are based.

■ CLINICAL EVALUATION

History

The meniscus is commonly injured in sports, but can occur as a sequela of age-related degeneration. In these cases there may be no trauma, but more typically, patients give a history of a twisting injury followed by pain. This acute episode may involve locking of the knee and moderate swelling. Recurrent episodes of pain and swelling are occasionally accompanied by complaints of mechanical symptoms such as catching, popping, or locking in the knee. The pain tends to localize along the joint line, especially with deep flexion and twisting motions.

Physical Examination

The patient is examined for signs of an effusion, loss of quadriceps bulk, and range of motion. Tenderness to palpation along either the medial or lateral joint line is among the most sensitive signs of a meniscal tear. The collateral and cruciate ligaments are assessed to determine whether additional injury is present. Special tests for assessing the meniscus, such as the McMurray or Apley tests, are not conclusive but can aid in the diagnosis. The McMurray provocative test is performed with the patient supine, the hip flexed to 90 degrees, and the knee in forced maximal flexion. The foot is grasped by the heel, the knee is steadied, and the joint line is palpated with the other hand. As the knee is slowly brought into extension, an external rotation stress will test the medial meniscus while an internal rotation stress tests the lateral meniscus. A positive test is a pain in the appropriate joint line accompanied by a thud or click. The hallmarks of a meniscal tear are presence of an effusion, joint line tenderness, as well as a positive McMurray test **(Fig 38-2)**.

Imaging

Evaluation of the meniscal tear should include routine anterior posterior (AP) and lateral x-rays of the knee. If degenerative changes are expected, standing views including a 45-degree flexion AP view should be performed to assess the

degree of joint space narrowing. Although not clinically indicated in all patients, magnetic resonance imaging (MRI) plays a valuable role in the evaluation of the full range of meniscal pathology including the primary diagnosis of a meniscal tear, the detection of a recurrent tear after resection or repair, and the demonstration of associated injuries and complications (23). Although it is usually not possible to identify menisci that are amenable to repair preoperatively, magnetic resonance imaging does show the relative locations of the tears and is able to determine the presence of a meniscal tear with an accuracy of over 90% (24,25). These results support reports in the literature that MRI is an accurate noninvasive technique for evaluating meniscal tears (26).

◼ INDICATIONS FOR MENISCAL REPAIR

The indications for meniscal repairs continue to be refined. Prior to making a determination regarding the reparability of a meniscal tear it is necessary to consider several factors including tear characteristics such as chronicity, size and appearance of the tear, medial versus lateral location, the presence of secondary tears, and whether associated with an anterior cruciate ligament injury. Patient factors such as patient age, activity, and compliance with rehabilitation also need to be considered in the algorithm of repair. The ultimate decision to repair or resect the meniscus depends on the combination of those factors and makes each case unique. Selection of an appropriate tear for repair precedes implant selection.

Given the vascularity of the meniscus, the peripheral, or red-red, tear is most amenable to repair, with good results also being reported in repair of tears in the red-white zone. Surgical repair of tears, which occur in the lateral meniscus, have a more favorable outcome, and thus have broader indications for repair. Short tears that are less than 2.5 cm long are easier and more amenable to repair than more extensive ones. The appearance of the meniscus is important as well, with the ideal tear being a vertical, longitudinal split. Flap, degenerative, and horizontal cleavage tears are not routinely repaired. In complex tears, all components are probed and assessed regarding the potential to heal. Rarely, all components of the complex tear are repaired, but more commonly, the central bucket handle portion is excised and the more peripheral aspects are sutured. No benefit has been shown with repairing horizontal cleavage tears, and radial tears of the middle part of the meniscus are best trimmed.

Repair of the meniscus in chronic and acute tears has long been studied, but the appearance and location remain the most important considerations. In an early study, Eggli et al. (27) found that tears repaired within 8 weeks of injury fared better, although others have found no difference in outcomes based on chronicity. Chronic bucket-handle tears will often deform with time and become difficult to reduce anatomically. Given that reduction is a prerequisite for fixing the meniscus, chronic

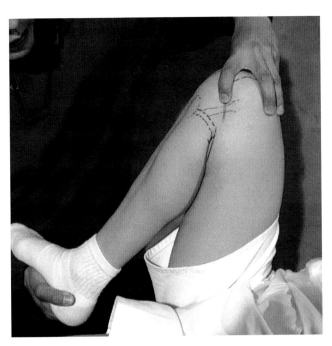

Fig 38-2. The McMurray test.

and deformed degenerative tears are best excised. The definition of a degenerative tear is one that shows signs of delamination, radial tears in the mid-portion of the bucket, and one that rolls when probed from the undersurface.

Special consideration must be given to the anterior cruciate ligament (ACL) injured knee, as it is known that meniscal repairs in the ACL deficient knee have a higher failure and re-tear risk (28). Given that the ACL deficient knee is also at risk of initiating tears and propagating smaller tears, ligament reconstruction should be considered seriously for the ACL deficient patient with a reparable meniscal tear (28,29). The effect of ACL transection on meniscal strain has been studied. The meniscus, in addition to transferring force across the joint, prevents tibial displacement on the femur if the ACL is injured. With a deficient ligament there is increased anterior-posterior tibial displacement, which contributes to increased strain in the meniscus (30). Clinically, cruciate instability has been found to contribute to higher failure rates for meniscal repairs, which can be obviated by concomitant ligament stabilization surgery (31). The hematoma and resultant fibrin clot which is created while reconstructing the ACL stimulates the healing in the meniscus. Consideration should still be given to meniscal repair in patients who refuse reconstruction of the anterior cruciate ligament, but the patient must be counseled regarding the higher rate of failure with this approach.

There is no specific age limit for performing meniscal repair. Meniscal repairs at the time of ACL reconstruction have been described in patients up to the age of 55. Historically, most authors recommended partial meniscectomy for patients with stable knees over age 45, but acceptable results with repairs have also been reported in this age group (32,33). Most importantly, the meniscal tear must have the characteristics which allow for successful repair, without evidence of fraying or degeneration.

Certain tears have been found to heal well without meniscal repair. As a result of the biologic stimulation and stability conferred to the knee following ACL reconstruction, certain tears may be neglected when identified at the time of ligament surgery. Short, stable tears of both medial and lateral menisci in the posterior aspect of the meniscus have been found to remain asymptomatic despite lack of treatment (34) or with only trephination (35). Fitzgibbon and Shelbourne's study (36) of 189 knees at follow up of one to nine years, confirms that certain lateral meniscal tears identified at the time of anterior cruciate ligament reconstruction can be left without removal or repair, and that they will remain asymptomatic. Specifically, posterior horn avulsion tears, asymptomatic vertical tears totally posterior to the popliteus tendon, and other complete and incomplete lateral meniscal tears (vertical longitudinal, radial, or anterior vertical), if stable at the time of anterior cruciate ligament reconstruction, can be left in situ without becoming clinically symptomatic. In a study by Shelbourne and Rask (37), over 94% of stable peripheral vertical medial meniscus tears treated with abrasion and trephination remain asymptomatic without stabilization. Talley and Grana (38)

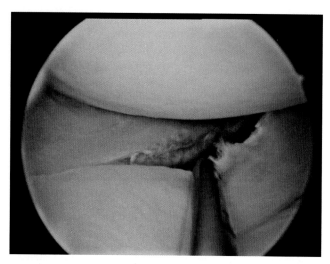

Fig 38-3. A reparable tear of the posterior horn of the medial meniscus.

concluded that although stable lateral meniscal tears healed well with only synovial abrasion, stable longitudinal medial meniscal tears have a higher propensity to fail over time by propagation of the tear, and may be better managed with meniscal repair.

In summary, the ideal reparable tear is a vertical one of the lateral meniscus, which occurs in the peripheral 3 mm of the red-red or red-white zone, and is being repaired with concomitant ACL reconstruction **(Fig 38-3)**.

■ TREATMENT OF MENISCAL INJURIES

Nonoperative

Meniscal tears are initially treated symptomatically with protected weight bearing, modified activity, ice, and nonsteroidal anti-inflammatory medications (NSAIDs). Some meniscal tears will become asymptomatic after several months of these interventions. The best activity for the patient during this period is to use the stationary bicycle and to avoid deep or full squatting exercises. If the patients are willing to modify their activities and have full motion and no pain or swelling, then conservative management of the tear may be successful. A locked knee, however, usually represents a displaced bucket handle tear and will need surgery acutely to restore motion.

Operative

If the patient continues to have pain, swelling and giving way, then operative intervention is indicated. If there is a degenerative flap tear, then meniscectomy is the only treatment **(Fig 38-4)**. The principle of meniscectomy is to remove any unstable fragments of meniscus, to contour the edges, and to trim the remaining rim so that it is stable to probing. If,

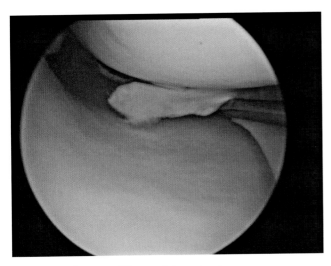

Fig 38-4. A flap tear of the medial meniscus.

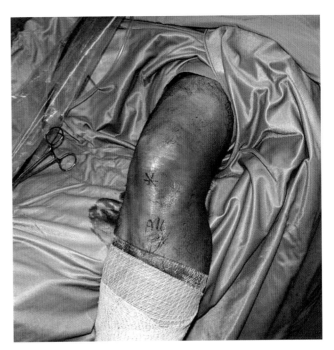

Fig 38-5. The set up for meniscal repair.

however, the meniscal tear is amenable to repair, this can be accomplished by means of various techniques and implants. The four major methods of repairing the meniscus are: open, arthroscopic outside-in, arthroscopic inside-out, or an arthroscopic all-inside technique. Prior to the widespread use of arthroscopy, open repair techniques were performed, but arthroscopic inside-to-outside approaches evolved to decrease the morbidity and enable access to areas that are difficult to reach with an open approach. An outside-to-inside approach was later popularized, as it minimized the risk to posterior neurovascular structures. Eventually, an all-inside technique for posterior horn tears was developed which obviates posterior capsular exposure, further reducing neurovascular risk. The following sections enumerate the advantages, indications, contraindications, complications, and results of each.

A variety of implants to address meniscal tears are commercially available to the arthroscopic surgeon. These include absorbable and nonabsorbable sutures, bio-absorbable arrows, tacks, and staples, as well as a number of repair-stimulating techniques such as trephination, rasping, and implantation of a fibrin clot. Most authors who advocate the use of sutures utilize nonabsorbable sutures. By providing longer lasting and more stable fixation, nonabsorbable sutures are believed to allow more complete remodeling of the meniscal repair tissue, which allows for improved healing rates (27). Menisci repaired with permanent sutures also had a lower incidence of clinical symptoms and a much lower failure rate (39).

■ SURGICAL TECHNIQUE

Patient Position and Diagnostic Arthroscopy

Patient positioning must allow circumferential access to the affected knee during meniscal repair. The leg should be prepped and draped to allow posteromedial and posterolateral incisions should they be required (Fig 38-5). This can be done

with the patient supine such that the break in the table is at the level of the tourniquet and can be flexed down to allow 90 degrees of knee flexion. Alternatively, a leg holder can be used that allows the surgeon to abduct the leg away from the operating table, allowing the knee to flex as needed for access. Diagnostic arthroscopy is performed using a 30-degree arthroscope and includes an evaluation of both menisci, the articular cartilage in the knee, and the cruciate ligaments. The menisci are probed on the inferior and superior surfaces to identify any tears. In assessing meniscal stability, it is important to realize that the lateral meniscus is normally more mobile than the medial meniscus (40). The definition of an unstable meniscal tear is one that is longer than half the length of the meniscus, and subluxes under the condyle when probed with a hook. Although a tourniquet may be used to improve visualization during the procedure, some surgeons prefer to leave it deflated for the diagnostic arthroscopy in order to assess the vascularity of the meniscal tear after rasping.

Repairs of the medial meniscus are usually done in some degree of extension, depending on the location of the tear, to allow for adequate visualization and access. On the lateral side, the greatest visualization is obtained with the knee flexed and the leg in the figure-of-four position. This position is also key in protecting the peroneal nerve, which lies posterior to the biceps femoris tendon and furthest from the joint capsule with the knee in flexion.

The Posteromedial and Posterolateral Incision

If performing an inside-out or outside-in repair of the meniscus, a "safety" incision is usually done on the appropriate side with the knee in flexion. In the inside-out technique, the incision is done just distal to the joint line, since the needles are passed in a cranio-caudal direction.

On the medial side, a 2 to 3 cm skin incision is performed posterior to the medial collateral ligament and then the fascia along the anterior border of the sartorius muscle is incised. The sartorius is retracted posteriorly, which protects the saphenous nerve and vein lying deep and towards the posterior border of the sartorius. Care should be taken to watch for the infrapatellar branch of the saphenous nerve, which penetrates the sartorius becoming superficial to the fascia near the joint line. With blunt dissection the interval between the posteromedial capsule and the medial head of the gastrocnemius is opened, just proximal to the semimembranosus tendon.

On the lateral side, the surgeon identifies the joint line, the lateral collateral ligament and the fibular head. With the knee at 90 degrees of flexion, an incision may be made posterior to the iliotibial band, again extending 3 cm distal from the joint line. This approach can then be continued with blunt dissection passing between the anterior aspect of the biceps femoris and the posterior aspect of the iliotibial band. If the superior lateral geniculate vessels are encountered, they can be coagulated. The biceps femoris is retracted posteriorly, protecting the peroneal nerve, which lies posterior and medial to the biceps tendon at this level. The lateral head of the gastrocnemius is identified and the dissection proceeds between the gastrocnemius and the capsule, where a retractor can be placed during the passage of sutures.

Preparing the Meniscus

The tear should be initially probed to determine if it is suitable for repair. The edges of the tear should be debrided of fibrous tissue with a rasp or a small shaver. Abrasion of the menisco-synovial junction is also believed to improve the rate of repair regardless of repair method (41,42). Animal studies in rabbits have shown that rasping a meniscal surface to repair a tear in the avascular zone stimulates vascular induction to the tear, resulting in meniscal healing. The cytokine network on the rasped meniscal surface appears to be the key to explaining the mechanism of vascular induction and meniscal healing by meniscal rasping (43). A technique of stimulation of the meniscal synovial border with electrocautery has been described by Pavlovich (44). The principle is to lightly "burn" the synovium to produce a healing response. Zhongnan et al. (45) demonstrated that the meniscus and the rim may be trephinated to produce vascular access channels. Trephination involves the creation of vascular access channels by removal of a core of tissue from the periphery of the meniscus adjacent to the tear, thus connecting the avascular portion of the meniscus to the peripheral blood supply. Zhang (46,47) continues to champion the technique, and has shown increased healing rates and decreased symptoms when trephination is performed during repair. Some authors believe that for symptomatic stable or incomplete meniscal tears, trephination without suturing may be sufficient, and

have shown good results while avoiding the complications associated with suturing (35,37).

Other techniques of biologic augmentation have been devised to improve healing rates. Arnoczky et al. (48) was the first to show that meniscal healing in the avascular zone of canine menisci can be enhanced by the use of a fibrin clot. Clinically, there have been favorable results with use of fibrin clot in repair of red-white meniscal tears (42,49–52). The technique involves withdrawal of 30 to 40 cc of the patient's blood by venipuncture, which is then placed in a sterile glass container and stirred with a glass rod for a few minutes until a well-organized firm fibrin clot is formed (51). After rinsing the clot in sterile saline to remove serum and red blood cells, it is tied to a previously placed repair suture that has been brought out of an anterior portal by means of a cannula. A probe can be used to position the clot between the meniscus and the tibia as the sutures are tensioned (53).

The sutures and bioabsorbable devices must be placed accurately to reduce the tear and hold it until it is healed. A common approach to large bucket handle tears is to use sutures in the middle segment to reduce and hold the bucket tear, and then use the bioabsorbable devices posterior horn region because it is more difficult to access and repair. In summary, for good results in meniscal repair, the principles of meniscal repair, namely that stimulation of circulation and proper reduction of the meniscus must be adhered to.

■ MENISCAL REPAIR TECHNIQUES

Open Meniscal Repair

Indications for open meniscal repair at the present time are somewhat limited. It could be used for very peripheral meniscal tears, such as meniscocapsular separation. In reality, the repair is performed open only in special circumstances, such as multi-ligament reconstruction after knee dislocation, and at the time of tibial plateau fixation.

A 3 to 5 cm incision is made longitudinally over the joint line and vertical sutures are placed from the capsule into the meniscus.

Inside-Out Repair

The arthroscopic inside-out suture repair originally described by Henning and Lynch (9) remains the gold standard by which other techniques are judged. A major advantage of this technique is its versatility, its ease of use, and the short learning curve. Excellent healing rates have been widely reported in the literature (54–64). The Zone-Specific method of inside-out meniscal repair was popularized by Rosenberg (63) in 1986, when he developed a single-lumen cannula system (Linvatec, Largo, FL) through which sutures could be passed to repair the meniscus. The system includes single-lumen cannulae with six different curvatures that allows the surgeon to direct the tip more easily to the left or right, as well as toward the anterior, middle, or posterior part of the meniscus. The cannulae have a 15-degree curve upward, which allows the cannula to be apposed against the meniscus and allows the needle to be passed parallel to the joint line from a slightly elevated portal. The shapes of the cannulae allow placement of the device around the tibial spines and femoral condyles, and direct the needles away from the important posterior neurovascular structures.

Tears are routinely repaired with the arthroscope in the ipsilateral anterior portal and the cannula coming in from the contralateral portal. The appropriate cannula is placed against the meniscus adjacent to the tear, allowing a 2-0 nonabsorbable suture attached on both ends to 10-inch needles to be passed across the tear. Prior to passing the suture, the needle can be used to spear the central part of the meniscal tear, thus reducing it anatomically. A safety incision is performed prior to passing the sutures through the capsule and a retractor is placed in this incision to guard the assistant from needle stick injury and to protect the neurovascular structures from the long needles. The retractor can be placed in such a fashion that it deflects the needles into the wound, aiding the assistant who retrieves them.

Commonly, after reducing and preparing the meniscus, the first stitch is placed on the superior surface of the peripheral rim. The cannula is then reoriented to lie against the superior surface of the central part of the meniscus. The other needle attached to the 2-0 nonabsorbable suture is passed through the meniscus, thus holding the tear well reduced with a vertical mattress stitch. Stitches are placed every 3 to 4 mm, alternating between the superior and inferior surfaces of the meniscus **(Fig 38-6)**. After they are in place, the sutures are tightened sequentially and tied over the capsule. The probe can be used to verify the reduction and fixation of the meniscus.

Modifications of the technique have also been described (64,65). These include use of flexible cannulae (Arthrex, Naples, FL), which uses a bender to modify the cannula to

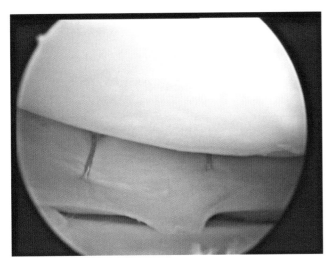

Fig 38-6. The inside out suture technique.

reach each meniscal tear. A reusable nitinol needle is then used to pass the suture. Another method described by Clancy and Graf allows the passage of two sutures through a double slotted cannula without needing to reposition. This, however, allows for the placement of only horizontal and not vertical mattress sutures. A device such as the SharpShooter Meniscal Repair System (Linvatec, Largo, FL) allows the surgeon to target and slowly advance the sutures in increments with one hand.

Outside-In Technique

The benefits of the outside-in meniscal repair technique include minimal equipment requirements, safety, and good visualization (66). The technique was originally described to minimize the chance of injury to the peroneal nerve during lateral meniscal repair. As well, it allows flexibility of placement and easier access in knees with a tight medial compartment, since it does not involve introduction of large rigid cannulae through the joint. Variations of the original technique have been described by several authors (67–69).

In outside-in meniscal repair, after preparing the meniscus, separate small incisions perpendicular to the joint line are made for each pair of sutures. Alternatively, to better protect the neurovascular structures, a single longitudinal incision can be made centered on the joint line after localizing the appropriate position by transilluminating with the arthroscope or placing a spinal needle so it passes adjacent to the tear. After spreading the subcutaneous tissue to expose the joint capsule, an 18-gauge spinal needle is placed across the meniscal tear from outside to inside under arthroscopic guidance. For posterior needle placement, the spinal needles may be curved to allow a safer passage. Occasionally, it is necessary to hold the meniscal tear reduced with a probe or obturator while passing the spinal needle across the tear. The stylet is removed and a suture is passed through the needle from outside the joint in. The sutures, usually 0 PDS, should be passed perpendicular to the meniscal tear at 3 to 5 mm intervals to increase the stability of the repair. A grasper introduced through the anterior portal holds the free intra-articular end of the suture and the needle is withdrawn. The intra-articular suture end is then pulled out through the anterior portal and three or four throws are tied creating a "mulberry" knot, which then sits on the articular surface of the tear after the suture is tensioned. Also described is bringing the free ends of two adjacent sutures out of the anterior portal, and then tying a square knot before pulling the suture back into the joint so the knot rests on the meniscal surface in a mattress-type suture. Alternatively, once across the meniscal tear, the free intra-articular end of the suture can be pulled back out through the meniscus with a second spinal needle or commercial snare device, creating a mattress suture. After all sutures have been placed across the tear, they are then tensioned and the meniscus is probed to assess the adequacy of the repair. If the tear is stable and well reduced, the sutures are then tied on the capsule (70).

All-Inside Techniques

Despite the excellent results obtained with inside-out and outside-in meniscal repair, disadvantages, such as the need for additional incisions, an assistant, and the risk for neurovascular damage, have led surgeons to develop an alternate technique. All-inside repairs were described for posterior horn tears by Morgan (71) using the Spectrum tissue repair system. With the advent of bioabsorbable devices and the relative speed and ease with which they are placed, this technique has largely been abandoned. Relative contraindications to all-inside repair include anterior horn tears, which are almost impossible to access, and meniscocapsular separation or lateral meniscal tears at the popliteal junction, since the devices used depend on a peripheral anchor.

Since the inception of all-inside repairs, four phases of repair techniques have been identified (72). The first phase refers to Morgan's technique (71), using a curved suture-hook passed through a posteromedial or posterolateral portal, which was twisted across the tear, allowing a suture to be passed and arthroscopically tied.

To improve on this, and better compress the tear, the second generation of devices, first reported by Albrecht-Olsen and co-workers, were rigid bioabsorbable implants, including darts, screws, and arrows **(Fig 38-7)**. Their ease of insertion led to an increase in the popularity of the meniscal repair, although concerns of complications such as chondral abrasion, loss of fixation, migration, and inflammation associated with degradation began to arise (73–82). Few prospective randomized trials were conducted to compare their efficacy to the gold standard of the inside-out repair with nonabsorbable vertical mattress sutures. Examples of these second generation devices include: the Linvatec BioStinger made of PLLA (Linvatec, Largo, FL), the Bionx Meniscal Arrow made of self-reinforced PLLA (Bionx

Implants, Blue Bell, PA), the Clearfix Meniscal Screw made of PLLA (Mitek Worldwide, Westwood, MA), the SD-sorb Staple made of a copolymer of PLLA and polyglycolide (Surgical Dynamics, Norwalk, CT), the Mitek Meniscal Repair System made of polydioxanone (Mitek Worldwide, Westwood, MA), the Arthrex Meniscus Dart made of PDLLA (Arthrex, Naples, FL), and the Arthrotec Meniscal Staple made of Lactosorb polymer (Biomet, Warsaw, IN).

The third phase of devices were developed to be implanted through the anterior portals, the best known of which was the T-Fix (Smith & Nephew, Andover, MA). This device required placement of two separate 2-0 monofilament sutures across the tear, which were attached to a 3 mm polyethylene bar driven through the tear into the periphery of the meniscus. The tensioning of the suture caused the bar to flip, resembling the letter "T," and anchor in the periphery. The meniscus could then be held reduced by tying together the two adjacent sutures over the surface of the meniscus with an arthroscopic knot-pusher. Disadvantages of this technique include the obligatory knot placement on the surface of the meniscus and the horizontal mattress configuration, which is less strong than vertical mattress sutures. Another disadvantage is the inability to consistently tension the knot, which compromised compression across the tear.

The fourth generation of devices has decreased the chance for chondral abrasion by combining a bioabsorbable anchor with a suture that can be tensioned on the surface of the meniscus. This allows the implant to deform with the meniscus when subjected to compressive loads. Cadaveric studies looking at the ease and safety of use identified some pitfalls with the initial designs. Even experienced surgeons had some difficulty correctly inserting the devices, causing the implants to be modified to provide easier deployment and a device limiting the depth of penetration. Examples of this generation of implants include the FasT-Fix (Smith & Nephew, Andover, MA), the Meniscal Stapler XLS (USS Sports Medicine, North Haven, CT) and the Rapid-Loc Meniscal Repair Device (Mitek Worldwide, Westwood, MA). Although long-term studies are pending, studies of initial fixation strength are promising and these fixation devices have become popular with arthroscopic surgeons (83).

■ MATERIALS USED IN FIXATION

Sutures

The advantage of using sutures in meniscal repair is that it has proven to be efficacious and cost effective. The disadvantages of using sutures in meniscal repair is that an accessory incision is necessary, it is more time-consuming, has a significant learning curve, and usually requires a second assistant. There is also the potential for needle stick injuries to the operating team, as well as the chance for neurovascular complications. The vertical loop suture was shown to be twice as strong as the horizontal loop suture, and the vertical-mattress

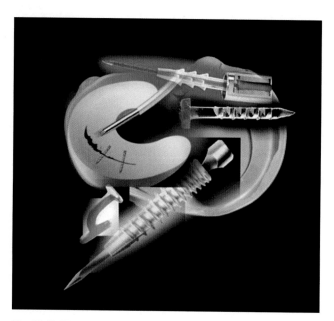

Fig 38-7. The initial rigid bioabsorbable meniscal fixators.

suture repair remains the gold standard by which other techniques are judged (84). Multiple vertical loops of nonabsorbable material placed 3 to 5 mm apart on the superior and inferior surface provides the best repair.

Bioabsorbable Devices

Bioabsorbable polymers are relatively new and now commonly used for meniscal repair (Fig 38-7). Biodegradable implants have been fashioned for meniscal fixation to simplify the technique and minimize neurovascular complications. Among the advantage of these implants is that meniscal tears, especially posterior horn tears, are easily and quickly repaired with little risk to the neurovascular structures.

The mechanical properties of these bioabsorbable implants vary depending on the polymer characteristics, as well as the size and shape of the implant. The chemical make-up, molecular weight, stereotactic orientation, and crystallinity are properties that contribute to the device's tensile strength, tensile modulus, bending strength, and bending modulus. In general, polylevolactic acid (PLLA), racemic polylactic acid (PDLLA), polydiaxonone (PDS), and polyglycolic acid (PGA) have an initial tensile strength of 30 to 70 MPa. The method of degradation of these implants is by hydrolytic degradation, eventually being released as carbon dioxide and water. The degradation occurs most rapidly near the center of the implant and progresses outward producing a mantle of polymer on the outside. Biocompatibility of these implants is controversial, as some materials have been found to cause a nonspecific tissue response with fibroblast activation and the appearance of inflammatory cells (85–88). Slow or intermediate degrading materials such as PDLLA, PLLA, or PLLA-co-PDLLA maintain their mechanical strength long enough to allow for tissue healing (89).

Not all of these devices are created equal. The original Biofix meniscal arrow introduced in 1993 (Bionix, Finland) was made with self-reinforced PLLA in 10, 13, and 16 mm lengths (90). When compared to a vertical loop suture of 2-0 Ethibond in fresh-frozen cadaveric menisci, the ultimate load to failure of the suture was much higher. The arrows failed by pulling out of the meniscus and permitted gapping at the repair site (91). In another study, single vertical loop suture again showed the highest overall pull-out strength, and the arrow was shown to have the same pullout strength as the horizontal loop suture (92). Although weaker than sutures, arrows should provide sufficient stability for meniscal healing, but the number of barbs engaged and angle of insertion are critical (93). The minimum pullout strength necessary for successful clinical use had not been established by these biomechanical studies. Several companies have since developed bioabsorbable implants for meniscal repair that address the shortcomings of the original meniscal arrow. Devices are now available that are strong yet flexible, cannulated for ease of reduction and placement, and have depth-limiting stops to protect extracapsular structures. It is, however, beyond the scope of this text to describe in detail the composition and insertion techniques of all the implants currently on the market.

A review of the literature shows that vertical mattress sutures remain the gold standard. They have better initial fixation strength and performance under cyclic loading than the horizontal sutures and knot-end techniques. Comparisons of the second and third generation bioabsorbable devices to the gold standard and to each other have not been conclusive. The most recent data suggest that the biomechanical performance of some fourth generation devices is nearly equivalent to current suture techniques (94). Of the second and third generation devices, the Linvatec Biostinger, Smith & Nephew T-Fix, Bionx Meniscus Arrow and two Arthrex Darts have separately been shown to have good initial fixation strength on load to failure, comparable to horizontal mattress suture techniques (94,95). Only the Bionx Arrow, Linvatec Biostinger, and Clearfix Screw have been shown to retain their initial strength through 24 weeks of hydrolysis time (95). Ultimately, the combination of a simplified surgical technique, high clinical healing rates (75%–92%) especially with concomitant ACL reconstruction, and relatively minor complications makes these devices attractive for properly indicated meniscal tears (96).

■ COMPLICATIONS OF MENISCAL REPAIR

Although rare, complications occur, even with appropriate preventive measures. Potential risks include damage to the peroneal nerve and popliteal vascular structures, failure of meniscal healing, and the usual complications of arthroscopy. Fortunately, most complications described have either resolved spontaneously or had satisfactory outcomes after appropriate treatment (97). Complications such as infection and thrombophlebitis can occur following any lower extremity surgery, and have been reported following arthroscopic meniscal repair. In a prospective 19-month study of complications in experienced arthroscopists, there was a lower incidence of complications in meniscal repair (1.29%), including both inside-out and outside-in techniques, than in meniscectomy (1.69%) (98,99).

Neurovascular injuries are among the more common complications, especially saphenous neuropathy, which patients usually describe as being only a minor nuisance (97). This has been reported for both inside-to-out and outside-to-in techniques. Some authors feel that these minor complications are likely underreported, as patients may only complain when asked specifically about the symptoms (100,101). Among other described neurovascular complications, was a case of a complete peroneal nerve palsy after lateral inside-out meniscus repair, despite having a posterior safety incision (102). A popliteal artery pseudoaneurysm has also been reported in the literature (103). Detailed knowledge of anatomy, as well as careful dissection and needle placement is key in avoiding neurovascular injuries.

Various cases of cyst formation have also been reported after meniscal repair. These include a case of meniscal cyst formation after all-inside meniscal repair (104). Another case of meniscal cyst formation after use of nonabsorbable sutures for meniscal repair has been described (105). As well, synovitis has been found to occur, even after suture repair (106). Since the introduction of bioabsorbable devices for meniscal repair, reports of chondral damage have been increasing (73,74,79). In theory, countersinking the head of the device, using a headless fixator, or using an implant that has no abrasive material on the surface of the meniscus, could decrease this incidence. There are also cases describing difficulty in deploying the bioabsorbable fixators (107), as well as reports of local complications related to device migration or prominence, and soft-tissue inflammation associated with absorption of the device (75,79,82,108,109). Inflammatory foreign-body reaction to bioabsorbable meniscal arrows has been described (110), as has a case of a cystic hematoma formation (111).

■ REHABILITATION

Despite the frequency with which meniscal repairs are performed, there continue to be varying recommendations with respect to motion and weight bearing in the early post-operative rehabilitation. There remains controversy, as well, with respect to when pivoting sports should be allowed. Basic science studies show that between flexion angles of 15 and 60 degrees the menisci are relatively immobile, but at the extremes of motion there is significant mobility. In knee flexion, the medial meniscus translates 5.1 mm posteriorly, while the excursion of the lateral meniscus is 11.2 mm (40). It may, therefore, be prudent to limit the extremes of flexion early after meniscal repair. Canine research has shown that immobilization may be detrimental to the healing of menisci by both decreasing collagen formation and maturation (112). Another reason given for starting early range of motion relates to the increased risk of arthrofibrosis with postoperative immobilization, particularly with concomitant ACL reconstruction (113).

With weight bearing, compressive forces are loaded across the menisci and are transmitted in the form of tensile forces across them. These hoop stresses are resisted by the structure of the meniscus, and therefore, the weight load in extension would tend to displace the edges of a transverse radial tear, but compress the edges of a vertical tear (33). Most meniscal tears are peripheral longitudinal tears with a vertical orientation, and theoretically, weight bearing should not have an adverse effect on healing after repair. This has been shown in clinical studies that support accelerated rehabilitation programs that allow weight bearing in the early postoperative phase (114–116).

Accelerated rehabilitation after meniscal repair was first popularized by Barber (115) in 1994, who published a comparison of outcomes between a "standard" rehabilitation program which limited weight bearing and motion for 6 weeks,

and an "accelerated" program permitting unlimited weight bearing and full motion. The clinical results between the two groups failed to show any difference and did not support the need for activity restriction in early rehabilitation. In Shelbourne's study (116) population, patients with adequate repair of the meniscal tears followed a rehabilitation program that also allowed immediate range of motion and weight bearing as tolerated. They achieved a clinical result comparable to patients who followed a restrictive rehabilitation program.

Although time to return to work or sport is also controversial, a conservative program would allow a return to pivoting sports at 6 months; however, in Barber and Click's study (115), the patients were allowed to return to pivoting sports after there was no effusion, full extension, and 120 degrees of motion. In this aggressively treated group (40 repairs) the failure rate was 10%, while in the restricted group (58 repairs) who were kept out of sport for 6 months, the failure rate was 19%.

No modification of an ACL reconstruction accelerated rehabilitation program is needed for meniscus repairs performed in conjunction with the reconstruction (117,118). In a study by Mariani et al. (119) 22 patients who underwent meniscal repair combined with ACL reconstruction were allowed immediate full range of motion and weight bearing. The low failure rate in the series suggested that an aggressive rehabilitation regimen may be prescribed without deleterious effects. This encourages patient and surgeon acceptance of the meniscus repair.

Outcomes

The outcome measures for various published studies differ in their definition of a successful repair. Although some use meniscal healing as verified by a second-look arthroscopy or imaging such as MRI or CT-arthrogram, others use functional outcome scores or questionnaires to confirm that there are no symptoms attributable to the repaired tear. Overall, clinical success rates are typically higher than the absolute rate of healing as determined by imaging or second-look arthroscopy. In fact, the true rate of anatomic failure as shown on second-look arthroscopy may be as high as twice the rate of clinical failure (120). Van Trommel et al. (121) has demonstrated that tears may be asymptomatic despite having only partially healed. Failure to heal the meniscus after repair may be due to several factors, including ACL-deficient status, poor surgical technique, poor selection of tear to repair, as well as reinjury. As well, the clinical relevance of biomechanical studies is unclear, as it has not been determined how much strength is required of devices for meniscal healing. The long-term implications of an anatomically failed but asymptomatic repair have not been established.

Open Repairs

There are few reports of results after open meniscal repairs. In a study of 30 patients and 33 open repairs at a mean follow up of over 10 years, DeHaven et al. (28) report a 79% long-term survival rate of the repaired menisci, as evidenced by clinical exam and weight-bearing radiographs. Increased retear rates were encountered in unstable knees.

Inside-Out Repairs

There have been excellent results reported with the inside-to-out meniscal repair technique. Miller's (122) early study consisted of 87 patients with 116 meniscus tears, 96 of which were repaired. Only nineteen patients (27%) had isolated meniscus injuries, and ligament-stabilizing procedures were done on all patients who had ACL-deficient knees. 79 repairs were assessed at a mean of 39 months (12 months to 5.5 years) and found to have a 91% success rate in retaining the meniscus. The study also concluded that the time from injury to repair did not affect meniscus healing, but that associated stabilization of ACL deficiencies is imperative in patients undergoing meniscus surgery.

Cannon and Vittori (123) have shown that lateral meniscal repairs fared better than medial repairs, and a smaller rim width yielded better overall healing. Patients with anterior cruciate ligament reconstruction did better than those with isolated meniscal repair, regardless of tear length. Older patients had better healing than younger ones, and acute repairs were more successful than repairs of chronic tears. In the study by Brown et al. (56), 92% of meniscal tears with rims of less than 4 mm no longer had symptoms after repair and returned to sport. Perdue et al. (54) looked at 63 patients who had their menisci repaired using the inside-out technique with malleable cannulae. Forty-five patients were available for clinical examination with a mean follow-up of 27 months. Tegner and Lysholm scores showed that clinical results were 64% excellent, 27% good, and 9% failure. In this study, age, gender, and length of the meniscal tear had no effect on clinical outcome.

In Ryu and Dunbar (124) study, 16 lateral and 15 medial menisci were repaired. The majority of the lesions (29 of 31) were in the red-red or red-white zones and were vertical bucket-handle tears of the posterior horn averaging 2.5 cm in length. Clinical healing was present in 27 (87%) of the 31 repaired menisci. Ventakatchalam et al. (125) and colleagues, retrospective study attempted to assess outcome and identify factors that might improve future clinical results. Of 60 meniscal repairs, the overall success rate was only 66.1%. Repair within 3 months of injury had a better prognosis than late repairs. Healing rates of atraumatic meniscus tears were much lower than for traumatic tears (42% vs. 73%). The isolated atraumatic medial meniscal tear appeared to do particularly poorly, with only 33% of those healing, and may be better treated by meniscectomy.

Shelbourne et al. (37) have shown us that repaired unstable peripheral vertical medial meniscus tears have a failure rate of 13.6%, with most retears occurring more than 2 years after repair. Of stable peripheral vertical medial meniscus tears treated with abrasion and trephination, most (94%) remained asymptomatic without stabilization. In a more recent publication of 155 patients with bucket-handle medial meniscal tears and anterior cruciate ligament tears, 56 menisci were repaired and 99 that were degenerative and crushed beyond repair were removed. At 6 to 8 years after surgery, functional outcome scores showed that patients with repaired degenerative tears had significantly lower subjective scores than those with nondegenerative tears (126).

Outside-In Repairs

Several studies have published results of meniscal tears repaired by the outside-to-in technique. An initial report by Morgan and Casscells (127) showed that at a mean follow-up of 18 months, 98% of 70 patients had an excellent clinical evaluation, with only one meniscus failing to heal. In a subsequent study by Morgan et al. (128), the failure rate was 16% out of 353 peripheral tears repaired. This failure rate was based on persistence of symptoms, and all failures were associated with ACL deficiency and tear location in the posterior horn of the medial meniscus. Seventy-four patients were assessed by second-look arthroscopy, and this showed that healed and partially healed menisci were found to be asymptomatic.

Van Trommel et al. (121) looked at the results of 51 patients at a mean of 14 months following meniscal repair. By second-look arthroscopy and/or imaging, 24% of menisci were not healed. Good results were obtained for tears in the middle and anterior portion of the medial meniscus, as well as all lateral meniscus tears, but poor healing with the outside-in technique was observed in patients with tears into the posterior horn of the medial meniscus. In a retrospective review of 41 knees which had undergone meniscal repair, Plasschaert et al. (129) found that 74% of repairs survived and did not need further surgery at a mean of 3.5 years. The average age of the patients was 25 years (12 to 38 years), and concomitant ACL reconstruction did not seem to impact significantly on the results.

Warren et al. (presented at AAOS, 2004) looked at the results of 90 repairs with a minimum follow-up of 3 years. They showed that 62 patients (69%) were asymptomatic and demonstrated a healed meniscus objectively by MRI, CT-arthrogram, or second-look arthroscopy. Sixteen patients were minimally symptomatic and had evidence of partial healing, while 12 patients (13%) had failure of healing. Additionally, 5 of 13 (38%) of repairs in ACL-unstable knees went on to fail repair, while 5 of 33 (15%) with ACL-stable knees failed to heal. This was contrasted with a 5% failure rate (2 of 38) in patients undergoing concomitant ACL reconstruction. Furthermore, 15% (11 of 72) medial menisci did not heal, while only 5% (1 of 18) lateral menisci failed the repair. A lower failure rate was also noted at the meniscocapsular junction (1 of 23 patients) as compared to the less vascular central third of the meniscus, where 4 out of 10 did not heal. Slightly less successful healing was more common when onset of injury was insidious, and there was a trend to partial healing only with increased age.

All-Inside Repair

Despite recent popularity and widespread availability of devices for all inside repair, few clinical studies have shown definitive long-term results with their use. At the present time, we do not know how much fixation is necessary for the meniscus to heal, and the biomechanical data continue to be encouraging. The literature is flooded with case reports of complications arising from the use of certain fixators, but most laboratory studies have shown that they are relatively safe to insert with respect to the important neurovascular structures.

In a prospective study of second look arthroscopies by the inventors of the Bionx Arrows, the arrows were no longer visualized at 3 to 4 months, and in 91% the menisci had gone on to heal (120). Ross et al. (74) found that clinical healing rates of approximately 90% could be expected with the Meniscal Arrow when the repair was performed in conjunction with ACL reconstruction. At a mean follow-up of 2.3 years, the clinical outcome of 29 out of 32 patients has been excellent. At a minimum follow-up of 2 years, Jones et al. (75) assessed the clinical outcomes of 39 meniscal repairs in 38 patients performed with the Meniscal Arrow. The overall clinical failure rate, which was defined as a need for reoperation, was only 7%.

Caborn et al. (130) reported on their use of the T-Fix implant in the repair of 55 menisci located in the red-red or red-white zones. Thirty-two patients (62%) underwent ACL reconstruction at the time of surgery. At a mean follow-up of 10.3 months (4 to 24 months), 96% (22 of 23) of patients having undergone isolated meniscal repair had excellent clinical results. Of the 32 patients who underwent concurrent ACL reconstruction, all had excellent clinical results. Barrett and co-workers reported on 21 meniscal repairs in 20 patients undergoing concurrent ACL reconstruction, at a minimum follow-up of 1 year. Clinically, four patients were symptomatic, but second-look arthroscopy revealed that three had healed, while one had not (131).

The results of all-inside repair have recently been reported by Ahn et al. (132). This study reported on the second look arthroscopy of 39 medial meniscal tears that were repaired associated with an ACL reconstruction. The technique was an all inside suture repair using the spectrum hook system, and two posteromedial portals to place and tie the sutures. The standard inside out repair was used for the mid portion of the meniscus tear. At the time of the second look (average 19 months after repair), 81% had healed, 15% had incomplete healing, and 2% had failed.

■ SUMMARY AND CONCLUSIONS

There is a growing belief based on animal and clinical studies that there is a direct relationship between the amount of meniscus removed and the eventual degree of degeneration in the knee. Although clinical studies indicate progressively improving outcomes of meniscal reconstruction, longer follow-up is needed to determine whether the natural history of joint degeneration can be altered. It is difficult to compare the results of meniscal repair in the literature because of the variety of repair techniques, as well as the patient and tear variables. We have, however, come a long way in delineating the factors that can promote or impair meniscal healing.

One of the best predictors for outcome has been shown to be the meniscal rim thickness and vascularity, with the most peripheral tears being favored. As well, lateral meniscal repairs have better results than medial meniscal repairs. It has also become clear than the menisci heal better when the anterior cruciate ligament is reconstructed concurrently, and that there are increased retear rates in unstable knees (28). The success of repairs in chronic versus acute tears remains a topic of some controversy, as does the role that the age of the patient plays. It is likely that these two factors come into play in the overall appearance of the injured meniscus because we know that degenerative and atraumatic tears have a poorer prognosis for healing. Based on these findings, an ideal candidate for meniscal repair would be a young individual with a traumatic, longitudinal, peripheral lateral meniscal tear that is 1 to 2 cm in length, repaired in conjunction with an ACL reconstruction

Long-term studies are needed to show the effects that preserving the meniscus has on protecting the articular surface of the knee. The all-inside meniscal repair devices will improve as surgeons look for faster, safer, and less invasive methods to achieve their goal. Techniques will continue to evolve to make meniscal repair easier and more successful. Future directions include biologic methods of restoring menisci, such as the delivery of growth factors to injured menisci and transplantation of autogenous fibrochondrocytes in meniscal defects. Other avenues of investigation include the use of cytokines to enhance meniscal healing and the potential to augment the repair by gene therapy techniques (51).

■ REFERENCES

1. Petrosini AV, Sherman OH. A historical perspective on meniscal repair. *Clin Sports Med.* 1996;15(3):445–453.
2. Annandale T. An operation for displaced semilunar cartilage. *Br Med J.* 1885;1:779.
3. Bland-Sutton J. *Ligaments: Their Nature and Morphology.* 2nd ed. London: JK Lewis; 1897.
4. Ikeuchi H. Meniscus surgery using the Watanabe arthroscope. *Orthop Clin North Am.* 1979;10(3):629–642.
5. Newman AP, Daniels AU, Burks RT. Principles and decision making in meniscal surgery. *Arthroscopy.* 1993;9(1):33–51.
6. Fukubayashi T, Kurosawa H. The contact area and pressure distribution pattern of the knee. A study of normal and osteoarthrotic knee joints. *Acta Orthop Scand.* 1980;51(6):871–879.
7. Walker PS, Erkman MJ. The role of the menisci in force transmission across the knee. *Clin Orthop.* 1975;(109):184–192.
8. Fairbank TJ. Knee joint changes after meniscectomy. *J Bone Joint Surg.* 1948;30B:664–670.
9. Henning CE, Lynch MA. Current concepts of meniscal function and pathology. *Clin Sports Med.* 1985;4(2):259–265.

10. Aglietti P, et al. A comparison between medial meniscus repair, partial meniscectomy, and normal meniscus in anterior cruciate ligament reconstructed knees. *Clin Orthop.* 1994;(307):165–173.

11. Johnson RJ, Kettlekamp DB, Clark W. Factors affecting late results after meniscectomy. *J Bone Joint Surg.* 1974;56A:719–729.

12. Ahmed AM, Burke DL. In-vitro measurement of static pressure distribution in synovial joints—Part I: Tibial surface of the knee. *J Biomech Eng.* 1983;105(3):216–225.

13. Baratz ME, Fu FH, Mengato R. Meniscal tears: the effect of meniscectomy and of repair on intraarticular contact areas and stress in the human knee. A preliminary report. *Am J Sports Med.* 1986;14(4):270–275.

14. Cox JS, Nye CE, Schaefer WW, et al. The degenerative effects of partial and total resection of the medial meniscus in dogs' knees. *Clin Orthop.* 1975;(109):178–183.

15. Sommerlath K, Gillquist J. The long-term course of various meniscal treatments in anterior cruciate ligament deficient knees. *Clin Orthop.* 1992;(283):207–214.

16. Howell JR, Handoll HH. Surgical treatment for meniscal injuries of the knee in adults. *Cochrane Database Syst Rev.* 2000;(2): CD001353.

17. Koski JA, et al. Meniscal injury and repair: clinical status. *Orthop Clin North Am.* 2000;31(3):419–436.

18. Cabaud HE, Rodkey WG, Fitzwater JE. Medial meniscus repairs. An experimental and morphologic study. *Am J Sports Med.* 1981;9(3):129–134.

19. Arnoczky SP, Warren RF. The microvasculature of the meniscus and its response to injury. An experimental study in the dog. *Am J Sports Med.* 1983;11(3):131–141.

20. Arnoczky SP, Warren RF. Microvasculature of the human meniscus. *Am J Sports Med.* 1982;10(2):90–95.

21. DeHaven KE. Decision making factors in the treatment of meniscal lesions. *Clin Orthop.* 1990;252:49–54.

22. Roeddecker K, Muennich U, Nagelschmidt M. Meniscal healing: a biomechanical study. *J Surg Res.* 1994;56(1):20–27.

23. Fitzgerald SW. Magnetic resonance imaging of the meniscus. Advanced concepts. *Magn Reson Imaging Clin N Am.* 1994;2(3): 349–364.

24. Mandelbaum BR, et al. Magnetic resonance imaging as a tool for evaluation of traumatic knee injuries. Anatomical and pathoanatomical correlations. *Am J Sports Med.* 1986;14(5):361–370.

25. Reicher MA, et al. Meniscal injuries: detection using MR imaging. *Radiology.* 1986;159(3):753–757.

26. Crues JV III, Ryu R, Morgan FW. Meniscal pathology. The expanding role of magnetic resonance imaging. *Clin Orthop.* 1990;(252):80–87.

27. Eggli S., et al. Long-term results of arthroscopic meniscal repair. An analysis of isolated tears. *Am J Sports Med.* 1995;23(6): 715–720.

28. DeHaven KE, Lohrer WA, Lovelock JE. Long-term results of open meniscal repair. *Am J Sports Med.* 1995;23(5):524–530.

29. Schmitz MA, Rouse LM Jr, DeHaven KE. The management of meniscal tears in the ACL-deficient knee. *Clin Sports Med.* 1996;15(3):573–593.

30. Hollis JM, Pearsall AW, Niciforos PG. Change in meniscal strain with anterior cruciate ligament injury and after reconstruction. *Am J Sports Med.* 2000;28(5):700–704.

31. Wickiewicz TL. Meniscal injuries in the cruciate-deficient knee. *Clin Sports Med.* 1990;9(3):681–694.

32. Noyes FR, Barber-Westin SD. Arthroscopic repair of meniscus tears extending into the avascular zone with or without anterior cruciate ligament reconstruction in patients 40 years of age and older. *Arthroscopy.* 2000;16(8):822–829.

33. Cannon WDJ. Arthroscopic meniscal repair. In: McGinty, JB, ed. *Operative arthroscopy.* New York: Raven Press; 1991.

34. Orfaly RM, McConkey JP, Regan WD. The fate of meniscal tears after anterior cruciate ligament reconstruction. *Clin J Sport Med.* 1998;8(2):102–105.

35. Fox JM, Rintz KG, Ferkel RD. Trephination of incomplete meniscal tears. *Arthroscopy.* 1993;9(4):451–455.

36. Fitzgibbons RES, KD. "Aggressive" nontreatment of lateral meniscal tears seen during anterior cruciate ligament reconstruction. *Am J Sports Med.* 1995;23(2):156–159.

37. Shelbourne KD, Rask BP. The sequelae of salvaged nondegenerative peripheral vertical medial meniscus tears with anterior cruciate ligament reconstruction. *Arthroscopy.* 2001;17(3):270–274.

38. Talley MC, Grana WA. Treatment of partial meniscal tears identified during anterior cruciate ligament reconstruction with limited synovial abrasion. *Arthroscopy.* 2000;16(1):6–10.

39. Barrett GR, et al. The effect of suture type on meniscus repair. A clinical analysis. *Am J Knee Surg.* 1997;10(1):2–9.

40. Thompson WO, et al. Tibial meniscal dynamics using three-dimensional reconstruction of magnetic resonance images. *Am J Sports Med.* 1991;19(3):210–215, discussion 215–216.

41. Henning CE, et al. Use of the fascia sheath coverage and exogenous fibrin clot in the treatment of complex meniscal tears. *Am J Sports Med.* 1991;19(6):626–631.

42. O'Meara PM. Surgical techniques for arthroscopic meniscal repair. *Orthop Rev.* 1993;22(7):781–790.

43. Ochi M, et al. Expression of cytokines after meniscal rasping to promote meniscal healing. *Arthroscopy.* 2001;17(7):724–731.

44. Pavlovich R. Hi-frequency electrical cautery stimulation in the treatment of displaced meniscal tears. *Arthroscopy.* 1998;14(6):566–571.

45. Zhongnan Z, Arnold JA, Williams T, et al. Repairs by trephination and suturing of longitudinal injuries in the avascular area of the meniscus in goats. *Am J Sports Med.* 1995;23(1):35–41.

46. Zhang Z, Arnold JA. Trephination and suturing of avascular meniscal tears: a clinical study of the trephination procedure. *Arthroscopy.* 1996;12(6):726–731.

47. Zhang Z, et al. Repairs by trephination and suturing of longitudinal injuries in the avascular area of the meniscus in goats. *Am J Sports Med.* 1995;23(1):35–41.

48. Arnoczky SP, Warren RF, Spivak JM. Meniscal repair using an exogenous fibrin clot. An experimental study in dogs. *J Bone Joint Surg Am.* 1988;70(8):1209–1217.

49. McAndrews PT, Arnoczky SP. Meniscal repair enhancement techniques. *Clin Sports Med.* 1996;15(3):499–510.

50. Henning CE, et al. Arthroscopic meniscal repair using an exogenous fibrin clot. *Clin Orthop.* 1990;(252):64–72.

51. Rodeo SA, Warren RF. Meniscal repair using the outside-to-inside technique. *Clin Sports Med.* 1996;15(3):469–481.

52. van Trommel MF, et al. Arthroscopic meniscal repair with fibrin clot of complete radial tears of the lateral meniscus in the avascular zone. *Arthroscopy.* 1998;14(4):360–365.

53. Cohen DB, Wickiewicz TL. Arthroscopic meniscal repair. *Oper Tech Sports Med.* 2003;11(2):91–103.

54. Perdue PS Jr, et al. Meniscal repair: outcomes and clinical follow-up. *Arthroscopy.* 1996;12(6):694–698.

55. Johannsen HV, et al. Arthroscopic suture of peripheral meniscal tears. *Int Orthop.* 1988;12(4):287–290.

56. Brown GC, Rosenberg TD, Deffner KT. Inside-out meniscal repair using zone-specific instruments. *Am J Knee Surg.* 1996; 9(3):144–150.

57. Cannon WD Jr. Arthroscopic meniscal repair. Inside-out technique and results. *Am J Knee Surg.* 1996;9(3):137–143.

58. Horibe S, et al. Second-look arthroscopy after meniscal repair. Review of 132 menisci repaired by an arthroscopic inside-out technique. *J Bone Joint Surg Br.* 1995;77(2):245–249.

59. Horibe S, et al. Results of isolated meniscal repair evaluated by second-look arthroscopy. *Arthroscopy.* 1996;12(2):150–155.

60. Rubman MH, Noyes FR, Barber-Westin SD. Arthroscopic repair of meniscal tears that extend into the avascular zone. A review of 198 single and complex tears. *Am J Sports Med.* 1998;26(1):87–95.

61. Spindler KP, et al. Prospective comparison of arthroscopic medial meniscal repair technique: inside-out suture versus entirely arthroscopic arrows. *Am J Sports Med.* 2003;31(6):929–934.

62. Stone RG, Frewin PR, Gonzales S. Long-term assessment of arthroscopic meniscus repair: a two- to six-year follow-up study. *Arthroscopy.* 1990;6(2):73–78.

63. Rosenberg TD, Scott SM, Coward DB, et al. Arthroscopic meniscal repair evaluated with repeat arthroscopy. *Arthroscopy.* 1986;2(1):14–20.

64. Ahn JH, Wang JH, Oh I. Modified inside-out technique for meniscal repair. *Arthroscopy.* 2004;20(suppl 2):178–182.

65. Graf B, Docter T, Clancy W Jr. Arthroscopic meniscal repair. *Clin Sports Med.* 1987;6(3):525–536.

66. Johnson LL. Meniscus repair: the outside in technique. In: Jackson DW, ed. *Reconstructive knee surgery.* New York: Raven Press; 1995.

67. Landsiedl F. Improved outside-in technique of arthroscopic meniscal suture. *Arthroscopy.* 1992;8(1):130–131.

68. Diment MT, DeHaven KE, Sebastianelli WJ. Current concepts in meniscal repair. *Orthopedics.* 1993;16(9):973–977.

69. O'Donnell JB, Ruland CM, Ruland LJ III. A modified outside-in meniscal repair technique. *Arthroscopy.* 1993;9(4):472–474.

70. Curl LA. Meniscal tear: arthroscopic outside-in repair. In: Craig EV, ed. *Clinical orthopaedics.* Philadelphia: Lippincott Williams & Wilkins; 1999:724–731.

71. Morgan CD. The "all-inside" meniscus repair. *Arthroscopy.* 1991;7(1):120–125.

72. Diduch DR, Poelstra KA. The evolution of all-inside meniscal repair. *Oper Tech Sports Med.* 2003;11(2):83–90.

73. Anderson K, et al. Chondral injury following meniscal repair with a biodegradable implant. *Arthroscopy.* 2000;16(7):749–753.

74. Ross G, Grabill J, McDevitt E. Chondral injury after meniscal repair with bioabsorbable arrows. *Arthroscopy.* 2000;16(7):754–756.

75. Jones HPL, Wilk MJ, Smiley RM, et al. Two-year follow-up of meniscal repair using a bioabsorbable arrow. *Arthroscopy.* 2002;18(1):64–69.

76. Seil R, et al. Chondral lesions after arthroscopic meniscus repair using meniscus arrows. *Arthroscopy.* 2000;16(7):E17.

77. Calder SJ, Myers PT. Broken arrow: a complication of meniscal repair. *Arthroscopy.* 1999;15(6):651–652.

78. Kumar A, Malhan K, Roberts SN. Chondral injury from bioabsorbable screws after meniscal repair. *Arthroscopy.* 2001;17(8):34.

79. Laprell H, Stein V, Petersen W. Arthroscopic all-inside meniscus repair using a new refixation device: a prospective study. *Arthroscopy.* 2002;18(4):387–393.

80. Miller MD, Kline AJ, Jepsen KG. "All-inside" meniscal repair devices: an experimental study in the goat model. *Am J Sports Med.* 2004;32(4):858–862.

81. Oliverson TJ, Lintner DM. Biofix arrow appearing as a subcutaneous foreign body. *Arthroscopy.* 2000;16(6):652–655.

82. Tsai AM, et al. Results of meniscal repair using a bioabsorbable screw. *Arthroscopy.* 2004;20(6):586–590.

83. Borden P, et al. Biomechanical comparison of the FasT-Fix meniscal repair suture system with vertical mattress sutures and meniscus arrows. *Am J Sports Med.* 2003;31(3):374–378.

84. Rimmer MG, et al. Failure strengths of different meniscal suturing techniques. *Arthroscopy.* 1995;11(2):146–150.

85. Bos RR, et al. Degradation of and tissue reaction to biodegradable poly(L-lactide) for use as internal fixation of fractures: a study in rats. *Biomaterials.* 1991;12(1):32–36.

86. Nordstrom P, et al. Tissue response to polyglycolide and polylactide pins in cancellous bone. *Arch Orthop Trauma Surg.* 1998;117(4–5):197–204.

87. Nordstrom P, et al. Tissue response to polyglycolide and polylevolactide pins in osteotomized cancellous bone. *Clin Orthop.* 2001;(382):247–257.

88. Anderson JM, Miller KM. Biomaterial biocompatibility and the macrophage. *Biomaterials.* 1984;5(1):5–10.

89. Bollom T, Meister K. Biodegradable materials. In: DeLee JC, Drez, D, Miller MD, eds. *DeLee & Drez's orthopaedic sports medicine: principles and practice.* Philadelphia: WB Saunders; 2002:196.

90. Albrecht-Olsen P, Kristensen G, Tormala P. Meniscus bucket-handle fixation with an absorbable Biofix tack: development of a new technique. *Knee Surg Sports Traumatol Arthrosc.* 1993;1(2):104–106.

91. Dervin GF, et al. Failure strengths of suture versus biodegradable arrow for meniscal repair: an in vitro study. *Arthroscopy.* 1997;13(3):296–300.

92. Albrecht-Olsen P, et al. Failure strength of a new meniscus arrow repair technique: biomechanical comparison with horizontal suture. *Arthroscopy.* 1997;13(2):183–187.

93. Boenisch UW, et al. Pull-out strength and stiffness of meniscal repair using absorbable arrows or Ti-Cron vertical and horizontal loop sutures. *Am J Sports Med.* 1999;27(5):626–631.

94. Barber FA, Herbert MA, Richards DP. Load to failure testing of new meniscal repair devices. *Arthroscopy.* 2004;20(1):45–50.

95. Arnoczky SP, Lavagnino M. Tensile fixation strengths of absorbable meniscal repair devices as a function of hydrolysis time. An in vitro experimental study. *Am J Sports Med.* 2001;29(2):118–123.

96. Farng E, Sherman O. Meniscal repair devices: a clinical and biomechanical literature review. *Arthroscopy.* 2004;20(3):273–286.

97. Austin KS. Complications of arthroscopic meniscal repair. *Clin Sports Med.* 1996;15(3):613–619.

98. Small NC. Complications in arthroscopic surgery performed by experienced arthroscopists. *Arthroscopy.* 1988;4(3):215–21.

99. Small NC. Complications in arthroscopic meniscal surgery. *Clin Sports Med.* 1990;9(3):609–617.

100. Austin KS, Sherman OH. Complications of arthroscopic meniscal repair. *Am J Sports Med.* 1993;21(6):864–868, discussion 868–869.

101. Sherman OH, et al. Arthroscopy—"no-problem surgery." An analysis of complications in two thousand six hundred and forty cases. *J Bone Joint Surg Am.* 1986;68(2):256–265.

102. Jurist KA, Greene PW III, Shirkhoda A. Peroneal nerve dysfunction as a complication of lateral meniscus repair: a case report and anatomic dissection. *Arthroscopy.* 1989;5(2):141–147.

103. Brasseur P, Sukkarieh F. [Iatrogenic pseudo-aneurysm of the popliteal artery. Complication of arthroscopic meniscectomy. Apropos of a case]. *J Radiol.* 1990;71(4):301–304.

104. Lombardo S, Eberly V. Meniscal cyst formation after all-inside meniscal repair. *Am J Sports Med.* 1999;27(5):666–667.

105. Choi NH, Kim SJ. Meniscal cyst formation after inside-out meniscal repair. *Arthroscopy.* 2004;20(1):E1–3.

106. Kelly JD, Ebrahimpour P. Chondral injury and synovitis after arthroscopic meniscal repair using an outside-in mulberry knot suture technique. *Arthroscopy.* 2004;20(5):E49–52.

107. Escalas F, et al. T-Fix anchor sutures for arthroscopic meniscal repair. *Knee Surg Sports Traumatol Arthrosc.* 1997;5(2):72–76.

108. Petsche TS, Selesnick H, Rochman A. Arthroscopic meniscus repair with bioabsorbable arrows. *Arthroscopy.* 2002;18(3):246–253.

109. Schneider F, Schroeder JH, Labs K. Failed meniscus repair. *Arthroscopy.* 2003;19(8):E93–96.

110. Menche DS, et al. Inflammatory foreign-body reaction to an arthroscopic bioabsorbable meniscal arrow repair. *Arthroscopy.* 1999;15(7):770–772.

111. Hechtman KS, Uribe JW. Cystic hematoma formation following use of a biodegradable arrow for meniscal repair. *Arthroscopy.* 1999;15(2):207–210.

112. Dowdy PA, et al. The effect of cast immobilization on meniscal healing. An experimental study in the dog. *Am J Sports Med.* 1995;23(6):721–728.

113. Cosgarea AJ, Sebastianelli WJ, DeHaven KE. Prevention of arthrofibrosis after anterior cruciate ligament reconstruction using the central third patellar tendon autograft. *Am J Sports Med.* 1995;23(1):87–92.

114. Ganley T, et al. The impact of loading on deformation about posteromedial meniscal tears. *Orthopedics.* 2000;23(6):597–601.

115. Barber FA. Accelerated rehabilitation for meniscus repairs. *Arthroscopy.* 1994;10(2):206–210.

116. Shelbourne KD, et al. Rehabilitation after meniscal repair. *Clin Sports Med.* 1996;15(3):595–612.

117. Barber FA, Click SD. Meniscus repair rehabilitation with concurrent anterior cruciate reconstruction. *Arthroscopy.* 1997;13(4):433–437.

118. Buseck MS, Noyes FR. Arthroscopic evaluation of meniscal repairs after anterior cruciate ligament reconstruction and immediate motion. *Am J Sports Med.* 1991;19(5):489–494.

119. Mariani PP, et al. Accelerated rehabilitation after arthroscopic meniscal repair: a clinical and magnetic resonance imaging evaluation. *Arthroscopy.* 1996;12(6):680–686.

120. Albrecht-Olsen P, et al. The arrow versus horizontal suture in arthroscopic meniscus repair. A prospective randomized study with arthroscopic evaluation. *Knee Surg Sports Traumatol Arthrosc.* 1999;7(5):268–273.

121. van Trommel MF, et al. Different regional healing rates with the outside-in technique for meniscal repair. *Am J Sports Med.* 1998;26(3):446–452.

122. Miller DB Jr. Arthroscopic meniscus repair. *Am J Sports Med.* 1988;16(4):315–320.

123. Cannon WD Jr, Vittori JM. The incidence of healing in arthroscopic meniscal repairs in anterior cruciate ligament-reconstructed knees versus stable knees. *Am J Sports Med.* 1992;20(2):176–181.

124. Ryu RK, Dunbar WH. Arthroscopic meniscal repair with two-year follow-up: a clinical review. *Arthroscopy.* 1988;4(3):168–173.

125. Venkatachalam, S.G., S. P.Harding, M. L., Review of the clinical results of arthroscopic meniscal repair. *Knee.* 2001;8(2):129–133.

126. Shelbourne KD, Carr DR. Meniscal repair compared with meniscectomy for bucket-handle medial meniscal tears in anterior cruciate ligament-reconstructed knees. *Am J Sports Med.* 2003;31(5):718–723.

127. Morgan CD, Casscells SW. Arthroscopic meniscus repair: a safe approach to the posterior horns. *Arthroscopy.* 1986;2(1):3–12.

128. Morgan CD, et al. Arthroscopic meniscal repair evaluated by second-look arthroscopy. *Am J Sports Med.* 1991;19(6):632–637, discussion 637–638.

129. Plasschaert F, Vandekerckhove B, Verdonk R. A known technique for meniscal repair in common practice. *Arthroscopy.* 1998;14(8):863–868.

130. Kocabey Y, et al. Patient outcomes following T-Fix meniscal repair and a modifiable, progressive rehabilitation program, a retrospective study. *Arch Orthop Trauma Surg.* 2004.

131. Barrett GR, Treacy SH, Ruff CG. Preliminary results of the T-fix endoscopic meniscus repair technique in an anterior cruciate ligament reconstruction population. *Arthroscopy.* 1997;13(2):218–223.

132. Ahn JH, Wang JH, Yoo JC. Arthroscopic all-inside suture repair of medial meniscus lesion in anterior cruciate ligament-deficient knees: results of second-look arthroscopies in 39 cases. *Arthroscopy.* 2004;20(9):936–45.

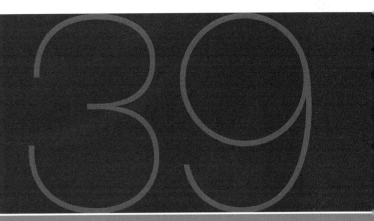

MENISCUS ALLOGRAFTS

WALTER R. SHELTON, MD

■ KEY POINTS

- The medial meniscus is a C-shaped triangular structure that is relatively more fixed than the lateral meniscus and is thicker posterior than anterior. The lateral meniscus is semi-circular, uniform from anterior to posterior, and more mobile.

- Candidates for meniscal allografts should be under 45 years old and have persistent pain after at least six months of conservative treatment following meniscectomy. The pain is usually oriented toward the side where the meniscus was removed.

- Extremity alignment and range of motion are critical when considering meniscus allograft surgery. Any abnormal valgus or varus or significant limitation of flexion or extension should be corrected prior to meniscus surgery.

- A cruciate deficient knee provides an opportunity to replace both the ligament and the meniscus with one surgery.

- Patients over age 45, with grade 4 arthritis, or with little or no pain are better suited for long-term conservative treatment.

- Meniscus allograft transplantation is a formidable procedure and complications can be significant. Deep vein thrombosis, post-surgical infection, and damage to articular surfaces are possible. Allografts also have the potential to transmit infectious diseases.

- Long-term data supporting the concept that a meniscus allograft will decrease the incidence of degenerative arthritis seen after meniscectomy is not yet available.

- Many insurance carriers still consider meniscal allograft surgery to be an experimental procedure and refuse to approve reimbursement.

- In rehabilitation, patients are started on full range of motion immediately. Patients usually go to one crutch at three weeks and are off crutches at six weeks, but are cautioned to avoid jumping, cutting, or running sports for at least six months.

■ BASIC SCIENCE

The anatomy of both the medial and lateral menisci have been well documented over the last 25 years. Recognition of their critical function of load distribution from femur to tibia has promoted investigation into every aspect of their makeup. The medial meniscus is a C shaped, triangular structure that is relatively more fixed than its counterpart and is thicker posterior than anterior **(Fig 39-1).** The lateral meniscus is semi-circular, uniform from anterior to posterior, and is more mobile. Both menisci attach to bone posteriorly

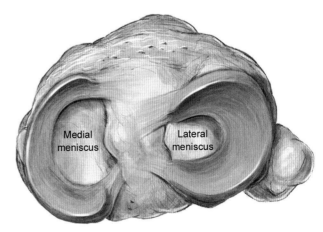

Fig 39-1. The medial and lateral menisci.

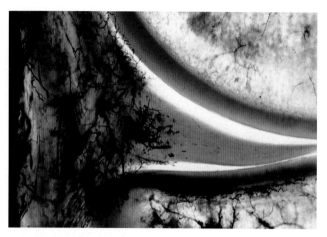

Fig 39-2. The blood supply of the meniscus.

at the back edge of the tibial spine. Anteriorly the medial meniscus inserts at the front edge of the tibial plateau; the lateral meniscus' anterior insertion is more posterior, opposite the anterior cruciate ligament (ACL) footprint. The lateral meniscus' capsular attachment is interrupted by the popliteus tendon in the posterolateral aspect of the joint.

Both menisci play a critical role in load-bearing and weight distribution from a relatively circular femoral condyle to a more flat tibial plateau. Pressure studies have shown that with normal menisci the load transmitted from the femur to the tibia throughout a full range of motion is evenly distributed over the tibial plateau. The lateral meniscus carries 70% of the load across the lateral compartment while the load is shared equally between meniscus and articular cartilage in the medial compartment. (The lateral meniscus is much more mobile than the medial meniscus.) (1) After meniscectomy the stress is highly concentrated toward the center of the tibial plateaus (2).

Most of the meniscus is composed of water. The remainder is made up of cells known as fibrochondrocytes and an extra-cellular matrix of proteoglycans. Blood supply of both menisci have been well documented by Arnoczky (Fig 39-2) and are composed of an outer one third that has an excellent blood supply (the red/red zone), a middle third where the blood supply becomes sparse (the red/white zone), and an inner third that is avascular (the white/white zone).

■ CLINICAL EVALUATION

Candidates for meniscal allografts should present with persistant pain at least 6 months after a meniscectomy. The pain is usually oriented toward the side of the joint where the meniscus was removed. Candidates should be relatively young (under the age of 45). They may present with swelling, uncommon after medial meniscectomy, but more of a persistent problem after lateral meniscectomy. Meniscectomy may exacerbate instability in a cruciate deficient knee, and concomitant meniscus replacement may enhance ligament reconstruction.

When considering meniscus allograft surgery, extremity alignment and range of motion are critical. Significant valgus or varus deformity or limitation of flexion or extension should be corrected prior to meniscus surgery. Routine long leg, standing x-rays should be obtained on all patients to assess alignment and arthritic changes within the knee. Magnetic resonance imaging (MRI) can assess the remaining meniscal rim and the presence of significant chondral damage.

Treatment algorithms should be formulated by a careful assessment of all findings including the history, physical findings, and imaging data. Patients without pain over the age of 45 or who have grade IV arthritis are not candidates for meniscus replacement.

■ TREATMENT

Patients should have at least 6 months of conservative treatment after total meniscectomy. Rehabilitation exercises, weight loss, nonsteroidal anti-inflammatory drugs (NSAIDS) to control pain and inflammation, and off loader bracing may be tried. The magnitude of the surgery and the potential of complications should be thoroughly explained and evaluated prior to any meniscus allograft. Patients better suited for other treatment options are over 45 years of age, with grade 4 arthritis, or those who have little or no pain.

■ OPERATIVE TREATMENT

Patients who meet the age, alignment, and motion criteria and have persistent postmeniscectomy pain after 6 months of conservative treatment may be considered for meniscus allograft replacement. A cruciate deficient knee provides an excellent opportunity to replace both the ligament and the meniscus with one surgery. Patients with significant varus or valgus mal-alignment should be corrected prior to a meniscus allograft. The two procedures are too extensive to be performed concomitantly.

Meniscus allografts are best accomplished with an arthroscopically assisted technique (3). Trimming retained meniscal fragments to achieve a stable rim and placement of bone tunnels using arthroscopic guides are easily achieved. A mini arthrotomy is required to place the meniscus and attached bony anchors into the joint.

Most medial meniscus allografts have been implanted with bone anchors at the anterior and posterior horns. A bone slot or keyhole is very difficult to accomplish on the medial side because the attachment of the anterior cruciate ligament on the tibia is at risk for disruption with the creation of a slot. The bone anchors are from 7 to 9 mm in diameter and 10 to 15 mm in length. Occasionally, a limited medial collateral release or a slight notchplasty of the intercondylar aspect of the femur is helpful in getting the posterior bone plug to the back of the joint. Care must be taken not to disrupt the femoral attachment of the posterial collateral ligament (PCL) and passage of the posterior bone plug through the intercondylar notch is easiest when the ACL is absent. After the meniscus has been introduced into the joint and the bone plugs have been seated, the meniscus is sutured peripherally, similar to the repair technique for a bucket-handle tear. Prior to insertion of the bone plugs, it is imperative to mark the anterior aspect of each plug so that once in place they can be oriented with proper rotation. Sutures passed through the tunnels can then be used to secure the bone plugs in their tunnels by tying the anterior and the posterior sutures together over a bridge of bone **(Fig 39-3)**.

Inserting a meniscus allograft without bone anchors by suturing the horns securely through drill holes would be technically easier. Biomechanical studies in cadaver knees show that meniscal allografts secured by bone anchors function similar to normal menisci in load distribution, whereas menisci sutured in without bone anchors tend to peripherally extrude and stresses are concentrated at the center of the tibial plateau.

The lateral meniscus can be inserted using a slot or keyhole technique **(Fig 39-4)**. This keeps the two horns of the lateral menisci attached by bone. The tibial attachment of the anterior cruciate ligament is more medial on the tibial plateau allowing enough room to develop a slot between the anterior and posterior horn attachments of the lateral meniscus. The centers of these bony attachments of the lateral menisci are

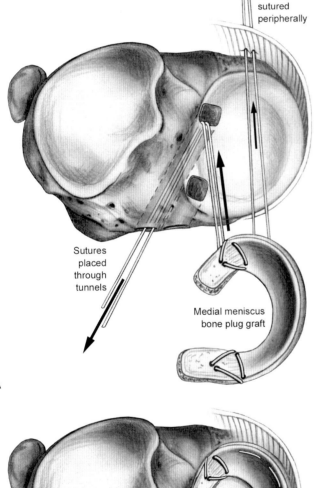

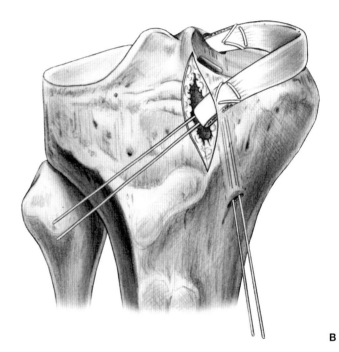

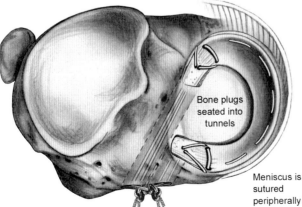

A

B

C Anterior and posterior sutures are passed through bone tunnels and sutured together over a bridge of bone

Fig 39-3. Medial meniscus insertion technique (cryolife).

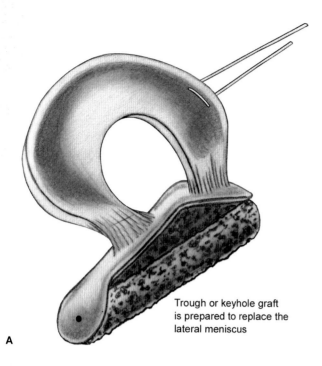

Trough or keyhole graft is prepared to replace the lateral meniscus

A

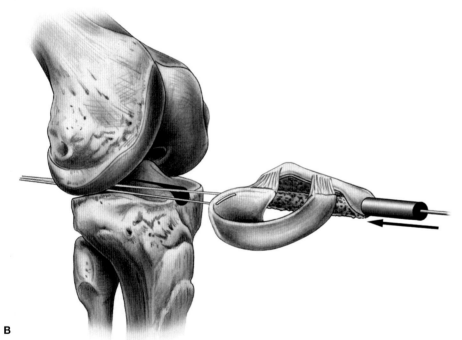

B

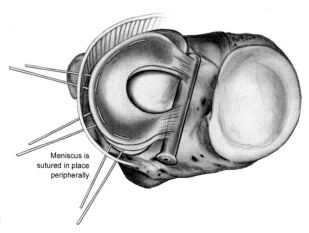

Meniscus is sutured in place peripherally

C

Fig 39-4. Lateral meniscus insertion—Keyhole technique (cryolife).

only about 2 cm apart. The use of a bone slot prevents merging tunnels, which is possible during concomitant ACL reconstruction. After inserting the lateral meniscus with its bone slot and securing it with either a pin or a screw, the periphery of the lateral meniscus can be sutured in an inside out method similar to repairing a bucket-handle tear of the lateral meniscus. It is important to accurately mark the tibial plateau at the anterior horn attachment of the old lateral meniscus to acutely position the new bone slot from anterior to posterior.

■ COMPLICATIONS, CONTROVERSIES, AND SPECIAL CONSIDERATIONS

Meniscus allograft transplantation is a formidable surgical procedure and complications can be significant. Deep vein thrombosis, post-surgical infection, and damage to articular surfaces are possible. Allografts also have the potential to transmit infectious diseases such as HIV, hepatitis, and sporoforms.

One particular problem seen with medial meniscus transplants is degenerative tears in the posterior horn (20% to 30% incidence at 3 years). High stresses placed on the posterior horn in flexion, its relatively large size, and the relative hypocellularity after graft maturation are thought to be the cause of these tears.

Another potential complication is graft shrinkage. Reports of 0% to 50% shrinkage have been presented (4). Shrinkage of the graft will decrease the ability of the meniscus to load transfer and thereby reduce its effectiveness.

Controversies

The most controversial aspect of meniscus transplantation is the absence of long term data supporting the concept that a meniscus allograft will decrease the incidence of degenerative arthritis seen after meniscectomy. The answer to this question will take well-designed studies of 10 to 20 years duration. Although it may seem logical to think that replacing a meniscus would decrease the likelihood of articular cartilage degeneration, it remains to be proven.

Special Considerations

In most areas, reimbursement issues can be a significant determent for meniscal allograft surgery. Many insurance carriers still consider it to be an experimental procedure and refuse to approve the procedure. Only long term follow-up with proven results will change this attitude.

Rehabilitation

Rehabilitation of meniscus allografts is identical the program for a bucket handle meniscus repair. Patients are

started on active full range of motion immediately. In line weight-bearing is allowed if firm fixation of the meniscus horns with bone plugs was achieved. Twisting, squatting, and rotational forces on the meniscus should be avoided. Patients usually go to one crutch at 3 weeks, are off crutches at 6 weeks, but are cautioned to avoid jumping, cutting, or running sports for at least 6 months.

■ CONCLUSIONS

Meniscus transplants have proven to be technically feasible and successful. Complete peripheral healing is seen in virtually all cases and bone anchors have been shown by pressure studies to prevent peripheral extrusion of the meniscus during weightbearing.

Special consideration should be given to potential hazards of meniscus allograft surgery. The procedure is technically demanding and damage to the articular surface is a real potential. The risk of transmittable diseases such as HIV, hepatitis, and sporoform infections must be explained to the patient in detail.

The best results are obtained in patients with minimal or no articular damage and normal alignment. One should question the advisability of doing a meniscus allograft in a patient with grade 4 arthritis or with significant varus or valgus alignment.

A meniscus allograft done in combination with an ACL or PCL reconstruction may be a helpful adjunct for enhancing stability. In most cases, the ligament and the meniscus allografts can be obtained from the same donor, thereby decreasing the risk of transmittable disease. The potential for meniscus shrinkage, the hypocellularity after cellular repopulation, and degenerative tears in the posterior horn of the medial meniscus at 3 to 5 years are all concerns. Replacing an absent meniscus with an allograft restores normal anatomy and biomechanics. If the allograft heals and does not shrink, the assumption that articular cartilage is being protected is logical but not yet proven by long term studies.

■ REFERENCES

1. Walker PS, Erkma MJ. The role of meniscus I force transmission across the knee. *Clin Orthop.* 1975;109:184–192.
2. Pablla GA Jr, Manning T, Snell E, et al. The effect of allograft meniscal replacement on intra-articular contact area and pressures in the human knee: a biomechanical study. *Am J Sports Med.* 1997;25:692–698.
3. Shelton WR, Dukes AD. Meniscus replacement with bone anchors: a surgical technique: *Arthroscopy.* 1994;10:324–327.
4. Stollsteiner OT, Shelton WR, Dukes A, et al. Meniscus allograft transplantation. A one- to five-year follow-up of 22 patients. *Arthroscopy.* 2000;16:343–347.

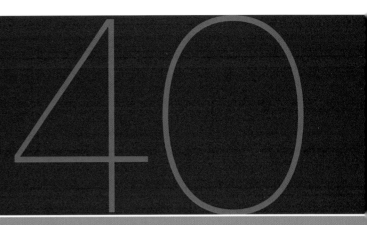

PATELLAR PROBLEMS IN ATHLETES

JEFFREY HALBRECHT, MD

■ KEY POINTS

- The patella is the largest sesamoid bone in the human body.
- Unlike most animals, humans often load the knee near full extension with the patella out of the confines of the trochlea and susceptible to instability.
- There are at least five bursas about the patella. The most clinically relevant is the subcutaneous prepatella bursa, which may become inflamed or infected.
- The patella articular cartilage is usually close to 5 mm thick, making it the thickest cartilage in the body.
- The medial patellofemoral ligament is the most important stabilizer of the patella to lateral translation.
- The physical examination of the patella is the most important part of the diagnostic workup and is often performed improperly. The knee is a kinetic chain and forces on the patella can be dramatically affected by anatomic derangements or asymmetries proximal or distal to the knee.
- There is evidence that bracing improves pain for patients with patellofemoral syndrome even if the brace does not appear to alter the biomechanical load on the patella.
- The standard imaging evaluation of patients with patellofemoral symptoms will include an anteroposterior (AP), lateral, and a 45-degree tangential view of the patella. The lateral view is useful to evaluate for loose bodies, patella alta or baja, and will reveal the presence of early degenerative changes with inferior or superior patella osteophytes.
- An acute dislocation of the patella is commonly confused with an anterior cruciate ligament (ACL) tear. The patient will present with a large hemarthrosis and will be tender to palpation along the medial retinaculum.

- When surgery is selected as the treatment option for patella dislocation, initial arthroscopic evaluation is recommended to confirm the diagnosis and address any loose chondral or osteochondral fractures.
- The treatment for recurring instability of the patella may differ from the treatment of an acute initial dislocation. Recurring instability may indicate a severe underlying anatomical dysplasia or predisposition that may require more aggressive treatment such as osteotomy of the tibial tubercle.
- One of the most common causes of anterior knee pain is the patella compression syndrome. This syndrome refers to excess pressure along the lateral facet of the patella, usually associated with a tight lateral retinaculum and radiographic evidence of patella tilt.
- Chondromalacia patients will present with pain, crepitus, and possibly a joint effusion. The history is usually that of insidious onset, although it may include a history of direct trauma such as a direct fall onto the patella or a blunt injury against a dashboard.

■ ANATOMY

The patella is the largest sesamoid bone in the human body (1), and like other sesamoid bones, most likely evolved as a mechanism to protect the quadriceps tendon from abrasion and to improve distribution of forces across the tendon (2). In addition, the patella acts to improve the biomechanical leverage of the quadriceps during extension, acting as a fulcrum (3) with greatest effect seen at 20 degrees of flexion (4).

Most animal species load the knee in a flexed position and have a well stabilized patella maintained within the confines of the trochlea throughout the range of motion. Humans, on the other hand, often load the knee near full extension with the patella out of the confines of the trochlea and are susceptible to instability. Interestingly, in greater apes the femoral diaphysis is straight and the trochlea is flat with no elevation of the lateral trochlea ridge and yet the patella remains stable due to the flexed angle of the knee in this species. In humans, the distal femur evolved into an obliquity angle of 8 to 10 degrees, necessitating the development of a deeper trochlea sulcus with an elevated lateral trochlear lip to stabilize the patella (5).

Bursas

There are at least five bursas about the patella **(Fig 40-1)**. The most commonly described is the subcutaneous prepatella bursa, which is the one that is most clinically relevant and may become inflamed or infected. The prepatellar tendon bursa can also rarely become clinically symptomatic. The intermediate and deep prepatellar bursa as well as the deep infrapatellar bursa are mostly just of anatomical interest. Recently, Dye et al. (6) have redescribed the three prepatella bursas as the prepatella subcutaneous bursa, the prepatella subfascial bursa, and prepatella sub aponeurotic bursa.

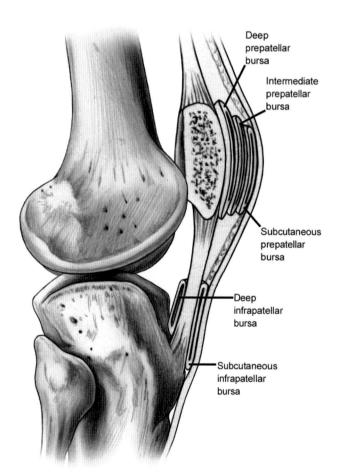

Fig 40-1. Location of bursae about the patella.

■ PATELLA ANATOMY

The typical patella is an asymmetrical sesamoid bone with a large flat lateral facet and a more sloped medial facet separated by the central ridge. A much smaller, more vertically shaped odd facet extends from the medial facet and makes contact with the medial trochlea only in maximum flexion **(Fig 40-2)**.

Different Shapes

Several authors have attempted to classify patella morphology into various shapes and types and correlate these types with the risk of patella chondromalacia and instability **(Fig 40-3)**. Wiberg (7) has described three basic types, and Baumgartl (8) has added a fourth and fifth with patella shape progressing from symmetrical medial and lateral facets (Type 1) to a vertical medial facet and flat lateral facet (Type 5). The Wiberg Type 2 is felt to be the most common type according to Hennsge (9).

Ratio of Patella to Tendon

The height of the patella relative to the trochlea can have functional significance and is easily measured with a simple lateral radiograph. The normal patella position can be measured in various ways, most commonly by comparing the patella length to the patella tendon length (10) **(Fig 40-4)**, although other methods have been described. A patella that sits too proximally, or patella alta, does not make as reliable contact with the trochlea and is often more mobile, resulting in an increased risk of instability. On the other hand, a low riding patella, or patella baja, can block knee flexion and place excessive loads on the patella, resulting in pain and progressive articular cartilage degeneration.

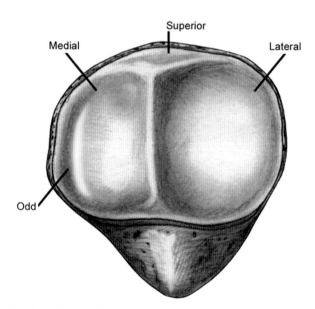

Fig 40-2. The patella has three articulating facets.

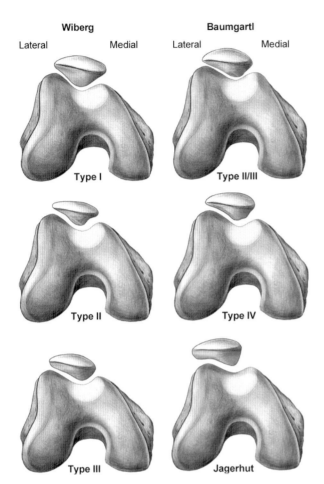

Fig 40-3. Classification of patella by morphology.

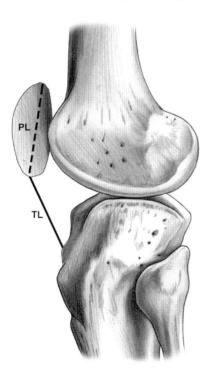

Fig 40-4. Measurement of patella position using the Insall-Salvati method. (From Insall J, Salvati E. Patella position in the normal knee joint. *Radiology*. 1971;101:101; with permission)

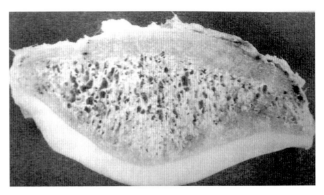

Fig 40-5. Patella articular cartilage is the thickest in the body, measuring close to 5 mm.

Cartilage Thickness

The patella articular cartilage is the thickest in the body and usually close to 5 mm thick (11). A recent study that carefully measured cartilage thickness of the patellofemoral (P/F) joint in 14 normal human knees using stereophotogrammetry and magnetic resonance imaging (MRI) revealed the average trochlea cartilage thickness to be 2.2 mm (+/−0.4) with a maximum of 3.7 mm, and the patella cartilage to be 3.3 mm (+/−0.6) with a maximum thickness of 4.6 mm (12) **(Fig 40-5)**.

■ BIOMECHANICS

Patellofemoral Contact Forces

The main biomechanical function of the patella is to lengthen the extension moment arm of the knee at full extension (13) **(Fig 40-6)**. Knee extension torque is the product of the quadriceps force multiplied by the length of the moment arm through which it acts. The patella shifts the quadriceps tendon anteriorly, increasing the length of the moment arm, and thus increasing knee extension torque.

Although frequently described as a pulley, the patella has been shown to function more like a balance beam. Depending upon the degree of knee flexion, the patella is free to tilt. This results in a variable force on the quadriceps and patella tendons depending upon flexion angle. Thus unlike a

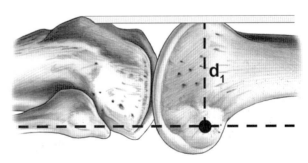

Fig 40-6. The patella serves to lengthen the extension moment arm of the knee in full extension.

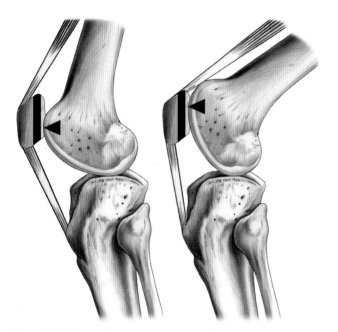

Fig 40-7. The patella acts as a balance beam as demonstrated by the striped bar. Change in patella tilt due to the balance beam effect results in changing lever arm length between the patella tendon and quadriceps tendon. As the lever arm decreases, force on the tendon increases, resulting in greater patella tendon force in extension and greater quadriceps tendon force in flexion.

pulley, where the force on the patella tendon and quadriceps tendon would be equal, the force on the patella tendon is greater near extension, while the force on the quadriceps is greater with knee flexion (14,15) **(Fig 40-7)**. This understanding is of great help in planning proper rehabilitation for injuries to the patella or quadriceps tendons.

The location of contact forces across the patella also varies depending upon knee flexion angle. Due to patella tilt, as well as a shifting moment arm, the distal patella is loaded more in lesser degrees of knee flexion, and the proximal patella is loaded more at greater degrees of knee flexion (16). Due to changing lever arms, quadriceps force and patella tendon force also vary with knee flexion angle, with greater quadriceps force occurring at high flexion angles **(Fig 40-8)**.

Patellofemoral compression force is the result of compression of the patella into the trochlea groove resulting from a combination of quadriceps and patella tendon forces. With standard weight bearing activities, maximum patella femoral contact force is thought to occur at approximately 70 to 80 degrees of knee flexion (17). As the knee flexes beyond this level, patella forces decreases as force is shifted onto the quadriceps tendon which begins to directly articulate with the trochlea. Although patellofemoral contact forces increase with knee flexion, the total contact area also increases with knee flexion. This distributes the forces over a greater contact area resulting in a less significant increase in force per sq mm, or contact pressure.

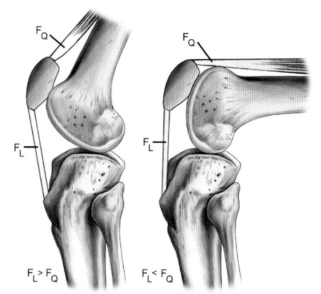

Fig 40-8. Maximum patella femoral contact force occurs at 70 to 80 degrees of flexion.

Patellofemoral contact force is generated by increased quadriceps torque. The quadriceps torque will increase based on the subject's body weight and the distance of the center of the body mass from the center of the knee joint (torque = force × distance). This has important implications for understanding how patients with patella disorders compensate their body position during stair climbing in order to unload the patella **(Fig 40-9)**.

Because patella pressure increases with knee flexion, the patella articular cartilage is thicker at its midpoint, where greatest contact pressure occurs.

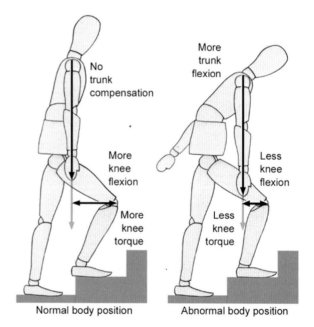

Fig 40-9. Patella femoral contact force is affected by body position, decreasing as patients forward flex at the hip during stair climbing.

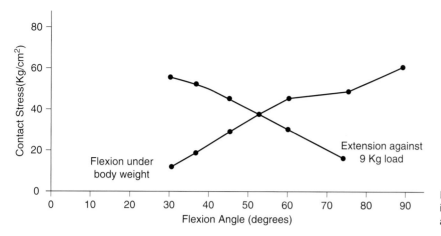

Fig 40-10. Patella femoral contact force increases four fold with leg extension exercises at 30 degrees.

Until now, we have been discussing the biomechanics of normal weight bearing or closed chain activities. With knee extension (open chain) exercises, the patellofemoral contact forces actually increase with extension rather than flexion, due to the application of weight so far from the knee joint and the increase lever arm. The resulting large contact force over the relatively small contact area present during knee extension results in excessive patellofemoral contact pressure (force per unit area). Performing a knee extension exercise at 30 degrees of flexion using a 20 pound weight will result in pressure that is four times that present during physiological loading (15) **(Fig 40-10)**.

Chondromalacia is thought to result from excessive patellofemoral contact pressure. After articular cartilage breakdown occurs, local contact pressure is reduced by up to 90%, resulting in concomitant increase in adjacent contact pressure of 90% (17). This may explain the often rapid progression of chondromalacia after it begins, and provides rationale for recommendation for activity modification for athletes with chondromalacia.

It is helpful to understand the relative patellofemoral forces associated with various activities. Various authors have evaluated these forces, with somewhat different conclusions based on experimental design. Reilly and Martens (18) showed that walking results in a PF force of 0.5 × body weight similar to straight leg raising **(Table 40-1)**. Stair climbing results in a force of 3.3 × body weight, and squatting in a whopping 7.6 × body weight. More recent studies have suggested that squatting may only increase forces to 3 × body weight (4,17,19). Jogging increases PF force to 6 × BW (20) and jumping to 12 × BW (20a).

Patella tracking is dependent upon a multitude of anatomic factors. Static factors include bony anatomy and ligamentous structures. Dynamic factors include muscular interaction and change in anatomical relationships related to range of motion of the knee. Static bony anatomy that contributes to PF stability includes the depth and shape of the trochlea, the shape of the patella, femoral anteversion, and tibial rotation, along with the relative valgus alignment of the femoral-tibial articulation.

TABLE 40-1	Patellofemoral Forces Associated with Physical Activity

BICYCLING: 1.2 × BW[a]
RISING FROM A CHAIR w ARMS: <3 × BW[b]
ISOKINETIC EXERCISES: Kaufman[c]

   60 deg/sec 5.1 BW at 70 deg
   180 deg/sec 4.9 BW at 80 deg

DAHLQUIST [d]

Squat–descent	7.6 BW at 140 deg	
Squat–rise	6.0 BW at 140 deg	

REILY AND MARTENS[e](18–119)

WALKING	0.5 bw	10 DEG
STRAIGHT LEG RAISE	0.5 bw	0 DEG
STAIRS (UP OR DOWN)	3.3 bw	60 DEG
SQUAT	7.6 bw	120 DEG

PF KINEMATICS

CONTRIBUTORS TO P/F STABILITY

[a] Eriscson MO, Nisell R. Tibiofemoral joint forces during ergometer cycling. *Am J Sports Med.* 1986;14(4):285–290
[b] Ellis MI, Sweedhom BB, Wright V. Forces in the knee joint whilst rising from a seated position. *J Biomed Eng.* 1984;6(2):113–120.
[c] Kaufman KR, et al. Dynamic joint forces during knee isokinetic exercise. *Am J Sports Med.* 1991;19(3):305–316.
[d] Dahlkvist NJ, et al. Forces during squatting and rising from a deep squat. *Eng Med.* 1982;11(2):69–76.
[e] Reilly DJ, Martens M. Experimental analysis of the quadriceps force and Patellofemoral joint reaction force for various activities. *Acta Orthop Scan.* 1972;43:126.

The Q angle is defined as the angle between the quadriceps mechanism and the patella tendon and is a helpful measure of patella tracking. The greater the anatomic valgus, or the greater external rotation present in the tibia, the larger the Q angle will be, resulting in laterally directed force vector **(Fig 40-11)**. Normal Q angle is typically considered to be <15 degrees. Increased femoral anteversion will also result in a high Q angle by causing internal rotation of the femur relative to the tibia.

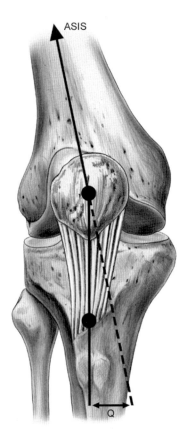

Fig 40-11. The Q angle is a helpful measure of patella tracking. There are differing opinions as to whether the Q angle is best measured in extension, 30 degrees, or 90 degrees of flexion.

From full knee extension to approximately 20 degrees of flexion, the patella rests superior to the trochlea groove, and is stabilized by a combination of ligamentous and muscular forces. Patella stability at this point is determined by overall quadriceps tension, with medial sided stability contributed by Vastus Medialis Obliquos (VMO) contracture and medial patella femoral ligament tension, and lateral stability contributed by the lateral retinaculum. After approximately 25 degrees of flexion, the patella becomes engaged in the trochlea groove and stability is maintained by bony congruity with the trochlea.

■ CONTRIBUTORS TO INSTABILITY

Disruption or distortion of any of the anatomic factors previously mentioned can result in patellofemoral instability.

Trochlea Dysplasia

Trochlea dysplasia is felt to be a contributor to patella instability, but is often difficult to measure accurately. A recent MRI study showed a 100% sensitivity and a 96% specificity when a criteria of <3 mm trochlea depth was utilized as a measurement, done 3 cm above the femorotibial articulation (21). Trochlea dysplasia is rare, and even when present, does

not usually require direct treatment. For patella instability associated with severe trochlea dysplasia, several procedures have been described to deepen the trochlea (trochleoplasty) including osteotomy and elevation of the lateral trochlea with bone grafting (22) or undermining and deepening of the trochlea groove (23). It is our experience that even in the presence of trochlea dysplasia, trochleoplasty is usually not necessary, and the vast majority of patella instability can be managed with either proximal soft tissue realignment, or osteotomy of the tibial tubercle

Medial Patellofemoral Ligament Insufficiency

Numerous studies have shown that the medial patellofemoral ligament (MPFL) is the most important stabilizer of the patella to lateral translation. Hautamaa et al. (24) showed in a cadaver biomechanical study that with serial sectioning, the MPFL contributes 50% of the patellofemoral stability (24) **(Fig 40-12)**. In a similar study, Desio et al. (25) showed that the MPFL contributes 60% of the stability, with the medial patellomeniscal ligament contributing an additional 1%. Clinical studies on patients with patella dislocation also seem to confirm this finding, with both surgical and MRI evidence of disruption of the MPFL after patella dislocation (26–28).

Excessive Femoral Anteversion

An increase in femoral anteversion will result in relative external rotation of the tibia. This will result in an increase in the Q angle and a tendency toward lateral tracking of the patella. Correction of patella malalignment in this situation can theoretically be accomplished through a femoral osteotomy. Because of the obvious invasiveness and risks, however, this procedure is not recommended. Treatment is directed at the relative external rotation of the tibia by osteotomizing the tibial tubercle and moving it medially to decrease the Q angle.

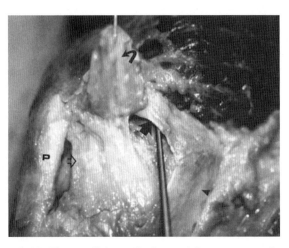

Fig 40-12. The medial patella femoral ligament contributes greater than 50% of the stability of the patella to lateral dislocation.

Excessive Tibial External Rotation

Excessive external rotation of the tibia will result in lateral displacement of the tibial tubercle and an increased Q angle. When felt to be the cause of patella instability, this can be corrected by osteotomy and medialization of the tubercle.

Weak Vastus Medialis Obliquos

The VMO is a distinct muscle grouping of the vastus medialis that has a distinct nerve supply (29) and whose fibers insert into the superior medial aspect of the patella at approximately 65 degrees to the longitudinal axis (16). There can be anatomic variation on the insertion site to the patella. The more medial the insertion, the more of a medial stabilizing effect. A more superior insertion changes the force vector, providing less medial stabilizing force, and may be a contributor to lateral instability. Weakness of the VMO removes a significant dynamic stabilizing influence on the patella. Strengthening of this muscle is an important component of any rehabilitation program. The VMO contracts maximally in the terminal range of extension, and can be best strengthened with terminal, short-arc extension exercises.

■ DIAGNOSING PATELLOFEMORAL PROBLEMS

Identifying the correct diagnosis is critical for the successful treatment of patella problems in the athlete. Typically, all patients complaining of anterior knee symptoms are lumped into a general category by physicians and therapists and treated with a standard, nonspecific, "patellofemoral" protocol. A careful history and physical examination is crucial before an effective focused and specific treatment plan can be initiated.

History

There are important questions that must be asked when evaluating a patient with anterior knee complaints. Important questions along with some common examples are presented as follows.

- Location: Identifying the exact location of symptoms is critical. Inferior pain will suggest patella tendonitis, while proximal pain could indicate quadriceps tendonitis or a partial tear. Superficial pain may suggest prepatella bursitis, or bursal scarring, while deeper pain would suggest an intra-articular etiology such as chondromalacia, a chondral defect of the trochlea, osteochondritis dissecans (OCD) of the patella, or peripatella synovitis.
- Sports History: What activities bring on symptoms? Pain with twisting activities would suggest possible patella instability; pain on stair climbing would suggest chronic myofascial pain [chondromalacia patella (CMP)], and pain with jumping sports would suggest patella tendonitis. Pain with kneeling might suggest prepatella bursitis.
- Duration: Anterior knee pain since adolescence, particularly in a female athlete, would suggest a developmental tracking abnormality. Recent knee pain from a traumatic fall on the patella might suggest a patella chondral defect or occult fracture.
- Timing of Symptoms: Occurs only during repetitive prolonged activity [plica, iliotibial band syndrome (ITBS)]; worse with prolonged sitting? ("movie sign") (CMP); aggravated by stair climbing (CMP); pain immediately upon kneeling (prepatella bursa).
- Past History: A past history of Osgood Schlatters could indicate residual pain from a persistent ossicle at the tibial tubercle. A history of previous patella dislocation might indicate the presence of a loose body, chondral injury, and of course persistent instability. A history of previous knee surgery might suggest painful scar tissue, catching/rubbing of adhesive bands, or scarring of the retropatella fat pad.
- Occupation: Patients who work on their knees such as carpenters and carpet layers often develop prepatella scaring and chronic bursitis.
- Trauma history: Try to elicit past history of seemingly unrelated trauma, such as fractures, leg length discrepancy (overload patella due to asymmetry); angular/rotational deformity (affecting patella alignment); chronic atrophy (weak quadriceps affects patella tracking), blunt trauma, thickened plica; scar; muscular injury (myositis, ossificans, chronic atrophy).
- Sport-specific history: Has there been any change in the frequency or duration of sports activity, such as training errors (excessive increase in mileage causing overuse); recent decrease in sports activity causing atrophy; VMO weakness (any change in equipment used in the patient's sport); new running shoes; change in playing/running surface (concrete vs wood or grass). Is the patient a bicycle rider (cleat position that affects knee rotation and bike frame/seat position that affects PF force); abrupt increased running distance, speed, times per week; or jumping sports, (think of patella tendonitis from overload) **(Fig 40-13)**.

■ PHYSICAL EXAMINATION

The physical examination of the patella is the most important part of the diagnostic workup and unfortunately is rarely performed properly. The first step in the proper evaluation of a patient with anterior knee complaints is to insist that they undress and put on a gown so that a complete examination of the lower extremities can be performed. The knee is a "kinetic chain" and forces on the patella can be dramatically affected by anatomic derangements or asymmetries proximal or distal to the knee.

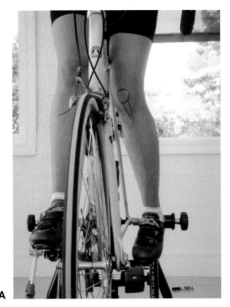
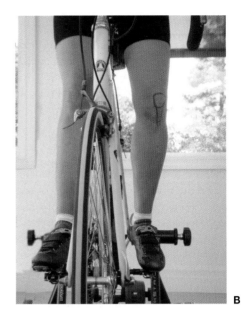

Fig 40-13. Improper bicycle and cleat positioning can cause patella femoral strain. **A:** Internal rotation of the cleat may cause strain to the lateral aspect of the patella femoral joint and the iliotibial band. **B:** External rotation of the cleat may cause strain to the medial aspect of the knee.

Standing Evaluation: Static

The patient must be asked to stand for the initial portion of the examination. Careful assessment of limb alignment and symmetry should be performed. This includes leg length assessment, pelvic balance, Q angle, varus-valgus alignment, knee recurvatum, flexion deformities, and foot position as it interacts with the floor during weight bearing **(Fig 40-14)**.

Limb Length

Limb length asymmetry can lead to excessive force on the anterior knee and is a common source of knee pain in runners due to the repetitive loading involved in this sport. Studies indicate that an asymmetry of up to 1 cm may be normal, but even subtle amounts of asymmetry may lead to problems in runners.

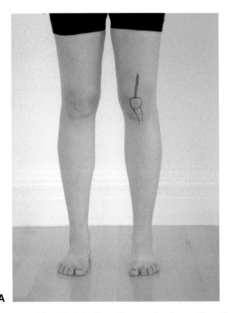
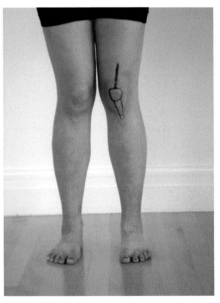

Fig 40-14. Standing evaluation with weight bearing is an important part of the patella examination. **A:** Patient demonstrating normal Q angle and alignment with normal foot pronation. **B:** Same patient showing increased Q angle and altered alignment as foot pronation is increased.

Alignment

Increased valgus knee angulation results in an increase in Q angle and can result in increased pressure on the lateral patella facet. Excessive varus may lead to medial joint overload and possible medial patella plica irritation. ITBS may be more common due to increased tension on the lateral aspect of the knee.

Recurvatum may cause anterior mensical abutment syndrome which can cause pain just medial to the medial border of the patella tendon (30). In addition recurvatum may indicate generalized ligamentous laxity and suggest a patella tracking abnormality.

A flexion deformity causes the patella to be fixed in the trochlea even in the heel strike phase of running resulting in excessive P/F pressure and chondral breakdown.

Measure leg length by assessing pelvic symmetry. A leg length discrepancy will cause an elevated hemi pelvis, a secondary flexible scoliosis, and may be a cause of knee pain in repetitive loading sports, particularly running.

Foot Position: The Role of Orthotics in Treating Patellofemoral Syndrome

Pronation

Excessive pronation of the foot leads to increased valgus of the knee and is thought to be one of the reasons why hyperpronation can cause patellofemoral pain (31–34) **(Fig 40-15)**. Authors have also suggested that prolonged pronation leads to external tibial rotation and thus increases the Q angle through this mechanism (33,34). To the contrary, however, other researchers believe that hyperpronation results in internal rotation of the tibia which would actually decrease the Q angle. Tiberio (35) has explained this

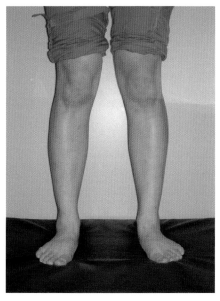

Fig 40-15. Excessive foot pronation can contribute to patella femoral pain.

discrepancy by suggesting that prolonged internal rotation of the tibia leads to compensatory internal rotation of the femur, which results in a secondary, relative increase in lateral tracking of the patella. This theory was also felt to be most plausible by Sims and Cavanagh (36). Another contributing factor is the effect of quadriceps activity during pronation. Electromyographic data show that the quadriceps begin contracting prior to heel strike and continue firing well into midstance, overlapping with the pronation phase of the gait cycle (37). The combination of the lateral tracking caused by pronation along with the increased patella compression associated with the increased quadriceps activity associated with the pronation phase of gait may best explain the deleterious effects of pronation in runners.

Use of Orthotics

Assuming that a relationship exists between excessive pronation and patellofemoral pain, the next controversy addresses the benefit of orthotics in controlling pronation and relieving patella femoral symptoms. A number of studies support the use of orthotics to alter lower extremity mechanics (38–40). James et al. (41) demonstrated that an orthosis corrects pronation in the injured foot to close to that of a normal foot without an orthosis.

Other studies have shown that mean pronation is reduced by a modest 2.5 degrees with the use of rigid orthotics, and only 1 to 2 degrees with semirigid devices (31,42–44). Soft orthotics may not alter maximal pronation at all (43), although other studies suggest that they do (45,46). Soft and semirigid orthotics may actually work by controlling maximal velocity of pronation rather than maximal degree of pronation (43). Although these studies suggest that correction of pronation is possible with an orthotic and that patella pain appears to be relieved by orthotic use in pronation runners, the complete scientific explanation for this effect is still lacking.

The scientific explanation for the association of pronation and patellofemoral pain remains vague; however, the clinical relationship of these two entities is supported by a number of studies.

Lutter (38) found that 77% of knee injuries in runners were associated with an abnormal foot position, of which 43% were hyperpronation. Of those runners with pronation related injuries, 28% had symptoms involving the patella, 15% had medial joint pain, and 57% had diffuse medial knee pain. Gross et al. (47) interviewed 347 runners of whom 12.6% had patellofemoral symptoms. Although data were not presented on the degree of pronation in these patients, 78% reported improvement of other with the use of orthotics. Similar benefits of orthotics have been reported by other authors (48).

More recent studies continue to support the benefit of orthotics to address patellofemoral pain **(Fig 40-16)**. Gross and Foxworth (49) have suggested that patients with patellofemoral pain may benefit from foot orthoses if they

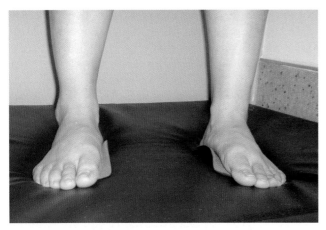

Fig 40-16. Orthotics may benefit patients with a combination of foot pronation and patella femoral symptoms.

also demonstrate signs of excessive foot pronation and/or a lower-extremity alignment profile that includes excessive lower-extremity internal rotation during weight bearing and increased Q angle. The mechanism for foot orthoses having a positive effect on pain and function for these patients may include a reduction in internal rotation of the lower extremity; a reduction in Q angle; reduced laterally directed soft tissue forces from the patellar tendon, the quadriceps tendon, and the iliotibial band; and reduced patellofemoral contact pressures and altered patellofemoral contact pressure mapping. Kuhn et al. (50) have shown that custom flexible orthotics can correct the Q angle in male subjects with hyperpronation. Saxena and Haddad (51) found that 76% of patients with chondromalacia and patellofemoral syndrome had significant improvement in pain after treatment with semirigid orthotics.

In summary, there appears to be satisfactory evidence to implicate hyperpronation as a cause of patellofemoral pain; however, one needs to consider other causes of pain before attributing symptoms to pronation alone. In combination with other treatments, we support the judicious use of semi-rigid orthotics in hyperpronators to relieve patellofemoral pain, and we have had success in our own clinical practice with this approach.

■ BRACING FOR PATELLOFEMORAL PAIN

The benefit of bracing for PF pain and instability is controversial; however, there appears to be good evidence that bracing improves pain for patients with patellofemoral syndrome, even if the brace does not appear to alter the biomechanical load on the patella (52) **(Fig 40-17)**. Another elegant study using dynamic MRI imaging has shown that at least one type of patella brace can objectively improve patella tracking (53). Another interesting study showed that a patella brace could be used prophylactically to prevent patella pain in patients embarking on a rigorous training program (54).

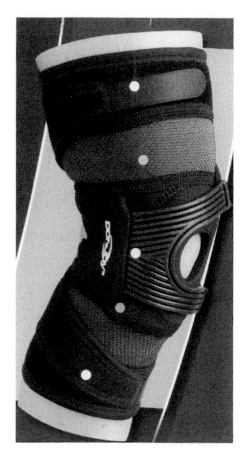

Fig 40-17. Patella bracing appears to benefit some patients with patella femoral pain.

Standing Evaluation: DYNAMIC

Single leg loading
Stresses P/F joint (Pain, crepitus)
Step up / step down

Several simple stress tests can be performed in the office to elicit PF symptoms and confirm a diagnosis of chondromalacia or PF compression syndrome. Have the patient stand on the affected leg and perform a single leg 30-degree knee bend with the examiners hand resting gently on the patella **(Fig 40-18)**. In the presence of chondromalacia, crepitus will be audible as well as palpable. With PF compression syndrome, pain may be elicited with this maneuver in the absence of crepitus. Another version of this stress test is to have the patient step down slowly from a step stool. Eccentric loading of the trailing leg will usually result in pain and crepitus. Concentric loading with a step up maneuver is somewhat less reliable. Unlike meniscal pain, patellofemoral symptoms will usually decrease with deep squatting as the patella disengages from the trochlea in maximal flexion.

Seated Evaluation:

Active ROM
Seated Q angle

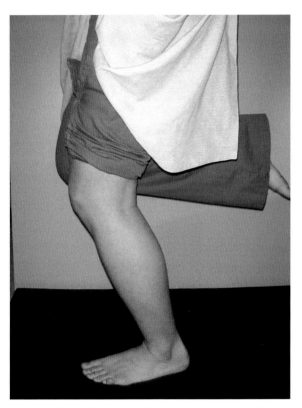

Fig 40-18. Single leg loading is a good stress test for patella femoral compression syndrome and chondromalacia.

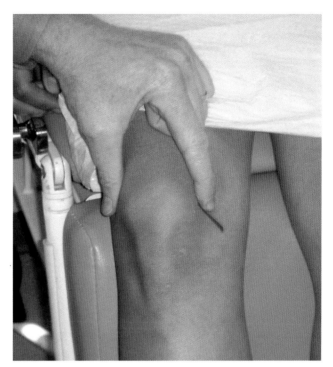

Fig 40-19. Careful examination may reveal a thickened painful plica snapping over the edge of the medial femoral condyle.

Seated evaluation is performed next. Have the patient sit with their legs over the edge of the examination table. Measure the seated "Q" angle, which some authors find more reliable than in the supine position. Have the patient actively extend the knee and evaluate for a "J" sign (a terminal lateral tracking of the patella as the knee approaches full extension). Palpate the patella once again for crepitus with active knee extension. This may be caused by articular cartilage irregularity similar to the crepitus elicited during single knee loading, or occasionally by lateral compression and pinching of synovium between the patella and lateral trochlea edge, resulting in "synovial crepitus" and pain that is localized laterally. With the patient in the seated position, the examiner should passively flex and extend the knee while palpating along the edge of the medial femoral condyle to evaluate for a symptomatic painful plica **(Fig 40-19)**.

Supine Evaluation: Passive

Inspection
Q angle
Swelling
Effusion
Old scars
Osgood Schlatters
Passive Rom (including hyperextension vs opp knee !!!)

Now have the patient lay supine. Measure the Q angle in this position. Measure leg length again from the anterior superior iliac spine (ASIS) to the medial mallelolus. Compare this to the standing assessment to determine if a true leg length discrepancy exists. Although standing assessment of leg length may be confused by associated scoliosis, muscular spasm, and posture, supine evaluation tends to eliminate the influence of these factors.

The knee should then be examined for a joint effusion. A fluid wave will indicate a small effusion (20 cc) while a bollatabel patella will suggest a more significant effusion (2,6,11,48,55–61).

Careful evaluation should be made of the prepatella tissues. Acute prepatella bursitis is easy to diagnose with swelling warmth and occasional erythema. A more subtle cause of prepatella symptoms may be due to scarring to the prepatella bursa resulting in thickened fibrous bands within the bursa that remain intermittently painful with direct loading activities such as kneeling.

Localized palpation should be performed over the bursa attempting to roll the thickened band under the examiner's finger which will recreate the patient's complaints.

The patella tendon is another source of potential pain and needs to be carefully evaluated. Inspection will usually reveal any evidence of old Osgood Schlatter's syndrome with obvious prominence of the tibial tubercle. Tenderness over the tubercle and occasionally a mobile painful ossicle will confirm the diagnosis **(Fig 40-20)**. Although most adults are not symptomatic from this entity, occasionally an old ossicle can reactivate and become symptomatic and needs to be kept in the differential of patella pain.

Patella tendonitis is best evaluated in the supine position. With the quadriceps relaxed, the examiner displaces the

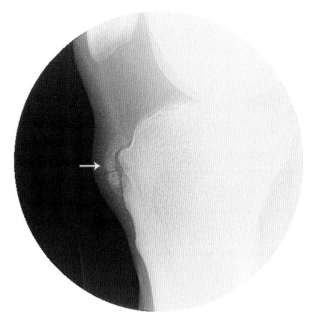

Fig 40-20. An old Osgood Schlatter's ossicle may become painful in adulthood.

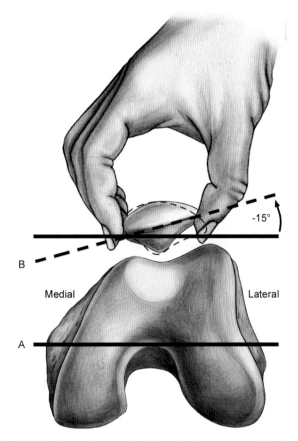

Fig 40-21. A positive patella tilt test is defined as inability to lift the lateral facet of the patella more than 15 degrees (or to neutral) and indicates a tight lateral retinaculum.

patella distally delivering the inferior pole of the patella to more direct examination. Direct palpation over the inferior pole of the patella will cause exquisite tenderness in patients with patella tendonitis. The findings must be compared to the opposite knee, however, because some discomfort during this maneuver is normal. A similar examination can be performed on the superior pole of the patella to rule out the much less common quadriceps tendonitis. In this case, the examiner displaces the patella proximally and palpates along the superior border of the patella.

The knee must also be inspected for old surgical scars. Peri patella pain can easily be caused by iatrogenic reasons. Some of the more common iatrogenic causes are scarring from an old arthroscopy portal that snaps against the edge of the patella tendon, saphenous neuroma (old meniscal repair incisions, ACL incisions), and retained hardware or sutures.

Instability Exam

The first step in evaluating a patient for instability is to inspect the knee during standing. Valgus alignment, foot pronation, and the presence of "squinting" patellae should be noted. The Q angle is an essential measurement for evaluating instability. Measurement is made from the ASIS to the center of the patella, and from the center of the patella to the tibial tubercle. This angle should be evaluated in extension as well as at 30 degrees and seated at 90 degrees. There is controversy regarding which evaluation is most useful, and there is significant intraobserver error reported (49). In my practice, the 0 and 30 degree Q angle is most helpful.

The lateral retinaculum is then assessed for tightness. If the examiner cannot lift the lateral edge of the patella 15 degrees, the patella tilt test is positive and indicates a

tight lateral retinaculum. The examiner should also attempt to translate the patella medially. Movement of less than 15 mm indicates a tight lateral retinaculum **(Fig 40-21)**.

Laxity of the medial retinaculum is then assessed by lateral translation of the patella and is compared to the opposite knee. Translation of more than 50% of the width of the patella is a sign of instability especially if this excursion is greater than the opposite knee. Subjective apprehension on the part of the patient with this maneuver indicates a positive "apprehension test" and also suggests instability.

The J sign indicates the presence of severe lateral translation of the patella in terminal extension of the knee and suggests instability. The patient is asked to actively extend the knee against gravity. As the patella disengages from the trochlea it jumps laterally making an inverted J.

Diagnosis: Imaging Studies

The standard evaluation of patients with patellofemoral symptoms will include an AP, lateral, and a 45-degree tangential view of the patella (referred to as a Merchant view) **(Fig 40-22)**. The AP view is rarely helpful but will reveal the presence of a bipartite patella or a patella fracture. The lateral view is useful to evaluate for loose bodies and patella alta or baja and will reveal the presence of early degenerative

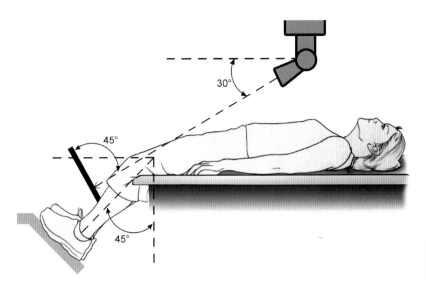

Fig 40-22. The 45 degree patella femoral view (*Merchant view*) is an extremely useful x-ray in evaluating the patella femoral joint.

changes with inferior or superior patella osteophytes. The lateral view will also reveal calcification or traction spurs associated with chronic patella/quadriceps tendonitis, and will demonstrate irregularity of the tibial tubercle associated with Osgood Schlatters disease. Trochlea depth and dysplasia may also be determined on the lateral view (62) **(Fig 40-23)**, although there is poor reproducibility and inter-observer reliability (63).

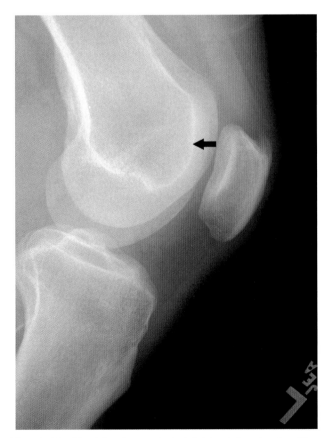

Fig 40-23. The lateral x-ray is helpful to determine trochlear depth (*see arrow*).

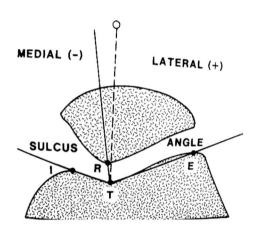

Fig 40-24. The congruence angle is one of the most useful measurements of patella alignment, and is measured by the difference between the angles formed by the bisector of the sulcus angle and a line from the apex of the sulcus angle to the central ridge. The more lateral, or positive, the angle, the greater the malalignment.

The Merchant view is useful to evaluate patella alignment. Various measurements can be performed on this x-ray that are useful in assessing patella tracking, including the congruence angle, tilt angle, and lateral translation **(Fig 40-24)**.

MRI evaluation has not been useful for the evaluation of patellofemoral complaints, although recent advances may make this test more valuable. Better magnets and enhanced cartilage imaging techniques have improved the ability of the MRI to pick up subtle changes of chondromalacia in the patella and trochlea **(Fig 40-25)**, and dynamic MRI evaluation is becoming available to evaluate patella tracking. At this time, however, MRI is not typically helpful for the diagnosis of patella instability, except in acute cases of patella dislocation where disruption of the medial patellofemoral ligament can be demonstrated. MRI findings also do not seem to correlate well to clinical findings

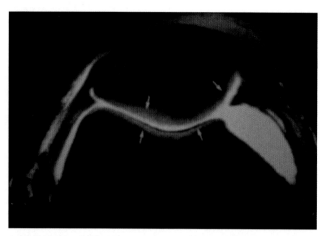

Fig 40-25. Newer MRI technology is improving the ability to image chondromalacia changes.

of patella tendonitis (64) or Plica syndrome (65). CAT scanning is occasionally useful to evaluate the patellofemoral joint in various degrees of flexion, when the standard 45 degree Merchant view does not demonstrate anticipated malalignment (66) **(Fig 40-26A)**.

Bone Scan

Scintigraphic evaluation can be a useful method to evaluate patients with patellofemoral pain (57) (Fig 40-26), although the findings are often nonspecific (67). Single photon emission computed tomography (CT) may be more sensitive and more accurate in localization of pathology (68). Bone scanning may be most useful in the diagnosis of complex regional pain syndrome (RSD) (69,70) or to identify malingerers **(Fig 40-27)**.

Other Diagnostic Testing

Injection

Judicious use of injections of xylocaine can be very helpful in localizing nonspecific knee pain. Occasionally, patients will have difficulty differentiating prepatella from retropatella pain. An intra-articular injection will help the patient differentiate the source of the pain. Similarly a localized injection into a painful area of prepatella bursal scar, or a painful arthroscopy portal can be quite useful. Other uses of a localized xylocaine injection include diagnosis of a saphenous.

Taping

When doubt exists regarding the presence of lateral patella compression syndrome (LPCS), a useful test to confirm the diagnosis is temporary patella taping **(Fig 40-28)**. A decrease in anterior knee pain should occur during squatting and stair climbing in response to taping to medialize the patella and will help confirm the diagnosis.

Taping appears to work by improving medial patella glide as a short term diagnostic tool, and has been shown to be of benefit before, but not after exercise (71) and may in fact only work by pain modulation from cutaneous stimulation (72).

■ PATELLA INSTABILITY

An acute dislocation of the patella may be described as a primary disruption of the patellofemoral relationship, where the patella is displaced out of the femoral sulcus. The direction of dislocation is most commonly lateral, although superior (73), medial (74), intra-articular (73), and vertical intercondylar (75) have also been described.

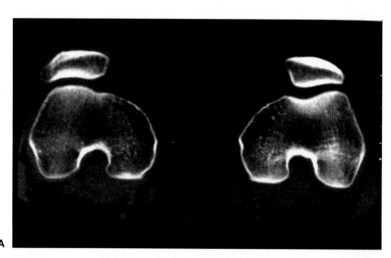

A

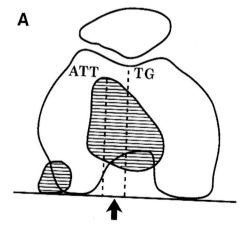

A

B

Fig 40-26. (A) CT scanning is useful to evaluate patella tracking in varying degrees of extension, and **(B)** may be used as an objective way to measure the true relationship of the tibial tubercle (*TT*) to the trochlear groove (*TG*), which is more accurate than the Q angle, using the TT-TG distance (abnormal is >15 mm).

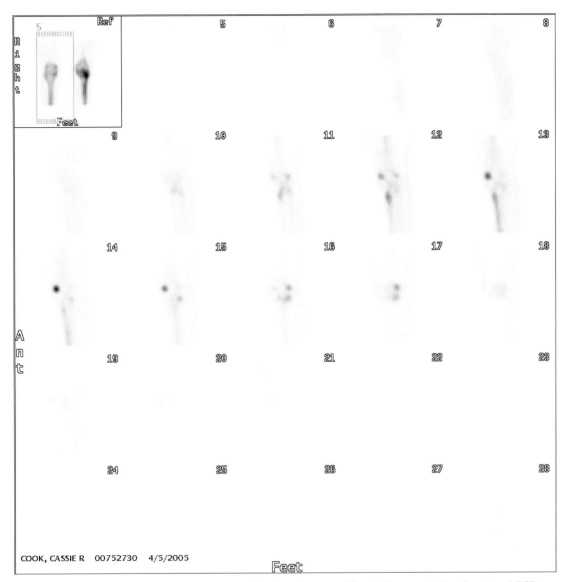

Fig 40-27. Bone scan may be useful in the evaluation of nonspecific patella complaints or to rule out RSD.

This chapter will deal only with the most common lateral patella dislocation **(Fig 40-29)**.

Acute Lateral Patella Dislocation

The incidence of acute dislocation of the patella is difficult to accurately assess and has only been addressed in a few studies. McManus et al. (76) reviewed the records of 94,875 pediatric visits to their emergency room over a 4-year period and found some evidence of patella dislocation in 55 (0.05%), although only 33 (0.03%) could be proven to be acute dislocations. Cash and Hughston (77) reported treating 399 patients with this disorder over a 30-year period (13.3 patients yearly). Castelyn and Handelberg (78) reported an incidence of acute patella dislocation of 2.44% in their series of knee injuries. More recently, Nietosvaara et al. (79) reported an incidence of acute patellar dislocation in 43 of 100, 000 adolescents per year (.04%).

Most reports in the literature agree that acute patella dislocation occurs in a young population, with an average age of approximately twenty most commonly reported (76,77); however, within this group, the incidence of redislocation appears to be significantly higher in patients who sustain their first dislocation at an earlier age (33,77). Although earlier studies suggested that females appeared to be at a higher risk for both acute and recurrent dislocation (33,80,81), more recent data suggest that the gender incidence may be equal (82).

The natural history of acute dislocation has been addressed in a number of studies. Hawkins (83) treated 20 patients conservatively (3 weeks of immobilization). At 40 months of average follow-up, 3 had redislocated (15%), 4 had apprehension or complaints of instability (20%), and 15 had pain associated with patellofemoral crepitis. Remarkably, 100% were able to return to work and recreational sports. Cofield (80) studied 48 patients with acute dislocations treated

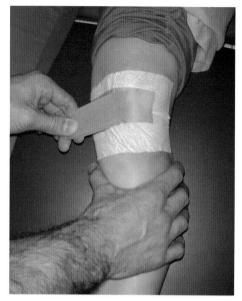

Fig 40-28. Patella taping can help temporarily relieve pain associated with lateral patella femoral compression syndrome.

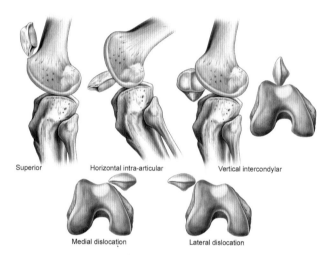

Superior   Horizontal intra-articular   Vertical intercondylar

Medial dislocation   Lateral dislocation

Fig 40-29. Five types of patella dislocation: **A:** Superior; patella caught on anterior femoral osteophyte. **B:** Horizontal intra-articular. **C:** Vertical intercondylar. **D:** medial. **E:** Lateral, most common type.

conservatively (closed reductions and immobilization for 1 to 6 weeks). Forty-four percent redislocated and 27% went on to need subsequent surgery. If subjective criteria are included, 52% were considered failures.

McManus et al. (76) reviewed 28 patients with acute dislocations: 21 were treated without surgery. Five patients redislocated and 11 were considered symptomatic. Cash Hughston (77) reported a redislocation rate of 20% to 43% among first time dislocators treated with immobilization alone, with the rate depending upon the presence of congenital predisposition (patellofemoral dysplasia). In a more recent study of 74 acute patella dislocations, Atkin et al. (82) reported that 58% of patients were still symptomatic during strenuous activities, at an early follow up of months (82). Review of the literature suggests that the natural history

of acute patellofemoral dislocation is that of a high percentage of redislocation (20% to 40%) and continued symptoms.

■ DIAGNOSIS

History

The diagnosis of acute dislocation of the patella is not difficult if the patella is acutely dislocated at the time of presentation; however, if the patella spontaneously reduces, the diagnosis may be difficult. The patient will often report that their knee gave way or "popped out of place" during a twisting activity. The patient may give a history of previous subluxation episodes or a history of dislocation of the opposite knee. Patients with generalized hyperlaxity may give a history of shoulder or ankle instability.

Understanding the mechanism of injury may be helpful in determining the diagnosis. Two mechanisms for acute lateral patella dislocation have been proposed—direct and indirect. The indirect mechanism of injury results from a powerful quadriceps contracture against an internally rotated femur (externally rotated tibia) and usually involves a sudden twisting motion on a firmly planted foot, such as a sudden change of direction playing soccer with cleats. The direct mechanism of dislocation involves a direct blow to the medial aspect of the patella, resulting from a fall or contact with another player during sports activity. A combination of these two mechanisms may contribute to a single injury **(Fig 40-30)**.

Physical Examination

Confusion with an ACL tear is common. The patient will usually present with a large hemarthrosis and will be tender to palpation along the medial retinaculum. There may also be tenderness along the lateral trochlea and medial patella from direct contact and shearing forces during the relocation phase of the injury. Often, however, the pain may be diffuse, and the diagnosis will remain in doubt. Demonstration of a hemarthrosis by needle aspiration, associated with tenderness along the medial retinaculum and subjective apprehension with lateral translation of the patella will help suggest the diagnosis. In the case of an osteochondral fracture, marrow fat globules may be evident in the knee aspirate.

Imaging

Radiographs are often normal with spontaneously reduced dislocations; however, the radiographs will be helpful if they reveal an osteochondral fracture fragment from the medial patella facet or lateral trochlea. An avulsion fracture of the retinaculum off the medial border of the patella is even more diagnostic. Teittge (84) suggested the use of an axial oblique view to better visualize this avulsion. The incidence of chondral and osteochondral fracture is up to 46% of patients with

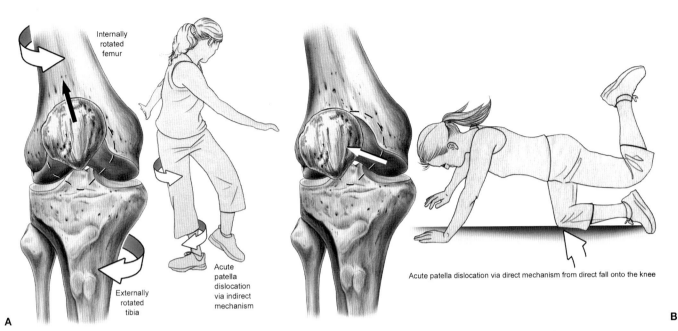

Fig 40-30. There are two mechanisms for acute patella dislocation. **A:** Indirect mechanism. Powerful quadriceps contracture imposed on an internally rotated femur (externally rotated tibia). **B:** Direct mechanism; direct blow to medial aspect of patella, usually by a direct fall onto the knee.

acute patella dislocation (85), although most of these are only visible by arthroscopic and MRI evaluation. Occasionally, the diagnosis can only be made by the demonstration of a torn medial retinaculum as seen by MRI **(Fig 40-31)**. In several studies, MRI was felt to be diagnostic in 81% to 87% of cases, while surgical evaluation was

diagnostic in confirming a torn medial retinaculum in 94% to 100% of cases (26–28).

Radiographs may also be helpful in revealing patella alta or dysplasia of the patella or trochlea.

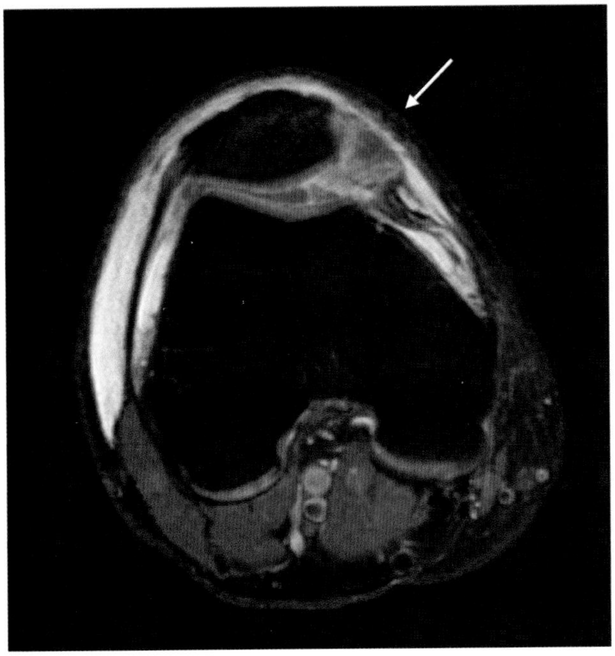

■ ACUTE DISLOCATION OF THE PATELLA

Nonoperative Treatment

The traditional treatment for acute patella dislocation has been nonoperative, although the exact method of treatment is controversial. Most studies in the literature recommend some sort of immobilization followed by an aggressive rehabilitation program (77,80,83); however, the benefit of immobilization following patellar dislocation has not been proven, and results after immobilization and early range of motion appear to be the same (77,80). Furthermore, there does not seem to be a correlation between length of immobilization and results (77,80,83).

Long-term results suggest that the natural history of nonoperative treatment of patellar instability is not as favorable as is commonly thought. In a group of 20 patients with acute dislocations treated conservatively, Hawkins et al. (83) reported a 20% incidence of ongoing instability, and a 15% incidence of pain and crepitus. In their series of 48 patients with acute dislocations, Cofield and Bryan (80) reported a 44% incidence of redislocation; 27% of these patients went on to subsequent surgery and, taking into account subjective criteria, 52% were considered failures.

Fig 40-31. MRI appearance of a torn medial retinaculum following a patella dislocation.

In 21 patients treated nonoperatively, McManus et al. (76) reported 5 redislocations and 11 patients who remained symptomatic. Cash and Hughston (77) reported a redislocation rate of 20% to 43% depending on anatomic evidence of dysplasia predisposing to instability.

Operative Treatment

With the advent of less invasive methods of treatment, and with more critical review of the results of nonoperative treatment, more authors are recommending surgical treatment (27,81,86,87).

Relative indications for surgical treatment of an acute patella dislocation include failure of conservative treatment, the presence of an osteochondral fracture (loose body), recurring instability, and significant residual malalignment on a postreduction Merchant view radiograph.

Arthroscopy

When surgery is selected as the treatment option, initial arthroscopic evaluation is recommended to confirm the diagnosis and address any loose chondral or ostechondral fractures. The exact method of stabilization is controversial, and numerous procedures have been advocated, both open and arthroscopic.

Lateral Release

Various surgical techniques have been proposed to correct patellar instability. Lateral release alone has been described, although results have been mixed, with a high incidence of recurring instability (88–90). Lateral release alone does not address the disrupted anatomy of the medial retinaculum and is not considered by most authors to be an effective treatment for true patellar instability or malalignment (subluxation) (91).

Medial Retinacular Repair and Reefing

When surgery is indicated for patellar instability, most authors have recommended some sort of proximal soft-tissue realignment. Complex surgical recommendations such as the extensive open reconstruction as described by Insall et al. (92) have fallen out of favor, and minimally invasive open procedures for direct anatomic repair of the medial retinaculum and medial patellofemoral ligament have become the preferred method of repair (87) **(Fig 40-32)**. Several arthroscopically assisted procedures have also been reported (93–95), as well as an all-inside arthroscopic method (85), which is our preferred technique at this time.

Whether to add a lateral release at the time of medial repair is controversial. Several authors routinely perform a lateral release at the time of medial repair (87) while others have shown no advantage to adding a lateral release (28) or individualize the decision based on tightness of the lateral

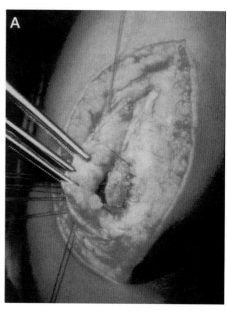

Fig 40-32. Extensive open reconstructions for patella dislocation have fallen out of favor due to higher risk of associated complications.

retinaculum (85). Our current recommendation is to base the decision on the tightness of the lateral retinaculum at the time of surgery, with a tendency toward recommending the lateral release if there is any doubt. An overly tight lateral retinaculum will inhibit proper realignment despite medial reefing, especially in more chronic cases of recurring instability.

Distal bony realignment procedures are reserved for patients with severe cases of malalignment, recurring instability, and a high Q angle, or for patients who have failed previous proximal soft-tissue realignments.

Arthroscopically Assisted Proximal Realignment

Initial recommendations for arthroscopic patella realignment consisted primarily of arthroscopically assisted techniques using a medial incision. Yamamoto (95) treated 30 acute patella dislocations with arthroscopic lateral release along with an arthroscopically assisted repair of the medial retinaculum. He recommended the transcutaneous passage of sutures through the retinaculum using a large curved needle, although the sutures were still tied through a medial skin incision. Only acute dislocations were treated. Reported results were excellent, with only one reported case of redislocation.

Small (94) reported a modified version of the Yamamoto technique, also utilizing an arthroscopically assisted method and a small medial incision **(Fig 40-33)**. Patients with acute and recurrent dislocations were included as well as patients with malalignment and subluxation. Results were good to excellent in 92.5% of their 24 patients (27 knees) according

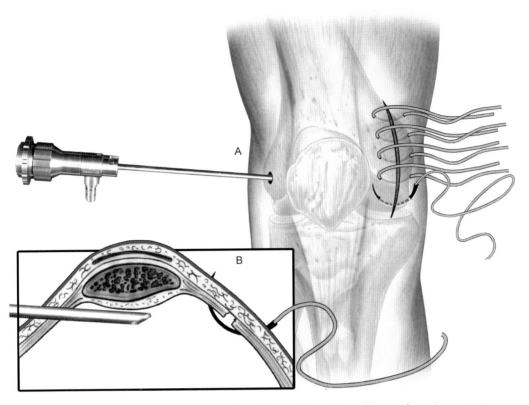

Fig 40-33. Arthroscopically assisted patella realignment is performed by passing sutures percutaneously and then making an incision to tie the sutures.

to a subjective questionnaire. There were two recurrent subluxations, one reoperation for arthrofibrosis, and one superficial infection.

Henry and Pflum (93) described an arthroscopically assisted technique using cannulated needles, but tied the sutures through a medial incision as well. No follow-up series or results were reported.

All-Arthroscopic Proximal Realignment

A number of authors have described entirely arthroscopic proximal realignment procedures, with good results (87,96–98). The author's technique for arthroscopic realignment is presented as follows, and our preferred method of treatment for patients with patella instability.

Surgical Technique: Arthroscopic Patella Realignment

Surgery is performed under general anesthesia with a thigh holder in place. A tourniquet is applied but rarely inflated. Before plication, a healing response is created along the medial retinaculum by gently shaving with a whisker blade **(Fig 40-34)** (Oratec, Menlo Park, CA).

Medial retinacular sutures are introduced percutaneously using an epidural needle (Tuohy Needle; Rusch, Deluth, GA). An epidural needle is essential because of the noncutting edge

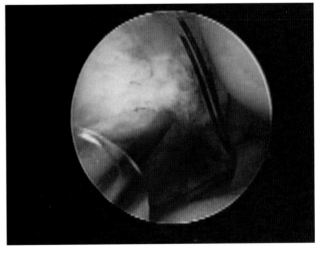

Fig 40-34. A healing response is created along the medial capsule in the area of the MPFL using a whisker blade.

on the inner bevel of the tip that prevents cutting of the suture. The needle is placed adjacent to the patella and a No. 1 PDS suture is passed manually through the needle and retrieved arthroscopically through an accessory superolateral portal **(Figs 40-35** and **40-36)**.

The needle is gently withdrawn from the retinaculum but not out of the skin. The needle is then redirected subcutaneously approximately 2 to 3 cm posteriorly and reinserted

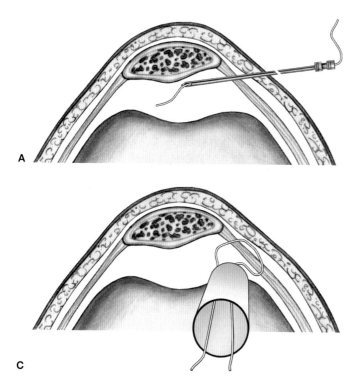

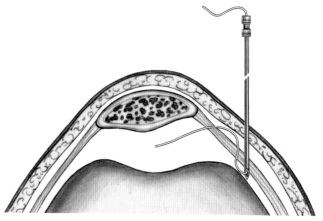

Fig 40-35. The authors preferred method of patella realignment is entirely arthroscopic. Sutures are inserted percutaneously, and tied arthroscopically avoiding an incision. **(A)** Percutaneous insertion of a #1 PDS suture **(B)**. Needle withdrawn to level of retinaculum and re-inserted **(C)**. Both limbs of suture withdrawn through accessory portal and tied arthroscopically.

through the retinaculum again. This creates a loop of suture that is retrieved again through the same accessory portal. The needle is then withdrawn completely and the process repeated until four to five sutures are in place. The sutures are retrieved through an accessory proximal lateral portal and clamped for later imbrication of the medial retinaculum. An arthroscopic lateral release is then performed with a standard electrocautery device. After the lateral release, the medial sutures are tied inside the joint from either the proximal lateral portal or the anteromedial portal using standard arthroscopic knot-tying techniques **(Fig 40-35C)**.

Rehab

Postoperative treatment involves a brace locked in full extension for 1 week, followed by physical therapy for 2 to 3 months. After the first week, the brace is unlocked to enable patients to begin range of motion exercises, but bracing is continued for 3 to 4 weeks until quadriceps strength returns. Patients are not allowed to flex past 90 degrees for 4 weeks, but may begin weight bearing immediately in the brace.

Results

In a recent review of our 5 year results (96), 93% of patients reported significant subjective improvement. The average Lysholm score improved from 41.5 to 79.3 ($P < .05$). Preoperative and postoperative radiographs were measured for congruence angle, lateral patellofemoral angle, and lateral patella displacement, and all showed significant

improvement postoperatively ($P < .05$) (Fig 40-36). There were no complications and no redislocations. Patients reported a significant improvement in pain, swelling, stair climbing, crepitus, and ability to return to sports ($P < .05$). Although the average Q angle in our study was 11 degrees, we have successfully performed this procedure on patients with Q angles up to 17 degrees. None of our patients required a second operation for debridement of scar tissue or manipulation. All patients regained full range of motion as compared with the opposite side.

Although we prefer an all arthroscopic method of proximal realignment, open and arthroscopically assisted proximal realignment procedures can also be effective in preventing recurring instability; however, these procedures are more frequently accompanied by the risk of joint stiffness and scar tissue.

■ RECURRING PATELLA INSTABILITY

The treatment for recurring instability of the patella may differ from the treatment of an acute initial dislocation. Recurring instability may indicate a severe underlying anatomical dysplasia or predisposition that may require more aggressive treatment such as osteotomy of the tibial tubercle or rarely the trochlea. In addition, patients with recurring disability may have damaged their MPFL to such a degree that a soft tissue reconstruction or augmentation is necessary. Decision making is complex in these cases and takes into account Q angle, anatomic valgus of

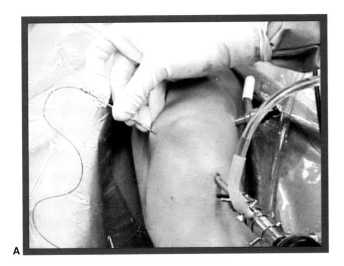

A

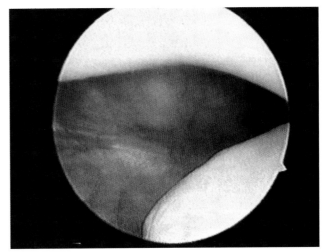

B

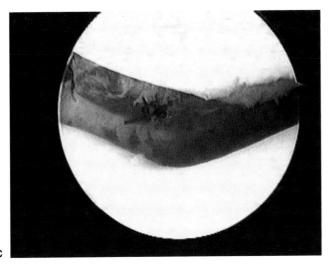

C

Fig 40-36. A: Intra-operative view of percutaneous insertion of suture. B: Appearance of patella prior to arthroscopic realignment. C: Appearance after realignment.

the knee, tibial tubercle external rotation, integrity of the MPFL, trochlea dysplasia, and history of previous surgical procedures.

Author's Recommendations

If the Q angle is less than 20 degrees, and the MPFL is intact, a proximal imbrication of the medial retinaculum is indicated along with release of a contracted lateral retinaculum, if present, similar to the treatment for acute dislocation previously described. This may be performed either open, or arthroscopically, depending upon the surgeon's preference. Some authors suggest adding a slight VMO advancement (91), although we have not found this necessary.

For skeletally immature patients regardless of the severity of the dysplasia, a soft tissue procedure is indicated rather than a bony procedure to avoid damage to the growth plate. In mild cases, a medial imbrication is appropriate. In severe cases, or for a failed imbrication, a semitendinosis transfer (Galeazzi procedure) (99), or reconstruction (100,101) may be warranted.

For adults with a more severe Q angle with dramatic external tibial torsion or femoral anteversion, a distal realignment with medialization of the tibial tubercle is appropriate. When both instability as well as chodral damage to the patella is present, a combined anteromedialization of the tubercle may be indicated, as described by Fulkerson (91) to both realign as well as biomechanically unload the patella (Fig 40-37). A trochlea osteotomy is rarely indicated, but should be considered in cases of failed previous realignment surgery with documented trochlea dysplasia. Care must be taken in placing too much emphasis on radiographic demonstration of trochlea dyplasia. Although some authors claim a correlation between radiographically demonstrated dysplasia and risk of dislocation (77,81), numerous other authors have attempted to correlate radiographic dysplasia to recurring dislocation and prognosis without success (33,82,83,102,103).

Reconstruction of the MPFL is an appropriate consideration for severe cases of recurring instability when the MPFL is attenuated (101,104) (Fig 40-38). Trochleoplasty has been described to deepen the trochlea by either undermining the

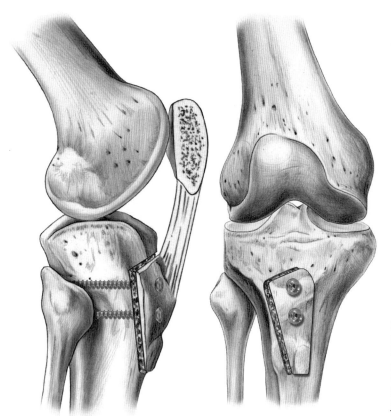

A

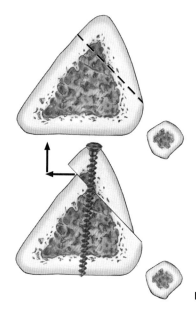

B

Fig 40-37. Tibial tubercle osteotomy technique as described by Fulkerson et al. The tubercle is shifted both medially **(A)** as well as anteriorly **(B)** by making an oblique cut. (From Fulkerson JP, Cautilli RA. Chronic patella instability: Subluxation and dislocation. In: Fox JM, Del Pizzo W, eds. *The patellofemoral joint.* New York: McGraw-Hill; 1993;135–147; with permission.

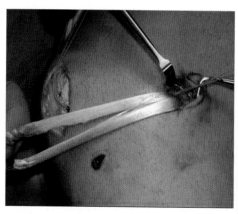

Fig 40-38. Reconstruction of the MPFL may be indicated for severe cases of instability when inadequate native tissue remains. Use of a hamstring allograft through minimal incisions can be very effective. (From Davis DK, Fithian DC. Techniques of medial retinacular repair and reconstruction. *Clin Orthop.* 2002;402:38–52 and Fithian D. Reconstruction of the medial Patellofemoral ligament (MPFL): relevant anatomy, indications, technique and rehabilitation. Washington, DC: AAOS Instructional Course; Feb 2005; with permission.)

sulcus, (23,105) or by osteotomizing and elevating the lateral trochlea wall (106); however, very little literature is available to determine the long term effect of these procedures, and there are biomechanical concerns that these procedures may increase contact pressure along the lateral facet of the patella (106). A recent study has shown poor clinical results with trochleoplasty, despite improvement in trochlea depth (107).

■ ANTERIOR KNEE PAIN

Patellofemoral Pain

Patellofemoral pain is the most common presenting complaint to the orthopedist's office and outnumbers the presentation of a PCL tear by 500:1 (108); however, the exact etiology of pain from patella femoral disorders is controversial. Cartilage is aneural and is not in itself a source of pain (58). Chondromalacia is present in 40% to 60% of patients at autopsy, and 20% to 50% at arthrotomy for other reasons (108); however, most often the area of chondromalacia is asymptomatic.

The most commonly accepted theory for pain related to chondromalacia is that there is abnormal pressure transmitted to the underlying nerve-rich subchondral bone through the area of injured cartilage (109); however, venous congestion in the subchondral bone as been proposed as an alternative theory, and has been proposed as the reason for success resulting from subchondral bone drilling (109).

In patients with patellofemoral pain, but normal appearing articular cartilage, it has been suggested that the pain results from inflamed synovium (58) or abnormal horizontal stresses from malalignment and resulting shear stress transmitted to the underlying subchondral bone (110).

In patients with pain associated with malalignment, the lateral retinaculum itself may be the source of pain, with demonstrated presence of fibroneuromatous degeneration and perineural fibrosus present on histologic evaluation of patients with patella pain at the time of lateral release (111).

Definitions

One of the frustrating aspects of evaluating and treating anterior knee pain is the confusing terminology in the literature. Patella femoral pain syndrome has been used as a catchall phrase for anterior knee pain. This phrase is nonspecific and will not be used in this chapter. Anterior knee pain has multiple specific causes and we will attempt to address these causes specifically.

A brief glossary of terminology will be helpful:

Patellofemoral pain syndrome: A nonspecific and generalized term for anterior knee pain.

Chondromalacia patella: A specific pathological term referring to articular cartilage damage.

Patella malalignment: A general term intended to indicate a disturbance in the articulation between the patella and trochlea. This term has been utilized to describe such disparate conditions as patella tilt, lateral tracking, subluxation, and dislocation.

Patella subluxation: Refers very specifically to lateral translation and instability of the patella without gross dislocation.

Patella instability: A general term that may suggest any subjective sense of patella instability, including subluxation or dislocation, or giving way due to chondromalacia.

Patella dislocation: A specific indication of actual complete dislocation of the patella.

Lateral patella compression syndrome: A specific entity referring to increased pressure along the lateral patella facet often associated with lateral patella tilt and a tight lateral retinaculum.

Patella hypertension or pressure syndrome: A specific entity that requires the presence of patella pain associated with a demonstrated increase in intraosseous patella pressure.

Other Causes of Anterior Knee Pain:

Prepatella bursitis
Patella tendonitis
Quadriceps tendonitis
Reflex sympathetic dystrophy (i.e., complex regional pain syndrome)
Infra-patella fat pad syndrome
Anterior meniscal impingement
Osgood Schlatters
Saphenous neuroma
Plica syndrome

Other chapters in this book will address overuse injuries and tendonitis conditions about the knee. The remainder of this chapter will focus on some of the other common causes of anterior knee pain related to the patella femoral articulation.

Lateral Patella Compression Syndrome

One of the most common causes of anterior knee pain is lateral patella compression syndrome (LPSC). This syndrome was originally described by Ficat in 1975 (112) and refers to excess pressure along the lateral facet of the patella, usually associated with a tight lateral retinaculum and radiographic evidence of patella tilt **(Fig 40-39)**.

This diagnosis should not be used in patients with actual lateral translation of the patella out of the trochlea groove, which is a sign of subluxation and is treated differently.

History

Patients will present with complaints of pain rather than instability. The pain often presents as a localized ache occurring after patella loading activities such as hiking, climbing, or running. Additional symptoms occur as the condition worsens. Chronic LPCS may lead to chondromalacia and crepitus often associated with a joint effusion following activities. The join effusion is most likely related to the breakdown and release of small particles of articular cartilage into the joint. A popliteal cyst will often occur as a result of the effusion and may be the presenting complaint in some patients. Many patients are unaware of the presence of crepitus and have a joint effusion as their first presenting complaint rather than pain or crepitation.

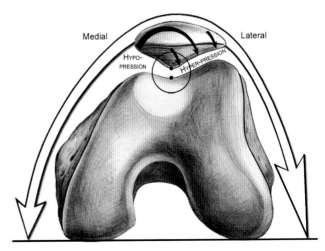

Fig 40-39. Lateral patella compression syndrome as originally described by Ficat in 1975 showing "hyper-pression" on the lateral patella facet. (From Ficat P, Ficat J, Bailleux A. Syndrome d'hyperpression externe de la rotule (SHPE). *Rev Chir Orthop.* 1975;61:39; with permission.)

Physical Exam

Patients with LPCS will often demonstrate foot pronation on standing evaluation. Q angle may be increased but is often normal. ITB is usually tight, and the lateral retinaculum must be tight by definition to cause lateral patella tilt. The patella will demonstrate a negative passive patella tilt test [the examiner will be unable to elevate the lateral facet of the patella at least to neutral (Fig 40-21)] and a medial patella glide of less than two quadrants (113). Lateral translation of the patella will reveal a stable MPFL with no apprehension sign. Medial translation of the patella should be at least one finger breadth (15 mm) in a normal knee. Anything less than this represents a tight lateral retinaculum (114).

Manual palpation over the patella will demonstrate crepitus with active range of motion of the knee when chondromalacia is present. Manual compression of the patella into the trochlea will often exacerbate the pain.

There may be tenderness over the lateral facet of the patella and along the lateral retinaculum in patients who are acutely inflamed.

Radiographs

A 45-degree tangential view of the patellofemoral joint will usually demonstrate patella tilt with a decreased lateral patellofemoral angle (Fig 40-40). Other signs that may present on this simple tangential view are increased subchondral sclerosis of the lateral facet as a result of chronic excess pressure and occasionally a traction osteophyte along the lateral facet.

CT, MRI

Rarely, a flexed knee CT scan may be necessary to demonstrate tilt in lesser degrees of knee flexion (115); however, in clinical practice this is rarely necessary. MRI is not usually

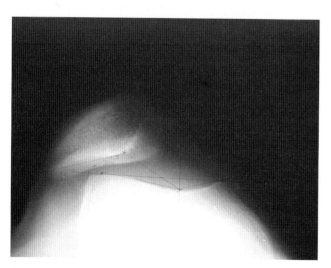

Fig 40-40. Merchant view of the patella showing severe lateral patella tilt.

helpful in making this diagnosis since the scan is taken in knee extension, although associated chondromalacia of the lateral facet may be demonstrated. Recent advances in dynamic MRI imaging may hold promise in the diagnosis of patella tilt and malalignment (116,117).

Treatment: Nonoperative

The mainstay of treatment for LPCS is nonoperative. In acutely inflamed knees, initial focus should be on relative rest, ice, and anti-inflammatory medication. When symptoms have subsided, treatment should focus on improving patella alignment. A rehabilitation program should be initiated which involves stretching of the tight lateral retinaculum and IT Band. VMO strengthening will help dynamically medialize the patella and unload the lateral facet. More specific details of patella rehabilitation will be discussed elsewhere in this textbook.

A unique treatment that may be effective in persistent cases of LPCS is the use of Calcitonin to disrupt the cycle of bone turnover in the subchondral bone. This treatment is most likely to be effective before articular cartilage breakdown begins. Nuclear medicine studies in patients with patellofemoral syndrome have demonstrated increased uptake on radionuclide studies (57,118,119). Nasal Calcitonin (Myacalcin) has been used anecdotaly to resolve pain in certain patients with this entity (Scott Dye, *personal communication*, 2004).

Surgical Treatment

As discussed previously, lateral retinacular release has been shown to be ineffective for the treatment of patella instability (89,90,120); however, it remains a mainstay of treatment for patella tilt causing LPCS. A severely tightened lateral retinaculum which has not responded to conservative treatment can be effectively treated with surgical release. When performed properly and for the correct diagnosis, a lateral retinacular release can be a highly effective procedure. Fulkerson showed that a lateral retinacular release effectively corrected lateral tilt using CT scanning before and after surgery (121).

Lateral retinacular release is best performed arthroscopically under direct vision with an electrocautery device, which reduces the risk of hemarthrosis and hastens the postoperative rehabilitation (61). Most authors recommend releasing the retinaculum from approximately 1 to 2 cm proximal to the patella to at least the anterolateral portal. Marumoto (30) showed that release inferior to the portal all the way to the tibial tubercle may be more effective. It is important to verify adequate release by demonstrating the ability to tilt the patella 90 degrees at the end of the procedure (Fig 40-41).

Paulos (113) has shown that patient selection is important with best results achieved in patients with a negative passive patella tilt test, a medial patella glide of less than two

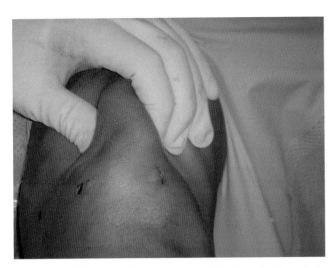

Fig 40-41. Following adequate release of the lateral retinaculum, the patella can be tilted 90 degrees.

quadrants, and a normal tubercle sulcus angle at 90 degrees of flexion.

When performed excessively or in a knee with no underlying lateral patella tilt, lateral release may result in medial subluxation, which can only be corrected with revision open lateral repair of the retinaculum (122).

Patella Hypertension Syndrome

Another explanation that has been espoused for anterior knee pain in younger patients is the patella hypertension syndrome. An increase in intraosseous pressure is thought to lead to patella pain even without evidence of chondromalacia or malalignment. Confirmation of this diagnosis requires intraosseous pressure measurement to confirm elevated intraosseous pressure as well as a positive response to an intraoperative "pain provocation test" under local anesthesia (123). In patients in whom conservative treatment has failed, treatment with extra-articular drilling to relieve the intraosseous pressure is recommended (123). Miltner (123) has shown an excellent response to drilling in 27 adolescent patients who demonstrated elevated intraosseous pressure, and a positive response to a "pain provocation test" under local anesthesia, with decreased intraosseous pressure and improved pain scores at follow up. Schneider reported similar results with 69 patients with 90% of patients reporting pain relief and 88% demonstrating decreased intraosseous pressure at 3 years (124).

Interestingly, drilling of the patella for anterior knee pain and chondromalacia was thought to be effective in older reports in the literature (125); however, drilling was historically performed through the articular cartilage and has mostly been abandoned in the United States except for the treatment of grade 4 chondromlacia to promote subchondral bleeding and fibrocartilage ingrowth. The concept that extra-articular drilling can be effective and that the benefit of drilling is to reduce intraosseous pressure is a newer and potentially significant contribution that merits further study.

It may very well be that the patella hypertension syndrome is simply a subset of the lateral patella compression syndrome previously described. Further study is needed to determine which patients may benefit from drilling alone and which patients will require release of the lateral retinaculum. Drilling alone, however, may be appropriate for a patient with no significant chondromalacia, and no significant lateral tilt or malalignment on imaging studies, who fails conservative treatment and demonstrates increased intraosseous pressure.

■ CHONDROMALACIA

One of the difficulties in treating patients with anterior knee pain is the confusion in terminology surrounding these patients. The term chondromalacia refers specifically to the pathological appearance of damaged articular cartilage. This damage may be present with or without knee pain and with or without patella malalignment or instability.

Although chondromalacia is often associated with pain, the etiology of this pain is unclear. Articular cartilage has no direct nerve supply, and therefore is not in and of itself a potential source of pain. Dye (58) has shown that the articular cartilage is not sensitive to stimulation, but that the adjacent synovium is the primary pain source. Certainly, the subchondral bone has nerve endings and is another likely source of pain from excessive load on an unprotected bone surface. Finally, the resulting effusion caused by articular breakdown may itself be a source of pain.

Etiology

Chondromalacia may be caused by repetitive normal biomechanical loading, a single traumatic episode, asymmetric overload caused by malalignment, or by arthritic conditions.

DIAGNOSIS

History

Patients will usually present with pain, crepitus, and possibly a joint effusion. The history is usually that of insidious onset, although may contain a history of direct trauma such as a direct fall onto the patella or a blunt injury against a dashboard.

Physical Examination

Chondromalacia has been classified into various types by a number of authors. The Outerbridge classification is still most useful for clinicians (126).

Stage 1 is softening, but no defect in the cartilage. Stage 2 is cracking or fissuring. Stage 3 is surface disruption with friable and unstable fragments. Stage 4 is disruption of the articular surface down to bone. The examiner will usually be able to elicit crepitus in Stage 3 to 4 chondromalacia. Stages 1 and 2 are difficult to confirm on physical examination. Crepitus may be elicited with the examiner's hand gently resting on the patient's patella during active flexion and extension. Sometimes, however, the examiner may be fooled by crepitation in terminal extension caused by synovial impingement in the suprapatellar pouch. A more accurate method of assessing chondromalacia may be to rest the examiner's hand gently on the patient's knee during single leg short arc squatting. If present, patella crepitus will usually be evident at approximately 30 degrees of loaded knee flexion.

Another test to confirm the presence of chondromalacia (CM) is called the patella compression test. In this test, the examiner manually compresses the patella into the trochlea during passive flexion and extension. An increase in symptoms or crepitus suggests CM of the patellofemoral joint. A further refinement of this test is to translate the patella medially and laterally under compression to determine the exact location of underlying chondromalacia (medial or lateral facet).

For complete accuracy, chondromalacia is best diagnosed under direct visual inspection at the time of arthroscopy. MRI is improving in its capability to evaluate chondromalacia; however, false readings are still quite common. Newer MRI cartilage imaging sequences (127) as well as MR arthrography may improve the accuracy of diagnosis (128).

Treatment

The appropriate treatment for chondromalacia depends on many associated factors. Most importantly, remember that the mere presence of crepitus or even the visual confirmation of chondromalacia does confirm that this is the cause of the patient's symptoms. Great care must be taken to correlate the location of the patient's symptoms with the anatomic location of chondromalacia before proceeding with treatment recommendations.

It is important to determine if the patient has isolated chondromalacia or if there is associated LPCS or instability. Patients with LPCS and chondromalacia should probably undergo a lateral release along with a chondroplasty for the chondromalacia, and patients with instability and chondromalacia should be considered for a stabilization procedure at the time of chondroplasty.

Conservative Treatment

Initial treatment for chondromalacia should involve treating any associated malalignment with rehabilitation techniques to strengthen the VMO and stretch the tight lateral retinaculum. Taping or bracing techniques to improve patella tracking and unload the area of chondromalacia may also be of benefit. Orthotics may be useful in patients with hyperpronation.

Oral nonsteroidal anti-inflammatory medication (NSAID) is useful to reduce inflammation and swelling associated with chondromalacia. Various nonprescription remedies for chondromalacia are currently available with limited scientific support for their benefit. The most popular of these is a combination of glucosamine and chondroitin sulfate. A number of studies have supported their benefit for use in arthritis, although their benefit for chondromalacia is still unclear. A meta-analysis review suggests that both glucosamine and chondroitin are highly beneficial in relieving symptoms as well as have an apparent structural benefit on joint space narrowing (129). These benefits seem to apply to patients with chondromalacia as well (130).

S-Adenosyl Methionine (SAMe) is another popular nonprescription supplement that has been shown to be as effective as a NSAID (Celebrex) in the treatment of osteoarthritis of the knee and anecdotally has been used to treat chondromalacia (131).

Decision Making

It is extremely important to try to understand the etiology of the chondromalacia. If a patient presents with Grade 3 chondromalacia of the central ridge of the patella with a history of a direct blow to this area, simple debridement would be appropriate. If a patient presents with a long history of progressive symptoms with lateral facet CM, a tight lateral retinaculum, and evidence of lateral patellar compression syndrome, a debridement plus a lateral retinacular release would be more appropriate. If a patient has a history of recurring patella dislocation or subluxation, a stabilization procedure along with arthroscopic debridement would be recommended. The location of the chondromalacia is important. If the patient has symptomatic medial facet chondromalacia, a stabilization procedure should be performed with caution to avoid creating excessive medially directed force on that facet by overtightening the medial retinaculum and MPFL **(Fig 40-42)**.

Surgical Treatment of CMP: Technical Aspects

Grade 1 and 2 chondromalacia is rarely treated directly, although some authors have recommended drilling to promote healing of these lesions (54). In our opinion these should be left alone in most situations. When symptomatic, grade 3 chondromalacia is treated with the intention of removing loose fragments of articular cartilage and stabilizing the remaining surface to minimize further chondral breakdown. Controversy has arisen regarding the most effective method for debriding and stabilizing the articular cartilage. Historically, mechanical debridement using a suction shaving device has been effective and is still the accepted gold standard; however, the advent of thermal methods of debridement have raised new questions. Thermal chondroplasty utilizes radiofrequency or bipolar heating methods to both debride and stabilize the chondral

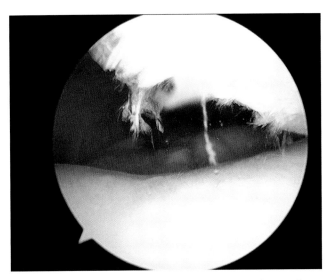

Fig 40-42. Chondromalacia of the medial facet of the patella as viewed arthroscopically. This finding is a contraindication to over-tightening of the medial retinaculum.

surface. Clinical studies have shown good results with these methods (132), perhaps surpassing results utilizing mechanical debridement (132). Concerns still remain regarding the long term safety of thermal techniques regarding potential collateral damage to adjacent chondrocytes (133,134) **(Fig 40-43)**.

At this point, based on our analysis of the existing literature and personal experience, if one is going to utilize thermal devices, it seems safest to utilize mechanical shaving devices to debulk the area of damaged cartilage by removing large unstable fragments of cartilage, and to utilize a thermal device to gently stabilize the remaining surface. A bipolar thermal device seems to be preferable to a monopolar device

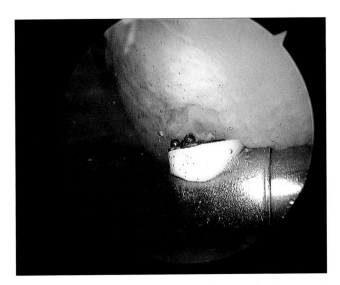

Fig 40-43. Thermal chondroplasty has demonstrated good short term results; however, concerns remain regarding long term results and chondrocyte viability.

so as to heat up a fluid layer just adjacent to the cartilage surface rather than directly touching the surface and risk burning the cartilage and should be used for brief periods with continuous arthroscopic fluid flow to prevent overheating. A temperature control probe should be utilized that prevents localized overheating and keeps the localized temperature below 60°C (135).

■ PLICA

There are a number of plicas in the knee, and most of them have been implicated as a cause of knee pain. The medial patella plica is by far the most common plica to become symptomatic. It originates on the superomedial wall of the knee joint and extends obliquely to insert on the medial portion of the infrapatellar fat pad. This plica is present in anywhere from 20% to 60% of knees in various studies (136,137); however, it is considered pathologic in 1/10 cases and in a maximum of 3% to 4% of arthroscopies (55,56) **(Fig 40-44)**.

Pathogenesis

The medial plica is felt to be an embryologic remnant caused by a remnant of the partially reabsorbed membrane that divides the knee embrologically. They are remnants of the mesenchymal tissue that occupies the space between the distal femoral and proximal tibial epiphyses in the 8-week-old embryo. The incomplete resorption leaves synovial pleats in most of the knee. The medial plica is usually asymptomatic; however, the plica can become thickened as a result of direct trauma such as a blow to the anteromedial knee from a dashboard injury or as a result of repetitive rubbing from sports activity. The thickened plica may then catch against the edge of the medial femoral condyle or patella causing clicking, catching, or simply pain.

History

Patients will present with anteromedial knee pain aggravated by activity. Unlike a meniscal injury, the pain is not usually aggravated by squatting or twisting activity, but is aggravated by repetitive flexion and extension activity.

Physical Examination

To confirm the diagnosis, the examiner should be able to feel a thickened cord just medial to the medial border of the patella and articular margin of the medial condyle. Firm palpation over this cord along with passive flexion and extension of the knee will usually recreate symptoms and confirm the diagnosis.

MRI will typically show the plica (138), but has not been helpful in differentiating an asymptomatic plica from a thickened symptomatic one.

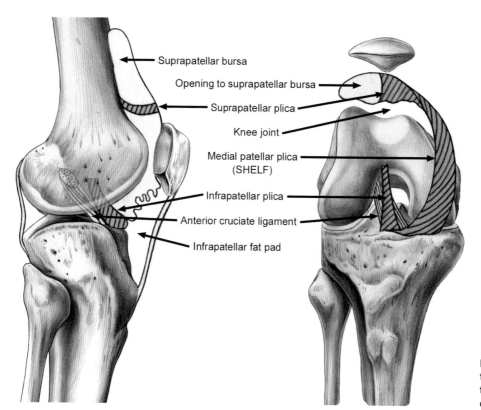

- Suprapatellar bursa
- Opening to suprapatellar bursa
- Suprapatellar plica
- Knee joint
- Medial patellar plica (SHELF)
- Infrapatellar plica
- Anterior cruciate ligament
- Infrapatellar fat pad

Fig 40-44. Anatomy of plicae about the knee. The medial patella plica is the most commonly implicated in clinical symptomatology.

Treatment: Nonoperative

Initial treatment should include stretching, ice, anti-inflammatory medication, and deep tissue releases, and mobilization over the plica region. Careful evaluation of anatomical and biomechanical factors may help correct the problem, such as correcting a leg length discrepancy with a lift or addressing hip tightness with a stretching program. Occasionally orthotics are useful to control foot pronation and improve knee alignment. Amatuzzi et al. (139) reported 40% good results and 20% average results with conservative treatment. Rovere and Adair (140) reported 73% relief of symptoms with injection of steroid; however, in our experience, injection has been much less effective.

Surgical Treatment

Arthroscopic resection of a symptomatic medial patella plica is usually successful (137). Dorchak et al. (55) reported an overall 75% success rate with plica excision. These results improved to 100% good/excellent results in patients who demonstrated associated findings of impingement against the trochlea ridge associated with chondromalacia.

■ ANTERIOR MENISCUS IMPINGEMENT SYNDROME

An uncommon cause of anterior knee pain described by McGuire et al. (141) is the anterior meniscus impingement

syndrome. In patients with knee hyperextension, the anterior horn of the meniscus can impinge against the anterior femoral condyle causing anteromedial knee pain. To confirm this diagnosis, patients should have impaction on the anterior medial femoral condyle by the leading edge of the medial meniscus, at least 5 degrees of knee hyperextension, and Outerbridge Grade 3 chondromlacia.

This syndrome typically occurs in female athletes after a specific hyperextension injury, often playing soccer. Initial treatment consists of bracing with a hinged knee brace that prevents hyperextension. If symptoms persist, arthroscopic debridement of the area of chondromalacia and associated synovitis may be warranted. Postoperative rehabilitation includes extension block bracing, hamstring strengthening, and closed-chain exercises.

■ REFERENCES

1. Holingshead HW. *Anatomy for Surgeons, vol 3: The Back and Limbs.* 2nd ed. Baltimore: Williams & Wilkins; 1990.
2. Dye Scott F. Patellofemoral anatomy, chapter 2. In: Fox JM, Del Pizzo W, eds. *The patellofemoral joint.* New York: McGraw-Hill; 1993.
3. Fu FH, Seel MJ, Berger R. Patellofemoral biomechanics, chapter 3. In: Fox JM, Del Pizzo W, eds. *The patellofemoral joint.* New York: McGraw-Hill; 1993.
4. Perry J, Antonelli D, Ford W. Analysis of knee joint forces during flexed knee stance. *J Bone Joint Surg.* 1975;57A:961.
5. Tardieu C, Dupont JY. The origin of femoral trochlear dyspalsia: comparative anatomy, evolution and growth of the patellofemoral joint. *Rev Chir Orthop Reparatrice Appar Mot.* 2001;87(4): 373–383.

6. Dye SF et al. Soft-tissue anatomy anterior to the human patella. *J Bone Joint Surg Am.* 2003;85A(6):1012–1017.

7. Wiberg G. Roentgenographic and anatomic studies on the femoropatellar joint. With special reference to chondromalacia patella. *Acta Orthop Scand.* 1941;12:319.

8. Baumgartl F. *Das Knieglenk.* Berlin: Springer Verlag; 1944.

9. Hennsge J. Arthrosid deformans des patella gleitweges. *Zentabl Chir.* 1962;32:1381.

10. Insall J, Salvati E. Patella position in the normal knee joint. *Radiology.* 1971;101:101.

11. JW (ed) Articular Cartilage and Knee Joint Function. New York: Raven; 1990.

12. Cohen ZA, et al. Templates of the cartilage layers of the Patellofemoral joint and their use in the assessment of osteoarthritic cartilage damage. *Osteoarthritis Cartilage.* 2003;11(8):567–79.

13. Kaufer H. Biomechanical function of the patella. *J Bone Joint Surg.* 1971;53A:1551–1560.

14. Buff HU, Jones LC, Hungerford DS. Determination of forces transmitted through the Patellofemoral joint. *J Biomech.* 1988;21:17.

15. Hungerford DS, Barry BS. Biomechanics of the Patellofemoral joint. *Clin Orthop.* 1979;144:9–15.

16. Huberti HH, Hayes WC, Stone JL, et al. Force ratios in the quadriceps tendon and ligamentum pateallae. *J Orthop Res.* 1984;2:49–54.

17. Hehne HJ. Biomechanics of the Patellofemoral joint and its clinical relevance. *Clin Orthop.* 1990;258:73.

18. Reilly DJ, Martens M. Experimental analysis of the quadriceps force and Patellofemoral joint reaction force for various activities. *Acta Orthop Scan.* 1972;43:126.

19. Ahmed AM, Burke DL, Hyder A. Force analysis of the patellar mechanism. *J Orthop Res.* 1987;5:69.

20. Flynn TW, Soutas-Little RW. Patellofemoral joint compressive forces in forward and backward running. *J Orthop Sports Phys Ther.* 1995;21(5):277–282.

20a. Ozguven HN, Berme N. An experimental and analytical study of impact forces during human jumping. *J Biomech.* 1988;21(12):1061–1066.

21. Pfirrmann CW, et al. Femoral trochlear dysplasia: MRI findings. *Radiology.* 2000;216(3):858–864.

22. Keene G, Marans HJ. Osteotomy for patellofemoral dysplasia. In: Fox JM, Del Pizzo W, eds. *The patellofemoral joint.* New York: McGraw Hill; 1993.

23. Peterson L, Karlsson J, Brittberg M. Patellar instability with recurrent dislocation due to Patellofemoral dysplasia. Results after surgical treatment. *Bull Hosp Joint Dis Othop Inst.* 1988;48(2):130–139.

24. Hautamaa PV, et al. Medial soft tissue restraints in lateral patellar instability and repair. *Clin Orthop.* 1998;349:174–182.

25. Desio SM, Burks RT, Bachus KN. Soft tissue restraints to lateral patellar translation in the human knee. *Am J Sports Med.* 1998;26(1):59–65.

26. Nomura E. Classification of lesions of the medial patellofemoral ligament in patellar dislocation. *Int Orthop.* 1999;23(5):260–263.

28. Sallay PI, et al. Acute dislocation of the patella. A correlative pathoanatomic study. *Am J Sports Med.* 1996;24(1):52–60.

27. Sanders TG, et al. Medial patellofemoral ligament injury following acute transient dislocation of the patella: MR findings with surgical correlation in 14 patients. *J Comput Assist Tomogr.* 2001;25(6):957–962.

29. Weinstabl R, et al. The extensor apparatus of the knee joint and its peripheral vasti. Anatomic investigation and clinical relevance. *Surg Radiol Anat.* 1989;11:17.

30. Marumoto JM, Jordan C, Akins R. A biomechanical comparison of lateral retinacular releases. *Am J Sports Med.* 1995;23(2):151–155.

31. Sims DS. The effect of a balanced foot orthosis on muscle function and foot pronation in compensated forefoot varus (masters thesis). Iowa City: University of Iowa; 1983.

32. Buchbinder MR, Napora NJ, Biggs EW. The relationship of abnormal pronation to chondromalacia of the patella in distance runners. *J Am Podiatric Assoc.* 1979;69:159.

33. Larsen E, Lauridsen F. Conservative treatment of patella dislocations: influence of evident factors on the tendency to redislocate and the therapeutic result. *Clin Orthop.* 1982;171:131.

34. Paulos L, et al. Patella malalignment: a treatment rational. *Phys Ther.* 1980;60:16–24.

35. Tiberio D. The effect of excessive subtalar joint pronation on patellofemoral mechanics: a theoretical model. *J Orthop Sports Phys Ther.* 1987;9:160.

36. Sims DS, Cavanagh PR. Selected foot mechanics related to the prescription of foot orthoses. In: Jahss MH, ed. *Disorders of the foot.* Philadelphia: WB Saunders; 1991:469–483.

37. Mann RA. Overview of foot and ankle biomechanics. In: Jahss MH, ed. *Disorders of the foot.* Philadelphia: WB Saunders: 1991;385–408.

38. Lutter LD. Foot related knee problems in the long distance runner. *Foot Ankle.* 1980;1:112–116.

39. Bates BT, et al: Foot orthoeic devices to modify selected aspects of lower extremity mechanics. *Am J Sports Med.* 1979;7:338–342.

40. Scranton PE, Pedegania LR, Whitesel JP. Alterations in support phase forces using supporting devices. *Am J Sports Med.* 1982;10:6–10.

41. James SL, Bates BT, Ostering LR. Injuries to runners. *Am J Sports Med.* 1978;6:40–50.

42. Rodgers MM, LeVeau BF. Effectiveness of foot orthotic devices used to modify pronation in runners. *J Orthop Sports Phys Ther.* 1982;4:86.

43. Smith LS, Clarke TE, et al. The effects of soft and semirigid orthoses upon rearfoot movement in running. *J Am Podiatr Assoc.* 1986;76:227.

44. Taunton JE, et al. A triplanar electrogoniometer investigation of running mechanics in runners with compensatory overpronation. *Can J Appl Sports Sci.* 1985;10:104.

45. Cavanagh PR, Clarke T, et al. An evaluation of the effect of orthotics on force distribution and rearfoot movement during running. Presented at the American Orthopedic Society for Sports Medicine Meeting. Lake Placid, NY: 1978.

46. Clarke TE, Fredrick EC, Hlavac HF. Effects of a soft orthotic device on rearfoot movement in running. *Podiatr Sports Med.* 1983;1:20.

47. Gross ML, Dvlin LB, Evanski PM. Effectiveness of orthotic shoe inserts in the long distance runner. *Am J Sports Med.* 1991;19:409–412.

48. Dugan RC, D'Ambrosia RD. The effects of orthotics in the treatment of selected running injuries. Proceedings of the Sixteenth Annual Meeting of the American Orthopedic foot and Ankle Society. *Foot Ankle.* 1986;6:313.

49. Gross MT, Foxworth JL. The role of foot orthoses as an intervention for patellofemoral pain. *Orthop Sports Phys Ther.* 2003;33(11):661–670.

50. Kuhn DR, Yochum TR, et al. Immediate changes in the quadriceps femoris angle after insertion of an orthotic device. *Manipulative Physiol Ther.* 2002;25(7):465–470.

51. Saxena A, Haddad J. The effect of foot orthoses on patellofemoral pain syndrome. *Am Podiatr Med Assoc.* 2003;93(4):264–271.

52. Powers CM, Ward SR, et al. Effect of bracing on patellofemoral joint stress while ascending and descending stairs. *Clin J Sports Med.* 2004;14(4):206–214.

53. Shellock FG, Mink JH, et al. Effect of a patellar realignment brace on patellofemoral relationships: evaluation with kinematic MR imaging. *J Magn Reson Imaging.* 1994;4(4):590–594.

54. Bently G. The surgical treatment of chondromalacia patella. *J Bone Joint Surg Br.* 1978;60(1):74–81.

55. Dorchak JD, et al. Arthroscopic treatment of symptomatic synovial plica of the knee. Long term followup. *Am J Sports Med.* 1991;19(5):503–507.

56. Dupont JY. Synovial plicae of the knee. Controversies and review. *Clin Sports Med.* 1997;16(1):87–122.

57. Dye SF, Boll DA. Radionuclide imaging of the patellofemoral joint in young adults with anterior knee pain. *Int Orthop.*1987; 11(1):29–33.

58. Dye SF, Vaupel GL, Dye CC. Conscious neurosensory mapping of the internal structures of the human knee without intra-articular anesthesia. *Am J Sports Med.* 1988;26(6):773–777.

59. Ellis MI, Sweedhom BB, Wright V. Forces in the knee joint whilst rising from a seated position. *J Biomed Eng.* 1984;6(2): 113–120.

60. Eriscson MO, Nisell R. Tibiofemoral joint forces during ergometer cycling. *Am J Sports Med.* 1986;14(4):285–290.

61. Ferkel RD. Lateral retinacular release. In: Fox JM, Del Pizzo W, eds. *The patellofemoral joint.* New York: McGraw-Hill; 1993:318.

62. Grelsamer RP, Tedder JL. The lateral trochlear sign. Femoral trochlear dysplasia as seen on a lateral view roentgenograph. *Clin Orthop.* 1992;(281):159–162.

63. Remy F, Chantelo C, Folntaine C, et al. Inter and intra observer reproducibility in radiographic diagnosis and classification of femoral trochlear dysplasia. *Surg Radiol Anat.* 1998; 20(4):285–289.

64. Shalaby M, Almekinders LC. Patellar tendonitis: the significance of magnetic resonance imaging findings. *Am J Sports Med.* 1999; 27(3):345–359.

65. Boles CA, Butler J, Lee JA, et al. Magnetic resonance characteristics of medial plica of the knee: correlation with arthroscopic resection. *J Comput Assist Tomogr.* 2004;28(3):397–401.

66. Schutzer SF, Rambsy GR, Fulkerson JP. Computed tomographic classification of patellofemoral pain patients. *Orthop Clin North Am.* 1986;17:235.

67. Fogelman I, et al. The "hot patella" is it any clinical significance? Concise communication. *J Nucl Med.* 1982;24:312.

68. Holder LE. Clinical radionuclide bone imaging. *Radiology.* 1990;176:607.

69. Kozin F, Soin JS, Ryan LM, et al. Bone scintigraphy in the reflex sympathetic dystrophy syndrome. *Radiology.* 1981; 138:437.

70. Ryan LM, et al. Bone scintigraphy in the reflex sympathetic dystrophy syndrome. *Radiology.* 1981;138:437.

71. Pfeiffer RP, DeBeliso M, Shea KG, et al. Kinematic MRI assessment of McConnell taping before and after exercise. *Am J Sports Med.* 2004;32(3):621–628.

72. Christou EA. Patellar taping increase vastus medialis oblique activity in the presence of patellofemoral pain. *J Electromyogr Kinesiol.* 2004;(4):495–504.

73. Friden T. A case of superior dislocation of the patella. *Acta Orthop Scand.* 58(4):429.

74. Larson RL, Jones OC. Dislocations and ligamentous injuries of the knee. In: Rockwood CA, Green DP, eds. *Fractures in adults.* 2nd ed. Philadelphia: Lippincott; 1984.

75. Kaufman I, Habermann ET. Intercondylar vertical dislocation of the patella. A case report. *Bull Hosp Joint Dis.* 1973;34:222.

76. McMannus MB, Rang M, Heslin J. Acute dislocation of the patella in children. *Clin Orthop.* 1979;139:88.

77. Cash JD, Hughston JC. Treatment of acute patella dislocation. *Am J Sports Med.* 1988;16:244.

78. Casteleyn PP, Handelberg F. Arthroscopy in the diagnosis of acute dislocation of the patella. *Acta Orthop Belg.* 1989;55:381.

79. Nietosvaara Y, Aalto K, Kallio PE. Acute patellar dislocation in children: incidence and associated osteochondral fractures. *J Pediatr Orthop.* 1994;14(4):513–515.

80. Cofield RH, Bryan RS. Acute dislocation of the patella: Results of conservative treatment. *J Trauma.* 1977;17:526.

81. Vainionpaa S, Laasonen E, Silvenoinen T, et al. Acute dislocation of the patella. A prospective review of operative treatment. *J Bone Joint Surg.* 1990;72:365.

82. Atkin DM, et al. Characteristics of patients with primary acute lateral patellar dislocation and their recovery within the first 6 months of injury. *Am J Sports Med.* 2000;28(4):472–479.

83. Hawkins RJ, Bell RH, Anisette G. Acute patella dislocations: The natural history. *Am J Sports Med.* 1986;14:117.

84. Teittge RA. Radiology of the Patellofemoral joint. Orthopedic Surgery Update Series. Princeton, NJ: Continuing Professional Education Center; 1985.

85. Harilainen A, Myllynen P. Operative treatment in acute patella dislocation. Radiologic predisposing factors, diagnosis and results. *Am J Knee Surg.* 1988;1:178.

86. Boring TH, O'Donoghue DH. Acute patella dislocation. Results of immediate surgical repair. *Clin Orthop.* 1978;136:182.

87. Ahmad CS, Stein BE, Matuz D, et al. Immediate surgical repair of the medial patellar stabilizers for acute patellar dislocation. A review of eight cases. *Am J Sports Med.* 2000;28(6):804–810.

88. Aglietti P, Pisaneschi A, De Baise P. Lussazione recidivante di rotula: Tre tipi trattamento chirurgico. *G Ital Ortop Traumat.* 1992;13:25.

89. Dandy DJ, Griffiths D. Lateral release for recurrent dislocation of the patella. *J Bone Joint Surg Br.* 1989;71:121.

90. Sherman OH, Fox JM, Sperling H, et al. Patellar instability: Treatment by arthroscopic electrosurgical lateral release. *Arthroscopy.* 1987;3:152.

91. Fulkerson JP, Cautilli RA. Chronic patella instability: Subluxation and dislocation. In: Fox JM, Del Pizzo W, eds. *The patellofemoral joint.* New York: McGraw-Hill; 1993:135–147.

92. Insall JN, Bullough PG, Burstein AH. Proximal tube realignment of the patella for chondromalacia patellae. *Clin Orthop.* 1979; 144:63.

93. Henry JE, Pflum FA Jr. Arthroscopic proximal patella realignment and stabilization. *Arthroscopy.* 1995;11:424–425.

94. Small NC. Arthroscopically assisted proximal extensor mechanism realignment of the knee. *Arthroscopy.* 1993;9:63–67.

95. Yamamoto RK. Arthroscopic repair of the medial retinaculum and capsule in acute patellar dislocations. *Arthroscopy.* 1986;2: 125–131.

96. Halbrecht JL. Arthroscopic patella realignment: an all-inside technique. *Arthroscopy.* 2001;17(9):940–945.

97. Haspl M, Cicak N, Klobucar H, et al. Fully arthroscopic stabilization of the patella. *Arthroscopy.* 2002;18(1)E2.

98. Fukushima K, et al. Patellar dislocation: arthroscopic patellar stabilization with suture anchors. *Arthroscopy.* 2004;20(7).

99. Letts RM, Davidson D, Beaule P. Semitendinosus tenodesis for repair of recurrent dislocation of the patella in children. *J Pediatr Orthop.* 1999;19(6):742–747.

100. Gomes J, Marcyz L, et al. Medial Patellofemoral ligament reconstruction with semitendinosus autograft for chronic patellar instability: a follow up study. *Arthroscopy.* 2004;20(2).

101. Fithian D. Reconstruction of the medial Patellofemoral ligament (MPFL): relevant anatomy, indications, technique and rehabilitation. Washington, DC: AAOS Instructional Course; Feb 2005.

102. Sanfridsson J, et al. Femorotibial rotation and the Q angle related to the dislocating patella. *Acta Radiol.* 2001;42(2):218–224.

103. Tsujimoto K, et al. Radiographic and computed tomographic analysis of the position of the tibial tubercle in recurrent dislocation and subluxation of the patella. *Am J Knee Surg.* 2000; 13(2):83–88.

104. Davis DK, Fithian DC. Techniques of medial retinacular repair and reconstruction. *Clin Orthop.* 2002;402:38–52.

105. Slocum B, Slocum TD. Trochlear wedge recession for medial patellar luxation. An update. *Vet Clin North Am Small Anim Pract.* 1993; Jul 23(4):869–875.

106. Kuroda R, et al. Distribution of Patellofemoral joint pressures after femoral trochlear osteotomy. *Knee Surg Sports Traumatol Arthrosc.* 2002;10(1):33–37.

107. Verdonk R, Jansegers E, Stuyts B. Trochleoplasty in dysplastic knee trochlea. *Knee Surg Sports Traumatol Arthrosc.* 2005; Jan 11. Epub ahead of print.

108. Beach W. Comprehensive approach to Patellofemoral pain instability and malalignment. ICL #203. AANA 23rd annual meeting. Orlando, FL: April 22–25, 2004.

109. Ficat P, Hungerford DS. *Disorders of the Patello-femoral Joint.* Baltimore: Williams & Wilkins; 1977.

110. Insall JN. Patella pain. *J Bone Joint Surg Am.* 1982;64A;147.

111. Fulkerson JP, Gossling HR. Anatomy of the knee joint lateral retinaculum. *Clin Orthop.* 1980;153:183.

112. Ficat P, Ficat J, Bailleux A. Syndrome d'hyperpression externe de la rotule (SHPE). *Rev Chir Orthop.* 1975;61:39.

113. Kolowich PA, Paulos LE, Rosenberg TD, et al. Lateral release of the patella: indications and contraindications; *Am J Sports Med.* 1990;18(4):359–365.

114. Merchant A. The lateral patellar compression syndrome. In: Fox JM, Del Pizzo W, eds. *The patellofemoral joint.* New York: McGraw-Hill; 1993:166.

115. Shea KP, Fulkerson JP. Preoperative computed tomography scanning and arthroscopy in predicting outcome after lateral retinacular release. *Arthropscopy.*1992;8(3):327–334.

116. O'Donnell P, Johnstone C, et al. Evaluation of patellar tracking in symptomatic and asymptomatic individuals by magnetic resonance imaging. *Skeletal Radiol.* 2004;26.

117. Harman M, Ipeksoy, et al. MR arthrography in chondromalacia patellae diagnosis on a low-field open magnet system. *Clin Imaging.* 2003;27(3):194–199.

118. Hejgaard N, Diemer H. Bone scan in the Patellofemoral pain syndrome. *Orthop Clin North Am.* 1986;17(2):249–262.

119. Butler-Manuel PA, Guy RL, et al. Scintigraphy in the assessment of anterior knee pain. *Acta Orthop Scan.* 1990;61(5):438–442.

120. Ahmad CS, Lee FY. An all-arthroscopic soft-tissue balancing technique for lateral patellar instability. *Arthroscopy.* 2001;17(50): 555–557.

121. Fulkerson JP, Schutzer SF, Rambsby GR, et al. Computerized tomography of the Patellofemoral joint before and after lateral release or realignment. *Arthroscopy.* 1987;3:19.

122. Teitge RA. Iatrogenic medial patellar dislocation. Presented at the 58th Annual Meeting of the American Association of Orthopedic Surgeons. Anaheim, CA: March 7–12, 1991.

123. Miltner O, Siebert CH, et al. Patellar hypertension syndrome in adolescence: a 455–459.

124. Schneider U, et al. A new concept in the treatment of anterior knee pain: patellar hypertension syndrome. *Orthopedics.* 2000. Jun 23(6):581–586.

125. McCarroll JR, O'Donoghue DH, Grana WA. The surgical treatment of chondromalacia of the patella. *Clin Orthop.* 1983;175: 130–134.

126. Outerbridge RE. The etiology of chondromalacia patella. *J Bone Joint Surg Br.* 1961;43B:752–757.

127. Macarini L, Perrone A, et al. Evaluation of patellar chondromalacia with MR: comparison between T-2 weighted FSE SPIR and GE MTC. *Radiol Med.* 2004;108(3):159–171.

128. Gagliardi JA, Chung EM, et al. Detection and staging of chondromalacia patellae: relative efficacies of conventional MR imaging, MR arthrography, and CT arthrography. *AJR AM J Roentgenol.* 1994;163(3):629–636.

129. Richy F, Bruyere O, Ethgen O, et al. Structural and symptomatic efficacy of glucosamine and chondroitin in knee osteoarthritis: a comprehensive meta-analysis. *Arch Intern Med.* 2003;163: 1514–1522.

130. Braham R, Dawson B, Goodman C, et al. The effect of glucosamine supplementation on people experiencing regular knee pain: *Br J Sports Med.* 2003;37(1):45–49.

131. Najm WI, Reinsch S, et al. S-Adenosyl methionine (SAMe) versus clecoxib for the treatment of ostoarthiris symptoms: a double blind cross over trial. *BMC Musculoskelet Disord.* 2004;26:5(1):6.

132. Uribe JW. Electrothermal chondroplasty—bipolar. *Clin Sports Med.* 2002;21(4):675–685.

133. Lu Y, Edwards RB III, Cole BJ, et al. Thermal chondroplasty with radiofrequency energy. An in vitro comparison of bipolar and monopolar radiofrequency devices. *Am J Sports Med.* 2001; 29(1):42–49.

134. Ryan A, et al. The effects of radiofrequency energy treatment on chondrocytes and matrix of fibrillated articular cartilage. *Am J Sports Med.* 2003;3:386–391.

135. Kaplan LK, Ionescu D, et al. Temperature requirements for altering the morphology of osteoarthritic and nonarthritic articular cartilage: in vitro thermal alteration of articular cartilage.

136. Patel D. Plica as a cause of anterior knee pain. *Orthop Clin North Am.* 1986;17:273.

137. Jackson RW, Marshall DJ, Fujisawa Y. The pathological medial shelf. *Orthop Clin North Am.* 1982;13:307.

138. Jee WH, et al. The Plica syndrome: diagnostic value of MRI with arthroscopic correlation. *J Comput Assist Tomogr.* 1998;22(5): 814–818.

139. Amatuzzi M, Fazzi A, Varella M. Pathologic synovial plica of the knee: Results of conservative treatment. *Am J Sports Med.* 1990;18:466.

140. Rovere GD, Adair DM. Medial synovial shelf plica syndrome. Treatment by intraplical steroid injection. *Am J Sports Med.* 1985;13:382.

141. McGuire DA et al. Meniscus impingement syndrome. *Arthroscopy.* 1996;12(6):675–679.

41

FRACTURES — TIBIAL PLATEAU, DISTAL FEMUR, PATELLA, AVULSIONS OF THE INTERCONDYLAR EMINENCE, OSGOOD-SCHLATTER DISEASE

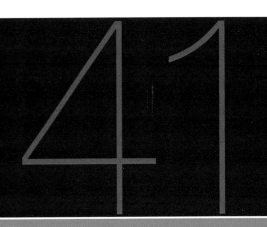

JAMES H. LUBOWITZ, MD, WYLIE S. ELSON, MD, DAN GUTTMAN, MD

■ KEY POINTS

Tibial Plateau Fractures

■ Fractures of the lateral tibial plateau are caused by a valgus force, such as the classic "bumper fracture" of a motor vehicle versus a pedestrian.

■ The mechanism of injury should be classified into high velocity and low velocity injuries. The former have more associated injuries.

■ The symptoms are pain, swelling, and difficulty in weight bearing.

■ The examination reveals swelling and lack of motion of the knee.

■ Imaging should include plain x-rays, CT scans with 3D reconstructions to view the bony injury, and MRI to evaluate the soft tissue injury.

■ Schatzker has classified six types of fracture pattern. Type 1 is a split fracture. Type 2 is a split and compression. Type 3 is central depression. Type 4 is a medial plateau fracture. Type 5 is a split of both condyles with or without compression. Type 6 is bicondylar with separation from the metaphysic.

■ The treatment goals are to restore joint stability, alignment, and congruity of the joint surface, while preserving motion of the joint.

■ Fractures that are stable in extension or peripheral with minimal displacement may be treated with immobilization and restricted weight bearing.

■ Arthroscopic reduction and internal fixation (ARIF) may be an alternative to open reduction and internal fixation (ORIF) in Schatzker Types 1 to 4.

■ ARIF is the definitive treatment for Type 3, central depression fractures.

■ Even in cases of ORIF, arthroscopy is a valuable adjunct to the diagnosis and treatment of other intra-articular pathology.

■ The disadvantages of arthroscopy is the problem of visualization due to the hemarthrosis and the potential for fluid extravasation into the muscle compartments of the lower leg.

■ The technique of repair requires the use of a tourniquet, a leg holder, traction on a fracture table, C-arm fluoroscopy, and the arthroscope.

■ The risk of fluid extravasation can be minimized by going dry during the reduction stage and by making an incision where the plate or screws will be placed to allow the fluid to escape.

■ The depressed fragments are elevated by placing a K-wire into the center of the fracture and using a tamp from below to overreduce the depressed joint surface.

■ The bone defect is filled with auto, allograft, or bone substitute.

■ Cannulated lag screws are used to buttress the elevated fragments in Type 3 fractures and to reduce and fixate the split fragments of Type 2 and 4.

■ For large fragments, a lateral buttress plate may be required.

■ Associated injuries to the meniscus (40%), the ACL (30%), and intercondylar eminence fractures may be dealt with at the same time.

Intercondylar Eminence Fractures

■ Intercondylar eminence fractures occur in youngsters and are an avulsion of the ACL from the tibia with a large bony fragment.

■ Myers and McKeever have classified the injuries into three types. Type 1 has minimal displacement of the fragment. Type 2 has displacement of the anterior third with a posterior hinge. Type 3 has total displacement of the fragment.

■ Type 1 may be treated with non-operative immobilization in extension.

■ Type 3 is treated surgically by ARIF with either screws or sutures placed around the fragment.

■ There is controversy about the treatment of Type 2. If there is adequate reduction with the knee in extension, then it may be treated conservatively.

■ If the fragment does not reduce completely, which may be due to the interposition of the transverse meniscal ligament, ARIF is indicated.

Fractures of the Distal Femur

■ These are often the result of high velocity injuries, and the ATLS guidelines recommend a complete assessment of the patient both clinically and radiologically.

■ The fractures should be imaged with plain x-rays to include the hip and pelvis.

■ Arteriography is recommended if there is suspicion of vascular injury.

■ The fractures are classified by the AO System into 3 types.

■ Conservative treatment is indicated for non-displaced or incomplete fractures, as well as gun shot wounds or severely infected wounds.

■ The goals of operative management are anatomic reduction, preservation of the blood supply, and stable internal fixation to allow early mobilization.

■ The fractures are managed according to the AO principles of anatomic reduction and fixation with 95* condylar blade plates, side plates and condylar screws, condylar buttress plates, intermeduallary rods, and external fixation as the fracture pattern dictates.

■ Injury to the femoral or popliteal artery occurs in 2% to 3% and demands high priority.

Fractures of the Patella

■ Fractures of the patella usually occur due to a direct blow, but may be due to a forceful contraction of the quadriceps muscle.

■ Displaced fractures with disruption of the extensor mechanism (unable to extend the knee) need operative intervention. This is about one third of all the patellar fractures.

■ Plain x-rays, AP, lateral, and Merchant views are required to evaluate the fractures.

■ Conservative treatment is recommended for fractures with minimal displacement and an intact extensor mechanism.

■ Operative treatment of a transverse fracture is by lag screw fixation and cerclage wiring.

■ Partial or total patellectomy may be required with severe comminution of the fracture fragments.

Osgood-Schlatter Disease

■ Repeated stress during growth may result in fragmentation of the appophysis of the tibial tubercle.

■ The diagnosis in the acute phase is clinical, as the radiological appearance is variable.

■ In most cases conservative activity modification results in healing after 7 months.

■ After growth is complete a separate ossicle may be present and imaged by plain x-rays.

■ If at the end of growth, symptoms persist for 1 to 2 years and x-rays show a separate ossicle, this may be surgically removed by splitting the patellar tendon longitudinally and removing the bony fragment.

This chapter presents evolving treatment options for fractures about the knee joint and how, in many cases, minimally invasive treatment alternatives reduce the extremes between open and closed management of these conditions. We will examine conditions where historical treatments were typically limited to cast immobilization and rest, but current recommendations are now being developed for some open treatments. In other cases, open surgical management is moving toward less invasive techniques with the help of modern technology.

The first two sections discuss treatment of tibial plateau fractures. In these cases, many injuries that were previously treated by cast immobilization, skeletal traction, or open reduction and internal fixation are now also considered favorable for arthroscopic management. The third section explores current recommendations for the treatment of fractures to the distal femur, which were typically treated with non-surgical methods in the past.

The fourth section explores the changing attitudes toward treatment of fractures of the patella. As our understanding of the function of the patella changes, management of this condition has changed to support the importance of maintaining the patella after fracture, as opposed to the historical treatment, which typically included patellectomy.

The final section in this chapter discusses new options for the treatment of Osgood-Schlatter Disease (OSD). Although OSD is typically self-limited and usually resolves with cessation of painful activity, some cases persist. This section discusses studies of open treatment for OSD in cases where there is evidence of fragmentation of the apophysis at presentation.

■ TIBIAL PLATEAU FRACTURES: INTRODUCTION

Traditionally, treatment methods for fractures of the tibial plateau included cast immobilization, skeletal traction, or open reduction and internal fixation. With the evolution of minimally invasive surgical techniques, arthroscopic treatment of tibial plateau fractures has proved a valuable adjunct to the open treatment of tibial plateau fractures

(1). Arthroscopic reduction and internal fixation (ARIF) of tibial plateau fractures has become the emerging state-of-the-art. This section describes our evolving understanding of ARIF of tibial plateau fractures.

Basic Science: Anatomy

The knee is the largest joint in the body. Knee function requires stability, range of motion in bending and rotation, and transmission of large muscular loads (2). The tibia is the major weight bearing bone of the knee joint. At its proximal articular surface, the tibia widens to form the medial and lateral condyles. Between the condyles, the intercondylar eminences serve as the sites of attachment for the fibrocartilaginous menisci and the anterior and posterior cruciate ligaments (3). The relatively flattened condylar portions of the proximal tibia comprise the weight bearing aspects of the tibial plateau. The medial and lateral tibial condyles articulate with corresponding medial and lateral femoral condyles. Anatomically, the medial tibial plateau is larger and stronger than the lateral tibial plateau (4). This finding may explain why fractures of the lateral condyle occur more frequently than medial condyle fractures (4).

Biomechanics

With regard to epidemiology, fractures of the tibial plateau constitute approximately 1% of all fractures (5) and generally result from trauma such as a fall or motor vehicle versus pedestrian accident. Approximately 5% to 10% of tibial plateau fractures are sports related (6) and this incidence is higher in skiers (5).

With regard to mechanism of injury, fractures involving the tibial plateau can result from medial, lateral, or axially directed forces. Forces directed medially (valgus force moment) are often classic "bumper fractures:" motor vehicle versus pedestrian accidents. More complex mechanisms involve combinations of both axial and varus or valgus directed forces. In most cases, the medial or lateral femoral condyle acts as an anvil imparting a combination of both shearing and compressive force to the underlying tibial plateau (4).

Clinical Evaluation: History and Physical Findings

A patient with a fracture of the tibial plateau generally presents with a painful swollen knee injured in some traumatic event (6). Usually, the patient is unable to bear weight on the affected leg (3), although this is not always the case (6). Occasionally, the patient can accurately describe the precise mechanism of injury, as in "bumper" injuries or accidents sustained playing football or soccer, during skiing, or in a fall. Often, however, this is not the case (3).

Despite the common inability to rely on a patient's history when determining the specific mechanism of injury of tibial plateau fractures, it is useful to ascertain the level of

force involved in the injury, specifically high-energy or low-energy forces (3). This is not a purely academic point; associated injuries such as fracture blisters, compartment syndromes, disruptions of the menisci or ligaments, or injuries to adjacent nerves and blood vessels occur most often in association with high-energy forces (3).

On examination of the affected extremity, one generally finds a distinct limitation of both active and passive knee motion because of pain and swelling. Additionally, voluntary or involuntary muscle guarding or spasm may make it difficult to evaluate the status of the ligaments or the extent of the fracture. Despite this limitation, an effort to examine the patient to determine associated ligamentous damage is recommended. In all cases, careful attention must be paid to peripheral pulses, neurological function, and the status of the compartments of the injured extremity. Any open wounds must be carefully evaluated to ascertain their relationship to the fracture site or joint space (3).

Imaging

Radiographic evaluation must include antero-posterior, lateral, and two oblique views. To assess the slope of the tibial plateau and the degree of articular depression, a 15-degree caudal tibial plateau view may also be helpful; however, measurement of the amount of depression of the fractured tibial plateau using standard radiographs may be inaccurate (In addition, standard radiographs are not considered the best studies to use in order to monitor healing after either closed or open management of tibial plateau fractures) (6). The extent and nature of bony or ligament injuries in association with fractures of the upper end of the tibia must be further evaluated using advanced studies (6).

Computed axial tomography (CT) combined with coronal and sagittal plane reconstructions provide precise information regarding the extent and pattern of both articular and extra-articular components of the fracture (6); however, CT is limited in that the soft tissues of the knee may not be visualized adequately (3).

Magnetic resonance imaging (MRI) is the examination of choice for soft tissue injuries in association with tibial plateau fracture. MRI is an especially valuable preoperative planning tool because the status of the menisci or ligaments is difficult to ascertain when pain prevents a reliable physical examination (7).

In summary, CT scanning is the standard for evaluating bony injury including articular depression, although MRI is the standard for evaluating associated soft tissue injury such as meniscal, ligamentous, or chondral injury in association with fractures of the tibial plateau.

Arteriography is a consideration when there is any alteration in the distal pulses and indicated in cases of knee dislocation or when the possibility of arterial injury is a concern (3). Schatzker Type IV, V, or VI tibial plateau fractures (discussed later), and injuries sustained as a result of high-energy trauma or in association with compartment syndrome should alert the surgeon to consider an arteriogram. Ultrasound evaluation is not recommended as an alternative to arteriography because ultrasound does not reliably detect intimal arterial damage (3).

Diagnostic arthroscopic evaluation allows direct visualization of the menisci, cruciates, and articular surfaces including the articular portion of the fracture site (1,3,8,9). In addition to a diagnostic role, arthroscopy may be used for treatment (discussed later) with a goal of allowing precise reduction of fracture fragments under direct visualization.

Decision Making Algorithms and Classification

The most commonly accepted classification scheme in current use is the Schatzker classification (10). This classification scheme owes a debt to the landmark work of Hohl and associates (11). The Schatzker classification (4,10) divides tibial plateau fractures into six types based upon the fracture pattern and fracture fragment anatomy:

- Type I is a wedge or split fracture of the lateral aspect of the plateau, usually as a result of valgus and axial forces. With this pattern, there is no compression (depression) of the wedge fragment because of strong underlying cancellous bone. This pattern is usually seen in younger patients.
- Type II is a lateral wedge or split fracture associated with compression. Mechanism of injury is similar to a Type I fracture, but the underlying bone may be osteoporitic and unable to resist depression or the forces may be greater.
- Type III is a pure compression fracture of the lateral plateau. As a result of an axial force, the depression is usually located laterally or centrally, but it may involve any portion of the articular surface.
- Type IV is a fracture that involves the medial plateau. Resulting from either varus or axial compression forces, the pattern may be either split or split and compression. As this fracture involves the larger and stronger medial plateau, the forces causing this type are generally greater than those associated with Types I, II, and III.
- Type V fractures include split elements of both the medial and lateral condyles and may include medial or lateral articular compression, usually as a result of a pure axial force occurring while the knee is in extension.
- Type VI is a complex, bicondylar fracture in which the condylar components separate from the diaphysis. Depression and impaction of the fracture fragments is the rule. This pattern results from high-energy trauma and diverse combinations of forces.

Treatment

The ultimate goals of tibial plateau fracture treatment are to re-establish joint stability, alignment, and articular congruity while preserving full range of motion. In such a case, painless knee function may be obtained and posttraumatic arthritis could be prevented (4,7).

Nonoperative

Not all fractures of the tibial plateau require surgery. The first challenge in the management of upper tibial fractures is to decide between non-operative or surgical techniques (6). Fractures that are stable in extension and are minimally displaced may be amenable to cast immobilization or bracing with early motion and delayed weight bearing (6). Other indications for non-operative management may include injuries to the peripheral (submeniscal) rim of the plateau and fractures in elderly, low demand, or osteoporotic patients (8).

Advantages of non-surgical treatment include a short hospital stay and no risk of sepsis (1); however, prolonged immobilization (greater than 2 or 3 weeks) can result in unacceptable joint stiffness (4). If traction is a viable option, good motion may be obtained but at the cost of a lengthy hospital stay, and at the risk of a pin tract infection (1). In addition, there is inadequate data regarding the amount of articular depression and displacement that may lead to posttraumatic arthritis (3). Finally, pain during recovery after closed treatment can be as severe as with open procedures, especially in cases with prolonged hemarthrosis (12).

When considering non-operative treatment, a CT scan of the affected extremity should be obtained as occult articular depression might change the plan from a closed to an open approach (6). As part of the closed treatment plan, patients should be followed with radiographs every 2 weeks for the first 6 weeks to monitor alignment and healing and activities should be restricted for 4 to 6 months (6). Possible complications of nonoperative treatment may include limited range of motion, pulmonary embolism, phlebitis, instability, and posttraumatic arthritis (12).

Operative

Open reduction and internal fixation (ORIF) using buttress plates and/or cancellous lag screws has been a mainstay for the treatment of displaced tibial plateau fractures. This technique may be applied to practically every type of tibial plateau fracture, so long as the soft tissue envelope permits surgical intervention (6).

Arthroscopy is accepted as a valuable adjunct in the treatment of some tibial plateau fractures such that the evolution of arthroscopy has complicated the debate concerning open versus non-operative management. Although open reduction and internal fixation has been the recent standard of care for displaced or compressed fractures (6), ARIF may represent a viable alternative to open surgery and may reduce morbidity associated with fracture repair (9,13). Arthroscopy is minimally invasive and more biologically benign than open reduction and internal fixation (7). In addition, arthroscopy allows for accurate fracture reduction while obviating the need for extensive operative exposure (12). In some regards, arthroscopy narrows the gap between the polar extremes of open versus non-operative management.

An additional advantage of arthroscopic treatment of tibial plateau fractures is the visualization of the entire articular surface without the extensive dissection required for traditional open reduction. Specifically, there is no need for meniscal detachment and repair when compared with open arthrotomy (7). The arthroscope allows for evacuation of hemarthrosis and any fracture debris (5). In addition, arthroscopic treatment of meniscal and ligamentous injuries is often superior to repair or reconstruction using large open incisions (5,7).

Arthroscopy may offer the advantages of rapid recovery with reduced pain, early full range of motion, improved fracture healing, and more complete and functional recovery (6,7, 12). Finally, patients with healed but symptomatic fractures can often benefit from arthroscopic intervention (17).

Indications

When articular compression or fracture displacement exists, surgery is required to restore joint congruity and alignment, to stabilize the knee, and to allow early joint motion (6,7). Recommendations regarding absolute indications for operative versus non-operative management vary. We believe that surgery is indicated for articular compression or fragment displacement greater than or equal to 4 mm. In addition, in cases of non-displaced but unstable fractures, rigid internal fixation may still be considered for active patients and athletes in whom early range of motion is a priority.

In our experience, the tibial plateau fracture patterns that may be most amenable to ARIF include Schatzker Types I to IV (fractures with split, split/compression, or pure compression) (10) as well as tibial intercondylar eminence avulsions (14), which are discussed separately in the following section. We acknowledge that percutaneous lag or buttress screws, percutaneous plates, or even open buttress plating may be required in such cases, and we specifically define ARIF as surgery where anatomic reduction and rigid internal fixation is achieved without a large or submeniscal arthrotomy.

More complex or higher-energy injury patterns (Schatzker Types V or VI) (10) may not be amenable to arthroscopic treatment (7,8). In addition, our recommendation is that although ARIF is the definitive treatment for Type III (central compression) fractures, ORIF may have advantages over ARIF in some Type I, II, and IV fractures. In cases where ORIF is preferred, arthroscopy remains useful both for diagnosis and for treatment of associated intra-articular pathology (7).

Potential disadvantages of ARIF or arthroscopic-assisted ORIF of tibial plateau fractures require consideration. Even with the use of a tourniquet, bleeding from the fracture site makes arthroscopy technically difficult. Although this challenge can be to some degree mitigated with the use of a pump, increased pump pressure compounds another problem: extravasation of arthroscopic fluid (15).

With the exception of isolated Type III compression fractures or intercondylar eminence avulsions, the tibial plateau fracture clefts are direct conduits linking the knee joint to the compartments of the leg. The complication of iatrogenic compartment syndrome requiring fasciotomy, always a concern in knee arthroscopy, is associated with traumatic or iatrogenic capsular disruption. This complication must be attentively considered in all cases of arthroscopic treatment of upper tibia fractures. Iatrogenic compartment syndrome requiring fasciotomy has occurred in the experience of the primary author (unpublished data).

A disadvantage of limited visualization of the submeniscal surface of the tibial articular surface has also been described (16). In our experience, specially designed meniscal (double hooked, self-retaining) retractors (Arthrex, Inc., Naples, FL) allow adequate visualization.

Timing

After confirming that the patient is otherwise stable, tibial plateau fractures may be addressed surgically without delay; however, a delay from seven to as long as 14 days could be permitted if circumstances dictate. Greater delays could result in early fracture healing, complicating the procedure.

In the case of open fractures, irrigation and debridement (I & D) is recommended on an urgent basis (as in the case of all fractures). Reduction with internal fixation may be performed at the time of I & D unless other issues (gross contamination or poor soft tissue coverage) suggests staged management could be preferred. Other exceptions to urgent treatment are similar, involving issues of soft tissue coverage, severe soft tissue swelling, or other medical or surgical patient issues. In such cases, temporary indirect external fixation with traction often facilitates staged definitive treatment.

Technique

Our recommended techniques represent modifications of techniques described by Caspari (17) and by Buchko and Johnson. (7). Operative treatment must be designed specifically for each fracture type (7). We recommend ARIF for central compression (Schatzker Type III) fractures, and we recommend consideration of ARIF for split and split compression fractures (Schatzker Types I, II and IV). Prior to surgery, an examination of the knee under anaesthesia may be of value for ligament evaluation (17).

We recommend the use of a circumferential leg holder and tourniquet. The fluoroscope (C-arm) is turned upside down so the flat (image acquiring) plate may be used as an operating table under the knee. Standard anterolateral (viewing) and anteromedial (instrumentation) portals are utilized. Often, the scope is placed anteromedially to view lateral fractures. The instrumentation or accessory portals may accommodate a hooked meniscal retractor (Arthrex, Inc.) in cases of peripheral and submeniscal pathology.

These blunt, double-hooked retractors may be used in a self-retaining mode with single-use, spring-loaded suction cup, which also prevent fluid extravasation.

Thorough lavage is required in order to remove hemarthrosis or grossly loose and small osteochondral fragments. When possible, reduction of the fracture may be performed in a dry field to decrease the risk of fluid extravasation and increased compartment pressures. In all cases, inflow pressure is kept to a minimum and the compartments are carefully and continuously palpated to assess pressure. This is especially important in split fractures where fluid extravasation occurs directly through the fracture lines. In cases of suspected increased pressures, formal measurement is recommended as is fasciotomy should frank compartment syndrome result.

Split fractures are reduced first. Reduction forceps are recommended, and sometimes an open incision (but not an arthrotomy) is required. Fluoroscopy may supplement the arthroscopic assessment of fracture reduction and is required for placement of wires for provisional split fracture reduction. For Type I fractures, percutaneous, cannulated lag screws may be placed over the wires. If mild fragment instability is suspected, a buttress screw, often used with a washer, is placed at the inferior apex of the split fragment. If greater instability or poor bone quality is of concern, buttress plates may be percutaneously placed or placed through traditional, extra-articular secondary incisions.

In Type II and Type IV fractures, compressed elements must be addressed prior to definitive fixation. Under arthroscopic guidance, an ACL guide with a modified spoon shaped tip (to mimic the curve of the femoral condyle) (Arthrex, Inc.) is used to place a 2.4 mm drill tipped guide pin (Arthrex, Inc.) in the center of the compressed fragment through a small incision in the proximal anteromedial tibial metaphysis. (A lateral approach muscle splitting can be considered for lateral fractures). A coring reamer is used to fully and circumferentially penetrate the tibial cortex while removing as little bone as possible. A cannulated tamp, specially angulated so the leading flat surface is parallel to the plateau (Arthrex, Inc.), is used to elevate the fracture site under direct arthroscopic visualization. Sometimes, it is helpful to over-reduce the fracture, and then place the knee through a range of motion to allow the femoral condyle to anatomically mold the tibial plateau. The underlying metaphyseal bone and cortical disc serve as autograft. In addition, the resulting cortical defect may be grafted using bone autograft, allograft, or bone substitute. Our current preference is freeze dried allograft croutons.

For most Type III patterns, cannulated screws may be introduced percutaneously, directly under the subchondral plate, to buttress the elevated fragments. In addition to the use of fluoroscopic guidance, the fracture guide wires may be placed while the cannulated tamp is still in place. If the wire hits the tamp, this directly confirms accurate screw placement beneath the compression fracture. The tamp may then be removed and the guide wire and ultimate cannulated screw(s) be placed using standard technique. In cases of Type II or Type IV fractures, similar cannulated lag screw techniques will buttress the compression and provide rigid internal fixation of the split fragment. A buttress screw or screw and washer can be additionally placed at the inferior apex of the split fragment. Again, if greater instability or poor bone quality is of concern, buttress plates may be percutaneously placed or placed through traditional, extra-articular secondary incisions.

Complications and Special Considerations

Associated injuries are common with fractures of the tibial plateau and may include injury to the menisci, ligaments, or articular surfaces of the femur, tibia, or patella (5). Although tibial plateau fractures may occur as isolated lesions, concurrent injuries are the rule (5). In cases of disruption of the lateral collateral ligament complex, injuries to the peroneal nerve or the popliteal vessels may be associated with greater frequency (4).

Up to 47% of knees with closed tibial plateau fractures have injuries of the menisci that may require surgical repair (18); it is difficult to predict the degree of meniscal injury based upon fracture pattern alone (6). Up to 32% of knees with tibial plateau fractures have complete or partial tears of the anterior cruciate (5).

The tibial intercondylar eminence is often avulsed in association with fractures of the tibial plateau (14). In addition, isolated tibial intercondylar eminence avulsion fractures may be considered a unique fracture. Tibial intercondylar eminence fractures are discussed in the following section.

Conclusions and Future Directions

Arthroscopy is a valuable tool for the assessment of tibial plateau fractures and is the treatment of choice for associated intra-articular pathology. In addition, ARIF of selected tibial plateau fractures allows achievement of anatomic reduction and rigid internal fixation with less morbidity than ORIF and with the advantage of superior visualization of the entire joint. We recommend ARIF for Type III fractures and consideration of ARIF for Types I, III, and IV. Some authors have applied ARIF to more complex (Type V or VI) fracture patterns. Published outcome studies of ARIF of tibial plateau fractures describe results that appear to equal outcomes of ORIF, but these studies suffer from extreme susceptibility bias. Future study of ARIF of tibial plateau fractures will require more rigorous descriptions of patient selection (inclusion and exclusion) criteria to allow comparison of arthroscopic and open treatment.

■ TIBIAL PLATEAU FRACTURES PART II—INTERCONDYLAR EMINENCE: INTRODUCTION

Orthopaedic treatment of fractures of the tibial plateau has undergone a dramatic evolution with the advent and widespread use of arthroscopy. In this section, fractures of the tibial intercondylar eminence will be given specific attention. As with other fractures within the knee joint, treatment modalities which were once limited to immobilization have broadened to include invasive types of procedures. The traditional open procedure to repair the tibial intercondylar eminence fractures has most recently given way to arthroscopic repair.

Basic Science: Anatomy

To review, the tibia serves as the major weight-bearing joint of the knee. Within the joint, the proximal tibia widens to form a shelf flanked by the medial and lateral condyles. This shelf is the intercondylar eminence which serves as the point of attachment for the menisci and the anterior and posterior cruciate ligaments (3).

Biomechanics

With regard to epidemiology, fractures isolated to the intercondylar eminence are most often seen in children and adolescents (20), although adults may be affected as well (19).

With regard to mechanisms of injury, a fracture of the tibial eminence is a consequence of ACL avulsion at its insertion on the tibia (21) and is an unusual occurrence in adults (16). In this specific scenario, the ACL is pulled from the tibia at the site of attachment with a piece of the bony tibial plateau. This particular problem is relatively common in children and equivalent to rupture of the ACL in adults. The underlying distinction between the pathology in children and adults is that children have a relative weakness of the incompletely ossified tibial eminence which fails before the relatively stronger ligament fails at times of pathology-inducing stress on the knee (22). This is all a consequence of greater elasticity of ligaments in the pediatric population (23).

Besides disrupting the ACL integrity, this fracture affects the articular surface of the tibia, as noted above. This fracture usually occurs between ages 8 and 14, and almost one half of these tibial eminence fractures are sequella of a fall from a bicycle (22). Though most commonly seen in the pediatric population, ACL avulsion fracture does happen in adults (23); however, with older patients, tibial eminence fractures are often combined with lesions of menisci, capsule, or collateral ligament (24).

Clinical Evaluation: History and Physical Findings

As with other fractures within the knee, patients with fractures involving the tibial eminence present with a painful swollen knee and usually cannot bear weight. The pain may make a thorough examination of ligaments impossible, but a complete neurologic and vascular examination must be obtained (3).

Imaging

Standard antero-posterior, lateral, and oblique radiographs are warranted when faced with injury to the knee. As discussed in the previous section, radiographs may be followed up with CT, MRI, and angiography as deemed clinically necessary.

As reviewed in the previous section, the utilization of the arthroscope for diagnosis allows direct visualization of the menisci, cruciates, articular surfaces, and the articular portion of the fracture site while minimizing extensive operative trauma (3).

Decision Making Algorithms and Classification

The most commonly cited classification system by Myers and McKeever summarizes three different fracture types, specific for the intercondylar eminence. Type I has minimal displacement of the anterior margin; Type II has displacement of the anterior third, with a posterior hinge intact; and Type III has total displacement of the fracture fragment (20).

In addition to this, Type III is sub-differentiated into Type III-A fractures which involve the ACL insertion only, and Type III-B fractures that include the entire intercondylar eminence (as proposed by Zifko and Gaudernak) (23).

One author, however, suggests that these classification schemes could be simplified into those that are displaced versus those that are nondisplaced (20).

Treatment

Nonoperative

The rule of thumb is that the treatment of tibial eminence fractures is based on their classification, with the underlying goal being total fracture reduction. Extension of the extremity may provide adequate reduction, but this is not a rule. If the fragment is not repositioned properly, the risk is the fracture will heal with the ACL in a relaxed position. It has been noted that younger children can compensate for some ACL instability as the skeleton grows, but that is not so with older children who lack this compensatory ability (63).

Most authors recommend treatment of Type I with nonoperative immobilization of the extremity in extension to maintain reduction. Aspiration of the hemarthrosis from a tense knee joint may also be beneficial (63).

Operative

Traditionally, open reduction and internal fixation was the norm, but like other tibial plateau fractures, fractures of the eminence can be very successfully assessed and treated using arthroscopy (20).

Indications. Type III injuries are treated with operative fixation (20,23). There is controversy concerning the treatment of the Type II fracture. Many authors recommend nonoperative treatment with cast immobilization (20). Other authors see the value of assessing the Type II fracture with the arthroscope because incarceration or impingement of the meniscus which prevents adequate fracture reduction, or because it can help to identify other intra-articular pathology that can be found only at operation. It is for these reasons that operative treatment (either open or arthroscopically) for both Type II and III lesions is suggested (24).

Timing

After confirming that the patient is otherwise stable, tibial intercondylar eminence fractures may be addressed surgically without delay. Although delays from 7 to as long as 14 days could be permitted if circumstances dictate, fibrous tissue and clot at the fracture site, arthrofibrosis and adhesions, and early fracture healing may complicate the procedure.

In the case of open fractures, irrigation and debridement (I & D) is recommended on an urgent basis (as in the case of all fractures). Reduction with internal fixation may be performed at the time of I & D unless other issues (gross contamination or poor soft tissue coverage) suggests staged management could be preferred. As with other tibial plateau fractures, exceptions to urgent treatment are similar, involving issues of soft tissue coverage, severe soft tissue swelling, or other medical or surgical patient issues; however, intercondylar eminence avulsions are generally low energy injuries (as compared to many tibial plateau fractures), and such exceptions as stated above are not common.

Technique

Specific techniques vary, but some caveats can be gleaned from the literature. One overlying consideration concerning any method of treatment for ACL avulsion is to achieve and maintain proper tension of the ligament at the time of repair. It must be cautioned that an over-reduction should be avoided so as to prevent excessive tightness of the ACL and thus limitation of full knee motion (23).

To reiterate, surgical treatment of eminence fractures is based upon the classification system, whether traditional open or arthroscopic management is performed. Options include non-absorbable suture repair of the ACL secured to the tibia via drill holes (22,63) or cannulated screw fixation (23).

After repair, the knee is placed through full range of motion to inspect the quality of the repair (21).

Complications and Special Considerations

Commonly, the meniscus is injured with fractures to the intercondylar eminence. In children, either the lateral or the medial meniscus may be affected. Injuries in adults have shown that the majority of ACL ruptures are associated with concomitant injuries to the meniscus (19). Intercondylar eminence fractures may be isolated, but as with other fractures to the tibia, injury patterns may include a combination of bone, chondral, meniscal, and ligamentous injuries (24).

Conclusions and Future Directions

As with the treatment of tibial plateau fractures in general, fractures of the tibial intercondylar eminence specifically are amenable to fixation using the aid of the arthroscope with successful outcomes.

■ FRACTURES OF THE DISTAL FEMUR: INTRODUCTION

Fractures of the distal femur are often very complex injuries (25). Before the 1970s, these fractures were usually treated with non-surgical methods (26) but the current trend involves operative fixation with internal stabilization, although this is still controversial (25).

With either a conservative or operative approach, management requires a complete understanding of anatomy and thorough diagnostic evaluation including radiographs. If surgical intervention is deemed appropriate, the use of appropriate fixation devices is critical (26).

Basic Science: Anatomy

Anatomically, the distal aspect of the femur corresponds to its lower third. As the femur progresses from superior to inferior, the bony shaft, or metaphysis, flares at the junction of the diaphysis and the metaphysis. This flaring culminates in the broad weight-bearing portion of the distal femur (27,28). Proximal to the flare, the supracondylar area comprises the distal 9 cm of the adult femur when measured from the inferior articular surface at the knee joint (26). At the knee, the femoral condyles flare so that posteriorly, they are wider when compared with the anterior portion (27).

We will focus on the supracondylar and metaphyseal portions of the distal femur, the areas between the distal diaphysis and the articular condyles of the femur (27,28).

On the anterior surface, the condyles articulate with the patella, whereas on the posterior aspect of the distal femur, the condyles make way for the intercondylar fossa, or notch, which provides attachment for the cruciate ligaments (26–28). On the lateral aspects of both condyles are the epicondyles, which act as points of attachment for each of the collateral ligaments (26). At the medial aspect of the knee lies the adductor tubercle (26,27).

At the knee, the femoral artery, which is a continuation of the iliac artery in the leg, runs between the extensor and adductor compartments in the medial aspect of the thigh. This large artery then transitions into the popliteal artery in the posterior thigh, approximately 10 cm proximal to the knee joint (27,29).

There are many muscles that act about the knee joint. The quadriceps are the collective term for the anterior thigh muscles that are made up of the vastus lateralus, vastus intermedius, vastus medialis, and rectus femoris. The posterior hamstrings are made up of the semimembranosus, semitendinosus, and biceps femoris (29).

It is the action of these muscles that causes fractures of the knee to behave in stereotypical ways: the hamstrings work to shorten the femur and the gastrocnemius pulls fragments posteriorly and adds rotation to the fragments (27,28).

Biomechanics

With regard to epidemiology, fractures of the distal femur have an estimated incidence of 4% to 7% of all femoral fractures (27) and are far less common than fractures of the femoral shaft or fractures at the hip (28). There are two distinct groups in which these fractures occur: young patients, especially male, due to high velocity forces such as motor vehicle accidents; and the elderly, especially females, due to low energy trauma, such as falls from a standing position (26,27).

With regard to mechanism of injury, as mentioned previously, fractures of the distal femur in young patients are usually the result of high-energy forces which result from motor vehicle accidents, motorcycle accidents, and falls from heights (27). The trauma is a result of axial loading with varus, valgus, or torsional forces exerted on the knee joint (26,28). The injury was most likely from force exerted on a flexed knee. These fractures in young patients are complicated in that they are often open and/or comminuted (27).

Given the high amount of energy required to cause distal femur fractures in young patients, it is likely that the injury is not isolated, but one of many problems for the trauma victim (25).

The other population presenting with a distal femur fracture is elderly as a result of falls from standing height, which involves considerably less energy and is often associated with osteoporosis (27).

Clinical Evaluation: History

Given the high amount of energy required to produce these fractures in young patients, and the likelihood of concomitant illness in elderly patients, ACLS/ATLS guidelines should be used in assessing any patient, even with low-energy injuries (29). Likewise, it is important to consider the patient's general medical condition, the presence of associated injuries, and pre-injury functional status (26) during the evaluation of such injuries.

Physical Findings

In the most general terms, supracondylar femur fractures will often present with femur shortening because of fracture segment displacement due to contraction of the leg muscles (27). As with any fracture, it is important to check the joint above and the joint below for bony abnormalities, as well as to evaluate distal pulses and to consider (thigh) compart-

ment syndrome (27). A systematic physical examination of affected extremity is indicated with special attention to assessing the soft tissues (25).

Not to be understated, it is best to have a high index of suspicion for other injuries of the body, including the head, chest, abdomen, and spine (25).

Imaging

Plain radiographs are the mainstay of initial imaging with standard antero-posterior and lateral radiographs. If possible, radiographs taken with the extremity held in traction may offer a better view. Oblique views help to evaluate fractures with intercondylar involvement (26,27). In accordance to ATLS protocols, radiographs are recommended to evaluate the pelvis and bilateral lower extremities in trauma situations, as deemed necessary (25).

Comparison radiographs of the unaffected extremity is helpful with surgical planning (27,29), as they help determine alignment and planning of plate or intramedullary nail size (26).

Beyond standard radiographs, computerized tomography is useful in delineating articular pathology (26,27) and magnetic resonance imaging is helpful in the assessment of ligament injuries (27).

As for arteriography, it is indicated for all suspected arterial injuries (27) as manifested in patients with diminished or absent pulses or bruit or even the suspicion of occult vascular injury including intimal disruptions of the arteries, which cannot be detected with manual palpation or ultrasound (28). In fact, some authors believe that all distal femur fractures with associated ligamentous injury should be evaluated with arteriography because of the high incidence of co-morbid arterial injuries (29).

Decision Making Algorithms and Classification

There are a number of classification methods in the literature that specifically address distal femur fractures; however, a universally accepted method of classification does not exist (28).

Neer and associates provide a three-part classification scheme in which fractures of Type I involve fragments in which the displacement is minimal. With Type II fractures, the condyles are displaced relative to femur shaft. In Type III fractures, there is an additional supracondylar component or there is comminution of the femoral shaft (29).

The classification scheme proposed by Seinsheimer is more involved: Four types of fractures are described and are further broken down into subtypes:

■ Type I fractures are non-displaced.
■ Type II fractures of the distal femur do not involve the intercondylar area and are sub-categorized into Type IIA for fractures with two pieces only and Type IIB for fractures which are comminuted.

- Type III fractures involve the intercondylar notch and one or both of the condyles are separated. Type IIIA has the medial condyle as the separated fragment and Type IIIB has the lateral condyle as the separated fragment. Type IIIC is when both condyles are separated from each other and from the femoral shaft.
- Type IV fractures involve the articular surface. Type IVA involves the medial condyle and Type IVB involves the lateral condyle. Type IVC fractures are complex and comminuted; they involve one condyle, the intercondylar notch, both condyles, or all three segments of the articular surface (29).

Finally, the AO/ASIF classification is also a subdivided system which emphasizes the position of the fractured fragment:

- Type A fractures are extra-articular with A1 being simple, A2 having the supracondylar portion in two parts, and A3 being comminuted.
- Type B fractures are unicondylar and thus intra-articular. Type B1 is a lateral condyle fracture with the fracture lying in the sagittal plane, whereas Type B2 is where the fracture of the medial condyle lies in the sagittal plane. Fractures of the subtype B3 involve the condyle lying in the coronal plane.
- Type C fractures are bicondylar in nature. Type C1 has no comminution. Type C2 has supracondylar comminution, with the articular surface made up of two major pieces. Type C3 has comminution involving the articular surface (26,29).

Treatment: Nonoperative

Historically, fractures involving the distal femur were managed with closed reduction and prolonged cast immobilization or traction (27), which required prolonged bed rest and was time consuming and expensive (28).

Current indications for nonoperative treatment include the presence of a non-displaced or incomplete fracture, some gunshot wounds, and severely infected wounds (aside from irrigation and debridement). Added to these, lack of adequate fixation devices and inexperience with surgical techniques are contraindications to operative management. Patient related factors such as significant underlying medical diseases or significant osteoporosis of the affected bone can sway the argument toward nonoperative management (28).

Times change, and so have the treatment options for patients with distal femur fractures. Depending on the fracture type and the individual patient, the decision of a nonoperative approach versus an operative one can now be made using strict criteria.

It must be maintained that the goals of nonoperative management are not for anatomical reduction per se, but to restore the natural length of the lower extremity and to restore axial alignment since the knee joint can tolerate less

than seven degrees of mediolateral mal-alignment (28). These fractures should be followed and assessed for signs of loss of reduction in the post injury period (30).

Treatment: Operative

As orthopaedic techniques have evolved, open reduction and internal fixation is now the treatment of choice for selected patients with fractures amenable to fixation. In its most basic sense, as outlined by the Swiss AO group, the goal for management of these fractures is anatomic reduction of the fracture with preservation of blood supply while providing stable internal fixation and early pain-free mobilization (27). Results of good to excellent in up to 60% to 80% of patients treated operatively have been achieved with the qualifier that careful operative technique is absolutely necessary (25), as the advantages of internal fixation can be offset by aggressive soft tissue dissection and periosteal stripping (31). At its best, successful surgery allows the patient to avoid the inherent complications of traction and prolonged bed rest or cast immobilization (25).

The pediatric population, who are affected with distal femur fractures more often due to increased participation with organized sports, are typically skeletally immature athletes. For this population, treatments should be customized to the individual's anatomy, including the difference in healing potential (32).

The surgical goals for the repair of a distal femur fracture are to restore the articular surface continuity and to re-establish anatomic alignment and limb length. An internal fixation device provides stability of the extremity and joint, thus allowing for early mobilization, rehabilitation of the knee, and prompt patient recovery (26,28).

Open reduction and internal fixation of this fracture type demands skill, thorough dissection and exposure, and is justified if the surfaces of the joint can be re-approximated. Mechanistically, the fixation is rigid internally in order to negate the need for any additional external stabilization. Once done, this stabilization allows for rapid extremity mobilization.

Tantamount to the above conditions, the soft tissues should be viable and allow for adequate injury and repair coverage (30).

Indications

Operative intervention is justified when a distal femur fracture cannot be externally reduced (25) and displaced fractures in the young should be surgically managed (28). Surgery is also indicated when the fracture is associated with vascular injury (25). Other indications for surgery are open fractures and fractures associated with current or impending compartment syndrome (26).

Fractures involving both distal femurs on the same patient are better internally fixed because of the inability of patients to tolerate bilateral lower extremity traction. Moreover, patients with head injuries who cannot lie still often require internal femur fracture fixation, as do patients with chest or abdominal injuries who cannot tolerate prolonged bed rest.

One other population for which operation should be considered is obese patients in whom prolonged bed rest with traction can result in increased risk of complications (25).

The contraindications for operative intervention with distal femur fractures include massive comminution, severe osteopenia, and/or inadequate facilities. Other contraindications are sepsis and infection or severely contaminated soft tissues that cannot be debrided well enough (25).

Timing

Except in the case of open fractures or neurovascular compromise, treatment should be delayed until the patient is medically and surgically stable. In cases of multitrauma, the general surgical team leader will determine whether surgical treatment of the distal femur may be performed during the initial operative intervention or delayed.

Technique

Over the years, several approaches for operative fixation have developed depending on fracture type and fixation method (29), with most fractures being managed operatively with screws, plates, or intramedullary nails (30).

Before surgery, the affected limb should be placed in traction with 5 to 15 pounds hung from a pin inserted into the proximal tibia. This frequently allows time for preoperative surgical planning and general medical and surgical stabilization (25).

1 95 degree condylar blade plate: Placement of this rigid fixation device requires 1.5–2 cm of uninterrupted distance from the articular surface. This is a fixed apparatus that is technically difficult to place because it requires secure attachment in the coronal, transverse, and sagittal planes, all at the same time (26). Although technically difficult, the broad plate allows for excellent resistance to torsional forces and is indicated with supracondylar and intercondylar femur fractures (30).

   Placement of this plate is prohibited in fractures that involve the articular surface and in cases where there is comminution of the lateral condyle (26).

2 Condylar screw and side plate: Unlike the condylar blade plate, the screw and plate are separate pieces, so they can be adjusted at the time of fixation of the fracture. Placement requires 4 cm of medial condyle to be intact (26). Technically the plate and screw are easier to apply than a blade plate and they can be adjusted on the operative field at the time of use (30).

3 Condylar buttress plate: This plate is indicated for comminuted fractures with intra-articular involvement, although it may prove to be weaker than the previous two procedures (26). Very low distal femur fractures with weakness after fixation may require the addition of

another plate placed medially for added strength (30). New, locking screw technology has improved the strength of these implant devices.

4 Intramedullary nailing: Some believe intramedullary nailing is superior to plating because there is load sharing between the bone and the intramedullary nail. This fixation is considered to be more anatomical. Intramedullary nails can be placed in an anterograde fashion for distal femur fractures that have at least 5 cm of distance from the fracture and the articular surface. Alternatively, retrograde nailing may be used for supracondylar fractures (26).

5 External fixators: These are rarely used, but are useful in severe open fractures with soft tissue or bone loss (26). The external fixator has the advantages of rapid placement, minimal dissection, and offers the ability to maintain the length of the extremity. On the other hand, problems with pin track infections, loss of knee motion, and loss of reduction when the apparatus is removed are potential adverse consequences (26,28). Ring fixators, which are used in the management of complex tibial fractures, have a limited role in the management of femur fractures and are thus rarely used, mostly because of their size and bulk. However, they are indicated for open condylar fractures with significant bone loss, in unstable multi-traumatized patients, and in patients with sepsis or burns.

Complications and Special Considerations

High-energy injuries are often complicated by intra-articular fracture and shaft comminution and are usually associated with multiple injuries associated with the forces required to cause the original femoral fracture (27). The position of the femur and hip at the time of injury dictates the incidence of associated injuries including fractures of the acetabulum, dislocations of the hip, and more proximal femur fractures (29).

In cases of unilateral fractures, concomitant injuries are present in approximately one third of patients in one estimation (30). Besides other fractures involving the femur, distal fractures are associated with tibial plateau fractures and ligamentous injuries occur in approximately 20% of cases. Associated ligament injuries are often not diagnosed preoperatively because the fracture obscures physical examination of the knee joint. The anterior cruciate ligament is most commonly injured in combination with a distal femur fracture (28).

Injuries to the femoral artery and disruption of popliteal artery occur in 2% to 3% of distal femur fractures (28). When associated with posterior dislocation of knee joint, arterial injury may occur in up to 40% of patients (27). The sciatic nerve is close to the popliteal artery, and this large nerve runs the risk of injury as well (29).

Statistically, open fractures make up 5% to 10% of distal femur fractures with the wound usually being anterior and with a high proportion associated with damage to extensor muscles and ligaments (28).

Distant from the fracture site, distal femur fractures are part of a constellation of multisystem trauma that also involves the head, chest, abdomen, and other parts of the skeleton (25).

In the pediatric population large forces are required to fracture the femur, and complications may be expected. Neurovascular damage at the time of the original injury and at the time of surgery must be considered (25).

Nonunion can occur in cases with significant bone loss and malunion may happen especially with closed reduction. In addition, infection is associated with high-energy mechanisms of injury, significant soft tissue stripping or devascularization, open fractures, or inadequate stabilization (29). Contracture, instability of the knee joint, thromboembolism, failure of a surgical implant, and re-fracture are other risks (25). Decreased knee motion is a complication that may be avoided with early knee motion and rehabilitation (29).

Conclusions and Future Directions

Open reduction and internal fixation is now the treatment of choice for displaced distal femur fractures. Careful planning, attention to associated medical or general surgical co-morbidity, and customization of treatment to the individual fracture pattern are keys to success. With a goal of early fixation achieving good alignment and joint continuity, successful treatment of the fracture may allow for rapid mobilization and recovery (26).

■ FRACTURES OF THE PATELLA: INTRODUCTION

In the field of orthopaedics, there is historical controversy about the function of the patella, especially regarding whether it is necessary to repair and or maintain the bone when it is injured or fractured. For many years, if the patella was fractured, it was simply removed. More recently, the importance of maintaining the patella after fracture is understood; total excision of the fractured patella often leads to permanent disability of the knee (33).

Although a fracture of the patella is somewhat uncommon, it has been learned over time that without operation to repair it, the fracture results in permanent joint pain, weakness of the quadriceps mechanism, and restriction in the range of motion of the knee joint (34).

Basic Science: Anatomy

The patella is the largest sesamoid bone in the body. It lies within the confines of the quadriceps tendon (33) in the anterior subcutaneous aspect of the knee joint (35).

The patella is an inverted triangle with the apex pointing distally. The proximal patella is the insertion site of the quadriceps muscles of the anterior thigh and the inferior portion gives rise to the patellar tendon with its insertion on the tubercle of the anterior tibia. The posterior aspect is mostly covered in cartilage and acts as the anterior boundary of the knee joint.

The patella serves to increase the mechanical strength of the quadriceps muscle at the knee by elevating the extensor mechanism off the knee joint proper. It also protects the femoral condyles from direct trauma. It receives its blood supply from anastomotic vessels that enter the bone through the mid-anterior aspect. This supply can be jeopardized during repair (or at the time of fracture) leading to avascular necrosis long after the original injury (33).

Biomechanics

With regard to epidemiology, patellar fractures make up approximately 1% of all skeletal injuries resulting from direct or indirect trauma (33,35). Affected individuals are usually within the 20- to 50-year-old age range and there is a higher incidence of males over females (33).

With regard to mechanism of injury, fractures of the patella can be caused by either direct trauma, indirect trauma, or a combination of the two. In cases involving direct trauma, the patella is fractured after hitting the knee on the dashboard in a motor vehicle accident, for example, or from a fall onto the patella itself. Indirect fractures are caused during a fall in which the quadriceps muscle, in an attempt to prevent the fall, contract with force that is stronger that the patella itself, thus causing the fracture. It is noted that most fractures are a combination of the direct and indirect mechanisms (33–35).

Another type of fracture is an osteochondral fracture, which can be a result of patellar dislocation (34).

Clinical Evaluation: History

As with all other suspected orthopaedic injury, assessment includes the history and physical to exclude other injuries sustained during the original trauma. Notice of the integrity of surrounding tissue and the neurovascular examination of the affected extremity is mandatory. The patient with a fractured patella will often complain of knee pain and localized tissue swelling will be evident.

Physical Findings

There are a few caveats specifically pertaining to patella fractures. On its most basic level, displaced fractures usually result in the inability to extend at the knee, although fractures that are not displaced often allow extension at the knee (34). This is because in fractures from direct trauma, there is usually little or no separation of the individual fragments, so the patient may be able to actively extend the limb at the knee against gravity. In contrast, fractures sustained from indirect trauma are the result of such a significant force that it not only causes bony fracture, but also leads to surrounding retinacular rupture. This causes separation of the bony fragments and the ability to actively extend the knee is lost (33).

Most authors agree that the inability to actively extend leg at the knee indicates disruption of the extensor mechanism and requires surgical intervention. However, if extension is limited by pain, aspiration of a hemarthrosis may relieve pressure and allow for extension, which provides evidence that the extensor mechanism is actually intact (35).

Imaging

Standard anteroposterior, lateral, and axial (Merchant) views are indicated after physical examination (35). The Merchant, or sunrise, view is a tangential radiograph of the patella taken with the knee flexed at 30 degrees (34) that helps to rule out vertical marginal fractures (33). Comparison radiographs of the contralateral knee may be be helpful in cases of patients with bipartite patellae, a congenital variant which can mimic an acute fracture on plain radiograph (34).

CT and MR may be indicated to further delineate anatomy (33) and a bone scan can be useful to detect a stress fracture, which is often difficult to diagnose otherwise (33).

Decision Making Algorithms and Classification

There is no widely accepted classification system for describing fractures of the patella. Some authors will differentiate based upon if the fracture is non-displaced versus displaced (35).

Other classification schemes separate fracture types based on the anatomy of the fracture. Transverse, stellate, comminuted, longitudinal or marginal, proximal or distal pole, and osteochondral are all descriptive terms used in identifying the anatomy of the patella fracture. It has been noted that of all these, fractures of the transverse type are the most common (33).

One classification system delineates transverse fractures from extensively displaced and comminuted fractures. Longitudinal, marginal, and avulsion fractures of the superior or inferior poles is another subclass. Finally, osteochondral fractures can be grouped together as they are usually associated with patellar dislocation (34).

Treatment: Nonoperative

When faced with a patient with a patella fracture, consideration must be given to nonoperative versus operative management. Fractures that are closed show minimal displacement and demonstrate an intact extensor retinaculum can be treated without operation (33,35). This approach dictates that the patient be fitted with long leg cast immobilization for 4 to 6 weeks. To maintain quadriceps muscle strength, straight leg raises are encouraged 1 to 2 days after cast placement (33).

It should be noted that closed methods often yield poor results because of lengthy immobilization, which results in peri-patellar muscle weakening despite leg raising exercises (33).

Treatment: Operative

Up to one third of all patellar fractures require surgery and around 20% are severely comminuted (33). With operative intervention, the goals are to re-establish continuity of the extensor mechanism, to preserve the function of the patella, and to reduce complications (33).

Indications

In contrast to the conservative approach, patella fractures that are open (a surgical emergency) and fractures that demonstrate fragment displacement of more that 2 to 3 mm are treated with operation with the aim being to restore the extensor mechanism and allow for stability for early mobilization (33–35).

Timing

Except in cases of open fractures or neurovascular compromise, surgical treatment of patellar fractures may be performed on an urgent (within 2 weeks) rather than emergent basis. Delay of greater than 14 days may result in knee joint arthrofibrosis as well as early fracture healing which may complicate the procedure.

Technique

If operation is indicated, the decision to be made at the time of surgery is between anatomical reduction of the fractured patella using wires and screws versus partial patellectomy versus total patellectomy (33,35).

Historically, a transverse incision was made over the affected patella, but now a vertical incision is preferred in the event that future operations are necessary (33).

In cases in which anatomic reduction is possible (simple fractures with minimal comminution), cerclage wiring in combination with Kirschner wire or lag-screw fixation provides for adequate fracture reduction. It has been noted that superior biomechanical strength is attained when the wires are placed on the tension side of the patella (anterior cortical surface) (33), specifically in regard to transverse fractures (34).

Partial patellectomy is indicated when the degree of comminution is such that the fragments cannot be stabilized easily with hardware. Non-viable fragments are removed and the remaining portions are re-approximated with the goal being reconstruction of as near normal anatomy as possible (33).

Lastly, total patellectomy is another operative option, but it carries a poorer prognosis and should be avoided if at all possible, except in cases involving severe comminution where no type of fixation would be adequate (34,35). If at all possible, attempts should be made to save at least the proximal or distal third of the patella for reconstruction (35).

If total patellectomy is indicated, the superceding goals are to reestablish the continuity of the reticula on the lateral and medial sides and to ensure that tracking of the extensor mechanism is normal (34).

After surgery, if adequate stable reduction of the patella has been achieved, active rehabilitation should be started early in the postoperative period and splinting maintained for up to one week (33). In cases involving severely comminuted fractures, immobilization for up to 6 weeks in a cast may be required (33,34). Similarly, partial patellectomy with tendon repair requires up to 4 weeks of cast immobilization (33).

Continuous passive motion machines can be used, if necessary; otherwise, it is recommended that quadriceps isometric exercises and active movement help to maintain thigh muscle tone during the rehabilitation. Full weight bearing is allowed only after there is radiographic evidence of fracture healing (33,34).

It is likely that maximal function of the knee does not occur until one year after surgery (34).

Complications and Special Considerations

Patellar fractures are generally associated with hemarthrosis (35) and can be associated with ipsilateral injuries to the femur, hip, and tibia (33).

There are a number of complications which occur with both conservative and operative management of patellar fractures. Although it is seen with both treatments, avascular necrosis is seen especially with operative repair. It is diagnosed months after repair with radiographic evidence of sclerosis of either the proximal or distal portion of the patella (33).

The occurrence of degenerative arthritis appears more likely in cases with severe comminution (33). In cases where rehabilitation was complicated with pain that limited movement, knee adhesions can develop but these can be released with arthroscopic lysis (33).

Fracture separation and dehiscence are uncommon. Refractures, although rare, can occur and usually are a result of minimal trauma (33). Atrophy of the quadriceps is seen after total patellectomy with resultant weakness of the extensor mechanism (33).

Conclusions and Future Directions

The understanding of the role of the patella and the disability that occurs after fracture and operative removal has led to improved operative techniques that allow for salvage of the smallest bone of the human knee. Experience shows that prognosis is good for operative repair (33), and most patients can walk without difficulty, though weakness when climbing stairs, walking downhill, and kneeling is common (33).

■ OSGOOD-SCHLATTER DISEASE: INTRODUCTION

Historically, Osgood-Schlatter Disease (OSD) has typically been managed with conservative treatments, as the majority of cases are self-limited; however, there are increasing numbers of orthopaedic treatments being evaluated for the management of cases in which OSD symptoms are chronic or debilitating. This section reviews the history of OSD,

discusses diagnostic techniques that identify possible related causes, and examines techniques to manage both its acute and chronic aspects.

Basic Science: Anatomy

In 1903, Osgood and Schlatter independently and simultaneously first described a disease that occurred near the tibial insertion of the patellar tendon (36). This disease was originally labeled as a "traction apophysitis." To fully appreciate the pathophysiology of OSD, it is necessary to review the normal anatomy and development of the adolescent knee. In the child, growth cartilage is located in three areas of the knee: the growth plate, the epiphysis (articular cartilage), and the apophysis (tendon insertion) (37).

OSD occurs at the tibial tuberosity. Development of the tibial tuberosity can be divided into the cartilaginous phase (0 to 11 years), the apophyseal stage (11 to 14 years), the epiphyseal stage (14 to 18 years), and the bony stage (>18 years). During the apophyseal stage, the anterior portion of the secondary ossification center of the tibial tubercle is a relatively weak membranous tissue. This area must handle the high tensile stress at the insertion of the ligamentum patellae fibers along the fibrocartilaginous physis (38). It is no coincidence that the onset of OSD occurs during this time.

Biomechanics

In addition to biomechanical forces, the growth process, especially as related to cartilaginous development, has been implicated in the etiology of OSD. During growth spurts, muscle tendon tightness increases around the joints with a subsequent loss in flexibility (39). At the knee joint this results in an increased tensile strength across the apophysis of the tibial tuberosity. Further increasing the tensile stress upon this fragile area is a high patellar position, patella alta. A high patella may increase the force transmitted from the quadriceps to the tibial tuberosity via the quadriceps tendon (40). Causality has not been established, however, because a high patella may be a complication of OSD (40) and other studies show an equivocal relationship depending on the index used to measure this height (41).

Histologically, deposition of fibrous tissue between the tuberosity and the anterior metaphysis correlates with increased traction at the tuberosity (42). This creates the perfect environment for overuse injury or repetitive microtrauma (43). In children, cartilage may be more susceptible to trauma than in adults' cartilage (44). Furthermore, the apophyseal cartilage is weaker than the surrounding tissue in children. The fibrocartilaginous physis is more resistant to traction than the secondary center of ossification during the apophyseal stage. This combination results in microavulsions and fractures at the secondary center of ossification. OSD is related to tiny avulsions secondary to this microtrauma and the body's attempts to heal. The fragment is typically the unossified portion of the cartilage from the anterior apophysis (45). If the fracture of the secondary ossification center fails to unite, an ossicle will form (46).

Epidemiological data correlates with the hypothesized pathophysiology. OSD typically occurs in adolescents during the growth spurt when the tibial tuberosity is at the apophyseal stage. For girls, this occurs from ages 10 to 12, and for boys, this occurs from ages 12 to 14 (45). Boys are typically affected more commonly in girls. OSD occurs more often in the active adolescent. This is further supported by the "take-off" or "kicking" leg being affected more often in unilateral cases (43).

Clinical Evaluation: History

Clinically, the history is very suggestive of OSD. During the acute phase of the disease, the afflicted individual will complain of a gradual onset of unilateral or bilateral knee pain with some associated swelling (38). The onset usually correlates with an episode of overuse such as athletic camps or practices on a hard wooden or cement floor (47).

The majority of individuals will report a variable limitation in activities such as inability to kneel without discomfort, but will still maintain the ability to move the knee and walk. Roughly half of presenting patients will give a clear history of trauma (45).

Physical Findings

On physical exam, tenderness of the anterior tibial tuberosity will be present (47). Pain will also occur in this area when the knee is straightened against resistance (48). Local swelling and prominence of the tibial tuberosity may be present (43,47). A roughening of the tuberosity or a prominent bony lump may result in an abnormal outline of the tibial tuberosity (47). Symptoms such as pain, heat, tenderness, local swelling, and prominence of the area of the tibial tuberosity are diagnostic of OSD (43). Imaging and lab tests are not necessary to confirm the diagnosis.

Imaging

Radiographic films are indicated when symptoms occur in an atypical pattern such as early onset of symptoms, long duration of symptoms, or unusual severity of symptoms. Radiographs are helpful to narrow the differential and rule out fractures, epiphysiolysis, tumors, and to estimate the developmental phase (49).

To rule in OSD, the radiographic of the lateral knee during the acute phase should reveal soft tissue swelling anterior to the tibial tuberosity and thickening of the infrapatellar fat pad and patellar tendon (43). Krause et al reviewed 50 radiographs during the acute phase; 44 revealed fragmentation of the epiphysis and soft tissue swelling, 28 revealed separated ossicles, and 20 had abnormally shaped tuberosities (47). Radiographs may show

fragments or small avulsions, which is important prognostic information as discussed previously; however, the absence of these fragments does not rule out the possibility of cartilaginous ossicles. In pre-operative radiographs, Glynn et al. found seven of thirteen with visible ossicles; however, the remaining six all had cartilaginous ossicles that were successfully removed during surgery (50).

In adults with symptomatic OSD, the presence of an irregularity of the tubercle with or without an ossicle formation will be present (51). In adults, the radiographs will not show the rounding of the infrapatellar fat pad or soft tissue swelling that is classic for the acute phase of OSD in adolescence (52).

Although controversial, as discussed earlier, a patella alta may be associated with OSD. Several ways exist to measure the patellar height radiographically (49). The Install-Savati method measures the ratio between the length of the patellar tendon and the patella (53). This method has been criticized because the insertion of the patellar ligament is often ill defined because of the anatomic alteration of the tibial tubercle (40). Furthermore, the inferior margin of the patella shows signs of apophysitis that makes measurement of the patellar length difficult and imprecise (40).

The Trickey-Blackbum-Peel Method measures the ratio between the perpendicular distance from the lowest margin of the patella to the tibial plateau and the length of the articular cartilage of the patella (54). The Trickey-Blackbum-Peel method is less than ideal because of variations secondary to the slope of the tibial plateau; measurement is also affected by the degree of development of the tibial epiphysis (40). The Caton-Deschamps index is a simple, reliable method that is not affected by skeletal maturation. It measures the ratio between the distal patella and the anterior superior tibia over the length of the patellar surface (55). In a prospective study, Aparicio et al found a strong association between OSD and patella alta (40).

Decision Making Algorithms and Classification

The natural history of OSD is typically self-limited and resolves with rest and cessation of activity that tends to exacerbate the pain. In one study, the acute phase of the illness lasted for 3.2 months following a period of rest. After 7.3 months, the adolescent typically returned to full athletic activities (43).

In a subset of individuals afflicted with OSD, however, symptoms persist far beyond the expected range. Krause et al. divided individuals in the acute phase into two groups based on the presence or absence of radiographic evidence of fragmentation of the apophysis at presentation. Those with no fragmentation did not have chronic symptoms and all had normal outline of the tibial tuberosity; those with fragmentation were more likely to have chronic symptoms and an abnormal outline of their tibial tuberosity (47). This study was retrospective; therefore classification at presentation is not accurate because fragmentation may occur later. The fragments may heal spontaneously via union with the tuberosity by forming a bridge or callous. Some fragments do not resolve; these are most likely to cause symptoms persisting into adulthood (45).

Treatment: Nonoperative

OSD is most often a self-limited condition; therefore, conservative treatments are typically utilized. Rest is most often the initial recommendation. The afflicted individual is instructed to avoid all physical activity that causes pain for approximately 2 months (43). This rest can be thought of as active or relative rest where swimming or bicycling is substituted for running, for example (37).

Historically, the recommendation of rest was taken to the extreme of a plaster cast. This option did little to affect the natural course of the disease or the final bone deformity of the tibial tuberosity (57). Furthermore, the plaster cast makes a tight, weak muscle tighter and weaker (37). Envelope braces that leave the patella open (Marshall or Palumbro) may have a role in the acute phase of the disease or when play is resumed (37).

An infrapatellar strap may be an effective means of shortening the acute phase of the disease. This is a slightly curved 2.5 cm vinyl padded band that is worn just below the patella during activities. It is hypothesized to work by limiting the pull of the quadriceps on the inflamed insertion of the patellar tendon. In one study, Levine et al. found that in a study of 24 knees, 19 had a definite improvement in 6 to 8 weeks. Despite the fact that no control group was utilized, this does appear to be a significantly shorter duration of the acute phase when contrasted with natural history studies of OSD (43). Injections of local anesthetic and steroid can also be used with a high success rate (57), but this option may offer only temporary resolution of pain and tenderness (45). In addition, steroid injection may weaken the patellar tendon resulting in risk of rupture. Steroid injections are therefore not recommended.

Treatment: Operative

Indications

Despite the reported success of conservative measures and the self-limited nature of OSD, some individuals may require surgery after failure of conservative options, severe pain, or severe disability. The timing for "failure" of conservative options appears variable. One study defined a "reasonable period of time" for treatment failure as an average of approximately 13 months before surgery was considered (38,45). Another study had an average duration of symptoms of 11 months (41). Glynn et al. performed surgery if symptoms did not improve after 3 months; operations performed prior to 3 months were more associated with a poor or fair outcome. The sample size, however, was very small (n = 5) (50). Another author would only consider surgery if the individual was interested in resuming athletics, and others were treated conservatively (45). A more rigorous

indication for surgery proposed by Kujala et al. is the presence of separate ossicles that persist and are symptomatic after ossification of the tibial tuberosity (43).

Timing

In general, OSD is self-limited. Surgery should only be considered in severe cases of greater that at least 12–24 months duration.

Technique

Because of the rarity of surgical treatment for OSD and the variety of surgical treatments employed over the years, comparison of techniques is difficult (41). Prior to the 1970s, various procedures were utilized with the common aim of expediting fusion of the apophyseal growth plate. Drilling the tubercle offered some pain relief in some, but did little to affect the final deformity (58). Autogenous bone peg insertion through the tubercle was associated with severe postoperative pain and an unsightly "knob" (38). Reattachment with fixation is no longer recommended because of association of postoperative pain, necessity of eventual removal, and the "knob" (41).

In 1967, Dunkerly described the excision of all intratendinous ossicles (59). In this technique, the fibers of the patellar tendon are split longitudinally and ossicles are palpated and removed with careful preservation of the tendon fibers and attachment.

A study from Glynn et al. compared the drilling technique with the excisional technique. This study was performed in a longitudinal fashion reflecting the evolution of techniques at their hospital. The final outcome of this study was reduction in symptoms of discomfort at the tibial tubercle and reduction of activity limitation. Of the 22 patients that received the drilling, 12 reported good or excellent results. Of the 22 patients that had pieces of bone or cartilage removed, 21 had good or excellent results (50). Another review by Binazzi et al. further supported excision of the ossicles with 93% of the population having good or excellent results (41). Residual postoperative complaints were minor and related to the natural outcome of OSD. The average postoperative time to resume full sporting activities was 3.8 months. No cases of genu recurvatum have been recorded in ossicle excision cases (45).

Despite the success rate of the above technique, patients should be instructed that excisions of the ossicles will not affect the final deformity of the tibial tubercle. To further address this potentially disfiguring symptom, a Thomson-Ferciot technique may be utilized to excise the prominence in addition to removing ossicles. In this technique, the medial and lateral tendons are released while the distal insertions are preserved to elevate the tendon from the tuberosity. The tuberosity is then reduced with an osteotome. Any osteocartilaginous material is then removed via the excisional technique. In one study, pain relief was seen in 95% of the patients, and a reduction in prominence was seen in 85.5% of the patients. Most patients returned to sporting activities in 15.2 weeks. Only minimal complications and no cases of genu recurvatum were reported (38).

It must be noted that despite a large sports medicine/knee practice, the chapter authors have little experience with surgical treatment of OSD.

Complications and Special Considerations

Complications not related to operative repair include persistence of symptoms into adult life. Some of these individuals develop diathrodial joint formation between an ossicle and the patellar ligament (60). By altering the amount of cartilage relative to fibrocartilage in the physis, OSD may be associated with avulsion fractures of the tibial tubercle (46). Some case reports comment on the relationship between OSD and genu recurvactum, but other authors believe that this may be related to Salter-Harris Type III epiphyseal injuries misdiagnosed as OSD (61). Other case reports document a relationship between OSD and tibia recurvatum and argue for routine screening of all individuals with OSD (62).

Conclusions and Future Directions

The understanding of the development of OSD and the possibility of the development of debilitating fragmentation has expanded treatment options in chronic cases of OSD. The current literature suggests that many months of conservative treatment, including rest and the use of an infrapatellar strap, should be recommended before consideration of more invasive treatments. In chronic and recalcitrant cases, however, surgical treatment may appear to improve the prognosis with regard to long-term pain management or deformity of the tibial tubercle.

■ REFERENCES

1. O'Dwyer KJ, Bobic VR. Arthroscopic management of tibial plateau fractures. *Injury.* 1992;23(4):261–264.
2. Clasby L, Young M. Management of sports-related anterior cruciate ligament injuries. *AORN J.* 1997;66(4):609–630.
3. Rockwood C, Green DP, Heckman JD, et al. eds. *Rockwood and Green's Fractures in Adults.* 4th ed. Philadelphia: Lippincott Williams & Wilkins; 1992.
4. Schatzker J. Tibial plateau fractures. In: Brower, ed. *Skeletal trauma.* 1st ed. Philadelphia: WB Saunders; 1992:1745–1768.
5. Gill TJ, Moezzi DM, Oates KM, et al. Arthroscopic reduction and internal fixation of tibial plateau fractures in skiing. *Clin Orthop Rel Res.* 2001;383:243–249.
6. McClellan RT, Comstock CP. Evaluation and treatment of tibial plateau fractures. *Curr Opin Orthop.* 1999;10(1):10–21.
7. Buchko GM, Johnson DH. Arthroscopy assisted operative management of tibial plateau fractures. *Clin Orthop Rel Res.* 1996;332:29–36.
8. Mills WJ, Nork SE. Open reduction and internal fixation of high-energy tibial plateau fractures. *Orthop Clin N Am.* 2002; 33(1):177–194.
9. Beaufils P, Cassard X, Hardy P. Arthroscopic treatment of tibial plateau fractures reported in 26 Cases. *J Bone Joint Surg Br.* 1999;81B(suppl II):155.
10. Schatzker J, McBroom R, Bruce D. The tibial plateau fracture. The Toronto experience. *Clin Orthop.* 1979;138:94–104.
11. Hohl M, Moore TM. Surgery of the musculoskeletal system, vol. 7. *Articular fractures of the proximal tibia.* New York: Churchill Livingstone; 1983.
12. Jennings JE. Arthroscopic management of tibial plateau fractures. *Arthroscopy.* 1985;1(3):160–168.
13. Lemon RA, Bartlett DH. Arthroscopic assisted internal fixation of certain fractures about the knee. *J Trauma.* 1985;25(4):355–358.
14. Meyers MH, McKeever FM. Fracture of the intercondylar eminence of the tibia. *J Bone Joint Surg.* 1959;41A:209–222.
15. Lobenhoffer P, Schulze M, Gerich T, et al. Closed reduction/percutaneous fixation of tibial plateau fractures: arthroscopic versus fluoroscopic control of reduction. *J Orthop Trauma.* 1999; 13(6):426–431.
16. Burnstein DB, Viola A, Fulkerson JP. Entrapment of the medial meniscus in a fracture of the tibial eminence. *Arthroscopy.* 1998;4(1):47–50.
17. Caspari RB, Hutton PM, Whipple TL, et al. The role of arthroscopy in the management of tibial plateau fractures. *Arthroscopy.* 1985;1(2):76–82.
18. Vangsness CT, Ghaderi B, Hohl M, et al. Arthroscopy of meniscal injuries with tibial plateau fractures. *J Bone Joint Surg.* 1994;76B(3):488–490.
19. McLennan JG. The role of arthroscopic surgery in the treatment of fractures of the intercondylar eminence of the tibia. *J Bone Joint Surg.* 1982;4(64B):477–480.
20. Chandler JT, Miller TK. Tibial eminence fracture with meniscal entrapment. *Arthroscopy.* 1995;11(4):499–502.
21. Berg EE. Comminuted tibial eminence anterior cruciate ligament avulsion fractures: failure of arthroscopic treatment. *Arthroscopy.* 1993;9(4):446–450.
22. Owens BD, Crane GK, Plante T, et al. Treatment of Type III tibial intercondylar eminence fractures in skeletally immature athletes. *Am J Orthop.* 2003;32(2):103–105.
23. Lubowitz JH, Grauer JD. Arthroscopic treatment of anterior cruciate ligament avulsion. *Clin Orthop Rel Res.* 1993;294:242–246.
24. Falstie-Jensen S, Sondergard Petersen PE. Incarceration of the meniscus in fractures of the intercondylar eminence of the tibia in children. *Injury.* 1984;15(4):236–238.
25. Mize RD. Supracondylar and articular fractures of the distal femur. In: Chapman MW, ed. *Operative orthopaedics.* 2nd ed. Philadelphia: JB Lippincott Co; 1993:651–662.
26. Placide RJ, Lonner JH. Fractures of the distal femur. *Curr Opin Orthop.* 1999;10(1):2–9.
27. Helfet, DL. Fractures of the distal femur. In: Browner BD, Jupiter JB, Levine AM, et al., ed. *Skeletal trauma.* 2nd ed. Philadelphia: WB Saunders; 1992:1643–1683.
28. Wiss DA. Supracondylar and intercondylar fractures of the femur. In: Rockwood C, Green DP, Heckman JD, et al., eds. *Rockwood and Green's fractures in adults.* 4th ed. Philadelphia: Lippincott Williams & Wilkins; 1992:1972–1999.
29. Sorkin AT, Helfet DL. Supracondylar and distal femur fractures. In: Insall JN, Scott WN, eds. *Surgery of the knee.* 3rd ed. Philadelphia: Churchill Livingstone; 2001:1239–1263.
30. Whittle AP. Fractures of the lower extremity. In: Canale ST, ed. *Campbell's operative orthopaedics.* 9th ed. Missouri: Mosby; 1998:2126–2132.
31. Seifert J, Stengel D, Matther G, et al. Retrograde fixation of distal femur fractures: results using a new nail system. *J Orthop Trauma.* 2003;17(7):488–495.
32. Pierz KA. Pediatric sports medicine. *Curr Opin Orthop.* 2003; 14(6):392–397.
33. Johnson EE. Fractures of the patella. In: Rockwood CA Jr, Green DP, eds. *Rockwood and Green's fractures in adults.* 4th ed. Philadelphia: Lippincott-Raven Publishers; 1996:1956–1970.

34. Bray TJ, Marder RA. *Patellar Fractures, Operative Orthopaedics.* 2nd ed. Philadelphia: JB Lippincott Co; 1993:663–670.

35. Whittle AP. Patella. In: Canale ST, ed. *Campbell's operative orthopaedics.* 9th ed. Missouri: Mosby; 1998:2111–2113.

36. Osgood RB. Lesions of the tibial tubercle occurring during adolescence. *Boston Med Surg J.* 1903;148:114–117.

37. Micheli LJ. Overuse injuries in children's sports: the growth factor. *Orthop Clin N Am.* 1983;14(2):337–360.

38. Flowers MJ, Bhadreshwar DR. Tibial tuberosity excision for symptomatic Osgood-Schlatter disease. *J Ped Orthop.* 1995;15:292–297.

39. Guerewitsch AD, O'Neill M. Flexibility of healthy children. *Arch Phys Ther.* 1944;25:216–221.

40. Aparicio G, Abril JC, Calvo E, et al. Radiologic study of patellar height in Osgood-Schlatter disease. *J Ped Orthop.* 1997;17:63–66.

41. Binazzi R, Felli L, Vaccari V, et al. Surgical treatment of unresolved Osgood-Schlatter lesion. *Clin Orthop Rel Res.* 1993;289:202–204.

42. Ogden JA, Hempton RF, Southwick WO. Development of the tibial tuberosity. *Anat Rec.* 1975;182:431–456.

43. Kujala UM, Kvist M, Heinonen O. Osgood-Schlatter's disease in adolescent athletes: retrospective study of incidence and duration. *Am J Sports Med.* 1985;13:236–241.

44. Bright RW, Burstein AH, Elmore SM. Epiphyseal plate cartilage — a biomechanical and histological analysis of failure modes. *J Bone Joint Surg.* 1974;56A:668–703.

45. King AG, Blundell-Jones G. A surgical procedure for the Osgood-Schlatter lesion. *Am J Sports Med.* 1981;9:250–253.

46. Ogden JA, Southwick WO. Osgood-Schlatter's disese and tibial tuberosity development. *Clin Orthop.* 1976;116:180–189.

47. Krause BL, Williams JPR, Catterall A. Natural history of Osgood-Schlatter disease. *J Ped Orthop.* 1990;10:65–68.

48. Cahill RB. Chronic orthopaedic problems in the young athlete. *J Sports Med.* 1973;1:36–39.

49. Crigler MW, Ridder HO. Soft tissue changes in x-ray diagnosis of the Osgood-Schlatter lesion. *Va Med.* 1982;109:176–178.

50. Glynn MK, Regan BF. Surgical treatment of Osgood-Schlatter's disease. *J Ped Orthop.* 1983;3:216–219.

51. Woolfrey BF, Chandler EF. Manifestations of Osgood-Schlatter disease in late teenage and early adulthood. *J Bone Joint Surg Am.* 1960;42:327–332.

52. Scotti DM, Sadhu VK, Heimberg F, et al. Osgood-Schlatter's disease—an emphasis on soft tissue changes in Roentgen diagnosis. *Skeletal Radiol.* 1979;4:21–25.

53. Aglietti P, Insall JN, Cerulli G. Patellar pain and incongruence, I: measurements of incongruence. *Clin Orthop.* 1983;176:217.

54. Blackburne JS, Peel TE. A new method of measuring patellar height. *J Bone Joint Surg.* 1977;59B:241.

55. Seil R, Muller B, Georg T, et al. Reliability and interobserver variability in radiological patellar height ratios. *Knee Surg Sports Traumatol Arthrosc.* 2000;8:231–236.

56. Ehrenborg G. The Osgood-Schlatter lesion, a clinical and experimental study. *Acta Chir Scand.* 1962;109(suppl):176–178.

57. Levine J, Kashyap S. A new conservative treatment of Osgood-Schlatter disease. *Clin Orthop Rel Res.* 1981;158:126–128.

58. Hogh J, Lund B. The sequelae of Osgood-Schlatter's disease in adults. *Inter Orthop.* 1988;12:213–215.

59. Cole JP. A study of Osgood-Schlatter disease. *Surg Gynecol Obstet.* 1937;65:55–67.

60. Dunkerley GE. Osgood-Schlatter and Sinding-Larsen-Johansson disease. *J Bone Joint Surg.* 1967;49B:591.

61. Christie MJ, Dvonch VM. Tibial tuberosity avulsion fracture in adolescents. *J Ped Orthop.* 1981;1:391–394.

62. Lynch MC, Walsh PJ. Tibia Recurvatum as a complication of Osgood-Schlatter's disease: A report of two cases. *J Ped Orthop.* 1991;11:543–544.

63. Canale ST. Fractures and dislocations in children. In: Canale ST, ed. *Campbell's operative orthopaedics.* 9th ed. Missouri: Mosby; 1998:2488.

TENDON DISORDERS

42

WILLIAM D. STANISH, MD, FRCSC, FACS, HORACIO YEPES, MD,
AMRO AL-HIBSHI, MBChB, FRCSC

■ KEY POINTS

- Chronic tendon disorders are widely called tendinosis.
- Inflammatory response to trauma seems most prevalent in tenosynovium and peritenon giving rise to the term 'peritendinitis.' Older patients with long-standing symptoms and a history of repetitive activity will be more likely to have tendinosis. Young patients with acute onset of symptoms will be more likely to have peritendinitis.
- Quadriceps tendon disorders may be silent on presentation. They are asymptomatic in the majority of cases, until a major traumatic event occurs. The mean age of the patient is older than 40 years old and the male to female ratio is from 6:1 to 10:1.
- In complete ruptures, a superficial prepatellar hematoma with a central gap is easily seen.
- Operative treatment is indicated for complete tears and partial tears involving more than 50% of the tendon. If enough of the tendon is present distally, the tendon can be repaired directly with non-absorbable sutures. If the tendon distally is not long enough to accept sutures securely, repair of the tendon to the patella is indicated.
- The four phases of jumper's knee are: Phase I, pain after activity; Phase II, pain during and after activity; Phase III, same as in Phase II, but with diminished performance; and Phase IV, complete rupture of the patellar tendon.
- Runner's knee is a condition that involves the lateral side of the joint with the iliotibial band rubs against the lateral epicondyle of the femur. It is most symptomatic when the patient is running downhill.

Injuries and disorders of the tendons around the knee can be a devastating problem for the athlete and his/her physician.

The accurate identification of these problems is extremely important to achieve proper treatment and rehabilitation. In this chapter we will review the basic science, clinical evaluation, and treatment of some of the common disorders involving the tendons in and about the knee in athletes.

■ BASIC SCIENCE

Anatomy

The tendons around the knee are of great importance for the stability of the joint. As muscle-tendon units, they function as primary movers of the knee joint. Knowledge of the anatomy is critical for the team physician. It helps the physician to understand the pathologic processes that he/she may encounter with different athletes suffering with tendon disorders.

The quadriceps group consists of four muscles that converge through a conjoined tendon to insert into the superior pole of the patella (1). Other than being a major part of the extensor mechanism and a stabilizer of the knee joint, the vastus medialis (with its oblique portion) and the vastus lateralis help maintain the patella centralized. The patella works to increase the effective lever arm of the quadriceps.

The hamstring group consists of the biceps femoris laterally and the semimembranosus and semitendinosus medially. Except for the short head of the biceps, they all span the hip and knee joints (1).

The pes anserinus is the tendinous insertion of the sartorius, gracilis, and semitendinosus muscles that insert into the anteromedial aspect of the proximal tibia. A bursa separates these structures from the medial collateral ligament.

729

The patellar tendon is closely related to the capsule, although its function is distinct from it. The tendon forms part of the extensor mechanism. The tendon extends in a slightly oblique fashion from the inferior pole of the patella to the tibial tuberosity. The infrapatellar bursa lies in close proximity to the patellar tendon (2–4).

The popliteus tendon lays posterolateral to the knee joint between the capsule and the synovial membrane. An area of bare tendon lies in contact with the lateral meniscus (2,5,6).

The iliotibial band is a thickened strip of the fascia lata that inserts into Gerdy's tubercle. The band lies anterior to the lateral femoral epicondyle in full knee extension. At 30 degrees of flexion, the iliotibial band translocates posterior to the epicondyle.

Biomechanics

There is a large gap between the stress that causes tendon failure and physiologic loads. The latter are reported to produce less than 4% strain (7). This is the "safe zone" of the stress-strain curve **(Fig 42-1)**. The safe zone represents the straightening of the crimped collagen fibers when the tendon is perfectly elastic and recovers its original length after the load is removed. At 4% to 8% strain, the collagen fibrils slide past one another. At 8% to 10% strain, the tendon begins to fail and resist less force. Tendon healing will be discussed in the next section on biology; the healed tendon may be up to 30% weaker biomechanically than the normal healthy tendon (8).

Biology of Healing

The body's response to any injury is an immediate inflammatory reaction. Tendinitis is the word used to describe inflammation of the tendon. A new concept has emerged for chronic tendon disorders. They are now widely called tendinosis. This refers to a degenerative condition of the tendon that seems to be related to both age and activity level. Histologically, surgical specimens show very few inflammatory cells and are more likely to show degeneration, with fatty mucoid and hyaline features. Inflammatory response to trauma seems most

prevalent in tenosynovium and peritenon giving rise to the term "peritendinitis." It is easier to understand these terms as points of a continuum rather than discrete clinical entities. In general, older patients with long standing symptoms and a history of repetitive activity will be more likely to have tendinosis. Young patients with acute onset of symptoms will be more likely to have peritendinitis. Tendonitis occurs when the tendon bears more load than it can withstand repeatedly. Damage and its sequelae inflammation and degeneration occurs. This can be due to excessive high loads across normal tendons or normal loads across degenerative tendons (8).

Tendons heal through three phases: inflammatory, reparative, and remodeling. The inflammatory response begins with the injury and may last from 2 to 7 days. Repair may start as early as 48 hours and last for 6 to 8 weeks. Remodeling starts from day 14 and may last up to one year (8).

■ CLINICAL EVALUATION

Disorders of the Quadriceps Tendon

History

Quadriceps tendon disorders may be silent on presentation. They are asymptomatic in the majority of cases, until a major traumatic event occurs. The mean age of the patient is usually older than 40 years. The male to female ratio is 6:1 to 10:1. The reduced tensile strength of the tendon is multifactorial. Aging and hypoxic degeneration of the tendon, combined with eccentric and compressive forces over the femoral condyles are proposed as risk factors for micro- and macroruptures. Injuries may also occur in younger athletes participating in high power sports such as basketball, high jump, volleyball, and weightlifting **(Fig 42-2)**. A chronic cycle of stiffness and pain with exercise may be experienced by the athlete, but in many cases no symptoms are experienced. In some cases, the history of quadriceps weakness and difficulties going down hill may bring the clinician a key for considering this pathology.

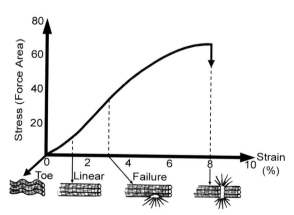

Fig 42-1. Typical stress-strain curve for tendon.

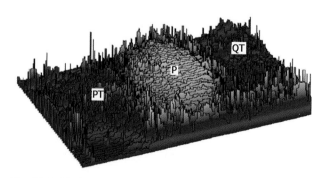

Fig 42-2. Digital map of the vasculature of quadriceps tendon (*QT*), patella (*P*), patellar tendon (*PT*). Hypovascular areas are noticed between 1.0 and 2.0 cm from the proximal insertion of the QT and in the central portion of the PT, correlating with the pattern of ruptures.

Patients experiencing ruptures commonly have an antecedent traumatic event with or without an eccentric force. Forceful quadriceps contraction within a degenerative and weak tendon in patients with rheumatologic or collagen diseases (as systemic lupus erythromatosus, rheumatoid arthritis, psoriasis, polyarteritis nodosa, or gout) may lead to rupture of the tendon. Patients with history of diabetes mellitus, hyperparathyroidism, uremia, chronic corticosteroid use, renal failure, or chronic acidosis are also at increased risk for developing non-traumatic ruptures. Cortisone injections lead to weakness of the tendon and increase the risk of non-traumatic ruptures. A complete medical history (including past history) should be obtained (9,10).

Physical Findings

Examination usually elicits tenderness and swelling in the central portion of the quadriceps tendon close to its insertion into the superior pole of the patella. Some patients experience the tenderness close to the musculotendinous junction. The commonest site of non-traumatic ruptures is between 1.0-2.0 cm from the insertion into the patella **(Fig 42-3)**. The commonest site for traumatic ruptures is at the insertion into the patella.

In our vascular laboratory, we have studied the vascular supply of the quadriceps tendon and patellar tendon using an injection technique of lead oxide gel and water. This mixture is injected into the femoral arteries. Angiograms of the tendons are created, and the density of vascularity is determined with image analyzer software. Our studies (paper in progress) identified a zone of hypovascularity within 2 to 3 cm from the insertion of the quadriceps into the patella (Fig 42-3). This finding correlates well with the site of clinical ruptures of the tendon.

In partial ruptures, the presence of a gap is not often easy to palpate. Partial tears might not be easily diagnosed initially until the size of the gap increases enough to be detected. Most patients with partial tears will still be able to perform straight leg raises.

In complete ruptures, a superficial prepatellar hematoma with a central gap is easily seen. The defect can get exaggerated if the patient is asked to perform active extension of the involved knee **(Fig 42-4)**. Failure to actively extend the knee and/or to straight leg raise indicate a complete tear of the tendon (9,10).

Imaging Modalities

These may include radiographs which are not specific for quadriceps tendon injury. With complete tears, patella infera (baja) may be identified **(Fig 42-5)**.

Magnetic resonance imaging (MRI) usually delineates the extent of the tear. MRI changes include signal change, hemorrhage, and edema **(Fig 42-6)**. MRI should be used to clarify the diagnosis, but not to diagnose the injury (9). Ultrasound imaging has been used to investigate the quadriceps tendon. We find that this modality is operator-dependent and not as reliable as MRI.

Treatment

Non-operative treatment is indicated for partial ruptures that involve less than 50% of the tendon. The knee should be immobilized in extension for 4 to 6 weeks. Weight bearing should be allowed as tolerated. Whenever the patient is able to perform pain-free straight leg raising, the immobilization should be discontinued. Protective braces and progressive eccentric strengthening exercises should allow the athlete a gradual functional return to his/her pre-injury level of activities.

Operative treatment is indicated for complete tears and partial tears involving more than 50% of the tendon. Early surgical repair has shown to be the best and most predictive approach to these problems. If enough tendon is present distally, the tendon can be repaired directly with non-absorbable sutures. If the tendon distally is not long enough to accept sutures securely, repair of the tendon to the patella is indicated. This is achieved with either suture anchors or with drill holes into the patella and passing the sutures through the holes (Fig 42-4). The latter option gives more secure and better rate of healing of the torn tendon. The repair is done preferably with no tourniquet, as the inflated tourniquet cuff leads the muscle and tendon to retract and move proximally. The repair should be tested intra-operatively with extension and flexion of the knee joint. The

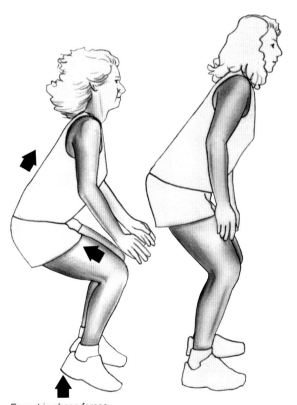

Eccentric phase forces
required to stand from a jump

Fig 42-3. The largest forces occur during the eccentric phase of landing from a jump.

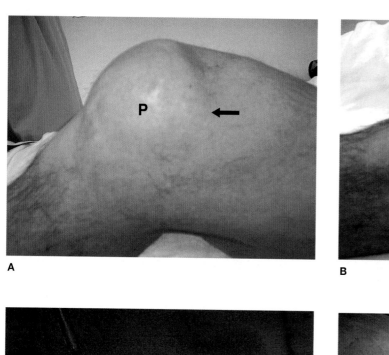
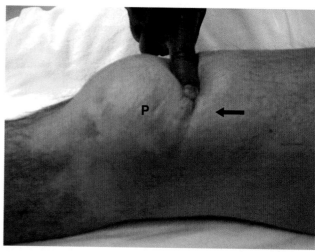

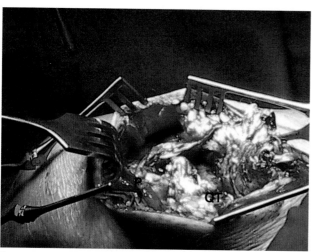
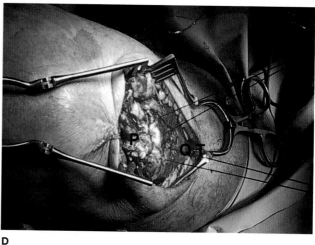

Fig 42-4. Patient with quadriceps tendon rupture. **A:** Notice the exaggeration of the defect with flexion of the knee. **B:** Deep palpation of the defect with the knee in extension. **C:** Intra-operative demonstration of the tear. **D:** Suture anchors have been placed in the superior pole of the patella, and the sutures have been passed through the quadriceps tendon. P, Patella; QT, Quadriceps Tendon.

repair can be augmented with either a circlage wire or a turned down triangular flap of quadriceps. In most cases of acute ruptures, these augmentations are not necessary. Attention should be paid intra-operatively to examine and repair the medial and lateral retinacula.

Postoperatively, the knee should be splinted in extension for 4 to 6 weeks. The patient must be instructed to perform straight leg raising exercises while in the splint. Weight bearing as tolerated should be encouraged immediately after the operation with the help of walking aids. After the splint is discontinued, progressive range of motion with active and active-assisted exercises should be encouraged. Eccentric strengthening exercises should be performed to prevent re-injury (9,11).

■ DISORDERS OF PATELLAR TENDON (JUMPER'S KNEE)

History

Pain on the patellar tendon close to the insertion into the inferior pole of the patella is experienced by the athlete with repetitive running, jumping, and kicking, specifically during an eccentric movement. Patellar tendon disorders are experienced mainly by patients younger than the age of 40 years. Jumping activities and powerful muscle contraction (eccentric loads) stress the tendon in sporting activities such as basketball, volleyball and weight lifting (Fig 42-2). Concentric forces may also cause pain when the athlete is

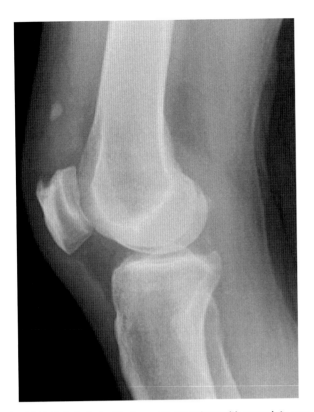

Fig 42-5. Patella baja. Radiograph of patient with complete rupture of quadriceps tendon. Notice the avulsed spur of bone.

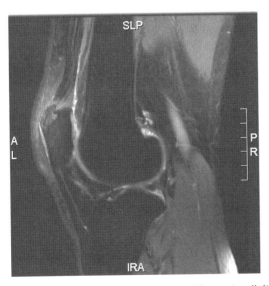

Fig 42-6. Incidental MRI finding of quadriceps tendinitis in patient suffering from meniscus tear. The patient had no symptoms associated with his quadriceps pathology.

lifting weights during open chain exercises. Pain may be felt during or after the activity. The problem can progress to a chronic painful syndrome, and the symptoms can be experienced even at rest (12,13).

Blazina et al. (14) developed a staging system for jumper's knee that divided this entity into four phases of progression:

> Phase I: Pain after activity
> Phase II: Pain during and after activity
> Phase III: Same as in phase II, but with diminished performance
> Phase IV: Complete rupture of the tendon

Stanish, Curwin, and Mandell devised the system shown in **Table 42-1** for symptom classification, similar to that used by other authors (15,16), Fox et al. 1975, and Perugia et al. 1976 (8). In advanced cases, partial and complete ruptures are seen. Poor vascularity, decreased capacity for healing, and structural changes of collagen and different proteins have been studied in attempts to explain the pattern of injuries of the tendon. Age appears to play a role in tendon failure. Patients over 25 years of age manifested in one study less severe pre-rupture symptoms than those less than 25 years (12,17). In adolescents, this condition was described independently by Sinding-Larsen and Johansson in 1921. It comprises a painful entity affecting the inferior pole of the patella. This can be accompanied by small fragmentation of the bone. Traction over the patellofemoral apparatus was proposed as an etiology. This entity is different from Osgood-Schlatter's disease (described initially by Paget in 1891), which affects the distal insertion of the patellar tendon into the tibial tuberosity (Fig 42-2).

In adults, ruptures are more commonly found at the proximal third and center of the tendon. They are manifested as an acute loss of extension accompanied by a painful noisy snap that can be recalled by the patient. The pattern of ruptures of the patellar tendon may be explained by the fact that the central portion of the tendon is more hypovascular decreasing the chances of healing after

TABLE 42-1	Classification of Patellar Disorder According to Pain
Level 1	No pain
Level 2	Pain with extreme exertion only; does not hinder sports performance and disappears when activity stops
Level 3	Pain with exertion, remains 1 to 2 hours afterward
Level 4	Pain during any athletic activity, lasts 4 to 6 hours afterward, increases throughout activity; performance level decreased
Level 5	Pain starts immediately after activity commences, causes withdrawal from activity
Level 6	Pain during daily activities; patient unable to participate in any sports

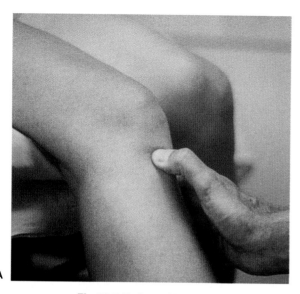

A

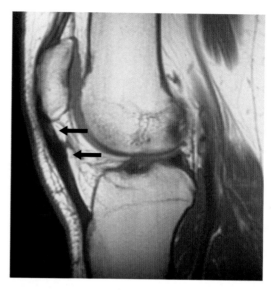

B

Fig 42-7 Patient with partial tear of the patellar tendon. **A:** Point of tenderness in the upper portion of the tendon. **B:** MRI of the tendon showing the tear.

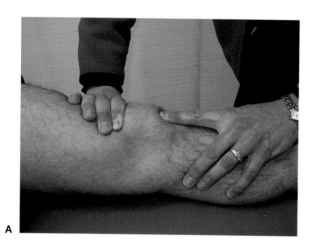

A

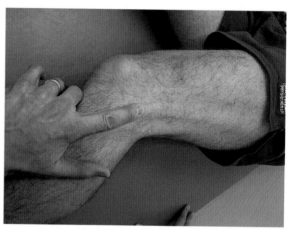

B

C

Fig 42-8. Common sites of tendinitis around the knee: **A:** Patellar tendon. **B:** Iliotibial band. **C:** Pes anserinus.

overusing the tendon (Fig 42-3). Some of the disorders which have been associated with patellar tendon ruptures are rheumatoid arthritis, systemic lupus erythematosus, gout, chronic renal failure, hyperparathyroidism, diabetes mellitus, and peripheral vascular disease.

Physical findings

The examiner can elicit tenderness over the tendon at its insertion into the inferior pole of the patella (12) **(Figs 42-7 and 42-8)**. With the patient lying in the supine position, the examiner displays upward pressure on the inferior pole of the patella. With the other hand, he/she should palpate the deep insertion of the tendon into the patella. This maneuver can elicit tenderness that simple palpation would not address. In some patients, soft tissue crepitus is noticed by applying gentle two-finger palpation over the paratenon-tendon unit in different angles of knee flexion. Pain may also be elicited by

asking the patient to perform active knee extension with or without resistance. In some acute cases, painful inhibition of the quadriceps muscle may be seen, preventing the athlete from reaching full active extension. Hamstring tightness and muscle imbalance should be examined **(Fig 42-9)**. These conditions can predispose to patellar tendon disorders.

Imaging Modalities

Plain x-rays might show calcification of the tendon in the case of chronic inflammation. With ruptured tendons, x-rays might show high riding patella (patella alta) (8). Ultrasound can be used to clarify the diagnosis, but not to diagnose. One study found an 18% incidence of degenerative changes in the control group (18). Ultrasound again is operator-dependent and is not as reliable as MRI. MRI has shown good correlation with clinical and histological findings. Tendinitis appears on MRI as increased signal intensity near the distal

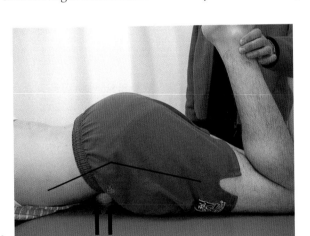

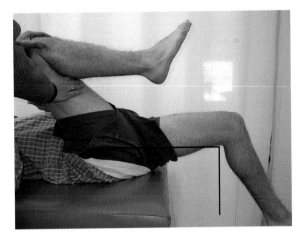

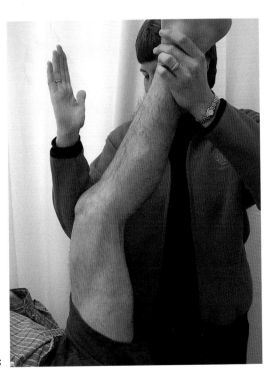

Fig 42-9. Different tests for muscle tightness. **A:** Quadriceps tightness. Notice flexion of the hip as the foot is pulled toward the buttock. **B:** Quadriceps tightness. With the contralateral hip flexed, the patient is unable to flex the affected knee to 90 degrees. **C:** Hamstring tightness. With the hip flexed to 90 degrees, the affected knee does not fully extend.

pole of the patella with an increased anteroposterior diameter of the proximal part of the tendon **(Fig 42-10)**. Lesions in the medial and central one third of the proximal tendon are also characteristic (19,20). The physician should be reminded that the role of MRI is confirmatory only, with clinical findings being paramount to treatment decisions.

Treatment

In most cases, treatment is nonsurgical. **Table 42-2** shows a general guideline for the treatment of jumper's knee, based on Blazina et al.'s (14) classification system. We cannot stress enough the importance, benefits, and value of the eccentric exercise program as shown in **Table 42-3** and (21) (**Figs 42-11** and **42-12**). The rate of failure of conservative treatment has been estimated between 16% and 33% for chronic cases. Eccentric exercise was not a part of the conservative treatment in these studies (8). In the rare cases of jumper's knees where non-operative treatment fails, surgical intervention in the form of debridement and resection of the degenerative portion is indicated (22) (**Figs 42-13** and **42-14**).

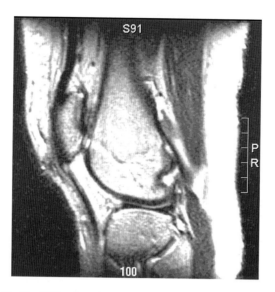

Fig 42-10. MRI of patient with jumper's knee. Notice the increased signal change anterior to the patellar tendon at the insertion into the lower pole of the patella.

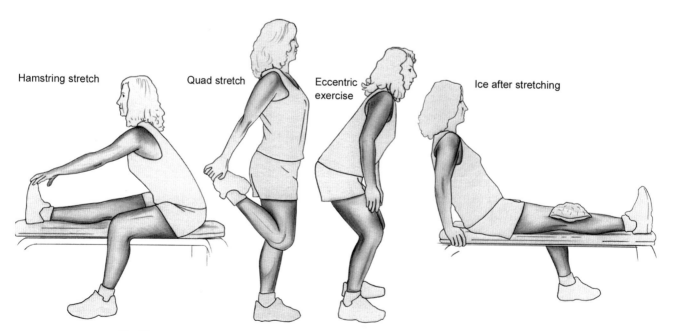

Fig 42-11. The stages of the exercise program: 1) stretch, 2) stretch quads, 3) eccentric exercise, and 4) ice (after stretching again).

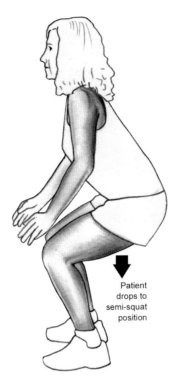

Fig 42-12. Patient drops to a semi-squatting position.

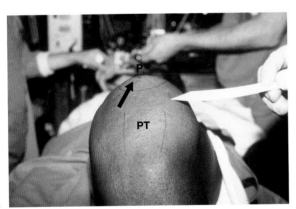

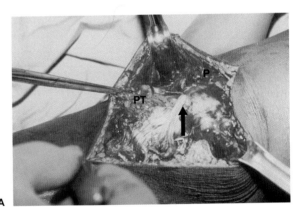

Fig 42-13. Intra-operative pictures of patient with ruptured patellar tendon. **A:** Defect is noticed inferior to the patella. **B:** After incision, the tear is being identified. P, Patella; PT, Patellar Tendon.

■ DISORDERS OF THE ILIOTIBIAL BAND (RUNNER'S KNEE, ILIOTIBIAL BAND SYNDROME)

Definition

This is a condition that involves the lateral side of the joint when the iliotibial band rubs against the lateral epicondyle of the femur.

History

Different factors have been blamed, including tightness and musculotendinous imbalances around the knee, excessive foot pronation and genu varus and overtraining. The pain arises from the iliotibial band that during flexion and extension of the knee rubs against the lateral epicondyle of the femur. If this structure lacks flexibility, it may cause local inflammation that is experienced by the athlete after running for prolonged periods of time. It is most symptomatic when running downhill. Its severity varies, but it can prompt the runner to stop.

Physical Findings

On physical exam, one can detect local swelling and tenderness over the iliotibial band anterior to the epicondylar origin of the lateral collateral ligament (Fig 42-8). The

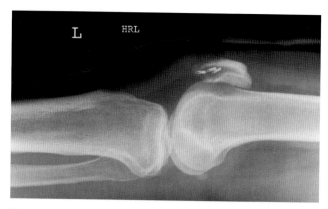

Fig 42-14. Postoperative radiograph of patient who had repair of ruptured patellar tendon. Notice the anchors in the lower pole of the patella.

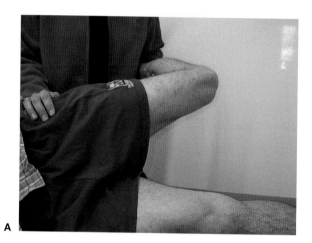

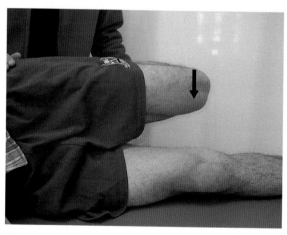

Fig 42-15. Ober test. **A:** While the patient is on the lateral position, the patient is asked to abduct the hip with the knee flexed. **B:** When asked to adduct the hip, patients with tight iliotibial band are not able to touch the examining table with the medial side of their affected extremities.

TABLE 42-2	Conservative Treatment Program for Patellar Tendinitis
Stage 1	Adequate warming up (5 to 10 minutes of push-ups, sit-ups, etc.)
	Ice after activity
	Local anti-inflammatory treatment and anti-inflammatory drugs for several weeks
	Physiotherapy, including isometric quadriceps exercises
	Elastic knee support
Stage 2	Same as stage 1
	Some form of heat before activity
	Period of rest
Stage 3	Same as stage 2 but also prolonged period of rest
	If conservative treatment fails, abstinence from sports or surgery
Stage 4	Primary repair of tendon

TABLE 42-3	Eccentric Exercise Program for Jumper's Knee

1. Warm-up
   a. General, whole-body warm-up
   b. Exercise not involving knee extension
   c. Sufficient when sweating is elicited

2. Stretching
   a. Static stretch of quadriceps and hamstrings
   b. Hold at least 30 seconds
   c. Repeat 3 times

3. Main program
   a. Squatting movements
   b. Focusing primarily on the rapid deceleration phase between downward and upward movement phase
      Week 1: No added resistance on days 1 and 2 (slow); days 3 to 7 (progressively faster)
      Week 2: Add resistance (10% body weight)
      Weeks 3 to 6: Add 4.5 – 13.5 kg progressively
   c. Do three sets of 10 repetitions once daily
   d. After 6 weeks, three sets of 10 three times weekly

4. Warm-down
   a. Static stretch as in item 2

5. Ice
   a. Ice on patellar tendon for 5 minutes after program

6. Optional support
   a. Apply tensor bandage support if desired

tenderness can be variable in different degrees of knee flexion. With the patient lying over the table in lateral position we can test for fascia lata and ilotibial band tightness, bringing the affected knee in 90 degrees of flexion, and testing it during different angles of hip flexion and extension, the knee should touch the table without producing pain

(Fig 42-15). Injuries to deeper structures such as the lateral meniscus should be ruled out; and the diagnostic key is to carefully palpate the joint line for tenderness, combining different maneuvers of lateral compartment compression and flexion.

Malalignment of the lower extremity such as in genu varus and excessive feet pronation may predispose the athlete to increased friction of the lateral knee structures. This condition can occur also if overtraining occurs without good warm up and stretching exercises.

Imaging Modalities

The diagnosis is mostly clinical, but high definition ultrasound and MRI will be helpful in ruling in/out internal pathology of the knee. Lateral meniscal degenerative ruptures and popliteal tendon tendonitis may also produce lateral knee pain.

Treatment

The patient may start ice massage and stretching exercises over the lateral structures of the thigh. Physical activities without pain are allowed. Running downhill or on very hard surfaces should be avoided. Proper stretching and warm up as well as periods of rest are encouraged. Short period of anti-inflammatory medication may be used.

In refractory cases steroid injections around the lateral epicondylar bursae can be useful but direct injection over the tendon should be avoided. If there is concomitant lower limb malalignment, orthotics may be prescribed.

■ REFERENCES

1. Brunet ME, Hontas RB. The thigh. In: DeLee JC, Drez D Jr, ed. *Orthopaedic sports medicine: Principles and practice.* Philadelphia: WB Saunders; 1994:1086–1112.
2. Stanish WD, Wood RM. Overuse injuries of the knee. In: Harries M, Williams C, Stanish WD, et al., ed. *Oxford textbook of sports medicine.* 2nd ed. Oxford: Oxford University Press; 1998:679–693.
3. Teider B, Marshall JL, Koslin B, et al. The anterior aspect of the knee joint. *J Bone Joint Surg.* 1981;63A:351–356.
4. Fulkerson JP, Hungerford DS. *Disorders of the Patellofemoral Joint.* Baltimore: Williams & Wilkins; 1990.
5. Last RJ. The popliteus muscle and the lateral meniscus. *J Bone Joint Surg.* 1950;32B:93–99.
6. Cohn AK, Mains DB. Popliteal hiatus of the lateral meniscus. *Am J Sports Med.* 1979;7:221–226.
7. Elliott D. Structure and function of mammalian tendon. *Biol Rev.* 1965;40:392–421.
8. Stanish WD, Curwin S, Mandell S. *Tendinitis: Its Etiology and Treatment.* New York: Oxford University Press; 2000.
9. Schenck RC Jr. Injuries of the knee. In: Bucholz RW, Heckman JD, ed. *Rockwood and Green's fractures in adults.* 5th ed. Philadelphia: Lippincott Williams & Wilkins; 2001:1843–1937.
10. Scuderi C. Ruptures of quadriceps tendon: Study of 20 tendon ruptures. *Am J Surg.* 1958;95:626–635.
11. Siwek KW, Rao JP. Ruptures of the extensor mechanism of the knee joint. *J Bone Joint Surg.* 1981;63A:932–937.
12. Nichols CE. Patellar tendon injuries. *Clin Sports Med.* 1992;11(4):807–813.
13. Roels J, Martens M, Muller JC, et al. Patellar tendinitis (jumper's knee). *Am J Sports Med.* 1978;6:362–368.
14. Blazina M, Kerlan R, Jobe F, et al. Jumper's knee. *Orthop Clin N Am.* 1973;4(3):665–678.
15. Fox et al. 1975.
16. Perugia et al. 1976.
17. Kelly DW, Carter VS, Jobe FW, et al. Patellar and quadriceps tendon ruptures—Jumper's knee. *Am J Sports Med.* 1984;12:375–380.
18. Khan K, Bonar F, et al. Patellar tendinosis (jumper's knee): Findings at histopathological examination, US and MR imaging. *Radiology.* 1996;200(3):821–827.
19. El-Khoury G, Wira L, et al. MR imaging of patellar tendinitis. *Radiology.* 1992;184(3):849–854.
20. McLoughlin R, Raber E, et al. Patellar tendinitis: MR imaging features, with suggested pathogenesis and proposed classification. *Radiology.* 1995;197(3):843–848.
21. Stanish WD, Rubinovich RM, Curwin S. Eccentric exercise in chronic tendinitis. *Clin Orthop.* 1986;208:65–68.
22. Karlsson J, Lundin O, Lossing IW, et al. Partial rupture of the patellar ligament: results after operative treatment. *Am J Sports Med.* 1991;19:403–408.

43

CHONDRAL INJURIES AND OSTEOARTHRITIS

43.1

CHONDRAL INJURIES IN THE KNEE

F. ALAN BARBER, MD, FACS

■ KEY POINTS

- Articular cartilage is a smooth, viscoelastic, hypocellular structure that provides a low coefficient of friction.
- The treatment of articular cartilage injury in the athlete presents several challenges. Most athletes want to return to full activity as soon as possible.
- Articular cartilage injury in the athlete can occur from shear forces associated with an anterior cruciate ligament (ACL) tear or blunt force trauma to the joint surface.
- If the articular cartilage is damaged, a defect may develop.
- The goal of treatment is to remove any tissue that is creating a problem and, when needed, to replace it with a tissue that not only fills the defect but also integrates well with the adjacent articular cartilage and does not deteriorate over time.
- Patients who present with chondral damage report various mechanisms of injury. These mechanisms often include a pivoting, twisting fall; a significant, direct impact on the knee; an ACL tear; or a patellar dislocation.
- Patients commonly report the onset of pain localized to one particular compartment or a persistent, dull, aching

pain that worsens after activity and may be most noticeable when the patient tries to fall asleep.

- The steps for a successful treatment program include effective communication with the patient, making an accurate diagnosis, and communicating the prognosis.
- Debridement of Outerbridge Type 3 and Type 4 lesions as a primary treatment is appropriate for smaller lesions, low-demand patients, and incidentally observed lesions with few symptoms. The best results seem to occur in younger patients with symptoms of less than 1 year in duration, a specific history of trauma, no previous surgery, little to no malalignment, and a low body mass index.
- Methods to treat defects in the articular cartilage by stimulating the subchondral marrow include penetrating the subchondral bone by drilling or microfracture and abrasion arthroplasty.
- Osteochondral autografting transfers a cylindrical plug of osteochondral material, including both normal articular cartilage with viable chondrocytes and the underlying attached viable subchondral bone from a nonarticulating portion of the joint, into an articular cartilage defect.

- The implantation of composite fresh cadaveric allografts is another technique to address full-thickness articular cartilage defects in the knee. One significant issue with allografts is that to optimize survival of the transplanted chondrocytes, the grafts should be implanted as soon after harvest as possible.
- Autologous chondrocyte implantation (ACI) is designed to address traumatic focal lesions of the weight-bearing surface, primarily of the femoral condyle. The technique attempts to replace a full-thickness articular defect with hyalinelike tissue. It is indicated for localized, symptomatic full-thickness articular cartilage lesions of at least 2 cm in diameter in young patients with good alignment, good stability, and nonarthritic joints. Patients must be able to comply with the rehabilitation protocol.

Articular cartilage injury is a sports-related injury commonly found at arthroscopic surgery. In a series of more than 31,000 arthroscopies, articular cartilage damage was found in 63% (1). The medial femoral condyle and the patellar surface were the most frequently injured sites (2). These lesions seem to be localized and limited in scope, but what they represent for the future of the knee may not be so innocuous.

The treatment of articular cartilage injury in the athlete presents several challenges. Not only does the average athlete wish to return to full activity as quickly as possible, but the assumption that this will happen as a normal course of seeking medical treatment sometimes raises unrealistic expectations. In addition, more individuals currently continue their athletic activities for a longer time, with the result that older patients are now included in the population sustaining articular cartilage damage.

The articular cartilage of the knee has a complex structure and plays a vital role in the normal athletic activity. Its function is to transmit loads uniformly across the joint and provide a smooth, low-friction, gliding surface. The lack of a vascular response and the relative absence of an undifferentiated cell population to respond to injury make damage to the articular cartilage a problem and limit its healing capacity. Localized full-thickness defects and contusions can cause significant symptoms and are especially problematic because of the potential for these lesions to progress. This is compounded by the natural environment of athletic participation in which the knee is subjected to repeated loading and the potential for violent contact with the ground or other participants.

Articular cartilage is a smooth, viscoelastic, hypocellular structure that provides a low coefficient of friction—estimated to be 20% of the friction seen with ice on ice (3)—and the ability to withstand significant recurring compressive loads. It has a large extracellular matrix composed principally of Type II collagen (60% of the dry weight of cartilage) (4,5). The collagen fibers provide form and tensile strength, and water gives it substance by comprising 75% to 80% of the extracellular matrix. The cellular component (chondrocytes) synthesizes and degrades proteoglycans and is the metabolically active portion of this structure.

Histologically, articular cartilage has four distinct zones: (a) a superficial (tangential) zone, (b) a middle (transitional) zone, (c) a deep (radial) zone, and (d) the calcified zone (Fig 43.1-1). The primary orientation of the collagen fibers in the superficial zone is parallel with the joint surface to resist compressive and sheer forces. This zone is the thinnest one, and it sometimes is referred to as the gliding zone. The surface layer, known as the lamina splendens, is cellfree and composed mainly of randomly oriented, flat bundles of fine collagen fibrils. Deep to the lamina splendens are more densely packed collagen fibers interspersed with elongated, oval chondrocytes oriented parallel to the articular surface. Little hyaluronic acid and few proteoglycan aggregates, but the highest water concentration, are found in this layer. This superficial zone acts as a barrier by limiting the penetration of large molecules, such as antibodies, into the deeper zone and preventing the loss of molecules from the cartilage into the synovial fluid.

The primary orientation of the middle (transitional) zone collagen fibers is parallel to the plane of joint motion, although some oblique fibers also are present. This layer resists compressive forces, and this zone has more proteoglycans and less water and collagen than the superficial zone. The chondrocytes are more spherical and have more cellular structures, suggesting a matrix synthesis function.

The deep (radial) zone fibers are perpendicular to the surface and resist both compressive and sheer forces. The collagen bundles are arranged in arcades known as the arcades of Benninghoff. These are not continuous (as once thought), and the collagen orientation is somewhat random. In this area, the chondrocytes are round and arranged in columns perpendicular to the joint surface. These cells possess many intracellular structures, and they appear to be very active with protein synthesis. The highest concentration of proteoglycans is found in this zone. The tidemark is located at the base of this zone and also resists sheer stress. It represents a zone of transition from the deep zone to the zone of calcified cartilage. It is an undulating hematoxophilic line, and collagen fibers from the deep zone penetrate this line directly into the calcified cartilage.

The calcified zone acts as an anchor between the articular cartilage and the subchondral bone. The deepest zone, it is a thin layer of calcified cartilage, creating a boundary with the underlying subchondral bone. The cells in this zone usually are smaller and surrounded by a cartilaginous matrix. Damage to any of these layers can alter the normal biomechanical properties of the articular cartilage and lead to progressive deterioration.

The articular cartilage injury that an athlete may sustain can occur from shear forces associated with an ACL tear or from blunt force trauma to the joint surface. This may result in the injury or death of articular chondrocytes. Experimentally, blunt trauma of greater than 25 N/mm^2 consistently results in articular chondrocyte death (6). This can play a role in the development of articular cartilage degeneration after injury, but such an injury may not be readily apparent at first.

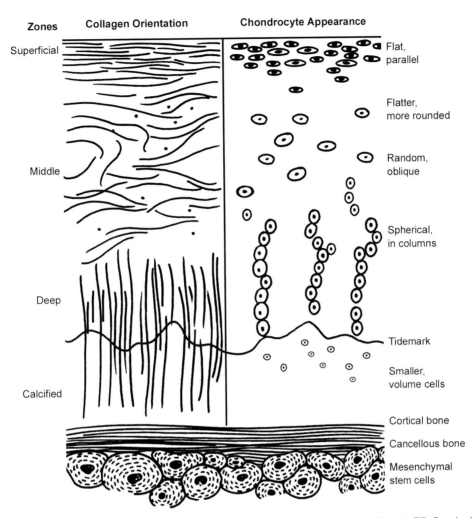

Fig 43.1-1. The basic structure of articular cartilage. (From Browne JE, Branch TP. Surgical alternative for treatment of articular cartilage lesions. *J Am Acad Orthop Surg.* 2000;8:180–189; with permission.)

Areas of chondral injury and subchondral bone edema (i.e., bruising) often are seen on magnetic resonance (MR) images depicting ACL tears. Arthroscopic biopsy of the articular cartilage overlying bone bruises demonstrates superficial articular chondrocyte death, matrix dehydration, and death of the subchondral osteocytes with empty lacuna (7). The inference is that the impact associated with an ACL tear also causes articular cell death in addition to injury to the underlying subchondral bone. The extent and implications of this injury may not be appreciated initially, which may be one explanation for the late appearance of degenerative change after ACL reconstruction.

If the articular cartilage is damaged, a defect may develop. Increased contact pressure is then placed on the edges of the articular cartilage defect and on any exposed subchondral bone. This leads to overloading and degeneration of the defect with an expansion of the lesion. As this situation progresses, the exposed bone contacts the opposing articular cartilage, leading to bipolar injury and, ultimately, a bone-on-bone lesion. The deteriorating cartilage will cause an inflammatory synovitis by the release of breakdown products, and the stress changes of the exposed subchondral bone will lead to venous congestion in the medullary cavity. These may result in chronic aching pain. The goal for the treatment of articular cartilage injury is to remove any tissue that is creating a problem and, when needed, to replace it with a tissue that not only fills the defect but also integrates well with the adjacent articular cartilage and does not deteriorate over time.

One of the challenges faced by the surgeon attempting to meet these goals is the lack of a blood supply or an endogenous source of new cells for the damaged articular cartilage. Spontaneous healing is very limited. Depending on the technique used for repair, the tissue produced may include fibrous tissue, degenerative hyalinelike tissue, fibrocartilage, and bone (8). The type of tissue created will determine the long-term clinical success or failure. Factors affecting the quality of the repair are the age of the patient, the lesion size, the depth of the lesion, any associated ligament instability or meniscus loss, any angular malalignment, and the acuteness of the injury when treatment occurs.

■ CLINICAL EVALUATION

History

Patients presenting with chondral damage report various mechanisms of injury. These mechanisms often include a pivoting or twisting fall, a significant direct impact on the knee, an ACL tear, or a patellar dislocation. The differential diagnosis of any patient presenting with a traumatic hemarthrosis also should include a traumatic chondral lesion. Sometimes, however, the patient remembers no clearly traumatic event and only reports pain with weight bearing.

Patients commonly report the onset of pain localized to one particular compartment or a persistent, dull, aching pain that worsens after activity and may be most noticeable when the patient tries to fall asleep. Loaded activities, such as running, stair climbing, rising from a chair, and squatting, aggravate these symptoms. Sitting for prolonged times, such as in an automobile, a theater, or an airplane, sometimes aggravates pain from a patellar lesion.

In addition to pain, the patient may complain of swelling, crepitus, and giving way, catching, and locking of the knee. These tend to be induced by activity but vary widely from patient to patient.

Physical Examination

Joint line tenderness or an effusion sometimes is present depending on the patient's activity before the evaluation. The alignment of the limb is important to evaluate; this includes looking for varus or valgus alignment, hyperextensile joints, or a flexion contracture.

For patellar or trochlear lesions, subpatellar crepitus, patellar grind, and pull-through sensitivity often are observed. Patellar maltracking, the Q angle, and tightness of the lateral retinaculum should be evaluated. Associated lesions should be considered, along with meniscal signs and joint instability.

Imaging

In the office, a standard radiographic evaluation should be performed. This includes a standing anteroposterior view of both legs in full extension to look for angular changes and to compare height of the joint space. If this view is not revealing, then a 45-degree flexion, posteroanterior, weight-bearing view to identify subtle joint space narrowing should be obtained. A non–weight-bearing lateral view with 45-degree flexion in which the posterior femoral condyles overlap, an axial view of both patellae to evaluate the patellar alignment, and an anteroposterior, knee-flexion view to outline the femoral intercondylar notch also should be obtained.

Magnetic resonance imaging can help to outline the surface of the articular cartilage and demonstrate localized, full-thickness lesions in a patient with otherwise normal standard radiographs. A layer of fluid or edema surrounding an articular cartilage lesion suggests that it is detached. The two most widely used imaging techniques are the T_1-weighted, fat-suppressed, three-dimensional spoiled gradient echo technique and the T_2-weighted, fast spin-echo technique. Software advances and newer MR imaging techniques with intravenous or intra-articular enhancement are continuing to improve the capability of MR imaging for the evaluation of articular cartilage.

Classification

Evaluating articular cartilage lesions is important to facilitate communication, to arrive at a prognosis, and to devise an appropriate treatment plan. An evaluation should consider not only the size and depth of the lesion but also its location, any damage to the subchondral bone, and any associated pathology in the knee, such as an ACL or meniscal tear. The most common classification used for articular cartilage lesions is that of Outerbridge (9). In this system, articular cartilage damage of grade 1 shows softening or blistering of the surface; grade 2 shows fibrillation or superficial fissures of less than 1 cm in diameter; grade 3 shows deeps fissuring extending to the subchondral bone, without exposed bone, and measuring more than 1 cm in diameter; and grade 4 shows exposed subchondral bone **(Fig 43.1-2)**. More recently, the Modified International Cartilage Repair Society Chondral Injury Classification System (10), or ICRS, has been developed. This system is based on the depth and amount of the cartilage injury. Using this system, ICRS grade 1 injuries are superficial, with a soft indentation or superficial fissures and cracks; ICRS grade 2 lesions involve less than half the cartilage depth; ICRS grade 3 lesions involve half or more of the cartilage depth, but not into the subchondral bone; and ICRS grade 4 lesions are osteochondral in extent.

Athletic injuries commonly injure the meniscal cartilage and, sometimes, the ACL as well. Injury to these structures can have a profound effect on the outcome of treatment of articular cartilage lesions. The meniscus cartilage functions to distribute loads more evenly across the joint surface, to improve cartilage nutrition, and to absorb shock. Loss of some or all of a meniscus can lead to osteoarthritis. This relationship makes preservation of the meniscus whenever possible a component of the treatment strategy to reduce articular cartilage injury. Continued ligamentous instability in the knee leads to additional articular and meniscal damage. When instability coexists with articular cartilage damage, the knee should be stabilized at the same time as the articular cartilage is repaired; otherwise, additional damage will compromise any articular cartilage procedure.

Any significant angular change in the leg (valgus or varus alignment) also should be corrected in conjunction with

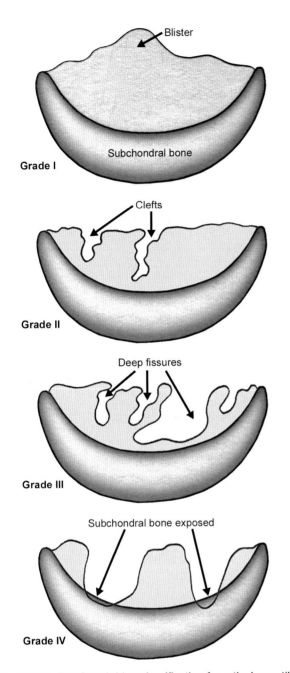

Fig 43.1-2. The Outerbridge classification for articular cartilage lesions. (From Browne JE, Branch TP. Surgical alternative for treatment of articular cartilage lesions. *J Am Acad Orthop Surg.* 2000;8:180–189).

articular cartilage surgery. If the malalignment is not corrected, then the articular cartilage will be subjected to increased pressures, and the result of the surgery will be compromised.

Decision-making Algorithms

Treatment algorithms depend on many factors, but size and depth of the associated lesions are paramount. In addition, if a

mobile fragment is associated with the lesion, then the possibility for reattachment exists only if the subchondral bone is viable. Some Outerbridge Type 4 lesions have associated bone loss. If the depth of loss is greater than 8 mm, then marrow-stimulating techniques and ACI are not suitable choices, and bone grafting to fill the defect should be performed either as part of an autograft or allograft procedure or as an independent initial step before ACI. **Table 43.1-1** outlines the treatment options based upon these factors.

■ TREATMENT

Nonoperative

At surgery, it is not uncommon to find a small area of Outerbridge Type 1 or Type 2 injury on a femoral condyle or tibial plateau that does not require any intervention. Small Type 3 lesions that are asymptomatic, especially in athletes participating in low-impact activities, can be observed and treated nonoperatively. Some painful Type 3 lesions may become asymptomatic once the acute synovitis resolves (11–13). A linear Type 3 lesion on the femoral condyle or tibial plateau **(Fig 43.1-3)** should be documented and the patient informed. Specific intervention should await the development of symptoms, particularly in a patient with another, more obvious reason for knee symptoms (e.g., torn meniscus or loose body). Long-term studies suggest that isolated chondral lesions of less than 1 cm in diameter have an excellent or good result without specific treatment and may be left alone (14). As long as these areas do not cause symptoms, intervention should be postponed.

Areas of what could be Outerbridge Type 3 damage observed at MR imaging also warrant a trial of nonoperative care. This includes a course of nonsteroidal anti-inflammatory drugs, physical therapy, activity modification, and possibly, bracing. Evaluating the particular position the athlete plays may provide opportunities for continued participation while "resting" the joint. Changes in the exercise program or technique also may prove to be helpful. Sometimes, the clinical symptoms amount to an overuse syndrome that a period of rest will resolve and are unrelated to small or superficial chondral abnormalities. Bracing options include patellar stabilizing braces for patellofemoral instability and load-shifting braces for angular unicompartmental damage that has not responded to surgical intervention and activity modification.

Other available medications include intra-articular injections of hyaluronic acid (15,16). On occasion, an intra-articular injection of steroid can be helpful. At this point, no conclusive evidence indicates that nutritional supplements are beneficial for the management of partial- or full-thickness chondral lesions.

Nonoperative treatment for an athlete often is chosen because of the particular sport's season. Operating on a player in the middle of his or her season can be a difficult choice, and surgery often is delayed until the season is over. This may be less than ideal. The future impact of this choice

TABLE 43.1-1

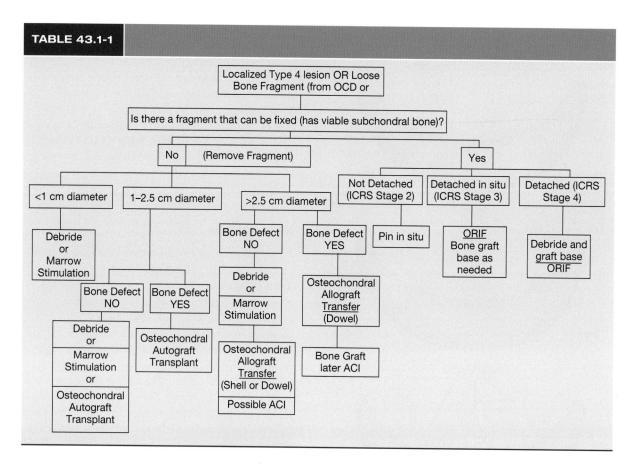

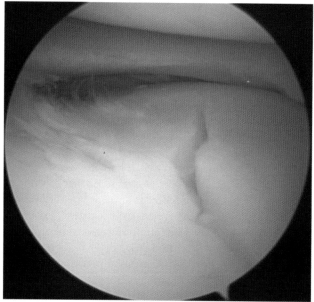

Fig 43.1-3. The linear cleft on the tibial surface is an Outerbridge Type 3 lesion that should be documented and observed.

may be profound to the athlete, however, and the decision should be made only after a candid and comprehensive discussion of the injury, its prognosis, and the potential consequences of the various treatment options by the physician with the athlete and, when appropriate, the athlete's family.

Operative Indications

The indications for surgical intervention include symptomatic Outerbridge Type 3 lesions that have failed an appropriate nonoperative trial, Type 4 areas, and damage associated with loose fragments. The goal of this surgery is to relieve the symptoms of pain, swelling, and catching, locking, and giving way as well as to stabilize the articular cartilage to prevent further deterioration and to remove unstable, loose fragments. Some lesions, such as unstable osteochondritis dissecans fragments with viable subchondral bone or fresh traumatic fragments with viable bone, can be treated by primary repair (i.e., refixation to the bone bed). Larger articular cartilage lesions (diameter, >2 cm), especially those with loose fragments, deserve immediate intervention, because the chances of successful nonoperative treatment are low but, if this condition is allowed to go untreated, the risks of more damage are high.

■ TECHNIQUES

Debridement

Debridement of Outerbridge Type 3 and Type 4 lesions as a primary treatment is appropriate for smaller lesions, low-demand patients, and incidentally observed lesions with few symptoms **(Fig 43.1-4)**. The best results seem to be in younger patients with symptoms of less than 1 year in duration, a specific history of trauma, no previous surgery, little to no malalignment, and a low body mass index (17). Debridement

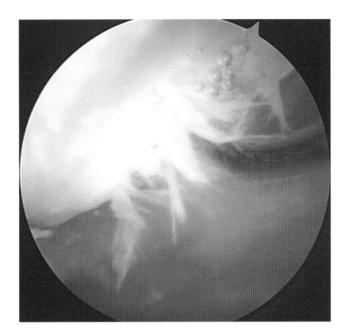

Fig 43.1-4. Debridement of Outerbridge Type 3 and Type 4 lesions is appropriate for smaller lesions, low-demand patients, and incidentally observed lesions with few symptoms.

should only remove unstable chondral fragments that may cause mechanical symptoms and that are likely to become detached with additional activity or trauma. One study reported good to excellent results in 23 consecutive soccer players treated for partial- and full-thickness chondral flaps by arthroscopic debridement with a 1-year follow-up (18). Mechanical debridement does not stimulate articular cartilage repair (19), and there is a risk that the adjacent hyaline cartilage can be damaged (19,20). With additional trauma, these other areas can proceed to osteoarthritis (21).

The technique for mechanical debridement uses a motorized shaver. A number of shaver blades are available, including an aggressive, open-faced shaver blade or a blade with small fenestrations (called a whisker blade) that is less likely to dig into normal material. The damaged articular cartilage should be probed to assess the extent of the softening and fragmentation. Only fragmented areas (i.e., Outerbridge Type 3) should debrided. The edges of Type 4 lesions that are unstable flaps also may be debrided. On occasion, the shaver blade may not be able to completely debride a flap of articular cartilage, and a basket punch is needed.

Once the extent and location of the lesion is appreciated, the shaver is inserted and brought into contact with the damaged articular cartilage. A little pressure on the shaver blade and a moderate amount of suction are required to perform this procedure. A back-and-forth, sweeping motion is used to remove the prominent fragments. When using the open-faced shaver blade, it is helpful to turn the blade on its side so that the open face is at a 90-degree angle to the articular cartilage surface. The suction will lift the fragments into the rotating shaver blade and amputate them. Additional portals may be needed (especially for the patella) to address all the damaged areas without digging excessively into the tissue. As

the debridement progresses, more pressure is placed on the shaver to remove the fragments to a stable base. Once a stable base is reached, debridement in that area is terminated. If thermal treatment is selected, it is applied to the area after the mechanical debridement is concluded.

The use of thermal techniques for treatment of Outerbridge Type 3 damage is currently under investigation **(Fig 43.1-5)**. The advocates of thermal articular cartilage treatment suggest that thermal treatment seals the cartilage, provides a smoother surface, and may prevent extension of the lesion **(Fig 43.1-6)**. Concerns about heat damage to the

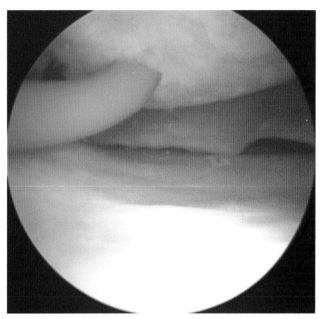

Fig 43.1-5. A monopolar thermal probe is used to treat Outerbridge Type 3 damage on the medial femoral condyle.

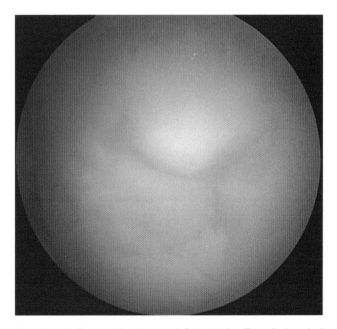

Fig 43.1-6. Thermal treatment of Outerbridge Type 3 chondral lesions seals the cartilage, provides a smoother surface, and may prevent the extension of the lesion.

adjacent, macroscopically undamaged articular cartilage and subchondral bone, however, have been raised. Treatment of the articular cartilage with heat causes immediate chondrocyte death and an overall decrease in proteoglycan levels (22,23). In addition, the type of heat application is significant. Bipolar devices penetrate 78% to 92% deeper that monopolar systems and reach the subchondral bone when a paintbrush pattern is used **(Fig 43.1-7)** (24). Currently, because of concerns about the safety and long-term benefits, radiofrequency treatment of articular cartilage has a limited role.

Debridement is a commonly performed procedure, and the postoperative treatment allows for an aggressive return to full activity. Weight bearing is allowed immediately after surgery, although crutches may be required for a day or two. An aggressive exercise program is allowed, and running can occur as early as 3 to 4 weeks after surgery if the swelling has resolved and if strength and pain permit. If full-thickness articular cartilage loss or extensive Outerbridge Type 3

damage exists over the weight-bearing areas, however, high-impact activities, such as running, should be avoided.

Marrow Stimulation (Drilling, Microfracture, Abrasion)

Methods to treat defects in the articular cartilage by stimulating the subchondral marrow include penetrating the subchondral bone by drilling or microfracture and the technique of abrasion arthroplasty. All of these techniques facilitate access to the vascular system and result in development of a fibrocartilage scar that deteriorates over time. The initial reports of open-abrasion arthroplasty were by Pridie (25), who observed that treated areas became covered by a fibrous scar and resulted in clinical improvement. Later, Johnson (26) advocated an arthroscopic variation of the technique called abrasion arthroplasty. This technique was principally indicated for extensive osteoarthritic knee surfaces. It required

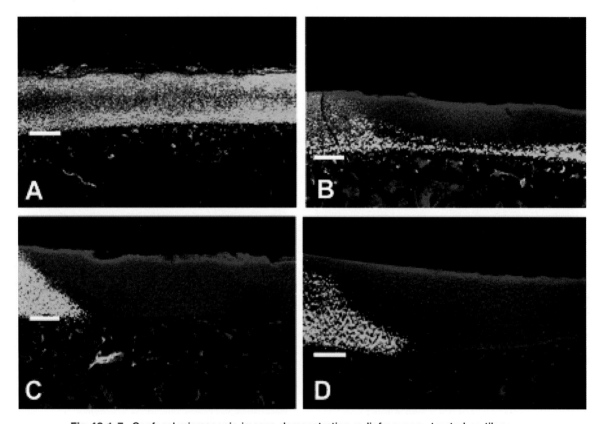

Fig 43.1-7. Confocal microscopic images demonstrating radiofrequency-treated cartilage surface (top of each image) and subchondral bone (bottom of each image) using a paintbrush pattern. The green dots indicate viable chondrocytes, and the red dots indicate dead chondrocytes. The white bars demonstrate the boundary between the cartilage and subchondral bone. **A:** Control. **B:** Oratec monopolar radiofrequency energy treatment caused immediate chondrocyte death, and penetration of cell death did not extend to subchondral bone. **C:** Mitek bipolar radiofrequency energy treatment caused immediate chondrocyte death, and penetration of cell death extended to subchondral bone in eight of eight specimens. **D:** ArthroCare bipolar radiofrequency energy treatment caused immediate chondrocyte death, and penetration of cell death extended to subchondral bone in eight of eight specimens. Original magnification, ×2). (From Lu Y, Edwards RB III, Cole BJ, et al. Thermal chondroplasty with radiofrequency energy. An in vitro comparison of bipolar and monopolar radiofrequency devices. *Am J Sports Med*. 2001;29:42–49; with permission.)

abrasion of the entire surface, removing 1 to 2 mm of bone in the involved area, followed by a period of non–weight bearing of up to 8 weeks. Most of the subjects were older, with degenerative arthritic changes, and some reports of this technique showed poor clinical outcomes. This technique has few advocates today, and it was controversial even at the height of its popularity (27–29).

For smaller, more localized areas, penetrating the subchondral bone by either a drill (30) or a pick is a common option **(Fig 43.1-8)** (31). This technique also provides a healing vascular response, leading to a fibrocartilage scar in the defect. Any chondral flaps are removed, and the calcified cartilage layer is lightly debrided, without damaging the underlying subchondral bone. Although the exact nature of the healing tissue is not known, the process by which this scar forms is thought to be through an influx of undifferentiated mesenchymal cells from the subchondral marrow. Of concern is that this tissue response can be both unpredictable and variable. In addition, it is unclear whether this repair tissue responds well to compression and shear loads and can withstand these stresses over time. The reported

clinical results indicate an 80% "improved" status at an average of 7 years after treatment (31).

Steadman et al. (31) advocates using variously angled picks for this technique. The use of picks to create perforations of the subchondral bone is, hypothetically, superior to other means of subchondral penetration for several reasons: (a) It generates less heat than drilling and, as a consequence, is less destructive to the bone; (b) the angled picks allow better access to various portions of the curved condyle; (c) there is a consistent depth of penetration; and (d) using the various angles of picks allows the holes to be perpendicular to the subchondral plate. The use of an angled pick permits easier access to the more posterior lesions, but questions remain regarding whether the depth and angle of penetration make any difference and whether, considering the cool aqueous environment, any significant heat difference exists between that created by the use of a pick and that created by use of a small, smooth drill.

The microfracture technique requires bed preparation by using a curette or full-radius shaver blade to remove any remaining fragments and tags of articular cartilage. At the lesion's margin, any loose fragments also are removed, and vertical walls of well-attached, healthy cartilage are created. The subchondral plate should not be penetrated, but the calcified cartilage layer above it should be removed with the curette. Using the set of picks and a mallet to impact them, multiple perforating holes are placed approximately 3 to 4 mm apart throughout the bed of the lesion. The pick limits the depth of penetration to approximately 4 mm **(Fig 43.1-9)**.

The indications for marrow stimulation techniques include grade 4 degenerative areas as well as focal traumatic lesions. Contraindications for this technique are areas with significant subchondral bone loss, malaligned knees, and noncompliant patients.

The required postoperative treatment of the microfracture technique is a continuous passive-motion device for up to 8 hours a day and non–weight bearing for up to 8 weeks. A stationary bicycle program begins 1 to 2 weeks after surgery. Full weight bearing is allowed at 8 weeks after surgery, followed by a progressive strengthening program. The rehabilitation program for the patellofemoral lesions is more aggressive. Recent reports raise questions about the necessity of partial weight bearing or continuous passive motion during the postoperative management of these procedures (32). Patients who did not use the continuous passive-motion device and who were allowed to bear weight immediately after surgery had no difference in outcome when compared to those patients who followed the more restrictive, standard protocol.

Osteochondral Autograft Transfer

Osteochondral autografting transfers a cylindrical plug of osteochondral material that includes normal articular cartilage with viable chondrocytes and the underlying attached viable subchondral bone from a nonarticulating portion of the joint into an articular cartilage defect. Several different equipment systems are available to accomplish this

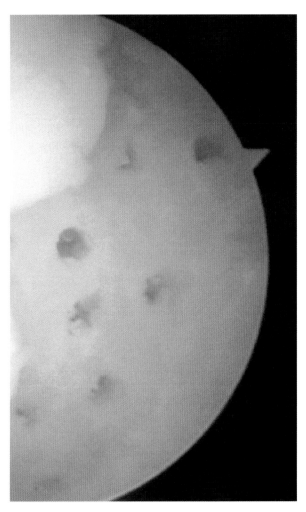

Fig 43.1-8. For smaller, more localized areas, penetrating the subchondral bone by either a drill or a pick is a common option.

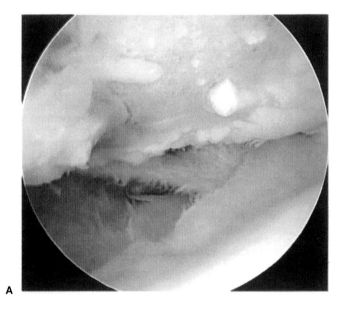

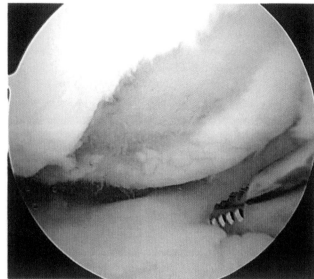

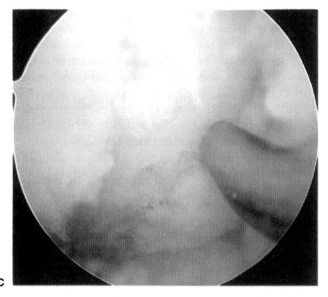

Fig 43.1-9. Microfracture of the femoral condyle in a patient with an acute ACL injury and chondral injury. **A:** Initial lesion. **B:** Debridement of the margins and calcified cartilage layer. **C:** Microfracture of the base using angled awls.

transfer, and various names are used, including COR (Depuy-Mitek, Norwood, MA), OATS, Arthrex, Naples, FL, and mosaicplasty (33–35).

Focal, symptomatic, full-thickness traumatic defects of the femoral condyle are the principal indication for this technique **(Fig 43.1-10)**. The lesion should be unipolar, between 1 and 2.5 cm in diameter, and in a stable joint. Any generalized osteoarthritic change and lesions in multiple sites are contraindications.

The advantages of the osteochondral autograft transplantation are that it provides noninflammatory healing with an arthroscopic technique, using three-dimensional, autologous material that is readily available, and can address lesions that also have bone loss. This single-step procedure carries a relatively low cost and can be done in an outpatient setting. The challenges of osteochondral autograft transplantation include the limit to the number of autograft plugs that can be

harvested from a single knee, making treatment of lesion greater than 2.5 cm in diameter difficult. The arthroscopic technique sacrifices material from one area to repair a defect in another area. Also, it is difficult to recreate an articular surface in a defect that is perfectly congruent with the adjacent convex femoral condyle.

The results of chondral osseous autograft transplantation were compared with abrasion arthroplasty, microfracture, and subchondral drilling of lesions between 1 and 9 cm^2. Subchondral bone penetration resulted in a deterioration of results over time. These marrow-stimulating procedures demonstrated improvements ranging from 48% to 62%, whereas the results from chondral osseous autograft transplantation remained between 86% and 90% at 5 years (35). Histological analysis of biopsy material from transplanted grafts has demonstrated living chondrocytes and osteocytes at 12 months after initial surgery (34).

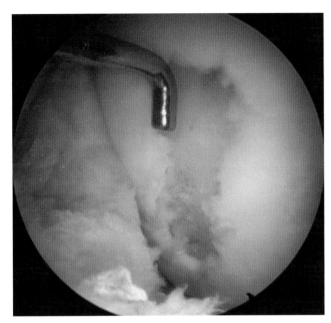

Fig 43.1-10. Focal symptomatic, full-thickness, traumatic defects of the femoral condyle are the principal indication for chondral osseous transplantation.

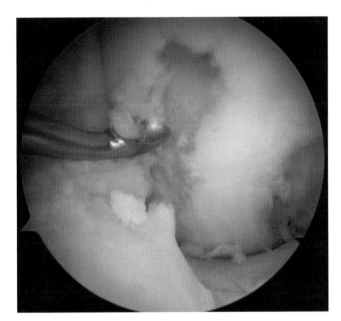

Fig 43.1-11. The defect base should be debrided of articular cartilage flaps and the margins of the lesion shaped with a curette to create vertical walls of healthy cartilage.

The technique requires careful evaluation and preparation of the lesion to determine the number of grafts that are needed. The defect base should be debrided of articular cartilage flaps and the margins of the lesion shaped with a curette to create vertical walls of healthy articular cartilage **(Fig 43.1-11)**. Various plug sizes are available, but the 6-mm diameter plug is the most commonly used. Once the size of the graft is determined, the Mitek/COR harvester is placed

against the prepared defect to determine the number of grafts that will be needed to repair the defect.

The amount of subchondral bone involvement and the size of the lesion are important. Taking a large graft from the femoral condyle for autologous repair should be done advisedly. With a larger lesion, the risk of secondary problems at the donor site is increased. It is important to consider the potential deleterious effects of what is called a "zone of influence" caused by the unsupported walls of a defect. In a goat study, even 6- $\times$ 6-mm defects were associated with deleterious changes in the adjacent osseous walls as well as in the surrounding articular cartilage. Progressive defect increase, development of a large cavity, and collapse of the surrounding subchondral bone and articular cartilage at the defect periphery occurred (36). This information suggests that grafts should not be large and that it is better to obtain two smaller grafts rather than one large graft. The effects of impact load also must be considered during surgical harvesting and transfer of osteochondral plugs—and kept to a minimum. Experimentally, blunt trauma of greater than 25 N/mm^2 consistently resulted in articular chondrocyte death (6). The recent development of a "back fill" prosthesis may offer a solution for the donor-site problem. One of these devices is composed of a copolymer of polyglycolide fibers, polylactide co-glycolide, and calcium sulfate, and it can be used to fill the donor site to support the adjacent wall; to serve as a scaffold for blood, marrow cells, and proteins; and to promote the healing of these defects **(Fig 43.1-12)**.

Harvesting of osteochondral plugs from the donor site can be an arthroscopic or an open procedure. Two commonly used donor sites are the superior lateral intercondylar notch **(Fig 43.1-13)** and the superior lateral femoral condyle above

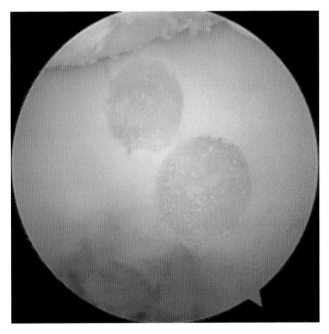

Fig 43.1-12. One backfill device is composed of polyglycolide fibers, polylactide co-glycolide, and calcium sulfate.

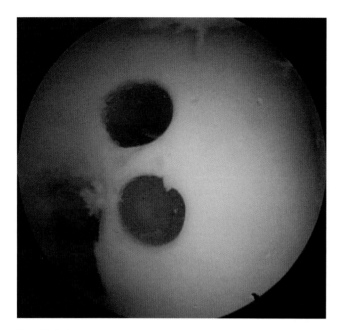

Fig 43.1-13. The superior lateral intercondylar notch is a common donor site.

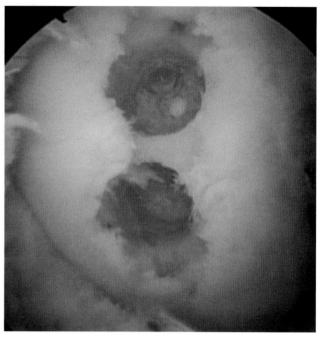

Fig 43.1-14. The drilled recipient sites should be placed immediately adjacent to the vertical articular wall of normal cartilage.

the linea terminalis. Regardless of the donor site, the COR harvester should be positioned perpendicular to the donor articular cartilage and impacted to the appropriate depth. Because the COR harvester has a tooth that undercuts the graft, a constant plug length can be obtained. The standard harvester provides an 8-mm plug length. The variable-depth harvester allows different lengths of grafts to be obtained. The consistent plug length permits drilling of the recipient site before graft harvest if needed.

Once the grafts are obtained, the first insertion site in the lesion is drilled. The drill should be placed immediately adjacent to the vertical articular wall of normal cartilage **(Fig 43.1-14)**. When drilling, it is important to keep the drill oriented perpendicular to the subchondral bone. Once the desired depth is achieved, the drill is removed, and then the debris is removed with the motorized shaver. Next, the harvested plug is inserted into the defect, keeping a vertical insertion orientation and being aware of any variation in the articular cartilage contour. The osteochondral autograft plug should not stand proud; if it is, then after the clear inserter is removed, use a tamp to adjust the height to match the adjacent articular cartilage surface **(Fig 43.1-15)**. Subsequent plugs are harvested and inserted using the same technique until the defect is filled.

The postoperative protocol for autograft transplantation includes immediate early motion and non–weight bearing for 3 weeks. These grafts are held in place by the press-fit design. They heal into position rapidly, and progressive weight bearing is allowed starting at 3 weeks and continuing to 6 weeks after surgery. Full weight bearing is permitted after 6 weeks. At that point, a progressive rehabilitation program can be initiated.

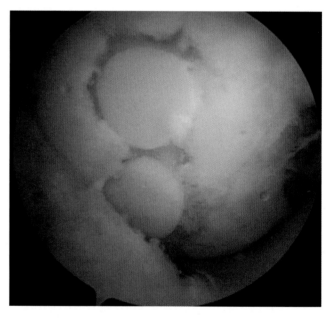

Fig 43.1-15. The osteochondral autograft plugs should be flush with the adjacent surface. A tamp can be used to adjust the height to match the adjacent articular cartilage level.

Osteochondral Allograft Transfer

The implantation of composite fresh cadaveric allografts is another technique to address full-thickness articular cartilage defects in the knee. These allografts come in various shapes and sizes, and they have both the intact articular cartilage and the subchondral bone as well. One significant issue with allografts is that to optimize the survival of the transplanted chondrocytes, the grafts should be implanted as soon after harvest as possible. They cannot be frozen, but they can be maintained at 4°C for up to 4 days and still retain 100% viability of the cartilage cells (37). This preserves the articular cartilage chondrocytes along with the cellular elements of the subchondral bone. Consequently, an antigenic exposure must be considered, along with a risk of viral transmission (37). As with osteochondral autograft transplantation, allograft transplantation is principally indicated for focal traumatic defects of the femoral condyle. In addition, these allografts are used for large osteochondral lesions, such as those seen with osteochondritis dissecans, osteonecrosis, large osteochondral fractures, and salvage procedures for cases in which other techniques have failed. Other applications include the treatment of full-thickness lesions on the patella and tibia.

Allograft reconstructions are recommended for use with lesions of greater than 3 cm in diameter and 1 cm in depth (37). These grafts are appropriate for lesions with substantial bone loss as well. A stable joint is required, and generalized osteoarthritic changes or lesions in multiple sites are contraindications. The advantages of the osteochondral allograft transplantation include the following: (a) Good documentation of the long-term results exists, (b) the technique is suitable for larger defect sizes, (c) no donor-site morbidity occurs, and (d) the defect configuration is not a limitation (38,39). Also, less concern exists about matching the articular cartilage contours. Typically, this is an open, rather than an arthroscopic, procedure, and although it is a single-step procedure, obtaining a well-matched donor femoral condyle requires careful preoperative planning and depends on donor availability.

The disadvantages of osteochondral allograft transplantation include the following: (a) An immune response must be considered, (b) transmission of disease may occur, (c) graft availability is limited, (d) rehabilitation is slower than with autografts, (e) cost is increased, and (f) the procedure is done on an inpatient basis. The process for insertion of an allograft starts by determining of the correct size requirements. A magnetic resonance image of the knee should be obtained, and this image often is sent to the tissue bank to aid in sizing an appropriate donor graft. Once a fresh graft is obtained, the surgery is scheduled as soon as possible. An arthroscopic procedure usually has been performed previously and any associated lesions already corrected.

Two types of allografts are available: dowel grafts **(Fig 43.1-16)**, and shell grafts. The procedure for using a dowel plug is similar to that of the osteochondral autograft transplantation, and it is best for well-defined lesions of up to 3.5 cm in diameter on the femoral condyle. A circular coring device is used to create a recipient site at the location of the lesion, and the donor plug is then press fit into this hole. For lesions with an irregular shape or contour, such as those on the patella, trochlear, or tibia, a shell graft works better.

Shell grafts are more technically challenging and require fixation. First, the defect is identified, and an outline is drawn around it using straight line. A regular geometric shape is

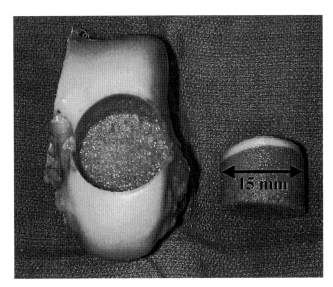

Fig 43.1-16. Allograft dowel graft for implantation into a femoral defect. (From Williams SK, Amiel D, Ball ST, et al. Prolonged storage effects on the articular cartilage of fresh human osteochondral allografts. *J Bone Joint Surg Am.* 2003;85:2111–2120; with permission.)

preferred, because it is easier to reproduce when cutting the graft by hand. As with other grafting techniques, vertical walls of normal articular cartilage adjacent to the lesion are created using a knife or curette. Once the recipient site has been prepared, a template is created using some readily available paper from the back table; this could be from a suture package or sterile cardboard. The template is cut to match the defect and then placed on the allograft. The allograft is marked with a pen, and the cuts are made. The shell graft should retain 5 mm of subchondral bone; it is better for the graft to be slightly larger than needed at first. The graft is carefully trimmed to the exact size using several trial fittings until the best match is achieved. The articular cartilage of the graft should fit flush with the adjacent normal articular cartilage. Biodegradable absorbable pins are used to fix the shell graft in place.

The postoperative protocol for allograft transplantation starts with extensive preoperative counseling and education regarding what to expect. Immediately after surgery, the patient should emphasize quadriceps activation and achieving full extension. A supervised physical therapy program should be included, along with use of a constant passive-motion machine and non–weight bearing for 6 to 12 weeks with dowel grafts, or non–weight bearing from 8 to 16 weeks for shell grafts. These ranges are dictated depending on the size and location of the grafts. Full activities may begin at 6 months for femoral condyle grafts and at 12 months for tibial plateau grafts. In either case, progression of activity is determined by radiographic evidence of healing.

Chondrocyte Implantation

Autologous chondrocyte implantation is a recently developed technique that addresses traumatic focal lesions on the weight-bearing surface, primarily of the femoral condyle (40,41). This technique attempts to replace a full-thickness articular cartilage defect with hyalinelike tissue. It is indicated for localized, symptomatic full-thickness articular cartilage lesions of at least 2 cm in diameter in younger patients with good alignment, good stability, and otherwise non-arthritic joints. The patient selected must be able to comply with the rehabilitation protocol. Lesions with bone loss of greater than 8 mm are not suitable until bone grafting of the defect is performed and completely healed. Multiple lesions are another contraindication. Any malalignment or ligament instability should be corrected at the time of ACI. Some authors have expanded the indications for ACI to include the patellofemoral surfaces, but ACI is not indicated for treatment of osteoarthritis, including bipolar bone-on-bone lesions. An opposing lesion with greater than grade 3 chondral damage also is a contraindication.

The ACI technique first requires the arthroscopic harvesting of 200 to 300 mg of viable autologous articular cartilage (40,41). A gouge or ring curette is used to take a 5- × 10-mm full-thickness segment of articular cartilage. The subchondral bone is not violated, which reduces the fibrovascular response. Harvest sites include the superior lateral or medial femoral condyle or the superior lateral intercondylar notch in an area that is nonarticulating with the tibia and that has limited patellar contact. The harvested articular cartilage is placed in a special, sterile container (provided by the company) filled with a culture medium. It is sent by an express mail carrier to Genzyme Corporation (Cambridge, MA) for processing. There, the cells are cultured and induced to increase in number and volume. This process requires as few as 3 weeks to complete, but it also can be temporarily suspended for use at a later time. When finished, a suspension of autologous chondrocytes containing 12 million cells per 0.4 mL of culture medium is prepared.

Once this step is complete, these cells are implanted several weeks later, in a separate procedure, through a medial or lateral parapatellar arthrotomy **(Fig 43.1-17)**. As with other cartilage repair procedures, clean vertical walls of normal articular cartilage are prepared adjacent to the lesion. Care should be taken not to penetrate the subchondral bone and to prevent bleeding into the defect. It is important that a wall of articular cartilage completely surround the lesion, creating a rim onto which the periosteum can be sewn. If that is not possible, small suture anchors sometimes may be used on a portion of the patch periphery. Bleeding must be completely controlled before proceeding to the next step. The defect is precisely measured, and a template is prepared using some sterile, disposable paper from the back table.

A medial tibial border incision is made, and the periosteum is exposed. The best harvest site for a periosteal graft is the proximal medial tibia, distal to the pes ancerine and the medial collateral ligament insertion. The periosteum is thicker on the posterior tibial cortex. Using sharp scissors and a wet sponge, remove the overlying fat and fascia from the periosteum before it is harvested. When ready for

harvesting, the periosteum should appear white and glistening. Periosteal atrophy may be found in older, obese patients who are inactive and smokers. If the proximal tibial periosteum is too thin and fragile, then the periosteum located immediately proximal to the articular surface of the distal medial or lateral femoral condyle may be used. This femoral periosteum requires a synovial incision and a subsynovial dissection. After harvesting a distal femoral periosteal graft, the synovium must be carefully repaired to its original location to avoid intra-articular bleeding. A piece of periosteum should be removed that is larger than the template that was created. Do not use an electrocautery for this process. Once harvested, the periosteum will tend to shrink; oversizing the periosteal patch by 2 mm in each direction is recommended. The periosteal patch should be kept moist, and a mark should be placed on the outer surface to distinguish it from the inner cambium layer, which should be sutured down to face the cells. Next, the tourniquet should be released and hemostasis obtained.

The periosteal patch is placed over the cartilage defect with the cambium layer down and trimmed to fit. It should be sutured to the adjacent, intact articular cartilage with #6-0 absorbable sutures on a P-1 cutting needle. First, suture the corners of the graft to the host cartilage to ensure a proper fit and graft tension. Next, trim any redundant periosteum from the graft with fine, sharp scissors. The periosteum should not overlap the adjacent articular cartilage. Proper periosteal graft tension should keep the graft taut and without wrinkles. A circumferential, watertight closure should be obtained except at the top of the lesion (where the cells will be inserted). The suture knots should be tied on the periosteal side rather than on the articular cartilage side and then cut with short tails. Injecting saline under the patch can test the watertight status. Once a watertight seal is confirmed, the saline is removed by aspiration through the remaining defect at the top of the patch, and the edges are sealed further with fibrin glue.

The autologous chondrocyte suspension should be carefully removed for the nonsterile vial after the cells are resuspended in the fluid by aspirating and injecting several times. An 18-gauge catheter attached to a syringe performs this step, and then the cells are carefully aspirated from the vial. The catheter attached to the syringe containing the cells is inserted through the defect at the top of the patch, and the cells are slowly injected into the lesion. The catheter is slowly removed, and the opening is closed with additional sutures and then sealed with fibrin glue.

The wounds are closed, and the knee is immobilized for 8 hours to allow the cells to adhere to the lesion base **(Fig 43.1-18)**. A review of the patients with between 2 and 9 years of follow-up demonstrated good to excellent results in 92% of isolated femoral condyle lesions, 65% of patellar lesions, and 89% of osteochondritis dissecans lesions (42). A concern about these initially published results, however, is that the reported success may have resulted from the natural history of partial-thickness chondral injuries or from the

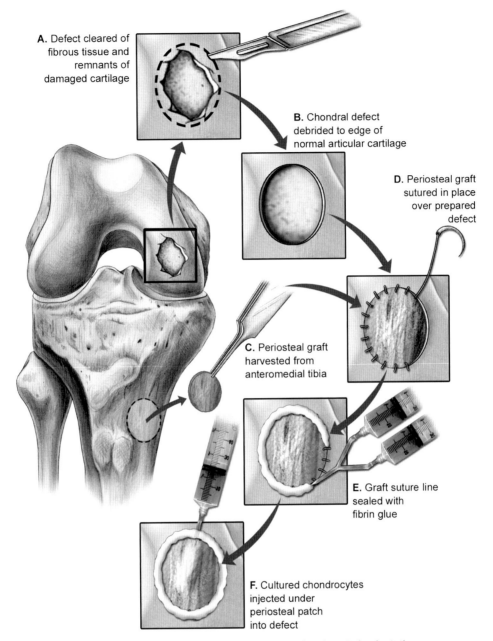

A. Defect cleared of fibrous tissue and remnants of damaged cartilage

B. Chondral defect debrided to edge of normal articular cartilage

D. Periosteal graft sutured in place over prepared defect

C. Periosteal graft harvested from anteromedial tibia

E. Graft suture line sealed with fibrin glue

F. Cultured chondrocytes injected under periosteal patch into defect

Fig 43.1-17. The technique for autologous chondrocyte implantation.

debridement performed as part of the procedure rather than from the chondrocyte transplantation (12). Underscoring these concerns is a recent comparison between ACI and microfracture, which showed significant clinical improvement in both groups at 2 years of follow-up. The SF-36 score, however, demonstrated significantly more improvement in the microfracture group than in the ACI group (43).

The rehabilitation program is a slow and gradual progression of activity. The basic principles are focused on maintaining mobility, protecting the graft, strengthening muscle, progressive weight bearing, and patient education. Postoperatively, the patient is required to use a continuous passive-motion machine 6 to 8 hours a day for up to 6 weeks.

Non–weight bearing or light-touch weight bearing is required for 6 weeks. Because patellofemoral contact pressures are maximized between 40 and 70 degree knee flexion, active knee flexion should avoid this range. The therapist should initiate patellofemoral mobilization early to avoid adhesions. By 6 weeks, full motion should be achieved, and weight bearing is progressed to full. Active knee extension should be avoided for the first 12 weeks. Strengthening exercises are started and progressed between 6 and 12 weeks. A return to full activity is delayed for 8 months. Recent clinical reports have not shown superior results at 2 years for ACI when compared to marrow-stimulating procedures, and they suggest that the healing that occurs in defects treated by ACI

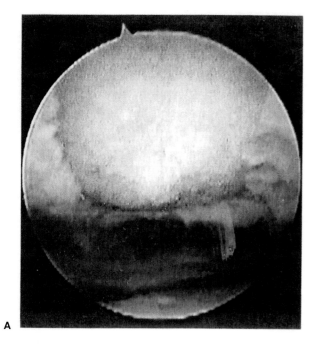

A

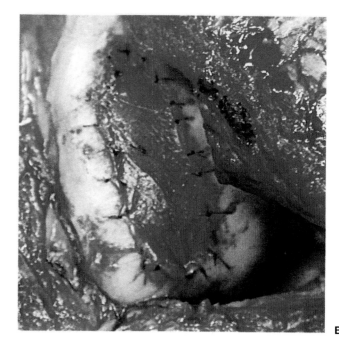

B

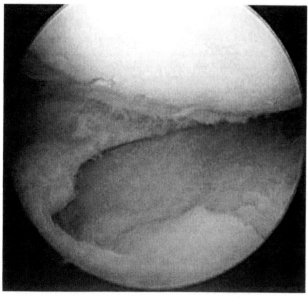

C

Fig 43.1-18. Clinical photographs of a full-thickness medial femoral condyle defect **(A)** after autologous chondrocyte implantation **(B)** and at arthroscopic reevaluation 18 months postoperatively **(C)**.

consists of fibrocartilage rather than hyaline articular cartilage (43,44). The clinical reports are mixed, however, when ACI is compared to osteochondral autograft transplantation (44,45), although patients undergoing ACI have a slower recovery. When compared to marrow-stimulating techniques, ACI seems to produce histologically similar tissue at the treated site (43).

■ REFERENCES

1. Curl WW, Krome J, Gordon ES, et al. Cartilage injuries: a review of 31,516 knee arthroscopies. *Arthroscopy.* 1997;13:456–460.
2. Bach BR Jr, Levy ME, Bojchuk J, et al. Single-incision endoscopic anterior cruciate ligament reconstruction using patellar tendon autograft. Minimum two-year follow-up evaluation. *Am J Sports Med.* 1998;26:30–40.
3. Mow VC, Ratcliffe A. Structure and function of articular cartilage and meniscus. In: Mow VC, Hayes WC, eds. *Basic orthopaedic biomechanics.* Philadelphia: Lippincott–Raven Publishers; 1997.
4. Buckwalter JA, Mankin HJ. Articular cartilage: tissue design and chondrocyte-matrix interactions. *Instr Course Lect.* 1998; 47:477–486.
5. Browne JE, Branch TP. Surgical alternatives for treatment of articular cartilage lesions. *J Am Acad Orthop Surg.* 2000;8:180–189.
6. Repo RU, Finlay JB. Survival of articular cartilage after controlled impact. *J Bone Joint Surg Am.* 1977;59:1068–1076.
7. Johnson DL, Urban WP Jr, Caborn DN, et al. Articular cartilage changes seen with magnetic resonance imaging–detected bone bruises associated with acute anterior cruciate ligament rupture. *Am J Sports Med.* 1998;26:409–414.
8. Nehrer S, Spector M, Minas T. Histologic analysis of tissue after failed cartilage repair procedures. *Clin Orthop.* 1999;365:149–162.

9. Outerbridge RE. The etiology of chondromalacia patellae. *J Bone Joint Surg Br.* 1961;43-B:752–757.

10. Brittberg M. Evaluation of cartilage injuries and cartilage repair. *Osteologie.* 2000;9:17–25.

11. Campbell CJ. The healing of cartilage defects. *Clin Orthop.* 1969;64:45–63.

12. Newman AP. Articular cartilage repair. *Am J Sports Med.* 1998;26:309–324.

13. Ghadially FN, Thomas I, Oryschak AF, et al. Long-term results of superficial defects in articular cartilage: a scanning electron-microscope study. *J Pathol.* 1977;121:213–217.

14. Messner K, Maletius W. The long-term prognosis for severe damage to weight-bearing cartilage in the knee: a 14-year clinical and radiographic follow-up in 28 young athletes. *Acta Orthop Scand.* 1996;67:165–168.

15. Snibbe JC, Gambardella RA. Use of injections for osteoarthritis in joints and sports activity. *Clin Sports Med.* 2005;24:83–91.

16. Wang CT, Lin J, Chang CJ, et al. Therapeutic effects of hyaluronic acid on osteoarthritis of the knee. A meta-analysis of randomized controlled trials. *J Bone Joint Surg Am.* 2004;86:538–545.

17. Harwin SF. Arthroscopic debridement for osteoarthritis of the knee: predictors of patient satisfaction. *Arthroscopy.* 1999;15:142–146.

18. Levy AS, Lohnes J, Sculley S, et al. Chondral delamination of the knee in soccer players. *Am J Sports Med.* 1996;24:634–639.

19. Kim HK, Moran ME, Salter RB. The potential for regeneration of articular cartilage in defects created by chondral shaving and subchondral abrasion. An experimental investigation in rabbits. *J Bone Joint Surg Am.* 1991;73:1301–1315.

20. Hunziker EB, Quinn TM. Surgical removal of articular cartilage leads to loss of chondrocytes from cartilage bordering the wound edge. *J Bone Joint Surg Am.* 2003;85(suppl 2):85–92.

21. Triantafillopoulos IK, Papagelopoulos PJ, Politi PK, et al. Articular changes in experimentally induced patellar trauma. *Knee Surg Sports Traumatol Arthrosc.* 2002;10:144–153.

22. Lu Y, Edwards RB III, Kalscheur VL, et al. Effect of bipolar radiofrequency energy on human articular cartilage. Comparison of confocal laser microscopy and light microscopy. *Arthroscopy.* 2001;17:117–123.

23. Lu Y, Hayashi K, Hecht P, et al. The effect of monopolar radiofrequency energy on partial-thickness defects of articular cartilage. *Arthroscopy.* 2000;16:527–536.

24. Lu Y, Edwards RB III, Cole BJ, et al. Thermal chondroplasty with radiofrequency energy. An in vitro comparison of bipolar and monopolar radiofrequency devices. *Am J Sports Med.* 2001;29:42–49.

25. Pridie KH. A method of resurfacing osteoarthritic knee joints. *J Bone Joint Surg Br.* 1959;41:618–619.

26. Johnson LL. Arthroscopic abrasion arthroplasty historical and pathologic perspective: present status. *Arthroscopy.* 1986;2:54–69.

27. Bert JM. Role of abrasion arthroplasty and debridement in the management of osteoarthritis of the knee. *Rheum Dis Clin North Am.* 1993;19:725–739.

28. Rand JA. Role of arthroscopy in osteoarthritis of the knee. *Arthroscopy.* 1991;7:358–363.

29. Friedman MJ, Berasi CC, Fox JM, et al. Preliminary results with abrasion arthroplasty in the osteoarthritic knee. *Clin Orthop.* 1984;182:200–205.

30. Mitchell N, Shepard N. The resurfacing of adult rabbit articular cartilage by multiple perforations through the subchondral bone. *J Bone Joint Surg Am.* 1976;58:230–233.

31. Steadman JR, Briggs KK, Rodrigo JJ, et al. Outcomes of microfracture for traumatic chondral defects of the knee: average 11-year follow-up. *Arthroscopy.* 2003;19:477–484.

32. Marder RA, Hopkins G, Timmerman LA. Arthroscopic microfracture of chondral defects of the knee: a comparison of two postoperative treatments. *Arthroscopy.* 2005;21:152–158.

33. Bobic V. Arthroscopic osteochondral autograft transplantation in anterior cruciate ligament reconstruction: a preliminary clinical study. *Knee Surg Sports Traumatol Arthrosc.* 1996;3:262–264.

34. Barber FA, Chow JC. Arthroscopic osteochondral transplantation: histologic results. *Arthroscopy.* 2001;17:832–835.

35. Hangody L, Kish G, Karpati Z, et al. Mosaicplasty for the treatment of articular cartilage defects: application in clinical practice. *Orthopedics.* 1998;21:751–756.

36. Jackson DW, Lalor PA, Aberman HM, et al. Spontaneous repair of full-thickness defects of articular cartilage in a goat model. A preliminary study. *J Bone Joint Surg Am.* 2001;83:53–64.

37. Shasha N, Aubin PP, Cheah HK, et al. Long-term clinical experience with fresh osteochondral allografts for articular knee defects in high demand patients. *Cell Tissue Bank.* 2002;3:175–182.

38. Fitzpatrick PL, Morgan DA. Fresh osteochondral allografts: a 6–10-year review. *Aust N Z J Surg.* 1998;68:573–579.

39. Ghazavi MT, Pritzker KP, Davis AM, et al. Fresh osteochondral allografts for post-traumatic osteochondral defects of the knee. *J Bone Joint Surg Br.* 1997;79:1008–1013.

40. Brittberg M, Lindahl A, Nilsson A, et al. Treatment of deep cartilage defects in the knee with autologous chondrocyte transplantation. *N Engl J Med.* 1994;331:889–895.

41. Brittberg M, Peterson L, Sjogren-Jansson E, et al. Articular cartilage engineering with autologous chondrocyte transplantation. A review of recent developments. *J Bone Joint Surg Am.* 2003;85(suppl 3):109–115.

42. Peterson L, Minas T, Brittberg M, et al. Two- to 9-year outcome after autologous chondrocyte transplantation of the knee. *Clin Orthop.* 2000;374:212–234.

43. Knutsen G, Engebretsen L, Ludvigsen TC, et al. Autologous chondrocyte implantation compared with microfracture in the knee. A randomized trial. *J Bone Joint Surg Am.* 2004;86:455–464.

44. Horas U, Pelinkovic D, Herr G, et al. Autologous chondrocyte implantation and osteochondral cylinder transplantation in cartilage repair of the knee joint. A prospective, comparative trial. *J Bone Joint Surg Am.* 2003;85:185–192.

45. Bentley G, Biant LC, Carrington RW, et al. A prospective, randomized comparison of autologous chondrocyte implantation versus mosaicplasty for osteochondral defects in the knee. *J Bone Joint Surg Br.* 2003;85:223–230.

43.2

OSTEOCHONDRITIS DISSECANS OF THE KNEE

■ DAWN L. SWARM, MD, ROBERT A. PEDOWITZ, MD, PhD

■ KEY POINTS

■ Traditionally, osteochondritis dissecans (OCD) is divided into juvenile (open physes) and adult (closed physes) formed based on skeletal maturity.

■ Typically, the skeletally immature patient initially is treated nonoperatively and has a better overall outcome.

■ Because operative intervention is the treatment of both adult OCD and an osteochondral fracture, most surgeons do not bother to differentiate the two.

■ The etiology of OCD remains unclear. Growth disorders, epiphyseal ossification abnormalities, endocrine imbalances, ischemia, genetic predisposition, and repetitive microtrauma have been theorized to be causes. In addition, OCD has been associated with other musculoskeletal abnormalities.

■ One common characteristic in patients with juvenile OCD is a high level of athletic activity.

■ The prevalence of OCD seems to be increasing, with the mean age decreasing and more females being affected. A contributing factor may be increased participation in higher competitive levels of organized sports by younger children.

■ In juvenile patients, the initial complaints are of vague, nonspecific, poorly localized anterior knee pain that worsens with activity and improves with rest. These symptoms are difficult to distinguish from those of patellar femoral syndrome.

■ Initial plain-film radiographs should include anteroposterior, lateral, and notch views of the knee, with an additional Merchant view if a patellar or trochlear lesion is expected. The notch view demonstrates the most common areas of OCD.

■ Comparison views should be obtained in pediatric and adolescent patients to prevent confusion with normal bone development.

■ Computed tomography provides bony detail of OCD lesions and are helpful in determining the size of the defect or if loose bodies are present.

■ Magnetic resonance imaging (MRI) can give an accurate estimation for the size of the lesion as well as the status of the cartilage and underlying bone.

■ The critical issue is to determine the stability of the lesion itself, if the cartilage over the lesion is intact or has fractured, and if the subchondral bone has separated from its base.

■ Any unstable lesion must be treated surgically.

■ Mechanical stabilization of fragments can be performed with a variety of devices, such as Kirshner wires, compression screws, bone pegs, bioabsorbable screws, and fibrin glues.

■ Fresh osteochondral allografting has been proposed as a viable option for treatment of osteochondral defects. Patient selection is critical to the success of this procedure. Patients should be active and well motivated, and any limb malalignment must be corrected before transplantation.

The term *osteochondritis dissecans*, or OCD, was first used by Konig in 1888, when he described loose bodies, or "corpora mobile," involving the articular surface of the joint. He initially speculated that these were caused by an inflammatory reaction that led to spontaneous necrosis of the subchondral bone and overlying cartilage (i.e., "dissecting inflammation") (1,2). Although Konig later retracted inflammation as the cause, the term is still commonly used today to describe the separation of an articular cartilage subchondral bone segment from the remaining articular cartilage (1,3–8).

Traditionally, OCD is divided into juvenile (open physes) and adult (closed physes) forms based on skeletal maturity (1,5,7). This distinction is useful in determining treatment options, because typically, the skeletally immature patient initially is treated nonoperatively and has a better overall outcome (1,3,5,7).

Some believe that adult OCD is a progression of an unresolved juvenile OCD lesion, but it is difficult to differentiate from a traumatic osteochondral fracture (1,4). Because operative intervention is the treatment of both adult OCD and an osteochondral fracture, however, most surgeons do not bother to differentiate the two (1).

■ ETIOLOGY/INCIDENCE

The etiology of OCD remains unclear, and multiple hypotheses have been proposed. Growth disorders, epiphyseal ossification abnormalities, endocrine imbalances, ischemia, genetic predisposition, and repetitive microtrauma have been theorized as causes (1–4,6–15). In addition, OCD has been associated with other musculoskeletal abnormalities, such as Legg-Calve-Perthes disease, ligamentous laxity, genu valgum, genu varum, tibial torsion, patellar malalignment, and Sinding-Larsen-Johansson and Osgood Schlatter disorders (3,16,17).

One common characteristic in patients with juvenile OCD is a high level of athletic activity (3,5,7,13,18,19). It is two- to threefold more common in males than in females, usually presenting between 10 and 20 years of age (5,8,13). It may be bilateral in up to one third of cases (4,13).

The incidence of OCD is unknown. Most published reports involve small numbers of patients referred to large centers, a lack of uniformity in the classification systems, and inconsistency in diagnosis and management (4,7).

The prevalence of OCD, however, seems to be increasing. A contributing factor may be increased participation in higher competitive levels of organized sports by younger children. Many children are engaged in organized sporting leagues year-round. The mean age is decreasing, and more females are involved. The advancement of arthroscopy and the widespread use of MRI also may have contributed to the increase in prevalence, because more patients with this disorder are being recognized (3,4).

■ LOCATION

Knee OCD lesions are seen most commonly (70% to 80%) in the "classic" or extended classic location (4,5,7,8,20). The classic site is the posterolateral aspect of the medial femoral condyle, and the extended classic site extends into the weight-bearing portion of the medial femoral condyle **(Fig 43.2-1)**. Inferocentral lateral condylar lesions are seen in 15% of cases (8,21,22). Lateral condylar lesions also have been associated with lateral discoid menisci (19,23–26). Patellar involvement is uncommon (<5%) but, when present, is located in the inferior pole. Femoral trochlear lesions account for less than 1% of cases (4,5,8,12,27,28).

■ CLINICAL FEATURES

In juvenile patients, the initial complaints are of vague, non-specific, poorly localized anterior knee pain that worsens with activity and improves with rest (18). These symptoms are difficult to distinguish from those of patellar femoral syndrome. A high index of suspicion should be maintained for active juvenile patients with these complaints (7). Other patients may be asymptomatic, with lesions being discovered incidentally when radiographs are obtained for unrelated reasons. In a European multicenter study of more than 500 juvenile cases of OCD, 32% of patients had no or little pain at the time of diagnosis (2).

In both the juvenile and adult forms, symptoms are preceded by trauma to the knee in from 40% to 60% of cases (5,29). Patients may complain of stiffness with or after activities and occasional swelling, and there may be tenderness over the affected condyle with the knee flexed. An unstable lesion may cause grinding, catching, or locking and, thus, a decrease in range or motion and/or an effusion. The patient may walk with an antalgic gait, externally rotating the involved lower extremity to prevent impingement of the lesion on the tibial spine when the lesion is in the classic location (1,4,5,13).

In 1967, Wilson (30) described a clinical test that is specific for diagnosing the classic medial femoral condyle lesion termed the *Wilson sign*. The test is performed by flexing the knee to 90 degrees, then slowly internally rotating the leg and extending it. Patients with a positive Wilson sign complain of pain at 30 degrees of flexion when the tibial spine abuts against the medial femoral condyle. The pain is relieved with external rotation (5,8,18,31). Unfortunately, however, this test is unreliable. Multiple studies found that from 70% to 75% of both juvenile and adult patients with OCD lesions had a negative Wilson sign during clinical evaluation (2,7,31).

Late findings include quadriceps weakness and atrophy (13). Both knees should be examined, because the condition is bilateral in from 20% to 30% of cases and involvement and because the magnitudes are not symmetrical (4,8,32).

■ DIAGNOSTIC STUDIES

Using the appropriate sequences and modalities will aid in the accurate assessment of the stability of OCD lesions and prevent unnecessary invasive procedures.

Plain-film Radiographs

Initial plain-film radiographs should include anteroposterior, lateral, and notch views of the knee, with an additional

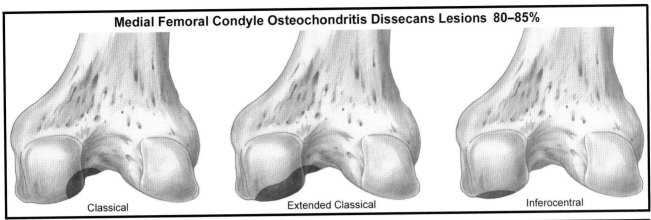

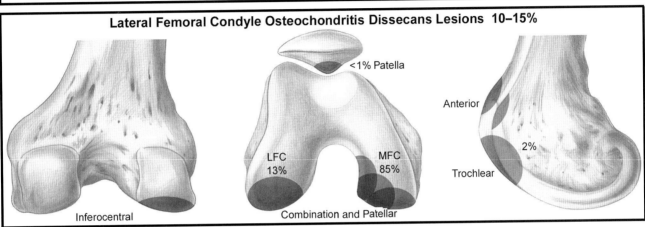

Fig 43.2-1. Common locations of osteochondritis dissecans lesions in the knee.

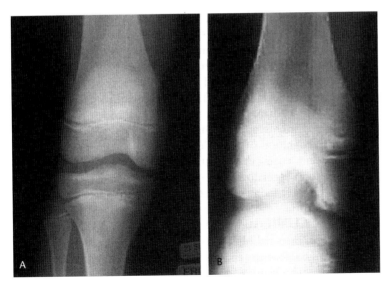

Fig 43.2-2. Anteroposterior **(A)** and notch **(B)** radiographs of a juvenile osteochondritis dissecans lesion of the medial femoral condyle. (From Flynn JM, Kocher MS, Ganley TJ. Osteochondritis dissecans of the knee. *J Pediatr Orthop.* 2004;24:434–443.)

Merchant view if a patellar or trochlear lesion is suspected. The notch view improves the yield, because it demonstrates the most common areas for OCD (1,10,11,13,27, 28,33) **(Fig 43.2-2)**. If the lateral view is scrutinized in the posterior half of the condyle, then the lesion usually can be identified. Characteristic findings include a well-circumscribed area of subchondral bone separated by a crescent-shaped,

sclerotic, radiolucent outline of the fragment. The lesion may be entirely radiolucent, but it often contains a central fragment of bone (7,8).

Comparison views should be obtained in pediatric and adolescent patients to prevent confusion with normal bone development or areas of irregular ossification (5,8,13). In younger children (age 7 to 12 years), irregularities of the distal femoral epiphyseal ossification center may simulate OCD. These irregularities, however, actually are benign anatomical variants of normal ossification. They are located on the posterior portion of the condyles and are best seen on a tunnel view, or posterior to a line coincident with the posterior femoral cortex intersecting the femoral condyle in the lateral view (4,5,7,13). An MRI may help to differentiate the two, and a bone scan will be normal in patients with irregular ossification variants.

A plain-film radiograph may localize the OCD lesion, rule out other bony pathology, and evaluate skeletal maturity, but routine radiographs are poor tools for determining the stability of the lesion or the state of the overlying cartilage (4,8,34). Therefore, additional studies are necessary to develop a treatment plan.

Scintigraphy

Technetium bone scans have been used to localize the lesion to a specific joint and to follow the progression of healing in juvenile patients, but it cannot delineate the state of the cartilage (4,7,15). Cahill and Berg (35) proposed that the degree of osseous uptake on bone scans was related to the regional blood flow or osteoblastic activity and, therefore, to the potential for healing. Those authors developed a protocol that included a bone scan for initial diagnosis with serial scans every 6 to 8 weeks to evaluate healing in the nonoperative patient as well as a qualitative classification scheme comprised of four stages. They used both scintigraphy and serial clinical examinations to follow the progress of healing. If three serial scans remain at the same stage, then healing of the lesion without surgery is doubtful.

To further evaluate the use of scintigraphy for the treatment of OCD, Paletta et al. (36) retrospectively reviewed the records of 12 patients and found that bone scans were 100% predictive for the prognosis of nonsurgical OCD management in six patients with open physes. A bone scan was less useful, however, in six patients with closed physes, showing a predictive value of only 33%.

The adolescent patient nearing skeletal maturity is the most difficult to treat. Bone scans do not seem to be a good method for determining treatment in this age group. In addition, the isotopic tracer remains in the area in question for a significant amount of time even after healing, which makes interpretation difficult (4). Serial bone scans have not been widely adopted. Possible reasons include the time required for the study, the need for intravenous access, the perceived risk of the isotope, and the emergence of MRI (4,7,15).

Computed Tomography

Computed tomography provides bony detail of OCD lesions and is helpful in determining the size of the defect or loose body, if present (8,37). Adding a contrast agent increases the accuracy and ability to stage OCD lesions. If the contrast agent infiltrates into the cleft, then the computed tomographic scan depicts a loose or unstable fragment (15). Because MRI provides more detailed information, however, computed tomography rarely is used in determining the treatment plan.

Magnetic Resonance Imaging

Magnetic resonance imaging provides more valuable information than many of the other diagnostic studies (4,8,38–40). It can give an accurate estimation for the size of the lesion as well as the status of the cartilage and underlying bone; thus, it has become a frequently ordered study for determining the stability of OCD lesions. The best MRI sequences for evaluating the OCD lesion and the surface cartilage are fast spin echo, proton density, and T_2 weighted (7,27,40) **(Fig 43.2-3)**.

The critical issue is determining the stability of the lesion itself, if the cartilage over the lesion is intact or fractured, and if the subchondral bone has separated from its base (7,20,41). A number of different staging systems have been proposed. Basically, the commonality of all the staging systems is determining the stability of the lesion to dictate treatment. All agree that a loose body or lesion in which the fluid completely surrounds the fragment is unstable. The difficulty lies in the questionable lesion that may have a low signal or incomplete line of fluid surrounding it.

De Smet et al. (38) retrospectively evaluated the MRIs of 14 patients with OCD to determine the value of MRI in depicting clinical outcome. Those authors described four MRI criteria for evaluating unstable OCD lesions on T_2-weighted images: (a) a line of high signal intensity at least 5 mm in length between the osteochondritic fragment and underlying bone; (b) a high signal line traversing the subchondral plate into the lesion, indicating an articular fracture; (c) a focal osteochondral defect filled with joint fluid; and (d) a 5 mm or larger, fluid-filled cyst deep to the lesion. Of these signs, a high signal line behind the fragment was the most predictive, being found in 72% of unstable lesions.

Similarly, Pill et al. (42) used the above criteria and clinical assessment in an attempt to predict the success of nonoperative treatment in patients with OCD. The most common MRI sign in patients who failed nonoperative treatment was a line of high signal intensity between the lesion and the subchondral bone. In addition, lesion size and skeletal maturity also were important predictors of failure of nonoperative treatment.

It has been suggested, however, that a high signal line may not necessarily represent synovial fluid and instability but, instead, a vascular granulation and healing response (4,5,10,43). The addition of intravenous contrast with gadolinium can distinguish enhanced granulation tissue from synovial fluid, which does not enhance (10). Comparing different sequences of the same images can be helpful in the final assessment. A high signal line on

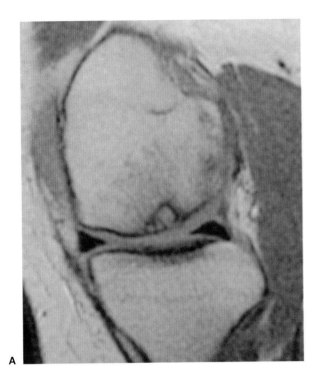

A

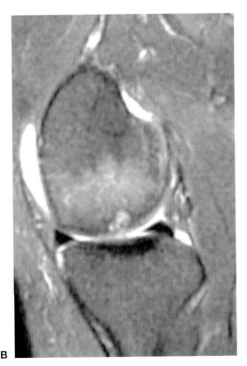

B

Fig 43.2-3. T1-weighted **(A)** and T2-weighted **(B)** magnetic resonance images of an osteochondritis dissecans lesion in the medial femoral condyle.

T_2-weighted images is more predictive of synovial fluid and, when accompanied by a breach in articular cartilage on T_1-weighted images, is more predictive of an unstable lesion (44). In addition, MRI–arthrography with gadolinium has been shown to have 100% predictive value in

determining the status of articular cartilage using gradient-echo techniques (40).

■ TREATMENT

Arthroscopy has enabled the orthopaedic surgeon to better diagnose, stage, and treat OCD lesions. The surfaces of the femoral cartilage must be carefully examined and probed to avoid missing an intact-appearing articular cartilage surface. A bluish-gray color often typifies an unstable cartilage lesion (8).

The treatment of OCD depends on the patient's age as well as on the lesion size, location, and stability (4,5,8,13). Regardless of age, any unstable lesion must be treated surgically. Lesions on the weight-bearing surface, lateral condyle, and greater than 1 cm in size tend to have less successful outcomes when treated nonoperatively (1,12,45,46). Overall, the age of the patient is the most significant factor, because regardless of conservative or operative interventions, skeletally immature patients have a better prognosis compared with their skeletally mature counterparts.

Most agree that initial nonoperative treatment is recommended for at least 3 to 6 months in a skeletally immature patient with a stable lesion (1,4,5,7,8,11,12,33,47,48). Reported healing rates range from 50% to 94% with nonsurgical treatment (2,3,7,9,38,39,43,49–51). Patients are followed with serial clinical examinations, radiographic evaluation, scintigraphy, or MRI (3,8,12,35). This recommendation is empirical, however, because no control studies have been reported and because follow-up have been limited in many studies.

Nonoperative treatments range from simple cessation of athletic activity to complete non–weight-bearing immobilization. In the past, some recommended cast immobilization, because many juvenile patients are noncompliant. Prolonged immobilization, however, leads to increased stiffness, atrophy, and degeneration of cartilage and decreases the healing potential (1,5,11,47,52).

Current recommendations for treatment of skeletally immature patients consist of a knee immobilizer, daily range-of-motion exercises, isometric muscle strengthening, nonweight bearing, and crutches for 6 to 8 weeks. Activity modification continues until healing is evident both radiographically and clinically (8). If no progression to healing is seen on radiographs after 6 months or if a lesion becomes unstable, arthroscopy is recommended (5,7,13).

■ EXTRACTION OF FRAGMENT

In the past, a common surgical treatment was simply to excise loose osteochondral fragments. More recent studies, however, have shown that the long-term results of both juvenile and adult patients are poor when treated with excision alone (11,26,53,54). Because of more extensive treatment options today, most would now agree that excision alone will result in a poor outcome. The addition of debridement or curettage of the crater has shown improved results in juvenile patients (11,55).

DRILLING

Drilling was one of the first surgical treatments described for treating OCD lesions that fail conservative management (56). Today, arthroscopic or open drilling, either alone or with various fixation methods, remains one of the most common operative interventions (5,7,47,57). Drilling is based on the theory that the lesion is basically a fracture nonunion and that penetration of the subchondral bone will initiate an inflammatory healing cascade and create channels for potential revascularization (1,5).

A number of studies have supported drilling as an effective treatment option, especially in the juvenile patient. Aglietti et al. (47) found a 95% radiographic healing rate after drilling 16 knees in 14 skeletally immature patients who failed conservative treatment at an average of 4.9 months after drilling. Similarly, Anderson et al. (9) found healing in 18 of 20 skeletally immature patients after transarticular drilling and in two of four skeletally mature patients with an average follow-up of 5 years.

Likewise, Kocher et al. (46) looked at the long-term follow-up of 30 knees in 23 skeletally immature patients treated with transarticular arthroscopic drilling after failing 6 months of conservative treatment. Those authors found radiographic healing in all patients at an average of 4 months after drilling.

A retrospective study by the French Society of Arthroscopy evaluated transarticular drilling in 17 skeletally immature patients and eight adult patients with stable lesions. That study noted 12 (of 17) radiographically healed lesions in the juvenile group but only two (of eight) radiographically healed lesions in the adult group (58).

Drilling options are either transarticular or retrograde through the epiphysis without articular penetration (1,8,45,47). Drilling through the epiphyses is technically challenging in terms of maintaining drill depth and accuracy of placement, and it may result in undesirable soft tissue injury. It does, however, allow the ability to graft bone (4,5). Transarticular drilling, although technically easier, creates articular channels that heal with fibrocartilage (5,9).

Recently, Kawasaki et al. (59) described another technique in which drilling is performed from the intercondylar bare area, thus eliminating further damage to the articular cartilage. Those authors operated on 16 knees of skeletally immature patients who failed conservative treatment at an average of 3 months. They found that all lesions healed by an average of 4 months as determined by standard radiographs and 7 months as determined by MRI. This may be a technique that warrants for further study.

REDUCTION OF FRAGMENT

Mechanical stabilization of the fragment can be performed with a variety of devices, such as Kirschner wires, compression screws, bone pegs, bioabsorbable screws, and fibrin glues. Many, however, require a second surgery for hardware removal.

Multiple smooth Kirschner wires have been used to reduce the fragment, although this method does not provide any compression (1,45,56,57,60). Bending the subchondral end of the Kirschner wire to correct this and provide compression has been described (3,52).

Herbert screws have been advocated for securing osteochondral fragments, because the different pitches in either end of the screw compress the fragment and the countersunk heads allow early motion without further risk of articular injury (1,61,62). Because of the relative stiffness of the screw as compared to the articular cartilage, screws that are not deeply embedded in bone should be removed (12). Because of the reported difficulty in removing the screw at a second arthroscopy because of fibrocartilage growth over the screw head, removal should be performed as early as possible (8).

Fixing OCD fragments with cannulated screws has been described as well. Screws must be removed before weight bearing, however, because prominent screw heads can abrade the opposing tibial articular surface (1,8,63–65). Cannulated screws may be easier to remove, but all types require a second surgery at 6 to 8 weeks after implantation. This second surgery, however, offers the advantage of gaining a "second look" at healing and assessing the stability of the fragment (3,8,65).

Kivisto et al. (66) reported the use of arthroscopically placed metal staples, which were thought not to require removal. In practice, broken staples were seen in 9 of 25 knees, and this method has been abandoned.

Bioabsorbable screws and rods have the advantages of providing compression, not requiring removal, and creating less artifact on MRI (67). Disadvantages include the cost of the implant, the strength of the implant, and reports of reactive synovitis and effusion (1,50,68–71). These implants do not degrade quickly, and they can retain their mechanical stiffness for many months. Loosening and failure of bioabsorbable screws that backed out, causing damage to adjacent articular surfaces, and unabsorbed screw heads as intra-articular loose bodies have been reported (68,72).

The OCD lesion may be fragmented, with small areas that are adherent but not adequately filling the defect. These areas can be augmented with bone grafts, such as tibial metaphyseal bone strips. The results of this technique have been fairly successful; patients have returned to strenuous activities without a second arthroscopy for screw or pin removal (67,70,73).

Often, the free fragment is either no longer present or in multiple pieces and unable to adequately cover the defect. A number of techniques have evolved to address this problem. One technique involves abrasion chondroplasty and microfracture. Others include osteochondral autografting, autologous chondrocyte implantation, and allografting.

Abrasion Chondroplasty and Microfracture

The theory behind both abrasion chondroplasty and microfracture is that penetration of the subchondral bone provides vascular access to the lesion and, thus, to the pluripotent stem cells, creating the potential for healing. Johnson (74) first described the abrasion arthroplasty technique, in which a bur is used to resect the bone by approximately 2 mm. Steadman et al. (75) popularized the microfracture technique, in which the bed of the lesion is first curetted through the calcified cartilage. The area is then penetrated with microfracture awls to a depth of approximately 4 to 5 mm at locations from 3 to 4 mm apart. Theoretically, the use of awls rather than a bur or power drills has the advantage of not creating heat necrosis. Postoperatively, the patient is non–weight bearing for 6 to 8 weeks and uses a continuous passive-motion machine for the same period of time. In both of these procedures, the goal is for the lesion to heal with fibrocartilage (7,74,76). Results from these techniques for large lesions, however, show deterioration with time because decreased fibrocartilage resilience and stiffness.

Microfracture results appear to be good in the short term, but many authors have questioned the long-term results (7). Steadman et al. (77) found that 80% of their patients who underwent microfracture for various cartilage lesions had improvement in their pain at 7-year follow-up.

Osteochondral Autograft

Osteochondral autografting and mosaicplasty involve the transplantation of autologous osteochondral plugs from non–weight-bearing portions of the knee to the osteochondral defect, thus filling the defect with hyaline cartilage (78–82). Autologous osteochondral grafts are harvested from the supracondylar ridge of the femur or intercondylar notch; the grafts have a diameter of up to 8.5 mm in diameter and a length of 10 to 15 mm (1). The grafts are then press fit into the defect. Fibrocartilage fills in between the plugs (1,80). Patients remain non–weight bearing for 6 to 8 weeks postoperatively. Retrospective studies and case reports have shown good to excellent clinical results from this procedure for treatment of osteochondral defects (63,78–80,82–87).

Harvesting the lateral patella facet as a donor site for transplantation to an OCD lesion in the femoral condyle also has been described. Studies have shown improved knee scores, incorporation of the grafts to surrounding bone on all radiographs, and minimal donor-site morbidity (88–90).

Potential disadvantages of mosaicplasty are donor-site morbidity, incongruent articular cartilage at graft sites, and loose bodies (83,88,91,92). Well-designed, long-term, prospective studies are needed to confirm the benefits and to delineate the complications of this technique.

Autologous Chondrocyte Implantation

Autologous chondrocyte implantation is a technique in which chondrocytes are harvested, expanded in vitro, and then reimplanted 2 to 6 weeks later under a periosteal patch to hold them contained within the defect (1,3,4,8). This can be used for treatment of lesions approximately 2 to 10 cm² (93).

Studies have shown good to excellent clinical results at follow-ups ranging from 2 to 10 years (94–98). Second arthroscopies and biopsies have revealed living, hyalinelike cartilage repair tissue (99,100). The new cartilage that formed was similar histologically to normal cartilage in that it had an abundance of type II collagen and a metachromatically stained matrix. This is important, because type II collagen is critical for the macromolecular framework of the extracellular matrix that gives articular cartilage its unique biomechanical properties (94,96,101,102).

In a prospective, randomized comparison trial, Bentley et al. (88) found autologous chondrocyte implantation to have significantly superior outcomes compared with autologous plugs for the treatment of osteochondral defects. Most of these osteochondral defects, however, were post-traumatic in origin. Disadvantages, however, include the cost of cell culture, the need for multiple surgical procedures, and tenuous fixation of the periosteum to the chondral surface.

Allograft

Fresh osteochondral allografting has been proposed as a viable option for treatment of osteochondral defects (12,22,93, 103–106). Instruments are used to adequately size and harvest the allograft, which is subsequently transplanted and secured by obtaining a tight press fit and using various fixation techniques, such as screws or bioabsorbable implants.

Grafts are transplanted fresh to maximize chondrocyte viability and usually are reserved for lesions of greater than 2 cm² (104). Initially, the grafts were implanted within a few days of donor death, but logistical issues and the time needed for tissue screening have led to an expanded period for implantation (now 2 to 3 weeks in some cases) without adversely affecting results (105–107). Sterilization methods have been explored to minimize the low risk of disease transmission. Unfortunately, the dose of radiation that is needed to be virucidal not only destroys the chondrocytes but also alters the properties of the graft material.

The immunological response to the allograft is another area of concern. Musculoskeletal allografts are capable of inducing both a cell-mediated response to the allograft surface antigens and humoral immune responses. Although these immune responses can occur, the clinical effects appear to be limited (78,105–107).

Patient selection is critical to the success of this procedure. Patients should be active and well motivated, and any limb malalignment must be corrected before transplantation. In addition, unipolar defects without any corresponding tibial lesions have better clinical outcomes (1,103,104).

The treatment of adult and adolescent patients who are nearing skeletal maturity and have OCD lesions remains controversial and an area for further research. Juvenile patients with OCD have a better outcome overall compared with their more skeletally mature counterparts. Treatment of the unstable lesion in all age groups, however, remains unclear. The infrequency of these lesions has given few surgeons extensive experience; consequently, prospective, randomized studies comparing different treatment modalities have not been performed. The pathophysiology, diagnosis, and treatment of OCD lesions will continue to be topics for further investigation.

■ REFERENCES

1. Cain EL, Clancy WG. Treatment algorithm for osteochondral injuries of the knee. *Clin Sports Med.* 2001;20:321–342.
2. Hefti F, Beguiristain J, Krauspe R, et al. Osteochondritis dissecans: a multicenter study of the European Pediatric Orthopedic Society. *J Pediatr Orthop B.* 1999;8:231–245.
3. Cahill BR. Osteochondritis dissecans of the knee: treatment of juvenile and adult forms. *J Am Acad Orthop Surg.* 1995;3: 237–247.
4. Flynn JM, Kocher MS, Ganley TJ. Osteochondritis dissecans of the knee. *J Pediatr Orthop.* 2004;24:434–443.
5. Robertson W, Kelly BT, Green DW. Osteochondritis dissecans of the knee in children. *Curr Opin Pediatr.* 2003;15:38–44.
6. Schenck RC, Goodnight JM. Current concept review— osteochondritis dissecans. *J Bone Joint Surg Am.* 1996;78:439–456.
7. Wall E, Von Stein D. Juvenile osteochondritis dissecans. *Orthop Clin North Am.* 2003;34:341–353.
8. Williams JS Jr, Bush-Joseph CA, Bach BR Jr. Osteochondritis dissecans of the knee. *Am J Knee Surg.* 1998;11:221–232.
9. Anderson AF, Richards DB, Pagnani MJ, et al. Antegrade drilling for osteochondritis dissecans of the knee. *Arthroscopy.* 1997;13:319–324.
10. Bohndorf K. Osteochondritis dissecans: a review and new MRI classification. *Eur Radiol.* 1998;8:103–112.
11. Federico DJ, Lynch JK, Jokl P. Osteochondritis dissecans of the knee: a historical review of etiology and treatment. *Arthroscopy.* 1990;6:190–197.
12. Garrett JC. Osteochondritis dissecans. *Clin Sports Med.* 1991;10: 569–593.
13. Glancy GL. Juvenile osteochondritis dissecans. *Am J Knee Surg.* 1999;12:120–124.
14. Koch S, Kampen WU, Laprell H. Cartilage and bone morphology in osteochondritis dissecans. *Knee Surg Sports Traumatol Arthrosc.* 1997;5:42–45.
15. Sanders RK, Crim JR. Osteochondral injuries. *Semin Ultrasound CT MR.* 2001;22:352–370.
16. Bramer JAM, Maas M, Dallinga RJ, et al. Increased external tibial torsion and osteochondritis dissecans of the knee. *Clin Orthop.* 2004;422:175–179.
17. Rowe SM, Chung JY, Moon ES, et al. Computed tomographic findings of osteochondritis dissecans following Legg-Calve-Perthes disease. *J Pediatr Orthop.* 2003;23:356–362.
18. Birk GT, DeLee JC. Osteochondral injuries. Clinical findings. *Clin Sports Med.* 2001;20:279–286.
19. Mizuta H, Nakamura E, Otsuka Y, et al. Osteochondritis dissecans of the lateral femoral condyle following total resection of the discoid lateral meniscus. *Arthroscopy.* 2001;17:608–612.
20. Hughes JA, Cook JV, Churchill MA, et al. Juvenile osteochondritis dissecans: a 5-year review of the natural history using clinical and MRI evaluation. *Pediatr Radiol.* 2003;33:410–417.
21. Bianchi G, Paderni S, Tigani D, et al. Osteochondritis dissecans of the lateral femoral condyle. *Chir Organi Mov.* 1999;84:183–187.
22. Garrett JC, Kress KJ, Mudano M. Osteochondritis dissecans of the lateral femoral condyle in the adult. *Arthroscopy.* 1992;8:474–481.
23. Matsumoto H, Suda Y, Otani T, et al. Meniscoplasty for osteochondritis dissecans of bilateral lateral femoral condyle combined with discoid meniscus: case report. *J Trauma.* 2000;49:964–966.
24. Mitsuoka T, Shino K, Hamada M, et al. Osteochondritis dissecans of the lateral femoral condyle of the knee joint. *Arthroscopy.* 1999;15:20–26.
25. Stanitski CL, Bee J. Juvenile osteochondritis dissecans of the lateral femoral condyle after lateral discoid meniscal surgery. *Am J Sports Med.* 2004;32:797–801.
26. Wright RW, McLean M, Matava MJ, et al. Osteochondritis dissecans of the knee: long term results of excision of the fragment. *Clin Orthop.* 2004;424:239–243.
27. Boutin RD, Januario JA, Newberg AH, et al. MR imaging features of osteochondritis dissecans of the femoral sulcus. *AJR Am J Roentgenol.* 2003;180:641–645.
28. Peters TA, McLean ID. Osteochondritis dissecans of the patellofemoral joint. *Am J Sports Med.* 2000;28:63–67.
29. Ewing JW, Voto SJ. Arthroscopic surgical management of osteochondritis dissecans of the knee. *Arthroscopy.* 1988;4:37–40.
30. Wilson JN. A diagnostic sign of osteochondritis dissecans of the knee. *J Bone Joint Surg Am.* 1967;49:477–480.
31. Conrad JM, Stanitski CL. Osteochondritis dissecans: Wilson's sign revisited. *Am J Sports Med.* 2003;31:777–778.
32. Arnold CA, Thomas DJ, Sanders JO. Bilateral knee and bilateral elbow osteochondritis dissecans. *Am J Orthop.* 2003;32:237–240.
33. Moti AW, Micheli LJ. Meniscal and articular cartilage injury in the skeletally immature knee. *Instr Course Lect.* 2003;52:683–690.
34. Browne RF, Murphy SM, Torreggiani WC, et al. Radiology for the surgeon: musculoskeletal case 30. Osteochondritis dissecans of the medial femoral condyle. *Can J Surg.* 2003;46:361–363.
35. Cahill BR, Berg BC. ^{99m}Technetium phosphate compound joint scintigraphy in the management of juvenile osteochondritis dissecans of the femoral condyles. *Am J Sports Med.* 1983;11:329–335.
36. Paletta GA, Bednarz PA, Stanitski CL, et al. The prognostic value of quantitative bone scans in knee osteochondritis dissecans. *Am J Sports Med.* 1998;26:7–14.
37. Mohr A, Heiss C, Bergmann I, et al. Value of micro-CT as an investigative tool for osteochondritis dissecans. *Acta Radiol.* 2003;44:532–537.
38. De Smet AA, Ilahi OA, Graf BK. Untreated osteochondritis dissecans of the femoral condyles: prediction of patient outcome using radiographic and MR findings. *Skeletal Radiol.* 1997;26:463–467.
39. Jurgensen I, Bachmann G, Schleicher I, et al. Arthroscopic versus conservative treatment of osteochondritis dissecans of the knee: value of magnetic resonance imaging in therapy planning and follow-up. *Arthroscopy.* 2002;18:378–386.
40. Kramer J, Stiglbauer R, Engel A, et al. MR contrast arthrography (MRA) in osteochondrosis dissecans. *J Comput Assist Tomogr.* 1992;16:254–260.
41. Loredo R, Sanders TG. Imaging of osteochondral injuries. *Clin Sports Med.* 2001;20:249–278.
42. Pill SG, Ganley TJ, Milam RA, et al. Role of magnetic resonance imaging and clinical criteria in predicting successful nonoperative treatment of osteochondritis dissecans in children. *J Pediatr Orthop.* 2003;23:102–108.
43. Yoshida S, Ikata T, Takai H, et al. Osteochondritis dissecans of the femoral condyle in the growth stage. *Clin Orthop Relat Res.* 1998;346:162–170.
44. O'Connor MA, Palaniappan M, Khan N, et al. Osteochondritis dissecans of the knee in children: a comparison of MRI and arthroscopic findings. *J Bone Joint Surg Br.* 2002;84:258–262.
45. Guhl JF. Arthroscopic treatment of osteochondritis dissecans. *Clin Orthop Relat Res.* 1982;167:65–74.
46. Kocher MS, Micheli LJ, Yaniv M, et al. Functional and radiographic outcomes of juvenile osteochondritis dissecans of the knee treated with transarticular arthroscopic drilling. *Am J Sports Med.* 2001;29:562–566.

47. Aglietti P, Buzzi R, Bassi PB, et al. Arthroscopic drilling in juvenile osteochondritis dissecans of the medial femoral condyle. *Arthroscopy.* 1994;10:286–291.
48. de Gauzy JS, Mansat C, Darodes PH, et al. Natural course of osteochondritis dissecans in children. *J Pediatr Orthop B.* 1999;8:26–28.
49. Cahill BR, Phillips MR, Navarro R. The results of conservative management of juvenile osteochondritis dissecans using joint scintigraphy. A prospective study. *Am J Sports Med.* 1989;17: 601–616.
50. Dervin GF, Keene GC, Chissell HR. Biodegradable rods in adult osteochondritis dissecans of the knee. *Clin Orthop.* 1998;356: 213–221.
51. Prakash D, Learmonth D. Natural progression of osteochondral defect in the femoral condyle. *Knee.* 2002;9:7–10.
52. Hughston JC, Hergenroeder PT, Courtenay BG. Osteochondritis dissecans of the femoral condyles. *J Bone Joint Surg Am.* 1984; 66:1340–1348.
53. Anderson AF, Pagnani MJ. Osteochondritis dissecans of the femoral condyles: long-term results of excision of the fragment. *Am J Sports Med.* 1997;25:830–834.
54. Twyman RS, Desai K, Aichroth PM. Osteochondritis dissecans of the knee: a long term study. *J Bone Joint Surg Br.* 1991;73: 461–464.
55. Aglietti P, Ciardullo A, Giron F, et al. Results of arthroscopic excision of the fragments in the treatment of osteochondritis dissecans of the knee. *Arthroscopy.* 2001;17:741–746.
56. Smillie I. Treatment of osteochondritis dissecans. *J Bone Joint Surg Br.* 1957;29:248–260.
57. Anderson AF, Lipscomb AB, Coulam C. Antegrade curettement, bone grafting and pinning of ostechondritis dissecans in the skeletally mature knee. *Am J Sports Med.* 1990;18:254–261.
58. Louisia S, Beaufils P, Katabi M, et al. Transchondral drilling for osteochondritis dissecans of the medial condyle of the knee. *Knee Surg Sports Traumatol Arthrosc.* 2003;11:33–39.
59. Kawasaki K, Uchio Y, Adachi N, et al. Drilling form the intercondylar area for treatment of osteochondritis dissecans of the knee joint. *Knee.* 2003;10:257–263.
60. Jaberi FM. Osteochondritis dissecans of the weight-bearing surface of the medial femoral condyle in adults. *Knee.* 2002;9:201–207.
61. Thomson NS. Osteochondritis dissecans and osteochondral fragments managed by Herbert compression screw fixation. *Clin Orthop Relat Res.* 1987;224:71–78.
62. Zuniga RJJ, Sagastibelza J, Lopez B, et al. Arthroscopic use of the Herbert screw in osteochondritis dissecans of the knee. *Arthroscopy.* 1993;9:668–670.
63. Cetik O, Bilen FE, Sozen YV, et al. A two-staged method for treatment of deep osteochondral lesions of the knee joint. *Arthroscopy.* 2001;17:E35.
64. Cugat R, Garcia M, Cusco X, et al. Osteochondritis dissecans: a historical review and its treatment with cannulated screws. *Arthroscopy.* 1993;9:675–684.
65. Johnson LL, Uitvlugt G, Austin MD, et al. Osteochondritis dissecans of the knee: arthroscopic compression screw fixation. *Arthroscopy.* 1990;6:179–189.
66. Kivisto R, Pasanen L, Leppilahtiv J, et al. Arthroscopic repair of osteochondritis dissecans of the femoral condyles with metal staple fixation: a report of 28 cases. *Knee Surg Sports Traumatol Arthrosc.* 2002;10:305–309.
67. Nakagawa T, Kurosawa H, Ikeda H, et al. Internal fixation for osteochondritis dissecans of the knee. *Knee Surg Sports Traumatol Arthrosc.* 2005;13:317–322.
68. Scioscia TN, Giffin JR, Allen CR, et al. Potential complication of bioabsorbable screw fixation for osteochondritis dissecans of the knee. *Arthroscopy.* 2001;17:E7.
69. Tuompo P, Arvela V, Partio EK, et al. Osteochondritis dissecans of the knee fixed with biodegradable self-reinforced polyglycolide and polylactide rods in 24 patients. *Int Orthop.* 1997;21:355–360.
70. Victoroff BN, Marcus RE, Deutsch A. Arthroscopic bone peg fixation in the treatment of osteochondritis dissecans in the knee. *Arthroscopy.* 1996;12:506–509.
71. Wouters DB, van Horn JR, Bos RR. The use of biodegradables in the treatment of osteochondritis dissecans of the knee: fiction or future. *Acta Orthop Belg.* 2003;69:175–181.
72. Friederichs MG, Greis PE, Burks RT. Pitfalls associated with fixation of osteochondritis dissecans fragments using bioabsorbable screws. *Arthroscopy.* 2001;17:542–545.
73. Navarro R, Cohen M, Filho MC, et al. The arthroscopic treatment of osteochondritis dissecans of the knee with autologous bone sticks. *Arthroscopy.* 2002;18:840–844.
74. Johnson LL. Arthroscopic abrasion arthroplasty historical and pathologic perspective: present status. *Arthroscopy.* 1986;2:54–69.
75. Steadman JR, Rodkey WG, Singleton SB, et al. Microfracture technique for full-thickness chondral defects: technique and clinical results. *Oper Tech Orthop.* 1997;7:300.
76. Breinan HA, Martin SD, Hsu HP, et al. Healing of canine articular cartilage defects treated with microfracture, a type II collagen matrix, or cultured autologous chondrocytes. *J Orthop Res.* 2000; 18:781–789.
77. Steadman JR, Briggs KK, Rodrigo JJ, et al. Outcomes of microfracture for traumatic chondral techniques of the knee: average 11 year follow-up. *Arthroscopy.* 2003;19:477–484.
78. Berlet GC, Mascia A, Miniaci A. Treatment of unstable osteochondritis dissecans lesions of the knee using autogenous osteochondral grafts (mosaicplasty). *Arthroscopy.* 1999; 15:312–316.
79. Chow JCY, Hantes ME, Houle JB, et al. Arthroscopic autogenous osteochondral transplantation for treating knee cartilage defects: a 2- to 5-year follow-up study. *Arthroscopy.* 2004;20:681–690.
80. Hangody L, Kish G, Karpati Z, et al. Mosaicplasty for the treatment of articular cartilage defects: application in clinical practice. *Orthopedics.* 1998;21:751–756.
81. Morelli M, Nagamori J, Miniaci A. Management of chondral injuries of the knee by osteochondral autogenous transfer (mosaicplasty). *J Knee Surg.* 2002;15:185–190.
82. Wang CJ. Treatment of focal articular cartilage lesions of the knee with autogenous osteochondral grafts. *Arch Orthop Trauma Surg.* 2002;122:169–172.
83. Jakob RP, Franz T, Gautier E, et al. Autologous osteochondral grafting in the knee: indications, results, and reflections. *Clin Orthop.* 2002;401:170–184.
84. Laprell H, Petersen W. Autologous osteochondral transplantation using the diamond bone-cutting system (DBCS): 6–12 years' follow-up of 35 patients with osteochondral defects. *Arch Orthop Trauma Surg.* 2001;121:248–253.
85. Marcacci M, Kon E, Zaffagnini S, et al. Use of autologous grafts for reconstruction of osteochondral defects of the knee. *Orthopedics.* 1999;22:595–600.
86. Nakagawa Y, Matsusue Y, Nakamura T. A novel surgical procedure for osteochondritis dissecans of the lateral femoral condyle: exchanging osteochondral plugs taken from donor and recipient sites. *Arthroscopy.* 2002;18:E5.
87. Yoshizumi Y, Sugita T, Kawamata T, et al. Cylindrical osteochondral graft for osteochondritis dissecans of the knee. *Am J Sports Med.* 2002;30:441–445.
88. Bentley G, Biant LC, Carrington RWJ, et al. A prospective, randomized comparison of autologous chondrocyte implantation versus mosaicplasty for osteochondral defects in the knee. *J Bone Joint Surg Br.* 2003;85:223–230.
89. Outerbridge HK, Outerbridge AR, Outerbridge RE. The use of a lateral patellar autologous graft for the repair of a large osteochondral defect in the knee. *J Bone Joint Surg Am.* 1995;77:65–72.
90. Outerbridge HK, Outerbridge RE, Smith DE. Osteochondral defects in the knee: a treatment using lateral patella autografts. *Clin Orthop.* 2000;377:145–151.

91. Ahmad CS, Guiney WB, Drinkwater CJ. Evaluation of donor site intrinsic healing response in autologous osteochondral grafting of the knee. *Arthroscopy*. 2002;18:95–98.

92. Kim SJ, Shin SJ. Loose bodies after arthroscopic osteochondral autograft in osteochondritis dissecans of the knee. *Arthroscopy*. 2000;16:E16.

93. Fox JA, Kalsi RS, Cole BJ. Update on articular cartilage restoration. *Tech Knee Surg*. 2003;2:2–17.

94. Brittberg M, Lindahl A, Nilsson A, et al. Treatment of deep cartilage defects in the knee with autologous chondrocyte transplantation. *N Engl J Med*. 1994;331:889–895.

95. Mandelbaum BR, Browne JE, Fu F, et al. Articular cartilage lesions of the knee. *Am J Sports Med*. 1998;8:208–212.

96. Peterson L, Brittberg M, Kiviranta I, et al. Autologous chondrocyte transplantation: biomechanics and long-term durability. *Am J Sports Med*. 2002;30:2–12.

97. Peterson L, Minas T, Brittberg M, et al. Treatment of osteochondritis dissecans of the knee with autologous chondrocyte transplantation: results at two to ten years. *J Bone Joint Surg Am*. 2003; 85:17–24.

98. Peterson L, Minas T, Brittberg M, et al. Two- to 9 year outcome after autologous chondrocyte transplantation of the knee. *Clin Orthop*. 2000;374:212–234.

99. Minas T, Peterson L. Advanced techniques in autologous chondrocyte transplantation. *Clin Sports Med*. 1999;18:13–14.

100. Minas T, Peterson L. Chondrocyte transplantation. *Oper Tech Orthop*. 1997;7:323.

101. Breinan HA, Minas T, Hsu HP, et al. Effect of cultured autologous chondrocytes on repair of chondral defects in a canine model. *J Bone Joint Surg Am*. 1997;79:1439–1451.

102. Hui JHP, Chen F, Thambyah A, et al. Treatment of chondral lesions in advanced osteochondritis dissecans: a comparative study of the efficacy of chondrocytes, mesenchymal stem cells, periosteal graft, and mosaicplasty (osteochondral autograft) in animal models. *J Pediatr Orthop*. 2004;24:427–433.

103. Bugbee WD, Convery FR. Osteochondral allograft transplantation. *Clin Sports Med*. 1999;18:67–75.

104. Garrett JC. Treatment of osteochondral defects of the distal femur with fresh osteochondral allografts: a preliminary report. *Arthroscopy*. 1986;2:222–226.

105. Shelton WR, Treacy SH, Dukes AD, et al. Use of allografts in knee reconstruction: I. Basic science aspects and current status. *J Am Acad Orthop Surg*. 1998;6:165–168.

106. Shelton WR, Treacy SH, Dukes AD, et al. Use of allografts in knee reconstruction: II. Surgical considerations. *J Am Acad Orthop Surg*. 1998;6:169–175.

107. Ball ST, Amiel D, Williams SK, et al. The effects of storage on fresh human osteochondral allografts. *Clin Orthop*. 2004;418: 246–252.

CARTILAGE TRANSPLANTATION

43.3

ALBERTO GOBBI, MD, RAMCES A. FRANCISCO, MD

■ KEY POINTS

- Properties that are unique to articular cartilage enable an almost frictionless joint movement and afford protection to the underlying bone from excessive load and trauma by dissipating the forces that are produced during movement.
- Within joints are two types of cartilage: fibrocartilage and hyaline cartilage. Fibrocartilage is an elastic cartilage, of which the menisci are composed. Hyaline cartilage is the tissue covering the extremities of the bones that make up the joint.
- Chondral defects of the knee commonly affect the medial femoral condyle. Once this protective layer of articular cartilage is compromised, subsequent trauma and excessive loading can accelerate the progression of wear and tear.
- Patients suffering from chondral injuries often find it difficult to recall a specific incident that triggered their symptoms. Swelling usually is present, and it can be accompanied by symptoms such as catching and clicking.
- A standard weight-bearing radiograph in full extension, a posteroanterior view at 45 degree flexion, and Merchant views remain the basic tools for establishing a diagnosis. Detection of malalignment requires a full-length standing film.
- The main indications for cartilage transplantation are symptomatic focal, full-thickness cartilage lesion (International Cartilage Repair Society [ICRS] grades III–IV) in the absence of significant arthritis in physiologically young patients (age 15 to 55 years).
- Surgical treatment should be considered when the patient's athletic involvement and daily activities are limited by the presence of chondral defects.

- Not all lesions can be addressed with a single technique. Retropatellar, tibial plateau, and posterior condylar lesions remain a challenge.

■ BASIC SCIENCE

Relevant Anatomy

Articular cartilage is a thin layer of specialized, connective tissue lining the articulations of diarthrodial joints. Properties that are unique to this tissue enable an almost frictionless joint movement and afford protection to the underlying bone from excessive load and trauma by dissipating the forces that are produced during movement.

The structural organization of articular cartilage can be divided into four major zones: (a) superficial, (b) middle, (c) deep, and (d) calcified (1,2). Each zone is distinctly structured, with cells and extracellular matrix (ECM) organized in specific patterns. The cells, known as chondrocytes, make up 1% to 2% of the total weight of the articular cartilage. On the other hand, the ECM, which makes up the rest of the cartilage, generally is composed of type II collagen, glycosaminoglycans, and proteoglycans.

Biomechanics

Within joints and, in particular, the knee, are two types of cartilage: fibrocartilage and hyaline cartilage. Fibrocartilage is an elastic or "fibrous" cartilage, of which the menisci are composed, whereas hyaline cartilage is the tissue covering the extremities of the bones that make up the joint. Hyaline cartilage has extremely important biomechanical functions, serving as a shock absorber as well as providing frictionless movement to the joint. Even though this layer of cartilage is only a few millimeters thick, it has a significant capacity for absorbing forces and for distributing loads to reduce stress on subchondral bone.

Chondral defects of the knee commonly affect the medial femoral condyle; once this protective layer of articular cartilage is compromised, subsequent trauma and excessive loading can accelerate the progression of the "wear and tear." Moreover, significant functional properties are lost, leading to further pathologic changes that can involve the surrounding cartilage and subchondral bone (2,3).

Biology

As early as 1743, Hunter (4) recognized that "articular cartilage lesions don't heal"; the limited intrinsic healing potential of articular cartilage is attributed to the presence of few and specialized cells with low mitotic activity. As the human body matures, the cell density, which influences the amount of ECM that is produced, declines further, limiting the capacity of articular cartilage to regenerate. Another property of articular cartilage that limits its reparative ability is that cartilage is avascular, and the absence of a vascular network prevents access by mesenchymal stem cells and macrophages, which normally would help in repairing tissues. Stem cells are responsible for the formation of new chondrocytes, whereas macrophages remove debris associated with damaged cartilage. Therefore, once injury occurs, surgical intervention may be necessary to repair of the resulting focal chondral defects and obtain good functional outcome.

■ CLINICAL EVALUATION

History

Patients suffering from chondral injuries often find it difficult to recall a specific incident that triggered their symptoms. Swelling usually is present in the affected knee but sometimes can be accompanied by mechanical symptoms, such as catching and clicking. A high index of suspicion for chondral injuries should be considered in patients who present with episodes of recurrent swelling in a knee that has effusion at the time of examination (5). In addition, Mandelbaum (6) emphasized that chondropenia (i.e., a process involving loss of cartilage volume and elevation of contact pressures over time, resulting in downward progression on the dose–response curve and eventual osteoarthritis formation) is a possible causative factor and should not be overlooked when encountering patients who present with these particular knee symptoms.

Physical Findings

Specific symptoms that are synonymous with chondral defects have been reported by several authors. Brittberg

et al. (7) and Ochi et al. (8) stressed that knee pain, locking, retropatellar crepitus, and swelling are among the prominent findings. Other authors, including Hangody et al. (9), mentioned that instability also could be present. Because signs and symptoms elicited during physical examination can mimic the presentation of other knee pathologies, the authors agree that correlation with other diagnostic modalities should be routine to increase the accuracy of diagnosis.

Imaging

Imaging modalities remain an essential part of the diagnosis, evaluation, and monitoring of articular chondral lesions. Advancements in this field have paralleled an increase in the accuracy of detecting lesions; however, a standard weight-bearing radiograph in full extension, a posteroanterior view at 45 degree flexion, and Merchant views remain the basics for diagnostics. Detection of malalignment requires a full-length standing film.

Among the diagnostic imaging modalities currently used, magnetic resonance (MR) imaging is the most accurate, with a reported sensitivity of 95% or greater (10–12). Aside from delineating the extent of the articular cartilage lesions, subchondral bone and associated ligament or meniscal injuries also can be assessed. The use of fast spin-echo (with or without fat suppression) and/or fat-suppressed (or water-selective excitation) spoiled-gradient echo images for better resolution has been recommended. Signal properties of articular cartilage are dependent on the following: (a) the MR pulse sequence used; (b) the cellular composition of collagen, proteoglycans, and water; (c) the orientation of collagen in different laminae of cartilage; and (d) an effective cartilage pulse sequencing (Potter).

Today, surgeons are using arthroscopy more extensively as a diagnostic tool. The benefit afforded by direct visualization of the extent of the defect (together with the information provided by MR imaging) significantly enhances the surgeon's capacity to plan the treatment necessary for addressing the pathology.

Decision-making Algorithms and Classification

The Outerbridge classification has been the traditional system, but recently, a more comprehensive system, the ICRS classification, has been adapted (13). In the ICRS system, normal cartilage is classified as ICRS 0 (normal). When visible fibrillation and/or slight softening on a rather intact surface is observed, the defect is classified as ICRS 1a, whereas with the presence of additional fissures/lacerations, the classification is ICRS 1b (nearly normal). Deeper defects that involve less than 50% of the cartilage thickness are classified as ICRS 2 (abnormal), and defects affecting more than 50% of the cartilage thickness are ICRS 3 (severely abnormal). Subgroupings in this class include the following: ICRS 3a, for defects that do not involve the calcified layer; ICRS 3b, for when the calcified layer is involved; ICRS 3c, for defects that extend down to, but not through,

TABLE 43.3.1	Treatment Guides for Simple Cartilage Lesions		
Location	**Size (cm^2)**	**Primary Treatment**	**Secondary Treatment**
Femoral condyle	<1	Debridement Marrow-stimulating techniques Osteochondral grafting	Marrow-stimulating techniques Osteochondral grafting
	≥1 to ≤2	Debridement Marrow-stimulating techniques Osteochondral grafting Autologous chondrocyte implantation	Osteochondral grafting Autologous chondrocyte implantation
	>2	Osteochondral grafting Autologous chondrocyte implantation Fresh allograft	Osteochondral grafting Autologous chondrocyte implantation Fresh allograft
Patellofemoral	<2	Physiotherapy Debridement Osteochondral grafting (trochlea) Autologous chondrocyte implantation	Osteochondral grafting (trochlea) Autologous chondrocyte implantation
	>2	Osteochondral grafting osteochondral Grafting (trochlea) Autologous chondrocute implantation	Osteochondral grafting (trochlea) Autologous chondrocyte implantation
Tibial plateau	<2	Debridement Marrow-stimulating techniques Autologous chondrocyte implantation	Marrow-stimulating techniques Autologous chondrocyte implantation
	>2	Bone grafting Autologous chondrocyte implantation	Bone grafting Autologous chondrocyte implantation

TABLE 43.3.2	Treatment Guides for Complex Cartilage Lesions		
Location	**Associated Pathology**	**Primary Treatment**	**Secondary Treatment**
Femoral condyle	ACL deficiency Meniscal tear/degeneration Malalignment	ACL reconstruction Meniscal repair/allograft transplantation Osteotomy (femoral/tibial) Osteochondral grafting Fresh allograft With option to carry out: Cartilage biopsy for ACI	Osteochondral grafting ACI Fresh allograft
Patellofemoral	Malalignment Instability	Physiotherapy Arthroscopic lateral release with or without medial plication Realignment procedures With option to carry out: Cartilage biopsy for ACI	Osteochondral grafting (trochlea) ACI Fresh allograft
Tibial plateau	Malalignment Instability	Osteotomy Marrow-stimulating techniques Bone grafting ACI	Bone grafting ACI

ACI, autologous chrondocyte implantation; ACL, anterior cruciate ligament.

the subchondral bone plate; and ICRS 3d, for blisters. Defects involving the subchondral bone are considered to be full-thickness lesions and are classified as ICRS 4.

Several options exist in the treatment of cartilage lesions; however, integrating these options into a comprehensive algorithm has not been easy. Any form of planned treatment should be based on patient characteristics and expectations, clinical symptoms, and type of lesions.

One algorithm proposed by Cole and Farr (14) and by Miller and Cole (15) presents an overview of a surgical decision scheme. In this algorithm, multiple options are presented for similar lesions without endorsing one specific treatment over the others.

In general, surgeons agree that parameters such as lesion size, depth, and associated issues (e.g., alignment as well as ligament and meniscal integrity) should be considered when planning the treatment of chondral defects. Furthermore, other factors related to the patient (e.g., age, genetic predisposition, level of activity, associated pathologies, and expectations) should not be overlooked.

To facilitate decision making when confronted with a particular case, a summary of cases and treatment options that can be encountered in practice is provided in **Tables 43.3.1** and **43.3.2**.

■ TREATMENT

Nonoperative

Symptomatic chondral lesions are not likely to revert to a previous subclinical state without an appropriate form of intervention or some degree of modification in activity level. It should be emphasized that these lesions commonly are associated with other knee pathologies; therefore, managing the problem nonoperatively, with activity modification, weight loss, physiotherapy, and pain medications, can provide symptomatic relief only for a limited period, and if pain relief is provided, how long the patient will remain symptom-free is not known. To compound the situation, most patients are relatively young and active; therefore, prescribing activity modification does not always sound appealing. Because outcome data regarding the natural course of these lesions are either incomplete or inconclusive, determining the appropriate treatment option is always a challenge.

Operative

Traditional techniques in the categories of palliative or reparative treatment options have demonstrated variable results. Lavage and chondroplasty can provide symptomatic pain relief with no actual formation of hyaline tissue; however, these techniques remove superficial cartilage layers, which include collagen fibers that are responsible for tensile strength, thus creating a cartilage tissue that is functionally inferior (16). Marrow-stimulation techniques, such as subchondral plate drilling or microfracture, have been reported to stimulate production of hyalinelike tissue with variable properties and durability compared to normal cartilage, but in many cases, these techniques tend to produce fibrocartilaginous tissue that will degenerate with time (17,18). Although osteochondral autologous transplantation and mosaicplasty can restore normal cartilage tissue, application is restricted to small defects, and some concerns exist regarding donor-site morbidity (18,19). On the other hand, autologous chondrocyte implantation, also known as the

Peterson technique, is capable of restoring normal cartilage tissue but requires two surgical procedures (12,20).

The apparent complexity of the Peterson periosteal technique and the possible complication of periosteal patch hypertrophy prompted surgeons to look for alternative techniques to enhance cell delivery and outcome. At present, the most promising seems to be tissue engineering, in which cells are combined with scaffolds to preform a given tissue. In general, the concept involves cultured autogenous or allogenous chondrocytes integrated in biodegradable and biocompatible scaffolds. Once cultivated on the scaffold, the chondrocytes must reacquire and maintain their chondrogenic phenotype to synthesize an ECM containing type II collagen, glycosaminoglycans, and proteoglycans, all of which are necessary to produce hyaline cartilage.

Scaffolds

Use of a three-dimensional scaffold for autologous chondrocyte culture was developed with the aim of improving both the biological performance of chondrogenic autologous cells as well as rendering the surgical technique easier, by avoiding use of the periosteal flap. A scaffold that is properly sized can be positioned directly into the articular defect under arthroscopic guidance. This technique offers the advantage of avoiding an open surgery, because the periosteal flap does not need to be harvested. Some technical limitations exist, however, including treatment of patellar lesions and posterior portions of femoral condyles or tibial plateau. It must be emphasized that these limits are common to all arthroscopic techniques and could be resolved, in part, with the development of new arthroscopic tools.

For some years now, different types of scaffolds with different matrices have been tested in animal models, and in some cases, human trials have been carried out to determine their efficacy in facilitating and promoting cartilage repair. These scaffolds can be divided according to their chemical nature into protein-based polymers (collagen, fibrin, and gelatin), carbohydrate polymers (hyaluronan, agarose, polylactic acid, polyglycolic acid, chitosan, and alginate), and artificial polymers (Teflon, Dacron, carbon fibers, polybutyric acid, and hydroxyapatite). Combination of these different polymers also are available.

Currently, the most common scaffolds are protein-based polymers composed of collagen fibers, but synthetic scaffolds are available that are not derived from animal tissues. The main problem with these synthetic scaffolds is that they are not "cell friendly," which means that these cells must be immersed in fibrin glue to keep them well attached to the scaffold surface. Fibrin glue, which facilitates cell adhesion to the scaffold, contains both recombinant human components and bovine proteins. Other carbohydrate polymer scaffolds use fetal calf serum for cell cultivation. The source should be selected carefully (samples coming from BSE-free countries are preferred) to avoid possible transmission of disease. Also, another challenge to overcome is demonstrating the consistent permanence of chondrocytes in situ after implantation.

The ideal scaffold should be biocompatible (i.e., not triggering any inflammatory response and not cytotoxic) and biodegradable (i.e., offering a temporary support to cells to promote replacement of a newly synthesized matrix and, possibly, to induce proliferation of the transplanted cells). The matrix also should be permeable to nutrients and provide firm adhesion to the surrounding edges of the cartilage wound so to promote integration. Furthermore, the scaffold must be reproducible, readily available, and versatile for repair and resurfacing (21). Hyaluronan (hyaluronic acid) is a naturally occurring, highly conserved glycosaminoglycan that is distributed widely in the body. Given its impressive multifunctional activity through its structural and biological role (22), it is an ideal molecule for tissue-engineering strategies in cartilage repair.

Through the chemical modification of hyaluronic acid, a scaffold can be obtained and processed into stable configurations to produce a variety of biodegradable structures having different physical forms and in vivo residence times. Extensive biocompatibility studies have demonstrated the safety of these biomaterials and their ability to be resorbed in the absence of an inflammatory response (23).

Three-dimensional, nonwoven scaffolds support in vitro growth of highly viable chondrocytes and promote expression of the original chondrogenic phenotype (24). Chondrocytes, previously expanded on plastic and seeded into the scaffold, produce a characteristic ECM that is rich in proteoglycans and express typical markers of hyaline cartilage, such as type II collagen and aggrecan (25,26). When implanted in full-thickness defects of the femoral condyle in rabbits, chondrocytes regenerated a cartilagelike tissue (27,28).

Indications

The main indications for cartilage transplantation are symptomatic focal, full-thickness cartilage lesion (ICRS grades III–IV) in physiologically young patients (age 15 to 55 years) without significant arthritis. Additional factors to consider include the patient's motivation and willingness to comply with the postimplantation rehabilitation regimen. Defect sizes ranging from 2 to 12 cm^2 have been shown to be favorable to regeneration. Osteochondritis dissecans is not a contraindication for cartilage transplantation as long as the bone loss does not exceed 8 mm (29). When bone loss is greater than 8 mm, initial bone grafting should be performed before implantation; otherwise, other techniques of repair can be used. When chondral lesions are located on the patella, associated pathologies, such as patellar malalignment, should be corrected before carrying out the transplantation to facilitate a successful outcome.

Timing

Surgical treatment should be considered when the patient's athletic involvement and daily activities are limited by the presence of these chondral defects. In certain cases, the treating surgeon will note that previous treatment with debridement, shaving, microfracture, or osteochondral autograft procedures has failed to provide relief. It also is important to note that many times, chondral lesions are found incidentally, when routine diagnostic arthroscopy is performed for other suspected knee pathologies.

Technique

Autologous chondrocyte implantation is carried out through the conventional arthrotomy approach. Recent advances in scaffold technology, however, have enabled surgeons to perform this technique arthroscopically.

This technique is a two-staged procedure. During an initial arthroscopy, the suitability of the lesion for repair is evaluated **(Fig 43.3-1)**. At the same time, cartilage from the edge of the lesion, the trochlea, or the intercondylar notch is obtained for in vitro replication **(Fig 43.3-2)**. Three to four weeks later, the cells are implanted into the defect with a medial or lateral parapatellar arthrotomy approach. To contain the cells within the defect, a periosteal patch is used. The patch is secured with a no. 6-0 PDS (polydioxanone) suture and is sealed watertight with fibrin sealant.

With the introduction of new scaffolds, this technique can now be carried out arthroscopically (30–32). To achieve this, the chondrocytes obtained from the biopsy performed during initial arthroscopy are seeded onto a three-dimensional biomaterial, where they will continue to proliferate and redifferentiate. During proliferation, chondrocytes organize in three dimensions to stimulate the synthesis of ECM molecules and to prevent the loss of cell phenotype. The time frame observed for this cultivation with respect to autologous chrondocyte implantation also is 3 to 4 weeks. At the time of graft implantation, the lesion is measured and mapped **(Fig 43.3-3)**, then prepared using a low-profile, cannulated drill that is maintained in place by a Kirschner guide wire (diameter, 0.9 mm) anchored in the bone **(Fig 43.3-4)**. A depth of 2 mm is observed while preparing the defect to

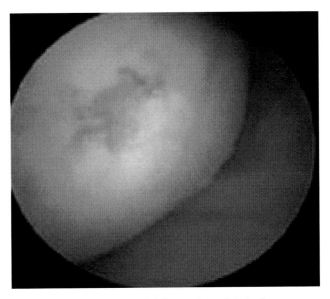

Fig 43.3-1. Grade III medial femoral condyle lesion as seen arthroscopically.

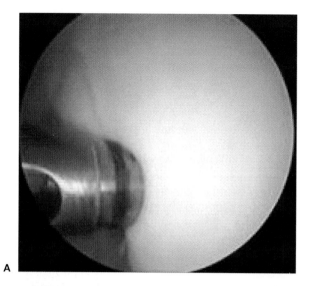

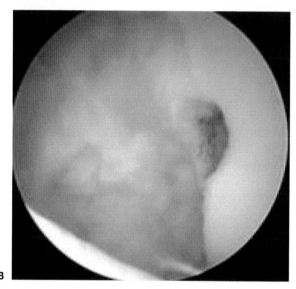

Fig 43.3-2. First phase of autologous chrondocyte implantation.
A: After evaluating the suitability of the lesion for chondrocyte
transplantation, grafts are harvested over the non–weight-bearing
areas of the knee (trochlear notch) or at the margins of the lesion.
B: Trochlear notch as it appears after obtaining the needed graft
for culture.

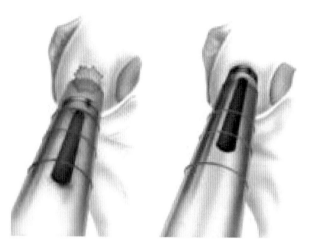

Fig 43.3-3. Second phase of autologous chrondocyte implantation.
Schematic demonstrating the measurement and mapping of the
lesion with the sharp ends of a customized graft-delivery system.
(Courtesy of Marcacci et al.)

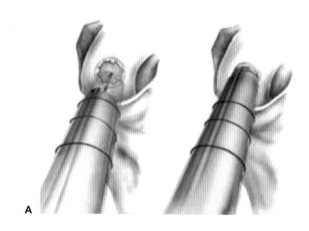

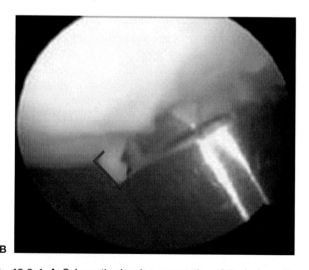

Fig 43.3-4. A: Schematic showing preparation of the lesion with a
low-profile, cannulated drill designed to avoid the subchondral
bone. (Courtesy of Marcacci et al.) **B:** Drilling of the defect to
remove fibrous and nonviable tissues. Marker indicates the low profile of the drill that prevents penetration of the subchondral surface.

avoid violating the subchondral bone plate. Once the defect
is completely devoid of fibrotic tissues, the hyaluronic acid
patch containing the cultured chondrocytes is obtained **(Fig
43.3-5)**. At this point, the knee joint is then drained of fluid,
and the scaffold is loaded in the delivery-system instrument
using the cannula to position the patch into the defect **(Fig
43.3-6)**. The intrinsic adhesive characteristics of the scaffold
assure its stability once positioned in the defect, and in the
majority of cases, no further fixation is needed. Graft position and stability are then verified with a probe and through
a range of knee movements before closure of the portals **(Fig
43.3-7)**. Otherwise, in large, uncontained defects and in the
patellofemoral compartment treated with open surgery,

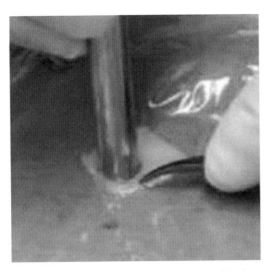

Fig 43.3-5. Preparing the specific size of graft (Hyalograft C) needed to cover the chondral defect with the sharp edge of the delivery system.

fibrin glue and/or other fixation systems maybe indicated to keep the graft in place (33).

Several reports from controlled trials in patients who were treated with use of these hyaluronic acid scaffolds have appeared (30,31). The largest collection of data (3,200 cases) using the scaffold in clinical practice, however, is represented by a multicenter observational study conducted at the Italian Orthopaedic Centers since 2001 (30,34,35).

■ EVALUATION OF OUTCOME

The outcome of cartilage transplantation can be assessed in several ways. The available means by which the integrity of the grafted area can be evaluated include clinical, histological, and mechanical/functional as well as imaging modalities (13,36,37).

Standard clinical evaluation is achieved with the International Knee Documentation Committee (IKDC) evaluation form endorsed by the ICRS (13). Objective data from the knee examination conducted by the surgeon is translated to knee scores, and subjective and functional scores are determined from questionnaires completed by the patients at designated intervals.

When indications are present, second-look arthroscopy can be performed. This provides an opportunity to visually inspect the grafted area; at this time, the graft can be assessed for depth of repair, integration to border zone, and macroscopic appearance. A corresponding numerical score (from 1 to 4) is ascribed to each evaluated parameter, and from these scores, a total score is obtained. The grafted area can be classified as grade I (12 points) when findings are normal, as grade II (8 to 11 points) when findings are nearly normal, as grade III (4 to 7 points) when findings are abnormal, and as grade IV (0 to 3 points) if severely abnormal morphological appearance is noted (12). Once evaluated, the surgeon has the option of obtaining core biopsy specimens from various areas of the graft for histological evaluation. Although regarded as the most precise manner of graft assessment, because it allows identification of the type of tissue formed (hyaline, hyalinelike, or fibrous tissue), biopsy is not applicable all the time (37).

Mechanical evaluation through indentometry also can be conducted at the time of second-look arthroscopy (36).

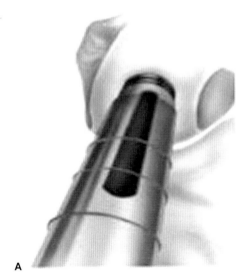

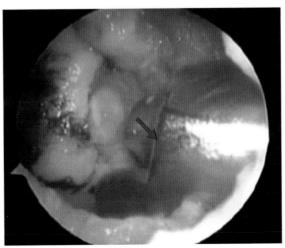

Fig 43.3-6. A: Schematic showing the graft being placed over the defect using the delivery system. (Courtesy of Marcacci et al.) **B:** Arrow pointing to the tamp inside the delivery system used to press fit the graft against the surface of chondral defect.

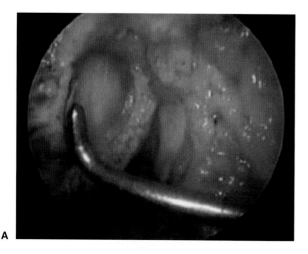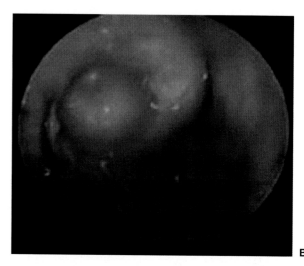

Fig 43.3-7. A: After the graft is placed, a probe can be used to check the position and adherence of the graft over the defect. **B:** Graft stability is tested before closure of portals by having the knee go through the full range of motion.

A measure of cartilage stiffness is obtained using a commercially available arthroscopic indentation instrument, which is pressed against the specific articular surface with a predefined force. The indenter force by which the articular surface resists the indentation indicates the degree of cartilage stiffness.

At present, to overcome the limitations on invasive means of evaluating the grafts after placement, noninvasive techniques, such as MR imaging and ultrasound, are being refined to accurately assess the status of cartilage repair. Recent studies by Burstein and Gray (10) and by Marinoni et al. (37) have demonstrated the use of delayed gadolinium-enhanced MR imaging of cartilage. This technique offers an improved morphological analysis as well as information regarding the biochemical composition and functional characteristics of the joint surface. Gadolinium contrast agent, when used, can penetrate the cartilaginous surface. Being similarly negatively charged as the glycosaminoglycans in cartilage, the contrast agent distributes itself at higher concentrations in areas where the glycosaminoglycan concentration is relatively low. This enables quantification of the glycosaminoglycan concentration by determining the distribution of gadolinium.

The other imaging modality that could be used to assess the status of the graft after placement is B-mode ultrasound, which can provide high-resolution images of the articular cartilaginous surface and subchondral bone, thereby allowing better assessment of structural changes in articular tissues secondary to degeneration or treatment with transplantation of autologous chondrocytes (36).

■ COMPLICATIONS AND SPECIAL CONSIDERATIONS

The most commonly cited complications of autologous chondrocyte implantation are graft hypertrophy and arthrofibrosis

(38). Graft hypertrophy has been noted to occur between 3 and 9 months postoperatively. Hypertrophy is thought to result from abrasion of the periosteal patch that overhangs from the margin of the defect. This problem is easily addressed with arthroscopic shaving and debridement of hypertrophic fibrous tissues. On the other hand, arthrofibrosis is more likely to be encountered as a complication when treating patellofemoral lesions. Therefore, early range-of-motion exercises are emphasized during physiotherapy to avoid this problem. Once arthrofibrosis sets in, however, manipulation under anesthesia can be done to address the problem, followed by arthroscopic debridement of fibrous tissue.

Tissue-engineered scaffolds have emerged as a consequence of the limitations encountered with the conventional technique of chondrocyte implantation. These scaffolds offer the possibility to circumvent some of the problems associated with periosteal harvest and other surgical complexities, but they, too, have complications that must be addressed.

Common to both techniques are documented cases of graft failure. A graft can delaminate or degenerate in certain situations; most reported cases have been complex and salvage lesions that somehow have extended the indications for this technique. Therefore, strict criteria for patient selection should be observed to decrease the possibility of such complications (39). Once encountered, however, treatment options include a repeat autologous chondrocyte implantation or, possibly, an osteochondral allograft procedure.

■ CONCLUSIONS AND FUTURE DIRECTIONS

A number of viable options have become available over the years to address problems of cartilage damage, and each technique has its advantages and disadvantages. Numerous studies are under way to clarify some of the questions that still remain unanswered regarding the long-term durability of these procedures and possible modifications that might achieve better results.

From an initial arthrotomy approach, some of the techniques can now be entirely performed arthroscopically. This modification has enabled surgeons to avoid possible intraoperative problems and to decrease operative time. By eliminating the need for an open procedure and harvesting of the periosteal flap, joint trauma is significantly reduced. Complications, such as graft hypertrophy and ossification, also are avoided with use of this three-dimensional hyaluronic acid scaffold.

At present, not all lesions can be addressed with a single technique. Retropatellar, tibial plateau, and posterior condylar lesions remain a challenge. Development of better instruments and introduction of new techniques in the near future will hopefully solve this dilemma.

In the future, use of a large number of heterologous chondrocytes or autologous mesenchymal progenitor cells in a temporary scaffold could be an improvement on currently available techniques. Researchers are exploring the possibility of manipulating stem cells in the laboratory to dedifferentiate into chondrocytes, which then can be integrated into a synthetic scaffold for later implantation. Once realized, benefits will include reduction of the technique to a "single" surgical procedure, because cells can be obtained on an outpatient basis with use of a bone marrow aspirator.

Biotechnology is progressing at a rapid pace, allowing the introduction of numerous products for clinical application. Carefully conducted, randomized, prospective studies for each of these innovations should be carried out, however, to validate its efficacy for cartilage regeneration.

■ REFERENCES

1. Mainil-Varlet P, Aigner T, Brittberg M, et al. Histological assessment of cartilage repair. A report by the Histology Endpoint Committee of the ICRS. *J Bone Joint Surg Am.* 2003;85(suppl 2): 45–57.
2. Poole R. What type of cartilage repair are we attempting to attain? *J Bone Joint Surg Am.* 2003;85(suppl 2):40–44.
3. Peterson L, Brittberg M, Kiviranta I, et al. Autologous chondrocyte transplantation. Biomechanics and long-term durability. *Am J Sports Med.* 2002;30:2–12.
4. Hunter W. On the structure and diseases of articulating cartilage. *Philos Trans R Soc Lond B Biol Sci.* 1743;9:277.
5. Miller M, Howard R, Plancher K. Treatment of chondral injuries and defects. In: *Surgical atlas of sports medicine.* Pennsylvania: WB Saunders; 2003:110–115.
6. Mandelbaum B. Articular cartilage repair: concepts and techniques 2004. In: *Instructional course materials.* AOSSM 2004 Annual Meeting, Quebec City, Canada; 2004:261–268.
7. Brittberg M, Peterson L, Sjogren-Jansson E, et al. Articular cartilage engineering with autologous chondrocyte transplantation. A review of recent developments. *J Bone Joint Surg Am.* 2003;85(suppl 3):109–115.
8. Ochi M, Adachi N, Nobuto H, et al. Articular cartilage repair using tissue engineering technique: novel approach with minimally invasive procedure. *Artif Organs.* 2004;28:28–32.
9. Hangody L, Kish G, Karpati Z, et al. Mosaicplasty for the treatment of articular cartilage defects: application in clinical practice. *Orthopedics.* 1998;21:751–756.
10. Burstein D, Gray M. New MRI techniques for imaging cartilage. *J Bone Joint Surg Am.* 2003;85(suppl):70–77.
11. Henderson IJ, Tuy B, Oakes B, et al. Prospective clinical study of autologous chondrocyte implantation and correlation with MRI at 3 and 12 months. *J Bone Joint Surg Br.* 2003;85:1060–1066.
12. Henderson I, Francisco R, Oakes B, et al. Autologous chondrocyte implantation for treatment of focal chondral defects of the knee: a clinical, arthroscopic, MRI and histologic evaluation at 2 years. *The Knee Journal.* 2005;12(3):209–216. Epub 2004;14.
13. Brittberg M, Winalski C. Evaluation of cartilage injuries and repair. *J Bone Joint Surg Am.* 2003;85(suppl 3):58–69.
14. Cole B, Farr J. Putting it all together. *Oper Tech Orthop.* 2001; 11:151–154.
15. Miller M, Cole B. Atlas of chondral injury treatment. *Oper Tech Orthop.* 2001;11:145–150.
16. McGinley BJ, Cushner FD, Scott WN. Debridement arthroscopy. 10-Year follow-up. *Clin Orthop.* 1999;367:190–194.
17. Gobbi A, Nunag P, Malinowski K. Treatment of full-thickness chondral lesions of the knee with microfracture in a group of athletes. *Knee Surg Sports Traumatol Arthrosc.* 2005;13(3):213–221.
18. Gobbi A, Francisco R, Allegra F, et al. Osteochondral lesions of the talus: randomized controlled trial comparing chondroplasty, microfrature, and osteochondral autograft transplantation. *Arthroscopy.* 2006;22(10):1085–1092.
19. Hangody L, Fules P. Autologous osteochondral mosaicplasty for the treatment of full-thickness defects of weight-bearing joints. *J Bone Joint Surg Am.* 2003;85(suppl 3):25–32.
20. Minas T, Peterson L. Advanced techniques in autologous chondrocyte transplantation. *Clin Sports Med.* 1999;18:13–44.
21. Hunziker E. Articular cartilage repair: basic science and clinical progress. A review of the current status and prospects. *Osteoarthritis Cart.* 2002:433–463.
22. Chen W, Abatangelo G. Functions of hyaluronan in wound repair. *Wound Repair Regen.* 1999;7:79–89.
23. Campoccia D, Doherty P, Radice M, et al. Semisynthetic resorbable materials from hyaluronan esterification. *Biomaterials.* 1998;19:2101–2127.
24. Brun P, Abatangelo G, Radice M, et al. Chondrocyte aggregation and reorganization into three-dimensional scaffolds. *J Biomed Mater Res.* 1999;46:337–346.
25. Aigner J, Tegeler J, Hutzier P, et al. Cartilage tissue engineering with novel nonwoven structured biomaterial based on hyaluronic acid benzyl ester. *J Biomed Mater Res.* 1998;42:172–181.
26. Grigolo B, Lisignoli G, Piacentini A, et al. Evidence for redifferentiation of human chondrocytes grown on a hyaluronan-based biomaterial (HYAFF 11): molecular, immunohistochemical, and ultrastructural analysis. *Biomaterials.* 2002;23:1187–1195.
27. Grigolo B, Roseti L, Fiorini M, et al. Transplantation of chondrocytes seeded on a hyaluronan derivative (HYAFF 11) into cartilage defects in rabbits. *Biomaterials.* 2001;22:2417–2424.
28. Solchaga LA, Yoo JU, Lundberg M, et al. Hyaluronan-based polymers in the treatment of osteochondral defects. *J Orthop Res.* 2000;18:773–780.
29. Peterson L, Minas T, Brittberg M, et al. Treatment of osteochondritis dissecans of the knee with autologous chondrocyte transplantation: results at two to ten years. *J Bone Joint Surg Am.* 2003;85(suppl 3):17–24.
30. Marcacci M, Zaffagnini S, Kon E, et al. Arthroscopic autologous chondrocyte transplantation: technical note. *Knee Surg Sports Traumatol Arthrosc.* 2002;10:154–159.
31. Nehrer S, Schatz K, Marlovits S, et al. Preliminary results of matrix-assisted chondrocyte transplantation using a hyaluronan matrix. ICRS Symposium, Toronto, Canada; 2002.

32. Sgaglione NA, Miniaci A, Gillogly SD, et al. Update on advanced surgical techniques in the treatment of traumatic focal articular cartilage lesions in the knee. *Arthroscopy.* 2002;18(suppl 1): 9–32.

33. Gobbi A, Berruto M, Francisco R, et al. Patellofemoral full-thickness chondral defects treated with Hyalograft-C: a clinical, arthroscopic, and histologic review. *Am J Sports Med.* 2006;34:(11) 1763–1773.

34. Marcacci M, Berruto M, Gobbi A, et al. Articular cartilage engineering with Hyalograft C. 3-year clinical results. *Clin Orthop Relat Res.* 2005;435:96–105.

35. Pavesio A, Abatangelo G, Borrione A, et al. Hyaluronan-based scaffolds (Hyalograft C) in the treatment of knee cartilage defects: clinical results. Tissue Engineering in Musculoskeletal Clinical Practice (AAOS). 2004;8:73–83.

36. Laasanen M, Toyras J, Vasara A, et al. Mechano-acoustic diagnosis of cartilage degeneration and repair. *J Bone Joint Surg Am.* 2003;85(suppl 3):78–84.

37. Marinoni E, Berruto M, Colombo E, et al. Delayed gadolinium-enhanced MRI of cartilage (dGEMRIC) evaluation compared with clinical and functional outcomes in three different ACI procedures: a three-year follow-up study. ICRS Symposium, Gent, Belgium, 2004.

38. Bentley G, Biant LC, Carrington RW, et al. A prospective, randomized comparison of autologous chondrocyte implantation versus mosaicplasty for osteochondral defects in the knee. *J Bone Joint Surg Br.* 2003;85:223–230.

39. Muellner T, Knopp A, Ludvigsen TC, et al. Failed autologous chondrocyte implantation. Complete atraumatic graft delamination after two years. *Am J Sports Med.* 2001;29:516–519.

HIGH TIBIAL OSTEOTOMY

43.4

■ TIM SPALDING, MB, BS, FRCS Orth, PRICE A.M. GALLIE, MB, BS, FRACS

■ KEY POINTS

- High tibial osteotomy remains one of the important options for surgical treatment of knee malalignment and angular deformity about the knee.
- Indications for surgery fall into two main groups: (a) for unloading a compartment suffering from early degenerative change, and (b) for controlling instability of the knee resulting from specific ligamentous laxities.
- The goal of osteotomy is to relieve pain, to improve function, and to slow down the degenerative process.
- Patients older than 60 years would be considered candidates for knee replacement, whereas patients younger than 50 years would be better suited for osteotomy with the intention of "buying time" before knee replacement is required. For patients between 50 and 60 years, a decision has to be made based on activity level, expectations, and degree of degeneration.
- A variety of fixation systems are commercially available for opening-wedge valgus high tibial osteotomy. All procedures, however, involve the same principles of exposure of the upper medial tibia; creation and opening of a controlled, incomplete osteotomy above the level of the tibial tuberosity while protecting posterior structures; and previous insertion of a plate-fixation device.
- The principle of closing-wedge osteotomy is to remove an appropriately sized wedge from the lateral aspect of the tibia above the tibial tubercle and to obtain accurate apposition of the bony surfaces, achieving union with stable fixation.
- The main advantages of opening-wedge osteotomy compared with closing-wedge osteotomy are as follows: (a) no

damage to the proximal tibia fibular joint and peroneal nerve, (b) easier to perform two-plane osteotomy, (c) no opening of the anterior compartment of the leg, (d) no alteration in the shape of the upper tibia, and (e) ease of correction intraoperatively.

- The disadvantages with respect to closing-wedge osteotomy are as follows: (a) use of a graft, (b) possible delayed union or nonunion of the osteotomy site, and (c) difficulty in managing large corrections.
- A concern regarding total knee replacement (TKR) after osteotomy is the additional difficulty of the procedure associated with the previous surgery in obtaining both adequate exposure and optimal soft tissue balancing during total knee arthroplasty.
- The main factors that affect outcome adversely are the following: (a) age older than 55 years, (b) extreme obesity, (c) lateral compartment osteoarthritis, (d) correction to less than 7 degrees valgus, not by (e) high adduction moment in walking, and (f) multiple previous operative procedures on the knee.

High tibial osteotomy remains one of the important options for surgical treatment of knee malalignment and angular deformity about the knee. The overall principle is to adjust the mechanical access of the lower limb such that the load is redistributed from one compartment to the other. High tibial osteotomy principally is indicated to correct varus alignment into valgus alignment, but it also can be used for the opposite correction. Indications for surgery fall into two main groups: (a) for unloading a compartment suffering from early degenerative change, and (b) for controlling instability of the knee resulting from specific ligamentous laxities.

Limb malalignment is recognized to accentuate the stress on the articular surface within the involved compartment, resulting in further loss of the articular surface cartilage and increased stress on the subchondral bone, leading in turn to further progressive increase in the degree of malalignment. The goal and aim of osteotomy is to relieve pain, to improve function, and to slow down the wear-and-tear degenerative process. This concept of buying time before possibly needing arthroplasty is an important issue that needs to be grasped by patients to justify the recovery period associated with osteotomy.

In addition to the basic principle of load distribution, recent reports have indicated that the quality of repair tissue after osteotomy can be influenced by combining osteotomy with cartilage repair surgery, including autologous chondrocyte transplantation, microfracture, or even meniscal transplant. The important aspects of the procedure of high tibial osteotomy include careful patient selection and assessment, accurate surgical technique to correct alignment, and prevention of complications.

This chapter outlines the biomechanical principles of osteotomy and correction of alignment in addition to the indications, surgical techniques, and current results of the two main procedures: (a) opening-wedge high tibial osteotomy and (b) closing-wedge high tibial osteotomy.

■ INDICATIONS

Valgus High Tibial Osteotomy for Medial Arthritis

Medial arthritis is the most common indication, with patients experiencing symptoms of medial compartment pain usually following earlier partial or total medial meniscectomy or chondral damage associated with chronic deficiency of the anterior cruciate ligament (ACL). Overload of the medial compartment also may result from malalignment caused by an extra-articular fracture malunion. Patients usually complain of localized, activity-related pain in the knee, usually described as pain felt on the medial aspect and radiating down the medial border of the tibia. Patients usually do not have patellofemoral symptoms, and range of movement generally is well maintained. The ideal indications for osteotomy in this group of patients are as follows: (a) age of 60 years or younger, (b) flexion to greater than 100 degrees with no significant loss of extension, and (c) low body mass index (i.e., <25).

The activity level of the patient is an important factor in deciding whether to perform osteotomy. Knee replacement has become an increasingly popular and successful procedure for management of arthritis in less active patients older than 60 years, in whom the knee arthroplastic implant would be expected to last from 20 to 25 years and, generally, outlive the patient. Patients older than 60 years who are particularly active or most patients younger than 60 years would be expected to require revision of a knee replacement, if

performed, because of a higher frequency of problems involving loosening or failure of the polyethylene tibial surface. In general, patients older than 60 years would be considered candidates for knee replacement, either total or unicompartmental, whereas patients younger than 50 years would be better suited for osteotomy with the intention of buying time before requiring knee replacement. For patients between 50 and 60 years of age, a decision must be made depending on activity level, expectations, and degree of degeneration.

It also should be recognized that rehabilitation following knee arthroplasty is quicker than that following osteotomy; hence, patients older than 60 years may be better suited for a procedure with a shorter period of rehabilitation and, perhaps, more complete relief of pain than can occur with osteotomy (1). Patients who are obese are do less well following osteotomy, achieving lower activity levels and poorer outcomes. A further relative contraindication to tibial osteotomy is significant laxity of the lateral collateral ligament.

Posterolateral Corner Instability

Patients with injury to the posterior cruciate ligament (PCL) and posterolateral corner of the knee are at risk of developing symptoms of instability, especially with preexisting physiological varus. The result is a lateral thrust to the knee on walking.

The terms *double varus* and *triple varus* (2–5) have been applied to the situation in which varus malalignment progresses over time following ACL deficiency in the physiologically varus knee or in which varus deformity follows medial arthrosis or medial meniscal injury. Progressive varus leads to stretching of the posterolateral structures, causing double varus, and with further time and repeated anterior translation of the tibia, stretching of the posterolateral structures occurs, leading to hyperextension and recurvatum (i.e., the so-called triple varus). In addition, the neuromuscular or proprioceptive control of the joint provided by the soft tissue structures may be lost when ligamentous disruption occurs. Loss of this control may then exacerbate the malalignment, leading to clinical symptoms of instability (2).

On its own, ligament repair and reconstruction has a low chance of success in controlling instability because of the persistence of deforming forces that stretch the lateral structures and repaired tissues. In this situation, osteotomy is indicated to reduce the lateral thrust, with the intention to shift the weight-bearing line from hip to ankle so that it passes through the lateral compartment. In this way, the knee, on heel strike, is pushed medially rather than laterally, reducing the symptom of instability. Any hyperextension can be corrected through the osteotomy by increasing the posterior slope of the tibia (discussed later in this chapter), which has the added benefit of helping to resist posterior translation forces on the tibia associated with PCL injury. It also is likely that with distraction by opening-wedge osteotomy some tightening of the lateral structures occurs, again helping to improve the laxity (2).

Patients who undergo this procedure generally are in the younger age group and more sporting, because injury usually follows sport or traffic accidents. Often, little evidence of degenerative change exists, and patients may well have experienced some benefit from using a brace, resisting the posterior and lateral thrust on walking.

■ RADIOGRAPHIC EVALUATION AND PREOPERATIVE PLANNING

The basis of osteotomy in the management of osteoarthritis around the knee is to correct the abnormal weight-bearing line or load-bearing line that passes from the center of the head of the femur to the center of the talus at the ankle joint **(Fig 43.4-1)**. Limb malalignment is accepted as a cause of increased stress on damaged articular cartilage, leading to pain, progressive loss of articular cartilage, and increasing angular deformity around the knee.

Brown and Amendola (6) reviewed the concept of radiographic evaluation and preoperative planning for high tibial

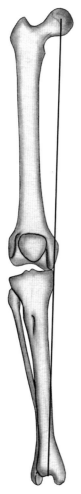

Fig 43.4-1. The weight-bearing line passes from the center of the femur to the center of the head of the talus at the ankle joint.

osteotomy in an excellent article. In this article, the authors established how most recommendations point toward the same degree of correction. Confusion lies in the definition of the axes around the knee, and current figures of correction are based on the analysis of papers reporting good long-term results. In 1985, Coventry (7) recommended a correction of anatomical valgus to between 8 and 10 degrees (normal is 5 to 7 degrees). In 1987, Hernigou et al. (8) recommended correction to between 3 and 6 degrees of valgus mechanical axis (lateral angle between the center of the knee and the head of the femur and the center of the tibia at the knee and the center of the ankle; normal is 180 degrees). In 1992, Dugdale et al. (9) recommended correction of the weight-bearing line (center of the head of the femur to center of the talus) to a point from 62% to 66% of the position across the tibia from medial to lateral. The weight-bearing line is reported as a deviation from the center of the knee in millimeters or as a percentage of the tibial plateau width, with convention directing that the medial edge of the medial compartment is indicated as 0% and the lateral edge of the lateral compartment as 100%. The term *weight-bearing line* generally is preferred to avoid confusion with the other angular axes that are defined around the knee. When the indication for osteotomy is for hyperextension thrust, then the objective is to correct the alignment to neutral, with the weight-bearing line passing through the knee at 50% medial to lateral. The intention is to eliminate the abnormal thrust on walking, while realizing that it does not eliminate the static ligamentous laxity (10).

Miniaci et al. (11) reported a method for planning closing-wedge osteotomy without use of tracing paper or a template. His method **(Fig 43.4-2)** is modified for the opening-wedge osteotomy as follows:

- The mechanical axis is drawn on the long leg alignment radiograph, passing from the center of the head of the femur to the center of the talus.
- The required mechanical axis is drawn on the radiograph, passing from the center of the head of the femur through a point 62% from medial to lateral on the tibial plateau. This indicates the new position where the center of talus needs to be and is marked on the radiograph.
- The hinge point on the lateral tibial cortex is marked, and a line is drawn from the hinge point to the new position on the talus as determined by the required mechanical weight-bearing line.
- The line representing the "old" position from the hinge point to the current position of the talus is drawn.
- The planned osteotomy is marked on the radiograph, and the length (*L*) is noted.
- This length *L* is marked on the new line between the hinge point and the new position of the talus.
- The height of the osteotomy plate used in the opening-wedge osteotomy is then measured using the two lines between the hinge point and the old ankle point and the new position of the talus.

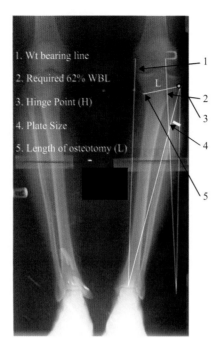

Fig 43.4-2. Planning for an opening-wedge osteotomy involves drawing the current weight-bearing line, drawing the weight-bearing line that is needed, and determining the hinge point, plate size, and length of the osteotomy.

1. Wt bearing line
2. Required 62% WBL
3. Hinge Point (H)
4. Plate Size
5. Length of osteotomy (L)

■ OPENING-WEDGE VALGUS HIGH TIBIAL OSTEOTOMY

The principle of an opening-wedge osteotomy is to perform an osteotomy from the medial side, above the level of the tibial tubercle, correcting the weight-bearing line through the knee while holding the osteotomy apart with a mechanical device either combined with or without bone graft. The methods of fixation include plate-and-screw fixation with or without synthetic, autogenous, or allogeneic bone graft; a technique involving hemicallotasis with external fixation; and application of an external frame with small-wire fixation devices.

Surgical Technique

A variety of fixation systems are commercially available, but all procedures involve the same principles of exposure of the upper medial tibia; creating and opening a controlled, incomplete osteotomy above the level of the tibial tuberosity while protecting posterior structures; and insertion of a plate-fixation device.

This section outlines the surgical technique using the Puddu plate-fixation device (Arthrex, Naples, FL) for the opening-wedge high tibial osteotomy **(Fig 43.4-3)** (12). The procedure is performed using tourniquet control on the upper thigh, and the leg is positioned supine on the operating table, with a foot bolster close to the foot such that the leg may be positioned in abduction and external rotation with

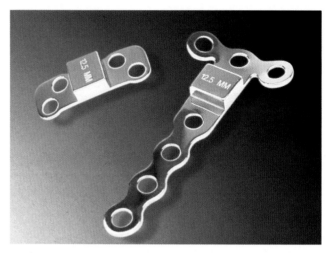

Fig 43.4-3. The Puddu plate fixation device for the opening-wedge high tibial osteotomy.

the knee at 45 to 60 degrees, thereby exposing the upper medial border of the tibia at the level at the knee joint.

Before skin draping, the center of the head of femur is localized using fluoroscopy control and marked with a cardiac monitor dot. This can then be easily palpated through the drapes to reduce radiation exposure. It also is important to undertake tight bandaging of the foot and ankle during draping to allow easy palpation of the center of the ankle of joint.

A skin incision is made on the anterior medial aspect of the tibia halfway between the tibial tubercle and the posterior medial border of the tibia. The incision is taken from the joint line superiorly to a position from 6 to 8 cm inferiorly.

The tibial tubercle is identified, and a longitudinal incision is made just medial to the patella tendon, identifying the important landmark of the junction of patella tendon on the tibial tubercle. A transverse incision in the periosteum and superficial fibers of the medial collateral ligament is made, starting from the superior border of the tubercle **(Fig 43.4-4)**. The periosteal elevator is then used to strip the tissue on the medial aspect of the tibia and around the posteromedial border, allowing insertion of a special, curved retractor to partially protect the vascular structures at the posterior aspect of the knee.

In this approach, the fibers of the deep medial collateral ligament remain attached to the tibia between this incision and the level of the joint line (Fig. 43.4-4). The superficial fibers of the medial collateral ligament, however, are divided down to bone.

The guide pin for the osteotomy is then inserted freehand, with the position checked by radiography, with the goal for it to be passing just superior to the tibial tubercle ending approximately 15 to 20 mm below the lateral aspect of the tibial plateau. These landmarks are used in the preparation for passing the guide pin. A finger is placed on the head of fibula and a lever retractor placed under the patella tendon to identify the superior part of tibial tubercle. The extrapolation of a line between these two points determines

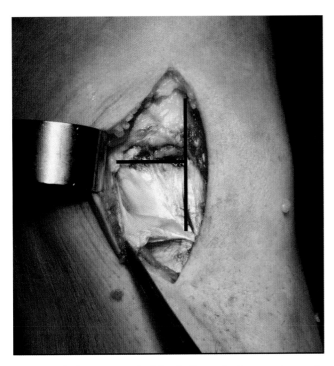

Fig 43.4-4. A transverse incision in the periosteum and superficial fibers of the medial collateral ligament.

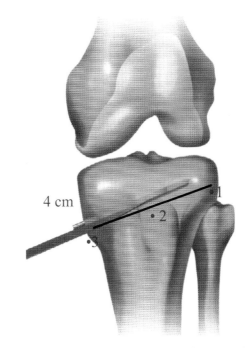

Fig 43.4-5. Positioning of the guide wire in an opening-wedge valgus high tibial osteotomy.

the start point for the guide wire, which usually is in the middle of the cleared space (Fig 43.4-5), approximately 4 cm below the joint line and midway from anterior to posterior. Take care to ensure that the head of fibula is in a normal anatomical relationship 10 to 15 mm below the joint line. In a patient with a high-lying fibular head, the articular portion of the superior tibiofibular joint usually remains 15 mm below the joint line, and this can be taken in to account during insertion of the wire.

Once the wire is inserted, the knee is moved into a supine position. Then an image is taken to confirm the position, and the wire is adjusted as necessary (Fig 43.4-6).

Osteotomy with the oscillating saw is performed by inserting the saw to a depth of approximately 20 to 30 mm less than the measured length of the guide wire (Fig 43.4-7). It is important to ensure that the oscillating saw is inserted from true medial to lateral, avoiding the temptation to make the osteotomy from anteromedial to posterolateral. The osteotomy is progressed using the thin, sharp osteotome that is supplied with the instrumentation (Fig 43.4-8), again taking care to insert the osteotome from true medial to lateral. The position of the advancing osteotome is assessed by radiography, aiming to end 1 cm short of the lateral tibial cortex. At this point, gentle valgus stress is applied to the tibia, and an assessment of the degree of opening is made. The osteotome is advanced until a relatively easy opening of the medial side is visible on valgus stressing of the knee. As a guide, it should comfortably open between 2 and 3 mm with gentle stress so that the wedge opener, when inserted, will not lead to any propagation of the osteotomy toward the joint surface or into the superior tibiofibular joint.

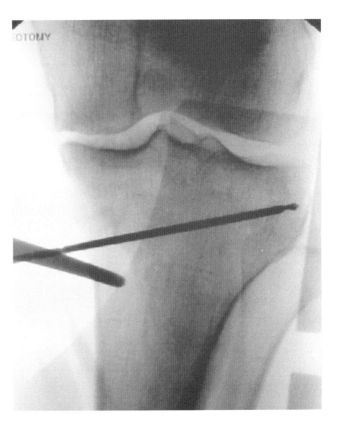

Fig 43.4-6. An image is taken to confirm the position of the wire and to adjust it if necessary.

The wedge opener is inserted and gently tapped into place, gradually increasing the opening of the osteotomy (Fig 43.4-9). Take care at this point to avoid heavy hammering,

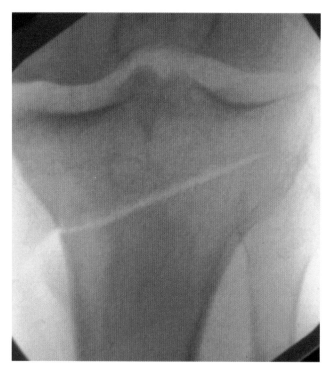

Fig 43.4-7. The oscillating saw is inserted to a depth of approximately 20 to 30 mm less than the measured length of the guide wire.

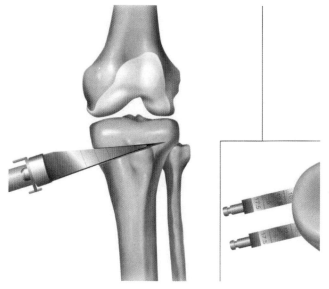

Fig 43.4-9. The wedge increases the opening of the osteotomy.

because the sudden impact may lead to unpredictable propagation of the osteotomy.

Once the osteotomy wedge opener is inserted to the point predicted by preoperative planning, the long leg alignment rod is applied from the palpable cardiac monitor dot marker over the hip joint to the center of the talus. Fine adjustments are then made to the wedge opener, allowing accurate positioning of the new weight-bearing line at a point 62% from medial to lateral **(Fig 43.4-10)**. This usually is halfway down the slope of the lateral tibial spine, which is very easily assessed on the fluroscopy screen.

Once the position has been found, the true height of opening is measured, and an appropriate plate is chosen, attached to a joystick, and inserted after removal of the handle of the wedge opener **(Fig 43.4-11)**. If the tibial slope is thought to have been affected by the osteotomy, then a sloped Arthrex plate can be used to compensate. This is best judged by remembering that the height of the osteotomy at the level of the tibial tubercle should be half that of the opening of the medial cortex. If this is not the case, then either the osteotomy must be repositioned to a more posterior aspect on the medial side or an appropriately sloped plate must be chosen.

The plate is held in place using four screws. It is best to insert a proximal screw while the wedge opener is still in place to ensure stability of the construct. The opener is then removed, allowing contact of the cortex on to the stepped plate. This is important, because the bone needs to rest on the plate rather than on the screws.

The usual combination of screws is a 6.5-mm, fully threaded, cancellous screw in the proximal tibial metaphysis, with the screws aimed into the good-holding cancellous bone under the tibial spines. Two cortical screws (4.5 mm) are used to hold the lower part of the plate, aiming transversely across the tibia onto the opposite cortex **(Fig 43.4-12)**.

If the space is 10 mm or greater, then a bone or synthetic graft is inserted into the open gap. This graft can be mixed with local bone graft harvested from the tibial metaphysis and diaphysis using a small osteotome. The final alignment position is confirmed by radiography, and the wound is closed over a single drain.

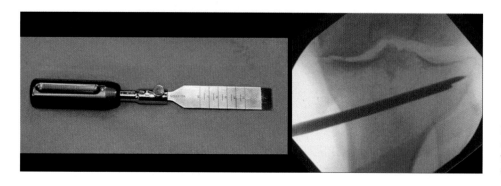

Fig 43.4-8. The thin, sharp osteotome is inserted to a position 1 cm short of the lateral tibial cortex.

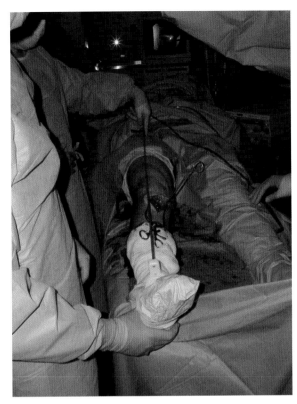

Fig 43.4-10. With the osteotomy wedge opener in place, the long leg alignment rod is applied over the hip joint to the center of the talus.

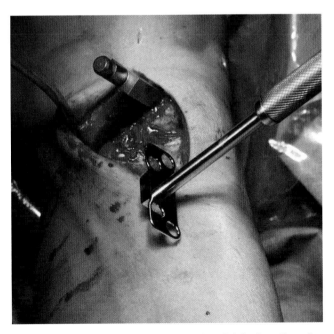

Fig 43.4-11. The plate is attached to a joystick for insertion after removal of the handle of the wedge opener.

Postoperative Rehabilitation

It is important to encourage the patient to limit weight bearing for a total of 2 months. Touch weight bearing is allowed for the first month and up to partial weight bearing

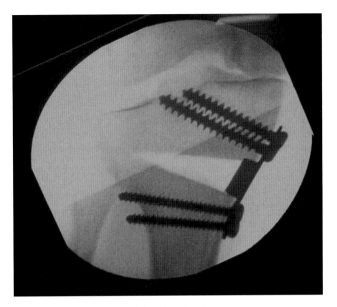

Fig 43.4-12. Screws hold the plate in place.

for the second month. If a large osteotomy is performed (≥15 mm), then touch weight bearing should remain until 2 months. The knee is protected in a hinged range-of-movement brace, allowing control of varus/valgus but freedom of flexion as tolerated. Full weight bearing can begin after 8 weeks if radiographs reveal satisfactory healing. It is important to encourage the patient not to go faster than the allowed rehabilitation schedule because of the potential for displacement of the fixation.

Results of Opening-wedge Osteotomy

The Puddu plate was developed as a simple fixation device (12) for the opening-wedge osteotomy and uses two screws proximally and two screws distally. Few results have been published in the literature, but Amendola et al. (13) have reported on their first 74 consecutive patients over a 2-year period. Their results indicate a 90% satisfaction rate and a realistic learning curve for the procedure. All osteotomies in this series were held by the first-generation Puddu plate, with one hole above and below the osteotomy. Intra-articular fracture as an extension of the osteotomy during the early part of the series was associated with a high osteotomy and too thick an osteotome. Modification of the technique prevented any further fracture. Four failures of fixation were reported; these failures were attributed to early, aggressive weight bearing and a vertical, unstable construct.

The same group also has reported their results with osteotomy for symptomatic hyperextension–varus thrust in 16 patients followed for a mean of 56 months (10,14). Again, the plate used was the two-hole, first-generation Puddu plate. The intended correction was to alter the weight-bearing line to a mean of 50% from medial to lateral, and the final correction achieved was a mean femorotibial axis of 6-degrees valgus and the weight-bearing line to 46%, representing a shift of 28%. Posterior tibial slope also was increased to correct hyperextension, with a mean increase of 7 degrees. Activity scores increased by two points on the Tegner and Lysholm score. The average decrease in the Blackburne–Peel ratio of patella height was 0.17, with two patients developing patella infera, but no correlation with the functional result was found. The authors reported one case of delayed union, which was treated by prolonged immobilization, and no cases of fracture, nonunion, or peroneal nerve palsy. Only 5 of the 17 patients required later reconstruction of the PCL.

Koshino et al. (15) reported successful use of a porous hydroxyapatite wedge in a series of 21 knees in 18 patients followed for an average of 78.6 months. All patients had relief of pain and improvement in functional activities of walking. No patient required conversion to TKR or experienced collapse of the graft. The procedure involved the use of external fixation for an average of 7 weeks. The fixation method was associated with pin-track infection, nonunion, and deep vein thrombosis.

Patella baja is a recognized complication of opening-wedge osteotomy (16), associated with immobilization following osteotomy. The complication is reduced if early mobilization is allowed, preventing tethering of the patella.

One of the criticisms of the four-hole Puddu plate is the limited stability that the plate offers in the sagittal plane (17). Spahn (18) reported a 43.6% complication rate following Puddu osteotomy. Modifications to the Puddu plate, using angle-stabilized locking bolts that eliminate the toggle of screws within a conventional plate, may improve fixation. This principle has been employed in the Tomofix plate (Stratec Medical, Synthes, Solothorn, Switzerland), which was developed in 2000 (19). In this device, eight locking bolts are used, with four proximal and four distal to the osteotomy. The osteotomy is biplanar, starting lower on the tibia and involving a vertical extension of the osteotomy behind the tibial tubercle. Lobenhoffer and Agneskirchner (17) reported six nonunions with loss of correction and implant failure out of 101 osteotomies using the Puddu plate, with all nonunions following a correction of 12.5 mm or greater. In 112 subsequent operations using the Tomofix plate, those authors reported no further cases of delayed union, loss of correction, or implant failure. The mean opening in both series was 11.6 cm. Staubli et al. (20), from the same group, reported only one delayed union in the first 92 osteotomies using the Tomofix plate; the mean correction was 9.2 degrees. In the cases of nonunion, technical errors in positioning of the plate were identified. In addition, in this series, no bone graft was used, and it was recommended that the plate not be removed before 12 months to avoid any recurrence of varus alignment. From the work of those authors, the technical aspects of performing opening-wedge osteotomy clearly remain important.

Stoffel et al. (21) tested the biomechanical properties of the four-hole Puddu plate without locking screws and of the Tomofix plate for a 15-mm gap in a synthetic, composite tibial bone. Before failing at the lateral cortex, both constructs tolerated axial and torsional loading at values higher than those that occur in normal walking. Once the lateral cortex had become unstable, rigidity substantially reduced. With the Puddu plate, the axial stiffness was reduced by 66% and the torsional rigidity by 78%, and with the Tomofix plate, the reductions were significantly less (47% and 54%, respectively). Use of locking screws may have the advantage of providing stability not only at the medial opening but also at the lateral hinge by virtue of their angular stability (21).

One proposed, novel modification to the technique is use of an anteroposteriorly directed, stress-relieving drill hole at the apex of the osteotomy to allow increased opening before fracture of the lateral cortex. In cadaver bones, the amount of opening increased from 6.7 to 10 degrees before developing fracture (22).

■ CLOSING-WEDGE OSTEOTOMY

The principle of closing-wedge osteotomy is to remove an appropriately sized wedge from the lateral aspect of the tibia above the tibial tubercle and to obtain accurate apposition of the bony surfaces, achieving union with stable fixation. The closing-wedge osteotomy originally was made popular by Coventry, and fixation was achieved using a step staple supported by an immobilization cast. New instrumentation has allowed more accurate cuts to be made, with the addition of better internal fixation devices allowing early movement of the knee. Several devices are commercially available, all of which essentially involve a small plate on the lateral aspect to obtain rigid fixation, with cancellous screws in the proximal tibia and cortical screws distally.

Surgical Technique

Exposure of the lateral tibial cortex is achieved through a longitudinal incision just lateral to the tibial tubercle. The anterior group of muscles are elevated off the tibia using a Cobb elevator to expose the superior tibiofibular joint. The anterior capsule of this joint is incised, and the articular surface of the fibula is excised, using an osteotome directed in the anteroposterior direction while avoiding damage to the peroneal nerve. The nerve does not need to be routinely exposed in the procedure.

Guide pins are placed across the joint to allow orientation, and the proximal tibia is drilled to measure the exact tibial width. Next, a calibrated drill and saw blade are then used to fashion the osteotomy approximately 2 cm below the joint line, stopping approximately 1 cm from the medial cortex. An oblique osteotomy is then fashioned, removing a bone wedge of a size based on preoperative indication and planning. Traditionally, the required angle of correction is calculated from the preoperative long leg alignment radiographs, and this is converted to a wedge size based on the tibial width (11). Some of the newer systems may allow progressive increases in the size of wedges to be taken, ensuring accurate correction on the operating table. To ensure good closure of the osteotomy site, it is important to remove all bone fragments. A compression-clamp device can be used to compress the osteotomy.

On completion, the anterior compartment fascia is closed over the plate as much as possible and a drain inserted.

Postoperative Rehabilitation

Because of the primary strong internal fixation, rehabilitation can be taken slightly faster than following opening-wedge osteotomy. Patients generally are allowed 50% weight bearing during the first 6 weeks, and full weight bearing should be easily tolerated by 12 weeks (23).

■ RESULTS OF OSTEOTOMY

High tibial osteotomy has a high success rate. A synopsis of the literature indicates that tibial osteotomy provides good relief of pain and restoration of function in approximately 80% to 90% of patients at 5 years and 50% to 65% at 10 years (24). The two main factors are appropriate correction of the femorotibial angle and proper selection of the patient (25–28). Naudie et al. (29) reported a joint survival rate of 80% in a 10-year follow-up study of 94 lateral closing-wedge osteotomies and 12 dome osteotomies in patients who were younger than 50 years. Holden et al. (30) reported 70% excellent or good results at 10 years in 51 patients.

Poor results have been associated with undercorrection or with failure to maintain valgus alignment (29,31,32).

Sprenger and Doerzbacher (33) reported on 10-year results related to postoperative alignment at 1 year. In this study, 90% of 41 knees that had retained a valgus alignment of between 8 and 16 degrees survived and were functioning well, but 45% of 28 knees with less than 8 degrees or greater than 16 degrees of valgus underwent a TKR. In this series, the authors reported a complication rate of 21% after closing-wedge high tibial osteotomy, including a 9% incidence of peroneal nerve palsy and 5% rate of nonunion (33).

Closing-wedge osteotomy in the chronically ACL-deficient knee has been associated with good functional results. Noyes et al. (4) reported a reduction of pain in 71%, elimination of "giving way" in 85%, and resumption of light recreational activities in 66% of patients. Dejour et al. (34) showed a 65% rate of return to leisurely sports activities and a 91% satisfaction rate.

■ OPENING- VERSUS CLOSING-WEDGE OSTEOTOMY

Advantages of Opening-wedge Osteotomy

The main advantages of opening-wedge osteotomy of the tibia compared with closing-wedge osteotomy include the following:

1 **Avoidance of damage to the proximal tibia fibular joint and peroneal nerve**. Closing-wedge osteotomy exposes this corner of the knee, where there is a significant risk of damage. Interference with the proximal tibia fibular joint is an essential part of the operation, but excision can lead to pain. Injury to the peroneal nerve also is recognized as a significant complication, with an incidence of up to 27% (17,35).

2 **Easier to perform a two-plane osteotomy**. If osteotomy is required to correct a hyperextension and varus alignment, then positioning the osteotomy more anterior than medial can result in the appropriate correction. This is useful for dealing with ACL or PCL insufficiency patterns.

3 **No opening of the anterior compartment of the leg**. Anterior compartment syndrome is a recognized, severe complication of closing-wedge osteotomy. This is avoided with opening-wedge osteotomy.

4 **No alteration in the shape of the upper tibia**. Closing-wedge osteotomy distorts the shape of the upper tibia, and this may interfere with later TKR.

5 **Ease of correction intraoperatively**. Most techniques involve radiographic control of the osteotomy and use of an alignment rod to predict positioning **(Fig 43.4-13)**. This usually is not possible with closing-wedge systems. Opening-wedge high tibial osteotomy requires only a single bone cut, which can be adjusted in both planes.

Disadvantages of Opening-wedge Osteotomy

The main disadvantages of opening-wedge osteotomy of the tibia compared with closing-wedge osteotomy include the following:

1 **Use of a graft**. Osteotomies of greater than 1 cm generally require use of a bone graft of some sort, either autogenous or synthetic. This can be expensive and can lead to morbidity from harvest of the iliac crest.

2 **Union of the osteotomy site**. Delayed union or nonunion is possible with opening-wedge osteotomy, but the exact incidence is unknown. Nonunion is uncommon with closing-wedge osteotomy.

3 **Management of large corrections**. Opening-wedge osteotomy probably is unsuitable for osteotomies that require an opening of greater than 15 mm, because fixation is difficult to hold with a four-hole plate system. Closing-wedge osteotomy, however, also can be difficult in such situations because of the distortion of upper tibial anatomy that the osteotomy creates.

■ EFFECT OF OSTEOTOMY ON THE TIBIAL SLOPE

Naudie et al. (10) reported that anterior opening-wedge osteotomy caused anterior tibial translation in the PCL-deficient knee, potentially restoring normal knee biomechanics.

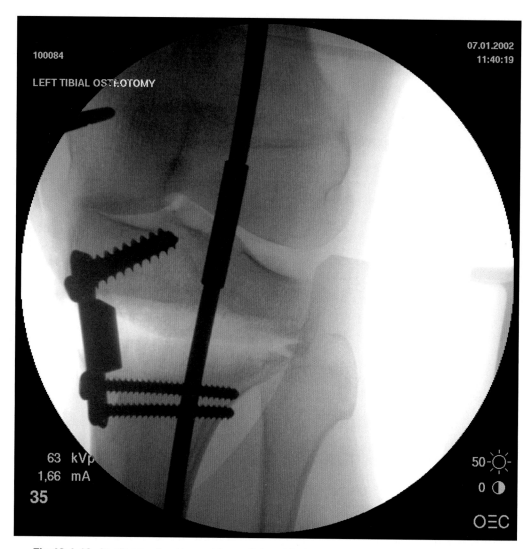

Fig 43.4-13. An alignment rod is used to predict positioning, which is checked by radiography.

Those authors reported that clinically, high tibial osteotomy in posterior instability in the presence of a posterolateral thrust improved subjective feelings of instability in 16 of 17 patients at a minimum follow-up of 2 years.

Giffin et al. (36) analyzed the effect of increasing tibial slope on knee kinematics and the in situ forces in the cruciate ligaments in more detail, and they showed that following an anterior opening-wedge osteotomy, an increase in tibial slope occurs that shifts the resting position of the tibia anteriorly relative to the femur. This anterior shift was present throughout the range of knee flexion, reaching a maximum of 3.6 mm in full extension, and was accentuated under axial loads. When the ACL and PCL were intact, however, the in situ forces in the ligaments were not altered, indicating that small changes in the slope associated with osteotomy are unlikely to cause issues with the ligaments. Still, the shift in position will have an effect on ligament deficiency. Increasing the tibial slope, which can easily be built into an anteromedial

opening-wedge osteotomy, should improve stability in the PCL-deficient knee by reducing the posterior tibial sag in this setting. Conversely, decreasing slope therefore may be protective in an ACL-deficient knee by reducing the force shifting the tibia forward. The clinical implication of this effect is that closing-wedge osteotomy, which has a tendency to reduce tibial slope, may be more suitable for use in the ACL-deficient knee. If opening-wedge osteotomy is the procedure of choice for the surgeon, then care must be taken not to increase the tibial slope inadvertently. In this scenario, use of the sloping version of the Puddu plate may be indicated.

Amendola (2) has suggested that in the management of a knee with multiple ligaments that are acutely injured, there also may be a role for correction of malalignment. Long-term results for ligament reconstruction in the knee with multiple injured ligaments have been inconsistent, and perhaps in some of these cases, it may be that pre-existing malalignment may have contributed to a poor result.

■ TOTAL KNEE REPLACEMENT AFTER OSTEOTOMY

Much debate exists concerning the results of TKR following high tibial osteotomy, particularly in regard to difficulties in surgical technique, complication rate, and long-term outcome (37). Some authors have indicated that the outcome may be more comparable to results after revision TKR, with long-term success rates of 80%, compared with 90% to 95% for uncomplicated primary TKR (38,39). In general, however, the older literature indicates a worse outcome for TKR after osteotomy (38–41) compared with that reported in more recent papers (42–44). The more recent evidence indicates that the long-term success rate following TKR may be only slightly reduced if surgery is undertaken after high tibial osteotomy (37).

Parvizi et al. (45) reported a slightly higher incidence of revision and radiolucent lines, and they identified male gender, increased weight, young age at the time of total knee arthroplasty, coronal laxity, and preoperative limb malalignment as risk factors for early failure. In another recent comparative study of 39 patients who had undergone bilateral total knee arthroplasty (44), the clinical and radiographic results for knees with and without a previous proximal tibial osteotomy were not substantially different at a mean follow-up of 8.7 years.

The main issue with TKR after osteotomy is the additional technical difficulty of the procedure, associated with the previous surgery, in obtaining both adequate exposure and optimal soft tissue balancing during total knee arthroplasty (38,46). Osteotomy may have resulted in altered anatomy of the upper tibia, patella baja, periarticular scarring, malalignment because of under- or overcorrection, and proximal tibial bone deficiency. Retained hardware also may contribute to the technical difficulty.

One of the main factors in assessing the outcome of arthroplasty following osteotomy, however, is the fact that patients who had sufficient symptoms to warrant osteotomy are a highly selected group. Parvizi et al. (45) observed that the majority of patients undergoing proximal tibial osteotomy are young, active, and frequently heavy men who are deemed to be too young for total knee arthroplasty (because of their unfavorable demographic status). In their series, the same factors affected outcome in patients who had not undergone osteotomy, and it is possible that failure to match for these differences in age, gender, and weight may account for the disparity in conclusions that have been reported in various other well-conducted studies (41,42,47–50).

Most of the published literature concerning this issue refers to arthroplasty following closing-wedge or dome osteotomies, and it could be argued that an opening-wedge osteotomy does not create the same change in the anatomy of the upper tibia that follows a closing-wedge osteotomy. As yet, little has been published in this area, but it does seem to be likely.

In particular, patella infera is a recognized complication of both closing- and opening-wedge osteotomy. In closing-wedge osteotomy, the resulting low patella is a function of patella ligament contracture following prolonged immobilization, whereas after opening-wedge osteotomy, it results from raising the joint line (16). Wright et al. (16) reported that 64% of 28 patients developed patella infera following opening-wedge osteotomy according to the criteria of a Blackburn–Peel ratio of less than 0.54, but no significant change in patella tendon length was noted. Tigani et al. (51), using the Caton method for measuring patella height and early mobilization following both opening- and closing-wedge osteotomy, showed that patellar "lowering" occurred more often with opening-wedge osteotomy that with closing-wedge osteotomy.

Gaasbeek et al. (52) recently described a technique of opening-wedge osteotomy performed at the level of the tibial tuberosity but keeping the tuberosity attached to the proximal part of the tibia, and those authors showed no patella infera as measured by the Caton index. They recommended that this technique be considered over traditional proximal tibial osteotomy when corrections of more than 10 degrees are required or in the presence of pre-existing patella infera.

■ FACTORS ASSOCIATED WITH POOR LONG-TERM OUTCOME AFTER OSTEOTOMY

The main factors that affect outcome adversely include the following: (a) age older than 55 years, (b) extreme obesity, (c) lateral compartment osteoarthritis, (d) correction to less than 7 degree of anatomical valgus, (e) high adduction moment in walking, and (f) multiple previous operative procedures on the knee (53,54).

As mentioned previously, the main factor is inadequate correction. Catani et al. (55), using gait analysis, assessed the biomechanical influence of insufficient correction following osteotomy, resulting in early failure, and noted that undercorrection does not reduce the adductor moment or the lateral thrust that normally is associated with varus alignment. The result is further overloading of the medial compartment and recurrence of the varus deformity. In combination with a high adductor moment, the quadriceps activity is increased in an attempt to stabilize the knee. The increase in muscle contraction causes increase in the compressive force on the medial side, leading to more rapid progression in arthritis (54). A further observation from this work is the compensatory pattern of "toe-out" walking, resulting in increased foot pronation and external rotation moment about the knee, thereby reducing loading in the medial compartment.

It is possible that computer-assisted navigation will help us to achieve the ideal postoperative alignment (56), but perhaps the most important recommendation is for patients to not be smokers at the time of osteotomy. W-Dahl and Toksvig-Larsen (57) showed that in smokers, the risk ratio was 2.7 for developing delayed union after osteotomy by hemicallotasis and 8.1 for pseudarthrosis. The risk for smokers developing complications was 2.5-fold greater than that in nonsmokers (57).

■ OSTEOTOMY IN COMBINATION WITH CARTILAGE REPAIR

The effect of osteotomy on regeneration and repair of the articular surface has been assessed by several authors. Odenbring et al. (58) showed surface regeneration in 9 of 14 overcorrected knees 2 years after osteotomy without any correlation between the clinical results and the arthroscopic stage at follow-up examination. Koshino et al. (59) showed a relationship between the stage of regeneration of knee articular cartilage and postoperative limb alignment, with more hyalinelike articular cartilage being found in the well-corrected knees. In addition, those authors reported more mature regeneration in patients with previously exposure of subchondral bone compared to that in patients who still had a layer of degenerate cartilage. It is believed that either the layer of old, degenerated cartilage interferes with new growth or that because no chondral bone is exposed, a limited healing response from the bone marrow occurs. Those authors proposed that if the degenerated cartilage could be shaved off completely, down to subchondral bone, in the weight-bearing portion of the medial femoral condyle at the time of initial osteotomy for knee osteoarthritis of less-advanced grade, then new cartilage regeneration could be expected in that area.

Sterett and Steadman (60) have reported on the addition of microfracture cartilage repair during distraction opening-wedge tibial osteotomy using an external fixator in the difficult group of young, active patients who have bare-bone degeneration. They discussed 33 of 38 patients, with a mean age of 51.3 years at a mean follow-up of 45 months. In this series, the entry criteria included a desired Tegner activity score of 4, which represents moderate work or recreational sports. The mean Tegner score achieved was 5, and the survivorship at 5 years was 84%, with revision high tibial osteotomy or arthroplasty been required as end points in two patients. The quality of the repair tissue was not assessed but the authors concluded that patients with varus malalignment and chondral surface lesions of the knee can be treated effectively with chondral resurfacing by microfracture and high tibial osteotomy.

■ SUMMARY

The role and place for osteotomy in the armamentarium of the knee surgeon has evolved in recent years. In part, this has resulted from the redefining of the role of arthroplasty, the good long-term results of which have lowered the age for when joint replacement is considered. This is especially true of unicompartmental replacement. Osteotomy has continued to have a role in the younger, more active individual with early degenerative change, maintaining the concept of buying time before potentially undergoing arthroplasty.

The second contributing factor has been the development of newer techniques. Closing-wedge osteotomy has become more accurate, and internal fixation has allowed earlier rehabilitation, avoiding the use of cast immobilization and reducing

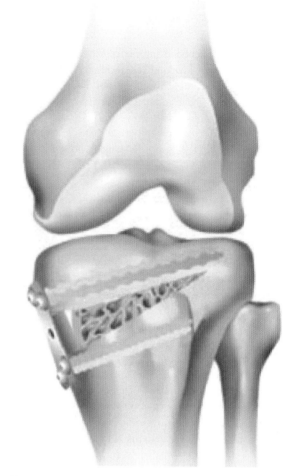

Fig 43.4-14. Opening-wedge osteotomy.

the tendency for patella infera. Opening-wedge osteotomy **(Fig 43.4-14)** has gained in popularity with its proposed advantages of less upper tibial deformation, reduced complication rate (especially for exposure of the lateral structures), and early mobilization. It remains to be seen whether this technique will lead to a reduction in the technical difficulty of knee replacement following closing-wedge osteotomy and improved implant survival.

Osteotomy remains important for the sports-orientated knee surgeon, especially when used in combination with other techniques for cartilage repair, meniscal salvage, or reconstruction, in which alignment is critical to long-term survival. Small yet important corrections of alignment can be easily undertaken with predictable results.

■ REFERENCES

1. Stukenborg-Colsman C, Wirth CJ, et al. High tibial osteotomy versus unicompartmental joint replacement in unicompartmental knee joint osteoarthritis: 7–10-year follow-up prospective randomized study. *Knee.* 2001;8:187–194.
2. Amendola A. The role of osteotomy in the multiple ligament injured knee. *Arthroscopy.* 2003;19(suppl 1):11–13.

3. Markoff KL, Bargar WL, Shoemaker SC, et al. The role of joint load in knee stability. *J Bone Joint Surg Am.* 1988;70:977–982.
4. Noyes FR, Barber-Westin SD, Hewett TE. High tibial osteotomy and ligament reconstruction for varus angulated anterior cruciate ligament-deficient knees. *Am J Sports Med.* 2000;28:282–296.
5. Hughston JC, Jacobsen KE. Chronic posterolateral rotatory instability of the knee. *J Bone Joint Surg Am.* 1985;67:351–359.
6. Brown GA, Amendola A. Radiographic evaluation and preoperative planning for high tibial osteotomy. *Oper Techn Sports Med.* 2000;5:2–14.
7. Coventry MB. Upper tibial osteotomy for osteoarthritis. *J Bone Joint Surg Am.* 1985;67:1136–1140.
8. Hernigou P, Medevielle D, Debeyre J, et al. Proximal tibial osteotomy for osteoarthritis with varus deformity: a ten- to thirteen-year follow up study. *J Bone Joint Surg Am.* 1987;69:332–354.
9. Dugdale TW, Noyes FR, Styer D. Preoperative planning for high tibial osteotomy. *Clin Orthop.* 1992;274:248–264.
10. Naudie D, Amendola A, Fowler P. Opening wedge high tibial osteotomy for symptomatic hyperextension–varus thrust. *Am J Sports Med.* 2004;32:60–70.
11. Miniaci A, Ballmer FT, Ballmer PM, et al. Proximal tibial osteotomy: a new fixation device. *Clin Orthop.* 1989;246:250–259.
12. Puddu G, Franco V, Cipolla M, et al. Opening wedge osteotomy—proximal tibia and distal femur. In: Jackson DW, ed. *Master techniques in orthopaedic surgery: reconstructive knee surgery.* 2nd ed. Philadelphia: Lippincott Williams & Wilkins; 2002:375–390.
13. Amendola A, Fowler PJ, Litchfield R, et al. Opening-wedge high tibial osteotomy using a novel technique: early results and complications. *J Knee Surg.* 2004;17:164–169.
14. Naudie D, Amendola A, Folwer P. Opening-wedge high tibial osteotomy for chronic posterior instability. Proceedings AOSSM Meeting, Keystone, CO, July 2001.
15. Koshino T, Murase T, Saito T. Medial opening-wedge high tibial osteotomy with use of porous hydroxyapatite to treat medial compartment osteoarthritis of the knee. *J Bone Joint Surg Am.* 2003;85:78–85.
16. Wright JM, Heavrin B, Begg M, et al. Observations on patellar height following opening wedge proximal tibial osteotomy. *Am J Knee Surg.* 2001;14:163–173.
17. Lobenhoffer P, Agneskirchner JD. Improvements in surgical technique of valgus high tibial osteotomy. *Knee Surg Sports Traumatol Arthrosc.* 2003;11:132–138.
18. Spahn G. Complications in high tibial (medial opening wedge) osteotomy. *Arch Orthop Trauma Surg.* 2004;124:649–653.
19. De Simone C. Staubli A. Neue fixationstechniken fur mediale open-wedge osteotomien der proximalen tibia. *Schweiz Med Wochenschr.* 2000;119–130.
20. Staubli AE, De Simoni C, Babst R, et al. TomoFix: a new LCP concept for open-wedge osteotomy of the medial proximal tibia—early results in 92 cases. *Injury.* 2003;34(suppl 2):B55–B62.
21. Stoffel K, Stachowiak G, Kuster M. Open-wedge high tibial osteotomy: biomechanical investigation of the modified Arthrex osteotomy plate (Puddu plate) and the TomoFix plate. *Clin Biomech.* 2004;19:944–950.
22. Kessler OC, Jacob HA, Romero J. Avoidance of medial cortical fracture in high tibial osteotomy: improved technique. *Clin Orthop.* 2002;395:180–185.
23. Hofmann AA, Cook TM. High tibial osteotomy: where did you go? *Orthopaedics.* 2003;26:949–950.
24. Amendola A. Unicompartmental osteoarthritis in the active patient: the role of high tibial osteotomy. *Arthroscopy.* 2003;19(suppl 1):109–116.
25. Berman AT, Bosacco SJ, Kirshner S, et al. Factors influencing long-term results in high tibial osteotomy. *Clin Orthop.* 1991;272:192–198.
26. Coventry MB, Ilstrup DM, Wallrichs SL. Proximal tibial osteotomy: a critical long-term study of eighty-seven cases. *J Bone Joint Surg Am.* 1993;75:196–201.
27. Nagel A, Insall JN, Scuderi GR. Proximal tibial osteotomy. A subjective outcome study. *J Bone Joint Surg Am.* 1996;78:1353–1358.
28. Insall JN, Joseph DM, Msika C. High tibial osteotomy for varus gonarthrosis. A long-term follow-up study. *J Bone Joint Surg Am.* 1984;66:1040–1048.
29. Naudie D, Bourne RB, Rorabeck CH, et al. Survivorship of the high tibial valgus osteotomy. A 10- to 22-year follow-up study. *Clin Orthop.* 1999;367:18–27.
30. Holden DL, James SL, Larson RL, et al. Proximal tibial osteotomy in patients who are fifty years old or less. A long-term follow-up study. *J Bone Joint Surg Am.* 1988;70:977–982.
31. Rudan JF, Simurda MA. High tibial osteotomy. A prospective clinical and roentgenographic review. *Clin Orthop.* 1990;255:251–256.
32. Yasuda K, Majima T, Tsuchida T, et al. A 10- to 15-year follow-up observation of high tibial osteotomy in medial compartment osteoarthrosis. *Clin Orthop.* 1992;282:186–195.
33. Sprenger TR, Doerzbacher JF. Tibial osteotomy for the treatment of varus gonarthrosis: survival and failure analysis to twenty-two years. *J Bone Joint Surg Am.* 2003;85:469–474.
34. Dejour H, Neyret P, Boileau P, et al. Anterior cruciate reconstruction combined with valgus tibial osteotomy. *Clin Orthop.* 1994;299:220–228.
35. Aydogdu S, Cullu E, Arac N, et al. Prolonged peroneal nerve dysfunction after high tibial osteotomy: pre- and postoperative electrophysiological study. *Knee Surg Sports Traumatol Arthrosc.* 2000;8:305–308.
36. Giffin JR, Vogrin T, Zantop T, et al. Effects of increasing tibial slope on the biomechanics of the knee. *Am J Sports Med.* 2004;32:376–382.
37. Scott N, Clarke H. The role of osteotomy 2003: defining the niche. *Orthopaedics.* 2004;27:975–976
38. Windsor RE, Insall JN, Vince KG. Technical considerations of total knee arthroplasty after proximal tibial osteotomy. *J Bone Joint Surg Am.* 1988;70:547–555.
39. Diduch DR, Insall JN, Scott WN, et al. Total knee replacement in young active patients. Long-term follow-up and functional outcome. *J Bone Joint Surg Am.* 1997;79:575–582.
40. Katz M, Hungerford DS, Krackow KA, et al. Results of total knee arthroplasty after failed proximal tibial osteotomy for osteoarthritis. *J Bone Joint Surg Am.* 1987;69:225–233.
41. Mont MA, Alexander N, Krackow KA, et al. Total knee arthroplasty after failed high tibial osteotomy. *Orthop Clin North Am.* 1994;25:515–525.
42. Nizard RS, Cardinne L, Bizot P, et al. Total knee replacement after failed high tibial osteotomy: results of a matched-pair study. *J Arthroplasty.* 1998;13:847–853.
43. Toksvig-Larsen S, Magyar G, Onsten I, et al. Fixation of the tibial component of total knee arthroplasty after high tibial osteotomy: a matched radiostereometric study. *J Bone Joint Surg Br.* 1998;80:295–297.
44. Meding JB, Keating EM, Ritter MA, et al. Total knee arthroplasty after high tibial osteotomy. A comparison study in patients who had bilateral total knee replacement. *J Bone Joint Surg Am.* 2000;82:1252–1259.
45. Parvizi J, Hanssen A, Spangehl M. Total knee arthroplasty following proximal tibial osteotomy: risk factors for failure. *J Bone Joint Surg Am.* 2004;86:474–479.
46. Scuderi GR, Windsor RE, Insall JN. Observations on patellar height after proximal tibial osteotomy. *J Bone Joint Surg Am.* 1989;71:245–248.
47. Ritter MA, Fechtman RA. Proximal tibial osteotomy. A survivorship analysis. *J Arthroplasty.* 1988;3:309–311.
48. Amendola A, Rorabeck CH, Bourne RB, et al. Total knee arthroplasty following high tibial osteotomy for osteoarthritis. *J Arthroplasty.* 1989;4(suppl):S11–S17.

49. Meding JB, Keating EM, Ritter MA, et al. Total knee arthroplasty after high tibial osteotomy. A comparison study in patients who had bilateral total knee replacement. *J Bone Joint Surg Am.* 2000;82:1252–1259.

50. Staeheli JW, Cass JR, Morrey BF. Condylar total knee arthroplasty after failed proximal tibial osteotomy. *J Bone Joint Surg Am.* 1987;69:28–31.

51. Tigani D, Ferrari D, Trentani P, et al. Patellar height after high tibial osteotomy. *Int Orthop.* 2001;24:331–334.

52. Gaasbeek RD, Sonneveld H, van Heerwaarden RJ, et al. Distal tuberosity osteotomy in open-wedge high tibial osteotomy can prevent patella infera: a new technique. *Knee.* 2004;11:457–461.

53. Pfahler M, Lutz C, Anetzberger H, et al. Long-term results of high tibial osteotomy for medial osteoarthritis of the knee. *Acta Chir Belg.* 2003;103:603–606.

54. Prodromos CC, Andriacchi TP, Galante JO. A relationship between gait and clinical changes following high tibial osteotomy. *J Bone Joint Surg Am.* 1985;67:1188–1194.

55. Catani F, Marcacci M, Benedetti MG, et al. The influence of clinical and biomechanical factors on the results of valgus high tibial osteotomy. *Chir Organi Mov.* 1998;83:249–262.

56. Keppler P, Gebhard F, Grutzner PA, et al. Computer aided high tibial open-wedge osteotomy *Injury.* 2004;35(suppl 1):S68–S78.

57. W-Dahl A, Toksvig-Larsen S. Cigarette smoking delays bone healing—a prospective study of 200 patients operated on by the hemicallotasis technique. *Acta Orthop Scand.* 2004;75:347–351.

58. Odenbring S, Egund N, Lindstrand A, et al. Cartilage regeneration after proximal tibial osteotomy for medial gonarthrosis. An arthroscopic, roentgenographic and histologic study. *Clin Orthop.* 1992;277:210–216.

59. Koshino T, Wada S, Ara Y, et al. Regeneration of degenerated articular cartilage after high tibial valgus osteotomy for medial compartmental osteoarthritis of the knee. *Knee.* 2003;10:229–236.

60. Sterett W, Steadman JR. Chondral resurfacing and high tibial osteotomy in the varus knee. *Am J Sports Med.* 2004:32:1243–1249.

43.5

UNICOMPARTMENTAL KNEE REPLACEMENT

JACK M. BERT, MD

■ KEY POINTS

- Hemiarthroplasty of the knee refers to the concept of placing a "spacer" in one half of the femoral tibial joint to prevent bone-on-bone apposition.

- The biomechanics and feel of a knee after unicompartmental knee arthroplasty (UKA) generally is closer to those of a normal knee than after total knee arthroplasty (TKA). In addition, studies have shown superior results for UKA compared to upper tibial osteotomy.

- The advantages of UKA are that it allows preservation of bone stock, improved range of motion, reduced blood loss, reduced inpatient stay, and decreased cost.

- The disadvantages of UKA in the past have revolved around poor instrumentation and design. The design of the undersurface macrostructure of the tibial component in UKA is critical to its ability to withstand shear and offset loading in the laboratory.

- Among the clinical indications for UKA are a patient with a relatively sedentary occupation, a patient who is not obese, and unicompartmental pain only.

- Improvements in prosthetic devices have allowed the addition two other types of patients: middle-aged patients with osteoarthritis who desire a reliable initial result with retention of both cruciates and easy revision to TKA if necessary, and geriatric patients who probably will not survive the life span of the UKA and who may have medical problems precluding a major reconstructive process.

Hemiarthroplasty of the knee was first described in the 1950s. It refers to the concept of placing a "spacer" in one half of the femoral tibial joint to prevent bone-on-bone apposition. McKeever (1) first introduced his Vitallium "tibial plateau" **(Fig 43.5-1)** in 1957. MacIntosh (2) followed with an "acrylic tibial plateau" **(Fig 43.5-2)** in 1958, which was followed in turn by Vitallium in 1964. MacIntosh (2) then presented his initial series in Switzerland in 1967 and published a series of patients in 1972 with "good results" in the "majority" of patients having a follow-up period of 6 years (3). The modern version of the hemiarthroplasty is the "unispacer" **(Figs 43.5-3** and **43.5-4)**, with a reported success rate of 67% to 80% after 2 years of follow-up (4, 4a).

During the early 1970s, the Gunston and polycentric unicompartmental arthroplasty (UKA) procedure was introduced **(Figs 43.5-5** and **43.5-6)**. The revision rate at 2 years for these early devices was approximately 10% (5,6). Multiple authors from 1973 to 1983 noted success rates varying between 37% and 92% from 2 to 8 years of follow-up (5–13). From 1987 to 1991, long-term results were published, with 87% to 90% survivorship at 13 to 16 years of follow-up (14–16).

From 1990 to 1993, several authors reported 90% to 96% fair to good results using a combination of metal-backed and all-polyethylene tibial components with 2 to 7 years of follow-up (17–21). This was the first time that obese patients were noted to have a 1.4-fold greater failure rate (18).

Multiple survivorship studies were reported from 1993 to 2003, with success rates from 87% to 98% noted at 6 to 14 years of follow-up (22–30). In one series, 83% of the failures resulted from progressive wear in the unresurfaced compartment (27).

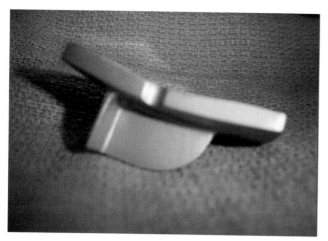

Fig 43.5-1. McKeever hemiarthroplasty prosthesis.

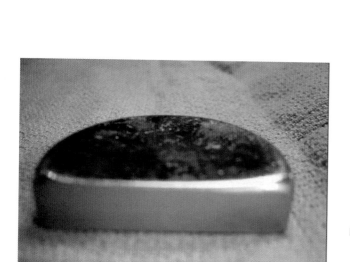

Fig 43.5-2. MacIntosh hemiarthroplasty prosthesis.

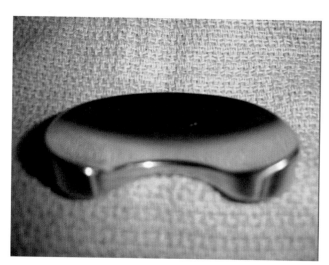

Fig 43.5-3. Unispace prosthesis.

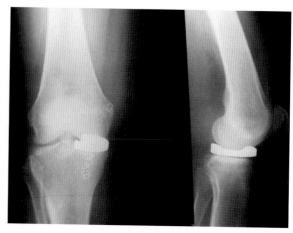

Fig 43.5-4. Radiographic views of a unispacer prosthesis.

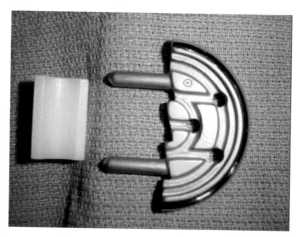

Fig 43.5-5. Polycentric unicompartmental prosthesis.

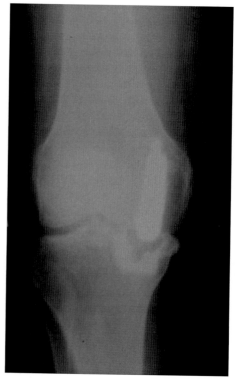

Fig 43.5-6. Radiographic view of a polycentric unicompartmental prosthesis.

■ ADVANTAGES AND DISADVANTAGES

Because of the resurgence in popularity of UKA, primarily as a result of the "mini-incision" technique (30), it is important to understand both the advantages and the disadvantages of this procedure compared to those of TKA and upper tibial osteotomy. The indications and contraindications for this procedure must be understood as well.

When comparing UKA to TKA in patients with a UKA in one knee and a TKA in the other, 75% of patients have noted that their UKA "feels closer to a normal knee" than their contralateral TKA **(Fig 43.5-7)**. The UKA knee had better range of motion and decreased blood loss compared to a TKA knee (31–33). In addition, because of only one third of the knee joint is being replaced, the biomechanics of a UKA knee are closer to those of a normal knee than to those of a TKA knee (17).

When comparing UKA to upper tibial osteotomy **(Fig 43.5-8)**, the UKA results in three different series with 3.5 to 15 years of follow-up were significantly superior. Specifically; 46%, 48%, and 65% success rates were found for upper tibial osteotomy, compared to 76%, 90%, and 88% for UKA, respectively (34–36).

The advantage of UKA is that it allows preservation of bone stock, improved range of motion, reduced blood loss, reduced inpatient stay, and decreased cost. In a community-based hospital registry in St. Paul, Minnesota, a review of 240 cases with 15 years of follow-up showed a mean range of motion of 127 degrees, a mean blood loss of 350 mL, and a mean length of stay of 2.8 days, compared to 5,200 TKAs with a mean length of stay of 4.5 days (37). The UKA is easy to revise (38) if excessive amounts of bone have not been removed **(Figs 43.5-9** and **43.5-10)**. In two

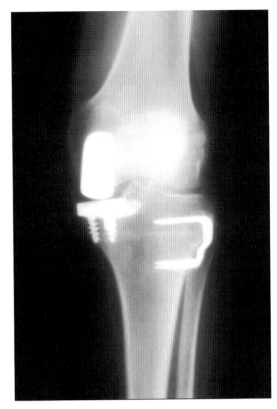

Fig 43.5-8. Upper tibial osteotomy followed by unicompartmental knee arthroplasty in the same patient.

published series with 7 to 10 years of follow-up, however, only 75% to 85% of patients had good to excellent results (39,40). In both studies, up to 75% of the patients had significant osseous defects **(Figs 43.5-11** and **43.5-12)**. In a personal series of 31 cases with a mean follow-up of 9.2

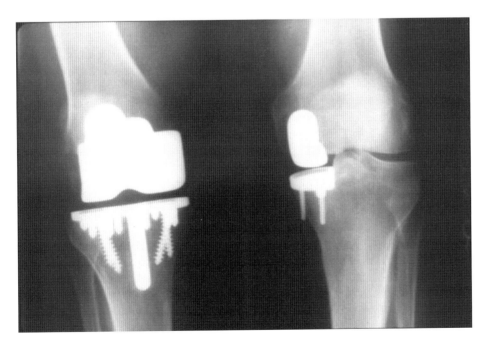

Fig 43.5-7. Total knee arthroplasty and contralateral unicompartmental knee arthroplasty in the same patient.

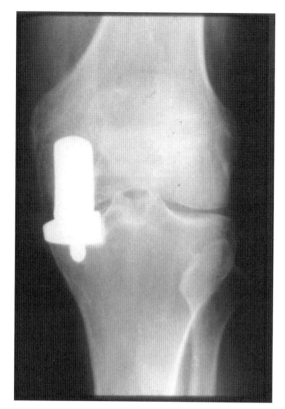

Fig 43.5-9. Painful unicompartmental knee arthroplasty revised to total knee arthroplasty with a 12-mm polytibial insert.

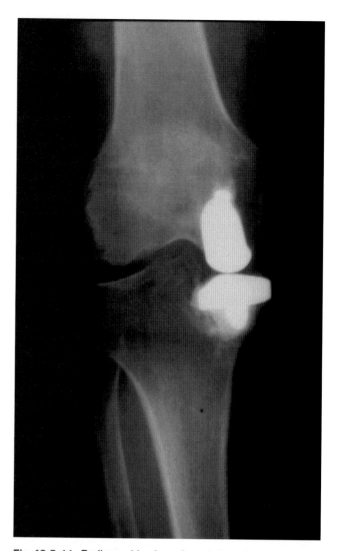

Fig 43.5-11. Radiographic view of a painful unicompartmental knee arthroplasty revised to total knee arthroplasty using an "older"-style tibial wedge augmentation.

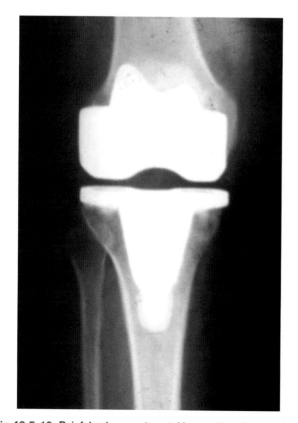

Fig 43.5-10. Painful unicompartmental knee arthroplasty revised to total knee arthroplasty with a 12-mm polytibial insert.

years, 96.3% had good to excellent results, but only 4% of these cases had significant osseous defects (41). Furthermore, in a study of 47 revision UKAs from a community-based registry in St. Paul, Minnesota, with 1.9 to 16 years of follow-up (mean follow-up, 9.4 years), survivorship was 94% (42). Also, in 1998. Lewold (43) noted that conversion to TKA after UKA is easier and more successful than conversion to TKA from upper tibial osteotomy.

The disadvantages of UKA in the past have included poor instrumentation and design (44), uncemented systems failures (40), and poor fixation. The design of the undersurface macrostructure of the tibial component in UKA is critical to its ability to withstand shear and offset loading in the laboratory (45,46). Compared to TKA, reduced survivorship has been reported with development of arthritis in the contralateral compartment **(Fig 43.5-13)**, resulting in early failure (26,27,29).

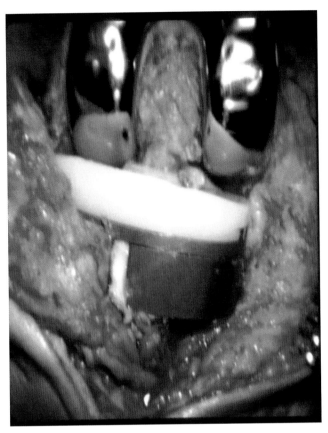

Fig 43.5-12. Painful unicompartmental knee arthroplasty revised to total knee arthroplasty using an "older"-style tibial wedge augmentation.

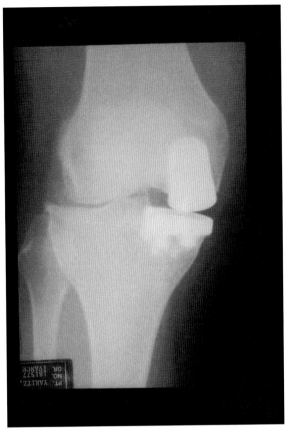

Fig 43.5-13. Progression of arthritis in the contralateral femoral tibial compartment.

■ INDICATIONS

The clinical indications for UKA are a patient with a relatively sedentary occupation, less than 10 degrees of varus deformity, range of motion of at least 90 degrees without a flexion contracture, medial instability only, a patient who is not obese, a diagnosis of osteoarthritis or posttraumatic arthritis, and most importantly, unicompartmental pain only (44). To clinically assess unicompartmental pain, the patient should have a positive "one finger test" **(Fig 43.5-14)**. This test is performed by having the patient point to the involved compartment with one finger when asked where the pain is. This is in contradistinction to the patient who performs a "knee grab" when asked where their pain is **(Fig 43.5-15)**; in other words, the patient cannot localize the pain to one area in the knee and literally grabs the entire knee when asked where the pain is. When this occurs, a TKA instead of a UKA should be performed. Therefore, UKA should not be performed on everyone with strictly unicompartmental disease if the remainder of the knee is symptomatic. In fact, when three different active knee surgeons were asked to determine which patients with osteoarthritis of the knee were suitable for UKA, only 6%, 15%, and 12% were considered to be appropriate candidates for UKA (47–49). Commonly accepted radiographic indications (50) for UKA are 50% unicompartmental joint space collapse (Ahlback I) and

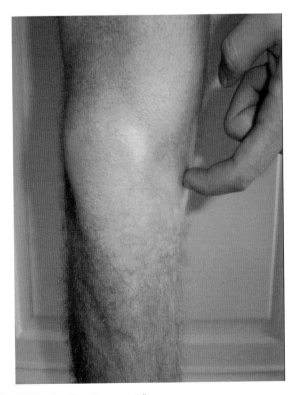

Fig 43.5-14. "One finger test."

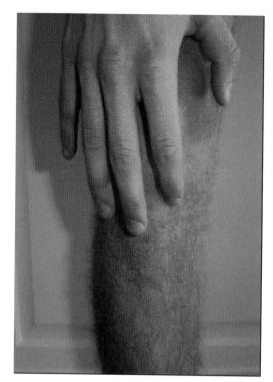

Fig 43.5-15. "Knee grab."

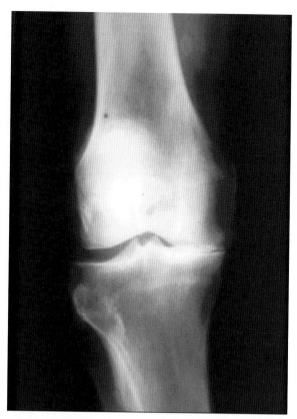

Fig 43.5-17. Standing radiograph shows Ahlback II changes indicating complete collapse of the medial joint space.

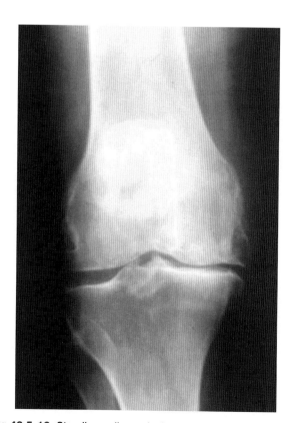

Fig 43.5-16. Standing radiograph shows Ahlback I changes indicating 50% collapse of the medial joint space.

complete collapse (Ahlback II) on standing radiographic views **(Figs 43.5-16** and **43.5-17)**.

Because of improvements in survivorship of UKA as a result of improved prosthetic devices and surgical technique, UKA should be considered in two additional patient categories. The first is the middle-aged patient with osteoarthritis who desires a reliable initial result with retention of both cruciates and easy revision to TKA if necessary. The second is the geriatric patient who most probably will not survive the life span of the UKA and who may have medical problems precluding a major reconstructive procedure such as a TKA (51). In this second patient category, UKA may improve the patient's lifestyle and reduce a significant amount of the patient's ambulatory and rest pain.

■ CONTRAINDICATIONS

Contraindications to UKA are rheumatoid arthritis, "nonlocalized" knee pain, decreased range of motion with a flexion contracture, active lifestyle (sports), obesity, knee instability with absence of the anterior cruciate ligament, and the patient with unrealistic expectations regarding the activity level and longevity of the prosthesis. Young heavy laborers must be educated regarding the limitations of a UKA, and this type of patient may be better served by an osteotomy. Radiographic contraindications are Ahlback IV changes **(Fig 43.5-18)**, consisting of joint space obliteration plus medial-lateral subluxation of 3 to 4 mm. Operative contraindications consist of moderately significant bi- or tricompartmental disease, contralateral Outerbridge Type 4 (52) changes on the femoral or tibial weight-bearing surfaces **(Fig 43.5-19)**, an absent anterior cruciate ligament, and greater than 10 degrees of varus deformity for medial compartment disease. An absent anterior cruciate ligament usually indicates more significant contralateral compartment changes precluding UKA. Patellofemoral disease is not a contraindication to UKA unless the patient has patellofemoral symptoms (53,54).

■ CAUSES OF FAILURES

Failures of UKA have many etiologies. In a series of 31 failed UKA cases published in 1997 (41), 35% had medial–lateral mismatch **(Fig 43.5-20)**, 19% had failed uncemented ingrowth **(Fig 43.5-21)**, 16% had malaligned tibial components **(Fig 43.5-22)**, 10% had failed cemented femoral components **(Fig 43.5-23)**, 10% had a failed tibial polyethylene

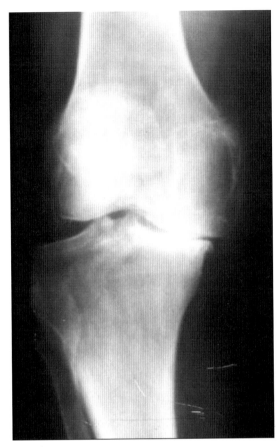

Fig 43.5-18. Radiograph shows Ahlback IV changes with medial–lateral subluxation.

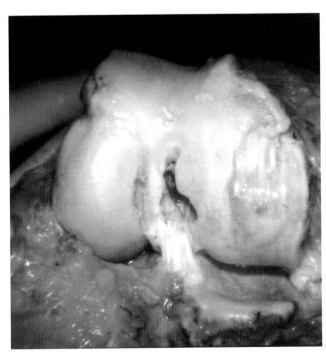

Fig 43.5-19. Outerbridge type 4 changes on the lateral femoral condyle with "kissing lesion" indicating medical–lateral instability.

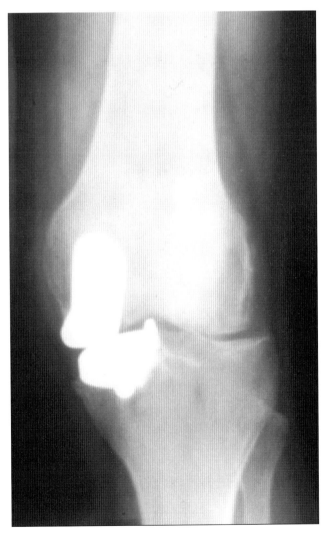

Fig 43.5-20. Medial–lateral mismatch of femoral and tibial components.

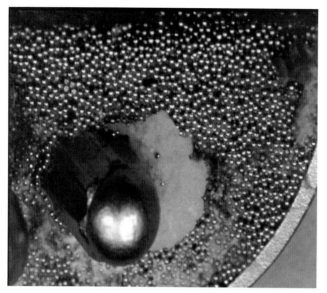

Fig 43.5-21. Lack of ingrowth into tibial base plate with failure of fixation.

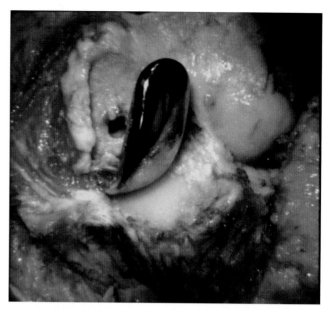

Fig 43.5-23. Failed cemented femoral component.

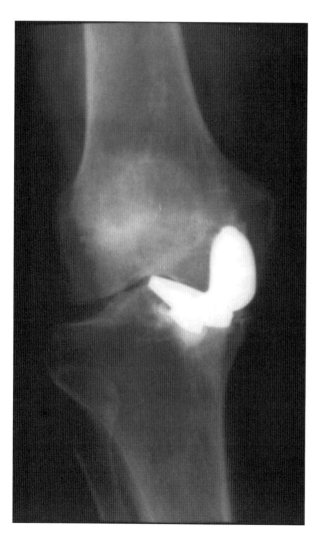

Fig 43.5-22. Malaligned tibial component.

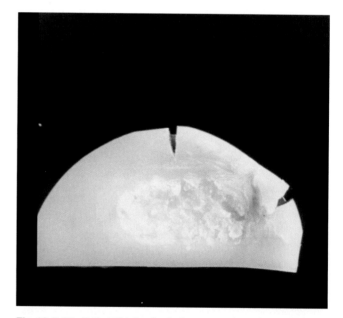

Fig 43.5-24. Failed tibial polyethylene component wear.

component because of wear **(Fig 43.5-24)**, and 10% had progressive, contralateral compartment osteoarthritis (Fig. 43.5-13). Refinements in UKA component design, however, have occurred during the past 30 years. It is important to have articulating geometry, which avoids increased surface-contact stresses. The articular surfaces between the components should have the ability to allow minor variations in medial and lateral placement of the components and afford the ability to accept a minor difference in rotational malignment during flexion and extension of the knee. Thus, the component articular surfaces cannot be severely constrained, nor should they be "flat on flat." Furthermore, it is imperative to use a system with a wide femoral component that will obviate medial–lateral mismatch (51). Finally, during placement of the prosthesis, the instrumentation used should not require significant resection of either femoral or tibial bone, because if significant bone resection occurs, revision arthroplasty will be difficult (39,40).

■ TECHNIQUE

The minimally invasive, limited-incision surgical technique involves an approximately 6- to 8-cm medial incision **(Fig 43.5-25)** for a medial compartment UKA extending from 1.5 cm inferior to the joint line approximately 5 to 6 cm superior along the medial edge of the patella. If possible, incising superiorly into more than 5 to 6 mm of the vastus medialis insertion should be avoided. The medial compartment is exposed, and a 1/4-inch Steinman pin is drilled into the intercondylar notch to retract the patella laterally and to facilitate what often is a very difficult exposure. Two self-retaining retractors are then used to help expose the medial compartment. An external tibial cutting jig is applied to the leg, and no more than 4 to 5 mm of bone is removed from the tibia. Bone should be removed laterally right up to the insertion of the anterior cruciate ligament. The tibial cut surface must be perpendicular to the shaft of the tibia, and most systems allow a 3 to 5 degree posterior inclination of the tibial component. The femoral

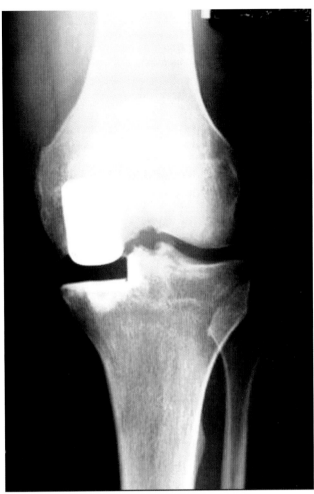

Fig 43.5-26. Postoperative view of a well-positioned, cemented unicompartmental knee arthroplasty.

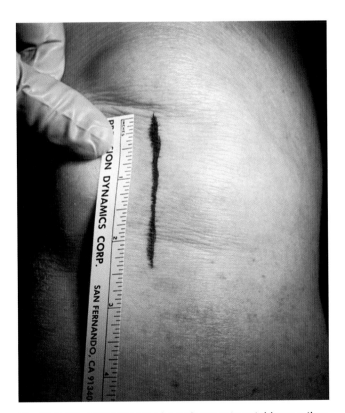

Fig 43.5-25. Minimally invasive unicompartmental knee arthroplasty incision.

surface is measured with a sizing device, and a cutting jig is applied to the femur. After cutting, burring, or rasping the surface down to cancellous bone, depending on the system being used, the trial femoral component is fit to the joint surface, and the fin slots are burred if necessary, and the femoral peg hole is drilled to accept the femoral component. It should be emphasized that regardless of the component and instrumentation system, the femoral component should always be lateralized on the femur to avoid medial–lateral mismatch during extension and flexion. Femoral components that are too small and/or narrow if medialized tend to maltrack and may sublux during extension, especially if a smaller, narrower tibial component is chosen for implantation. After preparing the bony cut surfaces with multiple drill holes pulse lavage, and drying, as has been recommended for TKA (55), the components should be cemented simultaneously, checked for appropriate tracking throughout flexion and extension, and the knee placed in full extension as the cement hardens. Care must be taken to make certain that all cement is removed from the joint despite the limited exposure afforded by this technique.

A hemovac drain should be placed before fascial and skin closure and a soft dressing placed. Most patients are discharged 24 to 48 hours after this procedure and use a cane for the first 2 weeks **(Fig 43.5-26)**.

■ CONCLUSION

Unicompartmental arthroplasty is a successful procedure in a moderately active, older patient with strictly unicompartmental pain who understands that the prosthesis is not going to last forever. It also is a reasonable procedure to perform in an elderly patient who is unable to medically tolerate a TKA. Limited incision techniques work well with appropriate instrumentation. The selection of prosthetic device should be based on logical design principles and tested biomechanical rationale. Remember that despite newer techniques of implantation, better instrumentation, and updated prosthetic devices, a UKA is still simply a UKA. The indications for this procedure are significantly different from those for a TKA.

The single most important factor for the success of this operation—and the most difficult factor to ascertain—is appropriate patient selection. A well-performed UKA in the wrong patient will eventually fail.

■ REFERENCES

1. McKeever DC. Tibial plateau prosthesis. *Clin Orthop*. 1960;18:86.
2. MacIntosh DL. Arthroplasty of the knee in rheumatoid arthritis using the hemiarthroplasty prosthesis. In: Chapcal G, ed. *Synovectomy and arthroplasty in rheumatoid arthritis: Second International Symposium*. Stuttgart: Theime Medical Publishers; 1967:79.
3. MacIntosh DL, Hunter GA. The use of the hemiarthroplasty prosthesis for advanced osteoarthritis and rheumatoid arthritis of the knee. *J Bone Joint Surg Am*. 1972;54:244.
4. Friedman M. The unispacer. *Arthroscopy*. 2003;19(10):120.
4a. Sisto D, Mitchell I. Unispacer arthroplasty of the knee. *J Bone Joint Surg Am*. 2005;87:1706.
5. Skolnick M, Peterson LF, Combs JJ. Polycentric knee arthroplasty—a two-year follow-up. *J Bone Joint Surg Am*. 1975;57:1033.
6. Skolnick M, Coventry M, Ilstrup D. Geometric total knee arthroplasty: a two-year follow-up study. *J Bone Joint Surg Am*. 1976;58:731.
7. Bae D, Guhl J, Keane S. Unicompartmental knee arthroplasty for single compartment disease. Clinical experience with an average 4 year follow-up study. *Clin Orthop*. 1983;176:233.
8. Laskin R. Unicompartmental tibiofemoral resurfacing arthroplasty. *J Bone Joint Surg Am*. 1978;60:182.
9. Cameron H, Hunter G, Welsh R, et al. Unicompartmental knee replacement. *Clin Orthop*. 1981;160:109.
10. Insall J, Aglietti P. A five to seven year follow-up of unicondylar arthroplasty. *J Bone Joint Surg Am*. 1980;62:1329.
11. Insall J, Walker P. Unicondylar knee replacement. *Clin Orthop*. 1976;120:83.
12. Marmor L. The modular knee. *Clin Orthop*. 1973;94:242.
13. Marmor L. Results of single compartment arthroplasty with acrylic cement fixation. A minimum follow-up of two years. *Clin Orthop*. 1977;122:181.
14. Marmor L. Unicompartmental arthroplasty of the knee with a minimum of 10 year follow up. *Clin Orthop*. 1988;228:171.
15. Scott R, Cobb A, Ewald P, et al. Unicompartmental knee arthroplasty: 8 to 12 year follow-up with survivorship analysis. *Clin Orthop*. 1991;271:96.
16. Rand J, Ilstrup D. Survivorship analysis of total knee arthroplasty: cumulative rates of survival of 9,200 total knee arthroplasties. *L Bone Joint Surg*. 1991;73:397.
17. Hodge W, Chandler H. Unicompartmental knee replacement: a comparison of constrained and unconstrained designs. *J Bone Joint Surg*. 1992;74:877.
18. Heck D, Marmor L, Gibson A, et al. Unicompartmental knee arthroplasty: a multicenter investigation with long-term follow-up evaluation. *Clin Orthop*. 1993;286:154.
19. Cobb A, Kozinn S, Scott R. Unicondylar or total knee replacement: the patient's preference. *J Bone Joint Surg Br*. 1990;72:166.
20. Sisto D, Blazina M, Heskiaoff D, et al. Unicompartmental arthroplasty for osteoarthrosis of the knee. *Clin Orthop*. 1993;286:149.
21. Rougraff B, Heck D, Gibson Z. A comparison of tricompartmental and unicompartmental arthroplasty for the treatment of gonarthrosis. *Clin Orthop*. 1991;273:157.
22. Cartier A, Kozinn S, Scott R. Unicompartmental knee arthroplasty surgery. *J Arthroplasty*. 1996;11:782.
23. Gresalmer R. Unicompartmental osteoarthritis of the knee. *J Bone Joint Surg*. 1995;77:278.
24. Kennedy W. Unicompartmental total knee arthroplasty of the knee: postoperative alignment and its influence on overall results. *Clin Orthop*. 1997;221:278.
25. Tabor O, Tabor O Jr. Unicompartmental arthroplasty: a long-term follow-up study. *J Arthroplasty*. 1998;13:378.
26. Squire M, Callaghan J, Goetz D, et al. Unicompartmental knee replacements: a minimum 15 year follow-up study. *Clin Orthop*. 1999;367:51.
27. Bert J. 10-Year survivorship of metal backed unicompartmental arthroplasty. *J Arthroplasty*. 1978;13:901.
28. Svard U, Price A. Oxford medial unicompartmental knee arthroplasty: a survival analysis of independent series. *J Bone Joint Surg Br*. 2001;83:191.
29. Gioe T, Bert J, Killeen K, et al. Analysis of unicompartmental arthroplasty in a community-based implant registry. *Clin Orthop*. 2003;416:111.
30. Repicci J. Benefits and limitations of the unicondylar knee prosthesis. *J Orthopedics*. 2003;26:274.
31. Newman J, Ackroyd C, Shah N. Unicompartmental or total knee replacement. Five year results of a prospective randomized trial of 102 osteoarthritic knee with unicompartmental arthritis. *J Bone Joint Surg Br*. 1998;80:862.
32. Laurencin C, Zelicof S, Scott R, et al. Unicompartmental versus total knee arthroplasty in the same patient: a comparative study. *Clin Orthop*. 1991;273:151.
33. Rougraff B, Heck D, Gibson A. A comparison of tricompartmental and unicompartmental arthroplasty for the treatment of gonarthrosis. *Clin Orthop*. 1991;273:157.
34. Karpman R, Volz R. Osteotomy vs. unicompartmental prosthetic replacement in the treatment of unicompartmental arthritis of the knee. *Orthopedics*. 1982;5:989.
35. Broughton N, Newman J, Bailey R. Unicompartmental replacement and high tibial osteotomy for osteoarthritis of the knee. *J Bone Joint Surg Br*. 1986;68:447.
36. Weale A, Newman J. Unicompartmental arthroplasty and high tibial osteotomy for osteoarthrosis of the knee: a comparative study with 12 to 17 year follow-up period. *Clin Orthop*. 1994;302:134–137.
37. Bert J. Analysis of unicompartmental arthroplasty in a community based registry. Scientific exhibit presented at AAOS, Dallas, Texas, February 13, 2002.
38. Mcauley J, Engh G, Ammeen D. Revision of failed unicompartmental arthroplasty. *Clin Orthop*. 2001;392:279.

39. Lai C, Rand J. Revision of failed unicompartmental total knee arthroplasty. *Clin Orthop.* 1993;287:193.
40. Padgett D, Stern S, Insall J. Revision total knee arthroplasty for failed unicompartmental replacement. *J Bone Joint Surg Am.* 1991;73:186.
41. Bert J, Smith R. Failures of metal-backed unicompartmental arthroplasty. *Journal of the Knee.* 1997;4:41.
42. Bert J. Long term survivorship of revision unicompartmental arthroplasty. Submitted for publication, December 2004.
43. Lewold L. Revision total knee arthroplasty after unicompartmental arthroplasty vs. upper tibial osteotomy. *Acta Orthop Scand.* 1998;71.
44. Bert J. Universal intramedullary instrumentation for unicompartmental knee arthroplasty. *Clin Orthop.* 1991;271:79.
45. Bert J, Koeneman J. A comparison of the mechanical stability of various unicompartmental tibial components. *J Orthop.* 1994; 17:559.
46. Derosa R, Bert J, Warwick B, et al. Evaluation of all-ultra-high molecular weight polyethylene unicompartmental tibial component cement fixation mechanisms. *J Bone Joint Surg Am.* 2202; 84(suppl A):102.
47. Stern S, Becker M, Insall J. Unicondylar knee arthroplasty: an evaluation of selection criteria. *Clin Orthop.* 1993;286:143.
48. Bramby S, Thornhill T. Unicompartmental osteoarthrosis of the knee. In: Laskin RS, ed. *Controversies in total knee replacement.* London: Oxford University Press; 2001:285.
49. Laskin R. Unicompartmental knee replacement. *Clin Orthop.* 2001;392:267.
50. Ahlback S. Osteoarthrosis of the knee: a radiographic investigation. Thesis. Karolinska Institute, Stockholm, Sweden; 1968.
51. Scott R. Unicompartmental total knee arthroplasty. In: Insall, Scott, eds. *Surgery of the knee,* Vol. 1. Philadelphia: Churchill Livingston; 2001:1621.
52. Outerbridge R. The etiology of chondromalacia of the patellae. *J Bone Joint Surg Br.* 1961;43:752.
53. Cartier P, Sanouiller J, Grelsamer R. Unicompartmental knee arthroplasty surgery. *J Arthroplasty.* 1996;11:782.
54. Corpe R, Engh G. A quantitative assessment of degenerative changes acceptable in the unoperated compartment of knees undergoing unicompartmental replacement. *Orthopedics.* 1990; 13:319.
55. Bert J, McShane M. Is it necessary to cement the tibial stem in cemented total knee arthroplasty? *Clin Orthop.* 1998;356:73.

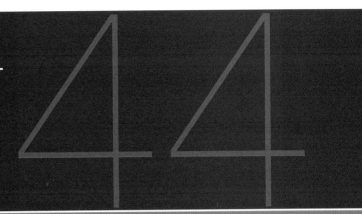

ANTERIOR CRUCIATE LIGAMENT RECONSTRUCTION WITH PATELLAR TENDON AUTOGRAFT: PRINCIPLES OF REHABILITATION

K. DONALD SHELBOURNE, MD, CAMIRON PFENNING, MD,
SCOTT E. LAWRANCE, MS, PT, ATC, CSCS

■ KEY POINTS

- The patellar ligament, more commonly referred to as the patellar tendon, is a strong, thick, fibrous band passing from the patella to the tibial tuberosity.
- The anterior cruciate ligament (ACL) provides stability against anterior stress applied to the tibia.
- The cruciate ligaments enable the knee to both roll and slide for maximum motion while still maintaining contact and stability.
- Most ACL injuries can be diagnosed with a careful patient history, emphasizing mechanism of injury, coupled with good physical examination technique. Diagnostic imaging or procedures usually are not necessary to establish the diagnosis of an ACL tear but can be useful when assessing menisci, subchondral bone, and other ligamentous structures.
- Although a variety of mechanisms can lead to an ACL tear, sports competition against another player that involves twisting, jumping, pivoting, cutting, and landing unpredictably, together with sudden changes in direction, exposes the ACL to injury.
- After an ACL tear, the patient will walk with a bent-knee gait if he or she is able to tolerate any weight-bearing activity. It also is common to observe that the patient will have difficulty lifting the leg onto the examining table.
- After examining the ACL, the other cruciate ligaments need to be assessed. Injury to the medial and/or lateral meniscus also is common when the ACL is torn, with a 69% incidence of meniscal injury after an acute ACL tear.
- If the diagnosis is still in question after a thorough history and a complete physical examination, the immediate approach involves reducing the athlete's pain and

swelling and then reevaluating a few days later. An ACL tear does not require immediate surgery; rather, it involves minimizing patient discomfort and restoring full range of motion, regardless of the ultimate treatment decision.

- With the appropriate rehabilitation process and long-term exercise program, many patients can maintain an active lifestyle with an ACL-deficient knee. This option is most appropriate for those individuals who do not participate in recreational sports activities or engage in other high-risk activities that involve twisting or rotational forces through the lower extremity.
- In athletes who choose nonoperative treatment or who want to complete their current season before reconstruction, it is crucial to evaluate the menisci before this type of therapy is allowed. A magnetic resonance imaging (MRI) evaluation is an excellent way to determine the status of the menisci.
- If surgery can be delayed without having episodes of instability, a preoperative rehabilitation program can be used and schedules adjusted to perform the surgery under more ideal conditions. This delay in surgery decreases postoperative complications.
- Postoperative rehabilitation begins in the operating room with placement of the patellar tendon graft. It is critical that full range of motion, including hyperextension, is achieved at this point to ensure that the graft has not been overtensioned, resulting in a captured joint that prevents full range of motion.
- Complications during rehabilitation are much easier to prevent than they are to treat. The patient needs to have a thorough understanding of the goals of each phase of rehabilitation.

This chapter focuses on ACL reconstruction with the patellar tendon autograft and rehabilitation for the ACL injury as well as the graft site. The patellar ligament, more commonly referred to as the patellar tendon, is a strong, thick, fibrous band passing from the patella to the tibial tuberosity.

■ BASIC SCIENCE

Anatomy

An understanding of normal knee anatomy is paramount when attempting ACL reconstruction and rehabilitation.

Bony Anatomy

The stability of the knee joint depends on the ligaments that connect the femur and the tibia as well as the surrounding muscles and their tendons. The knee consists of the tibiofemoral joint and the patellofemoral joint composed of three separate bones: (a) the femur superiorly, (b) the tibia inferiorly, and (b) the patella anteriorly. The bones are enclosed in the joint capsule, which is lined with synovium that produces synovial fluid to help protect and nourish the joints. The osseous structures involved in knee anatomy include the patella, the femoral condyles, and the tibial plateaus. The patella is a sesamoid bone that is wider at the proximal end than at the distal end and acts as a fulcrum to assist in extension of the quadriceps muscle. When the knee is extended and the quadriceps muscles are relaxed, the patella can be pushed both medially and laterally so that the underlying facets can be palpated.

Deep to the patellar tendon is the infrapatellar fat pad. The tibiofemoral joint has medial and lateral compartments, corresponding with the medial and lateral femoral condyles, which articulate with the medial and lateral tibial plateaus. In the patellofemoral joint, the patella articulates with the femoral trochlea only. The medial and lateral tibial plateaus are palpable just beneath their corresponding femoral condyles. Laterally, just below the tibial joint line, is the Gerdy tubercle, which is the attachment site for the iliotibial band.

Musculature

The musculature of the knee includes the quadriceps, sartorius, gracilis, and semitendinosus muscles. The quadriceps mechanism proximal to the patella consists of the vastus lateralis, rectus femoris, vastus intermedius, and vastus medialis. The vastus medialis obliquus, which is the most distal and medial part of the vastus medialis, consists of obliquely oriented fibers attached to the patella. Broad, fibrous medial and lateral patellar retinacula expand on both sides of the patella and attach to the iliotibial band laterally and to the vastus medialis obliquus medially. The quadriceps muscles function principally in extension, but the hamstrings are involved in the flexion mechanism. The sartorius, gracilis, and semitendinosus muscles help to protect the knee against rotatory and valgus stress.

Ligaments

Four major ligaments are involved in knee stability. The posterior cruciate ligament (PCL) provides stability against posterior stress applied to the tibia, and the ACL provides stability against anterior stress applied to the tibia. The lateral collateral ligament (LCL) provides lateral stability against varus stress, and the medial collateral ligament (MCL) provides medial stability against valgus stress. Although this chapter focuses primarily on ACL injuries, it is important to understand the interactions between all the ligaments of the knee joint (Fig 44-1).

The cruciate ligaments criss-cross within the center of the joint and join the femur and the tibia. The PCL originates on the lateral aspect of the medial femoral condyle and attaches behind the intercondylar area of the posterior surface of the tibia. When the knee is flexed and weight bearing, the PCL tightens and provides stabilization. On the other hand, the ACL originates on the tibial plateau both anterior and lateral to the medial tibial spine, and it inserts onto the medial aspect of the lateral femoral condyle. The ACL is composed of an anteromedial band and a posterolateral band, which are named based on their tibial attachment sites. When the knee is fully extended, the ACL is taut to prevent posterior displacement of the femur on the tibia and hyperextension of the knee joint. Medial stability is provided

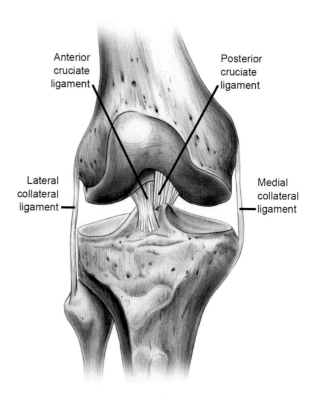

Fig 44-1. The knee joint and its major ligamentous structures.

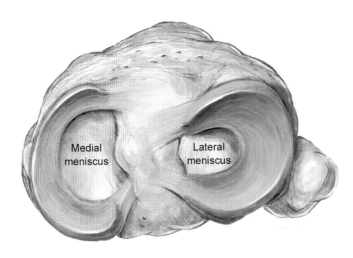

Fig 44-2. Superior view of the tibial plateau and menisci shows the size and shape of the lateral and medial menisci.

statically by the MCL. From anterior to posterior, the lateral structures of the knee are the iliotibial band, lateral capsule, popliteus, LCL, biceps femoris, and lateral head of the gastrocnemius. All these structures contribute to lateral stability. The superficial MCL runs from the medial epicondyle, crosses the joint line, and can be palpated medially, on the posterior half of the medial aspect knee. The deep MCL is not palpable as a discrete structure.

Menisci

The menisci are crescent-shaped, fibrocartilaginous structures that lie between the hyaline cartilage surfaces of the femur and the tibia. Inferiorly, the menisci attach to the tibia via the coronary ligaments. The lateral meniscus is nearly circular and covers more of the tibial articular surface than the medial meniscus does **(Fig 44-2)**.

Biomechanics of the Knee

The overall motion of the knee is controlled by interactions between ligaments, other supporting soft-tissue structures, and constraints of the articular surfaces. Unfortunately, when structures become damaged, the overall motion of the knee usually is altered. To understand injury mechanisms and to develop rehabilitation protocols for knee injuries, it is important to look at the basic biomechanics of the individual ligaments, the interaction between the ligaments, the role of the meniscus, and the functions of the patellofemoral joint.

The cruciate ligaments enable the knee to both roll and slide for maximum motion while still maintaining contact and stability. If knee flexion involved purely a sliding motion, then the femur would strike the posterior tibial plateau and limit flexion. Conversely, if knee flexion

involved only a rolling motion, then the femur would roll off the back of the tibia. Fortunately, the ACL and PCL enable the knee to perform important movements. Knee flexion is limited by a combination of ligaments as well as leg and thigh muscles, but extension is limited by the ligaments, the joint capsule posteriorly, and joint compression.

The ACL is the primary restraint against anterior tibial translational force, providing 85% of the anterior restraining force at 90 degree of flexion (1). The posterolateral bundle of the ACL is tight in extension, whereas the anteromedial bundle of the ACL in tight in flexion. The PCL provides 94% of restraint against posteriorly directed force at 90 degree of flexion. Together, the ACL and PCL are secondary stabilizers and provide some resistance to varus stress if the primary lateral structures have been disrupted.

The menisci are important for transmitting load across the knee and for distributing forces throughout the underlying articular cartilage. They increase the contact surface area between the round femoral condyles and the relatively flat tibial plateau on the medial side and the convex tibial plateau on the lateral side. When all or part of the meniscus is removed, the contact pressure between the femur and the tibial articular surfaces increases and may predispose patients to early joint surface wear (2). During normal walking, which causes knee-joint forces of two- to fourfold normal body weight, menisci bear 40% to 50% of the total load transmitted across the joint in extension and 85% of the compressive load at 90 degree of flexion. On the medial side, load is shared equally between the medial meniscus and the articular surfaces. The lateral meniscus, however, bears most of the lateral-side load transmission, making degenerative changes after a partial lateral meniscectomy more common than after a partial medial meniscectomy.

Depending on the type of activity, the forces across the patellofemoral joint vary. The patellofemoral joint increases the lever arm and, therefore, increases the efficiency of the quadriceps muscle. This joint also allows the quadriceps force to be transmitted around an angle without significant loss of energy from friction. In addition, the patellofemoral joint provides functional knee stability under load with the patella's opposing force against the distal femur.

■ CLINICAL EVALUATION

History

When clinically evaluating an athlete with an acute knee injury, it is helpful to obtain a clear and concise history and to perform a thorough and accurate physical examination. Most ACL injuries can be diagnosed with a careful history, emphasizing mechanism of injury, coupled with good physical examination techniques. Diagnostic imaging or procedures usually are not necessary to establish the diagnosis of an ACL tear but can be useful when assessing menisci, subchondral bone, and other ligamentous structures. In addition to listening to the athlete's recollection of the injury, encourage the athlete to include information such as his or her year in school, position played in the particular sport, additional athletic activities, and future athletic aspirations; this information will help to guide treatment decisions (3).

Although a variety of mechanisms can lead to an ACL tear, sports competition against another player that involves twisting, jumping, pivoting, cutting, and landing unpredictably, together with sudden changes in direction, expose the ACL to injury. Fetto and Marshall (4) described two basic mechanisms of injury: (a) a valgus force applied to a flexed knee with the leg in external rotation, and (b) hyperextension of the knee with the leg internally rotated. The incidence of ACL injury is higher among people who participate in high-risk sports, such as basketball, football, skiing, and soccer. For example, a college football player may have as much as a 16% chance of an ACL injury during his 4-year career (5). On the contrary, ACL tears are uncommon in hockey, because these athletes do not fix their feet to the ground. When comparing all sports, noncontact mechanisms account for more ACL tears than contact mechanisms do (6).

An ACL injury typically is described as a major, unexpected, traumatic event that forced the athlete to the ground. Athletes immediately indicate that they experienced a "big-deal" injury, and few will be able to continue participation in the game secondary to pain, swelling, and instability of the knee. In fact, in most cases, the officials will pause the game, and the athlete will require assistance getting off the field. Generally, no reason exists to perform a knee examination on the playing field; it is more important to recognize the typical patterns of injury to further direct evaluation and treatment.

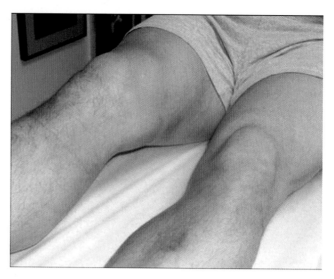

Fig 44-3. The patient's knee after an acute anterior cruciate ligament injury usually will develop a hemarthrosis and will lack full extension.

Frequently, an athlete will describe the injury as the sensation of hearing or feeling a "pop" when the knee "came apart" or "gave away." If evaluated within the first 12 hours after injury, the athlete often will have a hemarthrosis along with difficulty in weight-bearing activities. An athlete with an ACL injury likely will have difficulty achieving full knee extension, because the ACL stump does not fit in the intercondylar notch. The majority of knees that have a traumatic hemarthrosis (i.e., an intra-articular accumulation of blood in the joint) will have injury to the ACL (Fig 44-3) (7).

Most ACL injuries will be diagnosed based on the history described above. It is important, however, to broaden your knowledge about the minority of patients who may have atypical presentations. Some patients may suffer an ACL injury secondary to less significant trauma and only have a minimal hemarthrosis. Athletes with chronic ACL deficiency may describe intermittent locking or may explain situations involving multiple giving-way episodes before their most recent injury that prompted medical care. For these patients with a history of other knee injuries, it is important to delve further into their history to establish an accurate diagnosis before jumping immediately to a surgical procedure.

Physical Findings

Examination of a knee injury can be guided by the history to confirm the suspected diagnosis. After an ACL tear, the patient will walk with a bent-knee gait if he or she is able to tolerate any weight-bearing activity. The patient also commonly will have difficulty lifting the leg onto the examining table. After examining the patient's gait, both lower extremities must be entirely exposed and well supported beyond the heel to allow an accurate examination. Before examining the injured knee, the physician should obtain a baseline for comparison by first examining the uninjured knee, which also helps to gain the patient's confidence.

The athlete must be comfortable and relaxed during the examination. The Lachman test, which is the most reliable and reproducible examination method to confirm an ACL injury, should be performed first (8,9). If the Lachman test is performed correctly in an acute setting, it has a sensitivity of 87% to 98% for detecting an ACL tear. Allowing the hip to rotate externally and supporting the knee in slight flexion will facilitate relaxation. One hand should firmly grasp the femur while the other is positioned below the joint, grasping the tibia to allow anterior translation. A quick, firm motion pulling the tibia anteriorly while stabilizing the femur by pushing it posteriorly allows the examiner to appreciate the degree of translation and the quality of the end point. Increased translation and a soft or absent end point compared with an uninjured knee can confirm the ACL injury. It is more important to interpret the Lachman test as positive or negative than it is to quantify the amount of laxity **(Fig 44-4)**.

To perform the Lachman test correctly, the physician must practice and perform numerous knee examinations. Many inexperienced physicians will immediately begin the knee examination with the anterior drawer test (i.e., translation of the tibia forward relative to the femur with the knee in 90 degree of flexion). Torg et al. (10), however, found this test to be positive in only 50% of ACL injuries if the posterior horn of the medial meniscus and/or the posterior capsule were intact. The Lachman test, when performed accurately, is the physical diagnostic test of choice, but the flexion–rotation drawer test also can be performed acutely. This test also is less anxiety-provoking for the patient compared with the classic pivot–shift test. While the physician cradles the calf and flexes the knee, a posteriorly directed force on the tibia will cause reduction of the tibia as the femur rotates from an externally rotated position **(Fig 44-5)**.

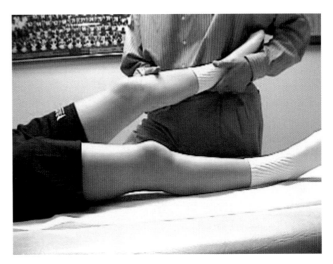

Fig 44-5. Flexion–rotation drawer examination: While cradling the calf and flexing the knee, a posteriorly directed force on the tibia will cause reduction of the tibia as the femur rotates from an externally rotated position.

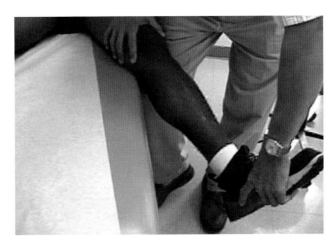

Fig 44-6. Medial collateral ligament testing is performed with the patient's leg relaxed and the thigh supported by the examination table. The examiner holds the foot with the lower leg off the side of the table and gently stresses the medial collateral ligament at 30° of knee flexion.

After examining the ACL, the MCL, LCL, and PCL need to be assessed for injury. Testing of the MCL and LCL is performed with the patient's leg relaxed and the thigh supported by the table. The physician holds the foot with the lower leg off the side of the table and gently stresses the MCL at 30 degree of flexion **(Fig 44-6)**. When testing the LCL, the examiner places a hand behind the knee and uses the other hand to hold the patient's foot and ankle to stress the LCL at 30 degree of flexion **(Fig 44-7)**. Compared to ACL injuries, PCL injuries are not as common or as disabling but are frequently misdiagnosed. The posterior drawer test is the most sensitive and specific for PCL injury (11). The posterior drawer is performed with the patient lying supine. The hip is flexed approximately

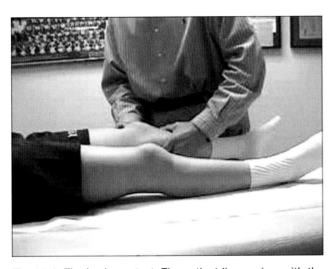

Fig 44-4. The Lachman test. The patient lies supine, with the heels fully supported on the table. External rotation and heel support are used to promote relaxation, which also allows the examiner to obtain a more accurate result.

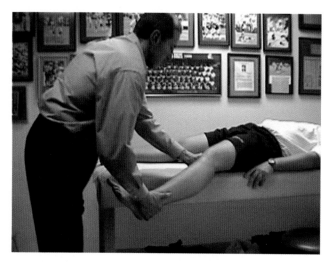

Fig 44-7. Lateral collateral ligament testing is performed with the patient's leg relaxed and the thigh supported by the examination table. The examiner places a hand behind the knee for support. The examiner's other hand holds the outside of the patient's foot and ankle to stress the lateral collateral ligament at 30° of flexion.

45 degrees, and the foot rests firmly on the evaluating surface. The examiner sits lightly on the patient's forefoot to stabilize the leg. The proximal calf muscles are cradled in the examiner's fingers both medially and laterally, with the thumbs resting on the tibial articular landmarks on either side of the patellar tendon. The amount of anterior tibial plateau projecting anterior to the femoral condylar surface is evaluated by direct palpation. The proximal tibia is pushed straight posteriorly with a firm and smooth motion, and the change in alignment of the tibial plateau in reference to the femoral condyles is evaluated **(Fig 44-8)**.

Injury to the medial and/or lateral meniscus is common when the ACL is torn, with a 69% overall incidence of meniscal injury after an acute ACL tear (3). The classic "O'Donoghue terrible triad," which is described as an ACL, MCL, and medial meniscal tear, is an unusual clinical entity among athletes (12). In fact, a triad of ACL, MCL, and lateral meniscal tear is more common in athletes with a combined injury (13). Meniscal trauma frequently occurs in association with ACL injury, but joint-line tenderness with an acute ACL tear does not necessarily indicate meniscal tears (14).

Imaging

Even though the diagnosis of an ACL injury usually can be established with the combination of a history and physical examination, four plain-film radiographic views are recommended for further assessment. Our routine examination includes a Rosenberg posteroanterior weight-bearing view in 45 degree of flexion (15), bilateral lateral views with 60 degree of knee flexion, and bilateral Merchant patellofemoral views (16). The Rosenberg view is used as a standard technique to better evaluate joint-space narrowing compared with an anteroposterior view. In addition, the posteroanterior view provides an accurate method for evaluating the intercondylar notch width of the femur. We have shown that the incidence of ACL tears is related to notch width as measured radiographically and have confirmed the correlation between our radiographic measurement and our measurement intraoperatively in a series of patients (17,18). We found no significant differences in the ACL tear rates between men and women with notch widths of equal size. Women, however, do tend to have narrower notch widths, which is a possible explanation for why the initial ACL tear rate is higher for women than for men (18).

Most often, plain-film radiographs of patients with an acute ACL injury are normal. In some patients, however, a Segond fracture (i.e., an avulsion fracture from the lateral capsule tearing off the tibia) is seen.

Unfortunately, many MRIs are ordered after an acute knee injury without any proven indication. The accuracy of diagnosing an ACL tear by MRI is high (19), but MRI is not necessary because of the dependability and precision of the history and physical examination. Management rarely is altered by MRI findings, but occasionally, the imaging may influence treatment decisions. At the time of an acute ACL injury, a displaced bucket-handle meniscal tear is uncommon. However, MRI can be useful in the chronic setting, when a patient cannot extend his or her knee after a new giving-way episode, in which a displaced bucket-handle meniscal tear is more common. In addition, MRI can be helpful when a meniscal injury is suspected in a skeletally immature athlete or when an athlete with a likelihood of future meniscal injury desires to return to play with a knee brace. Finally, in patients with chronic ACL deficiency, an MRI can be used to determine the etiology of extension loss.

Decision Making

If the diagnosis is still in question after a thorough history and a complete physical examination, the immediate approach involves reducing the athlete's pain and swelling and then reevaluating the knee a few days later. This approach often will avoid unnecessary, expensive diagnostic tests, such as MRI, examination under anesthesia, or arthroscopy. Fortunately, an acute ACL tear does not require immediate surgery; rather, involves minimizing patient discomfort and restoring full range of motion, regardless of the ultimate treatment decision. The only reason for doing acute ACL surgery would be when the lateral-side structures are injured, because no reliable reconstructive procedures exist for chronic lateral instability.

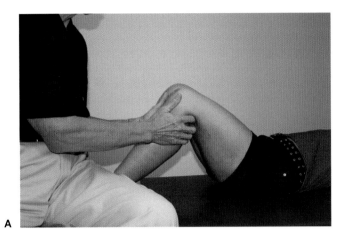

A

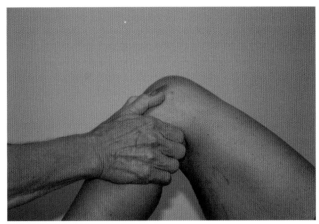

B

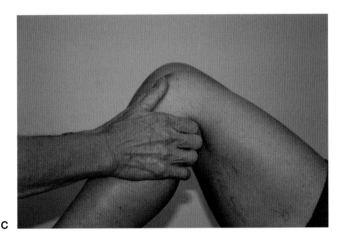

C

Fig 44-8. Posterior drawer examination. **A:** The hip is flexed, and the examiner sits lightly on the patient's forefoot to stabilize the leg. The examiner palpates the hamstring muscles to make sure the muscles are relaxed. **B:** The proximal calf muscles are cradled in the examiner's fingers, and the thumbs rest on the tibial articular landmarks on either side of the patellar tendon. **C:** The proximal tibia is pushed straight posteriorly with a firm and smooth motion, and the change in alignment of the tibial plateau in reference to the femoral condyles is evaluated.

■ TREATMENT

Although most individuals who sustain an ACL tear are active in some type of sports activity, their expectations after injury are very broad, depending on their stage of life. Adolescents and younger adults most often want to return to their preinjury sport or level of activity and are unable to do so with an unstable knee. Many older adults, however, may be willing to modify their activities to avoid further injury and, thus, the need for surgical intervention.

Nonoperative Treatment

Reconstruction of the ACL is an elective procedure for most individuals. With the appropriate rehabilitation process and long-term exercise program, many patients can maintain an active lifestyle with an ACL-deficient knee. This option is most appropriate for those individuals who do not partici-pate in recreational sports activities or engage in other high-risk activities that involve twisting or rotational forces through the lower extremity.

The natural history of a knee with an ACL injury is important to consider when determining whether a patient is an appropriate candidate for nonoperative treatment. We have found, as have other investigators, that younger, school-aged athletes with an untreated ACL injury will not be able to participate in most sports without an increased rate of the knee giving way and, thus, are at risk for significant intra-articular damage (20,21). Individuals who have multiple giving-way episodes have a high incidence of subsequent symptomatic meniscal and chondral injuries, with premature degeneration of the joint (22,23). Older patients have a less clearly defined course. In these patients, nonoperative treat-ment revolves around rehabilitation of presenting symptoms along with activity modification and a dedicated exercise program that maintains good knee function.

Although most school-aged athletes should undergo ACL reconstruction, there is a group, most often because of skeletal immaturity, that will not undergo ACL reconstruction once the knee has returned to a quiescent state. In this group, patient education and avoidance of high-risk sports are criti-cal. Following return of normal range of motion and strength, the athlete often receives a functional knee brace—with a warning that it will not prevent a giving-way episode if he or she returns to cutting and pivoting activities. Previously, knees of preadolescent athletes were stabilized by performing extra-articular reconstructions or primary repair of the ACL, thus avoiding open tibial and femoral growth plates and the poten-tial complication of growth disturbance. These procedures have not been shown to have better long-term results than those with nonoperative treatment (21,24). Therefore, we feel it is best to wait until the athlete has reached a level of skeletal maturity that allows intra-articular reconstruction when the risk of growth disturbance is minimal.

We use Tanner staging (25), allowing athletes to compare themselves to a series of drawings, along with menstrual history, recent growth history, height of the parents, and serial radiographs demonstrating blurring of the physes to determine when reconstruction is safe. The characteristics of Tanner stages 3 and 4 include the onset of menses, slowing of the preadolescent growth spurt, and radiographs demonstrating blurring of the physes. It is safe to proceed with an intra-articular reconstruction, with little fear of growth disturbance, as long as the procedure is performed so that bony blocks and fixation are not placed across the physes. This approach to surgery may result in the athlete missing one or two seasons of competition (usually at the junior-high level), but most patients usually are compliant with this plan, thus avoiding additional chondral and meniscal injuries. Our results using this criterion and performing an autogenous bone–patellar–bone reconstruction have resulted in no growth abnormalities and excellent clinical results (26).

For athletes who choose nonoperative treatment or who want to try to complete their current season before reconstruction, it is crucial to evaluate the menisci before allowing this course. Magnetic resonance imaging is an excellent way to determine the status of the menisci, because it is noninvasive and does not require ionizing radiation. If repairable meniscal tears are demonstrated, we advise the athlete not to return to play and, instead, to undergo ACL reconstruction at the time of meniscal repair because of the greater likelihood of meniscal healing and the prevention of further instability episodes. If no meniscal damage is present and full range of motion and strength have returned, we allow athletes to return to play if they are already involved in a low-risk sport or they play at a low-risk position in their sport (i.e., lineman in football) and it is their final year of competition. The risks must be discussed with the athlete and the family, with the stipulation that if the knee gives out, the athlete must stop participation. These situations are rare, however, and should be treated on a case-by-case basis.

As of this writing, no study has demonstrated that bracing an ACL-deficient knee will prevent episodes of instability when the athlete returns to cutting and pivoting sports, but several studies have shown a decrease in anterior tibial translation at low levels of force. If the athlete and family decide that they do not want to proceed with ACL reconstruction, it must be understood that activity modification (i.e., avoiding twisting, cutting, and deceleration activities) will be necessary to prevent giving-way episodes. If the athlete attains and maintains full range of motion and at least 90% strength of the contralateral lower-extremity strength, low-risk sports, such as running, bicycling, and swimming, can be performed.

Nonoperative treatment of an ACL injury can be successful if the patient is willing to modify his or her lifestyle to avoid additional giving-way episodes. For many patients, this is difficult to accomplish. Bonamo et al. (27) found that despite a regimented strengthening program, including sport-specific exercises, 40% of 79 recreational athletes who sustained an ACL tear and elected to have nonoperative treatment had to modify their athletic activity significantly to avoid giving-way episodes, but only 9 patients (11%) demonstrated excellent results. Hawkins et al. (20) and Andersson et al. (28) similarly found that 75% to 80% of prospectively followed, ACL-deficient patients who were treated nonoperatively could not return to level I or II sports activities, although most could participate in some lower-risk sports. In fact, Daniel et al. (29) found that an athlete's inability to return to sports is what brings that athlete to surgical treatment. Others have found that even with a mild grade of instability or with a patient who is relatively sedentary, half will fare poorly with nonoperative treatment (30). Both Warren (31) and Daniel et al. (29) found that the outcome of nonoperative treatment worsens as the severity of laxity increases, particularly in those who continue to participate in high-risk sports. Finally, studies do confirm that patients with chronic anterior instability develop meniscal tears (usually medial) with greater frequency and, in addition, are more likely to have chondral injuries compared with those having acute ACL injury.

Operative Indications

Although ACL reconstruction is an elective procedure, we advocate performing a reconstruction for those individuals who wish to maintain an active lifestyle involving high-risk sports, such as basketball or soccer. In addition, we advocate reconstruction for younger patients, regardless of lifestyle, because of the increased risk of future meniscal or chondral damage in the involved knee.

Surgical Technique

The procedure that is selected for ACL reconstruction must meet several criteria. It must have a high rate of successfully restoring normal stability and full motion, including hyperextension. Primary repair of the ACL by suturing together the ends of the torn ligament has not resulted in predictable stability and, thus, has been essentially abandoned (32). Thus, reconstruction of the native ACL has become the treatment of choice. Autogenous tissue that can be used includes patellar tendon (with bone attached both proximally and distally) and hamstring tendons, along with less frequently and more historically used tissues such as the iliotibial band and meniscus. Allograft tissue, sterilely prepared, also is used and is attractive to some surgeons, because they believe that the morbidity associated with autogenous patellar tendon harvest is reduced. Synthetic materials, such as Dacron and Gore-Tex (W.L. Gore and

Associates, Inc., Flagstaff, AZ), have been used in the past but now are of mostly historical interest, because multiple studies have shown unacceptably high rates of long-term failure as well as other complications secondary to wear of the material (33,34).

The ACL reconstruction technique performed by the senior author (K.D.S.) has been described in detail elsewhere (35). A medial miniarthrotomy is used, because we believe this procedure offers a reproducible method for obtaining excellent clinical results. The following discussion provides highlights of this technique, emphasizing several technical points that are crucial to the success of any ACL reconstructive procedure.

Impingement of the ACL graft within the intercondylar notch is one cause of limited extension and possible graft failure (36). Performing an adequate notchplasty is critical, because the space available for the native ACL may not be great enough for the 10-mm patellar tendon graft. Notch enlargement so that 10 mm exist between the lateral border of the PCL and the lateral wall of the notch will prevent lateral impingement of the graft.

The creation of bony tunnels in the tibia and femur independent of one another reduces the likelihood of tunnel placement error. Historically, the tibial tunnel has been placed anteriorly to reduce graft elongation with knee flexion. Anterior placement, however, can lead to graft failure and lack of full extension postoperatively because of notch impingement during knee extension (36,37). Placement of the tibial tunnel is illustrated **Figure 44-9.**

Correct placement of the femoral tunnel is technically the most difficult and clearly the most important aspect. Malposition of this tunnel is a common cause of failure after reconstruction (38). It is important to place the tunnel as deep in the notch as possible so that after reaming, 1 to 2 mm

of bone remain posterior to the tunnel. The tunnel should be positioned so that the graft will lie adjacent to the lateral border of the PCL. After reaming both the tibial and femoral tunnels, a straight guide pin should pass easily through the tibial tunnel, across the knee, and into the femoral tunnel of the knee in 30 degree of flexion. This step confirms correct placement of the tunnels after independently determining their location.

We use a polyethylene button to secure the sutures that have been placed through the bone plug. Along with the advantage of having the entire bony tunnel occupied by a bone plug, the buttons offer a distinct advantage when tensioning the graft. Adjustments in tension can be made a number of times if necessary after the knee is put through a full range of motion (including full flexion). This approach avoids the possibility of overtensioning the graft and capturing the joint. This form of fixation is weaker when tested against interference screws and staples in vitro (39), but very little tension should be on the graft when the knee is ranged from 0 to 120 degree. Patients rarely obtain greater motion before the end of 2 weeks, at which point bone healing in the tunnels should be progressing. We have not seen a failure of this fixation technique.

Other Techniques

It is important to mention that other techniques, including arthroscopic (40), arthroscopically assisted (24), and operating though the patellar tendon defect (41), can achieve excellent results. Clearly, the most important component in any of these techniques is correct, reproducible placement of the tibial and femoral tunnels. If correct placement cannot be achieved, then the reconstruction may be doomed to failure, regardless of what occurs during the postoperative period.

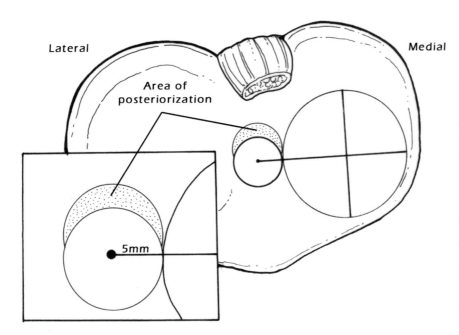

Fig 44-9. Tibial tunnel placement. A clock face is interposed on that portion of the medial tibial plateau that is visualized through the miniarthrotomy. The tunnel is drilled grossly. Then, the area of posteriorization is created for refinement of the position so that the back of the tunnel is just at the front slope of the tibial spine. A curette is used to position the medial and posterior wall of the tibial tunnel in the desired place. (From Shelbourne KD, Klootwyk TE. Two-incision mini-arthrotomy technique for anterior cruciate ligament reconstruction with autogenous patellar tendon graft. In: Vince KD, Fu FH, eds. *Technique in knee surgery*. Philadelphia: Lippincott Williams & Wilkins; 2001:73–82; with permission.)

Lateral   Medial

Area of posteriorization

5mm

Contralateral Patella Tendon Graft

When the patellar tendon graft is harvested from the contralateral knee, several minor changes in surgical routine are made. After drilling the femoral tunnel, the tourniquet is inflated on the contralateral leg, an incision is made, and the patellar tendon graft is harvested as described (35). The wound is infiltrated with 25 mL of 0.25% bupivacaine and is packed and compressed with an elastic bandage, after which the tourniquet is deflated. The donor patellar tendon graft is placed and secured in the ACL-reconstructed knee. The patella and tibial donor sites are packed with bone graft that is retrieved from drilling the tunnels. The patellar tendon defect is loosely closed, and both wounds are closed.

■ REHABILITATION

Our present philosophy concerning rehabilitation of ACL reconstructions has evolved significantly during the past 20 years by observing our patients and their results and then adapting our approach to improve the final outcome. Ideally, in a patient with an ACL-deficient knee undergoing an ACL reconstruction, we would like to end up with an ACL-stable knee that has full range of motion, strength, and normal function as compared to the opposite knee. Through our clinical research, we have discovered that our surgical technique, graft strength, and graft fixation are not limitations to early aggressive rehabilitation (42,43). We have adjusted our preoperative as well as our postoperative rehabilitation guidelines to minimize the postoperative morbidity so that the patient can obtain a good final result.

Many of the problems and complications that evolve from ACL reconstruction have resulted from two beliefs: (a) the need for immediate surgery following acute knee injuries, and (b) the belief that early postoperative limitations in knee motion, strengthening, and functional activities are necessary because of the weakness of both the ACL graft and the fixation of the graft. By analyzing our patients' results and documenting their nonprescribed activities during the early postoperative period, we have discovered that both of these beliefs are not true.

Stability results following ACL surgery are similar in acute and chronic cases, but acute surgery is associated with a much higher incidence of postoperative range-of-motion deficits (44). Therefore, if surgery can be delayed without the athlete having episodes of instability, we could allow a preoperative rehabilitation program and adjust family, social, and school schedules to perform the surgery under more ideal conditions. This delay in surgery has decreased postoperative complications and allowed the patient more control over the timing of their surgery.

During the early postoperative period, we have found that if certain problems are allowed to develop, those problems are difficult to eliminate in the long term. These problems are (a) lack of full knee hyperextension (equal to the opposite side) (45), (b) lack of good leg control, or (c)

hemarthrosis and swelling in the knee. Our present philosophy concerning rehabilitation is based on our close follow-up of all patients. Our goal remains to avoid short-term complications and to ensure no long-term deterioration of results.

In 1994, the senior author began using the patellar tendon graft from the contralateral knee for primary ACL reconstructive surgery. Previous, this method had been used for patients undergoing revision ACL surgery when the patellar tendon had already been harvested in the ACL-injured knee. We observed that patients recovered more quickly and more smoothly when the graft was harvested from the opposite knee (46). Therefore, we cautiously began using this approach with certain athletes who had a desire to return to sports quickly after surgery. Using the contralateral graft allows the rehabilitation to be divided between the two knees, with the ACL-reconstructed leg needing only to have postoperative swelling controlled and to regain full range of motion and the contralateral donor site needing only to rehabilitate the graft source extensor mechanism.

The remaining part of this chapter will present the rehabilitation programs that are used for both knees after ACL reconstruction with a contralateral patellar tendon graft and explain the philosophy for the rehabilitation. The principles presented can easily be applied to the use of an ipsilateral patellar tendon graft.

Preoperative Rehabilitation

It is essential that rehabilitation of an injury to the ACL begin immediately after the initial office evaluation. In an acutely torn ACL, a knee hemarthrosis and intra-articular inflammatory state occur. This hemarthrosis and inflammatory reaction cause the athlete to develop decreased range of motion and strength in the affected lower leg and also lead to gait compensations. Preoperative rehabilitation is divided into two areas of emphasis. First, the patient should have a resolution of swelling in the knee and the return of full range of motion of the knee and a normal gait. Second, the patient should be prepared mentally for the operative procedure and subsequent rehabilitation.

The initial emphasis after an acute injury to the ACL is to control and then decrease the amount of swelling and pain. We use the knee Cryo/Cuff (Aircast, Inc., Summit, NJ), which combines cold with compression **(Fig 44-10)**. The second area of rehabilitation after an acute ACL disruption is restoration of full range of motion, including full hyperextension equal to that of the noninjured knee. Obtaining full range of motion before surgery reduces the likelihood of motion problems postoperatively.

A habit of performing full hyperextension exercises is important to develop preoperatively so that the exercises are an easy part of the daily routine after surgery. Hyperextension is obtained by doing exercises such as towel stretches and prone hangs and using passive extension habits. Towel stretches are performed as a passive self-mobilization using

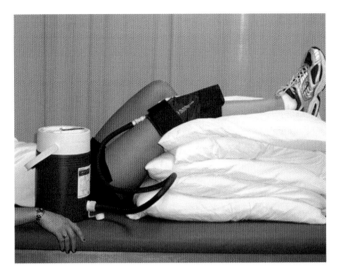

Fig 44-10. The Cryo/Cuff provides both compression and cold therapy to reduce swelling. When used in combination with elevation, this modality can effectively reduce any intra-articular effusion or hemarthrosis.

a towel looped around the midfoot. The ends of the towel are held in one hand, and the other hand is used to press and hold the thigh to the table. The towel is used to lift the heel of the affected lower extremity to end-range hyperextension by pulling the end of the towel upward, toward the shoulder, where it is held for a count of 5 seconds, and then the heel is lowered back to the table (Fig. 44-11). For patients who have decreased quadriceps muscle control, an active heel-lift exercise can easily be added to the towel stretch. The active heel lift is accomplished by contracting the quadriceps musculature after the towel stretch is performed, trying to keep the heel of the affected leg elevated without using the towel to hold it in the air. Following an acute injury, patients

often display some degree of quadriceps muscle inhibition, making a normal gait pattern difficult. It is important that the patient continue to try actively elevating the heel to the height of the passive stretch.

Passive extension in a seated position can be obtained by performing a heel prop on a towel or other type of bolster. The bolster should be high enough to elevate both the calf and the thigh of the effected extremity off the level of the table (Fig 44-12). A small weight can be added to the proximal tibia to facilitate full extension. The standing extension habit focuses on the patient's ability to stand on the affected leg with the knee in a fully hyperextended position. It is normal to stand on one leg with the knee locked into full hyperextension, and following an injury, patients tend to favor their injured leg and to stand on the nonaffected leg. To stand comfortably on one leg, patients must regain full hyperextension to rest on the passive joint structures. Forcing patients to stand on the affected lower extremity ensures that full hyperextension is regained and maintained (Fig 44-13).

Regaining knee flexion is achieved through performing wall slides and heel slides. Wall slides are performed while laying supine, with both legs extended up the wall. The heel of the injured leg is allowed to slide down the wall so that the knee is put into a flexed position, with assistance from the noninjured leg, until a stretch is felt in the knee. This is maintained for approximately 10 to 15 seconds, and then the leg is extended back to the starting position, where the quadriceps muscle is contracted and the leg is locked out for 5 seconds, after which the exercise is repeated. Heel slides are started once the patient has at least 90 degree of flexion. They are performed while in a long sitting position as the patient grasps the ankle of the involved extremity and passively pulls the leg into knee flexion. This is held for

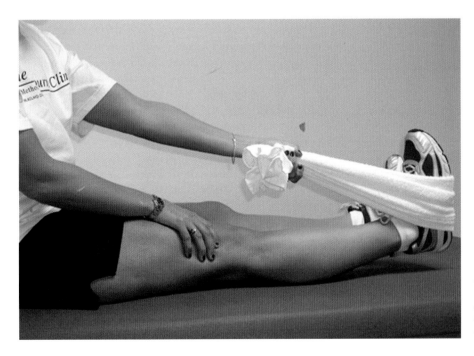

Fig 44-11. Towel stretch for knee extension. The towel is used to lift the heel of the affected lower extremity to end-range hyperextension by pulling the end of the towel upward and toward the shoulder.

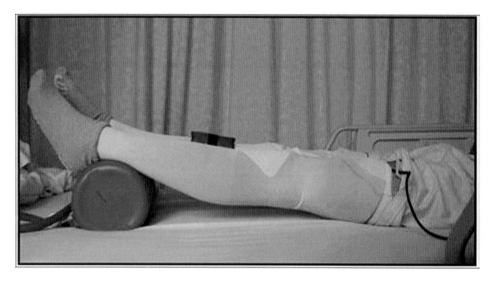

Fig 44-12. Heel-prop exercise: Both heels are propped on a bolster high enough so the thigh is elevated off the examination table or bed and the knee falls into passive hyperextension.

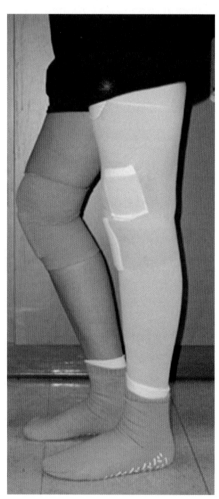

Fig 44-13. Standing with the knee locked out into hyperextension is a habit patients should use to keep from favoring the leg and to work continually on knee extension with everyday activities.

10 to 15 seconds, and then the leg is allowed to fully extend back to a resting position. Patients should be instructed to watch for compensation in the hip during these flexion exercises, because it is common for patients to substitute hip retraction in place of knee flexion when first trying to perform them. This should be avoided to maximize full flexion of the knee.

Gait training is performed for all patients, and full weight-bearing is allowed as tolerated initially. Crutches are used to assist ambulation if the patient exhibits an antalgic gait. Once a normal gait is obtained, patients are allowed to ambulate without the use of any assistive device or prophylactic braces. Once the patient has achieved full range of motion, good leg control, and a normal gait with minimal swelling, he or she can begin a low-impact strength and conditioning program until surgery. Appropriate activities include the use of a stationary bicycle, elliptical machine, or stair-stepping machine, along with closed kinetic chain strengthening exercises for the lower extremity, such as leg-press, hip-sled, and step-down exercises. Patient education regarding avoidance of high-risk activities that include twisting and rotation of the knee should be emphasized so that episodes of instability before surgery can be avoided.

We perform preoperative testing so that we can have objective measures for closely monitoring postoperative progress and for assisting the patient in setting performance goals. The testing includes KT2000 arthrometer (Medmetric, Inc., San Diego, CA) testing of anterior translation, isokinetic strength at 180 and 60 degree, and isometric leg-press tests. The single-leg-hop test is performed on the uninjured leg only. Strength is measured as a percentage of the involved lower extremity against that of the noninvolved lower extremity. Differences observed between the two lower extremities should be within 10% before surgery when using an ipsilateral patellar tendon graft source. If differences between the two legs are greater than 10%, a delay in surgery may be recommended so that the patient can work on strengthening the weaker lower extremity. When using a contralateral patellar tendon graft source, strength differences of greater than 10% are allowable as long as the patient has good quadriceps control and normal ambulation. These data are used again postoperatively, starting at 1 month, to compare the athlete's current status to his or her preoperative strength and function.

The overall goal of physical therapy during the preoperative phase is to control and decrease pain and swelling, to restore full range of motion, to aid in the resumption of a normal gait, and to initiate a strengthening program. By accomplishing these goals, the patient will present to the operating room for the reconstructive procedure with a normal-appearing and functioning knee except for the absence of the ACL.

Mental Preparation

The second important factor in the preoperative preparation for an ACL reconstruction is the mental preparation of the patient. The physician must explain the nature of the injury to the athlete and the family. The patient benefits from a detailed explanation of the operative procedure and the postoperative rehabilitation. The physical therapist also should review with the patient exactly what will be performed during all phases of the postoperative rehabilitation and how each phase of rehabilitation will be accomplished. The patient should approach the reconstructive procedure with a positive mental outlook. A "let's just get it over with" attitude is not acceptable and can lead to less-than-superior results even with perfect surgical and rehabilitation techniques. The patient should arrive in the operating room ready to go, with an attitude of looking forward to the reconstructive procedure and with an understanding of the postoperative rehabilitation.

Postoperative Rehabilitation

Phase I: Prevent hemarthrosis and regain ROM and leg control

Postoperative rehabilitation begins in the operating room after placement of the patellar tendon graft. It is critical that full range of motion, including hyperextension, is achieved at this point to ensure that the graft has not been overtensioned, resulting in a captured joint that prevents full motion. We strongly believe that the success of the operation mostly depends on correct graft placement and that the role of the physician and the physical therapist is to help guide the patient through the postoperative period to avoid complications without restricting the speed of the rehabilitation and the ultimate return to sports.

A local anesthetic is applied to the patellar tendon in the operating room. This allows for relatively painless flexion exercises to begin, permitting the tendon to remain at its full length. Later, heel-slide exercises and quadriceps muscle contractions during weight bearing and straight-leg raises will similarly draw the patella proximally and stretch the tendon to its full length. The combination of these two exercises decreases patellar tendon stiffness and contracture, which are processes that otherwise could occur after graft harvest and cause pain at the donor site.

Another important concept that we use, allowing the patient to fully participate in phase I rehabilitation, is the avoidance of narcotic medications during the perioperative period. Although occasional use of oral narcotic medication is needed for some patients, parenteral narcotics decrease a patient's ability to participate, both physically and cognitively, in their exercise program. With the use of a ketorolac infusion, continuous cold/compression therapy, supplemental oral nonnarcotic pain medication, and immediate motion, narcotics can be avoided altogether in most instances (47). A regimen focused on preventing rather than treating pain increases both patient participation and satisfaction. Finally, in the operating room, external drains are placed in the region of the fat pad. Along with leg elevation and cold/compression therapy, external drains decrease the incidence and volume of postoperative hemarthrosis. Patients are kept on 23-hour outpatient observation to prevent hemarthrosis and to allow initiation of immediate rehabilitation.

Before leaving the operating room, antiembolism stockings are placed on both lower extremities. A Cryo/Cuff is placed on the ACL-reconstructed knee, and an elastic sleeve with a frozen gel pack (Durasoft Patellar Tendon Wrap; DJ Orthopedics, Inc., Vista, CA) is placed over the contralateral donor side. Suprapatellar compression is not needed on the graft-donor knee, because graft harvest is an extra-articular procedure with no risk for an intra-articular effusion. As the patient arrives in the postoperative recovery area, the ACL-reconstructed leg is placed into a continuous passive-motion machine (CPM) set to move the knee from 0 to 30 degree. Continuous passive motion not only provides gentle motion but, more importantly, also elevates the lower leg. The graft-donor leg also is elevated on pillows to the same level to avoid increased strain on the lower back that can lead to lumbosacral pain. Both knees are elevated above the level of the heart **(Fig 44-14)**.

Phase-I rehabilitation continues on arrival to the outpatient observation unit, where targeted physical therapy begins. The patient and the family caregiver are provided with an exercise diary that outlines the rehabilitation exercises to be performed. Check marks or measurements are placed in boxes next to each exercise as they are completed. This practice aids in compliance by giving the patient a visual reference for specific exercises. Another additional benefit of performing preoperative rehabilitation is that the patient can become familiar with the postoperative exercises to be performed, thus reducing the chances of confusion or improper exercise technique.

We start with exercises for range of motion with CPM-assisted flexion for the ACL-reconstructed leg. The patient is instructed to maximally flex the CPM to 125 degree and then hold this position for a period of 3 minutes. The CPM is progressed to maximum flexion slowly and as tolerated by the patient. Heel slides are performed next for both the ACL-reconstructed leg and the contralateral donor-site leg. A yardstick is positioned next to the leg with the zero end lined up with the end of the heel. Next, the patient flexes the knee with the help of a towel looped under the thigh until further flexion becomes difficult. Terminal flexion is held for

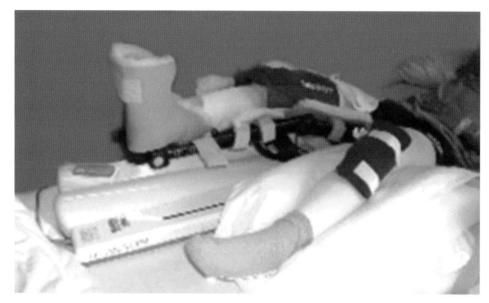

Fig 44-14. The anterior cruciate ligament–reconstructed leg is elevated in a continuous passive-motion machine, and the graft-donor knee is elevated on pillows.

1 minute. The number of centimeters that the heel has traveled is recorded; this number makes it easy for both the patient and the physical therapist to communicate changes in range of motion over the phone during the first week. Postoperative flexion in the contralateral graft-donor knee should be full and equal to preoperative measurements. The postoperative ACL-reconstructed leg flexion should immediately be approximately 110 to 120 degree.

Patients then prop both legs into extension with their heels resting on the Cryo/Cuff canister, allowing any hyperextension. A small, 2.5-pound weight is placed just distal to the incision on the ACL-reconstructed leg. This exercise is maintained for 10 minutes. Following heel props, our patients perform three to five knee-thunk exercises on each knee, in which they flex their knee to a height of several inches and then allow the leg to relax and "thunk" into hyperextension. Thunk exercises can be difficult for patients to perform on their ACL-reconstructed leg at first for fear of damaging the ACL reconstruction. Thus, thunk exercises typically are performed first on the graft-donor leg so that the patient understands how hyperextension feels. Five to 10 towel-stretch exercises are performed for each leg as described previously. Active heel-lift exercises are combined with the towel stretch to achieve good quadriceps control **(Fig 44-15)**.

Straight-leg raises for leg control are performed on both legs by having the patient first initiate a quadriceps muscle contraction and then focus on maintaining their knee locked out while lifting the leg so that the heel is 2 to 3 feet in the air above the mattress **(Fig 44-16)**. The Shuttle (Contemporary Design, Inc., Glacier, WA) is implemented on the graft-donor leg only, because it is meant to help regenerate and then strengthen the donor site. The Shuttle

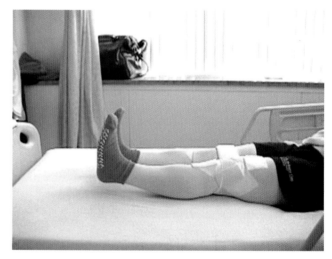

Fig 44-15. Active heel-lift exercise. The patient actively contracts the quadriceps muscle to bring the knee into hyperextension.

is a lightweight, low-resistance, portable leg-press machine **(Fig 44-17)**. Resistance is provided by the placement of weighted rubber cords, with each cord adding additional resistance. This weight is applied during both the concentric and the eccentric movements. Twenty-five repetitions with one cord (7 pounds) are then completed, with the emphasis on slow, controlled motion.

Following these exercises, the Cryo/Cuff and gel pack are applied to the ACL-reconstructed knee and graft-donor knee, respectively, and the ACL-reconstructed leg is placed back into the CPM set from 0 to 30 degree, with the graft-donor leg again propped up on pillows. The Cryo/Cuff water is changed once every waking hour to help control swelling and pain. The patient is confined to bed rest with the

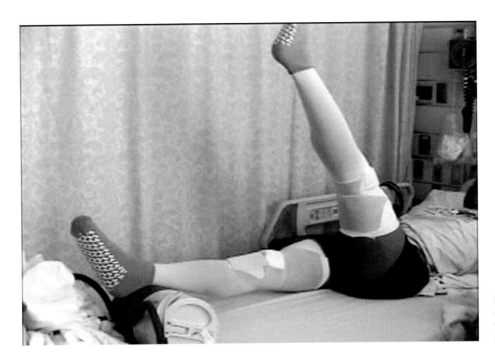

Fig 44-16. A patient with good quadriceps muscle control is able to lift the leg easily on the day of surgery.

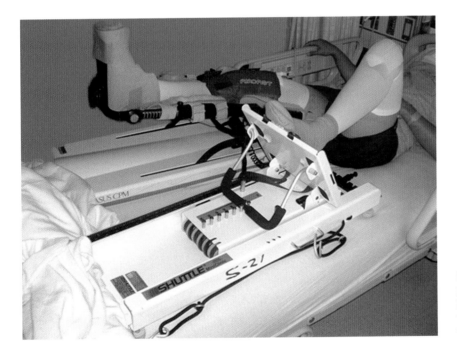

Fig 44-17. The Shuttle machine is a portable leg-press machine that provides low resistance. Patients use the machine for the contralateral leg to stimulate the graft-donor site immediately after surgery.

use of a portable urinal and bedpan if needed. The patient may ambulate at this time but does so at the risk of developing a hemarthrosis.

The drains are removed from both knees the following morning, and an identical set of exercises is performed. At the end of this session, the patient ambulates for the first time. This is accomplished carefully to avoid a fall. First, the patient sits at the edge of the bed, and when it is clear that he or she is steady and not dizzy, standing is encouraged. Standing is allowed for a few minutes, with the clinician close by to make sure that a vasovagal episode does not occur.

Next, the patient is instructed to shift his or her weight over to the ACL-reconstructed leg and to lock that leg into hyperextension with a quadriceps muscle contraction. The patient then ambulates to the door of the room and back, using small steps and focusing on a point high on the wall in the direction in which they are ambulating. Patients are allowed to ambulate fully weight bearing as tolerated; however, the use of crutches or a walker is allowed for patients who are unsteady on their feet and are at risk of falling.

Patients are released from the hospital the day after surgery. Before release from the hospital, however, each patient must demonstrate full extension of the ACL-reconstructed leg equal to that of the contralateral graft-donor leg, flexion of at least 110 degree on the ACL-reconstructed leg, full or near-full flexion of the graft-donor leg, the ability to lift both legs independently with quadriceps muscle contraction, the ability to ambulate independently, and a complete understanding of their home exercise program. Patients are advised that flexion may decrease from the previous day in the ACL-reconstructed knee, but the flexion that is obtained initially after surgery should return gradually after 2 to 3 days. In general, patients are counseled against pushing flexion too hard during this period, because maintaining full extension remains more important. Flexion in the contralateral graft-donor knee should remain full.

Following discharge from the hospital, patients are called at home daily for the first week to monitor progress and to answer any questions that might arise. The previous list of exercises is carried out five to six times daily with the exception of the Shuttle, which is used three times daily and on the contralateral donor leg only. Patients are instructed not to use the Shuttle during the first morning exercise session and, if the knee becomes too sore at the graft site or begins to lose flexion on daily measurements, to discontinue its use until further instructed by the physical therapist. Daily flexion measurements are made using the yardstick, measuring the distance the heel travels on both knees (Fig 44-18). Barring these events, patients are allowed to increase the number of repetitions that are performed during each session on a daily basis by up to 10 additional repetitions per day. When 100 repetitions become easy for the patient, an additional cord can be added for progressive resistance, but the number of repetitions is decreased to 50 per session. The patient is then allowed to begin progression up to 100 repetitions (again) with the increased weight. If flexion in the graft-donor leg starts to decrease (as measured by yardstick daily), the patient is advised to either decrease the shuttle exercise weight, frequency, or both until full flexion in that leg returns.

In the ACL-reconstructed leg, knee extension is emphasized more than flexion during this phase. If the amount of knee extension plateaus or decreases, then the amount of exercises to increase flexion should be decreased accordingly. Patients are warned that exercises will become more difficult at 2 or 3 days after surgery before gradually improving as a result of the body metabolizing the ketorolac medication from the hospital. During the first week after surgery, patients are allowed out of bed only two to three times daily for bathroom needs.

Phase II: Achieve knee symmetry

The first postoperative visit is at 1 week after surgery. The primary goal of the first week is full extension of the ACL-reconstructed leg; 110 degree of knee flexion is a secondary goal and represents the average flexion during this period. No patient, however, should have less than 90 degree of flexion. Full flexion is expected in the graft-donor knee.

Next, quadriceps muscle control is assessed. Each patient should be able to perform a straight-leg raise without a lag and an active heel lift, contracting the quadriceps muscle with the knee in a hyperextended position. The patient also should have sufficient control of the quadriceps muscle to ambulate stairs using only the handrail for balance. If

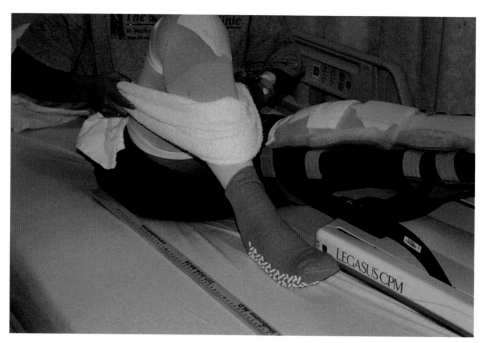

Fig 44-18. Knee-flexion evaluation. A yardstick is an easy tool for helping patients monitor knee flexion. Using the centimeter side, the zero end is placed at the heel, and the patient can flex the knee as far as he or she is able and then record the number of centimeters at the heel.

achieving an active heel lift through voluntary contraction is not possible, the condition may be the result of quadriceps muscle inhibition. (Treatment of this problem is discussed later in the chapter.)

If satisfactory goals have been achieved, the patient progresses to the intermediate phase of rehabilitation. Specific exercises during this phase are discussed below. Again, a diary with detailed instructions and spaces to record progress is provided to the patient. Rehabilitation remains unique to each leg. The patient continues to work on maintaining full extension of the ACL-reconstructed knee while concentrating on patellar tendon remodeling and regrowth in the graft-donor knee through strengthening exercises and maintaining full flexion. Leg control is emphasized bilaterally with gait and stance training.

Good knee-extension habits are again emphasized during this phase. Whenever sitting, the patient should be performing a heel prop to work on passive extension on the ACL-reconstructed leg. Whenever standing, weight should be shifted to the involved leg, locking the knee into hyperextension. Towel stretches are continued during this phase as well. The importance of fully symmetrical hyperextension cannot be overemphasized. If asymmetrical hyperextension is noted and not correctable by the end of this follow-up appointment, then a more vigorous technique to regain full extension is needed. (These techniques will be explained later in this chapter with regard to problems with rehabilitation.)

Flexion exercises also are implemented for the ACL-reconstructed knee, and the goal for the end of the second week is 120 degree. Exercises including heel slides and wall slides are routinely given. Flexion hangs (i.e., holding the posterior thigh with the hip flexed to 90 degree and allowing gravity to passively flex the knee) can be added at this point for patients with flexion of less than 120 degree. All range-of-motion exercises are performed two to four times a day during the intermediate phase.

During the second week, the CPM is discontinued, but cold/compression therapy continues. The cold/compression device is used by the patient as needed throughout the day to control swelling, and continued use throughout the night is encouraged but not required if the swelling is adequately controlled. Shuttle exercises for the contralateral graft-donor leg are progressed as described previously as long as the patient retains full flexion. Front step-down exercises are initiated at this point, and patients start with 50 repetitions three times per day on the 2-inch step. This is progressed in a manner similar to that of the Shuttle, until the patient is performing 100 repetitions on the 2-inch step. The patient independently advances this progression based on the amount of donor-site soreness. The step box is a hinged, foldable device allowing step exercises from heights up to 8 inches. While performing front step-down exercises, patients should focus on quality of form and technique rather than on quantity performed **(Fig 44-19)**. The patient balances on the graft-donor leg with the hands placed on his

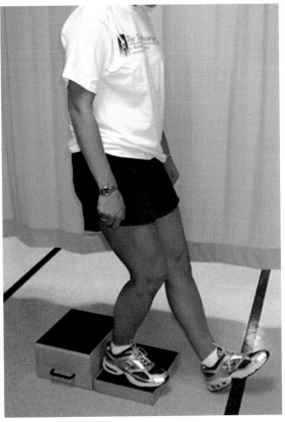

Fig 44-19. Step-down exercises. The patient balances on the graft-donor leg with his or her hands placed on the hips. Keeping the pelvis level, the heel of the opposite leg is lowered to the floor in front of the step box until it touches the floor.

or her hips, and the heel of the opposite leg is lowered to the floor in front of the step box until it touches the floor. It is important for the patient to keep the pelvis in a neutral position during the descent phase to prevent compensation from the hip musculature.

If patients continue to maintain good knee motion and to avoid joint effusion during the second postoperative week, they are allowed to increase the time they are upright by 1 to 2 hours per day. Patients usually can attend school or work half-days starting about 1.5 weeks postoperatively. By 10 to 12 days postoperatively, if motion remains good and effusion is not an issue, patients are allowed to be upright for a full day, with brief periods of elevated rest as needed.

The second postoperative visit takes place two weeks after surgery. Knee range of motion, gait, and quadriceps muscle control are again carefully examined. By this time, patients should report that they are back to performing their full normal activities of daily living both independently and without difficulty or other compensatory strategies. In the ACL-reconstructed knee, 120 degree of flexion are expected in addition to full extension. Effusion should be well controlled. Excessive effusion is indicative of an overly intense activity level and should be addressed immediately. Patients should be instructed to return to a decreased level of activity, with their leg elevated on pillows and continuous usage of the Cryo/Cuff until the swelling level has returned to an expected baseline amount of swelling. During this time, patients are still able to perform their range-of-motion exercises. Full flexion and extension in the graft-donor knee should be maintained. Normal gait should be demonstrated, and patients should be able to ambulate up and down stairs without holding the handrail.

The goal of rehabilitation between the second and fourth weeks is remodeling and regrowth of the donor patellar tendon through high-repetition, low-resistance exercise carried out several times daily. These exercises are essential to avoid long-term pain at the donor site. Patients are instructed in leg-press and knee-extension exercises as well as in continuation of the step-down exercises. Each exercise is performed only on the graft-donor leg. Typically, patients are asked to start with half their body weight or less for the leg-press exercise and with 2 to 5 pounds for the knee-extension exercise. These exercises can be performed every other day to ensure that the graft-donor site does not become overly sore. Three to five sets of 10 to 12 repetitions of each exercise usually are sufficient. The weight used for both exercises can be progressed slowly as the patient improves their strength. In our experience, patients can easily overexert themselves with either the leg press or the knee extensions and, thus, make the donor site sore. If the patient develops soreness that persists and does not decrease with cryotherapy, these exercises may need to be discontinued for a period of time. The most important thing is that the patient continues to demonstrate full graft-leg range of motion with continued improvement in strength without development of unrelenting donor-site pain.

Step-down exercises are progressed during this visit as the patient is able so that they provide an appropriate challenge. If the patient has maximized the number of repetitions during the second week (100 repetitions performed four to six times per day), then he or she is allowed to progress up to the 4-inch step; otherwise, the patient continues to progress on the 2-inch step. The number of repetitions is decreased to 50 on the 4-inch step, and the patient can progress this number back up to 100 repetitions per session as he or she is able. Once 100 repetitions are reached on the 4-inch step, the patient is allowed to go up to the 6-inch step, again reducing the number of repetitions performed to 50 and progressing that number as able. Soreness in the tendon should be relieved with cryotherapy, not interfere with normal gait or stairs, and be absent from the tendon before the next session. If the graft-donor leg becomes overly sore or if a decrease in knee flexion is noticed during exercises, the graft-donor leg strengthening intensity should be decreased until full flexion returns. Maintaining full extension of the ACL-reconstructed knee and making progress in flexion are vital. By the 1-month visit, the goal is for patients to be able to sit comfortably on his or her heels with the ankles in maximal plantarflexion, which is indicative of full knee flexion (Fig 44-20). Motion exercises for the ACL-reconstructed knee remain the same as

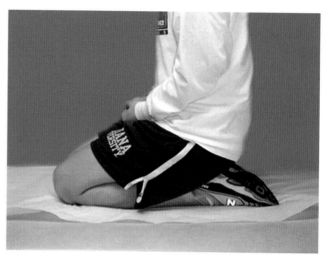

Fig 44-20. Achieving fully symmetrical flexion means that the patient should be able to kneel and sit back on the heels comfortably.

those during the first and second weeks. Extension habits are again reviewed and reinforced, because some patients have trouble integrating these into their daily routine.

Phase III: Advanced Strengthening

Four weeks after surgery, the patient returns for a full round of strength testing as well as KT2000 evaluation. The single-leg-hop test usually is not included in this visit, because most patients have not had their confidence fully return and are not ready to begin sports activities again. The results of these tests are helpful to assess the patient's progress over the previous four weeks and to develop a plan for further activity. At this point, the recovery of preoperative strength is not as important as symmetry between the ACL-reconstructed leg and the graft-donor leg. For a patient who is doing well, isokinetic strength in the graft-donor leg should be within 10% of that in the ACL-reconstructed knee.

The ability to return to activities between 4 and 8 weeks depends on the strength of the graft-donor knee, the presence of full motion in both knees, and the lack of an effusion in the ACL-reconstructed knee. If symmetrical quadriceps muscle strength (i.e., differences of less than 10% on testing) is achieved, the patient begins bilateral strengthening and conditioning exercises. Leg-press, knee-extension, and step-down exercises are continued for both legs, with the patient performing the exercises using each leg independently and continuing to progress the intensity by adding weight as able. Low-impact conditioning, including a stationary bike, Stairmaster, or elliptical trainer, is added. These activities need to be started very slowly and cautiously, however, because the amount of swelling in the ACL-reconstructed knee is being monitored. Typically, most patients tolerate starting with 10 minutes every other day and then increasing to between 20 and 30 minutes over the course of the next 4 weeks. Straight-line forward and backward jogging can be introduced, as can lateral slides and cross-overs. Shooting baskets or other individual, noncompetitive, sport-specific drills are performed as tolerated. No competitive situations are allowed at this time.

If asymmetry still exists between the two knees at examination, continued focused rehabilitation addressing the differences should be undertaken and activities restricted until the 8-week visit, when additional testing is performed and the patient is reevaluated for symmetry.

Phase IV: Return to Competition

No strict guidelines exist for when a patient may return to sports. Patients return to the clinic for regular follow-up testing and adjustment to their home exercise programs and activity level at their 2-, 4-, and 6-month visits. Rehabilitation continues to be monitored as patients return to their preoperative, fully competitive level of activity. Symmetry, in the form of equal strength, full range of motion, and joint effusion, are evaluated at each visit. Once symmetry between both knees is achieved, the level of activity can be increased slowly to include return to sports activities—but only on an every-other-day basis until the patient reaches 100% of the preoperative strength in both legs.

A typical progression for a basketball player who gains knee symmetry at 4 weeks postoperatively would be to return to individual, noncompetitive activities until the 2-month visit. If symmetry is still maintained and the patient has not had problems during the previous month with joint effusion, then he or she is allowed to start half-court activities in a two-on-two or three-on-three setting. When the patient has had sufficient practice time in a half-court setting to develop confidence in both knees, activities may progress to full-court activities every other day. Practicing on an every-other-day basis continues as the patient becomes stronger in both legs and can test at 100% of the preoperative, normal-strength values. Progression for other sports and activities can be similar, starting with an individual, noncompetitive level of activity and gradually progressing in both intensity and frequency of the sport contacts as long as symmetry between the knees is maintained for motion and strength.

Addressing Problems with Rehabilitation

As mentioned, the key to successful ACL reconstructive surgery is avoiding complications. Extensive experience has shown that these complications are much easier to prevent than to treat. The entire protocol described above has been created in an effort to avoid these complications while returning athletes to their sports both safely and expediently. Despite the best efforts from the surgeon and physical therapist, however, problems do arise, whether from noncompliance, deviation from principles, or physiology, and should be dealt with appropriately.

Lack of Knee Motion

No other complication has as much potential to create a poor outcome as lack of normal knee motion, hence the obvious emphasis in our rehabilitation protocol. Lack of normal knee motion is best prevented with a return to physiological normal range of motion during preoperative rehabilitation before ACL reconstruction. A return to full extension can be encouraged with the regimen presented above. In the patient for whom attaining full preoperative extension is difficult, discontinue all strengthening exercises and flexion exercises. The use of an Extension Board (O and P Associates, Indianapolis, IN) **(Fig 44-21)** or an Elite Seat (Kneebourne Therapeutics, Indianapolis, IN) **(Fig 44-22)** can be used to provide an increased mechanical stretch to the knee. Both devices passively stretch the knee into extension, compressing or forcing aside tissues in the intercondylar notch. The extension board is controlled with Velcro straps and requires a second person for correct use, whereas the Elite Seat works from a proximally controlled pulley and can be used independently by the patient. Both devices should be used under the supervision of a physical therapist to aid in attaining full extension.

Similar principles are used postoperatively. If full extension is difficult to achieve or not achievable at any point, the Elite Seat or Extension Board should be added immediately as an adjunct activity and the patient followed more closely until a full return of extension is demonstrated. Similarly, flexion and strengthening exercises are discontinued until full extension is achieved again. With close follow-up, a patient rarely requires additional intervention; however, a persistent asymmetry of extension is an indication for operative intervention.

Lack of knee flexion typically is easier to treat. In the absence of extension loss, aggressive flexion exercise should be instituted immediately if continued improvement is not noted as per the goals described above. As mentioned, persistent swelling can be the enemy of motion. If persistent effusion is problematic, then activity level and strengthening should be decreased, and use of the Cryo/Cuff increased, until a more normal state is achieved.

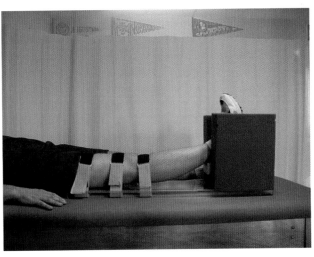

Fig 44-21. An Extension Board can be used to assist with obtaining full knee hyperextension.

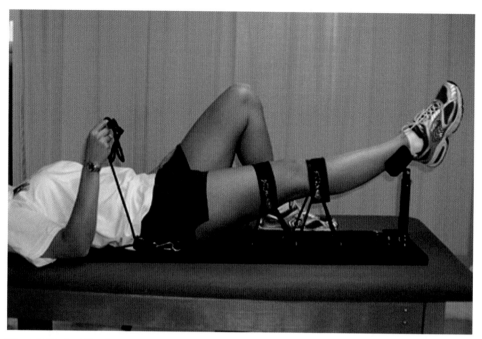

Fig 44-22. An Elite Seat allows the patient to recline completely, which relaxes the hamstrings. The patient uses a pulley control to increase the mechanical force for knee extension.

Quadriceps Inhibition

Occasionally, a patient will present postoperatively with poor quadriceps muscle function. This usually is the case if a patient is having difficulty with quadriceps muscle control before surgery. The hallmark of this condition is an inability to initiate quadriceps muscle contraction when the knee is brought into hyperextension. Normally, a patient should be able to use the quadriceps muscle to hold the knee in a hyperextended position. The examiner's hand, when placed between the table and the popliteal fossa, should feel increased pressure during this maneuver; however, the opposite will occur in the presence of quadriceps muscle inhibition. The patient will not be able to hold the affected foot off the examining table using the quadriceps muscle, and the examiner will feel decreased pressure under the popliteal fossa. More importantly, the lack of contraction will be visible. Clinically, this condition manifests itself in a poor gait pattern. Quadriceps muscle inhibition does not represent femoral nerve palsy, as it is often labeled.

Helpful exercises for correcting this phenomenon include the following: (a) stance and gait training, (b) step box training, (c) tubing exercises, and (d) neuromuscular manual stimulation. Stance and gait training includes using a mirror to help the patient visualize and understand the correct position of a hyperextended knee in stance as well as working on gait using a decreased step length and focusing on terminal extension during initial contact with overemphasized heel contact. Step-up box training involves standing on the affected leg and placing the noninvolved leg up onto an elevated surface (6 to 8 inches should be sufficient) and then back to the ground **(Fig 44-23)**. The patient must control the

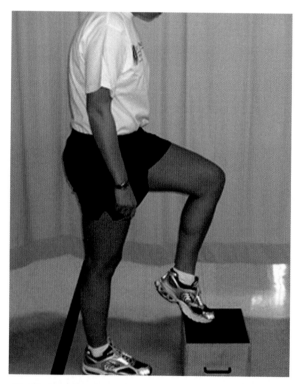

Fig 44-23. Step box training. The patient stands on the affected leg and lifts the noninvolved leg up onto an elevated surface (6–8 inches should be sufficient) and then back to the ground.

affected limb during stance while the other leg is moving, forcing the quadriceps muscle to activate and provide stability. This exercise also can be performed while standing on the noninvolved leg and lifting the involved foot onto the step to help with neuromuscular control of the lower extremity. Manual neuromuscular input may be useful in providing tactile stimulation and biofeedback to initiate quadriceps contraction during hyperextension.

Persistent Weakness

A contralateral graft is useful in preventing this complication. Occasionally, however, patients will present with persistent weakness of graft-donor leg strength, which may be exacerbated by donor-site tendon pain. It is important to keep in mind that this asymmetry cannot be remedied with bilateral exercises. Rather, decreasing bilateral strengthening activities and focusing on unilateral exercises, such as step-down, leg-press, and knee-extension exercises, are recommended. Donor-site tendon pain should guide the progression through these exercises.

Anterior Knee Pain

Much has been written about anterior knee pain following ACL reconstruction. Anterior knee pain is the best example of a complication best prevented. It is important to keep in mind that anterior knee pain is not a diagnosis; rather, it is a symptom. Donor-site tendon soreness, loss of motion, and weakness all may cause pain in the anterior knee. Indeed, some donor-site tendon soreness is universal and useful as a guide to progression through exercise. Early high-repetition and low-resistance exercise, immediate full flexion, and early weight bearing are essential in making this pain temporary. An injured tendon tends to become stiff and contracted if left alone or immobilized. Over an extended period of time, a stiff, contracted tendon can cause pain in the front of the knee because of a poor ability to transmit stress as well as its compressive effect on the patellofemoral joint. If given physiological stress while healing, tissues will heal with increased strength and improved collagen orientation (48). This same principle is applied to the donor patellar tendon. Frequent transmission of physiological loads and exercises designed to draw the tendon to its full length can ensure that the tendon heals as anatomically normal as possible in terms of strength and elasticity. Early donor-site soreness should not be confused with the more malignant, long-term entity caused by an unrehabilitated patellar tendon. Loss of motion or weakness should be treated as described above.

Another clinical entity that can contribute to anterior knee pain is a lack of quadriceps muscle flexibility. Even in the face of good knee flexion, the proximal quadriceps musculature can remain tight. This is best examined with the hip in extension and the patient lying prone. In this position, the heel should still easily reach the buttock. If the patient demonstrates a decrease in flexibility, appropriate stretching should begin.

Ipsilateral Patella Tendon Graft Rehabilitation

The evolution of our contralateral ACL-reconstruction rehabilitation protocol has impacted the way that we rehabilitate patients who have an ACL reconstruction with the patellar tendon graft taken from the same knee. In general, rehabilitation of an ACL reconstruction with an ipsilateral patellar tendon graft tends to be a bit slower for return to sports activity compared with the reconstruction process using a contralateral graft. This results from the conflicting processes of regaining full range of motion and achieving full strength in the same leg. By taking the donor-graft from the opposite knee, we can separate these two processes and speed rehabilitation.

Preoperative rehabilitation identical to that in the contralateral graft protocol is undertaken. The differences in rehabilitation begin following surgery. Rehabilitation exercises during the first postoperative week focus entirely on control of swelling, achieving good range of motion, and keeping good quadriceps control using exercises similar to those described above. No attempt is made during the first week to address rehabilitation of the donor site, because effective regrowth and remodeling of the tendon cannot be performed until the patient has full motion. All exercises performed during the first week are similar to those in the rehabilitation protocol described above, with the exception that the Shuttle is not used during this phase. During the 1-week visit, the patient should be able to demonstrate full hyperextension of the ACL-reconstructed knee, with flexion to 110° and good quadriceps control.

Patients continue to work toward full range of motion and increased leg control during the second postoperative week. The range-of-motion exercises used are again similar to those described above, including towel stretches and heel props for extension as well as heel slides and wall slides to help regain flexion. Proper extension habits also are emphasized, with appropriate attention given to correct stance and heel props when sitting. Leg-control exercises can be advanced to include knee-extension and step-down exercises. Knee-extension exercises are performed by slowly extending the knee until terminal extension is reached, after which the patient is instructed to squeeze the quadriceps muscle for a period of 4 to 5 seconds and then slowly lower the leg to the initial starting position. No weight is used for resistance initially, and patients are instructed to focus on the quality of the muscle contraction after achieving terminal knee extension. Step-down exercises are performed on the 2-inch step as described previously. Thirty to 50 repetitions of these exercises are performed three to four times per day and progressed as the patient is able.

Goals for returning to the clinic following the second week include normal gait and ambulation up and down stairs without using a handrail, full hyperextension, and flexion to 125 degrees. At this point, patients continue to work on knee range of motion, but light strengthening exercises can be added. Step-down exercises are progressed by the patient in a manner identical to that described for the contralateral graft protocol and performed three to four times daily.

When the patient returns for the 4-week visit, full range of motion is expected in the ACL-reconstructed knee. At this point, the patient can start aggressive strengthening exercises, including leg-press, knee-extension, and step-down exercises, as well as low-impact conditioning, such as a stationary bicycle, stairmaster, or elliptical trainer, following a strengthening protocol similar to that for the graft-donor leg in the contralateral rehabilitation protocol.

The patient continues to make regular visits for testing at 2, 4, and 6 months. When strength testing and the single-leg-hop test have returned to a level of 80% that of the opposite leg, light sports activities are allowed, including half-court activities in a noncompetitive situation. Patients continue to work on strengthening during this time and may need to take a day off after sports activities if the knee becomes sore. When patients test within 90% of the opposite leg's isokinetic strength and single-leg hop, full return to activity is allowed based on soreness and swelling in the knee. In our experience, most patients can begin aggressive strengthening after their 4-week visit and, usually, can start light sports activities at approximately 2 to 4 months. Full participation depends on equal isokinetic strength and single-leg hop, symmetrical range of motion, and controlled joint effusion, which usually can take 6 to 8 months following surgery.

■ COMPLICATIONS, CONTROVERSIES, AND SPECIAL CONSIDERATIONS

With the continued emphasis on and research concerning ACL injuries, surgery, and rehabilitation in recent years, many advances have been made in the care of the injury. As surgical and rehabilitative care techniques have improved, the once-dreaded, career-ending injury now has become a predictable result. Controversies still remain, however, regarding surgical technique, timing of surgery, rehabilitation principles and activities, and expected outcomes.

Should We Expect a "Normal" Knee after Reconstruction?

Several authors (29,49,50) have suggested that following an ACL reconstruction, a patient's knee will never be normal again. We believe that obtaining a normal knee after surgery is possible for any patient who has sustained an acute ACL rupture but still has intact cartilage and either normal menisci or meniscal tears that are repairable or can be left in situ. Our current clinical data support this theory (42,43). If we are able to replace the torn ACL with a graft that has been placed and tensioned properly and if the knee obtains full motion intraoperatively, then why should we not ultimately expect the knee to feel normal and to function normally postoperatively? If the anatomy is surgically restored, then the rehabilitation program should be able to help guide the knee back to its premorbid state. We believe

that the physician's philosophy—and the goal of ACL reconstruction—should be to attempt to return the patient's knee back to a normal state. If an excellent result is not the goal, then our behavior will respond accordingly, and we will be producing suboptimal results forever.

Controversy exists regarding what features make a knee "normal." If the features are not well understood, then it is difficult to design a rehabilitation protocol, because specific outcome goals are not be defined clearly. Most physicians agree that a normal knee is stable, has no effusion, shows good strength, and allows normal gait and functional activities. We suggest that the concept of symmetry between the legs should define what is normal for a knee. Normal people do not have legs that are unequal in the amount of range of motion, swelling, strength, or function. Those patients who seek treatment do so because of an asymmetry between their good knee and their bad knee. We base our concept of normal following ACL injury on what the contralateral knee looks like before surgery, and we then restore the person to that same level of range of motion, swelling, strength, and function. The controversies of defining a normal knee revolve around what is considered to be a full range of motion and a normal level of soreness.

Normal knees are not painless. Athletes with normal knees usually have some occasional symptoms associated with activity. Shelbourne and Nitz (51) reported a survey of 140 Division I college athletes with no history of knee injury. These athletes completed a modified Noyes questionnaire, which gives a total score from 0 to 100 points, with a score of 100 meaning that the athlete had no symptoms of pain, swelling, or instability and could participate in activities as desired. The average score was 94 points for football players, 90 for wrestlers, 90 for basketball players, and 95.2 for swimmers. These scores for athletes with normal knees would indicate that the young, athletic individual does not experience occasional symptoms that are noticeable.

Another controversy surrounding the evaluation of knees is the description of normal knee motion. Some authors describe normal range of motion as from 0 to 135 degree (52–54). Most individuals, however, have some degree of hyperextension in their knee that is normal for them. In a study of 889 high-school preseason athletes, 96% demonstrated some hyperextension, with an average of 5 degree hyperextension for men and 6 degree hyperextension for females (55). An understanding of normal knee motion is critical to the development of an ACL postoperative rehabilitation protocol that can restore normal function in each patient.

Having normal hyperextension is important for two reasons. First, it is necessary to allow the normal screw-home mechanism, which can only occur with full extension for that person, whether that is 0 degree of extension or 5 to 10 degree of hyperextension. Second, full hyperextension is important so that the knee will "feel normal." During stance, it is normal to stand on one leg with the knee locked out, relaxing the quadriceps musculature while still maintaining the upright position. If the knee does not hyperextend, then the patient will not be able to lock out the knee, and standing on that leg will require constant use of quadriceps, possibly resulting in anterior knee pain.

Most people have greater than 135 degree of knee flexion, which is a commonly cited amount of full flexion (52–54). A study by DeCarlo and Sell (55) found that the average knee flexion was 140 degree for men and 143 degree for women. Asymmetrical flexion is noticed by patients just as they notice asymmetrical extension—and especially by patients who are involved in running and jumping sports. As with extension, normal knee flexion should mean that the patient has achieved flexion equal to that of the opposite knee, not just 135 degrees.

Return to Activities

The return to activities and sports after ACL reconstruction is a much debated topic. Some surgeons believe in a time-based philosophy for allowing patients to return to activities. The time at which most surgeons release patients to playing sports is 6 months after surgery. This philosophy is based on the thought that 6 months is enough time to let the ACL graft mature and to have a low risk of reinjury. There is nothing magical about the 6-month time frame, however. Determining the exact time when patients return to activities is very difficult. Some patients begin to do some activities, such as shooting a basketball or dribbling a soccer ball, as early as 1 month after surgery. A person might begin doing some one-on-one sports drills at 2 months after surgery. Some patients are able to compete at 3 or 4 months after surgery, but they usually begin by playing part-time and building up to being able to play an entire competition. Once patients are back to playing full-time, they report that it takes 2 to 3 months before they feel totally back to normal. Our goal is for patients to have equal knee range of motion and equal strength in both legs before they return to fully competitive situations. To accomplish this goal, the patient must go through the progression described above. A defined time period cannot be used, because each patient and the demands of different sports are unique.

■ CONCLUSIONS AND FUTURE DIRECTIONS

Clinical research and medical improvements in the specialty of acute knee injuries are continuous processes involving patient observation and close follow-up. With the proper guidance, the future for an athlete suffering an ACL tear is promising, and most patients can anticipate returning to athletic activities safely and with a good long-term prognosis. In addition to perfecting the surgical technique of ACL reconstruction, both preoperative and postoperative guidelines must be updated on a regular basis to minimize surgical morbidity and to help provide the patient with a successful clinical outcome. The rehabilitative course after surgery can be smooth and predictable when the patient has a thorough understanding of the goals for each phase of rehabilitation. Return to athletics must be individualized, depending on the patient's lifestyle and goals. The continuous improvement during an ACL reconstruction–specific rehabilitation will help to ensure long-term stability and to fulfill the athlete's desire to have a knee that feels normal after surgery.

■ REFERENCES

1. Rosenberg A, Mikosz RP, Mohler CG. Basic knee biomechanics. In: Scott WN, ed. *The knee*. St. Louis: Mosby–Year Book; 1994:75–94.
2. Cox J, Cordell L. The degenerative effects of medial meniscus tears in dogs' knees. *Clin Orthop*. 1977;125:236–242.
3. Shelbourne KD, Foulk DA. *Principles and practice of orthopaedic sports medicine*. Philadelphia: Lippincott Williams & Wilkins; 2000:743–761.
4. Fetto JF, Marshall JL. The natural history and diagnosis of anterior cruciate ligament insufficiency. *Clin Orthop*. 1980;147:29–38.
5. Hewson GF Jr, Mendini RA, Wang JB. Prophylactic knee bracing in college football. *Am J Sports Med*. 1986;14:262–266.
6. Ray JM. A proposed natural history of symptomatic anterior cruciate ligament reconstruction. *Am J Sports Med*. 1992;20:519–526.
7. Noyes FR, Bassett RW, Grood ES, et al. Arthroscopy in acute traumatic hemarthrosis of the knee. *J Bone Joint Surg Am*. 1980;62:687–757.
8. Paessler HH, Michel D. How new is the Lachman test? *Am J Sports Med*. 1992;20:95–98.
9. DeHaven KE. Diagnosis of acute knee injuries with hemarthrosis. *Am J Sports Med*. 1980;8:9–14.
10. Torg JS, Conrad W, Kalen V. Clinical diagnosis of anterior cruciate instability in the athlete. *Am J Sports Med*. 1976;4:84–93.
11. Rubinstein RA Jr, Shelbourne KD, McCarroll JR, et al. The accuracy of the clinical examination in the setting of posterior cruciate ligament injuries. *Am J Sports Med*. 1994;22:550–557.
12. O'Donoghue DH. Surgical treatment of fresh injuries to the major ligaments of the knee. *J Bone Joint Surg Am*. 1950;32:721–738.
13. Shelbourne KD, Nitz PA. The O'Donoghue triad revisited. Combined knee injuries involving anterior cruciate and medial collateral ligament tears. *Am J Sports Med*. 1991;19:474–477.
14. Shelbourne KD, Martini DJ, McCarroll JR, et al. Correlation of joint line tenderness and meniscal lesions in patients with acute anterior cruciate ligament tears. *Am J Sports Med*. 1995;23:166–169.
15. Rosenberg TD, Paulos LE, Parker RD, et al. The forty-five degree posteroanterior flexion weight-bearing radiograph of the knee. *J Bone Joint Surg Am*. 1988;70:1479–1483.
16. Merchant AC, Mercer, RL, Jacobsen RH, et al. Roentgenographic analysis of patellofemoral congruence. *J Bone Joint Surg Am*. 1974;56:1391–1396.
17. Shelbourne KD, Davis TH, Klootwyk TE. The relationship between intercondylar notch width of the femur and the incidence of anterior cruciate ligament tears: a prospective study. *Am J Sports Med*. 1998;26:402–408.
18. Shelbourne KD, Facibene WA, Hunt JJ. Radiographic and intraoperative intercondylar notch width measurements in men and women with unilateral and bilateral anterior cruciate ligament tears. *Knee Surg Sports Traumatol Arthrosc*. 1997;5:229–233.
19. Fischer SP, Fox JM, Del Pizzo W, et al. Accuracy of diagnosis from magnetic resonance imaging of the knee. A multicenter analysis of one thousand and fourteen patients. *J Bone Joint Surg Am*. 1991;73:2–10.

20. Hawkins RJ, Misamore GW, Merritt TR. Follow-up of the acute nonoperated isolated anterior cruciate ligament tear. *Am J Sports Med.* 1986;14:205–210.

21. McCarroll JR, Rettig AC, Shelbourne KD. Anterior cruciate ligament injuries in the young athlete with open physes. *Am J Sports Med.* 1988;16:44–47.

22. Giove TP, Miller SJ, Kent MA, et al. Nonoperative treatment of the torn anterior cruciate ligament. *J Bone Joint Surg Am.* 1983;65:184–192.

23. McDaniel WJ, Dameron TB. Untreated ruptures of the anterior cruciate ligament. *J Bone Joint Surg Am.* 1980;62:696–705.

24. Diment MT, Sebastianelli WJ, DeHaven KE. Arthroscopically assisted anterior cruciate ligament reconstruction using a central-third patellar tendon autograft and two incisions. *Op Tech Sports Med.* 1993;1:45–49.

25. Tanner JM. *Growth at adolescence.* 2nd ed. Oxford: Blackwell Scientific Publications; 1962.

26. Shelbourne KD, Gray T, Wiley BV. Results of transphyseal anterior cruciate ligament reconstruction using patellar tendon autograft in Tanner stage 3 or 4 adolescents with clearly open growth plates. *Am J Sports Med.* 2004;32:1218–1229.

27. Bonamo JJ, Fay C, Firestone T. The conservative treatment of the anterior cruciate ligament-deficient knee. *Am J Sports Med.* 1990;18:618–623.

28. Andersson C, Odensten M, Gillquist J. Knee function after surgical or nonsurgical treatment of acute rupture of the anterior cruciate ligament: a randomized study with a long-term follow-up period. *Clin Orthop.* 1991;264:255–263.

29. Daniel DM, Stone ML, Dobson BE, et al. Fate of the ACL injured patients. A prospective outcome study. *Am J Sports Med.* 1994;22:632–644.

30. Clancy WG, Ray JM, Zontan DJ. Acute tears of the anterior cruciate ligament. Surgical versus conservative treatment. *J Bone Joint Surg Am.* 1983:65:184–192.

31. Warren RF. Meniscectomy and repair of the anterior cruciate ligament-deficient patients. *Clin Orthop.* 1990;252:55–63.

32. Engebretsen L, Svenningsen S, Benum P. Poor results of anterior cruciate ligament repair in adolescence. *Acta Orthop Scand.* 1998;59:684–686.

33. Barrett GR, Line LL, Shelton WR, et al. The Dacron ligament prosthesis in anterior cruciate ligament reconstruction. A four-year review. *Am J Sports Med.* 1993;21:367–373.

34. Paulos LE, Rosenberg TD, Grewe SR, et al. The GORE-TEX anterior cruciate ligament prosthesis. A long-term follow-up. *Am J Sports Med.* 1992;20:246–252.

35. Shelbourne KD, Rask BP. Anterior cruciate ligament reconstruction using a mini-open technique with autogenous patellar tendon graft. *Techniques in Orthopaedics.* 1998;12:221–228.

36. Howell SM, Clark JA. Tibial tunnel placement in anterior cruciate ligament reconstructions and graft impingement. *Clin Orthop.* 1992;283:187–195.

37. Howell SM, Berns GS, Farley RE. Unimpinged and impinged anterior cruciate ligament grafts: MR signal intensity measurements. *Radiology.* 1991;179:639–643.

38. Graf BK, Uhr F. Complications of intra-articular anterior cruciate ligament reconstruction. *Clin Sports Med.* 1988;7:835–848.

39. Kurosaka M, Yoshiya S, Andrish JT. A biomechanical comparison of different surgical techniques of graft fixation in anterior cruciate ligament reconstruction. *Am J Sports Med.* 1987;15:225–229.

40. Christian CA, Indelicato PA. Allograft anterior cruciate ligament reconstruction with patellar tendon: an endoscopic technique. *Op Tech Sports Med.* 1993;1:50–57.

41. an Meter CD, Sallay P, McCarroll JR. Anterior cruciate ligament reconstruction through the patellar tendon defect. *Op Tech Sports Med.* 1993;1:40–44.

42. Shelbourne KD, Gray T. Anterior cruciate ligament reconstruction with autogenous patellar tendon graft followed by accelerated rehabilitation. A two- to nine-year follow-up. *Am J Sports Med.* 1997;25:786–795.

43. Shelbourne KD, Gray T. Results of anterior cruciate ligament reconstruction based on the meniscal and articular cartilage status at the time of surgery: five- to fifteen-year evaluations. *Am J Sports Med.* 2000;28:446–452.

44. Mohtadi NG, Bogaert SW, Fowler PJ. Limitation of motion following anterior cruciate ligament reconstruction. A case control study. *Am J Sports Med.* 1991;19:620–625.

45. Shelbourne KD, Wilckens JH, Mollabashy A, et al. Arthrofibrosis in acute anterior cruciate ligament reconstruction. The effect of timing of reconstruction and rehabilitation. *Am J Sports Med.* 1991;19:332–336.

46. Shelbourne KD, O'Shea JJ. Revision anterior cruciate ligament reconstruction using the contralateral bone-patellar tendon-bone graft. *AAOS Instructional Course Lectures.* 2002;51:343–346.

47. Shelbourne KD, Liotta FJ, Goodloe SL. Preemptive pain management program for anterior cruciate ligament reconstruction. *Am J Knee Surg.* 1998;11:116–119.

48. Akeson WH. The response of ligaments to stress modulation and overview of the ligament heasssling response. In: Daniel DM, Akeson WH, OConner JJ, eds. *Knee ligaments. Structure, function, and repair.* New York: Raven Press; 1990:315–327.

49. Dye SF. The knee as a biologic transmission with an envelope of function. *Clin Orthop.* 1996;323:10–18.

50. Gillquist J. Repair and reconstruction of the ACL: is it good enough? *Arthroscopy.* 1993;9:68–71.

51. Shelbourne KD, Nitz P. Accelerated rehabilitation after anterior cruciate ligament reconstruction. *Am J Sports Med.* 1990;18:292–299.

52. Hunter RE, Mastrangelo J, Freeman JR, et al. The impact of surgical timing on postoperative motion and stability following anterior cruciate ligament reconstruction. *Arthroscopy.* 1996;12:667–674.

53. Majors RA, Woodfin B. Achieving full range of motion after anterior cruciate ligament reconstruction. *Am J Sports Med.* 1996;24:350–355.

54. Noyes FR, Barber-Westin SD. A comparison of results of acute and chronic anterior cruciate ligament ruptures of arthroscopically assisted autogenous patellar tendon reconstruction. *Am J Sports Med.* 1997;25:460–471.

55. DeCarlo MS, Sell K. Normative data for range of motion and single leg hop in high school athletes. *Journal of Sports Rehabilitation.* 1997;6:246–255.

LEG, ANKLE, AND FOOT

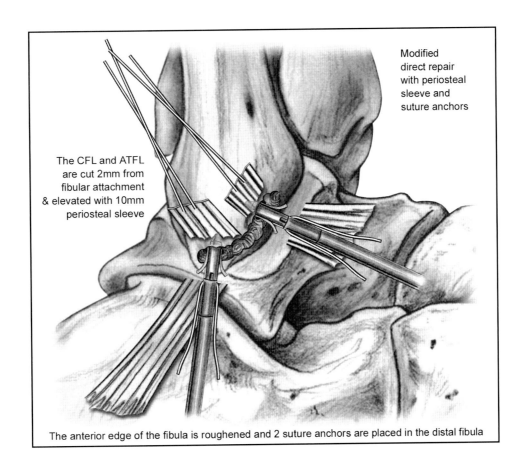

Modified direct repair with periosteal sleeve and suture anchors

The CFL and ATFL are cut 2mm from fibular attachment & elevated with 10mm periosteal sleeve

The anterior edge of the fibula is roughened and 2 suture anchors are placed in the distal fibula

LEG, ANKLE, AND FOOT: HISTORY, PHYSICAL, AND INVESTIGATIONS

45

KEVIN J. WING, MD, FRCSC, ALASTAIR YOUNGER, MSc, MBChB, FRCSC

■ KEY POINTS

■ By the end of the history, the examiner should know the functional restrictions of the patient and the specific areas of discomfort. The nature of the injury should be determined, if an isolated event. Insidious onset may be related to change in routine.

■ Changes in training routine or footwear can aggravate or cause a stress injury.

■ In an elite female athlete, it is appropriate to inquire about menstrual history, keeping in mind the female athlete triad of disordered eating, amenorrhea, and osteoporosis.

■ Determination of the absolute range of motion is less critical than assessment of loss of motion compared with the opposite side, as motion is very variable between patients.

■ The recent development of Multidetector-row computed tomography (CT) has dramatically improved the quality of foot and ankle images. The high resolution axial scans, in conjunction with sagital and coronal reformats, has improved the diagnosis and visualization of osteochondral lesions of the talar dome, arthritic joints, stress fractures, or small rim fractures.

We have added this chapter on the examination of the foot and ankle in the athlete. Most errors in the management of foot and ankle conditions in the athlete are caused by a poor history and physical, and the examination is not as well taught or thought out compared with other areas of the body. We hope you will learn from inclusion of this chapter.

■ HISTORY

By the end of the foot and ankle history, the examiner should know the functional restrictions of the patient and the specific areas of discomfort. The nature of injury should be determined, if an isolated event. Insidious onset may be related to changes in routine. Patients typically report one or a combination of pain, instability, and locking.

Pain

Patients should remove their socks and shoes prior to the history so they can indicate the area of discomfort or deformity. This seems to be a much more effective method of communication than verbal description.

Patients should describe the severity of their pain, as well as the quality, radiation, and timing. They should also describe any precipitating and relieving factors. The effect of hills and stairs should be determined (anterior and posterior ankle impingement). Subtalar or triple joint pathology and peroneal tendon problems may cause pain on uneven ground. The effects of anti-inflammatories or acetaminophen on their pain pattern should also be noted.

Instability

Instability most commonly affects the ankle joint. It is the result of laxity of the anterior talofibular ligament (ATFL). The calcaneal fibular ligament (CFL) is also frequently found to be deficient at the time of surgery.

The examiner should delineate between apprehension and true inversion sprains. The frequency of these episodes and the setting in which they occur should be assessed.

Locking

Locking in the foot and ankle may relate to an osteochondral defect or loose body within the ankle. Patients may find the symptoms hard to define compared to pain and instability.

Functional Restriction

The impact of the disability should be determined. Sports practiced prior to and since the onset of symptoms are recorded. Impact on specific sports and activities within sports (running, cutting, jumping, and so on) will determine the need for treatment.

Impact on employment should also be recorded.

Treatment to Date

Treatment to date may include physiotherapy, medication, surgery, bracing, or orthotics. Knowledge of prior treatment and its success or failure will allow the physician to plan an appropriate treatment strategy. For instability, specific treatment may include bracing and physiotherapy. Patients should bring in their braces and orthotics for review.

Change in Foot Shape

The onset of an acquired flat foot deformity or an acquired post-traumatic flat foot deformity is an important finding in the adult. We have found a series of patients with superficial deltoid injuries presenting with a planovalgus foot deformity. Patients with midfoot injuries (Lisfranc joint level) may also develop a flat foot deformity.

A progressive high arched (cavovarus) foot deformity is less common but significant symptom often associated with instability. This pertains more to the younger athlete encountering a neuromuscular disorder, such as Charcot Marie Tooth. Occasionally patients will develop a high arched foot after an acute injury to the talar neck. This can be missed or the nature of the injury underestimated. A painful locked foot with hindfoot varus and forefoot varus will result.

Previous Foot and Ankle Conditions

Prior injuries, such as high school injuries, may be only volunteered on specific questioning. Pre-existing deformities or family history of flat or high arched feet are also significant. Many of these deformities become more symptomatic with age.

Stress/Overuse Injuries

Changes in training routine or footwear can aggravate or cause a stress injury (1,2). A history of the exercise routine should be sought.

In an elite female athlete it is appropriate to inquire about menstrual history, keeping in mind the female athlete triad of disordered eating, amenorrhea, and osteoporosis (3).

Past Medical History

Recording the typical past medical history, past surgical history, current medications, and allergies must complete the history section. A patient filled form may be the most reliable screening method for obtaining details.

■ EXAM

The feet should already be exposed for the history. The height and weight should be recorded. Terminology should accurate: Because pronation and supination mean different things to different practitioners, we prefer to describe feet in general as flat, high arched, or neutral. More specific description of foot shape includes hindfoot varus and valgus, forefoot varus and valgus (inverted or everted toward or away from the midline), and forefoot abduction and adduction in the transverse plane. This is consistent terminology that most practitioners understand.

We use a nine-point physical exam that ensures that all of the relevant details in the physical exam are covered. These points are discussed in the following sections.

Exposure

The physical exam should be conducted with the patient dressed in shorts and a T-shirt, so that the alignment of the limb can be clearly seen (Fig 45-1).

Gait

A brief examination of gait requires a moderate sized exam room or corridor of at least 10 to 15 feet (3 to 5 m). The patient is asked to walk back and forth on three occasions, watching first the left foot and its posture in stance phase. On the return the position, the swing phase is watched. The routine is then repeated for the right foot. The patient is asked to heel walk out and toe walk back.

Inspection of Standing Posture

Standing posture starts with an observation of alignment with the patient facing the examiner and feet shoulder width apart. A "peek-a-boo" heel may be observed indicating hindfoot varus (Fig 45-2) (4). The weight bearing position of the toes (clawing, hallux valgus) is inspected.

After the patient turns around the posture is observed from behind. A quick screening exam of the back, pelvic alignment, and measurement of significant leg length discrepancy can be performed now. Focusing on the foot, the examiner can determine whether the heel is in neutral

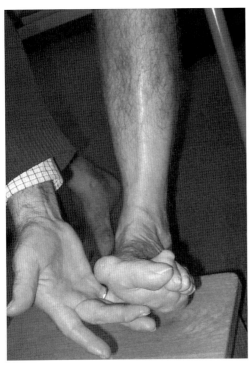

Fig 45-1. Exposure of the limb. The patient is pointing at the painful second metatarsal base.

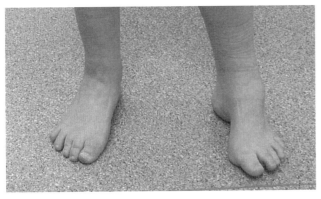

Fig 45-2. Peek a boo heel sign. A patient with Charcot Marie Tooth disease with a reconstructed foot on the right and preoperative foot on the left. The right appears well aligned, and the left has a peek a boo heel.

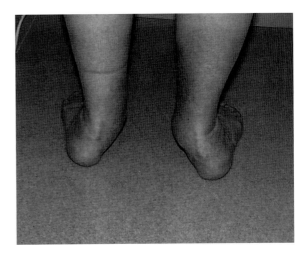

Fig 45-3. Too many toes sign.

Inspection of the Foot with the Patient Sitting

The patient is moved to a sitting position preferably on a slightly raised bed with the legs hanging over the edge and the examiner seated on a low stool. This allows optimal visualization of the leg, foot, and ankle.

The foot is examined for callosities that indicate areas of excessive load in the foot. Common sites include metatarsal heads, the lateral border of the foot (cavus foot), and over the interphalengeal joints (claw toes).

Any scars from previous surgeries or injuries are inspected and recorded. Their effect on any further surgery should be considered. They should be palpated and examined for any signs of infection.

Swelling may exist over a joint or tendon. Its location and extent should be recorded. If necessary, assessment of tibial rotation, length, varus, or valgus alignment may be relevant after fracture or growth arrest.

Palpation

Palpation is the critical part of examination. Determination of the areas of maximum tenderness and knowledge of the underlying anatomy will point to the diagnosis.

Joint swelling and osteophytic or post-traumatic bony changes at the joint margins should be noted.

The following joint margins should be palpated.

- Ankle joint: Anterior joint line, medial and lateral gutters **(Fig 45-4)**
- Subtalar joint: Sinus tarsi, middle facet of the subtalar joint
- Talonavicular joint
- Calcaneocuboid joint
- Navicular cuneiform joint
- Tarsal metatarsal joints 1–5
- Metatarsal phalangeal joints 1–5
- IP joints 1–5
- DIP joints 2–5

(three to six degrees) physiologic valgus. A flat foot will typically be associated with a hindfoot valgus and lateral displacement of the forefoot indicated by the "too many toes" sign (5) **(Fig 45-3).**

A single leg stance will assess proprioceptive control of the lower extremity. This can be made more vigorous by asking the patient to hop while on one leg. The patient can be asked to do a single leg heel raise to both ascertain proprioceptive control in plantarflexion, and that they reconstitute a normal longitudinal medial arch and have normal heel inversion as a result of tibialis posterior tendon function and a supple hindfoot (6).

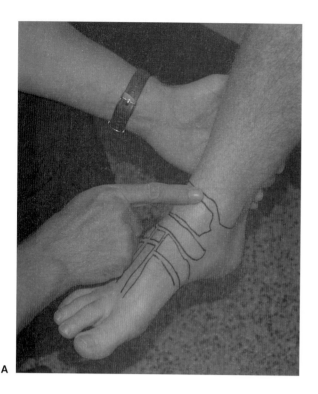

A

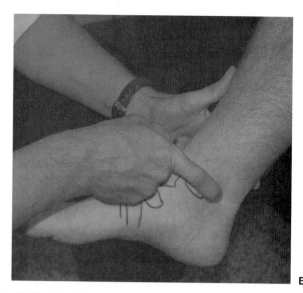

B

Fig 45-4. **A:** Anterior ankle joint margin palpation. **B:** Ankle joint margin palpation—posterior margin.

Tendon Palpation

Each tendon should be palpated along its course. Synovitis, pain, or nodularity may be demonstrated. The patient should actively contact the muscle against resistance. The prominent tendon can then be easily palpated and strength determined **(Fig 45-5)**.

Flexor Tendons

The Achilles tendon may suffer a paratendonopathy, a tendonopathy, insertional tendonitis, or have bursitis possibly aggrevated by a Hagelund deformity.

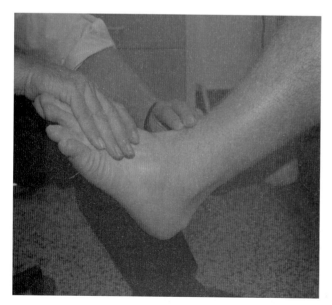

Fig 45-5. Tendon palpation—Tibialis Anterior.

A paratendonopathy (swelling of the tendon sheath without swelling of the tendon) will not move with dorsiflexion and plantarflexion of the foot, while an area of Achilles tendonopathy will move during palpation **(Fig 45-6)**.

Achilles tendon rupture can be acute or chronic. Most acute Achilles tendon ruptures can be palpated and a gap felt. A chronic insufficiency can be determined by excessive dorsiflexion on the affected side as dorsiflexion range in both ankles with the knees extended should be the same. Excessive dorsiflexion indicates a stretched out and functionally long tendon.

Flexor digitorum longus can be palpated behind and lateral to the tibialis posterior. Resisted flexion of the great toe can also demonstrate the flexor hallucis longus deep to the posterior tibial artery, which runs lateral to the flexor digitorum longus.

Extensor Tendons

The distal tibialis anterior tendon can be palpated for nodules or rupture during dorsiflexion of the ankle. Rupture of the tibialis anterior is often missed because of lack of specific examination. The tendon runs under and medial to the medial cuniform and first metatarsal. Extensor hallucis longus runs medial to the tibialis anterior and lateral to the dorsalis pedis artery. The common tendons of extensor digitorum lonugs run lateral to the artery. On the lateral border of the foot peroneus tertius goes down toward the base of the fifth metatarsal. All of the extensor tendons run deep to the extensor retinaculum making them hard to feel at the level of the ankle. The extensor tendons rupture less often than the flexor tendons, but are more commonly involved with benign lesions such as ganglions and pigmented villonodular synovitis (PVNS).

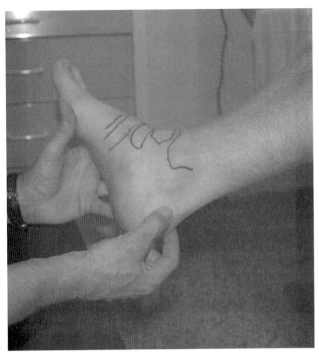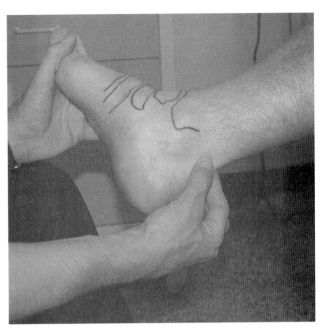

A   B

Fig 45-6. A: Achilles tendon palpation—calcaneal bursa. **B:** Achilles tendon palpation. The examiner should also palpate the insertion of the Achilles onto the calcaneus.

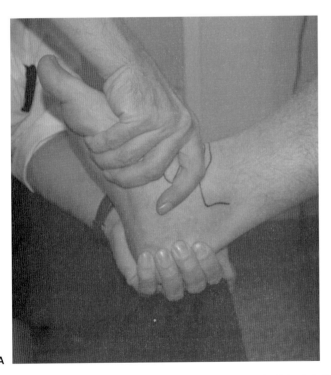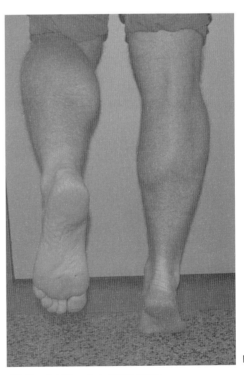

A   B

Fig 45-7. A: Ankle motion. The subtalar joint is held immobile with the right hand, and the talonavicular joint cupped with the left hand. The ankle is then dorsiflexed **(A)** and plantar flexed **(B)** with the left thumb palpating the joint margin. **B:** Ankle motion.

Peroneal Tendons

Peroneus brevis should be palpated along the posterior fibula and down to the fifth metatarsal. It is active in eversion and plantar flexion. The tendon may sublux or dislocate out of the peroneal groove. A cavus foot position can aggrevate tendonitis.

Peroneus longus lies posterior and medial to peroneus brevis. Resisted plantar flexion of the first ray will cause the intact tendon to contract. It can snap over brevis within the fibular groove or it can dislocate out around the fibula (7).

Range of Motion

Determination of absolute range of motion is less critical than assessment of loss of motion compared with the opposite side, as motion is very variable between patients.

The symptomatic joint as well as the joints above and below should be ranged in isolation. The surgeon should feel for crepitus and determine if isolated joint motion is associated with discomfort.

It takes practice to examine each joint in isolation. For example, for the ankle, the tibia is immobilized with the left hand while the talonavicular joint is cupped in the right hand. The talus is dorsiflexed and plantar flexed on the tibia, feeling for pain and crepitus **(Fig 45-7)**.

Ankle joint motion can be determined in degrees using a goniometer against the long axis of the tibia. The remainder of the joints in the foot's motion can be graded as normal, hypermobile, mild, or severe restriction.

Special Tests

Single Leg Stance and Toe Raise
This tests for active hindfoot inversion. While the patient goes onto their toes the examiner observes the hindfoot motion. The heel goes from valgus into varus. The motion

may be deficient in patients with no subtalar motion, an extreme planovalgus foot (the tibialis posterior tendon is not strong enough to pull the heel over), or patients with ruptured tibialis posterior tendons **(Fig 45-8)**.

Anterior Drawer
This tests for integrity of the anterior talofibular ligament. The examiner internally rotates and anterior translates the talus on the tibia. As joint laxity is variable between patients a side to side comparison is required **(Fig 45-9)**.

Inversion Stress Test
This tests for integrity of the calcaneofibular ligament. The examiner inverts the calcaneus and holds the tibia feeling for opening of the lateral side of the talus. Side to side comparison is required **(Fig 45-10)**.

Thompson Test
This test is used to determine if the Achilles tendon is intact. Squeezing the gastrocsoleus should cause the foot to plantar flex. If the Achilles is ruptured, the foot fails to plantar flex and the tendon is ruptured.

Mulder's Click
This is a test for Morton's neuroma. The examiner compresses the metatarsal heads while palpating for a click between the metatarsal heads. A Morton's neuroma will click between the metatarsal heads (8) **(Fig 45-11)**.

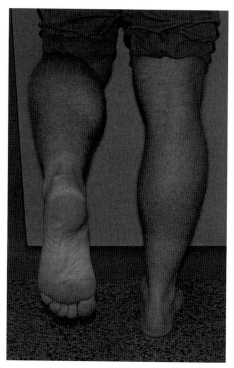
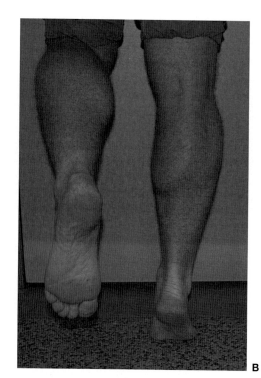

Fig 45-8. A: Single toe raise. The hindfoot rests in a neutral position. **B:** Single toe raise. After going up on tip toes the hindfoot goes into varus.

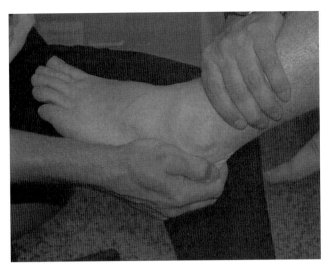

Fig 45-9. Anterior drawer. The right hand brings the calcaneus forward and into internal rotation. The left hand holds the tibia back. The ankle is kept in plantar flexion. The left index finger can be used to palpate the motion of the lateral talus.

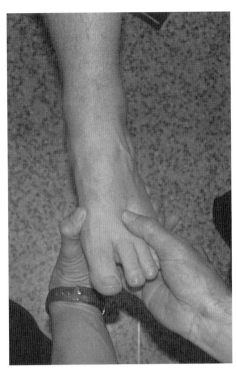

Fig 45-11. Mulder's click. The left hand compresses the metatarsal heads while the right hand palpates for a click in the second then third web space proximally.

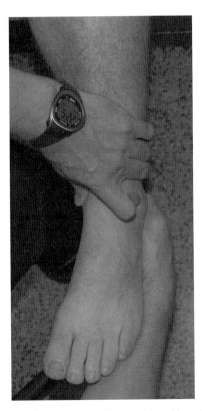

Fig 45-10. Inversion stress test. The right hand inverts the calcaneus. The left index finger palpates the lateral margin of the talus. The left hand immobilizes the tibia.

Tests for Syndesmosis Instability

A squeeze test compresses the tibia and fibula together demonstrating restoration of syndesmosis stability. During fibular translation, the fibula is manipulated in an anterior and posterior direction. During the external rotation test, the ankle is externally rotated in neutral dorsiflexion to see if the ankle opens. Pain rather than instability may be a more reliable end point (9,10).

Gastrocnemius Tightness

A tight gastrocnemius muscle can cause increased forefoot load. The tight heel cord also causes hindfoot varus because of the geometry of the ankle. Finally, the heel cord is often tight in planovalgus feet and may drive the flat foot deformity. A tight heel cord can therefore be part forefoot pain, ankle instability, and planovalgus foot deformity. The gastrocnemius muscle originates from the posterior femur and if tight will cause loss of dorsiflexion range with the knee extended. With the foot held in a normal arch position, the range of ankle dorsiflexion is measured with the knee flexed and extended **(Fig 45-12)**. Loss of ankle dorsiflexion at neutral or beyond indicates a tight gastrocnemius muscle. If the range of dorsiflexion remains the same with the knee flexed and extended, then the etiology is likely outside the heel cord and may represent either a soft tissue restraint in the ankle capsule or within the anterior ankle (11).

Coleman Block Test

In a high arched foot, the forefoot may drive the hindfoot position. In this case, the hindfoot varus will correct providing the midfoot is stable. Correction of the foot with a Coleman block test will tell the examiner that orthotic correction of the forefoot position is viable, and that some correction of the hindfoot can be expected if the forefoot is surgically corrected to a neutral position (12) **(Fig 45-13)**.

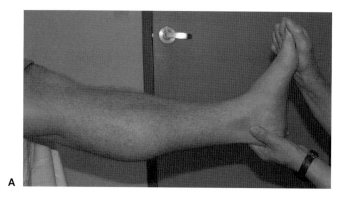

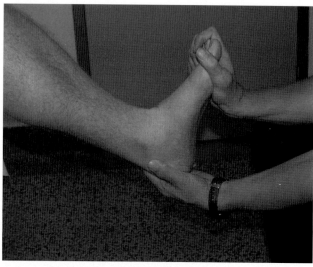

Fig 45-12. A: Gastrocnemius tightness. Dorsiflexion range with the knee extended. **B:** Gastrocnemius tightness. The foot is held in the inverted position and dorsiflexed.

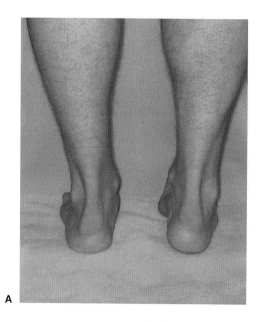

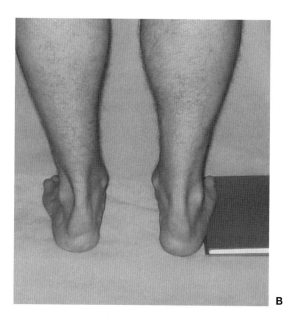

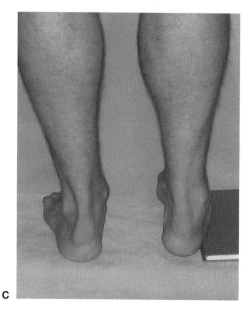

Fig 45-13. A: Coleman block test. A cavus foot with a plantar flexed first ray (forefoot valgus) and secondary hindfoot varus. **B:** Coleman block test. Correction with a flexible hindfoot after placement of a block laterally. **C:** Coleman block test. A rigid hindfoot not correcting with the block test.

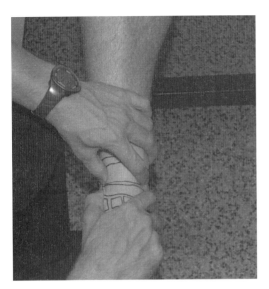

Fig 45-14. Talonavicular joint motion being examined for a patient with ankle pain.

Joints Above and Below the Symptomatic Joint

The surrounding joints are measured for pain, range of motion, and crepitus **(Fig 45-14)**.

Neuro Vascular Exam

Pulses are felt behind the medial maleolus (tibial artery) and in the dorsum of the foot (dorsalis pedis). Patients with a burning nature to their pain require testing along the courses of the nerves percussing for a Tinel's sign. Each dermatome is checked.

Monofilament examination (at 9 g) will determine if the patient has protective sensation (13). Reflexes complete the examination **(Fig 45-15)**.

■ INVESTIGATIONS

The ankle should be evaluated with standing anterior posterior (AP) and lateral **(Fig 45-16)**. A mortise view is indicated if syndesmosis instability is suspected, or to better image an osteochondral defect, but does not routinely need to be obtained (14). The foot should be evaluated with standing AP and lateral as well as nonweight-bearing oblique views, if indicated (45) **(Fig 45-17)**. Oblique views are helpful for tarsal coalitions, fractures of the talar neck, and assessment of midfoot fractures and arthritis. The calcaneal axial view can be helpful in situations of previous calcaneal fracture. A standing hindfoot alignment view is more reliable for assessment of hindfoot position, but requires specific training of radiology staff (16). Occasionally, stress views of the ankle can be helpful in documenting lateral ligament insufficiency.

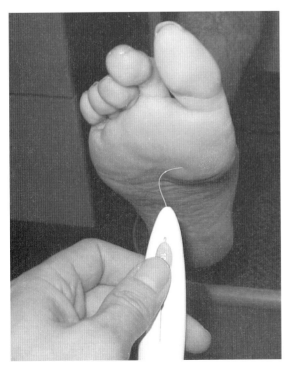

Fig 45-15. Monofilament test.

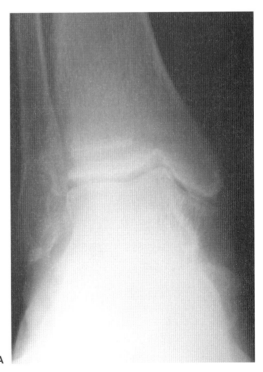

A

Fig 45-16. A: Correct views of the ankle for ankle pain. Standing AP of the ankle of a patient with recurrent lateral ankle instability for many years, subtalar pain, a medial osteochondral defect, and medial joint space narrowing. The joint space narrowing would not be apparent on a nonweight-bearing view. **B:** Correct views of the ankle for ankle pain. A standing mortise view of the same patient showing the lateral ankle joint line. **C:** Correct views of the ankle for ankle pain. The lateral view shows joint space narrowing in the posterior subtalar joint and anterior osteophytes in the ankle. The relationship of the osteophytes and range of motion would not be apparent without a weight-bearing film.

Fig 45-16. *(continued)*

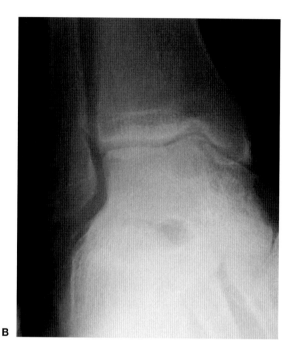

B

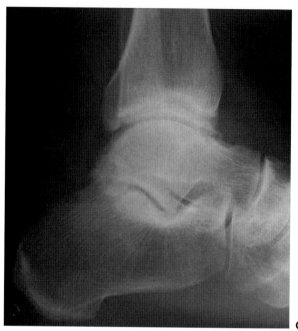

C

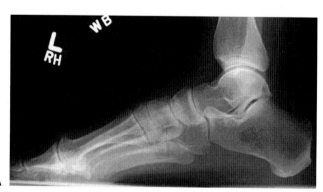

A

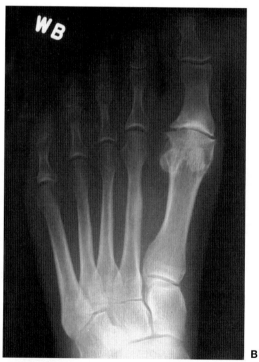

B

Fig 45-17. A: Correct views of the foot. A young runner with ongoing pain at the first MTP joint. The elevation of the first ray would not be apparent in a nonweight-bearing view, and the tarsometatarsal joints would not be correctly visualized. The relationship of the dorsal osteophytes in the first MTP joint with respect to motion would not be appreciated in a nonweight-bearing view. **B:** Correct views of the foot. A standing anteroposterior view of the same patient. The relationship between the first and second rays can be appreciated, and the midfoot joints can be visualized on a weight-bearing view.

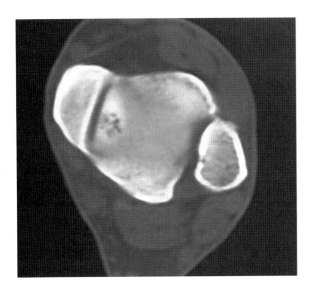

Fig 45-18. CT examination of an osteochondral defect.

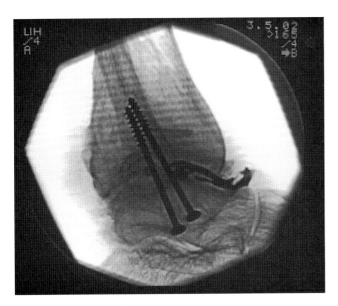

Fig 45-19. Joint injection.

The recent development of Multidetector-row computed tomography has dramatically improved the quality of foot and ankle images. The high resolution axial scans in conjunction with sagital and coronal reformats has improved the diagnosis and visualization of osteochondral lesions of the talar dome, arthritic joints, stress fractures, or small rim fractures (17) **(Fig 45-18).**

Nuclear medicine in the form of a technician three-phase bone scan is valuable for localizing stress fractures when plain x-ray or CT scans may be negative (18).

MRI continues to improve with greater magnet strengths. Visualization of pure cartilage defects and bone bruising is possible. Identifying early tendon pathology is also possible (19).

Ultrasound, although operator dependent, has improved its resolution dramatically and offers the advantage of dynamic imaging.

Image controlled joint injection can determine the origin of joint pain in patients with a unclear physical examination (20) **(Fig 45-19).**

■ REFERENCES

1. Coris EE, Lombardo JA. Tarsal navicular stress fractures. *Am Fam Physician.* 2003;67:85–90.
2. Meyer SA, Saltzman CL, Albright JP. Stress fractures of the foot and leg. *Clin Sports Med.* 1993;12:395–413.
3. Warren MP, Perlroth NE. The effects of intense exercise on the female reproductive system. *J Endocrinol.* 2001;170:3–11.
4. Manoli A II, Graham B. The subtle cavus foot, "the underpronator." *Foot Ankle Int.* 2005;26:256–263.
5. Johnson KA. Tibialis posterior tendon rupture. *Clin Orthop Relat Res.* 1983:140–147.
6. Churchill RS, Sferra JJ. Posterior tibial tendon insufficiency. Its diagnosis, management, and treatment. *Am J Orthop.* 1998; 27:339–347.
7. McConkey JP, Favero KJ. Subluxation of the peroneal tendons within the peroneal tendon sheath. A case report. *Am J Sports Med.* 1987;15:511–513.
8. Mastantuono M, Bassetti E, Di Giorgio L, et al. [Considerations on Mulder maneuver in a particular case of Civinini-Morton neuroma studied with cine magnetic resonance imaging]. *Radiol Med (Torino).* 1998;95:381–383.
9. Beumer A, Swierstra BA, Mulder PG. Clinical diagnosis of syndesmotic ankle instability: evaluation of stress tests behind the curtains. *Acta Orthop Scand.* 2002;73:667–669.
10. Beumer A, van Hemert WL, Swierstra BA, et al. A biomechanical evaluation of clinical stress tests for syndesmotic ankle instability. *Foot Ankle Int.* 2003;24:358–363.
11. Pinney SJ, Hansen ST Jr, Sangeorzan BJ. The effect on ankle dorsiflexion of gastrocnemius recession. *Foot Ankle Int.* 2002;23:26–29.
12. Fortin PT, Guettler J, Manoli A II. Idiopathic cavovarus and lateral ankle instability: recognition and treatment implications relating to ankle arthritis. *Foot Ankle Int.* 2002;23:1031–1037.
13. Smieja M, Hunt DL, Edelman D, et al. Clinical examination for the detection of protective sensation in the feet of diabetic patients. International Cooperative Group for Clinical Examination Research. *J Gen Intern Med.* 1999;14:418–424.
14. Brage ME, Rockett M, Vraney R, et al. Ankle fracture classification: a comparison of reliability of three x-ray views versus two. *Foot Ankle Int.* 1998;19:555–562.
15. Saltzman CL, Brandser EA, Berbaum KS, et al. Reliability of standard foot radiographic measurements. *Foot Ankle Int.* 1994;15:661–665.
16. Saltzman CL, el-Khoury GY. The hindfoot alignment view. *Foot Ankle Int.* 1995;16:572–576.
17. Bencardino JT, Rosenberg ZS. MR imaging and CT in the assessment of osseous abnormalities of the ankle and foot. *Magn Reson Imaging Clin N Am.* 2001;9:567–578, xi.
18. Brukner P, Bennell K. Stress fractures in female athletes. Diagnosis, management and rehabilitation. *Sports Med.* 1997; 24:419–429.
19. Lazarus ML. Imaging of the foot and ankle in the injured athlete. *Med Sci Sports Exerc.* 1999;31:S412–S420.
20. Lucas PE, Hurwitz SR, Kaplan PA, et al. Fluoroscopically guided injections into the foot and ankle: localization of the source of pain as a guide to treatment—prospective study. *Radiology.* 1997;204:411–415.

46

MUSCLE STRAINS AND CONTUSIONS

■ MICHAEL P. SWORDS, DO, DOUGLAS P. DIETZEL, DO

■ KEY POINTS

■ Muscle injuries occur in high-level athletes in active competition as well as nonathletes in the course of daily life. Pain and disability can lead to alteration in sports participation and can interfere with occupational and personal activities.

■ Muscles that cross multiple joints—the hamstrings, rectus femoris, gastrocnemius, and adductor magnus—are more susceptible to strain injury. The gastrocnemius crosses the knee, ankle, and subtalar joint before inserting on the posterior aspect of the calcaneus, making it more susceptible to injury than any other muscles of the leg.

■ A muscle strain occurs when tissue is only partially torn, although rupture involves a tear of all fibers of the muscle-tendon unit. Muscle strains usually occur as a result of a stretch. The two terms represent a continuum of the same injury.

■ Muscle strain often occurs while the muscle is controlling, or decelerating, joint range of motion during activity.

■ Most ruptures occur at a musculotendinous junction.

■ A history of blunt trauma is characteristic of muscle contusion and can be either debilitating at the time of injury or present later after further swelling has occurred.

■ History of previous muscle injury or strain is important as incomplete recovery may leave an athlete vulnerable to more severe injury in the future.

■ Magnetic resonance imaging (MRI) is often used to delineate muscle injuries. In muscle strains, MRI has documented subcutaneous location of bleeding, confirming the bleeding is not confined strictly to the injured muscle tissue. In contusions, bleeding is typically confined to the muscle itself.

■ Pain out of proportion to injury should heighten the suspicion of compartment syndrome.

■ The majority of muscle injuries do not require operative intervention. Acute compartment syndrome is an absolute surgical indication. Occasionally drainage of hematoma from contusion is necessary.

Muscle injuries form a large portion of any sports medicine or orthopaedic practice. These injuries occur in high-level athletes in active competition as well as nonathletes in the course of daily life. Pain and disability can lead to alteration in sports participation and can also interfere with occupational activities and personal interests.

■ BASIC SCIENCE

The muscular anatomy of the leg is divided into four compartments. The anterior compartment consists of the tibialis anterior, extensor hallicus longus, extensor digitorum longus, and peroneus tertius muscles as well as the deep peroneal nerve and anterior tibial artery. The peroneus longus, peroneus brevis muscles, and superficial peroneal nerve make up the contents of the lateral compartment. The superficial posterior compartment contains the gastrocnemius, soleus, plantaris muscles, and the sural nerve. Tibialis posterior, flexor digitorum longus, flexor hallicus longus muscles, the posterior tibial artery, and the tibial nerve are all found in the deep posterior compartment. The various compartments serve to control motion at the ankle and in the foot based on their anatomical location. Each specific muscle has its own function but generally speaking, muscles located in the anterior compartment provide dorsiflexion, muscles in the lateral compartment provide eversion, muscles in the deep posterior compartment provide plantar flexion and inversion in the foot, and muscles located in the superficial posterior compartment provide plantar flexion at the ankle. All muscles originate in the leg itself with the exception of the gastrocnemius, which originates on the posterior aspect of the femoral condyles, and the plantaris, which originates on the lateral femoral condyle. Muscles that cross multiple joints, the hamstrings, rectus femoris, gastrocnemius, and adductor magnus, are more susceptible to strain injury (1). The gastrocnemius crosses the knee, ankle, and subtalar joint before inserting on the posterior aspect of the calcaneus, making it more susceptible to injury than the other muscles of the leg (2).

Strain or rupture of the medial head of the gastrocnemius is often referred as "Tennis Leg." Initially this clinical entity was believed to be a strain of the plantaris muscle. The plantaris has a similar anatomical course to the gastrocnemius in the leg, but a review of the literature did not support rupture or strain of the plantaris as a clinical entity. Miller (3) reported on his surgical experience with tennis leg and found the gastrocnemius to be torn in every case while the plantaris was found to be intact. Although the overwhelming majority of muscular injuries to the leg are of the gastrocnemius, two surgically documented cases of plantaris rupture have been reported (4,5). Additionally, tear of the peroneus longus is a rare injury that has also been reported in the literature and should be kept in consideration when evaluating these injuries (6–8).

Muscle strains usually occur as a result of stretch. A muscle strain occurs when the tissue is only partially torn; rupture involves a tear of all the fibers of the muscle–tendon unit. The two terms represent a continuum of the same injury. Muscles are more prone to injury during eccentric contraction than during passive stretching alone (9). In eccentric contraction the length of the muscles increases over the course of contraction. Higher muscle forces can be seen during lengthening (10), which can be additive to forces due to the connective tissues (11). Muscle strain often occurs while the muscle is controlling, or decelerating, joint range of motion during activity. This is often the case in many higher speed sports including soccer, basketball, and football. The gastrocnemius muscle has the capability to restrict range of motion at the ankle, specifically dorsiflexion, if it is intrinsically tight. Most muscular injuries to the leg are isolated to the gastrocnemius muscle. They can either be acute sprains or rupture of the muscle itself. Most ruptures occur at the musculotendinous junction. The medial head is most commonly torn. The muscle belly of the medial head is larger than that of the lateral head. Additionally, the muscle fibers are fast twitch. Both are believed to contribute to the frequency of injury to the medial head of the gastrocnemius (12).

Muscle contusion is another frequently seen injury to the muscular structures of the leg. The injury is a result of direct blunt trauma. Contusion can occur to any muscular structure in the leg but is most commonly seen in the muscles of the anterior compartment. Local pain and swelling of the tissues are characteristic of this form of injury.

■ CLINICAL EVALUATION

History

It is important to gain an accurate history of the activity at the time of injury. It has been proposed that gastrocnemius strains occur more commonly in middle-age men who play tennis or jog (13). As stated previously, strain injuries are more common during higher speed activities and are associated with eccentric contraction. If it is a true muscle strain, or rupture, the athlete is usually unable to continue with the sporting activity and can clearly recall a specific moment of injury. Numerous authors have described a tearing sensation in the calf with sudden dorsiflexion of the ankle while extending the knee joint (3,14,15). A batsman in a cricket game sustained this injury while being filmed, and the analysis from the video agrees with this described mechanism of injury (16). Some athletes feel sudden pain during the athletic event which worsens later when at rest (17). Muscle strain injury differs from delayed onset muscle soreness which appears 12 to 34 hours after activity and is not related to an acute injury. History of previous muscle injury or strain is important as previous incomplete injury may leave an athlete more vulnerable to a more severe injury in the future. A history of blunt trauma is characteristic of muscle contusion and can be either debilitating at the time of injury or present later after further swelling has occurred.

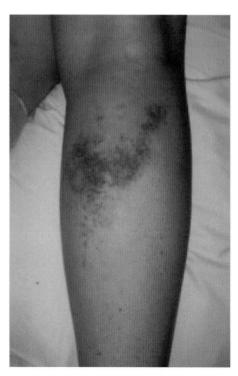

Fig 46-1. Swelling and ecchymosis centered on the midportion of the gastrocnemius muscle belly secondary to a contusion injury as a result of blunt trauma to the posterior aspect of the leg.

Physical Findings

Patients with strain injury or tearing of the gastrocnemius usually present with a significant amount of calf swelling and pain located in the posterior aspect of the leg. Tearing of the highly vascular muscle tissue can lead to significant hemorrhage and can occasionally mask any palpable defect in the acute injury period (13). Inability to perform a single heel raise should also raise suspicion of injury to the gastrocnemius (13). Pain can be present at various locations of the gastrocnemius including the upper portion of the muscle belly, the mid portion of the muscle belly, and the musculotendinous junction (17). All patients have an antalgic gait.

Ecchymosis may not be present initially but may develop over the following 24 hours **(Fig 46-1)**. Pain will be present with passive stretch of the gastrocnemius and with palpation of the medial head of the gastrocnemius. The possibility of compartment syndrome secondary to hemorrhage, while rare, has been reported in conjunction with this injury and must be considered. Pain out of proportion to injury should heighten the suspicion of a compartment syndrome. The contralateral foot should also be examined to assess for gastrocnemius equinus. Ankle dorsiflexion is assessed with the talonavicular joint held in neutral. Range of motion is assessed with the knee extended and with the knee straight. Gastrocnemius equinus exists if the ankle will not dorsiflex

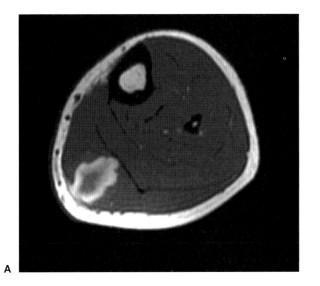

A

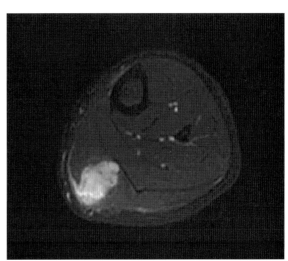

B

C

Fig 46-2. T1-weighted axial **(A)**, T2-weighted axial **(B)**, and T2-weighted sagittal **(C)** MR images show increased signal within the medial head of the gastrocnemius consistent with a partial tear proximal to the musculotendinous junction.

past neutral with the knee extended, but can dorsiflex past neutral with the knee in flexion. If the equinus does not correct with knee flexion, the equinus is a result of soleus contracture. Underlying gastrocnemius equinus increases the tension in the muscle and theoretically makes it more vulnerable to strain injury.

Imaging

When imaging is required, magnetic resonance imaging (MRI) is most often used to delineate muscle injuries. In strain injury MRI has documented subcutaneous location of bleeding, confirming that bleeding is not confined strictly to the injured muscle tissue [18]. Hematoma can form between the muscle tissue and the surrounding compartment [19]. In muscle contusion, bleeding is typically confined to the muscle itself [20,21]. MRI is effective at evaluating tears of the gastrocnemius [22] **(Fig 46-2)**. Ultrasound is also an effective modality for evaluating these injuries and can also be used to evaluate for the presence of deep venous thrombosis which can change, or complicate, the diagnosis and treatment [23,24]. Conventional radiographs are of little utility in evaluating these injuries.

■ TREATMENT

Early management consists of icing, elevation, and compression with an Ace bandage to limit swelling. If there are concerns for compartment syndrome, the patient should be monitored closely and compression is not advised. Cases of acute compartment syndrome should be treated by emergent fasciotomy. Patients presenting with large hematoma secondary to contusion should also be followed closely as occasionally drainage of the hematoma is required. Crutches or other ambulatory assist devices may be required initially. With a contusion, the injured muscle may be immobilized for a short period of time. It is important to immobilize the contused muscle in a stretched position to prevent scar formation and subsequent limitation of joint motion. Range of motion is initiated as soon as comfort allows. Imaging studies are obtained shortly after injury if the diagnosis is in doubt.

Nonoperative Treatment

The majority of injuries can be treated successfully with nonoperative management. Ice and compression are used in the early post injury period and physical therapy should be initiated early. Millar reported on nonoperative management of 720 strain injuries over a 12 year period. The treatment program was initiated within 48 hours of injury and consisted of ice, stretching, ultrasound, and isotonic exercises for antagonist muscles. The majority of patients had complete resolution of pain within the first week. Only 5% took longer than 3 weeks to recover. The rate of

recurrent injury was 0.7%. Delay in recovery was associated with presence of extensive bruising for days preceding treatment and noncompliance with the rehabilitation protocol. Shields reported on nonoperative treatment in 25 patients with 1 to 3 years follow up. The protocol is similar to that described by Millar with the addition of a neoprene calf sleeve for compression in the early post injury period and routine use of oral nonsteroidal anti-inflammatory medication (NSAID). A one-half inch heel lift was also placed in the shoe to reduce stretch on the injured tissues, as advocated by Froimson [15]. All patients were able to return to their sport of choice. Cybex II testing showed no difference in strength between injured and noninjured extremities. Contusion is also typically managed nonoperatively. Range of motion is started as soon as comfort allows. The active use of the injured muscle is allowed as tolerated. In severe contusion injuries rehabilitation can be lengthy and require participation in a physical therapy program focusing on range of motion early followed by muscle activation and strengthening.

Operative Treatment

The majority of injuries do not require operative intervention. Acute compartment syndrome is an absolute surgical indication. Most authors do not support operative treatment of gastrocnemius tears. [13,15,17,25]. Miller [3] advised operative treatment in patients who could not perform a single leg heel rise. In all reported cases the medial head of the gastrocnemius had pulled off at the musculotendinous junction and still had a small portion of tendon attached. The orientation of the tear was oblique. Suture was used for the repair in both of his operative cases and was described as quite simple. Occasionally drainage of hematoma from contusion is necessary.

■ RETURN TO ACTIVITY

Many patients with these injuries can benefit from physical therapy. Before returning to sport, the extremity should be pain free and motion at the knee and ankle should be full. Strength should be 90% of the uninjured extremity. Proprioception should also be evaluated when determining return to sport to prevent other injuries from occurring.

■ REFERENCES

1. Brewer BJ. Mechanism of injury to the musculotendinous unit. *Instr Course Lect.* 1960;17:354–358.
2. Anouchi Y, Parker R, Seitz W. Posterior compartment syndrome of the calf resulting from misdiagnosis of a rupture of the medial head of the gastrocnemius. *J Trauma.* 1987;27:678–680.
3. Miller W. Rupture of the musculotendinous juncture of the medial head of the gastrocnemius muscle. *Am J Sports Med.* 1977;5:191–193.

4. Mennen U. Rupture of the plantaris: does it exist? [letter]. *J Bone Joint Surg Am.* 1982;65:1030.

5. Hamilton W, Klostermeier T, Lim E, et al. Surgically documented rupture of the plantaris muscle: a case report and literature review. *Foot Ankle Int.* 1977;18:522–523.

6. Arciero R, Shishido N, Parr T. Acute anterolateral compartment syndrome secondary to rupture of the peroneus longus muscle. *Am J Sports Med.* 1984;12:366–367.

7. Davies JAD. Peroneal compartment syndrome secondary to rupture of the peroneus longus. A case report. *J Bone Joint Surg Am.* 1979;61:783–784.

8. Goodman M. Isolated lateral compartment syndrome. Report of a case. *J Bone Joint Surg Am.* 1980;62:834.

9. Zarins B, Ciullo JV. Acute muscle and tendon injuries in athletes. *Clin Sports Med.* 1983;2:167–182.

10. Stauber WT. Eccentric action of muscles: physiology, injury and adaptation. *Exerc Sports Sci Rev.* 1989;17:157–185.

11. Elftman H. Biomechanics of muscle. *J Bone Joint Surg Am.* 1966;48:363–377.

12. Sutro C, Sutro W. The medial head of the gastrocnemius: a review of the basis for partial rupture and for intermittent claudication. *Bull Hosp Jt Dis.* 1985;45:150–157.

13. Shields CI, Redix L, Brewster C. Acute tears of the medial head of the gastrocnemius. *Foot Ankle.* 1985;5:186–190.

14. Arner O, Lindholm A. What is tennis leg? *Acta Chir Scand.* 1958;116:73–77.

15. Froimson AI. Tennis leg. *JAMA.* 1969;209:415–416.

16. Orchard JW, Alcott E, Farhart P, et al. Exact moment of a gastrocnemius muscle strain captured on video. *Br J Sports Med.* 2002;36:222–223.

17. Millar AP. Strains of the posterior calf musculature ("tennis leg"). *Am J Sports Med.* 1977;7:172–174.

18. De Smet AA, Best TM. MR imaging of the distribution and location of acute hamstring injuries in athletes. *AJR Am J Roentgenol.* 2000;174:393–399.

19. Fornage BD, Tokuche DH, Segal P, et al. Ultrasonography in the evaluation of muscular trauma. *J Ultrasound Med.* 1983;2:549–554.

20. Rooser B. Quadriceps contusion with compartment syndrome: evacuation of hematoma in 2 cases. In: Anderson JL, George FJ, Shepard RJ, eds. *Year book of sports medicine.* Chicago: Year Book Medical Publishers; 1988.

21. Rothwell AG. Quadriceps hematoma: a prospective clinical study. *Clin Orthop.* 1982;171:97–103.

22. Menz M, Lucas G. MRI of a rupture of a medial head of the gastrocnemius muscle: a case report. *J Bone Joint Surg Am.* 1991;73:1260–1262.

23. Bianchi S, Martinoli C, Abdelwahab IF, et al. Sonographic evaluation of tears of the gastrocnemius medial head ("tennis leg"). *J Ultrasound Med.* 1998;17:157–162.

24. Delgado GJ, Chung CB, Lektrakul N, et al. Tennis leg: clinical US study of 141 patients and anatomic investigation of four cadavers with MR imaging and US. *Radiology.* 2002;224:112–119.

25. Leach R. Leg and foot injuries in racquet sports. *Clin Sports Med.* 1988;7:359–370.

CHRONIC COMPARTMENT SYNDROME

47

ROBERT A. PEDOWITZ, MD, PhD, DEREK W. WEICHEL, BS

■ KEY POINTS

- Compartment syndrome is a condition of elevated pressure within a space bounded by bone and/or fascia which results in decreased perfusion of tissues within the compartment.
- Chronic compartment syndrome (CCS) is the chronic exertional form of compartment syndrome, found as a result of sports or exercise.
- CCS is always associated with pain that occurs during exercise and with increased intracompartmental pressures.
- Patients with CCS often do not present with a classic set of symptoms. Therefore a high index of suspicion is required for patients with exertional extremity pain. The clinical examination is more effective in ruling out other possibilities than it is for providing a definitive diagnosis of CCS.
- Patients will almost always describe pain that is induced by exertion and resolves with rest. Elite athletes, as well as recreational athletes, involved in both running and non-running activities can suffer from CCS.
- Direct measurement of intracompartmental pressure remains the hallmark of objective assessment of both CCS and acute compartment syndrome (ACS).
- During measurement of pressure, the physician should avoid injecting large amounts of anesthetic into the compartment. However, the skin, subcutaneous tissue, and fascia can be anesthetized without fear of raising intracompartmental pressure.
- It is important that CCS patients reproduce their symptoms during diagnostic assessment. The patient needs to perform the specific exercise activity that causes the pain.
- Activity modification, taping, stretching, nonsteroidal anti-inflammatory administration (NSAID), and the use of

orthotics are included in nonsurgical management of CCS, but are rarely successful.
- Fasciotomy is advised for patients who want to return to full unrestricted activities and can be effective even after a delayed diagnosis.

Compartment syndrome can occur, either acutely [acute compartment syndrome (ACS)] or in a chronic exertional form [chronic compartment syndrome (CCS)] in sports and exercise. CCS should be in the differential diagnosis of any patient who presents with exertional extremity pain (1–4). Mubarak and Hargens (5) define compartment syndrome as a condition of elevated pressure within a space bounded by bone and/or fascia that results in decreased perfusion of tissues within the compartment. There have been many reports of compartment syndrome in both the upper and lower extremities (6–24). The pathophysiology of CCS is not yet fully understood; however, it can be treated surgically in the majority of cases. This chapter will address the pathophysiology and diagnosis of CCS.

■ ANATOMY

The anatomical features that are relevant to a discussion of compartment syndrome have been described previously (25). Local osseofascial anatomy defines the compartments of the body and it is useful to think of each compartment as a closed space. Each compartment has its own pressure-volume relationship. Factors that cause an increase in intracompartmental volume, such as hemorrhage or interstitial swelling, may lead to significant increases in intracompartmental pressure, since bone and fascia have little elasticity.

Extrinsic compression, such as a cast or tight dressing, can also lead to increased pressure within the compartment. In ACS, increased intracompartmental pressure leads to decreased perfusion, tissue ischemia, and a persistent vicious cycle of further swelling, etc. If the ischemia is prolonged, Volkman's ischemic contracture (25a) with myonecrosis, decreased extremity function, and permanent deformity may result.

Rarely, CCS will develop into ACS (26,27). Prolonged tissue ischemia is not typically associated with CCS. Intermittent elevation of compartment pressure is observed with exertion in CCS. CCS is always associated with pain that occurs during exercise and with increased intracompartmental pressures. However, the mechanism of pain production associated with CCS is still debated.

ACS or CCS can be seen in virtually any extremity or axial skeletal muscle; however, CCS is most commonly diagnosed in the four compartments of the leg. Anatomic dissections that revealed variable proximal and distal sub-compartments of the deep posterior compartment of the leg (28) support the claims made by some authors that the deep posterior compartment of the leg is subdivided into two or three sub-compartments (29,30). When making the diagnosis or considering surgical treatment, such variations in anatomy should be considered. The anterior, lateral, and superficial posterior compartments make up the remaining leg compartments.

The three compartments of the thigh are the anterior which includes the quadriceps, the posterior which includes the hamstrings, and the adductor groups. The upper arm also has three compartments which are the deltoid, the posterior which contains the triceps, and the anterior (biceps-brachialis). The volar and dorsal compartments make up the forearm; however, the mobile wad is considered to be functionally separate by some authors. The hand is made up of the interosseous groups, thenar, and hypothenar compartments. The carpal tunnel is typically considered to be a distinct compartment from both the forearm and the hand. The foot has lateral, medial, central, and intraosseous compartments.

The gluteal muscles are a functionally separate compartment. Remaining compartments include the paraspinal musculature and the muscles of the internal and external pelvis. The abdomen is also considered a functional compartment in which organ ischemia and severe morbidity may result from increased abdominal pressure (31,32). Improper placement of invasive intra-muscular pressure measurement devices can penetrate and damage neurovascular structures. Therefore, it is important to have a good understanding of the three dimensional anatomy of these muscular compartments.

Pathophysiology of Compartment Syndromes

It is understood that a common characteristic associated with compartment syndrome is elevated pressure within the osseofascial compartment which in the case of ACS causes ischemia and possible necrosis. However, the basic pathophysiology of this syndrome is still not completely understood. Capillary perfusion is required for healthy tissue. The

Starling equation defines the balance of extravascular and intravascular fluid dynamics that affect transcapillary flow (33). Permeability factors (capillary surface area and water conductivity), colloid osmotic factors (plasma and interstitial colloid osmotic pressures), and hydrostatic factors (intravascular and interstitial fluid pressures) are all included in the Starling equation (33). Because normotensive humans have a capillary blood pressure between 20 to 30 mm Hg, interstitial fluid pressures that rise much above 30 mm Hg may lead to a slow decrease in capillary perfusion. This is the point at which hypoperfusion starts but it may not be the threshold for overt compartmental necrosis. A clinician's clinical concern for compartment syndrome should be increased when interstitial pressure reaches 30 mm Hg in a normotensive individual. In a state of systemic hypoperfusion, the driving force for local perfusion is decreased which leads to decreased critical compartment pressure thresholds for tissue liability. This theory is supported by Arbabi et al. (34) who demonstrated that the neuromuscular abnormalities associated with compartment syndrome occur at lower compartment pressures when the compartment is also subjected to hypotension and hypoxia, suggesting that the signs and symptoms of compartment syndrome are related not only to the compartment pressures, but also to the compartment perfusion pressure.

The specific anatomic basis of microvascular dysfunction in compartment syndrome is not well understood. Early reports (35) suggested that increased intracompartmental pressure causes reflex arterial spasm with consequent tissue ischemia. However, Vollmar et al. (36) found that blood flow ceased in arterioles with increasing pressure on the vessel without any sign of spasm or collapse.

Other descriptions look at the effects of increased compartment pressure on the microvasculature. The theory which suggests that microvasculature occlusion occurs when the tissue pressure is greater than the arterial or transmural pressure was proposed by Burton (37) and Eaton et al. (38). These authors suggest that increased tissue pressure or decreased systemic blood pressure would lead to occlusion of the microvasculature.

It was proposed by Hargens et al. (39) that collapse and occlusion of the thin walled capillary vessels is caused by increased compartmental pressure. Normotensive dogs had intracapillary pressures between 20 to 30 mm Hg which correlates well with a compartmental pressure threshold of 30 mm Hg for observation of early ischemic changes associated with compartment syndrome. This concept has been challenged by Vollmar et al. (36) who found that capillaries did not collapse at high pressures even after they demonstrated cessation of blood flow.

The critical driving force for blood flow across the capillary bed is the arterial venous (A-V) pressure gradient. One theory is that a drop in the A-V gradient is caused by increased venous pressure due to the increased intracompartmental pressure (40). Birtles et al. (41) support the theory that the signs and symptoms associated with CCS are at least partially due to venous obstruction caused by the increased intracompartmental pressure. They found that healthy patients demonstrated increased muscle fatigability, pain, and size in the anterior tibialis muscle when fitted with a sphygmomanometer cuff just below the knee that was inflated to a pressure of 81 mm Hg to occlude venous outflow. These findings are supported by Zhang et al. (42) who demonstrated that the anterior compartment of the leg had decreased blood flow and perfusion pressure with thigh tourniquet induced venous stasis. The work by Vollmar et al. (36) also supports these findings as they observed venular vessels collapse, regardless of diameter, at much lower pressures than those needed to collapse arteriolar vessels. Upon venular collapse and cessation of venular outflow, there was still perfusion of the arteriolar segments of the vasculature. Similarly, as pressure on the vessel was slowly decreased from levels at which both arteriolar and venular blood flow had ceased, arteriolar blood flow resumed before venous drainage was evident. Vollmar et al. (36) concluded that impaired venous drainage with impaired capillary stasis, but not arteriolar ischemia, could be the main physiological component of compartment syndrome.

Researchers cannot agree on one common etiology of CCS. It is understood that intermittent elevation of tissue pressure occurs during exertion and reverses at rest in patients with CCS. Intramuscular pressures greater than 500 mm Hg have been measured during normal vigorous skeletal muscle contractions (43,44). Therefore, tissue perfusion must occur between muscle contractions. However, the intramuscular pressures between contractions are elevated with CCS, thereby preventing effective tissue perfusion.

Styf and Korner (45) suggested that occlusion of large vessels by local muscle herniation as they transverse the interosseous membrane causes CCS of the anterior leg (46). Martens and Moeyersoons (47) believe that the fascia in CCS patients is not as compliant as normal fascia and that it is not able to accommodate the increased muscle volume that normally occurs during exercise. According to Raether and Lutten (19), vigorous exercise may result in an intracompartmental volume increase up to 20% over the baseline. Detmer et al. (2) observed increased fascial thickness in 25 of 26 samples taken from legs of CCS patients. Similar results were reported by Garcia-Mata et al. (7) who found that the fascia of adolescent patients with CCS was thicker, enlarged, and harder than that of normal patients. It is not known if these abnormalities are the cause or the effect of chronically increased intramuscular pressures. Deirder et al. (6) observed similar changes in muscle size during exercise between control subjects and subjects with CCS suggesting that tight fascia may not be the cause of pain in these patients. Others (18,48–50) have observed a variety of anatomic abnormalities that could put an individual at risk for CCS. However, no unifying theme has emerged in these observations.

The role of muscle ischemia in CCS has been a surprisingly controversial subject. Amendola et al. reported that MR imaging did not reveal consistent ischemic changes in

patients with CCS. Similarly, nuclear magnetic resonance spectroscopy did not show ischemic changes in the majority of patients studied by Balduini et al. (51); however, a number of articles do support the theory that muscle ischemia is a significant factor in CCS. Takebayashi et al. (52) observed decreased Thallium201 distribution in muscle affected by CCS using SPECT imaging. In addition, Mohler et al. (53) observed greater relative deoxygenation, as well as delayed re-oxygenation, after exercise in patients with CCS using near infrared spectroscopy (NIRS). Van den Brand et al. (54) also noted greater relative deoxgenation during exercise in patients with CCS compared with normal subjects when measured with NIRS. Ota et al. (55) reported delayed muscular re-oxygenation in a patient with chronic exertional compartment syndrome following exercise. Breit et al. (56) observed oxygen levels in muscles subjected to exercise and external compression progressively decreased while it remained fairly constant in subjects with no compression. During recovery, it also took longer for the tissue oxygenation levels to return to baseline in subjects with external compression. Abraham et al. (57) observed limited maximal blood flow immediately after exercise which seemed to be caused by increased intracompartmental pressure in CCS patients; however, a delayed peak in hyperemia following exercise coincided with pain relief. New diagnostic methods may facilitate better understanding of the underlying etiology and pathophysiology of CCS.

Birtles et al. (58) observed greater delayed onset muscle soreness in patients who have CCS and suggested that this may be due to damage and inflammation of the connective tissue. However, Kalchmair et al. (59) observed several biological changes in the plasma during reperfusion following a period of ischemia which could also be related to this finding. They found increased histamine release immediately upon reperfusion which is kept in check by diamine oxidase (DO) for the first 60 minutes after which the DO is no longer able to metabolize all the histamine. The plasma monomine oxidase levels also remain consistently high throughout the reperfusion period.

■ DIFFERENTIAL DIAGNOSIS OF CCS

The differential diagnosis of CCS has been described previously (25). The signs and symptoms associated with CCS are very similar to those of other etiologies of exertional leg pain. According to the classification established by Detmer et al. (2), a stress fracture (Type I), medial tibial periostalgia (Type II), and CCS (Type III) are the most common diagnoses to consider in patients with exertional leg pain. Venous stasis, vascular or neurogenic claudication, tendonitis, nerve entrapment disorders, occult infection, metabolic bone disease, or neoplastic process are other possible diagnoses. Turnipseed (60) observed that 93% of cases of atypical claudication in adolescents and young adults were caused by CCS.

Some types of vascular abnormalities could be misdiagnosed as CCS. Intermittent distal ischemia can be caused by popliteal entrapment syndrome (61) or by constriction of the superficial femoral artery in the adductor canal (62). A subject with a popliteal artery aneurysm was originally misdiagnosed and treated with a fasciotomy for CCS in a case reported by Knight et al. (63). Studies including bone scintigraphy, magnetic resonance imaging, angiography, or electromyography may be needed to rule out other disorders in the process of making the correct diagnosis. Definitive diagnosis of CCS often requires the use of objective diagnostic methods.

CLINICAL PRESENTATION OF CCS

Patients with CCS often do not present with a classic set of symptoms and therefore a high index of suspicion is required for patients with exertional extremity pain. Although some of the described clinical presentations will be found in both upper and lower extremity CCS, most of the published information pertains to the lower leg.

Patients will almost always describe pain that is induced by exertion and resolves with rest. Elite athletes as well as recreational athletes involved in both running and nonrunning activities can suffer from CCS. Some reports state that the sex distribution is equal (2,3); others claim that it is more prevalent in males (47,64). More recent reports, however, observed a higher prevalence in females (65,66). Although CCS has been diagnosed in elderly patients and adolescents (3,7), it is usually seen in active, young adults.

Any patient who may have CCS should be carefully questioned about their pain which they may describe as cramping, muscle tightness, swelling, or a feeling of weakness or numbness. The symptoms may be achy, sharp, dull, or diffuse. Neuromuscular disorders such as slap foot or abnormal distal sensation during exercise may be described. A recent report found that 68% of patients with CCS had it bilaterally (66). The pain caused by CCS could be brought on with relatively light exertion or heavy exercise; however, each athlete usually has a consistent pattern of pain production in terms of duration of exercise. Their symptoms will also normally resolve over a consistent time period which may be minutes, hours, or rarely days after exertion. The clinical presentation may be complicated if other forms of exercise-induced extremity pain are also present. CCS has been described in the intraosseous compartments of the hand, dorsal, and volar forearm compartments, lumbar paraspinal muscles, the feet, and the thigh (6,8–11,16,18–24,48,67); however, it is most common in the leg.

The anterior and/or lateral compartments of the leg are most frequently involved. The least frequently involved compartment is the superficial posterior compartment, an observation that is probably related to its relatively greater natural compliance. CCS of the deep posterior compartment is a subject of controversy. Due to the fact that they were not able to demonstrate increased muscle relaxation pressures during or after exercise in the tibialis posterior or flexor digitorum longus muscles, Melberg and Styf (12) believed that CCS of the deep posterior compartment was extremely rare; however, other authors have reported 63 cases (47) and 15 cases (3) of CCS in the deep posterior compartment of the leg. Due to the fact that it is functionally and anatomically separated from the rest of the deep posterior compartment, Davey et al. (29) believed that the tibialis posterior compartment may be another site of CCS. Anatomic dissections have validated these concerns (28). It is not uncommon for a patient to have more than one compartment affected in the same limb (52). Any muscle compartment can be involved by CCS so a high index of suspicion is required. Although objective compartmental pressure measurements are very important for confirming the diagnosis, they may be problematic in atypical locations as pressure criteria for one compartment are not necessarily directly applicable to other muscle compartments.

A key component of the physical exam for CCS is to rule out other possibilities in the differential diagnosis. Ulmer (68) concluded that the presence of clinical findings was not as useful for making the diagnosis of compartment syndrome as the absence of findings was for excluding other diagnoses; however, he also observed that the probability that the patient has compartment syndrome increases significantly if three or more clinical findings are present simultaneously. Pedowitz et al. (3) observed an increased rate of fascial hernias in patients with CCS when compared to healthy subjects. Other authors have reported a 20% to 60% instance of fascial defects in patients with CCS (5,7,26,47,69). Normally, the neurovascular examination is normal; however, Rowden et al. (70) found through careful examination that patients who had CCS of the anterior compartment of the leg demonstrated decreased vibratory sensation in the deep peroneal distribution. In addition, these patients did not have normal postexercise potentiation of the peroneal motor amplitude. If the patient has any periosteal or bony tenderness, other etiologies of exertional leg pain are likely.

When subjected to various forms of exercise, several findings may suggest CCS but none are truly diagnostic variables. Deirdre et al. (71) observed that following 4 minutes of isometric exercise, patients with CCS had significantly more pain than a group of controls. The same study demonstrated that CCS patients have a slower recovery of voluntary force when at rest following 20 minutes of isometric exercise. Birtles et al. (58) observed that following eccentric exercise, patients with CCS do not appear to have greater pain, fatigue, or swelling; however, they may have increased delayed onset muscle soreness.

OBJECTIVE ASSESSMENT

As indicated by Pedowitz and Hargens (25), direct measurement of intracompartmental pressure remains the hallmark of objective assessment for both ACS and CCS and are still the gold standard when compared with newer methods. For the majority of compartments, intracompartmental pressure measurements can be obtained safely without much pain.

There are direct and indirect techniques for intracompartmental pressure measurement. A miniature pressure transducer is directed at the tissue level for direct techniques. There is transmission of fluid pressure from the muscle level to a remote transducer for the indirect techniques.

Fine needles were inserted into the interstitium and intermittent or continuous fluid injections kept the needle tip from occluding with the early methods of tissue pressure measurement. Excess fluid administration, however, can lead to false readings or even cause ACS. The use of the wick catheter for the clinical assessment of ACS was described by Mubarak et al. (72). Scholander et al. (73) originally described this technique in animal studies. To minimize tip occlusion and increase the surface area at the catheter tissue interface, the wick catheter uses Dexon fibers that are fixed at the tip of a fluid filled polyethylene catheter. With the creation of small slits in the polyethylene tubing catheter, the slit catheter soon replaced the wick catheter (74). The benefits of this catheter included the facts that it eliminated the risk of retained wick material and gave a more rapid response. These systems involved transmission of fluid pressure to a remote transducer. This transducer needed to be "zeroed" to the planned level of pressure measurement.

The introduction of a handheld device with the pressure transducer included (Stryker Surgical, Kalamazoo, Michigan) simplified the process of measuring intracompartmental pressure. In this system, the transducer is connected to a needle that has several side ports. These side ports help eliminate muscle occlusion of the needle. While this device is relatively simple to use, it can produce false readings if it is not applied carefully. Hutchinson and Ireland (75) described the appropriate use of the device and its application for making the diagnosis of CCS. Uliasz et al. (76) compared the Stryker Monitor with the IV pump method, which is a technique that utilizes slow infusion of normal saline through a needle (77), and found that they were equally acceptable methods for measuring intramuscular pressure. Sangwan et al. (78) recently described the effective, safe, and reproducible use of a saline manometer to measure compartment pressures. The benefits of this device include that it is cheap, easy to assemble, and is available to physicians at peripheral hospitals who may not have access to other technology.

A micro-capillary infusion technique for measuring intracompartmental pressure during exercise was described by Styf and Korner (46). A Teflon catheter (Atos Medical Inc., Moorby, Sweden) is utilized along with constant infusion of 0.2 cc per hour or less. The tip has many side holes which are kept open by the slow constant infusion. This system has a very high dynamic response for exercise studies. Unfortunately, the changing level of a hydrostatic fluid column causes artifacts that are difficult to control outside of the controlled laboratory condition.

Direct methods for measurement of intracompartmental pressure which use transducer tip catheters have the advantage of not being affected by variable height of the hydrostatic column. Good accuracy and dynamic characteristics were reported with the use of a transducer-tipped fiberoptic catheter by Crenshaw et al. (79); however, after exercise the catheter may underestimate muscle relaxation pressure and muscle rest pressure. A solid state transducer-tipped catheter system for the measurement of intracompartmental pressures has resulted from miniaturization techniques. A more recent study by Willy et al. (80) supported the use of a new electronic transducer-tipped catheter system for measurement of intracompartmental pressures. They found the device accurate and easy to use, not needing any calibration. They observed that it prevented hydrostatic pressure artifacts. Another advantage is the fact that it eliminates the need for fluid infusion. Long term monitoring is possible with this device without any need for manipulation. In addition, it can be used to measure compartment pressures intraoperatively. During exercise, this system provides dynamic responses and high-frequency recordings. This type of pressure-measurement device may become more commonplace in the future; however, the cost of such devices is somewhat prohibitive at this time.

For all forms of intracompartmental pressure measurement, a sterile technique and a small amount of local anesthesia should be used prior to catheter insertion (25). Although the physician should avoid injecting large amounts of anesthetic into the compartment, the skin, subcutaneous tissue, and fascia can be anesthetized without fear of raising the intracompartmental pressure. Care should be taken to avoid damaging the overlying and adjacent neurovascular anatomy. Techniques for catheter placement have been previously described (5).

It is important that the CCS patients exercise to elicit symptoms so that any changes in intracompartmental pressure can be observed. Intracompartmental pressure measurements can be taken before, during, and after exercise in these patients. The pressures that are recorded before and after exercise are static measurements. A high frequency response is needed to observe rapid changes in intramuscular pressure that are encountered during and between contractions with exercise. Most methods for measuring intracompartmental pressures during exercise that utilize transmission along the fluid column to a separate transducer have substantial artifact due to the changing hydrostatic columns. For this reason, most clinicians rely on static measurements taken before and after exercise to assist with making the diagnosis.

A number of recent articles have demonstrated that MR imaging may be a useful noninvasive tool for the diagnosis of chronic compartment syndrome. Eskelin et al. (81) found good correlation between post-exercise intracompartmental pressure and increased MR signal intensity following exercise in CCS patients and suggested that MR imaging may be used to assess the severity of the syndrome and for studying the pathology of CCS. A number of studies advocate the specific use of T2-weighted MR imaging and observed increased signal intensity in the affected compartments of the leg in patients with CCS with the use of this imaging technique (55,82–85). A similar increased signal was found in the extensor compartment muscles of the forearms in a patient with CCS of that compartment (9). For patients with any type of medial tibial pain, which may include CCS, Mattila et al. (86) recommend an MR imaging protocol consisting of axial STIR images with T1-weighted axial pre- and post-contrast images to depict any bone pathology as well as dynamic contrast enhanced imaging to detect periosteal edema and abnormal contrast enhancement inside a compartment. Other benefits of MR imaging include evaluation for other possible diagnoses in atypical cases and follow-up evaluation after definitive treatment (82). In the future, MRI may allow better delineation of the involved compartments, which could improve the specificity of surgical treatment (84).

Recently, several articles have been published supporting the use of Near-infrared spectroscopy (NIRS) as a noninvasive technique that may be used for the diagnosis of both acute and chronic compartment syndrome. This noninvasive technique assesses the relative concentration of oxygenated versus deoxygenated blood within the muscle based upon the different absorbance characteristics of oxyhemoglobin and deoxyhemoglobin. In an animal model, Garr et al. (87) found a correlation between tissue oxyhemoglobin levels measured by NIRS and compartment pressure, perfusion pressures, and neuromuscular dysfunction. In a simulated compartment syndrome with external compression, NIRS was able to detect changes in muscle oxygen concentration during exercise (56). Similarly, Hargens et al. (88) observed that NIRS can detect deoxygenation caused by abnormally elevated intramuscular pressure that resulted from external compression in exercising skeletal muscle. Van de Brand et al. (54) differentiated healthy legs from patients with CCS of the lower extremity with the use of NIRS. Mohler et al. (53) also observed greater deoxygenation of the muscles in the compartments affected with CCS during exercise and delayed recovery of oxygenation of the same muscles after cessation of exercise with the use of NIRS. The use of NIRS revealed a similar prolonged ischemia of the anterior compartment in CCS patients following exercise in a report by Ota et al. (55). The use of NIRS for the diagnosis of acute compartment syndrome has also been supported by recent literature (34,89). Giannotti et al. (89) state that NIRS is effective at measuring tissue oxygen saturation levels in the superficial posterior, anterior, and lateral compartments of the leg; however, the effectiveness of the device on other compartments remains to be tested. Although it is a promising tool, at this time there are no widely accepted diagnostic criteria that can be applied for NIRS in the clinical situation.

Other indirect methods may also be useful for making the diagnosis of CCS. 201T1 SPECT has been shown to define the four compartments of the lower leg and evaluate blood perfusion in each compartment. Further testing will be needed before it can be used reliably in making the diagnosis of CCS (52). With further testing, Laser Doppler Flowmetry, which measures blood flow in a compartment, may be a useful tool for understanding the pathophysiology of CCS and in making the diagnosis (57). Normal thermodiffusion values, which are a measure of tissue perfusion, are 20 ml/min 100 g; however, the values of ischemic muscle are below 10 ml/min 100 g, suggesting that this may be another way to monitor the tissue perfusion in patients who may have compartment syndrome (90). Recent studies suggest that with further development, 99Tcm-methoxyisobutyl isonitrile (MIBI) scintigraphy may be a useful tool for the diagnosis of compartment syndrome (91,92). Lynch et al. (93) demonstrated that a noninvasive ultrasonic pulsed phase locked loop (PPLL) device is able to detect fascial displacement caused by very small changes in intramuscular pressure (as little as 1 mm Hg). More research is needed to apply these findings to the clinical diagnosis of CCS. Finally, a noninvasive hardness measurement of the compartment with an EBI Noninvasive Compartment Evaluator 1000 (EBI Inc, Parsippany, NJ) is not recommended due to the low specificity and accuracy observed by Dickson et al. (94).

As Pedowitz and Hargens (25) pointed out, it is very important that CCS patients reproduce their symptoms during diagnostic assessments of CCS. While various exercise protocols have been described for this purpose, the patient may need to perform the specific activity that causes their pain (95). A false negative diagnosis could result if pressure measurements (or other parameters) are acquired without reproduction of the pain. To maximize the likelihood that the patient will be able to reproduce their symptoms during the evaluation, they should be asked to exercise in the days to weeks prior to their appointment so there is a relatively clear and predictable time sequence for eliciting symptoms on the day of testing.

■ DIAGNOSTIC CRITERIA FOR CCS

Pressure criteria for the diagnosis of CCS are described for pressures before, during, and after exercise; however, there is controversy regarding which criteria should be used. As stated previously, it is difficult to get accurate pressure measurements during running or other vigorous activity due to the need for transducers with high frequency response that are not affected by changes in hydrostatic columns. Normally, intramuscular pressures become extremely high during active muscle contractions. For this reason, mean intramuscular pressures and peak intramuscular pressures are not useful for diagnostic purposes. Patients with CCS have been found to have increased intramuscular pressures between contractions (96). This is the interval when muscle is actually perfused, analogous to myocardial perfusion that occurs during diastole. Styf et al. (96) observed that CCS patients complain of pain and swelling, which is associated with decreased muscle blood flow, when the muscle relaxation pressure is greater than 35 mm Hg. Some patients with "muscle hypertension syndrome" have generalized increased muscle tension at rest which makes the use of intramuscular pressure before exercise debatable according to Styf and Korner (50). In addition, some of these patients with muscle hypertension syndrome could be given a false positive diagnosis of CCS as they can also have elevated pressures after exercise due to their inability to relax.

Because it is relatively simple to measure resting pressures before and after exercise with the patient in a stationary position, the objective diagnosis of CCS has focused on these measurements. Pedowitz et al. (3) collected intracompartmental pressure measurements on 210 leg compartments of patients with exertional pain but who did not have CCS. Through these measurements, confidence intervals for diagnostic purposes were defined. Diagnostic pressures of ≥15 mm Hg at rest, ≥30 mm Hg 1 minute after exercise, and/or ≥20 mm Hg 5 minutes after exercise were felt to be diagnostic of CCS. Due to the unique physiological characteristics of specific compartments (related to local anatomy and compliance), the criteria did vary somewhat according to the specific leg compartment that was studied; therefore, unusual sites of CCS may not fit these criteria. A more recent report (97) in which the subjects did have CCS found the following criteria to be adequate for the diagnosis of CCS: a tissue pressure immediately after exercise >52 mm Hg OR a tissue pressure between 30 and 50 mm Hg immediately after exercise with a pressure >30 mm Hg 5 minutes after exercise OR a tissue pressure >20 mm Hg at rest and >30 mm Hg immediately after exercise. Turnipseed (66) used a measurement of greater than 25 mm Hg at rest or pressure that remained greater than 25 mm Hg after exercise as diagnostic for CCS. Taking into account the fact that a child's circulatory status is different from that of an adult, Garcia-Mata et al. (7) established criteria for the diagnosis of CCS in youth. They determined that a baseline intracompartmental pressure >10 mm Hg, a 1 minute post-exertion pressure >20 mm Hg, a 5 minute post exertion measurement >20 mm Hg, or a normalization time of intracompartmental pressure >15 minutes to be diagnostic for CCS.

Other investigators (46,74,96,98–101) have observed delayed return to baseline after cessation of exercise in patients with CCS. It should not take more than 10 minutes for intramuscular pressures to return to baseline following exercise and this fact could be useful in the assessment of CCS, and in most cases, pressures return to baseline values within 5 or 6 minutes. Two important facts to keep in mind when collecting these pressure measurements are that the joint position can significantly alter compartment pressure measurements (102) and that the pressure within one compartment is not always the same at all locations in that compartment (103).

Treatment of CCS

Conservative treatment may be tried for CCS as it is not a limb or life threatening condition. If it is not treated, however, it has been shown to cause atypical claudication in adolescents

and young adults (60). Activity modification and conditioning, taping, stretching, nonsteroidal anti-inflammatory administration, and the use of orthotics are included in the nonsurgical management of CCS; however, these are rarely successful at treating the condition.

Fasciotomy is advised for those patients who want to return to full unrestricted activities **(Figs 47-1** and **47-2)**. Fasciotomy can be an effective treatment for CCS even after a delayed diagnosis (9). Definitive treatment of CCS involves decompressive fasciotomy that may be performed through relatively limited skin incisions. There is some controversy, however, regarding the requisite size of the skin incision. Turnipseed (66) recommends open fasciotomies for CCS due to better outcomes and fewer complications. It should be emphasized that the length of dermotomy for CCS may be substantially less than the skin incision required for treatment of an acute compartment syndrome, where skin incisions need to be relatively generous. Several authors have previously described the details of decompression for the various compartments (5,104). More recently, several authors have described fasciotomy procedures for CCS using one (105), two (106,42), and three (55) small incisions. Decompression of the superficial peroneal nerve as it exits the fascial defect between the anterior and lateral compartments may be appropriate if there are signs of nerve compression/irritation at this level.

Good cosmetic result can be achieved whether multiple small incisions or one larger longitudinal dermotomy is used, but care must be taken to avoid injury to neurovascular structures because these methods are relatively "blind." Hutchinson et al. (107) concluded that optimal visualization of known structures could be achieved with either an endoscope technique or open technique to prevent neurovascular injury. It may be more difficult to decompress the deep posterior compartment when compared to the other three compartments of the leg. Due to the varied anatomy and sub-compartmentation of the deep posterior compartment, greater visualization and careful decompression are indicated in this area.

In patients who demonstrate signs and symptoms of CCS in only the anterior compartment, it does not appear to be necessary to perform both an anterior and lateral compartment fasciotomy. Schepsis et al. (108) found success rates of 90% regardless whether or not a lateral release was performed with the anterior compartment release. In addition, those who did not have the lateral compartment release avoided any damage to branches of the superficial peroneal nerve and were able to return to their activities significantly sooner. If there are questions regarding possible co-existent CCS of the lateral compartment, it is probably prudent to carefully release the lateral side to avoid persistent postoperative CCS symptoms.

After surgery, a light compressive dressing is placed over the incision and the patient is allowed to return to weight-bearing as tolerated. Garcia-Mata et al. (7) recommend weight bearing within 24 hours of the fasciotomy in adolescents. Gradual strengthening and return to sports are allowed after

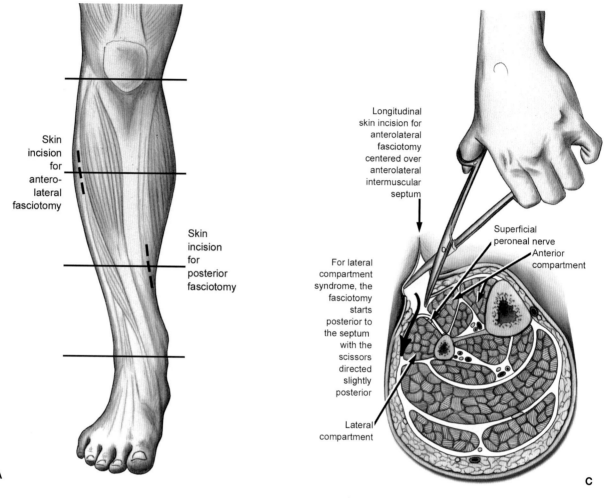

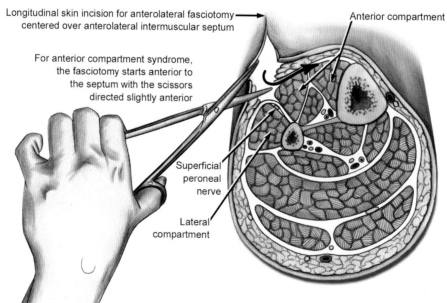

Fig 47-1. The anterolateral fasciotomy for chronic exertional compartment syndrome can be performed through a longitudinal skin incision centered over the anterolateral intermuscular septum. The skin incision should be at the junction of the proximal and middle third of the leg. In the anterior compartment, the fasciotomy should begin anterior to the septum, with scissors directed anteriorly, in order to avoid injury to the superficial peroneal nerve. In the lateral compartment, the fasciotomy should start posterior to the septum, with scissors directed slightly posterior.

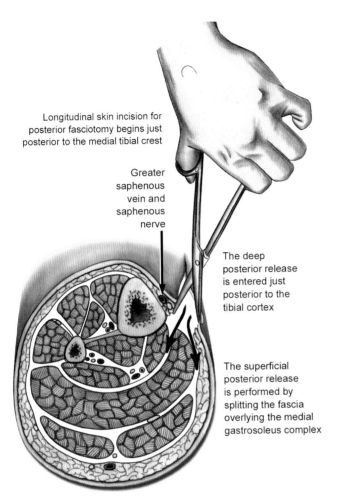

Longitudinal skin incision for posterior fasciotomy begins just posterior to the medial tibial crest

Greater saphenous vein and saphenous nerve

The deep posterior release is entered just posterior to the tibial cortex

The superficial posterior release is performed by splitting the fascia overlying the medial gastrosoleus complex

Fig 47-2. The posterior fasciotomy for chronic exertional compartment syndrome begins with a skin incision just posterior to the medial tibial crest, at the junction of the middle and distal third of the leg. Care should be taken to protect the saphenous nerve and vein. The superficial posterior release is performed by splitting the fascia overlying the medial gastrosoleus complex. The deep posterior compartment is entered just posterior to the tibial cortex. Scissors should be slightly open during the fasciotomy to avoid injury to perforating vessels and/or the posterior tibial neurovascular structures.

wound healing is achieved. Return to sports is typically possible within 1 to 2 months after fasciotomy.

The majority of patients demonstrate improved function, decreased pain, and return to a higher level of sports participation following a fasciotomy for CCS. Any adverse effects that the fasciotomy may have on muscle function are a theoretical concern. Garfin et al. (109) observed that the intact fascia does have an important biomechanical role for force production. With sufficient rehabilitation after a decompressive fasciotomy, however, most patients recover good strength in clinical situations. Recent literature reports success rates of 60% to 100% (7,8,60,65,97,108,110–3) after fasciotomy for the treatment of CCS in the upper and lower extremity. Those patients who underwent surgery for deep posterior compartment syndrome of the lower leg seemed to have less

favorable results compared to those who had anterior or lateral compartment fasciotomies (112). Slimmon et al. (113) observed that patients who underwent combined anterior and posterior compartment fasciotomies of the lower leg had worse outcomes compared to those who had an anterior or posterior fasciotomy alone. NIRS measurements have confirmed that oxygen saturation measurements both before and after exercise return to those of healthy individuals following fasciotomy, supporting the fact that this treatment is successful at reversing any ischemic complications (54).

Although uncommon, there are a number of complications related to fasciotomy for CCS. Turnipseed (66) reported excessive bleeding (1.4%), cellulitis (0.4%), seroma formation (2.7%), and recurrent compartment syndrome (3.9%) as complications following an open fasciotomy. Payne et al. (114) reported a case of a severed left saphenous nerve after fasciotomy for CCS of bilateral anterior compartments and the left deep posterior compartment. Hutchinson et al. (107) demonstrated that the superficial peroneal nerve and the saphenous vein are at risk for injury when a percutaneous release is used.

Incomplete decompression or an incorrect diagnosis may lead to poor results. The clinical situation should be carefully reviewed if fasciotomy fails to make sure that the patient was not misdiagnosed. If recurrent CCS is suspected, repeat diagnostic pressure studies may be needed. Scarring at the fasciotomy site can occasionally lead to a true recurrence of the syndrome. Repeat fasciotomy or partial fasciectomy may be considered in this situation.

■ CONCLUSION

CCS is a clinical concern because of the morbidity, pain, and decreased quality of life associated with it. The pathophysiology of this complex syndrome is still not fully understood and further research is needed in this area. The clinical examination may be better for eliminating other important diagnoses, as opposed to making the definitive diagnosis of CCS. Direct measurement of intracompartmental pressure both before and after exertion is still the gold standard for definitive diagnosis, although newer techniques are being developed that may assist clinicians in making the diagnosis noninvasively in the future. Nonsurgical treatment of CCS is usually not successful, thus decompressive fasciotomy is recommended if the patient wants to return to unrestricted, pain free activity.

■ REFERENCES

1. Abraham P, Leftheriotis G, Saumet JL. Laser doppler flowmetry in the diagnosis of chronic compartment syndrome. *J Bone Joint Surg Br.* 1998;80B:365–369.
2. Arbabi S, Brundage SI, Gentilello LM. Near-infrared spectroscopy: a potential method for continuous transcutaneous monitoring for compartmental syndrome in critically injured patients. *J Trauma.* 1999;47(5):829–833.

3. Balduini FC, Shenton DW, O'Connor KH, et al. Chronic exertional compartment syndrome: correlation of compartment pressure and muscle ischemia utilizing 31P-NMR spectroscopy. *Clin Sports Med*. 1993;12:151–165.

4. Birtles DB, Rayson MP, Casey A, et al. Venous obstruction in healthy limbs: a model for chronic compartment syndrome? *Med Sci Sports Exerc*. 2003;35(10):1638–1644.

5. Zhang Q, Styf J, Lindberg LG. Effects of limb elevation and increased intramuscular pressure on human tibialis anterior muscle blood flow. *Eur J Appl Physiol*. 2001;85:567–571.

6. Birtles DB, Rayson MP, Jones DA, et al. Effect of eccentric exercise on patients with chronic exertional compartment syndrome. *Eur J Appl Physiol*. 2003;88(6):565–571.

7. Boutin RD, Fritz RC, Steinbach LS. Imaging of sports-related muscle injuries. *Radiol Clin North Am*. 2002;40(2):333–362.

8. Breit GA, Gross JH, Watenpaugh DE, et al. Near-infrared spectroscopy for monitoring of tissue oxygenation of exercising skeletal muscle in chronic compartment syndrome model. *J Bone Joint Surg Am*. 1997;79A:838–843.

9. Burton AC. On the physical elquilibrium of small blood vessels. *Am J Physiol*. 1951;1674:319–329.

10. Carr D, Gilbertson L, Frymoyer J, et al. Lumbar paraspinal compartment syndrome. A case report with physiological and anatomic studies. *Spine*. 1985;10:816–820.

11. Cook S, Bruce G. Fasciotomy for chronic compartment syndrome in the lower limb. *ANZ J Surg*. 2002;72:720–723.

12. Crenshaw AG, Styf JR, Mubarak SJ, et al. A new "transducer-tipped" fiber optic catheter for measuring intramuscular pressures. *J Orthop Res*. 1990;8:464–468.

13. Darling RC, Buckley CJ, Abbott WM. Intermittent claudication in young athletes: popliteal artery entrapment syndrome. *J Trauma*. 1974;14:543–551.

14. Davey JR, Rorabeck CH, Fowler PJ. The tibialis posterior muscle compartment. An unrecognized cause of exertional compartment syndrome. *Am J Sports Med*. 1984;12:391–397.

15. Deirdre BB, Minden D, Wickes SJ, et al. Chronic exertional compartment syndrome: muscle changes with isometric exercise. *Med Sci Sports Exerc*. 2002;34(12):1900–1906.

16. Detmer DE. Chronic shin splints. Classification and management of medial tibial stress syndromes. *Sports Med*. 1986;3:436–446.

17. Detmer DE, Sharpe K, Sufit RL, et al. Chronic compartment syndrome: diagnosis, management, and outcomes. *Am J Sports Med*. 1985;13:162–170.

18. Dickson KF, Sullivan MJ, Steinberg B, et al. Noninvasive measurement of compartment syndrome. *Orthopedics*. 2003;26(12):1215–1218.

19. Eaton RG, Green WT, Stark HA. Volkmann's ischemic contracture in children. *J Bone Joint Surg Am*. 1965;47A:1289.

20. Edwards PD, Miles KA, Owens SJ, et al. A new noninvasive test for the detection of compartment syndromes. *Nucl Med Commun*. 1999;20:215–218.

21. Eskelin MKK, Lotjonen JMP, Mantysaari MJ. Chronic exertional compartment syndrome: MR imaging at 0.1T compared with tissue pressure measurement. *Radiology*. 1998;206:333–337.

22. Fontes D, Clement R, Roure P. Endoscopic aponeurotomy for chronic exertional compartmental syndrome of the forearm: report of 41 cases. *Chir Main*. 2003;22(4):186–196.

23. Fronek J, Mubarak SJ, Hargens AR, et al. Management of chronic exertional anterior compartment syndrome of the lower extremity. *Clin Orthop*. 1987;220:217–227.

24. Garcia-Mata S, Hidalgo-Ovejero A, Martinez-Grande M. Chronic exertional compartment syndrome of the legs in adolescents. *J Pediatr Orthop*. 2001;21:328–334.

25. Garfin SR, Tipton CM, Mubarak SJ, et al. Role of fascia in maintenance of muscle tension and pressure. *J Appl Physiol*. 1981;51:317–320.

25a. Mubarak SJ, Hargens AR. *Compartment Syndromes and Volkmann's Contracture*. Philadelphia: WB Saunders; 1981.

26. Garr JL, Gentilello LM, Cole PA, et al. Monitoring for compartmental syndrome using near-infrared spectroscopy: a noninvasive, continuous, transcutaneous monitoring technique. *J Trauma*. 1999;46(4):613–618.

27. Giannotti G, Cohn SM, Brown M, et al. Utility of near-infrared spectroscopy in the diagnosis of lower extremity compartment syndrome. *J Trauma*. 2000;48(3):396–399.

28. Goldie BS, Jones NF, Jupiter JB. Recurrent compartment syndrome and Volkmann contracture associated with chronic osteomyelitis of the ulna. *J Bone Joint Surg Am*. 1990;72A:131–133.

29. Goubier JN, Saillant G. Chronic compartment syndrome of the forearm in competitive motor cyclists: a report of 2 cases. *Br J Sports Med*. 2003;37(5):452–453.

30. Griffiths DL. Volkmann's ischaemic contracture. *Br J Surg*. 1940;28:239.

31. Hargens AR, Akeson WH, Mubarak SJ, et al. Fluid balance within the canine anterolateral compartment and its relationship to compartment syndromes. *J Bone Joint Surg Am*. 1978;60A:499–505.

32. Hargens AR, Pedowitz RA, Mohler LR, et al. Noninvasive diagnosis of exertional, anterior compartment syndrome using near-infrared spectroscopy. *Hefte zu der Unfallchirurg*. 1998;267:296–303.

33. Hargens AR, Villavicencio JL. Mechanics of tissue/lymphatic transport. In: Bronozino JD, ed. *Biomedical engineering handbook*. Boca Raton, FL: CRC Press, Inc; 1995:493–504.

34. Howard JL, Mohtadi NGH, Wiley JP. Evaluation of outcomes in patients following surgical treatment of chronic exertional compartment syndrome in the leg. *Clin J Sports Med*. 2000;10:176–184.

35. Hutchinson MR, Bederka B, Kopplin M. Anatomic structures at risk during minimal-incision endoscopically assisted fascial compartment releases in the leg. *Am J Sports Med*. 2003;31(5):764–769.

36. Hutchinson MR, Ireland ML. Chronic exertional compartment syndrome: gauging pressure. *Phys Sportsmed*. 1999;27(5):101–102.

37. Kalchmair B, Klocker J, Perkmann R, et al. Alterations in plasma amine oxidase activities in a compartment syndrome model. *Inflamm Res*. 2003;52(suppl 1):S67–S68.

38. Kitajima I, Tachibana S, Hirota Y, et al. One-portal technique of endoscopic fasciotomy: chronic compartment syndrome of the lower leg. *Arthroscopy*. 2001;17(8):E33.

39. Knight JL, Au K, Whitley MA. Popliteal aneurysm presenting as chronic exertional compartment syndrome. *Orthopedics*. 1997;20:166–169.

40. Kumar PR, Jenkins JP, Hodgson SP. Bilateral chronic compartment syndrome of the dorsal part of the forearm: the role of magnetic resonance imaging in diagnosis: a case report. *J Bone Joint Surg Am*. 2003;85A(8):1557–1559.

41. Kumar P, Salil B, Bhaskara KG, et al. Compartment syndrome: effect of limb position on pressure measurement. *Burns*. 2003;29(6):626.

42. Kutz JE, Singer R, Lindsay M. Chronic exertional compartment syndrome of the forearm: a case report. *J Hand Surg Am*. 1985;10A:302–304.

43. Kwiatkowski TC, Detmer DE. Anatomical dissection of the deep posterior compartment and its correlation with clinical reports of chronic compartment syndrome involving the deep posterior compartment. *Clin Anat*. 1997;10:104–111.

44. Lauder TD, Stuart MJ, Amrami KK, et al. Exertional compartment syndrome and the role of magnetic resonance imaging. *Am J Phys Med Rehabil*. 2002;81:315–319.

45. Leversedge FJ, Casey PJ, Seiler JG III, et al. Endoscopically assisted fasciotomy: description of technique and in vitro assessment of lower-leg compartment decompression. *Am J Sports Med*. 2002;30(2):272–278.

46. Lokiec F, Sievner I, Pritsch M. Chronic compartment syndrome of both feet. *J Bone Joint Surg Br*. 1991;73B:178–179.

47. Lynch JE, Heyman JS, Hargens AR. Ultrasonic device for the noninvasive diagnosis of compartment syndrome. *Physiol Meas.* 2004;25(1):N1-N9.

48. Mannarino F, Sexson S. The significance of intracompartmental pressures in the diagnosis of chronic exertional compartment syndrome. *Orthopedics.* 1989;12:1415–1418.

49. Manoli A. Compartment syndromes of the foot: current concepts. *Foot Ankle.* 1990;10:340–344.

50. Mars M, Hadley GP. Raised intracompartmental pressure and compartment syndromes. *Injury.* 1998;29(6):403–411

51. Martens MA, Moeyersoons JP. Acute and effort-related compartment syndrome in sports. *Sports Med.* 1990;9:62–68.

52. Matsen FA III, Clawson DK. The deep posterior compartmental syndrome of the leg. *J Bone Joint Surg Am.* 1975;57A:34–39.

53. Matsen FA III. Etiologies of compartment syndromes. In: *Compartmental syndromes.* New York: Grune and Stratton; 1980.

54. Mattila KT, Komu MES, Cahlstrom S, et al. Medial tibial pain: a dynamic contrast-enhanced MRI study. *Magn Reson Imaging.* 1999;17(7):947–954.

55. McDermott APG, Marble E, Yabsley RH, et al. Monitoring dynamic anterior compartment pressure during exercise: a new technique using the STIC catheter. *Am J Sports Med.* 1982;10:83–89.

56. Melberg PE, Styf J. Posteromedial pain in the lower leg. *Am J Sports Med.* 1989;17:747–750.

57. Mendelson S, Mendelson A, Holmes J. Compartment syndrome after acute rupture of the peroneus longus in a high school football player: a case report. *Am J Orthop.* 2003;32(10):510–512.

58. Micheli LJ, Solomon R, Solomon J, et al. Surgical treatment for chronic lower-leg compartment syndrome in young female athletes. *Am J Sports Med.* 1999;27(2):197–201.

59. Mohler LR, Styf JR, Pedowitz RA, et al. Intramuscular deoxygenation during exercise in patients who have chronic anterior compartment syndrome of the leg. *J Bone Joint Surg Am.* 1997;79A:844–849.

60. Mollica MB, Duyshart SC. Analysis of pre- and postexercise compartment pressures in the medial compartment of the foot. *Am J Sports Med.* 2002;30(2):268–271.

61. Mubarak SJ, Hargens AR. *Compartment Syndromes and Volkmann's Contracture.* Philadelphia: WB Saunders; 1981.

62. Mubarak SJ, Hargens AR, Owen CA, et al. The wick catheter technique for measurement of intramuscular pressure: a new research and clinical tool. *J Bone Joint Surg Am.* 1976;58A: 1016–1020.

63. Mubarak SJ. Surgical management of chronic compartment syndrome of the leg. *Oper Tech Sports Med.* 1995;3:259–266.

64. Mueller KL, Farley FA. Superficial and deep posterior compartment syndrome following high tibial osteotomy for tibia vara in a child. *Orthopedics.* 2003(5);26:513–514.

65. Myerson MS. Management of compartment syndromes of the foot. *Clin Orthop.* 1991;271:239–248.

66. Oseto MC, Edwards JZ, Acus RW III. Posterior thigh compartment syndrome associated with hamstring avulsion and chronic anticoagulation therapy. *Orthopedics.* 2004;27(2):229–230.

67. Ota Y, Senda M, Hashizume H, et al. Chronic compartment syndrome of the lower leg: a new diagnostic method using near-infrared spectroscopy and a new technique of endoscopic fasciotomy. *Arthroscopy.* 1999;15(4):439–443.

68. Owens S, Edwards P, Miles K, et al. Chronic compartment syndrome affecting the lower limb: MIBI perfusion imaging as an alternative to pressure monitoring: two case reports. *Br J Sports Med.* 1999;33:49–53.

69. Padhiar N, King JB. Exercise induced leg pain—chronic compartment syndrome. Is the increase in intra-compartment pressure exercise specific? *Br J Sports Med.* 1996;30:360–362.

70. Pedowitz RA, Hargens AR. Acute and chronic compartment syndrome. In: Garrett WE, Speer KP, Kirkendall DT, eds. *Principles and practice of orthopaedic sports medicine.* Philadelphia: Lippincott Williams & Wilkins; 2000.

71. Pedowitz RA, Hargens AR, Mubarak SJ, et al. Modified criteria for objective diagnosis of chronic compartment syndrome of the leg. *Am J Sports Med.* 1990;18:35–40.

72. Pedowitz RA, Toutounghi FM. Chronic exertional compartment syndrome of the forearm flexor muscles. *J Hand Surg.* 1988;13A: 694–696.

73. Pyne D, Jawad AS, Padhiar N. Saphenous nerve injury after fasciotomy for compartment syndrome. *Br J Sports Med.* 2003;37(6): 541–542.

74. Raether PM, Lutten LD. Recurrent compartment syndrome in the posterior thigh. *Am J Sports Med.* 1982;10:40–43.

75. Reeves ST, Pinosky ML, Byrne TK, et al. Abdominal compartment syndrome. *Can J Anaesth.* 1997;44:745–753.

76. Reid RL, Travis RT. Acute necrosis of the second interosseous compartment of the hand. *J Bone Joint Surg Am.* 1973;55A: 1095–1097.

77. Reneman RS. The anterior and the lateral compartmental syndrome of the leg due to intensive use of muscles. *Clin Orthop.* 1975;118:69–80.

78. Rominger MB, Lukosch CJ, Bachmann GF. MR imaging of compartment syndrome of the lower leg: a case control study. *Eur Radiol.* 2004; Apr 6 [Epub ahead of print].

79. Rorabeck CH, Castle GS, Hardie PC, et al. Compartmental pressure measurement: an experimental investigation using the slit catheter. *J Trauma.* 1981;21:446–449.

80. Rowdon GA, Richardson JK, Hoffman P, et al. Chronic anterior compartment syndrome and deep peroneal nerve function. *Clin J Sports Med.* 2001;11:229–233.

81. Rydholm U, Werner C, Ohlin P. Intracompartmental forearm pressure during rest and exercise. *Clin Orthop.* 1983;175: 213–215.

82. Sammarco GJ, Russo-Alesi FG, Munda R. Partial vascular occlusion causing pseudocompartment syndrome of the leg: a case report. *Am J Sports Med.* 1997;25:409–411.

83. Sangwan SS, Marya KM, Devgan A, et al. Critical evaluation of compartment pressure measurement by saline manometer in peripheral hospital setup. *Trop Doct.* 2003;33(2):100–103.

84. Schein M, Wittman DH, Aprahamian CC, et al. The abdominal compartment syndrome: the physiological and clinical consequences of elevated intra-abdominal pressure. *J Am Coll Surg.* 1995;180:745–753.

85. Schepsis AA, Gill SS, Foster TA. Fasciotomy for exertional anterior compartment syndrome: is lateral compartment release necessary? *Am J Sports Med.* 1999;27(4):430–435.

86. Scholander PF, Hargens AR, Miller SL. Negative pressure in the interstitial fluid of animals. *Science.* 1968;161:321–328.

87. Sejersted OM, Hargens AR, Kardel KR, et al. Intramuscular fluid pressure during isometric contraction of human skeletal muscle. *J Appl Physiol.* 1984;56:287–295.

88. Slimmon D, Bennell K, Brukner P, et al. Long-term outcome of fasciotomy with partial fasciectomy for chronic exertional compartment syndrome of the lower leg. *Am J Sports Med.* 2002; 30(4):581–588.

89. Soffer SR, Martin DF, Stanish WD, et al. Chronic compartment syndrome caused by aberrant fascia in an aerobic walker. *Med Sci Sports Exerc.* 1991;23:304–306.

90. Styf J. Chronic exercise-induced pain in the anterior aspect of the lower leg. *Sports Med.* 1989;7:331–339.

91. Styf J. Diagnosis of exercise-induced pain in the anterior aspect of the lower leg. *Am J Sports Med.* 1988;16:165–169.

92. Styf J. Pressure in the erector spinae muscle during exercise. *Spine.* 1987;12:675–679.

93. Styf J, Forssblad P, Lundborg G. Chronic compartment syndrome in the first dorsal interosseous muscle. *J Hand Surg.* 1987;12A:757–762.

94. Styf J, Lysell E. Chronic compartment syndrome in the erector spinae muscle. *Spine.* 1987;12:680–682.

95. Styf JR. Intramuscular pressure measurements during exercise. *Oper Tech Sports Med.* 1995;3:243–249.

96. Styf JR, Korner LM. Chronic compartment syndrome of the leg. Results of treatment by fasciotomy. *J Bone Joint Surg Am.* 1986;68A:1338–1347.

97. Styf JR, Korner LM. Diagnosis of chronic anterior compartment syndrome in the lower leg. *Acta Orthop Scand.* 1987;58:139–144.

98. Styf JR, Korner LM. Microcapillary infusion technique for measurement pressure during exercise, *Clin Orthop.* 1986;207:253–262.

99. Styf JR, Korner L, Suurkula M. Intramuscular pressure and muscle blood flow during exercise in chronic compartment syndrome. *J Bone Joint Surg Br.* 1987;69B:301–305.

100. Takebayashi S, Takazawa RS, Sasaki R, et al. Chronic exertional compartment syndrome in lower legs: localization and follow-up with Thallium-201 SPECT imaging. *J Nucl Med.* 1997;38(6):972–976.

101. Tompkins DG. Exercise myopathy of the extensor carpi ulnaris muscle: report of a case. *J Bone Joint Surg Am.* 1977;59A:407–408.

102. Turnipseed WD. Atypical claudication with overuse injury in patients with chronic compartment, functional entrapment, and medial tibial stress syndromes. *Cardiovasc Surg.* 2003;11(5):421–423.

103. Turnipseed WD. Diagnosis and management of chronic compartment syndrome. *Surgery.* 2002;132(4):613–619.

104. Turnipseed W, Detmer DE, Girdley F. Chronic compartment syndrome. An unusual cause for claudication. *Ann Surg.* 1989;210:557–562.

105. Uliasz A, Ishida JT, Fleming JK, et al. Comparing the methods of measuring compartment pressures in acute compartment syndrome. *Am J Emerg Med.* 2003;21(2):143–145.

106. Ulmar T. The clinical diagnosis of compartment syndrome of the lower leg: are clinical findings predictive of the disorder? *J Orthop Trauma.* 2002;16(8):572–577.

107. Uppal GS, Smith GC, Sherk HH, et al. Accurate compartment pressure measurement using the Intervenous Alarm Control (IVAC) Pump: a report of a technique. *J Orthop Trauma.* 1992;6:87–89.

108. Van den Brand JG, Verleisdonk EJ, van der Werken C. Near infrared spectroscopy in the diagnosis of chronic exertional compartment syndrome. *Am J Sports Med.* 2004;32(2):452–456.

109. Verleisdonk EJMM, van Gils A, van der Werken C. The diagnostic value of MRI scans for the diagnosis of chronic exertional compartment syndrome of the lower leg. *Skeletal Radiol.* 2001;30:321–325.

110. Verleisdonk EJ, Schmitz RF, van der Werken C. Long-term results of fasciotomy of the anterior compartment in patients with exercise-induced pain in the lower leg. *Int J Sports Med.* 2004;25(3):224–229.

111. Vollmar B, Westermann S, Menger MD. Microvascular response to compartment syndrome-like external pressure elevation: an in vivo fluorescence microscopic study in the hamster striated muscle. *J Trauma.* 1999;46(1):91–96.

112. Wallenstein R. Results of fasciotomy in patients with medial tibial stress syndrome or chronic anterior compartment syndrome. *J Bone Joint Surg Am.* 1983;65A:1252–1255.

113. Willy C, Gerngross H, Sterk J. Measurement of intracompartmental pressure with use of a new electronic transducer-tipped catheter system. *J. Bone Joint Surg.* 1999;81–A(2):158–168.

114. Zapletal Ch, Herzog L, Martin G, et al. Thermodiffusion for the quantification of tissue perfusion in skeletal muscle—clinical evaluation in standardized traumatological procedures with tourniquet and potential application in the diagnosis of compartment syndrome. *Microvasc Res.* 2003;66(2):164–172.

115. Amendola A, Rorabeck CH, Vellett D, et al. The use of magnetic resonance imaging in exertional compartment syndromes. *Am J Sports Med.* 1990;18:29–34.

116. Gold BS, Barish RA, Dart RC, et al. Resolution of compartment syndrome after rattlesnake envenomation utilizing noninvasive measures. *J Emerg Med.* 2003;24(3):285–288.

117. Zhang Q, Styf J, Lindberg LG. Effects of limb elevation and increased intramuscular pressure on human tibialis anterior muscle blood flow. *Eur J Appl Physiol.* 2001;85:567–571.

118. Hargens AR, Ballard RE. Basic principles for measurement of intramuscular pressure. *Oper Tech Sports Med.* 1995;3:237–242.

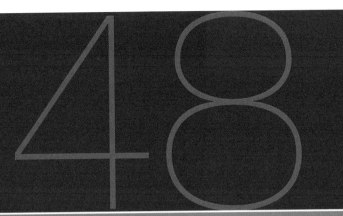

INSTABILITY OF THE ANKLE

■ MURRAY J. PENNER, MD, FRCSC

■ KEY POINTS

- Ankle instability, from the patient's perspective, is a sense of "giving way" or a feeling that the ankle is about to "give way."
- Ankle instability should be classified as either true- or pseudo-instability, with true instability composed of dynamic or static instability. Because aspects of all three may be present in one ankle, it is helpful to try to determine which component is currently predominant, and which component may have been the initial problem.
- Pseudo-ankle instability is a sensation of giving way, accompanied by, and often immediately preceded by an acute pain stimulus. Treatment is directed at the pain stimulus.
- Acute ankle instability is most often a result of a sprain of the lateral ankle ligament complex. Treatment is almost always nonsurgical, consisting of rest, ice, compression, and elevation, followed by rehabilitation. Most ankle sprains heal uneventfully, but about 20% lead to chronic ankle instability.
- Acute injury of the ankle ligaments is the most common injury associated with recreational and sports activities and the most common orthopedic injury overall. Sprains make up 75% of all ankle injuries, with the vast majority involving the lateral ankle ligaments.
- Ankle sprains make up 45% of all basketball injuries, 31% of all soccer injuries, and 25% of all running injuries.
- Surgical stabilization may be indicated in patients who have symptoms that are not restricted to risk activities and find problems with bracing and those that have had previous surgery that has removed some of the stabilizing structures.

■ DEFINING INSTABILITY

Ankle instability can be defined, from the patient's perspective, as a sensation of the ankle "giving way" under load, or a sense of apprehension that the ankle is about to "give way". These symptoms may be due to true ankle instability, as defined by objective signs of ankle joint laxity, or they may be due to pseudo-ankle instability, where objective findings of laxity are lacking. Distinction between these two is critical.

Pseudo-ankle instability is generally associated with a sensation of giving way, accompanied by, and often immediately preceded by, an acute pain stimulus in the ankle (Table 48-1). The sensation of the ankle giving way is the result of brief reflex inhibition of the ankle musculature, generally caused by the pain stimulus. This is analogous to a knee "buckling" on stairs as a result of patellofemoral chondromalacia. Treatment of pseudo-ankle instability is directed at treatment of the pain stimulus. There is often overlap between true and pseudo-ankle instability, with many of the lesions described in Table 48-1 often being found in association with, and often being caused by, objective ankle laxity.

The focus of this chapter is true ankle instability, from here on simply referred to as ankle instability.

Acute ankle instability occurs when the ankle is subjected to forces outside of "normal" loading conditions, causing subluxation of the talus in the ankle mortise. Most often, this occurs as the result of a plantarflexion and inversion stress, resulting in a sprain of the lateral ankle ligament complex (1). Treatment is almost always nonsurgical, consisting of rest, ice, compression, and elevation, followed by a rehabilitation program. Most acute sprains heal uneventfully, with no persistent symptoms; however, much like in the shoulder, where

TABLE 48-1	Lesions to Consider in Patients with Symptoms of Chronic Ankle Instability: Potential Causes of Pseudo-instability or Secondary Results of True Instability

- Bone
  - Fractures (missed or stress)
    - Lateral or posterior process talus
    - Anterior process calcaneus
    - 5th metatarsal base
    - Malleoli
  - Tarsal coalition
  - Anterior tibiotalar impingement
- Cartilage
  - Osteochondral lesions of talus and tibia
- Tendon
  - Os peroneum syndrome
  - Peroneal tendon instability
  - Peroneus longus tear
  - Peroneus brevis split/tear
- Soft tissue
  - Anterolateral ankle impingement (Bassett lesion)
  - Ankle synovitis
- Neurologic
  - Sural/superficial peroneal nerve neuroma
  - Charcot-Marie-Toothe Disease

acute dislocation is often the initiator of chronic recurrent shoulder instability, *acute* ankle sprains will lead to *chronic* ankle instability in as many as 20% of cases (2,3).

Chronic ankle instability has been divided into either functional or mechanical instability. Functional instability, as described by Freeman (2), is the subjective giving way of the ankle, as noted by the patient. To avoid confusion with pseudo-instability, functional instability is now more readily understood as true dynamic instability.

Dynamic instability is defined as insufficiency of the dynamic stabilizers of the ankle, allowing subluxation of the ankle joint while under "normal" loads, within the confines of stable ligamentous restraints. This may be brought about by primary neuromuscular (4) or tendon problems (5), or as the result of lower extremity mal-alignment that places the dynamic stabilizers at a comparative disadvantage (6). Demonstration of dynamic instability can be difficult in the clinical setting, and is often a diagnosis of exclusion, after pseudo-instability triggers and mechanical ligamentous laxity have been ruled out (7).

Mechanical instability has previously been defined as objectively documented hypermobility of the ankle joint, demonstrated with stress radiography (2). It can now be more concisely considered as true static instability or insufficiency of the static ligamentous stabilizers of the ankle. Currently, just as cruciate ligament insufficiency of the knee and gleno-humeral instability of the shoulder are diagnoses based on clinical examination, so, too, is static ankle instability.

Understanding of the definitions, or classification, of ankle instability is critical for understanding the condition, for focusing the evaluation of the unstable ankle, and for communication with other physicians and therapists.

In summary, ankle instability should be thought of as either true- or pseudo-instability, with true instability composed of dynamic or static instability. Because aspects of all three may be present in one ankle, it is helpful to try to determine which component is currently predominant, and which component may have been the initial problem. For example, a patient with a cavovarus foot may have dynamic instability due to malalignment; repetitive giving way may lead to osteochondral injury of the talar dome, resulting in a new pain stimulus, contributing to pseudo-instability. A subsequent major giving way episode may result in a severe sprain of the lateral ankle ligaments, potentially leading to static instability. Recognition of all of the components of such a patient's instability is important to avoid incomplete treatment of the condition.

Localizing Instability

Lateral ankle instability, where the tibio-talar joint gives way into hindfoot inversion, is by far the most common form of ankle instability (1). It is due to insufficiency of the lateral ankle stabilizers, dynamic or static. Not infrequently, a portion of this instability is due to inversion "laxity" of the subtalar joint (8,9). Rarely, this aspect can become the predominant aspect of the problem, and this is then primarily termed sub-talar instability (10).

Even more rarely described is medial ankle instability (11). This condition as an isolated entity remains somewhat controversial, although it has been described as occurring in conjunction with recalcitrant lateral instability and with adult acquired flat foot disorder (12). It is felt to be present when there is a sense of giving way into hindfoot eversion on a recurrent basis, usually associated with anteromedial ankle pain.

The Scope of Ankle Instability

Acute injury of the ankle ligaments is not only the most common injury associated with recreational and sports activities (13,14), but is also the most common orthopedic injury overall (15). Ankle sprains make up 75% of all ankle injuries, with the vast majority involving the lateral ankle ligaments (14). Reported rates of acute ankle sprains range from 7 to 37 per 1,000 people per year (3,16). The association with sports is very strong, with ankle sprains comprising 45% of all basketball injuries, 31% of all soccer injuries (14), and 25% of all running- and jumping-sport injuries overall (17). These injuries are most common among males, particularly between the ages of 20 and 30 years, though after age 40, where sporting mechanisms no longer dominate, women are more frequently injured (16). On a sport-specific basis, however, the incidence is approximately equal between males and females (14).

Most acute sprains go on to satisfactory recovery with nonoperative therapies. However, 20% to 40% of patients with acute sprains will have ongoing symptoms of instability (18). As a result, persistent instability of the ankle constitutes a major ongoing therapeutic problem.

This chapter describes the anatomy and biomechanics of the ankle and briefly touches on the most relevant aspects of the clinical evaluation of ankle instability. Current nonoperative and operative treatment options are then reviewed.

■ ANATOMY AND BIOMECHANICS

Underpinning the concept that differentiates ankle instability into static and dynamic subtypes is the fact that the mechanical function of the ankle is afforded by, and constrained by, both static and dynamic stabilizers. The static constraints are provided by the ankle ligaments and the osseous architecture of the joint itself, while the dynamic constraints are the tendons.

Osseous Architecture

Bony constraints are felt to contribute approximately 30% of the resistance to rotational forces about the ankle, with the remainder attributed to the soft tissues (19). The trapezoidal shape of the talus, wide anteriorly and narrow posteriorly, provides strong bony constraint to the tibio-talar joint in neutral flexion or dorsiflexion. But this also allows laxity of the talus within the mortise in plantarflexion, increasing dependence on the soft tissue constraints in this position, and increasing the risk of inversion injury (20).

Recent studies have shown that variations in the osseous anatomy of the ankle and hindfoot are a significant contributor to ankle lateral ankle instability. Van Bergeyk et al. (21) demonstrated a trend toward increased hindfoot varus on computed tomography (CT) scan in patients with chronic lateral instability when compared with controls. It is postulated that this configuration may increase varus forces about the ankle, increasing the likelihood that the soft tissue stabilizers will be overcome in inversion, resulting in giving way and recurrent sprains.

Berkowitz and Kim (22) have verified the earlier hypothesis of Scranton et al. (23) that posterior positioning of the fibula in relation to the ankle mortise is associated with, and potentially a cause of, lateral ankle instability. These studies put forward the concept of an "open ankle mortise," where posterior positioning of the fibula reduces the relative constraint of the fibula on the talus, possibly allowing increased internal rotation and inversion of the talus. This mechanism remains to be confirmed.

Static Stabilizers—Ligaments

Static instability of the ankle results from insufficiency of the static stabilizers of the ankle, namely the ligaments. Understanding the anatomy of these ligaments is important both for understanding the biomechanics of instability and for achieving satisfactory restoration of ankle and subtalar mechanics at the time of surgery.

The lateral ligament complex **(Fig 48-1)** is made up of the anterior talo-fibular ligament (ATFL), the calcaneo-fibular ligament (CFL), the posterior talo-fibular ligament (PTFL), and the lateral talo-calcaneal ligament (LTCL). The ATFL spans across the anterolateral ankle joint, blending with the anterior ankle capsule. Its origin on the anterior edge of the fibula is centered 10 mm proximal to the tip of the lateral malleolus. It inserts into the lateral talar neck, immediately distal to the articular surface, 18 mm above the subtalar joint (24). The PTFL originates from the posteromedial surface of the lateral malleolus, stretching transversely medially to insert broadly on the nonarticular posterior surface of the talus (20). The CFL does not originate at the tip of the lateral malleolus. Rather, it originates just below the ATFL origin on the anterior aspect of the fibula, 8.5 mm proximal to the fibular tip (24). It is directed plantar, posterior, and medial (deep to the peroneal tendons), attaching to the lateral aspect of the calcaneus, 13 mm distal to the subtalar joint. It spans both the ankle and subtalar joints and is aligned perpendicular to the posterior facet of the subtalar joint, but parallel to the

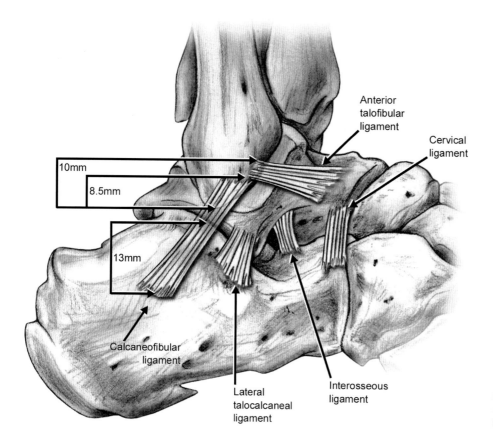

Fig 48-1. Anatomy of the major ligamentous stabilizers of the lateral ankle.

subtalar joint axis in the sagittal plane. The angle between the ATFL and CFL in the sagittal plane averages 105 degrees, ranging from 70 degrees to 140 degrees. The LTCL has a variable configuration. It is generally found as a rectangular or triangular structure, spanning the lateral subtalar joint just anterior to the CFL (24). Additional important stabilizers of the subtalar joint are the interosseous ligament (IL) (more deeply located in the sinus tarsi), the anteriorly located cervical ligament (CL), and the lateral root of the inferior extensor retinaculum (IER).

In dorsiflexion, the CFL is taut in a position nearing vertical, allowing it to function as a true collateral ligament resisting varus talar tilt (20). With plantarflexion, however, the axis of CFL, along with the axis of the subtalar joint, becomes more horizontal and tension in the CFL decreases. This results in the CFL being much less able to resist varus talar tilt in plantarflexion (24). The ATFL becomes taut and more vertical in plantarflexion, taking on the function of a true collateral ligament. It is in the plantarflexed position, where the osseous architecture of the ankle is least stabilizing and the CFL is disadvantaged, that the ATFL acts as the "sole" stabilizer, placing it at most risk for inversion injury.

Motion in the ankle and hindfoot, however, is more complex than simple sagittal plane flexion and frontal plane varus. It also includes rotation of the talus and hindfoot about the long axis of the tibia, as well as anterior/posterior translation

of the talus relative to the tibia (24). Cass and Settles confirmed that hindfoot inversion is always accompanied by obligatory external rotation of the tibia (relative to the hindfoot), and that this primarily occurs through the subtalar joint in intact ankles (25). They further showed that increased varus talar tilt is not necessarily seen after isolated release of the ATFL or CFL, as one might expect, though tilting occurs after release of both; however, external rotation of the tibia relative to the hindfoot is increased significantly with release of the ATFL, the CFL, or both. This increase in external tibial rotation does not occur through the subtalar joint (the site of normal tibial external rotation). Rather, it occurs between the talus and the tibia. This work strongly supports the concept that the kinematics of lateral ankle instability includes, at least in part, rotation as well as inversion. This concept fits well with the following observations: (a) true static instability can be seen in the absence of radiographically demonstrable talar tilt (24), (b) the anterior drawer test is primarily rotatory rather than translational (26), and (c) posterior fibular position (which, in effect, externally rotates or "opens" the ankle mortise) predisposes to lateral instability (22). The effect of this is seen in **Figure 48-2**. Here, opposing lesions on the lateral tibial and talar joint surfaces strongly suggest an injury mechanism where the lateral talar dome experienced edge-loading under the anterolateral tibial lip, a situation only possible with internal rotation of the talus within the mortise. Understanding of this rotational component is

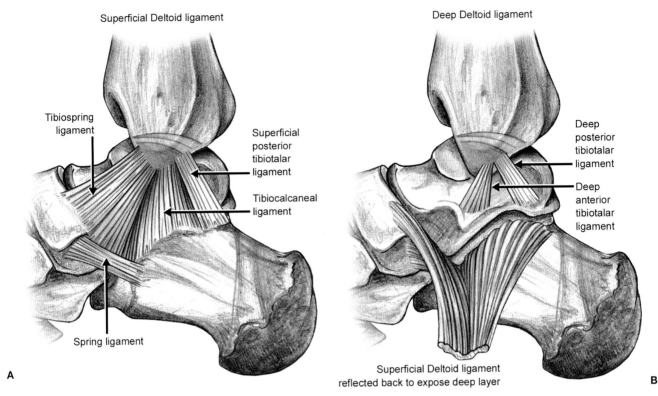

Fig 48-2. Anatomy of the medial ankle ligamentous stabilizers. **A:** Superficial deltoid ligament layer. **B:** Deep deltoid ligament layer. (Reprinted from Berquist TH. *Radiology of the Foot and Ankle.* 2nd ed. Philadelphia: Lippincott Williams & Wilkins; 2000: Fig. 1-46; with permission).

imperative in the assessment and treatment of lateral ankle instability and the associated lesions.

The subtalar joint is stabilized against inversion primarily by the CFL, with contributions by the LTCL, IL, CL, and IER (10). In neutral or dorsiflexion, where the CFL contribution to overall hindfoot inversion stability is maximal, the ankle is inherently more stable due to bony architecture, reducing the overall risk to the CFL. This likely explains why the CFL is rarely injured in isolation, usually being exposed to injury only when the ankle is in plantarflexion, a situation where the ATFL is most likely to be injured first. This relatively "protected" position of the CFL and the number of additional ligaments which stabilize the subtalar joint likely contribute to the relative rarity of isolated subtalar instability. The LTCL, IL, CL, and IER all act as subtalar stabilizers independent of subtalar or ankle position (27), suggesting that injury to these structures may occur in any position. Only the CFL demonstrates positional variance. It is most susceptible to isolated injury when inversion is imposed on the dorsiflexed hindfoot (28,29). It is this condition that is felt to be necessary to produce isolated subtalar instability (30). This has led some authors to suggest that the best indicator of isolated subtalar instability is a sense of giving way or apprehension when the foot is loaded and in neutral or dorsiflexion, rather than in the plantarflexed position typically associated with ankle instability (31).

The deltoid ligament is the medial stabilizer of the ankle joint **(Fig 48-3)**. Wide variations in the description of its anatomy have been reported. This is not surprising because large variation between specimens is typically noted. A recent study by Milner and Soames (32) described six different component bands of the deltoid ligament. They were divided into four superficial bands (tibiospring and tibionavicular [constant]; superficial posterior tibiotalar and tibiocalcaneal ligaments [nonconstant]), and two deep bands (deep posterior tibiotalar [constant]; deep anterior tibiotalar ligaments [nonconstant]). These findings are somewhat similar to the description of Boss and Hintermann (33), who found five distinct components, three lying superficial (tibiospring, tibiocalcaneal, superficial posterior tibiotalar ligament [nonconstant]) and two deep (deep posterior tibiotalar, deep anterior tibiotalar [nonconstant]). They did not find the tibionavicular to be a distinct ligament, but rather a strong fibrous layer of the ankle capsule. It appeared to be the largest portion of the superficial layer.

Instability of the medial ligaments remains poorly understood. So too does the relationship between instability, acquired flat foot syndrome, and ankle arthritis, although some authors have felt such a relationship exists (12). It has been shown, however, that the deltoid ligament does play a key role in coupling tibial rotation to ankle flexion (34). As a result, the competence of the deltoid ligament may influence not only

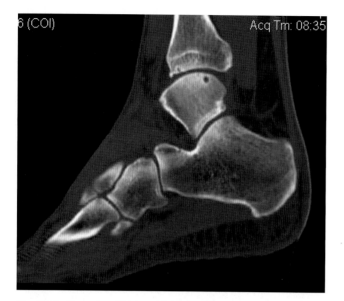

Fig 48-3. Opposing tibial and talar lateral osteochondral defects in a patient three years after severe inversion ankle sprain, as visualized on sagittal CT scan of the ankle. Such lesions appear to be caused by edge-loading of the talar dome by the anterolateral lip of the tibial plafond, a situation only possible where at least one component of the instability kinematics is internal rotation of the talus.

medial stability, but lateral stability as well, through this rotational coupling mechanism. External rotation of the leg has been shown by Rasmussen et al. (35,36) to selectively rupture the deep layers of the deltoid, while the superficial ligaments were the primary stabilizer against talar valgus tilt. Clinical medial ankle instability, where the patient senses giving way medially, is not always associated with radiologically or clinically apparent talar valgus tilt; however, it is associated with attenuation of the deltoid components, particularly the deep portion (12). In view of Rasmussen's findings, this suggests medial instability has a consistent rotational component, again hinting at a connection between medial and lateral ankle instability, as suggested by Hintermann et al. (12).

Dynamic Stabilizers—Tendons

The peroneal tendons are the dynamic stabilizers of the lateral ankle and subtalar joints. They provide the majority of the eversion force to the hindfoot, with 35% attributed to the peroneus longus (PL) and 25% to the peroneus brevis (PB) (37). Both also function as weak ankle plantarflexors, and the peroneus longus as a plantar flexor of the first ray, potentially inducing forefoot valgus, and secondarily, hindfoot varus. Both tendons run through a fibro-osseous tunnel behind the lateral malleolus, with soft tissue constraint provided by the superior and inferior peroneal retinacula proximally and distally. The floor of the tunnel is defined by the PTFL and the CFL. As the tendons emerge from the sheath near the peroneal tubercle on the lateral calcaneus, the PB continues to insert into the base of the fifth

metatarsal, while the PL turns under the cuboid, obliquely crossing the plantar midfoot to insert into the plantar base of the first metatarsal and medial cuneiform.

Although frank weakness of the peroneals has been suggested as a contributor to dynamic lateral ankle instability, this has not been demonstrated (38). Rather than invoking peroneal strength in general as the key to dynamic ankle stability, it is more helpful to consider dynamic ankle stability to be dependent on two factors: (a) the ability to avoid situations where the foot/ankle complex is forced into inversion past the limit that secures stability prior to loading with a compressive force, (b) and the ability, when the ankle is subject to an inversion torque, to prevent unstable situations from progressing to injury of the lateral ligaments and capsule of the ankle/foot complex (4). To put this another way, a person who does not get the ankle complex into situations of excessive plantar flexion and inversion is not at risk, and if the ankle has become subject to an inversion torque, injury can still be prevented if the reaction to counteract the inversion torque is sufficiently fast and powerful (4). The ability to position the foot to avoid injury is under neuromuscular control, and is subject to variation and errors in positioning. Konradsen et al. (39) have demonstrated significant increases in positioning errors after acute ankle inversion injury, even 12 weeks post-injury, suggesting a potential cause of increased susceptibility to recurrent instability. The ability of the peroneals to react quickly to counteract excessive inversion hinges on peroneal reaction time. This has been studied by a number of authors, with the majority indicating increased peroneal reaction time is typically present in patients with dynamic ankle instability (4). These factors form the basis for peroneal recruitment training and proprioception training for the treatment of ankle instability, both dynamic and static.

■ CLINICAL EVALUATION

Clinical evaluation is the key to diagnosis of ankle instability. The goal is to obtain a working diagnosis of instability by history, and use physical examination for confirmation and to rule out other associated injuries or diagnoses. Ultimately, the aim is to determine if the patient's complaint represents pseudo- or true-instability. If true instability is present, localizing the instability lesion to the lateral ankle, medial ankle or subtalar joint follows. Determining whether the instability is static or dynamic is then required.

History

Patients will most often report the onset of instability after an initial ankle spraining injury, although it is not unusual for multiple smaller injury episodes to be reported, rather than a single major sprain. Occasionally, no specific inciting injury will be present. Because lateral instability is by far the most common, most patients note the initial injury, and subsequent instability to be in inversion. Eversion symptoms suggest medial instability. The history of chronic instability includes symptoms of insecurity and apprehension of use of the ankle. Recurrent giving way or frank sprain injuries, possibly associated with falls, may be reported. Difficulty with jumping or walking on uneven surfaces or stairs is common. The sense of instability with the foot planted, as opposed to positioning in plantarflexion has been suggested as being more indicative of subtalar instability (31).

Although approximately 30% of patients will be asymptomatic between giving way episodes, the majority will report at least some symptoms between episodes (24). These may include chronic ankle pain (most often lateral), tenderness, or swelling. If such symptoms are present in the intervals between sprains, further diagnoses in addition to, or instead of, true instability should be considered (Table 48-1). The amount and effectiveness of prior treatments, including physiotherapy and ankle bracing, should be noted.

Physical Findings

Assessment of the ankle for instability includes evaluation of the knee and entire foot, as well. Lower extremity alignment, ankle and foot range of motion testing, localization of any tenderness, and tests of ankle stability and proprioception are required. Assessment of neurologic and vascular function and of the adjacent tissues for the presence of associated lesions (Table 48-1) completes the evaluation.

Assessment of alignment is done with the patient standing. Hindfoot varus may contribute to instability, and if present, must be considered in any treatment plan. Hindfoot valgus may be associated with medial instability or with tarsal coalition (which may present with recurrent instability). Flexibility of the hindfoot is thus important to note.

Direct ligamentous stability testing includes assessment of subtalar motion, talar tilt, and the anterior drawer test. Subtalar motion is difficult to isolate and quantify. Generally, comparison with the contralateral side is used to determine if laxity is present (20). Care must be taken to differentiate inversion due to subtalar motion from varus talar tilt, although this, too, can be difficult. To assess talar tilt, the ankle is placed in slight plantarflexion, and the hindfoot and midfoot should then be inverted as a unit, not allowing the forefoot to rotate medially. As the hindfoot is inverted, a sulcus may become visible or palpable at the anterolateral joint line of the ankle, and a perception of varus motion occurring above the level of the subtalar joint, between the tibia and talus, may be present. These findings suggest the presence of talar tilt (1).

The anterior drawer test is carried out with the lower leg hanging free, knee flexed. The ankle is slightly plantarflexed, and the tibia stabilized with one hand and the hindfoot and heel grasped with the other. The hindfoot is drawn forward with an anterior translation and internal rotation force. The talus will typically internally rotate with anterior translation, as an intact deltoid ligament will serve as a medial tether. The amount of anterior translation of the lateral side of the talus relative to the tibia is quantified and compared to the contralateral side (1). A difference of 5 mm is considered abnormal, as is an absolute value of 10 mm, although these values are difficult to specify with such detail (20). The tactile sensation of the presence and quality of an "end point" is often more important.

Proprioception deficits are part of dynamic instability and should be sought. Single-leg hopping and hop-turn maneuvers may demonstrate apprehension or frank giving way. The Romberg test, comparing single leg stance of the symptomatic side with the asymptomatic side, with eyes open and shut, is also an indicator of proprioception.

Imaging

A standard weight-bearing ankle x-ray series, with anteroposterior (AP), lateral, and mortise views, is required in all cases to ensure no major skeletal abnormalities are present, and to aid in ruling out associated lesions (Table 48-1).

Bone scans, CT scans, and magnetic resonance imaging (MRI) scans are not routinely required, but may be useful to identify associated pathology or potentially augment an equivocal physical examination.

Lateral tilt and AP translation stress x-rays have been widely reviewed (40). Their use remains controversial because only 40% of patients with radiological instability will have ankle instability symptoms and almost 40% of symptomatic patients will appear stable on stress x-rays (24). As such, definitive diagnosis is not based on stress x-rays, though they may be used as adjuncts to the whole clinical picture, when the contralateral ankle is used as a control.

■ TREATMENT

Nonoperative Treatment

Nonoperative modalities are the primary treatment for all forms of ankle instability, while treatment of the provocative lesion is the key in pseudo-instability.

Physiotherapy and mechanical supports are the mainstays of nonoperative treatment. Physiotherapy typically emphasizes proprioceptive training, peroneal recruitment, and peroneal strengthening. The role of proprioception and peroneal reaction time in reproducibly positioning the ankle safely, and detecting and countering abnormal ankle motion, makes these modalities useful both for dynamic and static instability patterns. Specific proprioception training has been well shown to reduce instability symptoms (41).

Augmentation of physiotherapy with mechanical supports is also recommended. Mild degrees of hindfoot malalignment can be addressed with orthotics or shoe modifications. Many patients with lateral instability, particularly running athletes with increased dynamic supination, will benefit from an external lateral heel wedge (20).

Ankle bracing or taping for activities with increased risk of ankle twisting is important. When used in conjunction with an appropriate physiotherapy program, most patients, including competitive athletes, will have a dramatic reduction in symptoms and require no further treatment (1). Taping of the ankle has been shown to have a greater stabilizing effect than lace-up bracing, though its effects deteriorate with time and stretching (42,43). Plastic stirrup-style braces have been shown to restrict inversion and eversion effectively (44).

Operative Treatment

General Indications

As noted previously, most patients will be successfully treated nonoperatively; however, a small percentage will continue to have symptoms despite appropriate therapy and bracing. In addition, some will have instability symptoms that are not restricted to risk activities, but that occur with simple activities of daily living. In such cases, even if bracing provides relief, some patients may find routine daily brace use impossible. Finally, some patients will have had previous surgical treatment that has failed, potentially removing some of the dynamic or static stabilizing structures that would be necessary for successful nonoperative treatment. Surgical stabilization is indicated in these groups of patients.

Surgical Techniques—Lateral Instability

The variety of surgical procedures that have been used for treatment of lateral ankle instability is considerable, with over eighty different techniques described in the literature (20). These techniques can be broadly divided into nonanatomic reconstructions, anatomic reconstructions, and additional procedures. The wide variability in techniques recommended in the literature can lead to confusion and difficulty in selecting a reconstructive technique. Recent studies have helped clarify these issues.

Nonanatomic Reconstructions. Nonanatomic reconstruction techniques typically involve creating a "checkrein" on the lateral aspect of the ankle through tenodesis of all or part of the peroneus brevis tendon. Three of the most common techniques described and modified are the Watson-Jones procedure, the Evans procedure, and the Chrisman-Snook procedure (11). Multiple biomechanical studies of these techniques have shown that they result in substantial alteration of ankle and subtalar joint kinematics, while producing variable degrees of stabilization and reduced range of motion (45–49). Long term follow-up reports have demonstrated increased rates of recurrent subjective instability, objective laxity on anterior drawer testing, and degenerative changes on x-ray for these techniques, when compared to anatomic reconstructions (50–52). As a result, these techniques are now primarily of historical interest, and anatomic reconstructions are strongly favored where technically feasible (24,50,53).

Anatomic Reconstructions. Anatomic reconstructions can be divided into either *direct repairs* (reefing the ATFL and CFL) or *anatomic ligament reconstructions* (augmentation of the ATFL and CFL with tendinous tissue). Both techniques are used by the author and are widely reported in the current literature. In principle, the simplest and least anatomically disruptive procedure that will attain the surgical goal should be the procedure that is selected. On this basis, the author's primary procedure for ankle stabilization is direct repair; however, this is often not feasible, as the lateral capsular tissues and the ATFL are often severely attenuated and insufficient for stable repair (1,54). Such tissue insufficiency may be present in patients with marked laxity on anterior drawer testing or subtalar inversion. If severe laxity is noted on clinical exam, or generalized joint laxity is present, an anatomic ligament reconstruction technique should be used, rather than direct repair, to avoid reliance on weak capsular tissues. In addition to patients with severe laxity, the author also favors anatomic ligament reconstruction in patients with failed previous reconstructions, as they, too, may be lacking in adequate tissue for repair.

Because direct repair relies solely on the holding strength of sutures for early strength and on adequate soft-tissue healing for late strength, there are some additional situations where direct repair may not be optimal. These situations typically arise when above average stresses are expected after surgery, either early or late. For example, when early return to activity is desired (e.g., professional athletes), immediate initiation of rehabilitation may be required, potentially exposing a direct repair to excessive stress early on. Alternately, excessive stresses may be anticipated later, after successful repair, in very large or obese patients, elite-level athletes at high risk for inversion injury, or patients with neurologic or peroneal muscle impairment. In these patients, anatomical ligament reconstruction with strong tissue and solid attachment to bone is recommended.

Direct Repair

Direct late repair of the lateral ankle ligaments was described by Brostrom (55) in 1966. His technique involved identifying the stretched ATFL and CFL, cutting them mid-substance, shortening them, and then directly repairing them, also in mid-substance. In 1980, Gould et al. (56) presented a modification of Brostrom's procedure. They augmented the direct repair by mobilizing the proximal edge of the lateral aspect of the extensor retinaculum and attaching it to the anterior aspect of the fibula, overlying the Brostrom repair. This has become known as the Brostrom-Gould procedure and is the most commonly used technique for direct repair **(Fig 48-4)**.

Others have further modified Brostrom's procedure. Additional methods of tissue augmentation have been described to deal with lateral tissues that are frequently inadequate for repair (57). As an alternative to augmentation,

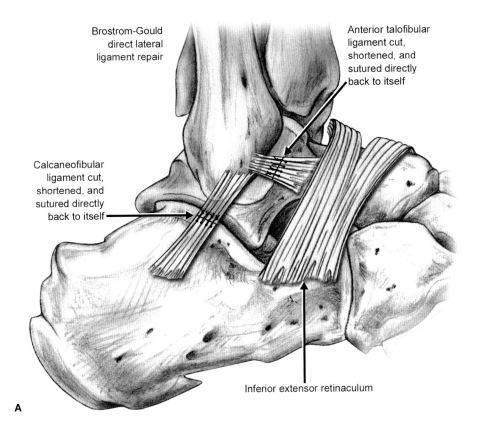

Brostrom-Gould direct lateral ligament repair

Anterior talofibular ligament cut, shortened, and sutured directly back to itself

Calcaneofibular ligament cut, shortened, and sutured directly back to itself

Inferior extensor retinaculum

A

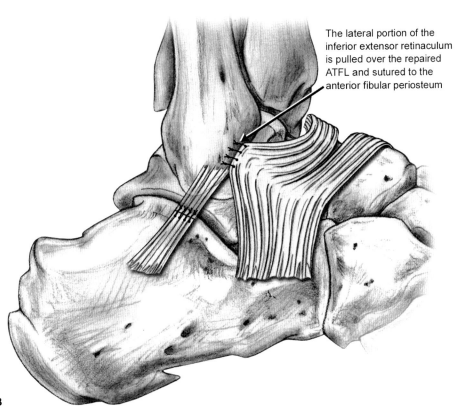

The lateral portion of the inferior extensor retinaculum is pulled over the repaired ATFL and sutured to the anterior fibular periosteum

B

Fig 48-4. The Brostrom-Gould direct lateral ligament repair. A: The ATFL and CFL are cut, shortened, and sutured directly. B: The lateral portion of the inferior extensor retinaculum is pulled over the repaired ATFL and sutured to the anterior fibular periosteum. ATFL, anterior talo-fibular ligament; CFL, the calcaneo-fibular ligament.

others have described variations in the specific site of shortening of the ligaments (58) and newer methods of fixation of the repair with suture anchors (59), all with the aim of improving repair strength in the face of potentially weak tissue. The author's preferred direct repair technique, described following, is similar to that described by Messer et al. (59), following the modification of Brostrom's repair described by Karlsson (58) in 1989, and including Gould's extensor retinaculum augmentation.

Surgical Technique—Direct Repair

The patient is positioned supine with a bolster behind the ipsilateral buttock. A thigh tourniquet is used. A bolster is placed behind the Achilles tendon, keeping the heel suspended to avoid forward pressure on the heel. A curvilinear incision, 3 to 4 cm in length, is made following the anterior border of the lateral malleolus, ending at the peroneal tendons. Branches of the sural and superficial peroneal nerves are protected. If peroneal tendon pathology is suspected pre-operatively, a postero-lateral curvilinear incision is used, following the course of the peroneal tendons, elevating the skin flap anteriorly to allow exposure of the ATFL. The proximal edge of the inferior extensor retinaculum is dissected out and tagged for later use. The capsule of the lateral ankle joint is then identified deeper in the incision, and the ATFL condensation within the capsule is found. Often, a discrete ATFL is not visible, and only attenuated capsular tissue is present. The CFL condensation in the capsule lies deep to the peroneal tendons near the tip of the lateral malleolus, and can be found with inferior retraction of the peroneals. The lateral capsule, including the ATFL and CFL, is divided 1 to 2 mm from its attachment to the fibula, rather than mid-substance as described by Brostrom (55). The proximal limb of the capsule is elevated subperiosteally off the fibula, creating a periosteal sleeve 10 mm in length. The anterior edge of the lateral malleolus is roughened with a rongeur and two 5.0 mm Bio-Corkscrew Suture Anchors (Arthrex Inc., Naples, FL) are inserted, one at the origin of the ATFL and the other just inferior, at the origin of the CFL, located as described earlier. Two #2 nonabsorbable sutures from the proximal suture anchor are placed into the ATFL, and two sutures from the distal anchor are placed into the CFL **(Fig 48-5A)**. With the foot in slight plantarflexion and eversion, the sutures are tied, shortening up the ligaments, and tightly securing them to the bone trough in the anterior fibula. The periosteal sleeve is then laid over top of the newly attached capsule and ligaments, and sutured to it in a "pants-over-vest" fashion, with #2 nonabsorbable suture **(Fig 48-5B)**. The proximal edge of the extensor retinaculum is then drawn to the fibula, and sutured onto the periosteal flap and capsule with #1 absorbable suture, completing the repair **(Fig 48-5C)**. The wound is irrigated and closed in layers. A bulky dressing is applied, and the ankle is splinted in slight plantarflexion and eversion.

Postoperative Management

The patient is kept in the splint and nonweight-bearing for 2 weeks. A below-knee walker boot is applied and used full-time, immobilizing the ankle in neutral position for 4 more weeks. Gentle physiotherapy is initiated at 6 weeks postoperatively, and the patient is weaned out of the walker boot over the next 2 to 4 weeks, using an ankle stirrup brace. Light activity is allowed after 10 weeks, and full activities after 3 months.

Clinical Results

Brostrom (55) reported an 80% success rate in 60 patients using his technique in 1966. In 1988, Karlsson et al. (60) reported good or excellent results in 87% of the 152 cases reported in their series using Brostrom's technique at an average of 6 years follow-up. The following year, Karlsson et al. (58) presented their new modification of Brostrom's technique, utilizing a periosteal flap. Good or excellent results were noted in 88% of their 60 patients, after 3.5 years. In 1991, Sjolin et al. (61) reported satisfactory results in 86% of their 28 patients, using a periosteal flap technique similar to that described by Karlsson. Hamilton et al. (62) reported on 28 Brostrom-Gould procedures in 1993. Excellent results were seen in 26 procedures, a good result in one, and a fair result in one. No complications, failures, or "stretch-outs" were reported after an average of 64.3 months. In 1996, Hennrikus (63) compared Karlsson's direct repair with the Chrisman-Snook procedure in a randomized, prospective trial with 40 patients and 29 month follow-up. Of the 19 Chrisman-Snook cases, three were excellent, 13 good, one fair, and two poor, based on functional results reported by the patients. In contrast, the direct repair cases had ten excellent, seven good, three fair, and one poor, with notably fewer complications. In 1997, Karlsson et al. (64) compared the Brostrom-Gould procedure with their periosteal flap modification of Brostrom's procedure in a prospective, randomized trial of 60 patients (64). At three years follow-up, 90% of the periosteal flap cases were deemed satisfactory, as were 83% of the Brostrom-Gould cases. This difference was not felt to be significant, and both groups had equal mechanical stability on x-ray evaluation. They concluded both variations of Brostrom's original technique were useful. Messer et al. (59) reported their results using the surgical technique described above, incorporating a periosteal sleeve, suture anchors, and extensor retinaculum augmentation. After 34.5 months follow-up, 20 of 22 patients (91%) reported good or excellent functional outcomes. Finally, in 2004, Chen et al. (65) reported on 56 cases using a periosteal flap technique. Good and excellent results were reported in 91.1%, based on the Ankle-Hindfoot Scale of the American Orthopedic Foot and Ankle Society (AOFAS) (66), with the average score improving from 71 preoperatively to 92 postoperatively.

Anatomic Ligament Reconstructions

In some situations, direct repair is not feasible or recommended, as noted earlier in this chapter. In these cases, using tendon graft to reconstruct the anatomic courses of the CFL and ATFL is recommended. Multiple anatomic ligament reconstruction techniques have been described, and these vary primarily in their choice of tendon, with peroneus brevis autograft being most commonly described (57,67–69), and semitendinosis (ST) (70), gracilis (54), plantaris (12), patellar tendon-bone (71), and palmaris longus (72) tendons also being used. Currently, there is little information available to guide the choice of tendon graft (73). Some authors advocate avoidance of peroneus brevis harvest, as the peroneals are the primary dynamic stabilizers of the lateral ankle (70). The author's preferred technique follows the procedure described recently by Coughlin et al. (54), with the addition of two modifications. First, the author uses ST tendon graft instead of gracilis, as used by Coughlin, because it is typically larger and stronger than gracilis. Use of either of the hamstring tendons offers the advantage of peroneal tendon preservation, with minimal donor site morbidity (70). Second, bio-absorbable interference screws are used to anchor the graft in bone, rather than graft loops through bone tunnels, providing immediate, secure fixation analogous to that used in anterior cruciate ligament reconstruction (74).

Surgical Technique—Anatomic Ligament Reconstruction

Patient positioning and set-up are the same as for direct repair. Unless peroneal tendon pathology is suspected, an anterior curvilinear incision is used, 5 to 10 mm anterior to the lateral malleolus, following its anterior border. The incision is carried posteriorly, crossing the peroneal tendons, taking care to avoid any damage to them, ending 5 to 10 mm posterior to the tendons, directly over the CFL insertion in the calcaneus. Care is taken to avoid the sural nerve. The proximal edge of the extensor retinaculum is mobilized and tagged. The lateral ankle capsule is identified. If the tissue is noted to be of good quality for repair, the surgeon can choose to carry out a direct repair as mentioned earlier in this chapter, if this option was deemed reasonable preoperatively. If the tissues are inadequate for direct repair alone, ligament reconstruction will follow as planned; however, in all but the most severely attenuated cases, the lateral capsule is still imbricated in mid-substance at this point, using the classic Brostrom technique.

The ST tendon is then harvested, using a 3 cm vertical incision, beginning 2 cm medial to the tibial tubercle and incising distally. The sartorius fascia is identified and the ST and gracilis tendons palpated deep to it. The fascia is incised in-line with the ST tendon for 3 to 4 cm, and the ST tendon, larger and more posteroinferior than gracilis, can then be hooked with a Lauer forceps, and pulled up into the

wound. The knee is maximally flexed, allowing a more of the tendon to be pulled into the wound. The fascial attachments along the ST tendon are divided, and the tendon palpated with a finger all the way to its musculotendinous junction. Often the junction is then visible, and the ST tendon can then be divided just distal to the junction with a scissor. Occasionally, a tendon-stripper is needed. The proximal end of the ST tendon is pulled into the wound and prepared with a Krackow stitch. The tibial attachment of the ST tendon is now detached from bone, and the tendon end trimmed. A graft length of 10 to 15 cm is routinely available. Graft diameter is measured, and is typically 5 to 7 mm.

The fibular bone tunnel is created next **(Fig 48-5)**. Drill holes are then placed in the fibula, the first in the anterior cortex at the ATFL attachment, centered 15 mm proximal to the fibular tip, and the second just anterior and proximal to the fibular tip. The holes are connected to create a tunnel in the fibula, using a curette. Care is taken to maintain a strong bone bridge. Drill size is dependent on graft size, most often 6 or 7 mm.

Drill holes for the talar and calcaneal attachments are made next. A 7 mm drill from the Bio-Tenodesis Screw System (Arthrex Inc., Naples, FL) is used to drill a 25 mm deep hole in the talar neck from lateral to medial, taking care to avoid penetration of the medial cortex. The hole is located in the middle of the ATFL insertion, just beyond the lateral articular cartilage. A similar drill hole is placed in the CFL attachment point to the lateral calcaneus, which is exposed with anterior retraction of the peroneals. It is centered in line with the posterior cortex of the fibula, approximately 12 to 15 mm below the subtalar joint line.

The ST graft is pulled through the fibular tunnel, from the fibular tip, and out the anterior hole. The free end of the graft at the fibular tip is passed deep to the peroneal tendons and grasped with the Bio-Tenodesis Screw inserter. The end of the tendon is seated deeply in the calcaneal hole, and a 7 mm Bio-Tenodesis screw inserted until flush. Solid purchase of the tendon within the calcaneus is confirmed. The foot is kept in slight flexion, and eversion, with the heel suspended, allowing the talus to "drop back" fully into the ankle mortise. The graft is now pulled taut with the Krackow sutures, tensioning the CFL portion of the reconstruction. The required length of tendon to fully seat in the talar hole is estimated, and the graft is cut to this length. This free end is grasped with the Bio-Tenodesis Screw inserter, and pushed into the talar drill hole. Tension can be adjusted manually with this system, and is set to be taut. A 7 mm Bio-Tenodesis screw is then inserted until flush, again confirming rigid fixation. Graft tension is confirmed and anterior drawer testing done to ensure stability. The ankle is moved through a range of motion to ensure the repair is isometric and that motion is not restricted. Subtalar inversion of 15 to 20 degrees is expected. The graft attachment points at the fibula, calcaneus, and talus are reinforced with absorbable suture to periosteum and capsule. The extensor retinaculum is

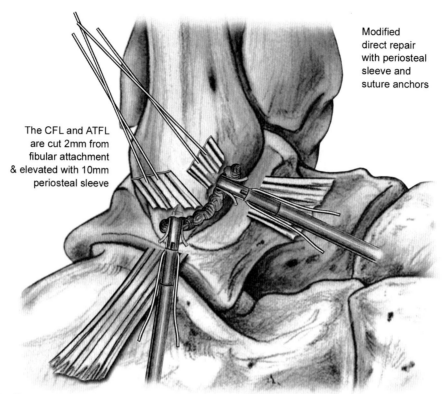

Modified direct repair with periosteal sleeve and suture anchors

The CFL and ATFL are cut 2mm from fibular attachment & elevated with 10mm periosteal sleeve

A   The anterior edge of the fibula is roughened and 2 suture anchors are placed in the distal fibula

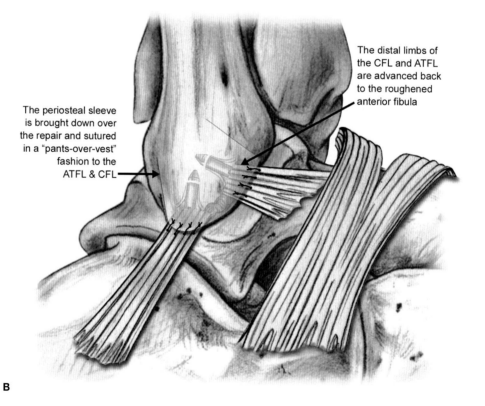

The distal limbs of the CFL and ATFL are advanced back to the roughened anterior fibula

The periosteal sleeve is brought down over the repair and sutured in a "pants-over-vest" fashion to the ATFL & CFL

B

Fig 48-5. The modified direct repair with periosteal sleeve and suture anchors. **A:** The ATFL and CFL are cut 1 to 2 mm from their fibular attachment. The fibular origins are elevated with a 10 mm periosteal sleeve off the lateral fibula. The anterior edge of the fibula is roughened and two suture anchors are placed in the distal fibula at the ATFL and CFL origins, and the distal limbs of the ATFL and CFL are advanced tightly approximated to the roughened anterior fibula. **B:** The periosteal sleeve is brought down over the repair and sutured in a "pants-over-vest" fashion to the ATFL and CFL.

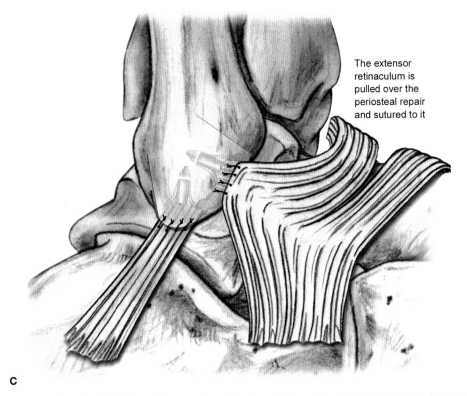

The extensor retinaculum is pulled over the periosteal repair and sutured to it

C

Fig 48-5. (*continued*) **C:** The extensor retinaculum is pulled over the periosteal repair and sutured to it. ATFL, anterior talo-fibular ligament; CFL, the calcaneo-fibular ligament.

advanced to the fibula, and attached to periosteum with nonabsorbable suture. The wound is irrigated and closed in layers. A bulky dressing is applied, and the ankle is splinted in slight plantarflexion and eversion.

Postoperative Management

The patient is kept in the splint and nonweight-bearing for 2 weeks. A below-knee walker boot is then used and weight-bearing initiated. A stirrup brace is used at night. Very gentle ankle range of motion is allowed. The boot is discontinued at 6 weeks postoperatively, and vigorous physiotherapy initiated. The stirrup brace is used for 3 more weeks and for vigorous activity thereafter. Return to activity is dependent on progress with physiotherapy, and anticipated between 9 and 12 weeks after surgery.

Clinical Results

Coughlin et al. (54) recently reported results using this technique without the author's modifications **(Fig 48-6)**. At an average of 23 months follow-up, 24 of 28 patients were rated

as excellent and 4 of 28 rated as good, using patient subjective self-assessment, visual analog pain assessment, and AOFAS and Karlsson scores. Talar tilt and anterior drawer were improved significantly, while ankle and subtalar motion were unaffected. No major complications were noted and minimal donor site morbidity was reported.

Capsulorrhaphy

Some authors have recently advocated the use of heat-induced modification of the lateral ankle ligaments and capsule as an alternative for treating patients with subjective instability symptoms and mild objective laxity (75). This technique has been used with variable success for treatment of shoulder instability. The procedure, typically performed arthroscopically, involves application of heat to tissue with a laser or radio-frequency heat probe. Heat applied in a controlled way to ligaments and capsular tissue, at approximately $65°C$, is thought to lead to denaturation of Type 1 collagen fibers and subsequent shrinkage, tightening the

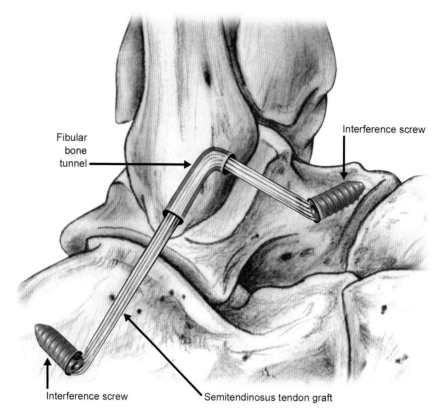

Fig 48-6. The modified Coughlin anatomic ligament reconstruction with free hamstring tendon graft. The semitendinosis tendon graft is passed through a bone tunnel in the distal fibula, with the inlet and outlet at the anatomic origins of the ATFL and CFL. The free graft is attached to the lateral calcaneus and lateral talar neck with interference screw fixation. ATFL, anterior talo-fibular ligament; CFL, the calcaneo-fibular ligamen

ligaments, and potentially reducing instability. In a small study of carefully selected patients with mild instability, this procedure has been reported to produce reasonable short term results (75); however, it currently remains investigational and is not used routinely.

■ ADDITIONAL PROCEDURES

Calcaneal Osteotomy

As noted earlier, varus hindfoot alignment may contribute to lateral ankle instability. Van Bergeyk et al. (21) suggested that failure to address malalignment may be a contributing factor in failed ligament reconstruction (21). Colville (1) has stated that correction of severe hindfoot varus deformities is important if recurrent instability is to be avoided after ligament reconstruction in patients with such malalignment; however, treatment of ankle instability with a lateralizing calcaneal osteotomy or valgus-inducing distal tibial osteotomy, either alone or together with ligament reconstruction, has not been reported in the literature. Nevertheless, hindfoot realignment utilizing a lateral sliding calcaneal osteotomy certainly seems

sensible in patients with gross varus malalignment on initial presentation, or any varus alignment after failed previous reconstruction attempts, and this is the author's practice.

Ankle Arthroscopy

Although wholly arthroscopic techniques for lateral ankle reconstruction have not been commonly reported or utilized, the use of ankle arthroscopy in association with ankle stabilization has been advocated (76). Komenda and Ferkel (76) observed intra-articular abnormalities, such as loose bodies, osteochondral lesions, and synovitis in 51 of 55 ankles examined arthroscopically prior to lateral ankle reconstruction. Such experience has led multiple other authors to recommend routine use of ankle arthroscopy for diagnosis and treatment of associated ankle pathology if preoperative assessment suggests it may be present (1,20). The author routinely performs ankle arthroscopy at the time of ligament reconstruction in all patients, except those with absolutely no clinical or radiologic findings suggestive of a pseudo-instability lesion (Table 48-1), who give a very clear history of having no pain between inversion episodes.

Although this approach seems reasonable, there are currently no studies documenting improved short or long term outcomes with this practice.

Surgical Techniques—Subtalar Instability

Subtalar instability is most commonly seen in combination with lateral ankle instability (10,77,78). In this setting, subtalar instability has been recognized for some time, and many authors have described techniques to stabilize the lateral subtalar joint in conjunction with lateral ankle stabilization. Clanton and Berson (78) advocated the use of the Brostrom-Gould direct repair of the CFL and ATFL for this problem, while others have recommended ligament reconstructions (79). Given that 10% to 25% of all lateral ankle instability cases may have associated subtalar instability (10), the high success rates of direct repairs and anatomic reconstructions for ankle instability suggest these techniques are also effective in dealing with the subtalar component of the instability problem.

Defining when the subtalar component becomes the primary component of the instability problem, or even the only component, is very difficult. Isolated subtalar instability has been described, but no consensus on etiology or diagnostic criteria exists, making reliable clinical diagnosis and differentiation from lateral ankle instability nearly impossible. As a result, it is difficult to utilize and compare the few reports describing treatment because it is not clear if the entities being treated are comparable. The difficulty in defining a real, reproducible diagnosis of isolated subtalar instability and differentiating it from lateral ankle instability (with or without a subtalar component), has led some authors to use the same procedure for treating all lateral instability. Recently, this has most commonly been the Brostrom-Gould technique. Others, however, have described procedures to reconstruct subtalar ligaments specifically, including the interosseous and cervical ligaments (80–82). Currently, in the absence of clear diagnostic criteria, no basis exists upon which to choose one surgical procedure over another for treatment of subtalar instability. Given this situation, the author currently considers subtalar instability to be a part of lateral ankle and hindfoot instability as a whole, even when it seems to be the major component. Although this perspective may need to be modified as more information becomes available, or when a diagnostic consensus can be reached, it currently leads the author to treat all lateral instability with the techniques outlined in the prior section.

Surgical Techniques—Medial Instability

Medial ankle instability has only recently received increasing attention in the literature. Similar to subtalar instability, no clear diagnostic criteria have been presented. Medial instability is thought to occur most commonly in conjunction with lateral instability and has been included in the overall concept of rotational instability of the ankle (83). Medial instability, however, is also felt to exist as an isolated entity, separate from lateral ankle instability and adult acquired flatfoot, at least initially (12). In these situations, the clinical findings are reported to be a sense giving way into eversion, most often with medial ankle pain and tenderness. In more obvious cases, frank deltoid ligament laxity may be sensed on anterior drawer testing. With loss of the medial deltoid "hinge," direct anterior talar translation, rather than antero-lateral translation and internal rotation, may be noted (34). Increased eversion may also be seen, typically with an external rotation component. Valgus talar tilt may be visible on stress radiographs, though much like in lateral instability, the correlation of this to symptoms is not clear.

In 2004, Hintermann et al. (12) reported on the clinical and surgical findings in 52 ankles which underwent surgical treatment for a preoperative diagnosis of medial ankle instability. They were careful to mention that cases of posterior tibial tendon dysfunction were not included in this series, although 60% had increased hindfoot valgus and 50% had a flattened longitudinal arch. All had an abnormal anterior drawer test. Valgus talar tilt greater than 5 degrees on stress x-rays was noted in 55%. They defined moderate instability as the ability to distract the tibial plafond–talar dome joint space between 2 to 5 mm on the medial aspect intra-operatively. Severe instability was defined as greater than 5 mm of distraction. Using these criteria, all patients with suspected medial instability preoperatively were noted to have moderate or severe medial instability on the medial aspect. They used direct repair with imbrication of the deltoid ligament in 94% and a free plantaris tendon graft for reconstruction of the deltoid ligament in 6%. Lateral ligament reconstruction was done in 69% of cases and spring ligament repair in 21%. Calcaneal lateral column lengthening osteotomy was added to 27% of cases. AOFAS hindfoot scores improved from an average of 42.9 to 91.6, with 90% scored as good or excellent at a mean of 4.4 years follow-up.

There are few other detailed reports of diagnosis and treatment of medial instability available. As a result, the author uses a similar approach to that outlined by Hintermann, treating all patients who require surgical intervention with arthroscopy for assessment, and then primary deltoid ligament repair, shortening and reattaching it with suture anchors to the medial malleolus. If the spring ligament is also seen to be lax, it is also imbricated. If the tissues are felt to be incompetent for adequate repair, augmentation with free tendon graft, using what Hansen has termed "expendable" tendons (84) (e.g., plantaris), seems warranted, though the author's current experience with this method is too limited to advocate. Sacrifice of part, or all, of the posterior tibial tendon, the major medial dynamic stabilizer, as described by Wiltberger and Mallory (85) in 1972, seems less than ideal.

■ CONCLUSION

Ankle instability encompasses many different aspects. Until recently, research has focused on the lateral ankle primarily, and treatment algorithms have become generally agreed upon, with anatomic repairs or reconstructions being favored. The relationship between "typical" lateral ankle instability and both subtalar and medial ankle instability is now being analyzed, and may lead to a more comprehensive understanding and treatment regimen for ankle and hind-foot instability as a whole. Even better understanding of normal and abnormal ankle and hindfoot kinematics, particularly in vivo, will be required to sort out etiologies and allow definition of diagnostic criteria. Meaningful comparison of different treatment techniques for these entities will only be possible after clear definitions of these entities are available.

■ REFERENCES

1. Colville MR. Surgical treatment of the unstable ankle. *J Am Acad Orthop Surg*. 1998;6:368–377.
2. Freeman MA. Instability of the foot after injuries to the lateral ligaments of the ankle. *J Bone Joint Surg Br*. 1965;47:669–677.
3. Kannus P, Renstrom P. Current concepts review: treatment for acute tears of the lateral ligaments of the ankle—operation, cast, or early controlled mobilization. *J Bone Joint Surg Am*. 1991;73:305–312.
4. Konradsen L. Sensori-motor control of the uninjured and injured human ankle. *J Electromyogr Kinesiol*. 2002;12:199–203.
5. Abraham E, Stokes S. Neglected ruptures of the peroneal tendons causing recurrent sprains of the ankle. *J Bone Joint Surg Am*. 1979;61:1247–1248.
6. Fortin PT, Guettler J, Manoli A. Idiopathic cavovarus and lateral ankle instability: recognition and treatment implications relating to ankle arthritis. *Foot Ankle Int*. 2002;23:1031–1037.
7. Hubbard TJ, Kaminski TW, Vander Griend RA, et al. Quantitative assessment of mechanical laxity in the functionally unstable ankle. *Med Sci Sports Exerc*. 2004;36:760–766.
8. Renstrom AF. Persistently painful sprained ankle. *J Am Acad Orthop Surg*. 1994;2:70–280.
9. Baker JM, Ouzounian TJ. Complex ankle instability. *Foot Ankle Clin*. 2000;5:887–896.
10. Keefe DT, Haddad SL. Subtalar instability: etiology, diagnosis, and management. *Foot Ankle Clin*. 2002;7:577–610.
11. Clanton TO. Athletic injuries to the soft tissues of the foot and ankle. In: Coughlin MJ, Mann RA, eds. *Surgery of the foot and ankle*. 7th ed. St. Louis: Mosby; 1999:1090–1209.
12. Hintermann B, Valderrabano V, Boss A, et al. Medial ankle instability: an exploratory, prospective study of fifty-two cases. *Am J Sports Med*. 2004;32:183–188.
13. Ekstrand J, Trapp H. The incidence of ankle sprains in soccer. *Foot Ankle*. 1990;11:41–44.
14. Garrick JG. The frequency of injury, mechanism of injury and epidemiology of ankle sprains. *Am J Sports Med*. 1977;5:241–242.
15. Sammarco VJ. Principles and techniques in rehabilitation of the athlete's foot: part III: rehabilitation of ankle sprains. *Tech Foot Ankle Surg*. 2003;2:199–207.
16. Holmer P, Sondergaard L, Konradsen L, et al. Epidemiology of sprains in the lateral ankle and foot. *Foot Ankle Int*. 1997;15:72–74.
17. Mack RP. Ankle injuries in athletes. *Clin Sports Med*. 1982;1:71–84.
18. Sammarco VJ. Complications of lateral ankle ligament reconstruction. *Clin Orthop*. 2001;391:123–132.
19. Stormont DM, Morrey BF, An K, et al. Stability of the loaded ankle. *Am J Sports Med*. 1985;13:295–300.
20. Berlet GC, Anderson RB, Davis WH. Chronic lateral ankle instability. *Foot Ankle Clin*. 1999;4:713–728.
21. Van Bergeyk AB, Younger A, Carson B. CT analysis of hindfoot alignment in chronic lateral ankle instability. *Foot Ankle Int*. 2002;23:37–42.
22. Berkowitz CP, Kim DH. Fibular position in relation to lateral ankle instability. *Foot Ankle Int*. 2004;25:318–321.
23. Scranton PE, McDermott JE, Rogers JV. The relationship between chronic ankle instability and variations in mortise anatomy and impingement spurs. *Foot Ankle Int*. 2000;21:657–664.
24. Hintermann B. Biomechanics of the unstable ankle joint and clinical implications. *Med Sci Sports Exerc*. 1999;31(suppl):S459–S469.
25. Cass JR, Settles H. Ankle instability: in vitro kinematics in response to axial load. *Foot Ankle*. 1994;15:134–140.
26. McCullough CJ, Burge PD. Rotatory stability of the load-bearing ankle: an experimental study. *J Bone Joint Surg Br*. 1980;6:460–464.
27. Stephens M, Sammarco G: The stabilizing role of the lateral ligament complex around the ankle and subtalar joints. *Foot Ankle*. 1992;13:130.
28. Solheim LF, Denstad TF. Chronic lateral instability of the ankle. *Acta Orthop Scand*. 1980;51:193–196.
29. Laurin CA, Quellet R, St-Jaques R. Talar and subtalar tilt: an experimental investigation. *Can J Surg*. 1968;11:270–279.
30. Brantigan JW, Pedeganna LR, Lippert FG. Instability of the subtalar joint. *J Bone Joint Surg Am*. 1977;59:321–324.
31. Frey C. Subtalar instability. AOFAS Advanced Techniques in Foot and Ankle Surgery Course, San Francisco, May 2002.
32. Milner CE, Soames RW. The medial collateral ligaments of the human ankle joint: anatomical variations. *Foot Ankle Int*. 1998;19:289–292.
33. Boss AP, Hintermann B. Anatomical study of the medial ankle ligament complex. *Foot Ankle Int*. 2002;23:547–553.
34. Hintermann B, Sommer C, Nigg BM. The influence of ligament transection on tibial and calcaneal rotation with loading and dorsi-plantarflexion. *Foot Ankle Int*. 1995;16:567–571.
35. Rasmussen O. Stability of the ankle joint. *Acta Orthop Scand*. 1985;211(suppl):56–78.
36. Rasmussen O, Kroman-Andersen C, Boe S. Deltoid ligament: functional analysis of the medial collateral ligamentous apparatus of the ankle joint. *Acta Orthop Scand*. 1983;54:36–44.
37. Clarke D, Kitaoka HB, Ehman RL. Peroneal tendon injuries. *Foot Ankle Int*. 1988;19:280–288.
38. Munn J, Beard DJ, Refshauge KM, et al. Eccentric muscle strength in functional ankle instability. *Med Sci Sports Med*. 2003;35:245–250.
39. Konradsen L, Olesen S, Hansen HM. Ankle sensorimotor control and eversion strength after acute ankle inversion injuries. *Am J Sports Med*. 1998;26:1–6.
40. Amendola A, Frost SCL. Is stress radiography necessary in the diagnosis of acute or chronic ankle instability? *J Sports Med*. 1999;9:40–45.
41. Freeman MA, Dean MR, Hanham IW. The etiology and prevention of functional instability of the foot. *J Bone Joint Surg Br*. 1965;47:678–685.
42. Bunch RP, Bednarski R, Holland D, et al. Ankle joint support: a comparison of reusable lace-on braces with taping and wrapping. *Physician Sportsmed*. 1985;13:59–62.
43. Fumich RM, Ellison AE, Guerin GJ. The measured effect of taping on combined foot and ankle motion before and after exercise. *Am J Sports Med*. 1981;9:165–170.

44. Gross MT. Effects of recurrent lateral ankle sprains on active and passive judgement of joint position. *Phys Ther.* 1987;10:67–69.

45. Bahr R, Pena F, Shine J, et al. Biomechanics of ankle ligament reconstruction: an in vitro comparison of the Brostrom repair, Watson-Jones reconstruction, and a new anatomic reconstruction technique. *Am J Sports Med.* 1997;25:424–432.

46. Colville MR, Marder RA, Zarins B. Reconstruction of the lateral ankle ligaments: a biomechanical analysis. *Am J Sports Med.* 1992;20:594–600.

47. Liu SH, Baker CL. Comparison of lateral ankle ligamentous reconstruction procedures. *Am J Sports Med.* 1994;22:313–317.

48. Hollis JM, Blasier RD, Flahiff CM, et al. Biomechanical comparison of reconstruction techniques in simulated lateral ankle ligament injury. *Am J Sports Med.* 1995;23:678–682.

49. Rosenbaum D, Becker HP, Wilke HJ, et al. Tenodeses destroy the kinematic coupling of the ankle joint complex. A three-dimensional in vitro analysis of joint movement. *J Bone Joint Surg Br.* 1998;80: 162–168.

50. Rosenbaum D, Becker HP, Sterk J, et al. Functional evaluation of the 10-year outcome after modified Evans repair for chronic ankle instability. *Foot Ankle Int.* 1997;18:765–771.

51. Rosenbaum D, Engelhardt M, Becker JP, et al. Clinical and functional outcome after anatomic and nonanatomic ankle ligament reconstruction: Evans tenodesis versus periosteal flap. *Foot Ankle Int.* 1999;20:636–639.

52. Krips R, van Dijk CN, Halasi PT, et al. Long-term outcome of anatomical reconstruction versus tenodesi for the treatment of chronic anterolateral instability of the ankle joint: a multicenter study. *Foot Ankle Int.* 2001;22:415–421.

53. Schmidt R, Cordier E, Bertsch C, et al. Reconstruction of the lateral ligaments: do the anatomical procedures restore physiologic ankle kinematics? *Foot Ankle Int.* 2004;25:31–36.

54. Coughlin MJ, Schenck RC Jr, Grebing BR, et al. Comprehensive reconstruction of the lateral ankle for chronic instability using a free gracilis graft. *Foot Ankle Int.* 2004;25:231–241.

55. Brostrom L. Sprained ankles: VI. Surgical treatment of "chronic" ligament ruptures. *Acta Chir Scand.* 1966;132:551–565.

56. Gould N, Seligson D, Gassman J. Early and late repair of lateral ligaments of the ankle. *Foot Ankle.* 1980;1:84–89.

57. Girard P, Anderson RB, Davis WH, et al. Clinical evaluation of the modified Brostrom-Evans procedure to restore ankle stability. *Foot Ankle Int.* 1999;20:246–252.

58. Karlsson J, Bergsten T, Lansinger O, et al. Surgical treatment of chronic lateral instability of the ankle: a new procedure. *Am J Sports Med.* 1989;17:268–274.

59. Messer TM, Cummins CA, Ahn J, et al. Outcome of the modified Brostrom procedure of chronic lateral ankle instability using suture anchors. *Foot Ankle Int.* 2000;21:996–1003.

60. Karlsson J, Bergsten T, Lansinger O, et al. Reconstruction of the lateral ligaments of the ankle for chronic lateral instability. *J Bone Joint Surg Am.* 1988;70:581–588.

61. Sjolin SU, Dons-Jensen H, Siimonsen O. Reinforced anatomical reconstruction of the anterior talofibular ligament in chronic anterolateral instability using a periosteal flap. *Foot Ankle.* 1991;12:15–18.

62. Hamilton WG, Thompson FM, Snow SW. The modified Brostrom procedure for lateral ankle instability. *Foot Ankle Int.* 1993;14:1–7.

63. Hennrikus WL, Mapes RC, Lyons PM, et al. Outcomes of the Chrisman-Snook and modified Brostrom procedures for chronic lateral ankle instability: a prospective, randomized comparison. *Am J Sports Med.* 1996;24:400–404.

64. Karlsson J, Eriksson BI, Bergsten T, et al. Comparison of two anatomic reconstructions for chronic lateral instability of the ankle joint. *Am J Sports Med.* 1997;25:48–53.

65. Chen CY, Huang PJ, Kao KF, et al. Surgical reconstruction for chronic lateral instability of the ankle. *Injury.* 2004;35: 809–813.

66. Kitaoka H, Alexander I, Adelaar R, et al. Clinical rating system for the ankle-hindfoot, midfoot, hallux, and lesser toes. *Foot Ankle Int.* 1994;5:349–353.

67. Sammarco GJ, Idusuyi OB. Reconstruction of the lateral ankle ligaments using a split peroneus brevis tendon graft. *Foot Ankle Int.* 1999;20:97–103.

68. Baltopoulos P, Tzagarakis GP, Kaseta MA. Midterm results of a modified Evans repair for chronic lateral ankle instability. *Clin Orthop.* 2004;422:180–185.

69. Colville MR, Grundel RJ. Anatomic reconstruction of the lateral ankle ligaments using a split peroneus brevis tendon graft. *Am J Sports Med.* 1995;23:210–213.

70. Paterson R, Cohen B, Taylor D, et al.. Reconstruction of the lateral ligaments of the ankle using semi-tendinosis graft. *Foot Ankle Int.* 2000;21:413–419.

71. Sugimoto K, Takakura Y, Kumai T, et al. Reconstruction of the lateral ankle ligaments with bone-patellar tendon graft in patients with chronic ankle instability: a preliminary report. *Am J Sports Med.* 2002;30:340–346.

72. Okuda R, Kinoshita M, Morikawa J, et al. Reconstruction for chronic lateral ankle instability using the palmaris longus tendon: is reconstruction of the calcaneofibular ligament necessary? *Foot Ankle Int.* 1999;20:714–720.

73. Bohnsack M, Surie B, Kirsch IL, et al. Biomechanical properties of commonly used autogenous transplants in the surgical treatment of chronic lateral ankle instability. *Foot Ankle Int.* 2002;23:661–664.

74. Clanton T, Penman M. Interference screw fixation of tendon transfers in the foot and ankle. *Foot Ankle Int.* 2002;23:355–356.

75. Berlet GC, Saar WE, Ryan A, et al. Thermal-assisted capsular modification for functional ankle instability. *Foot Ankle Clin.* 2002;7:567–576.

76. Komenda GA, Ferkel RD. Arthroscopic findings associated with the unstable ankle. *Foot Ankle Int.* 1999;20:708–713.

77. Karlsson J, Eriksson BI, Renstrom PA. Subtalar ankle instability. A review. *Sports Med.* 1997;24:337–346.

78. Clanton TO, Berson L. Subtalar joint athletic injuries. *Foot Ankle Clin.* 1999;4:729–743.

79. Chrisman OD, Snook GA. Reconstruction of lateral ligament tears of the ankle: an experimental study and clinical evaluation of seven patients treated by a new modification of the Elmslie procedure. *J Bone Joint Surg Am.* 1969;51:904–912.

80. Schon LC, Clanton TO, Baxter DE. Reconstruction for subtalar instability: a review. *Foot Ankle.* 1991;11:319–325.

81. Kato T. The diagnosis and treatment of instability of the subtalar joint. *J Bone Joint Surg Br.* 1995;77:401–406.

82. Pisani G. Chronic laxity of the subtalar joint. *Orthopedics.* 1996;19:431–437.

83. Hintermann B. Medial ankle instability. *Foot Ankle Clin.* 2003;8:723–738.

84. Hansen ST Jr. *Functional Reconstruction of the Foot and Ankle.* Philadelphia: Lippincott Williams & Wilkins; 2000.

85. Wiltberger BR, Mallory TM. A new method for reconstruction of the deltoid ligament of the ankle. *Orthop Rev.* 1972;1: 37–41.

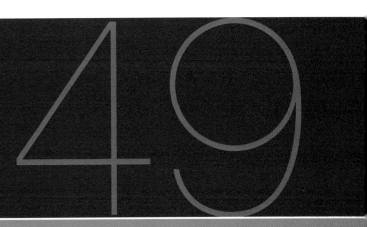

TREATMENT OF OSTEOCHONDRAL LESIONS OF THE TALAR DOME

■ JAMES W. STONE, MD

■ KEY POINTS

- Although osteochondral lesions can occur over any portion of the talar dome or the tibia, the talar lesions typically occur over the anterolateral or the posteromedial talar dome.
- Medial lesions tend to be deeper and cup shaped. Patients tend to present with more chronic symptoms of ankle pain, rather than acute injury. They are found to have an osteochondral lesion on plain radiograph or magnetic resonance imaging (MRI) of the ankle.
- Lateral lesions tend to be thinner and more wafer shaped. Patients frequently present with an acute injury and positive radiographic findings.
- In the absence of a discrete lesion on plain radiograph, MRI examination is the most appropriate follow-up examination for patients with persistent symptoms despite a period of nonoperative management.
- Treatment decisions are based upon the site and size of the lesion, the skeletal maturity of the patient, the quality of the articular cartilage, and the quality of the associated bone fragment.
- Surgical approaches include simple excision; excision with curettage; and excision, curettage, and drilling.
- Drilling of an intact lesion may be appropriate if arthroscopic evaluation reveals perfect articular cartilage congruity in the absence of a mobile subchondral bone fragment, particularly in the skeletally mature patient.
- Internal fixation is usually only appropriate for acute anterolateral lesions with a bone base which is sufficient to support internal fixation with pins or screws.
- Most of the lesions requiring surgical treatment are posteromedial in location, have poor quality articular cartilage, a loose bone fragment, necrotic bone beneath the lesion, and are poor candidates for healing with internal fixation. Excision of the loose fragment with treatment of the base by curettage, abrasion, or microfracture has been the most commonly recommended treatment for these lesions.
- Newer techniques such as osteochondral autograft, osteochondral allograft, and autologous chondrocyte transplantation are promising; however, long term results are unknown.

The term osteochondritis dissecans was originally applied to lesions of the talar dome of the ankle by Kappis (1) in 1922 referring to abnormalities of the articular cartilage and underlying subchondral bone which can result in fragment separation and loose body formation. Although the term might imply an inflammatory etiology for this lesion, no such association has been noted on pathologic examination of specimens. Indeed, most studies have suggested a traumatic etiology for the majority of these lesions (2–5). More generic terms such as flake fracture, transchondral fracture, or talar dome fracture have been used in the modern literature on the subject to reflect the fact that the etiology is uncertain in many cases. The most generic term, osteochondral lesion of the talar dome, will be used in this chapter.

■ ANATOMY

Although osteochondral lesions can occur over any portion of the talar dome or the tibia, the talar lesions typically occur over the anterolateral or the posteromedial talar dome. The medial lesions tend to be deeper and cup shaped whereas the lateral lesions tend to be thinner and more wafer shaped (2). The vast majority of lateral lesions are associated with a distinct traumatic episode and patients frequently present with an acute injury and positive radiographic findings. The patients with medial lesions tend to present with more chronic symptoms of ankle pain rather than an acute injury, and are found to have an osteochondral lesion on plain radiograph or magnetic resonance imaging (MRI) of the ankle. The more chronic nature of the medial lesions along with the absence of a definite traumatic association with many medial talar dome lesions supports the possibility that they are either due to low level repetitive trauma or perhaps to another cause such as avascular necrosis, steroid use, embolic event, endocrine abnormality, or hereditary factors (6). In addition, although the lateral lesions are usually unilateral, the medial lesions are found to be bilateral in up to 10% of patients (2).

ETIOLOGY

Most studies have suggested that the lesions are traumatic in nature. They can occur after a single specific injury, or be the result of repetitive microtrauma. The repetitive trauma events may be in the form of recurrent ankle sprains, where joint deformation causes direct impact of the talar dome on the adjacent tibia or talus. This is the theory supported by the early study of Berndt and Harty (3) where a small number of talar dome lesions were created in cadaver ankles by applying inversion or eversion forces combined with ankle dorsi or plantar flexion. The lateral talar dome lesion could be produced with a combination of ankle dorsiflexion and inversion. The medial lesion could be produced when the plantarflexed foot was subjected to an inversion force. Although their numbers were very small (only a total of three lesions were created in a total of 15 ankles), their study suggested that the lateral lesion resulted when the anterolateral talar dome impacted the articular surface of the fibula with the ankle in a dorsiflexed position. In contrast, when the externally rotated ankle was in a plantar flexed position, inversion of the joint resulted in physical contact of the posteromedial talar dome with the tibial articular surface. Stauffer (7) refined the biomechanical explanation of causation of these lesions, suggesting that relatively small tangential or shear forces resulted in bony fracture with the articular cartilage remaining intact, whereas failure of both bone and articular cartilage occurs with application of larger forces.

HISTORY

A patient with an osteochondral lesion of the talar dome will most commonly present with a chief complaint of ankle pain, sometimes poorly localized and nonspecific. The location of the patient's pain may not predict the location of the

lesion as patients with medial lesions not uncommonly complain of lateral joint pain. Although one might expect a loose lesion to cause mechanical symptoms, complaints of locking, catching, or swelling are less common, except when a lateral lesion has caused an acute loose body to be formed. Pain with weight bearing and a sensation of giving way are more common but nonspecific complaints. The patient will usually report a distinct episode of trauma when a lateral lesion is present, but with medial lesions there may be no specific injury or the common historical association of one or more ankle sprains in the past.

PHYSICAL FINDINGS

Swelling is commonly found in acute injuries, although it may be absent in chronic cases especially with medial lesions. Tenderness localized to the joint line may be noted in the plantar flexed ankle laterally in the case of an anterolateral talar dome lesion and posteromedially in the dorsiflexed ankle in the case of a posteromedial lesion. Either lesion may be associated with clinical evidence of joint laxity, so the examiner should compare the effected joint to the normal joint and check for evidence of anterior or lateral laxity. Because the history and physical examination findings are often nonspecific and the differential diagnosis includes multiple other entities such as tendonitis, instability, impingement lesions, neurological causes such as neuroma or tarsal tunnel syndrome, subtalar symptoms including os trigonum, a careful physical examination must be performed to assess these possibilities.

IMAGING

Plain radiographs are indicated in the evaluation of any patient with acute or chronic ankle pain. Routine views include anteroposterior (AP), lateral, and mortise views. In addition, the mortise view may be obtained in plantar flexion to better assess a posteromedial lesion or in dorsiflexion to assess an anterolateral lesion. The staging system proposed by Berndt and Harty (3) as applied by them combined both radiographic and surgical findings, but in the modern literature has been applied only to plain radiographic findings (Table 49-1).

In the absence of a discrete lesion on plain radiograph, MRI examination is the most appropriate follow-up examination for patients with persistent symptoms despite a period of nonoperative management. MRI is sensitive in detecting osteochondral lesions of the talar dome and may also aid in the evaluation of other soft tissue and bony entities on the differential diagnosis. If an osteochondral lesion is noted on plain radiographs, the MRI may be useful in evaluating the lesion itself for articular cartilage congruity, whether there is fluid signal beneath the bony fragment to suggest a loose lesion and to evaluate the degree of edema in the surrounding talus. Because the MRI is very sensitive in

TABLE 49-1	Berndt and Harty Classification: Osteochondral Lesions of the Talar Dome
Stage I	Small compression fracture
Stage II	Incomplete avulsion of fragment
Stage III	Complete avulsion of fragment without displacement
Stage IV	Avulsed fragment displaced within joint

From Berndt AL, Harty M. Transchondral fractures (Osteochondritis Dissecans) of the talus. *J Bone Joint Surg.* 1959;41A:988–1020; with permission.

TABLE 49-2	Anderson et al. MRI Classification: Osteochodral Lesions of the Talar Dome
Stage I	Subchondral trabecular compression
Stage II	Incomplete separation of fragment
Stage IIA	Formation of subchondral cyst
Stage III	Unattached, undisplaced fragment
Stage IV	Displaced fragment

From Anderson IF, Crichton KJ, Gratan-Smith T, et al. Osteochondral fractures of the dome of the talus. *J Bone Joint Surg.* 1989;71A:1143–1152; with permission.

detecting bone edema, it may actually overestimate the size of the lesion. Several classification schemes for MRI evaluation have been suggested (8). They tend to mimic the plain radiographic evaluation suggested by Berndt and Harty (3), but add the evaluation of the cystic component which is present in may of the osteochondral lesions **(Table 49-2)**. The MRI also has the advantage over both plain radiographs and

computed tomography (CT) scanning in its ability to detect the true Stage I lesion where the only finding may be edema in the body of the talus without a discrete bony lesion.

CT is the most precise means of evaluating the bone lesion itself. CT staging again mimics the plain radiographic and MRI evaluations and also incorporates evaluation of the cystic component (9) **(Fig 49-1)**. Primary axial and coronal

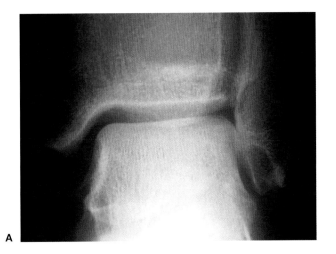
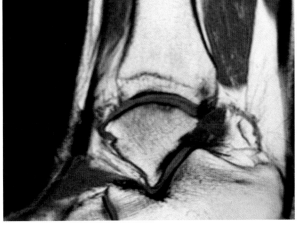
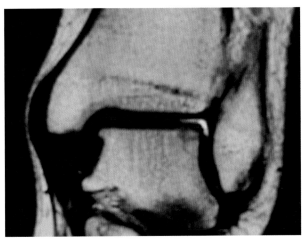
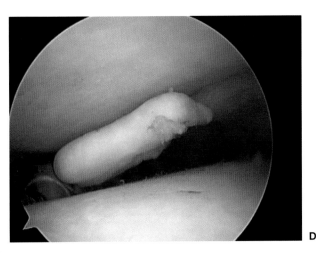

Fig 49-1. A: Anteroposterior radiograph of a patient with ankle pain. The lateral talar dome osteochondral lesion is difficult to evaluate. **B:** Lateral MRI examination more clearly delineates the lesion. **C:** Coronal MRI suggests that the bone fragment is nondisplaced. **D:** Intraoperative arthroscopic photograph shows a loose chondral body not predicted by the MRI scan.

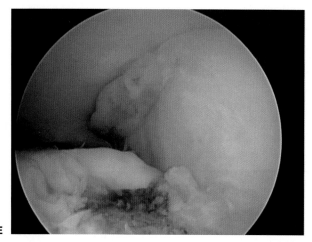

E

Fig 49-1. E: Intraoperative photograph showing the anterolateral talar dome lesion after debridement and abrasion of the base.

thin section CT scanning combined with sagittal reconstructions give the best bony detail.

■ CLINICAL DECISION MAKING

There is no universally accepted treatment algorithm for osteochondral lesions of the talar dome. This lack of consensus stems from several factors, including the absence of controlled, randomized studies comparing various treatment alternatives, lack of studies documenting the natural history of untreated lesions of various stages, the addition over time of new diagnostic modalities such as CT and MRI which have expanded our ability to define the lesions preoperatively, and the addition of arthroscopy to the surgeon's armamentarium. Treatment decisions are based upon the site of the lesion, the size of the lesion, the skeletal maturity of the patient, the quality of the articular cartilage, and the quality of the associated bone fragment.

The study of Tol et al. (10) highlights the difficulties in utilizing existing published studies to guide treatment of this disorder. The authors reviewed 32 articles published over a period of 32 years and found no randomized studies. Their analysis revealed nonoperative management to yield a success rate of 45%. Surgical approaches included simple excision (success rate 38%), excision with curettage (78% success rate), and excision, curettage, and drilling (success rate 85%).

Canale and Belding (11) supported the suggestions of Berndt and Harty (3) that nonoperative treatment is appropriate for Stage I and II lesions, in addition to Stage III medial lesions. Surgical intervention was advocated for Stage IV lesions and those other lesions which failed to respond to nonoperative management. Flick and Gould (5) advocated a more aggressive surgical approach, even including some Stage II lesions. More recently Ferkel et al. (2) have suggested nonoperative management for CT Stage I and II lesions **(Table 49-3)**, with surgical intervention for symptomatic CT Stage III and IV lesions. Multiple studies have documented poor correlation between preoperative plain radiographic studies and the results of actual arthroscopic evaluation of the articular cartilage and subchondral bone (12). In the absence of definitive studies suggesting otherwise, nonoperative management is suggested for all asymptomatic lesions, regardless of stage. Nonoperative management may include a period of nonweight-bearing with or without immobilization for 6 to 12 weeks. Arthroscopic evaluation is the appropriate initial surgical approach for symptomatic lesions which have failed to respond to nonoperative management or for symptomatic CT or MRI Stage III or IV lesions.

■ SURGICAL MANAGEMENT

Surgical options can be categorized into several groups:
I. Maintain the native articular cartilage
 a. Drilling intact lesion
 b. Open reduction/internal fixation acute fracture
II. Removal of lesion, with treatment of base (goal: fibrocartilage replacement of articular cartilage surface)
 a. Simple excision
 b. Excision with curettage or abrasion of base

TABLE 49-3	Ferkel and Sgaglione CT Classification: Osteochondral Lesions of the Talar Dome
Stage I	Cystic lesion within dome of talus, intact roof on all views
Stage IIA	Cystic lesion with communication to talar dome surface
Stage IIB	Open articular surface lesion with overlying nondisplaced fragment
Stage III	Undisplaced lesion with lucency
Stage IV	Displaced fragment

From Ferkel RD, Sgaglione NA. Arthroscopic treatment of osteochondral lesions of the talus: long term results. *Orthop Trans.* 1993–1994;17:1011; with permission.

c. Excision with drilling of base

d. Excision with microfracture of base

III. Replacement of articular cartilage with articular cartilage

a. Osteochondral autograft

b. Osteochondral allograft

c. Autologous chondrocyte transplantation

d. Other biologic matrix/chondrocyte applications

Drilling of an intact lesion may be appropriate if arthroscopic evaluation reveals perfect articular cartilage congruity in the absence of a mobile subchondral bone fragment, particularly in the skeletally mature patient (13–15). Drilling of an anterolateral lesion can be performed using a smooth Kirschner wire through the anterolateral portal. Most posteromedial lesions are difficult to approach from anterior, even with the ankle in maximum plantarflexion. They require either drilling via a transmalleolar approach or a transtalar approach where the lesion is approached from below with the wire introduced into the talus in the sinus tarsi (15). Either approach can be facilitated by using a commercially available drill guide for accuracy.

Internal fixation is usually only appropriate for acute anterolateral lesions with a bone base which is sufficient to support internal fixation with pins or screws. The fixation may be performed with metal fixation devices or with bioabsorbable pins or screws. Internal fixation of a displaced acute anterolateral lesion, especially one which has flipped such that the articular surface points toward the bony bed, requires a high level of arthroscopic expertise. It may be performed more easily, and with less damage to the articular cartilage, via a small anterolateral incision. Debridement of a lateral osteochondral lesion with treatment of the base is the appropriate treatment for more chronic lesions (Fig 49-2).

Most of the lesions requiring surgical treatment are posteromedial in location, have poor quality articular cartilage, a loose bone fragment, necrotic bone beneath the lesion, and are poor candidates for healing with internal fixation. Excision of the loose fragment with treatment of the base with curettage, abrasion, or microfracture has been the most commonly recommended treatment for these lesions. The goal of this procedure is to remove the loose body and to optimize conditions such that the lesion will fill in with fibrocartilage over a

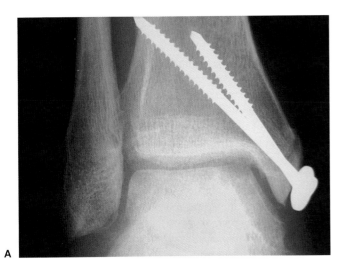

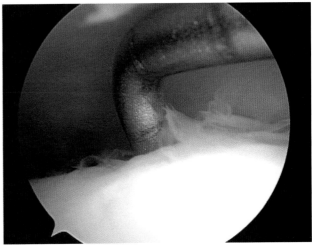

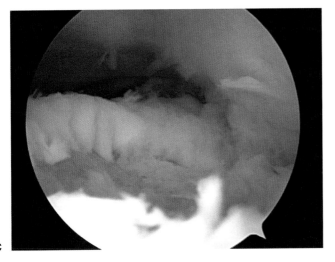

Fig 49-2 **A:** Anteroposterior radiograph in a patient referred after open debridement of an osteochondral lesion of the medial talar dome using a medial malleolar osteotomy failed to relieve symptoms. The osteotomy was performed poorly, too distal on the malleolus, probably limiting access to the lesion. **B:** Intraoperative arthroscopic photograph with probe on the loose medial talar dome lesion. **C:** Intraoperative arthroscopic photograph showing the lesion after debridement of the loose bone fragment and abrasion of the base.

stable bone base (Fig 49-2). For open surgery posteromedial lesions may be difficult to approach anteromedially even with ankle plantarflexion, and a medial malleolar osteotomy may be required. Arthroscopic approaches to these lesions have largely replaced open techniques because they can be performed with equal effectiveness and with less morbidity.

■ ARTHROSCOPIC TECHNIQUE

The patient is positioned supine on the operating table with the ipsilateral hip and knee flexed and supported by a padded leg holder **(Fig 49-3)**. This position allows the foot and ankle to hang free in a plantigrade position for sterile

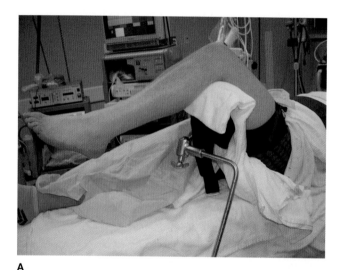

A

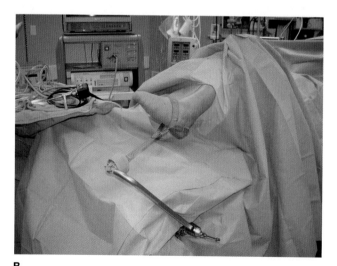

B

Fig 49-3 **A:** Intraoperative photograph shows the operative leg positioned with the hip and knee flexed and supported by a well padded leg holder. The foot hangs in a plantigrade position and is completely free for skin preparation and draping. **B:** This photograph shows the noninvasive ankle distraction applied to the operative ankle. This mechanism for distraction allows access to both anterior and posterior portals and allows ankle joint motion intraoperatively.

prep and drape. After draping, a commercially available noninvasive ankle joint distraction device is applied. This device provides efficient joint distraction while allowing intraoperative joint motion and access to both anterior and posterior portals.

Anatomic landmarks are outlined with a sterile marker and the locations for the anteromedial, anterolateral, and posterolateral portals are identified. Each portal is created by first incising the skin, then gently spreading the subcutaneous tissues with a mosquito hemostat to protect superficial nerves, and then the portal is completed with a blunt trochar to pierce the capsule. A 2.7 mm arthroscope with 30 degree viewing angle is used, with a 70 degree viewing arthroscope also available. Small joint instruments including probe, curettes, loose body forceps, shavers, and abraders are utilized.

The lesion is usually easily identifiable as a disruption in the smooth articular cartilage of the remainder of the talar dome. A probe is used to outline the lesion and to begin to elevate the abnormal articular cartilage and subchondral bone. After the lesion is elevated with probe, freer elevator, and/or curette, a loose body forceps is used to remove the major fragments. Smaller fragments and necrotic bone at the base of the lesion are completely removed using angled curettes until stable subchondral bone is identified. The edges of the lesion peripheral margin must be trimmed back with curettes until stable articular cartilage is present over the entire margin. It is most important to be certain that the entire lesion is removed, including that portion which is located on the vertical surface of the talus in the medial gutter. Failure to remove this unstable bone may result in a poor surgical result.

The base of the lesion should be treated so that bleeding subchondral bone can be demonstrated as the inflow pressure is reduced. There has been some controversy regarding the relative utility of abrasion, drilling, and microfracture techniques. There has been no definitive study comparing these techniques; therefore, abrasion alone is probably sufficient if bleeding bone is identified over the entire surface. This can be supplemented with drilling or microfracture technique if required to achieve a bleeding base.

A review of multiple studies suggests that traditional treatment with loose body excision and treatment of the base with abrasion, drilling, or microfracture yields good or excellent results in the near to medium term in the range of 70% to 100%, with most studies suggesting a range of 80% to 90% (16–20).

■ SURGICAL TECHNIQUES TO RESURFACE WITH ARTICULAR CARTILAGE

The fact that procedures which involve fragment removal alone can at best result in coverage with fibrocartilage, and the suggestion that results which appear satisfactory in the near to medium term probably deteriorate over time, have articular cartilage defects with viable articular cartilage. The technique of osteoarticular autograft popularized by Hangody et al. (21) for knee joint articular cartilage defects has been adapted for the ankle. The defect may be replaced by a single graft or multiple grafts in a mosaic pattern. The procedure requires obtaining the graft from the knee joint and transfer of the osteoarticular core to the ankle. Posteromedial lesions are difficult to approach anteriorly even with forced plantar flexion, although some may be approached in this way especially if grooving of the anterior tibia is utilized; however, most of these lesions require medial malleolar osteotomy to be performed. Several considerations regarding this procedure have not been addressed in long term studies including: a) potential donor site morbidity in the knee; b) morbidity of the medial malleolar osteotomy; c) results of mosaic versus single graft; d) how to approach the portion of the lesion on the vertical surface of the talus—ignore it and resurface only the weightbearing surface? Find a curved donor surface which matches the curvature of the talus? Use a mosaic technique including the vertical surface? How to deal with an associated talar cyst? Does knee articular cartilage of different thickness than normal ankle articular cartilage function similar to normal ankle cartilage?

Early studies with short term follow up have suggested a high percentage of good and excellent results in both primary patients and in patients who have failed previous surgery (21–27). It should be noted, however, that there are no comparative randomized studies available to compare the short and long term results of this technique to more traditional techniques.

Another means of replacing articular cartilage with articular cartilage is to utilize allograft (28). This technique has been used especially in the case of large defects, greater than 1.5 to 2.0 cm diameter and when a large cystic defect is present. Large area resurfacing of up to one half of the talar dome has been performed, but in small numbers. Fresh osteoarticular allograft material has a higher proportion of live chondrocytes compared to frozen grafts, but most surgeons do not have access to these grafts in their communities. The procedure remains investigational.

Autologous chondrocyte transplantation is another technique which attempts to replace the missing articular cartilage with articular cartilage (29–32). The procedure involves performing an initial procedure where articular cartilage is harvested from the knee, and then the chondrocytes are replicated in vitro using a proprietary technique resulting in 10 to 12 million viable cells. A second surgical procedure is performed where the lesion is generally approached using a medial malleolar osteotomy and the lesion is debrided, removing all abnormal cartilage and subchondral bone. A piece of periosteum harvested from the tibia is sized to the lesion and sutured at the margins using 6 to 0 absorbable suture. The chondrocyte solution is injected beneath the periosteum and then sealed with fibrin glue. The medial malleolar osteotomy is fixed internally with screws and the patient remains nonweight-bearing

for 8 to 12 weeks postoperatively. Similar to early reports with osteochondral autografts, short term follow up studies suggest good near term results. There are no comparative randomized studies comparing this technique with more traditional approaches, and it remains investigational.

One randomized study is available in the knee joint where autologous chondrocyte implantation was compared to simple microfracture for isolated femoral condyle defects (33). The study found no significant difference in macroscopic or pathologic results in the two groups. Clinical improvement was actually better in the microfracture group at two years postoperative.

Complications

Complications of arthroscopic surgery for osteochondral lesions of the talar dome related to the procedure itself include iatrogenic articular cartilage damage resulting from the arthroscope or instrumentation, neuroma at the level of the portal site, draining sinus formation, broken instruments, and superficial or deep infection (34–36). Deep vein thrombosis is a rare a complication of arthroscopic ankle surgery. Articular cartilage damage can be minimized by using small joint 2.7 mm arthroscopes, small joint instruments, and small joint motorized equipment. In addition, noninvasive joint distraction allows easier passage of instruments while avoiding the potential complications of invasive distraction which include pin tract infection, fracture through the pin sites, ligament injury, and neurovascular injury secondary to pin placement. Neuroma formation is avoided by careful attention to portal creation including incision through the skin only, subcutaneous tissue blunt spreading, and dull trochar use. Portals should be of sufficient size to allow easy passage of instruments rather than small portals with difficult instrument passage causing soft tissue damage. Instruments should be checked regularly for wear and replaced if necessary to avoid broken instruments. Draining sinus may be minimized by wound suturing and a limited period of postoperative immobilization. Prophylactic antibiotics may decrease the incidence of infection.

Persistent symptoms after technically adequate surgical treatment is a type of complication which should stimulate the operating surgeon to carefully review the history, physical examination, and diagnostic tests to be certain that the patient's pain was actually caused by the osteochondral abnormality and not by another less obvious cause on the differential diagnosis. In addition, chronic pain syndromes including reflex sympathetic dystrophy should be considered, diagnosed, and treated appropriately.

■ CONCLUSIONS

Asymptomatic osteochondral lesions of the talar dome can be treated nonoperatively and followed clinically and radiographically. Symptomatic Stage I and II lesions should undergo an initial period of nonoperative treatment with surgical intervention reserved for failures of conservative management. In general, symptomatic Stage III and IV lesions are approached surgically. Displaced lateral lesions with sufficient bone may be treated with internal fixation either open or arthroscopically. Medial lesions with intact articular cartilage, particularly in skeletally immature patients, may be treated with in situ drilling. Loose medial lesions are generally debrided and the base treated with abrasion, drilling, or microfracture.

The long term results of newer techniques such as osteochondral autograft, osteochondral allograft, and autologous chondrocyte transplantation are not known and randomized studies comparing these techniques to traditional techniques are needed.

Studies in Europe utilizing membrane bound chondrocytes which are transplanted as a layer are in early trials with promising results. None of these materials is currently clinically approved for use in the United States.

■ REFERENCES

1. Kappis M. Weitere Beitrage zur traumtisch—mechanischen Entstehung der "spontanen" Knorpelablosungen [More thoughts on traumatic and mechanical development of spontaneous osteochondritis dissecans]. *Dtsch Z Chir.* 1922;171:13–29.
2. Barnes CJ, Ferkel RD. Arthroscopic debridement and drilling of osteochondral lesions of the talus. *Foot Ankle Clin N Am.* 2003;8:243–257.
3. Berndt AL, Harty M. Transchondral fractures (Osteochondritis Dissecans) of the talus. *J Bone Joint Surg.* 1959;41A:988–1020.
4. Stone JW. Osteochondral lesions of the talar dome. *J Am Acad Orthop Surg.* 1996;4:63–73.
5. Flick AB, Gould N. Osteochondritis dissecans of the talus (transchondral fractures of the talus): review of the literature and new surgical approach for medial dome lesions. *Foot Ankle.* 1985;5:165–185.
6. Navid DO, Myerson MS. Approach alternatives for treatment of osteochondral lesions of the talus. *Foot Ankle Clin N Am.* 2002;7:635–639.
7. Stauffer RN. Intraarticular ankle problems. 115–142.
8. Anderson IF, Crichton KJ, Gratan-Smith T, et al. Osteochondral fractures of the dome of the talus. *J Bone Joint Surg.* 1989;71A:1143–1152.
9. Ferkel RD, Sgaglione NA. Arthroscopic treatment of osteochondral lesions of the talus: long term results. *Orthop Trans.* 1993–1994;17:1011.
10. Tol JL, Struijs PA, Bossuyt PM, et al. Treatment strategies in osteochondral defects of the talar dome: a systematic review. *Foot Ankle Int.* 2000;8:233–242.
11. Canale ST, Belding RH. Osteochondral lesions of the talus. *J Bone Joint Surg.* 1980;62A:97.
12. Pritsch M, Horoshovski H, Fariine I. Arthroscopic treatment of osteochondral lesions of the talus. *J Bone Joint Surg.* 1986;68A:862.
13. Kumai T, Yoshinori T, Higashiyama I, et al. Arthroscopic drilling for the treatment of osteochondral lesions of the talus. *J Bone Joint Surg.* 1999;81A:1229–1235.
14. Lahm A, Erggelet C, Steinwachs M, et al. Arthroscopic management of osteochondral lesions of the talus: results of drilling and

15. Taranow WS, Bisignani GA, Towers JD, et al. Retrograde drilling of osteochondral lesions of the medial talar dome. *Foot Ankle Int.* 1999;20:474–480.
16. Kelberine F, Frank A. Arthroscopic treatment of osteochondral lesions of the talar dome: a retrospective study of 48 cases. *Arthroscopy.* 1999;15:77–84.
17. Ogilvie-Harris DJ, Sarrosa EA. Arthroscopic treatment of osteochondritis dissecans of the talus. *Arthroscopy.* 1999;15:805–808.
18. Ogilvie-Harris DJ, Sarrosa EA. Arthroscopic treatment after previous failed open surgery for osteochondritis dissecans of the talus. *Arthroscopy.* 1999;15:809–812.
19. Parisien JS. Arthroscopic treatment of osteochondral lesions of the talus. *Am J Sports Med.* 1986;14:211–217.
20. Schuman L, Struijs PAA, van Dijk CN. Arthroscopic treatment for osteochondral defects of the talus: results at follow-up at 2 to 11 years. *J Bone Joint Surg.* 2002;84B:364–368.
21. Hangody L, Kish G, Modis L, et al. Mosaicplasty for the treatment of osteochondritis dissecans of the talus: two to seven year results in 36 patients. *Foot Ankle Int.* 2001;22:552–558.
22. Hangody L. The mosaicplasty technique for osteochondral lesions of the talus. *Foot Ankle Clin N Am.* 2003;8:259–273.
23. Hoser C, Bichler O, Bale R, et al. A computer assisted surgical technique for retrograde autologous osteochondral grafting in talar osteochondritis dissecans (OCD): a cadaveric study. *Knee Surg Sports Traumatol Arthrosc.* 2004;12:65–71.
24. Al-Shaikh RA, Chou LB, Mann JA, et al. Autologous osteochondral grafting for talar cartilage defects. *Foot Ankle Int.* 2002;23:381–389.
25. Assenmacher JA, Kelikian AS, Gottlob C, et al. Arthroscopically assisted autologous osteochondral transplantation for osteochondral lesions of the talar dome: an MRI and clinical follow-up study. *Foot Ankle Int.* 2001;22:544–551.
26. Scranton PE, Mcdermott JE. Treatment of type V osteochondral lesions of the talus with ipsilateral knee osteochondral autografts. *Foot Ankle Int.* 2001;22:380–384.
27. Sammarco GJ, Makwana NK. Treatment of talar osteochondral lesions using local osteochondral graft. *Foot Ankle Int.* 2002; 22:693–698.
28. Gross AE, Agnidis Z, Hutchison CR. Osteochondral defects of the talus treated with fresh osteochondral allograft transplantation. *Foot Ankle Int.* 2001;22:385–391.
29. Bazaz R, Ferkel RD. Treatment of osteochondral lesions of the talus with autologous chondrocyte implantation. *Tech Foot Ankle Surg.* 2004;3:45–52.
30. Giannini S, Buda R, Grigolo B, et al. Autologous chondrocyte transplantation in osteochondral lesions of the ankle joint. *Foot Ankle Int.* 2001;22:513–517.
31. Koulalis D, Schultz W, Heyden M. Autologous chondrocyte transplantation for osteochondritis dissecans of the talus. *Clin Orthop.* 2002;395:186–192.
32. Petersen L, Brittberg M, Lindahl A. Autologous chondrocyte transplantation of the ankle. *Foot Ankle Clin N Am.* 2003; 8:291–303.
33. Knutsen G, Engebretsen L, Ludvigsen TC, et al. Autologous chondrocyte implantation compared with microfracture in the knee. *J Bone Joint Surg.* 2004;86:455–464.
34. Barber FA, Click J, Britt BT. Complications of ankle arthroscopy. *Foot Ankle.* 1990;10:263–266.
35. Ferkel RD, Heath DD, Guhl JF. Neurological complications of ankle arthroscopy. *Arthroscopy.* 1996;12:200–208.
36. Small NC. Complications in arthroscopic surgery performed by experienced arthroscopists. Arthroscopy. 1988;4:215–221.

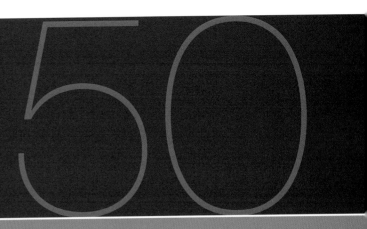

TENDON DISORDERS IN THE LOWER EXTREMITY

■ MARK A. GLAZEBROOK, MD, MSC, PhD, DIP SPORTS MED, FRCS(C)

■ KEY POINTS

- Achilles tendon disorders represent a small portion of tendon disorders in general, but are cited to be increasing in frequency in the modern world.
- The most common patient profile for Achilles tendon rupture is a male in his third or fourth decade of life that plays sports occasionally.
- Magnetic resonance imaging (MRI) is the gold standard for imaging musculoskeletal soft tissues, yielding the most detailed information about the midsubstance of the tendons and surrounding structures.
- Only short periods of immobilization are recommended in severe cases because prolonged immobilization is detrimental to tendon and muscle strength and worsens joint stiffness.
- The goal of treatment for tibial posterior tendon injuries is relief of symptoms, restoration of function, and prevention of progression of the disease. Early stages are usually treated nonoperatively. Late stages may require surgical treatment with debridement, tendon transfer, or various forms of arthrodesis.
- The primary function of the peroneal tendons is that of eversion and plantarflexion of the foot. The peroneus longus is also responsible for plantar flexion of the first metatarsal.
- Peroneal tendon instability often coexists with peroneal tendon disease and partial tears. Instability may be viewed as a continuum with frank traumatic dislocation at one end and subluxation within the peroneal groove at the other end. Traumatic dislocation is associated with sports, including skiing, soccer, football, ice skating, and gymnastics.

Tendon disorders about the foot and ankles are both a diagnostic and therapeutic challenge. Most disorders result from overuse with intrinsic and extrinsic factors contributing in a multifactorial manner. To understand and clinically manage tendon problems of the foot and ankle one must gain an understanding of the basic science of normal and diseased tendon including anatomy, biology, and biomechanics. Also, expertise and experience in clinical evaluation and treatment are essential. This chapter will begin with comprehensive discussions on the management of tendon disease in the foot and ankle.

■ BASIC SCIENCE

Tendon Anatomy

Collagen accounts for approximately 70% of the dry weight of a tendon (1) with 95% of this collagen being Type 1 (2). The tendon microstructure was described by Kastelic et al. (3). The endotenon is a mesh of loose connective tissue that encloses blood vessels, lymphatics, nerves, fibroblasts, and bundles of collagen fibers. The endotenon layer of the tendon is continuous with the muscles perimysium at the musculotendinous junction. The tendon has proprioceptive nerve endings at the musculotendinous junction and pain receptors ending in the peritendinous tissue. The mechanoreceptors include Pacini corpuscles (velocity sensors), Ruffini corpuscles (pressure sensors), and Golgi tendon organs (tension receptors).

Tendon Biology

Nondiseased Tendons

Approximately 95% of tendon's collagen is Type I, which is embedded in an extracellular matrix of proteoglycans. Elastin represents only a small portion (2). The biosynthesis of collagen begins with polypeptides that are synthesized and then hydroxylated and glycosylated. These polypeptides aggregate into a triple helix referred to as procollagen. The procollagen bundles are then secreted by the fibroblasts where they undergo extracellular modifications including hydrolysis of peptide bonds to form a collagen molecule (tropocollagen). The collagen molecule is the most fundamental unit of the hierarchical organization of the tendon as described by Kastelic et al. (3) **(Fig 50-1)**. Five of these tropocollagen units aggregate to form a microfibril. Intramolecular cross-links exist within the collagen molecules while intermolecular cross-links bind adjacent collagen molecules together. The microfibrils associate in a quartered staggered array (overlap by one-fourth) and are grouped into subfibrils, which in turn are grouped to form fibrils. The fibrillar collagens polymerize side-by-side and end-to-end into a long fibrillar aggregate or collagen fibers. The collagen fibrils are arranged longitudinally but have a wavy or crimped appearance (4,5) secondary to the helical structure of the underlying molecules.

The nondiseased tendon has well described histological features (6) including highly organized, tightly packed parallel collagen bundles (6,7) that stain pink-red (eosinophilic) with hematoxylin and eosin staining (7) **(Fig 50-2)**. The sparse nuclei are elongate and found interspersed between the collagen bundles (6,7).

Diseased Tendon

The terminology used to describe tendon disease is somewhat confusing and there is a lack of consistency in the literature (8,9). Some use the term tendonitis with the suffix

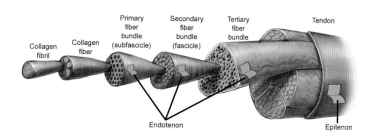

Fig 50-1. Hierarchical organization of the tendon. (Adapted from Stanish WD, Curwin S, Mandell S. *Tendinitis: Its etiology and treatment.* Oxford University Press; 2000:49–64; with permission.)

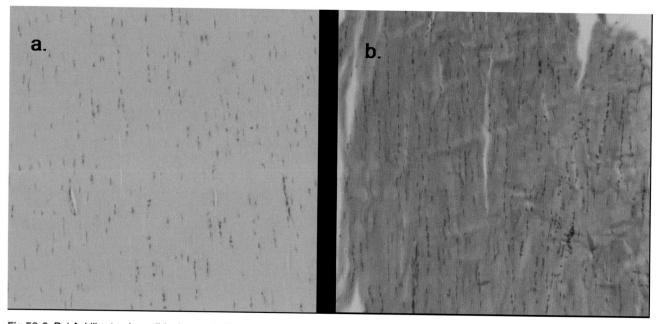

Fig 50-2. Rat Achilles tendons slide demonstrating normal **(A)** and diseased **(B)** histology features including more intense hematoxylin-eosin staining, increased cell numbers and less organized collagen.

"itis" denoting inflammation that is often the case when the paratenon is involved with or without involvement of the tendon itself. Others use the term tendinosis with "osis" denoting a degenerative process of the tendon itself that may be clinically asymptomatic with no evidence of an inflammatory infiltrate (12–16).

Descriptions of the histology of diseased tendons are derived from biopsies of human patients with subcutaneous rupture and human patients with chronic, localized tendon symptoms. These studies demonstrate many consistent features suggestive of a common pathological process that may represent a continuum with tendon rupture as the end-stage. The histopathological features include: disorganized collagen arrangement, increased number of cells, rounding of cell nuclei, variable collagen staining, and increased glycosaminoglycan content (13,17–20) **(Fig 50-3)**. These features may represent a healing response to repetitive microtrauma (21).

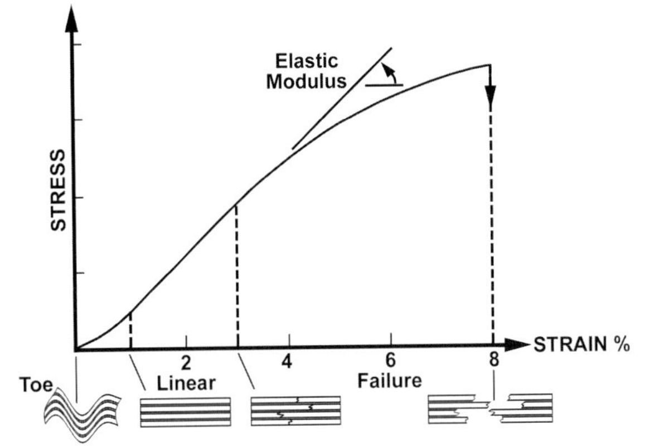

Fig 50-3. Stress and strain relationship of tendon. (Adapted from Stanish WD, Curwin S, Mandell S. *Tendinitis: Its etiology and treatment.* Oxford University Press; 2000:49–64; with permission.)

Tendon Biomechanics

The biomechanical response of the tendon to strain was reviewed by Stanish et al. (22) **(Fig 50-4)**. When the tendon is strained at low levels, the first response is a straightening of the wavy appearance of the collagen fibrils. This is represented by the "toe region" of the stress strain curve and results from the decreased elastic modulus as supplied by the elastic fiber component of the tendon (23).

As strain increases, the collagen fibers are engaged and the increased modulus of elasticity is reflected by the more linear portion of the tendon stress-strain curve. As long as the strain remains less than 4% the process is reversible due to the elastic recoil of the elastic component of the tendon. At strain levels of 4% to 8% the collagen fibrils slide past one another and the cross links begin to break (24). This results in microtrauma (molecular damage) to the tendon. The stress strain curve becomes linear as the tendon stiffens, and as collagen cross links begin to fail, the curve becomes convex and the tendon begins to rupture. At strains greater than 8% it is common for the tendon to fail or rupture completely. This represents the highest point on the stress-strain curve (ultimate tensile failure). The mechanical failure in the underlying collagen is not due to breakage of collagen molecules, but pulling apart of adjacent molecules, and it is generally believed that when the tendon fails it is most often a consequence of increased forces placed across abnormal tendon.

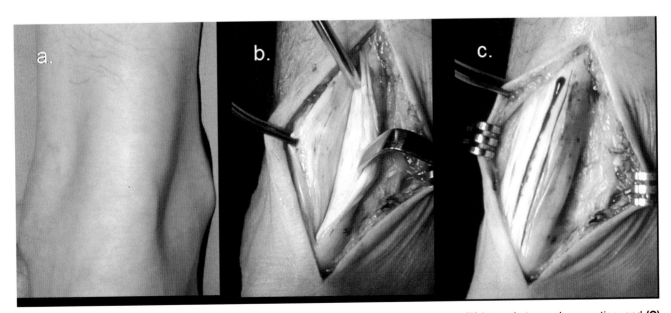

Fig 50-4. Pictures of human Achilles tendon disease showing: **(A)** swollen Achilles tendon, **(B)** intrasubstance degeneration, and **(C)** results of surgical debridement.

■ ACHILLES TENDON

Achilles tendon disorders represent a small portion of tendon disorders in general. Achilles disorders are cited to be increasing in frequency in the modern civilized world (13,14,25). Most disorders result from overuse with intrinsic and extrinsic factors contributing in a multifactorial manner. The end result is a diseased tendon that is both symptomatic and biomechanically inferior predisposed to catastrophic rupture.

Achilles Anatomy

A merging of the insertions of the gastrocneimus, which has its origin at the femoral condyle posteriorly, and the soleus, originating from the posterior superior aspect of the tibia and fibula, forms the Achilles tendon. The soleus component varies from 3 to 11 cm while the gastrocneimus varies from 11 to 26 cm (26). The confluence of these two tendons insert on the calcaneus posterior and inferior to the superior calcaneal tuberosity. The Achilles tendon rotates 30 to 150 degrees before its insertion point. This permits elongation and elastic recoil within the tendon allowing stored energy to be released during the appropriate phase of gait.

The blood supply of the Achilles arises from branches of the posterior tibial and peroneal arteries and is similar to that for other tendons surrounded by a paratenon as described by Mayer (27). Namely, it receives its blood from three sources: vessels in the musculotendinous junction, vessels in the surrounding connective tissue, and possibly from the osseous insertion vessels. A consistent decrease in the number of blood vessels in the mid portion of the Achilles tendon has been documented (28–30). This corresponds to the area identified by Kreuger-Franke et al. (31) as the most common site of rupture.

Achilles Tendon Biomechanics

Absolute force and the angular application of these forces play a role in the creation of Achilles tendon pathology. Peak forces of 3786 N have been measured within the Achilles tendon (32), which corresponds to a force that approximates six to eight times body weight during vigorous activities (30,33); however, the Achilles most commonly experience stresses that correspond to strains less than 4% (24) corresponding to a force of five times body weight (33).

Achilles Clinical Implications

Although the clinical presentation of an acute Achilles rupture may be a somewhat obvious chronic rupture or more subtle, Achilles pathology may present a diagnostic challenge. Achilles pathology may be categorized as insertional tendonitis involving the tendon-bone junction or noninsertional tendonitis involving the tendon proximal to its insertion (34).

Noninsertional tendonitis may involve the paratenon and/or the tendon itself. Involvement of either of these two components may occur in isolation or in combination (Fig 50-5) as classified by Puddu et al. (10).

Insertional Achilles tendon disease may also be subdivided into insertional calcific tendonitis, Haglunds deformity (referring to a prominent posterior superior tuberosity of the calcaneus), retrocalcaneal bursitis, precalcaneal bursitis, and calcaneal exostosis "pump bump" or "skaters heel."

Catastrophic rupture of the Achilles tendon (Fig 50-6) represents the final stage of Achilles tendon pathology. The most common patient profile for human Achilles tendon rupture would be that of a male in his third or fourth decade of life that plays sport occasionally. Men to women rupture rate has been reported from 2:1 to 12:1 (10,35,36). The mean age has been estimated between the 30's and 40's (17,18,31,36,37) with the left Achilles being ruptured more commonly than the right, probably reflecting right side dominance with left leg pushing off (38). The site of rupture has been reported to occur in the myotendinous junction in 12.1%, the insertion in 4.6%, and 3.5 cm proximal to the insertion in 83% (36).

History and Physical Examination

When approaching the patient with Achilles pathology it may be best to consider the continuum of pathology similar to that proposed by Puddu et al. (10). In the early phases, patients will complain of pain following strenuous activities that will usually progress to pain with regular activities and sometimes at rest. It is common for the patient to complain of pain and stiffness worse in the morning or after inactivity typical of "start-up pain" that may be a result of the paratendonitis adhesions.

Important information to gather includes first onset of symptoms paying particular attention to an episode of trauma. Activity related questions should include identifying changes in activity level to better delineate the repetitive overuse variables. Also, with respect to sporting activities that should gather information regarding warm-up, mileage, intensity, running surface, and shoe wear.

An acute rupture generally presents to the hospital emergency department with the classic history of sudden pain with an audible pop and a sensation of being struck by a fellow sportsman.

The physical examination begins with inspection of the patient's shoe wear and then lower limb weight-bearing alignment (anterior, posterior, and lateral). If possible, observation of gait should be performed as well. The most significant positive finding would be that of excessive hindfoot varus or valgus forcing the Achilles to course to its insertion point in a relatively shortened or contracted manner. Next, one should the subtalar joint in a neutral position while flexing and extending the knee to assess the extent of Achilles contracture.

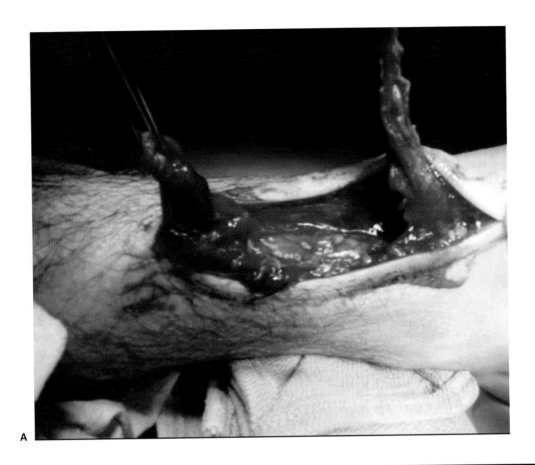

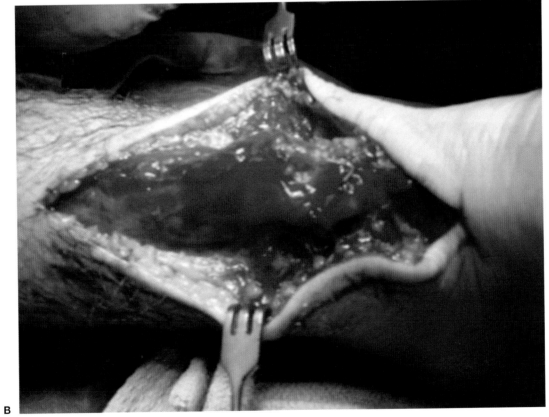

Fig 50-5. Pictures of human Achilles tendon disease showing: **(A)** traumatic rupture and **(B)** surgical repair.

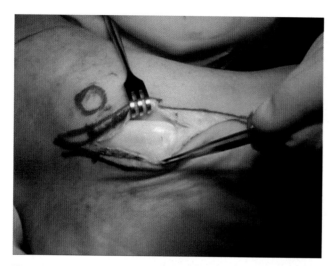

Fig 50-6. Picture of human diseased tibialis posterior tendon.

Localized findings may include gastrocneimus soleus wasting or localized swelling bruising or defect about the Achilles. Wasting of the gastrocneimus soleus complex is suggestive of a more severe affliction. Neurovascular examination should be documented as well as a detailed assessment of strength and range of motion. An inability to tip-toe walk may suggest chronic rupture, neurological problems, or pain that is inhibiting adequate muscular contraction.

The best way to further assess the Achilles tendon is with the patient in the prone position and feet hanging off the end of the examining table. This allows a systematic assessment of mechanical alignment, palpation of areas of tenderness, nodules, defects in the tendon, and crepitus, which are all hallmarks of Achilles pathology. Recreation of pain may be elicited with an eccentric contraction against resistance. Specialized tests include the Simmond's calf squeeze test (39) wrongly accredited to Thompson who described the test jointly with Doherty (40). This involves the examiner squeezing the patient's calf muscles while examining for a lack of plantar flexion compared to the contralateral side, a finding suggestive of Achilles rupture. Other tests for rupture that are for the most part unnecessary include Matles' test, the needle test, and Copeland's sphygmomanometer cuff test.

Laboratory Investigations

The only role for laboratory investigation would be for investigating underlying diseases or predisposing conditions that the clinician may be suspicious of. A good example of this would be that of serological testing for crystal arthropathy.

Imaging Studies

Plain x-ray films confirm any bony prominence such an exostosis visualized best on an axial view of the heel as a posterolateral prominence. Haglunds deformity is also easily depicted on the lateral view using the parallel pitch lines

where the tuberosity projects above the upper parallel pitch line and a Phillip and Fowler angle greater than 69 degrees. Distal calcification is easily identified near the Achilles insertion. Signs of Achilles rupture are evidenced by a loss of Kagers triangle or the retro calcaneal fat pad bound by the Achilles tendon, the calcaneus, and the deep toe flexors.

Ultrasound is useful for demonstrating bursal inflammation and any tendon degeneration. Some also use this for diagnosis of a rupture, but these entities should be diagnosed with clinical presentation. Lastly, MRI is the gold standard for imaging musculoskeletal soft tissues (17) yielding more detailed information about the midsubstance of the tendons and surrounding structures.

Nonoperative Treatment

Because Achilles pathology presents as a continuum with multifactorial etiology, it is important for the patient to be educated about the identification and various methods of controlling etiological factors to reduce the chance of progression. The obvious solution to excessive stress causing severe Achilles pathology rendering the patient unable to weight bear would be that of immobilization. It is recommended that only short periods (2 to 4 weeks) of immobilization be utilized in severe cases because prolonged immobilization is detrimental to tendon and muscle strength, articular cartilage, and worsens joint stiffness (13). This treatment is useful as the first phase of a broader treatment plan including other modalities below. With a partial Achilles rupture nonoperative treatment would include casting in plantar flexion for 3 weeks, followed by a dorsal block splint restricting dorsiflexion to some degree of plantar flexion. This is gradually increased to neutral by 6 weeks. The patient may be weight bearing in the splint over the last 2 weeks.

The use of professionally fashioned customized orthotics may relieve symptoms and provide a more biomechanical favorable condition to halt or reverse progression. The orthotics should correct flexible hindfoot malalignment in the coronal plain. As a generalized principle, shoe wear with a good sole and solid heel counter should be recommended to prevent excessive heel movement. Pump bump spacers may be utilized to unload pressure areas in the heel posteriorly. Also, a heel lift may unload the Achilles to some extent through decreased dorsiflexion angle at the ankle.

Although commonly used, injected or oral anti-inflammatory medications have not proven to be effective in clinical trials (41,42). Also one should be aware of the potential deleterious affects of Achilles injection.

Stretching is a very important part of nonoperative treatment regimes. An excellent daily routine would include standing backwards on a stair step for 5 minutes with the hindfoot overhanging the step. Commercial splints for stretching serve as an excellent adjunct for stretching. Night splints, although cumbersome, will provide one with a continuous minor stretch that reduces morning pain and stiffness.

After the inflammatory processes are under control with appropriate rest and stretching one may concentrate more on a strengthening program such as an eccentric exercise program proposed by Curwin and Stanish (43) in 1984. Eccentric strengthening causes a greater overall reduction in pain than the traditional concentric exercises (44).

Operative Treatment

Indications for surgery will vary depending on the severity of pathology and medical condition of the patient. In general one must consider all nonsurgical treatment modalities before surgery, for one can always operate at any time. One should be aware of negative prognostic patient factors specifically for outcomes in Achilles tendon surgery including diabetes mellitus, smoking, malnourishment, and generalized poor medical condition.

Achilles pathology may present at any stage from simple tendonitis to frank rupture thus accurate diagnosis will dictate surgical options. Noninsertional Achilles tendon disease that fails nonoperative treatment and Achilles rupture are the most common indication for surgical treatment. If the preoperative work up indicates that there is an intact tendon with disease in the mid-substance then consideration should be given to Achilles tendon debridement that includes excision of areas of tendon degeneration through a longitudinal incision (Fig 50-6). There are several case series, which report fair results after surgical treatment. (45,46,153–156).

Complete rupture of the Achilles may be treated operatively or nonoperatively. The proponents of operative treatment cite re-rupture rates as the main disadvantage of nonoperative treatment ranging from 0% to 5% (47). The proponents of nonoperative treatment cite complication rates as the main disadvantage of operative treatment ranging from 4.9% to 26.8% (47). In a meta-analysis by Lo et al. (48) it was concluded that operative treatment reduces the re-rupture rate over nonoperative treatment with minor and moderate complication rates being twenty times greater.

Thus, a tailored approach considering the concerns and health of the patient was recommended.

Operative treatment of a rupture may be subdivided into a primary repair versus reconstruction. The primary repair is the best option in the acute setting where ample tendon substance is available suitable for repair. Reconstruction is better reserved for the more chronic cases with excessive tendonosis or acute cases without adequate tendon that is repairable. The reconstruction may be performed though an Achilles turndown flap (48) if minimal defect is present or a more aggressive reconstruction procedure involving transfer of the flexor hallucis longus tendon (49). The percutaneous techniques are becoming more popular given the development of safer and user-friendlier surgical instrument devices. Although we have no experience with this technique one must consider the complications of sural nerve entrapment and a weaker repair leading to a higher re-rupture rate (50,51). Acute open repair is our method of choice **(Fig 50-7)** with end to end approximation of the tendon utilizing a suture technique similar to that of Jaakkola et al. (52).

Surgical treatment of insertional Achilles tendon disease that is directed at removal of the bony prominence if present and resection of calcification and inflamed bursal tissues. With Haglunds the posterosuperior calcaneal prominence must be completely removed and a second lateral incision in addition to the medial one is sometimes necessary to assure complete resection. Patients undergoing this surgical procedure must be cautioned about a prolonged recovery period sometimes taking 6 to 12 months for resolution of symptoms.

For simple posterolateral calcaneal exostosis (pump bump) only a small lateral approach is necessary for limited resection of the exostosis alone.

■ TIBIALIS POSTERIOR TENDON

The most common complaint of the population in general with respect to midfoot pain would include pain and disability from posterior tibialis tendon (PTT) disease causing

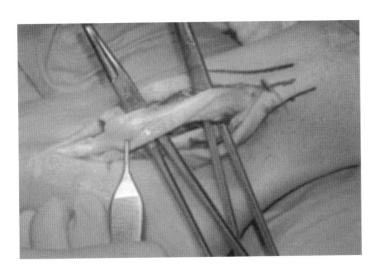

Fig 50-7. Picture of human diseased peroneal tendon.

dysfunction affecting the midfoot. Although this entity is not common in the athletic population it deserves mention because of the increased frequency in the general population and the increased frequency of missed diagnosis. In the athletic population pathologies associated with the PTT dysfunction include accessory navicular bones and navicular tuberosity fractures. These clinical conditions may progress to full blown PTT disease and medial arch collapse if not diagnosed and treated early.

Tibialis Posterior Tendon Anatomy

The PTT muscle takes its origin from the post aspect of the proximal one third of the tibia, fibula, and interosseous membrane and courses through the deep posterior compartment of the leg. Prior to its turn about the posterior aspect of the medial malleolus the PTT muscle converges to a very strong tendon which ultimately inserts principally on the navicular tuberosity but also on cuneiforms and bases of the second, third, and fourth metatarsals (53). The multiple insertions also blend the ligaments of the medial arch of the foot (54). The innervation arises from the tibial nerve while the blood supply is derived from the branches from the posterior tibial artery, periosteal vessels from the medial plantar artery of the posterior tibial artery, or the medial tarsal artery from the dorsalis pedis artery (55).

Tibialis Posterior Tendon Biomechanics

The primary function of the PTT is that of inversion and plantarflexion of the foot. This results in a locking of the midfoots transverse tarsal joints (talonavicular and calcaneocuboid) (56). The PTT also acts as an adductor of the forefoot at the midtarsal joint apposing the action of the peroneus brevis (54) and provides support for the longitudinal arch of the foot.

Tibialis Posterior Tendon Clinical Implications

The presenting complaint of PTT dysfunction is that of medial ankle pain and swelling and tenderness localized directly over the navicular tuberosity in the presence of underlying tuberosity fracture or accessory navicular. There is often coexisting lateral sinus tarsi pain (57). Physical examination of the patient demonstrates forefoot abduction (too many toes), midfoot pes planus (flat foot), and hindfoot valgus. Patients are usually able to perform the bilateral heel rising, but will lack the normal heel inversion if the PTT is dysfunctional. Single foot heel rising on the symptomatic limb is usually not possible or at least painful and weak. Lastly, some patients will come with a variety of custom or premanufactured foot orthotics and it is often useful to assess the patient standing in these to assess the medial arch support provided. A clinically useful classification would be that discussed by Johnson and Strom (58). This includes dividing the pathology according to deformity and whether or not it is correctable.

Stage 1 involves pain localized along the course of the PTT; Stage 2 represents a situation in which the PTT is diseased as in Stage 1 with the tendon being functionally incompetent resulting in medial arch collapse; Stage 3 has all the features of Stages 1 and 2 but the deformities are rigid and not passively correctable. Finally, Stage 4 includes the features of Stage 3 plus ankle joint incongruency.

Investigations

The only role for laboratory investigation would be to rule out underlying diseases or predisposing conditions (i.e., infection, inflammatory disease, neuropathy, or vasculopathy). Imaging studies are often not necessary to make the diagnosis of PTT disease because the clinical features discussed above are fairly consistent. Standing anteroposterior and lateral plain x-rays of the foot and ankle are most important for an objective assessment of the alignment of foot to identify pes planus. Hindfoot alignment views (59) are best for assessing hind foot valgus. Plain films will usually reveal the accessory navicular or tuberosity fracture. Bone scan followed by a CT is best for identifying subtle accessory navicular or tuberosity fracture. MRI is reserved for accessing posterior tibial tendon synovitis or intrasubstance tendon disease.

Treatment

The goal of treatment is relief of symptoms, restoration of function, and prevention of progression of the disease. Early stages usually mandate nonoperative treatment with activity modification, anti-inflammatory medication, physiotherapy, and medial arch support orthotics. Casting for 2 to 4 weeks may decrease inflammation and assist with accessory navicular or tuberosity fracture.

Late stages and resistant cases usually require orthopedic consultation for surgical treatment. Surgical options include tendon debridement in Stage 1 with or without a bony procedure such as a medial weight bearing axis shifting calcaneal osteotomy or lateral column lengthening procedure. The passively correctable flatfoot is treated with a combination of a soft tissue reconstruction of the PTT in an attempt to restore a function PTT with a bony procedure (above) to reverse deformity. The choices for reconstruction of the PTT include transfer of the flexor digitorum longus (FDL) or flexor hallucius longus (FHL). Stage 3 and 4 PTT dysfunction represents a therapeutic challenge in that the deformities are not passively correctable; thus, tarsal arthrodesis such as subtalar, talonavicular, and calcaneocuboid, and sometimes tibial calcaneal for Stage 4.

■ PERONEAL TENDONS

The major pathological conditions afflicting the peroneal tendons include disease afflicting the peritenon or tendon proper and shall be referred to as peroneal tendon disease.

Peroneal tendon disease secondary to trauma or stenosis is very common. Traumatic entities that may cause the peroneal tendons to become diseased include overuse with micro rupture or calcification, dislocation or subluxation, lateral malleolar fractures, calcaneal fractures, and inversion ankle injuries. Nontraumatic entities include inflammatory arthritis, infection, Os peroneum, congenital enlarged peroneal tubercle, or very rarely local tumors.

Peroneal Tendon Anatomy

The peroneal tendons include the peroneus longus and brevis with variably present accessory muscles (60) including peroneus quartus, peroneus accessories, and peroneus digiti minimi. The peroneus longus and brevis take their origin from upper two-thirds and lower two-thirds of lateral fibula and intermuscular septum respectively. The peroneus longus inserts on the lateral tubercle of the first metatarsal and the first cuneiform while the peroneus brevis inserts on the base of the fifth metatarsal. The nerve supply is from the superficial peroneal nerve while the blood supply (61) arises two posterolateral vincula, one for the peroneus longus tendon and one for the peroneus brevis tendon. These vincula are supplied by branches of the posterior peroneal artery.

Peroneal Tendon Biomechanics

The primary function of the peroneal tendons is that of eversion and plantarflexion of the foot. The peroneus longus is also responsible for plantar flexion of the first metatarsal. The superior peroneal retinaculum serves as the primary restraint to peroneal tendon subluxation. Other structures important in maintaining peroneal stability include a fibrocartilaginous ridge of the lateral malleolus and the retromalleolar sulcus (62).

Peroneal Tendon Clinical Implications

Peroneal Tendon Disease

The clinical presentation of peroneal tendon disease is usually that of clinical signs and symptoms of underlying inflammation in the area where the underlying tendon is afflicted most often posterior to the fibula. This includes swelling and tenderness exacerbated by resisted stretching of the tendons with a planter flexion inversion force. Patients may also exhibit a decrease in subtalar motion and subsequent difficulty with walking on uneven ground. The diagnosis may be confirmed with MRI (63), ultrasound (64), or local anesthetic injection (65).

Treatment of peroneal tendon disease should first be directed at the underlying cause of the pathology and the accepted strategies for other common tendonitis are indicated. These include activity modification (cast immobilization for a short period if necessary), icing, and antinflammtories. Orthotics and shoe wear modifications are sometimes helpful in certain situations. An example would

include decreasing calcaneal fibular impingement with a medial heel wedge. After inflammation is controlled, physiotherapy directed at strengthening and mobility should be instituted. Surgery should be reserved for resistant cases and again should address the underlying cause with or without a debridement of the diseased tendon. Often peroneal instability contributes to the diseased peroneals and therefore strong consideration should be given to a peroneal stabilization procedure concurrent with a debridement.

Partial or Complete Peroneal Tendon Ruptures

Occasionally a complete or partial tear of the peroneal tendons results from neglected or failed treatment of peroneal tendon disease. Indeed, primary traumatic rupture of the peroneal tendons is rare and requires a high index of suspicion (66). On the other hand, longitudinal split tears of the proneus brevis are more common and were investigated by Sobel et al. (67) who showed that peroneus brevis splits are the result of a dynamic mechanical insult at the fibular groove due to laxity of the superior peroneal retinaculum. Traumatic dislocation is associated with sports including skiing, soccer, football, ice-skating, and gymnastics.

The clinical presentation of partial ruptures of the peroneal tendons is similar to peroneal tendon disease with the possible addition of a history of ankle instability or repeated ankle sprains. Complete rupture is often indicated with a clinical presentation of increased hindfoot varus and pain and weakness with active eversion. In this clinical scenario the MRI is most useful to delineate the differential diagnosis of complete, partial, or no tear (68).

The treatment of ruptured peroneal tendons follows a similar course for that of peroneal tendon disease with or without tendinosis with the exception that one may be more aggressive to initiate surgical treatment. An acute rupture may benefit from early surgical intervention to promote rehabilitation and prevent re-rupture as with other tendons. With respect to partial or chronic tears a debridement and repair or reconstruction of the tendon will be indicated upon failure of nonoperative care.

Peroneal Instability

Peroneal tendon instability often coexists with peroneal tendon disease and partial tears (Fig 50-7). Instability may be viewed as a continuum with frank traumatic dislocation at one end and subluxation within the peroneal groove at the other end (69). Traumatic dislocation is associated with sports including skiing, soccer, football, ice-skating, and gymnastics; however, the chance of dislocation is most likely a direct reflection of predisposing anatomic factors that restrain the peroneal tendons from dislocation. Some of these factors include abnormal superior peroneal retinaculum, shallow fibular groove, and calcaneal varus.

The clinical presentation of patients with peroneal instability again may be similar to that of peroneal tendon disease and partial tears. Also, the patient may complain of a click or audible snap with or without pain. The subluxation or dislocation may be reproducible with resisted eversion and dorsiflexion and palpation of the tendons.

Nonoperative treatment includes immobilization and bracing techniques in an acute scenario with subsequent physiotherapy. More than often this treatment fails and a persistence of symptoms results in a surgical procedure. These include direct repair of retinaculum (70), rerouting procedures of the peroneal tendons (71), fibular sliding osteotomies (71), or fibular groove deepening procedures (72).

OTHER TENDONS OF THE FOOT AND ANKLE

When considering tendon problems about the foot and ankle one must consider all the clinical significant tendons in addition to the three major ones listed earlier in this chapter. These include the following tendons: flexor hallucis longus (FHL), flexor digitorum longus (FDL), tibialis anterior, extensor hallucis longus, extensor digitorum longus tendon, and intrinsic tendons. Although important when pathological, clinical presentation of these other tendon problems occurs less frequently than those of the Achilles, tibialis posterior, and peroneal tendons. Thus, in this section these other tendons will be considered collectively with mention made of particular common entities.

First, it should be stated that all tendons of the foot and ankle are subject to peritendonitis with or without tendinosis and this results in a clinical presentation of similar local inflammatory signs and symptoms. The treatment is fundamentally similar for all tendons and involves nonoperative measures to control inflammation, rehabilitation to reverse functional deficits, and possibly surgical intervention when nonoperative measures fail.

FHL tendon pathology most commonly results from overuse and is most prominent in dancers (73), sometimes runners (74), and the general population (75). The operative treatment to consider after failed nonoperative treatment should be directed at the factors causing the pathology and include a release of the FHL tendon sheath (76) with or without debridement. FDL tendon rupture is very rare (77). One isolated case report discovered by this review noted in association with FHL tendon pathology in a tennis player.

Tibialis anterior tendon pathology may progress to rupture resulting in weak dorsiflexion of the foot and often foot drop. Because this is a rare occurrence (78) it is often missed. Treatment is usually that of surgical repair or reconstruction but some reports suggest nonoperative treatment may suffice especially in the less active patients (79).

Extensor hallucis longus tendon pathology is rarely cited in the literature other than some case reports, one of which was associated with steroid injection (80). Extensor digitorum longus tendon pathology is equally rare and more often may become diseased from shoe wear and respond well to

nonoperative measures. A rupture, which is rare, will do well with surgical treatment.

Intrinsic tendons of the foot may become problematic if neurologically compromised or defunctioned as in missed compartment syndrome of the foot. The clinical result is usually that of flexion deformity of the toe responding well to flexor tendon release or transfer should nonoperative treatment fail.

REFERENCES

1. O'Brien M. Functional anatomy and physiology of tendons. *Clin Sports Med.* 1992;11(3):505–20.
2. Gross M. Chronic tendonitis: pathomechanics of injury, factors affecting the healing response and treatment. *J Orthop Sports Phys Ther.* 1992;16:248–261.
3. Kastelic J, Galeski A, Baer E. The multicomposite structure of tendon. *Connect Tissue Res.* 1978;6(1):11–23.
4. Gathercole LJ, Keller A, Shah JS, The periodic wave pattern in native tendon collagen: correlation of polarizing with scanning electron microscopy. *J Microsc.* 1974;102:95–105.
5. Diamant J, et al. Collagen; ultrastructure and its relation to mechanical properties as a function of ageing. *Proc R Soc Lond B Biol Sci.* 1972;180(60):293–315.
6. Perugia L, Ricciardi Pollini PT, Ippolito E. Ultrastuctural aspects of degenerative tendinopathy. *Int Orthop.* 1978;1:303–307.
7. Maffulli N, et al. Tenocytes from ruptured and tendinopathic achilles tendons produce greater quantities of type III collagen than tenocytes from normal achilles tendons. An in vitro model of human tendon healing. *Am J Sports Med.* 2000;28(4):499–505.
8. Maffulli N, Kahn KM. Clinical nomenclature for tendon injuries. *Med Sci Sports Exerc.* 1999;31(2):352–353.
9. Almekinders LC, Temple JD. Etiology, diagnosis, and treatment of tendonitis: an analysis of the literature. *Med Sci Sports Exerc.* 1998;30(8):1183–1190.
10. Puddu G, Ippolito E, Postacchini F. A classification of Achilles tendon disease. *Am J Sports Med.* 1976;4(4):145–150.
11. Backman C, et al. Chronic achilles paratenonitis with tendinosis: an experimental model in the rabbit. *J Orthop Res.* 1990;8(4):541–547.
12. Beskin JL, et al. Surgical repair of Achilles tendon ruptures. *Am J Sports Med.* 1987;15(1):1–8.
13. Kannus P, Jozsa L. Histopathological changes preceding spontaneous rupture of a tendon. A controlled study of 891 patients. *J Bone Joint Surg Am.* 1991;73(10):1507–1525.
14. Jozsa L, et al. Fine structural alterations of collagen fibers in degenerative tendinopathy. *Arch Orthop Trauma Surg.* 1984;103(1):47–51.
15. Cetti R, Junge J, Vyberg M. Spontaneous rupture of the Achilles tendon is preceded by widespread and bilateral tendon damage and ipsilateral inflammation: a clinical and histopathologic study of 60 patients. *Acta Orthop Scand.* 2003;74(1):78–84.
16. Arner O, Lindholm A, Orell SR. Histologic changes in subcutaneous rupture of the Achilles tendon; a study of 74 cases. *Acta Chir Scand.* 1959;116(5-6):484–490.
17. Arner O, LA. Subcutaneous rupture of the acchilles tendon: a study of 92 cases. *Acta Chir Scand Supp.* 1959;230:1–151.
18. Fox JM, et al. Degeneration and rupture of the Achilles tendon. *Clin Orthop.* 1975;107:221–224.
19. Astrom M, Rausing A. Chronic Achilles tendinopathy. A survey of surgical and histopathologic findings. *Clin Orthop.* 1995;(316):151–164.
20. Movin T, et al. Tendon pathology in long-standing achillodynia. Biopsy findings in 40 patients. *Acta Orthop Scand.* 1997;68(2):170–175.

21. Glazebrook M. Achilles tendon disease: development of an animal model and an investigation of histology, biochemistry and biomechanics. In: *Faculty of medicine.* Nova Scotia: Halifax; 2005.

22. Stanish WD, Curwin S, Mandell S. *Tendinitis: Its etiology and treatment.* Oxford University Press; 2000:49–64.

23. Roach M, Burton A. The reason for the shape of the distensibility curves of arteries. *Can J Biochem Physiol.* 1957;35:681–690.

24. Hess GP, et al. Prevention and treatment of overuse tendon injuries. *Sports Med.* 1989;8(6):371–384.

25. Hattrup SJ, Johnson KA. Chevron osteotomy: analysis of factors in patients' dissatisfaction. *Foot Ankle.* 1985;5(6):327–332.

26. Cummings EJ, et al. The structure of the calcaneal tendon (of achilles) in relation to orthopaedic surgery: with additional observations on the plantaris muscle. *Surg Gynaecol Obstetr.* 1946; 83:106–107.

27. Mayer L. The physiological method of tendon trasplantation. *Surg Gynaecol Obstetr.* 1916;22:183–197.

28. Kristensen JK, Andersen PT. Rupture of the Achilles tendon: a series and a review of literature. *J Trauma.* 1972;12(9):794–798.

29. Lagergren C, Lindholm A. Vascular distribution in the Achilles tendon: Angiographic and micrographic study. *Acta Chir Scand.* 1959;116:491–495.

30. Carr AJ, Norris SH, The blood supply of the calcaneal tendon. *J Bone Joint Surg Br.* 1989;71(1):100–101.

31. Krueger-Franke M, Siebert CH, Scherzer S. Surgical treatment of ruptures of the Achilles tendon: a review of long-term results. *Br J Sports Med.* 1995;29(2):121–125.

32. Fukashiro S, et al. In vivo Achilles tendon loading during jumping in humans. *Eur J Appl Physiol Occup Physiol.* 1995;71(5): 453–458.

33. Scheller AD, Kasser JR, Quigley TB. Tendon injuries about the ankle. *Orthop Clin North Am.* 1980;11(4):801–811.

34. Clain MR, Baxter DE. Achilles tendinitis. *Foot Ankle.* 1992;13(8):482–487.

35. Carden DG, et al. Rupture of the calcaneal tendon. The early and late management. *J Bone Joint Surg Br.* 1987;69(3):416–420.

36. Jozsa L, et al. The role of recreational sport activity in Achilles tendon rupture. A clinical, pathoanatomical, and sociological study of 292 cases. *Am J Sports Med.* 1989;17(3):338–343.

37. Boyden EM, et al. Late versus early repair of Achilles tendon rupture. Clinical and biomechanical evaluation. *Clin Orthop.* 1995(317);150–158.

38. Stein SR, Luekens CA Jr. Closed treatment of Achilles tendon ruptures. *Orthop Clin North Am.* 1976;7(1):241–246.

39. Simonds FA. The diagnosis of the ruptured achilles tendon. *Practitioner.* 1957;179:56–58.

40. Thompson TC, Doherty JH. Spontaneous rupture of tendon of Achilles: a new clinical diagnostic test. *J Trauma.* 1962;2: 126–129.

41. Astrom M, Westlin N. No effect of piroxicam on achilles tendinopathy. A randomized study of 70 patients. *Acta Orthop Scand.* 1992;63(6):631–634.

42. DaCruz DJ, et al. Achilles paratendonitis: an evaluation of steroid injection. *Br J Sports Med.* 1988;22(2):64–65.

43. Curwin SL, Stanish WD. *Tendonitis: its etiology and treatment.* Lexington, Toronto. Collamore Press; 1984.

44. Niesen-Vertommen SL, et al. The effect of eccentric versus concentric exercises in the management of Achilles tendonitis. *Clin J Sports Med.* 1992;2(2):109–113.

45. Amiel D, et al. The effect of immobilization on collagen turnover in connective tissue: a biochemical-biomechanical correlation. *Acta Orthop Scand.* 1982;53(3):325–332.

46. Clement DB, et al. Evaluation of performance following achilles tendon surgery in competitive runners. *IAAF.* 1992;7(2):33–37.

47. Waterston SW, Maffulli N, Ewen SW. Subcutaneous rupture of the Achilles tendon: basic science and some aspects of clinical practice. *Br J Sports Med.* 1997;31(4):285–298.

48. Lo IK, et al. Operative versus nonoperative treatment of acute Achilles tendon ruptures: a quantitative review. *Clin J Sport Med.* 1997;7(3):207–211.

49. Wapner KL, et al. Repair of chronic Achilles tendon rupture with flexor hallucis longus tendon transfer. *Foot Ankle.* 1993;14(8):443–449.

50. Klein J, Tiling T. [Tendon injuries in sports]. *Langenbecks Arch Chir Suppl Kongressbd.* 1991;473–476.

51. Rowley DI, Scotland TR. Rupture of the Achilles tendon treated by a simple operative procedure. *Injury.* 1982;14(3):252–254.

52. Jaakkola JI, et al. Achilles tendon rupture repair: biomechanical comparison of the triple bundle technique versus the Krakow locking loop technique. *Foot Ankle Int.* 2000;21(1):14–17.

53. Johnson KA. Tibialis posterior tendon rupture. *Clin Orthop.* 1983;177:140–147.

54. Mueller TJ. Acquired flatfoot secondary to tibialis posterior dysfunction: biomechanical aspects. *J Foot Surg.* 1991;30(1):2–11.

55. Frey C, Shereff M, Greenidge N. Vascularity of the posterior tibial tendon. *J Bone Joint Surg Am.* 1990;72(6):884–888.

56. Elftman H. The transverse tarsal joint and its control. *Clin Orthop.* 1960;16:41–46.

57. Anderson MW, et al. Association of posterior tibial tendon abnormalities with abnormal signal intensity in the sinus tarsi on MR imaging. *Skeletal Radiol.* 2000;29(9):514–519.

58. Johnson KA, Strom DE. Tibialis posterior tendon dysfunction. *Clin Orthop.* 1989(239):196–206.

59. Saltzman CL, el-Khoury GY. The hindfoot alignment view. *Foot Ankle Int.* 1995;16(9):572–576.

60. Sobel M, Levy ME, Bohne WH. Congenital variations of the peroneus quartus muscle: an anatomic study. *Foot Ankle.* 1990;11(2):81–89.

61. Sobel M, et al. Microvascular anatomy of the peroneal tendons. *Foot Ankle.* 1992;13(8):469–472.

62. Davis WH, et al. The superior peroneal retinaculum: an anatomic study. *Foot Ankle Int.* 1994;15(5):271–275.

63. Mota J, Rosenberg ZS. Magnetic resonance imaging of the peroneal tendons. *Top Magn Reson Imaging.* 1998;9(5):273–285.

64. Thermann H, et al. The use of ultrasonography in the foot and ankle. *Foot Ankle.* 1992;13(7):386–390.

65. Mizel MS, Michelson JD, Newberg A. Peroneal tendon bupivacaine injection: utility of concomitant injection of contrast material. *Foot Ankle Int.* 1996;17(9):566–568.

66. Kilkelly FX, McHale KA. Acute rupture of the peroneal longus tendon in a runner: a case report and review of the literature. *Foot Ankle Int.* 1994;15(10):567–569.

67. Sobel M, et al. The dynamics of peroneus brevis tendon splits: a proposed mechanism, technique of diagnosis, and classification of injury. *Foot Ankle.* 1992;13(7):413–422.

68. Major NM, et al. The MR imaging appearance of longitudinal split tears of the peroneus brevis tendon. *Foot Ankle Int.* 2000;21(6):514–519.

69. Harper MC. Subluxation of the peroneal tendons within the peroneal groove: a report of two cases. *Foot Ankle Int.* 1997;18(6):369–370.

70. Eckert WR, Davis EA Jr. Acute rupture of the peroneal retinaculum. *J Bone Joint Surg Am.* 1976;58(5):670–672.

71. Steinbock G, Pinsger M. Treatment of peroneal tendon dislocation by transposition under the calcaneofibular ligament. *Foot Ankle Int.* 1994;15(3):107–111.

72. Kollias SL, Ferkel RD. Fibular grooving for recurrent peroneal tendon subluxation. *Am J Sports Med.* 1997;25(3):329–335.

73. Sammarco GJ, Cooper PS. Flexor hallucis longus tendon injury in dancers and nondancers. *Foot Ankle Int.* 1998;19(6): 356–362.

74. Theodore GH, Kolettis GJ, Micheli LJ. Tenosynovitis of the flexor hallucis longus in a long-distance runner. *Med Sci Sports Exerc.* 1996;28(3):277–279.

75. Oloff LM, Schulhofer SD. Flexor hallucis longus dysfunction. *J Foot Ankle Surg.* 1998;37(2):101–109.

76. Lynch T, Pupp GR. Stenosing tenosynovitis of the flexor hallucis longus at the ankle joint. *J Foot Surg.* 1990;29(4): 345–348.

77. Drape JL, et al. Closed ruptures of the flexor digitorum tendons: MRI evaluation. *Skeletal Radiol.* 1998;27(11):617–624.

78. Patten A, Pun WK. Spontaneous rupture of the tibialis anterior tendon: a case report and literature review. *Foot Ankle Int.* 2000;21(8):697–700.

79. Trout BM, Hosey G, Wertheimer SJ. Rupture of the tibialis anterior tendon. *J Foot Ankle Surg.* 2000;39(1):54–58.

80. Poggi JJ, Hall RL. Acute rupture of the extensor hallucis longus tendon. *Foot Ankle Int.* 1995;16(1):41–43.

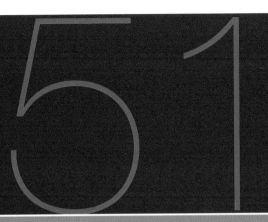

STRESS FRACTURES OF THE ATHLETIC LEG, ANKLE, AND FOOT

DONALD R. BOHAY, MD, FACS, JONATHAN P. CORNELIUS, MD, JOHN G. ANDERSON, MD

■ KEY POINTS

- Military personnel are more prone to stress fractures of calcaneus and metarsals. Athletic injured patients have more tibial stress fractures.
- Stress fractures are most common in running sports as vertical ground reaction forces are three times greater compared to walking.
- Fatigue fractures occur as a result of repetitive activity, when bone is subjected to abnormal stress.
- With the proper index of suspicion, stress fractures can be diagnosed early. In most cases, patients will return to their prior level of competition after nonoperative treatment.
- Patients with stress fractures give a classic history of insidious onset of pain in a localized area. The pain is exacerbated by repetitive activity and relieved by rest.
- A change in running surface or shoes occasionally relates to the onset of symptoms.
- Standing x-rays are the first line of imaging for these injuries. Most x-rays will initially be negative. A bone scan or magnetic resonance imaging (MRI) can be used for definitive diagnosis and may be positive within a few days of injury.
- Stress fractures of the sesamoids and phalanges, although uncommon, do occur.
- Fractures of the base of the second metatarsal may be seen in ballet dancers who are routinely in the en pointe position.
- Stress fractures of the cuboid are rare and occur in runners.
- Stress fractures of the navicular are common in basketball, football, and track and field athletes and difficult to diagnose and treat. Some cases require operative intervention.

- Calcaneal stress fractures are more common than those in the talus. Patients will present with pain and swelling on both sides of the heel. These injuries occur in the military and in dancers.
- Tibial shaft stress fractures are subdivided into fractures of the posterior and anterior tibia. Anterior tibial stress fractures are more problematic and should be considered for surgical intervention.

Stress fractures were originally described by Breithaupt (1), a Prussian military physician, in 1855. The observation was made after examination of soldiers with swollen, painful feet. From the first description of "march fractures," our current understanding of stress fractures has grown immensely. Military personnel are different from sports injured patients as they are more prone to stress fractures of the calcaneus and metatarsals (2). Athletic injured patients have more tibial stress fractures (3–5). Stress fractures are seen in 10% to 15% of sports medicine patients (5–7). Stress fractures are most common in running sports as vertical ground reaction forces are three times greater compared to walking (8). Insufficiency fractures are defined as fractures that occur in abnormal bone which has been subjected to normal stress, and will not be covered here. Fatigue fractures occur when normal bone is subjected to abnormal stress.

■ ANATOMY

Certain anatomical variants have been found to predispose patients to fatigue fractures. Pronated feet are implicated in tarsal and tibial stress fractures (4,7). An anatomic study by Giladi et al. (9) showed a high degree of external rotation of the hip and narrow tibiae predispose individuals to stress fractures of the lower extremity. Other anatomical variants found to increase chances of stress fracture are leg length inequality and excessive forefoot varus (8). Talocalcaneal and calcaneonavicular coalitions place the talus at risk of fatigue fracture (6). A rigid cavus foot will predispose the athlete to fatigue fracture (10).

Biomechanics

Fatigue fractures occur as a result of repetitive activity. One proposed etiology suggests that fatigued muscles fail causing higher strains (7). Bone is subjected to compressive and tensile forces. Muscle contraction converts tensile forces into compressive forces, a phenomenon referred to as stress shielding. This protects the bone and prevents injury. When muscles fatigue this protective process fails and microfractures accumulate (6). In addition, muscle fatigue is accompanied by changes in gait, which may also alter the force on bone.

In another proposed cause of stress fractures the repetitive pull of contracting muscles act on bones causing microfracture. This explains the presence of stress fracture in nonweight-bearing bones (6,7).

Pathophysiology

Wolff's Law of Transformation states bone undergoes cyclical stress and rest allowing it to remodel the bony architecture to optimally withstand its environment. Bone is subjected to stress microfractures. Cortical bone remodels initially by osteoclastic resorption at the level of the osteon. Bone loss peaks at 3 weeks. The resorption cavities are filled with lamellar bone by osteoblasts, producing the Haversian system. The cycle takes 3 months to complete. An imbalance of resorption and bone deposition leads to weakening of bone (11). On the tensile side of bone, osteons debond at the cement lines causing microfractures (10). On the compression side, oblique cracks and longitudinal splitting occurs through canalicular defects and the Haversian canals (7). In cancellous bone stress forms trabecular microfractures producing microcallus. These thickened trabeculae appear as sclerosis on x-rays. Stress fractures represent a continuum of injury and bony response. In this dynamic process, if the stress continues, the fatigue fracture may become complete and ultimately displaced (3).

History

Patients with stress fractures give a classic history of insidious onset of pain in a localized area. The pain is exacerbated by repetitive activity and relieved by rest. Symptoms persist from weeks to months. As the injury progresses, the pain will occur earlier and with greater intensity during activity. A training error may relate to the onset of symptoms. Training errors include changes in distance, intensity, or frequency of workout. On occasion there may be change in the running surface or shoes. Inadequate footwear can also

contribute. In athletes with exertional bone pain, 50% will have a stress fracture (7).

Physical Exam

Stress fractures will result in point tenderness over the affected bone. Patients will generally have a full range of motion at all joints, with normal muscle tone and function. Neurovascular function is normal. There may be some subtle soft tissue swelling in the foot. Running, walking, or toe walking may recreate the symptoms.

Imaging

Standing x-rays are the first line of imaging in these injuries. Most x-rays will initially be negative. Baseline films on presentation will allow recognition of radiographic changes later in the course of the injury. After several weeks long bones such as the metatarsals or tibia will show periosteal new bone formation or cortical break. Cancellous bone such as the calcaneus or tarsal bones will show medullary sclerosis. A bone scan is the investigation of choice, and it will be positive as early as 3 days after injury (7). The bone scan will be positive in all three phases with a focal intense area of uptake, even in the setting of normal x-ray findings (3). The bone scan is virtually 100% sensitive in diagnosing stress fractures, but its specificity is less than x-ray (4). Bone scan cannot distinguish stress fracture from neoplasm or infection (7). Computed tomography (CT) scans have a role in evaluation of navicular, calcaneal, tibial, and pediatric fatigue fractures. Magnetic resonance imaging (MRI) can also be a useful adjunct in some circumstances with negative films and equivocal bone scan.

Forefoot

Sesamoids

Stress fractures of the sesamoids, although uncommon, do occur. The sesamoids are subject to injury due to their positioning under the head of the first metatarsal. Up to 50% of body weight is born through the great toe complex (12). They impart mechanical advantage to the flexor hallucis brevis tendons by acting as a fulcrum. The medial sesamoid may be more frequently injured, although in one study the medial and lateral sesamoids were found to be involved equally (13,14).

Patients with stress fractures of the sesamoids will present with the classic history of a stress fracture. Patients will have pain standing on their toes or with dorsiflexion of the first toe. The differential diagnosis of pain in the first metatarsophalangeal joint includes sesamoiditis, chondromalacia, stress fracture, osteochondritis, turf toe, hallux valgus, medial plantar digital proper nerve syndrome, and bursitis (15,16).

Standing anteroposterior (AP) and lateral foot x-rays and a sesamoid view will evaluate the sesamoids (13). If a bipartite sesamoid is seen, a bone scan will be cold with a multipartite sesamoid and will show increased uptake with a stress fracture (15). In a histological study of the stress fractured sesamoid by

Van Hal et al. (14), the cellular structure of the stress fracture resembled a pseudoarthrosis (14).

Initial treatment of a stress fracture of a sesamoid involves 6 weeks of immobilization in a cast or walker boot. Diebold has immobilized the toe in flexion using a K wire to achieve bone healing. After 6 weeks the foot is re-examined and x-rays taken. If unhealed, surgery may be considered. Surgical excision of one sesamoid may be considered, particularly if the sesamoid is fragmented (14) **(Fig 51-1)**. If both sesamoids are excised the patient will have an unacceptable result of a cock-up-toe deformity, and this is highly discouraged (13). Partial excision of the smaller fragment can also be performed. Bone grafting of a well-defined fracture nonunion may be considered. If at the time of surgery there is no gross motion at the nonunion site, it is recommended that the nonunion be bone grafted. If there is gross motion the sesamoid should be excised as reported by Anderson et al. (12).

Phalanges

Although very rare, there are reported cases of stress fractures of the phalanges. In a series by Shiraishi et al. (16), there were reported three cases of stress fracture of the proximal phalanx of the great toe. These injuries were all seen in athletes who were involve in sports with repeated running and jumping, causing repetition of forced dorsiflexion of the great toe. The differential diagnosis of pain in the first metatarsophalangeal joint is discussed in the sesamoid section. X-rays revealed a fracture in all three cases. The patients were treated with complete cessation of training for 6 weeks (16).

Metatarsals

Stress fractures of the metatarsals are most likely to be seen in the second and third metatarsal shafts. A hypermobile first ray, short first ray and/or gastrocnemius equinus contracture are anatomical variations predisposing the athlete to fatigue fracture of the second metatarsal. A Morton foot, which has a second metatarsal longer than the first metatarsal, has been thought to predispose the athlete to these fractures; however, Drez et al. (17) found the Morton foot does not predispose to stress fractures of the metatarsals. These fractures will present with localized pain and tenderness. Initial x-ray findings may be inconclusive. If treated early patients will respond well to cessation of training. If there has been a delay in treatment with visible findings on x-ray, nonweight-bearing immobilization is recommended for 4 to 6 weeks until callus is seen **(Fig 51-2)** and the patient is asymptomatic.

Stress fractures of the first metatarsal are uncommon, accounting for between 1% and 10% of metatarsal stress fractures. They are predominantly seen in the cancellous proximal end of the bone. Initial x-ray will be negative, but early films will begin to show linear sclerosis at the site of injury. Bone scan will be diagnostic. The treatment is activity and shoe modification for 4 to 6 weeks (18).

Fractures of the base of the second metatarsal may be seen in ballet dancers who are routinely in the en pointe position. With the foot plantar flexed and the weight borne on the first and second phalanges, the leg forms a long lever arm with the forces concentrated at the second tarsometatarsal junction. The middle cuneiform acts as the keystone of this rigid arch, concentrating the force in the midfoot (19,20). The differential diagnosis in ballet dancers includes synovitis of Lisfranc's joint versus stress fracture. If plain films are negative, an MRI is recommended to obtain the proper diagnosis (20). Dancers may continue to perform with a diagnosis of synovitis, although a stress fracture will require cessation of dancing until asymptomatic. Patients will additionally require a fracture shoe or walking cast. A prompt recovery may be expected in the majority of patients (19).

Additional consideration must be given to stress fractures of the fifth metatarsal. Jones originally described the fracture sustained while dancing, but in can be seen in a wide variety of

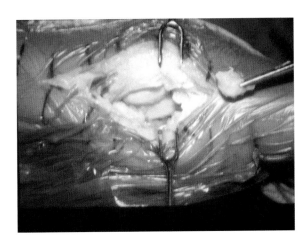

Fig 51-1. This is an intraoperative photograph of a college basketball player who sustained a stress fracture of his sesamoid and went on to have the fragment excised. (Photo courtesy Dr. P. Kolodziej.)

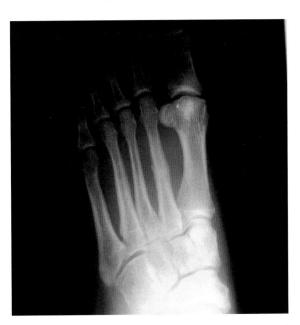

Fig 51-2. This x-ray was taken 4 weeks after presentation in a basketball player with forefoot pain.

athletes, especially basketball and football players (21). In the athlete this fracture may be seen acutely or in a chronic course. A stress fracture occurs 1.5 cm distal to the tuberosity of the fifth metatarsal in the metaphyseal-diaphyseal junction (10). These fractures occur at a watershed area for the blood supply and thus take a particularly long time to heal compared to the other metatarsals. The fracture may also reflect a cavus foot position with overload of the lateral border of the foot resulting in slow healing or refracture. Standing AP, lateral, and oblique x-ray views may show beaking and sclerosis at the lateral cortex **(Fig 51-3)**. Treatment involves 6 to 8 weeks of non-weight bearing. The athlete will be allowed to return to activity when asymptomatic. In the high performance athlete, refracture may be common; therefore, some surgeons may elect for early operative fixation to allow quicker return to competition and decreased risk of refracture. Surgery is indicated for symptomatic nonunion using intramedullary compression screw fixation and possible bone grafting (22). Consideration should be given to treatment of the underlying cavus foot. After operative fixation, the patient should be in a short leg cast for two weeks and then switched to a walking boot walker with progressive weight bearing for 3 to 4 weeks. The patient may progress to full activity 8 weeks postoperatively (23). The Jones fracture should not be confused with the dancer's fracture, which is an avulsion of the tuberosity of the fifth metatarsal **(Fig 51-4)**. These fractures do well with nonoperative treatment.

Midfoot

Cuboid

Stress fractures of the cuboid are rare and occur in runners. A case report of fatigue fracture of the cuboid occurring in collegiate athletes showed that, on presentation, the injury mimicked peroneal tendonitis (24). The cuboid is not subjected to the load bearing stresses of the medial column, and

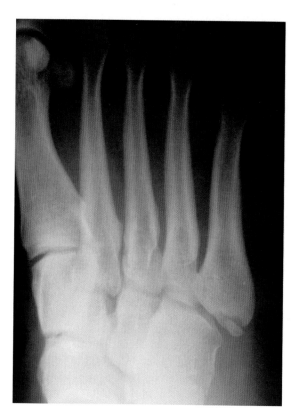

Fig 51-4. X-ray of the dancer's fracture.

therefore these injuries are uncommon. It should be suspected in the athlete with localized cuboid tenderness. Treatment consists of immobilization for 4 to 6 weeks followed by gradual return to activity. These fractures may have the potential to have a prolonged healing course, up to several months (24).

Cuneiform

Cuneiform stress fractures are also rare. Their location in the middle column of the foot predisposes them to compressive forces of weight bearing. The first cuneiform bears the most weight and is at greatest risk. The third cuneiform has articulations with six separate bones and may also be at risk. On x-ray, these will show as medullary sclerotic bands. These fractures follow with the classic history and imaging. Conservative treatment is recommended (25).

Navicular

Stress fractures in the navicular are common and difficult to diagnose and treat, with some cases requiring operative intervention. This entity was first described in 1970 by Towne et al. (26). These injuries are common in basketball, football, and track and field athletes. The diagnosis of navicular stress fracture may be difficult to make as the patient will complain of diffuse midfoot pain. The physical exam sign described by Khan is the "N" spot which is pain with direct pressure on the dorsal talonavicular articulation (27). Symptoms are reproducible with hopping on the affected foot in a plantar flexed position (28). Imaging should include plain films and

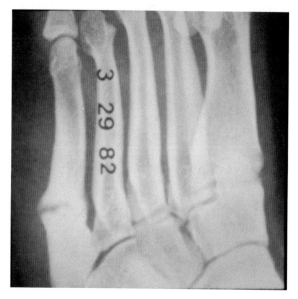

Fig 51-3. This is an x-ray of a patient with a chronic stress fracture of the fifth metatarsal. (Photo courtesy Dr. P. Kolodziej.)

bone scan. A CT scan will define the anatomy and displacement of the fracture (10). A linear sagittal fracture at the junction of the middle and lateral one-third of the navicular is the most common fracture pattern **(Fig 51-5)**. This occurs in the vascular watershed area in the navicular.

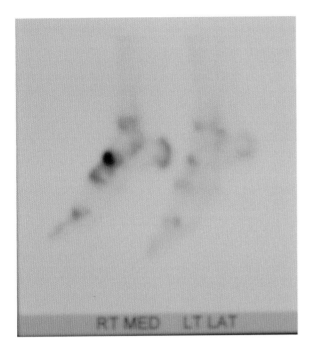

RT MED   LT LAT

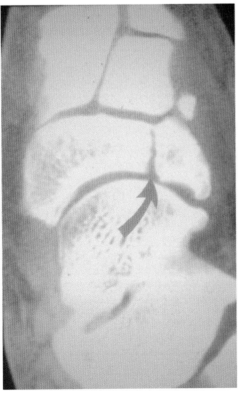

Fig 51-5. Bone scan and CT scan of a female collegiate basketball player with a stress fracture of her navicular. (Photo courtesy Dr. P. Kolodziej.)

Conservative therapy is the initial treatment. Quirk (29) describes a protocol of 6 weeks in a nonweight-bearing cast. The cast is removed after 6 weeks and the foot re-examined. If the "N" spot is still tender, the patient is recasted for 2 weeks. When asymptomatic, a gradual return to activity is initiated (29). Indications for surgical intervention include acute complete displaced fracture, delayed union, and nonunion.

An open reduction and internal fixation with a lag screw across the fracture, preferably from lateral to medial, is performed. In the acute setting this is sufficient. In the setting of delayed or nonunion, autologous bone grafting is recommended in addition to the lag screw fixation. Postoperatively the patient should be nonweight-bearing for 4 weeks, with gradual return to full weight bearing over the next 4 weeks. Return to full activity will require at least 3 months (23).

Hindfoot

Talus
Stress fractures of the talus are rare, but have been reported in the body, neck and lateral process (30,31,32). Talar neck fractures are reported in military literature, although lateral process fractures are more often seen in the athlete. The postulated mechanism of injury is excessive subtalar pronation and plantar flexion, causing the lateral process of the calcaneus to impinge on the lateral process of the talus. The diagnosis is often confused with severe sinus tarsi syndrome (30). Patients will present with chronic lateral ankle pain and decreased subtalar motion (31). CT scanning is important in the evaluation of any patient with decreased subtalar mobility. If a stress fracture is found the patient should be placed on 6 weeks of nonweight-bearing followed by gradual return to activity (30).

Calcaneus
Calcaneal stress fractures are more common than those in the talus. Patients will present with pain and swelling on both sides of the heel. These injuries occur in the military and in dancers (10). They will have pain with compression of the calcaneus from medial and lateral pressure. Patients will also have pain with toe walking and resisted plantar flexion (33). X-ray examination will reveal no changes initially, but after several weeks characteristic changes will be present. The fracture in the calcaneus occurs in cancellous bone, giving a band of sclerosis perpendicular to the long axis of the calcaneus. The fracture is generally located between the calcaneal tuberosity and the posterior articular surface for the talus (34). Calcaneal stress fractures are usually nondisplaced and treated by cessation of offending activity with a heel pad in the shoe until symptoms are resolved.

Leg

Fibula
Stress fractures of the fibula were originally described by Burrows (35) in 1948. He classified these injuries into two groups. The first was in young male runners with the fractures

occurring 6 centimeters proximal to the distal tip of the lateral malleolus and the second group with middle aged females sustaining fractures 3 centimeters proximal to the distal tip (35). These distal fibula fractures are most common, but occasionally there may be high fibula stress fractures seen in runners (36). If the fracture is nondisplaced, treatment consists of nonweight-bearing until asymptomatic, usually 4 to 8 weeks (37). Displaced fractures should be treated with open reduction and internal fixation.

Medial Malleolus

Stress fracture of the medial malleolus was described in 1975 by Devas (38). Shelbourne et al. (39) further described the injury as occurring at the junction of the medial malleolus and tibial plafond. Athletes will complain of pain over the medial malleolus and will have point tenderness. X-rays will demonstrate a vertical fissure at the junction of the medial malleolus and the tibial plafond. If fracture is visualized on x-ray, open reduction and internal fixation is recommended (39). If fracture is not visualized on plain film, but bone scan is positive, conservative therapy is warranted. In the case of nonunion, open reduction and internal fixation with bone grafting is indicated (40).

Tibial Shaft

The large majority of stress fractures are found in the tibial shaft, up to 73% in some studies (41). Tibial shaft stress fractures are subdivided into fractures of the posterior and anterior tibia. These two types vary greatly in their cause and treatment. Posterior fractures are more common and are caused by compressive forces. Anterior fractures are caused by tensile forces and harder to treat. Runners typically injure the posterior middle and distal third, although jumping athletes such as dancers, volleyball, and basketball players injure the anterior cortex. Transverse and oblique patterns are more common, although longitudinal and spiral patterns occur occasionally (37). Differential diagnosis includes medial tibial stress syndrome, peripheral nerve compression, and exercise induced compartment syndrome.

Bone scan of posterior fractures initially shows a diffuse uptake pattern and later shows a sharply marginated fusiform uptake pattern. After diagnosis, posterior stress fractures of the tibial shaft are treated with nonweight-bearing cast immobilization of 8 to 12 weeks. Pneumatic bracing may facilitate earlier return to sport (37).

Anterior stress fractures of the tibia present a very difficult rehabilitation problem. These fractures are more likely to progress to complete fracture or go on to nonunion compared to posterior tibial stress fractures (42). If x-ray demonstrates a solitary anterior cortical fracture, surrounded by sclerosis, this is representative of a nonunion that will progress to complete fracture and requires operative fixation (11). Poor blood supply and musculotendinous support in addition to tensile loads contribute to the delayed healing of this injury (37). Conservative therapy of this injury entails 6 months of no running or jumping, with graduated return to

sport. Electrical stimulation may be beneficial to healing as this is a tensile injury. Delayed or nonunions should have surgical intervention at 3 to 6 months (42). For undisplaced fractures the cortex is drilled to stimulate bone growth. In nonunion or complete fracture reamed intermedullary nailing with bone grafting is the treatment of choice. This difficult injury will take an average of nine months to heal (37).

Treatment

If initial x-rays are negative, the athlete should be placed on 2 weeks of rest from the offending activity. They may cross train during this time with swimming, cycling, water running, or other nonimpact cardiovascular exercises. After 2 weeks the patient should be re-examined. If symptomatic, a bone scan should be ordered at that time. If fatigue fracture is diagnosed, most will respond to restricted activity for 3 to 6 weeks (7).

■ CONCLUSION

Stress fractures of the lower extremity are commonly seen in the athletic population. Stress fractures of the navicular, fifth metatarsal, and anterior cortex of the tibial shaft are the most problematic to treat. Stress fracture should always be considered when evaluating and athlete with lower extremity pain. With the proper index of suspicion, these injuries can be diagnosed early in their course. In most cases with appropriate nonoperative treatment, patients will return to their prior level of competition.

■ REFERENCES

1. Breithaupt. Zur Pathologie des menschlichen fusses. *Med Zeitung.* 1855;24–169.
2. Schmidt Brudvig TJ, Gudger TD, Obermeyer L. Stress fractures in 295 trainees: a one year study of incidence as related to age, sex, and race. *Mil Med.* 1983;148:666–667.
3. Belkin SC. Stress fractures in athletes. *Orthop Clin North Am.* 1980;11(4):735–742.
4. Matheson GO, Clement DB, McKenzie DC, et al. Stress fractures in athletes. *Am J Sports Med.* 1987;15(1):46–58.
5. Bennell KL, Malcolm SA, Thomas SA, et al. The incidence and distribution of stress fractures in competitive track and field athletes. *Am J Sports Med.* 1996;24(2):211–217.
6. Verma RB, Sherman O. Athletic stress fractures: part I. History, epidemiology, physiology, risk factors, radiography, diagnosis, and treatment. *Am J Sports Orthop.* 2001;30(11):798–806.
7. Meyer SA, Saltzman CL, Albright JP. Stress fractures of the foot and leg. *Clin Sports Med.* 1993;12(2):395–413.
8. Korpelainen R, Orava S, Karpakka J, et al. Risk factors for recurrent stress fractures in athletes. *Am J Sports Med.* 2001;29(3):304–310.
9. Giladi M, Milgrom C, Simkin A, et al. Stress fractures. Identifiable risk factors. *Am J Sports Med.* 1991;19(6):647–652.
10. Eisele SA, Sammarco GJ. ICL, AAOS. Fatigue fractures of the foot and ankle in the athlete. *J Bone Joint Surg.* 1993;75:290–298.

11. Umans H, Pavlov H. Stress fractures of the lower extremities. *Semin Roentgenol*. 1994;29:176–193.

12. Anderson RB, McBryde AM Jr. Autogenous bone grafting of hallux sesamoid nonunions. *Foot Ankle Int*. 1997;18:293–296.

13. Hulkko A, Orava S, Pellinen P, et al. Stress fractures of the sesamoid bones of the first metatarsophalangeal joint in athletes. *Arch Orthop Traum Surg*. 1985;104:113–117.

14. Van Hal ME, Keene JS, Lange TA, et al. Stress fractures of the great toe sesamoids. *Am J Sports Med*. 1982;10:122–128.

15. Chisin R, Peyser A, Milgrom C. Bone scintigraphy in the assessment of the hallucal sesamoids. *Foot Ankle Int*. 1995;16:291–294.

16. Shiraishi M, Mizuta H, Kubota K, et al. Stress fracture of the proximal phalanx of the great toe. *Foot Ankle*. 1993;14:28–34.

17. Drez D Jr, Young JC, Johnston RD, et al. Metatarsal stress fractures. *Am J Sports Med*. 1980;8:123–125.

18. Lucas MJ, Baxter DE. Stress fracture of the first metatarsal. *Foot Ankle Int*. 1997;18:373–374.

19. O'Malley MJ, Hamilton WG, Munyak J, et al. Stress fractures at the base of the second metatarsal in ballet dancers. *Foot Ankle Int*. 1996;17:89–94.

20. Harrington T, Crichton KJ, Anderson IF. Overuse ballet injury of the base of the second metatarsal. *Am J Sports Med*. 1993; 21:591–598.

21. Jones R. Fracture of the base of the fifth metatarsal bone by indirect violence. *Ann Surg*. 1902;35:697–700.

22. Rettig AC, Shelbourne KD, Wilckens J. The surgical treatment of symptomatic nonunions of the proximal (metaphyseal) fifth metatarsal in athletes. *Am J Sports Med*. 1992;20:50–54.

23. Marder RA. Stress fractures. In: Chapman MW, ed. *Chapman's orthopaedic surgery*. 3rd ed. Philadelphia: Lippincott Williams & Wilkins; 2001:2485–2491.

24. Beaman DN, Roeser WM, Homes JR, Saltzman CL. Cuboid stress fractures: a report of two cases. *Foot Ankle*. 1993;14:525–528.

25. Meurman KOA, Elfving S. Stress fracture of the cuneiform bones. *Br J Radiol*. 1980;53:157–160.

26. Towne L, Blazina M, Cozen L. Fatigue fracture of the tarsal navicular. *J Bone Joint Surg*. 1970;52:376–378.

27. Khan K, Brukner P, Kearney C, et al. Tarsal navicular stress fractures in athletes. *Sports Med*. 1994;17:65–76.

28. Ostlie DK, Simons SM. Tarsal navicular fracture in a young athlete. *J Am Board Fam Pract*. 2001;14:381–385.

29. Quirk R. Stress fractures of the navicular. *Foot Ankle Int*. 1998;19(7):494–496.

30. Bradshaw C, Khan K, Brukner P. Stress fracture of the body of the talus in athletes demonstrated with computer tomography. *Clin J Sport Med*. 1996;6:48–51.

31. Motto S. Stress fracture of the lateral process of the talus-a case report. *Br J Sports Med*. 1993;27(4):275–276.

32. Black KP, Ehlert KJ. A stress fracture of the lateral process of the talus in a runner. A case report. *J Bone Joint Surg*. 1994;76A(3): 441–443.

33. Hopson CN, Perry DR. Stress fractures of the calcaneus in women marine recruits. *Clin Orthop Rel Res*. 1977;128:159–162.

34. Darby RE. Stress fractures of the os calcis. *JAMA*. 1967;200(13): 131–133.

35. Burrows HJ. Fatigue fractures of the fibula. *J Bone Joint Surg*. 1948;30B(2):266–279.

36. Miller MD, Marks PH, Fu FH. Bilateral stress fractures of the distal fibula in a 35 year old woman. *Foot Ankle Int*. 1994; 15(8):450–453.

37. Verma RB, Sherman O. Athletic stress fractures: part II. The lower body. *Am J Sports Orthop*. 2001;30:848–860.

38. Devas M. *Stress fractures*. Churchill Livingstone; 1975:93.

39. Shelbourne KD, Fisher DA, Rettig AC, et al. Stress fractures of the medial malleolus. *Am J Sports Med*. 1988;16:60–63.

40. Reider B, Falconiero R, Yurkofsky J. Nonunion of a medial malleolus stress fracture. *Am J Sports Med*. 1993;21:478–481.

41. Greaney RB, Gerber FH, Laughlin RL. Distribution and natural history of stress fractures in US Marine recruits. *Radiology*. 1983;146:339–346.

42. Rettig AC, Shelbourne KD, McCarroll JR, et al. The natural history and treatment of delayed union stress fractures of the anterior cortex of the tibia. *Am J Sports Med*. 1988;16:250–255.

52

LIGAMENTOUS LISFRANC JOINT INJURIES: LEG/ ANKLE/FOOT: MIDFOOT INJURIES, LISFRANC

■ MICHAEL S. ARONOW, MD

■ KEY POINTS

- The tarsometatarsal (TMT), or Lisfranc, joints consist of the five metatarsals and their articulation with the corresponding cuneiforms and cuboid.
- The first, second, and third TMT joints undergo slight dorsiflexion, plantarflexion, supination, and pronation motion that helps absorb shock; however, their principal function is to act as a rigid lever connecting the hindfoot to the forefoot.
- In a Lisfranc injury, there is instability, subluxation, or dislocation of the TMT joints secondary to ligament disruption often with associated bone fractures.
- In most displaced Lisfranc injuries, the relatively weak dorsal TMT ligaments are disrupted first, followed by rupture of stronger plantar and interosseus ligaments, which in conjunction with more substantial plantar soft tissue support, usually displaces the metatarsals dorsally.
- In severe injuries with dislocation of the TMT joints, there is pain, swelling, deformity, inability to bear weight, and occasionally neurovascular compromise.
- Visualization of the TMT joints is improved with the x-ray beam angled parallel to the TMT joint surfaces for the anteroposterior (AP) and 30 (degree) oblique views.
- An anatomic reduction of the TMT joints restoring articular congruity decreases the risk of arthritic pain and functional loss. Pure ligamentous injuries do not always heal and may cause long-term disability.
- Lisfranc injuries without subluxation on weight-bearing or stress x-rays are treated nonoperatively.
- Immediate intervention is required in the presence of open injuries, forefoot compartment syndrome, or

neurovascular compromise of the forefoot. Significant deformity and dislocation requires early reduction, preferably open reduction with fixation, to prevent further skin, soft tissue, or neurovascular compromise.

- Outcomes after Lisfranc injury improve with quality of TMT joint reduction. Factors causing poor outcome include high-energy injuries with increased initial articular and soft-tissue damage, delay in diagnosis, and possibly pure ligamentous injuries.

■ BASIC SCIENCE

Anatomy

The tarsometatarsal (TMT), or Lisfranc, joints consist of the five metatarsals and their articulation with the corresponding cuneiforms and cuboid. TMT joint stability comes from a combination of bone morphology, ligaments, and soft tissue support **(Fig 52-1)**. The second metatarsal base forms a keystone where it articulates with all three cuneiforms. The metatarsal bases, cuneiforms, and cuboid are wedge-shaped bones that form a stable roman arch configuration. Ligaments cross the TMT, naviculo-cuneiform, and intercuneiform joints. Ligaments connect the second through fifth metatarsal bases, but not the first and second. The strong interosseus Lisfranc's ligament connects the medial cuneiform to the medial second metatarsal base. There is a less strong plantar ligament from the medial cuneiform to the plantar aspect of the second and third metatarsal bases and a weaker still dorsal ligament from the medial cuneiform to the medial second metatarsal base (1,2). Additional plantar arch support comes from the

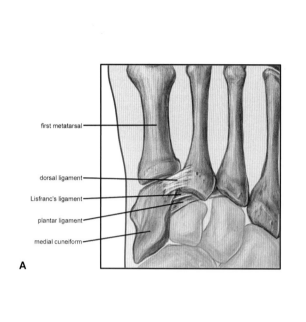

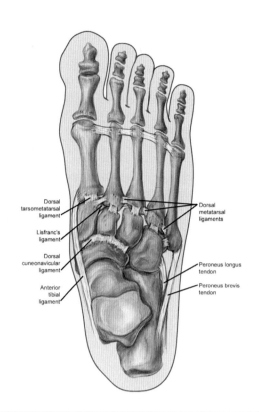

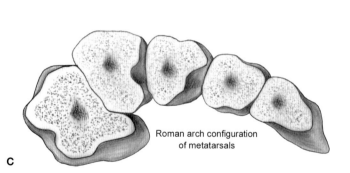

Roman arch configuration of metatarsals

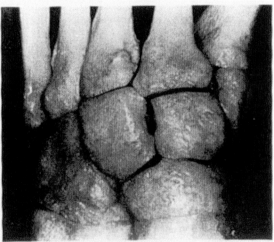

Fig 52-1. Anatomy of the tarsometatarsal joints.

intrinsic foot muscles, and the posterior tibial, anterior tibial, and peroneus longus tendons. The plantar fascia acts as a tie rod to support the arch.

Biomechanics

The first, second, and third TMT joints undergo slight dorsiflexion, plantarflexion, supination, and pronation motion that helps absorb shock; however, their principal function is to act as a rigid lever connecting the hindfoot to the forefoot. The fourth and fifth TMT joints have more motion which helps accommodate the forefoot on uneven terrain (3).

In a Lisfranc injury, there is instability, subluxation, or dislocation of the TMT joints secondary to ligament disruption and/or bone fractures. Lisfranc injuries occur by both direct and indirect mechanisms. Motor vehicle accidents and crush injuries are examples of direct injuries with dorsally or plantarly directed blows with a rotational component. The indirect mechanism of injury involves an axial force to a plantarflexed foot with subsequent rotation. Examples include a fall on the stairs, sports injuries when another player lands on the posterior heel of the plantarflexed foot, or with abduction of a foot fixed in a stirrup in equestrian and windsurfing injuries. In most displaced

Lisfranc injuries the relatively weak dorsal TMT ligaments are disrupted first, followed by rupture of stronger plantar and interosseus ligaments, which in conjunction with more substantial plantar soft tissue support, usually displaces the metatarsals dorsally.

■ CLINICAL EVALUATION

History and Physical Findings

In severe injuries with dislocation of the TMT joints there is pain, swelling, deformity, inability to bear weight, and occasionally neurovascular compromise. In subtle injuries there is usually pain, swelling, and tenderness, although it is usually less extensive and may be limited to the area over Lisfranc's ligament. Heel weight-bearing is painful, but often possible. There may be a *plantar ecchymosis sign* (4) in which there is ecchymosis of the plantar medial arch or a *gap sign* (5) in which there is diastasis between the hallux and second toe. There may be no deformity or loss of the medial longitudinal arch with weight-bearing only. Often the diagnosis is made late as the investigations are equivocal, or nonweight-bearing views obtained.

Imaging

Weight-bearing anteroposterior (AP), 30 degree oblique, and lateral views of the foot are taken with the ankle in dorsiflexion. For subtle injuries comparison views of the foot are performed at the same time. Visualization of the TMT joints is improved with the x-ray beam angled parallel to the TMT joint surfaces for the AP and 30 degree oblique views (about 17 degrees from perpendicular to the floor, which can be measured on the lateral x-ray). If x-rays do not show subluxation or dislocation, stress x-rays should be taken to rule out ligamentous instability. The cuboid and medial cuneiform are stabilized and then the AP view is repeated while abducting, adducting, and then divergently stressing the first and second metatarsals. Often a *fleck sign* (6) is seen, representing an avulsion fracture of the medial second metatarsal base at the attachment site of Lisfranc's ligament. Other fractures within the midfoot can occur, including a compression fracture of the cuboid. Magnetic resonance imaging (MRI) and computed tomography (CT) may show fractures not seen by plain x-ray, TMT joint subluxation, and Lisfranc ligament disruption (7). In a cadaver study, unlike computerized tomography, plain radiographs could not detect 1 mm of second TMT joint displacement and could not detect 2 mm of displacement 33% of the time (8). Because MRI or CT can rarely be obtained with simulated weight-bearing, however, TMT joint subluxation may be missed on these investigations. Bone scans can confirm TMT joint injury or sprain in the absence of TMT joint subluxation.

Decision Making Algorithms and Classification

After the diagnosis of a Lisfranc injury has been made by history, physical examination, and imaging studies, the amount of TMT or inter-cuneiform joint malalignment must be determined. While multiple criteria for "significant" displacement have been advocated, the amount of subluxation or displacement resulting in a poorer functional outcome has not been definitively determined. Athletes tolerate less displacement as they expect a higher level of function.

In most clinical studies, the indications for surgical intervention and the assessment of reduction are based on the distance between the lateral border of the first metatarsal and the medial border of the second metatarsal (6,9–19). The radiographic criteria for an anatomic reduction has ranged from a first-second metatarsal distance of ≤2 mm (6,9,11,15,16) to ≤5 mm (12,19). In two studies (11,14), the foot with a Lisfranc injury had a first-second metatarsal distance of between 2 to 5 mm, while the distance in the normal contralateral foot was noted to average either 1.3 mm (10) or range from to 1 to 5 mm (14). As the anatomy varies between different patients the assessment should be based on the opposite uninjured foot.

Although it more directly reflects disruption of Lisfranc's ligament, the distance between the lateral border of the medial cuneiform and the medial border of the second metatarsal has been used less commonly. In one study, MRI and weight-bearing x-rays were taken of both the injured and contralateral normal foot. The medial cuneiform-second metatarsal distance ranged from 2 to 5 mm on x-rays of the normal foot. On MRI, the distance ranged from 1 mm less to 3 mm more than the normal side in 18 patients with MRI-determined partial Lisfranc ligament tears, and was at least 2 mm greater than the uninjured foot in three patients with complete Lisfranc ligament ruptures (14).

Malalignment of the first and second TMT joints can be measured on the AP x-ray and the third and fourth TMT joints on the 30 degree oblique (20). The medial and lateral aspects of the first, second, and third metatarsal should line up with the medial and lateral aspects of the medial, intermediate, and lateral cuneiform, respectively. The medial aspect of the fourth metatarsal should line up with the medial aspect of the cuboid. In most displaced Lisfranc injuries at least one of the medial two TMT joints will be subluxed. The exception is isolated injuries to both the medial-intermediate intercuneiform and Lisfranc's ligaments in which only the medial cuneiform-second metatarsal distance and first-second metatarsal distance will be increased. Open reduction and internal fixation has been recommended for 2 mm or more displacement of any of the TMT joints (21). In cadavers, 1 mm of dorsolateral displacement of the second metatarsal produced an average of 13.1% decreased second TMT joint contact, 2 mm of dorsolateral displacement produced an average of 25.5% decreased second TMT joint contact, and 4 mm of dorsolateral displacement produced an average of 50.6% decreased second TMT joint contact (22).

On an AP abduction stress x-ray, a Lisfranc injury is likely if a line drawn tangential to the medial aspect of the medial cuneiform and navicular does not intersect the first metatarsal base (23).

On the lateral x-ray the dorsal and plantar aspects of the metatarsals should line up with the corresponding cuneiform or cuboid. Faciszewski et al. (11) found patients with flattening of the longitudinal arch had a poor prognosis and should undergo open reduction and internal fixation. They defined a flattened arch as when the medial cuneiform was plantar to the fifth metatarsal base or when the same distance was 1.5 mm greater than the normal foot. Myerson et al. (6) recommended open reduction if the lateral talo-first metatarsal angle was greater than 15 degrees. However, all three of these lateral x-ray findings may be occasionally seen in patients with asymptomatic, atraumatic flatfoot deformities.

■ LISFRANC INJURY CLASSIFICATION

The most commonly used classification system is Myerson et al.'s (6) modification of Hardcastle et al.'s (24) modification of Quenu and Kuss's (25) classification (Fig 52-2). There are three main types: Total Incongruity—all five metatarsals subluxing the same direction (Type A); Partial Incongruity—the first metatarsal subluxing medially (Type B_1) or one or more of the lateral four metatarsals subluxing laterally (Type B_2) with or without a component of dorsal/plantar subluxation; and Divergent—the first metatarsal subluxing medially and some (Type C_1) or all four (Type C_2) of the lateral four metatarsals subluxing laterally and/or dorsal/plantarly.

Nunley and Vertullo (26) described a midfoot sprain classification system for athletes. Stage I is a Lisfranc ligament sprain with no diastasis or arch height loss seen on weight-bearing radiographs but increased uptake on bone scintigrams. Stage II sprains have a 1 to 5 mm diastasis between the first and second metatarsals compared to the contralateral foot with no arch height loss. Stage III sprains have a first to second metatarsal diastasis greater than 5 mm and loss of arch height as described by Faciszewski et al. (11). Only Stage I and II sprains were reported on in their study.

■ TREATMENT

The goal of treatment is a pain-free functional foot. An anatomic reduction of the TMT joints restoring articular congruity should decrease the risk of developing painful arthritis and preserve function. The reduction should be maintained until ligamentous stability has been restored to preserve the height of the longitudinal arch. With rare exception (27), most studies show outcome after Lisfranc injury improves with better TMT joint reduction (6,9,10,12,13,15,16,19, 24,28–35). This stability may be obtained fairly quickly in incomplete ligament tears or after bone healing of large avulsion fractures attached to Lisfranc's ligament. Ligamentous stability takes longer or may not occur at all in patients with pure ligamentous injuries or a small Lisfranc's ligament avulsion fracture (32,33). As a principle of general trauma care, treatment should also minimize additional trauma to the soft tissues and articular surfaces.

Nonoperative Treatment

Lisfranc injuries without subluxation on weight-bearing or stress x-rays are treated nonoperatively. One protocol involves 6 weeks nonweight-bearing in a cast or removable brace followed by gradual increased activity and custom orthotic support. All seven patients in Nunley and Vertullo's study (26) with Stage I sprains had an excellent outcome with return to sport in 11 to 18 weeks using this protocol. Shapiro et al. (36) treated eight patients with subtle Lisfranc injuries and a 2 to 3 mm first-second metatarsal distance on weight-bearing x-rays. They allowed touch down weight-bearing in a cast or splint. All eight returned to athletics at an average of 13 weeks (range 6 to 20 weeks), were asymptomatic, and had no x-ray changes. In another study of collegiate football players with nonoperatively treated midfoot sprains, players with lateral midfoot tenderness had shorter

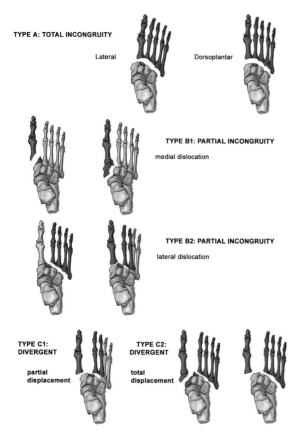

Fig 52-2. Lisfranc injury classification. (Reprinted from Myerson MS, Fisher RT, Burgess AR, et al. Fracture dislocations of the TMT joints: end results correlated with pathology and treatment. *Foot Ankle*. 1986;6:228; with permission.)

periods of disability than those with medial and global tenderness (37). At mean 30.8 month follow-up, thirteen athletes had no pain or swelling, five noted minor residual pain or stiffness after athletic activity, and one had ongoing pain requiring him to alter his recreational activity.

Low demand or high surgical risk patients with mild subluxation may also be treated nonoperatively. Many will do reasonably well with respect to pain and function and the remainder may benefit from late reconstruction.

Operative Treatment

Indications

Current standard of care dictates open or indirect reduction and surgical fixation for all displaced or unstable Lisfranc injuries.

I consider a medial cuneiform second metatarsal distance 2 mm or greater than the normal contralateral side, or greater than 2 mm metatarsal subluxation relative to the corresponding cuneiform or medial cuboid an indication for surgical reduction. Absolute surgical indications include open injuries, foot compartment syndrome, significant vascular injury, and irreducible dislocation secondary to interposed anterior tibial tendon, capsule, or bone fragments.

If an anatomic reduction can be obtained, closed reduction and percutaneous fixation is an acceptable option; however, most surgeons recommend open reduction to allow removal of interposed intra-articular capsule, cartilage, or bone fragments and to confirm the accuracy of reduction with direct visualization (9,13,15,21,29–34,38).

Primary TMT joint arthrodesis is indicated if there is severe articular cartilage damage making symptomatic post-traumatic arthritis likely. Some surgeons feel that primary TMT joint arthrodesis is also indicated in the presence of pure ligamentous Lisfranc injuries without fracture or with only a small *fleck sign*, given the normal limited motion of the medial three TMT joints and the risk of recurrent deformity and post-traumatic arthritis. Primary arthrodesis is indicated for late reconstruction of unrecognized symptomatic injuries. An attempt should be made to preserve the more mobile fourth and fifth TMT joints. If there is severe articular cartilage damage or peri-articular bone loss, a fourth and fifth TMT joint interpositional arthroplasty using the peroneus tertius or extensor digitorum brevis muscle belly is preferred over arthrodesis (39).

Timing

Immediate intervention is required in the presence of open injuries, forefoot compartment syndrome, or neurovascular compromise of the forefoot. Significant deformity and dislocation requires early reduction, preferably open reduction with fixation, to prevent further skin, soft tissue, or neurovascular compromise. Should significant soft tissue swelling or skin issues such as fracture blisters prevent safe open reduction, closed reduction should be performed to decrease deformity. Lesser deformities are addressed when the soft tissues are ready, ideally when abrasions and fracture blisters have healed over the future incision sites and the skin wrinkles. While surgery, particularly in the presence of associated fractures, is more difficult after 10 to 14 days post injury, open reduction and internal fixation may be performed 6 weeks or later if needed (32).

Technique

Fixation is recommended after open or closed reduction. Options include K-wires, screws, plates, and external fixation. Trans-articular screw fixation is considered the current treatment gold standard for the medial three TMT joints (9,13,15,17,18,21,29–33,38). Screws provide rigid fixation and can be placed percutaneously. They have a lower infection risk than K-wires; however, there are several disadvantages with screw fixation of Lisfranc injuries. Because the screws are trans-articular, their placement further damages the articular cartilage of the joints that an attempt is being made to preserve. Screw breakage can occur and removal can be technically difficult. This may be necessary as intra-articular broken screws may cause further joint damage. The fear of screw breakage may delay early rehabilitation, including weight bearing and range of motion exercises. Either the normal limited functional motion of these joints is eliminated (40), or a second operation for screw removal is required. Although this second operation can be avoided by using absorbable screws (21,38), these screws are less rigid than those made of metal, their insertion still damages the articular cartilage, and there may be a risk of further joint damage from the screw breakdown products.

K-wires can be inserted percutaneously, cause less joint damage than K-wires, are simple to insert, and can be removed in the clinic; however, K-wires can back out through bone causing loss of reduction. The K-wires may become infected and require removal before the ligaments are healed (29,30,32,38). Currently, K-wires are principally used for stabilizing the more mobile fourth and fifth TMT joints, which often are transfixed for as little duration as 6 weeks. They may be used for very comminuted fracture/dislocations that are not amenable to screw fixation (21). They also can be used after closed reduction when soft tissue swelling, skin quality, or patient morbidity makes the risk of open incisions too high.

Plates can rigidly stabilize TMT joints without further damaging the articular cartilage, can span comminuted fractures, and there is no risk of intra-articular screw breakage. Plates, however, require much larger soft tissue dissection for placement, are usually placed on the dorsal compression rather than tension side of the TMT joints, are more prominent, and may require a second operation for hardware removal.

External fixation is appropriate for Grade III open fractures, can be used to span significantly comminuted fractures, does not further damage the articular surfaces, and is easily removed. However, it is more difficult to obtain and maintain an anatomic reduction and usually there is less rigid joint fixation.

Screws, plates, and K-wires are often placed across the subluxable TMT joints, stabilizing the first, second, and/or third metatarsal to their corresponding cuneiform or in the case of the fourth and fifth metatarsal, to the cuboid. In cases of diastasis, fixation may also be placed from the medial cuneiform to the second metatarsal base and/or from the medial cuneiform to the intermediate cuneiform **(Fig 52-3)**.

Closed reduction of dislocations is aided by hanging the foot using mesh finger traps on the toes and manipulating the metatarsals into position. Reduction may be assisted with percutaneously placed clamps over the medial aspect of the medial cuneiform and the lateral aspect of the second metatarsal base. If an anatomic reduction can be confirmed by fluoroscopy, fixation may be achieved percutaneously using K-wires or cannulated screws.

Open reduction and internal fixation is performed through one or two dorsal longitudinal incision(s). The medial incision is made overlying the interval between the first and second TMT joints. The first TMT joint is exposed either medial to the extensor hallucis longus tendon or between the tendons of the extensor hallucis longus and extensor hallucis brevis. Care is taken to protect the adjacent branch of the dorsal medial cutaneous branch of the superficial peroneal nerve. Dissecting superficial to the dorsalis pedis artery and deep peroneal nerve, the second TMT joint is exposed in the interval between the extensor hallucis brevis muscle and the second toe extensor digitorum longus tendon. The incision is extensile proximally to the naviculo-cuneiform joint. If the third TMT joint cannot be accessed from this incision and remains displaced, a second dorsal longitudinal incision is made overlying the interval between

the third and fourth TMT joints. Taking care to avoid branches of the superficial peroneal nerve, the third and fourth TMT joints can be exposed by dissecting between the extensor digitorum longus tendons and splitting the extensor digitorum brevis muscle or going between its tendons. A transverse incision has also been described but is less extensile (41).

The TMT joints are inspected and hematoma, small comminuted bone and cartilage fragments, and interposed capsule removed. The second metatarsal is reduced with the aid of a clamp between its lateral base and the medial aspect of the medial cuneiform. After anatomic reduction is confirmed by direct visualization and fluoroscopy, the second metatarsal is stabilized to the cuneiforms with screws or a plate. If needed, the first and third TMT, intercuneiform, and naviculo-cuneiform joints are reduced and stabilized. The fourth and fifth TMT joints may need reduction and stabilization with percutaneously placed K-wires from the fifth metatarsal base, and (less commonly) the fourth metatarsal base, into the cuboid. The interosseus Lisfranc ligament and the dorsal capsular ligaments are repaired if possible. Attempts to reconstruct Lisfranc's ligament with autologous tendons such as the extensor digitorum longus, peroneus tertius, and plantaris, allograft tendons, periosteal flaps, and synthetic material have been described, but no published results are available.

Postoperative management involves 6 weeks in a non-weight-bearing cast followed by 6 to 10 weeks progressive weight-bearing in a CAM walker or orthotic. In athletes or reliable patients with stable fixation, consideration can be made for early motion and limited protected weight-bearing to decrease muscle atrophy, disuse osteopenia, and joint stiffness.

K-wires across the fourth and fifth TMT joints are usually removed 6 to 12 weeks postoperatively. Fixation of the first, second, and third TMT joints should ideally be left in place for at least 3 to 4 months to allow sufficient ligamentous healing. Earlier removal increases the risk of recurrent TMT joint subluxation. Whether or not the hardware should be removed after 3 to 4 months is controversial, as the risks of the second procedure may outweigh the benefits.

■ COMPLICATIONS AND SPECIAL CONSIDERATIONS

Outcomes after Lisfranc injury improve with quality of TMT joint reduction (6,9,10,12,13,15,16,19,24,28–35). Factors causing a poor outcome include high energy injuries with increased initial articular and soft tissue damage (30), delay in diagnosis (41), and possibly pure ligamentous injuries (33). The results of open or closed reduction and fixation of displaced Lisfranc injuries are better than those with no reduction or closed reduction without fixation (6,12,13,15,29–31).

An anatomic reduction does not guarantee a good result (6,9,15,17,19,30,33–35,38). Reasons for a less optimal result after anatomic reduction include concurrent local soft tissue

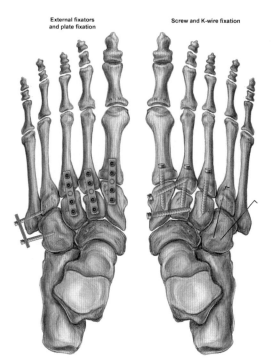

External fixators
and plate fixation

Screw and K-wire fixation

Fig 52-3. Lisfranc injury fixation methods.

or nerve injury, traumatic injuries to other parts of the body, inadequacy of ligamentous healing resulting in TMT sub-luxation after hardware removal, and TMT joint arthritis.

Lisfranc injuries are associated with neurovascular injury, compartment syndrome, infection, symptomatic and/or bro-ken hardware, post-traumatic arthritis, and residual defor-mity. Abduction and dorsiflexion of the TMT joints will cause loss of the longitudinal arch. This may be mistaken for or cause posterior tibial tendon dysfunction.

Poor outcomes occur when the TMT joints heal with residual displacement (6,9,10,12,13,15,16,19,24,28–35). This may be caused by misdiagnosis, inadequate reduction, or inadequate fixation.

Late conservative treatment of a symptomatic patient includes orthotic or brace support, anti-inflammatory med-ication, corticosteroid injection, and activity modification. Surgical options include reduction and fusion of the medial three TMT joints (43). With respect to significant arthritis of the more mobile fourth and fifth TMT joints, resection arthroplasty (39) is generally preferable to arthrodesis.

■ CONCLUSIONS AND FUTURE DIRECTIONS

Midfoot injuries require a high degree of suspicion to avoid missing a Lisfranc injury. Treatment should obtain and maintain anatomic reduction of the TMT joints. This pre-vents late arthritic change and preserves the arch of the foot.

The current gold standard treatment for displaced or unstable Lisfranc injuries is open reduction internal fixation with trans-articular metallic screw fixation for the medial three TMT joints and percutaneous K-wire fixation for the fourth and fifth. In the future there may be a greater role for absorbable fixation, primary arthrodesis, and ligament reconstruction.

■ REFERENCES

1. Kura H, Luo Z, Kitaoka H, et al. Mechanical behavior of the Lisfranc and dorsal cuneometatarsal ligamnets: In vitro biome-chanical study. *J Orthop Trauma*. 2001;15:107–110.
2. Solan M, Moorman C III, Miyamoto RG, et al. Ligamentous restraints of the second tarsometatarsal joint: a biomechanical evaluation. *Foot Ankle Int*. 2001;22:637–641.
3. Ouzounian T, Shereff MJ. In vitro determination of midfoot motion. *Foot Ankle*. 1989;10:140–146.
4. Ross G, Cronin R, Hauzenblas J, et al. Plantar ecchymosis sign: a clinical aid to diagnosis of occult Lisfranc tarsometatarsal injuries. *J Orthop Trauma*. 1996;10:119–122.
5. Davies MS, Saxby TS. Intercuneiform instability and the "gap" sign. *Foot Ankle Int*. 1999;20:606–629.
6. Myerson MS, Fisher RT, Burgess AR, et al. Fracture dislocations of the tarsometatarsal joints: End results correlated with pathol-ogy and treatment. *Foot Ankle*. 1986;6:225–242.
7. Peicha G, Preidler KW, Lajtai G, et al. Diagnostic value of con-ventional roentgen image, computerized and magnetic resonance

8. tomography in acute sprains of the foot. A prospective clinical study. *Unfallchirurg*. 2001;104:1134–1139.
8. Lu J, Ebraheim NA, Skie M, et al. Radiographic and computed tomographic evaluation of Lisfranc dislocation: a cadaver study. *Foot Ankle Int*. 1997;18:351–355.
9. Bloome DM, Clanton TO. Treatment of Lisfranc injuries in the athlete. *Tech Foot Ankle Surg*. 2002;1:94–101.
10. Cassebaum WH. Lisfrance fracture-dislocations. *Clin Orthop*. 1964;30:116–128.
11. Faciszewski T, Burks R, Manaster BJ. Subtle injuries of the lis-franc joint. *J Bone Joint Surg*. 1990;72A:1519–1522.
12. Goossens M, DeStoop N. Lisfranc's fracture-dislocations: etiology, radiology, and results of treatment. *Clin Orthop*. 1983;176:154–162.
13. Myerson MS. The diagnosis and treatment of injury to the tarsometatarsal joint complex. *J Bone Joint Surg*. 2001;81B: 756–763.
14. Potter H, Deland JT, Gusmer PB, et al. Magnetic resonance imaging of the Lisfranc ligament of the foot. *Foot Ankle Int*. 1998;19:438–445.
15. Rutledge EW, Templeman DC, deSouza LJ. Evaluation and treatment of Lisfranc fracture-dislocations. *Foot Ankle Clin*. 1999;4:603–615.
16. Schenk RC Jr, Heckman JD. Fractures and dislocations of the forefoot: operative and nonoperative treatment. *J Am Acad Orthop*. 1995;3:70–78.
17. Teng AL, Pinzur MS, Lomasney L, et al. Functional outcome following anatomic restoration of tarsal-metatarsal fracture dislo-cation. *Foot Ankle Int*. 2002;23:922–926.
18. Trevino SG, Kodros S. Controversies in tarsometatarsal joints. *Orthop Clin North Am*. 1995;26:229–238.
19. Wilppula E. Tarsometatarsal fracture-dislocation: Late results in 26 patients. *Acta Orthop Scand*. 1973;44:335–345.
20. Stein RE. Radiological aspects of the tarsometatarsal joints. *Foot Ankle*. 1983;3:286–289.
21. Thordarson DB. Lisfranc ORIF with absorbable fixation. *Tech Foot Ankle Surg*. 2003;2:21–26.
22. Ebraheim NA, Yang H, Lu J, et al. Computer evaluation of second tarsometatarsal joint dislocation. *Foot Ankle Int*. 1996;17:685–689.
23. Coss H, Manos RE, Buoncristiani A, et al. Abduction stress and AP weightbearing radiography of purely ligamentous injury in the tarsometatarsal joint. *Foot Ankle Int*. 1998;19:538–541.
24. Hardcastle PH, Reschauer R, Kutscha-Lissberg E, et al. Injuries to the tarsometatarsal joint. *J Bone Joint Surg*. 1982;64B:349–356.
25. Quenu E, Kuss G. Etude sur les luxations du metatarse. *Reb Chir*. 1909;39:281–336.
26. Nunley JA, Vertullo CJ. Classification, investigation, and man-agement of midfoot sprains: Lisfranc injuries in the athlete. *Am J Sports Med*. 2002;30:871–878.
27. Brunet JA, Wiley JJ. The late results of tarsalmetatarsal joint injuries. *J Bone Joint Surg*. 1987;69B:437–440.
28. Aitken AP, Poulson D. Dislocations of the tarsometatarsal joint. *J Bone Joint Surg*. 1963;45A:246–260.
29. Arntz CT, Hansen ST. Dislocations and fracture dislocations of the tarsometatarsal joints. *Orthop Clin North Am*. 1987;18:105–114.
30. Arntz CT, Veith RG, Hansen ST. Fractures and fracture-dislocations of the tarsometatarsal joint. *J Bone Joint Surg*. 1988;70A:173–181.
31. Buzzard BM, Briggs PJ. Surgical management of acute tar-sometatarsal fracture dislocation in the adult. *Clin Orthop*. 1998;353:125–133.
32. Chiodo C, Myerson M. Developments and advances in the diag-nosis and treatment of injuries to the tarsometatarsal joint. *Orthop Clin North Am*. 2001;32:11–20.
33. Kuo R, Tejwani N, DiGiovanni CW, et al. Outcome after open reduction and internal fixation of Lisfranc joint injuries. *J Bone Joint Surg*. 2000;82A:1609–1618.
34. Resch S, Stenstrom A. The treatment of tarsometatarsal injuries. *Foot Ankle*. 1990;11:117–123.

35. Wiss DA, Kull DM, Perry J. Lisfranc fracture-dislocations of the foot: a clinical-kinesiological study. *J Ortho Trauma*. 1988;1:267–274.

36. Shapiro MS, Wascher DC, Finerman GA. Rupture of Lisfranc's ligament in athletes. *Am J Sports Med*. 1994;22:687–691.

37. Meyer SA, Callaghan JJ, Albright JP, et al. Midfoot sprains in collegiate football players. *Am J Sports Med*. 1994;22:392–401.

38. Thordarson DB, Hurwitz G. PLA screw fixation of Lisfranc injuries. *Foot Ankle Int.*. 2003;23:1003–1007.

39. Berlet GC, Anderson RB. Tendon arthroplasty for basal fourth and fifth metatarsal arthritis. *Foot Ankle Int*. 2002;23:440–446.

40. Lakin RC, DeGnore LT, Pienkowski D. Contact mechanics of normal tarsometatarsal joints. *J Bone Joint Surg*. 2001;83A: 520–528.

41. Vertullo CJ, Easley ME, Nunley JA. The transverse dorsal approach to the Lisfranc joint. *Foot Ankle Int*. 2002;23:420–426.

42. Curtis MJ, Myerson M, Szura B. Tarsometatarsal joint injuries in the athlete. *Am J Sports Med*. 1993;21:497–502.

43. Sangeorgan BJ, Veith R, Hansen ST. Salvage of Lisfranc's tarsometatarsal joint by arthrodesis. *Foot Ankle Int*. 1990;10: 193–200.

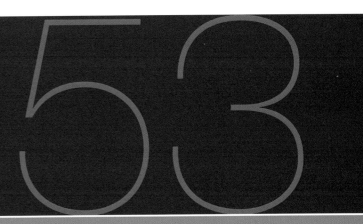

HALLUX VALGUS IN THE ATHLETE

WALTER J. PEDOWITZ, MD, DAVID I. PEDOWITZ, MD, MS

KEY POINTS

- First ray bunion deformity causes pain, difficulty with normal shoe wear, and loss of the normal biomechanical integrity of the forefoot in locomotion.
- Hallux valgus may result from a multitude of causes, which are divided into extrinsic and intrinsic events. The principal extrinsic cause is improperly fitted shoewear.
- Generally patients with hallux valgus have markedly reduced pain when they remove their shoes, while patients with hallux rigidus have pain with shoes on or off.
- Radiological studies for bunions should be done in the standing position. Any arthritis or deformity should be noted.
- Initial treatment of bunions should always be conservative. Continued pain after conservative care, split shoe requirements, and deformity that greatly interferes with lifestyle are appropriate reasons for operation.
- Bunion management in the high-performance athlete is challenging. Metatarsophalangeal (MTP) motion is essential in running, jumping, and dancing. Bunion surgery should be avoided in sprinters, high jumpers, pole vaulters, and ballet dancers because it will dramatically alter or terminate high performance.
- Interdigital or Morton's neuroma is an entrapment neuropathy of the plantar digital nerve, which is most common in the third intermetatarsal (IM) space. Trauma, bursal inflammation, a thickened IM ligament, a local ganglion cyst, or repetitive sports stress can cause it.
- "Turf toe" refers to a severe sprain of the first metatarsal phalangeal joint (MTPJ) without concomitant dislocation or injury to the sesamoid complex.

- Although most players have an uneventful return to athletics after a turf toe injury, management is facilitated by knowledge of the relevant anatomy, clinical signs, and the appropriate imaging in order to avoid chronic instability and/or pain.
- Regardless of the etiology, the patient with metatarsalgia usually presents with pain in the distal forefoot exacerbated by activity that is relieved by rest. Because metatarsalgia is merely a symptom of a number of foot and ankle disorders, examination should include the entire foot and ankle.

Management of first ray bunion deformity continues to attract great attention in the orthopedic community. It causes pain, difficulty with normal shoe wear and loss of the normal biomechanical integrity of the fore foot in locomotion. With well over 100 repairs described in the literature, the current central issues still remain: Where is the deformity, what forces have caused it, does it cause disability, does it need to be fixed, and if so how?

In this subset of individuals the active athlete needs special consideration. Will operative intervention allow continuation of the sport and enhance performance? Or, on the other hand, will improvement of anatomy interfere with function and are all sports the same?

BASIC SCIENCE

Stability, range of motion and weight transfer across the first metatarsophalangeal (MTP) joint are provided by the interplay of the capsular ligamentous sling and the intrinsic shape of the joint. The metatarsal head in this joint, however, has no actual muscle insertions; therefore, failure of the supporting

915

structures may lead to deviation. Initial stability is maintained through strong fan shaped collateral ligaments from the head of the metatarsal to the base of the proximal phalanx medially and laterally. Similar ligaments also extend from the metatarsal head to the medial and lateral sesamoids.

The sesamoids, located within the split tendon of the flexor hallucis brevis, articulate with the inferior surface of the metatarsal head on either side of the cresta and are further stabilized medially by the abductor hallucis and laterally by the adductor hallucis. These attachments coalesce under the MTP joint to form the strong plantar plate, which inserts onto the base of the proximal phalanx. The flexor hallucis longus passes just inferior to the plantar plate toward its insertion on the distal phalanx. The extensor hallucis brevis and longus are stabilized dorsally by the foot alignment of the MTP joint and insert into the proximal phalanx and distal phalanx, respectively. The shapes of the first MTP joint and first metatarsocuneiform (MTC) joint help determine stability as well. Opposing flat surfaces are inherently stable, whereas rounder joints are more easily deviated (1,2).

Hallux valgus may result from a multitude of causes, which are divided into extrinsic and intrinsic events. The principal extrinsic cause is related to shoes. The incidence of hallux valgus has been shown to be higher in shoe-wearing societies than in populations that do not wear shoes. Women's shoewear is often implicated as the cause of the high preponderance of hallux valgus found in females. In general, the outline of men's feet is comparable to the outline of men's shoes, resulting in no compression or constriction of the forefoot. Women's shoes, however, do not conform to the outer dimensions of the foot and are, on average, 1.2 cm narrower than the forefoot (3). In addition, as the height of the heel rises, the forefoot force increases

exponentially, driving the hallux into the narrow toe box of the shoe, leading to lateral deviation of the great toe (3–6).

Hypermobility of the first ray at the metatarsal cuneiform joint, metatarsus primus varus and abnormal metatarsal length are intrinsic causes of hallux valgus formation. Hyperpronation and/or relatively tight Achilles tendon leads to pronation of the first ray, causing stress on the medial aspect of the toe during normal gait.

With valgus deviation of the great toe, the pull of the adductor hallucis muscle causes lateral deviation of the base of the proximal phalanx on the metatarsal head, which pushes the first metatarsal into greater varus. The medial capsule is attenuated, and the lateral structures contract. The transverse metatarsal ligament anchors the sesamoids to the second metatarsal, thus the sesamoids stay in place while the head of the first metatarsal moves medially, flattening the cresta. The result is mechanical derangement of the first MTP joint, including a prominent medial eminence, lateral subluxation of the base of the proximal phalanx, dissociation of the first metatarsal sesamoid complex, pronation of the hallux, and an increased angle between the first and second metatarsals. Pronation of the hallux varies with axial rotation of the first metatarsal. With increasing pes planus pronation, the first metatarsal rotates longitudinally, the orientation of the first MTP joint becomes oblique in relation to the floor, great toe function markedly decreases, and weight bearing is transferred laterally. Some bunion deformities involve congruent joints, meaning that there is lateral deviation of the articular surface of the first MTP joint without significant sesamoid displacement, hallux rotation, or sequential progression of the hallux valgus **(Fig 53-1)**. Any attempt to move the proximal phalanx around on the articular surface of the metatarsal head would disrupt the normal joint relationship.

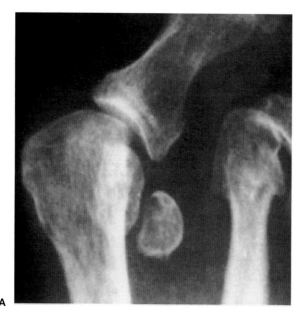
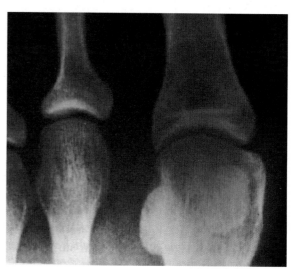

A   B

Fig 53-1. Incongruent joint **(A)** and congruent joints **(B)**. (From Pedowitz WJ. Bunion deformity. In: Pfeffer GB, Frey CC, eds. *Current practice in foot and ankle surgery.* New York: McGraw Hill; 1993:219–242; with permission.)

Lateral deviation of the great toe may also take place at the interphalangeal joint and is referred to as hallux valgus interphalangeus. This condition may be isolated or exist in conjunction with deviation at the MTP joint. All bunion deformities are not the same and a clear understanding and assessment of the underlying pathologic anatomy is critical to patient assessment.

■ CLINICAL FINDINGS

The bunion patient will complain of swelling, redness, and pain on the inner side of the foot at the level of the MTP joint. Pain is more pronounced when wearing shoes and will diminish barefoot. Patients complain that they have difficulty finding a good fit in shoes.

This deformity is dynamic and the patient should be evaluated in both the weight-bearing and nonweight-bearing position. In the standing position the degree of forefoot spread, great toe angulation, and lessor toe deformity should be documented. The clinician must note whether the toe pads make contact with the ground while standing. The hindfoot and longitudinal arch must be assessed while standing and during gait.

Special attention is given to the first MTP joint. Axial rotation, angular deformity, and dorsiflexion are carefully measured. Normal dorsiflexion of the great toe is 70. Any MTP arthritis as noted by pain on range of motion of the great toe associated with limited motion should be documented. Generally patients with hallux valgus have markedly reduced pain when they remove their shoes, while patients with hallux rigidus have pain with shoes on or off. Instability at the first MTC is also recognized as important but difficult to assess. The physician can manually manipulate the MTC joint of the first ray to assess laxity, and the presence of a callus under the second metatarsal head my reveal diminished weight bearing of the great toe.

Radiologic Studies

Radiological studies should be done in the standing position. Any arthritis or deformity should be noted and measurements should be calculated **(Fig 53-2)**.

Increased angulation of the MTC joint and greater roundness of the metatarsal head indicates greater instability; a facet between the base of the first and second metatarsals suggests greater rigidity. Special attention should be paid to the distal metatarsal angulation in anticipating the need for an osteotomy. Measurements taken from radiographs can vary from examiner to examiner; and slight deviations in the angle of the beam, placement of the cassette, and rotation of the foot can significantly affect accuracy; therefore, these studies should be used as clinical guides and not absolute indications for surgical care (7,8).

Nonoperative Treatment

Initial treatment should always be conservative. With mild deformity, a patient who is willing to compromise with a

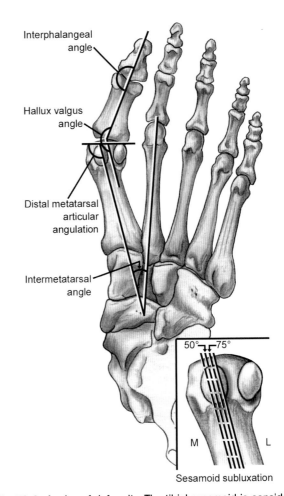

Fig 53-2. Angles of deformity. The tibial sesamoid is considered medial if 75% of its width is medial to the central line, lateral if 75% is lateral to the central line. Otherwise, the sesamoid is considered to be centrally located. (From Pedowitz WJ. Bunion deformity. In: Pfeffer GB, Frey CC, eds. *Current practice in foot and ankle surgery*. New York: McGraw Hill; 1993:219–242; with permission.)

properly fitting, low-heeled, extra-depth, or combined-last shoe, augmented with a good quality cushioned insole has a good chance to find comfort. With more significant deformity, a bunion last shoe with a broad toe box made of soft leather and a flexible sole will often relieve symptoms.

Continued pain after conservative care, split size shoe requirements (one foot greater in size than the other) and deformity that greatly interferes with lifestyle are appropriate reasons for operation. Cosmesis is not a realistic indicator and a risk benefit ratio needs to be assessed carefully. The American Orthopedic Foot and Ankle Society strongly condemns the cosmetic reconstruction of the foot.

■ BUNIONS IN THE ATHLETE

Bunion management in the high-performance athlete is a unique challenge. Running, jumping, and dancing can put 275% of body weight across the MTP joint and increase shear force 50%; excellent MTP motion is essential (9). Accurate correction of an obvious deformity can inadvertently cause decreased MTP motion and thus end a career. Bunion surgery should be avoided in sprinters, 400-m runners, high jumpers, pole vaulters, and ballet dancers (9). It should be made clear that surgical intervention may dramatically alter or terminate performance in the high performance athlete.

Extreme dorsiflexion, however, is less of a concern in middle and long-distance runners and cyclists. If conservative care fails and the deformity prevents performance without severe limiting pain, surgery should be done.

Bunions may also be symptomatic in the teen and preteen athlete. They are more likely to have an adducted foot with an increased distal metatarsal articular angulation. If possible, reconstruction should be delayed until skeletal maturity and because their unique deformity is more likely to require osteotomy.

Operative Intervention

A surgeon considering operative intervention in a symptomatic bunion should be skilled in assessing the type of bunion and able to match it to an operative procedure with a high rate of predictability and ease of salvage. A long first metatarsal, a long great toe, an adducted foot, and generalized ligamentous laxity are associated with higher rates of recurrence **(Fig 53-3)**.

Soft tissue realignment of the first MTP joint will only correct the intermetatarsal (IM) angle about 5 degrees. Combined with a medial eminence resection of the distal first metatarsal this will correct only a mild deformity.

A chevron osteotomy, which involves a medial capsulloraphy, chevron shaped osteotomy with about 4 mm of lateral displacement of the metatarsal head, will correct an IM angle up to 15 degrees. For an incongruent joint a medially based wedge is taken out of the osteotomy site to better align the joint **(Fig 53-4)**.

For greater angular deviation of the first metatarsal with significant hallux valgus, a distal soft tissue release involving proximal transfer of the adductor to the metatarsal neck, lateral sesamoid and IM ligament recession, and medial capsular reefing is combined with a proximal osteotomy of the first metatarsal to close the IM angle **(Fig 53-5)**; however, a proximal osteotomy will stiffen the forefoot and transfer force to the hindfoot and ankle in athletic pursuit.

With significant arthritis of the great toe MTP joint, arthrodesis will give the greatest chance of returning to sports including doubles tennis, jogging, golf, ballroom dancing, and cycling **(Fig 53-6)**. Silastic implants to the MTP joint have also been suggested for arthritis; however, it is generally thought that they will not hold up well or give the biomechanical support needed for active sports activity.

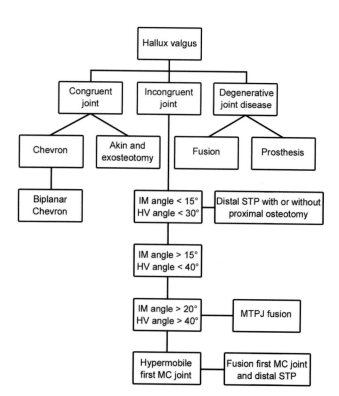

Fig 53-3. Algorithm for treatment decisions. IM, intermetatarsal; HV, hallux valgus; STP, soft tissue procedure, MTPJ, metarsophalangeal joint; MC, metatarsocuneiform. (Modified from Mann RA. Decision-making in bunion surgery. *Instr Course Lect.* 1990;39: 3–13; with permission.)

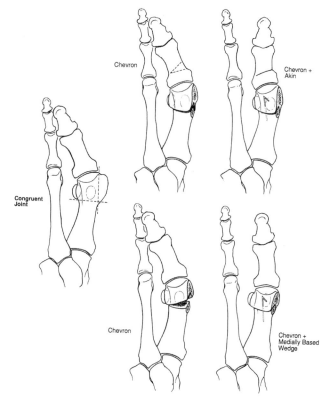

Fig 53-4. Management of the congruent joint. Chevron-Akin, biplane Chevron. (From Pedowitz WJ. Bunion deformity. In: Pfeffer GB, Frey CC, eds. *Current practice in foot and ankle surgery.* New York: McGraw Hill; 1993:219–242; with permission.)

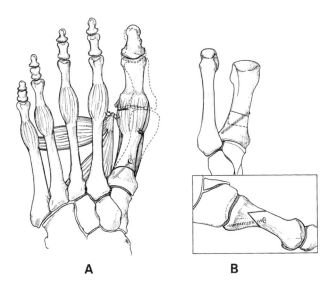

A   **B**

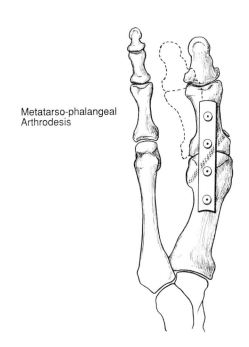

Metatarso-phalangeal
Arthrodesis

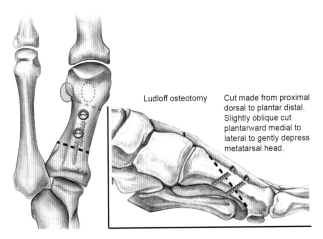

Ludloff osteotomy   Cut made from proximal
dorsal to plantar distal.
Slightly oblique cut
plantarward medial to
lateral to gently depress
metatarsal head.

Fig 53-5. A: Distal soft tissue procedure with proximal crecentic osteotomy. **B:** Proximal Chevron osteotomy. (From Pedowitz WJ. Bunion deformity. In: Pfeffer GB, Frey CC, eds. *Current practice in foot and ankle surgery*. New York: McGraw Hill; 1993:219–242; with permission.)

Fig 53-6. Metatarsophalangeal (MTP) arthrodesis. Alignment should be 15 degrees of valgus, 25 degrees of dorsiflexion in relation to the metatarsal shaft, and 15 degrees with respect to the plantar aspect of the foot. (From Pedowitz WJ. Bunion deformity. In: Pfeffer GB, Frey CC, eds. *Current practice in foot and ankle surgery*. New York: McGraw Hill; 1993:219–242; with permission.)

With documented instability of the MTC joint a distal soft tissue release plus a MTC arthrodesis is the procedure of choice **(Fig 53-7)**. The instability itself is recognized as being hard to determine. Plain radiographs showing a hyperacute MTC angle or a curved distal first cuneiform articulation are suggestive. Arthritis at the first MTC articulation is diagnostic. A callus under the second metatarsal head may indicate decreased weight bearing by the first ray.

■ INTERDIGITAL NEUROMA IN THE ATHLETE

Interdigital or Morton's neuroma is an entrapment neuropathy of the plantar digital nerve. Trauma, bursal inflammation, a thickened IM ligament, a local ganglion cyst, or

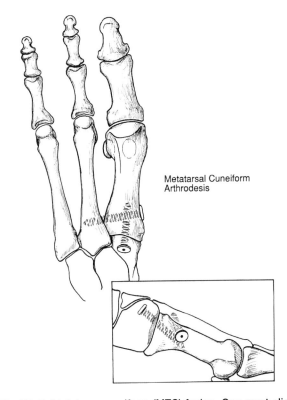

Metatarsal Cuneiform
Arthrodesis

Fig 53-7. Metatarsocuneiform (MTC) fusion. One must slightly flex and adduct the first metatarsal to obtain proper alignment. (From Pedowitz WJ. Bunion deformity. In: Pfeffer GB, Frey CC, eds. *Current practice in foot and ankle surgery*. New York: McGraw Hill; 1993;219–242; with permission.)

repetitive sports stress can cause it. Anatomically it usually involves a lateral branch of the medial plantar nerve and sometimes an additional branch from the lateral plantar nerve **(Fig 53-8)**.

Essential Anatomy

The third IM space is the most common site. It is the narrowest interspace, and there is a shift in mobility there as the third metatarsal has much less motion than the fourth.

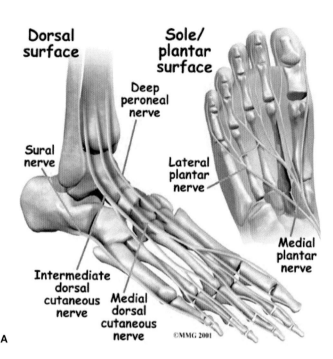

A

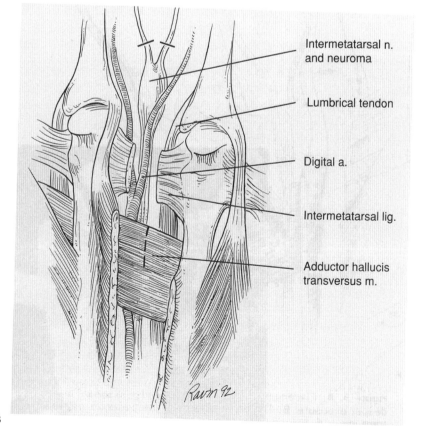

B

Fig 53-8. A: Nerves of the foot. **B:** Interdigital neuroma.

Neuromas occur less frequently at the second interspace and presence at the first or fourth interspace is extremely rare. Incidence is greater in women than in men, a fact attributed to their tendency to wear tighter, high-heeled shoes. With each centimeter rise in heel height, there is an exponential rise in forefoot pressure and the nerve becomes ever more stretched against the IM ligament.

The diagnosis is based on a history of plantar forefoot pain radiating to the tips of the toes. The pain is aggravated by tight shoewear and removing the shoe and massaging the foot often obtain relief. It also may radiate proximally.

The exam centers on careful palpation. The interspace will be painful and pressure will aggravate it. A click (Mulder's) may be felt. Sensory changes are variable. Make sure to evaluate the adjacent MTP join to rule out synovitis, which can mimic neuroma pain. Confusion can lead to unnecessary nerve excision, progressive synovitis, and eventual deviation and dislocation of the toe.

Plain films should be taken to rule out associated pathology. Magnetic resonance imaging (MRI) and ultrasound will reveal large lesions best; however this may be misleading. Lesion size cannot be correlated with clinical results after excision.

The pathology of the lesion is also confusing. Sections of neuroma nerve and non-neuroma nerve from similar interspaces are histomorphologically the same. The neuroma nerve is thicker and the non-neuroma nerve thinner but there is significant overlap. The need for MRI, ultrasound, or even pathology is therefore brought into question (10).

Conservative care involves wide comfortable laced shoes, low heels, and orthotic support to the interspace. A longitudinal arch support with a 3/16-inch metatarsal lift proximal to the second, third, and fourth metatarsal heads. In addition a rocker on the sole proximal to the metatarsal heads can also be helpful.

Administering a carefully placed injection will aid both in diagnosis and possible therapy. Local anaesthetic (0.05% bipivucaine and 1%-2% lidocaine both without epinephrine) plus depomedrol (40 mg) is injected into the interspace. The injection will be diagnostic in that relief of pain from the local anesthetic will help confirm the diagnosis. The cortisone may be therapeutic and 5% to 10% of patients may have cessation of symptoms after one to three injections. Greater than three injections are discouraged because of possible skin color change and atrophy of the local fat pad.

Ultimately 60% to 70% of patients request surgery after conservative care has failed (11). In the current literature three choices are available: neurolysis alone, excision through a dorsal approach, or excision through a plantar approach. The advantage with neurolysis is there is no residual neural stump to form a new neuroma and sensation is preserved.

With neurolysis a dorsal incision is created in the interspace and the IM ligament is severed. The nerve is neurolysed 3 cm proximal to the ligament. The wound is closed, a large bulky dressing applied, and the patient allowed to weight bear as tolerated. The sutures are removed and activity resumed with diminution of pain. Some authors have reported 70% to 80% good to excellent results (12).

The dorsal approach has the advantage of no plantar scar. Through a dorsal approach, the IM ligament is severed and the nerve identified. Too much proximal extension of the incision will jeopardize branches of the superficial nerve. The nerve stalk is pulled distally and sharply severed so that the remaining proximal end will lie 3 cm proximal to the ligament. Leave the fat pad alone.

Dorsiflexion of the foot will demonstrate retraction of the cut end. Failure to retract may indicate accessory branches (present 10% of the time), which must be excised to avoid failure. The same post-op regimen is applied as with neurolysis but the morbidity may be greater because of the nerve excision. One can expect 85% good to excellent results, although 35% will demonstrate some residual pain at the site of the resection and complain of minor shoewear problems (11).

A well-documented peer reviewed study has shown that a plantar approach can work with equal success to the dorsal approach (13). Weight bearing is avoided until the surgical wound has healed; however, one must be careful not to put the scar under the metatarsal head, and if a keloid scar forms on the weight-bearing surface of the foot a myriad of problems may develop.

The initial resection of a well-documented interdigital neuroma is a safe, well tolerated procedure with little morbidity and should pose no long-term problem for the active athlete.

Recurrent neuromas are rare but can cause great disability. Symptoms recur from poor initial resection, a bulb neuroma reforms in a tight space, lack of resection of accessory branches, or underappreciation of co-existent pathology (e.g., synovitis of the MTP joint). Careful repeated exams are critical to establishing an accurate diagnosis.

Initial conservative care should include adequate shoewear, ultrasound, physical therapy, and nerve modifying medication [e.g., tricyclics, selective serotonin reuptake inhibitors (SSRIs), anticonvulsants]. One should look for the possibility of Complex Regional Pain Syndrome 1 or 2.

With the failure of conservative care the nerve should be approached dorsally or plantar ward, adequate excision is essential and the end of the residual nerve should be implanted into bone. 20% to 40% will not improve with revision (14).

In summary, with interdigital neuroma, it is critical to make the diagnosis. Is it a neuroma, synovitis, or a bony deformity? Pursue conservative care. Excise through an approach you are comfortable with, and pursue revisions carefully.

■ TURF TOE

Originally described by Bowers and Martin (15) in 1976, the term "turf toe" refers to a severe sprain of the first metatarsal phalangeal joint (MTPJ) without concomitant dislocation or injury to the sesamoid complex. Likely due to a combination of modern more flexible athletic footwear and the use of a myriad of artificial playing surfaces, injuries to the first MTPJ have become well known to those treating athletic injuries of the foot and ankle. In fact, this injury is thought to be third in importance, only behind knee and ankle injuries, for lost time from sport (16).

Although turf toe injuries have been documented in ballet dancers, sprinters, rugby, and basketball players, it is most commonly associated with American football. The incidence of turf toe injuries has been estimated to be between 11% and 45% in active football players, and more common in linemen and wide receivers (17,18).

Basic Science: Anatomy

The bony anatomy of the first MTPJ has little inherent stability. Although the cam-shaped metatarsal head is mated with a like concave surface at the proximal phalanx, the majority of stability for this joint is conferred by the variety of surrounding soft tissue structures. Although the dorsal capsule is tenuous, the plantar capsule is thick and is essentially a condensation of tissue (with the medial and lateral metatarsosesamoid ligaments) forming the plantar plate. This plate is firmly anchored to the base of the proximal phalanx. Embedded in this structure are the two sesamoid bones, in the flexor hallucis tendon, which bear the majority of force during weight bearing through the great toe. Additional contributions to stability are made by the adductor and abductor hallucis tendon insertions, as well as the flexor hallucis brevis into the sesamoids. The normal first MTPJ has approximately 30 degrees of plantar flexion and 80 degrees of dorsiflexion (19).

Clinical Evaluation

History

The classic mechanism of injury is one of hyper-dorsiflexion of the first MTPJ with axial loading of the heel, while the foot is plantar flexed **(Fig 53-9)**. This combination of forces results in two primary injuries: a) a tearing of the capsular structures where they insert on the metatarsal neck; and b) a compression injury to the dorsal articular surface of the metatarsal head (Fig 53-9). Clinically, this is most often seen when one player has his foot firmly planted on the playing surface while another player lands on the back of his foot, forcing the first MTPJ into hyperextension (dorsiflexion). Hyperflexion, varus, and valgus mechanisms have also been described, but are less common.

Physical Findings

The usual presentation is one of swelling, erythema, tenderness to palpation, and painful range of motion of the first MTP joint. Chronic injuries may be characterized by deformity consisting of hammering and subluxation of the joint. Following a complete physical examination of the foot and ankle, mediolateral and dorsiplantarflexion stress evaluation of the first MTP joint should be performed to fully assess for the presence of any instability.

Imaging

Plain radiographs including weight-bearing anteriorposterior (AP), lateral, and oblique studies of the foot should be

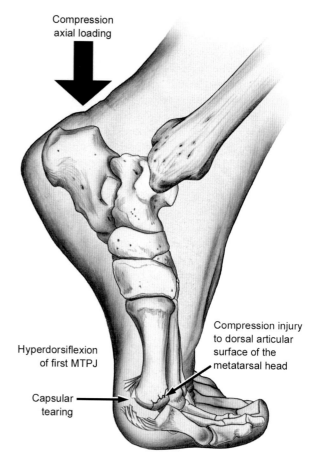

Fig 53-9. Turf toe.

obtained if a turf toe injury is suspected. Additionally, contralateral views are helpful in assessing for occult sesamoid fracture or proximal migration, which may mandate a slightly different treatment algorithm. On the AP view, the distance between the base of the proximal phalanx to the distal pole of either sesamoid must be within 3 mm of the sesamoid position on the contralateral side (20). These radiographs also allow the clinician to evaluate for intra- or extra-articular fractures, dislocations, and bony avulsions of the collateral ligaments. In the athlete, Anderson recommends MRI if the patient has a significant sprain or has radiographic abnormalities (21). This allows further characterization of the injury and evaluation of the soft tissues.

Decision Making and Treatment

A grading system originally described by Clanton and Ford (22) has been proposed that provides a useful classification of first MTP joint sprains based on physical exam findings to help guide treatment and assess prognosis **(Table 53-1)**. In general, the treatment of turf toe injuries is nonoperative, consisting of rest, ice, elevation, and compression. Grade I sprains often respond to a stiff insole, which limits first MTP joint motion. There is usually no loss of playing time

TABLE 53-1	Classification of Turf Toe Injuries 1			
	Signs and Symptoms	**Pathology**	**Treatment**	**Course**
Grade I	Plantar or medial tenderness Minimal swelling No ecchymosis	Intrasubstance stretch of capsular structures	Rest, ice, compression, elevation	May play with protection
Grade II	Diffuse tenderness Mild to moderate swelling Ecchymosis Decreased range of motion	Tear of capsular structures	Include buddy taping with above protocol	Up to 2 weeks loss of activity
Grade III	Severe diffuse tenderness, maximally dorsally Marked swelling and ecchymosis Marked decreased range of motion	Capsular tear with articular compression injury usually dorsally	Add immobilization until able to bear weight comfortably Use stiff forefoot insert to resist metatarsophalangeal joint dorsiflexion	3 to 6 weeks loss of activity

Modified from Clanton T, Butler J, Eggert A. Injuries to the MTP joints in athletes. *Foot Ankle Int*. 1986;7(3):162–176.

with a grade I sprain. Grade II sprains are characterized by disruption of the capsular structures of the first MTP joint and, therefore, require some degree of immobilization to facilitate healing. Buddy taping in addition to those modalities used for a grade I sprain usually allow athletes to return to play within 2 weeks. The addition of a bony compression injury, as seen in grade III sprains, often will require immobilization with a walking boot or short leg cast for greater than 3 weeks. After the athlete can achieve asymptomatic full weight bearing on the involved extremity (3 to 6 weeks) they may return to play. This individual will often benefit from a protective steel shank applied to an insole with or without strapping the hallux in slight plantarflexion. The use of a total contact insole with a Morton extension may also be helpful in preventing further injury.

Although most patients have an uneventful return to play following rest and modified levels of immobilization, operative intervention should be considered for the patient with a large capsular avulsion, an unstable joint, diastasis of a bipartite or sesamoid fracture, loose body, significant sesamoid retraction, or chronic cases which have been unresponsive to conservative care (21). When primary repair of the plantar plate and or the collateral ligaments is not possible, the abductor hallucis may be used to reinforce the plantar plate (21).

As with most lower extremity sports injuries, initial protected weight bearing is recommended until pain and swelling subside. After asymptomatic full weight bearing is achieved, activity can progress to running, cutting, and then to activities related to specific sports (i.e., blocking in American football). Clanton and Ford (23) found that regardless of the degree of sprain, full recovery generally required 4 weeks of conservative care. Anderson (21) determined that return to play was highly dependent upon the player's healing potential, level of discomfort, and their

position. This often correlated with pain-free dorsiflexion of 50 to 60 degrees of the first MTP joint.

■ CONCLUSIONS AND FUTURE DIRECTIONS

Turf toe remains a common condition in selected athletes and is being diagnosed more regularly as awareness of the injury increases. Ultimately, it is the early diagnosis and appropriate treatment that will limit the potential morbidity, disability, and loss of play due to this injury. Although most players will have an uneventful return to athletics, knowledge of the relevant anatomy, clinical signs, and the appropriate imaging is important to help prevent chronic instability and disability.

■ METATARSALGIA

Although forefoot disorders may affect athletes from a myriad of sports, the runner in particular, is often plagued by significant discomfort around the distal aspect of the lesser metatarsals during activity. Known as metatarsalgia, it may have primary or secondary causes.

Primary metatarsalgia results from aberrations in normal metatarsal anatomy, their relationship to each other, and the way they function with respect to the rest of the foot (24). The most common cause of primary metatarsalgia is thought to derive from a relatively long second or third metatarsal that extends past the "normal" cascade of the distal metatarsal contour **(Fig 53-10)**. As the longest bone in the cascade, this metatarsal is subjected to increased pressures and subsequently becomes symptomatic during the propulsive phase of gait (25). Hypermobility of the first ray can

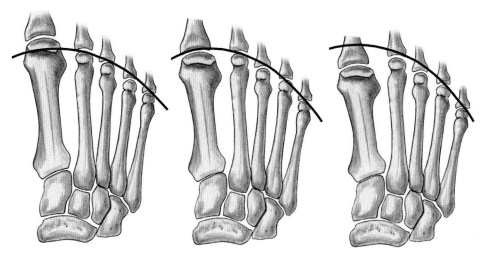

Fig 53-10. The three basic metatarsal cascades. (Modified from Viladot A. *Patologia del antegpieed*. Barcelona: Ediciones Toray; 1975.) (Modified from Viladot A. *Patologia* del *antegpie*. Barcelona: Ediciones Toray, 1975 – found in Myerson's book pg 360.)

also have the same result, as the loss of a medial buttress causes the transfer of force to more lateral structures (20).

A relatively plantarflexed lesser metatarsal, or one which is enlarged or irregularly shaped in comparison to adjacent metatarsals, can also be problematic for the athlete. In contrast to a long lesser metatarsal, which causes symptoms when the foot is fully loaded during push off, the metatarsal which is more prominent on the plantar surface tends to be more symptomatic during the stance phase of gait. This deformity can be primary or secondary to hammering of the toe distal to the metatarsal.

As a hammertoe begins to contract and elevate dorsally, the metatarsal head becomes more prominent on the ball of the foot. Plantar metatarsal head prominence can lead to increased pressures at that site resulting in pain, swelling, and an intractable plantar keratosis (IPK). Relative equinus of the forefoot, although not that common in the elite athlete, can also produce abnormal weight bearing and transfer of force to the metatarsals, resulting in a painful foot with activity (25).

When primary mechanisms appear unlikely the clinician should have a high index of suspicion for secondary causes of metatarsalgia. Those commonly seen include inflammatory or crystalline arthropathy, nerve entrapment (i.e., tarsal tunnel syndrome), interdigital neuroma, Freiberg's infraction, post-traumatic or post-surgical metatarsal deformity, and fat pad atrophy which may itself be primary or secondary to other metabolic disturbances.

Although the aforementioned causes of metatarsal pain are relevant to athletes and non-athletes, the presence of an Achilles tendon contracture or anterior ankle impingement deserve specific mention with regard to the runner because they both limit ankle dorsiflexion. Restriction of dorsiflexion at the ankle results in more force transfer to the forefoot, as the ankle is unable to accommodate the obligate dorsiflexion ordinarily seen during the gait cycle. To compensate, the subsequent over pull of the extensor digitorum longus leads to clawing of the lesser toes. A claw toe deformity (hyperextension of the MTP joint with concomitant distal hammer or mallet deformity) itself causes distal migration of the fat pads normally located under the metatarsal heads. As a consequence the uncovered metatarsal heads are exposed to increased pressures.

Basic Science

Force transmitted through the forefoot is significant during the gait cycle. While most data suggest the greatest force is transmitted through the hallux, Hennig and Rosenbaum (26) found the next greatest peak pressure to be under the head of the third metatarsal and Hughes et al. (27) found that forces beneath the second metatarsal head were second only to the hallux. Because intense running can generate forces from three to eight times body weight, even mild anatomic abnormalities, which might otherwise remain clinically silent, may lead to significant discomfort in the runner (24,16).

Anatomy

An appreciation for forefoot anatomy is essential when treating the athlete with suspected metatarsalgia. The *forefoot* itself begins just distal to the MTC and cuboid joints and extends distally to include the toes. In the sagittal plane the metatarsals are inclined in a distal-to-proximal fashion with decreasing degrees of inclination as one moves laterally (28). In that plane, one also finds that the MTP joints are normally dorsiflexed an average of 16 degrees (23).

Some of the more important intrinsic stabilizers of the forefoot are the IM ligaments. Located deep to the tendons of the dorsal interossei, these distinct structures extend between the heads of the metatarsals. Below these ligaments run the corresponding digital nerves and vessels (Fig 53-8B).

The "ball" of the foot is essentially a continuation of the sole of the foot, with longitudinal structures extending to the toes while traversing the MTP joints (21). The skin in this region is thick and is actually the distal insertion site for the plantar aponeurosis, which provides a fibrous tunnel for the flexor tendons and also inserts into the plantar plate (21). At the core of the ball of the foot is the phalangeal apparatus that consists of the proximal phalanx and the plantar plate which inserts into the base of the proximal phalanx and the sides of the metatarsal heads (28). Dorsally, the extensor apparatus broadens over the MTP joint while the interossei, digital nerves, and vessels flank the metatarsals along their length.

Clinical Evaluation

Regardless of the etiology, the patient with metatarsalgia usually presents with pain in the distal forefoot exacerbated by activity that is relieved by rest. Because metatarsalgia is merely a symptom of a number of foot and ankle disorders, examination should include the entire foot and ankle. The examination should begin with inspection for deformity (fixed or flexible), intrinsic atrophy, contracture, callosities, keratoses, or other skin changes. Active and passive range of motion should be noted especially at the ankle and the MTP joints.

After proximal lesions have been considered, a more focused distal exam is appropriate. The toes should be carefully examined for range of motion with the ankle in dorsiflexion, equinus, and also with weight bearing. Holding the metatarsal shaft with one hand and the proximal phalanx in the other allows one to assess for pain with or without instability by shifting the two bones dorsally and plantar. Examine each MTP joint individually to identify point tenderness, synovitis, or instability. Point tenderness may indicate a bone bruise, stress fracture, fat pad atrophy, IPK, Frieberg's infraction, or synovitis. A single depressed metatarsal head will show a discreet hard lesion while a symptomatic long metatarsal head will create a large broad callus (**Figs 53-11** and **53-12**).

The neurologic examination of the foot is especially important in patients with metatarsalgia because conditions such as nerve irritation, entrapment, and neuromas may produce the distal and plantar symptoms of metatarsalgia. Carefully palpate the interspaces, especially the third, looking for tenderness or fullness which may indicate a cyst or Morton's neuroma. If a neuroma is suspected a click may sometimes be heard when the foot is squeezed in a mediolateral direction while plantar pressure is applied to the third interspace (29). Paresthesia felt along the distribution of the medial and lateral plantar nerves when the nerve is palpated behind the medial malleolus may indicate tarsal tunnel syndrome. Finally, we advocate inspection of the patient's athletic

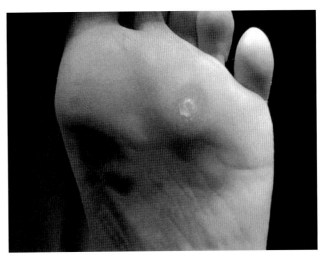

Fig 53-11. Painful IPK from single depressed metatarsal head. IPK, intractable plantar keratosis.

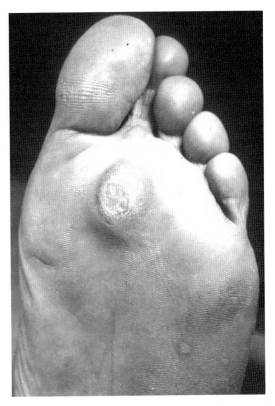

Fig 53-12. Large IPK from long second metatarsal. IPK, intractable plantar keratosis.

shoewear, as it often gives the examiner insight into the context in which the foot becomes symptomatic.

Imaging

Radiographic evaluation of the patient with metatarsalgia should always consist of plain AP, oblique, and lateral weight-bearing projections of the foot. On the AP view, the distal metatarsal cascade can easily be appreciated. Intrinsic

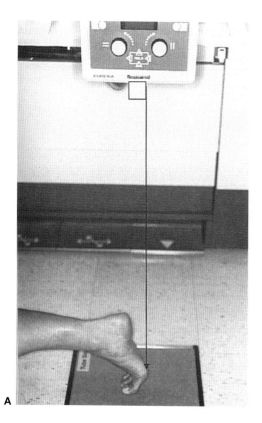

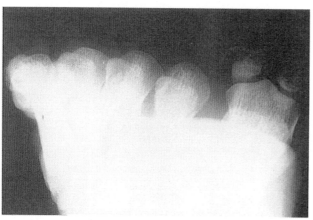

Fig 53-13. Axial view of the weight-bearing sesamoids (i.e., Lewis method). **A:** The patient is standing, and the toes are on the cassette with maximal dorsiflexion at the MTP joints and the knee flexed forward to bring the heel out of the beam's path. The beam is perpendicular to the cassette and centered on the first or third metatarsal head. **B:** This view was obtained with the beam centered on the third metatarsal head. (From Marks R. In: Myerson M, ed. *Foot and ankle disorders.*, Philadelphia: WB Saunders; 2000: 99; with permission.)

bony deformity, bony lesions, stress fractures, and Freiberg's infraction (adolescent ischemic necrosis of the epiphysis of the second metatarsal head) can also be appreciated on the AP view. The lateral image of the foot will allow one to identify the presence of sagittal metatarsal deformities, the degree of metatarsal inclination, and subtle or overt subluxation of the MTP joint. An axial weight-bearing view

(patient standing, toes on cassette in maximal dorsiflexion at the MTP joints, with the knee flexed forward) gives an excellent view of the metatarsal heads, their shape and position in relation to each other **(Fig 53-13)**.

Additional studies such as bone scan, computed tomography (CT), and MRI are often unnecessary in the evaluation of metatarsalgia but become important when secondary causes become more likely.

Treatment

Although operative treatment is occasionally necessary, conservative treatment is the rule in the management of metatarsalgia. Prior to suggesting surgery we recommend that the clinician consider that there may be a need to change the patient's shoewear, training surface, or training habits. Most runners who have minor foot problems will benefit from either changing brands of shoes or obtaining a new pair (15). When properly diagnosed, most metatarsalgia responds well to a period of ice, anti-inflammatory drugs, activity modification, and properly placed metatarsal pads with a shock-absorbing insert (for *both* the patient's athletic and daily shoewear). Additionally, flexible orthoses can often cool down the inflamed and painful foot with metatarsalgia **(Table 53-2)**.

When conservative measures have been exhausted, certain operative interventions have been found to be useful in alleviating the symptoms of metatarsalgia. If a claw toe is the offending deformity and has not responded to a metatarsal lift, surgical correction should be considered. Similarly a chronic interdigital neuroma should be resected. A tight Achilles tendon should be initially managed with heel-cord stretching while anterior ankle impingement often responds to debridement of anterior tibial or talar osteophytes. A hypermobile first ray or a long second metatarsal may be treated with MTP arthroplasty with removal of a small

TABLE 53-2	
Metatarsalgia or neuritic metatarsal pain from a neuroma	A longitudinal arch support with a 3/16th inch metatarsal lift proximal to the second, third, and fourth metatarsal heads; also possible to use a rocker bottom placed on the outer sole of the midsole of the shoe proximal to the metatarsal heads
Metatarsal calluses and blisters	An innersole to decrease friction, 1/8th inch metatarsal pad proximal to the affected areas; also possible to wear two pairs of socks and use a lubricant on the calluses prior to running; calluses should be debrided with a pumice stone

Modified from. Baxter DE. Running injuries. In: Jahss MH, ed. *Disorders of the foot and ankle, medical and surgical management.* 2nd ed. Philadelphia: WB Saunders; 1991.

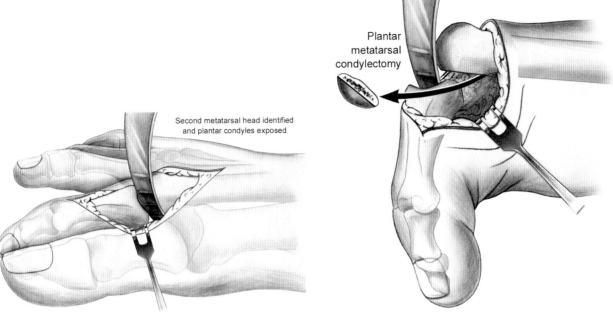

Second metatarsal head identified and plantar condyles exposed

Plantar metatarsal condylectomy

A

B

Fig 53-14. Plantar metatarsal condylectomy. The metatarsal head is freed from adjacent structures, and the plantar condyles are exposed **(A)**. The plantar condyles are removed with an osteotome **(B)**. Care is taken to keep the detached condyles from retracting deep into the plantar space.

amount of plantar condyle (24). When there is an isolated IPK below a prominent metatarsal head, plantar condylectomy is often curative **(Fig 53-14)**. Generally, metatarsal osteotomies and metatarsal head resection are not recommended in athletes as the results are less predictable and may result in transfer metatarsalgia (14).

■ REFERENCES

1. Bordelon RL. Evaluation and operative procedures for hallux valgus deformity. *Orthopedics*. 1987;10:38–44.
2. Mann RA. Decision-making in bunion surgery. *Instr Course Lect*. 1990;39:3–13.
3. Frey C, Thompson F, Smith J, et al. American orthopaedic foot and ankle society women's shoe survey. *Foot Ankle*. 1993;14:78–81.
4. Coughlin MJ, Thompson FM. The high price of high-fashion footwear. *Instr Course Lect*. 1995;44:371–377.
5. Frey CC. Trends in women's shoewear. *Instr Course Lect*. 1995;44: 385–387.
6. Seale KS. Women and their shoes: unrealistic expectations? *Instr Course Lect*. 1995;44:379–384.
7. Johnson KA. "What's a foot surgeon to believe?" *Foot Ankle*. 1992;13:508.
8. Scott G, Wilson DW, Bentley G. Roentgenographic assessment in hallux valgus. *Clin Orthop*. 1991;143–147.
9. Baxter DE, Zingas C. The foot in running. *J Am Acad Orthop Surg*. 1995;3:136–145.
10. Morscher E, Ulrich J, Dick W. Morton's intermetatarsal neuroma: morphology and histological substrate. *Foot Ankle Int*. 2000;21:558–562.
11. Coughlin MJ, Pinsonneault T. Operative treatment of interdigital neuroma. A long-term follow-up study. *J Bone Joint Surg Am*. 2001;83A:1321–1328.
12. Weinfeld SB, Myerson MS. Interdigital neuritis: diagnosis and treatment. *J Am Acad Orthop Surg*. 1996;4:328–335.
13. Richardson EG, Brotzman SB, Graves SC. The plantar incision for procedures involving the forefoot. An evaluation of one hundred and fifty incisions in one hundred and fifteen patients. *J Bone Joint Surg Am*. 1993;75:726–731.
14. Beskin JL, Baxter DE. Recurrent pain following interdigital neurectomy—a plantar approach. *Foot Ankle*. 1988;9:34–39.
15. Bowers KD Jr, Martin RB. Turf-toe: a shoe-surface related football injury. *Med Sci Sports*. 1976;8:81–83.
16. Riegler HF. Orthotic devices for the foot. *Orthop Rev*. 1987; 16:293–303.
17. Clanton TO, Butler JE, Eggert A. Injuries to the metatarsophalangeal joints in athletes. *Foot Ankle*. 1986;7:162–176.
18. Rodeo SA, O'Brien S, Warren RF, et al. Turf-toe: an analysis of metatarsophalangeal joint sprains in professional football players. *Am J Sports Med*. 1990;18:280–285.
19. Clanton TO. Etiology of injury to the foot and ankle. In: DeLee JC, Drez D, eds. *Orthopaedic sports medicine: principles and practice*. Philadelphia, PA: WB Saunders; 2003:2504–2511.
20. Baxter DE. Running injuries. In: Jahss M, ed. *Disorders of the foot and ankle, medical and surgical management*. 2nd ed. Philadelphia: WB Saunders; 1991.
21. Resch S. Functional anatomy and topography of the foot and ankle. In: Myerson MS, ed. *Foot and ankle disorders*. 1st ed. Philadelphia: WB Saunders; 2000:25–49.
22. Sarrafian SK. Functional characteristics of the foot and plantar aponeurosis under tibiotalar loading. *Foot Ankle*. 1987;8:4–18.
23. Joseph J. Range of movement in the great toe in men. *J Bone Joint Surg Br*. 1954;36:450.

24. Baxter DE. The foot in running. In: Coughlin M, Mann RA, ed. *Surgery of the foot and ankle*. 5th ed. St. Louis: Mosby; 1999: 1210–1224.

25. Dockery G. Evaluation and treatment of metatarsalgia and keratotic disorders. In: Myerson MS, ed. *Foot and ankle disorders*. 1st ed. Philadelphia: WB Saunders; 2000:359–377.

26. Hennig EM, Rosenbaum D. Pressure distribution patterns under the feet of children in comparison with adults. *Foot Ankle*. 1991;11:306–311.

27. Hughes J, Kriss S, Klenerman L. A clinician's view of foot pressure: a comparison of three different methods of measurement. *Foot Ankle*. 1987;7:277–284.

28. Sarrafian SK. *Anatomy of the foot and ankle: Descriptive, topographic, functional*. 2nd ed. Philadelphia: JB Lippincott; 1993.

29. Mann RA. Principles of examination of the foot and ankle. In: Coughlin MJ, Mann RA, eds. *Surgery of the foot and ankle*. 5th ed. St. Louis: Mosby; 1999:36–350.

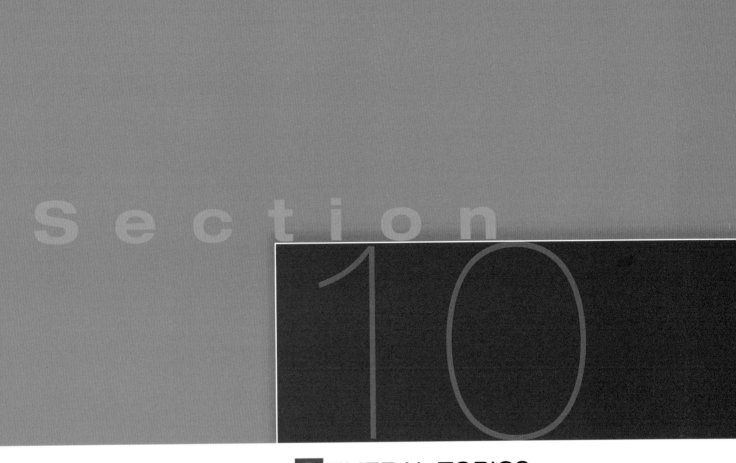

GENERAL TOPICS

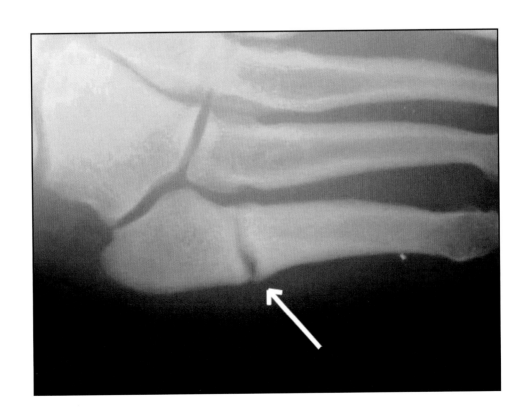

KURT P. SPINDLER, MD, MICHAEL S. GEORGE, MD, CHRISTOPHER C. KAEDING, MD, ANNUNZIATO AMENDOLA, MD

■ KEY POINTS

- Stress fractures behave differently according to their anatomical site and this must be considered when planning treatment.
- Stress fractures result from repeated microtrauma leading to a macrofracture, which occurs when the repetitive microtrauma exceeds bone regeneration.
- The three stages of fatigue failure are crack initiation, propagation along cement lines, and ultimate structural failure/complete fracture. Symptoms progress from insidious onset of pain with no definite history of trauma, to associated swelling and tenderness, then deformity with complete fracture.
- Predisposing factors include: increased activity, abnormal alignment, decreased vascularity, old age, poor nutrition, hormonal imbalance, and genetic factors.
- Radiographs lag behind bone scans by 1 to 2 weeks; bone scans are very sensitive but poor at monitoring bone healing; magnetic resonance imaging (MRI) has excellent sensitivity and displays precise extent of the injury; computed tomography (CT) scan best for bony detail and monitoring healing response. "Dreaded black line" in tibia represents a nonunion that should be treated operatively.
- In general, fractures on the tension side tend to progress to complete fractures and often require operative fixation. Fractures on the compression side tend to be stable and unite with activity modification. In addition, fractures in areas of poor vascularity have a high risk of nonunion and may require operative treatment.
- The tibial shaft is the most frequent of athletic stress fractures. The most common site is posteromedial or

compression side, which can be treated with rest and activity modification as well as pneumatic braces.
- Low-risk stress fractures are usually treated with activity modification and rest. Intermediate or high-risk fractures are treated with surgery if there is a clear fracture line on imaging or complete fracture. Intermediate or high-risk fractures are treated with a period of nonoperative management if no clear fracture line is visible on imaging. In all cases, default to surgical treatment if nonoperative therapy fails.

Stress fractures present a substantial concern to athletes in our society. Proper treatment of stress fractures is essential to avoid career ending injuries and unnecessary time off from athletics. Each anatomical site has unique healing characteristics and appropriate treatment strategies. Anatomical and physiological differences at each site affect the relative risk of complications. It is essential to understand the complex behavior of each stress fracture in order to effectively guide management.

■ PATHOPHYSIOLOGY OF STRESS FRACTURES

Fractures in athletes may occur as either acute fractures such as in a major trauma or chronic fractures such as in a stress fracture. An acute fracture is the result of a single loading event in which the applied stress exceeds the strength of the bone. A stress fracture is the accumulation of microtrauma that ultimately leads to the macrofracture of bone.

The normal healing response of bone produces a dynamic balance between tissue breakdown and osteosynthesis.

According to Wolff's law, stress loading of bone leads to bone remodeling and structural changes that dissipate the stress concentration in the bone. When osseous remodeling lags behind bone degradation, microfractures can accumulate and propagate. The fatigue life, or the number of cycles at a given applied load that leads to ultimate failure, may thus be exceeded in the absence of adequate healing of microfractures.

Fatigue failure of bone typically occurs in three stages. Crack initiation first occurs at areas of discontinuity in the bone, such as in the haversion canals, lacunae, and canaliculi. In the absence of healing, microfractures propagate along cement lines. Stress loading parallel to these cement lines results in faster crack advancement. Finally, continued crack propagation results in ultimate structural failure and complete fracture.

Many factors may predispose certain athletes to stress fractures. These fractures commonly occur in otherwise healthy athletes who increase their activity to the point where repetitive microtrauma exceeds bone regeneration. Abnormal anatomical alignment may cause excess stress on particular bony structures. Decreased bone vascularity either from previous injury or from certain medical conditions may decrease the healing response of bone. Old age, poor nutritional status, hormonal abnormalities, and genetic factors may also predispose certain athletes to stress fractures (1).

Diagnosis

Stress fractures usually present with an insidious onset of pain without a history of a specific traumatic event (2). In the early stages, pain may be present only during the inciting activity. As the process continues, pain occurs during simple activities of daily living and may be associated with diffuse swelling and tenderness to palpation. The final stage of stress fracture is advancement to complete fracture with pain and deformity.

Thorough patient evaluation should always include a detailed review of nutritional status, hormonal abnormalities, current medications, and other medical conditions and treatments. Osteopenia may result from certain medications such as corticosteroids that are commonly used in the treatment of asthma and other conditions. Special attention must be paid to the possibility of the female athletic triad consisting of amenorrhea, disordered eating, and osteoporosis.

Diagnostic imaging includes plain radiographs, bone scan, magnetic resonance imaging (MRI), and computed tomography (CT) scan. Fracture lines, sclerosis, and callus formation may be seen on plain radiographs, but usually do not appear until 1 to 3 weeks after the start of symptoms (3,4). Bone scan is very sensitive in the detection of stress fractures and usually displays changes 1 to 2 weeks before plain radiographs (5). Because bone scans remain positive for several months to over a year, they are not very useful for monitoring bony healing (3,5). MRI is very valuable in the detection of muscle and bone marrow edema and is as sensitive as bone scan in the detection of stress fractures. In addition, MRI allows precise anatomical detail and allows an excellent assessment of the extent of the injury (6,7). Bony

architecture is best viewed on CT scan, which can be used to determine cortical incontinuity and to assess periosteal reaction, bridging callus, and sclerosis.

Radiographic classification of stress fractures may be helpful in determining treatment. Type I stress fractures are subclinical fractures that are asymptomatic and are incidentally found on radiographs. These fractures are usually treated symptomatically. Type II fractures present with pain and are confirmed by bone scan or MRI, but are not evident on plain radiographs. These fractures are commonly referred to as bone strain, stress reaction, or early stress fracture. Type III fractures are symptomatic, nondisplaced fractures that can be seen on plain radiographs. Type IV fractures are displaced stress fractures that are usually treated operatively. Type V fractures are evident on plain radiographs as nonunions with sclerotic margins and no bridging callus formation. In the tibia, the "dreaded black line" heralds a type V fracture and should be treated operatively.

Stress fractures in different anatomical locations behave characteristically and should be considered individually. Suspected long bone fractures may best be evaluated by bone scans which offer a view of the entire extremity, while areas that require specific anatomical localization, such as the femoral neck, are better evaluated by MRI. A careful, systematic approach is critical to the proper diagnosis and treatment of stress fractures.

Treatment Principles

Specific anatomical locations may be classified as high, intermediate, or low risk based on the potential for the fractures to displace or exhibit poor healing. The likelihood of stress fracture complications is multifactorial. Fractures on the tension side of a bone have a predilection to progress to complete fractures because the stress load in tension tends to propagate the fracture lines. These fractures must be treated aggressively with strict nonweight-bearing in incomplete fractures and operative fixation in complete fractures. In contrast, compression side fractures tend to heal with activity modification alone because the stress load tends to approximate the fracture edges (Table 54-1).

Fractures that occur in watershed zones of poor vascularity must also be considered high risk (Table 54-2). These areas exhibit low healing potential and have a predilection for nonunion. A low threshold for operative treatment should be used in these troublesome areas.

Specific Fractures

Femoral Neck

Femoral neck stress fractures typically cause groin or hip pain, particularly at the extremes of motion. Diagnosis may be confirmed with either bone scan or MRI, although MRI may be more helpful in determining the exact anatomical location and extent of the fracture. Fracture appearance tends to be delayed 1 to 2 weeks on plain radiographs.

TABLE 54-1	**Classification of Stress Fractures**	
	High risk	**Low risk**
Stress Type	Tension	Compression
Natural History	Poor	Good
Management	*Aggressive*	*Conservative*
	Complete fx: Surgery	Symptomatic: Activity modification
	Incomplete fx: Strict NWB	Asymptomatic: No rx needed

TABLE 54-2	**Location of High Risk Stress Fractures**

High risk stress fractures

Femoral neck–superolateral
Femoral neck–inferomedial[a]
Patella
Anterior Tibial Diaphysis
Medial Malleolus[a]
Talus
Tarsal Navicular
Fifth Metatarsal
Sesamoids[a]

[a]Intermediate risk

Tension-side femoral neck stress fractures are high-risk fractures that occur in the superior portion of the neck. These fractures have a high risk of nonunion and avascular necrosis, which may have disastrous sequelae. Fractures that are not evident on plain x-rays may be treated with strict nonweight-bearing or with operative fixation depending on the extent of the injury. All superior femoral neck stress fractures that can be seen on plain x-rays should undergo operative fixation, typically with partially threaded 6.5 mm or 7.3 mm cannulated screws.

Compression-side femoral neck stress fractures occur in the inferior portion of the neck and are intermediate-risk **(Fig 54-1)**. Touch-down weight-bearing likely produces lower hip joint reactive forces than nonweight-bearing due to the reduction in hip abductor muscle tension, and is recommended for 6 weeks. Failed nonoperative treatment or propagation of the fracture requires operative intervention. Complete femoral neck fractures should always be treated with operative fixation to avoid complications.

Patella

Patellar stress fractures are high-risk fractures that occur in the anterocentral zone of the patella. Risk factors include knee flexion contracture, which increases the three-point bending forces on the patella, and previous harvest of bone-patellar-bone autograft for anterior cruciate ligament reconstruction, which creates stress risers in the patella. Nondisplaced fractures with an intact extensor mechanism tend to heal well with rest. Chronic or displaced fractures require open reduction internal fixation.

Tibial Shaft

Stress fractures of the tibial shaft represent 20% to 75% of all athletic stress fractures. The posteromedial diaphysis is the compression side of the tibia and is a low-risk region. Most tibial shaft stress fractures occur posteromedially and can usually be managed with activity modification. Pneumatic leg bracing has been shown to significantly reduce the time to return to full activity (8).

The anterior diaphysis is the tension side of the tibia and is a high-risk zone that is more prone to nonunion and displacement. The "dreaded black line" represents a cortical break and may progress to a complete fracture if left untreated **(Fig 54-2)**. These fractures rarely heal with conservative management and are best managed with operative intervention including intramedullary nail fixation and possibly bone grafting.

Medial Malleolus

Stress fractures of the medial malleolus are rare, intermediate-risk injuries that typically occur in running and jumping sports. Varus ankle malalignment may cause medial malleolar overload and contribute to the pathogenesis of medial malleolar stress fractures. Point tenderness and ankle effusions should raise suspicion for a stress fracture. The fracture line usually extends from the superomedial corner of the plafond toward the medial cortex of the medial malleolus. Low demand athletes may be treated with immobilization and nonweight-bearing (9). Open reduction and internal fixation or percutaneous screw fixation has been successfully used to treat complete fractures or stress fractures in high demand athletes, with return to full participation in 6 to 8 weeks (10).

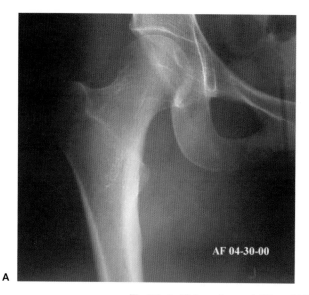
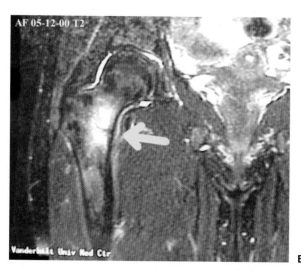

Fig 54-1. Plain radiograph **(A)** and MRI **(B)** of inferior femoral neck stress fracture.

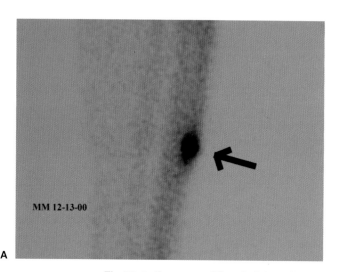
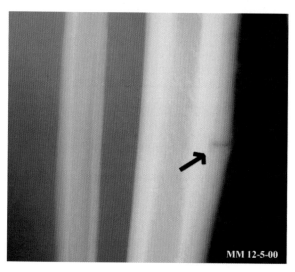

Fig 54-2. Bone scan **(A)** and plain radiograph **(B)** of tibial diaphyseal stress fracture. The plain radiograph exhibits the "dreaded black line."

Fibula

Fibular stress fractures usually occur approximately 5 cm proximal to the distal tip of the lateral malleolus, but may also occur proximally (11). These are rare, low-risk fractures that typically present with mild swelling, point tenderness, and pain with tibiofibular compression. Valgus hindfoot deformity may predispose to distal fibular overload and subsequent stress fracture. When diagnosed early, 3 to 6 weeks of rest followed by gradual return to activity leads to favorable results (10). Fibular stress fractures rarely require operative intervention.

Calcaneus

Calcaneal stress fractures are low-risk fractures that result from repetitive activities such as running and marching. The calcaneus is the most common site of stress fractures in female basic training soldiers, and is second only to metatarsal stress

fractures in male soldiers (12). Pain may be aggravated by toe walking and resisted plantar flexion. Swelling can be seen medially and laterally with pain on compression of the calcaneal tuberosity. In the early stages, diagnosis can be confirmed with bone scan or MRI. At 2 to 4 weeks, radiographs classically exhibit sclerotic lines oriented perpendicular to the trebecular stress lines. Activity modification and the use of cushioned heel inserts usually results in return to activity in 4 to 8 weeks.

Tarsal Navicular

Tarsal navicular stress fractures are high-risk fractures typically seen in runners and basketball players. Patients present with midfoot pain and tenderness along the medial longitudinal arch or dorsum of the foot. Predisposing factors include a short first metatarsal and long second metatarsal. Decreased motion in adjacent joints, such as in the case of a calcaneonavicular coalition or a large tibiotalar osteophyte, can cause transfer of stress to the navicular and may lead to stress fracture.

Stress fractures typically occur in the middle third of the navicular in the sagittal plane **(Fig 54-3)**. This region is a watershed zone of vascularity that faces high shear stresses during plantar flexion and pronation. Navicular stress fractures are difficult to diagnose, but can usually be detected on bone scan and MRI. Oblique and neutral dorsiflexion x-rays may also reveal abnormalities. CT scans must be taken in the plane of the navicular to properly assess the extent of the fracture line. A high index of suspicion must be maintained as diagnosis is often delayed 7 to 28 weeks (10).

Radiographic classification is helpful in determining the treatment of navicular stress fractures (13,14). Type I fractures involve only the dorsal cortex and can be treated with nonweight-bearing for 6 to 8 weeks, followed by protected weight-bearing and gradual return to activity (15–17). Type II fractures extend into the body of the navicular and can be treated with immobilization and nonweight-bearing for 6 to 8 weeks. Type III fractures involve both cortices and require operative treatment, usually with 4.0 to 4.5 mm partially threaded screws. Bone graft may be added in the face of sclerotic fracture margins. CT scan in the plane of the navicular is useful to follow bony healing.

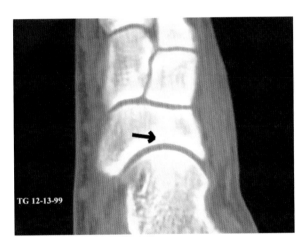

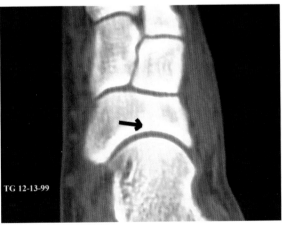

Fig 54-3. CT **(A)** and MRI **(B)** of navicular stress fracture.

Lesser Metatarsals (2 to 4)

Stress fractures of the second, third, and fourth metatarsals are low-risk injuries commonly seen in impact loading, running, and jumping athletes. Plain radiographs can usually diagnose these fractures, but bone scan and MRI may also be helpful. Lesser metatarsal stress fractures are usually successfully treated with activity modification alone.

Fifth Metatarsal

Football and basketball players, long distance runners, and military recruits commonly suffer from fifth metatarsal stress fractures (3,4,18). Patients present with dorsal foot swelling, localized tenderness, and pain with inversion of the foot. Plain radiographs may show a faint radiolucent line and callus formation at 1 to 2 weeks from the start of symptoms (4).

Classification of fractures of the proximal fifth metatarsal is critical in determining the appropriate treatment. Zone I fractures are avulsion fractures at the insertion of the peroneus brevis and lateral cord of the plantar fascia. These fractures enter the fifth metatarsal-cuboid articulation. Zone II fractures (Jones' fracture) extend into the articulation of the fourth and fifth metatarsals. Zone III fractures occur distal to the fourth metatarsal-fifth metatarsal articulation at the distal-most portion of the metaphysis. Most stress fractures occur in Zone III, although acute fractures can occur in this zone as well (3). Stress fractures typically start on the lateral (tension) side and progress medially. The poor vascularity of Zones II and III necessitates aggressive treatment of these fractures.

Zone III stress fractures can be initially treated in an above-knee nonweight-bearing cast, although conservative management has historically yielded poor results. Operative treatment of Zone II and III injuries achieves a more predictable outcome and earlier return to sports than conservative management (10,18,19). Surgical management usually consists of fluoroscopically guided percutaneous screw fixation. Pre-operative radiographs are used to determine the largest diameter screw that can be used (20). Usually a 4.5 or 6.5 mm screw with a length of 50 to 60 mm achieves good intramedullary fit and three-point cortical fixation **(Fig 54-4)**. Bone graft may be added in the case of a nonunion.

Results of operative treatment have been encouraging with return to activity at 6 to 12 weeks (16,18,19). Radiographic union should be confirmed prior to return to athletic activity in order to avoid nonunion (21). Complications of operative treatment include wound infection, nonunion, screw breakage, refracture, and hardware prominence.

Hallucal Sesamoids

Stress fractures of the hallucal sesamoids are intermediate-risk fractures that usually affect the tibial sesamoid. Cavus deformity or first metatarsal plantar flexion deformity may predispose patients to sesamoid stress fracture. Patients present with pain under the first metatarsal during weight bearing and toe-off. Plain radiographs may reveal a transverse or comminuted fracture. Jagged fracture margins differentiate sesamoid fractures from the smooth margins seen in bipartite

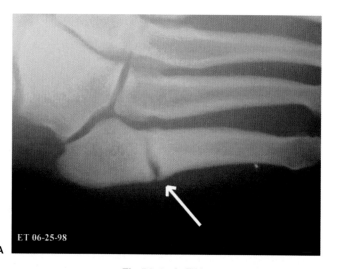

ET 06-25-98

A

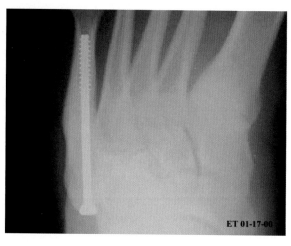

ET 01-17-00

B

Fig 54-4. A: Fifth metatarsal stress fracture. **B:** Healed fracture after operative fixation.

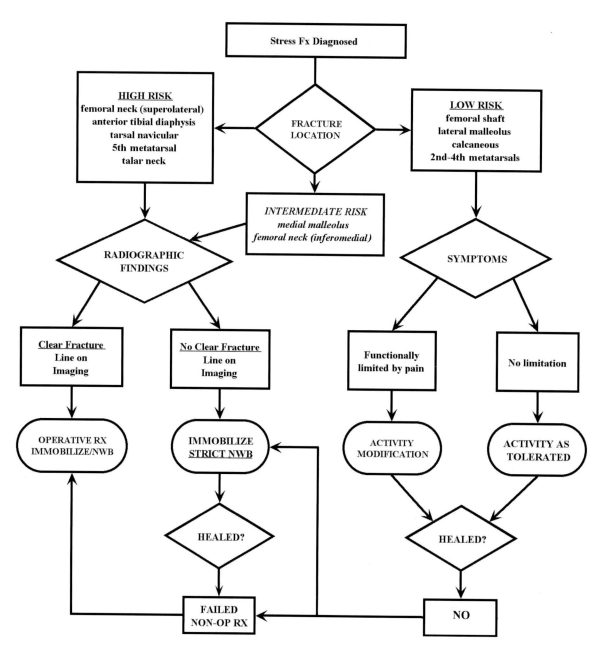

Fig 54-5. Stress fracture treatment algorithm.

sesamoids. The primary principle of treatment is to unload the first metatarsal with rest, immobilization, and stiff-soled orthotics with shock-absorbing wells. Complete resolution of symptoms may take up to 4 to 6 months (11). Operative intervention is indicated after failure of conservative management (22,23). Partial sesamoidectomy leads to good results with a high rate of return to competition (24). Complete sesamoidectomy can result in hallux varus or valgus deformity and weakness of the flexor hallucis brevis and should be avoided. First metatarsal dorsiflexion osteotomy or correction of cavus deformity may also be required.

Upper Extremity

Upper extremity stress fractures represent a minority of athletic stress fractures and are generally low-risk. Strain in the upper extremity may be created either by rotational torque or by axial loading. Stress fractures therefore occur differently in throwers (baseball and softball players, javelin throwers, and soccer goalies), swingers (golfers and tennis players), weight-bearers (gymnasts, cheerleaders, and divers), and weightlifters (power lifters and off-season lifters). In a review of upper extremity and rib stress fractures, the majority of fractures were seen in the shoulder girdle in throwers, lower ribs in swingers, distal to the elbow in weightbearers, and throughout the upper extremity in weightlifters (25). Most upper extremity stress fractures are successfully treated with activity modification and gradual return to activities.

Treatment Algorithm

A systematic approach must be followed in the treatment of athletic stress fractures **(Fig 54-5)**. An assessment of the risk of complications should be made based on anatomical location and vascular supply. In general, low-risk fractures can be treated symptomatically. Low-risk failures that fail nonoperative treatment should be considered for operative intervention. High-risk fractures with x-ray evidence of complete fracture should be treated aggressively with close monitoring or surgical fixation. Incomplete high-risk fractures may be treated with strict nonweight-bearing with a low threshold for operative treatment. A thorough understanding of the pathogenesis and behavior of stress fractures based on anatomical location and other risk factors is essential in the proper treatment of athletic stress fractures.

■ REFERENCES

1. Korpelainen R, Orava S, Karpakka J, et al. Risk factors for recurrent stress fractures in athletes. *Am J Sports Med*. 2001; 29(3): 304–310.
2. Matheson GO, Clement DB, McKenzie DC, et al. Stress fractures in athletes. A study of 320 cases. *Am J Sports Med*. 1987; 15(1):46–58.
3. Torg JS, Balduini FC, Zelco RR. Fractures of the base of the fifth metatarsal distal to the tuberosity. Classification and guidelines for non-surgical and surgical management. *J Bone Joint Surg Am*. 1984;66(2):209–214.
4. Boden BP, Osbahr DC. High-risk stress fractures. Evaluation and treatment. *J Am Acad Orthop Surg*. 2000;8:344–353.
5. Spitz DJ, Newberg AH. Imaging of stress fractures in the athlete. *Radiol Clin North Am*. 2002;40:313–331.
6. Lee JK, Yao L. Stress fractures: MR imaging. *Radiology*. 1988; 169:217–220.
7. Arendt EA, Griffiths HJ. The use of MR imaging in the assessment and clinical management of stress fractures of bone in high-performance athletes. *Clin Sports Med*. 1997;16:291–306.
8. Swenson EL Jr, DeHaven KE, Sebastianelli WJ, et al. The effect of a pneumatic leg brace on return to play in athletes with tibial stress fractures. *Am J Sports Med*. 1997;25:322–328.
9. Orava S, Karpakka J, Taimela S, et al. Stress fracture of the medial malleolus. *J Bone Joint Surg Am*. 1995;77:362–365.
10. Shelbourne KD, Fisher DA, Rettig AC, et al. Stress fractures of the medial malleolus. *Am J Sports Med*. 1988;16:60–63.
11. Meyer SA, Saltzman CL, Albright JP. Stress fractures of the foot and leg. *Clin Sports Med*. 1993;12:395–413.
12. Pester S, Smith PC. Stress fractures in the lower extremities of soldiers in basic training. *Orthop Rev*. 1992;21:297–303.
13. Pavlov H, Torg JS, Freiberger RH. Tarsal navicular stress fractures: Radiographic evaluation. *Radiology*. 1983;148:641–645.
14. Saxena A, Fullem B, Hannaford D. Results of treatment of 22 navicular stress fractures and a new proposed radiographic classification system. *J Foot Ankle Surg*. 2000;39:96–103.
15. Torg JS, Pavlov H, Cooley LH, et al. Stress fractures of the tarsal navicular: a retrospective review of twenty-one cases. *J Bone Joint Surg Am*. 1982;64:700–712.
16. Khan KM, Fuller PJ, Brukner PD, et al. Outcome of conservative and surgical management of navicular stress fracture in athletes: eighty-six cases proven with computed tomography. *Am J Sports Med*. 1992;20:657–666.
17. Khan KM, Brukner PD, Kearney C, et al. Tarsal navicular stress fracture in athletes. *Sports Med*. 1994;17(1):65–76.
18. DeLee JC, Evans JP, Julian J. Stress fracture of the fifth metatarsal. *Am J Sports Med*. 1983;11(5):349–353.
19. Mindrebo NK, Shelbourne D, Van Meter CD, et al. Outpatient percutaneous screw fixation of the acute Jones fracture. *Am J Sports Med*. 1993;21(5):720–723.
20. Wright RW, Fisher DA, Shively RA, et al. Refracture of proximal 5th metatarsal (Jones) fractures after intramedullary screw fixation in athletes. *Am J Sports Med*. 2000;28(5):732–736.
21. Larson CM, Almekinders LC, Taft TN, et al. Intramedullary screw fixation of Jones fractures: Analysis of failure. *Am J Sports Med*. 2002;30:55–60.
22. Richardson EG. Injuries to the hallucal sesamoids in the athlete. *Foot Ankle*. 1987;7:229–244.
23. Leventeen EO. Sesamoid disorders and treatment: an update. *Clin Orthop*. 1991;269:236–240.
24. Biedert R, Hintermann B. Stress fractures of the medial great toe sesamoids in athletes. *Foot Ankle Int*. 2003;24:137–141.
25. Sinha AK, Kaeding CC, Wadley GM. Upper extremity stress fractures in athletes: clinical features of 44 cases. *Clin J Sport Med*. 1999;9:199–202

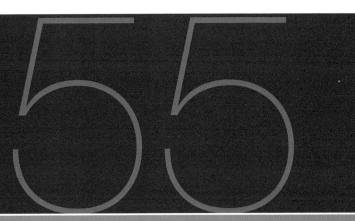

FEMALE ISSUES IN SPORT: RISK FACTORS AND PREVENTION OF ACL INJURIES

JEFFREY R. COUNTS, DO, LORI A. BOLGLA, PT, PhD, ATC, MARY LLOYD IRELAND, MD

■ KEY POINTS

- Anterior cruciate ligament (ACL) injuries are becoming more common and costly.
- The 15- to 45-year-old patient population is most likely to undergo an ACL reconstruction.
- The main function of the ACL is to limit anterior tibial translation on the femur.
- Although overall ACL injury rates for males and females are very similar, the rates do differ for specific sports. Studies have placed the rate of ACL injuries in female basketball players at 2.89 to 3.5 times higher than in males. The increased rate in female soccer players has been placed at 2.3 to 2.8 times that of males.
- Mechanics appear to contribute significantly to the ACL gender bias. Females generally exhibit greater knee valgus, femoral internal rotation, and femoral adduction on an externally rotated knee. Proximal instability from the trunk and hip results in greater knee valgus and knee external rotation, postures known to place increased strain on the ACL. Trunk instability, combined with limited knee flexion, further increases the risk of ACL injury because smaller knee flexion angle limits the hamstrings' ability to contract and prevent anterior tibial translation.
- Females with either a lower extremity or low back dysfunction have demonstrated greater side-to-side hip extension strength symmetry than males.
- Future studies should examine whether improvements in strength, proprioception, movement execution, or a specific combination of areas is most effective in preventing ACL injury. Those studies should also quantify the most appropriate time, duration, and intensity of participation in a prevention program relative to the competitive season.

Anterior cruciate ligament (ACL) injuries are one of the more serious injuries seen in sports medicine. Orthopaedic surgeons perform an estimated 100,000 ACL reconstructions (1) each year with an associated cost of approximately $1.7 billion (2). Furthermore, costs associated with conservative management of ACL injuries, postoperative rehabilitation, and long-term care of posttraumatic arthritis that may occur in certain situations further increase this financial burden. This has a huge economic impact. With today's current emphasis on staying fit, statistics suggest that these numbers will continue to rise in the future. Daniel and Fritschy (3) have reported ACL injury rates of one per 3,500 enrollees across a large managed care–insured population. The 15- to 45-year-old patient population, which encompasses nearly 47% of the entire U.S. population, is most likely to undergo an ACL reconstruction. Griffin et al. (4) have reported ACL injury projection rates specific to this population as one per 1,750.

Nearly 70% of all ACL injuries occur during sports participation (3). Typically, males sustain a higher absolute number of ACL injuries because of their greater sports participation (3). Since the passage of Title IX in 1972, the number of females competing in organized sports has increased. Surprisingly, overall ACL injury rates for males and females are very similar (implying no gender differences). However, these rates do differ when looking at specific sports (5). The National Collegiate Athletic Association (NCAA) (6) has reported that female basketball players sustained an ACL injury at a rate 2.89 times higher than male basketball players, and others (7–9) have reported injury rates as much as 3.5 times higher for female basketball players. Female soccer players have incurred similar rates of injury, with their reported injury rates ranging from 2.3 to 2.8 times greater than male players (7–9).

TABLE 55-1	Summary of Factors Contributing to ACL Injuries	
Intrinsic	**Extrinsic**	
ACL size	Kinetics	
Intercondylar notch size	Kinematics	
Structural alignment	Proprioception	
Tibial plateau orientation	Muscular activation	
Physiological laxity	Muscular strength	
Hormonal influences	and endurance	

2005, Mary Lloyd Ireland.

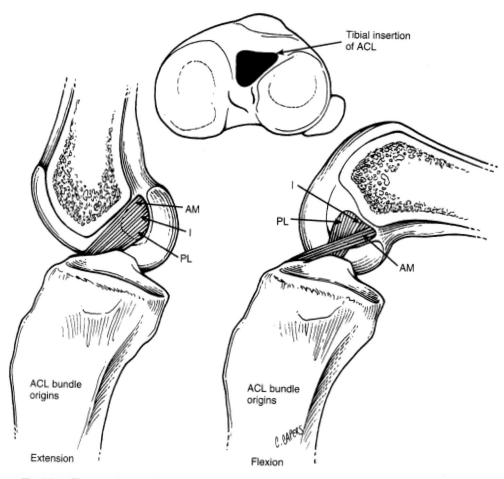

Fig 55-1. The anterior cruciate ligament (ACL) is divided into three bundles based on the tibial attachment: the anteromedial (AM), the intermediate (I), and the posterolateral (PL). With knee flexion, the posterior fibers loosen and the anteromedial fibers coil around the posterolateral ones. (From Baker CL, Flandry F, Henderson JM. *The Hughston Clinic Sports Medicine Book*. Baltimore: Williams & Wilkins; 1995.)

Basketball and soccer injuries usually result from a noncontact mechanism, which represents approximately 70% of all ACL injuries (4). Researchers (10) have described noncontact injuries occurring during two common movement patterns. First, injury may result during open cutting maneuvers. During the deceleration phase of a cutting maneuver, an athlete may exhibit an excessive knee valgus angle in combination with increased femoral internal rotation, resulting in an externally rotated knee. This combined loading has been shown to place a great amount of tension on the ACL that may lead to failure (11). ACL injury may also occur during the landing phase of a jumping maneuver in which the athlete is in a relatively upright position with minimal hip and knee flexion. In this position, greater quadriceps and less hamstring activation increases the forward translation of the tibia on the femur, which may result in an ACL injury (12).

Several factors may contribute to noncontact ACL injuries and can be classified as being intrinsic or extrinsic **(Table 55-1)** (13). Intrinsic factors are structural and physiological in nature, representing those features that clinicians cannot modify. They include the intercondylar notch width, ACL size, absolute pelvic width, femoral length, physiological laxity, and hormonal influences. Extrinsic factors are those that can be modified with therapeutic interventions and include biomechanical and neuromuscular influences. In this chapter, we will explain how all of these factors may lead to injury and present prevention program strategies that may decrease the risk of ACL injury in the female athlete.

■ ANATOMICAL OVERVIEW

The ACL is an intra-articular, extrasynovial ligament that primarily restrains anterior tibial translation on the femur. The ligament passes through the intercondylar notch from an anteromedial to a posterolateral direction. The ligament has attachments along the posteromedial wall of the lateral femoral condyle and just anterior to the medial tibial eminence. It consists of two distinct bands, although a third intermediate band has also been described (14). These bands are defined based on their tibial attachments and consist of anteromedial and posterolateral bundles **(Fig 55-1)**. As the knee moves, these bands provide differing stabilizing effects for the knee. When the knee is in full extension, the posterolateral bundle is tauter compared to the anteromedial bundle. As the knee flexes, the ACL assumes a relatively horizontal position. This position causes increased tightening of the anteromedial bundle and a loosening of the posterolateral bundle. One portion of the ACL remains under tension throughout the full range of motion, providing a continuous stabilizing effect for the knee.

■ INTRINSIC FACTORS

ACL and Intercondylar Notch Size

Since 1938, researchers (15) have theorized that a smaller intercondylar notch size may increase the risk of ACL injury. They believed that ACL injury results from an increased stretch over the inner margins of the femoral condyles, which may occur at positions near full knee extension where the ACL can abut the roof of the intercondylar notch. Therefore, athletes who have a smaller sized notch may be more susceptible to an ACL injury because of the

decreased space available within the intercondylar notch. Based on this relationship, researchers have investigated the correlation between intercondylar notch stenosis and ACL injury using plain radiographs, computed tomography (CT), and magnetic resonance imaging (MRI).

Plain Radiographs

Historically, physicians have assessed intercondylar notch size using plain radiographs. In an attempt to normalize notch size for comparison among subjects, Souryal et al. (16) developed the notch width index (NWI). This is defined as the ratio of the width of the intercondylar notch to the width of the distal femur at the level of the popliteal grove as seen on a tunnel view. They reported that high school athletes who sustained a noncontact injury had an NWI of 0.189 compared to 0.233 for those who injured their ACL during a contact mechanism. In a related study, Ireland et al. (17) reported that individuals who sustained an ACL injury had both smaller NWI and absolute notch width measurements, regardless of gender, than those individuals who did not injure their ACL ligament.

Researchers (18,19) have challenged the usefulness of the NWI. Shelbourne et al. (18) found that femoral bicondylar width increased as absolute femur length increased and believed that absolute notch width may be a more appropriate radiographic measurement. They reported a mean notch width of 16.9 mm and 14.5 mm, respectively, for noninjured males and females of similar height. For patients with unilateral ACL tears, the mean notch width decreased to 15.8 mm in males and 13.8 mm in females. The notch size decreased even more in those having bilateral ACL tears. For this subject cohort, males and females had average notch widths of 15.3 mm and 12.8 mm, respectively. Based on these findings, Shelbourne et al. (18) concluded that subjects with narrower absolute notch widths might possess a higher risk of injury.

Alternatively, others (20–23) have not found a relationship between notch size and incidence of ACL injury. The controversy in the literature may be due to limitations associated with plain radiographs that may influence measurement precision. Such factors include overlap and shadowing associated with plain radiographs and variation in knee position during radiography. Finally, plain radiographs only provide a two-dimensional view. Therefore, plain films may not adequately depict the true shape of the intercondylar notch and true relationship between the intercondylar notch and ACL size.

CT and MRI

More recently, researchers have analyzed the three-dimensional features of the intercondylar notch using more advanced imaging technology. Anderson et al. (24) collected CT images of the distal femur, created composite drawings of the intercondylar notch, and consistently identified five general shapes. Shapes ranged from an inverted "U" to a crested wave–shaped notch with a flattened superior medial corner. The crested wave shape resulted in a more stenotic notch. Patients with this morphology had a higher incidence of ACL injury, regardless of gender.

MRI has also been used to study the size of the intercondylar notch and the ACL. Davis et al. (25) reported a positive correlation between absolute intercondylar notch and ACL width. They also found that males exhibited larger notch and ACL widths than females. Other researchers have also compared ACL cross-sectional area between genders (19,26). In these studies, they reported larger ligaments in male subjects. They inferred that a smaller ligament may be weaker and more vulnerable to forces generated during certain athletic maneuvers. Some researchers have examined the strength of different sized ACL specimens and reported that a 14-mm ligament may withstand loads of up to 2,900 newtons (N), whereas a 10-mm ligament can only withstand loads up to 2,070 N (27). Few studies have examined this relationship, and more are needed to establish the relationship between ACL size and ligamentous strength.

Structural Alignment

Studies have shown that females tend to perform running and cutting activities with greater valgus angles and external abduction moments of the knee compared to males. Fung and Zhang (11) have shown that these actions may place greater strain on the ACL, and researchers have studied gender differences related to structural alignment. They have theorized that the structural malalignment that contributes to these movement patterns may increase the risk of ACL injury in the female athlete.

Conventional wisdom suggests that females have wider pelvises, which may lead to coxa varum, genu valgus, and increased rotational forces at the tibiofemoral joint. However, a study by Horton and Hall (28) found that, in absolute terms, females had smaller pelvic widths compared to male subjects. Subsequently, Livingston and Gahagan (29) examined pelvic width by calculating a hip width to femoral length ratio for males and females. Although females had smaller absolute pelvic widths, their hip width to femoral length was greater than in males. These authors concluded that the shorter femur length associated with female subjects increased the hip adduction required to position the feet under the center of mass of the body. This, in turn, may increase the knee valgus angle and, perhaps, the strain on the ACL. Therefore, the pelvic width to femoral length ratio might be more predictive of ACL injury than absolute pelvic width alone.

Loudon et al. (30) studied static structural faults that may be predictive of ACL injury. They reported that knee hyperextension, excessive navicular drop, and excessive subtalar joint pronation discriminated between females with and without ACL injury. They also determined that the presence of two or more structural faults may be more predictive of ACL injury than any one alone. For example, knee hyperextension in combination with tibial internal rotation can stretch the ACL over the lateral femoral condyle. During weight-bearing activities, subtalar pronation is coupled with tibial internal rotation (31). Therefore, excessive pronation can impart additional strain to the ACL, making it more vulnerable to injury. However, this study was retrospective in nature; it is unknown if these factors conclusively caused the ACL injury.

Tibial Plateau Orientation

The posterior slope of the tibial plateau has been suggested to contribute to ACL injury risk. This angle is formed by the tibial plateau in relation to the long axis of the tibia. The normal posterior slope ranges from 10 to 12 degrees. However, a steeper posterior slope may increase anterior tibial translation by placing the femur in a more posteriorly directed position relative to the tibia. Dejour and Bonnin (32) measured tibial slope and anterior tibial translation, using the radiological Lachman test, for the involved and uninvolved knee in subjects having a unilateral chronic ACL rupture. They then used linear regression analysis to determine the relationship between anterior translation and tibial slope. This analysis showed a 3.5-mm increase of anterior tibial translation for every 10-degree increase in tibial slope, and it was thought that a higher tibial slope may contribute to ACL injury. However, Meister et al. (33) measured posterior tibial slope in subjects diagnosed with and without ACL injury. Their results did not find differences in tibial slope between groups and were unable to validate this as a risk factor associated with ACL injury. Because limited research exists in this area, future investigations are needed to establish the possible relationship between tibial plateau orientation and ACL injury.

Physiological Laxity

The main function of the ACL is to limit anterior translation of the tibia on the femur. Failure occurs when the anterior load exceeds the strength of the ligament. Some researchers (34,35) have suggested that increased joint laxity results in excessive anterior tibial translation and ACL injury. Therefore, there has been some focus on the influence of both generalized joint laxity and ligamentous laxity on ACL injury.

Nicholas (36) originally reported a relationship between generalized joint laxity and knee injury in male football players. These relationships have also been compared between males and females in the context of understanding the gender bias in ACL injuries. Both Ostenberg and Roos (37) and Soderman et al. (38) have found generalized joint laxity to be a significant factor in the gender bias for ACL injury.

The KT-1000 Ligament Arthrometer (Med-Metric, San Diego, CA) has been used to assess gender differences in ligamentous laxity. Prior work has shown that collegiate female athletes have greater anterior tibial translation than their male counterparts (39–41). Furthermore, Uhorchack et al. (42) reported that females who exhibited ligamentous laxity values of one or more standard deviations above the mean were 2.7 times more likely to sustain a noncontact ACL injury than those with less laxity. This ligamentous laxity, in combination with a decreased intercondylar notch size, may further increase the likelihood of sustaining an ACL injury.

Hormonal Influences

Hormonal differences may further contribute to the ACL injury gender bias. Many studies have evolved from the earlier work of Liu et al. (43), who identified estrogen and progesterone receptors in human ACL cells. Estrogen is thought to decrease fibroblastic and collagen production (44), whereas progesterone has opposite effects (45). It has been hypothesized that cyclic changes, absolute level, and rate of hormonal change of estrogen and progesterone may affect ligament strength.

The menstrual cycle can be divided into the follicular, ovulatory, and luteal phases. Estrogen levels rise dramatically during the ovulatory phase and remain elevated throughout the luteal phase; progesterone levels remain relatively low until the luteal phase. These fluctuations may place the female athlete at greater risk of injury just prior to ovulation when estrogen levels are at their highest. Some researchers (46,47) have reported an association between high estrogen levels, ligament laxity, and ACL injury. However, in contrast, others (48–50) have not found this relationship. A limitation of many studies has been a smaller sample size and reliance on subjective history regarding the phase of menstrual cycle at the time of injury. Although researchers have documented hormone level using saliva and blood samples, larger scale studies are needed to better understand this relationship. Future studies should use common time intervals to define the menstrual phases; determine hormone levels based on urine, saliva, and serum; and report these levels both at the time of injury and at the beginning of the next period (51). Such information will help clinicians better determine the phase of the menstrual cycle and the length of time within the cycle that an injury occurred (51).

Oral contraceptive use further complicates this issue. Moller-Neilson and Hammar (52) reported that females who took an oral contraceptive pill (OCP) sustained fewer overall injuries than females who did not. Martineau et al. (53) reported a significant decrease in knee laxity in women who took an OCP. In stark contrast to these studies, an NCAA surveillance revealed higher injury rates prior to or immediately following menses regardless of OCP use. Therefore, at this point, there is a lack of consensus regarding the association between menstrual cycle phase, OCP use, and ACL injury.

■ EXTRINSIC FACTORS

Although anatomical and hormonal factors may play a role in injury risk, they are generally not modifiable. However, there are factors thought to be related to injury risk that may be amenable to change. These include movement patterns and forces (biomechanical factors) as well as the control of

muscular activity (neuromuscular factors). These factors will be discussed in the next sections.

Biomechanical Factors

Lower extremity kinematic differences between male and female athletes have been studied during many types of athletic maneuvers. Zeller et al. (54) examined gender differences during a single-legged squat and found that females demonstrated greater hip adduction and subtalar pronation compared to males. Females also maintained a valgus knee position throughout the task, while males remained in a more varus posture. These results showed that females moved toward knee valgus, a more risky knee position according to Hewett et al. (55), during a relatively low-demanding task **(Fig 55-2)**.

Malinzak et al. (56) evaluated gender differences in lower extremity kinematics during higher demanding activities of running, cross-cutting, and side-cutting. Compared to males, female athletes demonstrated greater knee valgus and less knee flexion angles during the stance phase of these maneuvers. Ferber et al. (57) conducted a study in recreational runners to identify gender differences in frontal- and transverse-plane knee and hip kinematics. As in the Malinzak et al. (56) study, females exhibited greater knee valgus angles, as well as greater hip adduction, hip internal rotation, and tibial external rotation angles compared to males.

Many noncontact ACL injuries occur during landing, and gender differences have been identified with these activities

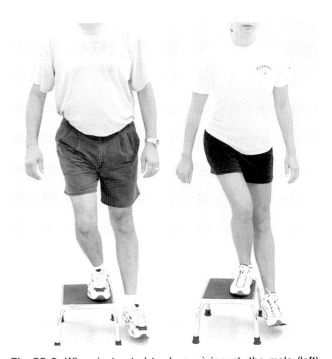

Fig 55-2. When instructed to do a minisquat, the male (left) demonstrates hip over knee over ankle alignment; the female (right) demonstrates femoral adduction and internal rotation and subsequent external rotation, valgus of the knee, and forefoot pronation. (Copyright 2001, M.L. Ireland.)

as well. Ford et al. (58) reported that high school female basketball players land in greater knee valgus than males during a drop vertical jump task. Lephart et al. (59) found that females performed landing activities with greater hip internal rotation, greater tibial external rotation, and less knee flexion than males. Fung and Zhang (11) have shown that combined tibial external rotation (that may result from increased femoral internal rotation) and knee valgus places high strain on the ACL.

Gender differences in kinetic variables have also been studied. Chappell et al. (60) showed that females generated greater external knee valgus moments during a vertical jump than males. More recently, Hewett et al. (61) assessed lower extremity kinetics in 205 healthy high school basketball, volleyball, and soccer athletes. They then followed them through two fall (soccer) and one winter (basketball) sports seasons and recorded any lower extremity injuries. They reported that females who went on to sustain an ACL injury exhibited 8-degree greater knee valgus angles than noninjured athletes. Injured athletes also had 2.5 times greater external knee abduction moments during landing and 20% higher ground reaction force during landing compared to noninjured females.

In general, females exhibit greater knee valgus, femoral internal rotation, and femoral adduction on an externally rotated knee, which Ireland (13) has described as the "position of no return." **Figure 55-3** compares optimal body alignment and muscle activity to this vulnerable position. A noteworthy point is that proximal instability (from the trunk and hip) results in greater knee valgus and knee external rotation, postures known to place increased strain on the ACL (11). This, in combination with limited knee flexion, further increases the risk of ACL injury because smaller knee flexion angles limit the hamstrings' ability to contract and prevent anterior tibial translation. In summary, mechanics appear to contribute significantly to the ACL gender bias.

Neuromuscular Factors

Although kinematic and kinetic patterns contribute to the ACL gender bias, neuromuscular factors are thought to also play a significant role. Studies have identified gender differences related to proprioception, muscular activation, and muscular strength and endurance. We believe that an understanding of these differences is paramount when developing and implementing ACL injury rehabilitation and prevention programs.

Proprioception

Proprioception, the recognition of joint motion and position during active and passive movements, is critical for normal joint function. The nervous system receives proprioceptive input from mechanoreceptors located in ligaments, such as the ACL. It uses this information to coordinate quadriceps

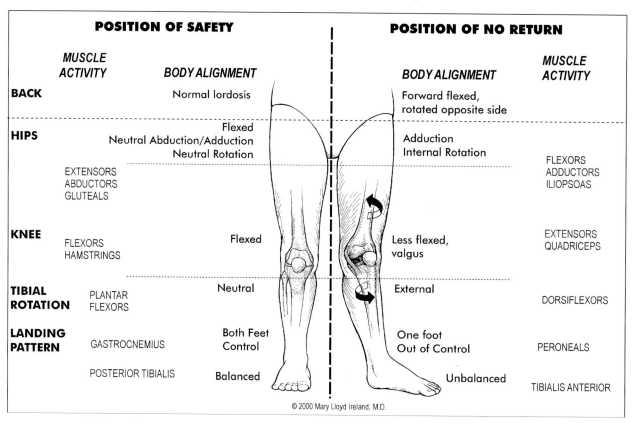

Fig 55-3. The position-of-no-return mechanism for ACL injury and the safe position. (Copyright 2002, M.L. Ireland.)

and hamstring co-contraction, which in effect stiffens and stabilizes the knee during dynamic activities. Therefore, diminished proprioception may alter knee musculature activation in such a way as to make the ACL more vulnerable to injury.

Gender differences may exist with respect to proprioception. Rozzi et al. (40) reported that females required longer time to detect motion during passive knee extension. This diminished proprioception suggests that the hamstring contraction required to counteract quadriceps activity may be delayed. Such a delay may be detrimental to the ACL because of the resultant anterior tibial shear force.

Muscular Activation

Regarding ACL injury risk, much attention has been focused on the balance between the quadriceps and hamstring activation. Hamstring activity helps prevent excessive anterior translation of the tibia. Wojtys et al. (62) reported that males can generate greater maximum isometric co-contraction of the quadriceps and hamstrings, resulting in significantly less anterior tibial translation, than females with similar knee laxity. During dynamic athletic maneuvers, it has been shown that males produce relatively higher peak flexor moments about the knee (2). However, females tend to perform landing maneuvers with predominant quadriceps activation, a pattern that may lead to excessive anterior tibial translation (12). Markolf et al. (63) found that an excessive quadriceps contraction causes increased tibial anterior translation during 0 to 30 degrees of knee flexion. As the knee approaches 45 degrees of flexion and beyond, the patella ligament's orientation changes and provides a posteriorly directed tibial force. Since females perform many demanding activities with limited knee flexion, they do not take advantage of the stabilizing influence knee flexion provides.

The focus of muscular activation in ACL injury has been on the knee. However, it is the hip musculature that has the greatest influence on frontal and transverse plane movements of the knee. Zeller et al. (54) were among the first researchers to examine gender differences in hip and knee muscle activity during a single-legged squat. They chose this activity because it simulated a common athletic position that required an individual to control body weight over a planted leg. As expected, in terms of kinematics, females performed a single-legged squat with greater hip adduction and knee valgus angles. With respect to electromyogram (EMG) activation, a multivariate analysis of variance for all muscle activity showed that females had higher overall activation than male subjects. When analyzing muscles separately, females demonstrated significantly greater rectus femoris amplitudes.

Studies for patellofemoral pain syndrome have shown that subjects with apparent quadriceps weakness require greater motor unit recruitment (higher activation) during stair climbing (64) and knee extension exercise (65). With respect to the Zeller et al. (54) study, greater hip activation demonstrated by females may reflect proximal weakness and account for greater hip adduction and internal rotation

(as discussed in Biomechanical Factors). Combined hip adduction and internal rotation can increase knee valgus which, when combined with rectus femoris activation, can impart a strong anterior tibial force on the knee and strain on the ACL. Additional studies are warranted to conclusively support the relationship between hip control and ACL injury.

Muscular Strength

Adequate quadriceps and hamstring muscle strength is required for normal knee function. Together, co-contraction of the knee musculature not only stiffens the knee but also attenuates ground reaction forces imparted through the lower extremity. Although male athletes exhibit overall greater knee strength than females (66), this bias does not occur until after puberty (55,67). During the adolescent growth spurt, males show dramatic increases in strength, power, and coordination, which is not similarly achieved by females (9,10,55). As a result, this difference may account for the increase in the postpubescent female ACL injury rates during this developmental stage. These findings support the importance of knee strength and its stabilizing effects.

Strength has also been significantly correlated with endurance, which, when decreased, results in early fatigue. Fatigue has been shown to lead to faulty movement patterns (68) and altered proprioception (69). Nyland et al. (70) evaluated the effect of fatigue on muscle activation in female basketball and volleyball athletes. As these athletes fatigued, they had delayed recruitment of the quadriceps and hamstring musculature and an acceleration of maximal knee flexion during running and rapid stopping maneuvers. Chappell et al. (71) examined the effect of lower extremity fatigue on knee kinematics and kinetics. They found that females demonstrated significantly higher peak proximal tibial anterior shear forces and external valgus moments and smaller knee flexion angles during landing from three stop-jump tasks. Based on these studies, it can be inferred that knee musculature fatigue may predispose the female athlete to knee injury.

The quadriceps and hamstrings are important knee stabilizers in the sagittal plane, but they play less of a role controlling frontal and transverse plane motion. Fortunately, the lumbopelvic musculature, referred to as the core, can influence these planes of motion. For example, the hip abductors control femoral adduction, and the hip external rotators control femoral internal rotation. Together, hip abductor and external rotator muscle strength may limit the amount of valgus strain placed on the knee.

As seen in the knee musculature, there appears to be a gender difference related to core strength. Females with either a lower extremity or low back dysfunction have demonstrated greater side-to-side hip extension strength asymmetry than males (72). Cahalan et al. (73) reported a 39% deficit in hip external rotation torque in females compared to males. Recently, Ireland et al. (74) have shown that females with anterior knee pain had significant hip abductor and external rotator muscle weakness. However, this study was cross-sectional in nature and was unable to assess cause and effect. To address this limitation, Leetun et al. (75) prospectively examined the association between core strength, endurance measures, and lower extremity injury in male and female collegiate athletes. Females generally exhibited lower measures of hip abduction, hip external rotation, and side bridging function. In addition, they were slightly weaker in their abdominal muscles. Over an entire competitive season, they found that athletes with weaker core muscles were more likely to incur a lower extremity injury. To date, limited literature exists regarding this association between core endurance and lower extremity injury. More prospective studies are needed to establish this relationship.

■ PREVENTION PROGRAMS

As the mechanisms of ACL injuries are being revealed, prevention programs are being developed. Some have stressed proper mechanics (76,77) and proprioception (77,78), whereas others have emphasized strengthening (2), conditioning (79), and neuromuscular training (2,80). Although each intervention has a primary focus and reported significant success, much overlap exists among programs, making it difficult to ascertain the most important factor. Based on the current state of knowledge, a prevention program should include all areas related to the neuromuscular, kinematic, and kinetic factors that are believed to increase the risk of ACL injury.

Beginning at the postpubescent developmental phase, females should engage in an aggressive knee and core neuromuscular rehabilitation program. Quadriceps and hamstring strength is needed to adequately support the knee and attenuate forces generated during high-demand activities. Core strength appears to be critical for proper hip and knee alignment. Proprioceptive training may further protect the female from injury because it allows her to anticipate external forces or loads applied to the knee. This anticipation, referred to as the feedforward mechanism, can help the athlete preactivate her muscles and develop movement patterns to protect the knee. Studies have shown that proprioception programs can significantly reduce the incidence of ACL injury (77,78,80).

Addressing these neuromuscular factors may help females develop proper kinematic and kinetic patterns during landing and cutting techniques. Henning and Griffis (81) have reported a significant reduction in ACL injury by training athletes to increase knee flexion during landing, avoiding a planted foot pivot, and using a three-step stop-deceleration. Furthermore, Hewett et al. (76) have shown that emphasis on minimizing knee varus and valgus alignment during these maneuvers can reduce injury. They also train their athletes to land softly to minimize external moments applied to the knee.

Clinicians can use both verbal and visual feedback to instruct the athlete on proper landing and cutting techniques. Hewett et al. (76) successfully used a prevention program that encouraged females to perform as many repetitions of plyometric drills as long as they used proper technique. However, the athletes were stopped when they exhibited signs of fatigue. Myklebust et al. (77) also implemented a training program where athletes were paired and provided each other with visual feedback on proper biomechanics. Using augmented feedback, Onate et al. (82) trained athletes to generate less ground reaction forces during a vertical jump. Together, these studies have found that feedback is an important component of an effective prevention program.

Finally, a prevention program should address sport-specific tasks. This component is very important because it will help train the female athlete to maintain optimal lower extremity alignment during more demanding activities. They should participate in a plyometric program that emphasizes landing in a more varus, flexed knee position **(Fig 55-4)**. Sport-specific agility drills may also be used to improve proprioception and biomechanics **(Figs 55-5 to 55-7)** (83). Finally, we cannot overemphasize that the female athlete

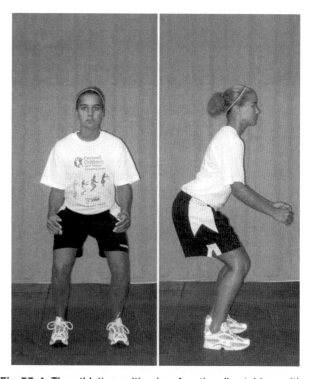

Fig 55-4. The athletic position is a functionally stable position with the knees comfortably flexed, shoulders back, eyes up, feet approximately shoulder width apart, and body mass balanced over the balls of the feet. The knees should be over the balls of the feet, and the chest should be over the knees. The athlete-ready position is the starting and finishing position for most of the training exercises. During some exercises, the finishing position is exaggerated with deeper knee flexion in order to emphasize the correction of certain biomechanical deficiencies. (From Myer GD, Ford KR, Hewett TE. Rationale and clinical techniques for anterior cruciate ligament injury prevention among female athletes. *J Athl Train.* 2004;39:352–364; permission pending.)

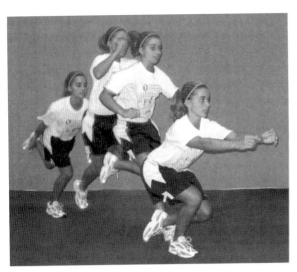

Fig 55-5. Single-leg hop and hold. The starting position is a semi-crouched position on a single leg. The athlete's arm should be fully extended behind her at the shoulder. She initiates the jump by swinging the arms forward while simultaneously extending at the hip and knee. The jump should carry the athlete up at an angle of approximately 45 degrees and attain maximal distance for a single-leg landing. She is instructed to land on the jumping leg with deep knee flexion (to 90 degrees) and to hold the landing for at least 3 seconds. Coach this jump with care to protect the athlete from injury. Start her with a submaximal effort on the single-leg broad jump so she can experience the level of difficulty. Continue to increase the distance of the broad hop as the athlete improves her ability to "stick" and hold the final landing. Have the athlete keep her visual focus away from the feet to help prevent too much forward lean at the waist. (From Myer GD, Ford KR, Hewett TE. Rationale and clinical techniques for anterior cruciate ligament injury prevention among female athletes. *J Athl Train*. 2004;39:352–364; permission pending.)

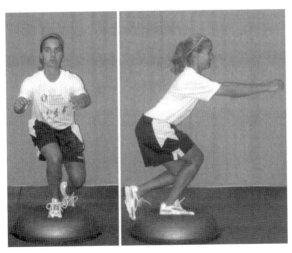

Fig 55-6. Single-leg balance. The balance drills are performed on a balance device that provides an unstable surface. The athlete begins on a device with a two-legged stance with feet shoulder width apart, in athletic position. As she improves, the training drills can incorporate ball catches and single-leg balance drills. Encourage the athlete to maintain deep knee flexion when performing all balance drills. (From Myer GD, Ford KR, Hewett TE. Rationale and clinical techniques for anterior cruciate ligament injury prevention among female athletes. *J Athl Train*. 2004; 39:352–364; permission pending.)

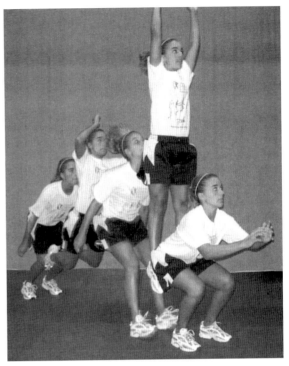

Fig 55-7. Jump, jump, jump, vertical jump. The athlete performs three successive broad jumps and immediately progresses into a maximum-effort vertical jump. The three consecutive broad jumps should be performed as quickly as possible and attain maximal horizontal distance. The third broad jump should be used as a preparatory jump that will allow horizontal momentum to be quickly and efficiently transferred into vertical power. Encourage the athlete to provide minimal braking on the third and final broad jump to ensure that maximum energy is transferred to the vertical jump. Coach the athlete to go directly vertical on the fourth jump and not move horizontally. Use full arm extension to achieve maximum vertical height. (From Myer GD, Ford KR, Hewett TE. Rationale and clinical techniques for anterior cruciate ligament injury prevention among female athletes. *J Athl Train*. 2004;39:352–364; permission pending.)

should practice proper deceleration techniques and prevent pivoting on a fixed foot (84).

In conclusion, recent studies have shown promising results with prevention programs. However, because the risk factors have not been clearly identified, additional prospective studies are required to determine the most critical aspect of a specific program. Additional information on prevention programs can be accessed at www.aclprevent.com and www.sportsmetrics.net.

■ CONCLUSION AND FUTURE DIRECTIONS

Females are known to be at higher risk than males for non-contact ACL injury in sports like basketball and soccer. Historically, research has focused on anatomic, physiological, and hormonal influences independent of each other. A review of the recent literature has not conclusively supported a single intrinsic factor responsible for injury. Future studies should examine the interdependence of these measures because a multifactorial approach may better explain the role of intrinsic factors on the ACL gender bias (85).

Fortunately, recent investigations have suggested that extrinsic factors might contribute more to the ACL gender bias. Studies on prevention programs have demonstrated that extrinsic factors are amenable to change and can reduce injury. Although these programs have had promising outcomes, it is inconclusive what specific changes they impart on the overall system. Future studies should examine whether improvement in strength, proprioception, movement execution, or a specific combination of areas is most effective in preventing ACL injury. Future investigations should also quantify the most appropriate time, duration, and intensity of participation in a prevention program relative to the competitive season (85).

■ REFERENCES

1. Huston LJ, Greenfield MVH, Wojtys EM. Anterior cruciate ligament injuries in the female athlete: potential risk factors. *Clin Orthop.* 2000;372:50–63.
2. Hewett TE, Lindenfeld TN, Riccobene JV, et al. The effect of neuromuscular training on the incidence of knee injury in female athletes. *Am J Sports Med.* 1999;27:699–705.
3. Daniel DM, Fritschy D. Anterior cruciate ligament injuries. In: DeLee JC, Drez D, eds. *Orthopedic sports medicine: principles and Practice.* Vol 2. Philadelphia: WB Saunders; 1994:1313–1361.
4. Griffin LY, Agel J, Albohm MJ, et al. Noncontact anterior cruciate ligament injuries: risk factors and prevention strategies. *J Am Acad Orthop Surg.* 2000;8:141–150.
5. Malone TR, Hardaker WT, Garrett WE, et al. Relationship of gender to anterior cruciate ligament injuries in intercollegiate basketball players. *J South Orthop Assoc.* 1993;2:36–39.
6. National Collegiate Athletic Association. *NCAA injury surveillance system summary.* Indianapolis, IN: National Collegiate Athletic Association; 2002.
7. Arendt E, Dick R. Knee injury patterns among men and women in collegiate basketball and soccer. NCAA data and review of the literature. *Am J Sports Med.* 1995;23:694–701.
8. Arendt E, Agel J, Dick R. Anterior cruciate ligament injury patterns among collegiate men and women. *J Athl Train.* 1999;34:86–92.
9. Miyasaka KC, Daniel DM, Stone ML, et al. The incidence of knee ligament injuries in the gender population. *Am J Knee Surg.* 1991;4:3–8.
10. Ireland ML, Gaudette M, Crook S. ACL injuries in the female athlete. *J Sport Rehabil.* 1997;6:97–110.
11. Fung DT, Zhang LQ. Modeling of ACL impingement against the intercondylar notch. *Clin Biomech.* 2003;18:933–941.
12. DeMorat G, Weinhold P, Blackburn T, et al. Aggressive quadriceps loading can induce noncontact anterior cruciate ligament injury. *Am J Sports Med.* 2004;32:477–483.
13. Ireland ML. The female ACL: why is it more prone to injury? *Orthop Clin N Am.* 2002;33:637–651.
14. Baker CL, Flandry F, Henderson JM. *The Hughston Clinic sports medicine book.* Baltimore: Williams & Wilkins; 1995.
15. Palmer I. On the injuries to the ligaments of the knee joint: a clinical study. *Acta Chir Scand.* 1938;53:1–28.
16. Souryal TO, Moore HA, Evans JP. Bilaterality in anterior cruciate ligament injuries: associated intercondylar notch stenosis. *Am J Sports Med.* 1988;16:449–454.
17. Ireland ML, Ballantyne BT, Little K, et al. A radiographic analysis of the relationship between size and shape of the intercondylar notch and anterior cruciate ligament injury. *Knee Surg Sports Traumatol Arthrosc.* 2001;9:200–205.
18. Shelbourne KD, Davis TJ, Klootwyk TE. The relationship between intercondylar notch width of the femur and the incidence of anterior cruciate ligament injury. A prospective study. *Am J Sports Med.* 1998;26:402–408.
19. Charlton WPH, St. John TA, Ciccotti MG, et al. Differences in femoral notch anatomy between men and women. A magnetic resonance imaging study. *Am J Sports Med.* 2002;30:329–333.
20. Schickendantz MS, Weiker GG. The predictive value of radiographs in the evaluation of unilateral and bilateral anterior cruciate ligament injuries. *Am J Sports Med.* 1993;21:110–113.
21. Herzog RJ, Silliman JF, Hutton K, et al. Measurements of the intercondylar notch by plain film radiography and magnetic resonance imaging. *Am J Sports Med.* 1994;22:204–210.
22. Teitz CC, Lind BK, Sacks BM. Symmetry of the femoral notch width index. *Am J Sports Med.* 1997;25:687–690.
23. Lombardo S, Sethi PM, Starkey C. Intercondylar notch stenosis is not a risk factor for anterior cruciate ligament tears in professional male basketball players. An 11-year prospective study. *Am J Sports Med.* 2005;33:29–34.
24. Anderson AF, Lipscomb AB, Liudahl KJ, et al. Analysis of the intercondylar notch by computed tomography. *Am J Sports Med.* 1987;15:547–552.
25. Davis TJ, Shelbourne KD, Klootwyk TE. Correlation of the intercondylar notch width of the femur to the width of the femur to the width of the anterior and posterior cruciate ligaments. *Knee Surg Sports Traumatol Arthrosc.* 1999;7:209–214.
26. Anderson AF, Dome DC, Gautam S, et al. Correlation of anthropometric measurements, strength, anterior cruciate ligament size, and intercondylar notch characteristics to sex differences in anterior cruciate ligament tear rates. *Am J Sports Med.* 2001;29:58–66.
27. Woo SL, Hollis JM, Adams DJ, et al. Tensile properties of the human femur-anterior cruciate ligament-tibia complex. The effects of specimen age and orientation. *Am J Sports Med.* 1991;19:217–225.
28. Horton MG, Hall TL. Quadriceps femoris muscle angle: normal values and relationships with gender and selected skeletal measures. *Phys Ther.* 1989;69:897–901.
29. Livingston LA, Gahagan JC. The wider gynaecoid pelvis-larger Q angles-greater predisposition to ACL injury relationship: myth or reality? *Clin Biomech.* 2001;16:951–952.
30. Loudon JK, Jenkins W, Loudon KL. The relationship between static posture and ACL injury in female athletes. *J Orthop Sports Phys Ther.* 1996;24:91–97.
31. Woodford-Rogers B, Cyphert L, Denegar CR. Risk factors for anterior cruciate ligament injury for high school and college athletes. *J Athl Train.* 1994;29:343–346.
32. Dejour H, Bonnin M. Tibial translation after anterior cruciate ligament rupture. Two radiological tests compared. *J Bone Joint Surg Br.* 1994;76:745–749.
33. Meister K, Talley MC, Horodyski MB, et al. Caudal slope of the tibia and its relationship to noncontact injuries to the ACL. *Am J Knee Surg.* 1998;11:217–219.
34. Acuasuso DM, Collantes EE, Sanchez-Guijo P. Joint hyperlaxity and musculoligamentous lesions: study of a homogenous age, sex, and physical exertion. *Br J Rheumatol.* 1993;32:120–122.
35. Lysens RJ, Ostyn MS, Auweele YV, et al. The accident-prone and overuse-prone profiles of the young athlete. *Am J Sports Med.* 1989;17:612–619.
36. Nicholas JA. Injuries to knee ligaments: relationship to looseness and tightness in football players. *JAMA.* 1970;212:2236–2238.
37. Ostenberg A, Roos H. Injury risk factors in female European football. A prospective study of 123 players during one season. *Scand J Med Sci Sports.* 2000;10:279–285.

38. Soderman K, Alfredson H, Pietila T, et al. Risk factors for leg injuries in female soccer players: a prospective investigation during one out-door season. *Knee Surg Sports Traumatol Arthrosc.* 2001;9:313–321.

39. Huston LJ, Wojtys EM. Neuromuscular performance characteristics in elite female athletes. *Am J Sports Med.* 1996;24:427–436.

40. Rozzi SL, Lephart SM, Gear WS, et al. Knee joint laxity and neuromuscular characteristics of male and female soccer and basketball players. *Am J Sports Med.* 1999;27:312–319.

41. Rosene JM, Fogarty TD. Anterior tibial translation in collegiate athletes with normal anterior cruciate ligament integrity. *J Athl Train.* 1999;34:93–98.

42. Uhorchak JM, Scoville CR, Williams GN, et al. Risk factors associated with noncontact injury of the anterior cruciate ligament. *Am J Sports Med.* 2003;31:831–842.

43. Liu S, Al-Shaikh RA, Panossian V, et al. Primary immunolocalization of estrogen and progesterone target cells in the human anterior cruciate ligament. *J Orthop Res.* 1996;14:526–533.

44. Liu SH, Al-Shaikh RA, Panossian V, et al. Estrogen affects the cellular metabolism of the anterior cruciate ligament. A potential explanation for female athletic injury. *Am J Sports Med.* 1997;25:704–709.

45. Yu W, Panossian V, Hatch J, et al. Combined effects of estrogen and progesterone on the anterior cruciate ligament. *Clin Orthop.* 2001;383:268–281.

46. Romani W, Patrie J, Curl LA, et al. The correlations between estradiol, estrone, estriol, progesterone, and sex hormone-binding globulin and anterior cruciate ligament stiffness in healthy, active females. *J Women's Health.* 2003;12:287–298.

47. Wojtys EM, Huston LJ, Lindenfeld TN, et al. Association between the menstrual cycle and anterior cruciate ligament injuries in female athletes. *Am J Sports Med.* 1998;26:614–619.

48. Karageanes SJ, Blackburn K, Vangelos ZA. The association of the menstrual cycle with the laxity of the anterior cruciate ligament in adolescent female athletes. *Clin J Sport Med.* 2000;10:162–168.

49. Slauterbeck JR, Fuzie SF, Smith MP, et al. The menstrual cycle, sex hormones, and anterior cruciate ligament injury. *J Athl Train.* 2002;37:275–280.

50. Belanger MJ, Moore DC, Crisco JJ, et al. Knee laxity does not vary with the menstrual cycle, before or after exercise. *Am J Sports Med.* 2004;32:1150–1157.

51. Murphy DF, Connolly DAJ, Beynnon BD. Risk factors for lower extremity injury: a review of the literature. *Br J Sports Med.* 2003;37:13–29.

52. Moller-Neilsen J, Hammar M. Women's soccer injuries in relation to the menstrual cycle and oral contraceptive use. *Med Sci Sports Exerc.* 1989;21:126–129.

53. Martineau PA, Al-Jassir F, Lenczner E, et al. Effect of the oral contraceptive pill on ligamentous laxity. *Clin J Sport Med.* 2004;14:281–286.

54. Zeller BL, McCrory JL, Kibler WB, et al. Differences in kinematics and electromyography activity between men and women during the single-legged squat. *Am J Sports Med.* 2003;31:449–455.

55. Hewett TE, Myer GD, Ford KR. Decrease in neuromuscular control about the knee with maturation in female athletes. *J Bone Joint Surg.* 2004;86-A:1601–1608.

56. Malinzak RA, Colby SM, Kirkendall DT, et al. A comparison of knee joint motion patterns between men and women in selected athletic tasks. *Clin Biomech.* 2001;16:438–445.

57. Ferber R, Davis IM, Williams DSI. Gender differences in lower extremity mechanics during running. *Clin Biomech.* 2003;18:350–357.

58. Ford KR, Myer GD, Hewett TE. Valgus knee motion during landing in high school female and male basketball players. *Med Sci Sports Exerc.* 2003;35:1745–1750.

59. Lephart SM, Ferris CM, Riemann BL, et al. Gender differences in strength and lower extremity kinematics during landing. *Clin Orthop.* 2002;401:162–169.

60. Chappell JD, Yu B, Kirkendall DT, et al. A comparison of knee kinetics between male and female recreational athletes in stop-jump tasks. *Am J Sports Med.* 2002;30:261–267.

61. Hewett TE, Myer GD, Ford KR, et al. Biomechanical measures of neuromuscular control and valgus loading of the knee predict anterior cruciate ligament injury risk in female athletes. *Am J Sports Med.* 2005;33:492–501.

62. Wojtys EM, Ashton-Miller JA, Huston LJ. A gender-related difference in the contribution of the knee musculature to sagittal-plane shear stiffness in subjects with similar knee laxity. *J Bone Joint Surg.* 2002;84-A:10–16.

63. Markolf KL, Burchfield DM, Shapiro MM, et al. Combined knee loading states that generate high anterior cruciate ligament forces. *J Orthop Res.* 1995;13:930–935.

64. Mohr KJ, Kvitne RS, Pink MM, et al. Electromyography of the quadriceps in patellofemoral pain with patellar subluxation. *Clin Orthop.* 2003;415:261–271.

65. Powers CM. Patellar kinematics. Part I: the influence of the vastus muscle activity in subjects with and without patellofemoral pain. *Phys Ther.* 2000;80:956–964.

66. Osternig LR, Caster BL, James R. Contralateral hamstring (biceps femoris) coactivation patterns and anterior cruciate ligament dysfunction. *Am J Sports Med.* 1995;27:805–808.

67. Kellis E, Tsitskaris GK, Nikopoulou MD, et al. The evaluation of jumping ability of male and female basketball players according to their chronological age and major leagues. *J Strength Cond Res.* 1999;13:40–46.

68. Wojtys EM, Bradford BW, Huston LJ. The effects of muscle fatigue on neuromuscular function and anterior tibial translation in healthy knees. *Am J Sports Med.* 1996;24:615–621.

69. Rozzi SL, Lephart SM, Fu FH. Effects of muscular fatigue on knee joint laxity and neuromuscular characteristics of male and female athletes. *J Athl Train.* 1999;34:106–114.

70. Nyland JA, Shapiro R, Stine RL, et al. Relationship between fatigued reaction forces, lower extremity kinematics, and muscle activation. *J Orthop Sports Phys Ther.* 1994;20:132–137.

71. Chappell JD, Herman DC, Knight BS, et al. Effect of fatigue on knee kinetics and kinematics in stop-jump tasks. *Am J Sports Med.* 2005;33:1022–1029.

72. Nadler SF, Malanga GA, DePrince M, et al. The relationship between lower extremity injury, low back pain, and hip muscle strength in male and female collegiate athletes. *Clin J Sport Med.* 2000;10:89–97.

73. Cahalan TD, Johnson ME, Liu S, et al. Quantitative measurements of hip strength in different age groups. *Clin Orthop.* 1989;246:136–145.

74. Ireland ML, Willson JD, Ballantyne BT, et al. Hip strength in females with and without patellofemoral pain. *J Orthop Sports Phys Ther.* 2003;33:671–676.

75. Leetun DT, Ireland ML, Willson JD, et al. Core stability measures as risk factors for lower extremity injury in athletes. *Med Sci Sports Exerc.* 2004;36:926–934.

76. Hewett TE, Stroupe AL, Nance TA, et al. Plyometric training in female athletes: decreased impact forces and increased hamstring torques. *Am J Sports Med.* 1996;24:765–773.

77. Myklebust G, Engebretsen L, Braekken IH, et al. Prevention of anterior cruciate ligament injuries in female team handball players: a prospective intervention study over three seasons. *Clin J Sport Med.* 2003;13:71–78.

78. Caraffa A, Cerulli G, Projetti M, et al. Prevention of anterior cruciate ligament injuries in soccer: a prospective controlled study of proprioceptive training. *Knee Surg Sports Traumatol Arthrosc.* 1996;4:19–21.

79. Heidt RS, Sweeterman LM, Carlonas RL, et al. Avoidance of soccer injuries with preseason conditioning. *Am J Sports Med.* 2000;28:659–662.

80. Mandelbaum BR, Silvers HJ, Watanabe DS, et al. Effectiveness of a neuromuscular training program in preventing anterior

cruciate ligament injuries in female athletes. *Am J Sports Med.* 2005;33:1003–1010.

81. Henning CE, Griffis ND. *Injury Prevention of the Anterior Cruciate Ligament* [Videotape]. Wichita, KS: Mid-America Center for Sports Medicine; 1990.

82. Onate JA, Guskiewicz KM, Sullivan RJ. Augmented feedback reduces jump landing forces. *J Orthop Sports Phys Ther.* 2001;31:511–517.

83. Giza E, Silvers HJ, Mandelbaum BR. Anterior cruciate ligament tear prevention in the female athlete. *Curr Sports Med Rep.* 2005;4:109–111.

84. Myer GD, Ford KR, Hewett TE. Rationale and clinical techniques for anterior cruciate ligament injury prevention among female athletes. *J Athl Train.* 2004;39:352–364.

85. Davis IM, Ireland ML. ACL injuries—the gender bias. *J Orthop Sports Phys Ther.* 2003;33:A2–A8.

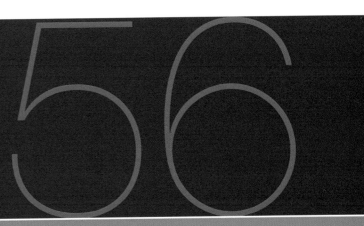

LIGAMENT INJURIES IN CHILDREN AND ADOLESCENTS

■ PATRICK S. BRANNAN, MD, HENRY G. CHAMBERS, MD

■ KEY POINTS

- Ligament injuries around the knee are unusual in children and adolescents but can present significant diagnostic and therapeutic challenges.
- Open physes, thick articular cartilage, and developmental issues complicate the care of the injured knee in childhood and adolescence.
- Several studies have documented the increased incidence of knee injuries, particularly to the anterior cruciate ligament (ACL), among females who play basketball and soccer.
- Children may present late with ligament or meniscal injuries because the initial examining physician underestimated the significance of the early physical examination findings.
- Because of the high incidence of fractures in children, at least anteroposterior and lateral radiographs of the knee should be obtained. A Merchant or sunrise view can be obtained to evaluate the patellofemoral joint, looking for osteochondral fractures of the patella or distal femur. A tunnel view should be obtained to evaluate the intercondylar notch and a possible osteochondral fracture.
- Arthroscopy should be considered as a diagnostic alternative for children who present with knee hemarthrosis.

Although rare in children and adolescents, ligament injuries around the knee present significant diagnostic and therapeutic challenges. The incidence and severity of the injury depends on the size of the child, their sport, and, as the adolescent approaches maturity, possibly even the sex of the child. In this chapter, the epidemiology of knee ligament injuries in children, unique physical examination findings, imaging challenges, and therapeutic approaches to the various ligament injuries are explored.

■ EPIDEMIOLOGY

There seems to be a spectrum of injuries to the knee in children. Younger children sustain metaphyseal fractures. Teenagers with low-energy trauma may experience anterior cruciate ligament (ACL) rupture, whereas those who have high-energy trauma may have physeal injuries (1). Fractures in the young child may be a representation of their small size and relatively lower energy imparted in sports. It has been postulated that increased ligamentous laxity (especially in children) would predispose to a greater injury rate. However, Grana and Moretz (2) found no correlation between ligamentous laxity and the occurrence or type of injury.

Alpine or downhill skiing is one of the most dangerous sports for children (3–5). Blitzer et al. (6) found that one fifth of skiing injuries were knee injuries. Deibert et al. (7) performed a large (>3 million skier visits), long-term (12 years) study of skiing injuries in children, adolescents, and adults. The medial collateral ligament injury rate in children from 1981 to 1987 was 20% (51 of 255 children), decreasing to 7% (19 of 273 children) for the period from 1987 to 1994. For adolescents, the rate was 9.6% (78 of 813 adolescents) in the first period and 8.8% (58 of 660 adolescents) in the second period. One ACL injury occurred between 1981 and 1987, and two occurred between 1987 and 1994. The adolescent age group had a 3.9% incidence of ACL tears in the first period and a 4.7% incidence in the second period. These findings compared with a 15.2% to 19% incidence for adults. The investigators felt that the overall 58% decrease in children's accidents was due to the use of properly functioning modern equipment (7). Although most of those who sustain snowboarding injuries are children and adolescents, the incidence of knee injury is significantly lower than for alpine skiing (8–11).

The quick stopping and direction in basketball and soccer predisposes the knee to ligamentous injuries. Several studies have documented the increased incidence of knee injuries among women who play basketball (12,13) and soccer (14,15). Gray et al. (16) reported a total of 19 ACL ruptures in female players compared with only four ACL injuries in male basketball players during the same period. Possible causative factors for this increase in ACL injuries in women may be extrinsic (i.e., body movement, muscular strength, shoe–surface interface, and skill level) or intrinsic (i.e., joint laxity, limb alignment, notch dimensions, and ligament size) (17,18). Additionally, others have suggested that differences in dynamic movement patterns and proximal muscle firing patterns play a role in the increased propensity for females to tear their ACL (19). Loudon et al. (20) found a significant correlation between ACL injuries and knee recurvatum, "navicular drop," and extrinsic subtalar pronation.

Football represents the leading cause of ACL tears in adolescents (21–24). In a survey of coaches from Kentucky, Stocker et al. (25) found an incidence of 0.055 knee injuries per player (257 knee injuries in 4,690 players). Volleyball also had a significant rate of ACL and medial collateral ligament injuries, with the most injuries caused from landing from a jump in the attack zone (26). Other sports commonly associated with ACL injuries include soccer (rate of 3.7 to 5.6 injuries per 1,000 hours and one ACL tear) (27) and wakeboarding (28).

■ PHYSICAL EXAMINATION

A high index of suspicion must be entertained when evaluating children or adolescents with knee injuries. Many children present late with ligamentous or meniscal injuries because the initial examining physician underestimated the significance of the physical examination findings and a hemarthrosis. Luhmann (29) found that ACL injuries, meniscal tears, and patellofemoral pathology accounted for 87% (48 of 55) of diagnoses of hemarthrosis in children 18 and younger. ACL pathology was much more common in males (13 of 16 diagnoses), whereas patellofemoral pathology was much more common in females (11 of 14 diagnoses). Overall, the differential diagnosis for a child with an acute hemarthrosis includes ACL tears, tibial spine avulsion fractures, patellar dislocations, osteochondral fractures, meniscal tears, physeal fractures of the distal femur, and medial collateral ligament tears (30). A posterior cruciate ligament (PCL) tear may not demonstrate a large hemarthrosis.

Associated injuries are not uncommonly found in children with ligamentous pathology. Twenty-six of 31 patients with ACL tears were found to have associated injuries

including meniscal tears, medial collateral ligament ruptures, and even femur fractures. Furthermore, there is a higher incidence of medial meniscal tears in children with chronic ACL tears (36%) (31).

ACL Injury

The standard physical examination techniques (e.g., Lachman, anterior drawer, pivot shift) used in evaluating adults have the same validity in children (32–34). Although children do have greater ligamentous laxity than adults, a side-to-side comparison usually aids in the diagnosis. Children are often more apprehensive than adults, and it can be difficult to perform these tests, particularly the pivot shift test. Physical examination of the child under general anesthesia increases its accuracy. Donaldson et al. (35) found that the pivot shift test was initially positive in only 35% of knees, increasing to 98% under general anesthesia. The Lachman test was equally sensitive to examination under anesthesia. The anterior drawer test was positive in 70% of knees, increasing to 91% under general anesthesia. Instrumented analysis (e.g., KT-1000 Ligament Arthrometer; Med-Metric, San Diego, CA) has a great advantage in the documentation and reproducibility of side-to-side differences. Newer testing equipment designed for children has been introduced and may further aid in the evaluation of children with ACL injuries.

Tibial Spine Avulsion Injuries

Tibial spine avulsion injuries manifest with a large hemarthrosis and with signs of an ACL injury (e.g., positive Lachman test, positive anterior drawer test). The meniscus (usually medial) may be entrapped in the fracture site. Mah et al. (36) found that, in nine of 10 displaced tibial spine fractures, there was interposition of the meniscus. The diagnosis is usually made by the anteroposterior and lateral radiograph results. Radiographs should be obtained as part of the examination of any knee in a child or adolescent with a hemarthrosis. A severe medial ligamentous injury also may be associated with a tibial spine fracture (37).

Patellar Dislocation

Often, the medical history of children is difficult to elicit. Even with ACL injuries, they say that their "knees dislocated." Patellar dislocations are frequently associated with a large hemarthrosis. Tenderness is experienced in the medial peripatellar region, and there is an occasional defect in the retinaculum. There may also be tenderness at the adductor tubercle, including a patellofemoral ligament tear.

Osteochondral Fractures

A twisting knee injury or a patellar dislocation can lead to a chondral or osteochondral fracture. A tense hemarthrosis with tenderness over either femoral condyle of a flexed knee may signify an osteochondral fracture. Radiographs, computed tomography (CT), or magnetic resonance imaging (MRI) can be used to help define the lesion and its extent. Chondral lesions are more common in children because the cartilage is thicker and therefore more prone to shear injury. Frequently, the diagnosis is made only at the time of arthroscopy.

Physeal Fractures

Physeal fractures are rare injuries of the distal femur. They must be distinguished from medial collateral ligament or lateral complex injuries in the child. There is usually a tense hemarthrosis with tenderness along the entire distal femur at the physis (i.e., adjacent to the upper pole of the patella or 2 to 3 cm above the joint line). If the fracture is limited to one condyle, tenderness will be greater at the involved physis. Laxity may be identified on varus or valgus stress testing. A diagnosis is usually made on the basis of plain radiographs. Occasionally, stress radiographs may be necessary to distinguish collateral ligament injury from physeal fractures. This is especially true in children and adolescents who have severe soft issue edema and ecchymosis.

The examiner must also be aware of the relationship between Salter Harris III fractures of the medial femoral condyle and ACL tears. Brone and Wroble (38) reported three cases of ACL tears associated with Salter Harris III fractures and found four other cases in the literature **(Fig 56-1)**.

Meniscal Tears

Meniscal tears are often associated with ACL tears, medial collateral ligament tears, or both and can lead to a significant hemarthrosis. Popping and especially locking of the knee in slight flexion are important symptoms. Joint line tenderness is very helpful if present, but its absence does not exclude a diagnosis of a meniscal tear. The McMurray test is nonspecific, but a positive result may suggest further investigation. In the very young child, clunking and increased laxity on the Lachman test may indicate a discoid meniscus.

Medial Collateral Ligament Injuries

Tenderness of the medial knee at the origin, midsubstance, or insertion of the medial collateral ligament aids in the diagnosis of a ligament strain (grade 1). With valgus stress applied to the knee in slight flexion, there may be opening of the joint with a good end point (grade 2). If the knee opens medially without an end point, there is a grade 3 tear with the possibility of a concomitant ACL tear. The children rarely have a large effusion, which differentiates this injury from a distal femoral physeal injury.

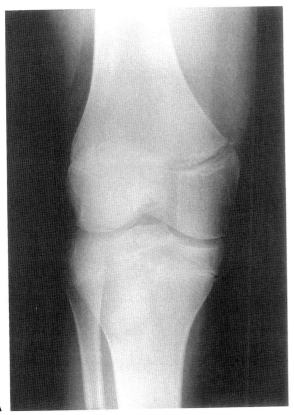
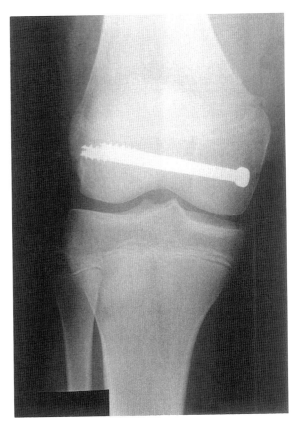

A   **B**

Fig 56-1. Salter Harris III fracture and after open reduction internal fixation.

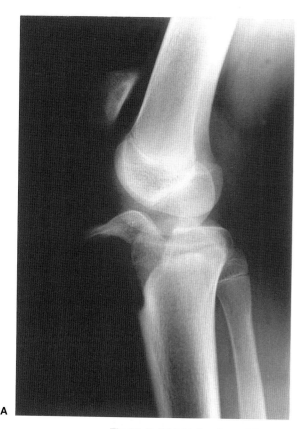
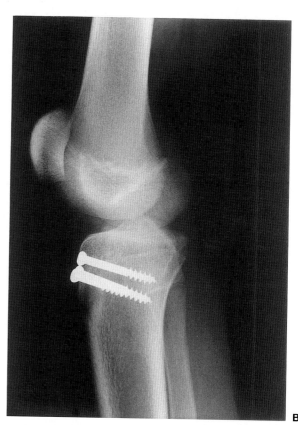

Fig 56-2. Tibial tubercle avulsion injury and after open reduction and internal fixation.

Tibial Tubercle Avulsion Injury

A large hemarthrosis occurs when there is an avulsion of the tibial tubercle with the patellar tendon. There is tenderness and edema over the entire surface of the knee, and crepitus may be present over the tibial tubercle. The patella is often high riding. This injury may be missed on a cursory examination because the finding of patella alta on the lateral radiograph is often subtle. In more extensive fractures, the fracture line may extend posteriorly into the knee joint and include the ACL **(Fig 56-2)**.

PCL and Posterolateral Complex Injuries

PCL tears are rare in children (39). The physical findings are the same as for adults. However, because of their rarity, the injury is often missed at first examination. It is usually diagnosed when the child or adolescent begins complaining of pain in the knee and medial joint line symptoms. Children have a higher incidence of bony avulsion fractures from the posterior tibia than adults. These fractures are amenable to open reduction and internal fixation.

■ IMAGING

Although the history and clinical examination suggest the diagnosis in most cases, imaging studies are often needed. Because of the high incidence of fractures in this age group,

at least anteroposterior and lateral radiographs of the knee should be obtained. It is also recommended that a Merchant or sunrise view be obtained to evaluate the patellofemoral joint, looking for osteochondral fractures from the patella or distal femur. A tunnel view should be obtained to evaluate the intercondylar notch and a possible osteochondral fracture. Occasionally, oblique radiographs of the knee are necessary to identify avulsion fractures at the medial and lateral margins of the proximal tibia.

MRI can be used to confirm the clinical diagnosis or to make the diagnosis if the clinical diagnosis is in question. Gelb et al. (40), however, found (in adult patients) that MRI was only 95% sensitive and 88% specific for the diagnosis of ACL tears relative to a 100% specificity and sensitivity for clinical examination. The results were even poorer for meniscal injuries (82% and 87%) and worse in articular surface damage (33%). They concluded that MRI is unnecessary in most knee disorders and not a cost-effective test (40–42). MRI does not appear to be helpful in the grading of medial collateral ligament tears (43). In studies in which MRI was used to evaluate knee injuries in children, investigations found that, although the MRI might aid in the diagnosis of the meniscal injuries, there was still a problem identifying the ACL because of its small size (44,45) or because of the poor sensitivity of MRI in finding an ACL tear (64%) (46). More recent studies have found MRI to be a helpful adjunct in the evaluation of knee injuries. Major et al. (47) found MRI to be 100% sensitive and specific for

ACL injuries and 93% sensitive and 95% specific for lateral meniscal injuries. Lee et al. (48) found a 95% sensitivity rate and 88% specificity rate for ACL injuries. Rangger et al. (49) suggested that MRI should be done in all cases in which the clinical diagnosis has been reduced to a suspected meniscal injury. MRI has also been effective in the diagnosis of posterolateral complex injuries of the knee (50) and is the only way to diagnose bone bruises or contusions (51,52).

The diagnosis of collateral ligament injuries can be very difficult. There is an inherent laxity in many children, and differentiation between ligamentous and physeal injuries is critical. The use of stress radiographs can be helpful. The best method of performing a radiographic stress test, especially if trying to distinguish between a medial collateral ligament injury and a Salter Harris I fracture of the distal femur, is to place the child supine and tie a belt or strap around the distal thighs with the knees slightly flexed (approximately 20 degrees) over a pillow. The feet are then abducted as the radiograph is taken **(Fig 56-3)**. The simple test differentiates medial collateral ligament tears, which open at the joint, from a Salter Harris I fracture, which opens at the physis. As previously stated, patients who have a physeal fracture often have a large hemarthrosis, which is not usually present in collateral ligament injuries. Other than its use in differentiating physeal fractures from medial collateral ligament tears, stress radiography seems to have little role in the evaluation of knee injuries in children. Although stress radiography is sensitive in the diagnosis of PCL tears, clinical examination or MRI provides sufficient information (53,54).

My approach to the use of imaging in children's knee injuries is to obtain anteroposterior, lateral, tunnel, and Merchant views of all injured knees. Comparison views may be necessary but are not ordered routinely. Knee pain in children may be referred from hip pathology such as Legg-Calve-Perthes syndrome or slipped capital femoral epiphysis, and if there is any doubt, anteroposterior and frog lateral pelvis radiographs should be obtained. Occasionally, the child is uncooperative or too uncomfortable to examine. An examination can be performed 7 to 10 days later. If there is

still a question of a ligamentous laxity injury or meniscal tear, an MRI scan can be ordered, with the realization that it may not be the definitive test. Rarely, when it is difficult to distinguish between physeal fractures and a medial collateral ligament tear, stress radiographs can be performed.

ROLE OF ARTHROSCOPY IN CHILDREN

After a complete clinical examination and appropriate injury studies, the diagnosis may still be in doubt. Several studies have addressed this problem in children with hemarthroses. Ure et al. (55) performed arthroscopy in 104 patients younger than 18 years old who had hemarthroses. They found that the most frequent diagnosis was patellar dislocation (45% of children and 29% of adolescents). The preoperative diagnosis was shown to be wrong or incomplete in 41% of the children and 24% of the adolescents, and in only 36% of the children were meniscal tears suspected before surgery. They concluded that every child with a hemarthrosis should have an arthroscopy. Faraj et al. (56) reported that clinical diagnosis and arthroscopic findings were compatible and correct in 61% of preadolescent patients. Matelic et al. (57) reported similar findings for 21 children, with osteochondral fractures found in 14 (67%) of the patients. The highest incidence of unsuspected pathologic findings from clinical examination and standard imaging, coupled with findings of additional pathology (i.e., meniscal tears, osteochondral and chondral fractures, and partial ACL tears), warrants considering diagnostic arthroscopy in all children who have an acute hemarthrosis (58–64).

TREATMENT OF LIGAMENT INJURIES IN CHILDREN

Collateral Ligament Injuries

Medial collateral ligament injuries often occur in conjunction with other ligamentous injuries (e.g., ACL), osteochondral fractures, or meniscal injuries (65). It was once thought that medial collateral ligament injuries could not occur before physeal closure. However, it is clear that medial collateral ligament tears do occur at the origin, midsubstance, or insertion of the ligament (66).

Earlier studies suggested that the injured medial collateral ligament needed to be repaired or at least immobilized, especially in the presence of an ACL tear (67,68). However, later studies suggest that treatment with a cast brace or prefabricated brace with free range of motion can lead to good or excellent results (69–72). Isolated tears of the medial collateral ligament should be treated by placing the knee in a range-of-motion brace set from 0 degrees to 90 degrees. After 10 to 14 days, the range of motion can be increased to full flexion. The brace is left in place for 4 to 6 weeks. The knee should be tested for laxity before allowing the child or adolescent to return to cutting activities.

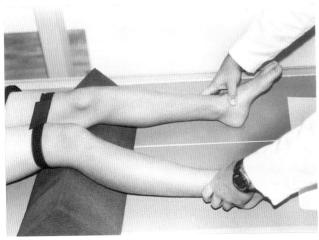

Fig 56-3. Technique for performing a stress radiograph to discriminate a medial collateral ligament tear from a physeal injury.

Lateral collateral injuries may have associated bony avulsions or even fibular physeal injuries. These physeal injuries are usually nondisplaced or minimally displaced but should be treated with immobilization in a knee immobilizer or cylinder cast. An ACL tear may be associated with a lateral collateral ligament tear. Associated posterolateral complex injuries must be completely excluded because they often require operative repair, even in children and adolescents.

PCL Injury

PCL injuries are rare injuries in children and are therefore often missed at the initial evaluation of a knee injury (73). It can be helpful to know the mechanism of injury, which is usually a fall on a flexed knee, a dashboard injury in a motor vehicle accident, or severe hyperextension (74,75). A PCL injury has been found in a 10-year-old child after a femur fracture (76). The degree of joint effusion is usually less than with an ACL tear, and evaluation of posterior laxity can be difficult in a child (77). PCL injuries may be associated with disability from degenerative disease of the medial joint compartment (78,79). There is no association between objective laxity and subjective knee scores or ability to return to sport (80).

Children have a higher incidence of bony avulsion injuries from the tibial insertion but may also have a bony avulsion from the femur. Anteroposterior, lateral, and oblique radiographs of the knee usually demonstrate the avulsion (81). Midsubstance tears can be identified with MRI **(Fig 56-4).**

The bony avulsion should be repaired with interepiphyseal sutures or screw fixation (82). Arthroscopies should be performed before prone positioning of the patient because of the high incidence of associated injuries (83). Because the repair of PCL injuries is controversial in adults, it may be prudent to treat the knee with physical therapy (range of motion) and strengthening combined with a PCL brace (keeping the knee in slight flexion) until the child is skeletally mature (84–88).

Combined PCL and posterolateral complex injuries are extremely difficult to treat in adults and in children. There are no natural history studies of children with this injury combination, and the most prudent approach is to perform any surgery (e.g., posterolateral repair, proximal advancement) that does not violate the physis of the femur, tibia, or fibula (89–91). Bracing until skeletal maturity with a reassessment of the functional laxity at that time should be the conservative approach.

Midsubstance ACL Tears

Although once thought to be rare in children and adolescents, the incidence of ACL tears seems to be rising because of increased awareness or increased sports participation (92,93). ACL tears have been found in children as young as 3 years old (94–96). It was once thought that most children would sustain a physeal injury rather than an ACL injury. Skak et al. (1) found that low-energy trauma was associated with ligamentous injuries and that high-energy trauma was associated with a physeal injury.

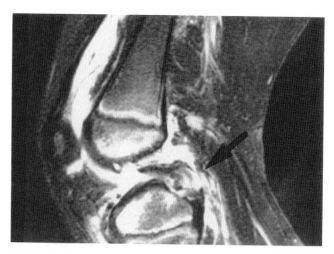

Fig 56-4. Magnetic resonance imaging of a 7-year-old child with a midsubstance posterior cruciate ligament tear.

The natural history of ACL injuries is not entirely predictable. Some children do well without an ACL, but others are unable to do even simple activities. Many early studies report that this can be a benign injury. However, longer follow-up demonstrates that there was a preponderance of fair to poor results (97–100). Clancy et al. (90) reported the significance of the pivot shift as a predictor of the need for ACL reconstruction. When the pivot shift test was not strongly positive, one half of the patients did well after treatment with a nonoperative program of functional rehabilitation. Patients with unstable knees (i.e., strongly positive pivot shift test result) had better results after reconstruction.

Several articles have evaluated the effect of ACL injuries in skeletally immature patients. Partial tears (<50%) in a skeletally immature individual (<14 years old) with normal or near-normal clinical exam findings may be managed conservatively (101). However, as in the adult population, nonsurgical management of ACL tears in skeletally immature individuals often leads to recurrent instability. Angel and Hall (58) reviewed 22 patients who had ACL tears at 51 months of follow-up. No patients were capable of returning to sports, 41% of the patients had associated pathology, and another 41% had or were recommended to have ACL reconstruction. Mizuta et al. (102) evaluated 18 patients who were skeletally immature and treated conservatively for a mean of 51 months. The modified Lysholm knee score showed one excellent, one good, eight fair, and eight poor results. Only one patient returned to her preinjury level of athletics. Fifty percent had meniscal tears, and radiographic evidence of ligamentous changes were found in 11 of 18 patients. Janarv et al. (103) reported similar findings, with 68% of their patients requiring ACL reconstruction because of the failure of conservative care. Pressman et al. (104) performed a long-term (5-year) retrospective review of 42 children and evaluated the efficacy of treatment and the clinical results of operative and nonoperative treatment. They found that intra-articular reconstruction provided the best outcome, which was confirmed by clinical examination and patient satisfaction outcome reports.

Besides the knee instability and inability to participate in sporting activities, there is an increased risk for meniscal tears. Williams et al. (105) found that 56% of their patients (13 of 24 patients) had coexistent meniscal tears. Graf et al. (106) reviewed 12 patients with midsubstance tears of the ACL and found that six patients had eight meniscal tears (four medial and four lateral). These young patients were braced and all developed "giving way" episodes (106).

The primary concern in treating ACL injuries in children is that the most successful reconstructions are intra-articular and require drill holes to be placed in the proximal tibia and distal femur. In children who are not skeletally mature, these drill holes must cross the growth plate or physis. If a bony bridge crosses the physis, a longitudinal or angular growth arrest may occur (107). This concern has provided the backdrop for the controversy surrounding the treatment of ACL injuries in children and adolescents.

There are four primary treatment options for the skeletally immature child or adolescent with an ACL tear: nonoperative; repair of the ligament tear; nonoperative treatment until the child is near or at skeletal maturity, at which time the ACL reconstruction is performed; or ACL reconstruction close to the time of injury, regardless of age. Controversy exists not only with regard to operative technique, but also with regard to initial management, operative indications, the effects of age and skeletal maturity, and the risk of growth disturbances.

Kocher et al. (108) conducted a survey with 187 questionnaires that were sent to clinicians who were members of the Herodicus Society or the ACL Study Group. Although questionnaire data were limited by being anecdotal and uncontrolled, they showed wide variability in physician preference regarding initial treatment for various prepubescent and adolescent patients, as well as surgical technique.

Nonoperative treatment does not have a good predictable outcome and carries the possibility of long-term instability, meniscal tears, and degenerative joint disease (99,106, 109–115). Another concern with nonoperative treatment is that this population of young athletes is often the most noncompliant group of patients.

Repair of the ACL

As in adults, it does not appear that repair of the ACL in children leads to a stable knee. Delee and Curtis (116) compared ACL repair in three children and found that there was a significant degree of ACL laxity at follow-up in two of the three patients. Engebretsen et al. (117) found that the knees were unstable in five of eight children after 3 to 8 years of follow-up after ACR repair and that all of the children had lower levels of activity.

■ ACL RECONSTRUCTION

The decision to perform an ACL reconstruction must take the following factors into account: the goals of the child, the ability to comply with possible preoperative and postoperative activity limitations, the ability to cooperate with the postoperative rehabilitation, the child's degree of skeletal maturity, the presence of an associated meniscal injury, and the extent to which the ACL instability is affecting the child's activities of daily living and sporting activities.

Assessment of Skeletal Maturity

Skeletal maturity can be assessed in several ways. In girls, age at menarche provides an important clue to their growth. Girls usually grow for approximately 18 months after menarche. An anteroposterior radiograph of the left hand can be taken to correlate with skeletal maturity using the Greulich and Pyle atlas (118). However, there is a large range of "normal" bone ages in the teenage years using this method. Plain radiographs of the knee can be used to subjectively rate the physis as "wide open" or "approaching maturity." The Tanner scale can be used to stage the sexual maturity of adolescents based on pubic hair and breast development in girls and pubic hair and penis or testes development in boys **(Table 56-1)**. This is often an embarrassing examination for teenagers, and even parents challenge its necessity. Assessment of a recent growth spurt or proximity in height to their parents or siblings can also be used to help assess skeletal maturity.

Patients can be considered skeletally immature if they meet the following criteria: anteroposterior and lateral radiographs with "wide open" physes, no adolescent growth spurt, patient significantly shorter than older siblings or parents (10 to 15 cm), and Tanner stage of 1 or 2. The child can be considered mature if he or she has radiographs demonstrating closing physes, has undergone an adolescent growth spurt, is of similar height to siblings and parents (within 2.5 to 5 cm), and has a Tanner stage of 4 or 5 (114).

ACL Reconstruction

When faced with a child with an ACL-deficient knee, many factors must be considered, including not only if and when a reconstruction should be performed, but also what type and technique. These include extra-articular and all epiphyseal reconstructions, as well as intra-articular techniques. Intra-articular techniques may be further divided into nontransphyseal reconstructions and transphyseal reconstructions.

Extra-articular Reconstruction

Nonanatomical extra-articular reconstructions are not recommended for the treatment of ACL injuries in the skeletally immature patient (119,120). The advantage of an extra-articular ACL reconstruction in a skeletally immature patient is that drilling across the physis is not required. However, studies demonstrate the recurrence of laxity because most extra-articular reconstructions are nonisometric. There is also a risk of growth disturbance secondary to placement of a fixation device near the physis.

In 1988, McCarroll et al. (113) reported 10 patients who received either an AO screw tenodesis of the iliotibial band

TABLE 56-1	Maturation in Adolescence		
Stage	Pubic hair	Genitalia	Breasts
Boys			
1	None	Prepubertal penis, testis, and scrotum	
2	Sparse, straight	Enlargement of testes and scrotum, no change in the size of the penis	
3	Darker, curling extends laterally	Enlargement of penis, testes, and scrotum	
4	Coarse, curly, does not extend to the thigh	Further growth of testes and scrotum. Increased breadth of penis	
5	Adult Type	Adult size and shape	
Girls			
1	None		Prepubertal, no breast tissue
2	Sparse, straight		Breast bud
3	Darker, curling		Breast mound and areola enlarge
4	Coarse, abundant		Breast enlarged, areola forms mound
5	Adult type, extends to medial thigh		Adult type, areola part of breast contour

Adapted from Tanner JM. *Growth at adolescence*, 2nd ed. Oxford, UK: Blackwell; 1960.

or a modified Andrews iliotibial band tenodesis. Five patients returned to sports without problems and five patients experienced episodes of giving way. Subsequent reports in 1994 reported deteriorating results, and the authors no longer recommend this extra-articular procedure (114). They recommend waiting until the child is almost skeletally mature and then performing the standard patellar tendon graft. Graf et al. (106) treated two patients with medial meniscal repair and modified Andrews iliotibial band tenodesis, and both experienced symptomatic instability.

According to some authors, extra-articular ACL reconstruction may serve a role in providing temporary stability until a child reaches skeletal maturity (121,122). Delee (121) recommends treating pediatric patients with a mild degree of instability with extra-articular repair. Delee (121) detaches the proximal origin of the iliotibial band, passes it behind the lateral collateral ligament, through a tunnel that lies superior to the distal femoral physis, and then back under the lateral collateral ligament to be attached by a screw to Gerdy's tubercle. Bergfeld's technique involves taking a portion of the infrapatellar tendon and passing it over the front of the tibia beneath the transverse ligament, over the lateral femoral condyle, and then attaching it above the distal femoral physis (121). Drez modified Bergfeld's technique by passing the graft through a groove in the tibial physis and then placing the graft in the over-the-top position of the femur through a second groove below the femoral physis (121). The tibial and femoral grooves allow a more posterior and anterior position of the graft, respectively. This places the graft in a more anatomical position.

Micheli et al. (122) describes a combination extra-articular and intra-articular technique that is a modification of MacIntosh and Darby's (123) 1976 described technique.

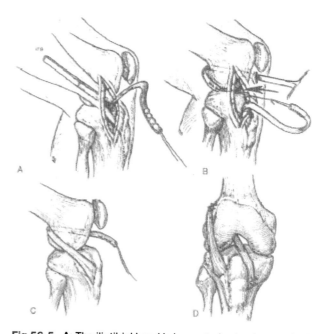

Fig 56-5. **A:** The iliotibial band is harvested subcutaneously. **B:** A hemostat is used to develop the "over-the-top" position. **C:** The graft is pulled through the "over-the-top" position and into the joint. The graft is sutured to the periosteum and intermuscular septum posteriorly. **D:** A hemostat is used to make a tunnel under the anterior horn of the medial meniscus. A small trough is made in the epiphysis and the graft is pulled through this trough and sewn into place in the periosteum. (From Micheli LJ, Rask B, Gerberg L. Anterior cruciate ligament reconstruction in patients who are prepubescent. *Clin Orthop Relat Res.* 1999;364:40–47. This figure was originally under Rask BP, Micheli LJ. The pediatric knee. In: Scott WN, ed. *The knee.* Vol 1. St Louis: Mosby-Year Book; 1994:229–275.)

Micheli's technique avoids the growth plate by passing the iliotibial band around the lateral femoral notch, through a notchplasty, and attaching it in an over-the-top position on the tibia. The graft is sutured medial to the tibial tubercle and proximally at the lateral femoral condyle. All 17 children were prepubescent (average chronological age, 11 years; average skeletal age, 10 years), and all patients were stable clinically and objectively by KT-1000 examination 66 months postoperatively **(Fig 56-5)**.

Intra-articular Reconstruction

As previously mentioned, most of the debate regarding the treatment of ACL injuries in children center on the potential of formation of a bone bridge across the physis. Several studies have been performed to determine the risk of drilling a graft tunnel across the physis. Guzzanti et al. (107) performed 21 semitendinosus reconstructions in rabbits through 2-mm tibial and femoral tunnels. No alteration in growth or axial deviation was found in the femur at 6 months. Two tibia subsequently developed axial deformity, and one shortened. Stadelmaier et al. (124) showed that, when a drill hole is placed across a physis and left unfilled, a bone bridge will form and growth arrest will occur. However, if the graft is filled with a soft tissue graft, normal growth continues. Drill holes should be filled with soft tissue grafts (124). Additionally, centrally placed holes are less likely to result in growth arrest and angular deformity than peripherally placed drill holes.

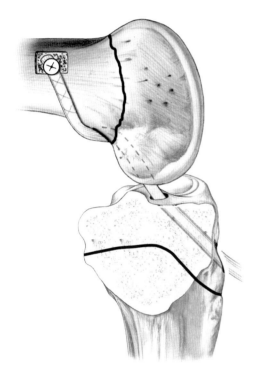

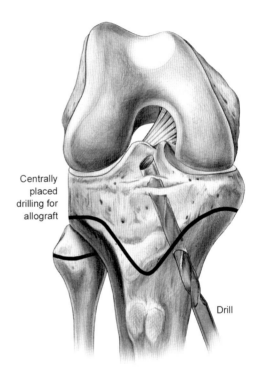

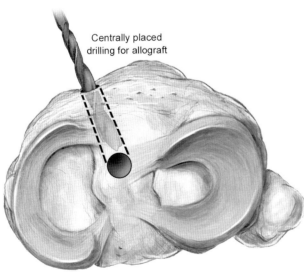

Fig 56-6. Over-the-top femoral position for placement of allograft. (From Andrews M, Noyes FR, Barber-Westin SD. Anterior cruciate ligament allograft reconstruction in the skeletally immature athlete. *Am J Sports Med.* 1994;22:48–54.)

Nontransphyseal intra-articular ACL reconstructions are an attempt to preserve the physis while providing a more anatomical reconstruction. Brief (125) developed a technique of ACL reconstruction without the use of transphyseal tunnels. The semitendinosus and gracilis tendons are left attached distally. They are passed into the knee joint under the anterior horn of the medial meniscus and attached to the lateral femoral condyle epiphysis by staples in the over-the-top position. Patients were a mean age of 17.2 years, and eight of nine patients were without symptoms of instability at the 3- to 6.5-year follow-up (125). Parker et al. (126) reported results of ACL reconstruction using hamstrings tendons placed in a groove in the tibia and over the top of the femur. Four of five patients returned to sports at 33 months of follow-up. Despite low risk to the physis, these techniques are nonanatomical and nonisometric. Additionally, there are no available long-term follow-up data.

Transphyseal intra-articular ACL reconstruction is the most anatomical and isometric of the above techniques. It is the treatment of choice in adults but is controversial in the skeletally immature. Most described transphyseal procedures have been used in children at or near skeletal maturity.

McCarroll et al. (113,114) reported on 60 patients who underwent patellar tendon graft reconstruction across the distal femoral and proximal tibial physes. Fifty-seven of 60 patients were at least 14 years old. Fifty-five of 60 patients were able to return to their original sports with no incidence of abnormal growth, giving way, or leg length discrepancy. The authors advised against using transphyseal techniques in any patient with significant growth remaining.

Andrews et al. (127) had good results using a 7-mm, centrally placed allograft (fascia lata or Achilles tendon) combined with an over-the-top femoral placement (Fig 56-6).

Seven of eight patients had good to excellent ratings, and one patient had a fair rating. KT-1000 arthrometer revealed a less than 3-mm side-to-side difference in five patients and a 3- to 5-mm difference in the remaining three patients. No patient had a clinically significant leg length discrepancy.

Lo et al. (128) evaluated five patients who had radiographically open physes. Three had reconstructions using hamstring tendons, and two had patellar tendon grafts. They used a 6-mm tibial drill hole and over-the-top positioning of the femur. After a mean of 7.4 years, they had no evidence of limb length discrepancy and less than 3 mm of anterior-posterior displacement on clinical examination of the knee.

Matava and Siegel (129) performed a retrospective review of eight skeletally immature patients who underwent hamstrings tendon autograft through distal femoral and tibial tunnels (7 to 9 mm). All eight patients returned to sports. No angular deformity or growth discrepancies were reported at 32 months of follow-up. One patient had an 8-mm side-to-side difference following an injury.

Aronowitz et al. (130) evaluated ACL reconstructions in adolescents with open physes and a skeletal age of at least 14 years. Nineteen patients underwent ACL reconstruction with Achilles tendon allograft across bone tunnels in the distal femur and tibia (9 to 10 mm). Sixteen of 19 patients returned to sports. Scanograms and long leg radiographs revealed no leg length discrepancies or angular deformities.

Bissen et al. (131) reported results of nine patients with "wide open" physes and a mean age of 13 years who underwent reconstruction using semitendinosus and gracilis tendon grafts passed through the tibial physis and over the top of the femoral tunnel. Seven patients had excellent results and returned to sports. No patients experienced clinically significant leg length discrepancy, angular deformity, or

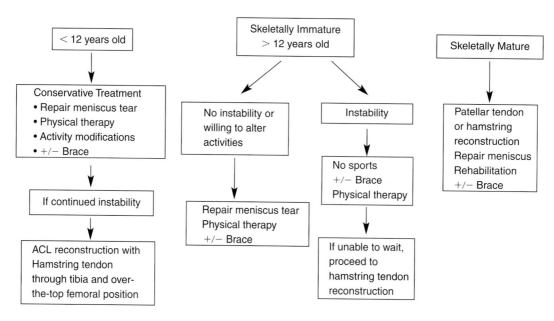

Fig 56-7. Algorithm for children with ACL tears.

radiographic evidence of physeal injury. Two grafts ruptured and were considered failures.

The survey by Kocher et al. (108) revealed an 11% incidence of growth disturbance (15 of 140 patients). There were eight cases of distal femoral valgus deformity, three cases of tibial recurvatum with arrest of the tibial tubercle apophysis, two cases of genu valgum without arrest, and two cases of leg length discrepancy. Associated risk factors included hardware across the lateral distal femoral physis, bone plugs across the distal femoral physis, large tunnels (12 mm), fixation across the tibial tubercle apophysis, lateral extra-articular tenodesis, and over-the-top femoral position.

Because of the possibility that a bone graft (from the bone-tendon-bone construct of the patellar tendon graft) might cause a growth arrest, many centers have been performing hamstring tendon ACL reconstructions. There is controversy about the best graft material (132,133), and there is much bias in the current literature **(Fig 56-7)**.

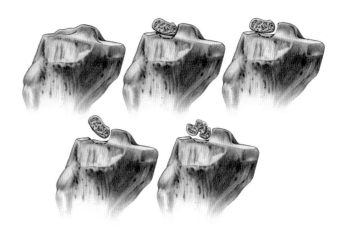

Fig 56-8. Classification of intercondylar eminence fractures.

■ TIBIAL SPINE INJURIES

The ACL is attached to the medial tibial spine, which is part of the tibial eminence. With stress, the incompletely ossified tibial eminence fails before the ligament through the cancellous bone of the subchondral plate (134). With this injury, the ACL is often stretched. The fracture may extend into the weight-bearing portion of the tibia (135), and the meniscus or intermeniscal ligament may be entrapped under the bony fragment (21,136,137).

Meyers and McKeever (138) classify these fractures as three basic types: Type I is nondisplaced, Type II is hinged or partially displaced, and Type III is completely displaced. Zaricznyj (139) added Type IV to include fractures with comminution of the fragment **(Fig 56-8)**.

The traditional teaching is that Type I and Type II fractures can be treated conservatively in slight flexion (20 degrees) (138,140,141), but McLennan (142,143) demonstrated that this position does not reduce the fracture fragment. Most surgeons agree that reductions should be performed in cases of Type III or IV fractures. However, the method and outcome of reduction is controversial. Treatment of Type III and IV fractures has included open or arthroscopically placed sutures or wire through the epiphysis and the ligament to hold the fragment in place (144–151), percutaneous Kirschner wire placement (142,143,152), and screw fixation (153–155). I prefer performing arthroscopy to evaluate the meniscus and transmeniscal ligament, evaluating the ability to reduce the fragment in a closed manner, and then performing a mini open arthrotomy to anatomically repair the fracture to the bed with a nonabsorbable suture through the epiphysis. This can certainly be done arthroscopically as well, but it is occasionally difficult to get the fat pad out of the way to anatomically reduce it **(Fig 56-9)**.

Outcome studies have demonstrated that, even with anatomical reduction and regardless of the technique of

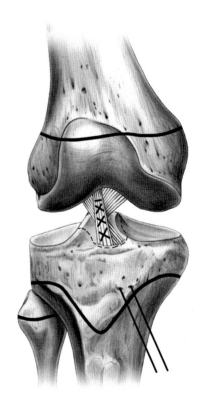

Fig 56-9. Method of fixation of intercondylar eminence fractures.

fixation, there is often residual laxity. Most of the patients are asymptomatic, however. Kocher et al. (155) found clinical and instrumented evidence of laxity in five of six patients but not subjective laxity. Willis et al. (156) found a 75% incidence of laxity as measured by the KT-1000 arthrometer. Smith (157) evaluated 12 patients who had open reduction and internal fixation and found that all had laxity. Others (103, 134,158,159) found similar laxity. The long-term (16 years) follow-up study by Janarv et al. (160) in 61 patients demonstrated good to excellent results in 87% of patients, but 38% had residual laxity. Molander et al. (161) did not find any laxity but did not use instrumented testing. McLennan (142) arthroscopically evaluated Type III fractures after they had healed and found there was often large (>3 mm) displacements. He concluded that, in his patients, there could be long-term morbidity with extension loss, chondromalacia, quadriceps weakness, and ligamentous instability; that the loss of reduction was common after closed reduction; that tibial spine fractures were not reduced by the femoral condyles; and that Type III fractures should have open reduction, ACL tensioning, internal fixation, and aggressive rehabilitation. In the rare case in which the bone block is so large that there is loss of full extension, a femoral notchplasty (Leuger) or an excision of a wedge of tibial bone can be performed (162).

■ CONCLUSIONS

The diagnosis and treatment of children's knee ligament injuries are challenging. Open physes, thick articular cartilage, and the developmental issues of childhood and adolescents combine to complicate the care of the injured knee. A careful history and physical examination, judicious use of the appropriate imaging technique, and knowledge of the pathoanatomy can lead the practitioner to the correct diagnosis and treatment.

■ REFERENCES

1. Skak SV, Jenson TT, Poulsen TD, et al. Epidemiology of knee injuries in children. *Acta Orthop Scand.* 1987;58:78–81.
2. Grana WA, Moretz JA. Ligamentous laxity in secondary school athletes. *JAMA.* 1978;240:1975–1976.
3. Garrick JG, Requa RK. Injury patterns in children and adolescent skiers. *Am J Sports Med.* 1979;7:245–248.
4. Shorter NA, Jensen PE, Harmon BJ, et al. Skiing injuries in children and adolescents. *J Trauma.* 1996;40:997–1001.
5. Ungerholm S, Engkvist O, Gierup J, et al. Skiing injuries in children and adults: a comparative study from an 8-year period. *Int J Sports Med.* 1983;4:236–240.
6. Blitzer CM, Johnson RJ, Ettlinger CF, et al. Downhill skiing injuries in children. *Am J Sports Med.* 1984;12:142–147.
7. Deibert MC, Aronsson DD, Johnson RJ, et al. Skiing injuries in children, adolescents, and adults. *J Bone Joint Surg Am.* 1998; 80:25–32.
8. Chow TK, Corbett SW, Farstad DJ. Spectrum of injuries from snowboarding. *J Trauma.* 1996;41:321–325.
9. Davidson TM, Laliotis AT. Snowboarding injuries, a four-year study with comparison with alpine ski injuries. *West J Med.* 1996;164:231–237.
10. Pigozzi F, Santori N, DiSalvo V, et al. Snowboard traumatology: an epidemiologic study. *Orthopedics.* 1997;20:505–509.
11. Sutherland AG, Homes JD, Myers S. Differing injury patterns in snowboarding and alpine skiing. *Injury.* 1996;27:423–425.
12. Baker MM. Anterior cruciate ligament injuries in the female athlete. *J Womens Health.* 1998;7:343–349.
13. Gomez E, DeLee JC, Farney WC. Incidence of injury in Texas girls' high school basketball. *Am J Sports Med.* 1996;24:684–687.
14. Micheli LJ, Metzl JD, Di Canzio J, et al. Anterior cruciate ligament reconstructive surgery in adolescent soccer and basketball players. *Clin J Sport Med.* 1999;9:138–141.
15. Giza E, Mithofer K, Farrell L, et al. Injuries in women's professional soccer. *Br J Sports Med.* 2005;39:212–216.
16. Gray J, Taunton JE, McKenzie DC, et al. A survey of injuries to the anterior cruciate ligament of the knee in female basketball players. *Int J Sports Med.* 1985;6:314–316.
17. Arendt E, Dick R. Knee injury patterns among men and women in collegiate basketball and soccer. NCAA date and review of literature. *Am J Sports Med.* 1995;23:694–701.
18. Hewett TE, Stroupe AL, Nance TA, et al. Plyometric training in female athletes. Decreased impact forces and increased hamstring torques. *Am J Sports Med.* 1996;24:765–773.
19. Ireland ML. The female ACL: why is it more prone to injury. *Orthop Clin North Am.* 2002;33:637–651.
20. Loudon JK, Jenkins W, Loudon KL. The relationship between static posture and ACL injury in female athletes. *J Orthop Sports Phys Ther.* 1996;24:91–97.
21. Chandler JT, Miller TK. Tibial eminence fracture with meniscal entrapment. *Arthroscopy.* 1995;11:499–502.
22. DeLee JC, Farney WC. Incidence of injury in Texas high school football. *Am J Sports Med.* 1992;20:575–580.
23. Halpern B, Thompson N, Curl WW, et al. High school football injuries: identifying the risk factors. *Am J Sports Med.* 1988; 16(suppl 1):S113–S117.
24. Pritchett JW. A claims-made study of knee injury due to football in high school athletes. *J Pediatr Orthop.* 1988;8:551–553.
25. Stocker BD, Nyland JA, Caborn DN, et al. Results of the Kentucky high school football knee injury survey. *J Ky Med Assoc.* 1997;95:458–464.
26. Ferretti A, Papandrea P, Conteduca F, et al. Knee ligament injuries in volleyball players. *Am J Sports Med.* 1992;20:203–207.
27. Schmidt-Olsen S, Jorgensen U, Kaalund S, et al. Injuries among young soccer players. *Am J Sports Med.* 1991;19:273–275.
28. Carson WG. Wakeboarding injuries. *Am J Sports Med.* 2004; 32:164–173.
29. Luhmann SJ. Acute traumatic knee effusions in children and adolescents. *J Pediatr Orthop.* 2003;23:199–202.
30. Eiskjaer S, Larson ST, Schmidt MB. The significance of hemarthrosis of the knee in children. *Arch Orthop Trauma Surg.* 1988;107:96–98.
31. Millett PJ, Willis AA, Warren RF. Associated injuries in pediatric and adolescent anterior cruciate ligament tears: does a delay in treatment increase the risk of meniscal tears. *Arthroscopy.* 2002; 18:955–959.
32. Clanton T, DeLee JC, Sanders B, et al. Knee ligament injuries in children. *J Bone Joint Surg Am.* 1979;61:1195–1201.
33. Jensen JE, Conn RR, Hazelrigg G, et al. Systematic evaluation of acute knee injuries. *Clin Sports Med.* 1985;4:295–312.
34. Sandberg R, Balkfors B, Henricson A, et al. Stability tests in knee ligament injuries. *Arch Orthop Trauma Surg.* 1986;106:5–7.
35. Donaldson WFD, Warren RF, Wickiewicz T. A comparison of acute anterior cruciate ligament examinations. Initial versus examination under anesthesia. *Am J Sports Med.* 1985; 13:5–10.
36. Mah JY, Adili A, Otsuka NY, et al. Follow-up study of arthroscopic reduction and fixation of Type III tibial-eminence fractures. *J Pediatr Orthop.* 1998;18:475–477.
37. Hayes JM, Masear VR. Avulsion fracture of the tibial eminence associated with severe medial ligamentous injury in an adolescent. A case report and literature review. *Am J Sports Med.* 1984;12: 330–333.
38. Brone LA, Wroble RR. Salter Harris III fracture of the medial femoral condyle associated with an anterior cruciate ligament tear. Report of three cases and review of the literature. *Am J Sports Med.* 1998;26:581–586.
39. MacDonald PB, Black B, Old J, et al. Posterior cruciate ligament injury and posterolateral instability in a 6-year-old child. A case report. *Am J Sports Med.* 2003;31:135–136.

40. Gelb HJ, Glasgow SG, Sapega AA, et al. Magnetic resonance imaging of knee disorders. Clinical value and cost effectiveness in a sports medicine practice. *Am J Sports Med.* 1996;24:99–103.

41. Kocabey Y, Tetik O, Isbell WM, et al. The value of clinical examination versus magnetic resonance imaging in the diagnosis of meniscal tears and anterior cruciate ligament rupture. *Arthroscopy.* 2004;20:696–700.

42. Luhmann SJ, Schootman M, Gordon JE, et al. Magnetic resonance imaging of the knee in children and adolescents. Its role in clinical decision making. *J Bone Joint Surg Am.* 2005;87:497–502.

43. Schweitzer ME, Tran D, Deely DM, et al. Medial collateral ligament injuries: evaluation of multiple signs, prevalence, and location of associated bone bruises, and assessment with MR imaging. *Radiology.* 1995;194:825–829.

44. King SJ. Magnetic resonance imaging of knee injuries in children. *Eur Radiol.* 1997;7:1245–1251.

45. King SJ, Carty HM, Brady O. Magnetic resonance imaging of knee injuries in children. *Pediatr Radiol.* 1996;26:287–290.

46. Zobel MS, Borrell JA, Liegel MJ, et al. Pediatric knee MR imaging: pattern of injuries in the immature skeleton. *Radiology.* 1994;190:397–401.

47. Major NM, Beard LN, Helms CA. Accuracy of MR imaging of the knee in adolescents. *Am J Sports Med.* 1998;180:17–19.

48. Lee K, Siegel MJ, Lau DM, et al. Anterior cruciate ligament tears: MR imaging-based diagnosis in a pediatric population. *Radiology.* 1999;213:697–704.

49. Rangger C, Klestil T, Kathrein A, et al. Influence of magnetic resonance imaging on indications for arthroscopy of the knee. *Clin Orthop.* 1996;330:133–142.

50. Ross G, Chapman AW, Newberg AR, et al. Magnetic resonance imaging for the evaluation of acute posterolateral complex injuries of the knee. *Am J Sports Med.* 1997;25:444–448.

51. Engebretson L, Arendt E, Fritts HM. Osteochondral lesions and cruciate ligament injuries. MRI in 18 knees. *Acta Orthop Scand.* 1993;64:434–436.

52. Snearly WN, Kaplan PA, Dussault RG. Lateral compartment bone contusions in adolescents with intact anterior cruciate ligaments. *Radiology.* 1996;195:205–208.

53. Harilainen A, Myllynen P, Rauste J, et al. Diagnosis of acute knee ligament injuries: the value of stress radiography compared with clinical examination, stability under anesthesia and arthroscopic or operative findings. *Ann Chir Gynaecol.* 1986;75:37–43.

54. McPhee IB, Fraser JG. Stress radiography in acute ligamentous injuries of the knee. *Injury.* 1981;12:383–388.

55. Ure BM, Tiling T, Roddecker K, et al. Arthroscopy of the knee in children and adolescents. *Eur J Pediatr Surg.* 1992;2:102–105.

56. Faraj AA, Schilders E, Martens M. Arthroscopic findings in the knees of preadolescent children: report of 23 cases. *Arthroscopy.* 2000;16:793–795.

57. Matelic TM, Aronsson DD, Boyd DW, et al. Acute hemarthrosis of the knee in children. *Am J Sports Med.* 1995;23:668–671.

58. Angel KR, Hall DJ. Anterior cruciate ligament injury in children and adolescents. *Arthroscopy.* 1989;5:197–200.

59. Harvell JC Jr, Fu FH, Stanitski CL. Diagnostic arthroscopy of the knee in children and adolescents. *Orthopedics.* 1989;12:1555–1560.

60. Haus J, Refior HJ. The importance of arthroscopy in sports injuries in children and adolescents. *Knee Surg Sports Traumatol Arthrosc.* 1993;1:34–38.

61. Kloeppel-Wirth S, Koltai JL, Dittmer H. Significance of arthroscopy in children with knee joint injuries. *Eur J Pediatr Surg.* 1992;2:169–172.

62. Stanitski CL, Harvell JC, Fu F. Observations on acute knee hemarthrosis in children and adolescents. *J Pediatr Orthop.* 1993;13:506–510.

63. Vahasarja V, Kinnuen P, Serlo W. Arthroscopy of the acute traumatic knee in children. Prospective study of 138 cases. *Acta Orthop Scand.* 1993;64:580–582.

64. Saciri V, Pavlovcic V, Zupanc O, et al. Knee arthroscopy in children and adolescents. *J Pediatr Orthop B.* 2001;10:311–314.

65. Garvin GJ, Munk PL, Vellet AD. Tears of the medial collateral ligament: magnetic resonance imaging findings and associated injuries. *Can Assoc Radiol J.* 1993;44:199–204.

66. Bradley GW, Shives TC, Samuelson KM. Ligament injuries in the knees of children. *J Bone Joint Surg Am.* 1979;61:588–591.

67. Hastings DE. The non operative management of collateral ligament injuries of the knee joint. *Clin Orthop.* 1980;147:22–28.

68. Lundberg M, Messner K. Long term prognosis of isolated partial medial collateral ligament ruptures. A ten-year clinical and radiographic evaluation of a prospectively observed group of patients. *Am J Sports Med.* 1996;24:160–163.

69. Mok DW, Good C. Non-operative management of acute grade III medial collateral ligament injury of the knee. A prospective study. *Injury.* 1989;20:277–280.

70. Petermann J, von Garrel T, Gotzen L. Non-operative treatment of acute medial collateral ligament injuries of the knee joint. *Knee Surg Sports Traumatol Arthrosc.* 1993;1:93–96.

71. Reider B. Medial collateral ligament injuries in athletes. *Sports Med.* 1996;21:147–156.

72. Reider B, Sathy MR, Talkington J, et al. Treatment of isolated medial collateral ligament injuries in athletes with early functional rehabilitation. A five-year follow-up study. *Am J Sports Med.* 1994;22:470–477.

73. Moyer RA, Marchetto PA. Injuries of the posterior cruciate ligament. *Clin Sports Med.* 1993;12:307–315.

74. Mayer PJ, Micheli LJ. Avulsion of the femoral attachment of the posterior cruciate ligament in an eleven-year-old boy. *J Bone Joint Surg Am.* 1979;61:431–432.

75. Sanders W, Wilkins K, Neidre A. Acute insufficiency of the posterior cruciate ligament in children. *J Bone Joint Surg Am.* 1980;62:129–131.

76. Goodrich A, Ballard A. Posterior cruciate ligament avulsion associated with ipsilateral femur fracture in a 10-year-old child. *J Trauma.* 1988;28:1393–1396.

77. Rubinstein RA, Shelboursneck A, McCarroll JR, et al. The accuracy of the clinical examination in the setting of posterior cruciate ligament injuries. *Am J Sports Med.* 1994;4:550–557.

78. Bickerstaff DR. Posterior cruciate ligament injuries. *Br J Hosp Med.* 1997;58:129–133.

79. Boynton MD, Tietjens BR. Long-term followup of untreated isolated posterior cruciate ligament deficient knee. *Am J Sports Med.* 1996;24:306–310.

80. Shelbourne KD, Davis TJ, Patel DV. The natural history of acute, isolated, nonoperatively treated posterior cruciate ligament injuries. A prospective study. *Am J Sports Med.* 1999;27:276–283.

81. Lobenhoffer P, Wunsch L, Bosch U, et al. Arthroscopic repair of the posterior cruciate ligament in a 3-year-old-child. *Arthroscopy.* 1997;13:248–253.

82. Satku K, Chew CN, Seow H. Posterior cruciate ligament injuries. *Acta Orthop Scand.* 1984;55:26–29.

83. Loos WC, Fox JM, Blazina ME, et al. Acute posterior cruciate ligament injuries. *Am J Sports Med.* 1981;9:86–92.

84. Fowler, PJ, Messieh SS. Isolated posterior cruciate ligament injuries in athletes. *Am J Sports Med.* 1987;15:553–557.

85. Hughston JC, Bowden JA, Andrews JR, et al. Acute tears of the posterior cruciate ligament. Results of operative treatment. *J Bone Joint Surg Am.* 1980;62:438–450.

86. Moore HA, Larson RL. Posterior cruciate ligament injuries. Results of early surgical repair. *Am J Sports Med.* 1980;8:68–78.

87. Richter M, Kiefer H, Hehl G, et al. Primary repair for posterior cruciate ligament injuries. An eight year follow-up of fifty-three patients. *Am J Sports Med.* 1996;24:298–305.

88. Strand T, Molster AO, Engesaeter LB, et al. Primary repair in posterior cruciate ligament injuries. *Acta Orthop Scand.* 1984;55:545–547.

89. Baker CL, Norwood LA, Hughston JC. Acute combined posterior cruciate and posterolateral instability of the knee. *Am J Sports Med.* 1984;12:204–208.

90. Clancy WG Jr, Ray JM, Zoltan DJ. Acute tears of the anterior cruciate ligament. Surgery versus conservative treatment. *J Bone Joint Surg Am.* 1980;70:1483–1488.

91. Noyes FR, Barber-Westin SD. Surgical restoration to treat chronic deficiency of the posterolateral complex and cruciate ligaments of the knee joint. *Am J Sports Med.* 1996;24:415–416.

92. Nottage WM, Matsuura PA. Management of compete traumatic anterior cruciate ligament tears in the skeletally immature patient: current concepts and review of literature. *Arthroscopy.* 1994;10:569–573.

93. Sullivan JA. Ligament injury of the knee in children. *Clin Orthop.* 1990;255:44–50.

94. Corso SJ, Whipple TL. Avulsion of the femoral attachment of the anterior cruciate ligament in a 3-year-old boy. *Arthroscopy.* 1996;12:95–98.

95. Eady JL, Cardenas CD, Sopa D. Avulsion of the femoral attachment of the anterior cruciate ligament in a seven-year-old child. A case report. *J Bone Joint Surg Am.* 1982;64:1376–1378.

96. Schaefer RA, Eilert RE, Gillogly SD. Disruption of the anterior cruciate ligament in a 4-year-old child. *Orthop Rev.* 1993;22:725–727.

97. Engstrom B, Gornitzka J, Johansson C, et al. Knee function after anterior cruciate ligament ruptures treated conservatively. *Int Orthop.* 1993;17:208–213.

98. Fetto JF, Marshall JL. The natural history and diagnosis of anterior cruciate ligament insufficiency. *Clin Orthop.* 1980;147:29–36.

99. Kannus P, Jaervinen M. Knee ligament injuries in adolescents: 8 year follow-up of conservative management. *J Bone Joint Surg Br.* 1988;70:772–776.

100. Sandberg R, Balkfors B, Nilsson B, et al. Operative versus nonoperative treatment of recent injuries to the ligaments of the knee. A prospective randomized study. *J Bone Joint Surg Am.* 1987;69:1120–1126.

101. Kocher MS, Micheli LJ, Zurakowski D, et al. Partial tears of the anterior cruciate ligament in children and adolescents. *Am J Sports Med.* 2002;5:697–703.

102. Mizuta H, Kubota K, Shiraishi M, et al. The conservative treatment of complete tears of the anterior cruciate ligament in skeletally immature patients. *J Bone Joint Surg Br.* 1995;77:890–894.

103. Janarv PM, Nystrom A, Werner S, et al. Anterior cruciate ligament injuries in skeletally immature patients. *J Pediatr Orthop.* 1996;16:673–677.

104. Pressman AE, Letts RM, Jarvis JG. Anterior cruciate ligament tears in children: an analysis of operative versus nonoperative treatment. *J Pediatr Orthop.* 1997;17:505–511.

105. Williams JS Jr, Abate JA, Fadale PD, et al. Meniscal and nonosseous ACL injuries in children and adolescents. *Am J Knee Surg.* 1996;9:22–26.

106. Graf BK, Lange RH, Fujisaki CK, et al. Anterior cruciate ligament tears in skeletally immature patients: meniscal pathology at presentation and after attempted conservative treatment. *Arthroscopy.* 1992;8:229–233.

107. Guzzanti V, Falciglia F, Gigante A, et al. The effect of intra-articular ACL reconstruction on the growth plates of rabbits. *J Bone Joint Surg Br.* 1994;76:960–963.

108. Kocher MS, Saxon HS, Hovis WD, et al. Management and complications of anterior cruciate ligament injuries in skeletally immature patients: survey of the Herodicus Society and the ACL Study Group. *J Pediatr Orthop.* 2002;22:452–457.

109. Barrick RL, Buckley SL, Bruckner JD, et al. Partial versus complete acute anterior cruciate ligament tears. The results of nonoperative treatment. *J Bone Joint Surg Br.* 1990;72:622–624.

110. Kannus P, Jarvinen M. Conservatively treated tears of the anterior cruciate ligament. Long-term results. *J Bone Joint Surg Am.* 1987;69:1007–1012.

111. Lehnert M, Eisenschenk A, Zeller A. Results of conservative treatment of partial tears of the anterior cruciate ligament. Long-term results. *Int Orthop.* 1993;17:219–223.

112. Lipcomb AB, Anderson AF. Tears of the anterior cruciate ligament in adolescents. *J Bone Joint Surg Am.* 1986;68:19–28.

113. McCarroll JR, Rettig AC, Shelbourne KD. Anterior cruciate ligament injuries in the young athlete with open physes. *Am J Sports Med.* 1988;16:44–47.

114. McCarroll JR, Shelbourne KD, Porter DA, et al. Patellar tendon graft reconstruction for midsubstance anterior cruciate ligament rupture in junior high school athletes. *Am J Sports Med.* 1994;22:478–484.

115. Shelbourne, KD, Patel DV, McCarroll JR. Management of anterior cruciate ligament injuries in skeletally immature adolescents. *Knee Surg Sports Traumatol Arthrosc.* 1996;4:68–74.

116. Delee JC, Curtis R. Anterior cruciate ligament insufficiency in children. *Clin Orthop.* 1983;172:112–118.

117. Engebretsen L, Svenningseen S, Beaum P. Poor results of anterior cruciate ligament repair in adolescents. *Acta Orthop Scand.* 1988;59:684–686.

118. Greulich W, Pyle S. *Radiographic atlas of skeletal development of the hand and wrist.* Stanford, CA: Stanford Press; 1959.

119. Pearl AJ, Bergfeld JA, eds. *Extraarticular reconstruction of the anterior cruciate ligament deficient knee: Part I. Validated statement summaries.* Champaign, IL: Human Kinetics Publishers;1992:1–11.

120. Larson RV, Ulmer T. Ligament injuries in children. *AAOS Instructional Course Lectures.* 2003;52:677–681.

121. Delee JC. Ligamentous injury of the knee. In: Stanitsky DL, DeLee JC, Drez D, eds. *Pediatric and adolescent sports medicine.* Philadelphia: WB Saunders Co; 1994:406–432.

122. Micheli LJ, Rask B, Gerberg L. Anterior cruciate ligament reconstruction in patients who are prepubescent. *Clin Orthop Relat Res.* 1999;364:40–47.

123. MacIntosh DL, Darby TA. Lateral substitution reconstruction. *J Bone Joint Surg Br.* 1976;58:142.

124. Stadelmaier DM, Arnoczky SP, Dodds J, et al. The effect of drilling and soft tissue grafting across open growth plates. A histologic study. *Am J Sports Med.* 1995;23:431–435.

125. Brief LP. Anterior cruciate ligament reconstruction without drill holes. *Arthroscopy.* 1991;7:350–357.

126. Parker AW, Drez D Jr, Cooper JL. Anterior cruciate ligament injuries in patients with open physes. *Am J Sports Med.* 1994;22:44–47.

127. Andrews M, Noyes FR, Barber-Westin SD. Anterior cruciate ligament allograft reconstruction in the skeletally immature athlete. *Am J Sports Med.* 1994;22:48–54.

128. Lo IK, Kirkley A, Fowler PJ, et al. The outcome of operatively treated anterior cruciate ligament reconstructions in the skeletally immature child. *Arthroscopy.* 1997;13:627–634.

129. Matava MJ, Siegel MJ. Arthroscopic reconstruction of the ACL with semitendinosus-gracilis autograft in skeletally immature adolescent patients. *Am J Knee Surg.* 1997;10:60–69.

130. Aronowitz ER, Ganley TJ, Goode JR, et al. Anterior cruciate ligament reconstruction in adolescents with open physes. *Am J Sports Med.* 2000;28:168–175.

131. Bisson LJ, Wickiewicz T, Levinson M, et al. ACL reconstruction in children with open physes. *Orthopedics.* 1998;21:659–663.

132. Aglietti P, Buzzi R, Zaccherotti G, et al. Patellar tendon versus double semitendinosus and gracilis tendons for anterior cruciate ligament reconstruction. *Am J Sports Med.* 1994;22:211–217.

133. Steiner ME, Hecker AT, Brown CH Jr, et al. Anterior cruciate ligament graft fixation. Comparison of hamstring and patellar tendon grafts. *Am J Sports Med.* 1994;22:240–246.

134. Wiley JJ, Baxter MP. Tibial spine fractures in children. *Clin Orthop.* 1990;255:54–60.

135. Pellacci F, Mignani G, Valdissi L. Fractures of the intercondylar eminence of the tibia in children. *Ital J Orthop Traumatol.* 1986;12:441–446.

136. Bursten DB, Viloa A, Fulkerson JP. Entrapment of the medial meniscus in a fracture of the tibial eminence. *Arthroscopy.* 1988;4:47–50.

137. Hunter RE, Willis JA. Arthroscopic fixation of avulsion fractures of the tibial eminence: technique and outcome. *Arthroscopy.* 2004;20:113–121.

138. Meyers MH, McKeever FM. Fracture of the intercondylar eminence of the tibia. *J Bone Joint Surg Am.* 1970;52:1677–1684.

139. Zaricznyj B. Avulsion fracture of the tibial eminence: treatment by open reduction and pinning. *J Bone Joint Surg Am.* 1977;59:1111–1114.

140. Driesson MJ, Winkelman PA. Fractures of the intercondylar eminence in childhood. *Neth J Surg.* 1984;36:69–72.

141. Oostvogel HJ, Klasen HJ, Reddingius RE. Fractures of the intercondylar eminence in children and adults. *Arch Orthop Trauma.* 1988;107:242–247.

142. McLennan JG. Lessons learned after second-look arthroscopy in Type III fractures of the tibial spine. *J Pediatr Orthop.* 1995;15:59–62.

143. McLennan JG. The role of arthroscopic surgery in the treatment of fractures of the intercondylar eminence of the tibia. *J Bone Joint Surg Br.* 1982;64:477–480.

144. Brunelli G. Fractures of the intercondylar tibial eminence. *Ital J Orthop Traumatol.* 1978;4:5–12.

145. Kogan MG, Marks P, Amendola A. Technique for arthroscopic suture fixation of displaced tibial intercondylar eminence fractures. *Arthroscopy.* 1997;13:301–306.

146. Matthews DE, Geissler WB. Arthroscopic suture fixation of displaced tibial eminence fractures. *Arthroscopy.* 1994;10:418–423.

147. Perez CL, Garcia SG, Gomez CF. The arthroscopic knot technique for fracture of the tibia in children. *Arthroscopy.* 1994;10:698–699.

148. Prince AR, Moyer RA. Arthroscopic treatment of an avulsion fracture of the intercondylar eminence of the tibia. Case report. *Am J Knee Surg.* 1995;8:114–116.

149. Shepley RW. Arthroscopic treatment of Type III tibial spine fractures using absorbable fixation. *Orthopedics.* 2004;27:767–769.

150. Ahn JH, Yoo JC. Clinical outcome of arthroscopic reduction and suture for displaced acute and chronic tibial spine fractures. *Knee Surg Sports Traumatol Arthrosc.* 2005;13:116–121.

151. Lehman RA Jr, Murphy KP, Machen MS, et al. Modified arthroscopic suture fixation of a displaced tibial eminence fracture. *Arthroscopy.* 2003;19:E6.

152. Bale RS, Banks AJ. Arthroscopically guided K-wire fixation for fractures of the intercondylar eminence of the tibia. *J R Coll Surg Edinb.* 1995;40:260–262.

153. Lubowitz JH, Grauer JD. Arthroscopic treatment of anterior cruciate ligament avulsion. *Clin Orthop.* 1993;294:242–246.

154. Mirbey J, Besancenot J, Chambers RT, et al. Avulsion fractures of the tibial tuberosity in the adolescent athlete. Risk factors, mechanism of injury, and treatment. *Am J Sports Med.* 1988;16:336–340.

155. Kocher MS, Foreman ES, Micheli LJ. Laxity and functional outcome after arthroscopic reduction and internal fixation of displaced tibial spine fractures in children. *Arthroscopy.* 2003;19:1085–1090.

156. Willis RB, Blokker C, Stoll TM, et al. Long term follow up of anterior tibial eminence fractures. *J Pediatr Orthop.* 1993;13:361–363.

157. Smith JB. Knee instability after fractures of the intercondylar eminence of the tibia. *J Pediatr Orthop.* 1984;4:462–464.

158. Bachelin P, Bugmann P. Active subluxation in extension, radiological control in intercondylar eminence fractures in childhood. *Z Kinderchir.* 1988;43:180–182.

159. Baxter MP, Wiley JJ. Fractures of the tibial spine in children. *J Bone Joint Surg Br.* 1988;70:228–230.

160. Janarv PM, Westblad P, Johannson C, et al. Long-term follow-up of anterior tibial spine fractures in children. *J Pediatr Orthop.* 1995;15:63–68.

161. Molander ML, Wallin G, Wilstad I. Fracture of the intercondylar eminence of the tibia: a review of 35 patients. *J Bone Joint Surg Br.* 1981;63:89–91.

162. Fyfe IS, Jackson JP. Tibial intercondylar fractures in children: a review of the classification and the treatment of malunion. *Injury.* 1981;13:165–169.

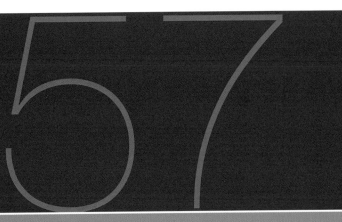

ENVIRONMENTAL ISSUES FOR THE ATHLETE

MARK D. BRACKER, MD, MARJORIE DELO, MD, ELISE T. GORDON, DO, CDR, MC, USN, JUDY R. SCHAUER, DO, CDR, MC, USN

■ KEY POINTS

■ Body temperature is maintained in a narrow range by an integrated system of internal and external processes.

■ Internal homeostasis is controlled by the hypothalamus, with the parasympathetic nervous system regulating sweat gland function and the sympathetic nervous system controlling changes in skin blood flow and vasodilatation.

■ Evaporation of sweat is the primary means of cooling once the environmental temperature exceeds 68°F.

■ A large number of medications can decrease the ability of the athlete's body to regulate internal temperature. Performance-enhancing supplements, such as ephedra, have been implicated as deleterious to the process.

■ The type of clothing worn and pre-existing medical conditions can also affect thermoregulation of the athlete.

■ An athlete who has acclimated to elevated temperature will need increased fluid intake because normal sweating rates may double.

■ Three primary heat illnesses—heat cramps, heat exhaustion, and heat stroke—are common to athletic populations.

■ In American high school athletics, heat stroke has been the third leading cause of death behind only head and neck trauma and cardiovascular disorders.

■ Individuals affected by heat cramps experience painful muscle contractions primarily in the arms, calves, and abdomen. Other symptoms include nausea, vomiting, fatigue, and lightheadedness.

■ Athletes with heat exhaustion present with symptoms of fatigue, inability to continue activity, mild confusion, nausea, vomiting, chills, piloerection, and profuse sweating.

■ It is imperative to begin treatment of heat exhaustion as soon as it is identified because this condition can progress to heat stroke, which is a medical emergency.

■ Symptoms of heat exhaustion and heat stroke are very similar, and therefore, on the field, efforts should be directed at cooling the patient immediately as though the patient has heat stroke. If in doubt, transporting the patient to the emergency department is the most prudent action.

■ Practices that may have contributed to the heat exhaustion episode (e.g., poor diet, insufficient fluids, etc.) should be examined, and corrective actions should be taken to prevent repeat occurrences.

■ Exertional heat stroke, a medical emergency, is defined by a core temperature greater than 104°F and severe central nervous system (CNS) disturbances, resulting in loss of homeostasis and damage to multiple organ systems.

■ In the field, a presumptive diagnosis of exertional heat stroke may be made when the patient is hot, environmental conditions are conducive to heat injury, and there are signs of moderate to severe CNS dysfunction.

■ CNS involvement is the hallmark, but the cardiovascular, integument, renal, splanchnic, and hepatic systems are also damaged by heat stroke.

■ People visit areas at altitudes greater than 2,500 m and engage in activities ranging from sedentary to strenuous. Physicians practicing in this setting should become familiar with the signs and symptoms of various high-altitude syndromes.

■ During ascent, increased sympathetic activity results in increased blood pressure, heart rate, cardiac output, and venous tone.

■ All of the acute mountain sickness syndromes are a result of neurohumoral and hemodynamic changes occurring when humans become hypoxic. First-line therapy, specifically descent and oxygen, is the same for any syndrome in the spectrum.

- High-altitude illness risk can be decreased through slow ascent and wise choice of sleeping altitude.
- Hypothermia and frostbite are the result of prolonged exposure to the elements without proper insulation, elemental protection, or energy stores.
- Exposure to cold conditions can lead to disease on a local or systemic level. Local disease ranges from frostnip, which does not cause permanent damage, to deep frostbite, which leads to irreversible damage to bones, joints, and muscle tissues. Systemic cold injury, or hypothermia, affects the entire body's metabolic and cellular function.
- Hypothermia refers to a decline in core temperature below 35°C.
- Winter sports enthusiasts and mountaineers are increasingly being treated for injury related to cold exposure.
- The risk of dying from hypothermia increases at the extremes of age.
- Emergency medical personnel can minimize injury from cold by rapidly removing the victims from further danger, insulating and immobilizing them, and transporting them to treatment facilities.

■ HEAT-RELATED ILLNESS

Recent high-profile deaths of high school, collegiate, and professional athletes from heat stroke have once again alerted physicians, athletic trainers, and coaches alike of the importance of recognizing and promptly treating heat-related illnesses (1,2).

Basic Science

Normal Human Temperature Regulation

Body temperature is maintained in a narrow range by an integrated system of internal and external processes. Internal thermal homeostasis is controlled by the hypothalamus, with the parasympathetic nervous system regulating sweat gland function and the sympathetic nervous system controlling changes in skin blood flow and vasodilatation (3) **(Fig 57-1)**. As environmental temperatures rise, blood flow is diverted to the skin, and sweat production increases (3,4). The rate of sweat production is affected by, among other factors, the acclimatization of the athlete being challenged. In general, a sweat rate of 1 to 2 L per hour with a sodium content of 65 mEq per L is achieved in the nonacclimatized individual (3,5). With the physiological changes of heat adaptation, the sweat rate increases to 3 to 4 L per hour, and the sodium concentration drops to 5 mEq per L (5).

Mechanisms of Heat Transfer

Available mechanisms of cooling include conduction, convection, radiation, and evaporation **(Fig 57-2)** (6). Conduction is the transference of heat from one body to another cooler one by direct contact. Air can act as an insulator to heat loss,

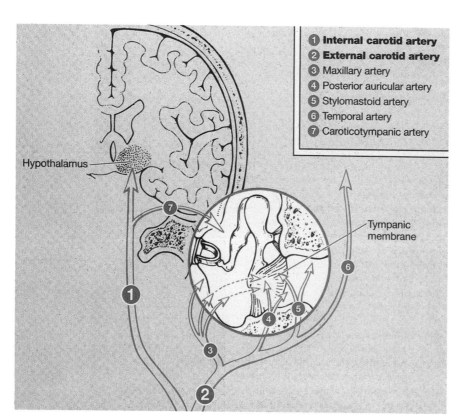

1. Internal carotid artery
2. External carotid artery
3. Maxillary artery
4. Posterior auricular artery
5. Stylomastoid artery
6. Temporal artery
7. Caroticotympanic artery

Hypothalamus

Tympanic membrane

Fig 57-1. The hypothalamus and parasympathetic nervous system regulate sweat gland function.

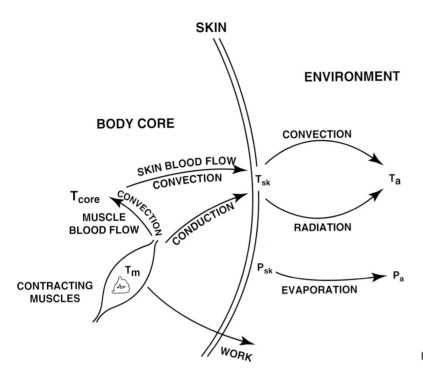

Fig 57-2. The mechanisms of cooling.

whereas water provides better conduction of heat, which is key in its use for immersion cooling.

Convection is transfer of heat to the surrounding circulating air. With elevated ambient temperatures, as when the air temperature is greater than the skin temperature, heat can actually be transferred to the skin.

Radiation is dispersal of heat in the form of infrared electromagnetic waves. These first three mechanisms are most useful for cooling when the ambient temperature is less than or equal to the skin temperature (3). In humans, by far the most important method of heat dissipation is evaporation (7). As sweat forms on the skin, surrounding warmer air evaporates the fluid, thus providing cooling. Evaporation of sweat is the primary means of cooling once the environmental temperature exceeds 68°F (20°C) (8,9). Each milliliter of evaporated sweat cools the body by 0.58 kcal (3); evaporative losses are influenced by wind current and clothing and, most importantly, by the relative humidity. Sweat that is not evaporated, as when there is elevated humidity, but instead rolls off and/or is absorbed by clothing does not provide the needed cooling.

Other Influences on Thermoregulation
The ability of the athlete to function in a hot environment is determined by many factors. Two of them, the physiological mechanisms available for cooling and acclimatization of the individual, have been mentioned. Also affecting thermoregulation of the athlete is the clothing worn, medications that are being used, and pre-existing medical illnesses. Recent National Collegiate Athletic Association (NCAA) guidelines support the gradual introduction of heavier uniform items such as full padding during the acclimatization process (10). Lighter clothing allows sweat to be wicked away from the body as it is more easily evaporated.

A large number of medications can decrease the ability of the athlete to regulate internal temperatures. These include antihistamines, anticholinergics, benzodiazepines, alpha-adrenergics, beta- and calcium blockers, neuroleptics, phenothiazines, diuretics, and tricyclic antidepressants (6, 11). In addition, drugs such as alcohol, cocaine, amphetamines, and ecstasy can adversely affect thermoregulation (4,6). Performance-enhancing supplements (e.g., ephedra) have also been implicated as deleterious to maintaining normal core temperatures (1). All medications and supplements must be identified to allow effective counseling with regard to performance and safety concerns.

Many pre-existing medical conditions can contribute to an individual's inability to adapt and function in a hot environment. These include alcoholism, anorexia, cardiac disease, cystic fibrosis, dehydration, diabetes insipidus, extremes of age, febrile illnesses, gastroenteritis, hypokalemia, obesity, poor conditioning, sleep deprivation, sunburn, and sweat gland dysfunction (3,4,6). Of note, anorexia (along with other eating disorders), dehydration, and gastroenteritis are conditions that are commonly observed in young populations. Coaches, athletic trainers, and physicians must be ready to identify those at risk. Furthermore, these multiple and diverse risk factors for heat illness highlight the importance of preparticipation screening as well as periodic medical updates to allow appropriate and individualized levels of play and/or activity in hot environments.

A history of previous heat injury has been listed as elevating the risk of subsequent heat illnesses. While it is true that activity modification is necessary as the athlete recovers from an illness, recent studies have not shown that an episode of heat injury universally predisposes to future episodes (12,13).

Acclimatization

Gradual acclimatization to a warm, humid environment is an important process in preventing heat-related illnesses. Normally taking 10 to 14 days to accomplish, it is a series of gradual physiological adaptations to heat that occurs with regular exposure to and exercise in a hot environment (13,14). Physiological changes that improve tolerance to heat include an increase in blood volume, an increase in sweat rate with a faster onset of sweating, a wider distribution of areas producing sweat, and a decrease in the sweat sodium concentration **(Fig 57-3)**.

There is a common misconception that, as the athlete acclimates to elevated temperature, there is a concomitant decrease in hydration requirement. The converse is true; normal sweating rates may double, thus significantly increasing the required fluid intake to maintain euhydration.

The significance of adequate hydration cannot be overemphasized. It has been estimated that for each 1% decrease in body weight secondary to dehydration, the core temperature increases by 0.15 to 0.2°C (7,15). Increased sweat rates add to the dehydrated state with hemodynamic instability resulting. Results of a recent study of high school athletes showed that over 60% began summer practice sessions in a dehydrated state, based on a initial urine-specific gravity of greater than 1.020 (16). Thirst is not a reliable indicator of volume status because a level of 2% to 3% dehydration is necessary to initiate this response (7). This level of dehydration is not uncommon with normal practice conditions and has also been noted to impair athletic performance. With thirst as the sole prompter of fluid ingestion, an athlete will only ingest one third to two thirds of fluid loss as sweat (17).

Measuring Heat Stress

Assessment of environmental conditions that increase risk of heat illnesses is another important step in injury prevention. A number of indices have been developed to attempt to define site-specific risk. One of the most widely known and used is the Wet Bulb Globe Temperature (WBGT) Index (13). Using three measurements to reflect dry temperature,

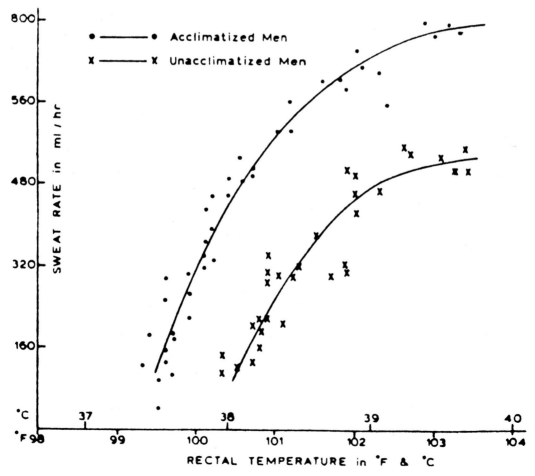

Fig 57-3. An increase in sweat rate improves heat tolerance.

humidity, and radiant heat effects and weighting them for importance, the generated score is correlated to a certain degree of danger from heat exposure. In this way, activities can be modified to reduce potential harm (18). The National Weather Index is another tool to evaluate heat exposure but is not specific to the area of play (4). While a WBGT meter is expensive, a more affordable method uses a sling psychrometer, and a free program is available on the internet (19).

Clinical Evaluation

Three primary heat illnesses are common to athletic populations: heat cramps, heat exhaustion, and heat shock. The actual incidence of the first two is not known because these are often treated on the field with referral for recalcitrant symptoms only. For the years of 1990 to 1995, there were 84 deaths among U.S. football players attributed to heat stroke (20). In 1995 alone, there were five heat-related deaths among American athletes (21). In American high school athletes, heat stroke has been listed as the third leading cause of death, following only head and neck trauma and cardiovascular disorders (22). Four teenage football players died in early August 2004 with heat-related illnesses as the probable cause (1).

With heat stroke being a largely preventable cause of death and the opinion of many that there is a continuum in the severity of heat illness symptoms, it is important to recognize the characteristics of each and act accordingly to prevent progression to a more hazardous condition.

Heat Cramps

With heat cramps, affected individuals experience painful muscle contractions primarily in the arms, calves, and abdomen, with inadequate electrolyte intake being the probable etiology. Athletes complain of extremity cramping in the most worked muscle groups and often after the activity has stopped. Other symptoms include nausea, vomiting, fatigue, and lightheadedness. Risk factors for heat cramps include the use of diuretics (as caffeinated beverages), unacclimatized state, and inadequate sodium intake. A classic study of workers in several industrial settings demonstrated four characteristics of heat cramps that are still valid: (a) contractions occur after sustained heavy effort in a hot environment; (b) affected individuals sweated profusely; (c) fluid replacement consisted of large volumes of water; and (d) cooling seemed to precipitate the spasms because they began after cessation of work (23).

Clinically, patients may appear ill and uncomfortable secondary to the cramping, and sweating will be noted. If measured, the rectal temperature would be below 104°F. Treatment involves removal of the patient to a cool environment, encouraged oral hydration with electrolyte-containing solutions, and stretching/massage of affected muscle groups. If fluid replenishment cannot be accomplished orally secondary to vomiting, parenteral hydration can be initiated. An athlete can return to play if, after treatment, he can successfully participate at the level expected for the sport and position played (24).

Heat Exhaustion

Athletes with heat exhaustion present with symptoms of fatigue, inability to continue activity, mild confusion, nausea, vomiting, chills, piloerection, and profuse sweating. Heat syncope may occur, but there is no major neurological impairment. Hypotension, hyperventilation, and elevated rectal temperatures are objective evidence for heat exhaustion.

Physiologically, affected athletes may be either volume depleted or sodium depleted, although there is often an overlap between the two types of heat exhaustion (4). Water-depleted heat exhaustion is most often observed in elderly populations (as a result of medications that affect hydration status) and in active individuals who are inadequately hydrated for the activity level and the environmental conditions.

Sodium-depleted heat exhaustion, on the other hand, is seen in unacclimatized persons who have overhydrated, taking in sufficient free water, but have not accounted for sodium losses in sweat by altering intake. Acclimatization increases sweat rates but concomitantly decreases sodium content in sweat.

Treatment of heat exhaustion depends on the type and degree of impairment. For mild heat exhaustion, in which the patient is hemodynamically stable, removal to a cool environment, removal of excess equipment and clothing, and replenishment of fluids orally are usually sufficient. Electrolyte/salt replacement is provided as needed (4).

Patients with more severe manifestations (hypotension, cardiac arrhythmias, or deteriorating mental status) or those unresponsive to conservative measures must be transported to emergency medical facilities. Although intravenous hydration may be initiated prior to transport, the volume of saline administered must be modest until electrolyte concentrations can be accurately measured. Heat exhaustion patients who are hypernatremic will need cautious hydration to avoid the cerebral edema caused by too rapid a correction.

It is imperative to begin the treatment of heat exhaustion as soon as it is identified because this condition can progress to heat stroke, which is a medical emergency. Because heat exhaustion and heat stroke symptoms are so similar and assessment of core temperatures may not be possible on the field, efforts should be directed at cooling the patient immediately as if the patient has heat stroke. If in doubt, transport to the emergency department is the most prudent action.

The athlete must be hydrated and asymptomatic before being allowed to return to the field, preferably after being cleared by a physician. In general, delaying return to play to the following day is preferable to allow recovery. Practices that may have contributed to the heat exhaustion episode, such as poor diet, insufficient fluids, and so on, should be examined, and corrective actions should be taken to prevent repeat occurrences. If the primary deficiency is one of not being acclimated, a practice and activity schedule should be engineered to ensure heat tolerance while maintaining conditioning (24).

Heat Stroke

Heat stroke, a medical emergency, is a failure of internal and external thermoregulatory mechanisms to control the cumulative effects of exogenous heat on endogenous systems, with a subsequent loss of homeostasis and damage to multiple organ systems (3,13,25,26). The mortality of this illness depends primarily on the degree of heat experienced and the duration of the temperature elevation. This again emphasizes the importance of early recognition and treatment. Typically, onset is acute, and a high index of suspicion concerning nonspecific presenting symptoms is needed.

Classic Heat Stroke. Two types of heat stroke are recognized and they differ in important aspects. The better known classic heat stroke occurs most often in the summer and usually during heat waves, which are defined as 3 or more days of air temperatures exceeding 90°F (27). The target populations are the elderly and those with chronic medical conditions and persons who are unable to seek cooler environments usually because of infirmities or financial constraints **(Table 57-1)**. The heat insult occurs over several days and results in hyperthermia, central nervous system (CNS) dysfunction, and anhidrosis. This last characteristic is a major distinction from exertional heat stroke, in which sweating, often profuse, continues. Between 1979 and 1999, 8,015 deaths were reported as heat related in the United States, with almost 50% occurring in the age group over 65 years old (27). Again, comorbidities contribute to the mortality of classic heat stroke. It is likely that the true incidence of this disease is higher because the resulting organ system failures (e.g., cardiovascular, renal, CNS) may be identified as the cause of death instead of the initiating heat injury.

Exertional Heat Stroke. Exertional heat stroke is defined by a core temperature greater than 104°F and severe CNS disturbances (see Table 57-1). Affected individuals are usually younger, more physically fit, and involved in physically challenging activities. For the 20% who have a prodromal syndrome, presentation may be similar to that of heat exhaustion (13). Symptoms may include dizziness, nausea and vomiting, frontal headache, confusion, drowsiness, disorientation, muscle twitching, ataxia, and psychiatric symptoms. More often, however, collapse is acute. Patients may experience syncope, seizures, and coma. Objectively, tachypnea, tachycardia, hypotension, and cardiac arrhythmias may be noted in addition to the elevated rectal temperatures. In the field, where a rectal probe may not be available, a presumptive diagnosis of exertional heat stroke may be made when the patient is hot, environmental conditions are conducive to heat injury, and there are signs of moderate to severe CNS dysfunction.

Immediate recognition of heat stroke is critical because no inherent internal thermoregulatory mechanism is adequate to combat the widespread effects. Although CNS involvement is the hallmark, other systems are also damaged, including the cardiovascular, integument, renal, splanchnic, and hepatic systems. The clinical picture has been likened to sepsis. A current theory for the global abnormalities seen postulates that, as skin blood flow increases to dissipate an ever increasing heat load, splanchnic circulatory support erodes to the point that gram-negative proteins are able to cross the blood–tissue barrier and cause decreased vascular resistance (28). It should be no surprise, given our unfolding knowledge that the inflammatory system involvement comprises multiple processes, that the current heat stress model attributes at least some of the tissue effects to circulating cytokines such as interleukin C. These modulators effect further changes, which serve to worsen the clinical situation.

With the normal shunting of blood from central to peripheral circulation exacerbated by pre-existing dehydration, the patient will demonstrate hemodynamic compromise via an elevated heart rate, a decreased blood pressure,

TABLE 57-1	Comparison of Symptoms of Classic and Exertional Heat Stroke	
Characteristic	**Classic**	**Exertional**
Age	Older	Young
Occurrence	Epidemic form	Isolated cases
Body temperature	Very high	High
Predisposing illness	Frequent	Rare
Sweating	Often absent	May be present
Acid–base disturbance	Respiratory alkalosis	Lactic acidosis
Rhabdomyolysis	Rare	Common
DIC	Rare	Common
Acute renal failure	Rare	Common
Hyperuricemia	Mild	Marked
Elevated muscle enzymes	Mild	Marked

DIC, disseminated intravascular coagulation.

and CNS compromise. It is not hard to appreciate, then, that the dehydrated or insufficiently hydrated athlete would be more susceptible to heat injury.

Treatment

The next critical step following recognition is immediate resuscitation and cooling (21,24–26). As with any emergency, attention to airway, breathing, and circulation is paramount. Simultaneously, cooling must be initiated, and the emergency medical system must be alerted.

Two basic methods presently advocated in the literature are cool water/ice immersion and evaporative cooling (13, 24,29). More easily accomplished in the field, evaporative cooling involves removing the outer equipment and clothing (attempting to preserve modesty), spraying water over the patient, and creating air currents/increasing air flow with the use of devices such as fans. An advantage to this method is that other aspects of resuscitation, such as airway support and cardiac monitoring, are not hindered by the measures used to cool the patient.

Cold water or ice immersion has been shown to produce a cooling rate twice that of evaporative cooling but is not usually available in a prehospital setting. The skin vasoconstriction achieved by immersion techniques serves to shift skin blood flow back to the central circulation and improves the hypotensive states. Other more traditional approaches such as packing the axilla and groin with ice packs have not been shown to be as effective.

If effective cooling and other resuscitative measures can be promptly initiated and appropriate medical support is available on scene, the rule of thumb is to cool first and then evacuate to a medical facility. Intravenous hydration with normal saline is also recommended. If repeat rectal temperatures show a decrease to the target goal of 101 to 102°F, the patient should still be transported to monitor status and evaluate organ system damage.

Complications and Special Considerations

Following exertional heat stroke, guidelines for returning the athlete to activity are similar to those for heat exhaustion. The patient may have suffered complications that would contraindicate further participation in hot environments. The permanence of heat illness susceptibility after heat stroke is controversial, with some studies implying there is no increased risk.

The athlete must be completely asymptomatic and all laboratory abnormalities must be resolved before return to play/activity is considered (24). The physician must provide activity clearance after a recovery time appropriate to the injury suffered and specific guidance on exercise allowed. In cooperation with the athletic trainer, a gradual acclimatization schedule must be developed to ensure maximal tolerance to elevated ambient temperatures.

Conclusion and Future Directions

Of course, the goal should be to prevent heat injury and illnesses before they happen. To this end, various groups including the NCAA and the National Athletic Trainers' Association (NATA) have issued guidelines on preventive measures. Education is the first step. Coaches and athletes alike must be informed as to proper evaluation and maintenance of hydration, as well as recognition and on-site management of heat-related illnesses.

Ensuring adequate hydration has been a focus of prevention and has been approached in various ways. First, the baseline weight of the athlete should be ascertained. Then, various techniques have been used to assess the change in hydration status with exercise and play. These include reweighing the athlete during and after practice, evaluation of urine-specific gravity, comparison of urine color to standardized charts, and actual measurement of urine output (17). Individuals should be able to determine their specific sweat rate and alter fluid/electrolyte intake to maintain homeostasis even during elevated ambient temperatures (17).

One recommendation is a buddy system where partners are educated on the symptoms of heat illnesses, know each other at baseline, and are alert to physical and mental status changes that may signal the onset of hyperthermic conditions (1).

Hydrating before, during, and after practice/activity has long been recognized as vital to encouraging adequate fluid intake. Although plain water is normally sufficient to replenish fluids, the addition of flavor and electrolytes has been demonstrated to increase voluntary hydration. Specific recommendations have been advanced to address hydration goals at various stages in activity. The current pre-exercise hydration regimen promotes ingestion of 500 mL of fluid 2 hours before exercise with the given provision that the athlete is already euhydrated (17).

Fluid intake during activity should be encouraged, with a minimum of 250 mL consumed every 20 minutes. This frequency is a general guideline and must be amended depending on the sport. Finally, replenishment of fluids after exercise should be determined by the weight lost, with the ideal being that the fluid volume ingested is equivalent to approximately 150% of weight change (17,30).

Prevention of heat injury is an ongoing process that begins with each new season. Background knowledge on heat illness should be explored with each athlete, and myths should be replaced with established and relevant facts. Only concerted teamwork with the athletes, coaches, athletic trainers, and providers can effectively alleviate heat-related morbidity and mortality.

■ HIGH ALTITUDE SYNDROMES

People visit areas at altitudes greater than 2,500 m every year and engage in activities ranging from sedentary (hanging out in the lodge) to active (e.g., biking, skiing, boarding) and strenuous (e.g., mountaineering). Physicians practicing in this setting should become familiar with the signs and symptoms of various high-altitude syndromes. In addition, trauma may occur concomitantly or as a result of high-altitude illness, making it necessary to recognize and treat both the orthopaedic injury and altitude-related illness in the same patient.

Most experts agree on the definitions of altitude (31):

- High Altitude: 1,500 to 3,500 m (4,921 to 11,483 feet). Most ski resorts in North America fall into this category. At these elevations, symptoms of acute mountain sickness (AMS) begin to appear.
- Very High Altitude: 3,500 to 5,500 m (11,483 to 18,045 feet). Symptoms of altitude illness often become severe and life threatening at these altitudes.
- Extreme High Altitude: >5,500 m (18,045 feet). Altitudes at which there is no permanent human habitation. These elevations serve primarily as venues for military activity and civilian recreation. This is the altitude at which physiological changes secondary to altitude exposure can overcome the human body's capability to acclimatize. Rapid death can occur at these altitudes to the unprepared and inexperienced. Mt. Everest, Mt. Kilimanjaro, and K2 are among some known extreme-altitude arenas.

Basic Science

Acclimatization to Altitude

Acclimatization to altitude is the process by which individuals gradually adjust to hypoxia and enhance their survival in this hostile environment. Successful acclimatization protects against altitude illness and improves sleep. Longer term acclimatization (days to weeks) primarily improves aerobic exercise capacity. As humans ascend in altitude, a series of physiological mechanisms respond to compensate for the dropping atmospheric partial pressure of oxygen.

Ventilatory Response. Initial changes within the pulmonary system occur via the hyperventilatory response (HVR) **(Fig 57-4)**. As the partial pressure of oxygen drops, ventilatory rate increases. This response is a function of the carotid body, which is located near the bifurcation of the common carotid artery in the neck, detecting a decrease in arterial oxygen saturation of blood. Eventually, increased ventilation will produce a respiratory alkalosis (hypocapnia). Alkalosis slows the central respiratory center, limiting any further increase in ventilatory rate, and increases renal excretion of bicarbonate, creating a relative metabolic acidosis **(Fig 57-5)**. As ascent continues, plasma bicarbonate concentration continues to decrease, creating additional stimulus of ventilation. A maximum HVR is reached by 4 to 7 days at a steady altitude. Physical conditioning does not change an individual's HVR; it is genetically determined (32).

Circulatory Response. During ascent, increased sympathetic activity results in increased blood pressure, heart rate, cardiac output, and venous tone. Bicarbonate diuresis by the kidneys, extra vascular fluid shift, and aldosterone suppression cumulatively cause a decrease in plasma volume and cardiac stroke volume. Acclimatization eventually returns resting heart rate to sea level values except at extreme high altitudes (>5,500 m).

The pulmonary circulation responds with an increase in pulmonary vascular resistance called the hypoxic pulmonary vasoconstriction response (HPVR). Pulmonary hypertension plays a role in high-altitude pulmonary edema (HAPE). Studies suggest that HPVR is not solely responsible for increased pulmonary vascular resistance. Oxygen administration alone does

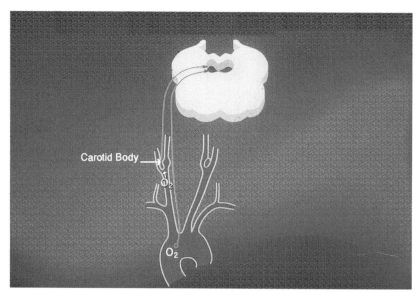

Fig 57-4. Hypoxic ventilatory response (HVR).

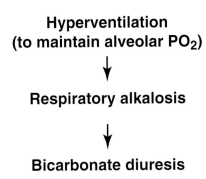

**Hyperventilation
(to maintain alveolar PO$_2$)**

$\downarrow$

Respiratory alkalosis

$\downarrow$

Bicarbonate diuresis

Fig 57-5. The physiology of acclimatization. PO$_2$, partial pressure of oxygen.

not entirely reverse the effects of HPVR, suggesting additional factors in several studies (33,34).

The product of cerebral blood flow (CBF) and arterial oxygen content determine oxygen delivery to the brain. As the barometric pressure drops, so does arterial oxygen saturation. Acclimatization attempts to preserve CBF. Hypoxia and hypocapnia have opposing responses within the cerebral circulation. The net balance of vasodilation due to hypoxia and vasoconstriction secondary to hypocapnia determine the CBF. Recent studies suggest that everyone with altitude exposure develops some degree of cerebral edema (33).

Hematopoietic. Erythropoietin is released into the blood stream within 2 hours of exposure to altitude. Immature red blood cells can be found within days. It takes weeks, however, to note an increase in the hematocrit. Studies evaluating iron supplementation for altitude adaptation have had mixed results; the greatest effect is usually seen in women (35).

The premise for live high–train low theories of exercise training results partially from this natural response to altitude (36). The increased red blood cell mass is capable of more oxygen-carrying capacity. This is the same effect as seen with blood doping and exogenous erythropoietin injections.

Sleep at Altitude. Sleep at altitude presents its own complications. Deep sleep periods (stages 3 and 4) are decreased with exposure to altitude (33). Research subjects demonstrate "periodic breathing" similar to Cheyne-Stokes breathing patterns in which rapid breathing is followed by periods of hypoventilation and apnea spells (37). This type of breathing pattern contributes to disturbed sleep and frequent waking.

Training and Exercise at Altitude. Exertion in any form becomes progressively more difficult upon ascent; with acclimatization, maximal oxygen uptake improves, but eventually hypoxemia limits muscle function and the ability to perform work. The live high–train low concept of conditioning introduced by Levine and Stray-Gunderson in 1997 capitalizes on improved oxygen-carrying capacity resulting from a high hematocrit.

Clinical Evaluation

Acclimatization is not a smooth process for every person; difficulties with physiological changes at altitude develop when neurohumoral and hemodynamic responses to hypoxia go beyond mere acclimatization. The exact pathophysiology resulting in AMS continues to be researched. It is generally agreed upon, however, that AMS represents a spectrum of illness. Abnormalities range from focal neurological syndromes and acute hypoxia to more life-threatening forms of AMS, such as high-altitude cerebral edema (HACE) and HAPE. Rate of ascent, final altitude reached, sleeping altitude, and individual physiology all contribute to determining who will develop altitude illness. Other risk factors include a previous history of high-altitude illness, residence at altitude below 900 m, level of exertion, and some cardiopulmonary conditions. Researchers have attempted to delineate what factors play a role in individual susceptibility for altitude syndromes, particularly HAPE. Interestingly, hypertension, coronary artery disease, and pregnancy are not risk factors for altitude syndromes. Men are more prone to HAPE but equally prone to AMS; genetic factors such as human leukocyte antigen alleles, angiotensin-converting enzyme, tyrosine hydroxylase, serotonin transporter, and endothelial nitric oxide genes have been evaluated without delineating a firm association between HAPE and genetic polymorphism (31,32,38). Level of physical fitness is not protective against high-altitude illness.

Treatment

All high-altitude syndromes are a result of neurohumoral and hemodynamic changes occurring when humans become hypoxic. First-line therapy, descent and oxygen, is the same for any syndrome in the spectrum. Utility of medical management and the agent used varies with the syndrome. Acetazolamide works best in AMS. Dexamethasone should be given in HACE. Furosemide can be helpful in HAPE. High-altitude headache responds well to a single dose of ibuprofen.

Other agents that have been studied have had inconsistent results. Theophylline recently has been found to be as effective as acetazolamide in AMS. This study gives a second treatment option for AMS for sulfa-allergic patients instead of acetazolamide. Angiotensin-converting enzyme (ACE) inhibitors have entered the discussion as a possible future treatment.

High Altitude Headache

Usually the first and most debilitating symptom experienced at altitude is headache. The proposed pathophysiology for headache starts with hypoxia triggering the trigeminal vascular system as well endothelial nitric oxide up-regulation (31).

Headache may precipitate other symptoms such as nausea, anorexia, and fatigue. It is important to be able to distinguish an exertional headache from AMS, particularly when decisions need to be made about whether or not to progress to higher altitude. Any headache present in the morning that is not easily relieved by nonnarcotic analgesics and associated with ataxia, confusion, or lethargy should be considered to be AMS. Ascent to higher elevation should not occur.

As with exertional headache, the treatment of high-altitude headache with a single dose of ibuprofen (400 to 600 mg) is usually effective (39). Common migraine headache therapies, such as sumatriptan, have had inconsistent results. Supplemental oxygen, if it is available, can provide relief of symptoms, as will descent to a lower elevation.

For prophylaxis, aspirin 325 mg given every 4 hours for a total of three doses decreases the incidence of headache (39). Acetazolamide (Diamox) 250 mg at bedtime may improve periodic breathing at night and decrease the incidence of morning headache. Acetazolamide is not recommended for people with known sulfa allergy.

AMS

The Lake Louise Consensus Group defined AMS as a headache in an unacclimatized individual who has recently arrived (within 6 to 10 hours) at 2,500 m plus one or more of the following: gastrointestinal symptoms (anorexia, nausea, or vomiting), insomnia, dizziness, and fatigue (38,40). Some people have been known to develop AMS as soon as 1 hour at altitude and even at elevations below 2,500 m. AMS is a clinical diagnosis often confused with a viral illness, hangover, dehydration, exhaustion, hypothermia, or even medication effects. AMS does not manifest a fever or myalgias, and dehydration responds quickly to fluid replacement. Exhaustion may closely mimic AMS with no clues to separate the two. Nothing is lost if the patient is treated for AMS as the potential for morbidity and mortality is much higher for untreated AMS.

Management of AMS depends on severity of symptoms as well as response to treatment. Descent and supplemental oxygen comprise the first-line treatment of AMS. Medical management includes acetazolamide, dexamethasone, and furosemide. Acetazolamide is a carbonic anhydrase inhibitor. It is thought to prevent and treat the symptoms of AMS by decreasing reabsorption of bicarbonate and sodium, resulting in a bicarbonate diuresis and metabolic acidosis. This serves to counter the effects of increased ventilation (HVR) with subsequent respiratory alkalosis. The diuretic effect of acetazolamide minimizes or prevents fluid retention and decreases antidiuretic hormone (ADH) secretion and cerebrospinal fluid production **(Fig 57-6)**. Acetazolamide decreases periodic breathing and maintains arteriolar oxygenation saturation during sleep. Mild symptoms of AMS respond well to acetazolamide (125 to 250 mg twice daily orally) in addition to halting ascent for 12 hours to 4 days. More moderate symptoms or no response to therapy requires descent until symptoms resolve. A 500- to 1,000-m decrease in altitude usually suffices. When descent is impossible or dangerous, supplemental oxygen and use of hyperbaric chamber devices, if available, can slow progression and/or facilitate acclimatization.

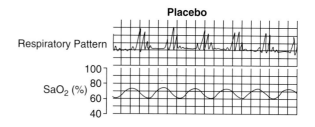

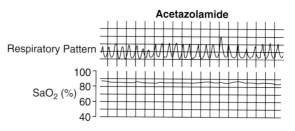

Fig 57-6. Respiratory patterns and arterial oxygen saturation (SaO_2%) with placebo and acetazolamide in two sleep studies of a subject at 4,400 m. (From Hackett PH, Roach RC. High altitude medicine. In: Auerbach PS, ed. *Wilderness medicine*. 4th ed. St. Louis: Mosby; 2001:2–43.)

Although acetazolamide is the first choice of treatment, dexamethasone has recently been shown to be as successful, if not more so, than acetazolamide in treatment of AMS. The caveat is that dexamethasone does not facilitate acclimatization as acetazolamide does. Patients experience symptoms of AMS once dexamethasone is discontinued. Onset of action is longer, within 12 hours (39), with dexamethasone. Dexamethasone 4 mg can be given every 6 hours orally, intramuscularly, or intravenously. The mechanism of action in dexamethasone in AMS and HACE is unknown.

Symptoms of nausea and vomiting can be treated with antiemetics such as prochlorperazine and promethazine. Avoid treating insomnia with sedative hypnotics. Zolpidem 10 mg orally can be very effective for insomnia without suppression of respiration. Remember, medication is the second choice in the treatment of AMS. Descent and oxygen are first-line therapies.

In the last few years, other therapies have been evaluated for their efficacy in treating AMS. Fischer et al. (37) demonstrated theophylline to be at least as effective as acetazolamide in normalizing high-altitude disordered breathing. Although theophylline may not replace acetazolamide, it can act as an alternate therapy, especially for those with sulfa allergy. Magnesium, however, did not prevent AMS and had only limited reduction in symptoms for those with established AMS (41). One last group of medications that has generated some interest is the ACE inhibitors. Although ACE inhibitors blunt the HPVR in humans, they also blunt erythropoietin release as well as the adaptive polycythemia (42). The role of ACE inhibitors in prevention or treatment of AMS or as a medication to be avoided in altitude exposure still merits evaluation.

Prevention starts with diminishing risk factors. Hackett and Roach (39) recommend the following for those with no altitude experience: avoid abrupt ascent to 2,500 m; allow 2 to 3 days to acclimatize before attempting further ascent; sleeping altitude should change by only 600 m daily above 2,500 m; and avoid alcohol and sedative hypnotics, which would exacerbate hypoxia during sleep through respiratory depression.

The number one medication recommendation for prophylaxis is acetazolamide (39). AMS prevention consists of acetazolamide 125 or 250 mg orally twice daily 24 hours prior to ascent and for 2 days during ascent (39,43,44). Dexamethasone is also a consideration for prevention (39,45). Symptoms of AMS return when dexamethasone has been discontinued. Ginkgo biloba 80 to 120 mg twice daily has demonstrated effectiveness in both prevention and symptom reduction in two controlled trials (39).

HACE

HACE is a severe, life-threatening encephalopathy that occurs in the setting of AMS or HAPE (31). Symptoms usually begin to develop within 1 to 3 days of altitude exposure and likely represent a progression of the same failure in acclimatization found with AMS. Patients suffering from HACE present with ataxic gait, severe lassitude, and altered mental status. Other neurological findings include retinal hemorrhages, hallucinations, seizures, cranial nerve palsy, hemiparesis, and hemiplegia.

Blood vessels within the CNS become progressively more permeable, resulting in vasogenic edema; the physical distance between nutrients and target cell increases, preventing diffusion of the necessary fuels for cerebral cell function (34,39,46). As the brain begins to swell, cerebrospinal fluid pressure increases dramatically, with pressure readings greater than 300 mm H_2O having been documented. As the brain is squeezed downward in the cranial vault, focal neurological findings may appear.

HACE must be recognized early and treated as a medical emergency. If unrecognized, a victim's condition may deteriorate rapidly, and irreparable damage may occur (47). Dexamethasone 4 to 8 mg should be started intravenously, intramuscularly, or orally with repeat dosing every 4 to 6 hours. Supplemental oxygen should be titrated to maintain oxygen saturation above 90%. Loop diuretics can be used to achieve a balance between intravascular volume for cerebral perfusion pressure and reducing brain edema. Comatose patients require definitive airway management and urinary output monitoring with bladder catheterization. Achieving high levels of care in the wilderness can only be accomplished with meticulous advanced planning and team leadership.

HAPE

HAPE has the highest mortality of all the high-altitude syndromes. Fortunately, HAPE is a noncardiogenic pulmonary edema that may be completely reversible if diagnosed and treated early (33). Patients with HAPE demonstrate increased pulmonary artery pressures as a result of exaggerated hypoxic ventilatory response **(Fig 57-7)**. Altitude research has demonstrated patterns of unequal perfusion within the lungs

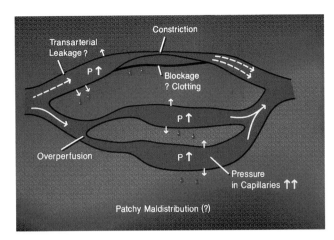

Fig 57-7. Patients with high altitude pulmonary edema (HAPE) demonstrate an increase in pulmonary artery pressures.

of individuals with HAPE; capillary leakage may occur secondary to increased vascular pressure resulting from the overperfusion (33). Mechanical and inflammatory causes of vascular permeability have been proposed (48). Early studies evaluating contents of bronchiolar lavage have documented increased leukocytes and other markers of inflammation. Recent studies, however, have challenged these findings and suggest that the inflammatory markers in bronchiolar fluid may not be as important as previously thought (49).

Patients present initially with symptoms of AMS, such as fatigue, weakness, and dyspnea on exertion. The most common time of presentation is the second night after rapid ascent to high altitude, but onset can take up to 4 days. Symptoms usually begin with a persistent dry cough that typically worsens at night. On examination, vital signs demonstrate elevated resting heart and respiratory rates. Nail bed and lip cyanosis is evident; lung examination is significant for rales initially in the right axilla and progressing to bilateral findings. Chest x-ray, if available, demonstrates patchy infiltrates, typically in the right middle and lower lobes.

Treatment of HAPE starts with descent and oxygen. Temporizing measures include nifedipine 10 mg orally at the onset, followed by 20- to 30-mg extended-release tablets every 12 hours. Nifedipine helps to decrease pulmonary artery pressures found in HAPE. A recent study examined the utility of salmeterol in preventing HACE (50). Beta-agonists increase the clearance of alveolar fluid from the alveolar space; however, there is no conclusive evidence for salmeterol use at this time. Nifedipine, however, is recommended as prophylaxis for those with previous history of HAPE (20 to 30 mg orally every 12 hours of extended-release formulation) (46).

Conclusion

High-altitude illness is a complex spectrum of neurological and pulmonary disorders that develop from a combination of neurohumoral and vasogenic responses to hypoxia. The exact mechanism for altitude syndromes is still being delineated. Decrease risk of high-altitude illness through slow ascent and wise choice of sleeping altitude. Consider acetazolamide, steroids, and nifedipine for prophylaxis in AMS, HACE, and HAPE, respectively. Although there are differences regarding the utility of medication management in AMS, HACE, and HAPE, all patients respond to descent and oxygen.

■ COLD INJURY: HYPOTHERMIA AND FROSTBITE

Exposure to cold conditions can lead to disease on a local or systemic level. Local disease ranges from frostnip, which does not cause any permanent tissue damage, to deep frostbite, which leads to irreversible damage to bones, joints, and muscle tissue. Systemic cold injury, or hypothermia, affects the entire body's metabolic and cellular function. Accidental hypothermia refers to a decline in core temperature below 35ºC (95ºF) secondary to exposure. Secondary hypothermia can occur as a result of medical conditions such as trauma, stroke, hypothyroidism, or sepsis.

Military history gives us some of the earliest and most extensive accounts of cold-induced injury. In 218 BC, Hannibal's army of 46,000 men lost nearly half of its troops to cold injury while crossing the Pyrenean Alps (51). George Washington left 10% of his army behind due to the brutal cold at Valley Forge during the winter of 1777 to 1778 (52). In World War II on the Eastern Front, 100,000 soldiers suffered frostbite, of whom 15,000 required amputation.

In more recent history, cold injury in developed nations became a problem for the urban destitute who had no protection from environmental insult. However, the increasing popularity of outdoor and extreme sports as well as mountain exploration is changing the population at risk. Winter sports enthusiasts and mountaineers are increasingly being treated for injury related to cold exposure. Movies such as *Everest*, directed by David Breashears, demonstrate the extremes to which the human bodies are being exposed. Endurance athletes are also at risk because energy depletion and fatigue substantially increase the incidence of cold injury. Medical support teams at marathons and triathlons frequently need to transport participants emergently for treatment of hypothermia.

Incidence and Prevalence

According to the *Morbidity and Mortality Weekly Report* published by the Centers for Disease Control and Prevention (CDC) in March, 2004, about 600 people die in the United Stated each year from accidental hypothermia (53). The morbidity and mortality of secondary hypothermia is unknown. Illness and death are usually attributed to the primary disorder. The deleterious effects of cold exposure on victims with underlying cardiovascular or neurological disease are largely underreported.

Hypothermia can occur in any season or geographical location. In 2001, approximately 71% of hypothermia-related deaths in the United States occurred between November and February.

The three states with the highest rates of death in descending order were Montana, Alaska, and New Mexico. The risk of dying from hypothermia increases at the extremes of age. There does not appear to be a difference in risk between sexes.

Frostbite only occurs in environments with temperatures below freezing. No comprehensive statistical data are available regarding frostbite injuries. Reports are much more predominant during military action or among winter sports enthusiasts and mountain explorers.

Definitions

Frostnip—transient numbness and tingling without permanent tissue damage

Superficial frostbite—cold injury to the skin and subcutaneous tissue causing pallor, edema, blistering, and desquamation

Deep frostbite—cold injury involving bone, joint, or muscle tissue resulting in hemorrhagic blistering, ulceration, or gangrene

Mild hypothermia—core temperature between 32 and 35°C (90 and 95°F)

Moderate hypothermia—core temperature between 28 and 32°C (82 and 90°F)

Severe hypothermia—core temperature below 28°C (82°F)

Pathophysiology of Cold Injury

Heat is exchanged with the environment via four routes: radiation, evaporation, convection, and conduction. Infrared **radiation** is exchanged with the environment at all temperatures due to the temperature gradient; clothing does not significantly affect loss of radiant energy. **Evaporation** causes heat and water losses via the skin and lungs. At elevation, deeper, more rapid breathing secondary to a drop in the atmospheric pressure of oxygen leads to increased heat loss from the lungs. **Convection** is the direct transfer of heat from the body to air currents, measured by wind chill. Convective heat loss is probably the greatest contributor to hypothermia in the wilderness and at elevation. This loss can be significantly reduced with proper clothing. **Conduction** is direct transfer of heat to an adjacent cooler object such as ice, snow, or water. Conductive heat loss plays a major role in hypothermia during cold water immersion. The thermal conductivity of water is 30 times greater than air. Cold injury occurs when the body is unable to protect itself against these heat losses.

The body's thermoregulatory priority is to maintain the core temperature. Early responses to cold stress are usually adaptive behaviors such as layering clothing or finding shelter. Subsequently, each organ system has physiological responses to temperature and metabolic insults **(Table 57-2)**.

Skin

Peripheral vasoconstriction occurs in response to cold stress. Thermal receptors, especially in the skin, signal the preoptic and anterior hypothalamic nuclei of cold exposure, and in

TABLE 57-2	Characteristics of Progressive Hypothermia		
Stage	**Core temperature**	**Physiological response**	**Clinical characteristics**
Mild	36–34°C (95–93.2°F)	Shivering, endocrine stimulation, vasoconstriction	Maximum shivering, amnesia, dysarthria, respiratory stimulation, judgment
Moderate	33–27°C (91.4–80.6°F)	Vasoconstriction, no shivering, decreased metabolic heat production	Stupor, cardiac arrhythmia, loss of reflexes and voluntary motion
Severe	26–9°C (78.8–48.2°F)	Heat conservation fails	Major and base disturbance, no corneal reflex, flat electroencephalogram, asystole

response, radiative heat loss is limited. Acral tissues, including the fingers, toes, ears, and nose, contain arteriovenous anastomoses, which shunt blood and drastically reduce blood flow. At 15°C (59°F), there is maximal vasoconstriction with minimal blood flow. Interestingly, when the temperature lowers to 10°C (50°F), cold-induced vasodilation (CIVD) occurs in 5- to 10-minute cycles (54). This is referred to as the "hunting" response. Eskimos, as well as Lapps and others of Nordic descent, are capable of more frequent and stronger CIVD responses.

Below 10°C, evidence of peripheral tissue damage becomes apparent. Microvascular spasm and leakage occur, and cutaneous sensation is lost. Radiation and conduction from deeper tissue prevent freezing until the surface temperature drops below 0°C (32°F). Frostbite occurs below 0°C.

Although controversy remains, there are two main phases of tissue damage. The first is architectural cell damage secondary to ice crystal formation; the second is reperfusion injury. Ice crystals form in the extracellular space. Water then exits the cell to maintain equilibrium. Dehydration, osmolarity disturbances, and electrolyte shifts lead to cellular collapse. Direct cell damage may also occur from the ice crystals. With rapid cooling, intracellular crystallization may occur initially. This is more detrimental to the cell.

As the extremity is rewarmed and blood flow returns, red cells sludge and form microthrombi, leading to microvascular collapse. Damaged endothelial cells allow leakage into the interstitial space, and arteriovenous shunting leads to further thrombosis and ischemia. The major determinate of tissue damage seems to be microvascular injury (55).

Nervous System

The initial response of the preoptic and anterior hypothalamus to cold exposure is sympathetic stimulation. This leads to peripheral and visceral vasoconstriction, hypertension, tachycardia, ileus, and bladder atony. The CNS induces shivering to

produce heat once the body temperature drops to 35°C (95°F). Initially, cerebral metabolism increases, but below 35°C, there is a linear decrease to allow neural protection. Clinically, this leads to loss of coordination, confusion, impaired judgment, slurred speech, and usually loss of consciousness below 30°C (86°F).

Cardiovascular

The initial cardiac response to cold stress is tachycardia and hypertension. As the temperature lowers, however, hypothermic bradycardia develops, and cardiac output progressively decreases. The conduction system is significantly more sensitive to cold than the myocardium, so the cardiac cycle lengthens, and re-entry arrhythmias can occur. Both atrial and ventricular arrhythmias are seen below 32.2°C (90°F). Independent electrical foci also develop, which can trigger abnormal rhythms. Below 25°C (77°F), ventricular fibrillation and asystole can occur spontaneously. Characteristic electrocardiogram (EKG) changes include the Osborne (J) wave, which is a slow positive deflection at the end of the QRS complex.

Respiratory

Following the initial stimulation of the respiratory drive, continued cold exposure leads to steady declines in respiratory rate and tidal volume. Below 30°C (86°F), respiratory rate is often between 5 and 10 breaths per minute. Bronchorrhea and suppression of the cough and gag reflex lead to an increased risk of aspiration pneumonia. Carbon dioxide retention increases, contributing to metabolic acidosis.

Renal

There is an initial cold diuresis often followed by oliguria or anuria. This may be secondary to a transient central hypervolemia following peripheral vasoconstriction, impairment of the kidneys' ability to concentrate, or an altered sensitivity to ADH. Cold water immersion and alcohol both increase the volume diuresed. In the immobile hypothermic patient, rhab-domyolysis is a risk and can lead to acute tubular necrosis.

Gastrointestinal

Ileus and gastric dilatation occur below 32°C. Hepatic function also declines, resulting in slowed metabolism of drugs or lactic acid. Gastric ulcerations and hemorrhagic pancreatitis can occur below 26.7°C (86°F).

Coagulation

Hypercoagulability similar to that of disseminated intravascular coagulation (DIC) develops during hypothermia or rewarming. Contributing factors include tissue thromboplastin release, circulatory collapse (described earlier), and the release of stress hormones. Viscosity is also increased secondary to diuresis and fluid shift into the extracellular space. Thrombocytopenia occurs, possibly secondary to direct bone marrow suppression or hepatic and splenic sequestration. Other changes include cryoglobulinemia and stiffening of red blood cells.

Risk Factors for Cold Injury

Factors increasing the risk of hypothermia or cold injury include extremes of age, malnutrition, fatigue, alcohol intoxication, drug overdose, and iatrogenic insult. Medical conditions that increase susceptibility include endocrine abnormalities, peripheral vascular disease or neuropathy, autoregulatory abnormalities, infection, dermatological conditions, and trauma (56).

Heat production is decreased both in infancy and in the elderly. Neonates have a large surface area to body mass ratio, as well as a minimal subcutaneous fat layer. They also lack behavioral defenses. The elderly have a diminished ability to sense cold as well as impaired physiological adaptive capabilities and slowed neuromuscular responses. Malnutrition decreases the subcutaneous protective fat layer as well as directly affecting thermoregulation. Fatigue causes a slowing of neuromuscular response and is often associated with fuel depletion, which increases vulnerability to cold injury.

Alcohol is the major cause of urban hypothermia. Ethanol directly impairs thermoregulation at any temperature. Intoxication leads to peripheral vasodilation, impaired shivering, and bizarre behaviors, which all contribute to cold injury risk. Typical medications used in overdose attempts such as barbiturates, benzodiazepines, phenothiazines, and tricyclic antidepressants can cause vasoconstriction and impaired thermoregulation (57). Removal of protective layers for complete trauma examination adds to other possible iatrogenic insult.

Endocrine disorders that lead to decreased metabolic rate such as hypothyroidism, hypopituitarism, and adrenal insufficiency can decrease heat production. Hypoglycemia is a risk secondary to insufficient fuel for endogenous heat production. Peripheral vascular disease significantly increases risk of cold injury to the extremities by compounding the compromise of peripheral blood flow. Peripheral neuropathy, such as in diabetes mellitus, also impedes the normal vasoconstriction

response. Central neurological abnormalities can affect hypothalamic function in response to cold stimuli. Some examples include autonomic neuropathy, spinal cord damage, and cerebrovascular accidents (CVA).

Systemic infections such as sepsis can alter the hypothalamic temperature set point and cause depression of the core temperature. Rashes or defects in the skin can contribute to cold injury secondary to radiation heat loss. Thermal injuries may lead to excessive skin losses of both moisture and heat. Trauma is definitely associated with a significantly increased risk of hypothermia. Core temperatures upon emergency room arrival usually are inversely proportional to the severity of injury (58). The direct relationship between hypothermia and trauma, however, is unclear and continues to be explored. The question remains of whether the hypothermia directly increases mortality or whether the more severely injured patients become hypothermic (59). Major trauma resulting in skull fractures, intracranial hemorrhage, or spinal cord injury directly affects hypothalamic function and the thermoregulatory system. Peripheral trauma, especially fracture, can contribute to hypothermia because of immobilization. Other consequences of trauma, such as massive blood loss and the resultant hypotension, dramatically affect the body's ability to maintain core temperature.

Other risk factors specific for frostbite include moisture, exposed skin, wind velocity, constricting garments, and previous cold injury. Wet skin will freeze at a higher temperature than dry skin. Many Arctic explorers leave their skin unwashed to protect from cold injury (60). A history of previous cold injury sensitizes an area such that subsequent cold exposure, even of lesser degree, causes more rapid tissue injury (61).

Clinical Evaluation

Hypothermia

The patient's history of environmental exposure can help add hypothermia to a medical differential. Hypothermia or cold injury should always be suspected in unconscious patients or trauma victims, either as a primary or secondary diagnosis. The conditions in which victims are discovered by rescue personnel should be considered, especially cold water immersion or outdoor exposure with wind chill. If possible, the circumstances and duration of exposure should be ascertained as well as any predisposing factors. Diagnosis can be straightforward when environmental exposure is obvious. However, mild disease can present with vague symptoms such as fatigue, nausea, and dizziness, and a high degree of clinical suspicion is important. Elderly or intoxicated patients often present with vague, nonspecific symptomatology.

Patients with mild hypothermia present with shivering and loss of complex motor function. They are able to walk, but they may be ataxic, speech may be slowed, and judgment may be impaired. Examination reveals tachycardia, tachypnea and hyperventilation, hyperreflexia, and cold diuresis.

Patients with moderate hypothermia may appear dazed and confused. They may have violent shivering or may have lost the shivering reaction and will have a flattened affect, loss of fine motor coordination, slurred speech, and irrational behavior. Paradoxical undressing is often observed at this stage. Examination findings include bradycardia, hypoventilation, and hyporeflexia. Cardiac arrhythmias can occur at this stage, including atrial fibrillation and junctional bradycardia.

Severely hypothermic patients may or may not be conscious. Examination reveals pale skin, dilated pupils, severely slowed respiratory rate with pulmonary edema, anuria, and abdominal distention. Heart sounds may be distant and muffled. Rate and rhythm range from bradycardia to ventricular fibrillation to asystole. All types of atrial and ventricular arrhythmias have been encountered below 32.2°C (90°F) (62).

Diagnosis rests upon measurement of core temperature. Many standard clinical thermometers are inaccurate below 35°C, so a low-reading glass or electronic thermometer must be used. A total-body survey should be conducted to evaluate for local cold injury and associated trauma.

Frostbite

Peripheral cold injury will be recognized upon full-body examination. Acral tissues are most commonly involved, including the fingers, toes, nose, and ears. Patients presenting with frostbite may complain of numbness and coldness of the involved extremity. If the patient arrives with the tissue still frozen, the extremity may appear white to yellow or mottled blue and may have no superficial sensation. The body part may appear frozen solid. With rewarming, hyperemia occurs, sensation returns, and blisters begin to form.

Upon initial evaluation, it can be difficult to predict the extent of peripheral tissue damage. Extent of tissue injury can be divided into superficial or deep, as described earlier, or into four separate degrees. Although these descriptions delineate the depth of tissue involvement, treatment of frostbite is similar regardless of degree. Prognosis, however, does significantly differ.

First-degree frostbite presents with numbness and erythema with a firm white to yellow plaque in the area of injury. Frequently, there is localized edema but no loss of tissue. Second-degree injury reveals superficial clear or white fluid-filled blisters on an erythematous base with localized swelling. Third-degree injury reveals deep hemorrhagic blisters. Third-degree frostbite symbolizes deep tissue damage to the reticular dermis and dermal vessels. Fourth-degree injury can present similarly to third-degree frostbite but is defined as damage completely through the dermal layer into the subcuticular tissue. Fourth-degree frostbite often involves bone and muscle tissue.

Treatment

Hypothermia

There is no consensus on the optimal treatment of hypothermia. General guidelines based on routine emergency medical technician and hospital practice as well as expert opinion are outlined in the following sections.

Hypothermia is a heterogeneous condition, so strategies to stabilize core temperature should be tailored to the specific scenario and associated injuries (63). Regardless of which methods are adopted, it is crucial to continue rescue efforts until death is confirmed after rewarming to 35°C. Patients who are cyanotic, cold, and stiff with dilated pupils and inaudible heart sounds have been successfully resuscitated (64). Remember the principle, "No one is dead until they're warm and dead." An exception to the rule would be if rescuers are in danger themselves from environmental exposure or natural disaster.

In the Field

Once a patient has been removed from an area of further potential danger, they should be rapidly examined, insulated from further exposure, and transported (65). Initial management should begin by establishing an airway, breathing, and circulation as well as determining core body temperature. In severe hypothermia, significant depression of respirations can occur, and patients may appear apneic. Respiratory rate should be averaged over 2 minutes. Peripheral pulses can be difficult to palpate in a severely vasoconstricted and bradycardic patient. At least 1 minute should be spent carefully palpating for a pulse.

If no evidence of perfusion can be found, cardiopulmonary resuscitation (CPR) should be initiated. If cardiac monitoring is available, identification of the rhythm and defibrillation of ventricular fibrillation should be done. Defibrillation attempts often are unsuccessful until core temperature is above 28°C (66). If this is the case, then active rewarming should begin with continued CPR en route to a treatment facility.

Wet clothing should be removed, and injuries should be stabilized in preparation for transport. In the case of immersion, gentle removal of the patient's clothing while supine is essential. Autonomic dysfunction occurs with hypothermia. If the patient attempts to sit or stand, severe hypotension can develop. Further heat loss can be prevented by covering the torso with blankets or insulating material.

If a treatment facility is close by, then time spent rewarming in the field may not be necessary. If a patient is shivering, they are producing endogenous heat. A mildly hypothermic patient may best be managed by drying, insulating, and transporting them. Surface heating would stop shivering and halt endogenous rewarming. Most rewarming methods available in the field supply less heat than shivering. If the patient is not shivering, then surface warming using the most effective means available is indicated. Intentionally maintaining hypothermia during transport should only be considered for patients with an isolated closed head injury (67).

Hypothermic patients must be handled carefully during transport. Below 32°C, the myocardium is irritable. Any jostling can potentially lead to cardiac arrhythmias. In general, the lower the core temperature is, the more likely that a mechanical disturbance could induce ventricular fibrillation.

Rewarming Methods

Rewarming techniques **(Fig 57-8)** are divided into passive external rewarming, active external rewarming, and active internal rewarming. **Passive external rewarming** is the treatment of choice for mild hypothermia. The patient is covered with blankets or insulating material or placed in a dry, insulated sleeping bag. Reduced heat loss and endogenous heat production lead to rewarming. For passive external rewarming to work, the patient must have physiological energy reserves sufficient for shivering or to increase the metabolic rate.

Active external rewarming is indicated for moderate to severe hypothermia. It could also be used in mildly hypothermic patients who fail passive external rewarming or have cardiovascular compromise. This method involves direct transfer of exogenous heat by applying warm blankets, chemical pads, hot water bottles, or forced warm air directly to the patient's skin. The Bair Hugger (Augustine Medical, Inc., Eden Prairie, MN) is a forced air rewarming system often used upon arrival to the emergency room (68). Body-to-body contact or hot water immersion has also been used but can interfere with resuscitation efforts. Afterdrop is a significant risk of active external rewarming.

Afterdrop refers to a continued decline in core temperature even after the patient has been removed from the cold environment. This phenomenon is felt to be multifactorial. Upon initial rewarming, peripheral vessels dilate, allowing central blood to perfuse cold extremities. Also, the blood pooled in the vasoconstricted extremities recirculates, causing cold blood to circulate through the core. Peripheral vasodilation also contributes to abrupt hypotension. Hypotension can lead to inadequate coronary perfusion and may explain fatal arrhythmias that have occurred during rewarming (69).

To minimize afterdrop, active tissue rewarming should begin with the trunk prior to the extremities. Contraction of peripheral muscles should be avoided to minimize muscular perfusion. Patients should be kept in the horizontal position when possible due to autonomic dysfunction and the risk of orthostatic hypotension. Combining active external

TABLE 57-3	Active Core Rewarming Options

Inhalation
Intravenous fluids
Irrigation
Peritoneal lavage
Thoracic cavity lavage
Extracorporeal
Diathermy

rewarming with active internal rewarming can also help minimize complications.

Surface burns are another risk during active external rewarming (70). The hypothermic patient is susceptible because of decreased peripheral sensation and reduced perfusion. Heating modalities should not be directly applied to bare skin, and skin should be monitored for early signs of damage. Forced air rewarming systems seem to minimize both afterdrop and thermal injury but are not always available in the field (71).

The most aggressive method of rewarming is **active internal rewarming (Table 57-3)**. It is usually reserved for moderate to severe hypothermia. Methods to directly transfer heat to the body core include heated intravenous infusion, inhalation of heated air, heated irrigation, diathermy, dialysis, and extracorporeal rewarming.

Heated (40 to 42°C) normal saline or lactated Ringer's (LR) with 5% dextrose can be given intravenously. This can be used during transport. The fluid bag may be placed beneath the patient's back to add infusion pressure. If peripheral access is difficult secondary to vasoconstriction, an intraosseous line may be placed. Blood products may also be heated prior to transfusion.

Inhalation of heated humidified air works primarily by preventing respiratory heat loss. One particular device is the Res-Q-Air (Res-Q Products, Quathiaski Cove, British Columbia, Canada), which is a portable air heater and humidifier that delivers air at 40 to 45°C (104 to 113°F) and functions at temperatures as low as −20°C (−4°F.) The rate of rewarming is enhanced with endotracheal tube intubation compared with delivery via a face mask (72). The rate of rewarming with heated inhalation therapy ranges from 1 to 2.5°C (1.8 to 4.5°F) per hour (73).

In the emergency department, heat can be transferred by irrigation fluid. Options include gastric, colonic, mediastinal/thoracic, bladder, or peritoneal lavage.

Extracorporeal rewarming consists of an arteriovenous or venovenous shunt in which blood is routed through a warming device and then returned to the patient. Techniques include hemodialysis, arteriovenous rewarming, venovenous rewarming, and cardiopulmonary bypass (CPB). CPB is three to four times faster than other active internal rewarming techniques and preserves oxygenation even with intermittent loss of cardiac activity (74). Peritoneal or hemodialysis can be used for rewarming and detoxification in cases of drug overdose or rhabdomyolysis. Diathermy, or transmission of heat by ultrasound

Hourly Rewarming Rates

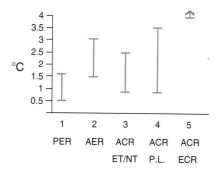

Fig 57-8. Rewarming methods. PER, passive external rewarming; AER, active external rewarming; ACR, active core rewarming; ECR, external core rewarming.

and low-frequency microwave radiation, is a technique being studied as an adjunct treatment for hypothermia.

Emergency Room Management. Upon arrival to the emergency department, hypothermia should be confirmed, and core temperature should be monitored with low-reading thermometers. Rectal temperature is the most practical but can lag behind core changes and can be influenced by cold lower extremities or feces. Tympanic or urine temperature seems to equilibrate quickly with the core. Esophageal temperature can also be accurate but will be affected by heated inhalation therapy. A Doppler may be necessary to access for pulse, and respirations should be averaged over 2 minutes because they may be irregular. The accuracy of certain routine measurements such as pulse oximetry and end-tidal carbon dioxide are unconfirmed in hypothermia, so they may not be a useful part of the initial assessment.

Simultaneously, any remaining clothing should be removed, and the patient should be wrapped in warm blankets. Unless the patient is able to protect their airway, intubation is necessary. Criteria for intubation in hypothermic patients are identical to criteria in normothermic patients (75). If not performed en route, intravenous access needs to be obtained, and cardiac monitoring should be initiated. An indwelling bladder catheter should be placed to monitor urinary output. Nasogastric tube should be considered in moderate to severe hypothermia to relieve gastric dilation secondary to poor motility.

If the patient is pulseless and no cardiac electrical activity can be identified, CPR should be continued or initiated. Again, resuscitation efforts should be continued until the patient is rewarmed to 35°C. Death can only be pronounced when lack of spontaneous breathing, cardiac electrical activity, and neural reflexes persist after rewarming.

Most atrial arrhythmias, including atrial fibrillation, convert spontaneously during rewarming. In these situations, focus should be directed toward correcting associated acid–base, fluid, and electrolyte abnormalities, which may trigger dysrhythmias. Intermittent supraventricular arrhythmias and ventricular extrasystoles can typically be ignored (77). Ventricular fibrillation is often refractory to therapy until core temperature is stable. Most antiarrhythmic medications have no effect or are unpredictable in hypothermia. Therefore, defibrillation should be reattempted once core temperature reaches 30°C. Bretylium (5 mg per kg) is the antiarrhythmic of choice for prophylaxis and treatment of ventricular fibrillation, but efficacy data are conflicting (76).

Mild hypothermics only require slow infusion of intravenous fluids. However, in moderate to severe hypothermia, patients are hypovolemic with hemoconcentrated blood. These patients should receive rapid fluid resuscitation with warmed normal saline with 5% dextrose. LR should be avoided because the cold liver is unable to metabolize lactate efficiently (73). Laboratory studies to be considered include blood sugar, arterial blood gas, complete blood count, electrolytes, amylase and lipase, coagulation profile, platelet count, creatine kinase, liver function, and a toxicology screen. Acid–base disturbances are

common, but there is no uniform pattern. The blood gas machine warms the blood. Because optimal values in hypothermia are unknown, typically values are uncorrected for temperature and compared with normothermic ranges. Serial blood gas and electrolyte levels should be drawn during rewarming.

Blood loss is often underestimated because viscosity of the blood increases with a fall in temperature. The hematocrit must be corrected for temperature. Glucose levels may be low, normal, or elevated. Frank pancreatitis often occurs in hypothermia. Coagulation abnormalities are common, as described earlier.

Imaging should be done based on the circumstances and physical examination. Any patient found unconscious should have head and spine imaging done prior to mobilization. Chest radiographs should be done to evaluate for aspiration pneumonia, and abdominal films should be taken to evaluate for gastrointestinal dilatation or pneumoperitoneum. Trauma patients should have appropriate imaging; however, core rewarming should begin immediately despite pending lab and radiology results.

Frostbite

Field Management. Frostbite is often associated with hypothermia **(Table 57-4)**. In this situation, priority is given to core rewarming and sustaining life when possible. Rewarming of peripheral tissue in the field is often impractical and should only begin if there is no risk of refreezing during transport. An example is to delay rewarming frostbitten toes if the patient needs to walk back to the rescue vehicle. Refreezing of damaged tissue leads to a significantly worse long-term prognosis. Wet and constrictive clothing should be removed, and affected areas should be placed in blankets or insulating material and immobilized.

Emergency Room Management. An accurate history of the conditions and duration of exposure should be taken upon arrival at the emergency department. The patient's medical history should be taken, focusing on any conditions that predispose the patient to peripheral tissue loss including a history of prior frostbite injury. Thawing should begin immediately.

TABLE 57-4	Factors That Increase the Risk of Frostbite Injury

Constricting clothing
Smoking
Atherosclerosis
Arthritis
Diabetes mellitus
Vasoconstrictive drugs
Previous cold injury
Immobilization
Hypothermia

Thawing is induced by immersion of the frozen or partially frozen tissue in circulating water warmed to between 40 and 42°C (104 and 108°F). Although other treatment methods have been proposed, rapid thawing in a warm water bath is still the consensus treatment for all degrees of frostbite (77). Typically after 10 to 30 minutes, a distal flush of erythema is seen in the involved tissue, and active motion is possible. Reperfusion of frozen tissue can be extremely painful; thus, intravenous analgesia is often indicated during rewarming. Patients may require intravenous fluid therapy as well because dehydration is often present after cold exposure. In patients with associated hypothermia or frostbite involving large surface areas, afterdrop is a risk of peripheral thawing. Core warming may need to be performed while the periphery is being thawed and cold, acidotic blood is recirculating through the core.

Rapid thawing will reverse the direct injury of ice crystal formation in affected tissue but will not prevent reperfusion injury. After thawing, the affected tissue should remain elevated to minimize edema. There is an increased risk of compartment pressure syndrome, and thus tissue pressure must be carefully monitored. Movement of the affected extremity should be encouraged to prevent venous stasis. Most patients with frostbite should be admitted to the hospital to ensure minimal tissue loss. Prognostic signs are provided in **Table 57-5**.

Blisters will form between 6 and 24 hours after rewarming (78). Clear blisters should be debrided to prevent prostaglandin and thromboxane present in the fluid from further damaging underlying tissue. Hemorrhagic blisters signify deep tissue injury. Thus, these blisters should be left intact to prevent converting the injury to full thickness. The fluid may be aspirated. Topical aloe vera should be applied to the blister sites, and sterile dressings should be applied.

Hospital Management. Ibuprofen should be administered to inhibit the arachidonic acid cascade and for its action of fibrinolysis **(Table 57-6)** (79). In severe frostbite injuries, intravenous penicillin should be administered to provide streptococcal prophylaxis. A tetanus booster may also be indicated if the patient has not received immunization within the prior 5 years. Whirlpool hydrotherapy for range of motion should be initiated early, as well as appropriate physical and occupational therapy.

Once patients are stabilized, they may be discharged and followed up weekly until wounds are stable. In cases of severe

TABLE 57-6	In-hospital Management
Debride clear blisters	
Hemorrhagic blisters are left intact	
Elevate, splint	
Tetanus	
Intravenous or intramuscular analgesics	
Ibuprofen 400 g every 12 hr	
Penicillin G 500,000 IU every 6 hr for 48–72 hr	
Hydrotherapy	

frostbite, gangrenous areas may not become demarcated for weeks to months. Patients should continue to keep area warm and elevated, and open areas should be covered with aloe vera and sterile dressings. Even patients with mild injury need to be aware that the damaged tissue is more susceptible to refreezing, and cold exposure should be minimized.

Early surgical management is only indicated if there is infection not responding to antibiotic therapy or if eschar is causing vascular constriction. Otherwise, surgical debridement or amputation is performed after the final demarcation between viable and nonviable tissue has been established. Amputation should never be performed until the line of demarcation is definitely formed to ensure salvage of the entire area of viable tissue. Some groups are advocating triple-phase bone scanning early after injury to define the extent of tissue damage and allow early debridement (80,81). However, this approach has not yet become standard care.

Sequelae. Healthy young patients can completely recover from hypothermia and have a fairly low mortality rate. Patients with predisposing conditions have a far worse prognosis. Long-term outcomes depend more on underlying risk factors than initial temperature at rescue or rewarming techniques. Overall mortality rates historically range from 30% to 80%; however, they have recently been closer to 30%.

Victims of frostbite often have long-term alteration of their sympathetic nerve function in the affected tissue. Nerve damage leads to increased cold sensitivity and risk of recurrent cold injury as well as excessive sweating, numbness, joint stiffness, and burning pain. With frostbite, the severity of long-term symptoms does correlate with the degree of initial injury. Dermatological evidence of injury includes skin pigment changes, nail irregularities, and certain cutaneous neoplasms. Bone reabsorption and subchondral defects also can develop months after cold injury, and in pediatric patients, there is concern for injury to the physis.

Conclusion and Future Directives

Hypothermia and frostbite are the result of prolonged exposure to the elements without proper insulation, elemental protection, or energy stores. Multiple medical, circumstantial, or social factors can predispose patients to cold injury.

TABLE 57-5	Prognostic Signs for Frostbite
Signs for Good Prognosis	**Signs for Poor Prognosis**
Sensation to pin prick	Hemorrhagic blebs
Normal skin color	Cyanosis
Clear vesicles	Frozen appearance

Emergency medical personnel can minimize injury by rapidly removing the victims from further danger, insulating and immobilizing them, and transporting them to definitive treatment facilities. Frostbite treatment is straightforward. The treatment of hypothermia, however, remains controversial. Treatment decisions will vary depending on associated injury and predisposing conditions.

Cold injuries are frequently preventable. Fibers such as dri-fit liners to wick moisture from the skin or Goretex to protect from wind chill and rain are now available. Drugs and alcohol should be avoided at high altitude or in freezing conditions. Athletes and mountaineers should be sure to take in adequate calories to maintain metabolic rate. The elderly, newborns, and those with predisposing conditions should be carefully observed to prevent chronic mild hypothermia. Although treatments are advancing and mortality is declining, prevention is the only dependable way to avoid sequelae of cold injury.

■ REFERENCES

1. Schnirring L. Heatstroke fatalities fan discussion. *Phys Sportsmed.* 2004;32:8–10.
2. Nelson C. Tackling the heat in the lethal summer of 2004. *Sports Med Dig.* 2004;26:85–88.
3. Gaffin SL, Moran DS. Pathophysiology of heat-related illnesses. In: Auerbach PS, ed. *Wilderness medicine.* 4th ed. St Louis: Mosby; 2001:240–289.
4. Wexler RK. Evaluation and treatment of heat-related illnesses. *Am Fam Physician.* 2002;65:2307–2314.
5. Allan J R. Influence of acclimatization on sweat sodium concentration. *J Appl Physiol.* 1971;30:708–712.
6. Barrow MW, Clark KA. Heat-related illnesses. *Am Fam Physician.* 1998;58:749–756, 759.
7. Coris EE, Ramirez AM, Van Durme DJ. Heat illness in athletes: the dangerous combination of heat, humidity, and exercise. *Sports Med.* 2004;34:9–16.
8. Werner J. Temperature regulation during exercise: an overview. In: Gisolfi CV, Lamb DR, Nadel ER, eds. *Perspectives in exercise science and sports medicine: Exercise, heat, and thermoregulation.* Dubuque, IA: Brown and Benchmark; 1993:49–77.
9. Luke A, Micheli L. Sports injuries: emergency assessment and field-side care. *Pediatr Rev.* 1999;20:291–301.
10. Nelson C. ACSM urges youth football coaches: avoid back-to-back two-a-days. *Sports Med.* 2004;26:87.
11. Olsen KR, Benowitz NL. Experimental and drug-induced hyperthermia. *Emerg Med Clin North Am.* 1984;2:459–474.
12. Armstrong LE, Leluca JP, Hubbard RW. Time course of recovery and heat acclimation ability of prior exertional heat stroke patients. *Med Sci Sports.* 1990;22:36.
13. Moran DS, Gaffin SL. Clinical management of heat-related illnesses. In: Auerbach PS, ed. *Wilderness medicine.* 4th ed. St Louis: Mosby; 2001:290–316.
14. Gisolfi CV. Influence of acclimatization and training on heat tolerance and physical endurance. In: Hales JRS, Richards DAB, ed. *Heat stress: physical Exertion and environment.* Amsterdam: Elsevier; 1987.
15. Montain SJ, Coyle EF. Influence of graded dehydration on hyperthermia and cardiovascular drift during exercise. *J Appl Physiol.* 1992;73:1340–1359.
16. Nelson C. New research focuses on acclimatization to heat. *Sports Med Dig.* 2004;26:89,92.
17. Casa DJ, Armstrong LE, Hillman SK, et al. National Athletic Trainer's Association position statement: fluid replacement for athletes. *J Athl Train.* 2000;35:212–224.
18. Mellion MB, Shelton GL. Safe exercise in the heat and heat injuries. In: Mellion MB, Walsh WM, Shelton GL, eds. *The team physician's handbook.* Philadelphia: Hanley and Belfus; 1997:151–165.
19. Nelson C. Downloadable "Heat Stress Advisor" invaluable, free. *Sports Med Dig.* 2004;26:96.
20. Tom PA, Garmel GM, Auerbach PS. Environment-dependent sports emergencies. *Med Clin North Am.* 1994;78:305–325.
21. Sandor RP. Heat illness on-site diagnosis and cooling. *Emergency.* 1997;25:35.
22. Lee-Chiong Jr TL, Stitt JT. Heatstroke and other heat-related illnesses: the maladies of summer. *Postgrad Med.* 1995;98:26–36.
23. Talbott JH. Heat cramps. *N Engl J Med.* 1935;302:777.
24. Binkley HM, Beckett J, Casa DJ, et al. National Athletic Trainer's Association position statement: Exertional heat illnesses. *J Alth Train.* 2002;37:329–343.
25. Bouchama A, Knochel JP. Medical progress: heat stroke. *N Engl J Med.* 2002;346:1978–1988.
26. Epstein Y, Moran DS, Shapiro Y, et al. Exertional heat stroke: a case series. *Med Sci Sports Exerc.* 1999;31:224–228.
27. Centers for Disease Control and Prevention. Heat-related deaths—Chicago, Illinois, 1996–2001, and United States, 1979–1999. *Morb Mortal Wkly Rep.* 2003;52:610–613.
28. Bouchama A, al-Sedairy S, Siddiqui S, et al. Elevated pyrogenic cytokines in heatstroke. *Chest.* 1993;104:1498–1502.
29. Costrini AM. Emergency treatment of exertional heatstroke and comparison of whole body cooling techniques. *Med Sci Sports Exerc.* 1990;22:15–18.
30. Fallowfield JL, Williams C. Carbohydrate intake and recovery from prolonged exercise. *Int J Sport Nutr.* 1993;3:150–164.
31. Groves BM, Reeves JT, Sutton JR, et al. Operation Everest II: elevated high altitude pulmonary resistance unresponsive to oxygen. *J Appl Physiol.* 1987;63:521–530.
32. Mortimer H, Patel S, Peacock A. The genetic basis of high-altitude pulmonary oedema. *Pharmacol Ther.* 2004;101:183–192.
33. Grissom CK, Elstad MR. The pathophysiology of high altitude pulmonary edema. *Wilderness Environ Med.* 1999;10:88–92.
34. Hackett PH. The cerebral etiology of high-altitude cerebral edema and acute mountain sickness. *Wilderness Environ Med.* 1999;10:97–109.
35. Friedman B, Jost J, Rating T, et al. Effects of iron supplementation on total body hemoglobin during endurance training at moderate altitude. *Int J Sports Med.* 1999;20:78–85.
36. Stray-Gundersen J, Chapman RF, Levine BD. "Living high-training low" altitude training improves sea level performance in male and female elite runners. *J Appl Physiol.* 2001;91:1113–1120.
37. Fischer R, Lang S, Leitl M, et al. Theophylline and acetazolamide reduce sleep-disordered breathing at high altitude. *Eur Respir J.* 2004;23:47–52.
38. Hultgren HN, Grover RF, Hartley LH. Abnormal circulatory responses to high altitude in subjects with a previous history of high altitude pulmonary edema. *Circulation.* 1971;54:759–770.
39. Hackett PH, Roach RC. High altitude medicine. In: Auerbach PS, ed. *Wilderness medicine.* 4th ed. St. Louis: Mosby; 2001:2–43.
40. Roach RC, Bartsch P, Oelz O, et al. Lake Louise AMS Scoring Consensus Committee. The Lake Louise acute mountain sickness scoring system. In: Sutton JR, Houston CS, Coates G, eds. *Hypoxia and molecular medicine.* Burlington VT: Charles S. Houston; 1993:272–274.
41. Dumont L, Lysakowski C, Tramer M, et al. Magnesium for the prevention and treatment of acute mountain sickness. *Clin Sci.* 2004;106:269–277.
42. Swenson E. ACE inhibitors and high altitude. *High Alt Med Biol.* 2004;5:92–94.

43. Basnyat B, Gertsch J, Johnson E, et al. Efficacy of low-dose acetazolamide (125 mg BID) for the prophylaxis of acute mountain sickness: a prospective, double-blind, randomized, placebo-controlled trial. *High Alt Med Biol.* 2003;4:45–52.

44. Carlston C, Swenson E, Ruoss S. A dose-response study of acetazolamide for acute mountain sickness prophylaxis in vacationing tourists at 12,000 feet (3630 m). *High Alt Med Biol.* 2004;5:33–39.

45. Basu M, Sawhney R, Kumar S, et al. Glucocorticoids as prophylaxis against acute mountain sickness. *Clin Endocrinol.* 2002;57:761–767.

46. Hackett PH, Roach RC. High altitude illness. *N Engl J Med.* 2001;345:107–114.

47. Schoene R. The brain at high altitude. *Wilderness Environ Med.* 1999;10:93–96.

48. Voelkel N. High-altitude pulmonary edema. *N Engl J Med.* 2002;346:1606–1607.

49. Swenson E, Maggiorini M, Mongovin S, et al. Pathogenesis of high-altitude pulmonary edema: inflammation is not an etiologic factor. *JAMA.* 2002;287:2228–2235.

50. Sartori C, Allemann Y, Duplain H, et al. Salmeterol for the prevention of high-altitude pulmonary edema. *N Engl J Med.* 2002;346:1631–1636.

51. Bracker MD. Environmental and thermal injury. *Clin Sports Med.* 1992;11:419–436.

52. Robson MC, Krizek TJ, Wray RC. Care of the thermally injured patient. In: *Management of surgical trauma.* Philadelphia: WB Saunders; 1979.

53. Center for Disease Control and Prevention. Hypothermia-related deaths—United States, 2003. *Morb Mortal Wkly Rep.* 2004;53:172–173.

54. Rosen P, Barkin R. *Emergency Medicine Concepts and Clinical Practice.* 4th ed. St. Louis: Mosby; 1998.

55. DelBeccaro RS, Robson MC, Heggers JP, et al. The use of specific thromboxane inhibitors to preserve the dermal microcirculation after burning. *Surgery.* 1980;87:137–141.

56. Biem J, Koehncke N, Classen D, et al. Out of the cold: management of hypothermia and frostbite. *CMAJ.* 2003;168:305–311.

57. Kallenback J, Bagg P, Feldman C, et al. Experience with acute poisoning in an intensive care unit: a review of 103 cases. *S Afr Med J.* 1981;59:587–589.

58. Bastow MD, Raulings J, Allison SP. Undernutrition, hypothermia, and injury in elderly woman with fractured femur: an injury response to altered metabolism? *Lancet.* 1983;1:14–146.

59. Gentilello LM, Jurkovich GJ, Stark MS, et al. Is hypothermia in the victim of major trauma protective or harmful? A randomized, prospective study. *Ann Surg.* 1997;226:439–447.

60. Lewis T. Observations on some normal and injurious effects of cold upon the skin and underlying tissues: III. Frostbite. *BMJ.* 1941;2:869.

61. Knize DM. *Cold Injury in Reconstructive Plastic Surgery: General Principles.* Vol 1. 2nd ed. Philadelphia: WB Saunders; 1977.

62. Duguid H, Simpson RG, Stowers JM. Accidental hypothermia. *Lancet.* 1961;2:1213–1219.

63. Danzl DF, Pozos RS, Hamlet MP. Accidental hypothermia. In: Auerback P, ed. *Management of wilderness and environmental emergencies.* 3rd ed. St. Louis: Mosby; 1995.

64. Lloyd EL. Hypothermia: the cause of death after rescue. *Alaska Med.* 1984;26:74–76.

65. Steinman A. Prehospital management of hypothermia. *Response.* 1987;6:18.

66. Mills WJ Jr. Accidental hypothermia: management approach. *Alaska Med.* 1980;22:9–11.

67. Marion DW, Penrod LE, Kelsey SF, et al. Treatment of traumatic brain injury with moderate hypothermia. *N Engl J Med.* 1997;336:540–546.

68. Hamilton RS, Paton BC. The diagnosis and treatment of hypothermia by mountain rescue teams: a survey. *Wilderness Environ Med.* 1996;7:37.

69. Harnett RM, O'Brien EM, Sias FR, et al. Initial treatment of profound accidental hypothermia. *Aviat Space Environ Med.* 1980;51:680–687.

70. Golden FS, Hervey GR, Tipton MJ. Circum-rescue collapse: collapse, sometimes fatal, associated with rescue of immersion victims. *J R Nav Med Serv.* 1991;77:139–149.

71. Samuelson T. Experience with standardized protocols in hypothermia, boom or bane? The Alaska experience. *Arctic Med Res.* 1991;50:28–31.

72. Rankin AC, Rae AP. Cardiac arrhythmias during rewarming of patients with accidental hypothermia. *Br Med J.* 1984;289:874–877.

73. Avidan MS, Jones N, Ing R, et al. Convection warmers—not just hot air. *Anaesthesia.* 1997;52:1073–1076.

74. Koller R, Schnider TW, Neidhart P. Deep accidental hypothermia and cardiac arrest rewarming with forced air. *Acta Anaesthesiol Scand.* 1997;41:1359–1364.

75. Miller JW, Danzl DF, Thomas DM. Urban accidental hypothermia: 135 cases. *Ann Emerg Med.* 1980;9:456–461.

76. Danzl DF, Pozos RS, Auerbach PS, et al. Multicenter hypothermia survey. *Ann Emerg Med.* 1987;16:1042–1055.

77. Jones AI, Swann IJ. Prolonged resuscitation in accidental hypothermia: use of mechanical cardio-pulmonary resuscitation and partial cardio-pulmonary bypass. *Eur J Emerg Med.* 1994;1:34–36.

78. Danzl DF, Pozos RS. Accidental hypothermia. *N Engl J Med.* 1995;332:1033.

79. Tintinalli JE, Ruiz E, Krome RL. *Emergency Medicine: A Comprehensive Study Guide.* 4th ed. New York: McGraw Hill; 1996.

80. Mills WJ Jr. Frostbite. *Alaska Med.* 1973;15:27–47.

81. Greenwald D, Cooper B, Gottlieb L. An algorithm for early treatment of frostbite with limb salvage directed by triple phase scanning. *Plast Reconstr Surg.* 1998;102:1069–1074.

TEAM PHYSICIAN ISSUES

58

58.1 TEAM PHYSICIAN ISSUES: PREPARTICIPATION EVALUATION

BERNIE LALONDE, MD

■ KEY POINTS

- The sports medicine team drives the preparticipation evaluation, deciding the content, frequency, personnel, and format to be used.
- Areas of emphasis change according to sport, such as concussion assessment for football.
- Adequate cardiovascular history includes questions on exertional chest pain, syncope, excessive shortness of breath, and/or fatigue with exercise; past or present detection of a murmur or increased blood pressure; and family history.
- The increase in number of female participants adds to the need to understand the unique needs of female athletes. Disordered eating, amenorrhea, and osteopenia/osteoporosis have been called the female athlete triad.
- Subtle, nonthreatening questions are recommended to try to identify eating disorders.

The preparticipation evaluation (PPE) has been the foundation of medical evaluation of athletes in some form or another for most Western countries. It varies from government-mandated obligations, such as in Italy, to selective evaluations of specific teams dependent largely on the idiosyncrasies of respective sports organizations. Such as it is, the PPE lacks uniformity and evidence-based validity. Nonetheless, it is a tool widely used in the sport medicine community. The sport medicine team largely drives this process. It decides the content, the frequency, the personnel, and the format to be used.

■ PURPOSE

Because the evidence is lacking, there are some who would argue that, based on the low yield of significant participation barring findings, the justification of such endeavors is weak at best. The majority would argue differently. One has to examine the overall purpose of the PPE to justify the energies expended. The following items represent some, but not all, of the suggested purposes of the PPE.

Uncover pre-existing life-threatening pathologies (i.e., cardiac abnormalities)

Establish a baseline for the general health of the athlete

Obtain knowledge of known medical problems

Obtain baseline neuropsychological testing

Obtain a relevant family history

Assess the pertinent musculoskeletal issues, past or present, to ensure that proper rehabilitation protocols have been adhered to

Record significant dietary concerns

Review allergies and strategies to prevent or intervene

Review drug and supplement history and fill in the appropriate Therapeutic Use Exemption forms for the respective governing bodies; the opportunity to counsel at this point is a very real one

Review immunization schedules and address inadequacies

Opportunity for sport medicine team to establish and develop a relationship with the athlete; this cannot be overstated

■ FREQUENCY

The timing and frequency of the PPE will be dictated by the sport involved, the level of competition, the sheer number of athletes, and the resources of that sport organization. When dealing with an elite international team, the sport medicine team of the Canadian Alpine Ski Team has twice-yearly assessments performed by a consortium of physicians, physiotherapists, trainers, sports vision experts, psychologists, nutritionists, and physiologists who congregate to discuss each individual athlete in great detail. This clearly represents one end of the spectrum. At the other end, one could foresee an entry-level assessment performed by a physician/therapist or other with reassessment on an ad hoc basis only. Entry-level evaluations could be more extensive, with scaled-down versions in subsequent years.

■ PERSONNEL

The choice of professional personnel to perform these tasks is largely decided by the concerned parties. It has varied from physicians, osteopaths, athletic therapists, physiotherapists, chiropractors, and nurses. The choice should be made with the notion in mind of the purpose and goals of the PPE. It is logical to assume that the head of that team be a sport medicine practitioner, primary care physician, orthopedic specialist, or osteopathic physician.

■ FORMAT

The individual physician in consort with his team will have to decide the content of the PPE. Certain areas of the

assessment need to be emphasized depending on the sport involved (e.g., concussion assessments would not be a priority in a sport like curling, whereas it has obvious importance in football). It is up to the team to insert into its PPE the necessary requirements to achieve the goals of the overall PPE.

How the team decides to obtain this information varies. Paper-based documents are on the way out. More sophisticated web-based approaches may be the wave of the future. The Stanford University group is just one example of a web-based approach (1). Visit www.stanford.edu/dept/sportsmed to see the Stanford University approach.

What behooves the physician charged with this task is to ascertain what and how the information is to be used. Carrying large busy folders with a traveling team is a thing of the past. Complete medical profiles can be transported on a computer, a disc, or a personal digital assistant (PDA), or they can even be web based. Central locations for storage can be a doctor's office in the case of a local or school-based team, a national team office in the case of a traveling team, or a trainer's/therapist's computer.

■ HISTORY

It still holds true, as Sir William Osler stated in his book, *The Principles and Practice of Medicine*, which was published initially in 1892 and subsequently often revised, that the patient will give you the diagnosis if you only listen.

Although the emphasis on its varying components may shift depending on the cohort on hand, the basic elements of history taking are the same for medicine in general: present history, past history, family history, systems review, allergy and medication history, dietary history, and psychological and social history.

There are elements of the history taking that do need particular emphasis in the athletic screening process, and these are discussed in the following sections.

Cardiovascular

The current state of cardiovascular screening has been expertly reviewed by various authors (2). Evidence-based medicine has not as yet answered the question of the most appropriate methodology to pursue in our quest of cardiovascular screening and the prevention of catastrophic events related to the heart. There are conflicting perspectives worldwide. The Italian experience, which is extensive in light of their federally mandated requirements for PPE for all athletes, would seem to favor a more aggressive investigative approach. The American model relies more heavily on the questionnaire approach and ponders the cost effectiveness of relying on the technology approach. The reader is referred to the thematic issue concerning PPE of the *Clinical Journal of Sport Medicine*, published in May 2004, for a more in-depth discussion of this contentious subject.

The European Society of Cardiology recently published a consensus statement outlining their position (3). It needs to be read in light of the consensus statement of the American Heart Association (AHA) (4). What the two positions do agree upon is the requirements of an adequate cardiovascular history, which should include the following:

■ Questions on exertional chest pain, syncope, excessive shortness of breath, and/or fatigue associated with exercise
■ Past or present detection of a murmur or increased blood pressure
■ Family history of premature death or significant disability from cardiovascular disease in close relatives less than 50 years old or specific knowledge of occurrences or certain conditions (i.e., hypertrophic cardiomyopathy, dilated cardiomyopathy, long QT, Marfan syndrome, or important arrhythmias)

The contentious issue is whether a 12-lead electrocardiogram (ECG) is warranted as a screening tool to help identify those individuals at risk for sudden death. The reader is encouraged to review the available evidence to institute his or her team's policy (3,4).

The experts do agree on the necessity of further testing if the preliminary screens yield positive results. Echocardiography, stress ECG, 24-hour Holter monitoring, biopsy, and or electrophysiological testing may be warranted. Positive results may warrant exclusion from that sport based on the 16th Bethesda Conference protocol on eligibility for competition among athletes (5).

Orthopaedic

In this area, one would think that the examination would outweigh the history taking elements of the PPE. The evidence would suggest otherwise (6). One must ask questions about the following topics:

■ Past history of significant orthopaedic issues such as fractures, ligament disruptions, surgeries, and major trauma
■ Recent issues of more immediate concern that may require institution of rehabilitation protocols with particular attention to injuries that have not been attended to
■ Use of braces, orthotic devices, and protective equipment

The subsequent examination will help fine tune the deficiencies, should they exist, of what has been identified in the history.

Head Injury

This continuously evolving area of interest has stimulated much scientific investigation along with the considerable interest amongst the press. The sport medicine team has a responsibility to document entry-level information along with ongoing concerns to best arrive at judgment decisions that may have to be made somewhere down the line. It has

become clear that previous guidelines for inclusion/exclusion may be inadequate based on the current knowledge of this area. Individualized protocols seem to be the norm of the day (7). To best achieve this, a thorough knowledge of past and present symptomatology appears to be essential.

There are several protocols that one can follow. A suggested form as outlined by McCrory (7) seems to fill the bill.

■ Specific information as to the number of previous concussions and their specific details are important. Date, circumstances, loss of consciousness, symptoms, duration, medical verification, and imaging are necessary components.
■ Use of protective equipment, such as helmets, and their current status are important.
■ Persistence of symptoms (e.g., dizziness, headache, nausea/vomiting, blurred vision, drowsiness, irritability, memory issues, sleep disturbances, concentration problems, feeling confused, balance issues, and light or noise sensitivity).

The First and Second International Conference on concussion in Sport held in 2001 and 2004, respectively (8,9), concluded that neuropsychological testing was the cornerstone of individual recovery assessment and the ultimate decision on returning that athlete to sport. There are numerous tools available for this testing, including paper and pencil approaches (e.g., McGill Ace, standardized assessment of concussion) and computerized web-based approaches (e.g., CogSport, ImPACT, ANAM, Headminders). The respective sport medicine team will have to make its decisions on the tools they use based on a variety of concerns that include accessibility, affordability, familiarity, and deliverability.

Pulmonary

The inclusion of a questionnaire for pulmonary concerns needs little justification in light of the prevalent nature of bronchoconstrictive disorders in our society. Among elite athletes at the summer Olympics in Sydney, exercise-induced bronchospasm (EIB) was reported in 21% of athletes (10). Endurance athletes and, in particular, winter athletes appear to be most affected. The following symptoms (particularly within the first 10 minutes after moderate to intense exercise) may help identify those suffering from this condition: chest tightness, shortness of breath, cough, and wheeze. However, EIB may be present in individuals without these symptoms.

Unfortunately questionnaires alone do not appear to capture all those affected. Some researchers consider these questionnaires to be unreliable (11). Holzer and Brukner (12) review the current state of the literature.

If the questionnaire alone is not sensitive enough on its own to identify those afflicted individuals, what else is available? There are two main types of tests available: direct and indirect. The direct tests, for example the methacholine challenge test, administer an agent that causes constriction. The indirect method (e.g., exercise challenge test, eucapnic voluntary hyperpnea challenge test, osmotic challenge test) results in the production of mediators that act on the airways and thus allow the measurement of airway parameters. There still exists controversy as to the accepted values for a positive test.

There is a continuously evolving recommendation for the requirements for documentation of EIB at the elite, Olympic level. One should refer to the respective sport organizations, the International Olympic Committee, or World Anti-Doping Agency (WADA) for a more up to date reference in this regard.

Female Athlete

North America has seen a dramatic increase in female participation in sports. Title IX of Education Amendments of 1972 in the United States and the Charter of Rights in Canada have played a major role in this regard. With this explosion, issues of unique needs of the female athlete have appeared. Among those are disordered eating, amenorrhea, and osteopenia/osteoporosis. This triad has been called the female athlete triad, and it comes with its own profile of morbidity and mortality. Rumball and Lebrun (13) have reviewed this area. Although standardization is lacking, there is an attempt to structure questionnaires in a nonthreatening way to obtain an honest and forthcoming manner.

A preparticipation task force has recommended subtle questions to identify eating disorders. Questions such as "How much of an issue is weight for you?", "How do you rate your diet?", "What do you consider your ideal weight?", "What do you do to control your weight?", "Do you worry about your weight?" are open-ended nonthreatening ways to obtain the information required.

The menstrual history should include questions as to the onset of menstruation, the frequency of present cycles, the duration of the cycle, time of last period, use of birth control pills, and previous treatment or diagnosis of anemia.

Inclusion of family history of osteoporosis, personal history of stress fractures, and sport training history might red flag the need for a more thorough investigation.

Drugs and Supplements

The PPE represents a unique opportunity to inquire about the athlete's past or present use of recreational, medically justified, or performance-enhancing substances. It also is the time to evaluate the need to complete forms that may be required by various governing bodies of sport. When dealing with international-level athletes, various drugs may have to be reported to WADA; WADA's forms may be downloaded from their web site (www.wada-ama.org).

The PPE also represents the time to address the thorny issue of supplementation with its inherent risks. Supplementation use has been an ever-increasing problem in doping because many of the substances represent unknown quantities with poor quality control of its contents.

Summary

Although this list of clinical history parameters represents the main issues to address, it is by no means exclusive. Each individual clinician in consort with his or her team must arrive at a decision as to the factors that are most important to identify through this process. Questions posed to the athlete as to personal goals and aspirations may reflect underlying psychological needs or deficiencies that require attention in a timely manner.

■ EXAMINATION

The history should have served its purpose of identifying those areas of greater concern. Coupled with the examination process, one should be well on the way to formulating decision-making processes for the athlete involved.

Cardiovascular

The AHA guidelines (5) recommend the following cardiovascular testing:

- Auscultation in both standing and supine positions
- Palpation of femoral pulses
- Recognition of the stigmata of Marfan syndrome (i.e., arm span to height ratio >1.05, scoliosis of >20 degrees, pectus carinatum, pectus excavatum requiring surgery, dislocated lens, aortic root enlargement, dissection of the aorta, mitral valve prolapse or regurgitation, etc.)
- Blood pressure (brachial, sitting)
- Pulse

Orthopedic

The 14-point examination presented in the Preparticipation Physical Evaluation Form appears to have endured. What is lacking is evidence-based validity for the process. The combination of the history and the 14-point evaluation would seem to allow for a more focused attention to identified deficiencies. Although rarely would one exclude an athlete from participation from sport on the basis of a singular finding, the PPE appears to serve its purpose in identifying restrictions and or weaknesses that need to be addressed prior to full clearance for return to competition. The old adage of full range of motion and full strength prior to returning to sport has served us all well. Form indeed does follow function.

Head Injury

The neurological examination rarely yields positive findings. Most deficits related to head injuries are of a cognitive nature and thus neuropsychological testing becomes the critical tool (7).

Visual Testing

To assume that all athletes arrive at a preseason screening with perfect or corrected vision is a bit of a jump in faith. It has been our custom at the Canadian Alpine Ski Team to ensure that all athletes have visual acuity testing and sport vision assessment every 2 years. Although no documentation exists to support our approach, it has been our opinion that such endeavors have helped the athlete in the critical area of sport vision. The ability to process images at high speeds can be a trained response, and correctional exercises have been instituted in those athletes found wanting. This is clearly not an exercise that all athletes or programs can afford but represents an area of increasing concern in the elite athlete.

Other Issues

The nature of this chapter precludes a thorough discussion of all issues germane to the topic of PPE. In the area of clinical examination, discussions of body habitus might assume increasing importance if one is dealing with potential eating disorders, and discussions of dermatological concerns that might be preeminent if one is dealing with a team where frequent and close body contact occurs (e.g., wrestling) have not been touched. This is not to minimize their importance. The emphasis on each area becomes the domain of the examining clinician. The sport medicine team must decide how it best uses the tools of history taking and clinical examination to achieve its goals.

Lab Screening

The area of lab screening for hematological abnormalities has been reviewed (14). One has to weigh the yield versus the cost involved. It would be hard to criticize the following: in male athletes, hemoglobin; and in female athletes, hemoglobin and ferritin. The nature of the group involved might dictate a more comprehensive investigation. A complete blood count might be more appropriate in the elite highly trained athlete. The decisions as to their nature and frequency should be made with a thorough knowledge of the area. The decision process as to when to treat is also a thorny one and requires education.

Report

The clinician involved may have to generate minimal documentation and merely complete an assertion of "fit to participate." The clinician involved with an elite team may have to sit down with a group of trainers, physiologists, psychologists, and so on, before formulating a plan of action. This in turn may have to be reviewed not only with the athlete but also the respective coach to ensure that all concerned are on the same page.

Nothing irritates athletes more than going through a process where the perception is that nothing has been gained. Writing down a synopsis of the findings and sitting down and discussing them with the concerned athlete goes a long way in establishing a path of communication and a much needed rapport that serves both the athlete and the medical team well.

■ REFERENCES

1. Peltz JE, Haskell WL, Matheson GO. A comprehensive and cost-effective preparticipation exam implemented on the World Wide Web. *Med Sci Sports Exerc.* 1999;31:1727–1740.
2. Wingfield K, Matheson GO, Meeuwisse WH. Preparticipation evaluation: an evidence-based review. *Clin J Sport Med.* 2004; 14:109–122.
3. Corrado, D. Pelliccia A, Bjornstad HH, et al. Cardiovascular preparticipation screening of young competitive athletes for prevention of sudden death: proposal for a common European protocol. Consensus Statement of the Study Group of Sport Cardiology of the Working Group of Cardiac Rehabilitation and Exercise Physiology and the Working Group of Myocardial and Pericardial Diseases of the European Society of Cardiology. *Eur Heart J.* 2005;26:516–524.
4. Maron BJ, Shirani J, Poliac LC, et al. Sudden death in young competitive athletes. Clinical, demographic, and pathological profiles. *JAMA.* 1996;276:199–204.
5. Maron BJ, Thompson PD, Puffer JC, et al. Cardiovascular preparticipation screening of competitive athletes. A statement for health professionals from the Sudden Death Committee (clinical cardiology) and Congenital Cardiac Defects Committee (cardiovascular disease in the young), American Heart Association. *Circulation.* 1996;94:850–856.
6. Gomez JE, Landry GL, Bernhardt DT. Critical evaluation of the 2-minute orthopedic screening examination. *Am J Dis Child.* 1993;147:1109–1113.
7. McCrory P. Preparticipation assessment for head injury. *Clin J Sport Med.* 2004;14:139–144.
8. Aubry M, Cantu R, Dvorak J, et al. Summary and agreement statement of the First International Conference on Concussion in Sport, Vienna 2001. Recommendations for the improvement of safety and health of athletes who may suffer concussive injuries. *Br J Sports Med.* 2002;36:6–10.
9. McCrory P, Johnston K, Meeuwisse W, et al. Summary and Agreement Statement of the 2nd International Conference on Concussion in Sport, Prague 2004. *Clin J Sport Med.* 2005; 15:48–55.
10. Corrigan B, Kazlauskas R. Medication use in athletes selected for doping control at the Sydney Olympics (2000). *Clin J Sport Med.* 2003;13:33–40.
11. Rundell KW, Im J, Mayers LB, et al. Self-reported symptoms and exercise-induced asthma in the elite athlete. *Med Sci Sports Exerc.* 2001;33:208–213.
12. Holzer K, Brukner P. Screening of athletes for exercise-induced bronchoconstriction. *Clin J Sport Med.* 2004;14:134–138.
13. Rumball JS, Lebrun CM. Preparticipation physical examination: selected issues for the female athlete. *Clin J Sport Med.* 2004; 14:153–160.
14. Fallon KE. Utility of hematological and iron-related screening in elite athletes. *Clin J Sport Med.* 2004;14:145–152.

RUNNING ON THE FIELD

RICHARD HAWKINS, MD

■ KEY POINTS

- When entering the field for an injury, the doctor and training staff are often required to make quick decisions.
- Prior contact with the team in other situations helps the doctor develop a rapport that is helpful in successful management of on-field injuries.
- Doctors might even be called on for dramatic treatment for those in life-threatening situations.
- On the professional sports level, there are often EMTs on hand to perform such tasks as intubation. Such personnel may not be available on the high school and other levels in which case the doctor may have to assume that responsibility or at least be able to resuscitate the patient appropriately.
- Training staff and doctors need to practice and be knowledgeable on the principles of resuscitation and on immobilization when it comes to head and neck injuries.
- Players who have sustained a head or neck injury may be found in an awkward position. The player should be left where found until it is determined that it is safe to roll the individual onto his back and proceed from there. If it is determined that a player has a significant head and/or neck injury, a strict protocol is followed to safely manage the situation.
- If the player complains that he can't move his arms or legs, it is assumed that he has a neck injury.
- For neck injuries in football and similar sports, the head is supported while the facemask is removed. The helmet is otherwise left in place during log rolling.

My friend Don Johnson has asked me to write a brief chapter for his textbook *Practical Sports Medicine and Arthroscopy* titled "Running on the Field." As it relates to running on the field, I've had the privilege of being head team physician for the Denver Broncos as well as the Colorado Rockies. Running on the field is frequent with injuries on the football team, but rarely with injuries on the baseball field. When there's an injury with the Denver Broncos, it's hard to miss the white (blond)-haired guy doctor running on to the field and I guess that's the reason I get the nod to write this chapter. The discussion in this chapter applies not only to a professional football team such as the Denver Broncos, but to other levels of play, such as college, high school, and other sports, such as soccer and basketball, among others. As team physicians, we work closely with the training staff, tending to injuries on the field of play. With the Denver Broncos, we take our lead from the training staff, which is responsible for communication to the coaching staff regarding players' injuries and removal from play. That may not always be the line of communication. It is important to appreciate that, in order to run on the field and care for injured athletes, the doctor needs a working relationship with the team, including training staff, players, even coaching staff and management. In order to develop such rapport, the doctor must be present in situations in which players and staff can get to know the medical personnel.

In going onto the field, the doctor and training staff are required to make decisions, often very quickly. They're the ones who are able establish a diagnosis on the field, and to what length this needs to be pursued depends on the circumstances and the situation. In most situations, the physician will perform a quick history and physical examination on the field, then evacuate the player to the sidelines for further examination, or even evacuate the player to the hospital for assessment in certain situations, such as a spinal cord injury. Unfortunately, doctors might be called upon for dramatic treatment on the field for those who may be in a life-threatening situation. ACLR training and knowledge is important, since one might have to resuscitate a player on the field. At the professional level, there are often EMT personnel to perform such tasks as intubation. Such personnel may not be available at the high school level, in which case the doctor may have to assume that responsibility, or at least be able to resuscitate the patient appropriately. Gratefully, these situations are rare.

In this chapter, we'd like to describe different situations in which a player goes down and outline the role of the doctor in each circumstance. In most circumstances, doctors and trainers are not allowed on the field until there is an appropriate stoppage of play, as indicated by the referee. I personally, however, have seen life-threatening situations in which as a physician I've moved very quickly to the scene before any whistle had blown. Training staff and doctors need to practice and be knowledgeable of the principles of resuscitation, and more important, the principles of immobilization, especially when it comes to care for the head-and-neck-injured player. In going on to the field, the physician often must rapidly assimilate knowledge about whether this represents a minor injury, moderate injury, or hopefully not a major potential life- or neurologically-worrisome injury. It is important that the doctors and trainers not get caught up in the excitement of the game and forget that their job is to watch carefully and be alert to situations in which players are injured.

With the Denver Broncos, the usual situation involves the training staff initially going on to the field, at a very fast clip, to attend to the downed player. The rapidity with which the doctor moves depends on circumstances. There is a debate as to whether doctors should always go on to the field with the training staff, particularly in football, or whether in fact these injuries should be handled by the training staff, who could then signal for the doctor if needed. We initially had this latter signaling situation with the Denver Broncos; however, it became clear there were many situations in which the doctors were required on the field to help establish a diagnosis and to initiate appropriate treatment for the downed player. Often the training staff is not comfortable in making the call, diagnosing, and treating certain injuries. For example, in the situation of a potential cervical spine injury, training staff often takes comfort in having a doctor make the call as to transport from the field. In some circumstances, if there is obviously a minor injury the doctor may not be required to attend to the player on the field. It is not uncommon for the doctor to roam the sidelines and be approached by the training staff to turn to a player who has found his way back to the bench, having sustained an injury such as a concussion, a burner or a stinger, or even a knee ligament injury. The time taken on the field to obtain a history and do a physical examination and institute appropriate treatment are very dependent upon the circumstances. It is important to take the appropriate time and not be rushed because of the urgency of removing the player from the field.

Subsequently, in this chapter we'll describe specific approaches to the patient with lower-extremity injury, the upper extremity injury, and the more serious head-and-neck injuries, along with their management and the role of the doctor on the field.

■ SITUATION: LOWER-EXTREMITY INJURY

When the player goes down, the whistle blows, the training staff and doctor go out on the field. What's the problem? Where does it hurt? How did it happen? A quick assessment leads to the tibia as an area of the problem. A quick palpation reveals a fracture. The diagnosis is made. At this point the doctor tells the training staff to bring on the splint and the wagon to transport the player safely off the field. From here it may be an x-ray in the facility or a direct transport to a nearly hospital facility, the location of which is predetermined and obviously well understood by all.

Such an examination on the field during this period of relative anesthesia will establish a diagnosis, for example, of an MCL or ACL ligament tear. Often during the initial moments after an injury, a player has little pain and allows medial opening or a Lackman to help establish this diagnosis. The player complains his knee twisted and he felt a pop. At this point the patient is carefully moved to the supine position for a quick examination of the knee. The diagnosis may be established at that point, or perhaps a questionable diagnosis, and if safe the patient is assisted off the field by the training staff in an upright manner. Once a player is transported to the sidelines, often pain sets in and examination becomes difficult, particularly with the uniform in place and sitting on a bench. The method in which the lower extremity injury is handled by the trainers is important to emphasize at this point, as they mobilize the player to an upright position. It is the role of the training and medical staff to get the patient from a supine to a sitting to an upright position, then transport him to the sidelines. The player sits, one trainer behind the player, the good knee fixed on the ground, the injured knee out and relaxed, another trainer in the front, and together the pull and the push from the trainers gets the player to the upright position. At that point the doctor and training staff all wait to see that conditions are reasonable for transport of the player to the sidelines (Fig 58.2-1). Further examination on the bench is now warranted, particularly to try to nail down the diagnosis more accurately. Transport to the dressing room may be warranted. The decision is then made about the injured regarding return to play. Always in these injuries the training staff informs the coaching staff that the player is out, at least temporarily, until further notice. ACL injuries can usually be diagnosed at the time of injury on the field with an efficient history and brief examination.

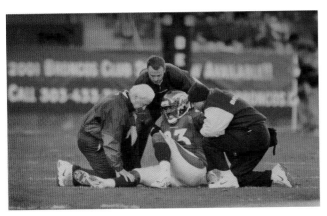

Fig 58.2-1. Preparing the player with lower-extremity injury for transport to the sidelines.

■ SITUATION: UPPER-EXTREMITY INJURY

The player goes down. Training staff and doctor go out on to the field to tend to the player with an upper-extremity injury. It may be a burner or stinger, dislocated shoulder, a dislocated elbow, or conceivably a fracture. The determination must be quick and accurate based on history and physical examination. A clearly dislocated elbow can be reduced on the field carefully, with not undue force but appropriate maneuvers. Similarly, a dislocated shoulder can be reduced carefully on the field in the upright position having the player bend over and gently pulling down the dependent arm. In some of these situations, transport to the sideline in an upright position with support is warranted for more definitive treatment. Before reduction, one must be careful that there is not an associated fracture, and that the diagnosis of dislocation of elbow or shoulder is accurate. An x-ray before reduction maneuvers would be safer if there is any doubt. Burners or stingers are very common in football players, and usually the diagnosis is very straightforward. On the field, the doctor needs to quickly clear the cervical spine and head, and be sure that this does represent a stinger. Frequently the player will have a history of this and know exactly what's going on. Sometimes one sees players coming off the field to the sidelines with their arm down beside them, to the side of the injury, a very characteristic pattern.

■ SITUATION: HEAD AND NECK INJURIES

Upon coming on the field of play, if he has sustained a head-and/or-neck injury, the player may be found in an awkward position. The player should be left where found until it is determined that it is safe to roll the individual onto his back and get him to a sitting, then subsequently standing position. If it is determined that the player has a significant head-and/or-neck injury, a strict protocol is followed to safely manage the situation.

The Head-Injured Unconscious Patient

If a player is unconscious we may have to deal with resuscitative efforts, keeping in mind there could be a cervical spine injury, and therefore treat the player accordingly. If there is need for resuscitation in the head-injured patient, we must with great expediency and care log roll the patient onto the back, support the head, and remove the face mask. This principle obviously applies in particular to football; face masks may not be present in situations such as soccer, basketball, etc. In the NFL, most trainers have power screwdrivers that allow quick removal of the screws from the face mask or large cutters. Normally, the helmet and chin straps are left in place, and the head supported. Longitudinal traction to support the legs is instituted. The patient may require intubation. If that expertise is not available, the patient could be ambu-bagged until transport. Transport from the field is described in the section on the neck-injured patient.

The Neck-Injured Patient (Spine)

If it is determined that the player has a neck injury, especially in the presence of any neurological findings, strict protocol should be followed. If the player complains that he can't move his legs, or arms, or both, it is assumed that he has a neck injury. The entire training and medical staff move into action to deal with this frightening situation. The aid of others, such as the coaching staff or players, may be required. The head is supported with minimal longitudinal traction, prompt removal of the face mask, leaving the chin strap and helmet in place, and appropriate log rolling, as directed by the leader. The leader, under these circumstances, should be the most experienced, either the head trainer and/or the doctor. One of the trainers and/or one of the medical staff is assigned to support the head, not with undue traction but keeping it stable, someone else supports and creates longitudinal traction of the lower extremities. The team leader then orchestrates the log rolling of this patient onto his back and careful transport simultaneously onto a board. The head and neck are then secured in position. Having followed this protocol, the player is then transported directly to the predetermined hospital. One of the medical staff accompanies the player in the ambulance to the hospital. The Denver Broncos have produced a videotape that is in the American Academy of Orthopaedic Surgeons library that goes over the protocol of the head and neck injured patient on the playing field. It is well worth having for those who look after such athletes and may find themselves in such a situation.

In summary, in running on to the field, the doctor must be prepared to make quick decisions, establish a diagnosis with limited history and physical examination, treat where applicable to the situation on the field, in a careful manner, and transport to the sidelines or to the hospital when indicated. Rapport with the players and the training and coaching staff is critical to successful management of such athletes. Experience and practice are wonderful teachers.

59

TRAVELING TEAM PHYSICIAN

■ CHADWICK PRODROMOS, MD

■ KEY POINTS

- The team physician and the head physician at most events other than marathons will generally be an orthopaedic surgeon because the vast majority of conditions needing medical attention are musculoskeletal injuries.
- The role of team physician often involves nontraditional compensation arrangements. Physicians can gain marketing benefits but often pay for advertising with the team. Physicians may provide some services for free but, in turn, will add more patients for services that are paid.
- The potential for conflict of interest exists. The team, which hires the physician, may want a player to return to action sooner than what is in the best interest of the athlete.
- A team physician is at greater risk for legal repercussions than an independent physician in the event of reinjury after an athlete's return.
- It is important for a team physician to have specialists available for referrals.
- Preparticipation physicals should include a written health history and an examination that follows the American College of Sports Medicine guidelines.
- If a significant question of fracture exists, an athlete should be sent for x-rays.
- Any loss of consciousness or orientation is reason to remove the athlete from that day's competition permanently.
- Generally, anesthetic or corticosteroid injections to strains, sprains, and minor fractures should be avoided. They can subject an athlete to greater damage by allowing a premature return to competition.

Basic Concept

Three basic functions underlie the team physician concept. The first and most important is the evaluation and treatment of injured athletes. The second is the provision of physician coverage at some athletic events, especially American football. The third is the arrangement of preparticipation physical examinations when necessary. With the exception of events such as marathons, the head or only team physician will generally be an orthopaedic surgeon since the vast majority of conditions needing medical attention are musculoskeletal injuries. The physician will then be responsible for providing consultants when needed. The arrangement logistics and intensity of involvement of the team physician vary by level (e.g., professional, collegiate, or high school) and by sport (e.g., American football vs. other sports).

Benefit to the Team

The basic benefit to the team of having a team physician derives from the time efficiency of having one physician, instead of many physicians, with whom to communicate. Secondary benefits to the team occur when the team physician provides reduced-price or free services to the team. Such services include any or all of the three described earlier (i.e., injury treatment, game coverage, and physicals). Secondary benefits can also include the physician buying advertising with the team or in some other direct or indirect manner providing cash flow to the team. The provision of discounted or free services to the team by the physician is common at all levels. Advertising or other payments, however, are more prevalent in professional teams, less so with college teams, and rare with high school teams.

Benefits to the Physician

Benefits to the team physician include the provision of patients for treatment for which services the physician will charge. Second, there may be marketing benefits to the physician of being associated with the team. Third, there may be direct payment to the physician, usually only at the professional or major college level, for provision of services. In recent times, these relationships have evolved toward the physician providing revenue to the team rather than receiving it from the team.

Conflict of Interest

There has always been an inherent conflict of interest in the team physician's role. This conflict arises from the team physician being hired by the administration of the team yet being the treating physician for the athlete. At times, the interest of the team in having the athlete play sooner after an injury may seem to conflict with the interest of the athlete in playing less soon so that they may heal more. The athlete or his or her family may suspect that the physician represents the team's interest more than the athlete's interest. This is particularly true if it is perceived that the physician receives benefit from the team that the physician may not want to jeopardize. This potential conflict is inherent in any situation in which an organization hires a physician to treat its members, whether in sports, occupational medicine, government, the military, or other areas. In such situations, it is increasingly common for the athlete to find a physician who is not hired by the team to render another opinion or take over care entirely. Pressure may indeed be exerted by a sports organization on the team physician to not "coddle" an athlete and allow them to play sooner. This is particularly true in American or Canadian football where injuries are common and playing with them is expected. In such situations, it is important that the physician and athletic trainer are united in their desire to protect the athlete from such administrative pressure. Even the most aggressive coach will usually defer to a reasoned presentation by the physician who is, of course, always the advocate of the injured athlete and not the team. In fact, the team physician will always be second guessed more and be more at risk for legal repercussions in the event of reinjury after the athlete's return than a perceived "independent" physician. The physician should further realize that his standing with the team may be jeopardized by his faithfulness to his medical principles on behalf of the athlete and not let this potential eventuality cloud his judgment.

Recent Changes in the Team Physician Concept

For several reasons, the team physician in the United States is evolving into a less influential position that it has traditionally been. With the increasing sophistication of sports medicine technology, there have come increased patient expectations. Professionals with salaries, collegiate athletes with scholarships, and high school athletes with potential scholarships want to maximize their chances of complete recovery for economic as well as enjoyment purposes. They are increasingly not content to entrust significant surgery to a physician selected by their organization rather than by themselves. For this reason, the modern team physician will spend more time coordinating care and less time delivering it than was true in the past. This may make the team physician concept less attractive to some practitioners. To others, the athletic environment involvement and perceived marketing benefits will continue to outweigh the time, financial, and potential legal liability costs.

Scope of Services

The team physician should be prepared to be at least as much of a triage officer as a treater. Some injuries, such as those to the face and head, should be referred to plastic and neurosurgical colleagues. Skin rashes and cardiac and respiratory problems are also common and are obviously beyond the scope of practice of an orthopaedic surgeon. However, in this era of increasing specialization, even many of the orthopaedic problems may need to be referred. Orthopaedic sports medicine subspecialists will typically handle all knee and shoulder problems. However, they may not be the best practitioner for a complicated hand or spine problem. Ultimately, it is important that the desire to treat the injured athlete not cause the practitioner to treat injuries for which he or she may not be the best available practitioner. It is extremely important that the head team physician have a cadre of specialists, whether within their own group or not, to which problems can be referred. The athletic trainer will feel comfortable referring such injuries to these affiliated doctors without needing to find the head team physician in each case.

Legal Liability

The dramatic increase in professional salaries has resulted in increased medical malpractice liability for the team physician at every level. Settlements and judgments at the professional level will potentially exceed the policy limits of team physicians due to the high salaries and potential lost wages involved. However, even the collegiate and high school athlete can lay claim to potentially high-lost earnings that could escalate malpractice judgments into seven figures. If the athlete demonstrated high potential at a lower level, the award may be nearly as high as if the athlete had in fact realized that potential. Furthermore, the adverse outcome leading to these judgments does not need to be as severe as in everyday life. An elite athlete who does not regain the ability to run or throw at an elite level, while being otherwise healthy and functioning normally, may lay claim to huge lost earnings.

Furthermore, juries may favor celebrity athletes in such proceedings. Jurors commonly obtain the autographs of plaintiff athletes after the conclusion of their trials. The legal liability risk has reached crisis proportions in the United States with no good answer in sight.

Preparticipation Physical

The orthopaedic surgeon will generally perform an orthopaedic exam and may or may not perform the entire physical exam. A written health history is very important. The physical exam should be complete and appropriate for the age of the athlete. The American College of Sports Medicine publishes a monograph with guidelines for middle school though college age athletes. The physical should follow American College of Sports Medicine guidelines. Even though the overwhelming majority of these athletes will be in perfect health, and few medical problems will be encountered, it is important that the exam not be done perfunctorily. Perhaps the most difficult area concerns attempts to detect silent heart disease. Some have advocated echocardiograms, but the cost of screening millions of athletes for these exceedingly rare problems is high, and echocardiograms are not routinely done at present. A complete blood count and dip-stick urinalysis may be cost-effective general screening devices. The orthopaedic team physician should always defer to a well-qualified internist conversant with the appropriate medical sports medicine literature regarding the appropriate scope of the preparticipation physical.

■ GAME COVERAGE PEARLS

General

Customarily, football is the only sport for which physician coverage is provided below the professional level. The most important principle of game coverage is to ensure that a potentially seriously injured athlete, who may feel little pain due to the heat of battle, not be allowed to return to competition if there is a question of serious injury. I have on numerous occasions seen athletes with acutely torn anterior cruciate ligaments (ACL) and hand, forearm, and ankle fractures vigorously arguing for return to play despite these injuries. If a significant question of fracture exists, the athlete should be sent for x-ray. In most cases, this will entail a trip to a local emergency room and the end of the athlete's participation for the day. In some venues, an x-ray will be able to be taken at the stadium such that the athlete would have time to resume playing if the x-ray were negative and the athlete had regained good function. There is tremendous pressure on the athlete to resume playing despite injury. It is up to the physician to protect the athlete from this pressure if the physician feels a serious problem may exist. The athlete will protest but relies on the physician to protect them if need be. Sometimes the athlete feels obliged to make a show of wishing to return so as not to be viewed as weak by their teammates, all the while expecting that the physician will keep him or her out of the game if the physician feels they should not return.

Emergency Services

Paramedics should either be in attendance or readily available at football games. In my opinion, physicians are less important at games than paramedics. The former generally deal with questions of who can play. The latter deal with issues of potential death and paralysis.

Head Injuries

Any loss of consciousness or orientation is reason to remove the athlete from that day's competition permanently. The athlete should have neurological consultation electively, and the recommendations of the neurologist should be followed regarding return to play on a subsequent day. Any signs of increased intracranial pressure such as nausea, any positive physical finding, such as pupillary abnormalities, and any persistence of mental status abnormalities are reasons for immediate dispensation to the local emergency room by ambulance.

Eye Injuries

Any persisting ocular symptoms, including pain or vision alteration, should result in the athlete receiving immediate emergency room evaluation.

Nose Injuries

Broken noses are less common in football than in wrestling and some other sports. Athletes may be able to return to play after a short layoff with a shield but should never be allowed to continue to play when the acute injury occurs.

Neck Injuries

Any significant neck pain, radicular pain, or extremity neurological physical finding should be treated by keeping the athlete flat on the ground and calling paramedics to apply a collar and transport the athlete to the emergency room on a stretcher. Great care must be taken to avoid moving the neck to avoid exacerbation of any neurological injury. It is extremely important that the athlete not be sat up if any question exists.

Chest Injuries

Collapsed lungs can occur as a result of blunt trauma, especially in football. Any athlete with any shortness of breath should be auscultated to make sure breath sounds exist in all lung fields. If there is any question, the athlete should be sent for chest x-ray. Collapsed lungs, rib fractures, and inter-costals muscle contusions can all produce chest tenderness and shortness of breath. Often only the auscultation will be able to differentiate them. If lung collapse has occurred, the athlete may need a chest tube. Breast contusions may cause scarring that should be noted with regard to future mammographic evaluations in the female athlete.

Stingers

Upper extremity weakness that does not completely resolve in a timely fashion after a head, neck, or shoulder blow is reason to remove the athlete from competition for that day. Elective workup can be conducted subsequently. Studies have shown that weakness from these injuries is often not transient as previously thought.

Shoulder Injuries

Dislocations, persisting or transient, are not uncommon. Beware of a transient dislocation being redislocated by a sideline exam. Athletes should be sent for x-ray in either case. Proximal humerus fractures can occur in adolescents and must not be manipulated in the mistaken belief that they are dislocations. It is acceptable to send a patient with a dislocated glenohumeral joint to the emergency room for treatment. An attempt at sideline reduction can be attempted with care if the diagnosis is secure.

Hand, Wrist, and Forearm

I have seen wrestlers and/or football players continue to play despite fractures including metacarpals, distal radii, radial shaft, and scaphoid. Dislocated fingers can be reduced on the sidelines if the diagnosis is clear. But displaced pha-langeal fractures can be worsened by attempted reduction of what was thought to be a dislocation. In all cases, x-rays should be taken if there is any question.

Abdominal Injuries

Significant injury to a viscus, such as a ruptured spleen (which I have seen in a hockey player checked over the boards), can occur as a result of blunt trauma. If any question exists, the athlete should be sent to the emergency room.

Groin Injuries

Severe testicular trauma occurs and should be treated emergently.

Hip/Femur

Hip dislocations are rare. Femur fractures are more common than hip fractures and can be accompanied by severe blood loss. Emergent treatment is indicated.

Knee Injuries

The athlete should be able to run, squat, and jump at full force with no pain before being allowed to return to play. The Lachman test should also be negative. If any of these conditions cannot be met, the athlete should be sent for x-ray and removed from competition. Acute ACL tears are often not particularly painful. Pain increases with later swelling. On more than one occasion, I have found a positive Lachman test on an injured football player with no ACL history and who had little pain, was able to run well, and wanted to return to play. The player and coach will want the player to return, and it is important to be resolute in preventing it. In a short period, pain and swelling will occur, and your decision will be validated.

Foot and Ankle

Distal fibular and metatarsal fractures are often played through by athletes in competition. If the exam suggests possible fracture, the athlete should be removed for x-rays. A high index of suspicion must be maintained.

Lacerations

In some settings, it may be appropriate to suture lacerations and return the athlete to play, especially on the professional level. For high school and most college athletes, the athlete should be removed from play and treated at the hospital. The orthopaedist should not attempt to suture facial lacerations, which should be sutured by a plastic surgeon.

Dental Injuries

Any teeth that are knocked out should be collected and sent to the emergency room with the athlete for treatment by the dentist.

Heat Injury

Athletes must be kept hydrated, although over hydration should be avoided because it has been linked to potentially serious dilutional electrolyte problems, particularly in runners. Athletes who feel weak in the heat, typically in summer football practice, should be removed from practice and medically evaluated. Renal failure from rhabdomyolysis is one sequela. Deaths occur every year in the United States, and a high index of suspicion for heat injury must be maintained.

Asthma

More athletes suffer from and play with asthma than in prior years. On-field medications must be maintained, and all players with known asthma should be monitored. The internal medicine or pulmonary specialist should be given full reign to design policy in this area. The athletic trainer must act in accordance with them.

Cardiac Event

Most hypotensive episodes are vasovagal, and blood pressure is restored almost instantly by laying the athlete supine and elevating the legs. The pulse should be simultaneously monitored. If the athlete does not immediately respond, appropriate resuscitation by the paramedics and physician should be carried out as preparation is made for hospital transfer. Fatal arrhythmia can occur from sternal cardiac contusion.

Specious Injury

It is axiomatic that athletes are injured more often toward the end of losing efforts. Even if an athlete does not seem objectively injured, if they feel injured, they should be removed. I have had one episode in which a professional football player feigned quadriplegia on national television, stating to me while prone that he could neither feel nor move his limbs after tackling with his helmet. However, x-rays and magnetic resonance imaging (MRI) were negative. This was later revealed by one of his teammates to be a premeditated effort to obtain an injury settlement. The physician, however, must always act in the belief that all claimed injuries are valid, which they usually are.

Other

In general, there is a tendency for injuries to be underdiagnosed and undertreated in the on-field setting. This is because the athlete's state of excitation tends to minimize symptomatic pain. It is important that the team physician err on the side of caution.

Nonplayer Injuries

The team physician is also called upon to treat injuries to spectators, cheerleaders, and others. I have been called upon to treat bee stings, fainting episodes, myocardial infarction, and a baby that fell 20 feet to the ground from bleachers (unharmed), among other problems. Be prepared for anything, and call the paramedics early and often.

On-field Etiquette

Allow the trainer to evaluate the injury first. Most fallen athletes will get up in short order without the team physician needing to attend to them. However, you should run (not walk) to the athlete if the trainer beckons or a short period passes without the athlete arising on his own and leaving the field. It is desirable to dress with proper neatness and decorum in part to help identify the physician from among the other sideline observers. Many team physicians will wear a jacket and tie.

Avoiding Physician Injury

Acromioclavicular separation has been called the "sideline shoulder" and may occur when the team doctor is knocked to the ground on the sideline by a player(s) running out of bounds. Especially in football, it is important to not get so wrapped up in the action that you forget to get out of the way.

■ INTERACTION WITH THE ATHLETIC TRAINER

The athletic trainer is a licensed health care professional dealing with the evaluation and prevention of injuries in athletes. He or she provides much more hands on care than the team physician. Depending on his level of experience, the athletic trainer may evaluate injuries with a very high level of skill. They are the most overworked, misunderstood, and underpaid of all health care professionals and are usually extremely dedicated. Injuries will be presented to the physician by the trainer when athletes are seen. It is important that the team physician understand the abilities and limitations of the given trainer so that physician may know how much he or she may rely on the trainer's findings (e.g., is his or her Lachman test reliable or unreliable?). All findings should be checked by the physician, but the exam of a skilled trainer may be good enough for the MRI to be ordered before rather than after the physician exam. The physician must always communicate directly with the trainer and not rely on the athlete to serve as a communication intermediary.

■ ON-SITE VISITS FOR INJURY EVALUATION

It is desired by many organizations that the team physician pay a weekly visit to the training room for injury evaluation. However, the quality of the evaluation is greatly inferior in this setting compared with the physician's office. The lack of x-ray in most such settings is the chief deficiency. The absence of materials for injections is another. Finally, the lack of medical records and of the physician's support staff to schedule tests, check records, and coordinate care is limiting. Some or all of these deficiencies can be addressed by attempting to expand the training room environment into a mini-clinic, but deficiencies will usually remain. It is far better for the trainer to transport athletes in a group to the physician's office where optimal care can be delivered. This should be explained to the trainer and organization. If they are resistive, the physician will have to decide whether the expenditure of time and inefficient working conditions are outweighed by whatever benefits he or she derives from the affiliation.

Injections of Acute Injuries

In general, anesthetic or corticosteroid injections of strains, sprains, and minor fractures should be avoided. There are rare cases where they may be provided without potential harm, and this should always be with the enthusiastic approval of the athlete. However, in general, analgesic or anti-inflammatory injections only subject the athlete to potentially greater damage to the affected area by allowing a prematurely high level of participation. In some environments, this may endanger the physician's standing with the team.

Medical Records

The hand-held recorder should be present in the training room and on the field. Ideally, duplicate records will be kept in the physician's office and by the trainer. Written notes to the trainer about the athlete are important, particularly concerning the question of return to play.

Nonorthopaedic Team Physicians

Nonorthopaedic doctors, osteopaths, and chiropractors, with or without formal subspecialty sports medicine training, often offer services at no charge at the subprofessional level for the perceived prestige of the affiliation. The orthopaedic sports medicine specialist may or may not wish to meet this standard for the opportunity of continuing in his position. The team may or may not perceive the more specialized skill of the orthopaedic sports medicine specialist to outweigh the greater availability of others.

Insurance Constraints

One of the greatest erosions of the team physician experience in the United States has occurred as a result of the growth of managed care. Two decades ago, the physician was free to treat the vast majority of injured team athletes. Currently at the high school and college level, the physician will be unable to treat many athletes because the physician is not in their health plan. Sometimes health plans can be changed but usually not without some frustration.

■ CONCLUSION

Team physician affiliations are generally enjoyable, may be a useful marketing device, and may generate revenue. Conversely, they are time consuming, they subject the practitioner to increased liability risk, and they may produce little net economic gain, particularly when time devoted is considered. Managed care, legal liability, and the growing perception by sports organizations that the team physician, rather than the team, benefits by the affiliation have eroded the experience. The appropriate desire of athletes to choose the best doctor for their problem has further diminished the importance of the position. If the orthopaedist chooses to serve, he or she must narrowly focus on the well-being of the athlete, whether or not his or her decisions are beneficial to the team. Despite the orthopaedist's desire to be helpful, he or she must also make sure the injured athlete is treated by the best available practitioner when there is a complicated problem.

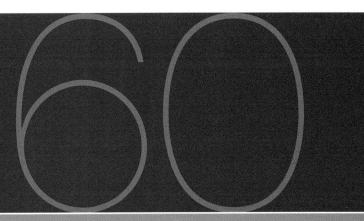

MASS PARTICIPATION EVENTS

60

HELEN D. IAMS, MD, MS, JAMES WILLIAMS, MD

■ KEY POINTS

■ Events with more than 1,000 participants are classified as mass participation events.

■ The medical care system at a sports event will need to manage a high volume of minor issues, while remaining prepared to quickly identify and treat life-threatening problems.

■ High-speed events have the potential for life-threatening trauma and require preparation for the management of such injuries.

■ Design of the medical system should begin months in advance and be based on the length and intensity of the event and the risk of catastrophic injury.

■ Physicians can help administrators plan a safer event. In hot climates, start times should be scheduled for early in the day or in the evening. In cold climates, events should start mid-day.

■ Identifying the risk of injury in hot weather is best done using a wet bulb globe thermometer.

■ Consideration needs to be given to where injuries are most likely to happen. Possible evacuation routes and traffic and pedestrian control need to be planned accordingly.

■ Costs can be minimized by borrowing supplies. Among the possible sources are the National Guard, American Red Cross, Coast Guard, and the National Ski Patrol.

■ The entire medical staff should have distinctive clothing or hats so that it can be easily identified by other race workers and athletes.

■ One physician needs to serve as medical director and is often so busy that he or she can not provide medical care. The medical director organizes and supervises the medical operations and serves as spokesperson in the case of an adverse event.

■ The physicians staffing a sports event need to have experience in managing the injuries that may be encountered. This makes orthopaedic surgeons, family physicians, and emergency physicians the most frequently recruited. Podiatrists are helpful at running events.

■ Ideally, liability is provided by the race administration. Physicians need to carefully review liability coverage before becoming involved.

Endurance sports events are growing in popularity and drawing increasingly large fields of participants. Events with over 1,000 participants, classified as mass participation events, have become common (1). Often, the race administration will ask local physicians to provide medical coverage for these events. Being able to fulfill this role requires that the physician understand the unique aspects of large sports events and how these aspects can affect medical care. Injury rates at mass sports events can be as high as 30%, necessitating a medical system that can handle a high volume of injuries (2). The medical staff may encounter a wide variety of injuries, from minor musculoskeletal pain to life-threatening trauma. The principles for providing medical care for athletes are the same whether the event is an Ironman or the local 5-km charity run. The medical care system at a sports event needs to be able to evaluate and treat injuries on site, to arrest the progression of serious injuries, to stabilize critical patients for transfer, and to minimize the impact of the event on the local emergency medical system (3). This chapter focuses on the special aspects of providing care for athletes. There is usually a separate medical team for spectators. If spectators are to be treated by the same medical staff, the medical staff will need to be larger and have more extensive supplies. Spectators present with a different spectrum of medical problems and tend to require more intensive care (1,4,5).

■ PLANNING

The medical director needs to design the medical care specifically for each sports event. The medical care system will need to manage a high volume of minor problems and yet still be able to quickly identify and treat life-threatening problems (2,5). Fortunately, serious problems, such as cardiac arrest and hyponatremia, are rare (6). The majority of injuries will be mild and self-limiting (7). For example, typical problems among athletes at the 1984 Olympics were minor musculoskeletal injuries, exercise-associated collapse, heat exhaustion, and dermatological complaints (4).

Different types of events will create different challenges for the medical team (8). Large venues, such as marathon courses, make it difficult to get medical personnel to injured athletes (9). Events that last over 4 hours have higher incidences of overhydration and hyponatremia (10). Extreme weather conditions increase the likelihood of injuries, and changing weather can create hazardous conditions in a short period of time. Courses that extend into remote areas tend to have poor access. High-speed events such as cycling, rollerblading, downhill skiing, or wheelchair races have the potential for life-threatening trauma and require the medical staff to be prepared to manage such injuries. Longer races have higher rates of injury but fewer entrants. Shorter races usually need less extensive medical care. However, catastrophic injuries can still happen even in shorter races, and there is a greater risk of heat illness with shorter, more intense events (2). Being prepared for all these tasks takes a significant amount of planning. Design of the medical system should begin months in advance of the competition.

The demographics of the athletes and their fitness levels will affect the injury rates. An event that encourages novices to participate requires special consideration as well. Novices often underestimate the amount of preparation they need, leaving them more prone to injuries and improper hydration (10). Smaller competitors, such as youth and women, are more at risk of developing hyponatremia and dehydration (6,11). Identifying the high-risk aspects of a particular competition will enable a physician to custom design an optimal medical care system.

■ SAFETY

Improving the safety of a competition involves more than just caring for injuries. Physicians can help race administration provide a safer event by considering factors such as the predicted weather, start times, and event regulations. Events should not be scheduled in extremely hot months, extremely humid months, or extremely cold months (12). If the date of the event cannot be moved to a safer season, the start time

should be moved to a safer time of day (3,7,12,13). In hot climates, start times should be scheduled for early in the day or in the evening. In cold climates, events should start midday. Event regulations can also increase athlete safety. For instance, requiring helmets for high-speed events in cycling and wheelchair races can decrease the incidence of serious head injuries (3). Other regulations, such as all medical personnel using universal precautions, can protect the volunteers as well as the athletes (12).

Course conditions need to be monitored during the event. The course may develop hazards such as dangerous water conditions in open water swims and poor traction in high-speed events. Changing environmental conditions can quickly create hazardous conditions for the athletes and volunteers (3). Temperature, humidity, and wind chill need to be monitored on site during the event because measurements made at a remote weather station may not reflect the conditions at the event (3,7,13,14). In cold weather, the wind chill dictates the risk of injury. The wind chill can be determined from the wind speed and the ambient temperature (12). Wind speeds can be estimated from observing the effect of the wind on nearby trees. If you can feel the wind on your face but trees are not moving, the wind speed is about 10 mph. If the small branches are moving, the wind speed is about 20 mph. Larger branches move at 30 mph, and entire trees will move in 40-mph winds (15). At 10°F and below, there is an increased chance of injury when the wind speed is 20 mph or greater. At −10°F, the likelihood of injury increases at wind speeds of 10 mph. There is a high likelihood of injury if the temperature is −20°F and the wind speed is over 30 mph (15).

Identifying the risk of injury in hot weather is best done using a wet bulb globe thermometer (WGBT) (12,13). WGBT readings take into account the combined effects of heat and humidity and thus are better indicators of environmental hazards than temperature alone **(Table 60-1)**. If a WGBT is not available, the risk of heat injury can be estimated using the local temperature and humidity readings and data published by the National Weather Service **(Table 60-2)** (16). If the risk of injury is high and the event cannot be rescheduled, the event can be modified to decrease the chance of heat injuries. For timed games, halftime can be increased, play times can be shortened, and more water breaks can be allowed (13,17). The game's regulations can be modified to allow unlimited substitutions during play (13). Arrangements can also be made to spray water on the athletes (13). As the risk of heat injury rises, more of these modifications should be used at the same time.

A cancellation policy for stopping or rescheduling the event should be developed and published in advance. Warm weather conditions posing high environmental risk for hyperthermia have been summarized by the American College of Sports Medicine (ACSM) (Table 60-1). Cross-country ski races should be canceled if the ambient temperature is below −4°F, even if there is no wind. This is because

TABLE 60-1	Risks of Environmental Injury	
Risk of Injury	**WBGT**	**Recommendations**
Moderate	<50°F	All participants at risk for hypothermia Very low risk for hyperthermia Windy, wet conditions increase risk of hypothermia
Low	50–65°F	Hyperthermia or hypothermia unlikely to occur
Moderate	65–73°F	Advise heat-sensitive participants to decrease intensity
High	73–82°F	All participants at risk for hyperthermia Advise heat-sensitive participants to withdraw
Extremely high	>82°F	Extreme risk for of hyperthermia for all participants Cancel, reschedule, or modify event if possible

Adapted from Armstrong LE, Epstein Y, Greenleaf JE, et al. American College of Sports Medicine position stand: heat and cold illnesses during distance running. *Med Sci Sports Exerc* 1996;28:i–x; and Elias SR, Roberts WO, Thorson DC. Team sports in hot weather: guidelines for modifying youth soccer. *Phys Sportsmed.* 1991;19:67–78.

TABLE 60-2	Estimating Heat Risk		
Humidity	**Moderate Risk**	**High Risk**	**Hazardous**
40%	90°F	100°F	110°F
50%	90°F	95°F	105°F
60%	85°F	95°F	105°F
70%	85°F	90°F	100°F
80% and up	85°F	90°F	95°F

National Weather Service. Heat Index. http://www.nws.noaa.gov/om/heat/index.shtml. Accessed October 10, 2006.

the wind chill generated by skiers moving at race speed creates a very high risk of cold injury (12). There should be a designated weather watcher to evaluate conditions as the day progresses. If hazardous conditions develop, the weather watcher must have the authority to stop the event.

Youth are at greater risk for heat collapse than adults. Youth do not tolerate the heat as well due to the fact that they do not sweat as much as adults and have less efficient body temperature control regulation. They also have a greater surface area to mass ratio, which causes them to gain proportionally more heat in a hot environment (18). It cannot be assumed that young athletes will understand how to pace themselves during activity in a hot and humid environment. Due to these factors, young athletes may need a modified cancellation policy (18).

A separate plan for lightning hazard must also be developed. The current recommendations are to stop the event for flash-to-bang times under 30 seconds and not to resume activity until 30 minutes after the last sighted lightning (19). Shelter for competitors in case of dangerous weather needs to be identified ahead of time.

■ ROUTE

The course itself will influence the types of injuries that occur and the ability of medical personnel to reach injured athletes. It needs to be closely inspected by the medical team before the event so that they can anticipate where problems may develop. Consideration needs to be given where injuries are most likely to happen, possible evacuation routes, and traffic and pedestrian control (3,5). Emergency vehicles will need routes to take medical staff to injured athletes and to take injured athletes to the local emergency room (1). Familiarity with the course will allow optimal placement of medical stations and ambulances. First aid stations need to be clearly identified and easily reached by medical staff and athletes. For road races, the main first aid station should be positioned adjacent to the finish line. For longer road races and large tournaments, multiple stations may be needed.

Some unique hazards may require additional attention (3,8). Large bodies of water may require spotters on the water (3). Triathlons need additional coverage in swim and transitions areas (20). Routes that include a downhill section increase the chances of wheelchair and cycling crashes (3). Fixed objects near high-speed courses need to be padded. These include telephone poles, trees, signs, and mail boxes. Cross-country ski courses and mountain bike courses often stretch through remote areas. Plans for getting emergency personnel to remote parts of the course need to be created ahead of time.

Athletes will need ready access to drinks during long events. Multiple hydration stations can be placed out on a course or at a tournament. Spacing of the stations should be such that athletes will have access to hydration every 15 to 20 minutes. For longer road events, specifically running events over 10 km, hydration stations need to be placed at the start and finish and approximately every 2 to 3 km along the course (12,21). These stations can be combined with the first aid stations (10). If a running course is shorter than 10 km, the drink station can be placed at the half-way point. If there are a large number of competitors, there may need to be more stations because large crowds can block access to the stations.

■ EQUIPMENT AND SUPPLIES

There is a standard set of equipment and supplies needed to provide general medical coverage for sports events **(Table 60-3)**. Additional supplies can be added for the specific range of injuries expected at each type of event. For instance, cycling races generate a significant number of abrasions and,

therefore, need a large supply of gauze pads and bandages. Suggestions of supplies for specific injuries are listed in **Table 60-4**. A particularly useful piece of equipment for endurance events is an iSTAT. An iSTAT can rapidly measure serum electrolytes and glucose on site. It can help differentiate between dehydration, hyponatremia, and hypoglycemia, conditions which have similar presentations (10).

The level of care to be provided on site must be decided well before the event (10). The presence of a critical care area and on-site triage significantly changes supply and ambulance needs. The budget for the medical system may limit the care that is provided on site. To keep costs down, some equipment can be borrowed. Often supplies can be borrowed from local

TABLE 60-3	Medical Supplies and Equipment

Equipment:

		Medications:
Alcohol pads	Oxygen	
Angiocath, 14 guage	Oral airways	Acetaminophen
Bandages and band-aids	Oral hydration fluids	Albuterol
Betadine swabs	Otoscope/ophthalmic scope	Afrin (for nose bleeds)
Blankets	Paper	Antihistamine
Blood pressure cuff	Patient instruction sheets	Aspirin
Buckets	Penlight	Dextrose
Cervical collar/spine board	Pens	Diazepam
Chairs	Pins	Epinephrine
Clipboards	Plastic bags	Glucagon
Cooler	Plastic wrap (to secure ice bags)	Magnesium sulfate
Cots	Pocket Venti-Mask	Morphine
Crutches	Pulse oximeter	Topical antibiotics
Cups	Protective equipment (gloves,	Toradol
Defibrillator	face shields)	ACLS medications
Elastic bandages	Razor, shaving cream	
Electrical source	Rectal thermometers	
Emesis basins	Reflex hammer	
Fans	Scalpel	
Gloves	Security fencing	
Glucometer	Sling	
Hand sanitizer	Steri-Strips/benzoin	
Heaters	Stethoscope	
Ice	Stretcher	
Intubation equipment	Spine board	
Immersion tubs	Splints	
iSTAT device	Suction device	
IV fluids	Tables	
IV starter kits	Tape	
Kling rolls	Tee shirts	
Knee immobilizer	Tongue depressors	
Nasal packing	Towels	
	Trauma shears	
	Wheelchair	

Adapted from Roberts WO. Mass-participation events. In: Lillegard WA, Butcher JD, Rucker KS, eds. *Handbook of sports medicine.* 2nd ed. Boston: Butterworth-Heinemann Publications; 1998:27–45; Cianca JC, Roberts WO, Horn D. Distance running: organizing of the medical team. In: O'Connor FG, Wilder RP, eds. *Text of running medicine.* New York: McGraw Hill; 2001:489–503; Roberts WO. Administration and medical management of mass participation endurance events. In: Mellion MB, Walsh WM, Madden C, et al, eds. *Team physician's handbook.* Philadelphia: Hanley & Belfus, Inc.; 2002:748–756; Armstrong LE, Epstein Y, Greenleaf JE, et al. American College of Sports Medicine position stand: heat and cold illnesses during distance running. *Med Sci Sports Exerc* 1996;28:i–x; Herring SA, Bergfeld JA, Boyajian-O'Neill LA, et al. Mass participation event management for the team physician: a consensus statement. http://www.newamssm.org/ MassParticipation.pdf. Accessed October 10, 2006; and Laird RH. Medical care at ultraendurance triathlons. *Med Sci Sports Exerc.* 1989;21:S222–S225.
IV, intravenous; ACLS, advanced cardiac life support.

TABLE 60-4	Supplies for Common Problems at Sporting Events
Injury	**Supplies**
Abrasions	Gauze pads, liquid soap, lidocaine solution, nonadhering dressings, Kerlex, tape, saline, and 50-cc syringe for irrigation
Asthma	Nebulizer or metered-dose inhaler albuterol, peak flow meter, pulse oximeter, stethoscope
Blisters	Moleskin, syringe, antibiotic ointment, band-aids
Chaffing	Petroleum jelly, band-aids
Cold injury	Warm shelter, blankets, dry clothes, rectal thermometer, heated fluids, heaters
Corneal abrasions	Blue light, fluorescein strips, eye pads
Contusion	Ice, plastic bags, plastic wrap to secure ice bags
Cramps	Oral fluids, intravenous (IV) diazepam (5 mg), IV magnesium (2–4 g)
Dehydration	Oral fluids, cots, iSTAT, IV fluids
Diabetes	Glucometer, glucose solutions
Exercise-associated collapse	Rectal thermometer, blood pressure cuff, cots, oral hydration fluids
Epistaxis	Afrin, 2 × 2 gauze pads or nasal packing
Heat illness	Rectal thermometer, ice, plastic bags, buckets, towels, cool fluids, fans, cots
Insect bites/stings	Epi-pens, topical Benadryl, oral antihistamine
Lacerations	Sterile instruments, sutures, syringes, sterile fields, sterile gloves, local anesthetic
Nausea, vomiting	Oral fluids, IV starter kit, IV fluids
Sprains	Ice, plastic bags, elastic bandages, splints, crutches, plastic wrap
Subungual hematomas	Syringe needle or hot cautery pen

Adapted from Herring SA, Bergfeld J, Boyd J, et al. Sideline preparedness for the team physician: a consensus statement. http://www.amssm.org/SidelinePrepare.html. Accessed October 10, 2006; Roberts WO. Exercise-associated collapse in endurance events: a classification system. *Phys Sportsmed.* 1989;17:49–55; Martinez JM, Laird R. Managing triathlon competition. *Curr Sports Med Rep.* 2003;2:142–146; Baker WM, Simone BM, Niemann JT, et al. Special event medical care: the 1984 Los Angeles summer Olympics experience. *Ann Emerg Med.* 1986; 15:185–190; Roberts WO. A 12 year profile of medical injury and illness for the Twin Cities Marathon. *Med Sci Sports Exerc.* 2000;32:1549–1555; and Cianca JC, Roberts WO, Horn D. Distance running: organizing of the medical team. In: O'Connor FG, Wilder RP, eds. *Text of running medicine.* New York: McGraw Hill; 2001:489–503.

organizations such as the National Guard, American Red Cross, Coast Guard, or the National Ski Patrol (12).

The medical stations will need to provide shelter from the environment. The main medical area can be placed in either a building or a tent **(Fig 60-1)**. For road races, this main medical station needs to be located adjacent to the finish area. For events such as soccer tournaments, consider a central location with good road access. There needs to be 250 to 1,500 square feet for each 1,000 participants (12). The main medical station should be stocked with the medical supplies listed in Table 60-3. Hazardous waste disposal and a sharps container will need to be provided. Include a portable toilet in medical area. Personal protective gear, such as gloves and eye protection, need to be readily available (25,26). Environmental conditions on race day will affect the needed supplies. Warmer weather means more heat-related injuries; usually this means

a greater need for cots, larger first aid areas, and more staff. Larger events will also need secondary stations spread across the course. Food and drinks need to be provided for the medical staff at each medical station. The entire medical staff will need distinctive clothing or hats so that they can be easily identified by other race volunteers and athletes (12).

The supplies at the hydration station depend on the nature of the event. Typically, athletes will need 6 to 12 oz of fluids every 20 to 30 minutes of activity and twice as much at the start and finish (12). For races that last less than 1 hour, water is usually sufficient for hydration. For longer events, electrolyte and water need to be available. In hot weather, the fluids should be cooled; in cold weather, they should be warmed. At each station, there should be 25% more cups available than participating athletes to allow for spillage (12).

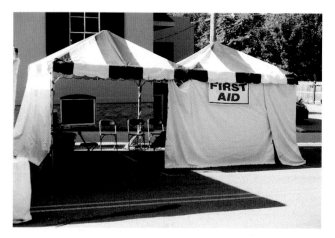

Fig 60-1. Medical stations need to be clearly identified and provide a protected and private area for treating injured athletes. Photo by Helen Iams.

■ MEDICAL STAFF

There will need to be one physician acting as the medical director. This person should be clearly identified early in the planning stages. It will be the medical director who organizes and supervises the medical operations during all phases of this process. The medical director has the final responsibility for all medical decisions, and if there is an adverse event, the medical director should be the medical spokesperson (3,12). The medical director is often so busy during the competition that he or she cannot actually provide medical care.

The medical director will need to recruit a variety of medical professionals. It is difficult to correctly predict how many health care professionals will be needed for a specific competition without previous experience. To estimate the size of the medical staff, first estimate the frequency and types of injuries that will occur. Using published injury rates, one can estimate injury rates for the event (1,2). Typically, endurance events have an injury rate of 5% (27). However, marathons and Ironmans have injury rates from 15% to 30% (27). Cycling races can have widely variable rates of injury, depending on the course, level of rider skill, and the weather conditions. This general injury estimate can then be modified for a specific event by considering the venue, type of activity, experience level of the athletes, and expected weather conditions.

ACSM has published general staffing recommendations for mass participation events (12). These recommendations are listed below. The numbers represent the number of professionals needed for each 1,000 competitors.

> Physicians: 1–2
> Podiatrists: 4–6
> Nurses: 2–4
> Physical therapists: 3–6
> Athletic trainers: 3–6
> Nonmedical assistants: 1–3
> Paramedics, emergency medical
technicians (EMTs): 1–4

The medical staff will often be treating injuries in less than optimal settings and sometimes under tight time constraints **(Fig 60-2)**. Therefore, the physicians staffing a sports event need to be experienced in managing the injuries that may be encountered. Typically, orthopaedic surgeons, family physicians, and emergency physicians are recruited. Podiatrists are especially helpful at running events such as marathons. There may be a need for rehabilitation specialists if wheelchair athletes are present (12). A variety of other professionals can be of great assistance in providing medical care at sports events. Physical therapists and athletic trainers are skilled in assessing injuries. They can work as mobile medical teams and assist in triage and in providing care in the medical tents. Chiropractors and massage therapists can also be helpful. Nonmedical volunteers can make operations in the medical tents more efficient. They can verify that documentation is filled out completely and run errands. After staffing a specific event for 2 to 3 years, more accurate projections for staffing needs can be made.

Ambulances and additional paramedics or EMTs are needed. There should be one ambulance for each 1,000 competitors (10). If an ambulance station is located near the race course, it may be possible to retain fewer ambulances for the race. However, another ambulance must be available if this ambulance is transporting an athlete to the local emergency room. Shorter courses may only need one ambulance at the

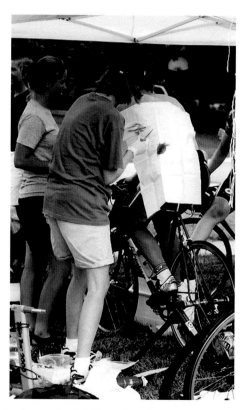

Fig 60-2. The medical staff needs to be prepared to treat a wide variety of injuries under less than optimal conditions. Photo by Paul Michna.

finish. Paramedics and EMTs should also be stationed along the course. Paramedics and EMTs can be recruited from local services such as local police and fire departments (12).

◼ LIABILITY

Liability coverage is always an issue for medical professionals. Ideally, the race administration will provide medical liability for all the medical volunteers. However, the administration may not have the financial resources to provide this coverage. Physicians need to carefully review their liability coverage before becoming involved. Some states have Good Samaritan laws with provisions that cover physicians volunteering at sporting events. However, not all states have these provisions. In this case, physicians will need to be sure that their personal malpractice insurance covers these activities (10,12,28).

◼ ORGANIZING THE MEDICAL STAFF

At endurance races, the majority of injured competitors will manage to finish the race but then immediately seek medical assistance. Therefore, most of the medical staff should be assigned to the finish area (12,20). The finish area staff should include physicians, nurses, athletic trainers, and physical therapists. A triage team should be organized to mingle among the finished racers looking for athletes on the verge of collapse. A suggested triage staff for a marathon would be one physician and 10 to 15 assistants (12). Nurses are ideal assistants for a triage team (29). Because cardiac arrests can happen, an arrest team should be identified ahead of time. The medical stations positioned along the race course should be staffed with a physician and a few medical assistants, such as athletic trainers, EMTs, and nurses. Ambulances should be stationed both at the main first aid tent and on the course. Generally, one ambulance for each 3,000 participants should be stationed at the finish line, and the remaining ambulances can be evenly distributed on the course (12).

Longer races will need a mobile medical staff. Depending on the type of race, mobile medical teams can be in automobiles or on bicycles. The mobile medical teams need to able to provide first aid and defibrillation. Paramedics and EMTs often make up the mobile teams. Automobile units on the course should be stocked with ice, towels, blood pressure cuff, intravenous fluids, a medical kit, an automatic external defibrillator (AED), blankets, oral rehydration fluids, and cups (12). Bicycle units should carry basic first aid equipment and an AED. Mobile units can initially be spaced throughout the race course (20). The medical staff can then be moved as the race progresses to provide optimal coverage (20). Arrangements need to be made to transport all competitors who are not able to finish the event (1,10). A final sweep vehicle needs to drive the course after it is closed to pick up any remaining athletes (12).

◼ PROTOCOLS

Developing medical care protocols can save time and confusion when an athlete presents with a serious problem. The protocols must be simple and not exceed the capabilities of the medical staff present. Specific protocols should be developed for commonly seen problems, such as asthma, exercise-associated collapse (30,31), hypoglycemia, and heat illness (11,21,30–33). Protocols should also be developed for rare but life-threatening issues, such as anaphylaxis, cardiac arrest (34–36), and hyponatremia (6,30,33,37,38). There must be provisions to protect the athletes' privacy, per Health Information Privacy Practice Act regulations (3,10). There may be instances when the ambulance should go directly to the local emergency room from the course, and a protocol should address these cases. The medical director should schedule staff meetings before the race to review all the protocols.

Medical personnel must have authority to assess athletes that they think are on the brink of collapse (12,22,32). The medical staff may wish to limit participation of an athlete about whom they have a concern (22). There need to be specific criteria for the medical staff to use to determine who can safely return to competition (22). Athletes need to know that the medical staff has this authority. At the same time, the staff needs to be sensitive to the implications of stopping competitors to examine them. The medical staff should be sufficiently aware of event regulations so that they do not accidentally disqualify an athlete in this way. It is helpful to publish the return to play criteria in advance (3,22). Other volunteers and course marshals need to know that medical staff have unlimited access to athletes and to all venues.

◼ COMMUNICATION

Having a smoothly running event requires close coordination between the medical staff, the security personnel, the emergency medical personnel, and the event administration (1). Effective communication needs to be established early (10). The medical director will need to be in contact with the race administration during the planning stages as well as on race day. The local emergency room needs to have advance notice of the date of the event and the expected injury rates. This will allow them to arrange for adequate staff on the day of the competition. When an injured athlete is being transferred to the local emergency room, the emergency room staff will need to be contacted directly to ensure safe transfer of care.

During the race, medical personnel need a simple means for reaching the medical director or dispatching ambulances to injured athletes on the course (1). Cell phones are a good option (12). However, there is always the problem of inadequate cell phone coverage, and providing cell phones can be expensive. A series of hand-held radios is an efficient means of communicating (12). A command center should be created where all race-day communication can be monitored. This center should be based in the main first aid area.

An ideal set-up for a command center is a main radio and a dedicated radio operator. The command center should have the phone numbers for the ambulances and the local emergency room. It is prudent to arrange for a hard-line phone in the main medical tent since radios and cell phones can fail. Communication should also be established with nonmedical volunteers and course marshals. This can make movement of medical personnel and injured athletes much easier.

Athletes need to be informed about the risks of participation, the environmental conditions that are expected, and the specific dangers on the course (3,12). It is important to begin communicating with the athletes well before the competition. They should also be provided with a description of the level of fitness needed to complete the event as well as information about overhydration, underhydration, and prevention strategies for these conditions (6). Athletes should be instructed to record important medical information, such as their name, contact information, and any medical problems, on the back of their race number (10,12). Athletes should also be advised to wear medical alert bracelets (3). Finally, the competitors need to know what medical services will be available and how to identify medical personnel. All of this can be accomplished by including medical information in registration packets, by posting the information on the event website, or by presenting it at a pre-event exposition (10).

On the day of the competition, communication with the athletes begins with a pre-race announcement by the medical director. This announcement should reiterate a description of the course hazards, locations of medical services, and cautions about pitfalls such as overhydrating or underhydrating (10,12). This announcement should also state the time at which services will stop being provided on the course. Athletes should be encouraged to get help for any participants who look ill. Plans need to be made to efficiently communicate weather hazards to athletes during the competition. Warning signs can be posted at hydration stations, and announcements can be made on the course. The ACSM has developed a flag system for communicating the risk of hyperthermia to competing athletes: black for extreme risk, red for high risk, yellow for moderate risk, green for low risk, and white for very low risk. Athletes will need to be notified of the significance of the flags in the pre-race literature. These flags can be posted throughout the course and be changed as weather conditions change during the event (12).

EVENT SET-UP

As soon as the course is secured, the first aid stations can be set up. Ideally, this will be the day before the race (10). The main first aid tent can be divided into minor care areas and critical care areas. Place an ambulance immediately adjacent to the critical care area (10). During the event, access to the medical stations should be restricted to only medical personnel and injured athletes. This restricted access will increase the efficiency of the medical care, promote confidentiality,

and aid in the control of hazardous wastes (10,12). This limited access should be enforced by security guards. Nonmedical staff at the first aid tent can provide information to family members about injured athletes.

There needs to be documentation of the medical care given during the event. The documentation can be simple and still contain the important data. For tracking purposes, the chart should include the competitor's name and race number. There should be a brief medical history and pertinent exam. The time the patient entered the tent and the time the athlete was discharged should also be recorded. All treatments should be recorded. The final diagnosis should be indicated as well as the disposition (20). A checklist of common findings and treatments can make completing the paperwork simpler and faster. Nonmedical volunteers can see that the records are completed before the athlete leaves the medical area.

POSTEVENT ANALYSIS

A postevent evaluation should be completed in the weeks following a race. This is an important step in improving the care for future events. The medical director should specifically review the strengths and weaknesses of the medical care provided, including an evaluation of the adequacy of the size of the staff and any problems that occurred. The findings should be summarized in a report that clarifies the problems and suggests solutions. By recalling what went well and what did not, the medical director will be able to make specific suggestions to improve the medical coverage.

SUMMARY

The variety and volume of injuries seen at mass participation sports events creates unique challenges not often seen outside an emergency room. An on-site medical team can greatly improve the safety of a sports event. Optimal care requires a comprehensive medical system, coordinated activities of a variety of medical professionals, and well-designed medical protocols. The key to having a smoothly running event is to begin planning months ahead of time. These activities take a significant investment of time and energy, often for no compensation besides a new tee shirt. However, providing care at sports events is tremendously rewarding and intellectually challenging, and it adds a new dimension to a physician's practice.

ACKNOWLEDGEMENT

Helen D. Iams is indebted to Barbara Fortune, a University of Wyoming librarian, for securing a large number of articles in a short period of time.

■ REFERENCES

1. Sanders AB, Criss E, Steckl P, et al. An analysis of medical care at mass gatherings. *Ann Emerg Med.* 1986;15:515–519.
2. Roberts WO. Mass-participation events. In: Lillegard WA, Butcher JD, Rucker KS, eds. *Handbook of sports medicine.* 2nd ed. Boston: Butterworth-Heinemann Publications; 1998:27–45.
3. Roberts WO. Administration and medical management of mass participation endurance events. In: Mellion MB, Walsh WM, Madden C, et al., eds. *Team physician's handbook.* Philadelphia: Hanley & Belfus, Inc.; 2002:748–756.
4. Baker WM, Simone BM, Niemann JT, et al. Special event medical care: the 1984 Los Angeles summer Olympics experience. *Ann Emerg Med.* 1986;15:185–190.
5. Michael JA, Barbera JA. Mass gathering medical care: a twenty-five year review. *Prehospital Disaster Med.* 1997;12:305–312.
6. Stuempfle KJ, Lehmann DR, Case HS, et al. Hyponatremia in a cold weather ultraendurance race. *Alaska Med.* 2002;44:51–62.
7. Roberts WO. A 12-year profile of medical injury and illness for the Twin Cities Marathon. *Med Sci Sports Exerc.* 2000;32:1549–1555.
8. Young C. Extreme sports: injuries and medical coverage. *Curr Sports Med Rep.* 2002;1:306–311.
9. DeLorenzo RA. Mass gathering medicine: a review. *Prehospital Disaster Med.* 1997;12:68–72.
10. Cianca JC, Roberts WO, Horn D. Distance running: organizing of the medical team. In: O'Connor FG, Wilder RP, eds. *Text of running medicine.* New York: McGraw Hill; 2001:489–503.
11. White JA, Pomfret D. Fluid replacement needs of well-trained male and female athletes during indoor and outdoor steady state running. *J Sci Med Sport.* 1998;1:131–142.
12. Armstrong LE, Epstein Y, Greenleaf JE, et al. American College of Sports Medicine position stand: heat and cold illnesses during distance running. *Med Sci Sports Exerc* 1996;28:i–x.
13. Elias SR, Roberts WO, Thorson DC. Team sports in hot weather: guidelines for modifying youth soccer. *Phys Sportsmed.* 1991;19:67–78.
14. Pearlmutter EM. The Pittsburgh Marathon: playing weather roulette. *Phys Sportsmed.* 1986;14:132–138.
15. Bangs CC, Boswick JA, Hamlet MP, et al. When your patient suffers frostbite. *Patient Care.* 1977;12:132–157.
16. National Weather Service. Heat Index. http://www.nws.noaa.gov/om/heat/index.shtml. Accessed October 10, 2006.
17. Sparling PB, Millard-Stafford M. Keeping sports participants safe in hot weather. *Phys Sportsmed.* 1999;27:27–34.
18. Bar-Or O. Climate and the exercising child: a review. *Int J Sports Med.* 1980;1:53.
19. Makdissi M, Brukner P. Recommendations for lightning protection in sport. *Med J Aust.* 2002;177:35–37.
20. Martinez JM, Laird R. Managing triathlon competition. *Curr Sports Med Rep.* 2003;2:142–146.
21. Casa DJ, Armstrong LE, Hillman SK, et al. National Athletic Trainers' Association position statement: fluid replacement for athletes. *J Athl Train.* 2000;35:212–224.
22. Herring SA, Bergfeld JA, Boyajian-O'Neill LA, et al. Mass participation event management for the team physician: a consensus statement. http://www.newamssm.org/MassParticipation.pdf. Accessed October 10, 2006.
23. Laird RH. Medical care at ultraendurance triathlons. *Med Sci Sports Exerc.* 1989;21:S222–S225.
24. Herring SA, Bergfeld J, Boyd J, et al. Sideline preparedness for the team physician: a consensus statement. http://www.amssm.org/SidelinePrepare.html. Accessed October 10, 2006.
25. American Academy of Pediatrics Committee on Sports Medicine and Fitness. Human immunodeficiency virus [acquired immunodeficiency syndrome (AIDS) virus] in the athletic setting. *Pediatrics.* 1991;88:640–641.
26. Becker KM, Moe CL, Southwick KL, et al. Transmission of Norwalk virus during a football game. *N Engl J Med.* 2000;343:1223–1227.
27. Jones BH, Roberts WO. Medical management of endurance events. In: Cantu RC, Micheli LJ, eds. *ACSM: Guidelines for the team physician.* Philadelphia: Lea and Febiger; 1991:266–286.
28. Parrillo SJ. Medical care at mass gatherings: considerations for physician involvement. *Prehospital Disaster Med.* 1995;10:273–275.
29. Thompson JM, Savoia G, Powell G, et al. Level of medical care required for mass gatherings: the XV Winter Olympic Games in Calgary, Canada. *Ann Emerg Med.* 1991;10:385–390.
30. Mayers LB, Noakes TD. A guide to treating Ironman triathletes at the finish line. *Phys Sportsmed.* 2000;28:8.
31. Roberts WO. Exercise-associated collapse in endurance events: a classification system. *Phys Sportsmed.* 1989;17:49–55.
32. Binkley HM, Beckett J, Casa DJ, et al. National Athletic Trainers' Association position statement: exertional heat illness. *J Athl Train.* 2002;37:329–343.
33. Speedy DB, Noakes TD, Kimber NE, et al. Fluid balance during and after an Ironman triathlon. *Clin J Sports Med.* 2001;11:44–50.
34. Thompson PD. The cardiovascular complications of vigorous physical activity. *Arch Intern Med.* 1996;156:2297–2302.
35. O'Connor FG, Kugler JP, Oriscello RG. Sudden death in young athletes: screening for the needle in the haystack. *Am Fam Physician.* 1998;57:2763–2770.
36. Johnson RJ. Sudden death during exercise. *Postgrad Med.* 1992;92:195–206.
37. Flinn SD, Sherer RJ. Seizure after exercise in the heat: recognizing life-threatening hyponatremia. *Phys Sportsmed.* 2000;28:9.
38. Hsieh M. Recommendations for treatment of hyponatremia at endurance events. *Sports Med.* 2004;34:231–238.
39. Wetterhall SF, Coulombier DM, Herndon JM, et al. Medical care delivery at the 1996 Olympic Games. *JAMA.* 1998;279:1463–1468.
40. American College of Sports Medicine. ACSM Position Stand: the prevention of thermal injuries during distance running. *Med Sci Sports.* 1987;19:529–533.

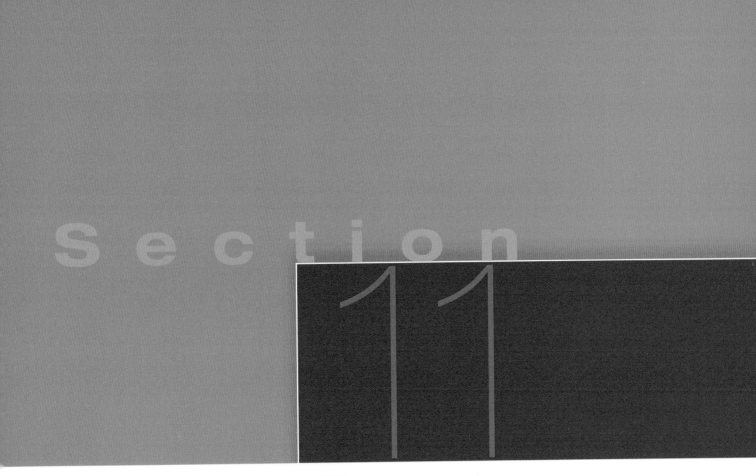

Section

11

APPENDICES

TEAM PHYSICIAN CONSENSUS STATEMENT

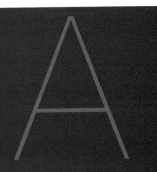

■ SUMMARY

The objective of the Team Physician Consensus Statement is to provide physicians, school administrators, team owners, the general public, and individuals who are responsible for making decisions regarding the medical care of athletes and teams with guidelines for choosing a qualified team physician and an outline of the duties expected of a team physician. Ultimately, by educating decision makers about the need for a qualified team physician, the goal is to ensure that athletes and teams are provided the very best medical care.

The Consensus Statement was developed by the collaboration of six major professional associations concerned about clinical sports medicine issues: American Academy of Family Physicians, American Academy of Orthopaedic Surgeons, American College of Sports Medicine, American Medical Society for Sports Medicine, American Orthopaedic Society for Sports Medicine, and the American Osteopathic Academy of Sports Medicine. These organizations have committed to forming an ongoing project-based alliance to "bring together sports medicine organizations to best serve active people and athletes."

This statement is not intended as a standard of care and should not be interpreted as such. It is only a guide and, as such, is of a general nature consistent with the reasonable, objective practice of health care.

Expert Panel

Stanley A. Herring, MD, Chair, Seattle, Washington
John A. Bergfeld, MD, Cleveland, Ohio
Joel Boyd, MD, Edina, Minnesota
William G. Clancy, Jr, MD, Birmingham, Alabama
H. Royer Collins, MD, Phoenix, Arizona
Brian C. Halpern, MD, Marlboro, New Jersey
Rebecca Jaffe, MD, Chadds Ford, Pennsylvania
W. Ben Kibler, MD, Lexington, Kentucky
E. Lee Rice, DO, San Diego, California
David C. Thorson, MD, White Bear Lake, Minnesota

■ TEAM PHYSICIAN DEFINITION

The team physician must have an unrestricted medical license and be an MD or DO who is responsible for treating and coordinating the medical care of athletic team members. The principal responsibility of the team physician is to provide for the well-being of individual athletes, enabling each to realize his/her full potential. The team physician should possess special proficiency in the care of musculoskeletal injuries and medical conditions encountered in sports. The team physician also must actively integrate medical expertise with other health care providers, including medical specialists, athletic trainers, and allied health professionals. The team physician must ultimately assume responsibility within the team structure for making medical decisions that affect the athlete's safe participation.

■ QUALIFICATIONS OF A TEAM PHYSICIAN

The primary concern of the team physician is to provide the best medical care for athletes at all levels of participation. To this end, the following qualifications are necessary for all team physicians:

- Have an MD or DO in good standing, with an unrestricted license to practice medicine
- Possess a fundamental knowledge of emergency care regarding sporting events
- Be trained in CPR
- Have a working knowledge of trauma, musculoskeletal injuries, and medical conditions affecting the athlete

In addition, it is desirable for team physicians to have clinical training/experience and administrative skills in some or all of the following:

- Specialty Board certification
- Continuing medical education in sports medicine
- Formal training in sports medicine (fellowship training, board-recognized subspecialty in sports medicine [formerly known as a certificate of added qualification in sports medicine])
- Additional training in sports medicine

- Fifty percent or more of practice involving sports medicine
- Membership and participation in a sports medicine society
- Involvement in teaching, research, and publications relating to sports medicine
- Training in advanced cardiac life support
- Knowledge of medical/legal, disability, and workers' compensation issues
- Media skills training

■ DUTIES OF A TEAM PHYSICIAN

The team physician must be willing to commit the necessary time and effort to provide care to the athlete and team. In addition, the team physician must develop and maintain a current, appropriate knowledge base of the sport(s) for which he/she is accepting responsibility.

The duties for which the team physician has ultimate responsibility include the following.

Medical Management of the Athlete

- Coordinate preparticipation screening, examination, and evaluation
- Manage injuries on the field
- Provide for medical management of injury and illness
- Coordinate rehabilitation and return to participation
- Provide for proper preparation for safe return to participation after an illness or injury
- Integrate medical expertise with other health care providers, including medical specialists, athletic trainers, and allied health professionals
- Provide for appropriate education and counseling regarding nutrition, strength and conditioning, ergogenic aids, substance abuse, and other medical problems that could affect the athlete
- Provide for proper documentation and medical record keeping

Administrative and Logistical Duties

- Establish and define the relationships of all involved parties
- Educate athletes, parents, administrators, coaches, and other necessary parties of concerns regarding the athletes
- Develop a chain of command
- Plan and train for emergencies during competition and practice
- Address equipment and supply issues
- Provide for proper event coverage
- Assess environmental concerns and playing conditions

■ EDUCATION OF A TEAM PHYSICIAN

Ongoing education pertinent to the team physician is essential. Currently, there are several state, regional, and national stand-alone courses for team physician education. There are also many other resources available. Information regarding team physician–specific educational opportunities can be obtained from the organizations listed to the right.

Team physician education is also available from other sources such as: sport-specific (*e.g.,* National Football League Team Physician's Society) or level-specific (*e.g.,* United States Olympic Committee) meetings; National Governing Bodies' (NGB) meetings; state and/or county medical societies meetings; professional journals; and other relevant electronic media (Web sites, CD-ROMs).

■ CONCLUSION

This Consensus Statement establishes a definition of the team physician and outlines a team physician's qualifications, duties, and responsibilities. It also contains strategies for the continuing education of team physicians. Ultimately, this statement provides guidelines that best serve the health care needs of athletes and teams.

■ RESOURCES

 American Academy of Family Physicians (AAFP) 11400 Tomahawk Creek Pkwy. Leawood, KS 66211-2672 1-800-274-2237; www.aafp.org

 American Academy of Orthopaedic Surgeons (AAOS) 6300 N. River Rd. Rosemont, IL 60018 1-800-346-AAOS; www.aaos.org

 American College of Sports Medicine (ACSM) 401 W. Michigan St. Indianapolis, IN 46202-3233 (317) 637-9200; www.acsm.org

 American Medical Society for Sports Medicine (AMSSM) 11639 Earnshaw Overland Park, KS 66210 (913) 327-1415; www.amssm.org

 American Orthopaedic Society for Sports Medicine (AOSSM) 6300 N. River Rd., Suite 200 Rosemont, IL 60018 (847) 292-4900; www.sportsmed.org

 American Osteopathic Academy of Sports Medicine (AOASM) 7611 Elmwood Ave., Suite 201 Middleton, WI 53562 (608) 831-4400; www.aoasm.org

Endorsed by:

American Academy of Podiatric Sports Medicine (AAPSM); www.aapsm.org
American Academy of Physical Medicine and Rehabilitation (AAPMR); www.aapmr.org
American Kinesiotherapy Association (AKA); www.akta.org

American Osteopathic Association (AOA); www.aoa-net.org

American Physical Therapy Association (APTA); www.spts.org

National Athletic Trainers Association (NATA); www.nata.org

National Strength and Conditioning Association (NSCA); www.nsca-lift.org

National Youth Sports Safety Foundation, Inc. (NYSSFI); www.nyssf.org

North American Spine Society (NASS); www.spine.org

Physiatric Association of Spine, Sports and Occupational Rehabilitation (PASSOR); www.aapmr.org/passor.htm

Supported by an unrestricted educational grant from Knoll Pharmaceuticals

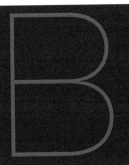

SUMMARY

The objective of the Sideline Preparedness Statement is to provide physicians who are responsible for making decisions regarding the medical care of athletes with guidelines for identifying and planning for medical care and services at the site of practice or competition. It is not intended as a standard of care and should not be interpreted as such. The Sideline Preparedness Statement is only a guide and, as such, is of a general nature, consistent with the reasonable, objective practice of the health care professional. Individual treatment will turn on the specific facts and circumstances presented to the physician at the event. Adequate insurance should be in place to help protect the physician, the athlete, and the sponsoring organization.

The Sideline Preparedness Statement was developed by a collaboration of six major professional associations concerned about clinical sports medicine issues; they have committed to forming an ongoing project-based alliance to "bring together sports medicine organizations to best serve active people and athletes." The organizations are: American Academy of Family Physicians, American Academy of Orthopaedic Surgeons, American College of Sports Medicine, American Medical Society for Sports Medicine, American Orthopaedic Society for Sports Medicine, and the American Osteopathic Academy of Sports Medicine.

CONSENSUS STATEMENT

Definition

Sideline preparedness is the identification of and planning for medical services to promote the safety of the athlete, to limit injury, and to provide medical care at the site of practice or competition.

Goal

The safety and on-site medical care of the athlete is the goal of sideline preparedness. To accomplish this goal, the team physician should be actively involved in developing an integrated medical system that includes:

- Preseason planning
- Game-day planning
- Postseason evaluation

PRESEASON PLANNING

Preseason planning promotes safety and minimizes problems associated with athletic participation at the site of practice or competition.

The team physician should coordinate:

- Development of policy to address preseason planning and the preparticipation evaluation of athletes
- Participation of the administration and other key personnel in medical issues
- Implementation strategies

Medical Protocol Development

It is essential that:

- Prospective athletes complete a preparticipation evaluation

In addition, it is desirable that:

- The preparticipation evaluation be performed by an MD or DO in good standing with an unrestricted license to practice medicine
- A comprehensive preparticipation evaluation form be used (e.g., the form found in the current edition of *Pre-Participation Physical Evaluation*)
- The team physician has access to all preparticipation evaluation forms
- The team physician review all preparticipation evaluation forms and determine eligibility of the athlete to participate
- Timely preparticipation evaluations be performed to permit the identification and treatment of injuries and medical conditions

Administrative Protocol Development

It is essential for the team physician to coordinate:

- Development of a chain of command that establishes and defines the responsibilities of all parties involved
- Establishment of an emergency response plan for practice and competition
- Compliance with Occupational Safety and Health Administration (OSHA) standards relevant to the medical care of the athlete
- Establishment of a policy to assess environmental concerns and playing conditions for modification or suspension of practice or competition
- Compliance with all local, state, and federal regulations regarding storing and dispensing pharmaceuticals
- Establishment of a plan to provide for proper documentation and medical record keeping

In addition, it is desirable for the team physician to coordinate:

- Regular rehearsal of the emergency response plan
- Establishment of a network with other health care providers, including medical specialists, athletic trainers, and allied health professionals
- Establishment of a policy that includes the team physician in the dissemination of any information regarding the athlete's health
- Preparation of a letter of understanding between the team physician and the administration that defines the obligations and responsibilities of the team physician

■ GAME-DAY PLANNING

Game-day planning optimizes medical care for injured or ill athletes.

The team physician should coordinate:

- Game-day medical operations
- Game-day administrative medical policies
- Preparation of the sideline "medical bag" and sideline medical supplies

Medical Protocol

It is essential for the team physician to coordinate:

- Determination of final clearance status of injured or ill athletes on game day prior to competition
- Assessment and management of game-day injuries and medical problems
- Determination of athletes' same-game return to participation after injury or illness
- Follow-up care and instructions for athletes who require treatment during or after competition
- Notifying the appropriate parties about an athlete's injury or illness

- Close observation of the game by the medical team from an appropriate location
- Provision for proper documentation and medical record keeping

In addition, it is desirable for the team physician to coordinate:

- Monitoring of equipment safety and fit
- Monitoring of postgame referral care of injured or ill athletes

Administrative Protocol

It is essential for the team physician to coordinate:

- Assessment of environmental concerns and playing conditions
- Presence of medical personnel at the competition site with sufficient time for all pregame preparations, and plan with medical staff of the opposing team for medical care of the athletes
- Introductions of the medical teams to game officials
- Review of the emergency response plan
- Checking and confirmation of communication equipment
- Identification of examination and treatment sites

In addition, it is desirable for the team physician to coordinate:

- Arrangements for the medical staff to have convenient access to the competition site
- A postgame review, and make necessary modifications of medical and administrative protocols

On-site Medical Supplies

The team physician should have a game-day sideline "medical bag" and sideline medical supplies. The following tables are lists of "medical bag" items and medical supplies for contact/collision and high-risk sports. Lightly shaded items are highly desirable; darker shaded items are desirable.

There are many different sports, levels of competition, and available medical resources that must all be considered when determining the on-site medical bag and sideline medical supplies.

■ POSTSEASON EVALUATION

Postseason evaluation of sideline coverage optimizes the medical care of injured or ill athletes and promotes continued improvement of medical services for future seasons.

The team physician should coordinate:

- Summarization of injuries and illnesses that occurred during the season
- Improvement of the medical and administrative protocols
- Implementation strategies to improve sideline preparedness

On-site Medical Bag

General	Cardiopulmonary	Head and Neck/Neurological
Alcohol swabs and povidone iodine swabs	Airway	Dental kit (e.g., cyanoacrylate, Hank's solution)
Bandage scissors	Blood pressure cuff	Eye kit (e.g., blue light, fluorescein stain strips, eye patch pads, cotton tip applicators, ocular anesthetic and antibiotics, contact remover, mirror)
Bandages: sterile/nonsterile, band-aids	Cricothyrotomy kit	Flashlight
Dextrose (50%) in water solution	Epinephrine 1:1,000 in a prepackaged unit	Pin or other sharp object for sensory testing
Disinfectant	Mouth-to-mouth mask	Reflex hammer
Gloves: sterile/nonsterile	Short-acting beta-agonist inhaler	
Large-bore angiocath for tension pneumothorax (14–16 gauge)	Stethoscope	
Local anesthetic/syringes/needles		
Paper and pen		
Sharps box and red bag		
Suture set/steri-strips		
Wound irrigation materials (e.g., sterile normal saline, 10–50 cc syringe)		
Benzoin	Advanced cardiac life support (ACLS) drugs and equipment	
Blister care materials	Intravenous fluids and administration set	
Contact lens case and solution	Tourniquet	
30% Ferric subsulfate solution (e.g., Monsel's for cauterizing abrasions and cuts)		
Injury and illness care instruction sheets for the patient		
List of emergency phone numbers		
Nail clippers		
Nasal packing materials		
Oto-ophthalmoscope		
Paper bags (for treatment of hyperventilation)		
Prescription pad		
Razor and shaving cream		
Rectal thermometer		
Scalpel		
Skin lubricant		
Skin staple applicator		
Small mirror		
Supplemental oral and parenteral medications		
Tongue depressors		
Topical antibiotics		

Sideline Medical Supplies		
General	**Cardiopulmonary**	**Head and Neck/Neurological**
Access to a telephone		Face mask removal tool *(for sports with helmets)*
Extremity splints		Semi-rigid cervical collar
Ice		Spine board and attachments
Oral fluid replacement		
Plastic bags		
Sling		
Blanket	Automated external defibrillator	Sideline concussion assessment protocol
Crutches		
Mouth guards		
Sling psychrometer and temperature/humidity activity risk chart		
Tape cutter		

Medical Protocol

It is essential for the team physician to coordinate:

- A postseason meeting with appropriate team personnel and administration to review the previous season
- Identification of athletes who require postseason care of injury or illness and encourage follow-up

In addition it is desirable for the team physician to coordinate:

- Monitoring of the health status of the injured or ill athlete
- Postseason physicals
- Off-season conditioning program

Administrative Protocol

It is essential for the team physician to coordinate:

- Review and modification of current medical and administrative protocols

In addition, it is desirable for the team physician to coordinate:

- Compilation of injury and illness data

■ CONCLUSION

This consensus statement outlines the essential and desirable components of sideline preparedness for the team physician to promote the safety of the athlete, to limit injury, and to provide medical care at the site of practice or competition. This statement was developed with the collaboration of six major professional associations concerned about clinical sports medicine issues: American Academy of Family Physicians, American Academy of Orthopaedic Surgeons, American College of Sports Medicine, American Medical Society for Sports Medicine, American Orthopaedic Society for Sports Medicine, and the American Osteopathic Academy of Sports Medicine.

Expert Panel

Stanley A. Herring, MD (Chair), Seattle, Washington
John Bergfeld, MD, Cleveland, Ohio
Joel Boyd, MD, Edina, Minnesota
Per Gunnar Brolinson, DO, Toledo, Ohio
Timothy Duffey, DO, Columbus, Ohio
David Glover, MD, Warrensburg, Mississippi
William A. Grana, MD, Oklahoma City, Oklahoma
Brian C. Halpern, MD, Marlboro, New Jersey
Peter Indelicato, MD, Gainesville, Florida
W. Ben Kibler, MD, Lexington, Kentucky
E. Lee Rice, DO, San Diego, California
William O. Roberts, MD, White Bear Lake, Minnesota

Resources

Ongoing education pertinent to the team physician is essential. Information regarding team physician specific educational opportunities can be obtained from the six participating organizations:

American Academy of Family Physicians
11400 Tomahawk Creek Parkway
Leawood, KS 66211-2672
(800)274-2237;
www.aafp.org

American Academy of Orthopaedic Surgeons
6300 North River Road
Rosemont, IL 60018
(800)346-AAOS; www.aaos.org

American Orthopaedic Society for Sports Medicine
6300 North River Road, Suite 200
Rosemont, IL 60018
(847)292-4900; www.sportsmed.org

American College of Sports Medicine
401 West Michigan Street
Indianapolis, IN 46202
(317)637-9200; www.acsm.org

American Medical Society for Sports Medicine
11639 Earnshaw
Overland Park, KS 66210
(913)327-1415; www.amssm.org

American Osteopathic Academy of Sports Medicine
7611 Elmwood Avenue, Suite 201
Middleton, WI 53562
(608)831-4400; www.aoasm.org

THE TEAM PHYSICIAN AND CONDITIONING OF ATHLETES FOR SPORTS: A CONSENSUS STATEMENT

SUMMARY

The objective of this Consensus Statement is to provide physicians who are responsible for the health care of teams with guidelines regarding conditioning for sports. This statement specifically addresses the role of exercise in conditioning. Nutrition and supplements are outside the scope of this statement. It is not intended as a standard of care and should not be interpreted as such. This statement is only a guide and, as such, is of a general nature, consistent with reasonable, objective practice of the health care professional. Individual conditioning issues will depend on the specific facts and circumstances presented to the physician.

Adequate insurance should be in place to help protect the athlete, the sponsoring organization, and the physician.

This Statement was developed by a collaboration of six major professional associations concerned with clinical sports medicine issues; they have committed to forming an ongoing project-based alliance to bring together sports medicine organizations to best serve active people and athletes. The organizations are: American Academy of Family Physicians, American Academy of Orthopaedic Surgeons, American College of Sports Medicine, American Medical Society for Sports Medicine, American Orthopaedic Society for Sports Medicine, and the American Osteopathic Academy of Sports Medicine.

Expert Panel

Stanley A. Herring, MD, Chair, Seattle, Washington
John A. Bergfeld, MD, Cleveland, Ohio
Joel L.Boyd, MD, Edina, Minnesota
Per Gunnar Brolinson, DO, Toledo, Ohio
Cindy J. Chang, MD, Berkeley, California
David W. Glover, MD, Warrensburg, Missouri
William A. Grana, MD, Tucson, Arizona
Peter Indelicato, MD, Gainesville, Florida
Robert J. Johnson, MD, Minneapolis, Minnesota
W. Ben Kibler, MD, Lexington, Kentucky
William J. Kraemer, PhD, CSCS, Muncie, Indiana

Joseph P. McNerney, DO, Vallejo, California
Robert M. Pallay, MD, Hillsborough, New Jersey
Jeffrey L. Tanji, MD, Sacramento, California

DEFINITION

Conditioning is a process in which stimuli are created by an exercise program performed by the athlete to produce a higher level of function.

GOAL

The goal of conditioning is to optimize the performance of the athlete and minimize the risk of injury and illness.

To accomplish this goal, the team physician should have knowledge of and be involved with:

- General conditioning principles
- Preseason issues
- In-season issues
- Off-season issues
- Available resources

GENERAL CONDITIONING PRINCIPLES

Specificity

Training adaptations are specific to the nature of the exercise stimulus (*e.g.*, muscle contraction type, mechanics, metabolic demand). Athletes are subject to specific demands in the performance of sport. Therefore, performance is dependent upon the individual athlete's ability to meet those demands.

Progressive Overload

A conditioning program should begin at a tolerable level of exercise and progress in intensity and volume toward a targeted goal for the individual athlete.

- Intensity is the percentage of the maximal functional capacity of the exercise mode (*e.g.*, percentage of maximal heart rate, percentage of one-repetition maximum).

■ Volume is the total amount of exercise performed in specific periods of time (*e.g.*, total distance run, total amount of weight lifted).

Prioritization

Priorities should be developed according to the individual's capabilities and sport-specific demands because not all elements of a conditioning program can be optimized at the same time, rate, or magnitude.

Periodization

Periodized training is planned variation in the total amount of exercise performed in a given period of time (intensity and volume of exercise). All periodization terminology describes either a certain type of training, a certain portion of a training cycle, or a certain length of time within a training cycle. Research supports periodization as an important corollary to the principle of progressive overload, as this type of planned variation is key to optimal physical development. Periodized training has shown greater improvements compared to low-volume, single-set training. Such training programs have been shown to be very effective during both short- and long-term training cycles, while reducing the risk of overtraining. Several combinations of variables may be manipulated in order to produce an adaptation specific to training goals.

Periodization Cycles

■ **Macrocycle:** an entire training year. For athletes, it is normally thought of as beginning and ending after the last competition of a season.
■ **Mesocycle:** a training period lasting 3 to 6 months.
■ **Microcycle:** a training period lasting 1 week or 7 days (can also relate to a training cycle of up to 4 weeks in length depending upon the program design).

■ TYPES OF PERIODIZATION PROGRAMS

Strength Training

■ **Linear Programs:** Linear programs address conditioning for sports with a limited number of competitions in-season and a well-defined off-season. Classic periodization methods utilize a progressive increase in the intensity and a decrease in the volume of exercise with small variations in each microcycle. The linear method is based on developing neuromuscular function and muscle hypertrophy, with concomitant improvements in strength and power. The linear method is repeated with each mesocycle as progress is made in the program. Rest between the training cycles (active recovery phase) allows for the needed recovery so that overtraining problems are reduced.

■ **Nonlinear (Undulating) Periodized Programs:** Nonlinear programs address conditioning for sports with long competitive seasons, multiple competitions, and year-round practice. The nonlinear program allows for variation in the intensity and volume within each 7- to 10-day cycle by rotating different protocols over the course of the training program. Typically, 3-month cycles are used before an active recovery phase. Nonlinear methods attempt to train the various components of the neuromuscular system within the same 7- to 10-day cycle. However, during a single workout, only one feature is trained on that day (*e.g.*, high-force strength, power, local muscular endurance).

Linear and nonlinear programs have been shown to accomplish similar training effects. Both are superior to constant-intensity and volume training programs. The key to workout success is variation. Different approaches can be used during the macrocycle to accomplish this training need.

Program Variables

Several variables may be periodized in order to alter the resistance-training stimulus to achieve the conditioning goal. Different combinations of these variables will create different workouts.

■ **Exercise Order:** the sequence in which exercises are performed during a training session (*e.g.*, large muscles before smaller ones and multi-joint exercises performed before single-joint exercises).
■ **Exercise Selection:** (*e.g.*, open- and closed-chain exercises, free weights, machines).
■ **Frequency:** the number of training sessions performed during a specific period of time.
■ **Intensity:** the percentage of the maximal functional capacity of the exercise as it relates to strength training.
■ **Load:** the amount of weight lifted per repetition or set as it relates to strength training.
■ **Muscle Action:** (*e.g.*, concentric, eccentric, and isometric).
■ **Repetition Speed:** varying resistive training speed from slow (strength development) to fast (power development) while utilizing the appropriate load.
■ **Rest Periods:** the amount of rest taken between sets, exercises, and/or repetitions.
■ **Volume:** the total number of repetitions performed during a training session as it relates to strength training.

■ AEROBIC CONDITIONING

Aerobic conditioning can be achieved with a multitude of programs (*e.g.*, interval training, continuous training) and modes of exercise (*e.g.*, running, cycling, swimming). It is important that the aerobic conditioning be specific to the sport. Conditioning should be progressive, periodized, prioritized, and compatible with other elements of the conditioning program and the practice sessions.

Sport-specific Conditioning

Sport-specific conditioning is the preparation of the athlete for unique physiological and biomechanical demands and the injury risks inherent in each sport.

- Physiological demands (*e.g.*, anaerobic/aerobic, environmental).
- Biomechanical demands (*e.g.*, throwing, running).
- Injury risks (*e.g.*, site-specific, traumatic, overload, age- and gender-specific).

Objectives of a sport-specific conditioning program are as follows.

Performance

Sports conditioning can be described as a pyramid of fitness and skills:

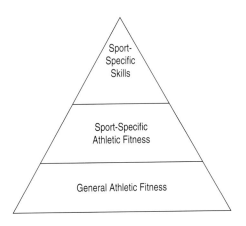

- **General athletic fitness** serves as a base for sport-specific fitness and includes total-body flexibility, total-body muscular strength and power, cardiorespiratory endurance, and body type, size, and structure.
- **Sport-specific athletic fitness** addresses physiological parameters, biomechanical actions, anatomical sites, and muscle activation patterns common or essential to the individual sport. These components are addressed through specific flexibility, strength balance, power/work, and aerobic/concentric training.
- **Sport-specific skill** is the ultimate goal. Optimal performance demands a refinement of unique training and skill acquisition.

Injury and Illness Prevention

Conditioning may decrease injury and illness by influencing sport-specific risk parameters (*e.g.*, acclimatization, site-specific flexibility, strength, balance, force production of muscle).

Components of a sport-specific conditioning program:

- An individualized **preconditioning evaluation** to determine a fitness profile for the purpose of entering a condi-

tioning program. This includes both a general and a sport-specific athletic fitness evaluation.
- A **periodized protocol** for the individual athlete that addresses the unique demands of that sport.
- An **evaluation process** to determine efficacy of the conditioning program.

■ CONDITIONING MODIFICATIONS

In certain populations, conditioning programs may need to be modified to optimize performance and minimize the risk of injury.

Youth

Physiological and biomechanical capabilities in young athletes are different from those of adults. Conditioning injuries in this population include physeal, apophyseal, joint injury, overload tendinitis, and unique susceptibility to environmental stressors.

Strength: Strength training programs are important for the young athlete. Strength gains in this population will be due to increases in recruitment and synchronization of muscle activation patterns. Strength training modifications for youth focus on proper supervision and lower intensity and volume, particularly during periods of rapid growth. As the athlete matures, gains in muscle mass will play a more significant role in strength increases.

Flexibility: Flexibility is traditionally included as a component of conditioning for youth; however, its benefit is unclear in this population.

Aerobics: Aerobic gains in this population are obtainable, but young athletes do not respond as effectively as adults.

Female Athletes

There are gender-related differences in muscle performance, particularly in the upper body. However, female athletes can obtain strength gains and aerobic gains in the same proportion as male athletes in a comparable training program. All female athletes should participate in a total-body conditioning program. The lower extremity and shoulder are frequent areas of injury in the female athlete. Strength deficits in these areas are more closely associated with injury in females than in males. In the female athlete's total-body resistance conditioning program, the upper body should always be emphasized. In addition, the female athlete at risk of unique sport-related injuries [*e.g.*, anterior cruciate ligament (ACL), ankle sprains] should participate in specific resistance conditioning programs. Proper conditioning programs to decrease ACL injuries particularly demonstrate these principles.

Multi-sport Athletes

With overlapping seasons, multi-sport athletes have unique conditioning challenges. Multi-sport athletes need to maintain their general athletic fitness base and focus their sport-specific conditioning toward their current sport. There is a distinct need for recovery between seasons; therefore, including an active recovery phase into the athletic participation and conditioning cycle is of particular importance to multi-sport athletes. Conditioning injuries may occur when an athlete tries to prepare simultaneously for two different sports.

Athletes Who Are Physically Challenged

Athletes who are physically challenged benefit from a conditioning program. Their program should be modified depending on the specific type of impairment and associated disability. Medical conditions in this population, such as temperature regulation, skin problems, cardiovascular function, and entrapment neuropathies, can affect or be affected by the conditioning process. A conditioning program for this population must also accommodate such unique concerns as access and equipment.

■ PRESEASON ISSUES

Network

The team physician should be involved in the network that integrates expertise regarding conditioning matters with certified strength and conditioning specialists (CSCS), the coaches, and other health care providers [which may include certified athletic trainers (ATC), physical therapists (PT), and medical specialists].

Education

Education of athletes and coaches about conditioning provides a framework for understanding the importance of such training for sports and will optimize sports performance and minimize the risk of injury and illness.

It is essential that the education furnished through the network provide athletes and coaches with:

- Instruction about the goals and content of the periodized preseason, in-season, and off-season conditioning programs.
- Instruction about needs for modification of the conditioning program.
- Medical information that affects the conditioning program.

In addition, it is desirable for:

- The entire network, including the team physician, to understand the goals and content of the periodized conditioning program.
- The entire network, including the team physician, to be involved in the educational process.

Conditioning Programs

It is essential for:

- The network to implement the proper periodized sport-specific conditioning programs.
- Medical information that affects the conditioning program to be made available to allow for appropriate program modification.

It is desirable for:

- The entire network, including the team physician, to monitor the conditioning program.
- The entire network, including the team physician, to be available to address concerns about the conditioning program.
- There to be an adequate facility for the conditioning program.
- The network to provide for proper documentation of individual conditioning programs.

■ IN-SEASON ISSUES

Network

The network should continue to integrate expertise regarding the conditioning program during the in-season.

Implementation of the In-season Conditioning Program

It is essential for:

- The network to implement the periodized in-season sport-specific conditioning program.

In addition, it is desirable for:

- The entire network, including the team physician, to monitor the in-season conditioning program.
- The entire network, including the team physician, to be available to address concerns about the in-season conditioning program.
- There to be an adequate facility for the in-season conditioning program.
- The network to provide proper documentation of individual conditioning programs.
- The team physician to observe the conditioning program.

Management and Rehabilitation of Injuries That Impact or Are a Result of Conditioning

The coordination of management and rehabilitation of injuries affecting conditioning is the duty of the team physician (as detailed in the Team Physician Consensus Statement, 2000).
It is essential for the team physician to:

- Be familiar with conditioning matters and the injuries that occur with conditioning.

- Coordinate the modification or cessation of a high-risk activity once identified.
- Coordinate the medical management of injury and illness.
- Coordinate rehabilitation of any conditioning injury or illness, focusing on return to conditioning with any modifications and return to play.

In addition, it is desirable for:

- The entire network, including the team physician, to be available to review conditioning matters.
- The entire network, including the team physician, to participate in the design of the reporting system for conditioning injuries.
- The entire network, including the team physician, to participate in injury surveillance to help identify practices that may be leading to increased rates of injury.
- The entire network, including the team physician, to develop proper documentation to identify and report conditioning injuries.

■ ISSUES

Review of Network and Conditioning Program

Off-season evaluation of the network and conditioning program established in the preseason promotes continued effectiveness. A timely meeting of the network should be held to review and modify the network and the conditioning program.

It is essential for the team physician to:
- Coordinate the evaluation of the possible role of the conditioning program in prevention or production of injuries.

In addition, it is desirable for the network to:

- Determine whether the conditioning program met the network's goals.
- Coordinate the development of an off-season conditioning program.
- Document and evaluate the sport-specific fitness level of each athlete.

Implementation of the Off-season Conditioning Program

The network should implement an active recovery phase followed by the proper, periodized, sport-specific off-season conditioning program.

■ AVAILABLE RESOURCES

Ongoing education pertinent to the team physician is essential. Information regarding team physician–specific educational opportunities is available from the six participating organizations:

American Academy of Family Physicians (AAFP) 11400 Tomahawk Creek Pkwy. Leawood, KS 66211-2672 1-800-274-2237; www.aafp.org

American Academy of Orthopaedic Surgeons (AAOS) 6300 N. River Rd. Rosemont, IL 60018 1-800-346-AAOS; www.aaos.org

American College of Sports Medicine (ACSM) 401 W. Michigan St. Indianapolis, IN 46202-3233 (317) 637-9200; www.acsm.org

American Medical Society for Sports Medicine (AMSSM) 11639 Earnshaw Overland Park, KS 66210 (913) 327-1415; www.amssm.org

American Orthopaedic Society for Sports Medicine (AOSSM) 6300 N. River Rd., Suite 200 Rosemont, IL 60018 (847) 292-4900; www.sportsmed.org

American Osteopathic Academy of Sports Medicine (AOASM) 7611 Elmwood Ave., Suite 201 Middleton, WI 53562 (608) 831-4400; www.aoasm.org

Also, specific information and education regarding conditioning issues is available from:

National Strength and Conditioning Association
PO Box 9908
Colorado Springs, CO 80932
1-800-815-6826; www.nsca-lift.org

■ REFERENCES

Suggested References

Baechle TR, Earle RW, eds. *Essentials of strength training and conditioning.* 2nd ed. Champaign, IL: Human Kinetics; 2000.

Chandler TJ, Kibler WB. *Muscle training in injury prevention. IOC encyclopedia of sports medicine—sports injuries.* London: Blackwell; 1993:252–261.

Faigenbaum AD, Kraemer WJ, Cahil B, et al. Youth resistance training: position statement paper and literature review. *Strength Cond.* 1996; 18:62–75.

Fleck SJ, Kraemer WJ. *Designing resistance training programs.* 2nd ed. Champaign, IL: Human Kinetics; 1997.

Kibler WB, Chandler J. Sport specific conditioning. *Am J Sports Med.* 1994;22:424–432.

Kibler WB, Livingston B. Closed-chain. rehabilitation for upper and lower extremities. *J Am Acad Orthop Surg.* 2001;9:412–421.

Komi PV. *Strength and power and sport.* Oxford: Blackwell Scientific Publications; 1992.

Kraemer, WJ, Faigenbaum AD, Bush JA, et al. Resistance training and youth: enhancing muscle fitness. In: Rippe JM, ed. *Lifestyle medicine.* Malden MA: Blackwell Science; 2000:626–637.

Kraemer WJ, Fleck SJ. *Strength training for young athletes*. Champaign, IL: Human Kinetics; 1993.

Kraemer WJ, Hakkinen K, eds. *Strength training for athletes*. Oxford: Blackwell Publishers, (In Press).

Kraemer WJ, Newton RU. *Training for muscular power: Clinics in sports medicine*. Philadelphia: W.B. Saunders Company; 2000: 341–368.

Kraemer WJ, Ratamess NA. *Physiology of resistance training: Current issues*. Philadelphia: W.B. Saunders Company; 2000:467–513.

Kraemer WJ, Ratamess NA, Rubin MR. Basic principles of resistance training. In: *Nutrition and the strength athlete*. Boca Raton, FL: CRC Press; 2000:1–29.

Kreider R, O'Toole M, Fry AC. *Overtraining in sport*. Champaign, IL: Human Kinetics; 1998.

Zatsiorsky V. *Science and practice of strength training*. Champaign, IL: Human Kinetics; 1995.

Suggested Journal References

Strength and Conditioning Journal. National Strength and Conditioning Association, Colorado Springs, CO (bimonthly)

Journal of Strength and Conditioning Research. National Strength and Conditioning Association, Colorado Springs, CO (quarterly)

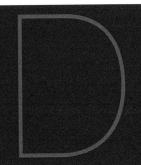

THE TEAM PHYSICIAN AND RETURN-TO-PLAY ISSUES CONSENSUS STATEMENT

■ SUMMARY

The objective of this Consensus Statement is to provide physicians who are responsible for the health care of teams with a decision process for determining when to return an injured or ill athlete to practice or competition. This statement is not intended as a standard of care and should not be interpreted as such. This statement is only a guide and, as such, is of a general nature consistent with the reasonable and objective practice of the health care professional. Individual decisions regarding returning an injured or ill athlete to play will depend on the specific facts and circumstances presented to the physician.

Adequate insurance should be in place to help protect the athlete, the sponsoring organization, and the physician. This statement was developed by the collaborative effort of six major professional associations concerned with clinical sports medicine issues; they have committed to forming an ongoing project-based alliance to "bring together sports medicine organizations to best serve active people and athletes." The organizations are: American Academy of Family Physicians, American Academy of Orthopaedic Surgeons, American College of Sports Medicine, American Medical Society for Sports Medicine, American Orthopaedic Society for Sports Medicine, and the American Osteopathic Academy of Sports Medicine.

Expert Panel

Stanley A. Herring, MD, Chair, Seattle, Washington
John A. Bergfeld, MD, Cleveland, Ohio
Joel Boyd, MD, Edina, Minnesota
Timothy Duffey, DO, Columbus, Ohio
Karl B. Fields, MD, Greensboro, North Carolina
William A. Grana, MD, Tucson, Arizona
Peter Indelicato, MD, Gainesville, Florida
W. Ben Kibler, MD, Lexington, Kentucky
Robert Pallay, MD, Hillsborough, New Jersey

Margot Putukian, MD, University Park, Pennsylvania
Robert E. Sallis, MD, Alta Loma, California

■ DEFINITION

"Return-to-play" is the process of deciding when an injured or ill athlete may safely return to practice or competition.

■ GOAL

The goal is to return an injured or ill athlete to practice or competition without putting the individual or others at undue risk for injury or illness.

To accomplish this goal, the team physician should have knowledge of and be involved with:

- Establishing a return-to-play process
- Evaluating injured or ill athletes
- Treating injured or ill athletes
- Rehabilitating injured or ill athletes
- Returning an injured or ill athlete to play

■ ESTABLISHING A RETURN-TO-PLAY PROCESS

Establishing a process for returning an athlete to play is an essential first step in deciding when an injured or ill athlete may safely return to practice or competition.

It is essential for the team physician to coordinate:

- Establishing a chain of command regarding decisions to return an injured or ill athlete to practice or competition
- Communicating the return-to-play process to player, family, certified athletic trainers, coaches, administrators, and other health care providers
- Establishing a system for documentation
- Establishing protocols to release information regarding an athlete's ability to return to practice or competition following an injury or illness

It is essential that the return-to-play process address the:

- Safety of the athlete
- Potential risk to the safety of other participants
- Functional capabilities of the athlete
- Functional requirements of the athlete's sport
- Federal, state, local, school, and governing body regulations related to returning an injured or ill athlete to practice or competition

■ EVALUATING INJURED OR ILL ATHLETES

Evaluation of an injured or ill athlete establishes a diagnosis, directs treatment, and is the basis for deciding when an athlete may safely return to practice or competition. Repeated evaluations throughout the continuum of injury or illness management optimize medical care.

It is essential that evaluation of an injured or ill athlete include:

- A condition-specific medical history
- A condition-specific physical examination
- Appropriate medical tests and consultations
- Psychosocial assessment
- Documentation
- Communication with the player, family, certified athletic trainer, coaches, and other health care providers

In addition, it is desirable that:

- The team physician coordinate evaluation of the injured or ill athlete

■ TREATING INJURED OR ILL ATHLETES

Treatment of an injured or ill athlete promotes the safe and timely return to practice or competition.

It is essential that treatment of the injured or ill athlete:

- Begin in a timely manner (see *Sideline Preparedness for the Team Physician: A Consensus Statement*, 2000)
- Follow an individualized plan, which may include consultations and referrals
- Include a rehabilitation plan
- Include equipment modification, bracing, and orthoses as necessary
- Address psychosocial issues
- Provide a realistic prognosis as to the safe and timely return to practice or competition
- Include continued communication with the player, family, certified athletic trainer, coaches, and other health care providers
- Include documentation

In addition, it is desirable that:

- The team physician coordinate the initial and ongoing treatment for the injured or ill athlete

■ REHABILITATING INJURED OR ILL ATHLETES

Comprehensive treatment includes proper rehabilitation of an injured or ill athlete, which optimizes the safe and timely return to practice or competition. The team physician should be involved in a network that integrates expertise regarding rehabilitation. This network should include certified athletic trainers, physical therapists, medical specialists, and other health care providers.

It is essential that the rehabilitation network:

- Coordinate the development of a rehabilitation plan that is designed to:
- Restore function of the injured part
- Restore and promote musculoskeletal and cardiovascular function, as well as overall well-being of the injured or ill athlete
- Provide sport-specific assessment and training, which can serve as a basis for sport-specific conditioning (see *The Team Physician and Conditioning of Athletes for Sports: A Consensus Statement*, 2001)
- Provide for continued equipment modification, bracing, and orthoses
- Continue communication with the player, family, rehabilitation network, and coaches concerning the athlete's progress
- Include documentation

In addition, it is desirable that:

- The team physician coordinate the rehabilitation program for the injured or ill athlete

■ RETURNING AN INJURED OR ILL ATHLETE TO PLAY

The decision for safe and timely return of an injured or ill athlete to practice or competition is the desired result of the process of evaluation, treatment, and rehabilitation.

It is essential for return-to-play that the team physician confirm the following criteria:

- The status of anatomical and functional healing
- The status of recovery from acute illness and associated sequelae
- The status of chronic injury or illness
- That the athlete pose no undue risk to the safety of other participants
- Restoration of sport-specific skills
- Psychosocial readiness

■ Ability to perform safely with equipment modification, bracing, and orthoses

■ Compliance with applicable federal, state, local, school, and governing body regulations

Prior to return-to-play, these criteria should be confirmed at a satisfactory level.

■ CONCLUSION

Using the information in this document allows the team physician to make an informed decision as to whether an injured or ill athlete may safely return to practice or competition.

The return-to-play process should be under the direction of the team physician whenever possible. While it is desirable that the team physician coordinate evaluating, treating, and rehabilitating the injured or ill athlete, it is essential that the team physician ultimately be responsible for the return-to-play decision.

Individual decisions regarding returning an injured or ill athlete to play will depend on the specific facts and circumstances presented to the team physician.

■ AVAILABLE RESOURCES

Ongoing education pertinent to the team physician is essential. Information regarding team physician-specific educational opportunities can be obtained from the six participating organizations:

American Academy of Family Physicians (AAFP)
11400 Tomahawk Creek Pkwy, Leawood KS 66211
800-274-2237; www.aafp.org

American Academy of Orthopaedic Surgeons (AAOS)
6300 N River Rd, Rosemont IL 60018
800-346-AAOS; www.aaos.org

American College of Sports Medicine (ACSM)
401 W Michigan St, Indianapolis IN 46202
317-637-9200; www.acsm.org

American Medical Society for Sports Medicine (AMSSM)
11639 Earnshaw, Overland Park KS 66210
913-327-1415; www.amssm.org

American Orthopaedic Society for Sports Medicine (AOSSM)
6300 N River Rd Suite 200, Rosemont IL 60018
847-292-4900; www.sportsmed.org

American Osteopathic Academy of Sports Medicine (AOASM)
7611 Elmwood Ave Suite 201, Middleton WI 53562
608-831-4400; www.aoasm.org

■ SUGGESTED REFERENCES

Adams, BB. Transmission of cutaneous infections in athletes. *Br J Sports Med.* 2000;34:413–414.

American College of Sports Medicine, American College of Cardiology, 26th Bethesda Conference. "Recommendations for competition in athletes with cardiovascular abnormalities." *Med Sci Sports Exerc.* 1994;26:S223–S283.

American Medical Society for Sports Medicine, American Academy of Sports Medicine. Human immunodeficiency virus and other blood-borne pathogens in sports. *Clin J Sports Med.* 1995;5: 199–204.

Cantu, RC. Return-to-play guidelines after a head injury. *Clin J Sports Med.* 1998;17:45–60.

Cantu RC. Stingers, transient quadriplegia and cervical spinal stenosis; return-to-play criteria. *Med Sci Sports Exerc.* 1997;29(7 Suppl): S233–S235.

Committee on Sports Medicine and Fitness. Cardiac dysrhythmias and sports. *Pediatrics.* 1995;95:786–789.

Goodman R, Thacker S, Soloman S, et al. Infectious disease in competitive sports. *JAMA.* 1994;271:862–866.

Herring SA. Rehabilitation of muscle injuries. *Med Sci Sports Exerc.* 1990;22:453–456.

Kibler WB, Herring SA, Press JM. *Functional rehabilitation of sports and musculoskeletal injuries.* Bethesda: Aspen Publishers; 1998.

Kibler WB, Livingston BP. Closed-chain rehabilitation for upper and lower extremities. *J Am Acad Orthop Surg.* 2001;9:412–421.

Maron BJ. Cardiovascular risks to young persons on the athletic field. *Ann Intern Med.* 1998;129:379–386.

Mellion MB, Walsh WM, Madden C, et al., eds. *Team physician's handbook,* 3rd ed. Philadelphia: Hanley & Belfus; 2002.

Mitten MJ, Mitten RJ. Legal considerations in treating the injured athlete. *J Orthop Sports Phys Ther.* 1995;21:38–43.

Preparticipation Physical Evaluation, 2nd ed. AAFP, AAP, AMSSM, AOSSM, AOASM. The Physician and Sportsmedicine. McGraw-Hill Healthcare; Minneapolis: 1997.

0195-9131/02/3301-1212/0
MEDICINE & SCIENCE IN SPORTS & EXERCISE®

FEMALE ATHLETE ISSUES FOR THE TEAM PHYSICIAN: A CONSENSUS STATEMENT

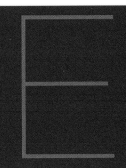

■ SUMMARY

This document provides an overview of select musculoskeletal and medical issues that are important to team physicians who are responsible for the medical care of female athletes. It is not intended as a standard of care and should not be interpreted as such. This document is only a guide and, as such, is of a general nature, consistent with the reasonable, objective practice of the health care professional. Individual treatment will turn on the specific facts and circumstances presented to the physician. Adequate insurance should be in place to help protect the physician, the athlete, and the sponsoring organization.

This statement was developed by a collaboration of six major professional associations concerned about clinical sports medicine issues; they have committed to forming an ongoing project-based alliance to bring together sports medicine organizations to best serve active people and athletes. The organizations are: American Academy of Family Physicians, American Academy of Orthopaedic Surgeons, American College of Sports Medicine, American Medical Society for Sports Medicine, American Orthopaedic Society for Sports Medicine, and the American Osteopathic Academy of Sports Medicine.

Expert Panel

Stanley A. Herring, MD, Chair, Seattle, Washington
John A. Bergfeld, MD, Cleveland, Ohio
Lori A. Boyajian-O'Neill, DO, Kansas City, Missouri
Timothy Duffey, DO, Columbus, Ohio
Letha Yurko Griffin, MD, PhD, Atlanta, Georgia
Jo A. Hannafin, MD, PhD, New York, New York
Peter Indelicato, MD, Gainesville, Florida
Elizabeth A. Joy, MD, Salt Lake City, Utah
W. Ben Kibler, MD, Lexington, Kentucky
Constance M. Lebrun, MD, London, Ontario, Canada
Robert Pallay, MD, Hillsborough, New Jersey
Margot Putukian, MD, University Park, Pennsylvania

■ DEFINITION

Female athletes experience musculoskeletal injuries and medical problems, resulting from and/or impacting athletic activity. Team physicians must understand the gender-specific implications of these issues.

■ GOAL

The goal is to assist the team physician in providing optimal medical care for the female athlete.

■ THE FEMALE ATHLETE AND ANTERIOR CRUCIATE LIGAMENT (ACL) INJURIES

It is essential that the team physician understand:

■ The female is at increased risk of ACL injury in multiple sports and activities
■ The anatomy, biomechanics, and mechanisms of injury of the ACL
■ Treatment strategies including surgical indications

It is desirable that the team physician:

■ Understand current prevention strategies
■ Coordinate a network to identify risk factors and implement treatment
■ Understand the potential long-term sequelae of ACL injury

Epidemiology

■ Noncontact ACL injury rate is two to 10 times higher in female athletes than in their male counterparts.
■ Examples of high-risk sports include basketball, field hockey, lacrosse, skiing, and soccer.

Physiology/Pathophysiology

■ Causes of noncontact ACL injuries may be multifactorial; proposed risks include environmental, anatomical, hormonal, biomechanical, and neuromuscular factors.

- Noncontact ACL injuries occur commonly during deceleration, landing, or cutting. At-risk positions during these maneuvers include knee extension, flat foot, and off-balance body position.

Evaluation and Treatment

It is essential that the team physician:

- Delineate the mechanism of the injury
- Conduct a comprehensive physical examination of the knee, including ACL assessment
- Know the indications for and utility of imaging techniques
- Know the indications for surgical consideration
- Facilitate early rehabilitation to improve strength, flexibility and neuromuscular control

It is desirable that the team physician:

- Review the results of imaging studies
- Understand the principles of the surgical management of the ACL injury

Prevention

It is essential that the team physician:

- Understand that neuromuscular factors may contribute to increased risk of noncontact ACL injuries and may be amenable to prevention with specific conditioning programs.
- Recognize that conditioning programs may need to be gender specific (see *The Team Physician and Conditioning of Athletes for Sports: A Consensus Statement*, 2001)

It is desirable that the team physician:

- Identify proposed risk factors during the preparticipation evaluation
- Coordinate a prevention program
- Educate athletes, parents, coaches, and other health care providers, including information about at-risk positions and game situations that are associated with ACL injury

■ THE FEMALE ATHLETE AND THE PATELLOFEMORAL JOINT

It is essential that the team physician understand:

- The anatomy and biomechanics of the patellofemoral joint
- The mechanisms of patellofemoral pain and dysfunction

It is desirable that the team physician:

- Coordinate the evaluation and treatment of athletes with patellofemoral problems
- Understand the potential long-term sequelae of patellofemoral pain and dysfunction

Epidemiology

- Patellofemoral problems occur frequently in female athletes.
- Patellofemoral pain and dysfunction result from macro-trauma and micro-trauma.

Physiology/Pathophysiology

- Normal patellofemoral mechanics involve a balance between bone alignment, articular cartilage, soft tissue (ligaments, muscles, tendons, fascia), and coordinated neuromuscular activation.
- Patellofemoral pain and dysfunction are multifactorial, including malalignment, articular cartilage lesions, instability, soft tissue factors, and psychosocial issues.
- Patellofemoral pain may occur in what appears to be a normal knee joint.
- Risk factors include:
  - Static and/or dynamic malalignment of the pelvis, hip, knee, ankle, and foot
  - Muscle weakness and/or imbalance and inflexibility
  - Altered patellar position and/or morphology
  - Trauma, overuse, and/or training errors

Evaluation and Treatment

It is essential that the team physician:

- Delineate key points relating to the history of the patellofemoral problem
- Conduct a specific examination for the patellofemoral problem
- Know the indications for and utility of imaging techniques
- Understand nonoperative management of patellofemoral problems, including patient education, activity modification, rehabilitation, bracing, orthoses, and medications

It is desirable that the team physician:

- Review the results of imaging studies
- Understand the principles of and indications for surgical management

Prevention

It is essential that the team physician:

- Know the risk factors for patellofemoral problems

It is desirable that the team physician:

- Identify risk factors during the preparticipation evaluation
- Implement a screening program for risk factors
- Educate athletes, parents, coaches, administrators, and health care providers

■ THE FEMALE ATHLETE AND SHOULDER CONDITIONS

It is essential that the team physician understand:

- The anatomy and biomechanics of the shoulder
- The mechanisms of shoulder injury and dysfunction

It is desirable that the team physician:

- Recognize that shoulder conditions may result from strength and flexibility imbalances or injuries elsewhere in the body
- Identify risk factors associated with shoulder conditions
- Coordinate the evaluation and treatment of shoulder conditions

■ EPIDEMIOLOGY

- Examples of high-risk sports include diving, gymnastics, swimming, tennis, throwing sports, and volleyball.
- Shoulder conditions result from macro-trauma and microtrauma.

■ PHYSIOLOGY/PATHOPHYSIOLOGY

- The integration of coordinated neuromuscular activation, capsular/ligament stiffness, and glenohumeral and scapulothoracic positioning is key to shoulder function.
- The female athlete's shoulder is at risk for injury due to increased biomechanical load, resulting from specific risk factors, including:
  - Increased joint laxity (translation)
  - Increased muscle and joint flexibility (range of motion)
  - Decreased upper body strength and poor posture
  - Acquired internal rotation deficits

■ EVALUATION AND TREATMENT

It is essential that the team physician:

- Delineate key points relating to the history of the shoulder condition
- Conduct a comprehensive examination for the shoulder condition, including assessment of range of motion, instability, rotator cuff pathology, and scapular dysfunction
- Know the indications and utility of imaging techniques
- Understand the principles of shoulder rehabilitation

It is desirable that the team physician:

- Evaluate strength and flexibility imbalances or injuries elsewhere in the body that may contribute to shoulder conditions
- Review the results of imaging studies
- Understand the principles of and indications for surgical management

Prevention

It is essential that the team physician:

- Know the risk factors for shoulder conditions

It is desirable that the team physician:

- Identify risk factors during the preparticipation evaluation
- Implement a screening program for risk factors
- Educate athletes, parents, coaches, administrators, and healthcare providers

■ THE FEMALE ATHLETE AND STRESS FRACTURES

It is essential that the team physician understand:

- A stress fracture in a female athlete can be an isolated injury or may indicate underlying medical and psychosocial problems. Therefore, evaluation and treatment must take into account the etiology of the stress fracture.
- Certain stress fractures are at high risk for complications and long-term sequelae.

It is desirable that the team physician:

- Coordinate, when necessary, multidisciplinary evaluation and treatment

Epidemiology

- Stress fractures occur frequently in female athletes.
- Some studies suggest a higher incidence of stress fractures in females, but there is little evidence to support a gender difference in stress fractures among trained athletes.
- Common anatomical areas include the foot, tibia, fibula, femur, and pelvis.

Physiology/Pathophysiology

- Stress fractures occur when bone is subjected to repetitive loads beyond its physiological capacity.
- An imbalance between bone resorption and deposition creates bone that may not withstand repetitive loads.
- Risk factors associated with stress fractures include:
  - Extrinsic factors [exercise (type, volume, and intensity), footwear]
  - Intrinsic musculoskeletal factors (muscle strength and balance, limb alignment)
  - Medical factors (osteopenia, osteoporosis, menstrual dysfunction, poor nutrition, disordered eating, and other psychosocial issues)

Evaluation and Treatment

It is essential that the team physician:

- Delineate key points relating to the history of the stress fracture
- Conduct a specific physical examination pertinent to the suspected stress fracture
- Identify potential underlying risk factors
- Know the indications for and utility of imaging techniques

- Identify stress fractures at high risk of complication and long-term sequelae
- Know the indications for surgical consideration
- Understand nonoperative management and rehabilitation

It is desirable that the team physician:

- Review the results of the imaging studies
- Understand the principles of and indications for surgical management
- Coordinate, when necessary, a multidisciplinary team approach to treatment

Prevention

It is essential that the team physician:

- Recognize there can be multiple risk factors for stress fractures

It is desirable that the team physician:

- Recognize risk factors during the preparticipation evaluation
- Implement a screening program for risk factors
- Educate athletes, parents, coaches, administrators, and health care providers

■ THE FEMALE ATHLETE AND OSTEOPENIA AND OSTEOPOROSIS

It is essential that the team physician understand:

- Osteopenia and osteoporosis can exist in the young female athlete
- These conditions have implications for athletic performance and long-term sequelae
- Disordered eating and menstrual dysfunction are common risk factors

It is desirable that the team physician understand:

- The evaluation and treatment of osteopenia and osteoporosis
- The importance of educating athletes, parents, coaches, administrators, and health care providers
- The value of prevention and early detection of osteopenia and osteoporosis

Epidemiology

- The incidence of osteopenia and osteoporosis in the female athlete is unknown.
- Several studies have demonstrated osteopenia and osteoporosis in young female athletes with menstrual dysfunction and/or eating disorders.
- The major determinant of adult bone mineral density (BMD) is bone mass achieved during adolescence and young adulthood. Osteoporosis-related fractures in later life are associated with significant morbidity and mortality.

Physiology/Pathophysiology

- Bone mass depends on the overall balance between resorption and deposition.
- Ninety percent of total bone mineral content is accrued by the end of adolescence, creating a window of opportunity to maximize BMD.
- Eighty percent of variance in BMD is attributed to genetic factors. Lean body mass, estrogen, exercise, and calcium intake are other important influences.
- Tobacco use, excessive alcohol consumption, certain medical conditions (e.g., renal disease, hyperparathyroidism), and medications (e.g., glucocorticoids) can negatively affect bone density.
- Athletes involved in impact sports and/or strength training routinely have higher site-specific BMD than athletes in nonimpact sports and nonathletes.
- The effect of impact activities and/or strength training is most pronounced during puberty and dependent upon intensity and volume of conditioning (see *The Team Physician and Conditioning of Athletes for Sports: A Consensus Statement*, 2001).

Evaluation and Treatment

It is essential that the team physician:

- Recognize risk factors for low BMD
- Know the indications for and the utility of imaging techniques
- Facilitate treatment for osteopenia and osteoporosis once identified

It is desirable that the team physician:

- Understand criteria for osteopenia [1 to 2.5 standard deviations (SD) below young adult mean BMD] and osteoporosis (> 2.5 SD below young adult mean BMD)
- Coordinate a screening process to identify athletes at risk
- Coordinate a comprehensive evaluation including assessment of menstrual status and nutritional intake, measurement of BMD, and laboratory testing as necessary
- Understand that multidisciplinary treatment may include restoration of normal menstrual cycles, optimization of physical activity and nutrition, psychological therapy, and pharmacological intervention.

Prevention

It is essential that the team physician understand:

- Optimal BMD is achieved by maintaining physiological estrogen levels, adequate nutrition, and load-bearing exercise
- The importance of prevention and early detection of osteopenia and osteoporosis

It is desirable that the team physician:

- Identify risk factors during the preparticipation evaluation

- Implement a screening program for risk factors, including information regarding strategies for maintaining optimal BMD and the effect of negative behaviors on BMD
- Educate athletes, parents, coaches, administrators, and healthcare professionals

THE FEMALE ATHLETE AND DISORDERED EATING

It is essential that the team physician understand:

- The importance of adequate nutrition in sports
- The spectrum of disordered eating and how it affects the female athlete
- Disordered eating can occur in any sport

It is desirable that the team physician understand:

- The evaluation and treatment of the athlete with disordered eating
- The importance of educating athletes, coaches, parents, administrators, and other health care providers
- The value of prevention and early detection of disordered eating

EPIDEMIOLOGY

- Disordered eating occurs on a spectrum. This ranges from calorie, protein, and/or fat restriction and pathogenic weight control measures (e.g., diet pills, laxatives, excessive exercise, self-induced vomiting) to classic eating disorders, such as anorexia nervosa (AN) and bulimia nervosa.
- Athletes in sports involving aesthetics, endurance, and weight classifications are at particular risk for the spectrum of disordered eating.
- Fifteen to 62% of college female athletes report a history of disordered eating.
- Eating disorders are psychiatric disorders with distortion of body image and significant nutritional and medical complications, including a mortality rate of 12% to 18% for untreated AN.
- Female athletes are at higher risk for developing eating disorders than the general population.

Physiology/Pathophysiology

- Nutritional and medical consequences of the spectrum of disordered eating include:
  - Nutritional deficiencies and electrolyte disturbances
  - Decreased BMD
  - Gastrointestinal problems (e.g., bleeding, ulceration, bloating, constipation)
  - Cardiovascular abnormalities (e.g., arrhythmias, heart block)

- Psychiatric problems (e.g., depression, anxiety, suicide)
- Risk factors include:
- Pressure to optimize performance and/or modify appearance
- Psychological factors, such as low self-esteem, poor coping skills, perceived loss of control, perfectionism, obsessive compulsive traits, depression, anxiety, and history of sexual/physical abuse
- Underlying chronic diseases related to caloric utilization (e.g., diabetes)

Evaluation and Treatment

It is essential that the team physician:

- Recognize risk factors for the spectrum of disordered eating
- Facilitate treatment once identified with a multidisciplinary approach as needed
- Understand the necessity of mental health treatment for eating disorders

It is desirable that the team physician:

- Coordinate a screening process to identify athletes at risk
- Understand a comprehensive evaluation includes assessment of nutrition, exercise behaviors, pathogenic weight control measures, and psychosocial factors, and additional laboratory and other diagnostic testing as necessary
- Understand treatment may involve a multidisciplinary approach (medical, mental health, and nutritional management), including parents, coaches, certified athletic trainers, physical therapists, and administrators.

Prevention

It is essential that the team physician understand:

- The importance of prevention and early detection of the spectrum of disordered eating

It is desirable that the team physician:

- Identify risk factors during the preparticipation evaluation
- Implement a screening program for risk factors, including information to dispel misconceptions about body weight, body composition, and athletic performance
- Educate athletes, parents, coaches, administrators and health care providers

THE FEMALE ATHLETE AND SELECTED MENSTRUAL DYSFUNCTION

It is essential that the team physician understand:

- The normal menstrual cycle and the spectrum of menstrual dysfunction
- The consequences of menstrual dysfunction on bone density and fertility

It is desirable that the team physician understand:

- The evaluation and treatment of the athlete with menstrual dysfunction
- The importance of educating athletes, parents, coaches, administrators, and health care providers about menstrual dysfunction
- The value of prevention and early detection of menstrual dysfunction

Epidemiology

- Menstrual dysfunction occurs in different forms:
  - Delayed menarche (onset of menstrual cycles after 16 years of age)
  - Secondary amenorrhea (absence of menses for 3 or more months after regular menses has been established)
  - Oligomenorrhea (six to nine cycles per year; cycle length greater than 35 days or less than 3 months)
  - Anovulation (absence of ovulation; may have regular menstrual bleeding)
  - Luteal phase deficiency (cycle length may be normal, but there are decreased progesterone levels)
- In the athlete, menstrual dysfunction is at least two to three times more common than in the nonathlete; 10% to 15% have amenorrhea or oligomenorrhea.

Physiology/Pathophysiology

- Normal menstrual cycle depends on intact hypothalamic-pituitary-ovarian (HPO) axis and normal pelvic organ function.
- The etiology of menstrual dysfunction is multifactorial, including body weight and body composition, nutrition, training, previous menstrual function, and psychosocial factors.
- The energy drain hypothesis states that energy expenditure exceeds stored and consumed energy, leading to disruption of the HPO axis.
- Intense exercise alone does not necessarily cause menstrual dysfunction, provided there is adequate caloric intake for the energy needs.
- Consequences of menstrual dysfunction may include lower levels of estrogen and/or progesterone, lower BMD, and higher incidence of stress fractures and infertility.
- Effects of lower levels of estrogen on BMD are not completely reversible; therefore, early detection and treatment of menstrual dysfunction is important.

Evaluation and Treatment

It is essential that the team physician:

- Understand menstrual dysfunction related solely to exercise is a diagnosis of exclusion
- Recognize risk factors for and implications of menstrual dysfunction

- Facilitate treatment of these conditions once identified, with a multidisciplinary approach as necessary

It is desirable that the team physician:

- Coordinate a screening program to identify athletes at risk
- Understand that a comprehensive evaluation includes assessment for other causes of menstrual dysfunction; detailed menstrual, nutrition, and medication history; laboratory testing; and additional diagnostic testing as necessary.
- Understand that treatment may include increasing caloric intake, decreasing energy expenditure, hormone supplementation, and psychotherapy as necessary

Prevention

It is essential that the team physician understand:

- The importance of prevention and early detection of menstrual dysfunction

It is desirable that the team physician:

- Identify risk factors during the preparticipation evaluation
- Implement a screening program for risk factors, including information about the importance of normal menstrual function
- Educate athletes, parents, coaches, administrators, and health care providers

■ THE FEMALE ATHLETE AND PREGNANCY/CONTRACEPTION

The majority of team physicians do not provide obstetrical care for female athletes, nor do they offer specific contraceptive counseling. Prenatal and postpartum care in the United States is generally carried out by an obstetrician/gynecologist and/or family medicine physician. Team physicians may defer to the specific expertise of the physician(s) providing primary obstetric care but can coordinate and collaborate in the management of sports-related injuries and illnesses.

It is essential that the team physician:

- Recognize the signs and symptoms of pregnancy
- Understand that absolute and relative contraindications to exercise throughout pregnancy exist
- Understand the importance of family planning and contraception

It is desirable that the team physician understand:

- Basic physiological changes associated with pregnancy and the postpartum period
- Sport-specific risks and benefits of exercise in pregnancy and exercise prescription

■ The effects of certain medications on maternal and fetal health
■ Medical and obstetrical conditions affecting participation and performance
■ Specific considerations in the pregnant athlete, including nutritional needs, environmental risks, appropriate use of imaging, and contraindications for physical therapy modalities
■ Contraceptive methods and alternatives, at-risk behaviors for unplanned pregnancy, and sexually transmitted diseases (STDs)

Epidemiology

■ Exercise throughout pregnancy is generally safe but must be carefully monitored and limitations applied as necessary.
■ Benefits of exercise throughout pregnancy include:
  ■ Avoidance of excessive weight gain, improved balance, and decreased back pain
  ■ Improved well-being, energy levels, and sleep patterns
  ■ Improved labor symptoms and facilitation of postpartum recovery
■ Risks include environmental exposure, dehydration, hypoxia, and uterine trauma
■ Contraceptive methods have different efficacies, potential side effects, and risks for STDs.
  ■ In certain populations, there may be a positive association between oral contraceptive use and BMD.
  ■ Use of injectable depot medroxyprogesterone acetate may lead to amenorrhea, lower estrogen levels, and decreased BMD.
■ Unplanned pregnancy and/or presence of STDs indicates high-risk behavior

Physiology/Pathophysiology

■ Physiological changes that may affect exercise throughout pregnancy include:
  ■ Musculoskeletal changes including weight gain
  ■ Medical changes including increased heart rate, cardiac output, blood volume, and respiratory rate
■ The goals of exercise throughout pregnancy are to maintain or improve pre-existing levels of maternal fitness without undue risk to the mother or the developing fetus
■ Pregnancy increases nutritional needs for calories, iron, calcium, and folic acid
■ Exercise in the supine position after 16 weeks should be avoided due to potential great vessel compression

Evaluation and Treatment

It is essential that the team physician understand:

■ There are specific issues of the female athlete in terms of pregnancy and contraception

It is desirable that the team physician:

■ Facilitate obstetric care and treatment, including referral
■ Understand evaluation includes a medical examination, nutritional assessment, and ongoing assessment of absolute and relative contraindications to exercise throughout pregnancy and the postpartum period
■ Understand treatment may include the limitation of physical activity as pregnancy progresses and that discussion with others (i.e., health care providers, parents, coaches, and certified athletic trainers) may be necessary

Prevention

It is essential that the team physician understand:

■ The importance of family planning and contraceptive options for the athlete
■ The implications of pregnancy and postpartum for training and competition

It is desirable that the team physician:

■ Implement a screening and education program for athletes at risk for pregnancy, including information regarding safe sexual practices, family planning, and contraceptive options.
■ Educate athletes, parents, coaches, administrators, and health care providers as to the benefits and risks of exercise throughout pregnancy and the postpartum period.

■ AVAILABLE RESOURCES

Ongoing education pertinent to the team physician is essential. Information regarding team physician-specific educational opportunities can be obtained from the six participating organizations:

American Academy of Family Physicians (AAFP)
11400 Tomahawk Creek Pkwy
Leawood, KS 66211
(800)-274-2237; www.aafp.org

American Academy of Orthopaedic Surgeons (AAOS)
6300 N River Rd
Rosemont, IL 60018
(800)-346-AAOS; www.aaos.org

American College of Sports Medicine (ACSM)
401 W Michigan St
Indianapolis, IN 46202
(317)-637-9200; www.acsm.org

American Medical Society for Sports Medicine (AMSSM)
11639 Earnshaw
Overland Park, KS 66210
(913)-327-1415; www.amssm.org

American Orthopaedic Society for Sports Medicine (AOSSM)
6300 N River Rd, Suite 500
Rosemont, IL 60018
(847)-292-4900; www.sportsmed.org

American Osteopathic Academy of Sports Medicine (AOASM)
7611 Elmwood Ave, Suite 201
Middleton, WI 53562
(608)-831-4400; www.aoasm.org

■ SELECTED READINGS

Anderson AF, Dome DC, Gautam S, et al. Correlation of anthropometric measurements, strength, anterior cruciate ligament size, and intercondylar notch characteristics to sex differences in anterior cruciate ligament tear rates. *Am J Sports Med.* 2001;29:58–66.

Arendt E, Dick R. Knee injury patterns among men and women in collegiate basketball and soccer: NCAA data and review of the literature. *Am J Sports Med.* 1995;23:694–701.

Chappell JD, Yu B, Kirkendall DT, et al. A comparison of knee kinetics between male and female recreational athletes in stop-jump tasks. *Am J Sports Med.* 2002;30:261–267.

Griffin LY, Agel J, Albohm MJ, et al. Noncontact anterior cruciate ligament injuries. *J Am Acad Orthop Surg.* 2000;8:141–150.

Hewett T, Lindenfeld TN, Riccobene JV, et al. The effect of neuromuscular training on the incidence of knee injury in female athletes. A prospective study. *Am J Sports Med.* 1999;27:699–706.

Huston L, Wojtys EM. Neuromuscular performance characteristics in elite female athletes. *Am J Sports Med.* 1996;24:427–436.

Rozzi SL, Lephart SM, Gear WS, et al. Knee joint laxity and neuromuscular characteristics of male and female soccer and basketball players. *Am J Sports Med.* 1999;27:312–319.

Wojtys EM, Huston LJ, Boynton MD, et al. The effect of the menstrual cycle on anterior cruciate ligament injuries in women as determined by hormone levels. *Am J Sports Med.* 2002;30:182–188.

Patellofemoral Joint

Arroll B, Ellis-Pelger E, Edwards A, et al. Patellofemoral pain syndrome: a critical review of the clinical trials on non-operative therapy. *Am J Sports Med.* 1997;25:207–212.

Baker MM, Juhn MS. Patellofemoral pain syndrome in the female athlete. *Clin Sports Med.* 2000;19:315–320.

Crossley K, Bennell K, Green S, et al. Physical therapy for patellofemoral pain: a randomized, double-blinded, placebo-controlled trial. *Am J Sports Med.* 2002;30:857–865.

Kowall MG, Kolk G, Nuber GW, et al. Patellar taping in the treatment of patellofemoral pain: a prospective randomized study. *Am J Sports Med.* 1996;24:61–66.

Malone T, Davies G, Walsh WM. Muscular control of the patella (review). *Clin Sports Med.* 2002;21:349–362.

Natri A, Kannus P, Jarvinen M. Which factors predict the long term outcome in chronic patellofemoral pain syndrome? A prospective follow-up study. *Med Sci Sports Exerc.* 1998;30:1572–1577.

Shoulder

Chandler TJ, Kibler WB, Uhl TL, et al. Flexibility comparisons of junior elite tennis players to other athletes. *Am. J. Sports Med.* 18:134–136,1990.

Griffin LY. The female athlete. In: Renstrom P, ed. *The IOC book on sports injuries: Principles of prevention and care.* London: Blackwell; 1993.

Hannafin JA. Upper extremity injuries: shoulder. In: Garret WE, ed. *Women's health in sports and exercise.* Rosemont, IL: AAOS;2001.

Kibler WB, Chandler TJ, Uhl T, et al. A musculoskeletal approach to the preparticipation physical examination: preventing injury and improving performance. *Am J Sports Med.* 1989;17:525–531.

Kibler WB. Rehabilitation of shoulder and knee injuries. In: Garrett WE, ed. *Women's health in sports and exercise.* Rosemont, IL: AAOS; 2001.

Stress Fractures

Barrow GW, Saha S. Menstrual irregularity and stress fractures in collegiate female distance runners. *Am J Sports Med.* 1988;16:209–216.

Bennell KL, Malcolm SA, Thomas SA, et al. Risk factors for stress fractures in track and field athletes: a twelve-month prospective study. *Am J Sports Med.* 1996;24:810–818.

Boden BP, Osbahr DC, Jimenez C. Low-risk stress fractures. *Am J Sports Med.* 2001;29:100–111.

Myburgh KH, Hutchins J, Fataar AB, et al. Low bone density in an etiologic factor for stress fractures in athletes. *Ann Intern Med.* 1990;113:754–759.

Nattiv A, Armsey TD, Jr. Stress injury to bone in the female athlete. *Clin Sports Med.* 1997;16:197–224.

Disordered Eating

Beals KA, Manore MM. Disorders of the female athlete triad among collegiate female athletes. *Int J Sport Nutr.* 2002;12:281–293.

Biller BMK, Saxe V, Herzog DB, et al. Mechanisms of osteoporosis in adult and adolescent women with anorexia nervosa. *J Clin Endocrinol Metab.* 1989;68:548–554.

Rigotti NA, Neer RM, Skates SJ, et al. The clinical course of osteoporosis in anorexia nervosa. *JAMA.* 1991;265:1133–1138.

Rosenblum J, Forman S. Evidence-based treatment of eating disorders. *Pediatrics.* 2002;14:379–383.

Sundgot-Borgen J. Risk and trigger factors for the development of eating disorders in female elite athletes. *Med Sci Sports Exerc.* 1994;26:414–419.

Sundgot-Borgen J. Eating disorders. In: Drinkwater B, ed. *Women in sport,* London: Blackwell; 2000:364–376.

Walsh JME, Wheat ME, Freund K. Detection, evaluation and treatment of eating disorders: the role of the primary care physician. *J Gen Intern Med.* 2000;15:577–590.

Menstrual Dysfunction

ACSM Position Stand on the female athlete triad. *Med Sci Sports Exerc.* 1997;29:1–9.

Drinkwater BL, Nilson K, Chestnut CH III, et al. Bone mineral content of amenorrheic and eumenorrheic athletes. *N Engl J Med.* 1984;311:277–281.

Drinkwater BL, Bruemmer B, Chestnut CH III. Menstrual history as a determinant of current bone density in young athletes. *JAMA.* 1990;263:545.

Drinkwater BL, Nilson K, Ott S, et al. Bone mineral density after resumption of menses in amenorrheic athletes. *JAMA.* 1986;256:380–382.

Loucks AB, Verdun M, Heath EM, et al. Low energy availability, not the stress of exercise, alters LH pulsatility in exercising women. *J Appl Physiol.* 1998;84:37.

American Academy of Pediatrics. Committee on Sports Medicine and Fitness. Medical concerns in the female athlete. *Pediatrics.* 2000;106:610–613.

Zanker CL, Swaine IL. The relationship between serum oestradiol concentration and energy balance in young women distance runners. *Int J Sports Med.* 1998;19:104–108.

Bone Issues

Gibson J. Osteoporosis. In: Drinkwater B, ed. *Women in sport.* London: Blackwell; 2000:391–406.

Hawker GA, Jamal SA, Ridout R, et al. A clinical prediction rule to identify premenopausal women with low bone mass. *Osteoporos Int.* 2002;13:400–406.

Kanis JA. Diagnosis of osteoporosis. *Osteoporos Int.* 1997;7:S108–S116.

Kanis JA, Melton LJ, Christiansen C, et al. The diagnosis of osteoporosis. *J Bone Miner Res.* 1994;9:1137–1141.

Khan K, Mckay P, Kannus P, et al. *Physical activity and bone health.* Champaign, IL: Human Kinetics; 2001.

Lindsay R, Meunier P. Osteoporosis: review of the evidence for prevention, diagnosis and treatment and cost-effectiveness analysis status report. *Osteoporos Int.* 1998;4(Suppl):S1–S88.

Modlesky CM, Lewis RD. Does exercise during growth have a long-term effect on bone health? *Exerc Sport Sci Rev.* 2002;30: 171–176.

Myburgh KH, Bachrach LK, Lewis B, et al. Low bone mineral density at axial and appendicular sites in amenorrheic athletes. *Med Sci Sports Exerc.* 1993;25:1197–1202.

Recker RR, Davies KM, Hinders SM, et al. Bone gain in young adult women. *JAMA.* 1992;268:2403–2408.

Rencken M, Chesnut CH, Drinkwater BL. Decreased bone density at multiple skeletal sites in amenorrheic athletes. *JAMA.* 1996;276: 238–240.

Scholes D, Lacroix AX, Ott SM, et al. Bone mineral density in women using depot medroxyprogesterone acetate for contraception. *Obstet. Gynecol.* 1999;93:233–238.

Pregnancy/Contraception

Araujo D. Expecting questions about exercise and pregnancy? *Phys Sportsmed.* 1997;25: April.

Artal R, O'Toole M. Guidelines of the American College of Obstetricians and Gynecologists for exercise during pregnancy and the postpartum period. *Br J Sports Med.* 2003;37:6–12.

Exercise during pregnancy and the postpartium period. ACOG Technical Bulletin Number 189, February 1994. *Int J Gynaecol Obstet.* 1994;45:65–70.

Kardel, KR, Kase T. Training in pregnant women: effects on fetal development and birth. *Am J Obstet Gynecol.* 1988;178:280–286.

Penttinen J, Erkkola R. Pregnancy in endurance athletes. *Scand. J Med Sci Sports.* 1997;7:226–228.

Page numbers followed by *f* indicate figures; those followed by *t* indicate tables.

Rotator interval (RTI)
  anatomy of, 150f, 151
  biomechanics of, 175
  collagen of, 275
  removal of, 280
Rough endoplasmic reticulum (RER), collagen
      synthesized in, 7
RS ligament. *See* Radioscaphoid ligament
RTC. *See* Rotator cuff
RTq ligament. *See* Dorsal radiotriquetral
      ligament
Ruffini endings, in meniscus, 16
Runner's knee. *See* Iliotibial band syndrome
Running on the field
  examples of, 994–995, 995f
  as team physician issue, 993–995

S

Sacrolemma, 38, 38f
Safety Toward Other Players (STOP), for
      cervical spine injury reductions, 55,
      55f, 64
Salmeterol, for HAPE, 977
SALT lesion. *See* Superior acetabular
      labral tear
Samsung Medical Center (SMC) knot, in
      arthroscopy, 300, 301f
Sarcomere
  contraction regulation, 42–43, 43f
  of muscle, 40f, 41, 43f
Sarcoplasmic reticulum (SR)
  calcium release from, 40–41
  lateral sac system of, 40–41
  longitudinal and T tubules in, 40–41
  skeletal muscle contraction and, 40–41
  of muscle, 806
Sartorius, anatomy of, 806
SC joint. *See* Sternoclavicular joint
SC ligament. *See* Scaphocapitate ligament
Scaffolds, for knee cartilage transplant,
      772–773
Scaphocapitate (SC) ligament, 388
Scaphoid nonunion advanced collapse (SNAC),
      in SLAC, 400
Scapholunate advanced collapse (SLAC)
  clinical evaluation of, 401
  management of, 401–402
    proximal row carpectomy, 402
    total wrist arthrodesis, 402
    total wrist arthroplasty, 402
  pathophysiology of, 400–401, 401f
  of wrist, 387, 400
Scapholunate (S-L) ligament, 388
  instability of, 387, 389, 389f
  in SLAC, 400
Scaphotrapeziotrapezoid (STT) ligament, 388
Scapula
  anatomy and biomechanics of, 105–106,
      105f, 108–109, 145–147, 146f, 324–327
  description of, 105–106, 106f
  dyskinesis of, 105–106, 326–327, 326t
  evaluation of, 107, 107f, 109–111, 110f
  glenoid cavity from, 147
  muscles from, 202
  projections of, 146
  scapular winging, 108–111

in shoulder dysfunction, 325–327, 326t, 327f
in shoulder function, 324–325, 325f
Scapula Stabilizing System (S3) device,
      328, 328f
Scapular rotators, for shoulder stability,
      175–176, 176f
Scapular winging, 108–111
  anatomy and biomechanics of, 108–109
  clinical evaluation of, 109–111, 110f
    history, 109
    physical examination, 109–110, 110f
  treatment of, 111
Scapulohumeral muscle group, 323–324
Scapulothoracic articulation, anatomy
      and biomechanics of, 145, 148f, 149
Scapulothoracic injuries, 105–108
  rehabilitation of, 330t–332t
SCC. *See* Sideline concussion checklist
Schwannoma, of hand, 426
Sciatica, 74
Scintigraphy, of OCD, 762
Scottie dog, 81–82, 81f–82f
Screw home mechanism, of knee, 626–627
Second-impact syndrome
  CTBI and, 136
  dangers of, 134
  overview of, 131, 136
Self assembly, of collagen, 6
Semimembranosus, 619
Semitendinosis muscles, 642
  anatomy of, 806
Septic arthritis, hip arthroscopy for, 468–469
Serratus anterior, of axioscapular muscle group,
      323–324
Sesamoids
  anatomy of, 916
  stress fracture of, 900–901, 901f
SGHL. *See* Superior glenohumeral ligament
Short lateral ligament, of posterolateral corner,
      627
Short radiolunate (short RL) ligament, 388
short RL ligament. *See* Short radiolunate
      ligament
Shoulder
  anatomy and biomechanics of, 145–156,
      324–327
  articulations of, 145, 148–149, 148f
  bones of, 145–148, 146f
  cartilage of, 243–251
  dynamic restraints of, 151–153
  female athletes and, 1036–1037
    clinical evaluation of, 1037
    epidemiology of, 1037
    physiology of, 1037
    treatment of, 1037
  fractures of, 259–271
  impingement of, 161–168
  instability of, 171–195
  kinetic chain of, 323–324
    failure of, 326–327, 327f
  muscles of, 323
  nerve injuries of, 153–154
  rehabilitation of, 323–334
    goal of, 323, 327
    phases of, 329–333, 330t–334t
    postoperative, 333–334, 333t–334t
    principles of, 327–329, 328f

repair of, 259
stiffness of (*See* Adhesive capsulitis)
thermal treatment for, 295–298
in throwing injuries, 310–316
  history, 310
  physical examination for, 311
  types of, 311–316
Shoulder cartilage, 243–251
  injury to
    biologic, 243–244
    mechanical, 243–244
  lesions of, 244–246
    diagnosis of, 245–246
    types of, 244–245
  osteoarthritis and, 244–245, 247–251,
      249f–250f
  overview of, 243–244
  repair of, 243
    allograft tissues for, 247
    autologous tissues for, 246–247
    goal of, 243, 246
    prosthetic components for, 247, 248f
    subchronal bone perforation,
      249, 250f
Shoulder impingement, 161–168
  anatomy and pathophysiology of,
      162–163, 162f
  diagnosis of, 163–164
  incidence of, 163–167
  overview of, 161–162, 162f
  physical exam of, 163, 164f
  postoperative management of, 168
  in throwing injury, 312–314
  treatment for
    complications of, 168
    non-operative, 165
    operative, 165–167, 165f–167f
    results of, 167–168
Shoulder instability, 171–195
  anatomy of, 172, 172f
  biomechanics of
    dynamic stability factors, 175–176, 176f
    IGHL, 173, 173f, 175, 175f
    MGHL, 173–174, 173f
    posterior capsule, 175
    RTI, 175
    SGHL, 173–174
    static stability factor, 173, 173f
  categorization of, 171, 178, 178t
  clinical evaluation of, 178–184
    degree and direction of, 179
    frequency and etiology of, 178–179
    history for, 179–180
    imaging for, 182–183
    physical findings of, 180–182, 180f–182f
  lesions and, 176–178
    Bankart lesions, 176–177, 176f
    capsular lesions, 177
    Hill Sachs lesions, 178, 178f
    skeletal lesions, 177, 177f
    superior labral lesions, 177–178
  overview of, 172
  surgery for, 184–193
    anesthesia for, 184
    arthroscopy, 184–186, 185f–186f
    complications and pitfalls of, 193–195
    open, 186–188, 187f